. This book is due for return not later than the last
date stamped below, unless recalled sooner.

# CRC Handbook
## of
# Sample Size Guidelines
## for
# Clinical Trials

Author

**Jonathan J. Shuster, Ph.D.**

Professor of Statistics, University of Florida
Gainesville, Florida

and

Co-Principal Investigator
Pediatric Oncology Group Statistical Office
St. Louis, Missouri

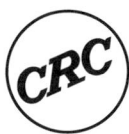

CRC Press
Boca Raton    Ann Arbor    Boston

**Library of Congress Cataloging-in-Publication Data**

Shuster, Jonathan, J., 1943 —
   Handbook of sample size guidelines for clinical trials / author,
Jonathan J. Shuster.
        p. cm.
   Includes bibliographies and index.
   ISBN 0-8493-3542-6
   1. Drugs — Testing — Statistical methods. 2. Clinical trials — Statistical methods. 3. Sampling (Statistics).
I. Title. [DNLM: 1. Clinical Trials — methods. 2. Research Design.
3. Statistics. QV 771 S562h]
RM301.27.S58 1990.
610′.72 — dc20
DNLM/DLC
 for Library of Congress                                                                89-17267
                                                                                              CIP

   Direct all inquiries to CRC Press, Inc., 2000 Corporate Blvd., N.W., Boca Raton, Florida, 33431.

© 1990 by CRC Press, Inc.

International Standard Book Number 0-8493-3542-6

Library of Congress Card Number 89-17267

Printed in the United States

# PREFACE

This book is primarily designed as a guide for physicians and biostatisticians working in clinical trials, where the primary objective is survival (or disease-free survival or progression-free survival etc). It will also be useful as a supplement to text material in courses dealing with biostatistics.

To project patient needs of a trial, the physician needs to provide "planning parameters". These include endpoints (eg 3 year survival); minimum difference the trial is to be sensitive to (eg 50% control vs 65% experimental); patient accrual rate (eg 55 patients per year are expected to be accrued); precision measures ("ALPHA" = probability of falsely concluding experimental therapy has efficacy given that it has none: typically .05) ("POWER" = probability of correctly concluding the experimental therapy has efficacy when the minimum difference is as above: typically .8 or .9 depending on the field); and anticipated rate of patient losses for non-study related reasons called "LOSSES TO FOLLOW-UP".

This Handbook is organized into three Chapters, an Appendix, and Tables. CHAPTER 1, *"How to Use the Sample Size Tables"*, is designed for users who simply want to know how many patients they need. This section is therefore a "Cookbook" approach, including a worksheet for obtaining the appropriate sample size for the trial. CHAPTER 2, *"Design and Analysis of Randomized Clinical Trials"*, is a non-technical discussion of the major elements of such trials. This section may be helpful for the user wishing to write a clinical protocol or a clinical research grant. A blueprint for protocol construction is included. CHAPTER 3, *"Derivation of the Statistical Results"*, contains a heuristic derivation of the statistical methods presented in CHAPTER 2. One full year of Calculus-based Mathematical Statistics is sufficient background to understand the material in CHAPTER 3. In addition, this Chapter contains some simple results on multiple comparisons and stratified analysis (in non-technical language). APPENDIX I contains a fairly detailed review of Mathematical Statistics, thereby making the text self-contained with respect to CHAPTER 3.

Summary of What you need to read:


1.    Cookbook: Give me the sample size needed. (CHAPTER 1)

2.    Clinicians: Help me write my Research Protocol. (CHAPTERS 1 and 2. For a discussion of "losses to

follow-up'', the reader might also consult Section 3.10 of CHAPTER 3. If the study has more than two treatments, see Section 3.12 of CHAPTER 3. Although that Section is far more technical than CHAPTER 2, most clinical investigators should be able to follow the main ideas. If after reading CHAPTER 2, ''stratification'' is contemplated, see Section 3.13 of CHAPTER 3.)

3.    Biostatisticians: Entire text material.

Extensions and Limitations: While the major scope of this Handbook is for two treatment randomized trials, CHAPTER 3 (Section 3.12) does contain methods for the design and analysis of trials involving three or more treatments. This Handbook is limited in scope to therapeutic comparisons involving survival (or disease-free survival or progression-free survival, etc) as the primary endpoint. Analysis of prognostic factors are not discussed.

*NOTE:* In any Clinical Trial, it is in everyone's best interest that a team of researchers be assembled at the planning stage. This team should consist of clinical researchers, a biostatistician, and computer scientists. Laboratory researchers are often important members of the team.

# THE AUTHOR

**Jonathan J. Shuster, Ph.D.,** is currently a Professor in the Department of Statistics, University of Florida, Gainesville, Florida. He serves as Co-Principal Investigator of the Statistical Coordinating Center of the Pediatric Oncology Group, which at any time has at least 75 active multi-center clinical trials in childhood cancer. Apart from cancer, he has participated in major collaborative projects in Ophthalmology and Urology. He has published over 80 articles in methodologic research and in medical applications. His major statistical research interests include the design and analysis of clinical trials and of large epidemiologic studies.

Dr. Shuster has served on numerous NIH Study Sections including the Epidemiology and Disease Control Study Section #1 (1986—90). He served as Chair of that Study Section for the 1989—1990 fiscal year. It is largely through service on these study sections that Dr. Shuster recognized the need for this book.

In addition to his research efforts, Dr. Shuster has been active in teaching. He has taught service statistics courses to students in the health sciences, as well as elementary, intermediate, and advanced courses in statistics.

Dr. Shuster received his Ph.D. degree from McGill University, Montreal, Canada in 1969. Since then, he has been at the University of Florida. As of the spring of 1990, he had received nearly $10 million in grants, mostly from the National Institutes of Health.

The author wishes to express his appreciation to many kind friends who directly contributed to this project, most notably to Dr. Jim Boyett, to Dr. Dick Scheaffer, and especially to Dr. Jeff Krischer.

This book is dedicated to Isobel and Samuel Shuster, parents of the author, on the occasion of their golden wedding anniversary.

# TABLE OF CONTENTS

Chapter 1

## HOW TO USE THE SAMPLE SIZE TABLES

**Introduction**

It is vital that a clinical trial has a reasonable chance of achieving its objectives. Small negative studies could be harmful, as they might not have had adequate power to find important differences. Researchers might falsely conclude from the completed trial that a new therapy lacks efficacy. Freiman et al (1978) reviewed a large number of published negative studies and concluded that the vast majority were not adequately sensitive to clinically meaningful differences. To avoid this problem, clinical trials must be well designed, and must have sufficient numbers of patients to answer the study question.

In order to use the sample size tables, the user must supply several values called parameters. The worksheet, Figure 2, will be helpful. Before getting too formal, let us have a glance at a "Statistical Consideration" of a research protocol. At first, it probably will look quite technical, but we shall unravel the details.

## STATISTICAL CONSIDERATION

"Historically, the Institute has been able to accrue 125 patients per year with newly diagnosed X-disease. Based on our prior studies, the three year survival rate is expected to be about 60% on the standard therapy (or control therapy). In order to detect a 15% improvement under the experimental therapy (three year survival of 75%), at "alpha"=.05 (one-sided) and 80% "power", a sample size of 204, half randomly assigned to each treatment, will be needed. This calculation assumes exponential survival with all patients followed to death or termination point of the study. Allowing for a 10% loss to follow-up, a figure consistent with past history, a revised sample size of 227 (1.8 years of accrual) is needed. Patients will be followed until death, loss to follow-up, or the completion of the study (up to 4.8 years). The logrank test will be used to make the treatment comparison."

## 1.1     Identification of Parameters

(1)     Minimum Planned Follow-up: At how many years will the key survival comparison be made?

3 years

(2)     Annual Accrual

125 Patients per year

(3)     Expected Accrual thru Minimum Follow-up

125 X 3=375 (This parameter is used in tables)

(4)     PCONT=Planning value for survival thru the minimum follow-up period (In this case 3 years) under the CONTROL treatment.

.6 (ie 60%) (This parameter is used in tables)

(5)     DEL=Planning value of improvement under the experimental treatment at the endpoint (ie at three years in this case.)

.15 (ie 15%) (This parameter is used in tables)

(6)     ALPHA=Chance of falsely concluding experimental therapy is superior to the control, when in fact it is equivalent to the control. In most studies, a value of .05 (ie 5%) is used. There is no special reason to pick this value other than standardization. For further discussion, see Chapter 2, especially as to one-sided versus two-sided tests. See also the footnote at the conclusion of the chapter.

.05 (ie 5%) (This value is used in the tables)

(7) POWER=Chance of correctly concluding that the experimental therapy is superior to the control, when in fact the planning values (4) and (5) are correct. The most common values for power are 80% and 90% depending on the field. This is discussed further in Chapter 2 and in the footnote at the end of this chapter.

.80 (ie 80%) (This value is used in the tables)

(8) FACT (for factor). This asks the following question. Consider a typical day before and after the endpoint. A value of FACT is the ratio of the instantaneous death rate after the endpoint to that before the endpoint. The exponential distribution implies a value of 1.0. If you consider patients cured after three years, you would use a value of 0. However, the tables can be used for intermediate situations. For example, you might consider that the typical day more than three years out carries half the risk of the typical day less than three years out. In that case, you would use a value of FACT=.5 (or 50%). A value of

FACT=BIN is for comparison only. This gives the sample size required if you only looked the "Binary" event of surviving three years or not surviving three years. The comparison would ignore time of death and all data collected after the patient had made it to the three year point. This comparison is distinct from the logrank test and carries a different sample size. This alternate and less powerful test is discussed in Chapter 2 under the name "Kaplan-Meier." If you browse through the tables, you will note that for many situations, the FACT=.00 and FACT=BIN sample size requirements are very close. When FACT=.00, no deaths are expected after the endpoint.

FACT=1.0 (Exponential) (This value is used in the tables)

## SUMMARY

(3) EXPECTED ACCRUAL THRU MINIMUM FOLLOW-UP=375

(4) PCONT=.60

(5)    DEL=.15

(6)    ALPHA=.05 (One-sided)

(7)    POWER=.80

(8)    FACT=1.0

To look up the sample size, we start from ALPHA and POWER. These are coded as follows:

To look up the sample size, on the basis of (6) and (7), we shall employ the TABLE 7. This is arranged in order of increasing expected accrual (3). Once the chart for ALPHA=.05, POWER=.80, and EXPECTED ACCRUAL=375 is located, locate the PCONT=.60 row and the DEL=.15 column.

The following six sample sizes:204,211,220,231,245, and 235 correspond respectively to FACT=1.0,.75,.50,.25,.00, and BIN. Since our FACT=1.0, we use

Sample Size= 204

The statistical section inflated the sample size to adjust for 10% losses to follow-up, for a total of 227 patients. By dividing by the accrual rate of 125 patients per year, this means that the accrual is expected to take 1.8 years, (22 months) and the study will require 4.8 years to complete.

*** Footnote on one-sided vs two-sided tests. In situations where you wish to compare two treatments, neither of which can be viewed as a control, you should run a two-sided test. Basically, you proceed exactly as above but replace the value of ALPHA by ALPHA/2. If the above study consisted of two experimental therapies, we would use ALPHA=.025. (TABLE 5) For the 45% vs 60% comparison, we would use PCONT=.45 and DEL=.15, with FACT=1.0. This would require 282 patients. For the 60% vs 75% comparison, we would use PCONT=.60 and DEL=.15 with FACT=1.0. This would require 250 patients. To be safe, we take the larger of these two numbers, 282. Allowing for 10% loss to follow-up, the final sample size would be 313 (2.5 years of accrual).

*** Further Reading. The sample size results of this handbook are similar to those of Schoenfeld (1981), Rubinstein et al. (1981), and especially Lachin (1981, where his equations (25) and (26) are employed). Another interesting method is due to Halpern and Brown (1987), who offer a computer program which can simulate the properties of the logrank statistic under any survival distributions provided by the user.

Finally, a method of Sposto and Sather(1985) is useful in some applications. That method yields similar results to those of this handbook.

# REFERENCES

1. **Freiman, J. A., Chalmers, T. C., Smith H., and Keubler, R.,** The importance of beta, the type II error and sample size in the design and interpretation of the randomized controlled trial, *N. Engl. J. Med.,* 299, 690, 1987.

2. **Halpern, J. and Brown, B. W.,** Designing clinical trials with arbitrary specification of survival functions for the log rank or generalized Wilcoxon test, *Control. Clin. Trials,* 8, 177, 1987.

3. **Lachin, J.,** Introduction to sample size determination and power analysis for clincial trials. *Control. Clin. Trials,* 2, 93, 1981.

4. **Rubinstein, L. V., Gail, M. H., and Santner, T. J.,** Planning the duration of a comparitive clinical trial with loss to follow-up and a period of continued observation, *J. Chron. Dis.,* 34, 469, 1981.

5. **Schoenfeld, D.,** The asymptotic properties of nonparametric tests for comparing survival distributions, *Biometrika,* 68, 316, 1981.

6. **Sposto, R. and Sather, H. N.,** Determining the duration of comparitive clinical trials while allowing for cure, *J. Chron. Dis.,* 38, 683, 1985.

FIGURE 1. Codes For Tables

ALPHA=.005  and POWER=.80 TABLE 1

ALPHA=.005  and POWER=.90 TABLE 2

ALPHA=.01   and POWER=.80 TABLE 3

ALPHA=.01   and POWER=.90 TABLE 4

ALPHA=.025  and POWER=.80 TABLE 5

ALPHA=.025  and POWER=.90 TABLE 6

ALPHA=.05   and POWER=.80 TABLE 7

ALPHA=.05   and POWER=.90 TABLE 8

FIGURE 2. Worksheet For Sample Size Determination

One-Sided Studies

50% assigned to each treatment.

(1)    Expected Annual Accrual     _____(Patients)

* (2)    Endpoint (? Year Survival) Minimum Planned Follow-up     _____(Years)

(3)    Expected Accrual thru Minimum Follow-up     _____(1)X(2)

(4)    PCONT (Control Planning Survival Probabilty to Endpoint)     _____(Decimal)

(5)    DEL (Planned improvement in Survival to Endpoint under     _____(Decimal)
Experimental Treatment)

(6)    ALPHA=Probability of concluding experimental therapy superior  _____(Decimal)
when it is equivalent to control

(7)    Power=Probability of correctly concluding experimental therapy  _____(Decimal)
superior when DEL is as in (5)

(8)    FACT=Ratio of instantaneous death rate after the endpoint     _____(Decimal)
to that before the endpoint

From (6) and (7), use FIGURE 1 to identify table code. Next, use (3) to identify chart. CONT and DEL identify row and column. This identifies six sample sizes, one for each of five values of FACT and one for binary comparison.

(9)    Identify Initial Sample Size     _____(Patients)

(10)    Estimated Fraction to be Lost to Follow-up     _____(Decimal)

(11)    Subtract number in (10) from 1.0     _____(Decimal)

(12)    Final Sample Size (9) divided by (11)     _____(Patients)

(13)    Accrual Period (12) divided by (1)     _____(Years)

(14)    Total Study Duration (2) + (13)     _____(Years)

FIGURE 3.  Modifications of Figure 2

1:     FOR TWO-SIDED TESTS

(A)    Replace ALPHA by ALPHA/2 in (6).

(B)    Replace PCONT by the lower of the two planning survival probabilities in (4)

(C)    Replace DEL by the difference between the two planning survival probabilities in (5).

(D)    Proceed as in Figure 2.  (You may have to do this twice if the planning survival probability is known for one of the experimental therapies while the other is planned at from DEL worse to DEL better.  If this is the case, do both calculations and use the larger of the two sample sizes.)

---

2:     FOR UNEQUAL PATIENT ALLOCATION (ie not a 50-50 randomization) (Valid for allocations from 33% to 67%)

(A)    Find the sample size as if the allocation was 50-50 using FIGURE 2 (and FIGURE 3-1 if needed)

(B)    Adjust as Follows

Allocation 2:1(67%) or 1:2(33%),Multiply result in (A) by 9/8

Allocation 3:2(60%) or 2:3(40%),Multiply result in (A) by 25/24

Allocation X:Y,Multiply result in (A) by $(X+Y)(X+Y)/(4XY)$

Note that this sample size is always higher than a 50-50  allocation.

Chapter 2

# DESIGN AND ANALYSIS OF RANDOMIZED CLINICAL TRIALS

This Chapter is a concise, non-technical introduction to the design and analysis of randomized clinical trials. For more detail, at a non-technical level, the reader is referred to the following excellent references: Pocock (1983), Buyse et al. (1984), and Meinert (1986). While the Tables of this volume apply to very specific types of trials, they are in fact applicable to the majority of major definitive trials run today. We shall discuss clinical trials in a more general framework, but restrict our analytic considerations to randomized trials. We shall discuss the trials under each of their four basic steps:

1. Formulate a therapeutic research question
2. Design a trial to answer this question
3. Conduct the trial as planned
4. Analyze the data and report the results

## 2.1 Formulation of the Therapeutic Question

This part of the trial is more medical than statistical. The question might be, for example, "Can Beta-Blocker X improve survival of newly diagnosed myocardial infarction patients over that of the standard Beta-Blocker Y?" This is the type of question which can form the starting point of a clinical trial. Note that there are two competing therapies proposed for this trial. While this book is devoted to two treatment trials, Section 3.12 provides extended use for more complicated questions involving three or more competing therapies.

Note that the research question is very loosely worded at this point. There will be considerable work to convert this question into a truly testable hypothesis.

### 2.1.1. One-Sided vs. Two-Sided Question

An important component of your research question is whether your question is "one-sided" or "two-sided". The following discussion will help make this determination.

When you conduct a clinical trial, you will usually put on trial one of the following statements

1. One-Sided Statement: The new (test) therapy is superior to the standard; or

2. One of the two therapies is superior to the other, but you have no vested interest as to which.

## Sample One-Sided Questions

Drug companies, developing a new drug, are generally interested in one-sided questions. Their product may only be marketable if they can prove beyond a reasonable doubt that their product is superior to the standard. The competing therapies have asymmetrical interest.

Again, if any scientific researcher is considering the efficacy of adding a toxic agent to a standard regimen, and comparing this to the standard regimen alone, a one-sided question results. After the study is over, one would use the new therapy only if it proved to be significantly better than the standard. Whether the efficacies were not significantly different or the toxic agent had significantly reduced the efficacy, one would make the management decison not to use this toxic agent for future patients.

## Sample Two-Sided Questions

There may be two standard therapies that are in widespread use, but no one really knows which is superior. The scientific issue here is simply, which is the better therapy? Interest is symmetric.

In some diseases, ther may be no known effective therapy. One might wish to test two new experimental therapies. Here too, a two-sided question is clear.

One-sided questions need fewer subjects than two-sided questions of equal precision. The "Zone of proof beyond a reasonable doubt" is concentrated in the zone where the test outperforms the control treatment. The two-sided question must create two such zones, one corresponding to superiority of each treatment. Consequently, the region of superiority of each given treatment must be smaller in the two-sided question corresponding to the one-side question of the same precision.

The one-sided vs. two-sided question must be spelled out in advance as a vital part of the research question. Clearcut rationale for asymmetric interest must be given. In point of fact, most trials conducted in the medical school environment should be two-sided, unless there is a compelling reason for asymmetry.

## 2.2 Design of the Clinical Trial

In order to conduct a valid clinical trial, it is vital to develop a complete plan for its conduct. A manual of operations, called a "Protocol", should be written with the following elements:

A. Objectives of the Study (What you hope to accomplish.)

B. Background Information (Literature review of prior therapy and outcome. Include your own experience as well.)

C. Rationale (Why you feel you have good prospects to achieve your objectives.)

D. Patient Eligibility (A Precise definition as to who can participate in the trial.)

E. Treatment Plans (Full description of how patients will be treated under each competing therapy. This must include contingency plans for complications.)

F. Off-Study Requirements (Full description of events that place the patient off study. For example, patient may go off study at time of recurrence of disease, allergic reaction to the drug, or death.)

G. Data Submission Requirements (This describes the schedule of follow-up, the medical tests required and their timing, and the description and timing of the data form submission.)

H. Statistical Consideration. (This describes the actual design, including the endpoint of the study, whether stratification and randomization will be used, plans for interim and final analysis, and sample size projections. If the study is a "masked design", this is also discussed in this Section.)

I. Study Monitoring (A committee called the Data Safety and Monitoring Committee should be listed along with their meeting schedules and responsibilities.)

J. Appendix (This should include blank copies of all data forms and the informed consent form. Instructions on forms completion should also be included.)

K. Database Documentation (While this may not be a formal part of the protocol, it is a critical element of the design. A protocol cannot be compromised by turnover in computer staff.)

This author was once sent a computer tape of a trial completed some six years earlier, in order to re-analyze the data. Unfortunately, the senders lacked documentation of the data. Despite our best efforts, we could not crack the code with enough confidence to complete any analysis.

## 2.2.1 Statistical Considerations

In planning a trial, there are a number of issues that need to be considered in (H) above. First, the eligibility conditions define the "Target Population". This is the hypothetical pool of past, present, and future patients with well defined characteristics. Note that the actual patients who participate in the study are considered to be a representative sample from this target population. Our ultimate conclusions will be directed to the target population not to the sample. Of course, we use the sample data to make an inference about this target population. Such inferences are subject to sampling error, since only a portion of the target population has been sampled. This is much like the use of voter surveys to project election results.

Answers to the following question are needed to formulate the statistical consideration.

**What is the single primary variable upon which the major comparison will be based?**

It is essential to pin down a primary variable up front. If this is not specified, the data may be analyzed in a wide variety of ways, leading to investigator selection bias. Each analysis carries a sampling error, and hence the more analyses one performs, the greater the cumulative error effect. To control this, a primary single analysis should be specified. Others can be done, but as strictly secondary analysis. Example primary variables might be three year remission, five year survival, two year peak intra-ocular pressure below 23 mm hg, etc.

As mentioned in the Introduction, there are two types of primary variables considered in this Handbook. The first type is "Censored Survival Data". Time is measured from entry onto the study until failure, termination of the study, or loss to follow-up. The last occurs if the patient exercises his or her option to quit the study. The only survival information available are (1) the time from entry to last follow-up and (2) the patient status at last follow-up. The data are censored (or more precisely, right censored), since for survivors, we do not know their true survival times, although we do know that they survived at least a given number of days (eg 655+ days). The second type of data in which these sample size tables can be used is binary data (yes/no). For example, a study on operative deaths (whether or not the patient died during surgery), is not concerned with time of death, but only whether or not the patient survived the surgical procedure. Unlike the censored survival situation, follow-up is short and equivalent for all patients. In a censored survival study, involving a three year patient accrual phase plus a two year minimum follow-up (a five year total study), patients have a potential follow-up of from two to five years. The risk of a study death among earlier entries is higher than that among later entries, since the early entries are at risk longer. This needs to be taken into account in the analysis. The operative death problem is quite different. The only data used in that analysis is whether or not the patient survived surgery.

**Will the study be randomized?**

This is a controversial topic. Let us suppose that you plan to compare two therapies. You may have considerable experience with one of the therapies (the "control" or "standard") and little experience on the other (the "experimental" or "test"). You may ask, "Why not simply recruit patients to the experimental regimen and compare these to the existing control patients?" This is called an "Historical Control Study". There are both advantages and disadvantages of such a strategy. Historical control studies often require fewer patients than randomized studies, and hence can often be completed in less time and at less cost than concurrently controlled studies. Unfortunately, however, historical control studies cannot be viewed as definitive scientific evidence about the relative merits of the competing therapies. You cannot adequately attribute differences (or lack of differences) in outcome with differences in efficacy. Subtle changes in any of the following can hopelessly confound the results of an historical control trial: Changes in referral pattern, changes in personnel, changes in diagnostic techniques, changes in concomitant care, changes in public awareness programs, etc. In addition, the trial may have been motivated by disappointing results under the standard therapy. Disappointment is more likely when the sampling error under the historical control is negative than it would be if the sampling error is positive. In other words, suppose the true success rate is 60% under the standard. A 50% observed success rate in your sample of 50 historical patients could provide greater motivation to conduct a study than a 70% observed success rate.

One advantage of historical control studies, not often mentioned in publications, is the issue of gaining informed consent. It is very difficult to approach a patient in order to gain consent for randomization. Uncertainty in a physician can undermine the confidence of the patient. However, in truth, the same uncertainty is generally present in the historical control study, although it is often downplayed.

Finally, historical control studies are fully justified if the historical control success rate is virtually zero. In such cases, you are unwilling to subject patients to a hopeless therapy. Even here, however, there is no unanimous agreement among scientists. For example, in 1986, randomized studies were conducted in AIDS patients, using a control known to offer no hope for survival. Surprisingly, there was a strong moral argument for the randomization. Since only a limited number of patients were approved for initial testing of new agents, a randomized design could treat as many patients as a non-randomized design. Further, by careful interim comparison of treatment vs. control patients, the randomized study offers the best way to study non-fatal events. For additional information on randomized vs. historical controls, see Zelen (1983), Shuster et al. (1985), Pocock (1983), Gehan (1978 and 1982), Peto et al. (1976), Diehl and Perry(1986), and Dupont (1985). These articles present all sides of the issues.

In summary, a randomized study is recommended very strongly, except perhaps when the historical success rate is near zero. However, if you consider a randomized study and determine that the required sample size is too large, an historical control study might be considered. Prior to doing so, however, the possibility of running a randomized study with additional institutions should be seriously considered.

**Note:** Randomization is a more complex topic than one might at first believe. It is important that the investigator cannot predict what therapy the next patient will be assigned. The purpose of randomization is threefold. First, it prevents unconscious bias in treatment assignment as compared to non- randomized assignment. Second, the framework of statistical analysis relies on randomization. Finally, a properly set up randomization procedure offers an audit trail of treatment assignments. This protects the investigator if the results of a study are questioned by a review group or by journal editors.

**Randomization Methods**

Some randomization techniques are discussed in Pocock (1983, Chapter 5). Figure 4 presents a table of randomized treatment assignments, based on "simple randomization". Each successive entry is an independent flip of an unbiased coin (50% probability of heads). Heads represents treatment 1, while tails represents treatment 2. Figure 5 represents an alternate design, with "random length permuted blocks". The following is the mechanism for Figure 5. First, a balanced coin is flipped. If the coin is heads, then we generate a random "word" consisting of three 1's and three 2's. Each of the possible 20 words consisting of three 1's and three 2's has an equal chance of occurring. If the coin lands tails, then we generate a random word consisting of two 1's and two 2's. Each of the following six equally likely words is drawn: 1122, 1212, 1221, 2112, 2121, 2211 This procedure is repeated, until the figure is completed. These figures provide the serial assignment of treatments for successive patients.

Simple randomization (Figure 4) is very simple to employ, but may lead to rather substantial differences in the number of patients assigned to each therapy. To illustrate, after 813 randomizations in Figure 4, there are 443 patients assigned to Treatment #1 and 370 assigned to treatment #2, for a net difference of 73 patients. This is the peak difference over the 1200 patient assignments. The random length permuted blocks procedure keeps the numbers well balanced throughout the study, while it is quite unpredictable to the investigator, especially if the exact mechanism of randomization is masked. Randomization is discussed further under stratification and institutional balancing below.

**Will the study be stratified?**

Are there key "risk factors" that need to be balanced "prospectively" or "retrospectively"? There is always concern that a randomized design will place a disproportionate number of poor risk patients on one of the treatments. If one has historical information about such risk factors, they might be planned for in two ways. First, we may wish to stratify the trial prospectively. That is, we shall define patient subgroups according to the risk factors, and essentially run independent trials within each subgroup. Using random length permuted blocks within each subgroup, we can maintain good balance of the treatments across each stratum. This is a good design feature, but it comes at a price. Over stratification can reduce the precision. Peto et al. (1976) estimate that the effective sample size of the study is reduced by one for each stratum you create, as compared to the luckily perfectly balanced randomized trial. For example, a trial stratified on age group (4 levels), sex (2 levels), smoking history (3 levels), and serum cholesterol (3 levels) would create 4 X 2 X 3 X 3 = 72 strata. Clearly, a poorly designed study could be so heavily stratified that there would be very few patients in any one stratum. The purpose of stratification is to compare like patients with like patients. However, stratification limits the possibility of comparison, as the following example illustrates. Suppose that there are 100 patients, 50 in stratum 1 and 50 in stratum 2. Suppose that 50 are assigned to each treatment. The un-stratified design allows 50 treatment #1 patients each to be compared to 50 treatment #2 patients (2500 comparisons). The stratified design eliminates half of these, namely patients in different strata and different treatments. Clearly, there is a trade-off. We recommend only very limited stratification, based on important proven risk factors, be made.

The second method to deal with stratification is to adjust for the risk factors retrospectively in the analysis. This method is discussed in CHAPTER 3.13. The reader is further referred to Peto et al. (1977). No within-stratum balancing is done, but imbalances are corrected for in the analysis.

**If the study is a multi-center study, will institutional balancing be used?**

When conducting a multi-institutional study, especially if it is conducted by a large number of institutions, each with a relatively small number of patients, one should consider balancing the randomization within institutions. While it seems that this might create too many strata, especially if the study is also stratified according to risk factors, a method called "Marginal Balancing" can be used to avert this problem. Basically, marginal balancing, as discussed in Shuster et al. (1985), works as follows. Assign the patient according to prior assignments for the institution and stratum as follows:

Priority #1: Check how many patients have been assigned to each treatment at this institution. If the difference between the number of assignments exceeds the maximum allowable margin, (say 2), assign the treatment that has been assigned less often at that institution. For example, if at X-Hospital, 7 patients are on Treatment #1 and 4 patients are on Treatment #2, and the maximum allowable margin for randomization is 2, the next patient at this institution must receive Treatment #2.

Priority #2: Applies only if Priority #1 has not forced a treatment assignment. For the patient's stratum, check the number of patients assigned to each treatment. If the difference exceeds the maximum allowable margin for randomization, assign the less used treatment. (Note that the stratum maximum margin need not match that of the institution.)

Priority #3: Applies only if Priorities #1 and #2 have not forced a treatment assignment. Assign treatment according to the next unused entry on the random length permuted block assignment sheet. (For example, Figure 5.)

Bookkeeping: After each patient assignment, it is necessary to update the number of patients assigned to each therapy by institution and stratum. In addition, the assignment should be recorded on the random length permuted block assignment sheet by crossing off the first available entry matching the assigned treatment. This will be the next entry if Priority #3 applies.

Marginal balancing keeps institutions and strata balanced. It also keeps the overall study balanced because of the permuted blocks. One of the advantages of marginal balancing is that the study can be analyzed as if it was a single institutional study. In other words, one can ignore the stratification effect of institution in the analysis. This is especially important in studies conducted by a large number of institutions with a large number of strata. In practice, the "error" one makes in treating the study as a single institutional study is in the conservative direction. That is, there will be a slight tendency to underestimate the significance of the differences between the treatments (overestimate the "P-values"). However, this error is rarely of practical significance.

Marginal balancing is also important for non-statistical reasons in studies where some institutions contribute small numbers of patients. Each institution should gain experience on both therapies. Without institutional balancing, there is more than a 12% chance that an institution contributing four patients will place all four on the same treatment.

**If the study is multi-institutional, will centralized randomization be employed?**

Centralized randomization is strongly recommended for all multi-center trials. Clearly, if marginal balancing is used, a central office must have up-to-the-minute information on all prior treatment assignments. There are more important considerations, however. The integrity of the study is best insured through centralized randomization. No patient can get onto the study without contact with the central office. Eligibility can be verified by standardized criteria prior to acceptance of the patient. Without centralized randomization, the study is open to the possibility that early failures may never be placed on the study. Individual investigators may overlook the important task of forwarding the information on such patients to the central office. With centralized registration and randomization, patients must be put on study before starting treatment. Registration and randomization need not be done at the same time. Some studies will have both treatments identical for the first 6-12 weeks, followed by a divergence. All participants should be registered at the time of treatment start, but a callback for randomization should occur at the time when the treatments diverge. This callback will in fact improve the precision of the comparison, since the major comparison will be based on outcomes after the divergence point. Failures before the divergence point are not part of the study question, although they are vital to the estimation of the efficacy of each therapy. The treatment differences must occur after the divergence point, but the overall success rate of each therapy is measured from the start of treatment. You have the luxury of using all patients (regardless of assigned therapy) to assess the efficacy of the therapy from its starting point to the divergence point.

**Will the study be masked (blinded)?**

It is a good experimental technique to mask the identity of the treatment from both the patient and the investigator. (The more common term is blinded, but as one with experience in ophthalmic trials, your author considers that designation is a bit short sighted.) Masking is an especially important consideration if (1) patient psychological factors may be involved, (2) the response measurements involve subjective judgement on the part of the physician or the patient, or (3) the treatment can be put in a masked form, ethically and logistically. Contra-indications for masking include possible discomfort to the control patient; the need for the physician to perform expensive and/or painful medical tests to monitor one of the treatments and its side-effects; and the ability to mask the therapy. It would be unethical to perform sham surgery on a patient in order to mask the true procedure.

Some masking is better than no masking. For example, if it is unethical to mask the treating physician, it might be possible to have the critical observations made by a colleague who is indeed masked as to the treatment identity. A vital consideration in masked studies is that the master code, indicating who got each treatment, be securely maintained. More than one masked study has failed because the master code was lost! If such a loss occurs, nothing can be done to recover.

**What methods of analysis will be used?**

This will be discussed further in Section 2.4. However, the statistical section must spell out the exact statistical details as to what methodology will be used.

This needs to be specified in the protocol, as a protection to the investigators. Journal reviewers can sometimes criticize a study on the basis that it was not analyzed according to the design of the study. The best protection against this contingency is to submit a copy of the protocol with the manuscript. Often, the protocol itself undergoes peer review, and hence, there is strong support for your analysis.

**What patients will be included in the analysis?**

In most studies, there will be some severe violations of the protocol, often for reasons beyond the control of the investigators. The question one might pose is, "Will the major comparison be based on all compliant patients, or on all eligible patients?" There is now fairly unanimous agreement that the most convincing scientific analysis is based on all eligible patients. Once a patient is deemed to meet the entry requirements, that patient is included in the major analysis, whether or not the patient complies with the assigned protocol. This is often called "The intent to treat principal". Many journals have published policy that the major analysis must consist of all patients who meet the eligibility conditions, whether or not they comply with the protocol. Two important editorials supporting this point are

Zelen (1983) and Simon and Wittes (1985). As soon as subjective judgement is allowed to enter the picture, the potential for bias arises. Other analysis can be done as secondary evidence. However, severe bias can be induced by eliminating non-compliant patients. Compliance can have a strange relationship to treatment, apart from merely a disproportionate number of non- compliers within the two treatment groups. Non-compliers on one treatment may be at increased risk, while non-compliers on the other treatment may be at decreased risk. The "intent to treat principal" also implies that patients are analyzed on the treatment to which they were assigned, even if they actually received the other therapy! This may seem to be invalid at first glance, but it is the only way to prevent bias. The argument is that the Intent to Treat Principal closely resembles the real world application of the treatment. Poor compliance to a protocol will adversely affect its success. It is vital to keep track of compliance, but the major analysis should not utilize compliance. For additional detail on this topic, see Shuster et al (1985), Simon and Wittes (1985), and Haynes and Dante (1987).

### What are the plans for interim analysis?

When conducting a long-term trial, there is considerable motivation to look at the results to date to see if the question can be answered early. Such a plan for example led to the early closure of the Multi-Institutional Osteosarcoma Trial of Link et al. (1986). That protocol specified times for interim analysis as well as conditions which would lead to early termination of the study. It needs to be pointed out that the decision to close a study early should be based on very compelling evidence. Generally speaking, the more interim analyses that are conducted, the greater the risk of false-positive results. If interim analyses are to be conducted, they should be conducted at a very small P-value as compared to a one-time final analysis. This can be put into a formal statistical methodology called "Group Sequential Methods" or in a more informal way, where the critical P-value is a small fraction of the final planning P-value. (eg .005 for interim analysis vs. .05 for the final planned analysis.) For more information on this topic see Armitage (1975), O'Brien and Fleming (1979) , and Tsiatis and Rosner (1985).

In any case, the protocol should spell out exactly when interim analyses will be conducted, and how decisions based on interim analyses will be made. If an interim analysis does in fact suggest that the study be terminated, the decision should not be made until the data have been reviewed carefully by the "Data Safety and Monitoring Committee". See Section 2.2.(I) discussed earlier.

## 2.3 Conduct of the Trial

Once the trial is opened to patient accrual, there are many elements which are required to ensure that the trial meets its objectives. Each institution must obtain annual approval from its Institutional Review Board (IRB) in order to register patients on the study. In order to place any patient on the trial, informed written consent must be obtained. The risks and benefits of the competing therapies must be explained as well as the objectives of the study. If the trial is randomized, the patient should know this before the treatment is assigned. There are some pre-consent randomization designs. See Zelen (1979 and 1982), Smith (1983), and Fletcher (1985) for more details. Such designs are highly controversial as these references point out. The vast majority of studies assume randomization after consent, unless the patient is incapable of giving informed consent, Abramson et al. (1985).

The patient becomes part of the trial as soon as consent is obtained. Further, once treatment is assigned, the patient is a part of that treatment group, regardless of whether or not the patient complies with the therapy. The investigator is ethically bound to follow the therapy as prescribed in the protocol, unless there is overwhelming evidence that violating the protocol is in the patient's best health interest. The patient assumes no legal commitment to follow the protocol, but does so in the spirit of physician-patient relationship.

### Data Submission

It is the responsibility of each investigator to fully comply with all data submission requirements of the trial. Even the world's most outstanding statistician is limited by the quality and quantity of data submitted by the investigators. Even small amounts of missing data can bias a study.

### Interim Analysis

A well-written protocol has provisions for interim analysis. However, it is important that while the trial is accruing patients, this information should be restricted to the Data Safety and Monitoring Committee. Investigators should not see interim treatment comparisons while patient accrual is ongoing. The committee is charged with the responsibility of determining if randomization remains ethical. With open reporting, selection bias could result from individualized analysis on the part of the investigators.

In some situations, it may be important to mask the treatment comparisons until all patients have completed therapy. For example, suppose that Treatment A consists of two years of Beta-Blocker X, while Treatment B consists of two years of Beta-Blocker Y, from the time of myocardial infarction. If an unblinded interim analysis shows a trend in favor of B, some investigators may want to switch their A patients to B. This could compromise the entire trial. The decision to switch or not switch should be in the hands of the Data Safety and Monitoring Committee, not the individual investigator.

**Protocol Amendments**

Once a protocol is actively accruing patients, amendments should be resisted. However, even the most carefully written protocols are not immune to unexpected results. For example, one might encounter toxicities, that had not occurred in pilot studies. Counter measures would have to be written into the protocol. If the counter measure has efficacy implications on one or both treatments, then the amendment may have the effect of forcing the investigators to start the accrual process over. The patients already accrued would not be used in the comparison of the treatments. Each amendment has to be sent back to the IRBs for approval. In addition, the Statistical Consideration and Consent Form will need modifications to incorporate these amendments. Amendments must be handled with as much precision as the original protocol.

## 2.4 Analysis and Reporting of the Trial

Upon completion of the accrual phase and minimum projected follow-up on all patients, the final analysis phase begins. The first step is to acquire all possible delinquent and missing information. Next, the analysis is completed as prescribed in the Statistical Consideration. Finally, the results of the trial are submitted for publication in a refereed medical journal.

### 2.4.1. Crucial Elements

The analysis described in the statistical section must be employed in the analysis. The sample size calculation only applies to the statistical methods detailed in the protocol.

**Definition of P-value:** The methodology of the statistical consideration provides an ordering of the possible outcomes in terms of how well they support a difference between the treatments (one-sided or two sided as specified in the design.) The P-value is interpreted as follows: Suppose that you repeated this study in another universe where the treatments were in fact equivalent. What is the maximum probability of observing evidence of a difference in this repetition that is as least as convincing as that observed in the actual trial? (The answer is the P-Value.) For example, suppose that the observed success rate of the test treatment was 46/84 while that in the control treatment was 34/81. The statement, which we shall discuss in more detail below is, "P = .05 one-sided." That is, if we repeated our protocol in a population where the success rates are equal, then there is at most a 5% chance of observing a difference of 12.8% or more in favor of the test treatment. (46/84-34/81 = .128=12.8%).

## Methods of Analysis of Clinical Trial Data

We shall discuss three methods of analysis of clinical trial data. These include Sections 2.4.2, Binomial Comparison; 2.4.3, Kaplan-Meier Comparison, and 2.4.4, Logrank Comparison.

### *2.4.2 Binomial Comparison*

The Binomial Comparison is applied to trials where the outcome is binary: Success or Failure. The following properties must be satisfied, at least conceptually, in order to apply this methodology:

P1: Trials are "INDEPENDENT". That is, the outcome of a given patient is not influenced by the outcome of any other patient. This methodology should not be used for matched studies, since the outcome of one patient will have more predictive value on the matched patient than it would on any other patient.

P2: The "Success Probability" within a given treatment is the same from patient to patient. That is, without knowing the patient characteristics in advance, the probabilities of success in the first, second, third, ... patients assigned to the given treatment are equal. For censored survival studies where patients enter serially and where the study is analyzed at a fixed point in time, this assumption is violated. Early entries are at risk for a longer period than later entries, and hence, have lower success rates than later entries. Of course, the success rate of each treatment need not be the same.

### *2.4.2.1  Large Sample Methodology*

Let N1=Sample Size for the Standard or Control Therapy

S1=Number of Successes in the Control Sample

F1=Number of Failures in the Control Sample

P1=S1/N1=Fraction of Successes in the Control Sample.

Let N2=Sample Size for the Test Therapy

S2=Number of Successes in the Test Sample

F2=Number of Failures in the Test Sample

P2=S2/N2=Fraction of Successes in the Test Sample.

The difference in Success rates is P2-P1. We also need a quantity called the "Estimated Variance of P2-P1", denoted by:

$$V=\{P1(1\text{-}P1)/N1\}+\{P2(1\text{-}P2)/N2\}$$

The test statistic for which a decision about the therapies is based is:

$$Z=(P2\text{-}P1)/SE$$

where

$$SE=SQRT(V) \qquad\qquad (SQRT=Square\ Root)$$

The approximate "P-value" associated with Z is obtained from FIGURE 6 for one-sided comparisons and from FIGURE 7 for two- sided comparisons. The intuitive interpretation of the P-value is given in Section 2.4.1.

### 2.4.2.2 Confidence Intervals

Another more descriptive way to report the above information is via a CONFIDENCE INTERVAL. A "One-Sided Confidence Interval" is reported for DEL, the true target population difference in success rates, as:

$$DEL >P2\text{-}P1\text{-}W\ SE$$

where W is selected from Figure 8 according to the desired confidence. The intuitive interpretation of the Confidence Interval is given below Figure 8.

A "Two-Sided Confidence Interval" is reported as:

$$P2-P1+W \text{ SE} > DEL > (P2-P1)-W \text{ SE}$$

where W is selected from Figure 9 according to the desired confidence. The intuitive interpretation of the Confidence Interval is given below Figure 9.

### 2.4.2.3 Numerical Example (Test)

Suppose that the Control therapy had N1=81 patients of whom S1=34 were successes and F1=47 were failures. We have P1=34/81=0.420. Suppose further that the Test therapy had N2=84 patients of whom S2=46 were successes and F2=38 were failures. Hence, P2=46/84=0.548.

To calculate V, note that 1-P1=1-.420=.580 and 1-P2=1-.548=.452.

$$V=\{(.420)(.580)/81\}+\{(.548)(.452)/84\}=\{.2463/81\}+\{.2477/84\} =0.00304+0.00295=.00599$$

$$SE=SQRT(V)=.0774$$

and

$$P2-P1=.548-.420=.128$$

Hence,

$$Z=.128/.0774=1.653$$

From Figure 6, this translates to a P-Value of slightly less than 0.05, for a one-sided test. Had this been a two-sided study, we see from Figure 7 that the two-sided P-value is slightly less than 0.10. Finally, if the Experimental and Test labels had been reversed so that the Experimental group had 34 successes in 81 patients while the Control group had 46 successes in 84 patients, the One-Sided P-Value would have been approximately 0.95.

### 2.4.2.4 Numerical Example (One-Sided Confidence Interval)

If one was to construct a 95% One-Sided Confidence Interval for DEL, the target difference in success rates, one would employ FIGURE 8:

$$DEL > .128 - 1.645\{.0774\} = .128 - .127 = .01$$

That is, DEL > .01 with 95% confidence.

Notice that the value of Zero, the point of equal efficacy, lies just outside the confidence interval. (Had the P-value been greater than 0.05, Zero would have appeared within the confidence interval. The two-sided confidence interval will illustrate this.)

### 2.4.2.5 Numerical Example (Two-Sided Confidence Interval)

Had this been a two-sided question, a 95% two-sided confidence interval would be obtained from Figure 9 as follows:

$$.128 + 1.96\{.0774\} > DEL > .128 - 1.96\{.0774\}$$

That is .28 > DEL > -.02 with 95% confidence.

Had this been a two-sided experiment, the outcome would not have achieved statistical significance at the conventional .05 level. However, we are highly confident that the Test treatment ranges from trivially inferior to vastly superior. The value in the confidence region most favorable to the control treatment represents only a 2% advantage to the control. The confidence interval allows a management decision to prefer the test treatment for future patients, despite the fact that conventional significance of the two-sided trial was not achieved. The P-Value alone does not allow this type of management logic.

### 2.4.2.6 Small Sample Methodology

In order to apply the Large Sample Methodology, the following rules of thumb are often used:

Each of the following four quantities are greater than 5.0:

$N1(S1 + S2)/(N1 + N2)$ = "Expected Successes for Control"

$N1(F1 + F2)/(N1 + N2)$ = "Expected Failures for Control"

$N2(S1 + S2)/(N1 + N2)$ = "Expected Successes for Test "

$N2(F1 + F2)/(N1 + N2)$ = "Expected Failures for Test "

The term "Expected" refers to the idealized distribution of the actual patient results to the two groups, where the success rate would be the same in both treatment groups. There is nothing magic about the number 5.0. However, the approximations seem to be "adequate" at this number of patients.

Generally speaking, if a randomized clinical trial is designed to be sensitive to clinically relevant differences, the approximations made for large samples will be valid. However, in very small trials with low power, exact methods are needed. The two most widely used methods are Fisher's Exact Test and the Exact Unconditional Z Test. We shall discuss these briefly. For more detail, the reader should consult Armitage (1971), Suissa and Shuster (1985), and Shuster (1988).

**Fisher's Exact Test**

In the numerical example above, imagine that we have a deck of cards, distributed as follows: 80 Cards are labeled SUCCESS and 85 Cards are labeled FAILURE, for a total of 165 cards. Now suppose that we randomly distribute the cards to two players called Control and Test (81 to Control and 84 to Test). What is the probability of distributing 46 or more successes to the Test player? In other words, if we repeated the experiment on a different target population, where in fact the control and test therapies were equivalent, and if we happened to again get a total of 80 Successes and 85 Failures, what is the likelihood of obtaining evidence at least as convincing as that observed in favor of the test therapy? The answer is P=.068. (The approximation had P=.05 one-sided)

Note that this is not a true P-value, since the additional proviso is made that in the replication of the experiment, you must match the total number of successes with that observed (80). We call such a P-Value "an Exact Conditional P-Value" to remind us that it was calculated under an added artificial condition.

A two-sided analogue of Fisher's Exact Test is also possible. The observed difference in success rates was P2-P1=.128.

If we had seen 44 successes in 81 controls and 36 successes in 84 test (keeping the total successes at 80), then the difference in success rates would have been .115; while the difference between 45/81 vs 35/84 is .139. On a two-sided basis, if the test group is dealt either (A) 46 or more successes or (B) 35 or fewer successes, the evidence in favor of a difference would be at least as strong as that observed (.128).The probability that either (A) or (B) occurs in redeals is:

$$P=.120 \text{ (Conditional) vs } P=.10 \text{ (2-sided approx.)}$$

The P-value requires the same condition in the replication of matching total successes to that observed. Thus, this is not a true P-value, but rather a conditional one.

**Exact Unconditional P-Value**

The Exact Unconditional Z-test works as follows. The observed Z value was 1.653. What is the probability that if we had 81 independent success/failure observations for control and 84 success/failure observations for test, with the success rate identical for both control and test, that we would observe a Z-value of at least 1.653? The answer may depend on the value of that common success rate. The exact unconditional Z-test maximizes this probability over all possible identical values for the success rates (from 0 to 1). According to the definition, this yields the P-value. A microcomputer program (including hardware requirements), to perform the calculations is described in Shuster (1988). The one-sided version considers values above the observed Z of 1.653 in favor of the test treatment, while the two-sided version considers values above the observed value of 1.653 in favor of either treatment.

The exact unconditional P-values are .057 (vs approximation of .05 one-sided) and .108 (vs approximation of .10 two-sided). These agree remarkably well.

As Suissa and Shuster (1985) point out, the Exact Unconditional Z-Test generally outperforms Fisher's Exact Test. (Requires fewer patients for trials.)

*2.4.3 Kaplan-Meier Comparison (Large Sample)*

The Kaplan-Meier (1958) methodology is designed to estimate the probability of surviving for a given number of years, utilizing "Censored Survival Data". Unlike the Binomial methods above, the Kaplan-Meier technique recognizes the possibility that patients' times at risk will be unequal. However, the Kaplan-Meier technique makes the very important assumption that the prognosis of a patient who withdraws from the study is the same as that of a patient of the same "age" who remains on the study. This means for example, that the prognosis of a patient who was lost to follow-up after 6 months on the test therapy is the same after the six month point as that of a patient still on the test therapy at six months. It is therefore clear that in many studies, the validity of the Kaplan-Meier method rests heavily on obtaining virtually complete follow-up on all patients. Note that the above assumption is reasonable for patients whose follow-up is short, but current. For example, it is reasonable to assume that if a patient entered the study six months before it was to be analyzed he/she has the same outlook post six months as that of a patient who entered the study on the first day the study opened, four years prior to the analysis.

For each treatment, the Kaplan-Meier curve provides an estimate of the true probability of surviving at least T-days. The true probability represents the hypothetical target population of all past, present, and future patients who meet the eligibility conditions of the study. The estimate is based on the sample of patients assigned to the given treatment. It is subject to sampling error, since the actual sample assigned to the treatment is assumed to be a conceptual random sample from the target population. It also could be subject to selection biases, if the sample of patients cannot be viewed as a conceptual random sample from the target population. A good example where selection bias can occur, is where there is selective participation by some institutions in a multi-center trial. For example, institution X agrees only to place their advanced patients on a study.

### 2.4.3.1 Assumptions Underlying the Kaplan-Meier Curve

P1. All observations are "INDEPENDENT". That is, the outcome of a given patient is not influenced by that of another.

P2. Given the treatment assignment, the survival probability distribution of each patient over time is the same from trial to trial. In other words, patient prognosis on the test treatment is the same for early entries in the trial as later entries. The same holds true within the control treatment.

P3. The loss to follow-up rate is very small. Otherwise, we assume that patient losses are not in any way influenced by the patient's prognosis. Failure of this assumption is especially serious if one of the therapies is more toxic, leading to vastly differing withdrawal rates between the treatments.

*Comment:* Withdrawals for toxicity probably violate this assumption. It is therefore vital to keep track of study losses to toxicity.

### 2.4.3.2 Calculation of the Kaplan-Meier Curve

The Kaplan-Meier curve starts at DAY 0 at a value of 1.00(100%). On each succeeding day, we compute the value from the preceding day as follows:

Let     R=Number of patients left at risk on that day(At Risk)

         F=Number of patient failures on that day (Deaths)

$$KM=KM \text{ (on previous day) } X \text{ (R-F) / R} \tag{1}$$

The estimate is easily justified intuitively as follows. The estimate is built on a day-to-day basis, using the data for each day. To survive 100 days, a patient has to survive day 1, day 2,...., day 100. The logical estimate of the probability of surviving a given day, assuming that the patient was alive at the start of that day, is (R-F)/R, the ratio of the number of patients who survived that day to the number at risk on that day. The Kaplan-Meier estimate for day 100 is simply the product of the (R-F)/R values for days 1,2,3,...,100. An analogy to successive taxes will further motivate the multiplication. Imagine that you wish to send $1000 to a relative in Angola. The money is routed as follows. First it goes to Canada, which extracts 1%. Next, it goes to Cuba, which takes 13% of the balance. Finally, it goes to Angola, which charges 16% of what is left. We see that 99% survives the first taxation; of that, 87% survives the second taxation; and of that, 84% survives the final levy.

$$\text{Surviving Gift}=\$1000X.99X.87X.84=\$723.49$$

1. Canada: 1% of $1000.00 tax ; 99% of $1000=$990 survives

2. Cuba : 13% of $990.00 tax ; 87% of $ 990=$861.30 survives

3. Angola: 16% of $861.30 tax:84% of $861.30=$723.49 survives.


Note that the KM value in (1) stays the same as the previous day, unless at least one failure occurs. We shall demonstrate the curve concept for the Control Treatment (See Figures 10 and 11).


### 2.4.3.3 Numerical Example: See Figures 10 and 11.

#### Control Kaplan-Meier Curve

On Day 1, F=2 and R=186 and hence (R-F)/R=184/186.

On Day 2, only 184 patients are at risk, two having been lost on day 1. For Day 2, F=1 and R=184 and hence (R-F)/R=183/184.

On Days 3-6, no failures occurred and hence (R-F)/R=1.000.

On Day 7, F=1 and R=183, and hence (R-F)/R=182/183.

On Days 8-11, no failures occurred and hence (R-F)/R=1.000.

On Day 12, no failure occurred, but one survivor had only 12 days of follow-up. Here too, F=0 and hence (R-F)/R=1.000.

On Days 13-15, no failures occurred and hence (R-F)/R=1.000.

On Day 16, F=1 and R=181, and hence (R-F)/R=180/181.

This process continues to day 3454.

On Day 1, KM=184/186=.98925.

On Day 2, KM=.98925X183/184=.98387.

On Days 3-6, KM stays at .98387, but on Day 7,

KM=.98387X182/183=.97850

On Days 8-15, KM stays at .97850, but on Day 16

KM=.97850X181/182=.97309

This process continues to day 3454.

Wouldn't a computer be nice? There are many excellent programs for both mainframe computers and micro-computers.

### 2.4.3.4 Standard Error

A second important quantity relative to the Kaplan-Meier Curve is the "Standard Error". This latter quantity is used to obtain confidence intervals for fixed term survival as well as for comparison of fixed term survival for two competing treatments. There are several forms of the standard error, but the most convenient is due to Peto et al (1977, Statistical Note 6).

For a given day,

$$SE=KM \text{ } SQRT\{(1-KM)/RX\} \tag{2}$$

With KM as in (1) above. RX is the number at risk at the start of the following day. [Some users replace RX by the value of R from (1). However, in nearly all cases, the alternate SE is virtually identical to that of (2).]

One-sided and two-sided approximate confidence intervals can be obtained (using W from Figures 8 and 9 respectively) for a single fixed term survival as: True Survival >KM-(W SE) One-Sided Upper (Figure 8)

| True Survival <KM+(W SE) | One-Sided Upper (Figure 8) |
| True survival <KM+(W SE) | One-Sided (Lower Figure 8) |
| KM-(W SE) <True Survival <KM+(W SE) | Two-Sided (Figure 9) |

From Figure 11, at three years, we see that KM=51.6%(.516) for the Control Group. RX=91, the number at risk at the start of Year 4, ie the next day. Note that there was no failure in the control group (Figure 10) at day 365*3=1095. Hence, R may be taken as the number at risk at the start of year 4 (Interval 3-4 Years), that is, R=91. In this case, the alternate SE is the same as that computed in (2).

$$SE= .516 \text{ } SQRT \text{ } \{(1-.516)/91$$

$$= .516 \text{ } SQRT \text{ } (.484/91)$$

$$= .516 \text{ SQRT } (.005319)$$

$$= .516 \text{ X } .0729$$

$$= .038 \text{ (or 3.8\% as per Figure 11)}$$

A One-sided 95% confidence interval for three-year survival is:

True control 3-year survival>.516-1.645X.038=.453

A Two-sided 95% confidence interval for three-year survival is:

.516-1.96X.038<True Control 3-year survival<.516+1.96X.038

that is between .442 and .590.

### 2.4.3.5 The Kaplan-Meier Comparison of Two Treatments

For the desired fixed term (eg 3 years), the following quantities are obtained: Control Group: KM1 and SE1, the Kaplan-Meier estimate and Standard Error at the desired time. Test Group: KM2 and SE2, the Kaplan-Meier estimate and Standard Error at the desired time.

Calculation of approximate P-value:

Let

$$Z = (KM2-KM1)/SQRT(SE1^2 + SE2^2) \tag{3}$$

Utilize Figure 6 (One-sided) or Figure 7 (Two-sided) to obtain the P-value.

In the numerical example of Figures 10 and 11, taken at three years,

KM1=.516 SE1=.038

KM2=.589 SE2=.036

$$Z=(.589-.516)/SQRT(.038^2 + .036^2)$$

$$=.073/SQRT(.001444+.001296)$$

=.073/SQRT(.002740)

=.073/.0523

=1.39

From Figure 6, the approximate P-value is .085, one-sided. (Had this been a two-sided comparison, the approximate P-value would have been .18. See Figure 7.)

## 2.4.3.6 Confidence Intervals for Difference in Fixed-Term Survival

Confidence Intervals for the difference in Fixed Term Survival can also be constructed. As in the Binomial example, they can be important in management decisions.

KM2-KM1 = Estimated difference in True survival at prescribed times (eg 3 years)

SED=SQRT($SE1^2+SE2^2$ ) is the Standard Error of this difference

A one-sided confidence interval is obtained using W from Figure 8 as:

True difference in fixed survival>(KM2-KM1) - W SED

A two-sided confidence interval is obtained using W from Figure 9 as:

(KM2-KM1) - W SED <True Difference <(KM2-KM1) + W SED

A one-sided 95% confidence interval in the numerical example of Figures 10 and 11 at three years is: (see calculation of Z above)

True difference in three year survival>(.073)-1.645 X.0523

> - .013

The corresponding two-sided 95% confidence interval at three years is:

$$-.030 = .073 - 1.96 \times .0523 < \text{True Difference} < .073 + 1.96 \times .0523 = .176$$

As in the binomial case, the practical implication of the confidence interval over that of the P-value alone is clear. With high confidence, we can state that the test treatment has from a 3.0% disadvantage to a 17.6% advantage in three year survival, when compared to that of the control. If disadvantages of the order of 3% are not considered to be clinically significant, then the test therapy is preferred, even though conventional significance at P<.05 was not achieved.

### 2.4.4 Logrank Test

By far the most common method of comparing treatments in censored survival experiments is via the logrank test. Justification for the name is somewhat technical. (Interested readers might refer to Section 5 of Peto and Peto (1972) for the rationale behind the name). The major difference between the Kaplan-Meier and Logrank tests concern the question which each asks. The Kaplan-Meier comparison asks if the survival probabilities differ at one and only one pre-specified point in time (eg 5 Years). The logrank test asks if the survival curves differ. In other words, the logrank comparison looks at the entire available spectrum of time and attempts to distinguish between the treatments on the basis of overall performance in terms of survival.

For each day, starting the clock at randomization, the data used is:

N1=Number of patients on the control therapy at risk at the start of that day.

F1=Number of control therapy patients who fail on that day.

N2=Number of patients on the test therapy at risk at the start of that day.

F2=Number of test therapy patients who fail on that day.

If we are asking the question: Are the therapies equivalent in terms of survival, we would expect that given the total number of failures on that day, that they would tend to be distributed to treatment groups in proportion to the number at risk in that group. We calculate

$$E1=N1(F1+F2)/(N1+N2) \text{ and } E2=N2(F1+F2)/(N1+N2)$$

The Logrank test looks at F1 vs. E1 and F2 vs. E2 across days. Suppose that when one adds across days, the F1 total vastly exceeds the E1 total. That is, the control therapy has many more failures than one would expect for equivalent therapy. One would infer that the hypothesis of equivalence was in doubt, and accept the hypothesis that the test therapy was superior. Conversely, fewer than expected failures on the control therapy would lead to inferred superiority of the control therapy.

In order to formalize this into a statistical test, a quantity, V is calculated for each day as follows. Suppose a deck of (N1+N2) cards has (F1+F2) failures. If we shuffle this deck and assign N1 to player "Control" and N2 to player "Test", we would expect on average E1 failures to be assigned to "Control" and E2 to "Test". The quantity V is the "Variance" in the number assigned, that is the AVERAGE SQUARED DIFFERENCE between the randomly dealt assignment and the EXPECTED ASSIGNMENT.

If N1+N2>1 then

$$V=N1N2(F1+F2)(N1+N2-F1-F2)/\{(N1+N2)(N1+N2)(N1+N2-1)\}$$

If N1+N2 = 1 then V=0.

The logrank statistic is defined as:

$$Z=\{Sum(F1)-Sum(E1)\}/SQRT\{Sum(V)\} \ ,$$

where Sum is taken over each day for which patients are on study.

An approximate P-value is obtained from Figure 6 for one-sided tests and from Figure 7 for two-sided tests.

### 2.4.4.1 Important Observations with Respect to the Logrank Test

Prior to studying a particular example, we note the following:

1. Days on which no failure occurs make no contribution to Z. On such days, F1=0, E1=0 (since F1+F2=0), and V=0. Hence, the sum can be restricted to days on which failures occur.

2. If either N1=0 (only test patients left on that day) or N2=0 (only control patients left on that day), no contribution to Z is made. Clearly, if N1=0, then F1=0, E1=0, and V=0. If N2=0 then clearly the number of test therapy failures on the day (F2) is zero. This further implies from the above formulas that E1=F1 and V=0. The contribution to the Sum(F1) is counterbalanced by that to Sum(E1). Hence, such days have no impact on either the numerator or denominator of Z.

3. On many studies, only one failure will occur on any given day. If this occurs,

$$V=N1N2/\{(N1+N2)(N1+N2)\}=E1E2. \text{ (One Failure)}$$

4. E1+E2=F1+F2. (See formulas).

5. Provided that relatively few failures occur on any given day, an excellent approximation for Sum(V) is

$$\text{Sum(V)} \doteq \text{Sum(E1)Sum(E2)}/\{\text{Sum(E1)+Sum(E2)}\}$$

$$\doteq \text{Sum(E1)Sum(E2)/(Total Number of Deaths)}$$

### 2.4.4.2 Numerical Example

Suppose that the control group survival (in days) is:

20,49+,122,245,301,332+,355+,378,398,402+,455,467+

while the experimental group survival is:

28+,122,255+,301+,344+,366,388+,409+,444+,477+,500,553+,

the survival in a randomized study of 24 patients. Only values followed by + indicate surviving patients.

The following table is a worksheet for the logrank test. Only days on which failures occur are included.

| Day | N1 | F1 | N2 | F2 | E1 | E2 | V |
|---|---|---|---|---|---|---|---|
| 20 | 12 | 1 | 12 | 0 | .500 | .500 | .250 |
| 122 | 10 | 1 | 11 | 1 | .952 | 1.048 | .474 |
| 245 | 9 | 1 | 10 | 0 | .474 | .526 | .249 |
| 301 | 8 | 1 | 9 | 0 | .471 | .529 | .249 |
| 366 | 5 | 0 | 7 | 1 | .417 | .583 | .243 |
| 378 | 5 | 1 | 6 | 0 | .455 | .545 | .248 |
| 398 | 4 | 1 | 5 | 0 | .444 | .556 | .247 |
| 455 | 2 | 1 | 3 | 0 | .400 | .600 | .240 |
| 500 | 0 | 0 | 2 | 1 | .000 | 1.000 | .000 |
| Sum | | 7 | | 3 | 4.113 | 5.887 | 2.200 |

$$Z=(7-4.113)/SQRT(2.200)=2.887/1.483=1.95$$

From Figure 6, this translates to a one-sided P=0.026.

**Sample calculation for day 122** — As can be seen from the data, there were 10 Control and 11 Test Patients alive at the start of Day 122. (Of the 12 controls, two did not reach day 122. One died at day 20 and another is alive but has only reached day 49.) (Of the 12 test patients, one is alive but has only reached day 28.) As can be seen from the data, one patient in each group failed on Day 122, and hence. F1=1 and F2=1. From the formulas for E1 and E2:

$$E1=N1(F1+F2)/(N1+N2)= (10X2)/21=20/21=.952$$
$$E2=N2(F1+F2)/(N1+N2)= (11X2)/21=22/21=1.048$$
$$V=N1N2(F1+F2)(N1+N2-F1-F2)/\{(N1+N2)(N1+N2)(N1+N2-1)\}$$
$$=(10X11X2X19)/(21X21X20)=4180/8820=.474$$

All other entries in the above table had only one failure on the day and hence for THOSE DAYS ONLY,E1=Proportion of patients on Control, E2=Proportion of patients on test, and V=E1E2.

### 2.4.4.3 *Footnotes to Numerical Example and the Logrank Test*

1. The approximation of Sum(V) in the above example is

$$Sum(V) \doteq Sum(E1)Sum(E2)/\{Sum(E1)+Sum(E2)\}$$

$$\doteq 4.113 \text{X} 5.887/(4.113+5.887) = 2.421$$

Had we used this approximation, we would have obtained:

$$Z \doteq 2.887/SQRT(2.421) = 2.887/1.556 = 1.86$$

instead of Z=1.95.

2. For large trials, despite the simplicity of the ideas, a computer would be most helpful in completing the analysis.

3. The validity of the approximate P-values depends on the accuracy of the "Normal Approximations". Generally speaking, for most applications, the approximations are acceptable if Sum(E1) and Sum(E2) both are five or more. The above example would be a borderline case.

As a check on the validity of the above one-sided P-value, we ran a small simulation study as follows. For each of 250 allocations, 12 patients were randomly reallocated to either the "Control" and 12 to the "Test" group. Using the same survival data, 4 of these reallocations had Z at least 1.95 in favor of the "Test" group. If there really was no target difference between the therapies, then any hypothetical allocation of the 24 patients into groups of 12 would be equally likely. Thus, of the 251 allocations (including the actual one), 5 (including the actual one) were 1.95 or higher. This yields a P-Value of about .020, one-sided. While as pointed out in Shuster and Boyett (1979) that this is a legitimate Exact "Conditional" P-value, it should be viewed as an approximation to complete enumeration of the 2.7 million possible reallocations of the 24 patients into two groups of 12.

A review of the definition of P-Values will be needed to grasp the next paragraph. See Section 2.4.1 (Crucial Elements).

Conditional P-values, as mentioned in the Section on Fisher's Exact Test, are similar to other P-values, except that they impose artificial restrictions on the replication process used in our definition of P-Value. For this simulation study, the restrictions are that the same 24 outcomes are obtained, and the actual replicated treatment assignment is randomly picked from the 251 assignments (250 from simulation study plus the actual observed assignment.).

4. For trials involving more than one treatment, see Section 3.12 of CHAPTER 3. Note that "Z sub ALPHA" and "Z sub BETA" are the upper 100ALPHA% and upper 100BETA% point of the Standard Normal Distribution (Figure 6).

5. If the trial is stratified, the analysis can be conducted as per CHAPTER 3, Section 3.13. This is a non-technical Section, but the notation is slightly different.

## Corresponding Values for Each Stratum

|  | **CHAPTER 2** | **CHAPTER 3 (Section 3.13)** |
|---|---|---|
| Failures on treatment #1 | **Sum(F1)** | O |
| Expected failures on treatment #1 | **Sum(E1)** | X |
| Variance | **Sum(V)** | V |

### *2.4.4.4 Proportional Hazards and the Logrank Test*

While the logrank test is valid for testing the equality of two survival curves, it has large sample optimality properties, see Peto and Peto (1972), for the "proportional hazard" situation defined below. The sample size tables of this Handbook are computed under this model.

**Proportional Hazards Model Assumption**

Under a proportional hazards model, we assume that hazard ratio, the ratio of instantaneous death rates (Control:Test), does not depend on the time on test. To make this assumption concrete, suppose that the probability that an individual alive 6 months post randomization has a 1/1000 chance of dying on the next day under the test therapy and a 2/1000 chance of dying on the next day under the control therapy. Considering a day as an instant, the ratio of instantaneous death rates is:

$$(2/1000) / (1/1000)=2.0 \text{ at 6 months}$$

While the treatment specific instantaneous death rates are allowed to change over time in the proportional hazards model, the ratio is assumed to be constant over time. If the instantaneous death rate for the test group is 1/3000 at 2 years , we assume it is 2/3000 (double) at 3 years in the control group, since otherwise the ratio at 6 months would not be the same as that at 2 years.

This assumption is only used in obtaining the sample size tables. Failure of this assumption does not render the logrank test invalid as a device to compare the equality of two survival distributions.

## REFERENCES

1. **Abramson, N. S., Meisel, J. D., and Safer, P.,** Deferred consent: a new aproach for resuscitation on comatose patients, *JAMA,* 255, 2466, 1986.

2. **Armitage, P.,** *Statistical Methods in Medical Research,* Blackwell Scientific, Oxford, England, 1971.

3. **Armitage, P.,** *Sequential Medical Trials,* Blackwell Scientific, Oxford, England, 1975.

4. **Buyse, M. E. , Staquel, M., and Sylvester, R. J.,** *Cancer Clinical Trials: Methods and Practise,* Oxford University Press, England, 1984.

5. **Diehl, L. F. and Perry, D. J.,** A comparison of randomized concurrent controls with matched historical controls: are historical controls valid?, *J. Clin. Oncol.,* 4, 114, 1986.

6. **Dupont, W.,** Randomized vs. historical clinical trials: are the benefits worth the cost?, *Am. J. Epidemiol.,* 122, 940, 1985.

7. **Fletcher R. H.,** Clinical trials, randomized consent and estimation (letter and response), *J. Chron. Dis.,* 37, 953, 1984.

8. **Gehan, E. A.,** Comparative clinical trials with historical controls, *Biomedicine,* 28 (Special issue), 13, 1978.

9. **Gehan, E. A.,** Randomized or historical control groups in cancer clinical trials: are historical controls valid?, *J. Clin. Oncol.,* 4, 1024, 1986.

10. **Haynes, R. B. and Dantes, R.,** Patient compliance and the conduct and interpretation of therapeutic trials, *Controlled Clin. Trials,* 8, 12, 1987.

11. **Kaplan E. L. and Meier, P.,** Nonparametric estimation from incomplete observatons, *J. Am. Stat Assoc.,* 53, 447, 1958.

12. **Link, M. P., Goorin, A. M., Miser, A. W. Green, A., Pratt, C., Belasco, J. B., Pritchard, J., Malpas, J. S., Baker, A. R., Kirkpatrick, J. A., Ayala, A. G., Shuster, J. J., Abelson, H. T., Simone, J. V., and Vietti, T. J.,** The effect of adjuvant chemotherapy on relapse-free survival in patients with osteosarcoma of the extremity, *N. Engl. J. Med.,* 314, 1600, 1986.

13. **Meinert, C. L.,** *Clinical Trials: Design, Conduct, and Analysis,* Oxford University Press, New York, 1986.

14. **O'Brien, P. C. and Fleming, T. R.,** A multiple testing procedure for clinical trials, *Biometrics,* 35, 549, 1979.

15. **Peto, R. and Peto, J.,** Asymptotically efficient rank invariant test procedures, *J. R. Stat. Soc. Ser. A,* 135, 185, 1972. (With discussion.)

16. **Peto, R., Pike, M. C., Armitage, P., Breslow, N. E., Cox, D. R., Howard, S. V., Mantel, N., McPherson, K., Peto, J., and Smith, P. G.,** Design and analysis of randomized clinical trials requiring prolonged observation of each patient. I. Introduction and design, *Br. J. Cancer,* 34, 585, 1976.

17. **Peto, R., Pike, M. C., Armitage, P., K., Peto, J., Breslow, N. E., Cox, D. R., Howard, S. V., Mantel, N., McPherson, K., Peto, J., and Smith, P. G.,** Design and analysis of randomized clinical trials requiring pro-longed observation of each patient. II. Analysis and examples, *Br. J. Cancer,* 35, 1, 1977.

18. **Pocock, S. J.,** *Clinical Trials: A Practical Approach,* John Wiley & Sons, New York, 1983.

19. **Shuster, J. J.,** EXACTB and CONF : Exact unconditional procedures for binomial data, *American Statistician,* 42, 234, 1988.

20. **Shuster, J. J. and Boyett, J. M.,** Nonparametric multiple comparison procedures, *J. Am. Stat. Assoc.,* 74, 379, 1979.

21. **Shuster, J. J., Krischer, J. P. , and Boyett, J. M.,** Ethical issues in cooperative cancer therapy trials from a statistical viewpoint. I. A general overview, *Am. J. Pediatr. Hematol./Oncol.,* 7, 57, 1985.

22. **Shuster, J. J., Krischer, J. P., and Boyett, J. M.,** Ethical issues in cooperative cancer therapy trials from a statistical viewpoint. II. Specific issues, *Am. J. Pediatr. Hematol./Oncol.,*7, 64, 1985.

23. **Simon, R. and Wittes, R. E.,** Methodologic guidelines for reports of clinical trials, *Cancer Treatment Rep.,* 69, 1, 1985.

24. **Smith, W.,** Randomization and optimal design (with discussion by M. Zelen), *J. Chron. Dis.* 36, 609 1983. (Discussion 613—614; Rejoinder 615.)

25. **Suissa, S. and Shuster, J. J.,** Exact unconditional sample sizes for the 2 ×.2 binomial trial, *J. R. Stat. Assoc.,* 53, 447,1971.

26. **Tsiatis, A. A. and Rosner, G. L.,** Group sequential tests with censored survival data adjusting for covariates, *Biometrika,* 72, 365, 1985.

27. **Zelen, M.,** New design for randomized clinical trials, *N. Engl. J. Med.,* 300,1242, 1978.

28. **Zelen, M.,** Strategy and alternate randomized design in cancer clinical trials, *Cancer Treatment Rep.,* 66, 1095, 1982.

29. **Zelen, M.,** Guidelines for publishing papers on cancer clinical trials: responsibilities of Editors and Authors, *J. Clin. Oncol.,* 1. 154, 1983.

**FIGURE 4. Simple randomization for 1200 patients.**

```
122112222211111121112111221212112222111212211212
>>>>>>>>>>>>>>>>>>>>>>>>>>>>>>>>>>>>>>>>>>>>>>>>>>
211121122111222122211221112111221212111212111221
>>>>>>>>>>>>>>>>>>>>>>>>>>>>>>>>>>>>>>>>>>>>>>>>>>
122121121212221112211221221222122221122212 1222112
>>>>>>>>>>>>>>>>>>>>>>>>>>>>>>>>>>>>>>>>>>>>>>>>>>
211111212121111211112222121212222221111122112111
>>>>>>>>>>>>>>>>>>>>>>>>>>>>>>>>>>>>>>>>>>>>>>>>>>
111212222121211122211211122122122112211211 2112122
>>>>>>>>>>>>>>>>>>>>>>>>>>>>>>>>>>>>>>>>>>>>>>>>>>
111112111112221122111221222112122112221111 11222122
>>>>>>>>>>>>>>>>>>>>>>>>>>>>>>>>>>>>>>>>>>>>>>>>>>
222211111221222222111112111211112122122121212111
>>>>>>>>>>>>>>>>>>>>>>>>>>>>>>>>>>>>>>>>>>>>>>>>>>
222122221121212111221121221121112112222222111121
>>>>>>>>>>>>>>>>>>>>>>>>>>>>>>>>>>>>>>>>>>>>>>>>>>
112112121111111121221121212122112122221211211 22212 1
>>>>>>>>>>>>>>>>>>>>>>>>>>>>>>>>>>>>>>>>>>>>>>>>>>
211212121111211121221121211111122121211122111122
>>>>>>>>>>>>>>>>>>>>>>>>>>>>>>>>>>>>>>>>>>>>>>>>>>
212211211221212212212111122211111112111221211222
>>>>>>>>>>>>>>>>>>>>>>>>>>>>>>>>>>>>>>>>>>>>>>>>>>
211222212121222121111121211111212222111221211122
>>>>>>>>>>>>>>>>>>>>>>>>>>>>>>>>>>>>>>>>>>>>>>>>>>
112121112112211111212112122112122211122111211 1211211
>>>>>>>>>>>>>>>>>>>>>>>>>>>>>>>>>>>>>>>>>>>>>>>>>>
122112222112222222111122211111121211211222121 1211211
>>>>>>>>>>>>>>>>>>>>>>>>>>>>>>>>>>>>>>>>>>>>>>>>>>
111121111211122122212111112222121111211112121 11111
>>>>>>>>>>>>>>>>>>>>>>>>>>>>>>>>>>>>>>>>>>>>>>>>>>
111222221112122222121111212111121222211111111221
>>>>>>>>>>>>>>>>>>>>>>>>>>>>>>>>>>>>>>>>>>>>>>>>>>
222212211112121112211222112222222221221122112 1122
>>>>>>>>>>>>>>>>>>>>>>>>>>>>>>>>>>>>>>>>>>>>>>>>>>
212112221221121122112222111111221112121212222222
>>>>>>>>>>>>>>>>>>>>>>>>>>>>>>>>>>>>>>>>>>>>>>>>>>
111212211121222211222221121222221211221112121212
>>>>>>>>>>>>>>>>>>>>>>>>>>>>>>>>>>>>>>>>>>>>>>>>>>
222212222122112112222222222211211222111222211221
>>>>>>>>>>>>>>>>>>>>>>>>>>>>>>>>>>>>>>>>>>>>>>>>>>
122112221112221112212211111121211121221122221111
>>>>>>>>>>>>>>>>>>>>>>>>>>>>>>>>>>>>>>>>>>>>>>>>>>
111211221211221222122222122122112121221111112111
>>>>>>>>>>>>>>>>>>>>>>>>>>>>>>>>>>>>>>>>>>>>>>>>>>
211121211121112212222111111121222111212211111122112
>>>>>>>>>>>>>>>>>>>>>>>>>>>>>>>>>>>>>>>>>>>>>>>>>>
211211211112221111222221121112112222221112122222
>>>>>>>>>>>>>>>>>>>>>>>>>>>>>>>>>>>>>>>>>>>>>>>>>>
```

**FIGURE 5. Random length permuted block lengths of four or six patients.**

```
22111221212122121121211212112212212112112112212212 2112
>>>>>>>>>>>>>>>>>>>>>>>>>>>>>>>>>>>>>>>>>>>>>>>>>>>>
21111222122112121211221212211221121221112212121211
>>>>>>>>>>>>>>>>>>>>>>>>>>>>>>>>>>>>>>>>>>>>>>>>>>>>
22122122111212211122112221112122221121112212212 2211
>>>>>>>>>>>>>>>>>>>>>>>>>>>>>>>>>>>>>>>>>>>>>>>>>>>>
21212112122212112111222121221121122111221222 1211
>>>>>>>>>>>>>>>>>>>>>>>>>>>>>>>>>>>>>>>>>>>>>>>>>>>>
11212212212211122211221211121221212 2112121212211
>>>>>>>>>>>>>>>>>>>>>>>>>>>>>>>>>>>>>>>>>>>>>>>>>>>>
12121221122111221212212121211221121212122 121211112221
>>>>>>>>>>>>>>>>>>>>>>>>>>>>>>>>>>>>>>>>>>>>>>>>>>>>
21122211221211221112211212222111212 12111122 21221
>>>>>>>>>>>>>>>>>>>>>>>>>>>>>>>>>>>>>>>>>>>>>>>>>>>>
22112221112212112211112212121221122211122 11121122
>>>>>>>>>>>>>>>>>>>>>>>>>>>>>>>>>>>>>>>>>>>>>>>>>>>>
12221121121222112212212111222122111212 22211111112
>>>>>>>>>>>>>>>>>>>>>>>>>>>>>>>>>>>>>>>>>>>>>>>>>>>>
2222112122111121222112221112211211212211 21221221
>>>>>>>>>>>>>>>>>>>>>>>>>>>>>>>>>>>>>>>>>>>>>>>>>>>>
12112222211111222221111122112122212112 2111222211
>>>>>>>>>>>>>>>>>>>>>>>>>>>>>>>>>>>>>>>>>>>>>>>>>>>>
12112212121222111212111222121221112211 22221111122
>>>>>>>>>>>>>>>>>>>>>>>>>>>>>>>>>>>>>>>>>>>>>>>>>>>>
2121222111111222112122121221212121212121 21122112
>>>>>>>>>>>>>>>>>>>>>>>>>>>>>>>>>>>>>>>>>>>>>>>>>>>>
12212121112212211222112112221112212222 11122121111
>>>>>>>>>>>>>>>>>>>>>>>>>>>>>>>>>>>>>>>>>>>>>>>>>>>>
12222112212121211212122111212211212212 1122111222
>>>>>>>>>>>>>>>>>>>>>>>>>>>>>>>>>>>>>>>>>>>>>>>>>>>>
22211121221121212112112122221211211122 2111222112
>>>>>>>>>>>>>>>>>>>>>>>>>>>>>>>>>>>>>>>>>>>>>>>>>>>>
21112221212221111122211122112212221122 2111221211
>>>>>>>>>>>>>>>>>>>>>>>>>>>>>>>>>>>>>>>>>>>>>>>>>>>>
22121121211221212112122211221122211122 1211112122
>>>>>>>>>>>>>>>>>>>>>>>>>>>>>>>>>>>>>>>>>>>>>>>>>>>>
11122222112122211111221212121121221122 1221112222
>>>>>>>>>>>>>>>>>>>>>>>>>>>>>>>>>>>>>>>>>>>>>>>>>>>>
11212112111222221112121212121211222112 1221222112
>>>>>>>>>>>>>>>>>>>>>>>>>>>>>>>>>>>>>>>>>>>>>>>>>>>>
21112222112121212112121212211222211111 1222112212
>>>>>>>>>>>>>>>>>>>>>>>>>>>>>>>>>>>>>>>>>>>>>>>>>>>>
22112112211212121121221221112211222121 1212112122
>>>>>>>>>>>>>>>>>>>>>>>>>>>>>>>>>>>>>>>>>>>>>>>>>>>>
21121221121122212121121212212121112211 21212 22111122
>>>>>>>>>>>>>>>>>>>>>>>>>>>>>>>>>>>>>>>>>>>>>>>>>>>>
21122211211112221221221211212111221222 1112121212
>>>>>>>>>>>>>>>>>>>>>>>>>>>>>>>>>>>>>>>>>>>>>>>>>>>>
22211121211121221122212112212121112221 2111221122
>>>>>>>>>>>>>>>>>>>>>>>>>>>>>>>>>>>>>>>>>>>>>>>>>>>>
```

## FIGURE 6. One-sided P-values for normal curves.

| IF Z WITHIN: P= | **** | IF Z WITHIN: P= | **** | IF Z WITHIN: P= | **** | IF Z WITHIN: P= | **** | IF Z WITHIN: P= |
|---|---|---|---|---|---|---|---|---|
| > 3.090: .001 | **** | 3.090 & 2.878: .002 | **** | 2.878 & 2.748: .003 | **** | 2.748 & 2.652: .004 | **** | 2.652 & 2.576: .005 |
| 2.576 & 2.512: .006 | **** | 2.512 & 2.457: .007 | **** | 2.457 & 2.409: .008 | **** | 2.409 & 2.366: .009 | **** | 2.366 & 2.326: .010 |
| 2.326 & 2.257: .012 | **** | 2.257 & 2.197: .014 | **** | 2.197 & 2.144: .016 | **** | 2.144 & 2.097: .018 | **** | 2.097 & 2.054: .020 |
| 2.054 & 2.014: .022 | **** | 2.014 & 1.977: .024 | **** | 1.977 & 1.943: .026 | **** | 1.943 & 1.911: .028 | **** | 1.911 & 1.881: .030 |
| 1.881 & 1.852: .032 | **** | 1.852 & 1.825: .034 | **** | 1.825 & 1.799: .036 | **** | 1.799 & 1.774: .038 | **** | 1.774 & 1.751: .040 |
| 1.751 & 1.728: .042 | **** | 1.728 & 1.706: .044 | **** | 1.706 & 1.685: .046 | **** | 1.685 & 1.665: .048 | **** | 1.665 & 1.645: .050 |
| 1.645 & 1.598: .055 | **** | 1.598 & 1.555: .06 | **** | 1.555 & 1.514: .065 | **** | 1.514 & 1.476: .07 | **** | 1.476 & 1.440: .075 |
| 1.440 & 1.405: .08 | **** | 1.405 & 1.372: .085 | **** | 1.372 & 1.341: .09 | **** | 1.341 & 1.311: .095 | **** | 1.311 & 1.282: .100 |
| 1.282 & 1.227: .11 | **** | 1.227 & 1.175: .12 | **** | 1.175 & 1.126: .13 | **** | 1.126 & 1.080: .14 | **** | 1.080 & 1.036: .15 |
| 1.036 & 0.994: .16 | **** | 0.994 & 0.954: .17 | **** | 0.954 & 0.915: .18 | **** | 0.915 & 0.878: .19 | **** | 0.878 & 0.842: .20 |
| 0.842 & 0.806: .21 | **** | 0.806 & 0.772: .22 | **** | 0.772 & 0.739: .23 | **** | 0.739 & 0.706: .24 | **** | 0.706 & 0.674: .25 |
| 0.674 & 0.643: .26 | **** | 0.643 & 0.613: .27 | **** | 0.613 & 0.583: .28 | **** | 0.583 & 0.553: .29 | **** | 0.553 & 0.524: .30 |
| 0.524 & 0.496: .31 | **** | 0.496 & 0.468: .32 | **** | 0.468 & 0.440: .33 | **** | 0.440 & 0.412: .34 | **** | 0.412 & 0.385: .35 |
| 0.385 & 0.358: .36 | **** | 0.358 & 0.332: .37 | **** | 0.332 & 0.305: .38 | **** | 0.305 & 0.279: .39 | **** | 0.279 & 0.253: .40 |
| 0.253 & 0.228: .41 | **** | 0.228 & 0.202: .42 | **** | 0.202 & 0.176: .43 | **** | 0.176 & 0.151: .44 | **** | 0.151 & 0.126: .45 |
| 0.126 & 0.100: .46 | **** | 0.100 & 0.075: .47 | **** | 0.075 & 0.050: .48 | **** | 0.050 & 0.025: .49 | **** | 0.025 & 0.000: .50 |
| 0.000 & -.025: .51 | **** | -.025 & -0.05: .52 | **** | -0.05 & -.075: .53 | **** | -.075 & -0.1: .54 | **** | -0.1 & -.126: .55 |
| -.126 & -.151: .56 | **** | -.151 & -.176: .57 | **** | -.176 & -.202: .58 | **** | -.202 & -.228: .59 | **** | -.228 & -.253: .60 |
| -.253 & -.279: .61 | **** | -.279 & -.305: .62 | **** | -.305 & -.332: .63 | **** | -.332 & -.358: .64 | **** | -.358 & -.385: .65 |
| -.385 & -.412: .66 | **** | -.412 & -0.44: .67 | **** | -0.44 & -.468 : .68 | **** | -.468 & -.496: .69 | **** | -.496 & -.524: .70 |
| -.524 & -.553: .71 | **** | -.553 & -.583: .72 | **** | -.583 & -.613: .73 | **** | -.613 & -.643: .74 | **** | -.643 & -.674: .75 |
| -.674 & -.706: .76 | **** | -.706 & -.739: .77 | **** | -.739 & -.772: .78 | **** | -.772 & -.806: .79 | **** | -.806 & -.842: .80 |
| -.842 & -.878: .81 | **** | -.878 & -.915: .82 | **** | -.915 & -.954: .83 | **** | -.954 & -.994: .84 | **** | -.994 & -1.04: .85 |
| -1.04 & -1.08: .86 | **** | -1.08 & -1.13: .87 | **** | -1.13 & -1.17: .88 | **** | -1.17 & -1.23: .89 | **** | -1.23 & -1.28: .90 |
| -1.28 & -1.34: .91 | **** | -1.34 & -1.41: .92 | **** | -1.41 & -1.48: .93 | **** | -1.48 & -1.55: .94 | **** | -1.55 & -1.64: .95 |
| -1.64 & -1.75: .96 | **** | -1.75 & -1.88: .97 | **** | -1.88 & -2.05: .98 | **** | -2.05 & -2.33: .99 | **** | -2.33 > : 1 |

### FIGURE 7. Two-sided P-values for normal curves; ignore sign of Z + VS -.

| IF Z WITHIN: P= | **** | IF Z WITHIN: P= | **** | IF Z WITHIN: P= | **** | IF Z WITHIN: P= | **** | IF Z WITHIN: P= |
|---|---|---|---|---|---|---|---|---|
| > 3.291: .001 | **** | 3.291 & 3.090: .002 | **** | 3.090 & 2.968: .003 | **** | 2.968 & 2.878: .004 | **** | 2.878 & 2.807: .005 |
| 2.807 & 2.748: .006 | **** | 2.748 & 2.697: .007 | **** | 2.697 & 2.652: .008 | **** | 2.652 & 2.612: .009 | **** | 2.612 & 2.576: .010 |
| 2.576 & 2.512: .012 | **** | 2.512 & 2.457: .014 | **** | 2.457 & 2.409: .016 | **** | 2.409 & 2.366: .018 | **** | 2.366 & 2.326: .020 |
| 2.326 & 2.290: .022 | **** | 2.290 & 2.257: .024 | **** | 2.257 & 2.226: .026 | **** | 2.226 & 2.197: .028 | **** | 2.197 & 2.170: .030 |
| 2.170 & 2.144: .032 | **** | 2.144 & 2.120: .034 | **** | 2.120 & 2.097: .036 | **** | 2.097 & 2.075: .038 | **** | 2.075 & 2.054: .040 |
| 2.054 & 2.034: .042 | **** | 2.034 & 2.014: .044 | **** | 2.014 & 1.995: .046 | **** | 1.995 & 1.977: .048 | **** | 1.977 & 1.960: .050 |
| 1.960 & 1.919: .055 | **** | 1.919 & 1.881: .060 | **** | 1.881 & 1.845: .065 | **** | 1.845 & 1.812: .070 | **** | 1.812 & 1.780: .075 |
| 1.780 & 1.751: .080 | **** | 1.751 & 1.722: .085 | **** | 1.722 & 1.695: .090 | **** | 1.695 & 1.670: .095 | **** | 1.670 & 1.645: .100 |
| 1.645 & 1.598: 0.11 | **** | 1.598 & 1.555: 0.12 | **** | 1.555 & 1.514: 0.13 | **** | 1.514 & 1.476: 0.14 | **** | 1.476 & 1.440: 0.15 |
| 1.440 & 1.405: 0.16 | **** | 1.405 & 1.372: 0.17 | **** | 1.372 & 1.341: 0.18 | **** | 1.341 & 1.311: 0.19 | **** | 1.311 & 1.282: 0.20 |
| 1.282 & 1.254: 0.21 | **** | 1.254 & 1.227: 0.22 | **** | 1.227 & 1.200: 0.23 | **** | 1.200 & 1.175: 0.24 | **** | 1.175 & 1.150: 0.25 |
| 1.150 & 1.126: 0.26 | **** | 1.126 & 1.103: 0.27 | **** | 1.103 & 1.080: 0.28 | **** | 1.080 & 1.058: 0.29 | **** | 1.058 & 1.036: 0.30 |
| 1.036 & 1.015: 0.31 | **** | 1.015 & 0.994: 0.32 | **** | 0.994 & 0.974: 0.33 | **** | 0.974 & 0.954: 0.34 | **** | 0.954 & 0.935: 0.35 |
| 0.935 & 0.915: 0.36 | **** | 0.915 & 0.896: .037 | **** | 0.896 & 0.878: 0.38 | **** | 0.878 & 0.860: 0.39 | **** | 0.860 & 0.842: 0.40 |
| 0.842 & 0.824: 0.41 | **** | 0.824 & 0.806: 0.42 | **** | 0.806 & 0.789: 0.43 | **** | 0.789 & 0.772: 0.44 | **** | 0.772 & 0.755: 0.45 |
| 0.755 & 0.739: 0.46 | **** | 0.739 & 0.722: 0.47 | **** | 0.772 & 0.706: 0.48 | **** | 0.706 & 0.690: 0.49 | **** | 0.690 & 0.674: 0.50 |
| 0.674 & 0.659: 0.51 | **** | 0.659 & 0.643: 0.52 | **** | 0.643 & 0.628: 0.53 | **** | 0.628 & 0.613: 0.54 | **** | 0.613 & 0.598: 0.55 |
| 0.598 & 0.583: 0.56 | **** | 0.583 & 0.568: 0.57 | **** | 0.568 & 0.553: 0.58 | **** | 0.553 & 0.539: 0.59 | **** | 0.539 & 0.524: 0.60 |
| 0.524 & 0.510: 0.61 | **** | 0.510 & 0.496: 0.62 | **** | 0.496 & 0.482: 0.63 | **** | 0.482 & 0.468: 0.64 | **** | 0.468 & 0.454: 0.65 |
| 0.454 & 0.440: 0.66 | **** | 0.440 & 0.426: 0.67 | **** | 0.426 & 0.412: 0.68 | **** | 0.412 & 0.399: 0.69 | **** | 0.399 & 0.385: 0.70 |
| 0.385 & 0.372: 0.71 | **** | 0.372 & 0.358: 0.72 | **** | 0.358 & 0.345: 0.73 | **** | 0.345 & 0.332: 0.74 | **** | 0.332 & 0.319: 0.75 |
| 0.319 & 0.305: 0.76 | **** | 0.305 & 0.292: 0.77 | **** | 0.292 & 0.279: 0.78 | **** | 0.279 & 0.266: 0.79 | **** | 0.266 & 0.253: 0.80 |
| 0.253 & 0.240: 0.81 | **** | 0.240 & 0.228: 0.82 | **** | 0.228 & 0.215: 0.83 | **** | 0.215 & 0.202: 0.84 | **** | 0.202 & 0.189: 0.85 |
| 0.189 & 0.176: 0.86 | **** | 0.176 & 0.164: 0.87 | **** | 0.164 & 0.151: 0.88 | **** | 0.151 & 0.138: 0.89 | **** | 0.138 & 0.126: 0.90 |
| 0.126 & 0.113: 0.91 | **** | 0.113 & 0.100: 0.92 | **** | 0.100 & 0.088: 0.93 | **** | 0.088 & 0.075: 0.94 | **** | 0.075 & 0.063: 0.95 |
| 0.063 & 0.050: 0.96 | **** | 0.050 & 0.038: 0.97 | **** | 0.038 & 0.025: 0.98 | **** | 0.025 & 0.013: 0.99 | **** | 0.013 & 0.000: 1.00 |

**FIGURE 8. Values for W in one-sided confidence intervals for approximately normally distributed estimates.**

| CONFIDENCE INTERVAL: | ABOVE | ESTIMATE - W | SE | (UPPER CI) |
|---|---|---|---|---|
| CONFIDENCE INTERVAL: | BELOW | ESTIMATE + W | SE | (LOWER CI) |

| W | Confidence (%) |
|---|---|
| 0.84 | 80 |
| 1.282 | 90 |
| 1.645 | 95 |
| 2.33 | 99 |

Note: SE = Estimated standard deviation of the estimate, = "Standard Error"

Interpretation: Before the study is conducted, the probability that the true value of the parameter being estimated falls below the estimate + 1.654 standard error is about 95%. Thus, after the study is over, we have 95% confidence in the confidence statement. Note that once the study has been completed, the "game is over" and probability is no longer applicable.

**FIGURE 9. Values for W in two-sided confidence intervals for approximately normally distributed estimates.**

| CONFIDENCE INTERVAL: | ESTIMATE - W | SE | (LOWER LIMIT) |
|---|---|---|---|
| TO | ESTIMATE + W | SE | (UPPER LIMIT) |

| W | Confidence (%) |
|---|---|
| 1.282 | 80 |
| 1.654 | 90 |
| 1.96 | 95 |
| 2.58 | 99 |

Note: SE = Estimated standard deviation of the estimate, = "Standard Error"

Interpretation: Before the study is conducted, the probability that the true value of the parameter being estimated falls between the estimate ± 1.96 standard error is about 95%. Thus, after the study is over, we have 95% confidence in the confidence statement. Note that once the study has been completed, the "game is over" and probability is no longer applicable.

**FIGURE 10. Survival in randomized pediatric cancer trial entries are in days with + to indicate survivors.**

## TREATMENT 1 — CONTROL THERAPY

| | | | | | | | | | |
|---|---|---|---|---|---|---|---|---|---|
| 1 | 1 | 2 | 7 | 12+ | 16 | 21+ | 43 | 47+ | 48 |
| 53 | 74 | 105 | 120 | 120 | 131 | 140 | 155+ | 172 | 195 |
| 195 | 209 | 237 | 252 | 256 | 265 | 287 | 309+ | 348 | 351 |
| 353 | 361 | 364 | 365 | 371 | 377 | 377 | 391 | 396 | 398 |
| 398 | 404 | 413 | 413 | 414 | 431 | 436 | 445 | 449 | 456 |
| 462 | 464 | 495 | 506 | 514 | 523 | 553 | 571 | 571 | 595 |
| 605+ | 605 | 617 | 629 | 641 | 650 | 671 | 700 | 766 | 769 |
| 772 | 795 | 801 | 802 | 804 | 828 | 844 | 870 | 874 | 898 |
| 908 | 932 | 949 | 964 | 973 | 977 | 984 | 1004 | 1028 | 1035 |
| 1047 | 1048 | 1062 | 1068 | 1084+ | 1158+ | 1173+ | 1195+ | 1321 | 1330 |
| 1367 | 1372 | 1442 | 1476 | 1514+ | 1559 | 1602 | 1639 | 1671 | 1678 |
| 1680 | 1690 | 1758 | 1777 | 1793 | 1797 | 1807+ | 1824 | 1861+ | 1922 |
| 1923+ | 1929 | 1935+ | 1946+ | 1952+ | 1984+ | 1987+ | 1992+ | 1993+ | 2019 |
| 2028+ | 2042+ | 2064+ | 2082+ | 2088+ | 2090 | 2110+ | 2122+ | 2129+ | 2166 |
| 2186+ | 2236 | 2245 | 2247+ | 2249+ | 2277+ | 2293+ | 2306+ | 2308+ | 2352 |
| 2353+ | 2353+ | 2405+ | 2436+ | 2464+ | 2465+ | 2491+ | 2501 | 2544+ | 2546 |
| 2580+ | 2605+ | 2630+ | 2640+ | 2667+ | 2674+ | 2678+ | 2684+ | 2693+ | 2733 |
| 2763+ | 2764+ | 2766+ | 2772+ | 2843+ | 2847+ | 2878+ | 2897+ | 2919+ | 2919 |
| 3018+ | 3037+ | 3047+ | 3070+ | 3074+ | 3454+ | | | | |

## TREATMENT 2 — TEST THERAPY

| | | | | | | | | | |
|---|---|---|---|---|---|---|---|---|---|
| 2 | 4 | 12 | 14 | 15 | 21 | 28 | 32 | 41 | 44 |
| 75 | 75 | 83+ | 98 | 98 | 104 | 104 | 133 | 139 | 206 |
| 213 | 215 | 223+ | 234 | 244 | 285+ | 285 | 290 | 313 | 318 |
| 319+ | 322+ | 349 | 357 | 371 | 372 | 375 | 381 | 390 | 394 |
| 424 | 436 | 443+ | 443 | 443 | 444 | 466+ | 475 | 479 | 514 |
| 531+ | 537 | 560 | 564 | 586 | 609 | 623 | 633 | 646 | 648 |
| 656 | 662 | 669 | 704 | 709 | 716 | 720 | 721 | 723 | 748 |
| 750 | 753 | 758 | 764 | 772 | 772 | 774 | 779 | 854+ | 888 |
| 893 | 912 | 952 | 959 | 959 | 960 | 980+ | 996 | 1000 | 1003 |
| 1039 | 1049 | 1053 | 1094 | 1176 | 1196 | 1213 | 1227+ | 1231 | 1245 |
| 1248+ | 1255+ | 1256 | 1274 | 1290 | 1331 | 1415 | 1433 | 1554 | 1572 |
| 1665+ | 1690 | 1700 | 1714+ | 1727+ | 1727 | 1767+ | 1772+ | 1779+ | 1779 |
| 1829 | 1835+ | 1842 | 1847 | 1848 | 1871+ | 1880+ | 1886+ | 1905+ | 1912 |
| 1914 | 1922+ | 1939 | 1961+ | 1983+ | 1987+ | 1992+ | 2003 | 2004+ | 2009 |
| 2029+ | 2051+ | 2051+ | 2058 | 2063+ | 2067+ | 2072+ | 2079+ | 2087+ | 2089 |
| 2121+ | 2145+ | 2154+ | 2155+ | 2174+ | 2195+ | 2196+ | 2213+ | 2241+ | 2254 |
| 2310+ | 2329+ | 2381+ | 2414+ | 2418+ | 2423+ | 2441 | 2447+ | 2453+ | 2497 |
| 2523+ | 2526+ | 2545+ | 2548+ | 2554+ | 2560+ | 2583+ | 2589+ | 2605+ | 2657 |
| 2671+ | 2697+ | 2714+ | 2714+ | 2719+ | 2723+ | 2730+ | 2736+ | 2744+ | 2746 |
| 2771 | 2772+ | 2815+ | 2841+ | 2863+ | 2863+ | 2876+ | 2928+ | 2957+ | 2959 |
| 2972+ | 3010+ | 3017+ | 3139+ | 3244+ | 3310+ | 3337+ | | | |

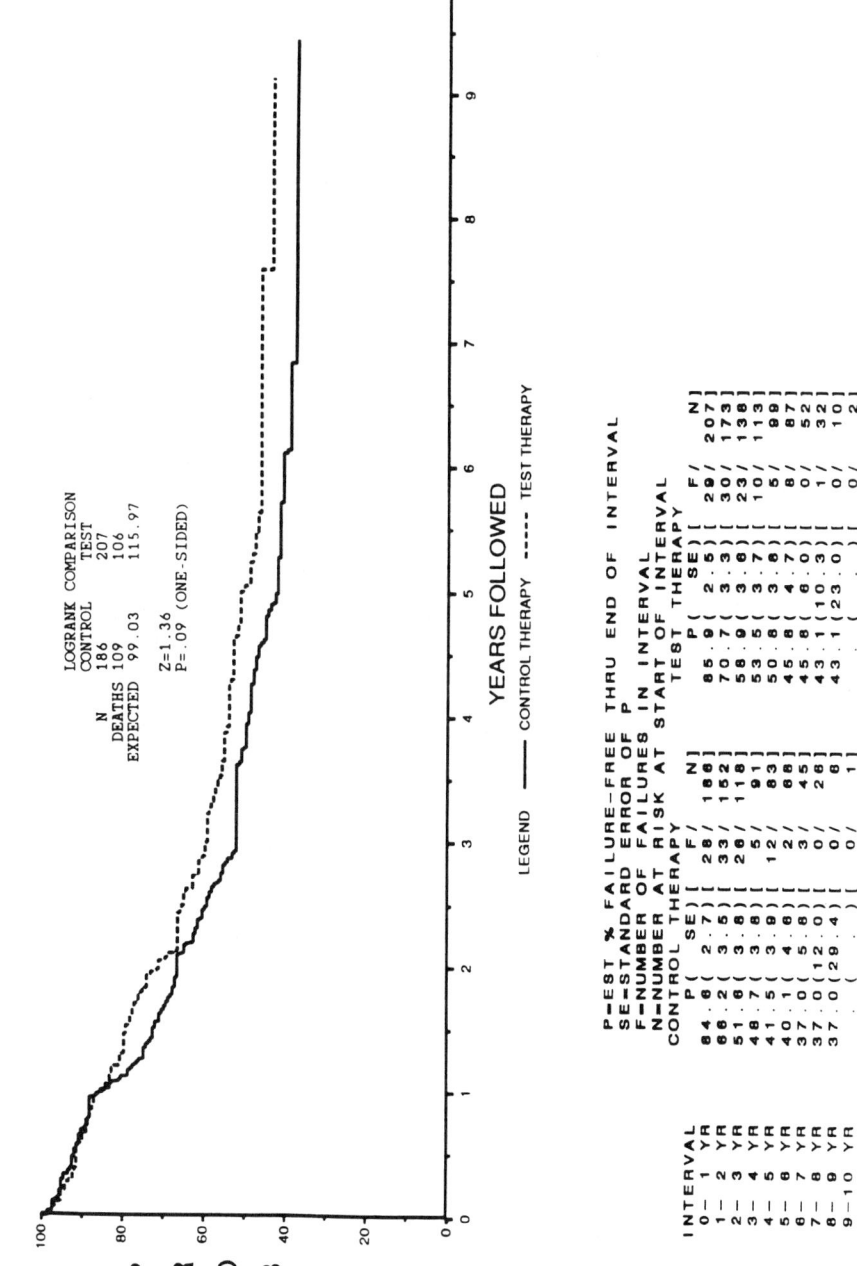

FIGURE 11. Survival comparison. See Figure 10 for raw data.

Chapter 3

# DERIVATION OF THE STATISTICAL RESULTS

In this section, we shall demonstrate the plausibility of the large sample results, while pointing to the gap in the derivation. The mathematical sophistication of a formal proof is well beyond the scope of this Handbook. The aim of this partial derivation is to keep the mathematical level at that of a reader who has completed one year of Mathematical Statistics. More advanced readers are referred to Crowley (1974) and Breslow and Crowley (1974) for complete derivations.

To avoid complicated "stochastic processes", we shall initially make the following artificial assumption. Imagine that for each treatment there is a potentially infinite source of patients. Imagine further that for treatment 1, we shall pick sample sizes of $N_1$ day #1's, $N_2$ day #2's, $N_3$ day #3's, etc. Similarly, for treatment 2, we shall pick sample sizes of $M_1$ day#1's, $M_2$ day #2's, $M_3$ day#3's, etc. For each day, j, we shall restrict our analysis to the first $N_j$ patients on treatment 1 at risk on day j and the first $M_j$ patients on treatment 2 at risk on day j. We assume that the $M_j$ and $N_j$ are selected in advance.

Of course, this not a practical way to conduct a trial. The best we usually can do in practice is to pick $N_1$ and $M_1$. The fate of the patient forces the actual values of the remaining N's and M's to be random. Further, since the recruitment process has staggered entry, the actual N's an M's are hard to control. Nonetheless, our artificial method of restricting the analysis allows us to treat the sample sizes (N's and M's) as fixed, and the outcomes on each treatment by day combination as independent binomial variables. The gap in applying the large sample results, as if the actual day-specific sample sizes were in fact planned, can be closed by more advanced "stochastic process" methodology. Intuitively, the percent error caused by using the actual sample sizes versus the non-random sample sizes equated to the expected sample sizes is negligible.

In summary, we shall prove our results under this artificial assumption. We shall argue that the results hold in general on the basis of intuition.

The attached notation chart will be useful in the derivations. Further, Appendix I gives a review of mathematical statistics topics used in the derivation of our results.

| NOTATION CHART | | |
|---|---|---|
| | TREATMENT 1 | TREATMENT 2 |
| 1. j | Patient Day # | Patient Day # |
| 2. Patients at Risk at Start of Day j | $N_j$ | $M_j$ |
| 3. Failures on Day j | $F_j$ | $G_j$ |
| 4. Probability of Surviving Day j given alive at start of Day j | $P_j$ | $R_j$ |
| 5. Probability of Failing on Day j given alive at start of Day j | $Q_j$ | $T_j$ |
| 6. Estimate of Parameter in 4 | $\hat{P}_j = (N_j\text{-}F_j)/N_j$ | $\hat{R}_j = (M_j\text{-}G_j)/M_j$ |
| 7. Estimate of Parameter in 5 | $\hat{Q}_j = F_j/N_j$ | $\hat{T}_j = G_j/M_j$ |
| 8. Cumulative Probability of Surviving at Least k days | $S_k = \prod\limits_{j=1}^{k} P_j$ | N/A |
| 9. Estimate of $S_k$ (Kaplan-Meier) | $\hat{S}_k = \prod\limits_{j=1}^{k} \hat{P}_j$ | N/A |
| 10. $D_k$ (Estimate Error of $\hat{S}_k$) | $D_k^2 = S_k^2 \sum\limits_{j=1}^{k} \left\{ Q_j/(P_j N_j) \right\}$ | N/A |
| 11. $\hat{D}_k$ (Estimate of $D_k$)(Greenwood) | $\hat{D}_k^2 = \hat{S}_k^2 \sum\limits_{j=1}^{k} \left\{ \hat{Q}_j/(\hat{P}_j N_j) \right\}$ | N/A |
| 12. $E_j$ = Expected Failures (Logrank) | $E_j = (F_j + G_j)\left\{ N_j/(N_j + M_j) \right\}$ | |

## 3.1 Derivation of the Large Sample Distribution of the Logrank Statistic

Consider the following null Hypothesis:

$H_0$ : Treatment 1 has the same survival curve as Treatment 2.

In terms of the parameters in item 4 of the Notation Chart, this is equivalent to

$$H_0 : P_j = R_j \text{ for all j}$$

The "logrank" test is sensitive to

$$H_0 : P_j = R_j \text{ for all j}$$

against

$$H_A^1 : P_j > R_j \text{ for all j} \qquad \text{(Treatment 2 Superior)}$$

or

$$H_A^2 : P_j < R_j \text{ for all j} \qquad \text{(Treatment 1 Superior)}$$

or a two sided alternative

$$H_A^3 : H_A^1 \text{ or } H_A^2.$$

When mixed behavior occurs under $H_A$, some $P_j < R_j$ while other $P_j > R_j$, the logrank test may not have good performance.

Structurally, we compute the following quantities relevant to Treatment 1:

$$O = \sum_j F_j \qquad \text{(observed failures on Treatment 1),} \qquad (1.1)$$

$$X = \sum_j E_j \qquad \text{(expected failures on Treatment 1),} \qquad (1.2)$$

where

$$E_j = \frac{(F_j + G_j)N_j}{N_j + M_j} \qquad (1.3)$$

and

$$SE^2 = \sum_j \frac{N_j M_j (F_j + G_j)(N_j + M_j - F_j - G_j)}{(N_j + M_j)^2 (N_j + M_j - 1)}. \qquad (1.4)$$

If $N_j + M_j = 1$, then the $j^{th}$ term in (1.4) is defined as zero. The logrank statistic is

$$Z = \frac{O - X}{SE} \tag{1.5}$$

which under mild regularity conditions is asymptotically standard normal under $H_0$.

Note: If we interchange the definition of Treatment 1 and Treatment 2, all we do is change the sign of Z.

---

> The P-value is obtained from (1.5) and Figure 6 or Figure 7,
>
> depending on the Alternative Hypothesis.

---

**Large Sample Result (Logrank)**

If the assumptions below hold, then Z given in (1.5) is asymptotically standard normal.

Assumptions:

(a)     $\sum_j \dfrac{N_j M_j P_j Q_j}{N_j + M_j} \to \infty.$

(b)     No day is a "wipeout." There exists a positive number $\delta < 1$ such that

$P_j > 1 - \delta$     for all j.

This is equivalent to bounding the failure rates away from one,

i.e., $Q_j < \delta$     for all j.     $(Q_j = 1 - P_j)$

Plan of the Proof:

Step 1:  Representation of Numerator of Z.

$$\text{Prove} \qquad O - X = \sum_j \frac{(M_j F_j - N_j G_j)}{N_j + M_j} \qquad\qquad (1.6)$$

with

$F_j$     Binomial with Parameters $N_j$ and $Q_j$

$G_j$     Binomial with Parameters $N_j$ and $T_j$

and     $\left\{F_j\right\}, \left\{G_j\right\}$ mutually independent.

Step 2:

$$\frac{O - X}{V} \xrightarrow{D} N(0, 1)$$

where

$$V^2 = \sum_j \frac{N_j M_j P_j Q_j}{N_j + M_j}. \qquad\qquad (1.7)$$

See A93 for a definition of convergence in distribution ($\xrightarrow{D}$).

Step 3:  If Y is binomial with parameter Q and sample size N, then for $P = 1 - Q$

$$E\left\{Y(N-Y)\right\} = N(N-1)PQ$$

and

$$\text{Var}\left\{Y(N-Y)\right\} \le N(N-1)^2 PQ.$$

Step 4:  Show

$$\frac{SE^2}{V^2} \xrightarrow{P} 1.$$

Step 5:  Complete the proof.

Show that Z, defined in (1.5) converges in distribution to the standard normal.

Proof of Step 1:

$$O - X = \sum_j F_j - \sum_j E_j$$

$$= \sum_j F_j - \sum_j \frac{(F_j + G_j)N_j}{N_j + M_j}$$

$$= \sum_j \left\{ F_j - \frac{(F_j + G_j)N_j}{N_j + M_j} \right\}$$

$$= \sum_j \left\{ \frac{(N_j + M_j)F_j - (F_j + G_j)N_j}{N_j + M_j} \right\}$$

$$= \sum_j \frac{(M_j F_j - N_j G_j)}{N_j + M_j}. \qquad (1.8)$$

Now    $F_j$ is Binomial with parameters $N_j$ and $Q_j$

$G_j$ is Binomial with parameters $M_j$ and $T_j$

from the model assumed in the introduction to Chapter 3. This completes Step 1.


Proof of Step 2:

Let us represent the $F_j$ and $G_j$ as Bernoulli Random Variables, and apply the central limit theorem for Bernoulli variables.

$$F_j = \sum_{i=1}^{N_j} Y_{ij_1}$$

$$G_j = \sum_{i=1}^{M_j} Y_{ij_2}$$

with $Y_{ij_\ell} = 1$ or $0$ depending respectively on whether for treatment $\ell$, the $i^{th}$ patient trial on day j results in a failure or survival.

From (1.8),

$$O - X = \sum_j \sum_{i=1}^{N_j} \frac{M_j Y_{ij_1}}{N_j + M_j} - \sum_j \sum_{i=1}^{M_j} \frac{N_j Y_{ij_2}}{N_j + M_j} \tag{1.9}$$

Using (1.9) and the null hypothesis $Q_j = T_j$ we have

$$E(O-X) = \sum_j \sum_{i=1}^{N_j} \frac{M_j Q_j}{N_j + M_j} - \sum_j \sum_{i=1}^{M_j} \frac{N_j T_j}{N_j + M_j}$$

$$= \sum_j \frac{N_j M_j}{N_j + M_j} (Q_j - T_j) = 0;$$

$$Var(O-X) = \sum_j \sum_{i=1}^{N_j} \frac{M_j^2}{(N_j + M_j)^2} P_j Q_j + \sum_j \sum_{i=1}^{M_j} \frac{N_j^2}{(N_j + M_j)^2} R_j T_j$$

$$= \sum_j \left\{ \frac{M_j^2 N_j + N_j^2 M_j}{(N_j + M_j)^2} \right\} P_j Q_j \qquad \left( P_j Q_j = R_j T_j \right)$$

$$= \sum_j \frac{N_j M_j}{N_j + M_j} P_j Q_j$$

$$= V^2. \qquad \left( \text{From } (1.7) \right)$$

We wish to apply the Central Limit Theorem for Bernoulli Variables: (Condition 2), See **A107**

Let

$$b_{ijk} = \frac{M_j}{N_j + M_j} \qquad k = 1$$

$$= \frac{-N_j}{N_j + M_j} \qquad k = 2$$

From (1.9)

$$O - X = \sum_j \sum_{i=1}^{N_j} b_{ij1} Y_{ij1} + \sum_j \sum_{i=1}^{M_j} b_{ij2} Y_{ij2}$$

with

$$\sum_j \sum_{i=1}^{N_j} b_{ij1}^2 P_j Q_j + \sum_j \sum_{i=1}^{M_j} b_{ij2}^2 P_j Q_j = V^2.$$

Now $\qquad\qquad V^2 \to \infty.$ $\qquad\qquad\qquad\qquad\qquad$ $\left(\text{Assumption (a)}\right)$

To apply condition 2 of **A107** we must show

$$\frac{W}{V^3} \to 0 \text{ where}$$

$$W = \sum_j \sum_{i=1}^{N_j} |b_{ij1}|^3 Q_j + \sum_j \sum_{i=1}^{M_j} |b_{ij2}|^3 Q_j. \tag{1.10}$$

Now $\qquad \displaystyle\sum_j \sum_{i=1}^{N_j} |b_{ij1}|^3 Q_j = \sum_j \frac{N_j M_j^3}{(N_j + M_j)^3} Q_j$

and $\qquad \displaystyle\sum_j \sum_{i=1}^{N_j} |b_{ij2}|^3 Q_j = \sum_j \frac{M_j N_j^3}{(N_j + M_j)^3} Q_j.$

Thus

$$W = \sum_j \sum_{i=1}^{N_j} |b_{ij1}|^3 Q_j + \sum_j \sum_{i=1}^{M_j} |b_{ij2}|^3 Q_j = \sum_j \frac{N_j M_j (N_j^2 + M_j^2) Q_j}{(N_j + M_j)^3}.$$

Now since $(N_j + M_j)^2 \geq N_j^2 + M_j^2$

$$W \leq \sum_j \frac{N_j M_j Q_j}{(N_j + M_j)}.$$

From assumption (b), $P_j > 1 - \delta$ with $\delta$ fixed. Hence

$$W \leq \frac{1}{1-\delta} \sum_j \frac{N_j M_j Q_j P_j}{(N_j + M_j)} = \frac{V^2}{1-\delta}$$

That is, since $V^2 \to \infty$

$$\frac{W}{V^3} < \frac{1}{(1-\delta)V} \to 0.$$

$\Big($The other condition 2 postulates are clearly satisfied since $Q_j < \delta$ (bounded away from one) and

$|b_{ijk}| \leq 1.$ $\Big)$

This completes the proof of step 2.

Proof of Step 3:

Let Y be binomial with sample size N and parameter Q. Let P = 1-Q.

For now, let N > 1.

$$
\begin{aligned}
E\Big(Y(N\text{-}Y)\Big) &= \sum_{y=0}^{N} y(N\text{-}y)\binom{N}{y}Q^y P^{N\text{-}y} \\[2mm]
&= N(N\text{-}1)PQ \sum_{y=1}^{N\text{-}1} \binom{N\text{-}2}{y\text{-}1}Q^{y\text{-}1}P^{(N\text{-}2)\text{-}(y\text{-}1)} \\[2mm]
&= N(N\text{-}1)PQ \sum_{j=0}^{N\text{-}2} \binom{N\text{-}2}{j}Q^j P^{N\text{-}2\text{-}j} \\[2mm]
&= N(N\text{-}1)PQ.
\end{aligned}
$$
(1.11)

Note: if N=1, formula (1.11) holds since both sides equal zero.

Similarly, if for now N > 2,

$$
\begin{aligned}
E\Big(Y(Y\text{-}1)(N\text{-}Y)\Big) &= N(N\text{-}1)(N\text{-}2)PQ^2 \sum_{j=0}^{N\text{-}3}\binom{N\text{-}3}{j}Q^j P^{N\text{-}3\text{-}j} \\[2mm]
&= N(N\text{-}1)(N\text{-}2)PQ^2.
\end{aligned}
$$
(1.12)

$$
\begin{aligned}
E\Big(Y(N\text{-}Y)(N\text{-}Y\text{-}1)\Big) &= N(N\text{-}1)(N\text{-}2)P^2Q \sum_{j=0}^{N\text{-}3}\binom{N\text{-}3}{j}Q^j P^{N\text{-}3\text{-}j} \\[2mm]
&= N(N\text{-}1)(N\text{-}2)P^2Q.
\end{aligned}
$$
(1.13)

If N = 1 or 2 (1.12) and (1.13) hold since both sides are zero.

If for now N > 3,

$$E\Big(Y(Y\text{-}1)(N\text{-}Y)(N\text{-}Y\text{-}1)\Big) \;=\; N(N\text{-}1)(N\text{-}2)(N\text{-}3)P^2Q^2 \sum_{j=0}^{N\text{-}4}\binom{N\text{-}4}{j}Q^j P^{N\text{-}4\text{-}j}$$

$$= N(N\text{-}1)(N\text{-}2)(N\text{-}3)P^2Q^2. \tag{1.14}$$

If N = 1, 2, or 3 (1.14) holds since both sides equal zero.

$$E\Big(Y^2(N\text{-}Y)^2\Big) = E\Big\{Y(Y\text{-}1)(N\text{-}Y)(N\text{-}Y\text{-}1)\Big\} + E\Big\{Y(Y\text{-}1)(N\text{-}Y)\Big\}$$

$$+ E\Big\{Y(N\text{-}Y)(N\text{-}Y\text{-}1)\Big\} + E\Big\{Y(N\text{-}Y)\Big\}. \tag{1.15}$$

The above is obtained by writing

$$Y^2(N\text{-}Y)^2 = Y(N\text{-}Y)\Big\{(Y\text{-}1)+1\Big\}\Big\{(N\text{-}Y\text{-}1)+1\Big\}.$$

Substitution of (1.11) - (1.14) into (1.15)

$$E\Big\{Y^2(N\text{-}Y)^2\Big\} = N(N\text{-}1)(N\text{-}2)(N\text{-}3)P^2Q^2 + N(N\text{-}1)(N\text{-}2)\Big\{PQ^2 + Q^2P\Big\} + N(N\text{-}1)PQ$$

$$= N(N\text{-}1)(N\text{-}2)(N\text{-}3)P^2Q^2 + N(N\text{-}1)(N\text{-}2)PQ(P+Q) + N(N\text{-}1)PQ$$

$$= N(N\text{-}1)(N\text{-}2)(N\text{-}3)P^2Q^2 + N(N\text{-}1)^2PQ. \tag{1.16}$$

$$\Big[E\big\{Y(N\text{-}Y)\big\}\Big]^2 = N^2(N\text{-}1)^2P^2Q^2. \tag{1.17}$$

Hence subtracting (1.17) from (1.16) yields:

$$\text{Var}\{Y(N\text{-}Y)\} = N(N\text{-}1)\{(N\text{-}2)(N\text{-}3) - N(N\text{-}1)\}P^2Q^2 + N(N\text{-}1)^2PQ$$

$$\leq N(N\text{-}1)^2PQ. \tag{1.18}$$

This competes the proof of step 3.

Proof of Step 4:

Under the null hypothesis $(F_j + G_j)$ are independent binomials with respective sample sizes $(N_j + M_j)$ and respective parameters $Q_j$.

From (1.4) and (1.11) successively,

$$
\begin{aligned}
E(SE^2) &= \sum_j \frac{N_j M_j E\{(F_j + G_j)(N_j + M_j - F_j - G_j)\}}{(N_j + M_j)^2 (N_j + M_j - 1)} \\
&= \sum_j \frac{N_j M_j (N_j + M_j)(N_j + M_j - 1)P_j Q_j}{(N_j + M_j)^2 (N_j + M_j - 1)} \\
&= \sum_j \frac{N_j M_j P_j Q_j}{N_j + M_j} = V^2.
\end{aligned}
\tag{1.19}
$$

from (1.4) and (1.18) successively,

$$
\begin{aligned}
\text{Var}(SE^2) &= \sum_j \frac{N_j^2 M_j^2 \text{Var}\{(F_j + G_j)(N_j + M_j - F_j - G_j)\}}{(N_j + M_j)^4 (N_j + M_j - 1)^2} \\
&\leq \sum_j \frac{N_j^2 M_j^2 (N_j + M_j)(N_j + M_j - 1)^2 P_j Q_j}{(N_j + M_j)^4 (N_j + M_j - 1)^2} \\
&\leq \sum_j \frac{N_j^2 M_j^2}{(N_j + M_j)^3} P_j Q_j
\end{aligned}
$$

Now since $\quad \dfrac{N_j M_j}{(N_j + M_j)^2} \leq .25,$

$$\text{Var}(\text{SE}^2) \leq .25 \sum_j \frac{N_j M_j P_j Q_j}{N_j + M_j} = .25 V^2. \tag{1.20}$$

From Chebyshev's Theorem A51, (1.19) and (1.20), we have

$$P\left[\left|\frac{\text{SE}^2}{V^2} - 1\right| > \epsilon\right] = P\left[|\text{SE}^2 - V^2| > \epsilon V^2\right]$$

$$\leq \frac{\text{Var}(\text{SE}^2)}{\epsilon^2 V^4} \leq \frac{1}{4\epsilon^2 V^2} \to 0.$$

$V \to \infty$ by (1.7) and assumption (a).

That is, from the definition of covergence in probability

$$\frac{\text{SE}^2}{V^2} \xrightarrow{P} 1.$$

This complete the proof of step 4.

Proof of Step 5:

From step 2, we have

$$\frac{O - E}{V} \xrightarrow{D} N(0,1).$$

From step 4 and Appendix A98,

$$\frac{V}{\text{SE}} \xrightarrow{P} 1.$$

Hence by Slutzky's multiplicative theorem, Appendix A105,

$$\frac{O - E}{\text{SE}} = \left(\frac{O - E}{V}\right) \frac{V}{\text{SE}} \xrightarrow{D} N(0,1).$$

This completes the proof.

## 3.2   Derivation of the Large Sample Distribution of the Kaplan-Meier Statistic

Refer to the Treatment 1 column of the Notation Chart.

Large Sample Results

Assumptions:

(a)   The sample size on day j, $N_j$ are non-increasing:

$$N_1 \geq N_2 \geq N_3 \geq \ldots$$

(b)   No day is a "wipeout". There exists a positive constant $\delta < 1$ such that $P_j$, the probability of surviving day j is:

$$P_j \geq 1 - \delta \qquad \text{for all j.}$$

(c)   There is a minimum hazard on any given day. There exists a constant $c > 0$ such that

$$Q_j > c \qquad \text{for all j.}$$

Note that c can be small.

(d)   $D_k \rightarrow 0.$                    (See Notation chart item 10)

(e)   $N_k D_k \rightarrow \infty.$

Conclusions:

(1)   $\dfrac{\hat{S}_k - S_k}{D_k} \xrightarrow{D} N(0,1).$          (Standard Normal)

(2)   $\dfrac{\hat{S}_k - S_k}{\hat{D}_k} \xrightarrow{D} N(0,1).$

Note:  The limiting process can involve $Q_j$ (the probability of failure on day j given patient was alive at the start of day j), k (the day number at which survival is evaluated), as well as $N_j$ (the number of patients at risk at the start of day j.)

$\hat{S}_k$ is given in item 9 of the Notation Chart, $S_k$ in item 8, $D_k$ in item 10, and $\hat{D}_k$ in item 11. The arrow represents the limiting distribution (approximate distribution).  See Appendix **A93**.

Plan of Proof:

Step 1:  Show that

$$\hat{S}_k - S_k = H_k + I_k,$$

where

$$H_k = S_k \sum_{j=1}^{k} (\hat{P}_j - P_j)/P_j,$$

and

$$I_k = S_k \sum_{j=1}^{k} \left(\hat{S}_{j-1} - S_{j-1}\right)\left(\hat{P}_j - P_j\right)/\left(S_{j-1}P_j\right),$$

with

$$\hat{S}_0 = S_0 = 1.$$

Step 2:  Show

$$\frac{H_k}{D_k} \xrightarrow{D} N(0, 1). \qquad \text{(Standard Normal)}$$

Step 3:  Show

$$\frac{I_k}{D_k} \xrightarrow{P} 0.$$

Step 4:  Show

$$\frac{\hat{S}_k - S_k}{D_k} \xrightarrow{D} N(0,1). \qquad \text{(Standard Normal)}$$

Step 5:  Show

$$\frac{\hat{D}_k}{D_k} \xrightarrow{P} 1.$$

Step 6:  Show

$$\frac{\hat{S}_k - S_k}{\hat{D}_k} \xrightarrow{D} N(0,1). \qquad \text{(Standard Normal)}$$

Before formally conducting the proof, some rationalization might be in order. First, Central Limit Theorems apply to sums. Hence, we would like to write $\left(\hat{S}_k - S_k\right)$ as a sum. The astute reader might ask, "Why not take logs?" This would work if each $\hat{P}_j$ was asymptotically normal. However, most of the applications will have a large $N_j$ and a small $Q_j$ ($P_j$ near one). In these situations, the $\hat{P}_j$ may not be well approximated by normality.

The decomposition in Step 1 is motivated as follows.

Lemma (Product Difference to Summation):

Let

$$A_0 = 1 \qquad \text{and} \qquad A_j = a_1 a_2 \cdots a_j = \prod_{i=1}^{j} a_i,$$

$$B_0 = 1 \qquad \text{and} \qquad B_j = b_1 b_2 \cdots b_j = \prod_{i=1}^{j} b_i$$

with each $b_i \neq 0$.  Then

$$A_k - B_k = B_k \sum_{j=1}^{k} \frac{A_{j-1}(a_j - b_j)}{B_j}.$$

Proof:  By adding and subtracting common terms,

$$A_k - B_k = (a_1 b_2 \cdots b_k - b_1 b_2 \cdots b_k) + (a_1 a_2 b_3 \cdots b_k - a_1 b_2 \cdots b_k)$$

$$+ (a_1 a_2 a_3 b_4 \cdots b_k - a_1 a_2 b_3 \cdots b_k) + \cdots + (a_1 a_2 \cdots a_k - a_1 a_2 \cdots a_{k-1} b_k)$$

$$= \sum_{j=1}^{k} \left( \frac{A_j B_k}{B_j} - \frac{A_{j-1} B_k}{B_{j-1}} \right).$$

The term
$$b_{j+1} \cdots b_k = \frac{b_1 \cdots b_k}{b_1 \cdots b_j} = \frac{B_k}{B_j} \, ,$$

which produces the above sum.

Now
$$A_j = a_j A_{j-1}$$

and
$$B_{j-1} = \frac{B_j}{b_j}.$$

Substitution in the sum yields
$$A_k - B_k = B_k \sum \frac{A_{j-1}}{B_j} (a_j - b_j).$$

The completes the proof of the Lemma.

Proof of Step 1:

First, we apply the Lemma with

$$a_j = \hat{P}_j \qquad\qquad\qquad b_j = P_j$$

$$A_j = \hat{S}_j = \prod_{i=1}^{j} \hat{P}_j \qquad\qquad B_j = S_j = \prod_{i=1}^{j} P_j.$$

This yields
$$\hat{S}_k - S_k = S_k \sum_{j=1}^{k} \frac{\hat{S}_{j-1}}{S_j} (\hat{P}_j - P_j).$$

But since $S_j = S_{j-1} P_j$, this further reduces to

$$\hat{S}_k - S_k = S_k \sum_{j=1}^{k} \frac{\hat{S}_{j-1}(\hat{P}_j - P_j)}{S_{j-1} P_j}. \qquad\qquad (2.1)$$

Now since $\hat{S}_{j-1} = S_{j-1} + (\hat{S}_{j-1} - S_{j-1})$, equation (2.1) can be rewritten as

$$\hat{S}_k - S_k = S_k \sum_{j=1}^{k} \frac{(\hat{P}_j - P_j)}{P_j} + S_k \sum_{j=1}^{k} \frac{(\hat{S}_{j-1} - S_{j-1})(\hat{P}_j - P_j)}{S_{j-1}P_j}$$

$$= H_k + I_k. \qquad\qquad \text{(See Statement of Step 1).}$$

This complete the proof of Step 1.

Proof of Step 2: To prove normality, we shall apply the Central Limit Theorem for Bernoulli variables, See **A107**. Note that

$$(\hat{P}_j - P_j) = -(\hat{Q}_j - Q_j)$$

where $\qquad\qquad \hat{Q}_j = 1 - \hat{P}_j$ and $Q_j = 1 - P_j$.

Now $\qquad\qquad$

$$H_k = -S_k \sum_{j=1}^{k} \frac{(\hat{Q}_j - Q_j)}{P_j}$$

$$= -S_k \sum_{j=1}^{k} \sum_{i=1}^{N_j} \frac{(Y_{ij} - Q_j)}{(N_j P_j)}, \qquad\qquad (2.2)$$

where $Y_{ij}$ $i = 1 \ldots N_j$, $j = 1 \ldots k$ are independent Bernoulli random variables with

$$P(Y_{ij} = 1) = Q_j$$

$$P(Y_{ij} = 0) = P_j = 1 - Q_j.$$

Let

$$V_k^2 = \text{Var}\left(\frac{\sqrt{N}\, H_k}{D_k}\right),$$

where

$$N = N_k D_k.$$

From (2.2),

$$V_k^2 = \sum_{j=1}^{k} \sum_{i=1}^{N_j} b_{ij}^2 P_j Q_j$$

where

$$b_{ij} = -\frac{\sqrt{N} S_k}{N_j P_j D_k}.$$

Hence

$$V_k^2 = \frac{NS_k^2}{D_k^2} \sum_{j=1}^{k} \sum_{i=1}^{N_j} \frac{Q_j}{N_j^2 P_j}$$

$$= \frac{NS_k^2}{D_k^2} \sum_{j=1}^{k} \frac{Q_j}{N_j P_j} = \frac{ND_k^2}{D_k^2}$$

$$= N.$$

Note that under our assumption (e), $N = N_k D_k \to \infty$ and hence $V_k^2 \to \infty$.

We next show that

$|b_{ij}|$ is bounded.

$$|b_{ij}| = \frac{\sqrt{N} S_k}{N_j P_j D_k}$$

$$= \frac{\sqrt{N_k D_k} S_k}{N_j P_j D_k}$$

$$\leq \frac{S_k}{P_j \sqrt{N_k D_k}} \qquad\qquad N_k \leq N_j$$

$$\leq \frac{S_k}{(1-\delta) \sqrt{N_k D_k}}. \qquad\qquad P_j \geq 1 - \delta \text{ by assumption (b)}$$

Now since $N_k D_k \to \infty$

$$\frac{1}{\sqrt{N_k D_k}} \to 0$$

and hence there exists $B \geq 0$:

$$\frac{1}{\sqrt{N_k D_k}} < B.$$

Thus,

$$|b_{ij}| < \frac{S_k}{(1-\delta)B} \qquad \text{throughout the limiting process.}$$

Further, the $Q_j = 1 - P_j \leq 1 - \delta < 1$ are bounded away from one. $\Big(\text{Assumption (b)}\Big)$. To obtain condition 2 of the Central Limit Theorem, (**A107**) we must show

$$\frac{\sum\limits_{j=1}^{k}\sum\limits_{i=1}^{N_j} |b_{ij}|^3 Q_j}{V_k^3} \to 0.$$

Now

$$\sum_{j=1}^{k}\sum_{i=1}^{N_j} \frac{|b_{ij}|^3 Q_j}{V_k^3} = \frac{N^{3/2}S_k^3}{N^{3/2}D_k^3}\sum_{j=1}^{k}\frac{Q_j}{N_j^2 P_j^3} \qquad \Big(\text{uses } V_k^2 = N\Big)$$

$$\leq \frac{S_k^3}{(1-\delta)^2 N_k D_k^3}\sum_{j=1}^{k}\frac{Q_j}{N_j P_j} \qquad (\text{Since } N_j \geq N_k,\ P_j \geq 1 - \delta)$$

$$\leq \frac{S_k D_k^2}{(1-\delta)^2 N_k D_k^3} = \frac{S_k}{(1-\delta)N_k D_k}$$

$$\to 0. \qquad \Big(\text{Since } N_k D_k \to \infty \text{ per assumption (e)}\Big)$$

Hence, from Appendix **A107**

$$\frac{\sqrt{N}H_k}{D_k V_k} \xrightarrow{D} N(0,1).$$

However, since $V_k^2 = N$, (as shown above)

$$\sqrt{N}\, \frac{H_k}{D_k V_k} = \frac{H_k}{D_k}$$

and hence

$$\frac{H_k}{D_k} \xrightarrow{D} N(0,1).$$

This completes step 2.

<u>Proof of Step 3</u>:  First note that $I_k$ is a linear combination of terms

$$B_j = \left(\hat{S}_{j-1} - S_{j-1}\right)\left(\hat{P}_j - P_j\right). \qquad (2.3)$$

We shall use the independence of $\hat{P}_1, \ldots, \hat{P}_k$ to obtain the means, variances, and covariances of the B's.  See A45 and A46.

(a)    $E(B_j) = 0$

Proof:    $E(B_j) = E\left(\hat{S}_{j-1} - S_{j-1}\right) E\left(\hat{P}_j - P_j\right).$      ($\hat{S}_{j-1}$ and $\hat{P}_j$ are independent)

Since $\hat{P}_j$ is the binomial estimate of $P_j$, (a) is clear.

(b)    $Var(B_j) = Var(\hat{S}_{j-1}) Var(\hat{P}_j)$

$$= \left[ \prod_{i=1}^{j-1} \left\{ P_i^2 + \frac{P_i Q_i}{N_i} \right\} - S_{j-1}^2 \right] \frac{P_j Q_j}{N_j}$$

Proof:    Note that $E(\hat{S}_{j-1}) = E(\hat{P}_1 \ldots \hat{P}_{j-1}) = E(\hat{P}_1) \cdots E(\hat{P}_{j-1}) = P_1 \cdots P_{j-1} = S_{j-1}.$

$$Var(B_j) = E(B_j^2) \qquad \left( \text{Since } E(B_j) = 0 \right)$$

$$= E\left[ \left(\hat{S}_{j-1} - S_{j-1}\right)^2 \left(\hat{P}_j - P_j\right)^2 \right]$$

$$= E\left[ \left(\hat{S}_{j-1} - S_{j-1}\right)^2 \right] E\left[ \left(\hat{P}_j - P_j\right)^2 \right] \qquad (\text{Independence})$$

$$= \text{Var}\left(\hat{S}_{j-1}\right)\text{Var}\left(\hat{P}_j\right). \tag{2.4}$$

Now
$$\text{Var}\left(\hat{S}_{j-1}\right) = E\left(\hat{P}_1^2, \hat{P}_2^2, ..., \hat{P}_{j-1}^2\right) - \left\{E\left(\hat{S}_{j-1}\right)\right\}^2$$

$$= E\left(\hat{P}_1^2\right) \cdots E\left(\hat{P}_{j-1}^2\right) - S_{j-1}^2$$

$$= \prod_{i=1}^{j-1} \left\{P_i^2 + \frac{P_i Q_i}{N_i}\right\} - S_{j-1}^2, \tag{2.5}$$

since
$$\text{Var}\left(\hat{P}_i\right) = E\left(\hat{P}_i^2\right) - \left[E\left(\hat{P}_i\right)\right]^2 \qquad \text{implies}$$

$$E\left(\hat{P}_i^2\right) = \left[E\left(\hat{P}_i\right)\right]^2 + \text{Var}\left(\hat{P}_i\right) = P_i^2 + \frac{P_i Q_i}{N_i}.$$

Also
$$\text{Var}\left(\hat{P}_j\right) = \frac{P_j Q_j}{N_j}. \tag{2.6}$$

Upon substituting (2.5) and (2.6) in (2.4), the result (b) holds.

(c)     $\text{Cov}\left(B_i, B_j\right) = 0.$            $i \neq j$

Proof:

Since
$$E(B_i) = E(B_j) = 0$$

$$\text{Cov}(B_i, B_j) = E(B_i B_j).$$

Now if $j < i$,

$$\text{Cov}(B_i, B_j) = E\left[\left(\hat{S}_{i-1} - S_{i-1}\right)\left(\hat{P}_i - P_i\right)\left(\hat{S}_{j-1} - S_{j-1}\right)\left(\hat{P}_j - P_j\right)\right]$$

$$= E\left(\hat{P}_i - P_i\right) E\left[\left(\hat{S}_{i-1} - S_{i-1}\right)\left(\hat{S}_{j-1} - S_{j-1}\right)\left(\hat{P}_j - P_j\right)\right],$$

since $\left(\hat{S}_{i-1} - S_{i-1}\right)\left(\hat{S}_{j-1} - S_{j-1}\right)\left(\hat{P}_j - P_j\right)$ depends only on $\hat{P}_1, \ldots, \hat{P}_{i-1}$ and is therefore independent of $\hat{P}_i$. Now $E\left(\hat{P}_i - P_i\right) = 0$ and hence $\mathrm{Cov}(B_i, B_j) = 0$.

The result follows in a similar fashion if $i < j$.

Next, we shall evaluate the mean and variance of $I_k$.

$$I_k = S_k \sum_{j=1}^{k} \frac{\left(\hat{S}_{j-1} - S_{j-1}\right)\left(\hat{P}_j - P_j\right)}{S_{j-1} P_j}$$

$$= S_k \sum_{j=2}^{k} \frac{B_j}{S_{j-1} P_j} \quad,$$

since $\hat{S}_0 = S_0 = 1$ and $B_j = \left(\hat{S}_{j-1} - S_{j-1}\right)\left(\hat{P}_j - P_j\right)$.

Using linear combinations per A45 and the fact that $\mathrm{Cov}\,(B_i, B_j) = 0$

$$E(I_k) \quad = S_k \sum_{j=2}^{k} \frac{E(B_j)}{S_{j-1} P_j} = 0$$

$$\mathrm{Var}(I_k) = S_k^2 \sum_{j=2}^{k} \frac{\mathrm{Var}(B_j)}{S_{j-1}^2 P_j^2}.$$

$$= S_k^2 \sum_{j=2}^{k} \frac{\left[\prod_{i=1}^{j-1}\left\{P_i^2 + \frac{P_i Q_i}{N_i}\right\} - S_{j-1}^2\right]}{S_{j-1}^2} \frac{Q_j}{N_j P_j}.$$

Since

$$S_{j-1} = \prod_{i=1}^{j-1} P_i,$$

$$\mathrm{Var}(I_k) = S_k^2 \sum_{j=2}^{k} \left[\prod_{i=1}^{j-1}\left\{1 + \frac{Q_i}{N_i P_i}\right\} - 1\right] \frac{Q_j}{N_j P_j}. \qquad (2.8)$$

Now applying the Lemma on converting products to sums, we see

$$\prod_{i=1}^{j-1}\left\{1 + \frac{Q_i}{N_i P_i}\right\} - 1 = \sum_{i=1}^{j-1} A_{i-1}\frac{Q_i}{N_i P_i} \tag{2.9}$$

where

$$A_0 = 1$$

$$A_i = \prod_{\ell=1}^{i}\left\{1 + \frac{Q_\ell}{N_\ell P_\ell}\right\} < A_j \quad i < j$$

$$\mathrm{Var}(I_k) < S_k^2 \sum_{j=2}^{k} A_j\left(\sum_{i=1}^{j-1}\frac{Q_i}{N_i P_i}\right)\frac{Q_j}{N_j P_j} \le \frac{A_k D_k^4}{S_k^2}. \tag{2.10}$$

The above follows since $A_j \le A_k$ for $j \le k$ and the definition of $D_k^2$ in the Notation Chart.

Consider (2.9) with $j = k$.

$$A_k - 1 = \sum_{i=1}^{k} A_{i-1}\frac{Q_i}{N_i P_i}$$

$$< A_k \sum_{i=1}^{k}\frac{Q_i}{N_i P_i} = \frac{A_k}{S_k^2} D_k^2.$$

From assumption (d), $D_k \to 0$ and hence if we are sufficiently far in the limiting process,

$$1 \le A_k \le \frac{S_k^2}{S_k^2 - D_k^2}.$$

Hence from (2.10):

$$\mathrm{Var}(I_k) < \frac{D_k^4}{S_k^2 - D_k^2}. \tag{2.11}$$

By Chebyshev's Theorem, Appendix A51, for any small challenge number $\epsilon > 0$,

$$P\left[|I_k| > \epsilon D_k\right] < \frac{\mathrm{Var}(I_k)}{\epsilon^2 D_k^2}$$

$$< \frac{D_k^4}{\epsilon^2 D_k^2\left(S_k^2 - D_k^2\right)} \qquad \left(\text{by (2.11)}\right)$$

$$< \frac{D_k^2}{\epsilon^2 \left( S_k^2 - D_k^2 \right)}$$

$$\rightarrow 0. \qquad \qquad \text{Since } D_k^2 \rightarrow 0 \left( \text{Assumption (e)} \right)$$

That is,

$$P\left[ |\frac{I_k}{D_k}| > \epsilon \right] \rightarrow 0$$

for any arbitrary $\epsilon > 0$. From the definition of convergence in probability (Appendix A92), this completes step 3.

Proof of Step 4:  From steps 1, 2, 3

$$\frac{\hat{S}_k - S_k}{D_k} = \frac{H_k + I_k}{D_k} = \frac{H_k}{D_k} + \frac{I_k}{D_k}$$

$$\frac{H_k}{D_k} \xrightarrow{D} N(0,1) \qquad \frac{I_k}{D_k} \xrightarrow{P} 0.$$

By Slutsky's Theorem, Appendix A104, $\frac{\hat{S}_k - S_k}{D_k}$ has some limiting distribution as $\frac{H_k}{D_k}$, that is

$$\frac{\hat{S}_k - S_k}{D_k} \xrightarrow{D} N(0, 1).$$

This completes step 4.

Proof of Step 5:  This is similar to Step 3, but considerably more involved. This itself is proved by a series of steps, which we shall call "tasks". The ultimate goal is to show that

$$\frac{\hat{D}_k}{D_k} \xrightarrow{P} 1$$

To avoid working with random variables in the denominator we shall consider

$$\hat{U}_k = \frac{\hat{D}_k^2}{\hat{S}_k}$$

$$= \hat{S}_k \sum_{j=1}^{k} \left\{ \frac{\hat{Q}_j}{(N_j \hat{P}_j)} \right\} \tag{2.12}$$

and

$$U_k = \frac{D_k^2}{S_k}$$

$$= S_k \sum_{j=1}^{k} \left\{ \frac{Q_j}{(N_j P_j)} \right\}.$$

The large picture of Step 5 is to prove that

$$\frac{\hat{U}_k}{U_k} \xrightarrow{P} 1.$$

Tasks are as follows:

Task 5.1: (See Notation Chart)

Let
$$Y_j = \frac{\hat{S}_k \hat{Q}_j}{\hat{P}_j} = \hat{P}_1 \hat{P}_2 \cdots \hat{P}_{j-1} \, \hat{Q}_j \, \hat{P}_{j+1} \cdots \hat{P}_k. \tag{2.13}$$

Show
$$E(Y_j) = \frac{S_k Q_j}{P_j}$$

and hence

$$E(\hat{U}_k) = U_k. \tag{2.14}$$

Task 5.2: Show that

$$\text{Var}(Y_j) = \frac{S_k^2}{P_j^2} \left[ \left\{ Q_j^2 + \frac{P_j Q_j}{N_j} \right\} G_j + \frac{P_j Q_j}{N_j} \right] \tag{2.15}$$

where

$$G_j = \left\{ \prod_{\substack{i=1 \\ i \neq j}}^{k} \left( 1 + \frac{Q_i}{N_i P_i} \right) \right\} - 1. \tag{2.16}$$

Task 5.3:

Show that

$$G_j \leq \left( 1 + G_j \right) \sum_{\substack{i=1 \\ i \neq j}}^{k} \frac{Q_i}{N_i P_i}. \tag{2.17}$$

Task 5.4:

Show that if we are sufficiently far enough in the limiting process, there exists a constant $B_0$ such that for all $j \leq k$

$$\mathrm{Var}(Y_j) < B_0 D_k^2. \tag{2.18}$$

Task 5.5

Show that if we are sufficiently far enough in the limiting process, there exists a constant $B_1$ such that

$$\mathrm{Var}(\hat{U}_k) < B_1 D_k^6.$$

Task 5.6

Show        $$\frac{\hat{U}_k}{U_k} \xrightarrow{P} 1.$$

Task 5.7

Show        $$\frac{\hat{S}_k}{S_k} \xrightarrow{P} 1.$$

Task 5.8

Show        $$\frac{\hat{D}_k}{D_k} \xrightarrow{P} 1.$$

<u>Proof of Task 5.1:</u>

From (2.13) and the independence of the members of the product,

$$E(Y_j) = E\left(\hat{P}_1\hat{P}_2\cdots\hat{P}_{j-1}\hat{Q}_j\hat{P}_{j+1}\cdots\hat{P}_k\right)$$

$$= E(\hat{P}_1)E(\hat{P}_2)\cdots E(\hat{P}_{j-1})E(\hat{Q}_j)E(\hat{P}_{j+1})\cdots E(\hat{P}_k)$$

$$= P_1P_2\cdots P_{j-1}Q_jP_{j+1}\cdots P_k$$

$$= \frac{S_kQ_j}{P_j}.$$

$$E(\hat{U}_k) = E(\Sigma Y_j/N_j)$$

$$= \Sigma E(Y_j/N_j)$$

$$= S_k\Sigma\frac{Q_j}{N_jP_j} = U_k.$$

This completes task 5.1.

<u>Proof of Task 5.2:</u>

$$Y_j - E(Y_j) = \hat{Q}_j\prod_{\substack{i=1\\i\neq j}}^{k}\hat{P}_i - Q_j\prod_{\substack{i=1\\i\neq j}}^{k}P_i$$

$$= \hat{Q}_j\left\{\prod_{\substack{i=1\\i\neq j}}^{k}\hat{P}_i - \prod_{\substack{i=1\\i\neq j}}^{k}P_i\right\} + (\hat{Q}_j - Q_j)\prod_{\substack{i=1\\i\neq j}}^{k}P_i$$

$$= \text{Term 1} \qquad\qquad + \text{Term 2.}$$

Note that from independence $E(\text{Term 1}) = 0$, $E\big\{(\text{Term 1})(\text{Term 2})\big\} = 0$, and $E(\text{Term 2}) = 0$.

From A45 and A44,

$$\begin{aligned} \text{Var}(Y_j) &= \text{Var}(\text{Term 1}) + \text{Var}(\text{Term 2}) + 2\,\text{Cov}(\text{Term 1}, \text{Term 2}) \\ &= E(\text{Term 1}^2) + E(\text{Term 2}^2). \end{aligned} \qquad (2.19)$$

By independence and the fact that from A43,

$$\text{Var}(T) = E\Big[\big\{T - E(T)\big\}^2\Big] = E(T^2) - \big\{E(T)\big\}^2,$$

$$\begin{aligned} E(\text{Term 1}^2) &= \left(Q_j^2 + \frac{P_j Q_j}{N_j}\right)\left\{ \prod_{\substack{i=1 \\ i \neq j}}^{k}\left(P_i^2 + \frac{P_i Q_i}{N_i}\right) - \prod_{\substack{i=1 \\ i \neq j}}^{k} P_i^2 \right\} \\ &= \frac{S_k^2}{P_j^2}\left(Q_j^2 + \frac{P_j Q_j}{N_j}\right)\left\{ \prod_{\substack{i=1 \\ i \neq j}}^{k}\left(1 + \frac{Q_i}{N_i P_i}\right) - 1 \right\} \\ &= \frac{S_k^2}{P_j^2}\left(Q_j^2 + \frac{P_j Q_j}{N_j}\right)G_j \qquad \big(\text{see } (2.16)\big) \end{aligned}$$

$$\begin{aligned} E(\text{Term 2}^2) &= \frac{P_j Q_j}{N_j} \prod_{\substack{i=1 \\ i \neq j}}^{k} P_i^2 \\ &= \frac{S_k^2}{P_j^2}\frac{P_j Q_j}{N_j}. \end{aligned}$$

From (2.19).

$$\text{Var}(Y_j) = \frac{S_k^2}{P_j^2}\left\{\left(Q_j^2 + \frac{P_j Q_j}{N_j}\right)G_j + \frac{P_j Q_j}{N_j}\right\}$$

This completes Task 5.2

Proof of Task 5.3:

$$G_j = \prod_{\substack{i=1 \\ i \neq j}}^{k} \left(1 + \frac{Q_i}{N_i P_i}\right) - 1.$$

This is a difference of products, to which we shall apply the product to summation lemma with

$$a_i = 1 + \frac{Q_i}{N_i P_i} \qquad\qquad b_i = 1$$

$$A_0 = 1 \qquad\qquad A_i = \prod_{\substack{\ell \leq i \\ \ell \neq j}} a_\ell \quad i \neq j \qquad A_j = A_{j-i}$$

$$B_0 = 1 \qquad\qquad B_i = b_1 b_2 \cdots b_i = 1.$$

$$G_j = \sum_{\substack{i=1 \\ i \neq j}}^{k} A_{i-1} \frac{Q_i}{N_i P_i}. \qquad\qquad (2.20)$$

Now since $a_i \geq 1$

$$A_{i-1} \quad \leq \prod_{\substack{i=1 \\ i \neq j}}^{k} a_i = \prod_{\substack{i=1 \\ i \neq j}}^{k} \left\{1 + \frac{Q_i}{N_i P_i}\right\}$$

$$\leq 1 + G_j \qquad\qquad \left(\text{see } (2.16)\right).$$

Substituting in (2.20), we have

$$G_j \leq \left(1 + G_j\right) \sum_{\substack{i=1 \\ i \neq j}}^{k} \frac{Q_i}{N_i P_i}.$$

This completes Task 5.3

Proof of Task 5.4:

First note that since $0 \leq \hat{Q}_j \leq 1$

$$E(\hat{Q}_j^2) = Q_j^2 + \frac{P_j Q_j}{N_j} \leq 1. \qquad\qquad (2.21)$$

Substitution of (2.17) and (2.21) into (2.15) yields

$$\text{Var}(Y_j) \leq \frac{S_k^2}{P_j^2}\left[\left(1 + G_j\right)\sum_{\substack{i=1 \\ i \neq j}}^{k} \frac{Q_i}{N_i P_i} + \frac{P_j Q_j}{N_j}\right]. \tag{2.22}$$

Now since $P_j \leq 1$, $\dfrac{P_j Q_j}{N_j} \leq \dfrac{Q_j}{P_j N_j}$.

Substitution into (2.22) yields

$$\text{Var}(Y_j) \leq \frac{S_k^2}{P_j^2}\left[\sum_{i=1}^{k} \frac{Q_i}{N_i P_i} + G_j \sum_{\substack{i=1 \\ i \neq j}}^{k} \frac{Q_i}{N_i P_i}\right]$$

$$\leq \frac{S_k^2}{P_j^2}\left[\left(1 + G_j\right)\sum_{i=1}^{k} \frac{Q_i}{N_i P_i}\right] \tag{2.23}$$

Returning once again to (2.17), we note

$$G_j \quad \leq \left(1 + G_j\right)\sum_{\substack{i=1 \\ i \neq j}}^{k} \frac{Q_i}{N_i P_i}$$

$$\leq \left(1 + G_j\right)\sum_{i=1}^{k} \frac{Q_i}{N_i P_i}. \tag{2.24}$$

Now since from assumption (d),

$$D_k^2 = S_k^2 \sum_{i=1}^{k} \frac{Q_i}{N_i P_i} \to 0$$

and hence

$$\sum_{i=1}^{k} \frac{Q_i}{N_i P_i} \to 0. \qquad\qquad \left(S_k \text{ is fixed}\right)$$

Hence we can find for any constant $\epsilon$, a critical point along the limiting process such that once we have passed this point,

$$\sum_{i=1}^{k} \frac{Q_i}{N_i P_i} < \epsilon.$$

That is, from (2.24)

$$G_j < (1 + G_j)\epsilon \qquad\qquad (2.25)$$

Since $\epsilon$ is arbitrary, let us select its value as

$$\epsilon = .5. \qquad\qquad (2.26)$$

This implies

$$G_j < \frac{\epsilon}{1 - \epsilon} = 1, \qquad\qquad (2.27)$$

as long as we are sufficiently far enough in the limiting process.

Substituting (2.27) into (2.23), we have

$$\text{Var}(Y_j) \leq \frac{2S_k^2}{P_j^2} \sum_{i=1}^{k} \frac{Q_i}{N_i P_i}.$$

Finally, from assumption (b), $P_j \geq 1 - \delta > 0$

$$\text{Var}(Y_j) \leq \frac{2S_k^2}{(1-\delta)^2} \sum_{i=1}^{k} \frac{Q_i}{N_i P_i} = \frac{2D_k^2}{(1-\delta)^2}.$$

As long as we are sufficiently far enough along the limiting process, we can use

$$\text{Var}(Y_j) \leq B_0 D_k^2,$$

where

$$B_0 = \frac{2}{(1-\delta)^2} .$$

This bound does not depend on j. This completes Task 5.4.

Proof of Task 5.5:

From (2.12) and (2.13)

$$\hat{U}_k = \sum_{j=1}^{k} Y_j/N_j \,.$$

From Appendix A45,

$$\text{Var}(\hat{U}_k) = \sum_{j=1}^{k} \frac{\text{Var}(Y_j)}{N_j^2} + 2 \sum_i \sum_{i<j} \frac{\text{Cov}(Y_i, Y_j)}{N_i N_j} \,. \qquad (2.28)$$

Now from Appendix A50,

$$\text{Cov}(Y_i, Y_j) \leq \sqrt{\text{Var}(Y_i)\text{Var}(Y_j)}. \qquad (2.29)$$

Substitution of (2.29) into (2.28) yields

$$\text{Var}(\hat{U}_k) \leq \sum_{i=1}^{k} \frac{\text{Var}(Y_j)}{N_j^2} + 2 \sum_{i<j} \frac{\sqrt{\text{Var}(Y_i)\text{Var}(Y_j)}}{N_i N_j}$$

$$\leq \left\{ \sum_{j=1}^{k} \frac{\sqrt{\text{Var}(Y_j)}}{N_j} \right\}^2 \,. \qquad (2.30)$$

Substitution of (2.18) into (2.30) yields

$$\text{Var}(\hat{U}_k) \leq B_0 D_k^2 \left[ \sum_{j=1}^{k} \left\{ \frac{1}{N_j} \right\} \right]^2 \qquad (2.31)$$

From assumption (c), there exists a constant $c > 0$:

$$Q_j > c$$

That is,

$$\frac{Q_j}{P_j} = \frac{Q_j}{1 - Q_j} > \frac{c}{1 - c},$$

and hence

$$\frac{1 - c}{c} \left( \frac{Q_j}{P_j} \right) > 1. \tag{2.32}$$

Substitution into (2.31) yields

$$\text{Var}(\hat{U}_k) \leq \frac{B_0 D_k^2 (1-c)^2}{c^2} \left\{ \sum_{j=1}^{k} \frac{Q_i}{N_i P_i} \right\}^2$$

$$< \frac{B_0 D_k^2 (1-c)^2}{c^2} \frac{D_k^4}{S_k^4} \qquad \text{(See Notation Chart-10)}$$

$$< B_1 D_k^6,$$

where

$$B_1 = \frac{B_0 (1-c)^2}{c^2 S_k^4}.$$

This completes Task 5.5.


Proof of Task 5.6:

From (2.14) and Chebyshev's Theorem A51,

$$P\left[ \left| \frac{\hat{U}_k}{U_k} - 1 \right| > \epsilon \right] = P\left[ |\hat{U}_k - U_k| > \epsilon U_k \right]$$

$$< \frac{\text{Var}(\hat{U}_k)}{\epsilon^2 U_k^2}$$

$$< \frac{S_k^2 B_1 D_k^6}{\epsilon^2 D_k^4} \qquad \text{(Task 5.5 and Def of } U_k\text{)}$$

$$< \frac{S_k^2 B_1 D_k^2}{\epsilon^2} \to 0. \qquad \left( D_k^2 \to 0 \text{ by assumption (b)} \right)$$

This completes Task 5.6.

Proof of Task 5.7:

From Step 4,

$$\frac{\hat{S}_k - S_k}{D_k} \xrightarrow{D} N(0,1).$$

Since from Assumption (d), the asymptotic standard deviation, $D_k \to 0$, it follows that

$$\hat{S}_k \xrightarrow{P} S_k.$$

This completes Task 5.7.

Proof of Task 5.8:

By definition

$$\hat{D}_k^2 = \hat{S}_k \hat{U}_k \quad \text{and} \quad D_k^2 = S_k U_k.$$

Hence from Tasks 5.6 and 5.7 and Appendix A101,

$$\frac{\hat{D}_k^2}{D_k^2} = \left(\frac{\hat{S}_k}{S_k}\right)\left(\frac{\hat{U}_k}{U_k}\right) \xrightarrow{P} 1.$$

Hence from A98,

$$\frac{\hat{D}_k}{D_k} \xrightarrow{P} 1.$$

This completes Step 5.

Proof of Step 6:

$$\frac{\hat{S}_k - S_k}{\hat{D}_k} = \frac{\hat{S}_k - S_k}{D_k}\left(\frac{D_k}{\hat{D}_k}\right).$$

Now since $$\frac{\hat{S}_k - S_k}{D_k} \to N(0,1) \qquad \text{(Step 4)}$$

and $$\frac{D_k}{\bar{D}_k} \overset{P}{\to} 1 \qquad \text{(Step 5 and Appendix A98)}$$

we apply the product version of Slutsky's Theorem (Appendix **A105**) to conclude that

$$\frac{\hat{S}_k - S_k}{\hat{D}_k} \to N(0,1).$$

This completes the proof.  (You thought it would last forever.)

### 3.2.1    Difference Between Kaplan-Meier Curves

Suppose we have two independent Kaplan-Meier Estimators

Treatment 1:

$$\frac{\hat{S}_k - S_k}{D_k} \overset{D}{\to} N(0,1),$$

$$\frac{\hat{S}_k - S_k}{\hat{D}_k} \overset{D}{\to} N(0,1),$$

$$\frac{\hat{D}_k}{D_k} \overset{P}{\to} 1,$$

$$D_k \overset{P}{\to} 0.$$

Treatment 2:

$$\frac{\hat{S}_k^* - S_k^*}{\hat{D}_k^*} \overset{D}{\to} N(0,1),$$

$$\frac{\hat{S}_k^* - S_k^*}{\hat{D}_k^*} \overset{D}{\to} N(0,1),$$

$$\frac{\hat{D}_k^*}{D_k^*} \xrightarrow{P} 1,$$

$$D_k^* \xrightarrow{P} 0.$$

In addition, assume

$$\frac{D_k}{D_k^*} \to c. \qquad \text{(a constant)}$$

Then from **A108** and **A109**,

$$\frac{\left(\hat{S}_k - \hat{S}_k^*\right) - \left(S_k - S_k^*\right)}{\sqrt{D_k^2 + D_k^{*2}}} \xrightarrow{D} N(0,1) \qquad\qquad (2.33)$$

and

$$\frac{\left(\hat{S}_k - \hat{S}_k^*\right) - \left(S_k - S_k^*\right)}{\sqrt{\hat{D}_k^2 + \hat{D}_k^{*2}}} \xrightarrow{D} N(0,1). \qquad\qquad (2.34)$$

## 3.3    Exponential Survival

In this section, we shall introduce methods for analysis of exponential survival data. Curiously, we discuss these methods despite the practical fact that we would rarely be in a position to assume exponentiality in the analysis of a clinical trial.

We introduce the methods for the following reasons. (1) We shall be able to show that the logrank and exponential comparisons of the treatments have nearly the same power when the data are in fact exponentially distributed; (2) Planning of clinical trials is generally done under "Proportional Hazards Models", which implies that by a single monotonic increasing transformation, the failure distribution of both therapies can be converted to exponential. The logrank test remains the same under monotonic increasing transformations; (3) Derivation of power and sample size for trials can be done in a straight forward manner for exponential survival. Because of (1), these calculations will apply to the logrank as well. Due to (2), the calculations can be extended to proportional hazards models.

This section will cover the following topics:

(A)   Introduction to the Exponential Distribution

The key element is that

$P_j$ = Probability of Surviving Day j, given patient is on Treatment 1 and is alive at the start of day j, is the same for all j. That is, $P_j$ does not depend on j.

Similarly $R_j$ the corresponding value for Treatment 2 does not depend on j.

(B)   Estimation of the difference in daily failure rates.

$Q - T = (1-P) - (1-R)$

where $P_j \equiv P$ and $R_j \equiv R$.

Because of (A),

$$\hat{Q} = \frac{\text{Total failures on Treatment } \#1}{\text{Total days on Test for Treatment } \#1}$$

Similarly,

$$\hat{T} = \frac{\text{Total failures on Treatment } \#2}{\text{Total days on Test for Treatment } \#2}$$

Next, we shall obtain the large sample distribution properties of $(\hat{Q} - \hat{T})$. Unlike the logrank test, this will be done under the "alternate and null hypotheses." The logrank properties were restricted to the null hypothesis.

(C)   Relate the logrank test to the exponential test when exponentiality holds. We shall see that the logrank test will have only slightly less power than the exponential test. The power loss will have no practical impact. (Section 3.4)

(D)   Derive the sample size for exponential survival under given "planning parameters." (Sections 3.5, 3.6, and 3.7)

(E)   Extend the derivation to "proportional hazard models." (Sections 3.8 and 3.9)

(F)   Relate the derivation to the sample size tables. (Section 3.11)

**(A)  Introduction to the Exponential Distribution**

The reader is first referred to the Appendix A70 - A76.

Note that if the "hazard rate" for Treatment #1 is $\lambda_1$, then under Treatment #1

$$P_j = P\left[\text{Survive day j}|\text{alive at start of day j}\right]$$

$$= \frac{P\left[\text{Survive at least j+1 days}\right]}{P\left[\text{Survive at least j days}\right]}$$

$$= \frac{\exp\left[-\lambda_1(j+1)\right]}{\exp\left[-\lambda_1 j\right]} = e^{-\lambda_1},$$

i.e., $P_j$ does not depend on j.

Similarly, $R_j$ does not depend on j, where $R_j$ is defined in a similar manner to $P_j$, except for Treatment #2.

**(B)  Estimates of Failure Rates and Their Asymptotic Properties**

If the survival distribution for each treatment is exponential, then a significant simplification of the survival analysis can be achieved.  Under exponential survival, each day carries the same risk, regardless of how long the patient has survived.

Let us consider the following (See Notation Chart)

$$F = \sum_j F_j = \text{Total failures on Treatment \#1.}$$

$$N = \sum_j N_j = \text{Total days on test for Treatment \#1.}$$

$$G = \sum_j G_j = \text{Total failures on Treatment \#2.}$$

$$M = \sum_j M_j = \text{Total days on test for Treatment \#2.}$$

$$Q = Q_j \text{ (Same for all j)} = \text{Probability of failing on Treatment \#1 on any}$$
$$\text{day given alive at start of day.}$$

$T = T_j$ (Same for all j) = Probability of failing on Treatment #2 on any

day given alive at start of day.

$$\hat{Q} = F/N = \frac{\text{Total Failures on Treatment \#1}}{\text{Time on test for Treatment \#1}}$$

$$\hat{T} = G/M = \frac{\text{Total failures on Treatment \#2}}{\text{Time on test for Treatment \#2}}$$

Provided that $0 < Q < 1$ and $0 < T < 1$ are fixed, $N \to \infty$, $M \to \infty$ with $\frac{NQ(1-Q)}{MT(1-T)} \to c$ then

$$\frac{(\hat{Q} - \hat{T}) - (Q - T)}{\sqrt{\dfrac{Q(1-Q)}{N} + \dfrac{T(1-T)}{M}}} \to N(0, 1) \tag{3.1}$$

and

$$\frac{(\hat{Q} - \hat{T}) - (Q - T)}{\sqrt{\dfrac{\hat{Q}(1-\hat{Q})}{N} + \dfrac{\hat{T}(1-\hat{T})}{M}}} \to N(0, 1). \tag{3.2}$$

Further, if the probability of failure on any day is small, but NQ and MT are large,

$$\frac{(\hat{Q} - \hat{T}) - (Q - T)}{\sqrt{\dfrac{Q}{N} + \dfrac{T}{M}}} \text{ is approximately } N(0,1)$$

and

$$\frac{(\hat{Q} - \hat{T}) - (Q - T)}{\sqrt{\dfrac{\hat{Q}}{N} + \dfrac{\hat{T}}{M}}} \text{ is approximately } N(0, 1).$$

Proof of (3.1) and (3.2):

We shall prove normality of $\hat{Q}$ and $\hat{T}$ and apply **APPENDIX A108 and A109**.

We shall appeal to the Central Limit Theorem for Bernoulli random variables using subscripts

$i$ = trial number

$j$ = day number

$k$ = treatment number

$Y_{ijk}$ = 1 or 0 depending upon whether the $i^{th}$ trial on treatment $k$ - day $j$

results in a failure or not.

$$N\hat{Q} = \sum_{j} \sum_{i=1}^{N_j} Y_{ij1} \tag{3.3}$$

$$M\hat{T} = \sum_{j} \sum_{i=1}^{M_j} Y_{ij2} \tag{3.4}$$

with
$$N = \Sigma N_j \quad \text{and} \quad M = \Sigma M_j.$$

To prove normality of $\hat{Q}$, we apply A107-1. If we let $b_{ij} = 1$ in (3.3), and note that

$$E(Y_{ij1}) = Q.$$

$$\text{Var}(N\hat{Q}) = \sum_{j} \sum_{i=1}^{N_j} Q(1-Q)$$

$$= NQ(1-Q).$$

and
$$\sum_{j} \sum_{i=1}^{N_j} b_{ij}^3 = \sum_{j} \sum_{i=1}^{N_j} 1 = N.$$

$$\frac{\Sigma b_{ij}^3}{\left[\text{Var}(N\hat{Q})\right]^{3/2}} = \frac{\left[Q(1-Q)\right]^{-\frac{3}{2}}}{\sqrt{N}} \to 0.$$

This yields all conditions of A107-1, that is

$$\frac{N\hat{Q} - NQ}{\sqrt{NQ(1-Q)}} = \sqrt{N}\ \frac{(\hat{Q} - Q)}{\sqrt{Q(1-Q)}} \xrightarrow{D} N(0,1). \qquad (3.5)$$

Similarly,

$$\sqrt{M}\ \frac{(\hat{T} - T)}{\sqrt{T(1-T)}} \xrightarrow{D} N(0,1). \qquad (3.6)$$

We apply Appendix **A108** directly to obtain (3.1).

To prove (3.2), note that (3.5) implies

$$\hat{Q} \xrightarrow{P} Q$$

and hence by **A98**

$$\sqrt{\hat{Q}(1-\hat{Q})} \xrightarrow{P} \sqrt{Q(1-Q)}.$$

By **A95**,

$$\frac{\sqrt{\hat{Q}(1-\hat{Q})}}{\sqrt{Q(1-Q)}} \xrightarrow{P} 1\ .$$

That is,

$$\frac{\sqrt{\left\{\hat{Q}(1-\hat{Q})/N\right\}}}{\sqrt{\left\{Q(1-Q)/N\right\}}} \xrightarrow{P} 1\ .$$

Similarly

$$\frac{\sqrt{\left\{\hat{T}(1-\hat{T})/M\right\}}}{\sqrt{\left\{T(1-T)/M\right\}}} \xrightarrow{P} 1\ .$$

The conditions for A109 have been established and from A109, (3.2) follows.

This proves the major results.

The final findings are obtained by replacing $1 - Q$, $1 - T$, $1 - \hat{Q}$, and $1 - \hat{T}$ by one, in the standard error terms.

As is illustrated in the example below, the percentage error in doing so is extremely small.

Suppose that the one year survival rates are 50% on treatment 1 and 75% on treatment 2. That is,

$$(1-Q)^{365} = .50 \quad \text{and} \quad (1-T)^{365} = .75.$$

Hence

$$Q = .0019 \quad \text{and} \quad T = .00079.$$

$$\frac{Q}{N}(1-Q) = \frac{Q}{N}(.9981).$$

$$\frac{T}{M}(1-T) = \frac{T}{M}(.99921).$$

$$\frac{Q}{N} + \frac{T}{M} > \frac{Q(1-Q)}{N} + \frac{T(1-T)}{M}.$$

Thus, the simplified standard error $\sqrt{\frac{Q}{N} + \frac{T}{M}}$ overestimates $\sqrt{\frac{Q(1-Q)}{N} + \frac{T(1-T)}{M}}$.

Also,

$$.9981\left(\frac{Q}{N} + \frac{T}{M}\right) < \frac{Q(1-Q)}{N} + \frac{T(1-T)}{M}$$

and hence

$$\sqrt{.9981}\sqrt{\frac{Q}{N} + \frac{T}{M}} < \sqrt{\frac{Q(1-Q)}{N} + \frac{T(1-T)}{M}}.$$

That is, the percentage error is less than

$$100\left(1 - \sqrt{.9981}\right)\% = 0.095\%$$

In general, by the above argument, the percent error is less than

$$B = 100\left\{1 - \sqrt{1 - \text{MAX}(Q, T)}\right\}.$$

The following chart illustrates the bound on the percent error:

**CHART**
**Bound on Error by Removing (1-Q) and (1-T) terms from Standard Error of**
$$(\hat{Q} - \hat{T})$$

| Inferior one year Survival | Bound on Error of Standard Normal Statistic |
|---|---|
| 1% | 0.63% |
| 2% | 0.54% |
| 5% | 0.41% |
| 10% | 0.31% |
| 25% | 0.19% |
| 50% | 0.095% |
| 75% | 0.039% |

Each entry is less than 1%.

## 3.4     Application of the Logrank Test When Survival is Exponential

If we knew that survival was indeed exponential we would compare the survival by the exponential test, rather than the logrank test. In practice, we can never be certain that survival is exponential.

A key question is how much better is the exponential test than the logrank test when we do have exponential data. It will turn out that the logrank test does almost as well as the exponential test. The margin of superiority of the exponential test is so slight, that the logrank test should be preferred even when the exponential assumption seems reasonable. The reason is that power loss is minimal, while the logrank analysis gives a valid comparison, irrespective of the underlying survival curve.

First, we shall study the numerator of the logrank Statistic: (See Notation Chart)

$$O - X = \sum_j F_j - \sum_j E_j$$

$$= \sum_j \left( M_j F_j - N_j G_j \right) / \left( N_j + M_j \right) \qquad \left( \text{See } (1.6) \right)$$

$$= \sum_j M_j N_j \left( \hat{Q}_j - \hat{T}_j \right) / \left( N_j + M_j \right), \tag{4.1}$$

where
$$\hat{Q}_j = F_j / N_j \quad \text{and} \quad \hat{T}_j = G_j / M_j.$$

Let
$$U_j = M_j N_j / \left( N_j + M_j \right) \tag{4.2}$$

and
$$W_j = U_j / \sum_i U_i. \tag{4.3}$$

That is,
$$U_j = \left( \sum_i U_i \right) W_j.$$

$$O - X = \left[ \sum U_i \right] \sum_j W_j \left( \hat{Q}_j - \hat{T}_j \right).$$

$$\text{Var}(O\text{-}X) = \left[ \sum U_i \right]^2 \sum_j W_j^2 \left\{ \frac{Q_j(1-Q_j)}{N_j} + \frac{T_j(1-T_j)}{M_j} \right\}.$$

The logrank statistic can therefore be rewritten as

$$Z = \frac{\sum W_j \left( \hat{Q}_j - \hat{T}_j \right)}{\sqrt{\hat{V}\text{ar}(O\text{-}X) / \left[ \sum U_i \right]^2}}. \tag{4.4}$$

The denominator is simply a standard error, and hence the key is the numerator in determining precision. (The null hypothesis is used to estimate the variance in the denominator.)

Note the numerator is a weighted average: (to estimate Q - T)

$$\text{Num} = \sum_j W_j \left( \hat{Q}_j - \hat{T}_j \right) = \sum_j W_j \hat{Q}_j - \sum_j W_j \hat{T}_j.$$

From (4.3) the weights, $W_j$, sum to unity.

The optimal exponential estimator would employ

$$\hat{Q} - \hat{T} = \sum_j \frac{N_j \hat{Q}_j}{N} - \sum_j \frac{M_j \hat{T}_j)}{M},$$

(minimizing the variance of $\hat{Q} - \hat{T}$).

Let us consider

$$W_j^* = \frac{N_j}{N} \text{ with } N = \Sigma N_j. \tag{4.5}$$

$$\text{Var}(\sum_j W_j \hat{Q}_j) = \text{Var}\left(\sum_j \left\{W_j^* + \left(W_j - W_j^*\right)\right\}\hat{Q}_j\right)$$

$$= \sum_j W_j^{*2}\text{Var}(\hat{Q}_j) + 2\sum_j W_j^*(W_j - W_j^*)\,\text{Var}(\hat{Q}_j)$$
$$+ \sum_j (W_j - W_j^*)^2 \text{Var}(\hat{Q}_j)$$

$$= \sum_j \frac{N_j^2}{N^2}\frac{Q(1-Q)}{N_j} + 2\sum_j \frac{N_j(W_j - W_j^*)Q(1-Q)}{NN_j}$$

$$+ \sum_j (W_j - W_j^*)^2 \frac{Q(1-Q)}{N_j}$$

$$= \frac{Q(1-Q)}{N^2}\Sigma N_j + 2\frac{Q(1-Q)}{N}\Sigma(W_j - W_j^*) + Q(1-Q)\Sigma\frac{(W_j - W_j^*)^2}{N_j}.$$

Since $\Sigma N_j = N$, $\Sigma W_j = \Sigma W_j^* = 1$, and $N_j = NW_j^*$,

$$\text{Var}\left(\Sigma W_j \hat{Q}_j\right) = \frac{Q(1-Q)}{N}\left[1 + 0 + \frac{\Sigma\left(W_j - W_j^*\right)^2}{W_j^*}\right]$$

$$= \text{Var}(\hat{Q})\left\{1 + \frac{\Sigma\left(W_j - W_j^*\right)^2}{W_j^*}\right\}. \tag{4.6}$$

Case 1:  If $N_j = M_j$ for all j then

$$U_j \quad = \frac{N_j M_j}{N_j + M_j} = \frac{N_j}{2}. \qquad \left(\text{From (4.2)}\right)$$

$$\sum U_i \quad = \frac{\sum N_j}{2} = \frac{N}{2}.$$

$$W_j \quad = \frac{U_j}{\sum U_i} = \frac{N_j/2}{N/2} = \frac{N_j}{N} = W_j^*. \qquad \left(\text{See (4.3) and (4.5)}\right)$$

$$\text{Var}\left(\sum W_j \hat{Q}_j\right) = \text{Var}(\hat{Q}). \qquad \left(\text{See (4.6)}\right)$$

Similarly,     $$\text{Var}\left(\sum W_j \hat{T}_j\right) = \text{Var}(\hat{T}).$$

Case 2:  If $N_j = aM_j$ for all j and a constant $a > 0$,

then     $$U_j \quad = \frac{N_j M_j}{N_j + M_j} = \frac{aM_j^2}{aM_j + M_j}.$$

$$= \frac{a}{1+a} M_j = \frac{N_j}{1+a}$$

$$\sum U_j = \frac{\sum N_j}{1+a} = \frac{N}{1+a}.$$

Hence     $$W_j = \frac{U_j}{\sum U_i} = \frac{N_j}{N}.$$

   Hence

$$\text{Var}\left(\sum_j W_j \hat{Q}_j\right) = \text{Var}(\hat{Q})$$

and similarly $\text{Var}\left(\sum W_j \hat{T}_j\right) = \text{Var}(\hat{T})$.

This implies full efficiency of the logrank test, in case 2.

In a randomized trial, it turns out that the $N_j$ and $M_j$ stay close enough together so as not to make a practical difference in terms of efficiency.

This is illustrated in the following abbreviated example where Treatment #2 seems to have a decided edge in terms of sample size. See (4.2), (4.3), (4.5), (4.6).

| Day | $N_j$ | $M_j$ | $U_j$ | $W_j$ | $W_j^*$ | $(W_j - W_j^*)^2 / W_j^*$ |
|---|---|---|---|---|---|---|
| 1 | 25 | 25 | 12.50 | .1694 | .1894 | .0021 |
| 2 | 20 | 23 | 10.70 | .1450 | .1515 | .0003 |
| 3 | 19 | 23 | 10.40 | .1409 | .1439 | .0001 |
| 4 | 17 | 22 | 9.59 | .1299 | .1288 | .0000+ |
| 5 | 16 | 22 | 9.26 | .1255 | .1212 | .0002 |
| 6 | 14 | 20 | 8.24 | .1116 | .1061 | .0003 |
| 7 | 11 | 18 | 6.82 | .0924 | .0833 | .0010 |
| 8 | 10 | 17 | 6.30 | .0853 | .0756 | .0012 |
| Total | 132 | 170 | 73.81 | | | .0052 |

$$U_j = \frac{N_j M_j}{N_j + M_j}.$$

$$W_j = \frac{U_j}{\sum U_i}.$$

$$\mathrm{Var}\left(\Sigma W_j \hat{Q}_j\right) = 1.0052 \ \mathrm{Var}(\hat{Q}).$$

Similarly, it can be shown that by switching rolls of Treatments #1 and #2:

$$\mathrm{Var}\left(\Sigma W_j \hat{T}_j\right) = 1.0086 \ \mathrm{Var}(\hat{T}).$$

$$\text{Var}\left[\Sigma W_j(\hat{Q}_j - T_j)\right] = \text{Var}\left[\Sigma W_j \hat{Q}_j\right] + \text{Var}\left[\Sigma W_j \hat{T}_j\right]$$

$$= 1.0052 \text{ Var}(\hat{Q}) + 1.0086 \text{ Var}(\hat{T})$$

$$< 1.0086\left\{\text{Var}(\hat{Q}) + \text{Var}(\hat{T})\right\}$$

$$< 1.0086 \text{ Var }(\hat{Q} - \hat{T}).$$

The "relative efficiency" of the logrank test compared to the binomial test, the ratio of variances, is greater than

$$(1.0086)^{-1} = .9915.$$

This implies from A130 that the Exponential Test with 99.15% of the patients in each time frame is less efficient than the logrank test with the actual arrival pattern.

## 3.5     Exponential Survival with a Poisson Accrual Process

Up to now, we have treated the number at risk at the start of each day as fixed. In this section, we take another look at exponential survival under a Poisson accrual process. The results will be almost identical to the fixed daily sample size, but considerable added insight will be obtained. Initially, consider Treatment #1 only. The notation will be as follows:

| | |
|---|---|
| Number of calendar days of patient accrual | s |
| Days from closure to accrual to analysis | t |
| Total duration of the trial in days | s+t |
| Expected daily accrual rate (Treatment #1)* | A   (For Now) |
| Daily population failure rate (Treatment #1) | Q |
| Total time on test (Treatment #1) | N |
| Total failures on Treatment #1 | F |
| $\hat{Q}$ | F/N |

Note: s = number of days from the opening of the trial until closure to accrual.

*Later, we shall set the accrual rate at (.5A) for each treatment.

---

Results for the one sample problem Poisson Arrival, Exponential Survival

(1) $\quad \dfrac{\sqrt{As}}{B}\left[\dfrac{F}{N} - Q\right] \xrightarrow{D} N(0, 1)$

where $\quad B^2 = Q^2\left[1 - \dfrac{1}{Qs}\left\{e^{-Qt} - e^{-Q(s+t)}\right\}\right]^{-1}$ $\hspace{3cm}$ (5.1)

(2) $\quad \dfrac{N}{\sqrt{F}}\left[\dfrac{F}{N} - Q\right] \xrightarrow{D} N(0, 1)$

---

Plan of the Proof

Step 1.

First, we shall condition on N(s), the number of patients accrued to time s.

We shall represent, conditional that N(s) = n,

$$\frac{F}{n} - \frac{QN}{n}$$

as a sample mean of independent, identically distributed random variables

$$U_j = V_j - QW_j,$$

where

$$V_j = 1 \text{ if patient j dies during study}$$

and
$$= 0 \text{ otherwise,}$$

$$W_j = \text{time on test for patient j}$$

$$= \text{time from arrival to death or closure (earlier of two).}$$

The index j represents a randomly selected patient from the n.

$$F = \Sigma V_j.$$

$$N = \Sigma W_j.$$

$$F - NQ = \Sigma U_j = \Sigma(V_j - QW_j).$$

Step 2: Show that given $N(s) = n$,

$$E(U_j) = 0.$$

$$Var(U_j) = 1 - \frac{1}{Qs}\left\{e^{Qt} - e^{-Q(s+t)}\right\} = \sigma^2. \tag{5.2}$$

Step 3: Show that given $N(s) = n \rightarrow \infty$,

$$\frac{\Sigma U_j}{\sqrt{n}} \xrightarrow{D} N(0, \sigma^2)$$

where $\sigma^2$ is given in (5.2).

Step 4: Show that conditionally , as $n \rightarrow \infty$

$$\sqrt{n}\left[\frac{F}{N} - Q\right] \xrightarrow{D} N(0, B^2).$$

$B^2$ is defined in (5.1).

Step 5: Show that as $As \rightarrow \infty$,

$$\frac{n}{As} \xrightarrow{P} 1,$$

and hence conditionally as $n \rightarrow \infty$,

$$\sqrt{As} \left[\frac{F}{N} - Q\right] \xrightarrow{D} N(0, B^2).$$

Step 6:  Show that

$$\hat{B}^2 = \frac{nF}{N^2}$$

satisfies $\qquad\qquad \frac{\hat{B}^2}{B^2} \xrightarrow{P} 1 \qquad\qquad$ (conditionally as $n \rightarrow \infty$),

and hence as $n \rightarrow \infty$,

$$\frac{N}{\sqrt{F}} \left[\frac{F}{N} - Q\right] \xrightarrow{D} N(0, 1).$$

Note that the conditional distributions and statistics in Steps 5 and 6 do not depend on n, and hence they are valid asymptotic unconditional distributions.

Proof of Step 1:

From our study of the Poisson Process, **A143** we know that given $N(s)$, the number of patients accrued to time s, is equal to n, the arrival times form a random sample from the uniform distribution over the interval from 0 to s.

We need to study the variable

$$\frac{F}{n} - \frac{QN}{n} \tag{5.3}$$

That is,

$$\frac{F - QN}{n}.$$

Now, this can be viewed as the mean of the following independent identically distributed random variables:  $U_j$, $j = 1, 2, \ldots, n$ with

$$U_j = V_j - QW_j.$$

$V_j = 1$ (death on study), 0 (survival) and $W_j =$ time on test.

For each j, independently generate the following two independent random variables:

$$X_j = \text{Arrival time, uniform on the interval 0 to s}$$

$$Y_j = \text{Survival, exponential with hazard Q (Mean 1/Q).}$$

Note that since the trial ends at s+t, the time at risk is $(s+t - X_j)$.

If $\qquad\qquad Y_j \le s+t-X_j$, then $V_j = 1$ $\qquad$ (patient dies during trial)

and $\qquad\qquad W_j = Y_j$ $\qquad\qquad\qquad$ (time on test of patient j is $Y_j$).

If $\qquad\qquad Y_j > s+t - X_j$ then

$\qquad\qquad\qquad V_j = 0$ $\qquad\qquad\qquad$ (patient lives to end of trial)

and $\qquad\qquad W_j = s+t - X_j$ $\qquad\qquad$ (time on test of patient j is $s+t - X_j$).

Prior to reading the next body of material, it will be helpful to review Gamma integrals (Appendix A82 and A77).

By independence, and the fact that $V_j$ and $W_j$ are functions of $X_j$ and $Y_j$, we have

$$E(V_j) = 0 \, P(V_j = 0) + 1 \, P(V_j = 1)$$

$$= \tfrac{1}{s} \int_0^s \int_0^{s+t-x} Qe^{-Qy} dy dx$$

$$= \tfrac{1}{s} \int_0^s \left[ 1 - e^{-Q(s+t-x)} \right] dx$$

$$= 1 - \tfrac{1}{Qs} \left\{ e^{-Qt} - e^{-Q(s+t)} \right\}. \qquad\qquad (5.4)$$

$$E(W_j) = \tfrac{1}{s} \int_0^s \left[ \int_0^{s+t-x} yQe^{-Qy} dy + \int_{s+t-x}^\infty (s+t-x)Qe^{-Qy} dy \right] dx$$

$$= \frac{1}{s} \int_0^s \left[ \frac{1}{Q} \left\{ 1 - e^{-Q(s+t-x)} - Q(s+t-x)e^{-Q(s+t-x)} \right\} + (s+t-x)e^{-Q(s+t-x)} \right] dx$$

$$= \frac{1}{Qs} \int_0^s \left\{ 1 - e^{-Q(s+t-x)} \right\} dx$$

$$= \frac{1}{Q} \left[ 1 - \frac{1}{Qs} \left\{ e^{-Qt} - e^{-Q(s+t)} \right\} \right] \tag{5.5}$$

For inference purposes, we shall need the second moments.

$$E\left( (V_j - QW_j)^2 \right) = E(V_j^2) - 2QE\left( V_j W_j \right) + Q^2 E\left( W_j^2 \right). \tag{5.6}$$

This will be greatly simplified when we show

$$Q^2 E\left( W_j^2 \right) = 2QE\left( V_j W_j \right). \tag{5.7}$$

$$E\left( V_j W_j \right) = \frac{1}{s} \int_0^s \left[ \int_0^{s+t-x} y Q e^{-Qy} dy \right] dx$$

$$= \frac{1}{Qs} \int_0^s \left\{ 1 - e^{-Q(s+t-x)} - Q(s+t-x)e^{-Q(s+t-x)} \right\} dx. \tag{5.8}$$

$$E\left( W_j^2 \right) = \frac{1}{s} \int_0^s \left\{ \int_0^{s+t-x} y^2 Q e^{-Qy} dy + \int_{s+t-x}^\infty (s+t-x)^2 Q e^{-Qy} dy \right\} dx. \tag{5.9}$$

We study

$$\int_0^{s+t-x} y^2 Q e^{-Qy} dy = \frac{2}{Q^2} \int_0^{s+t-x} \frac{Q^3}{2} y^2 e^{-Qy} dy$$

$$= \frac{2}{Q^2} \left\{ 1 - e^{Q(s+t-x)} - (s+t-x)Q e^{-Q(s+t-x)} - \frac{(s+t-x)^2}{2} Q^2 e^{-Q(s+t-x)} \right\}.$$

Also,

$$\int_{s+t-x}^{\infty} (s+t-x)^2 Q e^{-Qy} dy = (s+t-x)^2 e^{-Q(s+t-x)}.$$

Substituting these into (5.9), the first expression for $E\left(W_j^2\right)$ yields (after cancellation)

$$E\left(W_j^2\right) = \frac{2}{Q^2 s} \int_0^s \left\{ 1 - e^{-Q(s+t-x)} - (s+t-x) Q e^{-Q(s+t-x)} \right\} dx$$

$$= \frac{2}{Q} E\left(V_j W_j\right), \qquad \text{by (5.8).}$$

Hence,

$$E\left(\left(V_j - Q_j W_j\right)^2\right) = E\left(V_j^2\right) - 2QE\left(V_j W_j\right) + Q^2 E\left(W_j^2\right)$$

$$= E\left(V_j^2\right) - 2QE\left(V_j W_j\right) + \frac{2Q^2 E\left(V_j W_j\right)}{Q}$$

$$= E\left(V_j^2\right).$$

However, $V_j$ takes on only values of 0 or 1. Hence $V_j^2 = V_j$.

That is, from (5.6) and (5.4)

$$E\left(\left(V_j - Q_j W_j\right)^2\right) = E\left(V_j\right) = 1 - \frac{1}{Qs}\left\{e^{Qt} - e^{-Q(s+t)}\right\}.$$

Summary for Step 2.

We have shown the following properties of the $V_j$ and $W_j$ given the number of arrivals in the time interval from 0 to s

$$E(V_j) = QE(W_j) = 1 - \frac{1}{Qs}\left\{e^{Qt} - e^{-Q(s+t)}\right\}. \tag{5.10}$$

$$E\left(\left\{V_j - QW_j\right\}^2\right) = 1 - \frac{1}{Qs}\left\{e^{Qt} - e^{-Q(s+t)}\right\}. \tag{5.11}$$

Hence $U_j = V_j - QW_j$ satisfies

$$E(U_j) = 0,$$

$$\text{Var}(U_j) = 1 - \frac{1}{Qs}\left\{ e^{Qt} - e^{-Q(s+t)} \right\} = \sigma^2.$$

This completes Step 2.

Proof of Step 3.

Suppose that the number of arrivals, n, is sufficiently large to apply the central limit theorem on the $V_j$'s:

$$\sqrt{n}\ \frac{\Sigma\left\{ U_j - E(U_j) \right\}}{n}$$

$$= \frac{\Sigma U_j}{\sqrt{n}} \qquad \text{(From Step 2)}$$

$$\xrightarrow{\ D\ } N(0,\ \sigma^2). \qquad \text{(Central Limit Theorem A106 and Step 2).}$$

This completes Step 3.

Proof of Step 4.

$$\sqrt{n}\left[ \frac{F}{N} - Q \right] = \sqrt{n}\left\{ \frac{\sum_{j=1}^{n} V_j/n}{\sum_{j=1}^{n} W_j/n} - Q \right\}$$

$$= \frac{1}{\Sigma(W_j/n)}\left\{ \Sigma U_j/\sqrt{n} \right\}$$

$$= \frac{1}{E(W_j)}\left\{ \sum_j U_j/\sqrt{n} \right\} + \left[ \frac{1}{\Sigma W_j/n} - \frac{1}{E(W_j)} \right]\sum_j U_j/\sqrt{n}. \qquad (5.12)$$

By the Central Limit Theorem, **A106**,

$$\sqrt{n}\left\{\Sigma\frac{W_j}{n} - E(W_j)\right\} \xrightarrow{D} N\left(0, \text{Var}(W_j)\right)$$

and hence

$$\Sigma\frac{W_j}{n} - E(W_j) \xrightarrow{P} 0.$$

$\sqrt{n}\left[\frac{F}{N} - Q\right]$ is the sum of two components:  $\left(\text{See (5.12)}\right)$

a.    $$\frac{1}{E(W_j)}\left\{\sum_j U_j/\sqrt{n}\right\} \xrightarrow{D} N\left(0, \frac{\sigma^2}{\left[E(W_j)\right]^2}\right)$$

and

b.    $$\left[\frac{1}{\left[\Sigma W_j/n\right]} - \frac{1}{E(W_j)}\right]\sum_j U_j/\sqrt{n} \xrightarrow{P} 0.$$

Hence, by Slutzky's Theorem **A104**,

$$\sqrt{n}\left[\frac{F}{N} - Q\right] \xrightarrow{D} N\left(0, \frac{\sigma^2}{\left[E(W_j)\right]^2}\right) \tag{5.13}$$

By (5.10),

$$QE(W_j) = 1 - \frac{1}{Qs}\left\{e^{-Qt} - e^{-Q(s+t)}\right\}$$

$$= \sigma^2, \qquad\qquad \left(\text{See (5.2)}\right)$$

and hence

$$E(W_j) = \frac{\sigma^2}{Q}. \tag{5.14}$$

Substitution (5.14) into (5.13) yields

$$\sqrt{n}\left[\frac{F}{N} - Q\right] \xrightarrow{D} N\left(0, \frac{Q^2}{\sigma^2}\right). \tag{5.15}$$

Since

$$\sigma^2 = 1 - \frac{1}{Qs}\left\{e^{Qt} - e^{-Q(s+t)}\right\},$$

we see from (5.1), that

$$B^2 = \frac{Q^2}{\sigma^2}.$$

and hence from (5.15), the proof of Step 4 is complete.

Proof of Step 5.

Since n is Poisson with parameter As, we have from **A62**,

$$E(n) = As \quad \text{and} \quad Var(n) = As.$$

$$P\left[|\frac{n}{As} - 1| > \epsilon\right] = P\left[|n - As| > \epsilon As\right]$$

$$< \frac{Var(n)}{\epsilon^2 A^2 s^2} \quad \text{(Chebyshev Theorem A51)}$$

$$< \frac{As}{\epsilon A^2 s^2} = \frac{1}{\epsilon As}$$

$$\rightarrow 0 \quad \text{as As} \rightarrow \infty.$$

(It does not matter whether A is fixed and $s \rightarrow \infty$, or s is fixed and $A \rightarrow \infty$, or whether simply $As \rightarrow \infty$ on any path.) Thus

$$\frac{n}{As} \xrightarrow{P} 1.$$

Since

$$\sqrt{As}\left[\frac{F}{N} - Q\right] = \left\{\sqrt{n}\left[\frac{F}{N} - Q\right]\right\}\sqrt{\frac{As}{n}},$$

and since

$$\sqrt{\frac{As}{n}} \xrightarrow{P} 1, \qquad\qquad \text{(Appendix A98)},$$

Slutzky's Multiplicative Theorem, **A105**, and step 4 yield

$$\sqrt{As}\left[\frac{F}{N} - Q\right] \xrightarrow{D} N(0, B^2).$$

This completes Step 5.

Proof of Step 6:

Let

$$\hat{B}^2 = \frac{nF}{N^2}$$

$$= \frac{n}{F}\left(\frac{F}{N}\right)^2 \qquad\qquad (5.16)$$

Now since from Step 5:

$$\sqrt{As}\left(\frac{F}{N} - Q\right) \xrightarrow{D} N(0, B^2),$$

as $As \to \infty$

$$\frac{F}{N} \xrightarrow{P} Q. \qquad\qquad (5.17)$$

Now given n,

$$F = \Sigma V_j \qquad\qquad \text{(See Definition of } V_j \text{ in Step 1)}$$

is a sum independent identically distributed random variables. From (5.10), (5.1), and (5.2)

$$E(V_j) = 1 - \frac{1}{Qs}\left\{e^{-Qt} - e^{-Q(s+t)}\right\} = \frac{Q^2}{B^2}. \tag{5.18}$$

Since $V_j$ is Bernoulli,

$$\text{Var}(V_j) = E(V_j)\left\{1 - E(V_j)\right\}.$$

Given n is sufficiently large,

$$\sqrt{n}\left\{\frac{F}{n} - E(V_j)\right\} \xrightarrow{D} N\left(0, \text{Var}(V_j)\right),$$

and hence

$$\frac{F}{n} - E(V_j) \xrightarrow{P} 0.$$

That is, from **A95**,

$$\frac{F}{nE(V_j)} \xrightarrow{P} 1.$$

from (5.18),

$$\frac{B^2 F}{nQ^2} \xrightarrow{P} 1. \tag{5.19}$$

From Step 4, $F/(NQ) \xrightarrow{P} 1$. Application of **A98 and A101** to (5.17) and (5.19) yields,

$$\frac{nF}{N^2 B^2} = \left(\frac{nQ^2}{B^2 F}\right)\left(\frac{F}{NQ}\right)^2 \xrightarrow{P} 1. \tag{5.20}$$

Now

$$\frac{N}{\sqrt{F}}\left[\frac{F}{N} - Q\right] = \frac{\sqrt{n}}{B}\left[\frac{F}{N} - Q\right]\left\{\frac{NB}{\sqrt{nF}}\right\}.$$

From Slutzky's Multiplicative Theorem **A105** and (5.20)

$\frac{N}{\sqrt{F}}\left[\frac{F}{N} - Q\right]$ has the same asymptotic distribution as

$$\frac{\sqrt{n}}{B}\left[\frac{F}{N} - Q\right]$$

which is N(0, 1) from Step 4.

This completes the proof.

## 3.6    Extension to the Two-Sample Problem

Here the accrual rate is A/2 to each treatment, G is the number of failures on Treatment #2, M is the total time on test for Treatment #2. T is the daily failure rate on Treatment #2. We have by the one sample results (halving the accrual rate):

$$\sqrt{(.5A)s}\left[\frac{F}{N} - Q\right] \xrightarrow{D} N(0, B^2)$$

with

$$B^2 = Q^2\left[1 - \frac{1}{Qs}\left\{e^{-Qt} - e^{-Q(s+t)}\right\}\right]^{-1}.$$

$$\sqrt{(.5A)s}\left[\frac{G}{M} - T\right] \xrightarrow{D} N(0, C^2)$$

with

$$C^2 = T^2\left[1 - \frac{1}{Ts}\left\{e^{-Tt} - e^{-T(s+t)}\right\}\right]^{-1}$$

Hence

$$\sqrt{(.5A)s}\left[\left(\frac{F}{N} - \frac{G}{M}\right) - (Q - T)\right] \xrightarrow{D} N(0, B^2 + C^2),$$

Since from A142, each accrual process is independent, and A108 can be applied.

Now from the previous section, Steps 5 and 6

$$\frac{B^2/(.5As)}{F/N^2} \xrightarrow{P} 1$$

and

$$\frac{C^2/(.5As)}{G/M^2} \xrightarrow{P} 1.$$

Hence from the Appendix A103,

$$\frac{(B^2 + C^2)/(.5As)}{(F/N^2) + (G/M^2)} \xrightarrow{P} 1.$$

By applying A109, the following "Block" holds:

---

Results for Poisson Entry, Exponential Survival

(1) $$\frac{\sqrt{(.5As)}}{\sqrt{B^2 + C^2}}\left[\frac{F}{N} - \frac{G}{M} - (Q - T)\right] \xrightarrow{D} N(0, 1).$$

(2) $$\left[\frac{F}{N} - \frac{G}{M} - (Q - T)\right]\frac{1}{\sqrt{(F/N^2) + (G/M^2)}} \xrightarrow{D} N(0, 1).$$

(3) $$\frac{(B^2 + C^2)/(.5As)}{\sqrt{(F/N^2) + (G/M^2)}} \xrightarrow{P} 1.$$

$A$ = total accrual rate ($A/2$ to each treatment).

$$B^2 = Q^2\left[1 - \frac{1}{Qs}\left\{e^{-Qt} - e^{-Q(s+t)}\right\}\right]^{-1}.$$

$$C^2 = T^2\left[1 - \frac{1}{Ts}\left\{e^{-Tt} - e^{-T(s+t)}\right\}\right]^{-1}.$$

---

s = Accrual period. (Calendar time)

t = Time from end of accrual to analysis.

Q = Population daily failure rate on Treatment #1.

T = Population daily failure rate on Treatment #2.

F = Failures on Treatment #1 (observed).

G = Failures on Treatment #2 (observed).

N = Total time on test for Treatment #1 (total patient days).

M = Total time on test for Treatment #2.

---

Comparison with the fixed daily sample size version. The asymptotic result of section 3.3 was:

$$\frac{\hat{Q} - \hat{T} - (Q - T)}{\sqrt{\dfrac{\hat{Q}}{N} + \dfrac{\hat{T}}{M}}} \xrightarrow{D} N(0, 1). \qquad \text{(Approximately)}$$

Since $\hat{Q} = F/N$ and $\hat{T} = G/M$, this result is identical to (2) above.

---

<u>Sample size derivation</u> for exponential survival with Poisson Accrual.

Please consult Appendix A130(1) and A135, as well as template on final conclusions for Poisson entry above. We shall identify each term in A130:

$$H_0: \theta = Q - T = 0. \qquad\qquad (\theta_0 = 0)$$

$$H_A: \theta = Q - T = \theta_1 > 0. \qquad \text{(One-sided)}$$

$$\hat{\theta} = (F/N) - (G/M).$$

$$SE = \sqrt{(F/N^2) + (G/M^2)}.$$

$$S = \sqrt{(B^2 + C^2)/(.5As)}.$$

Hence the necessary sample size for Type I error $\alpha$ and Type II error $\beta$ (Power 1 - $\beta$) satisfies

$$S = \frac{Q - T}{(Z_\alpha + Z_\beta)}.$$

This is solved by bisection. See block below for full definition of terms.

---

Sample Size Equation for Poisson Accrual and Exponential Survival:

Two sample trial with 50% allocation to each treatment. One-sided Test Calculation. (Replace $\alpha$ by $\alpha/2$ for two-sided test.)

$$\frac{B^2 + C^2}{(.5As)} = \frac{(Q - T)^2}{(Z_\alpha + Z_\beta)^2} \tag{6.1}$$

A = Total accrual rate.

s = Total calendar time of accrual.

t = Time from end of accrual to analysis (minimum follow-up time).

Q = Daily failure rate on Treatment #1 (under $H_A$).

T = Daily Failure Rate on Treatment #2 (under $H_A$).

$\alpha$ = Probability of a Type I error (Reject $H_0$ when true).

$Z_\alpha$ = Upper $100\alpha\%$ point of the standard normal distribution.

$\beta$ = 1 - Power = Probability of a Type II error (Reject $H_A$ when true).

$Z_\beta$ = Upper $100\beta\%$ point of the standard normal

$$B^2 = Q^2 \left[ 1 - \frac{1}{Qs} \left\{ e^{-Qt} - e^{-Q(s+t)} \right\} \right]^{-1}. \tag{6.2}$$

$$C^2 = T^2 \left[ 1 - \frac{1}{Ts} \left\{ e^{-Tt} - e^{-T(s+t)} \right\} \right]^{-1}. \tag{6.3}$$

See Section 3.10 regarding losses to follow-up.

---

Tables for exponential survival appear in this volume under FACT = 1.0.

## 3.7     Exponential Survival with "Up-Front" Accrual

In rare instances, it is possible to accrue all patients at day 1 and follow them for t years.

We derive the distributional properties from the Poisson Arrival as follows:

Let the accrual period s → 0.

Let the accrual rate A → ∞,

with As → n (large).

From this, we shall obtain the analogous one sample and two sample results. Recall that

$$B^2 = Q^2 \left[ 1 - \frac{1}{Qs} \left\{ e^{-Qt} - e^{-Q(s+t)} \right\} \right]^{-1}.$$

By L'Hospital's rule, letting the accrual period s → 0

$$\lim_{s \to 0} \frac{e^{-Qt} - e^{-Q(s+t)}}{Qs} = \lim_{s \to 0} \frac{Qe^{-Q(s+t)}}{Q} = e^{-Qt}.$$

Hence

$$B^2 \to Q^2 \left[ 1 - e^{-Qt} \right]^{-1} \qquad \text{as } s \to 0.$$

This limit is used as the $B^2$ value in the variance formula.

Results for the One Sample Problem with Exponential Survival and Up Front Accrual:

(1) $\quad \dfrac{\sqrt{n}}{B}\left[\dfrac{F}{N} - Q\right] \xrightarrow{D} N(0, 1),$

where

$\quad Q$ = Daily failure rate.

$\quad n$ = Number of patients treated.

$\quad F$ = Observed failures.

$\quad N$ = Total time on test.

$\quad B^2 = Q^2\left[1 - e^{-Qt}\right]^{-1}.$

$\quad t$ = Time from accrual to analysis (follow-up time).

(2) $\quad \dfrac{N}{\sqrt{F}}\left[\dfrac{F}{N} - Q\right] \xrightarrow{D} N(0, 1).$

(3) $\quad \dfrac{N/\sqrt{F}}{\sqrt{n}/B} \xrightarrow{P} 1.$

Results for the Two Sample Problem with Exponential Survival and Up Front Entry:

(1)    $$\frac{\sqrt{.5n}}{\sqrt{B^2 + C^2}} \left[ \frac{F}{N} - \frac{G}{M} - (Q - T) \right] \xrightarrow{D} N(0, 1)$$

(2)    $$\left[ \frac{F}{N} - \frac{G}{M} - (Q - T) \right] \frac{1}{\sqrt{(F/N^2) + (G/M^2)}} \xrightarrow{D} N(0, 1)$$

(3)    $$\frac{(B^2 + C^2)/(.5n)}{\left[ (F/N^2) + (G/M^2) \right]} \xrightarrow{P} 1$$

with    $n$ = Total patient accrual ($n/2$ to each treatment).

$$B^2 = Q^2 \left[ 1 - e^{-Qt} \right]^{-1}$$
$$C^2 = T^2 \left[ 1 - e^{-Tt} \right]^{-1}.$$

$t$ = Time from start of study to analysis (follow-up time)

$Q$ = Population failure rate on Treatment #1.

$T$ = Population Failure rate on Treatment #2.

Sample Size Equation for Up Front Accrual and Exponential Survival: Two sample trial with 50% allocation to each treatment. One-sided Test Calculation. (Replace $\alpha$ by $\alpha/2$ for two-sided test.)

$$\frac{B^2 + C^2}{.5n} = \frac{(Q - T)^2}{(Z_\alpha + Z_\beta)^2}. \tag{7.1}$$

n = Total number of patients.

t = Time from start of study to analysis (follow-up time).

Q = Daily failure rate (Treatment #1).

T = Daily failure rate (Treatment #2).

$\alpha$ = Probability of a Type I error (Reject $H_0$ when true).

$\beta$ = Probability of a Type II error (Reject $H_A$ when true).

$Z_\alpha$ = Upper $(100\alpha)\%$ point of the standard normal distribution.

$Z_\beta$ = Upper $(100\beta)\%$ point of the standard normal distribution.

$$B^2 = Q^2\left[1 - e^{-Qt}\right]^{-1} \tag{7.2}$$

$$C^2 = T^2\left[1 - e^{-Tt}\right]^{-1}. \tag{7.3}$$

See Section 3.10 regarding losses to follow-up

This formula also can be used when patients are entered in any fashion, but followed for a period t, not longer.

The tables for up front accrual are in this volume under FACT = 0.

## 3.8    Proportional Hazard Models and the Exponential Distribution

Let $F_j(x)$ be the cumulative distribution of survival for treatment j, j = 1, 2 respectively.

$$F_j(x) = P\left[X_j \leq x\right] \qquad \text{(See A20)}$$

The logrank test is defined for testing the null hypothesis

$$H_0: F_1(x) = F_2(x) \quad \text{for all x.}$$

The alternative is typically for the one-sided case:

$$H_A: F_1(x) \leq F_2(x) \quad \text{for all x} \quad \text{(Treatment #1 Superior)}$$

The proportional hazard formulation adds structure to $H_A$ as follows:

$$H_A: \left\{1 - F_2(x)\right\} = \left\{1 - F_1(x)\right\}^\theta. \tag{8.1}$$

If the distributions have continuous densities represented by $f_1$ and $f_2$ respectively, then (8.1) can be considered as follows

$$F_2(x) = 1 - \left[\int_x^\infty f_1(t)dt\right]^\theta. \tag{8.2}$$

Differentiating both sides with respect to x yields for $\theta \neq 1$ (Chain rule)

$$F_2'(x) = f_2(x) = \theta f_1(x)\left[\int_x^\infty f_1(t)dt\right]^{\theta-1},$$

i.e.

$$f_2(x) = \theta f_1(x)\left\{1 - F_1(x)\right\}^{\theta-1}.$$

$$\frac{f_2(x)}{\left[1 - F_1(x)\right]^\theta} = \frac{\theta f_1(x)}{1 - F_1(x)}. \tag{8.3}$$

That is, from (8.1)

$$\frac{f_2(x)}{1 - F_2(x)} = \frac{\theta f_1(x)}{1 - F_1(x)} \tag{8.4}$$

Now if $\theta = 1$, (8.4), still holds.

From Appendix A75 which defines the Hazard Rate, the alternate hypothesis (8.1) states that the hazard rates are proportional. That is, the ratio of hazards is independent of time. If and only if $\theta < 1$, then Treatment #2 has a lower failure rate than Treatment #1.

The following result relates proportional hazards in a rather remarkable way to the exponential.

Theorem 8.1:

Let

$$1 - F_1(x) = \left[1 - G(x)\right]^{\gamma} \tag{8.5}$$

and

$$1 - F_2(x) = \left[1 - G(x)\right]^{\gamma + \theta}, \tag{8.6}$$

where $G(x)$ is a known distribution but $\gamma$ and $\theta$ are unknown.

Let us transform the time scale x by

$$y = -\log\left\{1 - G(x)\right\}. \tag{8.7}$$

In this time scale, let $Y_1$ and $Y_2$ represent random variables of survival times on Treatments #1 and #2 respectively.

Then $Y_1$ and $Y_2$ are respectively exponential with hazards $\gamma$ and $(\gamma + \theta)$.

Proof:

From the Appendix A89,

$$Y_1 \text{ has density } \frac{f_1(x)}{(dy/dx)}.$$

Now from (8.7),

$$\frac{dy}{dx} = \frac{G'(x)}{1 - G(x)}.$$

From Appendix A21 and (8.5)

$$f_1(x) = \gamma\left\{1 - G(x)\right\}^{\gamma-1} G'(x).$$

That is, $Y_1$ has density

$$h_1(y) = \gamma\left\{1 - G(x)\right\}^{\gamma} \qquad 0 < G(x) < 1.$$

But $1 - G(x) = e^{-y}$ $\left(\text{See } (8.7)\right)$ and hence $Y_1$ has density

$$h_1(y) = \gamma e^{-\gamma y} \qquad y > 0.$$

Similarly, replacing $\gamma$ by $(\gamma + \theta)$ in the above yields the fact that $Y_2$ has density

$$h_2(y) = (\gamma + \theta)e^{-(\gamma+\theta)y} \qquad y > 0.$$

This completes the proof.

This transformation converts a proportional hazard problem to an exponential problem.

## 3.9 Considerations in Planning a Trial Under Proportional Hazards: Putting It All Together

Suppose you wished to plan a trial with the following endpoints:

|  |  |
|---|---|
| Annual Accrual: | 150 patients per year. |
| Two Year Survival: | 40% Control (Treatment #1). |
|  | 50% Experimental (Treatment #2). |
| Alpha: | .05 (one-sided). |
| Power: | 80%. |
| Distribution: | Exponential (For Now). |

A total of 300 patients are expected to be accrued through the two year endpoint, and hence from the sample size Tables (FACT = 1.0), 541 patients (3.6 years of accrual) are required. The trial would require an additional two years of follow-up.

As we have seen in Section 3.4, the power loss in the use of the logrank test as opposed to the exponential test would be of no practical concern.

However, the key issue one faces is non-exponentiality.

In answering this question, let us first consider an alternate study where the accrual is up front (or similarly if we only use the first two years of patient data.) Suppose further that you were willing to assume proportional hazards. Then the power loss caused by lack of knowledge of G would be minimal, since

(a)     There exists a monotonic transformation to convert the data to exponential.

(b)     The logrank test is invariant under monotonic transformations.

(c)     From Theorem 8.1 the exponential parameters do not involve G.

(d)     The logrank and exponential tests have virtually the same power, when exponentiality holds.

\* The distribution G plays no role in planning this alternate study under proportional hazards and the planning endpoints.

In the actual setting of follow-up to the end of the study, the key sample size planning issue is what happens to patients after surviving to the endpoint of the study.

In the above example, the study is planned for 3.6 years of accrual plus 2 years of follow-up for a total of 5.6 years. Patients are at risk from 2.0 to 5.6 years.

To accommodate this in a quantitative way, we shall consider attaching exponential survival past the endpoint, but with a lower hazard. Proportional hazards are still assumed. More sophisticated assumptions would result in contingencies too numerous to tabulate.

The derivations will be conducted as follows:

|              | Daily Hazard Before t | Daily Hazard After t $(d \geq 0)$ |
|--------------|:---------------------:|:---------------------------------:|
| Treatment #1 | Q                     | dQ                                |
| Treatment #2 | T                     | dT                                |

Non-Exponentiality before the endpoint t will have virtually no impact on the power.

> NOTE: If d=0, no failures will occur after t, and we can use up front accrual results for design and analysis.

If $d > 0$, then the following transformation produces exponentiality under both treatments, with respective hazards Q and T. (Y is transformed time, X is original time.)

$$Y = X \qquad \qquad \text{if } X \leq t$$
$$= t + d(X\text{-}t) \qquad \text{if } X > t,$$

since for $x > t$, and treatment 1

$$P[X > x] \quad = P[X > t]P[X > x|X > t]$$

$$= e^{-Qt}e^{-dQ(x\text{-}t)}$$

$$= e^{-Q[t+d(x\text{-}t)]}$$

Setting $Y = t + d(X\text{-}t)$ and $y = t+d(x\text{-}t)$ yields exponentiality with hazard Q for $Y > t$.

Since it was assumed for $Y \leq t$, exponentiality holds for Y.

Based on exponential considerations, we would estimate Q by

$$\hat{Q} = \frac{\text{Total Failures}}{\text{Total accumulated time on test in Y-scale}}$$

Following the same derivation as seen in Section 3.5, "Exponential Survival with a Poisson Accrual

Process," the following results are obtained:

Let

$F_1$    = Number of failures occurring prior to patient time on test t.

$N_1$    = total accumulated time on test accrued by patients prior to t. (Clock only is on while patient is at risk less than t.)

$F_2$    = Number of failures occurring after patient time on test t.

$N_2$    = total accumulated time on test accrued by patients after t. (Clock starts for patient after t.)

with other notation per page 96.

Let

$$\hat{Q} = \frac{F_1 + F_2}{N_1 + dN_2}$$

be the exponential estimate of Q on the basis of the transformation to exponential. Then

$$\frac{\hat{Q} - Q}{V} \xrightarrow{D} N(0, 1), \tag{9.1}$$

where
$$V^2 = \frac{Q^2}{As} \left[ 1 - \frac{e^{-Qt}}{dQs} \left\{ 1 - e^{-dQs} \right\} \right]^{-1}. \tag{9.2}$$

Before proving this result, note that

(a)    If $d = 1$, we obtain the result for exponentials (5.1).

(b)    If $d \to 0$, by L'Hospital's rule

$$V^2 \to \frac{Q^2}{As} \left[ 1 - e^{-Qt} \right], \tag{9.3}$$

which agrees with the Up Front Accrual results in Section 3.7.

Proof: Although the proof can be derived exactly as in the exponential case, once $E(U_j)$ and $Var(U_j)$ are obtained, we shall outline an alternate proof.

Step 1: Show

$$\hat{Q} = \frac{F_1}{N_1} W_1 + \frac{F_2}{dN_2} W_2$$

where

$$W_1 = \frac{N_1}{N_1 + dN_2}$$

and

$$W_2 = \frac{dN_2}{N_1 + dN_2} = 1 - W_1.$$

Step 2: Apply results for Up Front Accrual to show

$$\frac{\left(\frac{F_1}{N_1} - Q\right)}{V_1} \xrightarrow{D} N(0, 1),$$

where

$$V_1^2 = \frac{Q^2}{As(1 - e^{-Qt})}$$

$$= \frac{Q}{E(N_1)}. \tag{9.4}$$

Step 3: Apply results for Poisson Accrual with minimum follow-up $t = 0$ to show that

$$\frac{\left(\frac{F_2}{dN_2} - Q\right)}{V_2} \xrightarrow{D} N(0, 1),$$

where

$$V_2^2 = \frac{Q^2}{As\ e^{-Qt}} \left[1 - \frac{1}{(dQs)}\left\{1 - e^{-dQs}\right\}\right]^{-1}$$

$$= \frac{Q}{dE(N_2)}. \tag{9.5}$$

This distribution holds independently of that of Step 2.

NOTE ON STEP 3: From the appendix on Poisson Processes, since patients must survive at least t to accrue time past t, arrivals past time t is a Poisson process with arrival rate

$$Ae^{-Qt} = A \; P[\text{Survival at least } t].$$

The "clock" for this process starts at calendar time t.

Step 4: Based on the already established results,

$$\frac{N_1}{E(N_1)} \xrightarrow{P} 1$$

and

$$\frac{N_2}{E(N_2)} \xrightarrow{P} 1.$$

Step 5: Show that

$$\frac{Q^* - Q}{V} \xrightarrow{D} N(0, 1)$$

where

$$Q^* = \frac{V_2^2}{V_1^2 + V_2^2}\left(\frac{F_1}{N_1}\right) + \frac{V_1^2}{\left(V_1^2 + V_2^2\right)}\left(\frac{F_2}{dN_2}\right)$$

and $V^2$, $V_1^2$, and $V_2^2$ are given in (9.2), (9.4), and (9.5) respectively.

Step 6: Apply Step 4 and Slutzky's Theorem to show

$$\frac{\hat{Q} - Q}{V} \xrightarrow{D} N(0, 1).$$

Footnote:

It is readily seen that

$$V^2 = \left( \frac{1}{V_1^2} + \frac{1}{V_2^2} \right)^{-1}$$

$$= \left( \frac{E(N_1)}{Q} + \frac{dE(N_2)}{Q} \right)^{-1} \tag{9.6}$$

Now from (5.10),and Step 1 of Section 3.5

$$E(N_1) = \frac{E(F_1)}{Q}$$

and

$$E(N_2) = \frac{E(F_2)}{dQ}$$

Thus,

$$V^2 = \left( \frac{E(F_1) + E(F_2)}{Q^2} \right)^{-1} = \frac{Q^2}{\text{Expected Failures}}$$

for this reason, power is connected by many authors to the expected number of failures. If one has proportional hazards, and the expected number of failures per group is fixed, exponentiality is not a factor in the power of the logrank test.

---

Sample Size Equation for Poisson Accrual and Piecewise Exponential Survival:

Two sample trial with 50% allocation to each treatment. One-Sided Test Calculation (Replace $\alpha$ by $\alpha/2$ for Two-Sided Test.)

$$\frac{B^2 + C^2}{(.5As)} = \frac{(Q - T)^2}{(Z_\alpha + Z_\beta)^2} \tag{9.7}$$

A = Total accrual rate.  (.5A to each treatment).

s = Total calendar time of accrual

t = Time from end of accrual to analysis (minimum follow-up time).

d = Hazard rate after t:  Hazard Rate Before t (ratio) (FACT in Sample Size Tables)

$Q$ = Daily failure rate on Treatment #1 (under $H_A$) to time t.

$T$ = Daily failure rate on Treatment #2 (under $H_A$) to time t.

$\alpha$ = Probability of a Type I error (Reject $H_0$ when true).

$Z_\alpha$ = Upper $100\alpha\%$ point of the standard normal distribution.

$\beta$ = 1 - Power = Probability of a Type II error (Reject $H_A$ when true).

$Z_\beta$ = Upper $100\beta\%$ point of the standard normal

$$B^2 = \frac{Q^2}{As}\left[1 - \frac{e^{-Qt}}{(dQs)}\left\{1 - e^{-dQs}\right\}\right]^{-1}. \qquad (9.8)$$

$$C^2 = \frac{T^2}{As}\left[1 - \frac{e^{-Tt}}{(dTs)}\left\{1 - e^{-dTs}\right\}\right]^{-1}. \qquad (9.9)$$

See Section 3.10 regarding losses to follow-up.

Tables for this Piecewise Exponential Model appear for

$d$ = "FACT" = 0 (up front accrual) $\left(\lim_{d \to 0}\right)^*$

    = .25 (75% hazard reduction)

    = .50 (50% hazard reduction)

    = .75 (25% hazard reduction)

    = 1.00 exponential.

Increased hazard after t is not expected in any real clinical trial.

$\left(* \text{ See } (9.2) \text{ and } (9.3)\right)$

## 3.10   Losses to Follow-Up and Sample Size Adjustment

The calculations of our sample size formulas assume no losses to follow-up (completing losses). (Patients quitting the study or failing due to non-study related cause are "lost to follow-up".)

The validity of a trial can be compromised by such losses, unless that are "uninformative." (Rubinstein et al. (1981) provide a formal method to adjust for such uninformative losses to follow-up.) We shall employ a less formal approach.

If a loss is <u>uninformative</u>, then the prognosis of the patient, given the treatment and time of removal from follow-up is presumed to be identical to patients, who stay on study and who are on that treatment, from the corresponding time onward.

### EXAMPLE 10.1

A patient, who has completed therapy, moves with her parents to a region where follow-up cannot be maintained. This patient had been followed for 27 months, and was on Treatment #2. This seems to be an uninformative loss to follow-up. It seems reasonable to believe that the patient's prognosis has not been altered by the move.

### EXAMPLE 10.2

In a study of coronary heart disease (CHD) a patient on Treatment #2 died at 25 months from a Non-CHD cause. If the major analysis is to be based on CHD events, then this patient is censored at 25 months. The patient would be counted in all days prior to death and would not be considered a CHD failure. We are forced to assume that the loss is uninformative, but this might not be a valid assumption. For example, if the patient died of renal failure, it might be indicative of poor vascular function. The CHD outlook of such a patient, assuming that the patient had survived the renal failure, might be much worse than other patients.

In clinical trials, site specific endpoints are especialiy prone to bias caused by competing losses. If one treatment has a greater tendency for such losses than the other, it might be difficult or impossible to interpret the results of the trial. Even in studying mortality, if one treatment is more toxic than the other, that treatment may lose more patients to follow-up than the other, compromising the trial.

Aggressive follow-up is a requirement of all clinical trials. External references can help keep track of participants. The National Death Index (National Center for Health Statistics) can help identify which losses have survived or died, provided that proper identifiers are collected.

For planning a study, although losses to follow-up are included in the analysis up to the time they leave the study, and therefore in theory reduce the variance of the statistics, it is recommended that the study be planned as if these patients contribute nothing. This is a bit conservative if losses are indeed uninformative.

---

**Adjustment for Losses to Follow-Up**

Let

$N_u$ = Sample Size obtained in the Table (Unadjusted).

Based on the length of time needed to accrue $N_u$ patients let

L = Fraction of patients expected to be lost to follow-up.

Then the adjusted sample size is

$$N_A = \frac{N_u}{1 - L}.$$

For example, if

$$N_u = 513$$

$$L = .1 \qquad\qquad (10\% \text{ to be lost to follow-up})$$

$$N_A = \frac{513}{1 - .1} = \frac{513}{.9} = 570$$

The recommended trial size is 570.

## 3.11    Interpretation of the Tables

The sample size tables are obtained from (9.7) for Poisson Accrual, (7.1) for Up Front Accrual, and A133 for the Kaplan-Meier (Binomial). A computer routine readily solves (9.7) and (7.1) by bisection.

The parameters for the Table are identified with (9.7) and (7.1) as follows (the term minimum follow-up is t, the planned endpoint).

(a)    Expected Accrual Through Minimum Follow-up = At

= (Accrual Rate)(Minimum Follow-up).

(b)    PCONT    $= e^{-tQ}$          (t = endpoint duration in days) (Q under $H_A$)

= Control Anticipated Survival Rate at time t, under $H_A$.

(c)    DEL  $= e^{-tT} - e^{-tQ}$          (T, Q under $H_A$)

= Difference between anticipated survival rates at time t

(d)    ALPHA = $\alpha$. (If two-sided, replace $\alpha$ by $\alpha/2$).

(e)    POWER = $1 - \beta$.

(f)    FACT = d

= Hazard rate after t:  Hazard rate before t.

## 3.12    Multi-Treatment Trials (3+ Treatments)

NOTE:  This section reflects the majority position among statisticians, but is not universally accepted.

Generally, there are several types of multi-treatment trials, with different objectives. We shall discuss the four most common. It is rarely practical to use more than three or four treatments.

*3.12.1 Type A*

The treatments in this type of trial are generally as follows: (3 treatment case)

Control

Control + X

Control + Y

The experimental questions are:

(1)    Is X efficacious?

(2)    Is Y efficacious?

In this trial, assume that comparison of (Control + X) versus (Control + Y) is not a primary objective.

This type of trial would be conducted to learn what component of therapy may have efficacy. Hopefully, this experience will lead to a future trial, incorporating one or both of X and Y.

This type of trial should be designed exactly as a two treatment trial, except that the accrual per comparison is only two thirds that of a two treatment study.

$$\text{ACCRUAL THROUGH minimum follow-up} = \text{Atx} \qquad (12.1)$$

A = Annual Accrual Rate.

t = Minimum Follow-up (Endpoint).

$x = \dfrac{2}{\text{Number of Treatments}}.$ \qquad (2/3 in our case)

The analysis would compare Control versus Control + X by a one-sided logrank test and Control versus Control + Y by a one-sided logrank test.

Controversy:  Some statisticians insist on controlling the overall error rate of the study, by adjusting the P-Value through a formal "multiple comparison" procedure.  We believe that such adjustment is not appropriate for the stated objectives of the trial, however.

- Had you done the two trials sequentially

| | | | |
|---|---|---|---|
| Control | versus | Control + X | (Trial 1) |
| Control | versus | Control + Y | (Trial 2) |

you would not have made such an adjustment.

- Why should data on the Control + Y group influence the efficacy comparison involving X?

### 3.12.2 Type B

The treatments for this type of trial are generally as follows:  (3 treatment case).

Control

Control + X

Control + X + Y

The experimental questions are

(1)    Is X efficacious?

(2)    Is Y efficacious over and above X?

Here, the only adjustment centers around the accrual rate, which is handled as in Type A.

The following numerical example might be helpful.

| | |
|---|---|
| Accrual Rate: | 150 patients per year |
| Planning two year survival: | 40% (Control) |
| | 55% (Control + X) |
| | 65% (Control + X + Y) |

FACT = .50 (Post two year hazard = 50% of Pre two-year hazard)

ALPHA = .05 (one-sided)

POWER = .80

MINIMUM FOLLOW-UP = 2 years

Effective Accrual Rate = 100 per comparison per year (200 through minimum follow-up)

From the tables, assuming negligible losses to follow-up we have:

Sample Size: 231 (Control versus Control + X)

437 (Control + X versus Control + X + Y)

In practice, we would run the trial as follows:

- Three-way randomization until 231 patients on Control or Control + X.

- Two-way randomization thereafter, with no controls. The first question will only utilize the 231 Control versus Control + X patients accrued in the three-way randomization.

In terms of total accrual time, at 150 patients per year, the three-way randomization would take about 2.3 years to accrue 346 patients (231 to question 1). It would take about 1.4 years to accrue the remaining 206 patients to answer the second question.

Technical Note: The accrual to the second experimental question was not Poisson, but skewed slightly toward later accrual. Thus it might be instructive to look at the second question assuming a two-way randomization throughout. (Accrual of 300 patients through the minimum follow-up.) This would require a sample of 467 (rather than 437). The actual trial has a greater expected follow-up than this hypothetical trial. Purists can either extend accrual by 30 in the two-way randomization, or extend follow-up about three additional months on the actual setup to achieve the power objective.

## 3.12.3    Type C

(All Two-Way Comparisons) The experimental questions here are

(1)    Is there a difference between X and Y?

(2)    Is there a difference between X and Z?

(3)    Is there a difference between Y and Z?

If these are your questions and you are willing to treat these as three distinct trials, then the only adjustments that would be made would be

(a)    Replace ALPHA by ALPHA/2.  (two-sided tests)

(b)    Effective accrual per comparison through minimum follow-up is two-thirds of the actual accrual through minimum follow-up.

However if you wish to find the best treatment, then multiple comparisons are needed.  In fact, the concept of power changes.  Our sample size tables cannot be used to handle this situation, but can give conservative approximations.

The following example gives conservative sample sizes.

| | |
|---|---|
| Annual Accrual: | 225 per year (150 per comparison). |
| Minimum Follow-up: | 2 years. |
| Two Year Survival: | 50% versus 50% versus 70%. |
| FACT: | 1.0 Exponential. |
| ALPHA: | (.05)/3 = .0167 (two sided). |
| POWER: | 90% (two specific comparisons with the best treatment). |

You are going to infer that two treatments differ if the P-Value for comparing these treatments is less than .0167 (two-sided).

When there is in fact no difference between the treatments there is less than a 5% chance of falsely declaring a difference.  (3 comparisons × .0167).

Your study will be successful if each comparison with the truly best treatment has a P-Value of below .0167 favoring the truly best treatment.

Since for each of the two comparisons with the truly best treatments there is a 10% chance of failing to declare superiority of the truly best treatment is at most a 20% chance of failing to declare the truly best treatment superior to one or both competitors.  (At least 80% overall power to achieve your goal.)

Now the sample size is based on these parameters

$$Z_\alpha = 2.40 \qquad \text{(Figure 7)}$$

($Z_\alpha = 2.40$ corresponds to two-sided P-Value = .0167) and

$$Z_\beta = 1.28. \qquad \text{(Figure 6)}$$

Note that the sample size equation (9.7) depends on $Z_\alpha$ and $Z_\beta$ only through their sum $Z_\alpha + Z_\beta$.

The following approximation greatly increases the use of the tables:

---

Non-Tabulated $Z_\alpha$ and $Z_\beta$

Actual $(Z_\alpha + Z_\beta) = U_A$

Table $(Z_\alpha + Z_\beta) = U_T$ $\qquad$ (Fairly Close to $U_A$)

Sample Size from Table $= N_T$

Recommended Sample Size $= N_A$

$$N_A = N_T \frac{U_A^2}{U_T^2} \qquad\qquad (12.2)$$

---

This approximation is evident in (7.1) and (9.7).

For our tables we have

| ALPHA | POWER | BETA | $(Z_\alpha + Z_\beta) = U_T$ |
|---|---|---|---|
| .005 | .8 | .20 | 3.42 |
| .005 | .9 | .10 | 3.86 |
| .01 | .8 | .20 | 3.17 |
| .01 | .9 | .10 | 3.61 |
| .025 | .8 | .20 | 2.80 |
| .025 | .9 | .10 | 3.24 |
| .05 | .8 | .20 | 2.48 |
| .05 | .9 | .10 | 2.92 |

In the actual application,

$$U_A = 2.40 + 1.28 = 3.68.$$

This yields for ACCRUAL THROUGH MINIMUM FOLLOW-UP of 300, PCONT = .50, DEL = .20, FACT = 1.0, ALPHA = .01, and POWER = .9, a sample size of $N_T$ = 252 per comparison (126 per treatment). From (12.2)

$$N_A = \frac{(3.68)^2 \, 252}{(3.61)^2} = 262.$$

That is, 131 patients per treatment are required for a total of 393.

### 3.12.4 Type D

(2×2 Factorial Design)  This is designed as follows:

Control

Control + X

Control + Y

Control + X + Y

The major therapeutic questions are usually

(1)    Is X efficacious?

(2)    Is Y efficacious?

Generally speaking, if one is willing to assume that no "qualitative interaction" between X and Y exists, then you can collapse this to <u>two</u> two-treatment questions.  That is, if you believe that if X is efficacious, it will be efficacious whether or not Y is used, you may pool the groups without X and the groups with X for the comparison, (assuming that the randomization is about 25% to each treatment). Most statisticians would "stratify" the analysis as discussed in Section 3.13.

X Comparison:  (Control) and (Control + Y) versus (Control + X) and (Control + X + Y)

Y Comparison:  (Control) and (Control + X) versus (Control + Y) and Control + X + Y)

In the absence of qualitative interaction, the Type D trial allows you to answer two questions for the price of one.

A test for Qualitative Interaction appears in Gail and Simon(1985).

## 3.13   Stratified Logrank Test

Often in clinical trials, investigators worry about imbalance in important prognostic groups. For example, it may be known that the extent of disease at baseline, as measured by lesion size, is highly predictive of outcome. Lesions below 5 cm in diameter have excellent prognosis, while lesions over 10 cm in diameter have a terrible prognosis.

The trial can be conducted in two ways:  Prospective Stratification or Retrospective Stratification.

(A)   Prospective Stratification

Conduct the study as if three trials were going on. Each trial will assign about equal numbers of patients to each treatment. Populations for Trials 1, 2, and 3 are respectively.

Stratum 1:   Patients with lesions less than 5 cm in diameter.

Stratum 2:   Patients with lesions 5 - 10 cm in diameter.

Stratum 3:   Patients with lesions over 10 cm in diameter.

The analysis for comparing outcomes in a two treatment trial is as follows: (Illustration for three strata.)

| Stratum | Observed Failures on Treatment #1 | Expected Failures on Treatment #1 | Variance |
|---------|-----------------------------------|-----------------------------------|----------|
| 1 | $O_1$ | $X_1$ | $V_1$ |
| 2 | $O_2$ | $X_2$ | $V_2$ |
| 3 | $O_3$ | $X_3$ | $V_3$ |
| Total | $O_T$ | $X_T$ | $V_T$ |

$$Z = \frac{O_T - X_T}{\sqrt{V_T}}$$
(13.1)

The P-Value is obtained from the standard normal table (Figure 6 or Figure 7) depending upon whether the comparison is one-sided or two-sided.

---

In summary, add the observed failures on Treatment #1 ($O_T$), the expected failures on Treatment #1 ($X_T$), and the variances ($V_T$). Compute Z as per (13.1) and determine the approximate P-Value from Figure 6 or Figure 7.

---

NOTE: As long as the number of strata is fairly small relative to the number of patients, prospective stratification has minimal impact on sample size requirements.

The sample size tables of this volume should be viewed as slightly conservative for use in prospectively stratified trials. That is, the sample size calculation slightly overestimates the true needs, since prospective stratification creates greater risk factor homogeneity between the groups than could be expected by chance. However, if the trial was conducted as a randomized study without using prospective stratification, the stratum specific percent of patients assigned to each treatment will still approach 50% as the sample size increases to infinity. In other words, for large trials with few strata, the benefit of stratification is more psychological than real.

(B)   Retrospective Stratification

Patients would be randomized as if the trial was not stratified, but then the results would be analyzed as if the trial was stratified. This is a perfectly valid procedure. In practice, with a large sample size and few retrospective strata, the sample size requirements for the post stratified analysis are slightly less than those obtained in the tables, and slightly more than the Prospectively Stratified Trial. The sample size tables are therefore conservative, but only slightly so.

Retrospective Stratification is very useful for exploratory analysis. For example, if you conduct a trial and discover that the two treatment groups have a serious imbalance in an important prognostic category, you may wish to rerun the analysis, adjusting for this imbalance via retrospective stratification. If this analysis qualitatively agrees with the planned analysis, then the final results arc supported. However, in the rare case that they disagree, the analysis still provides important insight as to an explanation of the difference or lack of a difference between the treatments.

*3.13.1 Advice on Stratification*

1.   If used at all, limit the number of strata to a small number. When you stratify, the efficacy comparison only compares patients within the same strata.

The following is illustrative

Stratum 1:   10 patients assigned to Treatment #1

10 patients assigned to Treatment #2

Stratum 2:   10 patients assigned to Treatment #1

10 patients assigned to Treatment #2

In the stratified trial, the outcome of each Treatment #1 patient is compared to only 10 Treatment #2 patients, while the unstratified trial has 20 Treatment #2 patients to compare with each Treatment #1 patient. If you overstratify, the lack of ability to compare more than offsets the homogeneity created.

2.   If you have stratum specific therapeutic questions, you must calculate sample size needs for each stratum separately. This could lead to a very much larger trial, than one where stratification is used only as a balancing tool.

3.   If limited stratification is used to balance the randomization, the sample size requirements will be well approximated by the tables of this volume, derived for non-stratified studies.

## 3.14 Intuitive Justification Why the Logrank Test and Kaplan-Meier Estimation for Actual Accrual Process Behave in the Limit in the Same Way as the Fixed Binomial Assumption

Consider the distribution on Day j given the history of the trial up to day j. In other words, if we had the trial results for all patients' day 1, day 2, ..., day j-1, we would know $N_j$ and $M_j$ the number of patients at risk at the start of day j. Given this information, $F_j$ and $G_j$ are binomial with respective sample sizes $N_j$ and $M_j$ and respective failure rates $Q_j$ and $T_j$. This <u>conditional</u> distribution is identical to the unconditional distribution of the fixed binomial case.

$$E\left(\frac{F_j}{N_j} \mid \text{Past History of Trial}\right) = Q_j \qquad (N_j \neq 0)$$

$$\text{Var}\left(\frac{F_j}{N_j} \mid \text{Past History of Trial}\right) = \frac{Q_j P_j}{N_j} \qquad (N_j \neq 0)$$

As an estimate of $Q_j$, if we can ignore the possibility that $N_j = 0$, we can say, $F_j/N_j$ is unbiased for $Q_j$ and is uncorrelated with its past history.

Consider an alternate trial where we shall preselect $N_j$ as

$$N_j^* = E(N_j) \qquad \text{(rounded to an integer)}$$

If $N_j \geq N_j^*$ we shall use the actual first $N_j^*$ day j's of the trial.

If $N_j \leq N_j^*$ we shall add an additional $(N_j^* - N_j)$ day j's (independent trials with failure rate $Q_j$).

Although it is difficult to prove at the mathematical level of this text, it is intuitively clear that $N_j/N_j^* \overset{P}{\to} 1$ as $N_j^* \to \infty$ and hence the <u>fraction</u> of overlapping data coverages to 100% as the $N_j^* \to \infty$.

In other words, it can be shown that the large sample distributions under the actual process and artificial fixed binomial accrual are identical. The non-overlapping data is an insignificant percentage.

### 3.15 Alternate Standard Error for the Kaplan-Meier Estimator

$\Big($Peto et al (1977)$\Big)$

The following estimator for $D_k$ in 10 of the Notation chart of Chapter 3 is often used to obtain the standard error of the Kaplan-Meier estimator, $\hat{S}_k$.

$$D_k^* = \hat{S}_k\left\{(1 - \hat{S}_k)/N_{k+1}\right\}^{\frac{1}{2}} \tag{15.1}$$

This is not completely rigorous but has a number of desirable properties. Some intuitive justification will be shown below.

Advantages over Greenwood Formula (Notation Chart item 11).

(a)    Can be computed from the Kaplan-Meier estimate at time k and the number of patients at risk at time k+1. It does not require a summation.

(b)    It agrees well with the Greenwood Formula except in the right hand portion of the curve where the fraction censored is high.

(c)    The standard error increases in the plateau portion of a curve as patients are censored. The Greenwood Formula has a standard error that changes only at times where failures occur. This leads to unrealistically low estimates of standard error by Greenwood's Formula for situations where few patients are at risk.

Disadvantages over Greenwood's Formula

(d)    $\dfrac{\hat{S}_k - S_k}{D_k^*}$ is not in theory asymptotically standard normal. It is close to standard normal where the sample size is large and the fraction censored before k is small. We shall see in Theorem 15.1 that the use of $D_k^*$ is conservative ($\hat{D}_k \leq D_k^*$).

(e)    If one wishes to make statements such as "We are 95% confident that the three year survival is <u>less</u> than x", then the Greenwood standard error is superior, even in plateaus. This is because survival curves are monotonically decreasing functions. Hence, if you are 95% confident that the two year survival is below 83%, you are certainly 95% confident that the three year survival is below 83%, whether or not there is a large fraction of patients censored between two and three years. If the two to three year interval is a plateau, for example, the upper limit of the 95% confidence interval for the alternate standard error will be higher at three years than at two years, while that of Greenwood's formula will remain fixed.

Intuitive justification of the alternative standard error:

<u>Theorem 15.1</u>:  $D_k^* \geq \hat{D}_k$

<u>Proof</u>:  From item 9 of the Notation Chart at the beginning of Chapter 3,

$$1 - \hat{S}_k = 1 - \prod_{j=1}^{k} \hat{P}_j. \tag{15.2}$$

Now, by applying the lemma on converting a difference of products to a sum (Section 3.2) with

$$a_j = 1 \quad \text{and } b_j = \hat{P}_j,$$

we have

$$1 - \hat{S}_k = \hat{S}_k \sum \frac{(1-\hat{P}_j)}{\hat{S}_j}$$

$$= \hat{S}_k \sum \frac{\hat{Q}_j}{\hat{S}_{j-1} \hat{P}_j}. \tag{15.3}$$

Now,

$$\frac{\hat{S}_k}{\hat{S}_{j-1}} = \frac{\hat{P}_1 \cdots \hat{P}_k}{\hat{P}_1 \cdots \hat{P}_{j-1}} = \hat{P}_j \cdots \hat{P}_k. \tag{15.4}$$

Now from the <u>actual</u> accrual process,

$$N_{j+1} = N_j - F_j - W_j$$

where

$N_j$ = Number of Patients at risk at start of day j,

$F_j$ = Failures on Day j,

$W_j$ = Competing "withdrawals" on Day j.

The $W_j$ include patients who are alive with time of risk j, as well as those who quit alive on day j.

$$\hat{P}_j = \frac{N_j - F_j}{N_j} \geq \frac{N_j - F_j - W_j}{N_j} = \frac{N_{j+1}}{N_j}. \tag{15.5}$$

As long as the $W_j$ are small percentages of $N_j$, approximate equality holds.

By substituting (15.5) into (15.4) we have

$$\frac{\hat{S}_k}{\hat{S}_{j-1}} \geq \prod_{i=j}^{k} \frac{N_{i+1}}{N_i} = \frac{N_{k+1}}{N_j}. \tag{15.6}$$

Substituting (15.6) in (15.3) yields

$$1 - \hat{S}_k \geq N_{k+1} \sum_j \frac{\hat{Q}_j}{N_j \hat{P}_j}. \tag{15.7}$$

Hence

$$\frac{(1 - \hat{S}_k)}{N_{k+1}} \geq \sum_j \frac{\hat{Q}_j}{N_j \hat{P}_j}. \tag{15.8}$$

That is,

$$D_k^* = \hat{S}_k\left\{\frac{(1 - \hat{S}_k)}{N_{k+1}}\right\}^{\frac{1}{2}}$$

$$\geq \hat{D}_k = \hat{S}_k\left\{\sum_j\frac{\hat{Q}_j}{N_j\hat{P}_j}\right\}^{\frac{1}{2}} \tag{15.9}$$

and approximate equality holds as long as the withdrawal rates are small fractions of the $N_j$.

Summary:

The use of $D_k^*$ instead of $\hat{D}_k$ is <u>conservative</u>. The formula will underestimate the precision of the estimator $\hat{S}_k$, but only slightly if the fraction of competing withdrawals is small.

### 3.16    Connection Between Kaplan-Meier and Binomial

Note that if there are no censored patients to day k, under <u>actual accrual</u>, $N_{j+1} = N_j - F_j$ and

$$\hat{P}_j = \frac{N_{j+1}}{N_j}.$$

This yields from the Notation Chart:

$$\hat{S}_k = \prod_{j=1}^{k}\frac{N_{j+1}}{N_j}$$

$$= \frac{N_2}{N_1}\frac{N_3}{N_2}\cdots\frac{N_{k+1}}{N_k} = \frac{N_{k+1}}{N_1}. \tag{16.1}$$

To evaluate $\hat{D}_k^2$, note hat

$$\hat{Q}_j = 1 - \hat{P}_j = \frac{N_j - N_{j+1}}{N_j}$$

and hence

$$\frac{\hat{Q}_j}{\hat{P}_j N_j} = \frac{N_j - N_{j+1}}{N_{j+1} N_j} = \frac{1}{N_{j+1}} - \frac{1}{N_j}$$

$$\sum_{j=1}^{k} \frac{\hat{Q}_j}{\hat{P}_j N_j} = \sum_{j=1}^{k} \left( \frac{1}{N_{j+1}} - \frac{1}{N_j} \right)$$

$$= \left( \frac{1}{N_2} - \frac{1}{N_1} \right) + \left( \frac{1}{N_3} - \frac{1}{N_2} \right) + \cdots + \left( \frac{1}{N_{k+1}} - \frac{1}{N_k} \right)$$

$$= \frac{1}{N_{k+1}} - \frac{1}{N_1} = \frac{N_1 - N_{k+1}}{N_1 N_{k+1}}$$

Hence

$$\hat{D}_k^2 = \hat{S}_k^2 \sum_{j=1}^{k} \frac{\hat{Q}_j}{\hat{P}_j N_j}$$

$$= \frac{N_{k+1}^2}{N_1^2} \frac{(N_1 - N_{k+1})}{N_1 N_{k+1}}$$

$$= \frac{N_{k+1}(N_1 - N_{k+1})}{N_1^3}$$

$$= \frac{\hat{S}_k(1 - \hat{S}_k)}{N_1} \qquad (16.2)$$

$\hat{D}_k^2$ is the binomial estimate of variance when there are no competing losses.

Studies based on the Kaplan-Meier are planned using the Tables with Binomial (BIN) value for FACT. Adjustments can be made for anticipated losses to follow-up. (See A133 for details).

## REFERENCES

1. **Crowley, J.,** Asymptotic normality of a new nonparametric statistic for use in organ transplant studies, *J. Am. Statist. Assoc.,* 69, 1006, 1974.

2. **Breslow, N. E. and Crowley, J.,** A large sample study of the life table and product limit estimates under random censorship, *Ann. Statist.* 2, 437, 1974.

3. **Gail, M. and Simon, R.,** Testing for qualitative interactions between treatment effects and patient subsets, *Biometrics,* 41, 361, 1985.

4. **Greenwood, M.,** *The Errors of Sampling of the Survivorship Tables, Reports on Public Health and Statistical Subjects,* Her Majesty's Stationery Office, London, 1926, 33.

5. **Kaplan, E. L. and Meier, P.,** Nonparametric estimation from incomplete observations, *J. Am. Statist. Assoc.,* 53, 447, 1958.

6. **Peto, R., Pike, M. C., Armitage, P., Breslow, N. E., Cox, D. R., Howard, S. V., Mantel, N., McPherson, K., Peto, J., and Smith, P. G.,** Design and analysis of randomized clinical trials requiring prolonged observation of each patient, II. Analysis and example, *Br. J. Canc.,* 35, 1, 1977.

7. **Rubinstein, L. V., Gail, M. H., and Santner, T. J.,** Planning the duration of a comparitive clinical trial with loss to follow-up and a period of continued observation, *J. Chron. Dis.,* 34, 469, 1981.

# APPENDIX I

# A REVIEW OF MATHEMATICAL STATISTICS

In order to follow the material in Chapter 3, it is assumed that the reader has a working knowledge of undergraduate mathematical statistics at a level of one of the following texts: Mendenhall, Scheaffer, and Wackerly (1986), Fraser (1976), Mood, Graybill, and Boes (1974), or Hogg and Craig (1978).

In order that this book be self contained, this appendix will list definitions and results. For convenient reference each is assigned a number.

A.1 Sample Space(s) (Definition): The set of all possible outcomes of an experiment (study or observation process). This is denoted by S.

A.2 Event (Definition): A subset of the Sample Space.

A.3 Union of Events: $E_1 \cup E_2$ (Definition) An event consisting of outcomes in one or both of $E_1$, $E_2$. (Unites the two events into a larger event).

This definition extends to multi-events $E_1 \cup E_2 \cup E_3$ etc.

A.4 Intersection of Events: $E_1 E_2$ (Definition) An event consisting of outcomes common to $E_1$ and $E_2$. To qualify for membership in $E_1 E_2$, the outcome must be in both event $E_1$ and event $E_2$.

This definition extends to multi-events $E_1 E_2 E_3$ etc.

A.5 Complement of Event: ($\bar{E}$) (Definition) The complement of the event E, denoted by $\bar{E}$, consists of all outcomes in the sample space that are not in the event E. (E and $\bar{E}$ have no outcomes in common, and together make up the sample space $E \cup \bar{E} = S$).

A.6 Null Event: ($\emptyset$) (Definition) The Event which contains no outcomes in the sample space is called the null Event ($\emptyset = \bar{S}$).

A.7 Mutually Exclusive Events (Definition): The events $E_1$ and $E_2$ are mutually exclusive if they have no outcomes in common. $E_1 E_2 = \emptyset$.

This definition extends to multi-events $E_1$, $E_2$, ..., $E_n$ as $E_i E_j = \emptyset$ for every i,j $1 \leq i < j \leq n$.

A.8   <u>Probability</u> (Definition) P is called a probability if

   (a)   P assigns a number $P(E)$ to every event in S with $0 \leq P(E) \leq 1$.

   (b)   If $E_1, E_2, \ldots, E_n$ are mutually exclusive events $P(E_1 \cup E_2 \cup \cdots \cup E_n) =$

   $P(E_1) + P(E_2) + \cdots + P(E_n)$

   (c)   $P(S) = 1$ where $S = $ Sample Space

<u>Probability Results</u> (Consequences)

A.9   (a)   $P(\emptyset) = 0$

A.10 (b)   $P(\bar{E}) = 1 - P(E)$

A.11 (c)   $P(E_1 \cup E_2) = P(E_1) + P(E_2) - P(E_1 E_2)$

A.12 <u>Conditional Probability</u> $\left( P(E_1 | E_2) \right)$ (Definition)

   The probability that $E_1$ occurs <u>given</u> that $E_2$ has occurred is denoted by

$$P(E_1 | E_2) = \frac{P(E_1 E_2)}{P(E_2)} \qquad \left( P(E_2) > 0 \right)$$

A.13 <u>Independence of two Events</u> (Definition)

   Events $E_1$ and $E_2$ are independent if $P(E_1 E_2) = P(E_1) P(E_2)$.

A.14 <u>Independence of two events</u> (Consequence)

   Provided that $P(E_2) > 0$, then events $E_1$ and $E_2$ are independent if and only if

$$P(E_1 | E_2) = P(E_1)$$

i.e. conditional and unconditional probability agree.

The proof is straight forward and is therefore omitted.

A.15 <u>Mutual Independence of Several Events</u> (Definition)

   Events $E_1$, $E_2$, $\ldots$, $E_n$ are mutually independent if for every subset $\left\{ j_1, j_2, \ldots, j_k \right\}$ of the integers $\{1, 2, \ldots, n\}$

$$P(E_{j_1} E_{j_2} \ldots E_{j_k}) = P(E_{j_1}) P(E_{j_2}) \cdots P(E_{j_k})$$

A.16 <u>Random Variable</u> (Definition)

A random variable assigns a number to each outcome in the sample space S. That is, if X is a random variable, then for each sample point s in S, X assigns a number X(s).

A.17 <u>Random Vector</u> (Vector of Random Variables) (Definition)

A random vector, Y, of dimension k is a k-dimensional vector of random variables

$$(X_1, X_2, \ldots, X_k) = Y$$

A.18 <u>Cumulative Distribution Function of a Random Variable</u> (cdf) (Definition)

The cumulative distribution function of the random variable X, denoted by $F_X(x)$, is

$$F_X(x) = P[X \leq x] \qquad -\infty < x < \infty$$

The cumulative distribution function is a plot of the probability that the random variable X takes on numerical value less than or equal to the number x. This is plotted over all real numbers, x.

A.19 <u>Discrete Random Variables</u> and <u>Probability Mass Function</u> (Definition)

A random variable X is "discrete" if the cumulative distribution is of the form

$$F_X(x) = \sum_{y:\, y \leq x} f_X(y)$$

y: y≤x refers to a <u>finite</u> set of <u>possible</u> values of the random variable X that assign values x or less and $F_X(x) \to 1$ as $x \to \infty$.

The function $f_X(y) = P[X=y]$ is called the <u>probability mass function</u>. This mass function will be zero except at a discrete set of values. (*This is not the most general definition, but it will meet our needs.*)

A.20 <u>Continuous Random Variables</u> and <u>Probability Density Function</u> (Definition)

A random variable X is "continuous" if the cumulative distribution is of the form

$$F_X(x) = \int_{-\infty}^{x} f_X(y)\,dy$$

with $F_X(x) \to 1$ as $x \to \infty$.

For the purpose of this volume, we shall assume that $f_X(y)$ has at most a finite number of discontinuities.

$f_X(y)$ is called the <u>probability density function</u>.

A.21 Relation between Cumulative Distribution and Probability Density Function (Consequence)

At each continuity point of $F_X(x)$,

$$f_X(x) = F'_X(x)$$

That is, the probability density is the derivative of the cumulative distribution function.

Proof:       $F_X(x+h) - F_X(x) = \int_x^{x+h} f_X(y)dy$

$$= hf_X(\xi) \quad \text{for some } \xi: \ x \le \xi \le x+h$$

The above follows from the Mean Value Theorem of Calculus.

If we divide both sides by h and let $h \to 0$, the result follows.

A.22 Cumulative Distribution Function for Random Vectors (Definition)

We shall write this in terms of two random vectors, but the extension to several dimensions is clear.

A random vector $X = (X_1, X_2)$ has cumulative distribution denoted by $F_X$:

$$F_X(x_1, x_2) = P(X_1 \le x_1, X_2 \le x_2)$$

A.23 Multivariate Analogues of Mass Function and Density (Definition)

(a)    $X_1, X_2$ discrete

$$f_X(x_1, x_2) = P\big[X_1 = x_1, X_2 = x_2\big]$$

$$F_X(x_1, x_2) = \sum_{\substack{y_1 \le x_1 \\ y_2 \le x_2}} f_X(y_1, y_2)$$

$f_X(x_1, x_2)$ is the joint probability mass function of $X_1, X_2$

(b)    $X_1, X_2$ continuous

$$F_X(x_1, x_2) = \int_{-\infty}^{x_1} \int_{-\infty}^{x_2} f_X(y_1, y_2)dy_2 dy_1$$

$f_X(x_1, x_2)$ is the joint probability density of $X_1, X_2$

Note:  at continuity points of $(x_1, x_2)$,

$$f_X(x_1, x_2) = \frac{\partial^2 F_X(x_1, x_2)}{\partial x_1 \partial x_2}$$

(c)  $X_1$ discrete, $X_2$ continuous

$$F_X(x_1,x_2) = \sum_{y_1 \leq x_1} \int_{-\infty}^{x_2} f_X(y_1,y_2)dy_2$$

$f_X(x_1,x_2)$ is the <u>joint probability mass-density</u> of $X_1$, $X_2$

A.24 <u>Marginal Distributions</u> (Definition and Consequences)

Here, we also study two variables $X_1$, $X_2$ but the extension to several variables is clear.

$$P\big[X_1 \leq x_1\big] \quad = \quad \lim_{x_2 \to \infty} P\big[X_1 \leq x_1, \, X_2 \leq x_2\big]$$

$$= \quad \lim_{x_2 \to \infty} F_X(x_1,x_2)$$

We denote this by the Marginal Cumulative Distribution of $X_1$:

$$F_{X_1}(x_1) \quad = \quad \lim_{x_2 \to \infty} F_X(x_1,x_2)$$

$$= \int_{-\infty}^{x_1}\left\{\int_{-\infty}^{\infty} f_X(y_1,y_2)dy_2\right\}dy_1 \quad X_1,X_2 \text{ continuous}$$

$$= \sum_{y_1 \leq x_1}\left\{\sum_{\text{all } y_2} f_X(y_1,y_2)\right\} \quad X_1,X_2 \text{ discrete}$$

$$= \sum_{y_1 \leq x_1}\left\{\int_{-\infty}^{\infty} f_X(y_1, y_2)dy_2\right\} \quad X_1 \text{ discrete, } X_2 \text{ continuous}$$

$$= \int_{-\infty}^{x_1}\left\{\sum_{\text{all } y_2} f_X(y_1, y_2)\right\}dy_1 \quad X_1 \text{ continuous, } X_2 \text{ discrete}$$

A25. If $X_2$ is <u>discrete</u>,

$$f_{X_1}(x_1) = \sum_{\text{all } y_2} f_X(x_1, y_2) \quad \text{is}$$

called the <u>Marginal density of $X_1$</u> if $X_1$ is <u>continuous</u>, or <u>Marginal Mass function of $X_1$</u> if $X_1$ is <u>discrete</u>.

A26. If $X_2$ is continuous

$$f_{X_1}(x_1) = \int_{-\infty}^{\infty} f_X(x_1, y_2) dy_2 \quad \text{is}$$

called the Marginal density of $X_1$ if $X_1$ is continuous, or Marginal Mass function of $X_1$ if $X_1$ is discrete.

A27. Conditional Distributions (Definition and Consequences).

The Conditional Mass function ($X_2$ discrete) or conditional density ($X_2$ continuous) of $X_2$ given $X_1 = x_1$ is defined by

$$f_{X_2|X_1}(x_2|x_1) = \frac{f_X(x_1, x_2)}{f_{X_1}(x_1)}$$

If $X_1$ is continuous, the above definition only applies to continuity points of $f_{X_1}(x_1)$ and $f_X(x_1, x_2)$.

Notes: (a)    If $X_1$ and $X_2$ are discrete, then by the definitions of conditional probability and marginal probability mass function (See A12 and A25)

$$f_{X_2|X_1}(x_2|x_1) = P\left[X_2 = x_2 | X_1 = x_1\right]$$

(b)    If $X_1$ and $X_2$ are continuous, $(x_1, x_2)$ is a continuity point of $f_X$, and $\Delta_1$ and $\Delta_2$ are small:

$$P\left[x_1 < X_1 < x_1 + \Delta_1, x_2 < X_2 < x_2 + \Delta_2\right] \simeq \Delta_1 \Delta_2 f_X(x_1, x_2)$$

$$P\left[x_1 < X_1 < x_1 + \Delta_1\right] \simeq \Delta_1 f_{X_1}(x_1)$$

$$P\left[x_2 < X_2 < x_2 + \Delta_2 | x_1 < X_1 < x_1 + \Delta_1\right] \simeq \frac{\Delta_2 f_X(x_1, x_2)}{f_{X_1}(x_1)}$$

That is, in the limit, as $\Delta_1 \to 0$ and $\Delta_2 \to 0$,

$$f_{X_1|X_2}(x_2|x_1) = \frac{f_X(x_1, x_2)}{f_{X_1}(x_1)}$$

behaves as a density, reflecting the appropriate conditional probability.

(c)  Similar analogues can be developed for mixed continuous-discrete random variables.

A28. <u>Conditioning on an Event</u> (consequence)

In the case of a continuous $X = (X_1, X_2)$ one may wish to find the conditional distribution of

$X_2$ given $X_1 < x_1$ rather than specifying an exact value of $x_1$.

$$P\left(X_2 < x_2 | X_1 < x_1\right) \quad = \frac{P\left[X_1 < x_1, X_2 < x_2\right]}{P\left[X_1 < x_1\right]}$$

$$= \frac{F_{X_1, X_2}(x_1, x_2)}{F_{X_1}(x_1)}$$

$$P\left[X_2 < x_2 | X_1 < x_1\right] \quad = \frac{\int_{-\infty}^{x_2}\left\{\int_{-\infty}^{x_1} f_X(y_1, y_2)dy_1\right\}dy_2}{F_{X_1}(x_1)}$$

This is the conditional cumulative distribution of $X_2$ given that $X_1 < x_1$.

Differentiating both sides with respect to $x_2$ yields the conditional density at continuity points:

$$f_{X_2|X_1}\left(x_2|X_1 < x_1\right) = \frac{\int_{-\infty}^{x_1} f_X(y_1, x_2)dy_1}{F_{X_1}(x_1)}$$

A29. Independence of Random Variables (Definition)

Random variables $X_1$ and $X_2$ are independent if for every $x_1$, $x_2$

$$F_X(x_1, x_2) = F_{X_1}(x_1)F_{X_2}(x_2)$$

That is, for every $x_1$, $x_2$ the events

$E_1$ that $\quad X_1 \leq x_1$ and

$E_2$ that $\quad X_2 \leq x_2$ are independent.

A30. Independence of Random Variables (Consequence)

Independence is equivalent to

$$f_X(x_1, x_2) = f_{X_1}(x_1)f_{X_2}(x_2)$$

with f the mass or density function depending on whether the random variable is discrete or continuous.

The proofs are straight forward.

A31. Independence of Several Random Variables (Definition and Consequence)

Either of these definitions imply independence

$$F_X(x_1, x_2, ..., x_k) = P\left[X_1 \leq x_1, X_2 \leq x_2, ..., X_k \leq x_k\right]$$
$$= F_{X_1}(x_1) F_{X_2}(x_2) ... F_{X_k}(x_k) \quad \text{for all } (x_1, ..., x_k)$$

or

$$f_X(x_1, ..., x_k) \quad = f_{X_1}(x_1) f_{X_2}(x_2) ... f_{X_k}(x_k) \quad \text{for all } (x_1, ..., x_k)$$

A32. <u>Random Samples</u> (<u>Independently Identically Distributed Random Variables</u>)

(<u>IID random variables</u>) (Definition)

Random variables $X_1$, $X_2$, ..., $X_k$ are independent identically distributed if they are independent and each $X_j$ has the same cumulative distribution:

$$F_{X_j}(x) = F(x) \qquad \text{Same for all j.}$$

$$F_X(x_1, ..., x_k) = F(x_1)\, F(x_2) \, ... \, F(x_k)$$

or sufficiently

$$f_X(x_1, ..., x_k) = f(x_1)\, f(x_2) \, ... \, f(x_k).$$

## EXPECTED VALUE OF A FUNCTION OF A RANDOM VECTOR
### (Definition)

A33. (a)     Univariate

Let g(X) be a function of the random variable X.  g(X) has <u>expectation</u> denoted by $E\big(g(X)\big)$

$$E\big(g(X)\big) \quad = \int_{-\infty}^{\infty} g(x) f_X(x) dx \qquad \text{(Continuous Case)}$$

$$= \sum_{\text{all x}} g(x) f_X(x) \qquad \text{(Discrete case)}$$

$f_X$ is the probability density for continuous X or the probability mass function for discrete X.

A34. (b)     Multivariate

Let g(X) be a function of the random vector $X = (X_1, X_2)$.  g(X) has expectation

$$E\big(g(X)\big) = \int_{-\infty}^{\infty}\int_{-\infty}^{\infty} g(x_1, x_2) f_X(x_1, x_2) dx_2 dx_1 \qquad \text{(Continuous case)}$$

with $f_X(x_1, x_2)$ the joint density of $X_1$, $X_2$.

Discrete components will involve sum instead of integral.

## SPECIAL UNIVARIATE FUNCTIONS (Definitions)

We shall only write these for the continuous case, but they apply in similar fashion to the discrete case too.

A35. (a)    $g(X) = X$                             (The <u>population mean</u> of X)

We generally denote the mean by $\mu$

$$\mu = E(X) = \int_{-\infty}^{\infty} x f_X(x) dx$$

A36. (b)    $g(X) = (X-\mu)^2$                       (The <u>population variance</u> of X)

We generally denote the population variance, the average squared deviation about the mean as $\sigma^2$

$$\begin{aligned} \text{Var}(X) \quad &= E\big[(X-\mu)^2\big] \\ &= \int_{-\infty}^{\infty} (x-\mu)^2 f_X(x) dx \\ \text{where} \quad \mu &= E(X) \end{aligned}$$

A37. (c)    $g(X) = e^{tX}$                          (The <u>moment generating function</u> of X)

We generally denote this by $M_X(t)$

$$M_X(t) = \int_{-\infty}^{\infty} e^{tx} f_X(x) dx$$

## A38. SPECIAL MULTIVARIATE FUNCTION

$$g(X) = (X_1 - \mu_1)(X_2 - \mu_2) \qquad \text{(\underline{Population Covariance})}$$

where $\mu_1 = E(X_1)$    $\mu_2 = E(X_2)$

$$\text{Cov}(X_1, X_2) = \int_{-\infty}^{\infty} \int_{-\infty}^{\infty} (x_1 - \mu_1)(x_2 - \mu_2) f_X(x_1, x_2) dx_2 \, dx_1$$

## RESULTS ON EXPECTATIONS (Consequences)

A39. (a)   Expectation of a constant is a constant.

If $g(X) = C$    for all X,

$$E\big(g(X)\big) = C$$

A40. (b)   If C is a constant,

$$E\big(Cg(X)\big) = CE\big(g(X)\big)$$

A41. (c)   Additivity of Expectation

$$E\big\{g_1(X) + g_2(X)\big\} = E\big\{g_1(X)\big\} + E\big\{g_2(X)\big\}$$

A42. (d)   $E\big\{ \sum_{j=1}^{k} a_j g_j(X) \big\} = \Sigma a_j E\big\{g_j(X)\big\}$

A43. (e)   Shortcut formula for Variance

$$\sigma^2 = E\big((X - \mu)^2\big) = E(X^2) - \mu^2$$

where $\mu = E(X)$

A44. (f)    Shortcut formula for covariance

$$\text{Cov}(X_1, X_2) = E\{(X_1 - \mu_1)(X_2 - \mu_2)\} \qquad \text{(Definition)}$$

$$= E(X_1 X_2) - \mu_1 \mu_2 \qquad \text{(Consequence)}$$

Proof (f)

$$(X_1 - \mu_1)(X_2 - \mu_2) = X_1 X_2 - \mu_1 X_2 - \mu_2 X_1 + \mu_1 \mu_2$$

Take expectation on both sides and apply (d) and (a) above.

A45. (g)    Linear Combinations (Consequence)

Let $Y = \sum_{j=1}^{k} a_j X_j$

Then $E(Y) = \sum_{j=1}^{k} a_j \mu_j$    where $\mu_j = E(X_j)$

and $\text{Var}(Y) = \sum_{j=1}^{k} a_j^2 \text{Var}(X_j) + 2 \sum_{j=2}^{k} \sum_{i=1}^{j-1} a_i a_j \text{Cov}(X_i, X_j)$

Proof (g):    The expectation of Y is obtained from (d) above.

$$\text{Var}(Y) = E\{Y - E(Y)\}^2 = E\left(\left\{\sum_{j=1}^{k} a_j(X_j - \mu_j)\right\}^2\right)$$

$$= \text{Desired Result by (d) above.}$$

A46. (h)    If $X_1$, $X_2$ are independent, then

$$\text{Cov}(X_1, X_2) = 0$$

Proof (h):

$$E(X_1 X_2) = \int_{-\infty}^{\infty} \int_{-\infty}^{\infty} x_1 x_2 f_X(x_1 x_2) dx_2 dx_1$$

$$= \int_{-\infty}^{\infty} \int_{-\infty}^{\infty} x_1 x_2 f_{X_1}(x_1) f_{X_2}(x_2) dx_2 dx_1 \qquad \text{(independence)}$$

$$= \int_{-\infty}^{\infty} x_1 f_{X_1}(x_1) dx_1 \int_{-\infty}^{\infty} x_2 f_{X_2}(x_2) dx_2$$

$$= \mu_1 \mu_2$$

From (f) above, $\quad \text{Cov}(X_1, X_2) = 0$

(i) Expectation and Variance for classical statistics for independent identically distributed random variables.

Let $X_1, X_2, ..., X_n$ be independent identically distributed random variables with

$$E(X_j) = \mu \quad \text{and} \quad \text{Var}(X_j) = \sigma^2$$

Let $\quad \bar{X} = \dfrac{\sum\limits_{j=1}^{n} X_j}{n}$ $\hfill$ (Sample Mean)

$$S^2 = \dfrac{\sum\limits_{j=1}^{n} (X_j - \bar{X})^2}{(n-1)} \hfill \text{(Sample Variance)}$$

A47. Then $\ E(\bar{X}) = \mu$

A48. $\quad \text{Var}(\bar{X}) = \dfrac{\sigma^2}{n}$

A49. $\quad E(S^2) = \sigma^2$

Proof (i): To prove the results for $\bar{X}$, we apply (g) above with $a_j = (\tfrac{1}{n})$. By independence $\text{Cov}(X_i, X_j) = 0$. This yields $E(\bar{X}) = \mu \quad$ and $\quad \text{Var}(\bar{X}) = \dfrac{\sigma^2}{n}$

$$S^2 = \dfrac{\left\{ \Sigma X_j^2 - n\bar{X}^2 \right\}}{(n-1)} \hfill (*)$$

From the shortcut formula

$$\sigma^2 = E(X_j^2) - \mu^2 \text{ implies } E(X_j^2) = \sigma^2 + \mu^2$$

and $\quad \text{Var}(\bar{X}) = E(\bar{X})^2 - \left\{ E(\bar{X}) \right\}^2$

i.e. $\quad \dfrac{\sigma^2}{n} = E(\bar{X})^2 - \mu^2.$

Hence $E(\bar{X})^2 = \mu^2 + \dfrac{\sigma^2}{n}.$

Taking expectation in $(*)$ yields:

$$E(S^2) = \frac{\left\{n\sigma^2 + n\mu^2 - n\mu^2 - \sigma^2\right\}}{(n-1)} = \sigma^2.$$

A50. (j)    $\left|\text{Cov}\left(X_1, X_2\right)\right| \leq \left\{\text{Var}(X_1)\,\text{Var}(X_2)\right\}^{\frac{1}{2}}.$

Proof (j):    $\text{Var}\left(X_1 + tX_2\right) = \text{Var}(X_1) + 2t\,\text{Cov}\left(X_1, X_2\right) + t^2\text{Var}(X_2).$

Since Var $(\ ) \geq 0$, we obtain the result by successively letting $t = \pm\sqrt{\dfrac{\text{Var}(X_1)}{\text{Var}(X_2)}}.$

Note that this implies

$$-1 \leq \rho = \frac{\text{Cov}\left(X_1, X_2\right)}{\left\{\text{Var}(X_1)\,\text{Var}(X_2)\right\}^{\frac{1}{2}}} \leq 1.$$

A51. (k)    Chebyshev Theorem (Consequence)

Let X be a random variable with mean $\mu$ and variance $\sigma^2$. Then for any $\epsilon > 0$

$$P\left[|X-\mu| \geq \epsilon\right] \leq \frac{\sigma^2}{\epsilon^2}.$$

Proof: We shall prove the result in the continuous case

$$\sigma^2 \;=\; \int_{-\infty}^{\infty} (x-\mu)^2 f_X(x)dx$$

$$\geq \int_{|x-\mu|\geq\epsilon} (x-\mu)^2 f_X(x)dx$$

$$\geq \int_{|x-\mu|\geq\epsilon} \epsilon^2 f_X(x)dx$$

$$\geq \epsilon^2 P\left[|X-\mu|\geq\epsilon\right].$$

Divide both sides by $\epsilon^2$ to obtain the result.

A52. (l)    "Consistency of $\bar{X}$" (Consequence)

If $X_1$, $X_2$, ... are independent, identically distributed random variables with mean $\mu$ and variance $\sigma^2$, then for any $\epsilon > 0$

$$P\left[|\bar{X}_n - \mu| > \epsilon\right] \to 0 \quad \text{as } n \to \infty$$

where $\bar{X}_n = \dfrac{\left(X_1 + \cdots + X_n\right)}{n}$.

In lay terms, this is the "Law of Averages".

Proof: From **A47** and **A48** above,

$$E(\bar{X}) = \mu \quad \text{and} \quad \text{Var}(\bar{X}) = \frac{\sigma^2}{n}.$$

By Chebyshev's Theorem (k)

$$P\left[|\bar{X} - \mu| > \epsilon\right] \leq \frac{\text{Var}(\bar{X})}{\epsilon^2} = \frac{\sigma^2}{n\epsilon^2} \to 0 \quad \text{as } n \to \infty.$$

## MOMENT GENERATING FUNCTIONS (Consequences)

$$M_X(t) = E\left(e^{tX}\right)$$

A53. (a)    If two cumulative distributions differ, then they have different moment generating functions. (The moment generating function uniquely identifies the distribution. In fact, we only need to identify the moment generating function in an open interval about t=0.)

See Fraser (1976, pages 544–546).

A54. (b)    Provided the moment generating function is defined in a neighborhood of $t = 0$, then

$$E(X^n) = \lim_{t \to 0} M_X^{(n)}(t)$$

(The $n^{\text{th}}$ derivative of $M_X(t)$ with respect to t is taken, and then $t \to 0$.)

See Fraser (1976, page 233).

A55. (c)   $M_X(t) = 1 + \sum\limits_{j=1}^{\infty} \dfrac{E(X^j)t^j}{j!}$

See Fraser (1976, page 233).

A56. (d)   If $X_1$, $X_2$, ..., $X_n$ are independent random variables with respective moment generating functions

$$M_{X_j}(t) \quad j = 1, ...,n$$

and

$$Y = \sum\limits_{j=1}^{n} a_j X_j$$

with $a_j$'s constant.  Then Y has moment generating function

$$M_Y(t) = \prod\limits_{j=1}^{n} M_{X_j}(a_j t)$$

Proof (d):

$$e^{tY} \qquad = e^{t\Sigma a_j X_j} = \prod\limits_{j=1}^{n} e^{ta_j X_j}$$

$$E(e^{tY}) \qquad = \prod\limits_{j=1}^{n} E\left(e^{ta_j X_j}\right) \qquad \text{by independence}$$

$$= \prod\limits_{j=1}^{n} M_{X_j}(a_j t) \qquad \text{by definition.}$$

## SPECIAL DISTRIBUTIONS
### BINOMIAL DISTRIBUTION (Discrete)

A57. (a)   Probability Mass Function of the binomial distribution

$$f(x) = \binom{n}{x} p^x (1-p)^{n-x} \quad x = 0, 1, ..., n \quad 0 < p < 1$$

where

$$\binom{n}{x} = \dfrac{n!}{x!(n-x)!}$$

$$a! = a(a-1)...1$$

$$0! = 1$$

A58. (b)   Mean and Variance

$\mu = np$

$\sigma^2 = np(1-p)$

A59. (c)   Moment Generating Function

$$M_X(t) = \left\{pe^t + (1-p)\right\}^n$$

A60. (d)   How it arises in the real world.

If X is the number of observed failures, in a sample of n <u>independent</u> trials, each with probability of failure, p, then X has the Binomial Probability Mass Function above.

## POISSON DISTRIBUTION (Discrete)

A61. (a)   Probability Mass Function of the Poisson distribution.

$$f(x) = \frac{\lambda^x e^{-\lambda}}{x!} \qquad x = 0,1,2,\dots \qquad \lambda > 0$$

A62. (b)   Mean and Variance

$\mu = \lambda$

$\sigma^2 = \lambda$

A63. (c)   Moment Generating Function

$$M_X(t) = \exp\left\{\lambda(e^t - 1)\right\}$$

A64. (d)   How it arises in the real world.

### Approximation to Binomial

If in the binomial, n is large and p is small with $np = \lambda$, then the Poisson distribution will provide an excellent approximation to the binomial distribution.

More formally, if $n \to \infty$ and $p \to 0$ with $np \to \lambda > 0$

$$\binom{n}{x}p^x(1-p)^{n-x} \to \frac{\lambda^x e^{-\lambda}}{x!} \qquad x = 0,1,2,\dots$$

## UNIFORM DISTRIBUTION (Continuous)

A65. (a)     Probability Density Function of the uniform distribution.

$$f(x) = \frac{1}{B-A} \quad A < x < B$$

A66. (b)     Mean and Variance

$$\mu = (A+B)/2$$

$$\sigma^2 = (B-A)^2/12$$

A67. (c)     Moment Generating Function

$$M_X(t) = \frac{1}{\{(B-A)t\}} \left\{ e^{Bt} - e^{At} \right\}$$

A68. (d)     How it arises in the real world

Roundoff error

A69. (e)     Cumulative Distribution

$$F(x) = \frac{x-A}{B-A} \quad A < x < B$$

## EXPONENTIAL DISTRIBUTION (Continuous)

A70. (a)     Probability Density Function of the exponential distribution

$$f(x) = \lambda e^{-\lambda x} \quad x > 0$$

A71. (b)     Mean and Variance

$$\mu = (1/\lambda)$$

$$\sigma^2 = (1/\lambda)^2$$

A72. (c)     Moment Generating Function

$$M_X(t) = \frac{\lambda}{\lambda - t} \quad t < \lambda$$

A73. (d)   How it arises in the real world

- As survival time data - see (f) below

A74. (e)   Cumulative Distribution

$$F(x) = 1 - e^{-\lambda x} \qquad x > 0$$

A75. (f)   Memoriless Property (Constant Hazard)

Let $s > 0$ and $t > 0$ and let X have the exponential distribution.

$$P[X > t] = 1 - F(t) = e^{-\lambda t}$$

$$P[X > t + s | X > s] = \frac{P[X > t + s, \ X > s]}{P[X > s]}$$

$$= \frac{P[X > t + s]}{P[X > s]} = \frac{e^{-\lambda(t+s)}}{e^{-\lambda s}}$$

$$= e^{-\lambda t}$$

The exponential distribution would imply that an s-year old individual has the same outlook as a newborn, in terms of future life.

The "Hazard Rate" defined as

$$H(x) = \frac{f(x)}{1 - F(x)} \qquad x > 0$$

$$= \frac{\lambda e^{-\lambda x}}{e^{-\lambda x}} = \lambda$$

$H(x)dx$ is the instantaneous probability of failure between x and x+dx, given survival of at least x.

A76. Constant Hazard implies exponentiality, since if

$$\frac{f(x)}{1 - F(x)} = \lambda \qquad\qquad\qquad x > 0$$

$$\int_0^t \frac{f(x)dx}{1 - F(x)} = \lambda t$$

$$\log\left\{1 - F(0)\right\} - \log\left\{1 - F(t)\right\} = \lambda t$$

Now $F(0) = 0$ for a survival distribution, and hence

$$1 - F(t) = e^{-\lambda t}$$

## GAMMA DISTRIBUTION (Continuous)

A77. (a)   Probability Density of gamma distribution.

$$f(x) = \frac{\lambda^{\alpha} x^{\alpha-1} e^{-\lambda x}}{\Gamma(\alpha)} \qquad\qquad x > 0,\ \alpha > 0,\ \lambda > 0$$

$$\Gamma(\alpha) = \int_0^{\infty} x^{\alpha-1} e^{-x} dx$$

Note: if $\alpha$ is an integer, n

$$\Gamma(n) = (n-1)!$$

A78. (b)   Mean and Variance

$$\mu = (\alpha/\lambda)$$

$$\sigma^2 = (\alpha/\lambda^2)$$

A79. (c)   Moment Generating Function

$$M_X(t) = \left\{\lambda/(\lambda - t)\right\}^{\alpha} \qquad\qquad t < \lambda$$

A80. (d)   How it arises in the real world

- If $\alpha = 1$, note that we obtain the exponential distribution

- Let $X_1, X_2, \ldots, X_n$ be independent, identically distributed exponential random variables

with parameter $\lambda$.

Let $S = X_1 + X_2 + \cdots + X_n$

Then S has the Gamma Distribution with parameters $\alpha = n$ and $\lambda$.

Proof From A72 and A56, S has moment generating function

$$M_S(t) = M_{X_1}(t)\, M_{X_2}(t) \ldots M_{X_n}(t)$$

$$= \left\{\frac{\lambda}{(\lambda - t)}\right\}^n.$$

From the uniqueness property of Moment Generating Functions A53, and by A79, the result holds.

A81.     The "chi-square" Distributions are special Gamma Distributions with

$$\alpha = (\text{Degrees of Freedom})/2$$

$$\lambda = \tfrac{1}{2}$$

A82. (e)     Cumulative Distribution (Integer $\alpha$ only)

Let $\alpha = n$ (an integer)

$$F(x) = 1 - \sum_{j=0}^{n-1} \frac{(\lambda x)^j e^{-\lambda x}}{j!}$$

Proof Differentiation of both sides yields result. (See A21.).

Note: Clear cut connection between Poisson Distribution and Gamma Distribution.

## NORMAL DISTRIBUTION (Continuous)

A83. (a)     Probability Density of normal distribution

$$f(x) = \frac{1}{\sigma\sqrt{2\pi}} \exp\left\{-(x-\mu)^2/2\sigma^2\right\} \qquad\qquad -\infty < x < \infty$$

A84. (b)     Mean and Variance

We have so denoted the two parameters $\mu$ and $\sigma^2$ ($\pi = 3.1416$).

A85. (c)     Moment Generating Function

$$M_X(t) = \exp\left(\mu t + \tfrac{1}{2}\sigma^2 t^2\right)$$

A86. (d)    Cumulative Distribution

No closed form, but the usual notation is

$F(x) = \Phi\left(\frac{x-\mu}{\sigma}\right)$ with

$\Phi(t) = \int_{-\infty}^{t} \frac{1}{\sqrt{2\pi}} \exp(-t^2/2) dt$

$\Phi$ is called the "Standard Normal" cumulative distribution, often denoted by N(0,1).

A87. (e)    Difference of independent normal random variables is normal.

Let $X_1$, $X_2$, be independent normally disributed random variables with respective means $\mu_1$ and $\mu_2$ and respective variances $\sigma_1^2$ and $\sigma_2^2$. Then $(X_1 - X_2)$ is normal with mean $\mu_1$-$\mu_2$ and variance $\sigma_1^2 + \sigma_2^2$.

Proof:

$$E\left(e^{t(X_1-X_2)}\right) = E(e^{tX_1})E(e^{-tX_2}) \qquad\qquad \text{Independence}$$

$$= \exp\left(\mu_1 t + \tfrac{1}{2}\sigma_1^2 t^2\right) \exp\left(-\mu_2 t + \tfrac{1}{2}\sigma_2^2 t^2\right) \qquad \text{by (c)}$$

$$= \exp\left\{(\mu_1\text{-}\mu_2)t + \tfrac{1}{2}(\sigma_1^2+\sigma_2^2)t^2\right\}$$

$X_1$-$X_2$ has the moment generating function of a normal random variable with mean $(\mu_1$-$\mu_2)$ and variance $\sigma_1^2 + \sigma_1^2$. The result follows from A53.

A88 (f)    How it arises in the real world.

-The Central Limit Theorem

Let $X_1$, $X_2$, ..., $X_n$, be a sequence of independent, identically distributed random variables with mean $\mu$ and variance $\sigma^2$. Let $\bar{X}_n = (X_1 + \cdots + X_n)/n$. then

$$P\left[\sqrt{n}\ (\bar{X}_n - \mu)/\sigma < x\right] \to \Phi(x)$$

This result is proved for the special case where the moment generating function exists in A106.

## A89. TRANSFORMATIONS (CONTINUOUS VARIABLES) (Consequence)

Let $X = (X_1, ..., X_n)$ be a vector of continuous random variables with joint probability density

$$f_X(x_1, ..., x_n)$$

Let $Y = (Y_1, ..., Y_n)$ where $Y_j = g_j(X_1, ..., X_n)$ $j=1,2,...,n$ be a $1-1$ function of X. That is, no two different X vectors produce the same Y vector. Let $K = K(X)$ be the matrix function whose $i^{th}$ row, $j^{th}$ column is

$$K_{ij}(X) = \frac{\partial g_j}{\partial x_i}(X) \qquad 1 \le i \le n, \quad 1 \le j \le n$$

Then Y has joint density

$$f_Y(y_1, ..., y_n) = \frac{f_X(x_1, ..., x_n)}{|\det(K)|}$$

with

$$\det(K) = \text{Determinant}$$

$$|\ | = \text{Absolute value}$$

$$y_j = g_j(x_1, ..., x_n)$$

The reader is referred to Hogg and Craig (1978) for further details, but an example might be helpful.

## A90. Example

Let $X_1, X_2, ..., X_n$ be independent exponential random variables with common parameter $\lambda$.

$$f_X(x_1, ..., x_n) = \lambda^n \exp\left\{-\lambda(x_1 + \cdots + x_n)\right\} \qquad x_j > 0$$

Let

$$Y_1 = X_1$$

$$Y_2 = X_1 + X_2$$

$$Y_j = X_1 + \cdots + X_j$$

$$\vdots$$

$$Y_n = X_1 + \cdots + X_n$$

Note    $$X_1 = Y_1$$

$$X_2 = Y_2 - Y_1$$

$$X_3 = Y_3 - Y_2$$

$$\vdots$$

$$X_n = Y_n - Y_{n-1}$$

Hence, the value of the X's is uniquely determined by the Y's.

$$y_j = g_j(x_1, \ldots, x_n) = x_1 + \cdots + x_j$$

$$\frac{\partial g_j}{\partial x_i} = 1 \qquad\qquad i \le j$$

$$= 0 \qquad\qquad i > j$$

$$K = \begin{bmatrix} 1 & 0 & 0 & \cdots & 0 \\ 1 & 1 & 0 & \cdots & 0 \\ 1 & 1 & 1 & 0 & 0 \\ \vdots & \vdots & \vdots & \vdots & \vdots \\ 1 & \cdots & \cdots & \cdots & 1 \end{bmatrix}$$

$$\det(K) = 1$$

$$f_y(y_1, \ldots, y_n) = \lambda^n \exp\left\{-\lambda(x_1 + \cdots + x_n)\right\}$$

$$= \lambda^n \exp\left\{-\lambda y_n\right\}$$

Now the range of the y's is obtained from the range of x's as

$$0 < x_1 < x_1 + x_2 < x_1 + x_2 + x_3 \cdots$$

$$0 < y_1 < y_2 < \cdots < y_n < \infty.$$

CONVERGENCE

A91. <u>Limit of a Sequence</u> (Definition)

Let $A_1$, $A_2$, ..., $A_n$, ... be a sequence of constants. We say that $A_n$ converges to the constant A,

$(A_n \to A)$ if for every $\epsilon > 0$, there exists a number $N = N(\epsilon)$ such that whenever

$$n > N, \quad |A_n - A| < \epsilon.$$

In other words, you challenge me with a tiny number $\epsilon$. I find a large N such that

$$|A_n - A| < \epsilon \text{ for all } n > N.$$

This can be done for every $\epsilon > 0$.

Example:   $A_n = 1/n$                    $A = 0$

$N(\epsilon) = 1/\epsilon$

A92. <u>Convergence in Probability</u> (Definition)

Let $X_1$, $X_2$, ..., $X_n$... be a sequence of random variables. We say that $X_n$ converges in probability to the constant C

$$X_n \xrightarrow{P} C$$

If for every $\epsilon > 0$

$$P\left(|X_n - C| > \epsilon\right) \to 0 \text{ as } n \to \infty$$

In other words, regardless of what small "challenge number" $\epsilon$ you provide, the probability that $X_n$ is within $\epsilon$ of C goes to one.

A93. <u>Convergence in Distribution</u> (Definition)

Let $X_1$, $X_2$, ... be a sequence of random variables with respective cumulative distributions

$$F_1(x), F_2(x), ..., F_n(x), ...$$

We say that

$$F_n \to F \text{ in distribution}$$

if

$$F_n(x) \rightarrow F(x) \qquad \text{at every continuity point of x.}$$

This is denoted by $F_n \xrightarrow{D} F$ or $X_n \xrightarrow{D} F$.

**A94.** <u>Convergence in Distribution</u> (Consequence)

Let $X_1$, $X_2$, ... be a sequence of random variables with respective cumulative distributions

$F_1(x)$, $F_2(x)$, ... and respective Moment Generating Functions

$$M_1(t), M_2(t), \ldots$$

Suppose that

$$M_n(t) \rightarrow M(t)$$

in a neighborhood of t=0 and M(t) is the Moment Generating Function of F(x). Then $F_n \xrightarrow{D} F$.

The proof is beyond the intended scope of the book. Interested readers might refer to

Fraser (1976, pages 248 and 558-560.)

<u>Convergence in Probability</u> (Consequence)

**A95. (i)**    If        $X_n \xrightarrow{P} x$

and        $Y_n = cX_n$            c constant

Then        $Y_n \xrightarrow{P} cx$

**A96. (ii)**    If        $X_n \xrightarrow{P} x$

and        $Y_n \xrightarrow{P} 0$

then        $X_n Y_n \xrightarrow{P} 0$

**A97. (iii)**    If        $X_n \xrightarrow{P} x$            and    $x \neq 0$,

then        if $Y_n = 1/X_n$

$Y_n \xrightarrow{P} (1/x)$

A98. (iv)   If   $X_n \xrightarrow{P} x$   and g is continuous at x

then   $g(X_n) \xrightarrow{P} g(x)$

Proofs:

(i)   If $c = 0$, then $Y_n = 0 = cx$ for all n and the result is immediate

If $c \neq 0$

$$P\big[|Y_n - cx| > \epsilon\big] = P\Big[|X_n - x| > \frac{\epsilon}{|c|}\Big] \to 0 \quad \text{since } X_n \xrightarrow{P} x$$

That is, $Y_n \xrightarrow{P} cx$

(ii)   The event that $|X_n Y_n| < \epsilon$ contains the intersection of the events

$|X_n - x| < \epsilon$   (event $A_n$)

and   $|Y_n| < \frac{\epsilon}{|x| + \epsilon}$   (event $B_n$)

$\Big($Event $A_n$ implies that $|X_n| < |x| + \epsilon$ and hence $A_n$ and $B_n$ together imply $|X_n Y_n| < \epsilon.\Big)$

$\quad P(A_n B_n) \quad = P(A_n) - P(A_n \bar{B}_n)$

$\qquad\qquad\qquad \geq P(A_n) - P(\bar{B}_n)$

Now   $P(A_n) \to 1$   since $X_n \xrightarrow{P} x$

and   $P(\bar{B}_n) \to 0$   since $Y_n \xrightarrow{P} 0$.

Hence $P(A_n B_n) \to 1$.

$$P\big[|X_n Y_n| < \epsilon\big] \geq P\big(A_n B_n\big) \to 1 \text{ as } n \to \infty.$$

(iii)   This is an important special case of (iv).

(iv)   Given $\epsilon > 0$, there exists a $\delta > 0$ such that whenever $|y - x| < \delta$, $|g(y) - g(x)| < \epsilon$.

Above is the definition of continuity.

Therefore, the event that $|g(X_n) - g(x)| < \epsilon$ contains the event $A_n$, that $|X_n - x| < \delta$. But

$$P\big[A_n\big] = P\big[|X_n - x| < \delta\big] \to 1 \qquad \text{(Convergence in P)}$$

Convergence in Probability (Consequence)

Let $X_n \xrightarrow{P} x$ and $Y_n \xrightarrow{P} y$. Then

A99. (v) $X_n + Y_n \xrightarrow{P} x+y$

A100. (vi) $X_n - Y_n \xrightarrow{P} x-y$

A101. (vii) $X_n Y_n \xrightarrow{P} xy$

A102. (viii) $X_n / Y_n \xrightarrow{P} x/y$          if $y \neq 0$

**Proofs:**

(v)    The event that $|X_n + Y_n - x - y| < \epsilon$ contains the event that both $|X_n - x| < \frac{\epsilon}{2}$ and $|Y_n - y| < \frac{\epsilon}{2}$.

$$P\left[|X_n - x| < \tfrac{\epsilon}{2}, \ |Y_n - y| < \tfrac{\epsilon}{2}\right] = P\left[|X_n - x| < \tfrac{\epsilon}{2}\right] - P\left[|X_n - x| < \tfrac{\epsilon}{2}, \ |Y_n - y| \geq \tfrac{\epsilon}{2}\right]$$

$$\geq P\left[|X_n - x| < \tfrac{\epsilon}{2}\right] - P\left[|Y_n - y| \geq \tfrac{\epsilon}{2}\right] \to 1 - 0 = 1 \text{ as } n \to \infty.$$

i.e.,    $P\left[|X_n + Y_n - x - y| < \epsilon\right] \to 1$

(vi)    By (i), $-Y_n \xrightarrow{P} -y$. Apply (v) to get desired result.

(vii)   $X_n Y_n - xy = X_n(Y_n - y) + (X_n - x)y$

      Now by (ii),     $X_n(Y_n - y) \xrightarrow{P} 0$

      and by (i),      $(X_n - x)y \xrightarrow{P} 0$

      Hence, by (v)    $X_n Y_n - xy \xrightarrow{P} 0$

(viii)  By (iii)  $\frac{1}{Y_n} \xrightarrow{P} \frac{1}{y}$. Results hold by (vii) above.

A103.  Convergence in Probability (Consequence)

If  $\frac{A_n}{B_n} \xrightarrow{P} 1$

$\frac{C_n}{D_n} \xrightarrow{P} 1$

with  $A_n, B_n, C_n, D_n > 0$

then  $\frac{A_n + C_n}{B_n + D_n} \xrightarrow{P} 1$

Proof:  Let $\epsilon > 0$, $\delta > 0$. Then there exists $N_1 > 0$ and $N_2 > 0$,

$$n > N_1 \Rightarrow P\left[1 - \epsilon < \left(\frac{A_n}{B_n}\right) < 1 + \epsilon\right] > 1 - \frac{\delta}{2}$$

$$n > N_2 \Rightarrow P\left[1 - \epsilon < \left(\frac{C_n}{D_n}\right) < 1 + \epsilon\right] > 1 - \frac{\delta}{2}$$

$$n > \max(N_1, N_2) \Rightarrow P\left[B_n(1 - \epsilon) < A_n < B_n(1 + \epsilon)\right] > 1 - \frac{\delta}{2}$$
$$P\left[D_n(1 - \epsilon) < C_n < D_n(1 + \epsilon)\right] > 1 - \frac{\delta}{2}.$$

The event

$$1 - \epsilon < \frac{A_n + C_n}{B_n + D_n} < 1 + \epsilon$$

includes the intersection of the events

$$B_n(1 - \epsilon) < A_n < B_n(1 + \epsilon)$$

with  $D_n(1 - \epsilon) < C_n < D_n(1 + \epsilon)$  and hence

$$P\left[1 - \epsilon < \frac{A_n + C_n}{B_n + D_n} < 1 + \epsilon\right] > 1 - \delta.$$

Since $\epsilon$ and $\delta$ are arbitrary, the desired result holds.

A104.  Convergence in Distribution (Consequence)

Slutzky's Theorem

Let $X_1, X_2, \ldots$ be a sequence of random variables with cumulative distributions

$F_1$, $F_2$, ..., with $X_n \xrightarrow{D} F$.

Let $Y_n$ be a sequence of random variables with $Y_n \xrightarrow{P} 0$.

Then if $Z_n = X_n + Y_n$, and if we denote the cumulative distribution of $Z_n$ by $G_n$, then

$$Z_n \xrightarrow{D} F \qquad (G_n \xrightarrow{D} F)$$

Note: We shall prove the result under the mild restriction that $F(x)$ has "isolated

discontinuities." That is, at each point $x_0$ such that $F$ has a jump at $x_0$, there exists

an $h > 0$ such that $F$ is continuous in the intervals $(x_0 - h, x_0)$ and $(x_0, x_0 + h)$.

Continuous distributions and discrete distributions over the integers have this property.

[A discrete distribution over the rational numbers is pathological, and does not have this

property.]

Proof:   Let x be a continuity point of $F$ and let

$A_n$ be the event that $X_n \leq x - \delta$

$B_n$ be the event that $Y_n \leq \delta$

$C_n$ be the event that $X_n + Y_n \leq x$.

Since $C_n$ contains the intersection of $A_n$ and $B_n$

$$G_n(x) = P(C_n) \geq P(A_n B_n)$$

$$\geq P(A_n) - P(A_n \bar{B}_n)$$

$$\geq P(A_n) - P(\bar{B}_n)$$

$$G_n(x) \geq F_n(x - \delta) - P(Y_n > \delta) \tag{1}$$

Similarly, if      $A_n^*$ is the event that $X_n > x + \delta$

$B_n^*$ is the event that $Y_n > -\delta$

$C_n^*$ is the event that $X_n + Y_n > x$

$C_n^*$ contains the intersection of $A_n^*$ and $B_n^*$ and hence

$$1 - G_n(x) \geq 1 - F_n(x + \delta) - P(Y_n \leq -\delta)$$

i.e.,       $$G_n(x) \leq F_n(x + \delta) + P(Y_n \leq -\delta) \tag{2}$$

Combining (1) and (2) we have

$$F_n(x-\delta) - P(Y_n > \delta) \leq G_n(x) \leq F_n(x+\delta) + P(Y_n \leq -\delta). \qquad (3)$$

Since discontinuities are isolated, we can restrict our attention to $\delta < h$, where F is continuous in the interval $(x-h, x+h)$.

In (3), as $n \to \infty$ $\qquad F_n(x+\delta) \to F(x+\delta)$

$$F_n(x-\delta) \to F(x-\delta)$$

by convergence in distribution.

Also, $\qquad P(Y_n > \delta)$ and $P(Y_n \leq -\delta) \to 0$

since $\qquad Y_n \xrightarrow{P} 0$.

Hence: $\qquad \lim_{n \to \infty} \left\{ F_n(x-\delta) - P(Y_n > \delta) \right\} = F(x-\delta)$

and $\qquad \lim_{n \to \infty} \left\{ F_n(x+\delta) + P(Y_n \leq -\delta) \right\} = F(x+\delta)$.

Let $\epsilon > 0$ be arbitrary. Then there exists $N_1 = N_1(\epsilon, \delta)$ and $N_2 = N_2(\epsilon, \delta)$ such that whenever $n > N_1$

$$G_n(x) \geq F_n(x-\delta) - P(Y_n > \delta) > F(x-\delta) - \epsilon$$

and whenever $n > N_2$

$$G_n(x) \leq F_n(x+\delta) + P(Y_n \leq -\delta) < F(x+\delta) + \epsilon.$$

That is, whenever $n > \text{Max}(N_1, N_2)$

$$F(x-\delta) - \epsilon < G_n(x) < F(x+\delta) + \epsilon. \qquad (4)$$

Finally, from the continuity of F at x, there exists $\delta_0$ such that

$$|F(x) - F(y)| \leq \epsilon \qquad\qquad \text{whenever}$$

$$|x-y| < \delta_0.$$

From (4), we have whenever

$$n > \text{Max} \left\{ N_1(\epsilon, \delta_0), N_2(\epsilon, \delta_0) \right\}$$

$$F(x) - 2\epsilon < G_n(x) < F(x) + 2\epsilon.$$

Since $\epsilon$ is arbitrary, we conclude that

$$G_n(x) \to F(x) \qquad \text{as } n \to \infty.$$

This completes the proof.

A105. Slutzky's Theorem for Products (Consequence)

Let $X_n \xrightarrow{D} F$ and $Y_n \xrightarrow{P} 1$

then $Z_n = X_n Y_n \xrightarrow{D} F$

Note: We shall prove the result under the same isolated discontinuity assumption as the previous result.

Proof: It is clear that

$$X_n Y_n = X_n + X_n(Y_n\text{-}1)$$

If we can show

$$X_n(Y_n\text{-}1) \xrightarrow{P} 0$$

the desired result is immediate from the previous result.

Suppose we are challenged with two small number, $\delta$ and $\epsilon$.

First, since F is a proper distribution we can find a real number B such that both B and -B are continuity points of F and

$$F(B) - F(\text{-}B) > 1\text{-}\delta$$

Let $A_n$ be the event that $\text{-}B < X_n \le B$ and $B_n$ be the event that $|Y_n\text{-}1| < \epsilon/B$.

The event that $|X_n(Y_n\text{-}1)| < \epsilon$ contains the intersection of $A_n$ and $B_n$.

$$P(A_n B_n) = P(A_n) - P(A_n \bar{B}_n)$$

$$\ge P(A_n) - P(\bar{B}_n)$$

$$\ge F_n(B) - F_n(\text{-}B) - P(\bar{B}_n)$$

$$\to F(B) - F(\text{-}B) \quad \text{as } n \to \infty$$

$$> 1\text{-}\delta.$$

i.e., since we can make $\delta$ as close to zero as we wish, and since $|X_n(Y_n\text{-}1)| < \epsilon$ whenever $A_n B_n$ holds,

$$|X_n(Y_n\text{-}1)| \xrightarrow{P} 0.$$

This completes the proof.

A106. Central Limit Theorem for Independent, Identically Distributed Random Variables

Let $X_1, X_2, \ldots, X_n \cdots$ be independent, identically distributed random variables with mean $\mu$, variance $\sigma^2$, and moment generating function $M_X(t)$.

Then $Z_n = \dfrac{n^{\frac{1}{2}}(\bar{X}_n - \mu)}{\sigma} \xrightarrow{D} N(0,1)$ where $\bar{X}_n = \dfrac{(X_1 + \cdots + X_n)}{n}$ and $N(0,1)$ is the standard normal distribution.

Proof. It is seen from **A56 and A40** that $Z_n$ has moment generating function

$$M_{Z_n}(\theta) = \left[ M_X\!\left(\tfrac{\theta}{\sigma\sqrt{n}}\right) \right]^n \exp\!\left[\tfrac{-\sqrt{n}\,\mu\theta}{\sigma}\right].$$

We need to show (See **A94 and A85**) that

$$M_{Z_n}(\theta) \to e^{\theta^2/2} \qquad \text{in a neighborhood of } \theta = 0.$$

That is, we must show

$$K_n(\theta) = \log M_{Z_n}(\theta) \to \frac{\theta^2}{2} \qquad \text{in a neighborhood of } \theta = 0. \tag{0}$$

$$K_n(\theta) = n \log M_X\!\left(\tfrac{\theta}{\sigma\sqrt{n}}\right) - \frac{\sqrt{n}\,\mu\theta}{\sigma} \tag{1}$$

By Taylor's Theorem, there exists $\theta^*$: $|\theta^*| < |\theta|$

$$K_n(\theta) = K_n(0) + \theta K_n'(0) + \frac{\theta^2}{2} K_n''(0) + \frac{\theta^3}{6} K_n'''(\theta^*). \tag{2}$$

From (1), and the fact that $M_X(0) = E\!\left(e^{0 X_n}\right) = 1$, we see that $K_n(0) = 0$

$$K_n'(\theta) = \frac{\sqrt{n}}{\sigma} \frac{M_X'\{\theta/(\sigma\sqrt{n})\}}{M_X\{\theta/(\sigma\sqrt{n})\}} - \frac{\sqrt{n}\,\mu}{\sigma} \tag{3}$$

$$K_n''(\theta) = \frac{1}{\sigma^2}\left[\frac{M_X''\{\theta/(\sigma\sqrt{n})\}}{M_X\{\theta/(\sigma\sqrt{n})\}} - \frac{\left[M_X'\{\theta/(\sigma\sqrt{n})\}\right]^2}{\left[M_X\{\theta/(\sigma\sqrt{n})\}\right]^2}\right] \tag{4}$$

$$K_n'''(\theta) = \frac{1}{\sqrt{n}\sigma^3}\left[\frac{M_X'''\{\theta/(\sigma\sqrt{n})\}}{M_X\{\theta/(\sigma\sqrt{n})\}} - \frac{3M_X''\{\theta/(\sigma\sqrt{n})\}M_X'\{\theta/(\sigma\sqrt{n})\}}{\left[M_X\{\theta/(\sigma\sqrt{n})\}\right]^2}\right.$$

$$\left. + \frac{2\left[M_X'\{\theta/(\sigma\sqrt{n})\}\right]^3}{\left[M_X\{\theta/(\sigma\sqrt{n})\}\right]^3}\right] \tag{5}$$

$$K_n(0) = 0 \tag{6}$$

$$K_n'(0) = \frac{\sqrt{n}}{\sigma}\frac{M_X'(0)}{M_X(0)} - \frac{\sqrt{n}}{\sigma}\mu = 0 \tag{7}$$

$$K_n''(0) = \frac{1}{\sigma^2}\left[E(X_j^2) - \mu^2\right] = \frac{\sigma^2}{\sigma^2} = 1 \tag{8}$$

$$K_n'''(\theta^*) \to 0 \text{ as shown below.} \tag{9}$$

Let

$$L_n(y) = \frac{M_X'''(y)}{M_X(y)} - \frac{3M_X''(y)M_X'(y)}{\left[M_X(y)\right]^2} + \frac{2\left[M_X'(y)\right]^3}{\left[M_X(y)\right]^3}.$$

Now

$$K_n'''(\theta^*) = \frac{1}{\sqrt{n}\sigma^3}L_n\{\theta^*/(\sigma\sqrt{n})\}$$

and $L_n(y) \to E(X_j^3) - 3\mu E(X_j^2) + 2\mu^3$ as $y \to 0$, a finite quantity. Hence

$$\lim_{n\to\infty}K_n'''(\theta^*) = \lim_{n\to\infty}\left(\frac{1}{\sqrt{n}\sigma^3}\right)\lim_{n\to\infty}L_n\{\theta^*/(\sigma\sqrt{n})\} = 0. \tag{10}$$

From (2), (6), (7), (8) and (10) we have

$$K_n(\theta) \to \theta^2/2 \quad \text{as } n \to \infty.$$

This completes the proof, as the requirement of equation (0) has been met.

A107.   A Central Limit Theorem for Sums of Bernoulli Random Variables

Let $X_j$, $j = 1, 2, ..., n$ be independent Bernoulli Random Variables (i.e., Binomial with sample size 1) with mass function

$$\begin{aligned} f_j(x) \quad &= 1 - p_j \quad & x = 0 \\ &= p_j \quad & x = 1 \\[1em] &= 0 \quad & \text{elsewhere.} \end{aligned}$$

Let $b_j$, $j = 1, 2, ...$ be constants and

$$S_n = \sum_{j=1}^{n} b_j X_j$$

$$M_n = \sum_{j=1}^{n} b_j p_j$$

$$V_n^2 = \sum_{j=1}^{n} b_j^2 p_j (1 - p_j)$$

and

$$Z_n = \frac{S_n - M_n}{V_n}$$

Without loss of generality in what follows, the $b_j$, $p_j$ (and hence $X_j$) may be functions of n. We dropped the subscript n for ease of notation.

A107-1 Condition 1:

If $V_n \to \infty$

and

$$\frac{\sum_{j=1}^{n} |b_j|^3}{V_n^3} \to 0 \text{ as } n \to \infty.$$

then

$$Z_n \xrightarrow{D} N(0,1) \quad \text{(Standard Normal)}.$$

A107-2 Condition 2:

If the $b_j$ and $p_j$ are bounded:

$$p_j < p_0 < 1 \text{ and } |b_j| < B$$

and           $V_n \to \infty$

and if

$$\frac{\sum_{j=1}^{n} |b_j|^3 p_j}{V_n^3} \to 0 \quad \text{as } n \to \infty$$

then

$$Z_n \xrightarrow{D} N(0,1).$$

This is designed to cover cases where $p_j \to 0$.

**Proof.** Let

$$K_n(\theta) = \log E\left(e^{\theta Z_n}\right) \tag{0}$$

the log of the moment generating function of $Z_n$.

It is readily seen by independence that

$$K_n(\theta) = \sum_{j=1}^{n} \left\{ \log\left[ (1-p_j) + p_j e^{b_j \theta / V_n} \right] - \frac{b_j p_j \theta}{V_n} \right\} \tag{1}$$

To prove normality, we need to show that

$$K_n(\theta) \rightarrow \frac{\theta^2}{2} \quad \text{as } n \rightarrow \infty$$

in a neighborhood of $\theta = 0$.

By Taylor's Theorem, there exists a $\theta^*$ such that $|\theta^*| \leq |\theta|$ with

$$K_n(\theta) = K_n(0) + \theta K_n'(0) + \frac{\theta^2}{2}K_n''(0) + \frac{\theta^3}{6}K_n'''(\theta^*). \qquad (2)$$

$$K_n'(\theta) = \sum_{j=1}^{n} \frac{b_j p_j}{V_n} \left\{ \frac{1}{(1-p_j)e^{-b_j \theta/V_n} + p_j} - 1 \right\}. \qquad (3)$$

$$K_n''(\theta) = \sum_{j=1}^{n} \frac{b_j^2 p_j(1-p_j)}{V_n^2} \frac{e^{-b_j \theta/V_n}}{\left\{(1-p_j)e^{-b_j \theta/V_n} + p_j\right\}^2}. \qquad (4)$$

$$K_n'''(\theta) = 2\sum_{j=1}^{n} \frac{b_j^3 p_j(1-p_j)^2 e^{-2b_j \theta/V_n}}{V_n^3 \left\{(1-p_j)e^{-b_j \theta/V_n} + p_j\right\}^3} - \sum_{j=1}^{n} \frac{b_j^3 p_j(1-p_j)e^{-b_j \theta/V_n}}{V_n^3 \left\{(1-p_j)e^{-b_j \theta/V_n} + p_j\right\}^2}. \qquad (5)$$

Clearly, $K_n(0) = 0$ $\left(\text{Substitute } \theta = 0 \text{ in (1)}\right)$.

By substituting $\theta = 0$ in (3), we see that

$$(1 - p_j)e^{-b_j \theta/V_n} + p_j = (1 - p_j)e^0 + p_j$$
$$= 1.$$

Hence $\qquad\qquad K_n'(0) = 0.$

Similarly, from (4),

$$K_n''(0) = \sum_{j=1}^{n} \frac{b_j^2 p_j(1 - p_j)}{V_n^2} = \frac{V_n^2}{V_n^2} = 1.$$

To prove <u>Condition 1</u>, consider in (5)

$$\frac{p_j}{(1 - p_j)e^{-b_j\theta/V_n} + p_j} \le 1,$$

and

$$\frac{(1 - p_j)e^{-b_j\theta/V_n}}{(1 - p_j)e^{-b_j\theta/V_n} + p_j} \le 1.$$

Hence

$$|K_n'''(\theta)| < 3\,\frac{\Sigma|b_j|^3}{V_n^3} \tag{6}$$

Since the right hand side of (6) converges to zero, convergence to zero of $K_n'''(\theta)$ is assured.

From (2)

$$K_n(\theta) \to \frac{\theta^2}{2}$$

and hence

$$E\left(e^{\theta Z_n}\right) \to e^{\theta^2/2} \quad n\to\infty.$$

That is from **A94**,

$$Z_n \xrightarrow{D} N(0,1) \text{ under condition 1.}$$

For <u>Condition 2</u>, note that since $V_n \to \infty$ there exists for given $V_0 > 0$, a number N such that whenever

$$n > N, \quad V_n > V_0.$$

Now working with (5) we see

$$\frac{1}{(1 - p_j)e^{-b_j\theta/V_n} + p_j} \le \frac{1}{(1 - p_j)e^{-b_j\theta/V_n}} \le \frac{e^{|b_j\theta|/V_n}}{1 - p_j} \le \frac{e^{|B\theta|/V_0}}{1 - p_0} \quad n > N,$$

also

$$\frac{(1 - p_j)e^{-b_j\theta/V_n}}{(1 - p_j)e^{-b_j\theta/V_n} + p_j} \leq 1.$$

Hence for $n > N$, Condition 2 and (5) yield

$$|K_n'''(\theta)| < \frac{3e^{|B\theta|/V_0}}{1 - p_0}\left\{\frac{\sum_{j=1}^{n}|b_j|^3 p_j}{V_n^3}\right\} \qquad \text{for } n > N$$

$$\to 0.$$

Hence $\qquad K_n(\theta) \to \dfrac{\theta^2}{2}$

and hence $\qquad E\left(e^{\theta Z_n}\right) \to e^{\theta^2/2},$

and hence from A94,

$$Z_n \xrightarrow{D} N(0,1) \quad \text{under Condition 2.}$$

A107-EX    Example:

$$p_j = p_j(n) = \frac{1}{\sqrt{n}}$$

$$b_j = 1$$

$$V_n^2 = n\left(\frac{1}{\sqrt{n}}\right)\left(1 - \frac{1}{\sqrt{n}}\right) = \sqrt{n} - 1$$

$$b_j^3 = 1 \text{ and } \Sigma b_j^3 = n$$

$$\frac{\Sigma b_j^3}{V_n^3} = \frac{n}{\left\{\sqrt{n}-1\right\}^{\frac{3}{2}}} \sim n^{\frac{1}{4}} \quad \text{(Condition 1 fails, since this does not go to zero).}$$

$$\frac{\Sigma b_j^3 p_j}{V_n^3} = \frac{\sqrt{n}}{\left\{\sqrt{n-1}\right\}^{\frac{3}{2}}} \to 0 \quad \text{(Condition 2 succeeds)}.$$

**A108    Asymptotic Normality of a Difference**

Suppose $X_n$ and $Y_n$ are independent with

$$\frac{X_n - \mu_n}{\sigma_n} \overset{D}{\to} N(0, 1)$$

$$\frac{Y_n - \nu_n}{\lambda_n} \overset{D}{\to} N(0, 1)$$

$$\frac{\sigma_n}{\lambda_n} \to c$$

where $\mu_n$, $\nu_n$, $\sigma_n$, $\lambda_n$ are constants.

Then     $\dfrac{(X_n - Y_n) - (\mu_n - \nu_n)}{\sqrt{\sigma_n^2 + \lambda_n^2}} \overset{D}{\to} N(0, 1)$

Proof:

$$\frac{X_n - \mu_n}{\sqrt{\sigma_n^2 + \lambda_n^2}} = \frac{X_n - \mu_n}{\sigma_n \sqrt{\left(1 + \dfrac{\lambda_n^2}{\sigma_n^2}\right)}}.$$

Now since $\dfrac{\lambda_n^2}{\sigma_n^2} \to c^{-2}$,

Slutzky's Multiplicative Theorem **A105** implies

$$\frac{X_n - \mu_n}{\sqrt{\sigma_n^2 + \lambda_n^2}} \quad \text{and} \quad \frac{X_n - \mu_n}{\sigma_n \sqrt{1 + c^{-2}}}$$

have the same asymptotic distribution. That is

$$\frac{X_n - \mu_n}{\sqrt{\sigma_n^2 + \lambda_n^2}} \xrightarrow{D} N\left(0, \frac{1}{1+c^{-2}}\right).$$

Similarly,

$$\frac{Y_n - \nu_n}{\sqrt{\sigma_n^2 + \lambda_n^2}} = \frac{Y_n - \nu_n}{\lambda_n \sqrt{1 + \dfrac{\sigma_n^2}{\lambda_n^2}}} \xrightarrow{D} N\left(0, \frac{1}{1+c^2}\right)$$

From A87,

$$\frac{(X_n - Y_n) - (\mu_n - \nu_n)}{\sqrt{\sigma_n^2 + \lambda_n^2}} \xrightarrow{D} N\left(0, \frac{1}{1+c^2} + \frac{1}{1+c^{-2}}\right)$$

But

$$\frac{1}{1+c^2} + \frac{1}{1+c^{-2}} = \frac{1}{1+c^2} + \frac{c^2}{1+c^2} = 1$$

Therefore

$$\frac{(X_n - Y_n) - (\mu_n - \nu_n)}{\sqrt{\sigma_n^2 + \lambda_n^2}} \xrightarrow{D} N\left(0, 1\right)$$

A109.  Asymptotic Normality of a Difference

If in addition to the conditions of **A108**, we have consistent estimators

$$\frac{\hat{\sigma}_n}{\sigma_n} \xrightarrow{P} 1$$

$$\frac{\hat{\lambda}_n}{\lambda_n} \xrightarrow{P} 1$$

Then

$$\frac{(X_n\text{-}Y_n) - (\mu_n\text{-}\nu_n)}{\sqrt{\hat{\sigma}_n^2 + \hat{\lambda}_n^2}} \xrightarrow{D} N\left(0, 1\right)$$

Proof:  By **A98**,

$$\frac{\hat{\sigma}_n^2}{\sigma_n^2} \xrightarrow{P} 1$$

$$\frac{\hat{\lambda}_n^2}{\lambda_n^2} \xrightarrow{P} 1.$$

Hence by **A103**,

$$\frac{\hat{\sigma}_n^2 + \hat{\lambda}_n^2}{\sigma_n^2 + \lambda_n^2} \xrightarrow{P} 1.$$

Again using **A98**, this yields

$$\frac{\sqrt{\hat{\sigma}_n^2 + \hat{\lambda}_n^2}}{\sqrt{\sigma_n^2 + \lambda_n^2}} \xrightarrow{P} 1.$$

Finally, from **A108** snd Slutsky's Theorem (Products), **A105**, the desired result holds.

## STATISTICAL INFERENCE

A110 <u>Estimator of a Parameter</u> (Definition)

A random variable, whose observed value will estimate a parameter.

Example: The sample mean is an estimator of the population mean.

If the parameter is $\theta$, then the estimator is denoted by $\hat{\theta}$

A111 <u>Unbiased Estimator</u> (Definition)

$\hat{\theta}$ is "unbiased" for $\theta$ if $E(\hat{\theta}) = \theta$

A112 <u>Consistent Estimator(s)</u> (Definition)

Let $\hat{\theta}_1, \hat{\theta}_2, \ldots$ be a sequence of estimators of $\theta$. $\hat{\theta}_n$ is "consistent" for $\theta$ if

$$\hat{\theta}_n \xrightarrow{P} \theta.$$

(More formally, this is called "weakly consistent".)

A113 <u>Maximum Likelihood Estimator</u>

$\hat{\theta}$ is said to be the Maximum Likelihood Estimator of $\theta$ if the probability of the observed sample (discrete case) or joint density of the observed sample (continuous case) is maximized at $\theta = \hat{\theta}$.

This is a technique to obtain estimators of $\theta$. In many applications, they are consistent, asymptotically normal, with optimal asymptotic variance.

We shall not make use of these estimators directly, but we include the definition for the sake of completeness.

A114   <u>Confidence Interval</u> (Definition)

Consider two estimators $\hat{\theta}_L < \hat{\theta}_U$ such that the <u>pre-experiment</u> probability

$$P\left[\hat{\theta}_L < \theta < \hat{\theta}_U\right] = (1 - \alpha).$$

We say that

$$\left(\hat{\theta}_L, \hat{\theta}_U\right)$$

form a $100(1-\alpha)\%$ confidence interval for $\theta$.

After the data has been collected, probability no longer applies. $\hat{\theta}_L$, $\theta$, and $\hat{\theta}_U$ are simply three numbers. We do have $100(1-\alpha)\%$ confidence in our procedure to capture the true $\theta$. [The analogy is the following. Before playing a key ball game, Team A was believed to have a 90% chance of defeating team B. You might consider betting on the outcome. Even if you did not know the true result, but you did know that the game was over, you would not bet on the game.]

## HYPOTHESIS TESTING (*P*-values)

A115   <u>Null Hypothesis</u> (Definition)

A statement corresponding to an <u>unsuccessful</u> outcome of an experiment or study. This is generally expressed in terms of parameters. The objective of the study will be achieved if we can reject the null hypothesis in favor of the alternate hypothesis below. We denote this by $H_0$.

A116   <u>Alternate Hypothesis</u> (Definition)

A statement corresponding to a successful outcome of an experiment or study. We denote this by $H_A$.

A117    Example (i):

Suppose you wish to determine which of two therapies is better in terms of five year survival. Since it is inconceivable that the five year survival under each therapy is exactly equal, the goal of the study is to find out which is better. The null hypothesis would be that the five year survival of each therapy is exactly the same. The alternative hypothesis is that there is a difference.

$$H_0 : P_5 = Q_5 \quad \text{versus} \quad H_A : P_5 \neq Q_5$$

with $P_5$ and $Q_5$ the five year survival under treatment A and treatment B respectively. If you can conclude beyond a reasonable doubt that one of the treatments is superior to the other (reject $H_0$), your research question will have been answered. If you fail to reject $H_0$, you do not conclude that the treatments are equal in terms of five year survival, but rather, that the data are inconclusive.

This is called a two tailed test. The burden of evidence is always placed on rejecting $H_0$ in favor of $H_A$.

A118    Example (ii):

Suppose that you wish to determine if the addition of a drug to a "standard" treatment improves five year survival, over the standard treatment alone. You wish to place the burden of proof on showing that the addition of the drug has efficacy. In this situation, we have

$$H_0 : P_5 \leq Q_5 \quad \text{versus} \quad H_A : P_5 > Q_5$$

In such situations, if you cannot demonstrate beyond a reasonable doubt that $P_5$, the five year survival of the "experimental" therapy (standard plus drug) is greater than $Q_5$, the five year survival of the "control" therapy (standard alone), then the drug is considered unproven in terms of efficacy, over and above the standard.

This is called a <u>one tailed test</u>. The burden of proof is to show a difference in a specified direction.

Note: Some authors will write the one-tailed test as

$$H_0 : P_5 = Q_5 \text{ (instead of } H_0 : P_5 \leq Q_5) \quad \text{versus} \quad H_A : P_5 > Q_5$$

This is the most difficult situation among the candidates, where the more general $H_0$ is true, to distinguish $H_0$ from $H_A$. For example, it is harder to distinguish between hypotheses for situation (A) below than situation (B):

Situation (A):  $P_5 = Q_5 = .20$    versus    $P_5 = .20 \ Q_5 = .10$

Situation (B):  $P_5 = .10 \ Q_5 = .20$    versus    $P_5 = .20 \ Q_5 = .10$

**A119**   <u>Test Statistic</u> (Definition)

A quantity, calculated from the data, upon which the hypothesis test will be based. (The test statistic is simply the value of a random variable.)

**A120**   <u>P-Value</u> (Definition)

The maximum probability that in a replication of the study where the <u>null hypothesis is true</u>, that the test statistic would be at <u>least as "extreme"</u> as the observed test statistic (from the actual study.)

**A121**   <u>Two-Tailed Example</u> :

Suppose you wanted to determine which of two candidates is preferred. We might sample N = 400 individuals and assume that p = true proportion favoring A and 1-p = true proportion favoring B. Our hypotheses are

$$H_0 : p = .50 \quad \text{versus} \quad H_A ; p \neq .50$$

The test statistic generally used is

$$Z = 2\sqrt{n}(\hat{p} - .50)$$

where $\hat{p}$ is the fraction of the sample favoring A.

"Extreme" values for Z simply means large absolute values, since the larger $|Z|$ is, the stronger the evidence against $H_0$.

Under $H_0$, Z has an approximate standard normal distribution (see A107).

If for example, $\quad \hat{p} = \frac{176}{400} = .440$,

$$Z = -2.40.$$

The p-value, as obtained from Figure 7, is $p = .018$. This provides strong evidence against $H_0$, and in favor of Candidate B.

A122    One-Tailed Example:

Via a randomized trial, a drug company wishes to show that their experimental agent combination can place a higher proportion of relapsed acute lymphocytic leukemia patients into remission than can the standard agent combination. If $P_E$ and $P_S$ are the experimental and standard remission rates respectively, we wish to test

$$H_0 : P_E \leq P_S \quad \text{versus} \quad H_A : P_E > P_S.$$

The test statistic used will be

$$Z = \frac{\hat{P}_E - \hat{P}_S}{\sqrt{\left\{\frac{\hat{P}_E(1-\hat{P}_E)}{N_E} + \frac{\hat{P}_S(1-\hat{P}_S)}{N_S}\right\}}}$$

where $\hat{P}_E$ and $\hat{P}_S$ are the fraction of patients achieving a remission on the experimental and standard agents respectively, and $N_E$ and $N_S$ are the corresponding sample sizes.

It is readily shown from results taken in our Appendix A107, A108, and A109, that if $P_E = P_S$, the hardest case in $H_0$ to distinguish from $H_A$, then Z is asymptotically standard normal.

Suppose that the observed value of Z is

$$Z = 0.37.$$

From Figure 6, this yields a p-value of $P = 0.36$. This value is certainly in the reasonable doubt range, and hence, we cannot reject $H_0$ in favor of $H_A$.

The study should be viewed as <u>inconclusive</u> as far as whether or not the experimental combination is superior.


A123    <u>Standard Reasonable Doubt Thresholds</u>:

The most widely used standard of doubt is a p-value of $P = .05$. In many fields, values below .05 are considered to be conclusive while values above are considered inconclusive.

Other than standardization, there is no logical basis for the 5% figure.


A124    <u>Planning a Study</u> (Sample Size Determination)

In planning a study, there are several ingredients needed in order to evaluate the sample size.

These include        - Null Hypothesis

- Alternative Hypothesis

- Test Statistic


A125            - "Type I Error." ($\alpha$) Threshold p-value where you consider the dividing line
                between reasonable doubt and beyond reasonable doubt lies.) (This is usually
                denoted by $\alpha$.)

A126      - "Planning Parameters." Under the alternate hypothesis, specify the parameters so that distributional properties of the test statistic can be evaluated. Generally, this involves specifying the smallest detectable difference of interest to the investigators, and other quantities such as accrual rate, "nuisance" parameters, and minimum follow-up time.

A127      - "Type II Error."$(\beta)$ Specify the probability of failing to reject the null hypothesis, when the planning parameters represent the true target population conditions. (This is usually denoted by $\beta$.)

A128      - "Power" = 1 - Type II Error = probability of rejecting the null hypothesis when the planning parameters represent the true target population conditions. (This is usually denote by $\prod$.)

A129.    The most common situation is the following: We shall show this as one-sided.

$$H_0: \theta = \theta_0 \text{ (or } H_0 : \theta \leq \theta_0) \quad\quad \text{versus} \quad\quad H_A : \theta > \theta_0$$

$$\text{Test Statistic: } Z = \frac{\hat{\theta} - \theta_0}{SE}$$

with SE = "Standard Error" of $\hat{\theta}$, (estimated standard deviation of $\hat{\theta}$), calculated from the data and $Z \sim N(0,1)$ approximately, when $H_0$ is true.

To plan a study, enough information must be supplied to obtain an approximate distribution of Z under $H_A$.

This may involve specification of nuisance parameters.

For example, suppose that the planner of the acute lymphocytic leukemia study had come to you prior to conducting the study saying $\Big(\text{see Chapter 2, Section 2.1.1}\Big)$

"The study needs to be sensitive to a 10% difference. Type I Error should be $\alpha =$

.05 and Type II Error should be $\beta = .20$.  I want equal sample sizes in each group."

$$H_0 : P_E - P_S = 0 \quad \text{versus} \quad H_A : P_E - P_S = .10$$

Test Statistic:

$$Z = \frac{\hat{P}_E - \hat{P}_S}{\sqrt{\left\{ \frac{\hat{P}_E(1-\hat{P}_E)}{N_E} + \frac{\hat{P}_S(1-\hat{P}_S)}{N_S} \right\}}}$$

where     $N = N_E + N_S =$ Total Sample Size

$N_E =$ Number assigned to Experimental Therapy

$N_S =$ Number assigned to Standard Therapy.

Z is approximately standard normal under $H_0$, but the approximate distribution of Z under $H_A$ depends heavily on the actual values of $P_E$ and $P_S$, not just the difference.  The planner needs to provide values for both $P_E$ and $P_S$ under $H_A$ to compute the sample size.

"Jumping ahead" somewhat, the required sample size in each group is: $\left( \text{See formal derivation} \right.$ in A132$\left. \right)$.

$$N_E = N_S = 617.5 \left\{ P_E(1-P_E) + P_S(1-P_S) \right\}$$

$$= 56 \quad P_S = 0, P_E = .1 \quad \text{(lowest possible value)}$$

$$= 306 \quad P_S = .45, P_E = .55 \quad \text{(highest possible value)}$$

It is much easier to distinguish 0 from 10% than it is to distinguish 45% from 55%.

A130   Sample Size Determination

The following derivation has not been developed in any text, yet is the basic background to nearly every sample size derivation. The ideas will look peculiar at first glance, but will make perfect sense once some examples are considered.

Consider the hypothesis:

$$H_0 : \theta = \theta_0 \quad \text{versus} \quad H_A : \theta = \theta_1 > \theta_0.$$

Let us set a Type I Error $\alpha$ and Power $(1-\beta)$ (Type II Error $\beta$). Suppose that $\alpha + \beta < 1$.

Let us assume that we have statistics $\hat{\theta}$ and SE such that SE $> 0$,

(a)   $\quad P\left[\dfrac{\hat{\theta} - \theta_0}{SE} > Z_\alpha\right] \simeq \alpha$ under $H_0$

and

(b)   $\quad P\left[\dfrac{\hat{\theta} - \theta_1}{SE} - \dfrac{(Z_\alpha + Z_\beta)(SE - S)}{SE} > -Z_\beta\right] \simeq 1 - \beta$ under $H_A$,

with S, a function of the parameters of the distribution under $H_A$ satisfying the implicit sample size equation:

$$S = \frac{\theta_1 - \theta_0}{Z_\alpha + Z_\beta} \qquad\qquad (1). \text{ [KEY EQUATION]}$$

($Z_\alpha$ and $Z_\beta$ are generally the upper $(100\alpha)\%$ and $(100\beta)\%$ points of the standard normal distribution, but this derivation holds in general.)

Then

$$P\left[\frac{\hat{\theta} - \theta_0}{SE} > Z_\alpha\right] \simeq 1-\beta \text{ under } H_A.$$

That is, if S is given as per the (1) [key equation], then the rejection region

$$\hat{\theta} > \theta_0 + Z_\alpha SE$$

has approximate Type I Error $\alpha$ and Power $1 - \beta$.

Proof:

This is simply a straight forward substitution for S in (b):

$$(1-\beta) \simeq P\left[\frac{\hat{\theta} - \theta_1}{SE} - \frac{(Z_\alpha + Z_\beta)(SE - S)}{SE} > -Z_\beta\right] \qquad (\text{under } H_A)$$

$$= P\left[\frac{\hat{\theta} - \theta_1 + (Z_\alpha + Z_\beta)S}{SE} - (Z_\alpha + Z_\beta) > -Z_\beta\right]$$

$$= P\left[\frac{\hat{\theta} - \theta_1 + (\theta_1 - \theta_0)}{SE} > Z_\alpha\right] \qquad (Z_\alpha + Z_\beta)S = \theta_1 - \theta_0$$

$$= P\left[\frac{\hat{\theta} - \theta_0}{SE} > Z_\alpha\right] \qquad (\text{under } H_A)$$

That is, the Type I and Power requirements are approximately met when equation (1) holds.

Note:  S is the asymptotic standard deviation of the statistic under $H_A$, and may contain nuisance parameters.  [SE usually has the same form as S, except population values under $H_A$ (from S) are replaced by consistent estimators to obtain SE.]

A131   Extension to the two-sided test

For the two-sided test, we can replace $\alpha$ by $\alpha/2$ can utilize the equation

$$S = \frac{|\theta_1 - \theta_0|}{Z_{\alpha/2} + Z_\beta}$$

This implies two calculations, one for each alternative

$$H_A : \theta = \theta_1 = \theta_0 + \Delta \quad (\Delta > 0) \quad \text{and} \quad H_A : \theta = \theta_1 = \theta_0 - \Delta \quad (\Delta > 0)$$

The larger resulting sample size would be used.

A132    Example 1:  Two Sample Independent Binomial with Equal Sample Sizes

The following notation will be used:

|  | Treatment 1 | Treatment 2 |
|---|---|---|
| Failure Rate | Q | T |
| Sample Size | N | N |
| Failures in Sample | F | G |
| Estimated Failure Rate | $\hat{Q} = F/N$ | $\hat{T} = G/N$ |

$\theta = Q - T$

$H_0 : \theta = 0$

$H_A : \theta = \theta_1 > 0$

$\hat{\theta} = \hat{Q} - \hat{T}$

$$SE = \sqrt{\frac{\hat{Q}(1-\hat{Q})}{N} + \frac{\hat{T}(1-\hat{T})}{N}}$$

$$S = \sqrt{\frac{Q(1-Q)}{N} + \frac{T(1-T)}{N}}$$

For large N, we know

(i)    $\dfrac{\hat{\theta} - 0}{SE} \to N(0,1)$              under $H_0$

(ii)   $\dfrac{S}{SE} \xrightarrow{P} 1$              under $H_A$

(iii)  $\dfrac{\hat{\theta} - \theta_1}{SE} \to N(0,1)$              under $H_A$

The approximation (a) of **A130** follows from (i), while from (ii), (iii) and Slutsky's theorem (A104), we have the approximation (b) of **A130**.

To obtain the sample size, we use

$$S = \frac{\theta_1 - \theta_0}{Z_\alpha + Z_\beta}.$$

Squaring both sides yields

$$\frac{Q(1-Q)}{N} + \frac{T(1-T)}{N} = \frac{(\theta_1 - \theta_0)^2}{(Z_\alpha+Z_\beta)^2} = \frac{(Q-T)^2}{(Z_\alpha+Z_\beta)^2}$$

That is, <u>each</u> sample size must be

A133
$$N = \frac{\left[Q(1-Q)+T(1-T)\right](Z_\alpha+Z_\beta)^2}{(Q-T)^2}$$

The two-tailed version of this formula appears in Pocock 1983, page 125.

A134    Example 2:

Let $Q = .7$ $T = .5$ in example 1, with $\alpha = .05$ and $\beta = .20$ (80% power), then

$$N = \frac{\left[.21 + .25\right](1.645 + .84)^2}{(.2)^2} = 71 \qquad \text{(each treatment)}$$

How good are these approximations? The exact binomial probability that the left hand term in assumption (a) exceeds 1.645 is 5.2% under $H_0$ (common $Q = T = .7$), while the exact binomial probability that the left hand term in assumption (b) exceeds -.84 is exactly 79.5% under $H_A$. These are very close to the asymptotic values of 5% and 80% respectively. For an exact approach to the two sample binomial problem see Suissa and Shuster (1985).

In the binomial example, we used a standard error valid under $H_0$ and $H_A$. We did not pool the proportions in the calculation.

A135  Summary of Sufficient Conditions to Apply the Sample Size Methodology

(1)    $\dfrac{(\hat{\theta} - \theta)}{SE}$    is asymptotically normal under $H_0$, $\theta = \theta_0$.

(2)    $\dfrac{(\hat{\theta} - \theta)}{SE}$    is asymptotically normal under $H_A$, $\theta = \theta_1$.

(3)    $\dfrac{S}{SE} \xrightarrow{P} 1$    under $H_A$.

(4)    SE    is calculated from the data.

(5)    S    is calculated from the parameters under $H_A$.

Note:  This methodology will be employed to derive the sample size requirements for clinical trials, analyzed via censored survival analysis.

## A136. THE POISSON PROCESS

## INTRODUCTION

The Poisson Arrival Process is a logical model for patient accrual. The arrival rate (accrual rate), A, represents the expected number of patients to be accrued per unit time. The number of patients accrued in t units of time has a Poisson Distribution, with mean (At). Finally, conditional on the accrual of exactly n patients to time t, the n accrual times are uniformly distributed over the interval from 0 to t.

This will be an appropriate model for the accrual process of many clinical trials. First, there is a time scale, denoted by t. The Poisson process is simply a count $N(t)$ of the number of patient entries up to time t.

Let us assume that we have a very large population of K patients. Assume that for a small interval of time of length $\Delta t$ that the number of entries is binomial with sample size K and probability of incidence of disease

$$\frac{A\Delta t}{K}.$$

That is, the expected number of entries is $A\Delta t$, which is proportional to the length of $\Delta t$.

A137    <u>A is called the arrival rate or accrual rate</u>

We shall further assume that the number of entries in non-overlapping intervals are independent events. This may seem artificial, but is generally a reasonable assumption. The number of patients who develop the disease and leave the population will be a negligible fraction of K. The net effect of other departures and arrivals will also generally be a negligible fraction of K.

## PLAN OF DERIVATION OF PROPERTIES

A138    (1) Divide the time scale from 0 to t into M intervals

$$0, \Delta t, 2\Delta t, ..., M\Delta t = T \quad M = T/\Delta t.$$

A139    (2) Prove that as $K \rightarrow \infty$ and $\Delta t \rightarrow 0$ the probability that every interval has no more than one arrival goes to one. Hence, we can consider (in the limit) that each interval will have either 0 or 1 arrival.

A140    (3) Prove that as $K \rightarrow \infty$ and $\Delta t \rightarrow 0$

$$P\left[N(t) = x\right] \rightarrow (At)^{x} e^{-At}/x! \quad x = 0, 1, ...$$

that is, N(t) is Poisson with mean At.

A141     (4) Prove that the waiting time between arrivals is exponential with parameter A.

A142     (5) Suppose we have a Poisson Process (with arrival rate A) where arrivals are assigned by independent flips of a fair coin to treatment 1 and treatment 2. Then the two processes $N_1(t)$, the number of patients assigned to Treatment 1 by time t and $N_2(t)$, the number of patients assigned to Treatment 2 by time t are independent Poisson Processes with common arrival rates A/2.

A143     (6) In a Poisson process, given that r entries occur by time t, the entry times are uniformly distributed over the time interval from zero to t.

Proofs:

    Prior to proving the results, two lemmas will be derived for later use.

A144     <u>Lemma A:</u>

    Let $0 < |y| < 1$. Then there exists $z : |z| \le |y|$ and $\log(1+y) = y - \dfrac{y^2}{2(1+z)^2}$

Proof:     This is simply Taylor's Theorem applied to the second derivative

$$f(y) = \log(1+y) \qquad\qquad\qquad f(0) = 0$$

$$f'(y) = \tfrac{1}{1+y} \qquad\qquad\qquad f'(0) = 1$$

$$f''(y) = \frac{-1}{(1+y)^2}$$

    Taylor's theorem states that there exists a $z : |z| \le |y|$ with
$$f(y) = f(0) + yf'(0) + \frac{y^2}{2}f''(z)$$

A145    <u>Lemma B:</u>

Let $A_n \to \infty$ and $B_n \to \infty$ with $\dfrac{A_n}{B_n} \to 1$ as $n \to \infty$

$$W_n = \left(1 + \frac{x}{B_n}\right)^{A_n} \to e^x \text{ as } n \to \infty.$$

**Proof:**   Since $B_n \to \infty$, there exists N such that whenever $n > N$, $|x/B_n| < \frac{1}{2}$. We shall work exclusively with $n > N$ so that logs are defined, and $x/B_n$ is bounded away from -1.

Let $Y_n = \log W_n = A_n \log(1 + \frac{x}{B_n})$.

From Lemma A (A144), there exists $z_n : |z_n| \le |x/B_n|$

$$Y_n = \frac{A_n x}{B_n} - \frac{A_n x^2}{2B_n^2(1+z_n)^2}. \qquad\qquad (*)$$

$$\frac{A_n x}{B_n} \to x \quad \text{ since } A_n/B_n \to 1$$

We show that second term of $(*)$ goes to zero.

Recall that $B_n \to \infty$ and $A_n/B_n \to 1$.   Hence

$$0 < \frac{A_n x^2}{B_n^2(1+z_n)^2} \le \frac{4}{B_n}\left(\frac{A_n}{B_n}\right) x^2 \to 0,$$

which implies

$$\frac{A_n x^2}{2B_n^2(1+z_n)^2} \to 0.$$

That is,

$$Y_n = \log(W_n) \to x.$$

That is        $W_n = e^{Y_n} \to e^x$.

We now return to the major derivation of results.

Proofs: (Main results)

First, we shall prove (2), that in the limit, multiple entries in any interval become impossible.

For a given interval, the probability of zero or one entry is obtained from the binomial distribution as

$$C = \left(1 - \frac{A\Delta t}{K}\right)^K + \frac{KA\Delta t}{K}\left(1 - \frac{A\Delta t}{K}\right)^{K-1} \qquad \text{(See A136)}$$

$$= \left(1 - \frac{A\Delta t}{K}\right)^{K-1}\left\{1 - \frac{A\Delta t}{K} + \frac{KA\Delta t}{K}\right\}$$

$$= \left(1 - \frac{A\Delta t}{K}\right)^{K-1}\left\{1 + \left(\frac{K-1}{K}\right)A\Delta t\right\}.$$

By independence, the probability of 0 or 1 entry in all M intervals is

$$C^M = \left(1 - \frac{A\Delta t}{K}\right)^{M(K-1)}\left\{1 + \left(\frac{K-1}{K}\right)A\Delta t\right\}^M.$$

Now $\Delta t = T/M$ and hence

$$C^M = \left(1 - \frac{AT}{MK}\right)^{M(K-1)}\left\{1 + \frac{(K-1)}{KM}AT\right\}^M$$

We apply Lemma B to each term

$$\left(1 - \frac{AT}{KM}\right)^{M(K-1)} \rightarrow e^{-AT}$$

Since M(K-1) and MK $\to \infty$ with $\dfrac{M(K-1)}{MK} \to 1$.

Also

$$\left\{1 + \frac{(K-1)AT}{KM}\right\}^M \to e^{AT}$$

since $M \to \infty$, $\dfrac{KM}{(K-1)} \to \infty$ with $\dfrac{M(K-1)}{KM} \to 1$.

That is, $C^M \to e^{-AT}e^{AT} = 1$. Thus (2) holds.

In the limit, we can ignore the possibility of multiple arrivals. This will help prove (3).

The probability of zero and one arrivals respectively in a single interval are

$$P_0 = \left(1 - \frac{A\Delta t}{K}\right)^K \text{ and } P_1 = A\Delta t\left(1 - \frac{A\Delta t}{K}\right)^{K-1}.$$

The probability of r arrivals to time t is simply binomial

$$D_r = \binom{M}{r}P_0^{M-r}P_1^r$$

$$= \binom{M}{r}\left(1 - \frac{A\Delta t}{K}\right)^{K(M-r)}(A\Delta t)^r\left(1 - \frac{A\Delta t}{K}\right)^{(K-1)r}$$

$$= \binom{M}{r}\left(1 - \frac{AT}{MK}\right)^{MK-r}\left(\frac{AT}{M}\right)^r \qquad\qquad (\Delta t = T/M)$$

$$= \left[\frac{M(M-1)(M-2)\cdots(M-r+1)}{M^r}\right]\frac{(At)^r}{r!}\left[1 - \frac{AT}{MK}\right]^{MK-r}. \qquad (**)$$

Now as $M \to \infty$, $K \to \infty$

$$\frac{M(M-1)\cdots(M-r+1)}{M^r} \to 1$$

and by Lemma B, and the fact that MK$\to\infty$ implies MK-r $\to\infty$ with (MK-r)/MK$\to$1,

$$\left[1 - \frac{AT}{MK}\right]^{MK-r} \to e^{-AT}.$$

That is, substituting in (**) the probability of r arrivals to time t,

$$D_r \to \frac{(AT)^r e^{-AT}}{r!}$$

This completes the proof of (3).

To prove (4), let us first look at the first arrival and show the time is exponential.

In order to have an arrival before time t, we must have $N(t) \geq 1$, that is, at least one arrival prior to time t.

$$
\begin{aligned}
P(\text{Arrival prior to time t}) &= P\Big((N(t) \geq 1\Big) \\
&= 1 - P\Big(N(t) = 0\Big) \\
&= 1 - (AT)^0 e^{-AT}/0! \\
&= 1 - e^{-At}
\end{aligned}
$$

The cumulative distribution of $T_1$, the time to the first arrival satisfies (see A74)

$$P\left[T_1 < t\right] = 1 - e^{-At} \qquad \text{(exponential)}$$

Now let $T_r$ be the time of the $r^{th}$ arrival. From the independent interval binomial construction, the number of arrivals in the next t units of time, given $T_r$ is Poisson with parameter At. $\left(T_{r+1} - T_r \text{ is the time between the } r^{th} \text{ and } (r+1)^{th} \text{ arrival.}\right)$

Hence

$$P\left(T_{r+1} - T_r < t | T_r\right) = P(\text{at least one arrival in t units of time})$$

$$= 1 - P(\text{no arrivals in t units of time})$$

$$= 1 - e^{At} \qquad \text{(exponential)}$$

This does not depend on $T_r$.

Hence, successive arrival times are independent identically distributed exponential random variables with parameter A.

To prove (5), it is clear from the structure discussed in **A136 - A138** that each of $N_1(t)$ and $N_2(t)$ is a Poisson Process with accrual rate $(A/2)$. Further, the number of arrivals in a given interval to Treatment 1 and number of arrivals to a second interval (mutually exclusive of the first) are mutually independent events, since the overall process

$$N(t) = N_1(t) + N_2(t)$$

is constructed that way.

To complete the proofs, we need to show the somewhat surprising result that $X_1$, the number of patients assigned to Treatment 1 in a given interval is statistically independent of $X_2$, the number of patients assigned to Treatment 2 in the same interval.

Assuming the interval is of length $t_1$

$$P\big[X_1 = x_1, X_2 = x_2\big] = \frac{(At)^{x_1+x_2} e^{-At}}{(x_1+x_2)!} \binom{x_1+x_2}{x_1} (.5)^{x_1+x_2}$$

$$= \left[\frac{(At/2)^{x_1} e^{-At/2}}{x_1!}\right]\left[\frac{(At/2)^{x_2} e^{-At/2}}{x_2!}\right]$$

$$= P\big[X_1 = x_2\big]P\big[X_2 = x_2\big]$$

Hence $X_1$ and $X_2$ are independent as required.

**Proof of (6)**

Since successive arrival times are independent, identically distributed, exponential random variables, the joint distribution of the successive times between arrivals of the first (r+1) patients is

$$f(x_1, \ldots, x_{r+1}) = \prod_{j=1}^{r+1} \left( Ae^{-Ax_j} \right) \qquad \text{(exponential densities)}$$

$$= A^{r+1} e^{-A\sum_{j=1}^{r+1} x_j} \qquad x_1 > 0, \; x_2 > 0, \ldots$$

Note that this is only a function of

$$T_{r+1} = \sum_{j=1}^{r+1} x_j \text{ the total elapsed time until the } (r+1)^{st} \text{ arrival.}$$

Now we make a transformation (1-1)

$$T_1 = x_1$$
$$T_2 = x_1 + x_2$$
$$\vdots$$
$$T_r = x_1 + \cdots + x_r$$
$$T_{r+1} = (x_1 + x_2 + \cdots + x_{r+1}).$$

Since the Jacobian (see **A89** and **A90**), is unity,

the joint distribution of

$T_1, \ldots, T_{r+1}$ is

$$g(T_1, \ldots, T_{r+1}) = A^{r+1} e^{-AT_{r+1}} \qquad 0 < T_1 < T_2 < \cdots < T_{r+1}.$$

Let U be the event that exactly r arrivals have occurred by time t.

The conditional density of $(T_1, \ldots, T_r)$ given U is

$$g(T_1, \ldots, T_r | U) = \frac{\int_t^\infty g(T_1, \ldots, T_{r+1}) dT_{r+1}}{P(U)}.$$

Once the $T_1, \ldots, T_r$ with $T_r < t$ are fixed, U occurs only if $T_{r+1} > t$.

$$P(U) = P(\text{Exactly r arrivals to time t})$$

$$= \frac{(At)^r e^{-At}}{r!} \qquad \text{(Poisson Process)}.$$

$$\int_t^\infty g(T_1, \ldots, T_{r+1}) dT_{r+1} = A^{r+1} \int_t^\infty e^{-AT_{r+1}} dT_{r+1}$$

$$= A^r e^{-At}$$

Hence, the conditional density of $T_1, \ldots, T_r$ given U is

$$g(T_1, \ldots, T_r|U) = r! t^r \qquad 0 < T_1 < \cdots < T_r < t$$

That is, the ordered arrival times are uniformly distributed from zero to t. (This conditional density does not depend on the values of the T's provided they are ordered as above.)

This completes the discussion of the Poisson Process.

## REFERENCES

1. **Fraser, D. A. S.**, *Probability and Statistics: Theory and Applications*, Duxbury Press, Boston, 1976.

2. **Hogg, R. V. and Craig, A. T.**, *Introduction to Mathematical Statistics*, Macmillan, New York, 1978.

3. **Mendenhall, W., Scheaffer, R. L., and Wackerly, D. D.**, *Mathematical Statistics with Applications*, Duxbury Press, Boston, 1986.

4. **Mood, A. M., Graybill, F. A., and Boes, D. C.**, *Introduction to the Theory of Statistics*, McGraw-Hill, New York, 1974.

5. **Suissa, S. and Shuster, J. J.**, Exact unconditional sample sizes for the 2 × 2 binomial trial, *J. R. Statist. Soc., Ser. A*, 148, 315, 1985.

# APPENDIX II

## TABLE OF CONTENTS

## TABLE 1: ALPHA= 0.005 POWER= 0.8    EXPECTED ACCRUAL THRU MINIMUM FOLLOW-UP= 30

| | | DEL=.10 | | | DEL=.15 | | | DEL=.20 | | | DEL=.25 | | | DEL=.30 | | |
|---|---|---|---|---|---|---|---|---|---|---|---|---|---|---|---|---|
| FACT= | | 1.0 .75 | .50 .25 | .00 BIN | 1.0 .75 | .50 .25 | .00 BIN | 1.0 .75 | .50 .25 | .00 BIN | 1.0 75 | .50 .25 | .00 BIN | 1.0 .75 | .50 .25 | .00 BIN |
| PCONT=*** | | | | | REQUIRED NUMBER OF PATIENTS | | | | | | | | | | | |
| 0.05 | *** | 245 | 246 | 265 | 142 | 144 | 155 | 100 | 101 | 109 | 78 | 79 | 84 | 64 | 65 | 69 |
| | *** | 245 | 248 | 409 | 143 | 146 | 216 | 101 | 103 | 138 | 78 | 81 | 97 | 65 | 66 | 72 |
| 0.1 | *** | 386 | 388 | 444 | 204 | 206 | 236 | 134 | 136 | 155 | 99 | 101 | 113 | 78 | 80 | 89 |
| | *** | 387 | 393 | 584 | 205 | 211 | 289 | 135 | 140 | 176 | 100 | 104 | 119 | 79 | 83 | 86 |
| 0.15 | *** | 498 | 502 | 609 | 250 | 254 | 307 | 158 | 162 | 193 | 113 | 117 | 137 | 87 | 90 | 105 |
| | *** | 499 | 508 | 736 | 251 | 261 | 351 | 159 | 168 | 208 | 114 | 122 | 138 | 88 | 95 | 98 |
| 0.2 | *** | 580 | 585 | 755 | 282 | 287 | 368 | 173 | 179 | 226 | 122 | 127 | 157 | 92 | 97 | 117 |
| | *** | 581 | 595 | 865 | 283 | 298 | 403 | 175 | 188 | 234 | 124 | 134 | 153 | 94 | 103 | 107 |
| 0.25 | *** | 631 | 639 | 879 | 300 | 308 | 419 | 182 | 190 | 252 | 126 | 133 | 172 | 95 | 101 | 127 |
| | *** | 634 | 653 | 970 | 303 | 322 | 444 | 185 | 202 | 255 | 129 | 142 | 164 | 97 | 108 | 113 |
| 0.3 | *** | 656 | 666 | 980 | 307 | 318 | 459 | 184 | 195 | 272 | 127 | 136 | 183 | 95 | 102 | 133 |
| | *** | 659 | 685 | 1052 | 311 | 336 | 475 | 188 | 209 | 269 | 130 | 147 | 171 | 98 | 111 | 117 |
| 0.35 | *** | 656 | 669 | 1056 | 305 | 318 | 488 | 182 | 194 | 285 | 125 | 135 | 189 | 93 | 102 | 136 |
| | *** | 661 | 694 | 1110 | 309 | 341 | 496 | 186 | 212 | 278 | 129 | 149 | 175 | 97 | 111 | 119 |
| 0.4 | *** | 636 | 652 | 1108 | 294 | 311 | 506 | 175 | 190 | 292 | 120 | 133 | 192 | 90 | 100 | 136 |
| | *** | 641 | 684 | 1145 | 300 | 338 | 507 | 181 | 211 | 281 | 125 | 147 | 175 | 94 | 110 | 117 |
| 0.45 | *** | 598 | 619 | 1134 | 276 | 297 | 512 | 166 | 183 | 292 | 114 | 128 | 190 | 85 | 96 | 134 |
| | *** | 605 | 659 | 1157 | 284 | 329 | 507 | 172 | 206 | 278 | 119 | 143 | 171 | 89 | 107 | 113 |
| 0.5 | *** | 548 | 574 | 1134 | 255 | 280 | 506 | 154 | 174 | 286 | 107 | 121 | 184 | 80 | 91 | 128 |
| | *** | 557 | 623 | 1145 | 264 | 315 | 496 | 161 | 198 | 269 | 112 | 137 | 164 | 84 | 102 | 107 |
| 0.55 | *** | 489 | 522 | 1109 | 231 | 259 | 490 | 141 | 162 | 274 | 98 | 113 | 174 | 73 | 84 | 120 |
| | *** | 500 | 579 | 1110 | 241 | 297 | 475 | 149 | 187 | 255 | 104 | 129 | 153 | 78 | 95 | 98 |
| 0.6 | *** | 425 | 466 | 1059 | 205 | 236 | 462 | 127 | 149 | 255 | 89 | 104 | 160 | 66 | 77 | 109 |
| | *** | 439 | 530 | 1052 | 217 | 276 | 444 | 136 | 173 | 234 | 95 | 119 | 138 | 71 | 87 | 86 |
| 0.65 | *** | 362 | 409 | 983 | 180 | 212 | 423 | 113 | 134 | 230 | 79 | 93 | 142 | 59 | 68 | 95 |
| | *** | 379 | 478 | 970 | 192 | 251 | 403 | 121 | 157 | 208 | 85 | 107 | 119 | 63 | 77 | 72 |
| 0.7 | *** | 302 | 354 | 882 | 155 | 186 | 372 | 98 | 117 | 198 | 68 | 80 | 120 | . | . | . |
| | *** | 321 | 424 | 865 | 167 | 223 | 351 | 106 | 138 | 176 | 73 | 92 | 97 | . | . | . |
| 0.75 | *** | 248 | 300 | 757 | 130 | 159 | 311 | 82 | 99 | 161 | . | . | . | . | . | . |
| | *** | 267 | 366 | 736 | 142 | 192 | 289 | 89 | 116 | 138 | . | . | . | . | . | . |
| 0.8 | *** | 198 | 246 | 607 | 105 | 129 | 239 | . | . | . | . | . | . | . | . | . |
| | *** | 217 | 305 | 584 | 115 | 155 | 216 | . | . | . | . | . | . | . | . | . |
| 0.85 | *** | 150 | 190 | 432 | . | . | . | . | . | . | . | . | . | . | . | . |
| | *** | 166 | 235 | 409 | . | . | . | . | . | . | . | . | . | . | . | . |

TABLE 1: ALPHA= 0.005 POWER= 0.8    EXPECTED ACCRUAL THRU MINIMUM FOLLOW-UP= 40

| | | DEL=.10 | | | DEL=.15 | | | DEL=.20 | | | DEL=.25 | | | DEL=.30 | | |
|---|---|---|---|---|---|---|---|---|---|---|---|---|---|---|---|---|---|
| FACT= | | 1.0 .75 | .50 .25 | .00 BIN | 1.0 .75 | .50 .25 | .00 BIN | 1.0 .75 | .50 .25 | .00 BIN | 1.0 75 | .50 .25 | .00 BIN | 1.0 .75 | .50 .25 | .00 BIN |
| PCONT=*** | | | | | REQUIRED NUMBER OF PATIENTS | | | | | | | | | | | |
| 0.05 | *** | 245 | 247 | 265 | 143 | 144 | 155 | 101 | 102 | 109 | 78 | 80 | 84 | 65 | 66 | 69 |
| | *** | 246 | 249 | 409 | 143 | 147 | 216 | 101 | 104 | 138 | 79 | 81 | 97 | 65 | 67 | 72 |
| 0.1 | *** | 387 | 390 | 444 | 205 | 208 | 236 | 135 | 138 | 155 | 100 | 102 | 113 | 79 | 81 | 89 |
| | *** | 388 | 395 | 584 | 206 | 213 | 289 | 136 | 142 | 176 | 101 | 106 | 119 | 80 | 84 | 86 |
| 0.15 | *** | 499 | 504 | 609 | 251 | 256 | 307 | 159 | 164 | 193 | 114 | 119 | 137 | 88 | 92 | 105 |
| | *** | 501 | 513 | 736 | 253 | 265 | 351 | 161 | 171 | 208 | 116 | 124 | 138 | 90 | 96 | 98 |
| 0.2 | *** | 581 | 588 | 755 | 283 | 291 | 368 | 175 | 183 | 226 | 124 | 130 | 157 | 94 | 100 | 117 |
| | *** | 584 | 601 | 865 | 286 | 304 | 403 | 178 | 193 | 234 | 126 | 137 | 153 | 96 | 105 | 107 |
| 0.25 | *** | 634 | 643 | 879 | 303 | 313 | 419 | 185 | 194 | 252 | 129 | 137 | 172 | 97 | 104 | 127 |
| | *** | 637 | 662 | 970 | 306 | 330 | 444 | 188 | 207 | 255 | 132 | 146 | 164 | 100 | 111 | 113 |
| 0.3 | *** | 659 | 672 | 980 | 311 | 324 | 459 | 188 | 200 | 272 | 130 | 140 | 183 | 98 | 106 | 133 |
| | *** | 664 | 697 | 1052 | 316 | 346 | 475 | 192 | 217 | 269 | 134 | 152 | 171 | 101 | 114 | 117 |
| 0.35 | *** | 661 | 677 | 1056 | 309 | 326 | 488 | 186 | 201 | 285 | 129 | 141 | 189 | 97 | 106 | 136 |
| | *** | 666 | 710 | 1110 | 315 | 353 | 496 | 192 | 221 | 278 | 133 | 154 | 175 | 100 | 115 | 119 |
| 0.4 | *** | 641 | 663 | 1108 | 300 | 321 | 506 | 181 | 198 | 292 | 125 | 139 | 192 | 94 | 104 | 136 |
| | *** | 649 | 704 | 1145 | 307 | 353 | 507 | 187 | 220 | 281 | 130 | 153 | 175 | 98 | 114 | 117 |
| 0.45 | *** | 605 | 633 | 1134 | 284 | 309 | 512 | 172 | 192 | 292 | 119 | 134 | 190 | 89 | 100 | 134 |
| | *** | 615 | 683 | 1157 | 293 | 345 | 507 | 180 | 216 | 278 | 125 | 150 | 171 | 94 | 111 | 113 |
| 0.5 | *** | 557 | 591 | 1134 | 264 | 293 | 506 | 161 | 183 | 286 | 112 | 128 | 184 | 84 | 95 | 128 |
| | *** | 569 | 651 | 1145 | 275 | 333 | 496 | 170 | 208 | 269 | 119 | 144 | 164 | 89 | 106 | 107 |
| 0.55 | *** | 500 | 542 | 1109 | 241 | 274 | 490 | 149 | 172 | 274 | 104 | 120 | 174 | 78 | 89 | 120 |
| | *** | 515 | 611 | 1110 | 253 | 315 | 475 | 158 | 197 | 255 | 111 | 136 | 153 | 82 | 99 | 98 |
| 0.6 | *** | 439 | 490 | 1059 | 217 | 252 | 462 | 136 | 159 | 255 | 95 | 110 | 160 | 71 | 81 | 109 |
| | *** | 457 | 564 | 1052 | 230 | 294 | 444 | 145 | 183 | 234 | 101 | 125 | 138 | 75 | 90 | 86 |
| 0.65 | *** | 379 | 435 | 983 | 192 | 228 | 423 | 121 | 143 | 230 | 85 | 99 | 142 | 63 | 72 | 95 |
| | *** | 399 | 513 | 970 | 206 | 269 | 403 | 130 | 166 | 208 | 91 | 112 | 119 | 67 | 80 | 72 |
| 0.7 | *** | 321 | 381 | 882 | 167 | 201 | 372 | 106 | 126 | 198 | 73 | 86 | 120 | . | . | . |
| | *** | 344 | 457 | 865 | 181 | 240 | 351 | 114 | 146 | 176 | 78 | 97 | 97 | . | . | . |
| 0.75 | *** | 267 | 326 | 757 | 142 | 173 | 311 | 89 | 106 | 161 | . | . | . | . | . | . |
| | *** | 290 | 398 | 736 | 154 | 206 | 289 | 96 | 123 | 138 | . | . | . | . | . | . |
| 0.8 | *** | 217 | 269 | 607 | 115 | 140 | 239 | . | . | . | . | . | . | . | . | . |
| | *** | 237 | 332 | 584 | 125 | 166 | 216 | . | . | . | . | . | . | . | . | . |
| 0.85 | *** | 166 | 208 | 432 | . | . | . | . | . | . | . | . | . | . | . | . |
| | *** | 183 | 256 | 409 | . | . | . | . | . | . | . | . | . | . | . | . |

## TABLE 1: ALPHA= 0.005 POWER= 0.8    EXPECTED ACCRUAL THRU MINIMUM FOLLOW-UP= 50

|  |  | DEL=.10 | | | DEL=.15 | | | DEL=.20 | | | DEL=.25 | | | DEL=.30 | | |
|---|---|---|---|---|---|---|---|---|---|---|---|---|---|---|---|---|
| FACT= | | 1.0 .75 | .50 .25 | .00 BIN | 1.0 .75 | .50 .25 | .00 BIN | 1.0 .75 | .50 .25 | .00 BIN | 1.0 75 | .50 .25 | .00 BIN | 1.0 .75 | .50 .25 | .00 BIN |
| PCONT=*** | | | | | REQUIRED NUMBER OF PATIENTS | | | | | | | | | | | |
| 0.05 | *** | 246 | 247 | 265 | 143 | 145 | 155 | 101 | 103 | 109 | 79 | 80 | 84 | 65 | 66 | 69 |
|  | *** | 246 | 250 | 409 | 144 | 147 | 216 | 102 | 105 | 138 | 79 | 82 | 97 | 65 | 67 | 72 |
| 0.1 | *** | 388 | 391 | 444 | 205 | 209 | 236 | 136 | 139 | 155 | 100 | 103 | 113 | 80 | 82 | 89 |
|  | *** | 389 | 398 | 584 | 207 | 215 | 289 | 137 | 144 | 176 | 102 | 107 | 119 | 81 | 85 | 86 |
| 0.15 | *** | 500 | 506 | 609 | 252 | 259 | 307 | 160 | 166 | 193 | 115 | 120 | 137 | 90 | 94 | 105 |
|  | *** | 502 | 517 | 736 | 255 | 268 | 351 | 163 | 173 | 208 | 117 | 126 | 138 | 91 | 97 | 98 |
| 0.2 | *** | 583 | 591 | 755 | 285 | 294 | 368 | 177 | 186 | 226 | 125 | 132 | 157 | 96 | 101 | 117 |
|  | *** | 586 | 608 | 865 | 288 | 309 | 403 | 180 | 196 | 234 | 128 | 140 | 153 | 98 | 107 | 107 |
| 0.25 | *** | 636 | 648 | 879 | 305 | 318 | 419 | 187 | 198 | 252 | 131 | 140 | 172 | 99 | 106 | 127 |
|  | *** | 640 | 671 | 970 | 310 | 337 | 444 | 191 | 212 | 255 | 135 | 150 | 164 | 102 | 113 | 113 |
| 0.3 | *** | 662 | 678 | 980 | 314 | 331 | 459 | 191 | 205 | 272 | 133 | 144 | 183 | 100 | 109 | 133 |
|  | *** | 668 | 709 | 1052 | 320 | 355 | 475 | 197 | 222 | 269 | 137 | 156 | 171 | 104 | 117 | 117 |
| 0.35 | *** | 665 | 686 | 1056 | 314 | 334 | 488 | 191 | 207 | 285 | 132 | 145 | 189 | 99 | 109 | 136 |
|  | *** | 672 | 725 | 1110 | 321 | 364 | 496 | 197 | 227 | 278 | 137 | 158 | 175 | 103 | 118 | 119 |
| 0.4 | *** | 647 | 674 | 1108 | 305 | 330 | 506 | 186 | 205 | 292 | 129 | 143 | 192 | 97 | 107 | 136 |
|  | *** | 656 | 722 | 1145 | 314 | 364 | 507 | 193 | 227 | 281 | 135 | 158 | 175 | 101 | 117 | 117 |
| 0.45 | *** | 612 | 646 | 1134 | 291 | 320 | 512 | 178 | 200 | 292 | 124 | 139 | 190 | 93 | 104 | 134 |
|  | *** | 624 | 705 | 1157 | 302 | 358 | 507 | 186 | 224 | 278 | 130 | 155 | 171 | 97 | 114 | 113 |
| 0.5 | *** | 566 | 608 | 1134 | 272 | 305 | 506 | 168 | 191 | 286 | 117 | 133 | 184 | 88 | 99 | 128 |
|  | *** | 580 | 676 | 1145 | 284 | 347 | 496 | 177 | 216 | 269 | 124 | 149 | 164 | 92 | 109 | 107 |
| 0.55 | *** | 511 | 562 | 1109 | 250 | 286 | 490 | 156 | 180 | 274 | 109 | 125 | 174 | 81 | 92 | 120 |
|  | *** | 529 | 637 | 1110 | 264 | 330 | 475 | 166 | 205 | 255 | 116 | 140 | 153 | 86 | 102 | 98 |
| 0.6 | *** | 453 | 511 | 1059 | 227 | 265 | 462 | 143 | 167 | 255 | 100 | 115 | 160 | 74 | 84 | 109 |
|  | *** | 474 | 592 | 1052 | 242 | 308 | 444 | 152 | 191 | 234 | 106 | 130 | 138 | 78 | 93 | 86 |
| 0.65 | *** | 394 | 458 | 983 | 203 | 240 | 423 | 128 | 151 | 230 | 89 | 103 | 142 | 66 | 75 | 95 |
|  | *** | 418 | 541 | 970 | 218 | 283 | 403 | 137 | 174 | 208 | 95 | 116 | 119 | 69 | 82 | 72 |
| 0.7 | *** | 338 | 404 | 882 | 178 | 213 | 372 | 112 | 133 | 198 | 77 | 89 | 120 | . | . | . |
|  | *** | 363 | 485 | 865 | 192 | 252 | 351 | 121 | 153 | 176 | 82 | 100 | 97 | . | . | . |
| 0.75 | *** | 285 | 348 | 757 | 151 | 183 | 311 | 94 | 112 | 161 | . | . | . | . | . | . |
|  | *** | 309 | 423 | 736 | 164 | 216 | 289 | 102 | 127 | 138 | . | . | . | . | . | . |
| 0.8 | *** | 232 | 289 | 607 | 123 | 149 | 239 | . | . | . | . | . | . | . | . | . |
|  | *** | 255 | 353 | 584 | 133 | 174 | 216 | . | . | . | . | . | . | . | . | . |
| 0.85 | *** | 179 | 223 | 432 | . | . | . | . | . | . | . | . | . | . | . | . |
|  | *** | 196 | 271 | 409 | . | . | . | . | . | . | . | . | . | . | . | . |

TABLE 1: ALPHA= 0.005 POWER= 0.8    EXPECTED ACCRUAL THRU MINIMUM FOLLOW-UP= 60

| | | DEL=.10 | | | DEL=.15 | | | DEL=.20 | | | DEL=.25 | | | DEL=.30 | | |
|---|---|---|---|---|---|---|---|---|---|---|---|---|---|---|---|---|---|
| FACT= | | 1.0 .75 | .50 .25 | .00 BIN | 1.0 .75 | .50 .25 | .00 BIN | 1.0 .75 | .50 .25 | .00 BIN | 1.0 75 | .50 .25 | .00 BIN | 1.0 .75 | .50 .25 | .00 BIN |
| PCONT=*** | | | | | REQUIRED | NUMBER | OF | PATIENTS | | | | | | | | |
| 0.05 | *** | 246 | 248 | 265 | 143 | 146 | 155 | 101 | 103 | 109 | 79 | 81 | 84 | 65 | 67 | 69 |
| | *** | 247 | 251 | 409 | 144 | 148 | 216 | 102 | 105 | 138 | 80 | 82 | 97 | 66 | 68 | 72 |
| 0.1 | *** | 388 | 393 | 444 | 206 | 211 | 236 | 136 | 140 | 155 | 101 | 104 | 113 | 80 | 83 | 89 |
| | *** | 390 | 400 | 584 | 208 | 217 | 289 | 138 | 145 | 176 | 102 | 107 | 119 | 81 | 85 | 86 |
| 0.15 | *** | 502 | 508 | 609 | 254 | 261 | 307 | 162 | 168 | 193 | 117 | 122 | 137 | 91 | 95 | 105 |
| | *** | 504 | 521 | 736 | 256 | 271 | 351 | 164 | 175 | 208 | 119 | 127 | 138 | 92 | 98 | 98 |
| 0.2 | *** | 585 | 595 | 755 | 287 | 298 | 368 | 179 | 188 | 226 | 127 | 134 | 157 | 97 | 103 | 117 |
| | *** | 588 | 614 | 865 | 291 | 313 | 403 | 183 | 199 | 234 | 130 | 142 | 153 | 100 | 108 | 107 |
| 0.25 | *** | 639 | 653 | 879 | 308 | 322 | 419 | 190 | 202 | 252 | 133 | 142 | 172 | 101 | 108 | 127 |
| | *** | 643 | 679 | 970 | 313 | 343 | 444 | 194 | 216 | 255 | 137 | 152 | 164 | 104 | 115 | 113 |
| 0.3 | *** | 666 | 685 | 980 | 318 | 336 | 459 | 195 | 209 | 272 | 136 | 147 | 183 | 102 | 111 | 133 |
| | *** | 672 | 720 | 1052 | 324 | 362 | 475 | 200 | 227 | 269 | 140 | 158 | 171 | 106 | 119 | 117 |
| 0.35 | *** | 669 | 694 | 1056 | 318 | 341 | 488 | 194 | 212 | 285 | 135 | 149 | 189 | 102 | 111 | 136 |
| | *** | 677 | 739 | 1110 | 326 | 372 | 496 | 201 | 232 | 278 | 141 | 161 | 175 | 106 | 120 | 119 |
| 0.4 | *** | 652 | 684 | 1108 | 311 | 338 | 506 | 190 | 211 | 292 | 133 | 147 | 192 | 100 | 110 | 136 |
| | *** | 663 | 739 | 1145 | 321 | 374 | 507 | 198 | 233 | 281 | 139 | 161 | 175 | 104 | 119 | 117 |
| 0.45 | *** | 619 | 659 | 1134 | 297 | 329 | 512 | 183 | 206 | 292 | 128 | 143 | 190 | 96 | 107 | 134 |
| | *** | 633 | 724 | 1157 | 309 | 369 | 507 | 192 | 230 | 278 | 134 | 158 | 171 | 100 | 116 | 113 |
| 0.5 | *** | 574 | 623 | 1134 | 280 | 315 | 506 | 174 | 198 | 286 | 121 | 137 | 184 | 91 | 102 | 128 |
| | *** | 591 | 697 | 1145 | 293 | 358 | 496 | 183 | 223 | 269 | 128 | 153 | 164 | 95 | 111 | 107 |
| 0.55 | *** | 522 | 579 | 1109 | 259 | 297 | 490 | 162 | 187 | 274 | 113 | 129 | 174 | 84 | 95 | 120 |
| | *** | 542 | 661 | 1110 | 274 | 342 | 475 | 172 | 212 | 255 | 120 | 144 | 153 | 89 | 104 | 98 |
| 0.6 | *** | 466 | 530 | 1059 | 236 | 276 | 462 | 149 | 173 | 255 | 104 | 119 | 160 | 77 | 87 | 109 |
| | *** | 490 | 617 | 1052 | 252 | 320 | 444 | 159 | 197 | 234 | 110 | 133 | 138 | 81 | 95 | 86 |
| 0.65 | *** | 409 | 478 | 983 | 212 | 251 | 423 | 134 | 157 | 230 | 93 | 107 | 142 | 68 | 77 | 95 |
| | *** | 435 | 566 | 970 | 228 | 294 | 403 | 143 | 179 | 208 | 99 | 119 | 119 | 72 | 84 | 72 |
| 0.7 | *** | 354 | 424 | 882 | 187 | 223 | 372 | 117 | 138 | 198 | 80 | 92 | 120 | . | . | . |
| | *** | 381 | 508 | 865 | 201 | 262 | 351 | 126 | 157 | 176 | 86 | 102 | 97 | . | . | . |
| 0.75 | *** | 300 | 366 | 757 | 159 | 192 | 311 | 99 | 116 | 161 | . | . | . | . | . | . |
| | *** | 326 | 444 | 736 | 173 | 225 | 289 | 106 | 131 | 138 | . | . | . | . | . | . |
| 0.8 | *** | 246 | 305 | 607 | 129 | 155 | 239 | . | . | . | . | . | . | . | . | . |
| | *** | 269 | 370 | 584 | 140 | 181 | 216 | . | . | . | . | . | . | . | . | . |
| 0.85 | *** | 190 | 235 | 432 | . | . | . | . | . | . | . | . | . | . | . | . |
| | *** | 208 | 284 | 409 | . | . | . | . | . | . | . | . | . | . | . | . |

## TABLE 1: ALPHA= 0.005 POWER= 0.8    EXPECTED ACCRUAL THRU MINIMUM FOLLOW-UP= 70

| | | DEL=.10 | | | DEL=.15 | | | DEL=.20 | | | DEL=.25 | | | DEL=.30 | | |
|---|---|---|---|---|---|---|---|---|---|---|---|---|---|---|---|---|
| FACT= | | 1.0 .75 | .50 .25 | .00 BIN | 1.0 .75 | .50 .25 | .00 BIN | 1.0 .75 | .50 .25 | .00 BIN | 1.0 75 | .50 .25 | .00 BIN | 1.0 .75 | .50 .25 | .00 BIN |
| PCONT=*** | | | | | REQUIRED NUMBER OF PATIENTS | | | | | | | | | | | |
| 0.05 | *** | 246 | 249 | 265 | 144 | 146 | 155 | 102 | 104 | 109 | 79 | 81 | 84 | 66 | 67 | 69 |
| | *** | 247 | 252 | 409 | 145 | 149 | 216 | 102 | 105 | 138 | 80 | 82 | 97 | 66 | 68 | 72 |
| 0.1 | *** | 389 | 394 | 444 | 207 | 212 | 236 | 137 | 141 | 155 | 102 | 105 | 113 | 81 | 83 | 89 |
| | *** | 391 | 403 | 584 | 209 | 218 | 289 | 139 | 146 | 176 | 103 | 108 | 119 | 82 | 86 | 86 |
| 0.15 | *** | 503 | 511 | 609 | 255 | 263 | 307 | 163 | 170 | 193 | 118 | 123 | 137 | 91 | 95 | 105 |
| | *** | 505 | 525 | 736 | 258 | 274 | 351 | 165 | 177 | 208 | 120 | 128 | 138 | 93 | 99 | 98 |
| 0.2 | *** | 586 | 598 | 755 | 289 | 301 | 368 | 181 | 190 | 226 | 128 | 136 | 157 | 98 | 104 | 117 |
| | *** | 590 | 620 | 865 | 293 | 317 | 403 | 185 | 201 | 234 | 131 | 143 | 153 | 101 | 109 | 107 |
| 0.25 | *** | 641 | 657 | 879 | 311 | 326 | 419 | 192 | 205 | 252 | 135 | 145 | 172 | 103 | 110 | 127 |
| | *** | 646 | 687 | 970 | 316 | 348 | 444 | 197 | 219 | 255 | 139 | 154 | 164 | 106 | 116 | 113 |
| 0.3 | *** | 669 | 691 | 980 | 321 | 341 | 459 | 198 | 213 | 272 | 138 | 150 | 183 | 104 | 113 | 133 |
| | *** | 676 | 730 | 1052 | 329 | 369 | 475 | 204 | 230 | 269 | 143 | 161 | 171 | 108 | 120 | 117 |
| 0.35 | *** | 673 | 702 | 1056 | 322 | 348 | 488 | 198 | 217 | 285 | 138 | 152 | 189 | 104 | 114 | 136 |
| | *** | 683 | 752 | 1110 | 332 | 380 | 496 | 205 | 237 | 278 | 144 | 164 | 175 | 108 | 122 | 119 |
| 0.4 | *** | 658 | 694 | 1108 | 316 | 346 | 506 | 195 | 216 | 292 | 136 | 150 | 192 | 102 | 112 | 136 |
| | *** | 670 | 754 | 1145 | 327 | 383 | 507 | 203 | 238 | 281 | 142 | 164 | 175 | 106 | 121 | 117 |
| 0.45 | *** | 626 | 672 | 1134 | 304 | 338 | 512 | 188 | 211 | 292 | 131 | 147 | 190 | 98 | 109 | 134 |
| | *** | 642 | 742 | 1157 | 317 | 379 | 507 | 197 | 235 | 278 | 138 | 161 | 171 | 103 | 118 | 113 |
| 0.5 | *** | 583 | 638 | 1134 | 287 | 325 | 506 | 179 | 203 | 286 | 125 | 141 | 184 | 93 | 104 | 128 |
| | *** | 602 | 717 | 1145 | 301 | 368 | 496 | 189 | 228 | 269 | 132 | 156 | 164 | 98 | 113 | 107 |
| 0.55 | *** | 532 | 595 | 1109 | 267 | 307 | 490 | 167 | 192 | 274 | 117 | 133 | 174 | 87 | 97 | 120 |
| | *** | 555 | 682 | 1110 | 282 | 352 | 475 | 177 | 217 | 255 | 123 | 147 | 153 | 91 | 106 | 98 |
| 0.6 | *** | 478 | 548 | 1059 | 244 | 285 | 462 | 154 | 179 | 255 | 107 | 122 | 160 | 79 | 89 | 109 |
| | *** | 504 | 638 | 1052 | 261 | 330 | 444 | 164 | 202 | 234 | 114 | 136 | 138 | 83 | 97 | 86 |
| 0.65 | *** | 423 | 496 | 983 | 220 | 261 | 423 | 139 | 162 | 230 | 96 | 110 | 142 | 70 | 79 | 95 |
| | *** | 451 | 587 | 970 | 236 | 303 | 403 | 149 | 184 | 208 | 102 | 121 | 119 | 74 | 85 | 72 |
| 0.7 | *** | 368 | 441 | 882 | 194 | 232 | 372 | 122 | 143 | 198 | 83 | 95 | 120 | . | . | . |
| | *** | 396 | 528 | 865 | 210 | 271 | 351 | 131 | 161 | 176 | 88 | 104 | 97 | . | . | . |
| 0.75 | *** | 313 | 383 | 757 | 166 | 199 | 311 | 103 | 119 | 161 | . | . | . | . | . | . |
| | *** | 341 | 462 | 736 | 180 | 232 | 289 | 110 | 134 | 138 | . | . | . | . | . | . |
| 0.8 | *** | 258 | 319 | 607 | 135 | 161 | 239 | . | . | . | . | . | . | . | . | . |
| | *** | 283 | 385 | 584 | 146 | 186 | 216 | . | . | . | . | . | . | . | . | . |
| 0.85 | *** | 199 | 246 | 432 | . | . | . | . | . | . | . | . | . | . | . | . |
| | *** | 218 | 295 | 409 | . | . | . | . | . | . | . | . | . | . | . | . |

## TABLE 1: ALPHA= 0.005 POWER= 0.8    EXPECTED ACCRUAL THRU MINIMUM FOLLOW-UP= 80

| | | DEL=.10 | | | DEL=.15 | | | DEL=.20 | | | DEL=.25 | | | DEL=.30 | | |
|---|---|---|---|---|---|---|---|---|---|---|---|---|---|---|---|---|
| FACT= | | 1.0 .75 | .50 .25 | .00 BIN | 1.0 .75 | .50 .25 | .00 BIN | 1.0 .75 | .50 .25 | .00 BIN | 1.0 75 | .50 .25 | .00 BIN | 1.0 .75 | .50 .25 | .00 BIN |
| PCONT=*** | | | | | | REQUIRED NUMBER OF PATIENTS | | | | | | | | | | |
| 0.05 | *** | 247 | 249 | 265 | 144 | 147 | 155 | 102 | 104 | 109 | 80 | 81 | 84 | 66 | 67 | 69 |
| | *** | 248 | 253 | 409 | 145 | 149 | 216 | 103 | 106 | 138 | 80 | 82 | 97 | 66 | 68 | 72 |
| 0.1 | *** | 390 | 395 | 444 | 208 | 213 | 236 | 138 | 142 | 155 | 102 | 106 | 113 | 81 | 84 | 89 |
| | *** | 392 | 405 | 584 | 210 | 220 | 289 | 140 | 146 | 176 | 104 | 109 | 119 | 82 | 86 | 86 |
| 0.15 | *** | 504 | 513 | 609 | 256 | 265 | 307 | 164 | 171 | 193 | 119 | 124 | 137 | 92 | 96 | 105 |
| | *** | 507 | 529 | 736 | 259 | 276 | 351 | 167 | 178 | 208 | 121 | 129 | 138 | 94 | 100 | 98 |
| 0.2 | *** | 588 | 601 | 755 | 291 | 304 | 368 | 183 | 193 | 226 | 130 | 137 | 157 | 100 | 105 | 117 |
| | *** | 593 | 625 | 865 | 295 | 320 | 403 | 186 | 203 | 234 | 133 | 144 | 153 | 102 | 110 | 107 |
| 0.25 | *** | 643 | 662 | 879 | 313 | 330 | 419 | 194 | 207 | 252 | 137 | 146 | 172 | 104 | 111 | 127 |
| | *** | 650 | 695 | 970 | 319 | 352 | 444 | 199 | 221 | 255 | 141 | 155 | 164 | 107 | 117 | 113 |
| 0.3 | *** | 672 | 697 | 980 | 324 | 346 | 459 | 200 | 217 | 272 | 140 | 152 | 183 | 106 | 114 | 133 |
| | *** | 681 | 740 | 1052 | 333 | 374 | 475 | 207 | 233 | 269 | 145 | 163 | 171 | 109 | 121 | 117 |
| 0.35 | *** | 677 | 710 | 1056 | 326 | 353 | 488 | 201 | 221 | 285 | 141 | 154 | 189 | 106 | 115 | 136 |
| | *** | 689 | 763 | 1110 | 337 | 386 | 496 | 209 | 240 | 278 | 146 | 166 | 175 | 110 | 123 | 119 |
| 0.4 | *** | 663 | 704 | 1108 | 321 | 353 | 506 | 198 | 220 | 292 | 139 | 153 | 192 | 104 | 114 | 136 |
| | *** | 677 | 768 | 1145 | 333 | 390 | 507 | 207 | 242 | 281 | 145 | 167 | 175 | 108 | 123 | 117 |
| 0.45 | *** | 633 | 683 | 1134 | 309 | 345 | 512 | 192 | 216 | 292 | 134 | 150 | 190 | 100 | 111 | 134 |
| | *** | 651 | 758 | 1157 | 323 | 387 | 507 | 202 | 239 | 278 | 141 | 164 | 171 | 105 | 120 | 113 |
| 0.5 | *** | 591 | 651 | 1134 | 293 | 333 | 506 | 183 | 208 | 286 | 128 | 144 | 184 | 95 | 106 | 128 |
| | *** | 613 | 734 | 1145 | 309 | 377 | 496 | 193 | 232 | 269 | 135 | 158 | 164 | 100 | 115 | 107 |
| 0.55 | *** | 542 | 611 | 1109 | 274 | 315 | 490 | 172 | 197 | 274 | 120 | 136 | 174 | 89 | 99 | 120 |
| | *** | 568 | 700 | 1110 | 290 | 361 | 475 | 182 | 221 | 255 | 127 | 149 | 153 | 93 | 107 | 98 |
| 0.6 | *** | 490 | 564 | 1059 | 252 | 294 | 462 | 159 | 183 | 255 | 110 | 125 | 160 | 81 | 90 | 109 |
| | *** | 518 | 657 | 1052 | 269 | 339 | 444 | 169 | 206 | 234 | 117 | 138 | 138 | 85 | 98 | 86 |
| 0.65 | *** | 435 | 513 | 983 | 228 | 269 | 423 | 143 | 166 | 230 | 99 | 112 | 142 | 72 | 80 | 95 |
| | *** | 465 | 606 | 970 | 244 | 311 | 403 | 153 | 187 | 208 | 105 | 123 | 119 | 75 | 86 | 72 |
| 0.7 | *** | 381 | 457 | 882 | 201 | 240 | 372 | 126 | 146 | 198 | 86 | 97 | 120 | . | . | . |
| | *** | 411 | 546 | 865 | 217 | 278 | 351 | 135 | 164 | 176 | 90 | 106 | 97 | . | . | . |
| 0.75 | *** | 326 | 398 | 757 | 173 | 206 | 311 | 106 | 123 | 161 | . | . | . | . | . | . |
| | *** | 354 | 477 | 736 | 186 | 238 | 289 | 113 | 136 | 138 | . | . | . | . | . | . |
| 0.8 | *** | 269 | 332 | 607 | 140 | 166 | 239 | . | . | . | . | . | . | . | . | . |
| | *** | 294 | 398 | 584 | 151 | 190 | 216 | . | . | . | . | . | . | . | . | . |
| 0.85 | *** | 208 | 256 | 432 | . | . | . | . | . | . | . | . | . | . | . | . |
| | *** | 227 | 304 | 409 | . | . | . | . | . | . | . | . | . | . | . | . |

## TABLE 1: ALPHA= 0.005 POWER= 0.8    EXPECTED ACCRUAL THRU MINIMUM FOLLOW-UP= 90

| | | DEL=.10 | | | DEL=.15 | | | DEL=.20 | | | DEL=.25 | | | DEL=.30 | | |
|---|---|---|---|---|---|---|---|---|---|---|---|---|---|---|---|---|---|
| FACT= | | 1.0 .75 | .50 .25 | .00 BIN | 1.0 .75 | .50 .25 | .00 BIN | 1.0 .75 | .50 .25 | .00 BIN | 1.0 75 | .50 .25 | .00 BIN | 1.0 .75 | .50 .25 | .00 BIN |
| PCONT=*** | | | | | REQUIRED NUMBER OF PATIENTS | | | | | | | | | | | |
| 0.05 | *** | 247 | 250 | 265 | 145 | 147 | 155 | 102 | 104 | 109 | 80 | 81 | 84 | 66 | 67 | 69 |
|  | *** | 248 | 254 | 409 | 146 | 150 | 216 | 103 | 106 | 138 | 81 | 83 | 97 | 66 | 68 | 72 |
| 0.1 | *** | 390 | 397 | 444 | 209 | 214 | 236 | 138 | 143 | 155 | 103 | 106 | 113 | 82 | 84 | 89 |
|  | *** | 393 | 407 | 584 | 211 | 221 | 289 | 140 | 147 | 176 | 104 | 109 | 119 | 83 | 86 | 86 |
| 0.15 | *** | 505 | 515 | 609 | 257 | 267 | 307 | 165 | 172 | 193 | 119 | 125 | 137 | 93 | 97 | 105 |
|  | *** | 508 | 532 | 736 | 261 | 278 | 351 | 168 | 180 | 208 | 122 | 129 | 138 | 95 | 100 | 98 |
| 0.2 | *** | 590 | 605 | 755 | 293 | 306 | 368 | 184 | 194 | 226 | 131 | 139 | 157 | 100 | 106 | 117 |
|  | *** | 595 | 630 | 865 | 298 | 323 | 403 | 188 | 205 | 234 | 134 | 145 | 153 | 103 | 110 | 107 |
| 0.25 | *** | 646 | 667 | 879 | 316 | 334 | 419 | 196 | 210 | 252 | 138 | 148 | 172 | 105 | 112 | 127 |
|  | *** | 653 | 702 | 970 | 322 | 356 | 444 | 202 | 223 | 255 | 142 | 157 | 164 | 108 | 118 | 113 |
| 0.3 | *** | 675 | 703 | 980 | 328 | 351 | 459 | 203 | 219 | 272 | 142 | 154 | 183 | 107 | 116 | 133 |
|  | *** | 685 | 749 | 1052 | 336 | 379 | 475 | 209 | 236 | 269 | 147 | 164 | 171 | 111 | 122 | 117 |
| 0.35 | *** | 682 | 717 | 1056 | 330 | 359 | 488 | 204 | 224 | 285 | 143 | 156 | 189 | 108 | 117 | 136 |
|  | *** | 694 | 774 | 1110 | 341 | 392 | 496 | 212 | 243 | 278 | 149 | 168 | 175 | 111 | 124 | 119 |
| 0.4 | *** | 668 | 713 | 1108 | 326 | 359 | 506 | 202 | 224 | 292 | 141 | 156 | 192 | 106 | 116 | 136 |
|  | *** | 684 | 781 | 1145 | 338 | 397 | 507 | 211 | 245 | 281 | 147 | 169 | 175 | 110 | 124 | 117 |
| 0.45 | *** | 640 | 694 | 1134 | 315 | 352 | 512 | 196 | 220 | 292 | 137 | 152 | 190 | 102 | 113 | 134 |
|  | *** | 659 | 772 | 1157 | 329 | 394 | 507 | 206 | 243 | 278 | 143 | 166 | 171 | 107 | 121 | 113 |
| 0.5 | *** | 600 | 664 | 1134 | 299 | 340 | 506 | 187 | 212 | 286 | 131 | 147 | 184 | 97 | 108 | 128 |
|  | *** | 623 | 750 | 1145 | 315 | 384 | 496 | 198 | 236 | 269 | 137 | 160 | 164 | 102 | 116 | 107 |
| 0.55 | *** | 552 | 624 | 1109 | 280 | 323 | 490 | 176 | 201 | 274 | 123 | 138 | 174 | 91 | 101 | 120 |
|  | *** | 579 | 717 | 1110 | 297 | 368 | 475 | 187 | 225 | 255 | 129 | 151 | 153 | 95 | 108 | 98 |
| 0.6 | *** | 501 | 579 | 1059 | 259 | 302 | 462 | 163 | 187 | 255 | 113 | 128 | 160 | 83 | 92 | 109 |
|  | *** | 530 | 674 | 1052 | 276 | 346 | 444 | 173 | 210 | 234 | 119 | 140 | 138 | 87 | 99 | 86 |
| 0.65 | *** | 447 | 528 | 983 | 234 | 276 | 423 | 147 | 170 | 230 | 101 | 114 | 142 | 73 | 81 | 95 |
|  | *** | 478 | 622 | 970 | 251 | 318 | 403 | 157 | 191 | 208 | 107 | 125 | 119 | 77 | 87 | 72 |
| 0.7 | *** | 393 | 472 | 882 | 208 | 246 | 372 | 129 | 150 | 198 | 88 | 99 | 120 | . | . | . |
|  | *** | 424 | 562 | 865 | 223 | 284 | 351 | 138 | 167 | 176 | 92 | 107 | 97 | . | . | . |
| 0.75 | *** | 337 | 411 | 757 | 178 | 211 | 311 | 109 | 125 | 161 | . | . | . | . | . | . |
|  | *** | 366 | 491 | 736 | 192 | 243 | 289 | 116 | 138 | 138 | . | . | . | . | . | . |
| 0.8 | *** | 279 | 343 | 607 | 145 | 170 | 239 | . | . | . | . | . | . | . | . | . |
|  | *** | 305 | 409 | 584 | 155 | 194 | 216 | . | . | . | . | . | . | . | . | . |
| 0.85 | *** | 216 | 264 | 432 | . | . | . | . | . | . | . | . | . | . | . | . |
|  | *** | 235 | 312 | 409 | . | . | . | . | . | . | . | . | . | . | . | . |

TABLE 1: ALPHA= 0.005 POWER= 0.8    EXPECTED ACCRUAL THRU MINIMUM FOLLOW-UP= 100

| | DEL=.10 | | | DEL=.15 | | | DEL=.20 | | | DEL=.25 | | | DEL=.30 | | |
|---|---|---|---|---|---|---|---|---|---|---|---|---|---|---|---|
| FACT= | 1.0 .75 | .50 .25 | .00 BIN | 1.0 .75 | .50 .25 | .00 BIN | 1.0 .75 | .50 .25 | .00 BIN | 1.0 75 | .50 .25 | .00 BIN | 1.0 .75 | .50 .25 | .00 BIN |
| PCONT=*** | | | | | | | REQUIRED NUMBER OF PATIENTS | | | | | | | | |
| 0.05 *** | 247 | 250 | 265 | 145 | 147 | 155 | 103 | 105 | 109 | 80 | 82 | 84 | 66 | 67 | 69 |
| *** | 248 | 254 | 409 | 146 | 150 | 216 | 104 | 106 | 138 | 81 | 83 | 97 | 67 | 68 | 72 |
| 0.1 *** | 391 | 398 | 444 | 209 | 215 | 236 | 139 | 144 | 155 | 103 | 107 | 113 | 82 | 85 | 89 |
| *** | 394 | 408 | 584 | 212 | 222 | 289 | 141 | 148 | 176 | 105 | 109 | 119 | 83 | 86 | 86 |
| 0.15 *** | 506 | 517 | 609 | 259 | 268 | 307 | 166 | 173 | 193 | 120 | 126 | 137 | 94 | 97 | 105 |
| *** | 510 | 535 | 736 | 262 | 280 | 351 | 169 | 180 | 208 | 123 | 130 | 138 | 95 | 100 | 98 |
| 0.2 *** | 591 | 608 | 755 | 294 | 309 | 368 | 186 | 196 | 226 | 132 | 140 | 157 | 101 | 107 | 117 |
| *** | 597 | 635 | 865 | 300 | 325 | 403 | 190 | 206 | 234 | 135 | 146 | 153 | 104 | 111 | 107 |
| 0.25 *** | 648 | 671 | 879 | 318 | 337 | 419 | 198 | 212 | 252 | 140 | 150 | 172 | 106 | 113 | 127 |
| *** | 656 | 708 | 970 | 325 | 360 | 444 | 204 | 225 | 255 | 144 | 158 | 164 | 109 | 118 | 113 |
| 0.3 *** | 678 | 709 | 980 | 331 | 355 | 459 | 205 | 222 | 272 | 144 | 156 | 183 | 109 | 117 | 133 |
| *** | 689 | 757 | 1052 | 340 | 383 | 475 | 212 | 238 | 269 | 149 | 166 | 171 | 112 | 123 | 117 |
| 0.35 *** | 686 | 725 | 1056 | 334 | 364 | 488 | 207 | 227 | 285 | 145 | 158 | 189 | 109 | 118 | 136 |
| *** | 699 | 784 | 1110 | 345 | 397 | 496 | 215 | 246 | 278 | 151 | 170 | 175 | 113 | 125 | 119 |
| 0.4 *** | 674 | 722 | 1108 | 330 | 364 | 506 | 205 | 227 | 292 | 143 | 158 | 192 | 107 | 117 | 136 |
| *** | 691 | 793 | 1145 | 343 | 403 | 507 | 214 | 249 | 281 | 149 | 170 | 175 | 112 | 125 | 117 |
| 0.45 *** | 646 | 705 | 1134 | 320 | 358 | 512 | 200 | 224 | 292 | 139 | 155 | 190 | 104 | 114 | 134 |
| *** | 668 | 786 | 1157 | 335 | 400 | 507 | 209 | 246 | 278 | 146 | 168 | 171 | 108 | 122 | 113 |
| 0.5 *** | 608 | 676 | 1134 | 305 | 347 | 506 | 191 | 216 | 286 | 133 | 149 | 184 | 99 | 109 | 128 |
| *** | 633 | 765 | 1145 | 322 | 391 | 496 | 201 | 239 | 269 | 140 | 162 | 164 | 103 | 117 | 107 |
| 0.55 *** | 562 | 637 | 1109 | 286 | 330 | 490 | 180 | 205 | 274 | 125 | 140 | 174 | 92 | 102 | 120 |
| *** | 590 | 732 | 1110 | 304 | 375 | 475 | 191 | 228 | 255 | 132 | 153 | 153 | 97 | 109 | 98 |
| 0.6 *** | 511 | 592 | 1059 | 265 | 308 | 462 | 167 | 191 | 255 | 115 | 130 | 160 | 84 | 93 | 109 |
| *** | 542 | 689 | 1052 | 282 | 352 | 444 | 177 | 213 | 234 | 121 | 141 | 138 | 88 | 100 | 86 |
| 0.65 *** | 458 | 541 | 983 | 240 | 283 | 423 | 151 | 174 | 230 | 103 | 116 | 142 | 75 | 82 | 95 |
| *** | 490 | 637 | 970 | 258 | 324 | 403 | 160 | 193 | 208 | 109 | 126 | 119 | 78 | 88 | 72 |
| 0.7 *** | 404 | 485 | 882 | 213 | 252 | 372 | 133 | 153 | 198 | 89 | 100 | 120 | . | . | . |
| *** | 436 | 576 | 865 | 229 | 289 | 351 | 141 | 169 | 176 | 94 | 108 | 97 | . | . | . |
| 0.75 *** | 348 | 423 | 757 | 183 | 216 | 311 | 112 | 127 | 161 | . | . | . | . | . | . |
| *** | 378 | 504 | 736 | 197 | 247 | 289 | 118 | 140 | 138 | . | . | . | . | . | . |
| 0.8 *** | 289 | 353 | 607 | 149 | 174 | 239 | . | . | . | . | . | . | . | . | . |
| *** | 315 | 419 | 584 | 159 | 197 | 216 | . | . | . | . | . | . | . | . | . |
| 0.85 *** | 223 | 271 | 432 | . | . | . | . | . | . | . | . | . | . | . | . |
| *** | 243 | 319 | 409 | . | . | . | . | . | . | . | . | . | . | . | . |

## TABLE 1: ALPHA= 0.005 POWER= 0.8    EXPECTED ACCRUAL THRU MINIMUM FOLLOW-UP= 110

| | | DEL=.05 | | | DEL=.10 | | | DEL=.15 | | | DEL=.20 | | | DEL=.25 | | |
|---|---|---|---|---|---|---|---|---|---|---|---|---|---|---|---|---|
| FACT= | | 1.0 .75 | .50 .25 | .00 BIN | 1.0 .75 | .50 .25 | .00 BIN | 1.0 .75 | .50 .25 | .00 BIN | 1.0 75 | .50 .25 | .00 BIN | 1.0 .75 | .50 .25 | .00 BIN |
| PCONT=*** | | | | REQUIRED NUMBER OF PATIENTS | | | | | | | | | | | | |
| 0.05 | *** | 698 | 700 | 746 | 248 | 251 | 265 | 145 | 148 | 155 | 103 | 105 | 109 | 80 | 82 | 84 |
| | *** | 698 | 706 | 1285 | 249 | 255 | 409 | 146 | 150 | 216 | 104 | 106 | 138 | 81 | 83 | 97 |
| 0.1 | *** | 1271 | 1278 | 1439 | 392 | 399 | 444 | 210 | 216 | 236 | 140 | 144 | 155 | 104 | 107 | 113 |
| | *** | 1274 | 1291 | 2033 | 394 | 410 | 584 | 212 | 222 | 289 | 142 | 148 | 176 | 105 | 110 | 119 |
| 0.15 | *** | 1758 | 1769 | 2109 | 507 | 519 | 609 | 260 | 270 | 307 | 167 | 174 | 193 | 121 | 126 | 137 |
| | *** | 1762 | 1790 | 2687 | 511 | 538 | 736 | 264 | 281 | 351 | 170 | 181 | 208 | 123 | 131 | 138 |
| 0.2 | *** | 2133 | 2150 | 2721 | 593 | 611 | 755 | 296 | 311 | 368 | 187 | 197 | 226 | 133 | 141 | 157 |
| | *** | 2139 | 2182 | 3247 | 599 | 639 | 865 | 302 | 328 | 403 | 191 | 207 | 234 | 136 | 147 | 153 |
| 0.25 | *** | 2393 | 2416 | 3256 | 650 | 675 | 879 | 320 | 340 | 419 | 200 | 214 | 252 | 141 | 151 | 172 |
| | *** | 2400 | 2462 | 3714 | 659 | 714 | 970 | 328 | 363 | 444 | 206 | 227 | 255 | 145 | 159 | 164 |
| 0.3 | *** | 2540 | 2572 | 3703 | 682 | 714 | 980 | 333 | 359 | 459 | 207 | 224 | 272 | 146 | 157 | 183 |
| | *** | 2551 | 2634 | 4088 | 693 | 765 | 1052 | 343 | 387 | 475 | 214 | 241 | 269 | 150 | 167 | 171 |
| 0.35 | *** | 2586 | 2627 | 4055 | 690 | 732 | 1056 | 338 | 368 | 488 | 210 | 230 | 285 | 147 | 160 | 189 |
| | *** | 2600 | 2710 | 4368 | 705 | 794 | 1110 | 350 | 402 | 496 | 218 | 248 | 278 | 152 | 171 | 175 |
| 0.4 | *** | 2542 | 2596 | 4308 | 679 | 731 | 1108 | 334 | 370 | 506 | 208 | 230 | 292 | 145 | 160 | 192 |
| | *** | 2560 | 2703 | 4555 | 698 | 804 | 1145 | 348 | 408 | 507 | 217 | 251 | 281 | 152 | 172 | 175 |
| 0.45 | *** | 2423 | 2492 | 4462 | 653 | 715 | 1134 | 325 | 364 | 512 | 203 | 227 | 292 | 141 | 157 | 190 |
| | *** | 2446 | 2628 | 4649 | 676 | 798 | 1157 | 340 | 406 | 507 | 213 | 249 | 278 | 148 | 169 | 171 |
| 0.5 | *** | 2244 | 2332 | 4514 | 616 | 687 | 1134 | 310 | 353 | 506 | 194 | 220 | 286 | 135 | 151 | 184 |
| | *** | 2273 | 2501 | 4649 | 642 | 778 | 1145 | 327 | 397 | 496 | 205 | 242 | 269 | 142 | 163 | 164 |
| 0.55 | *** | 2021 | 2133 | 4464 | 571 | 650 | 1109 | 292 | 336 | 490 | 183 | 209 | 274 | 127 | 142 | 174 |
| | *** | 2059 | 2337 | 4555 | 601 | 746 | 1110 | 310 | 381 | 475 | 194 | 231 | 255 | 134 | 154 | 153 |
| 0.6 | *** | 1773 | 1913 | 4312 | 521 | 605 | 1059 | 270 | 315 | 462 | 170 | 194 | 255 | 117 | 131 | 160 |
| | *** | 1821 | 2150 | 4368 | 553 | 703 | 1052 | 288 | 358 | 444 | 180 | 216 | 234 | 123 | 142 | 138 |
| 0.65 | *** | 1517 | 1686 | 4059 | 468 | 554 | 983 | 246 | 288 | 423 | 154 | 177 | 230 | 105 | 118 | 142 |
| | *** | 1576 | 1948 | 4088 | 502 | 651 | 970 | 263 | 329 | 403 | 164 | 196 | 208 | 111 | 127 | 119 |
| 0.7 | *** | 1269 | 1463 | 3706 | 414 | 497 | 882 | 219 | 257 | 372 | 135 | 155 | 198 | 91 | 101 | 120 |
| | *** | 1340 | 1737 | 3714 | 447 | 588 | 865 | 235 | 294 | 351 | 144 | 171 | 176 | 96 | 109 | 97 |
| 0.75 | *** | 1043 | 1248 | 3253 | 357 | 434 | 757 | 188 | 221 | 311 | 114 | 129 | 161 | . | . | . |
| | *** | 1120 | 1518 | 3247 | 388 | 515 | 736 | 202 | 251 | 289 | 121 | 142 | 138 | . | . | . |
| 0.8 | *** | 841 | 1039 | 2702 | 297 | 362 | 607 | 152 | 178 | 239 | . | . | . | . | . | . |
| | *** | 917 | 1287 | 2687 | 323 | 428 | 584 | 163 | 199 | 216 | . | . | . | . | . | . |
| 0.85 | *** | 655 | 828 | 2053 | 230 | 278 | 432 | . | . | . | . | . | . | . | . | . |
| | *** | 722 | 1035 | 2033 | 249 | 325 | 409 | . | . | . | . | . | . | . | . | . |
| 0.9 | *** | 467 | 596 | 1308 | . | . | . | . | . | . | . | . | . | . | . | . |
| | *** | 518 | 741 | 1285 | . | . | . | . | . | . | . | . | . | . | . | . |

## TABLE 1: ALPHA= 0.005 POWER= 0.8    EXPECTED ACCRUAL THRU MINIMUM FOLLOW-UP= 120

| | DEL=.05 | | | DEL=.10 | | | DEL=.15 | | | DEL=.20 | | | DEL=.25 | | |
|---|---|---|---|---|---|---|---|---|---|---|---|---|---|---|---|
| FACT= | 1.0 .75 | .50 .25 | .00 BIN | 1.0 .75 | .50 .25 | .00 BIN | 1.0 .75 | .50 .25 | .00 BIN | 1.0 75 | .50 .25 | .00 BIN | 1.0 .75 | .50 .25 | .00 BIN |
| PCONT=*** | | | | REQUIRED NUMBER OF PATIENTS | | | | | | | | | | | |
| 0.05 *** | 698 | 701 | 746 | 248 | 251 | 265 | 146 | 148 | 155 | 103 | 105 | 109 | 81 | 82 | 84 |
| *** | 699 | 707 | 1285 | 249 | 256 | 409 | 147 | 151 | 216 | 104 | 107 | 138 | 81 | 83 | 97 |
| 0.1 *** | 1272 | 1279 | 1439 | 393 | 400 | 444 | 211 | 217 | 236 | 140 | 145 | 155 | 104 | 107 | 113 |
| *** | 1274 | 1293 | 2033 | 395 | 411 | 584 | 213 | 223 | 289 | 142 | 148 | 176 | 106 | 110 | 119 |
| 0.15 *** | 1759 | 1771 | 2109 | 508 | 521 | 609 | 261 | 271 | 307 | 168 | 175 | 193 | 122 | 127 | 137 |
| *** | 1763 | 1794 | 2687 | 513 | 541 | 736 | 265 | 283 | 351 | 171 | 182 | 208 | 124 | 131 | 138 |
| 0.2 *** | 2135 | 2153 | 2721 | 595 | 614 | 755 | 298 | 313 | 368 | 188 | 199 | 226 | 134 | 142 | 157 |
| *** | 2141 | 2188 | 3247 | 601 | 643 | 865 | 304 | 330 | 403 | 193 | 208 | 234 | 137 | 147 | 153 |
| 0.25 *** | 2395 | 2420 | 3256 | 653 | 679 | 879 | 322 | 343 | 419 | 202 | 216 | 252 | 142 | 152 | 172 |
| *** | 2403 | 2470 | 3714 | 662 | 720 | 970 | 330 | 366 | 444 | 207 | 228 | 255 | 146 | 160 | 164 |
| 0.3 *** | 2543 | 2577 | 3703 | 685 | 720 | 980 | 336 | 362 | 459 | 209 | 227 | 272 | 147 | 158 | 183 |
| *** | 2554 | 2646 | 4088 | 697 | 772 | 1052 | 346 | 391 | 475 | 217 | 242 | 269 | 152 | 168 | 171 |
| 0.35 *** | 2589 | 2635 | 4055 | 694 | 739 | 1056 | 341 | 372 | 488 | 212 | 232 | 285 | 149 | 161 | 189 |
| *** | 2605 | 2725 | 4368 | 710 | 802 | 1110 | 353 | 406 | 496 | 220 | 250 | 278 | 154 | 172 | 175 |
| 0.4 *** | 2547 | 2606 | 4308 | 684 | 739 | 1108 | 338 | 374 | 506 | 211 | 233 | 292 | 147 | 161 | 192 |
| *** | 2566 | 2722 | 4555 | 704 | 814 | 1145 | 353 | 412 | 507 | 220 | 253 | 281 | 153 | 173 | 175 |
| 0.45 *** | 2429 | 2505 | 4462 | 659 | 724 | 1134 | 329 | 369 | 512 | 206 | 230 | 292 | 143 | 158 | 190 |
| *** | 2454 | 2652 | 4649 | 683 | 809 | 1157 | 345 | 411 | 507 | 216 | 251 | 278 | 150 | 170 | 171 |
| 0.5 *** | 2252 | 2348 | 4513 | 623 | 697 | 1134 | 315 | 358 | 506 | 198 | 223 | 286 | 137 | 153 | 184 |
| *** | 2284 | 2529 | 4649 | 651 | 790 | 1145 | 333 | 402 | 496 | 208 | 245 | 269 | 144 | 165 | 164 |
| 0.55 *** | 2032 | 2153 | 4464 | 579 | 661 | 1109 | 297 | 342 | 490 | 187 | 212 | 274 | 129 | 144 | 174 |
| *** | 2073 | 2370 | 4555 | 610 | 759 | 1110 | 315 | 386 | 475 | 197 | 234 | 255 | 136 | 156 | 153 |
| 0.6 *** | 1786 | 1937 | 4312 | 530 | 617 | 1059 | 276 | 320 | 462 | 173 | 197 | 255 | 119 | 133 | 160 |
| *** | 1838 | 2186 | 4368 | 564 | 716 | 1052 | 294 | 363 | 444 | 183 | 218 | 234 | 125 | 144 | 138 |
| 0.65 *** | 1533 | 1714 | 4059 | 478 | 566 | 983 | 251 | 294 | 423 | 157 | 179 | 230 | 107 | 119 | 142 |
| *** | 1597 | 1987 | 4088 | 513 | 663 | 970 | 269 | 334 | 403 | 166 | 198 | 208 | 112 | 128 | 119 |
| 0.7 *** | 1289 | 1493 | 3706 | 424 | 508 | 882 | 223 | 262 | 372 | 138 | 157 | 198 | 92 | 102 | 120 |
| *** | 1364 | 1776 | 3714 | 457 | 600 | 865 | 240 | 298 | 351 | 146 | 173 | 176 | 97 | 110 | 97 |
| 0.75 *** | 1065 | 1279 | 3253 | 366 | 444 | 757 | 192 | 225 | 311 | 116 | 131 | 161 | . | . | . |
| *** | 1146 | 1555 | 3247 | 397 | 525 | 736 | 206 | 254 | 289 | 122 | 143 | 138 | . | . | . |
| 0.8 *** | 863 | 1068 | 2702 | 305 | 370 | 607 | 155 | 181 | 239 | . | . | . | . | . | . |
| *** | 942 | 1321 | 2687 | 331 | 436 | 584 | 166 | 202 | 216 | . | . | . | . | . | . |
| 0.85 *** | 675 | 852 | 2053 | 235 | 284 | 432 | . | . | . | . | . | . | . | . | . |
| *** | 744 | 1063 | 2033 | 256 | 330 | 409 | . | . | . | . | . | . | . | . | . |
| 0.9 *** | 482 | 613 | 1308 | . | . | . | . | . | . | . | . | . | . | . | . |
| *** | 534 | 760 | 1285 | . | . | . | . | . | . | . | . | . | . | . | . |

## TABLE 1: ALPHA= 0.005 POWER= 0.8    EXPECTED ACCRUAL THRU MINIMUM FOLLOW-UP= 130

|  |  | DEL=.05 | | | DEL=.10 | | | DEL=.15 | | | DEL=.20 | | | DEL=.25 | | |
|---|---|---|---|---|---|---|---|---|---|---|---|---|---|---|---|---|
| FACT= | | 1.0 .75 | .50 .25 | .00 BIN | 1.0 .75 | .50 .25 | .00 BIN | 1.0 .75 | .50 .25 | .00 BIN | 1.0 75 | .50 .25 | .00 BIN | 1.0 .75 | .50 .25 | .00 BIN |
| PCONT=*** | | | | | REQUIRED | NUMBER OF | PATIENTS | | | | | | | | | |
| 0.05 | *** | 698 | 701 | 746 | 248 | 252 | 265 | 146 | 148 | 155 | 103 | 105 | 109 | 81 | 82 | 84 |
|  | *** | 699 | 708 | 1285 | 250 | 256 | 409 | 147 | 151 | 216 | 104 | 107 | 138 | 81 | 83 | 97 |
| 0.1 | *** | 1273 | 1280 | 1439 | 393 | 401 | 444 | 211 | 218 | 236 | 141 | 145 | 155 | 105 | 108 | 113 |
|  | *** | 1275 | 1295 | 2033 | 396 | 413 | 584 | 214 | 224 | 289 | 143 | 149 | 176 | 106 | 110 | 119 |
| 0.15 | *** | 1760 | 1773 | 2109 | 510 | 523 | 609 | 262 | 273 | 307 | 169 | 176 | 193 | 122 | 127 | 137 |
|  | *** | 1764 | 1798 | 2687 | 514 | 543 | 736 | 266 | 284 | 351 | 172 | 183 | 208 | 125 | 131 | 138 |
| 0.2 | *** | 2136 | 2156 | 2721 | 596 | 617 | 755 | 299 | 315 | 368 | 189 | 200 | 226 | 135 | 142 | 157 |
|  | *** | 2143 | 2194 | 3247 | 604 | 647 | 865 | 305 | 332 | 403 | 194 | 210 | 234 | 138 | 148 | 153 |
| 0.25 | *** | 2397 | 2424 | 3256 | 655 | 683 | 879 | 324 | 345 | 419 | 203 | 217 | 252 | 144 | 153 | 172 |
|  | *** | 2406 | 2479 | 3714 | 665 | 725 | 970 | 333 | 368 | 444 | 209 | 230 | 255 | 148 | 160 | 164 |
| 0.3 | *** | 2546 | 2583 | 3703 | 688 | 725 | 980 | 339 | 366 | 459 | 211 | 229 | 272 | 148 | 160 | 183 |
|  | *** | 2558 | 2657 | 4088 | 701 | 779 | 1052 | 349 | 394 | 475 | 219 | 244 | 269 | 153 | 169 | 171 |
| 0.35 | *** | 2593 | 2642 | 4055 | 698 | 745 | 1056 | 344 | 376 | 488 | 215 | 235 | 285 | 150 | 163 | 189 |
|  | *** | 2610 | 2740 | 4368 | 715 | 811 | 1110 | 357 | 410 | 496 | 223 | 252 | 278 | 156 | 173 | 175 |
| 0.4 | *** | 2552 | 2615 | 4308 | 689 | 747 | 1108 | 342 | 379 | 506 | 213 | 236 | 292 | 149 | 163 | 192 |
|  | *** | 2573 | 2741 | 4555 | 710 | 823 | 1145 | 357 | 417 | 507 | 223 | 256 | 281 | 155 | 174 | 175 |
| 0.45 | *** | 2435 | 2517 | 4462 | 665 | 733 | 1134 | 334 | 374 | 512 | 209 | 232 | 292 | 145 | 160 | 190 |
|  | *** | 2463 | 2675 | 4649 | 691 | 820 | 1157 | 350 | 415 | 507 | 219 | 254 | 278 | 152 | 172 | 171 |
| 0.5 | *** | 2260 | 2364 | 4514 | 630 | 707 | 1134 | 320 | 363 | 506 | 200 | 225 | 286 | 139 | 154 | 184 |
|  | *** | 2295 | 2557 | 4649 | 660 | 802 | 1145 | 338 | 407 | 496 | 211 | 247 | 269 | 146 | 166 | 164 |
| 0.55 | *** | 2042 | 2173 | 4464 | 587 | 672 | 1109 | 302 | 347 | 490 | 190 | 214 | 274 | 131 | 146 | 174 |
|  | *** | 2086 | 2402 | 4555 | 620 | 771 | 1110 | 321 | 391 | 475 | 200 | 236 | 255 | 137 | 157 | 153 |
| 0.6 | *** | 1799 | 1961 | 4312 | 539 | 628 | 1059 | 281 | 325 | 462 | 176 | 200 | 255 | 121 | 134 | 160 |
|  | *** | 1855 | 2221 | 4368 | 574 | 728 | 1052 | 299 | 368 | 444 | 186 | 220 | 234 | 127 | 145 | 138 |
| 0.65 | *** | 1549 | 1741 | 4059 | 487 | 577 | 983 | 256 | 299 | 423 | 160 | 182 | 230 | 108 | 120 | 142 |
|  | *** | 1617 | 2024 | 4088 | 523 | 675 | 970 | 274 | 338 | 403 | 169 | 200 | 208 | 114 | 129 | 119 |
| 0.7 | *** | 1309 | 1522 | 3706 | 433 | 519 | 882 | 228 | 267 | 372 | 140 | 159 | 198 | 94 | 103 | 120 |
|  | *** | 1387 | 1813 | 3714 | 467 | 610 | 865 | 244 | 302 | 351 | 149 | 174 | 176 | 98 | 110 | 97 |
| 0.75 | *** | 1087 | 1307 | 3253 | 375 | 453 | 757 | 196 | 229 | 311 | 118 | 133 | 161 | . | . | . |
|  | *** | 1170 | 1591 | 3247 | 406 | 534 | 736 | 210 | 257 | 289 | 124 | 144 | 138 | . | . | . |
| 0.8 | *** | 884 | 1095 | 2702 | 312 | 378 | 607 | 158 | 183 | 239 | . | . | . | . | . | . |
|  | *** | 965 | 1353 | 2687 | 339 | 444 | 584 | 169 | 204 | 216 | . | . | . | . | . | . |
| 0.85 | *** | 693 | 875 | 2053 | 241 | 290 | 432 | . | . | . | . | . | . | . | . | . |
|  | *** | 764 | 1089 | 2033 | 261 | 335 | 409 | . | . | . | . | . | . | . | . | . |
| 0.9 | *** | 496 | 629 | 1308 | . | . | . | . | . | . | . | . | . | . | . | . |
|  | *** | 549 | 777 | 1285 | . | . | . | . | . | . | . | . | . | . | . | . |

TABLE 1: ALPHA= 0.005 POWER= 0.8　　EXPECTED ACCRUAL THRU MINIMUM FOLLOW-UP= 140

| PCONT= | | DEL=.05 | | | DEL=.10 | | | DEL=.15 | | | DEL=.20 | | | DEL=.25 | | |
|---|---|---|---|---|---|---|---|---|---|---|---|---|---|---|---|---|
| FACT= | | 1.0 / .75 | .50 / .25 | .00 / BIN | 1.0 / .75 | .50 / .25 | .00 / BIN | 1.0 / .75 | .50 / .25 | .00 / BIN | 1.0 / 75 | .50 / .25 | .00 / BIN | 1.0 / .75 | .50 / .25 | .00 / BIN |
| | | REQUIRED NUMBER OF PATIENTS | | | | | | | | | | | | | | |
| 0.05 | *** | 698 | 702 | 746 | 249 | 252 | 265 | 146 | 149 | 155 | 104 | 105 | 109 | 81 | 82 | 84 |
| | *** | 700 | 709 | 1285 | 250 | 256 | 409 | 147 | 151 | 216 | 104 | 107 | 138 | 81 | 83 | 97 |
| 0.1 | *** | 1273 | 1281 | 1439 | 394 | 403 | 444 | 212 | 218 | 236 | 141 | 146 | 155 | 105 | 108 | 113 |
| | *** | 1276 | 1297 | 2033 | 397 | 414 | 584 | 214 | 224 | 289 | 143 | 149 | 176 | 106 | 110 | 119 |
| 0.15 | *** | 1761 | 1775 | 2109 | 511 | 525 | 609 | 263 | 274 | 307 | 170 | 177 | 193 | 123 | 128 | 137 |
| | *** | 1766 | 1802 | 2687 | 516 | 546 | 736 | 267 | 285 | 351 | 173 | 183 | 208 | 125 | 132 | 138 |
| 0.2 | *** | 2138 | 2159 | 2721 | 598 | 620 | 755 | 301 | 317 | 368 | 190 | 201 | 226 | 136 | 143 | 157 |
| | *** | 2145 | 2200 | 3247 | 606 | 651 | 865 | 307 | 333 | 403 | 195 | 210 | 234 | 139 | 148 | 153 |
| 0.25 | *** | 2399 | 2428 | 3256 | 657 | 687 | 879 | 326 | 348 | 419 | 205 | 219 | 252 | 145 | 154 | 172 |
| | *** | 2409 | 2487 | 3714 | 668 | 730 | 970 | 335 | 370 | 444 | 211 | 231 | 255 | 149 | 161 | 164 |
| 0.3 | *** | 2549 | 2589 | 3703 | 691 | 730 | 980 | 342 | 369 | 459 | 213 | 230 | 272 | 150 | 161 | 183 |
| | *** | 2562 | 2668 | 4088 | 705 | 785 | 1052 | 352 | 397 | 475 | 220 | 245 | 269 | 154 | 169 | 171 |
| 0.35 | *** | 2597 | 2650 | 4055 | 702 | 752 | 1056 | 348 | 380 | 488 | 217 | 237 | 285 | 152 | 164 | 189 |
| | *** | 2615 | 2754 | 4368 | 720 | 818 | 1110 | 360 | 413 | 496 | 225 | 254 | 278 | 157 | 174 | 175 |
| 0.4 | *** | 2556 | 2625 | 4309 | 694 | 754 | 1108 | 346 | 383 | 506 | 216 | 238 | 292 | 151 | 164 | 192 |
| | *** | 2579 | 2759 | 4555 | 716 | 832 | 1145 | 361 | 420 | 507 | 225 | 257 | 281 | 156 | 175 | 175 |
| 0.45 | *** | 2442 | 2530 | 4462 | 672 | 742 | 1134 | 338 | 379 | 512 | 211 | 235 | 292 | 147 | 161 | 190 |
| | *** | 2471 | 2697 | 4649 | 698 | 829 | 1157 | 354 | 420 | 507 | 221 | 256 | 278 | 153 | 173 | 171 |
| 0.5 | *** | 2268 | 2380 | 4514 | 638 | 717 | 1134 | 325 | 368 | 506 | 203 | 228 | 286 | 141 | 156 | 184 |
| | *** | 2305 | 2584 | 4649 | 668 | 812 | 1145 | 342 | 411 | 496 | 214 | 249 | 269 | 147 | 167 | 164 |
| 0.55 | *** | 2052 | 2193 | 4464 | 595 | 682 | 1109 | 307 | 352 | 490 | 192 | 217 | 274 | 133 | 147 | 174 |
| | *** | 2100 | 2433 | 4555 | 629 | 781 | 1110 | 325 | 395 | 475 | 203 | 238 | 255 | 139 | 158 | 153 |
| 0.6 | *** | 1812 | 1984 | 4312 | 548 | 638 | 1059 | 286 | 330 | 462 | 179 | 202 | 255 | 122 | 136 | 160 |
| | *** | 1872 | 2255 | 4368 | 583 | 739 | 1052 | 304 | 372 | 444 | 189 | 222 | 234 | 128 | 146 | 138 |
| 0.65 | *** | 1565 | 1767 | 4059 | 496 | 587 | 983 | 261 | 303 | 423 | 162 | 184 | 230 | 110 | 121 | 142 |
| | *** | 1638 | 2059 | 4088 | 532 | 685 | 970 | 278 | 342 | 403 | 171 | 201 | 208 | 115 | 130 | 119 |
| 0.7 | *** | 1327 | 1549 | 3706 | 441 | 528 | 882 | 232 | 271 | 372 | 143 | 161 | 198 | 95 | 104 | 120 |
| | *** | 1410 | 1849 | 3714 | 476 | 620 | 865 | 248 | 305 | 351 | 151 | 176 | 176 | 99 | 111 | 97 |
| 0.75 | *** | 1107 | 1335 | 3253 | 383 | 462 | 757 | 199 | 232 | 311 | 119 | 134 | 161 | . | . | . |
| | *** | 1194 | 1624 | 3247 | 415 | 542 | 736 | 213 | 260 | 289 | 126 | 145 | 138 | . | . | . |
| 0.8 | *** | 904 | 1120 | 2702 | 319 | 385 | 607 | 161 | 186 | 239 | . | . | . | . | . | . |
| | *** | 988 | 1383 | 2687 | 346 | 450 | 584 | 172 | 206 | 216 | . | . | . | . | . | . |
| 0.85 | *** | 711 | 897 | 2053 | 246 | 295 | 432 | . | . | . | . | . | . | . | . | . |
| | *** | 784 | 1113 | 2033 | 266 | 339 | 409 | . | . | . | . | . | . | . | . | . |
| 0.9 | *** | 510 | 645 | 1308 | . | . | . | . | . | . | . | . | . | . | . | . |
| | *** | 563 | 793 | 1285 | . | . | . | . | . | . | . | . | . | . | . | . |

## TABLE 1: ALPHA= 0.005 POWER= 0.8     EXPECTED ACCRUAL THRU MINIMUM FOLLOW-UP= 150

| | | DEL=.05 | | | DEL=.10 | | | DEL=.15 | | | DEL=.20 | | | DEL=.25 | | |
|---|---|---|---|---|---|---|---|---|---|---|---|---|---|---|---|---|
| FACT= | | 1.0 .75 | .50 .25 | .00 BIN | 1.0 .75 | .50 .25 | .00 BIN | 1.0 .75 | .50 .25 | .00 BIN | 1.0 75 | .50 .25 | .00 BIN | 1.0 .75 | .50 .25 | .00 BIN |
| PCONT=*** | | REQUIRED NUMBER OF PATIENTS | | | | | | | | | | | | | | |
| 0.05 | *** | 698 | 703 | 746 | 249 | 253 | 265 | 146 | 149 | 155 | 104 | 106 | 109 | 81 | 82 | 84 |
| | *** | 700 | 710 | 1285 | 250 | 257 | 409 | 147 | 151 | 216 | 105 | 107 | 138 | 82 | 83 | 97 |
| 0.1 | *** | 1274 | 1282 | 1439 | 395 | 404 | 444 | 212 | 219 | 236 | 142 | 146 | 155 | 105 | 108 | 113 |
| | *** | 1277 | 1299 | 2033 | 398 | 415 | 584 | 215 | 225 | 289 | 143 | 149 | 176 | 107 | 110 | 119 |
| 0.15 | *** | 1762 | 1777 | 2109 | 512 | 527 | 609 | 264 | 275 | 307 | 170 | 178 | 193 | 123 | 128 | 137 |
| | *** | 1767 | 1806 | 2687 | 517 | 548 | 736 | 268 | 286 | 351 | 173 | 184 | 208 | 126 | 132 | 138 |
| 0.2 | *** | 2139 | 2162 | 2721 | 600 | 623 | 755 | 302 | 318 | 368 | 191 | 202 | 226 | 137 | 144 | 157 |
| | *** | 2147 | 2206 | 3247 | 608 | 654 | 865 | 309 | 335 | 403 | 196 | 211 | 234 | 140 | 149 | 153 |
| 0.25 | *** | 2401 | 2432 | 3256 | 660 | 691 | 879 | 328 | 350 | 419 | 206 | 220 | 252 | 146 | 155 | 172 |
| | *** | 2411 | 2495 | 3714 | 671 | 734 | 970 | 337 | 372 | 444 | 212 | 232 | 255 | 149 | 161 | 164 |
| 0.3 | *** | 2552 | 2594 | 3703 | 694 | 735 | 980 | 344 | 371 | 459 | 215 | 232 | 272 | 151 | 162 | 183 |
| | *** | 2566 | 2679 | 4088 | 709 | 791 | 1052 | 355 | 399 | 475 | 222 | 247 | 269 | 156 | 170 | 171 |
| 0.35 | *** | 2601 | 2658 | 4055 | 706 | 758 | 1056 | 350 | 383 | 488 | 219 | 238 | 285 | 153 | 165 | 189 |
| | *** | 2620 | 2769 | 4368 | 725 | 825 | 1110 | 364 | 416 | 496 | 227 | 256 | 278 | 158 | 175 | 175 |
| 0.4 | *** | 2561 | 2635 | 4308 | 699 | 761 | 1108 | 349 | 387 | 506 | 218 | 240 | 292 | 152 | 165 | 192 |
| | *** | 2586 | 2777 | 4555 | 722 | 840 | 1145 | 364 | 424 | 507 | 227 | 259 | 281 | 158 | 176 | 175 |
| 0.45 | *** | 2448 | 2542 | 4462 | 677 | 750 | 1134 | 342 | 383 | 512 | 214 | 237 | 292 | 148 | 163 | 190 |
| | *** | 2479 | 2719 | 4649 | 705 | 839 | 1157 | 358 | 423 | 507 | 224 | 257 | 278 | 155 | 173 | 171 |
| 0.5 | *** | 2276 | 2396 | 4514 | 644 | 726 | 1134 | 329 | 373 | 506 | 206 | 230 | 286 | 142 | 157 | 184 |
| | *** | 2316 | 2610 | 4649 | 676 | 822 | 1145 | 347 | 415 | 496 | 216 | 251 | 269 | 149 | 168 | 164 |
| 0.55 | *** | 2062 | 2212 | 4463 | 603 | 691 | 1109 | 311 | 356 | 490 | 195 | 219 | 274 | 134 | 148 | 174 |
| | *** | 2113 | 2462 | 4555 | 637 | 791 | 1110 | 330 | 399 | 475 | 205 | 239 | 255 | 140 | 159 | 153 |
| 0.6 | *** | 1825 | 2006 | 4312 | 556 | 648 | 1059 | 290 | 335 | 462 | 181 | 204 | 255 | 124 | 137 | 160 |
| | *** | 1888 | 2287 | 4368 | 592 | 749 | 1052 | 308 | 376 | 444 | 191 | 223 | 234 | 130 | 146 | 138 |
| 0.65 | *** | 1581 | 1792 | 4059 | 505 | 596 | 983 | 265 | 307 | 423 | 164 | 186 | 230 | 111 | 122 | 142 |
| | *** | 1657 | 2092 | 4088 | 541 | 695 | 970 | 283 | 346 | 403 | 174 | 203 | 208 | 116 | 131 | 119 |
| 0.7 | *** | 1346 | 1576 | 3706 | 450 | 537 | 882 | 236 | 274 | 372 | 145 | 163 | 198 | 96 | 105 | 120 |
| | *** | 1431 | 1882 | 3714 | 485 | 629 | 865 | 252 | 308 | 351 | 152 | 177 | 176 | 100 | 111 | 97 |
| 0.75 | *** | 1127 | 1361 | 3253 | 390 | 470 | 757 | 203 | 235 | 311 | 121 | 135 | 161 | . | . | . |
| | *** | 1216 | 1656 | 3247 | 423 | 550 | 736 | 216 | 262 | 289 | 127 | 146 | 138 | . | . | . |
| 0.8 | *** | 923 | 1144 | 2702 | 325 | 392 | 607 | 164 | 188 | 239 | . | . | . | . | . | . |
| | *** | 1009 | 1411 | 2687 | 353 | 456 | 584 | 174 | 207 | 216 | . | . | . | . | . | . |
| 0.85 | *** | 728 | 917 | 2053 | 251 | 299 | 432 | . | . | . | . | . | . | . | . | . |
| | *** | 802 | 1136 | 2033 | 271 | 343 | 409 | . | . | . | . | . | . | . | . | . |
| 0.9 | *** | 522 | 659 | 1308 | . | . | . | . | . | . | . | . | . | . | . | . |
| | *** | 577 | 808 | 1285 | . | . | . | . | . | . | . | . | . | . | . | . |

TABLE 1: ALPHA= 0.005 POWER= 0.8 EXPECTED ACCRUAL THRU MINIMUM FOLLOW-UP= 160

| | | DEL=.05 | | | DEL=.10 | | | DEL=.15 | | | DEL=.20 | | | DEL=.25 | |
|---|---|---|---|---|---|---|---|---|---|---|---|---|---|---|---|
| FACT= | 1.0 .75 | .50 .25 | .00 BIN | 1.0 .75 | .50 .25 | .00 BIN | 1.0 .75 | .50 .25 | .00 BIN | 1.0 75 | .50 .25 | .00 BIN | 1.0 .75 | .50 .25 | .00 BIN |
| PCONT=*** | | | | REQUIRED NUMBER OF PATIENTS | | | | | | | | | | | |
| 0.05 *** | 699 | 703 | 746 | 249 | 253 | 265 | 147 | 149 | 155 | 104 | 106 | 109 | 81 | 82 | 84 |
| *** | 700 | 711 | 1285 | 251 | 257 | 409 | 148 | 151 | 216 | 105 | 107 | 138 | 82 | 83 | 97 |
| 0.1 *** | 1274 | 1284 | 1439 | 395 | 405 | 444 | 213 | 220 | 236 | 142 | 146 | 155 | 106 | 109 | 113 |
| *** | 1277 | 1302 | 2033 | 399 | 416 | 584 | 216 | 226 | 289 | 144 | 150 | 176 | 107 | 111 | 119 |
| 0.15 *** | 1763 | 1779 | 2109 | 513 | 529 | 609 | 265 | 276 | 307 | 171 | 178 | 193 | 124 | 129 | 137 |
| *** | 1768 | 1810 | 2687 | 519 | 550 | 736 | 269 | 287 | 351 | 174 | 184 | 208 | 126 | 132 | 138 |
| 0.2 *** | 2141 | 2165 | 2721 | 601 | 625 | 755 | 304 | 320 | 368 | 193 | 203 | 226 | 137 | 144 | 157 |
| *** | 2149 | 2212 | 3247 | 610 | 657 | 865 | 310 | 336 | 403 | 197 | 212 | 234 | 140 | 149 | 153 |
| 0.25 *** | 2403 | 2437 | 3256 | 662 | 695 | 879 | 330 | 352 | 419 | 207 | 221 | 252 | 146 | 155 | 172 |
| *** | 2414 | 2503 | 3714 | 674 | 739 | 970 | 339 | 374 | 444 | 213 | 233 | 255 | 150 | 162 | 164 |
| 0.3 *** | 2554 | 2600 | 3703 | 697 | 740 | 980 | 346 | 374 | 459 | 217 | 233 | 272 | 152 | 163 | 183 |
| *** | 2570 | 2690 | 4068 | 713 | 796 | 1052 | 357 | 402 | 475 | 224 | 248 | 269 | 157 | 171 | 171 |
| 0.35 *** | 2605 | 2665 | 4055 | 710 | 763 | 1056 | 353 | 386 | 488 | 221 | 240 | 285 | 154 | 166 | 189 |
| *** | 2625 | 2783 | 4368 | 730 | 832 | 1110 | 367 | 419 | 496 | 229 | 257 | 278 | 159 | 176 | 175 |
| 0.4 *** | 2566 | 2645 | 4308 | 704 | 768 | 1108 | 353 | 390 | 506 | 220 | 242 | 292 | 153 | 167 | 192 |
| *** | 2593 | 2795 | 4555 | 728 | 848 | 1145 | 368 | 427 | 507 | 229 | 261 | 281 | 159 | 177 | 175 |
| 0.45 *** | 2454 | 2555 | 4462 | 683 | 758 | 1134 | 345 | 387 | 512 | 216 | 239 | 292 | 150 | 164 | 190 |
| *** | 2488 | 2741 | 4649 | 712 | 847 | 1157 | 362 | 427 | 507 | 226 | 259 | 278 | 156 | 174 | 171 |
| 0.5 *** | 2284 | 2411 | 4514 | 651 | 734 | 1134 | 333 | 377 | 506 | 208 | 232 | 286 | 144 | 158 | 184 |
| *** | 2327 | 2635 | 4649 | 683 | 831 | 1145 | 351 | 418 | 496 | 218 | 252 | 269 | 150 | 169 | 164 |
| 0.55 *** | 2073 | 2231 | 4464 | 611 | 700 | 1109 | 315 | 361 | 490 | 197 | 221 | 274 | 136 | 149 | 174 |
| *** | 2127 | 2491 | 4555 | 646 | 801 | 1110 | 334 | 403 | 475 | 208 | 241 | 255 | 142 | 159 | 153 |
| 0.6 *** | 1838 | 2028 | 4312 | 564 | 657 | 1059 | 294 | 339 | 462 | 183 | 206 | 255 | 125 | 138 | 160 |
| *** | 1905 | 2318 | 4368 | 601 | 758 | 1052 | 313 | 379 | 444 | 193 | 225 | 234 | 131 | 147 | 138 |
| 0.65 *** | 1597 | 1816 | 4059 | 513 | 606 | 983 | 269 | 311 | 423 | 166 | 187 | 230 | 112 | 123 | 142 |
| *** | 1677 | 2125 | 4088 | 550 | 704 | 970 | 287 | 349 | 403 | 176 | 204 | 208 | 117 | 131 | 119 |
| 0.7 *** | 1364 | 1601 | 3706 | 457 | 546 | 882 | 240 | 278 | 372 | 146 | 164 | 198 | 97 | 106 | 120 |
| *** | 1453 | 1914 | 3714 | 493 | 637 | 865 | 256 | 311 | 351 | 154 | 178 | 176 | 101 | 112 | 97 |
| 0.75 *** | 1146 | 1386 | 3253 | 398 | 477 | 757 | 206 | 238 | 311 | 123 | 136 | 161 | . | . | . |
| *** | 1238 | 1686 | 3247 | 430 | 557 | 736 | 219 | 265 | 289 | 129 | 147 | 138 | . | . | . |
| 0.8 *** | 942 | 1168 | 2702 | 332 | 398 | 607 | 166 | 190 | 239 | . | . | . | . | . | . |
| *** | 1030 | 1437 | 2687 | 359 | 462 | 584 | 177 | 209 | 216 | . | . | . | . | . | . |
| 0.85 *** | 744 | 936 | 2053 | 256 | 304 | 432 | . | . | . | . | . | . | . | . | . |
| *** | 820 | 1157 | 2033 | 276 | 347 | 409 | . | . | . | . | . | . | . | . | . |
| 0.9 *** | 534 | 673 | 1308 | . | . | . | . | . | . | . | . | . | . | . | . |
| *** | 589 | 822 | 1285 | . | . | . | . | . | . | . | . | . | . | . | . |

## TABLE 1: ALPHA= 0.005 POWER= 0.8    EXPECTED ACCRUAL THRU MINIMUM FOLLOW-UP= 170

| | DEL=.05 | | | DEL=.10 | | | DEL=.15 | | | DEL=.20 | | | DEL=.25 | | |
|---|---|---|---|---|---|---|---|---|---|---|---|---|---|---|---|
| FACT= | 1.0 .75 | .50 .25 | .00 BIN | 1.0 .75 | .50 .25 | .00 BIN | 1.0 .75 | .50 .25 | .00 BIN | 1.0 75 | .50 .25 | .00 BIN | 1.0 .75 | .50 .25 | .00 BIN |

PCONT=***                     REQUIRED NUMBER OF PATIENTS

| PCONT | 1.0/.75 | .50/.25 | .00/BIN | 1.0/.75 | .50/.25 | .00/BIN | 1.0/.75 | .50/.25 | .00/BIN | 1.0/75 | .50/.25 | .00/BIN | 1.0/.75 | .50/.25 | .00/BIN |
|---|---|---|---|---|---|---|---|---|---|---|---|---|---|---|---|
| 0.05 *** | 699 | 704 | 746 | 249 | 253 | 265 | 147 | 149 | 155 | 104 | 106 | 109 | 81 | 82 | 84 |
| *** | 701 | 711 | 1285 | 251 | 258 | 409 | 148 | 152 | 216 | 105 | 107 | 138 | 82 | 83 | 97 |
| 0.1 *** | 1275 | 1285 | 1439 | 396 | 406 | 444 | 214 | 220 | 236 | 143 | 147 | 155 | 106 | 109 | 113 |
| *** | 1278 | 1304 | 2033 | 399 | 417 | 584 | 216 | 226 | 289 | 144 | 150 | 176 | 107 | 111 | 119 |
| 0.15 *** | 1764 | 1781 | 2109 | 514 | 531 | 609 | 266 | 277 | 307 | 172 | 179 | 193 | 124 | 129 | 137 |
| *** | 1770 | 1813 | 2687 | 520 | 552 | 736 | 270 | 288 | 351 | 175 | 185 | 208 | 126 | 133 | 138 |
| 0.2 *** | 2142 | 2167 | 2721 | 603 | 628 | 755 | 305 | 322 | 368 | 194 | 204 | 226 | 138 | 145 | 157 |
| *** | 2151 | 2217 | 3247 | 612 | 660 | 865 | 312 | 338 | 403 | 198 | 212 | 234 | 141 | 150 | 153 |
| 0.25 *** | 2405 | 2441 | 3256 | 664 | 698 | 879 | 332 | 354 | 419 | 209 | 222 | 252 | 147 | 156 | 172 |
| *** | 2417 | 2511 | 3714 | 677 | 743 | 970 | 341 | 376 | 444 | 215 | 234 | 255 | 151 | 163 | 164 |
| 0.3 *** | 2557 | 2606 | 3703 | 700 | 744 | 980 | 349 | 377 | 459 | 218 | 235 | 272 | 153 | 163 | 183 |
| *** | 2574 | 2701 | 4088 | 716 | 801 | 1052 | 360 | 404 | 475 | 225 | 249 | 269 | 157 | 171 | 171 |
| 0.35 *** | 2608 | 2673 | 4055 | 714 | 769 | 1056 | 356 | 389 | 488 | 222 | 242 | 285 | 155 | 167 | 189 |
| *** | 2630 | 2797 | 4368 | 734 | 838 | 1110 | 370 | 422 | 496 | 231 | 258 | 278 | 160 | 176 | 175 |
| 0.4 *** | 2571 | 2655 | 4308 | 709 | 775 | 1108 | 356 | 394 | 506 | 222 | 244 | 292 | 154 | 168 | 192 |
| *** | 2599 | 2813 | 4555 | 734 | 855 | 1145 | 371 | 430 | 507 | 231 | 262 | 281 | 160 | 177 | 175 |
| 0.45 *** | 2460 | 2567 | 4462 | 689 | 765 | 1134 | 349 | 390 | 512 | 218 | 241 | 292 | 151 | 165 | 190 |
| *** | 2496 | 2762 | 4649 | 718 | 855 | 1157 | 366 | 430 | 507 | 228 | 260 | 278 | 157 | 175 | 171 |
| 0.5 *** | 2292 | 2427 | 4513 | 657 | 743 | 1134 | 337 | 381 | 507 | 210 | 234 | 286 | 145 | 159 | 184 |
| *** | 2338 | 2660 | 4649 | 690 | 839 | 1145 | 355 | 422 | 496 | 221 | 254 | 269 | 151 | 169 | 164 |
| 0.55 *** | 2083 | 2249 | 4464 | 618 | 709 | 1109 | 319 | 364 | 490 | 199 | 223 | 274 | 137 | 150 | 174 |
| *** | 2140 | 2518 | 4555 | 653 | 810 | 1110 | 338 | 406 | 475 | 210 | 242 | 255 | 143 | 160 | 153 |
| 0.6 *** | 1851 | 2050 | 4312 | 571 | 666 | 1059 | 298 | 342 | 462 | 185 | 208 | 255 | 126 | 139 | 160 |
| *** | 1921 | 2348 | 4368 | 609 | 767 | 1052 | 317 | 383 | 444 | 195 | 226 | 234 | 132 | 148 | 138 |
| 0.65 *** | 1612 | 1840 | 4059 | 520 | 614 | 983 | 273 | 315 | 423 | 168 | 189 | 230 | 113 | 124 | 142 |
| *** | 1695 | 2155 | 4088 | 558 | 712 | 970 | 290 | 352 | 403 | 177 | 205 | 208 | 118 | 132 | 119 |
| 0.7 *** | 1381 | 1626 | 3706 | 465 | 554 | 882 | 243 | 281 | 372 | 148 | 166 | 198 | 98 | 106 | 120 |
| *** | 1473 | 1944 | 3714 | 501 | 645 | 865 | 259 | 313 | 351 | 156 | 179 | 176 | 102 | 112 | 97 |
| 0.75 *** | 1164 | 1410 | 3253 | 404 | 485 | 757 | 209 | 240 | 311 | 124 | 137 | 161 | . | . | . |
| *** | 1258 | 1715 | 3247 | 437 | 564 | 736 | 222 | 266 | 289 | 130 | 147 | 138 | . | . | . |
| 0.8 *** | 960 | 1190 | 2702 | 337 | 404 | 607 | 168 | 192 | 239 | . | . | . | . | . | . |
| *** | 1049 | 1462 | 2687 | 365 | 467 | 584 | 179 | 210 | 216 | . | . | . | . | . | . |
| 0.85 *** | 759 | 955 | 2053 | 260 | 308 | 432 | . | . | . | . | . | . | . | . | . |
| *** | 836 | 1177 | 2033 | 280 | 350 | 409 | . | . | . | . | . | . | . | . | . |
| 0.9 *** | 545 | 685 | 1308 | . | . | . | . | . | . | . | . | . | . | . | . |
| *** | 602 | 835 | 1285 | . | . | . | . | . | . | . | . | . | . | . | . |

TABLE 1: ALPHA= 0.005 POWER= 0.8    EXPECTED ACCRUAL THRU MINIMUM FOLLOW-UP= 180

| | | DEL=.05 | | | DEL=.10 | | | DEL=.15 | | | DEL=.20 | | | DEL=.25 | | |
|---|---|---|---|---|---|---|---|---|---|---|---|---|---|---|---|---|---|
| FACT= | | 1.0 .75 | .50 .25 | .00 BIN | 1.0 .75 | .50 .25 | .00 BIN | 1.0 .75 | .50 .25 | .00 BIN | 1.0 75 | .50 .25 | .00 BIN | 1.0 .75 | .50 .25 | .00 BIN |
| PCONT=*** | | | | REQUIRED NUMBER OF PATIENTS | | | | | | | | | | | | |
| 0.05 | *** | 699 | 704 | 746 | 250 | 254 | 265 | 147 | 150 | 155 | 104 | 106 | 109 | 81 | 83 | 84 |
| | *** | 701 | 712 | 1285 | 251 | 258 | 409 | 148 | 152 | 216 | 105 | 107 | 138 | 82 | 83 | 97 |
| 0.1 | *** | 1275 | 1286 | 1439 | 397 | 407 | 444 | 214 | 221 | 236 | 143 | 147 | 155 | 106 | 109 | 113 |
| | *** | 1279 | 1306 | 2033 | 400 | 418 | 584 | 217 | 226 | 289 | 145 | 150 | 176 | 107 | 111 | 119 |
| 0.15 | *** | 1765 | 1783 | 2109 | 515 | 532 | 609 | 267 | 278 | 307 | 172 | 180 | 193 | 125 | 129 | 137 |
| | *** | 1771 | 1817 | 2687 | 521 | 554 | 736 | 271 | 289 | 351 | 175 | 185 | 208 | 127 | 133 | 138 |
| 0.2 | *** | 2144 | 2170 | 2721 | 605 | 630 | 755 | 306 | 323 | 368 | 194 | 205 | 226 | 139 | 145 | 157 |
| | *** | 2153 | 2223 | 3247 | 614 | 663 | 865 | 313 | 339 | 403 | 199 | 213 | 234 | 141 | 150 | 153 |
| 0.25 | *** | 2407 | 2445 | 3256 | 667 | 702 | 879 | 334 | 356 | 419 | 210 | 223 | 252 | 148 | 157 | 172 |
| | *** | 2420 | 2519 | 3714 | 679 | 747 | 970 | 343 | 378 | 444 | 216 | 235 | 255 | 152 | 163 | 164 |
| 0.3 | *** | 2560 | 2612 | 3703 | 703 | 749 | 980 | 351 | 379 | 459 | 219 | 236 | 272 | 154 | 164 | 183 |
| | *** | 2577 | 2712 | 4088 | 720 | 806 | 1052 | 362 | 406 | 475 | 227 | 250 | 269 | 158 | 172 | 171 |
| 0.35 | *** | 2612 | 2680 | 4055 | 717 | 774 | 1056 | 359 | 392 | 488 | 224 | 243 | 285 | 156 | 168 | 189 |
| | *** | 2635 | 2811 | 4368 | 739 | 844 | 1110 | 372 | 424 | 496 | 232 | 259 | 278 | 162 | 177 | 175 |
| 0.4 | *** | 2576 | 2664 | 4308 | 713 | 781 | 1108 | 359 | 397 | 506 | 224 | 245 | 292 | 156 | 168 | 192 |
| | *** | 2606 | 2830 | 4555 | 739 | 862 | 1145 | 374 | 433 | 507 | 233 | 263 | 281 | 161 | 178 | 175 |
| 0.45 | *** | 2467 | 2580 | 4462 | 694 | 772 | 1134 | 352 | 394 | 512 | 220 | 243 | 292 | 152 | 166 | 190 |
| | *** | 2505 | 2783 | 4649 | 724 | 863 | 1157 | 369 | 433 | 507 | 230 | 262 | 278 | 158 | 176 | 171 |
| 0.5 | *** | 2300 | 2442 | 4513 | 664 | 750 | 1134 | 340 | 384 | 506 | 212 | 236 | 286 | 147 | 160 | 184 |
| | *** | 2348 | 2684 | 4649 | 697 | 847 | 1145 | 358 | 425 | 496 | 223 | 255 | 269 | 153 | 170 | 164 |
| 0.55 | *** | 2093 | 2267 | 4464 | 624 | 717 | 1109 | 323 | 368 | 490 | 201 | 225 | 274 | 138 | 151 | 174 |
| | *** | 2153 | 2545 | 4555 | 661 | 818 | 1110 | 342 | 409 | 475 | 212 | 244 | 255 | 144 | 161 | 153 |
| 0.6 | *** | 1863 | 2071 | 4312 | 579 | 674 | 1059 | 302 | 346 | 462 | 187 | 210 | 255 | 128 | 140 | 160 |
| | *** | 1937 | 2376 | 4368 | 617 | 776 | 1052 | 320 | 386 | 444 | 197 | 227 | 234 | 133 | 148 | 138 |
| 0.65 | *** | 1628 | 1863 | 4059 | 528 | 622 | 983 | 276 | 318 | 423 | 170 | 191 | 230 | 114 | 125 | 142 |
| | *** | 1714 | 2184 | 4088 | 566 | 720 | 970 | 294 | 354 | 403 | 179 | 206 | 208 | 119 | 132 | 119 |
| 0.7 | *** | 1398 | 1650 | 3706 | 472 | 562 | 882 | 246 | 284 | 372 | 150 | 167 | 198 | 99 | 107 | 120 |
| | *** | 1493 | 1973 | 3714 | 508 | 652 | 865 | 262 | 316 | 351 | 157 | 180 | 176 | 102 | 113 | 97 |
| 0.75 | *** | 1182 | 1433 | 3253 | 411 | 491 | 757 | 211 | 243 | 311 | 125 | 138 | 161 | . | . | . |
| | *** | 1279 | 1742 | 3247 | 444 | 570 | 736 | 225 | 268 | 289 | 131 | 148 | 138 | . | . | . |
| 0.8 | *** | 977 | 1211 | 2702 | 343 | 409 | 607 | 170 | 194 | 239 | . | . | . | . | . | . |
| | *** | 1068 | 1486 | 2687 | 370 | 472 | 584 | 181 | 211 | 216 | . | . | . | . | . | . |
| 0.85 | *** | 774 | 972 | 2053 | 264 | 312 | 432 | . | . | . | . | . | . | . | . | . |
| | *** | 852 | 1196 | 2033 | 284 | 353 | 409 | . | . | . | . | . | . | . | . | . |
| 0.9 | *** | 556 | 697 | 1308 | . | . | . | . | . | . | . | . | . | . | . | . |
| | *** | 613 | 847 | 1285 | . | . | . | . | . | . | . | . | . | . | . | . |

## TABLE 1: ALPHA= 0.005 POWER= 0.8    EXPECTED ACCRUAL THRU MINIMUM FOLLOW-UP= 190

| | | DEL=.05 | | | DEL=.10 | | | DEL=.15 | | | DEL=.20 | | | DEL=.25 | | |
|---|---|---|---|---|---|---|---|---|---|---|---|---|---|---|---|---|---|
| FACT= | | 1.0 .75 | .50 .25 | .00 BIN | 1.0 .75 | .50 .25 | .00 BIN | 1.0 .75 | .50 .25 | .00 BIN | 1.0 75 | .50 .25 | .00 BIN | 1.0 .75 | .50 .25 | .00 BIN |
| PCONT=*** | | | | | | REQUIRED NUMBER OF PATIENTS | | | | | | | | | | |
| 0.05 | *** | 700 | 705 | 746 | 250 | 254 | 265 | 147 | 150 | 155 | 104 | 106 | 109 | 81 | 83 | 84 |
|  | *** | 701 | 713 | 1285 | 252 | 258 | 409 | 148 | 152 | 216 | 105 | 107 | 138 | 82 | 83 | 97 |
| 0.1 | *** | 1276 | 1287 | 1439 | 397 | 407 | 444 | 215 | 221 | 236 | 143 | 147 | 155 | 106 | 109 | 113 |
|  | *** | 1280 | 1308 | 2033 | 401 | 419 | 584 | 217 | 227 | 289 | 145 | 150 | 176 | 108 | 111 | 119 |
| 0.15 | *** | 1766 | 1785 | 2109 | 516 | 534 | 609 | 268 | 279 | 307 | 173 | 180 | 193 | 125 | 130 | 137 |
|  | *** | 1772 | 1821 | 2687 | 523 | 555 | 736 | 272 | 289 | 351 | 176 | 185 | 208 | 127 | 133 | 138 |
| 0.2 | *** | 2145 | 2173 | 2721 | 606 | 633 | 755 | 307 | 324 | 368 | 195 | 206 | 226 | 139 | 146 | 157 |
|  | *** | 2155 | 2228 | 3247 | 616 | 666 | 865 | 314 | 340 | 403 | 200 | 214 | 234 | 142 | 150 | 153 |
| 0.25 | *** | 2409 | 2449 | 3256 | 669 | 705 | 879 | 335 | 358 | 419 | 211 | 224 | 252 | 149 | 157 | 172 |
|  | *** | 2423 | 2527 | 3714 | 682 | 750 | 970 | 345 | 379 | 444 | 217 | 235 | 255 | 153 | 163 | 164 |
| 0.3 | *** | 2563 | 2617 | 3703 | 706 | 753 | 980 | 353 | 381 | 459 | 221 | 237 | 269 | 155 | 165 | 183 |
|  | *** | 2581 | 2722 | 4088 | 724 | 811 | 1052 | 364 | 408 | 475 | 228 | 251 | 269 | 159 | 172 | 171 |
| 0.35 | *** | 2616 | 2688 | 4055 | 721 | 779 | 1056 | 361 | 395 | 488 | 225 | 245 | 285 | 157 | 169 | 189 |
|  | *** | 2640 | 2824 | 4368 | 743 | 850 | 1110 | 375 | 426 | 496 | 234 | 260 | 278 | 162 | 177 | 175 |
| 0.4 | *** | 2581 | 2674 | 4308 | 718 | 787 | 1108 | 362 | 400 | 506 | 226 | 247 | 292 | 157 | 169 | 192 |
|  | *** | 2612 | 2846 | 4555 | 744 | 868 | 1145 | 377 | 435 | 507 | 235 | 264 | 281 | 162 | 179 | 175 |
| 0.45 | *** | 2473 | 2592 | 4462 | 700 | 779 | 1134 | 355 | 397 | 512 | 222 | 245 | 292 | 154 | 167 | 190 |
|  | *** | 2513 | 2803 | 4649 | 730 | 870 | 1157 | 373 | 436 | 507 | 232 | 263 | 278 | 159 | 176 | 171 |
| 0.5 | *** | 2308 | 2457 | 4514 | 670 | 758 | 1134 | 344 | 388 | 506 | 214 | 238 | 286 | 148 | 161 | 184 |
|  | *** | 2359 | 2707 | 4649 | 704 | 855 | 1145 | 362 | 428 | 496 | 225 | 256 | 269 | 154 | 171 | 164 |
| 0.55 | *** | 2103 | 2285 | 4464 | 631 | 725 | 1109 | 326 | 372 | 490 | 203 | 227 | 274 | 139 | 152 | 174 |
|  | *** | 2167 | 2571 | 4555 | 668 | 826 | 1110 | 345 | 412 | 475 | 214 | 245 | 255 | 145 | 161 | 153 |
| 0.6 | *** | 1876 | 2091 | 4312 | 586 | 682 | 1059 | 305 | 349 | 462 | 189 | 211 | 255 | 129 | 140 | 160 |
|  | *** | 1953 | 2404 | 4368 | 624 | 783 | 1052 | 324 | 388 | 444 | 199 | 229 | 234 | 134 | 149 | 138 |
| 0.65 | *** | 1642 | 1885 | 4059 | 535 | 630 | 983 | 279 | 321 | 423 | 172 | 192 | 230 | 115 | 126 | 142 |
|  | *** | 1732 | 2213 | 4088 | 573 | 728 | 970 | 297 | 357 | 403 | 181 | 207 | 208 | 120 | 133 | 119 |
| 0.7 | *** | 1415 | 1672 | 3706 | 478 | 569 | 882 | 249 | 287 | 372 | 151 | 168 | 198 | 99 | 108 | 120 |
|  | *** | 1512 | 2001 | 3714 | 515 | 659 | 865 | 265 | 318 | 351 | 159 | 181 | 176 | 103 | 113 | 97 |
| 0.75 | *** | 1199 | 1456 | 3253 | 417 | 498 | 757 | 214 | 245 | 311 | 126 | 139 | 161 | . | . | . |
|  | *** | 1298 | 1768 | 3247 | 450 | 576 | 736 | 227 | 270 | 289 | 132 | 148 | 138 | . | . | . |
| 0.8 | *** | 993 | 1231 | 2702 | 348 | 415 | 607 | 172 | 195 | 239 | . | . | . | . | . | . |
|  | *** | 1086 | 1509 | 2687 | 376 | 476 | 584 | 182 | 213 | 216 | . | . | . | . | . | . |
| 0.85 | *** | 788 | 989 | 2053 | 268 | 315 | 432 | . | . | . | . | . | . | . | . | . |
|  | *** | 868 | 1214 | 2033 | 288 | 356 | 409 | . | . | . | . | . | . | . | . | . |
| 0.9 | *** | 567 | 709 | 1308 | . | . | . | . | . | . | . | . | . | . | . | . |
|  | *** | 624 | 859 | 1285 | . | . | . | . | . | . | . | . | . | . | . | . |

## TABLE 1: ALPHA= 0.005 POWER= 0.8    EXPECTED ACCRUAL THRU MINIMUM FOLLOW-UP= 200

| | | DEL=.05 | | | DEL=.10 | | | DEL=.15 | | | DEL=.20 | | | DEL=.25 | | |
|---|---|---|---|---|---|---|---|---|---|---|---|---|---|---|---|---|---|
| FACT= | | 1.0 .75 | .50 .25 | .00 BIN | 1.0 .75 | .50 .25 | .00 BIN | 1.0 .75 | .50 .25 | .00 BIN | 1.0 75 | .50 .25 | .00 BIN | 1.0 .75 | .50 .25 | .00 BIN |
| PCONT=*** | | | | | REQUIRED NUMBER OF PATIENTS | | | | | | | | | | | |
| 0.05 | *** | 700 | 705 | 746 | 250 | 254 | 265 | 147 | 150 | 155 | 105 | 106 | 109 | 82 | 83 | 84 |
| | *** | 702 | 714 | 1285 | 252 | 258 | 409 | 149 | 152 | 216 | 105 | 107 | 138 | 82 | 83 | 97 |
| 0.1 | *** | 1277 | 1288 | 1439 | 398 | 408 | 444 | 215 | 222 | 236 | 144 | 148 | 155 | 107 | 109 | 113 |
| | *** | 1281 | 1310 | 2033 | 402 | 420 | 584 | 218 | 227 | 289 | 145 | 151 | 176 | 108 | 111 | 119 |
| 0.15 | *** | 1767 | 1787 | 2109 | 517 | 535 | 609 | 268 | 280 | 307 | 173 | 180 | 193 | 126 | 130 | 137 |
| | *** | 1773 | 1824 | 2687 | 524 | 557 | 736 | 273 | 290 | 351 | 177 | 186 | 208 | 128 | 133 | 138 |
| 0.2 | *** | 2147 | 2176 | 2721 | 608 | 635 | 755 | 309 | 325 | 368 | 196 | 206 | 226 | 140 | 146 | 157 |
| | *** | 2157 | 2234 | 3247 | 618 | 668 | 865 | 316 | 341 | 403 | 200 | 214 | 234 | 143 | 151 | 153 |
| 0.25 | *** | 2412 | 2454 | 3256 | 671 | 708 | 879 | 337 | 360 | 419 | 212 | 225 | 252 | 150 | 158 | 172 |
| | *** | 2426 | 2535 | 3714 | 685 | 754 | 970 | 346 | 381 | 444 | 218 | 236 | 255 | 153 | 164 | 164 |
| 0.3 | *** | 2566 | 2623 | 3703 | 709 | 757 | 980 | 355 | 383 | 459 | 222 | 238 | 272 | 156 | 166 | 183 |
| | *** | 2585 | 2733 | 4088 | 727 | 815 | 1052 | 367 | 410 | 475 | 229 | 252 | 269 | 160 | 173 | 171 |
| 0.35 | *** | 2620 | 2695 | 4055 | 725 | 784 | 1056 | 364 | 397 | 488 | 227 | 246 | 285 | 158 | 170 | 189 |
| | *** | 2645 | 2838 | 4368 | 747 | 855 | 1110 | 377 | 428 | 496 | 235 | 261 | 278 | 163 | 178 | 175 |
| 0.4 | *** | 2586 | 2684 | 4308 | 722 | 793 | 1108 | 364 | 403 | 506 | 227 | 249 | 292 | 158 | 170 | 192 |
| | *** | 2619 | 2863 | 4555 | 749 | 875 | 1145 | 380 | 438 | 507 | 236 | 265 | 281 | 163 | 179 | 175 |
| 0.45 | *** | 2479 | 2604 | 4462 | 705 | 786 | 1134 | 358 | 400 | 512 | 224 | 246 | 292 | 155 | 168 | 190 |
| | *** | 2521 | 2822 | 4649 | 736 | 876 | 1157 | 376 | 438 | 507 | 233 | 264 | 278 | 160 | 177 | 171 |
| 0.5 | *** | 2316 | 2472 | 4514 | 676 | 765 | 1134 | 347 | 391 | 506 | 216 | 239 | 286 | 149 | 162 | 184 |
| | *** | 2369 | 2729 | 4649 | 711 | 862 | 1145 | 365 | 430 | 496 | 226 | 258 | 269 | 155 | 171 | 164 |
| 0.55 | *** | 2113 | 2303 | 4464 | 637 | 732 | 1109 | 330 | 375 | 490 | 205 | 228 | 274 | 140 | 153 | 174 |
| | *** | 2180 | 2596 | 4555 | 675 | 833 | 1110 | 349 | 415 | 475 | 215 | 246 | 255 | 146 | 162 | 153 |
| 0.6 | *** | 1888 | 2111 | 4312 | 592 | 689 | 1059 | 308 | 352 | 462 | 191 | 213 | 255 | 130 | 141 | 160 |
| | *** | 1968 | 2430 | 4368 | 631 | 791 | 1052 | 327 | 391 | 444 | 201 | 230 | 234 | 135 | 149 | 138 |
| 0.65 | *** | 1657 | 1906 | 4059 | 541 | 637 | 983 | 283 | 324 | 423 | 174 | 193 | 230 | 116 | 126 | 142 |
| | *** | 1749 | 2240 | 4088 | 580 | 735 | 970 | 300 | 359 | 403 | 182 | 208 | 208 | 121 | 133 | 119 |
| 0.7 | *** | 1431 | 1695 | 3706 | 485 | 576 | 882 | 252 | 289 | 372 | 153 | 169 | 198 | 100 | 108 | 120 |
| | *** | 1531 | 2027 | 3714 | 522 | 665 | 865 | 268 | 320 | 351 | 160 | 181 | 176 | 104 | 113 | 97 |
| 0.75 | *** | 1216 | 1477 | 3253 | 423 | 504 | 757 | 216 | 247 | 311 | 127 | 140 | 161 | . | . | . |
| | *** | 1317 | 1792 | 3247 | 456 | 581 | 736 | 230 | 272 | 289 | 133 | 149 | 138 | . | . | . |
| 0.8 | *** | 1009 | 1250 | 2702 | 353 | 419 | 607 | 174 | 197 | 239 | . | . | . | . | . | . |
| | *** | 1103 | 1531 | 2687 | 381 | 480 | 584 | 184 | 214 | 216 | . | . | . | . | . | . |
| 0.85 | *** | 802 | 1005 | 2053 | 271 | 319 | 432 | . | . | . | . | . | . | . | . | . |
| | *** | 882 | 1231 | 2033 | 291 | 359 | 409 | . | . | . | . | . | . | . | . | . |
| 0.9 | *** | 577 | 720 | 1308 | . | . | . | . | . | . | . | . | . | . | . | . |
| | *** | 635 | 870 | 1285 | . | . | . | . | . | . | . | . | . | . | . | . |

## TABLE 1: ALPHA= 0.005 POWER= 0.8    EXPECTED ACCRUAL THRU MINIMUM FOLLOW-UP= 225

|  |  | DEL=.05 | | | DEL=.10 | | | DEL=.15 | | | DEL=.20 | | | DEL=.25 | | |
|---|---|---|---|---|---|---|---|---|---|---|---|---|---|---|---|---|
| FACT= |  | 1.0 .75 | .50 .25 | .00 BIN | 1.0 .75 | .50 .25 | .00 BIN | 1.0 .75 | .50 .25 | .00 BIN | 1.0 75 | .50 .25 | .00 BIN | 1.0 .75 | .50 .25 | .00 BIN |
| PCONT=*** |  | REQUIRED NUMBER OF PATIENTS | | | | | | | | | | | | | | |
| 0.05 | *** | 701 | 706 | 746 | 251 | 255 | 265 | 148 | 150 | 155 | 105 | 106 | 109 | 82 | 83 | 84 |
|  | *** | 703 | 716 | 1285 | 253 | 259 | 409 | 149 | 152 | 216 | 106 | 107 | 138 | 82 | 84 | 97 |
| 0.1 | *** | 1278 | 1291 | 1439 | 399 | 410 | 444 | 216 | 223 | 236 | 144 | 148 | 155 | 107 | 110 | 113 |
|  | *** | 1283 | 1315 | 2033 | 404 | 422 | 584 | 219 | 228 | 289 | 146 | 151 | 176 | 108 | 111 | 119 |
| 0.15 | *** | 1769 | 1791 | 2109 | 520 | 539 | 609 | 270 | 282 | 307 | 175 | 182 | 193 | 126 | 131 | 137 |
|  | *** | 1777 | 1833 | 2687 | 527 | 560 | 736 | 275 | 291 | 351 | 178 | 186 | 208 | 128 | 134 | 138 |
| 0.2 | *** | 2150 | 2184 | 2721 | 612 | 640 | 755 | 311 | 328 | 368 | 198 | 208 | 226 | 141 | 147 | 157 |
|  | *** | 2162 | 2247 | 3247 | 623 | 674 | 865 | 318 | 343 | 403 | 202 | 215 | 234 | 144 | 151 | 153 |
| 0.25 | *** | 2417 | 2464 | 3256 | 676 | 716 | 879 | 341 | 363 | 419 | 214 | 227 | 252 | 151 | 159 | 172 |
|  | *** | 2433 | 2554 | 3714 | 691 | 761 | 970 | 350 | 384 | 444 | 220 | 237 | 255 | 155 | 165 | 164 |
| 0.3 | *** | 2573 | 2637 | 3703 | 716 | 767 | 980 | 360 | 388 | 459 | 225 | 241 | 272 | 157 | 167 | 183 |
|  | *** | 2594 | 2758 | 4088 | 735 | 825 | 1052 | 371 | 413 | 475 | 232 | 253 | 269 | 162 | 174 | 171 |
| 0.35 | *** | 2629 | 2714 | 4055 | 734 | 796 | 1056 | 369 | 403 | 488 | 230 | 249 | 285 | 160 | 171 | 189 |
|  | *** | 2658 | 2870 | 4368 | 758 | 867 | 1110 | 383 | 433 | 496 | 239 | 263 | 278 | 165 | 179 | 175 |
| 0.4 | *** | 2598 | 2708 | 4308 | 733 | 806 | 1108 | 371 | 409 | 506 | 231 | 252 | 292 | 160 | 172 | 192 |
|  | *** | 2635 | 2903 | 4555 | 761 | 888 | 1145 | 387 | 443 | 507 | 240 | 268 | 281 | 165 | 180 | 175 |
| 0.45 | *** | 2495 | 2634 | 4462 | 717 | 801 | 1134 | 365 | 407 | 512 | 228 | 250 | 292 | 157 | 169 | 190 |
|  | *** | 2542 | 2869 | 4649 | 750 | 892 | 1157 | 383 | 444 | 507 | 237 | 267 | 278 | 163 | 178 | 171 |
| 0.5 | *** | 2336 | 2508 | 4514 | 690 | 781 | 1134 | 354 | 398 | 507 | 220 | 243 | 286 | 151 | 164 | 184 |
|  | *** | 2396 | 2783 | 4649 | 726 | 878 | 1145 | 373 | 436 | 496 | 230 | 260 | 269 | 157 | 172 | 164 |
| 0.55 | *** | 2138 | 2346 | 4464 | 653 | 749 | 1109 | 338 | 382 | 490 | 209 | 232 | 274 | 143 | 155 | 174 |
|  | *** | 2212 | 2654 | 4555 | 691 | 850 | 1110 | 356 | 420 | 475 | 219 | 249 | 255 | 148 | 163 | 153 |
| 0.6 | *** | 1919 | 2159 | 4312 | 608 | 707 | 1059 | 316 | 360 | 462 | 195 | 216 | 255 | 132 | 143 | 160 |
|  | *** | 2006 | 2492 | 4368 | 648 | 807 | 1052 | 335 | 396 | 444 | 204 | 232 | 234 | 137 | 150 | 138 |
| 0.65 | *** | 1693 | 1958 | 4059 | 557 | 654 | 983 | 290 | 331 | 423 | 177 | 196 | 230 | 118 | 128 | 142 |
|  | *** | 1792 | 2303 | 4088 | 597 | 750 | 970 | 307 | 365 | 403 | 186 | 210 | 208 | 122 | 134 | 119 |
| 0.7 | *** | 1470 | 1747 | 3706 | 500 | 591 | 882 | 259 | 295 | 372 | 156 | 172 | 198 | 102 | 109 | 120 |
|  | *** | 1576 | 2089 | 3714 | 537 | 679 | 865 | 274 | 324 | 351 | 163 | 183 | 176 | 105 | 114 | 97 |
| 0.75 | *** | 1256 | 1527 | 3253 | 436 | 517 | 757 | 222 | 252 | 311 | 130 | 142 | 161 | . | . | . |
|  | *** | 1361 | 1850 | 3247 | 470 | 593 | 736 | 235 | 275 | 289 | 135 | 150 | 138 | . | . | . |
| 0.8 | *** | 1047 | 1296 | 2702 | 364 | 430 | 606 | 178 | 200 | 239 | . | . | . | . | . | . |
|  | *** | 1145 | 1581 | 2687 | 392 | 490 | 584 | 188 | 216 | 216 | . | . | . | . | . | . |
| 0.85 | *** | 834 | 1042 | 2053 | 280 | 326 | 432 | . | . | . | . | . | . | . | . | . |
|  | *** | 917 | 1271 | 2033 | 299 | 365 | 409 | . | . | . | . | . | . | . | . | . |
| 0.9 | *** | 600 | 745 | 1308 | . | . | . | . | . | . | . | . | . | . | . | . |
|  | *** | 659 | 895 | 1285 | . | . | . | . | . | . | . | . | . | . | . | . |

TABLE 1: ALPHA= 0.005 POWER= 0.8    EXPECTED ACCRUAL THRU MINIMUM FOLLOW-UP= 250

| | | DEL=.05 | | | DEL=.10 | | | DEL=.15 | | | DEL=.20 | | | DEL=.25 | | |
|---|---|---|---|---|---|---|---|---|---|---|---|---|---|---|---|---|
| FACT= | | 1.0 .75 | .50 .25 | .00 BIN | 1.0 .75 | .50 .25 | .00 BIN | 1.0 .75 | .50 .25 | .00 BIN | 1.0 75 | .50 .25 | .00 BIN | 1.0 .75 | .50 .25 | .00 BIN |
| PCONT=*** | | | | | REQUIRED NUMBER OF PATIENTS | | | | | | | | | | | |
| 0.05 | *** | 701 | 708 | 746 | 252 | 256 | 265 | 148 | 151 | 155 | 105 | 107 | 109 | 82 | 83 | 84 |
| | *** | 703 | 717 | 1285 | 253 | 259 | 409 | 149 | 152 | 216 | 106 | 108 | 138 | 82 | 84 | 97 |
| 0.1 | *** | 1280 | 1294 | 1439 | 401 | 412 | 444 | 217 | 224 | 236 | 145 | 149 | 155 | 108 | 110 | 113 |
| | *** | 1284 | 1319 | 2033 | 405 | 423 | 584 | 220 | 229 | 289 | 147 | 151 | 176 | 109 | 112 | 119 |
| 0.15 | *** | 1772 | 1796 | 2109 | 522 | 542 | 609 | 272 | 283 | 307 | 176 | 182 | 193 | 127 | 131 | 137 |
| | *** | 1780 | 1842 | 2687 | 530 | 564 | 736 | 277 | 293 | 351 | 179 | 187 | 208 | 129 | 134 | 138 |
| 0.2 | *** | 2154 | 2191 | 2721 | 616 | 645 | 755 | 314 | 331 | 368 | 199 | 209 | 226 | 142 | 148 | 157 |
| | *** | 2167 | 2260 | 3247 | 627 | 679 | 865 | 321 | 345 | 403 | 204 | 216 | 234 | 144 | 152 | 153 |
| 0.25 | *** | 2422 | 2474 | 3256 | 682 | 722 | 879 | 344 | 367 | 419 | 217 | 229 | 252 | 152 | 160 | 172 |
| | *** | 2439 | 2572 | 3714 | 697 | 768 | 970 | 354 | 386 | 444 | 222 | 239 | 255 | 156 | 165 | 164 |
| 0.3 | *** | 2580 | 2651 | 3703 | 723 | 775 | 980 | 364 | 392 | 459 | 228 | 243 | 272 | 159 | 168 | 183 |
| | *** | 2604 | 2782 | 4088 | 743 | 834 | 1052 | 376 | 417 | 475 | 234 | 255 | 269 | 163 | 174 | 171 |
| 0.35 | *** | 2639 | 2732 | 4055 | 742 | 807 | 1056 | 374 | 408 | 488 | 233 | 252 | 285 | 162 | 173 | 189 |
| | *** | 2670 | 2901 | 4368 | 767 | 878 | 1110 | 388 | 437 | 496 | 241 | 265 | 278 | 167 | 180 | 175 |
| 0.4 | *** | 2611 | 2731 | 4309 | 743 | 819 | 1108 | 377 | 415 | 506 | 234 | 254 | 292 | 162 | 174 | 192 |
| | *** | 2652 | 2940 | 4555 | 773 | 901 | 1145 | 393 | 447 | 507 | 243 | 270 | 281 | 167 | 181 | 175 |
| 0.45 | *** | 2511 | 2663 | 4462 | 729 | 814 | 1134 | 372 | 413 | 512 | 231 | 253 | 292 | 159 | 171 | 190 |
| | *** | 2563 | 2913 | 4649 | 763 | 905 | 1157 | 389 | 449 | 507 | 241 | 269 | 278 | 164 | 179 | 171 |
| 0.5 | *** | 2356 | 2543 | 4514 | 703 | 796 | 1134 | 361 | 404 | 507 | 224 | 246 | 286 | 153 | 165 | 184 |
| | *** | 2422 | 2833 | 4649 | 740 | 893 | 1145 | 379 | 441 | 496 | 234 | 262 | 269 | 159 | 173 | 164 |
| 0.55 | *** | 2163 | 2386 | 4464 | 666 | 765 | 1109 | 344 | 388 | 490 | 213 | 235 | 274 | 145 | 156 | 174 |
| | *** | 2243 | 2709 | 4555 | 706 | 865 | 1110 | 363 | 425 | 475 | 223 | 251 | 255 | 150 | 164 | 153 |
| 0.6 | *** | 1949 | 2204 | 4312 | 622 | 722 | 1059 | 323 | 366 | 462 | 199 | 219 | 255 | 134 | 144 | 160 |
| | *** | 2043 | 2549 | 4368 | 663 | 822 | 1052 | 341 | 401 | 444 | 208 | 234 | 234 | 139 | 151 | 138 |
| 0.65 | *** | 1727 | 2005 | 4059 | 571 | 669 | 983 | 296 | 336 | 423 | 180 | 199 | 230 | 120 | 129 | 142 |
| | *** | 1832 | 2361 | 4088 | 611 | 764 | 970 | 314 | 369 | 403 | 189 | 212 | 208 | 124 | 135 | 119 |
| 0.7 | *** | 1508 | 1795 | 3706 | 514 | 605 | 882 | 264 | 300 | 372 | 158 | 174 | 198 | 103 | 110 | 120 |
| | *** | 1618 | 2145 | 3714 | 551 | 692 | 865 | 280 | 328 | 351 | 165 | 184 | 176 | 106 | 114 | 97 |
| 0.75 | *** | 1293 | 1574 | 3253 | 449 | 529 | 757 | 227 | 256 | 311 | 132 | 143 | 161 | . | . | . |
| | *** | 1402 | 1902 | 3247 | 482 | 604 | 736 | 239 | 278 | 289 | 137 | 151 | 138 | . | . | . |
| 0.8 | *** | 1082 | 1337 | 2702 | 374 | 440 | 607 | 182 | 203 | 239 | . | . | . | . | . | . |
| | *** | 1182 | 1626 | 2687 | 402 | 498 | 584 | 191 | 218 | 216 | . | . | . | . | . | . |
| 0.85 | *** | 864 | 1076 | 2053 | 287 | 332 | 432 | . | . | . | . | . | . | . | . | . |
| | *** | 949 | 1306 | 2033 | 307 | 370 | 409 | . | . | . | . | . | . | . | . | . |
| 0.9 | *** | 621 | 768 | 1308 | . | . | . | . | . | . | . | . | . | . | . | . |
| | *** | 681 | 917 | 1285 | . | . | . | . | . | . | . | . | . | . | . | . |

## TABLE 1: ALPHA= 0.005 POWER= 0.8     EXPECTED ACCRUAL THRU MINIMUM FOLLOW-UP= 275

| | | DEL=.05 | | | DEL=.10 | | | DEL=.15 | | | DEL=.20 | | | DEL=.25 | | |
|---|---|---|---|---|---|---|---|---|---|---|---|---|---|---|---|---|
| FACT= | | 1.0 .75 | .50 .25 | .00 BIN | 1.0 .75 | .50 .25 | .00 BIN | 1.0 .75 | .50 .25 | .00 BIN | 1.0 75 | .50 .25 | .00 BIN | 1.0 .75 | .50 .25 | .00 BIN |
| PCONT=*** | | | | | | | REQUIRED NUMBER OF PATIENTS | | | | | | | | |
| 0.05 | *** | 702 | 709 | 746 | 252 | 256 | 265 | 149 | 151 | 155 | 105 | 107 | 109 | 82 | 83 | 84 |
| | *** | 704 | 718 | 1285 | 254 | 260 | 409 | 150 | 153 | 216 | 106 | 108 | 138 | 83 | 84 | 97 |
| 0.1 | *** | 1281 | 1297 | 1439 | 402 | 414 | 444 | 218 | 224 | 236 | 145 | 149 | 155 | 108 | 110 | 113 |
| | *** | 1286 | 1324 | 2033 | 407 | 425 | 584 | 221 | 229 | 289 | 147 | 151 | 176 | 109 | 112 | 119 |
| 0.15 | *** | 1774 | 1801 | 2109 | 525 | 545 | 609 | 274 | 285 | 307 | 177 | 183 | 193 | 128 | 132 | 137 |
| | *** | 1783 | 1849 | 2687 | 533 | 566 | 736 | 278 | 294 | 351 | 180 | 188 | 208 | 130 | 134 | 138 |
| 0.2 | *** | 2158 | 2199 | 2721 | 619 | 650 | 755 | 316 | 333 | 368 | 201 | 210 | 226 | 143 | 148 | 157 |
| | *** | 2171 | 2273 | 3247 | 631 | 683 | 865 | 323 | 347 | 403 | 205 | 217 | 234 | 145 | 152 | 153 |
| 0.25 | *** | 2427 | 2485 | 3256 | 686 | 729 | 879 | 347 | 370 | 419 | 218 | 231 | 252 | 154 | 161 | 172 |
| | *** | 2446 | 2590 | 3714 | 703 | 774 | 970 | 357 | 389 | 444 | 224 | 240 | 255 | 157 | 166 | 164 |
| 0.3 | *** | 2587 | 2665 | 3703 | 729 | 783 | 980 | 368 | 396 | 459 | 230 | 245 | 272 | 160 | 169 | 183 |
| | *** | 2613 | 2805 | 4088 | 750 | 842 | 1052 | 380 | 420 | 475 | 237 | 256 | 269 | 164 | 175 | 171 |
| 0.35 | *** | 2648 | 2751 | 4055 | 750 | 816 | 1056 | 379 | 412 | 488 | 236 | 254 | 285 | 164 | 174 | 189 |
| | *** | 2683 | 2930 | 4368 | 776 | 887 | 1110 | 393 | 440 | 496 | 244 | 267 | 278 | 168 | 180 | 175 |
| 0.4 | *** | 2623 | 2754 | 4308 | 752 | 830 | 1108 | 382 | 420 | 506 | 237 | 257 | 292 | 164 | 175 | 192 |
| | *** | 2668 | 2976 | 4555 | 783 | 912 | 1145 | 398 | 451 | 507 | 246 | 271 | 281 | 169 | 182 | 175 |
| 0.45 | *** | 2527 | 2692 | 4462 | 740 | 827 | 1134 | 378 | 419 | 512 | 234 | 255 | 292 | 161 | 172 | 190 |
| | *** | 2584 | 2955 | 4649 | 775 | 917 | 1157 | 395 | 453 | 507 | 244 | 270 | 278 | 166 | 180 | 171 |
| 0.5 | *** | 2376 | 2577 | 4513 | 715 | 809 | 1134 | 367 | 410 | 506 | 227 | 248 | 286 | 155 | 167 | 184 |
| | *** | 2447 | 2879 | 4649 | 753 | 905 | 1145 | 385 | 446 | 496 | 237 | 264 | 269 | 160 | 174 | 164 |
| 0.55 | *** | 2188 | 2425 | 4463 | 679 | 779 | 1109 | 351 | 394 | 490 | 216 | 237 | 274 | 147 | 158 | 174 |
| | *** | 2273 | 2759 | 4555 | 720 | 877 | 1110 | 369 | 430 | 475 | 226 | 252 | 255 | 152 | 165 | 153 |
| 0.6 | *** | 1978 | 2247 | 4312 | 635 | 736 | 1059 | 329 | 371 | 462 | 202 | 221 | 255 | 135 | 145 | 160 |
| | *** | 2078 | 2602 | 4368 | 677 | 834 | 1052 | 347 | 405 | 444 | 210 | 235 | 234 | 140 | 152 | 138 |
| 0.65 | *** | 1760 | 2050 | 4059 | 584 | 683 | 983 | 302 | 341 | 423 | 183 | 201 | 230 | 121 | 130 | 142 |
| | *** | 1870 | 2414 | 4088 | 625 | 776 | 970 | 319 | 373 | 403 | 191 | 213 | 208 | 125 | 135 | 119 |
| 0.7 | *** | 1543 | 1840 | 3706 | 526 | 618 | 882 | 270 | 304 | 372 | 161 | 175 | 198 | 104 | 111 | 120 |
| | *** | 1657 | 2197 | 3714 | 564 | 703 | 865 | 285 | 331 | 351 | 167 | 185 | 176 | 107 | 115 | 97 |
| 0.75 | *** | 1328 | 1616 | 3253 | 460 | 540 | 757 | 231 | 259 | 311 | 134 | 145 | 161 | . | . | . |
| | *** | 1441 | 1949 | 3247 | 494 | 613 | 736 | 244 | 280 | 289 | 139 | 152 | 138 | . | . | . |
| 0.8 | *** | 1114 | 1375 | 2702 | 384 | 449 | 607 | 185 | 205 | 239 | . | . | . | . | . | . |
| | *** | 1217 | 1667 | 2687 | 411 | 505 | 584 | 194 | 220 | 216 | . | . | . | . | . | . |
| 0.85 | *** | 891 | 1107 | 2053 | 293 | 338 | 432 | . | . | . | . | . | . | . | . | . |
| | *** | 978 | 1337 | 2033 | 313 | 374 | 409 | . | . | . | . | . | . | . | . | . |
| 0.9 | *** | 641 | 789 | 1308 | . | . | . | . | . | . | . | . | . | . | . | . |
| | *** | 701 | 936 | 1285 | . | . | . | . | . | . | . | . | . | . | . | . |

## TABLE 1: ALPHA= 0.005 POWER= 0.8    EXPECTED ACCRUAL THRU MINIMUM FOLLOW-UP= 300

| | | DEL=.05 | | | DEL=.10 | | | DEL=.15 | | | DEL=.20 | | | DEL=.25 | | |
|---|---|---|---|---|---|---|---|---|---|---|---|---|---|---|---|---|
| FACT= | | 1.0 / .75 | .50 / .25 | .00 / BIN | 1.0 / .75 | .50 / .25 | .00 / BIN | 1.0 / .75 | .50 / .25 | .00 / BIN | 1.0 / 75 | .50 / .25 | .00 / BIN | 1.0 / .75 | .50 / .25 | .00 / BIN |
| PCONT=*** | | | | | | | REQUIRED NUMBER OF PATIENTS | | | | | | | | | |
| 0.05 | *** | 703 | 710 | 746 | 253 | 257 | 265 | 149 | 151 | 155 | 106 | 107 | 109 | 82 | 83 | 84 |
| | *** | 705 | 720 | 1285 | 254 | 260 | 409 | 150 | 153 | 216 | 106 | 108 | 138 | 83 | 84 | 97 |
| 0.1 | *** | 1282 | 1299 | 1439 | 403 | 415 | 444 | 219 | 225 | 236 | 146 | 149 | 154 | 108 | 110 | 113 |
| | *** | 1288 | 1328 | 2033 | 408 | 426 | 584 | 222 | 229 | 289 | 148 | 152 | 176 | 109 | 112 | 119 |
| 0.15 | *** | 1777 | 1806 | 2109 | 527 | 548 | 609 | 275 | 286 | 307 | 178 | 184 | 193 | 128 | 132 | 137 |
| | *** | 1786 | 1857 | 2687 | 535 | 569 | 736 | 280 | 295 | 351 | 180 | 188 | 208 | 130 | 134 | 138 |
| 0.2 | *** | 2161 | 2206 | 2721 | 622 | 654 | 755 | 318 | 335 | 368 | 202 | 211 | 226 | 144 | 149 | 157 |
| | *** | 2176 | 2285 | 3247 | 635 | 687 | 865 | 325 | 348 | 403 | 206 | 217 | 234 | 146 | 152 | 153 |
| 0.25 | *** | 2432 | 2495 | 3256 | 691 | 734 | 879 | 350 | 372 | 419 | 220 | 232 | 252 | 154 | 161 | 172 |
| | *** | 2453 | 2606 | 3714 | 708 | 780 | 970 | 360 | 391 | 444 | 225 | 241 | 255 | 158 | 166 | 164 |
| 0.3 | *** | 2594 | 2679 | 3703 | 735 | 791 | 980 | 371 | 399 | 459 | 232 | 247 | 272 | 162 | 170 | 183 |
| | *** | 2623 | 2827 | 4088 | 757 | 849 | 1052 | 383 | 422 | 475 | 238 | 257 | 269 | 166 | 176 | 171 |
| 0.35 | *** | 2658 | 2769 | 4055 | 757 | 825 | 1056 | 383 | 416 | 488 | 238 | 256 | 285 | 165 | 175 | 189 |
| | *** | 2695 | 2958 | 4368 | 784 | 895 | 1110 | 397 | 443 | 496 | 246 | 268 | 278 | 169 | 181 | 175 |
| 0.4 | *** | 2635 | 2777 | 4308 | 761 | 840 | 1108 | 387 | 424 | 506 | 240 | 259 | 292 | 165 | 176 | 192 |
| | *** | 2684 | 3009 | 4555 | 793 | 921 | 1145 | 403 | 455 | 507 | 248 | 273 | 281 | 170 | 183 | 175 |
| 0.45 | *** | 2542 | 2719 | 4462 | 750 | 838 | 1134 | 383 | 423 | 512 | 237 | 257 | 292 | 163 | 173 | 190 |
| | *** | 2604 | 2994 | 4649 | 786 | 928 | 1157 | 400 | 457 | 507 | 246 | 272 | 278 | 168 | 181 | 171 |
| 0.5 | *** | 2396 | 2610 | 4513 | 726 | 822 | 1134 | 373 | 415 | 506 | 230 | 251 | 286 | 157 | 168 | 184 |
| | *** | 2472 | 2923 | 4649 | 765 | 917 | 1145 | 391 | 449 | 496 | 239 | 265 | 269 | 162 | 175 | 164 |
| 0.55 | *** | 2212 | 2462 | 4463 | 691 | 791 | 1109 | 356 | 399 | 490 | 219 | 239 | 274 | 148 | 159 | 174 |
| | *** | 2303 | 2806 | 4555 | 732 | 889 | 1110 | 375 | 433 | 475 | 228 | 254 | 255 | 153 | 166 | 153 |
| 0.6 | *** | 2006 | 2287 | 4312 | 648 | 749 | 1059 | 334 | 376 | 462 | 204 | 223 | 255 | 137 | 146 | 160 |
| | *** | 2111 | 2651 | 4368 | 689 | 846 | 1052 | 352 | 409 | 444 | 213 | 237 | 234 | 141 | 152 | 138 |
| 0.65 | *** | 1792 | 2092 | 4059 | 596 | 695 | 983 | 307 | 346 | 423 | 186 | 202 | 230 | 122 | 130 | 142 |
| | *** | 1906 | 2463 | 4088 | 637 | 787 | 970 | 324 | 376 | 403 | 193 | 214 | 208 | 126 | 136 | 119 |
| 0.7 | *** | 1576 | 1882 | 3706 | 537 | 629 | 882 | 274 | 308 | 372 | 163 | 177 | 198 | 105 | 111 | 120 |
| | *** | 1694 | 2244 | 3714 | 576 | 712 | 865 | 289 | 334 | 351 | 169 | 186 | 176 | 108 | 115 | 97 |
| 0.75 | *** | 1361 | 1656 | 3253 | 470 | 550 | 757 | 235 | 262 | 311 | 135 | 146 | 161 | . | . | . |
| | *** | 1477 | 1993 | 3247 | 504 | 621 | 736 | 247 | 282 | 289 | 140 | 152 | 138 | . | . | . |
| 0.8 | *** | 1144 | 1411 | 2702 | 392 | 456 | 607 | 188 | 207 | 239 | . | . | . | . | . | . |
| | *** | 1250 | 1704 | 2687 | 419 | 511 | 584 | 197 | 221 | 216 | . | . | . | . | . | . |
| 0.85 | *** | 917 | 1136 | 2053 | 299 | 343 | 432 | . | . | . | . | . | . | . | . | . |
| | *** | 1005 | 1366 | 2033 | 319 | 378 | 409 | . | . | . | . | . | . | . | . | . |
| 0.9 | *** | 659 | 808 | 1308 | . | . | . | . | . | . | . | . | . | . | . | . |
| | *** | 720 | 954 | 1285 | . | . | . | . | . | . | . | . | . | . | . | . |

## TABLE 1: ALPHA= 0.005 POWER= 0.8    EXPECTED ACCRUAL THRU MINIMUM FOLLOW-UP= 325

| | | DEL=.05 | | | DEL=.10 | | | DEL=.15 | | | DEL=.20 | | | DEL=.25 | |
|---|---|---|---|---|---|---|---|---|---|---|---|---|---|---|---|
| FACT= | 1.0 .75 | .50 .25 | .00 BIN | 1.0 .75 | .50 .25 | .00 BIN | 1.0 .75 | .50 .25 | .00 BIN | 1.0 75 | .50 .25 | .00 BIN | 1.0 .75 | .50 .25 | .00 BIN |

PCONT=***                REQUIRED NUMBER OF PATIENTS

| PCONT | | DEL=.05 1.0/.75 | .50/.25 | .00/BIN | DEL=.10 1.0/.75 | .50/.25 | .00/BIN | DEL=.15 1.0/.75 | .50/.25 | .00/BIN | DEL=.20 1.0/75 | .50/.25 | .00/BIN | DEL=.25 1.0/.75 | .50/.25 | .00/BIN |
|---|---|---|---|---|---|---|---|---|---|---|---|---|---|---|---|---|
| 0.05 | *** | 703 | 711 | 746 | 253 | 257 | 265 | 149 | 151 | 155 | 106 | 107 | 109 | 82 | 83 | 84 |
| | *** | 706 | 721 | 1285 | 255 | 261 | 409 | 150 | 153 | 216 | 106 | 108 | 138 | 83 | 84 | 97 |
| 0.1 | *** | 1284 | 1302 | 1439 | 405 | 416 | 444 | 220 | 226 | 236 | 146 | 150 | 155 | 109 | 111 | 113 |
| | *** | 1290 | 1331 | 2033 | 409 | 427 | 584 | 222 | 230 | 289 | 148 | 152 | 176 | 110 | 112 | 119 |
| 0.15 | *** | 1779 | 1811 | 2109 | 529 | 550 | 609 | 276 | 287 | 307 | 179 | 184 | 193 | 129 | 132 | 137 |
| | *** | 1790 | 1864 | 2687 | 538 | 571 | 736 | 281 | 295 | 351 | 181 | 188 | 208 | 131 | 135 | 138 |
| 0.2 | *** | 2165 | 2213 | 2721 | 626 | 658 | 755 | 320 | 337 | 368 | 203 | 212 | 226 | 144 | 149 | 157 |
| | *** | 2181 | 2296 | 3247 | 639 | 690 | 865 | 327 | 349 | 403 | 207 | 218 | 234 | 147 | 153 | 153 |
| 0.25 | *** | 2438 | 2505 | 3256 | 696 | 740 | 879 | 353 | 375 | 419 | 222 | 233 | 252 | 156 | 162 | 172 |
| | *** | 2460 | 2623 | 3714 | 713 | 785 | 970 | 362 | 392 | 444 | 227 | 241 | 255 | 159 | 167 | 164 |
| 0.3 | *** | 2602 | 2693 | 3703 | 741 | 798 | 980 | 375 | 402 | 459 | 234 | 248 | 272 | 163 | 171 | 183 |
| | *** | 2632 | 2849 | 4088 | 764 | 855 | 1052 | 387 | 424 | 475 | 240 | 258 | 269 | 167 | 176 | 171 |
| 0.35 | *** | 2667 | 2786 | 4055 | 765 | 833 | 1056 | 387 | 420 | 488. | 241 | 257 | 285 | 167 | 176 | 189 |
| | *** | 2708 | 2985 | 4368 | 792 | 903 | 1110 | 401 | 446 | 496 | 248 | 269 | 278 | 171 | 182 | 175 |
| 0.4 | *** | 2647 | 2799 | 4308 | 770 | 850 | 1108 | 391 | 428 | 506 | 242 | 261 | 292 | 167 | 177 | 192 |
| | *** | 2700 | 3041 | 4555 | 802 | 930 | 1145 | 407 | 458 | 507 | 251 | 274 | 281 | 171 | 183 | 175 |
| 0.45 | *** | 2558 | 2746 | 4462 | 760 | 849 | 1134 | 388 | 428 | 512 | 240 | 259 | 292 | 164 | 174 | 190 |
| | *** | 2624 | 3031 | 4649 | 796 | 937 | 1157 | 405 | 460 | 507 | 249 | 273 | 278 | 169 | 181 | 171 |
| 0.5 | *** | 2415 | 2642 | 4514 | 736 | 833 | 1134 | 378 | 419 | 506 | 233 | 253 | 286 | 158 | 169 | 184 |
| | *** | 2496 | 2964 | 4649 | 776 | 927 | 1145 | 396 | 453 | 496 | 242 | 267 | 269 | 163 | 176 | 164 |
| 0.55 | *** | 2235 | 2498 | 4463 | 703 | 803 | 1109 | 362 | 403 | 490 | 222 | 242 | 274 | 150 | 160 | 174 |
| | *** | 2332 | 2850 | 4555 | 744 | 900 | 1110 | 380 | 437 | 475 | 231 | 255 | 255 | 154 | 166 | 153 |
| 0.6 | *** | 2034 | 2326 | 4312 | 659 | 761 | 1059 | 340 | 380 | 462 | 207 | 225 | 255 | 138 | 147 | 160 |
| | *** | 2143 | 2697 | 4368 | 701 | 856 | 1052 | 357 | 412 | 444 | 215 | 238 | 234 | 142 | 153 | 138 |
| 0.65 | *** | 1822 | 2132 | 4059 | 608 | 706 | 983 | 312 | 350 | 423 | 188 | 204 | 230 | 123 | 131 | 142 |
| | *** | 1941 | 2509 | 4088 | 649 | 796 | 970 | 328 | 379 | 403 | 195 | 215 | 208 | 127 | 136 | 119 |
| 0.7 | *** | 1608 | 1922 | 3706 | 548 | 639 | 882 | 278 | 311 | 372 | 165 | 178 | 198 | 106 | 112 | 120 |
| | *** | 1730 | 2288 | 3714 | 586 | 721 | 865 | 293 | 336 | 351 | 171 | 187 | 176 | 109 | 116 | 97 |
| 0.75 | *** | 1392 | 1693 | 3253 | 479 | 559 | 757 | 238 | 265 | 311 | 137 | 147 | 161 | . | . | . |
| | *** | 1511 | 2033 | 3247 | 513 | 628 | 736 | 250 | 284 | 289 | 141 | 153 | 138 | . | . | . |
| 0.8 | *** | 1173 | 1444 | 2702 | 400 | 463 | 606 | 190 | 209 | 239 | . | . | . | . | . | . |
| | *** | 1281 | 1738 | 2687 | 427 | 516 | 584 | 199 | 222 | 216 | . | . | . | . | . | . |
| 0.85 | *** | 941 | 1162 | 2053 | 305 | 348 | 432 | . | . | . | . | . | . | . | . | . |
| | *** | 1030 | 1392 | 2033 | 324 | 381 | 409 | . | . | . | . | . | . | . | . | . |
| 0.9 | *** | 676 | 825 | 1308 | . | . | . | . | . | . | . | . | . | . | . | . |
| | *** | 737 | 970 | 1285 | . | . | . | . | . | . | . | . | . | . | . | . |

TABLE 1: ALPHA= 0.005 POWER= 0.8     EXPECTED ACCRUAL THRU MINIMUM FOLLOW-UP= 350

| | | DEL=.05 | | | DEL=.10 | | | DEL=.15 | | | DEL=.20 | | | DEL=.25 | | |
|---|---|---|---|---|---|---|---|---|---|---|---|---|---|---|---|---|---|
| FACT= | | 1.0 .75 | .50 .25 | .00 BIN | 1.0 .75 | .50 .25 | .00 BIN | 1.0 .75 | .50 .25 | .00 BIN | 1.0 75 | .50 .25 | .00 BIN | 1.0 .75 | .50 .25 | .00 BIN |
| PCONT=*** | | REQUIRED NUMBER OF PATIENTS | | | | | | | | | | | | | | |
| 0.05 | *** | 704 | 712 | 746 | 254 | 258 | 265 | 150 | 152 | 155 | 106 | 107 | 109 | 82 | 83 | 84 |
| | *** | 707 | 722 | 1285 | 255 | 261 | 409 | 150 | 153 | 216 | 106 | 108 | 138 | 83 | 84 | 97 |
| 0.1 | *** | 1285 | 1305 | 1439 | 406 | 418 | 444 | 220 | 226 | 236 | 147 | 150 | 155 | 109 | 111 | 113 |
| | *** | 1292 | 1335 | 2033 | 411 | 428 | 584 | 223 | 230 | 289 | 148 | 152 | 176 | 110 | 112 | 119 |
| 0.15 | *** | 1782 | 1815 | 2109 | 531 | 553 | 609 | 278 | 288 | 307 | 179 | 185 | 193 | 129 | 133 | 137 |
| | *** | 1793 | 1871 | 2687 | 540 | 573 | 736 | 282 | 296 | 351 | 182 | 189 | 208 | 131 | 135 | 138 |
| 0.2 | *** | 2169 | 2220 | 2721 | 629 | 662 | 755 | 322 | 338 | 369 | 204 | 213 | 226 | 145 | 150 | 157 |
| | *** | 2186 | 2307 | 3247 | 642 | 693 | 865 | 329 | 351 | 403 | 208 | 218 | 234 | 147 | 153 | 153 |
| 0.25 | *** | 2443 | 2515 | 3256 | 700 | 745 | 879 | 355 | 377 | 419 | 223 | 234 | 252 | 156 | 163 | 172 |
| | *** | 2467 | 2638 | 3714 | 718 | 789 | 970 | 365 | 394 | 444 | 228 | 242 | 255 | 159 | 167 | 164 |
| 0.3 | *** | 2609 | 2706 | 3703 | 747 | 804 | 980 | 378 | 405 | 459 | 236 | 249 | 272 | 164 | 171 | 183 |
| | *** | 2642 | 2869 | 4088 | 769 | 861 | 1052 | 390 | 426 | 475 | 242 | 259 | 269 | 167 | 176 | 171 |
| 0.35 | *** | 2676 | 2804 | 4055 | 772 | 841 | 1056 | 391 | 423 | 488 | 243 | 259 | 285 | 168 | 176 | 189 |
| | *** | 2720 | 3010 | 4368 | 799 | 910 | 1110 | 405 | 448 | 496 | 250 | 270 | 278 | 172 | 182 | 175 |
| 0.4 | *** | 2659 | 2821 | 4308 | 778 | 859 | 1108 | 395 | 432 | 506 | 245 | 262 | 292 | 168 | 178 | 192 |
| | *** | 2716 | 3071 | 4555 | 811 | 938 | 1145 | 411 | 460 | 507 | 253 | 275 | 281 | 173 | 184 | 175 |
| 0.45 | *** | 2573 | 2773 | 4462 | 769 | 859 | 1134 | 392 | 432 | 512 | 242 | 261 | 292 | 165 | 175 | 190 |
| | *** | 2644 | 3065 | 4649 | 806 | 946 | 1157 | 409 | 463 | 507 | 251 | 274 | 278 | 170 | 182 | 171 |
| 0.5 | *** | 2434 | 2672 | 4514 | 747 | 843 | 1134 | 382 | 423 | 507 | 235 | 255 | 286 | 160 | 170 | 184 |
| | *** | 2520 | 3002 | 4649 | 786 | 936 | 1145 | 400 | 456 | 496 | 244 | 268 | 269 | 164 | 176 | 164 |
| 0.55 | *** | 2258 | 2532 | 4464 | 713 | 814 | 1109 | 366 | 407 | 490 | 224 | 243 | 274 | 151 | 160 | 174 |
| | *** | 2359 | 2892 | 4555 | 755 | 909 | 1110 | 384 | 440 | 475 | 233 | 256 | 255 | 155 | 167 | 153 |
| 0.6 | *** | 2060 | 2362 | 4312 | 670 | 771 | 1058 | 344 | 384 | 462 | 209 | 227 | 255 | 139 | 148 | 160 |
| | *** | 2174 | 2740 | 4368 | 712 | 865 | 1052 | 362 | 415 | 444 | 217 | 239 | 234 | 143 | 153 | 138 |
| 0.65 | *** | 1851 | 2170 | 4059 | 618 | 716 | 983 | 316 | 353 | 423 | 190 | 206 | 230 | 125 | 132 | 142 |
| | *** | 1974 | 2551 | 4088 | 659 | 805 | 970 | 332 | 381 | 403 | 197 | 216 | 208 | 128 | 136 | 119 |
| 0.7 | *** | 1638 | 1959 | 3706 | 558 | 649 | 882 | 282 | 314 | 372 | 166 | 179 | 198 | 107 | 112 | 120 |
| | *** | 1763 | 2329 | 3714 | 596 | 729 | 865 | 297 | 338 | 351 | 172 | 188 | 176 | 109 | 116 | 97 |
| 0.75 | *** | 1422 | 1728 | 3253 | 488 | 567 | 757 | 242 | 267 | 311 | 138 | 148 | 161 | . | . | . |
| | *** | 1543 | 2070 | 3247 | 521 | 634 | 736 | 253 | 286 | 289 | 142 | 153 | 138 | . | . | . |
| 0.8 | *** | 1200 | 1475 | 2702 | 407 | 469 | 607 | 193 | 211 | 239 | . | . | . | . | . | . |
| | *** | 1310 | 1770 | 2687 | 434 | 521 | 584 | 201 | 223 | 216 | . | . | . | . | . | . |
| 0.85 | *** | 964 | 1187 | 2053 | 310 | 352 | 432 | . | . | . | . | . | . | . | . | . |
| | *** | 1054 | 1417 | 2033 | 328 | 384 | 409 | . | . | . | . | . | . | . | . | . |
| 0.9 | *** | 691 | 841 | 1308 | . | . | . | . | . | . | . | . | . | . | . | . |
| | *** | 753 | 984 | 1285 | . | . | . | . | . | . | . | . | . | . | . | . |

## TABLE 1: ALPHA= 0.005 POWER= 0.8    EXPECTED ACCRUAL THRU MINIMUM FOLLOW-UP= 375

| | | DEL=.05 | | | DEL=.10 | | | DEL=.15 | | | DEL=.20 | | | DEL=.25 | |
|---|---|---|---|---|---|---|---|---|---|---|---|---|---|---|---|---|
| FACT= | 1.0 .75 | .50 .25 | .00 BIN | 1.0 .75 | .50 .25 | .00 BIN | 1.0 .75 | .50 .25 | .00 BIN | 1.0 75 | .50 .25 | .00 BIN | 1.0 .75 | .50 .25 | .00 BIN | |

PCONT=***                     REQUIRED NUMBER OF PATIENTS

| PCONT | | .05 (1.0/.75) | .05 (.50/.25) | .05 (.00/BIN) | .10 (1.0/.75) | .10 (.50/.25) | .10 (.00/BIN) | .15 (1.0/.75) | .15 (.50/.25) | .15 (.00/BIN) | .20 (1.0/75) | .20 (.50/.25) | .20 (.00/BIN) | .25 (1.0/.75) | .25 (.50/.25) | .25 (.00/BIN) |
|---|---|---|---|---|---|---|---|---|---|---|---|---|---|---|---|---|
| 0.05 | *** | 704 | 713 | 746 | 254 | 258 | 265 | 150 | 152 | 155 | 106 | 107 | 109 | 83 | 83 | 84 |
|  | *** | 707 | 723 | 1285 | 256 | 261 | 409 | 151 | 153 | 216 | 107 | 108 | 138 | 83 | 84 | 97 |
| 0.1 | *** | 1287 | 1307 | 1439 | 407 | 419 | 444 | 221 | 227 | 236 | 147 | 150 | 155 | 109 | 111 | 113 |
|  | *** | 1294 | 1338 | 2033 | 412 | 429 | 584 | 223 | 230 | 289 | 149 | 152 | 176 | 110 | 112 | 119 |
| 0.15 | *** | 1784 | 1820 | 2109 | 533 | 555 | 609 | 279 | 289 | 307 | 180 | 185 | 193 | 130 | 133 | 137 |
|  | *** | 1796 | 1878 | 2687 | 542 | 575 | 736 | 283 | 297 | 351 | 182 | 189 | 208 | 131 | 135 | 138 |
| 0.2 | *** | 2173 | 2227 | 2721 | 632 | 665 | 755 | 324 | 340 | 368 | 205 | 213 | 226 | 145 | 150 | 157 |
|  | *** | 2191 | 2317 | 3247 | 645 | 696 | 865 | 331 | 351 | 403 | 209 | 219 | 234 | 148 | 153 | 153 |
| 0.25 | *** | 2448 | 2525 | 3256 | 704 | 749 | 879 | 358 | 379 | 419 | 224 | 235 | 252 | 157 | 163 | 172 |
|  | *** | 2474 | 2653 | 3714 | 722 | 793 | 970 | 367 | 395 | 444 | 229 | 242 | 255 | 160 | 167 | 164 |
| 0.3 | *** | 2616 | 2720 | 3703 | 752 | 810 | 980 | 380 | 407 | 460 | 237 | 250 | 272 | 165 | 172 | 183 |
|  | *** | 2651 | 2888 | 4088 | 775 | 866 | 1052 | 392 | 428 | 475 | 243 | 260 | 269 | 168 | 177 | 171 |
| 0.35 | *** | 2686 | 2821 | 4055 | 778 | 848 | 1056 | 394 | 426 | 488 | 244 | 260 | 285 | 169 | 177 | 189 |
|  | *** | 2732 | 3034 | 4368 | 807 | 916 | 1110 | 408 | 450 | 496 | 251 | 271 | 278 | 173 | 183 | 175 |
| 0.4 | *** | 2672 | 2842 | 4308 | 786 | 867 | 1108 | 399 | 435 | 506 | 247 | 264 | 292 | 169 | 178 | 192 |
|  | *** | 2731 | 3100 | 4555 | 819 | 945 | 1145 | 415 | 463 | 507 | 254 | 276 | 281 | 174 | 184 | 175 |
| 0.45 | *** | 2589 | 2798 | 4462 | 778 | 868 | 1134 | 396 | 435 | 512 | 244 | 263 | 292 | 167 | 176 | 190 |
|  | *** | 2663 | 3098 | 4649 | 815 | 954 | 1157 | 413 | 465 | 507 | 253 | 275 | 278 | 171 | 182 | 171 |
| 0.5 | *** | 2453 | 2701 | 4513 | 756 | 853 | 1134 | 387 | 427 | 506 | 237 | 256 | 286 | 161 | 170 | 184 |
|  | *** | 2543 | 3039 | 4649 | 796 | 945 | 1145 | 404 | 458 | 496 | 246 | 269 | 269 | 165 | 177 | 164 |
| 0.55 | *** | 2281 | 2564 | 4464 | 723 | 824 | 1109 | 371 | 411 | 490 | 226 | 245 | 274 | 152 | 161 | 174 |
|  | *** | 2386 | 2930 | 4555 | 765 | 918 | 1110 | 388 | 442 | 475 | 235 | 257 | 255 | 156 | 167 | 153 |
| 0.6 | *** | 2086 | 2397 | 4312 | 680 | 781 | 1059 | 348 | 388 | 462 | 211 | 228 | 255 | 140 | 149 | 160 |
|  | *** | 2204 | 2780 | 4368 | 722 | 874 | 1052 | 366 | 417 | 444 | 219 | 240 | 234 | 144 | 154 | 138 |
| 0.65 | *** | 1879 | 2206 | 4059 | 628 | 726 | 983 | 320 | 356 | 423 | 192 | 207 | 230 | 125 | 133 | 142 |
|  | *** | 2005 | 2591 | 4088 | 669 | 813 | 970 | 336 | 383 | 403 | 199 | 217 | 208 | 129 | 137 | 119 |
| 0.7 | *** | 1667 | 1994 | 3706 | 567 | 657 | 882 | 286 | 317 | 372 | 168 | 180 | 198 | 107 | 113 | 120 |
|  | *** | 1795 | 2367 | 3714 | 605 | 736 | 865 | 300 | 340 | 351 | 174 | 188 | 176 | 110 | 116 | 97 |
| 0.75 | *** | 1450 | 1761 | 3253 | 496 | 574 | 757 | 244 | 270 | 311 | 139 | 148 | 161 | . | . | . |
|  | *** | 1573 | 2105 | 3247 | 529 | 640 | 736 | 256 | 287 | 289 | 143 | 154 | 138 | . | . | . |
| 0.8 | *** | 1226 | 1503 | 2702 | 413 | 475 | 606 | 195 | 212 | 239 | . | . | . | . | . | . |
|  | *** | 1337 | 1799 | 2687 | 440 | 525 | 584 | 203 | 224 | 216 | . | . | . | . | . | . |
| 0.85 | *** | 985 | 1210 | 2053 | 314 | 355 | 432 | . | . | . | . | . | . | . | . | . |
|  | *** | 1076 | 1439 | 2033 | 332 | 386 | 409 | . | . | . | . | . | . | . | . | . |
| 0.9 | *** | 706 | 856 | 1308 | . | . | . | . | . | . | . | . | . | . | . | . |
|  | *** | 768 | 997 | 1285 | . | . | . | . | . | . | . | . | . | . | . | . |

## TABLE 1: ALPHA= 0.005 POWER= 0.8    EXPECTED ACCRUAL THRU MINIMUM FOLLOW-UP= 400

| | | DEL=.05 | | | DEL=.10 | | | DEL=.15 | | | DEL=.20 | | | DEL=.25 | | |
|---|---|---|---|---|---|---|---|---|---|---|---|---|---|---|---|---|
| FACT= | | 1.0 .75 | .50 .25 | .00 BIN | 1.0 .75 | .50 .25 | .00 BIN | 1.0 .75 | .50 .25 | .00 BIN | 1.0 75 | .50 .25 | .00 BIN | 1.0 .75 | .50 .25 | .00 BIN |
| PCONT=*** | | | | | REQUIRED NUMBER OF PATIENTS | | | | | | | | | | | |
| 0.05 | *** | 705 | 714 | 746 | 254 | 258 | 265 | 150 | 152 | 155 | 106 | 107 | 109 | 83 | 83 | 84 |
| | *** | 708 | 724 | 1285 | 256 | 261 | 409 | 151 | 153 | 216 | 107 | 108 | 138 | 83 | 84 | 97 |
| 0.1 | *** | 1288 | 1310 | 1439 | 408 | 420 | 444 | 222 | 227 | 236 | 148 | 151 | 155 | 109 | 111 | 113 |
| | *** | 1296 | 1342 | 2033 | 413 | 429 | 584 | 224 | 231 | 289 | 149 | 152 | 176 | 110 | 112 | 119 |
| 0.15 | *** | 1787 | 1824 | 2109 | 535 | 557 | 609 | 280 | 290 | 307 | 180 | 186 | 193 | 130 | 133 | 137 |
| | *** | 1800 | 1884 | 2687 | 544 | 576 | 736 | 284 | 297 | 351 | 183 | 189 | 208 | 132 | 135 | 138 |
| 0.2 | *** | 2176 | 2234 | 2721 | 635 | 668 | 755 | 325 | 341 | 368 | 206 | 214 | 226 | 146 | 151 | 157 |
| | *** | 2196 | 2327 | 3247 | 648 | 699 | 865 | 332 | 352 | 403 | 210 | 219 | 234 | 148 | 153 | 153 |
| 0.25 | *** | 2454 | 2535 | 3256 | 708 | 754 | 879 | 360 | 381 | 419 | 225 | 236 | 252 | 158 | 164 | 172 |
| | *** | 2481 | 2667 | 3714 | 727 | 797 | 970 | 369 | 397 | 444 | 230 | 243 | 255 | 161 | 167 | 164 |
| 0.3 | *** | 2623 | 2733 | 3703 | 757 | 815 | 980 | 383 | 410 | 459 | 238 | 252 | 272 | 166 | 173 | 183 |
| | *** | 2661 | 2907 | 4088 | 781 | 871 | 1052 | 395 | 430 | 475 | 244 | 260 | 269 | 169 | 177 | 171 |
| 0.35 | *** | 2695 | 2838 | 4055 | 784 | 855 | 1056 | 397 | 428 | 488 | 246 | 261 | 285 | 170 | 178 | 189 |
| | *** | 2745 | 3057 | 4368 | 813 | 922 | 1110 | 411 | 452 | 496 | 253 | 272 | 278 | 173 | 183 | 175 |
| 0.4 | *** | 2684 | 2863 | 4308 | 793 | 875 | 1108 | 403 | 438 | 506 | 249 | 265 | 292 | 170 | 179 | 192 |
| | *** | 2747 | 3128 | 4555 | 826 | 952 | 1145 | 418 | 465 | 507 | 256 | 277 | 281 | 174 | 185 | 175 |
| 0.45 | *** | 2604 | 2822 | 4462 | 786 | 876 | 1134 | 400 | 438 | 512 | 246 | 264 | 292 | 168 | 177 | 190 |
| | *** | 2682 | 3130 | 4649 | 823 | 962 | 1157 | 417 | 468 | 507 | 254 | 276 | 278 | 172 | 183 | 171 |
| 0.5 | *** | 2472 | 2729 | 4514 | 765 | 862 | 1134 | 391 | 430 | 506 | 239 | 258 | 286 | 162 | 171 | 184 |
| | *** | 2566 | 3073 | 4649 | 805 | 952 | 1145 | 408 | 461 | 496 | 248 | 270 | 269 | 166 | 177 | 164 |
| 0.55 | *** | 2303 | 2596 | 4464 | 732 | 833 | 1109 | 375 | 415 | 490 | 228 | 246 | 274 | 153 | 162 | 174 |
| | *** | 2412 | 2967 | 4555 | 774 | 925 | 1110 | 392 | 445 | 475 | 236 | 258 | 255 | 157 | 167 | 153 |
| 0.6 | *** | 2111 | 2430 | 4312 | 689 | 791 | 1059 | 352 | 391 | 462 | 213 | 230 | 255 | 141 | 149 | 160 |
| | *** | 2233 | 2818 | 4368 | 732 | 881 | 1052 | 369 | 420 | 444 | 221 | 241 | 234 | 145 | 154 | 138 |
| 0.65 | *** | 1906 | 2240 | 4059 | 637 | 735 | 983 | 324 | 359 | 423 | 193 | 208 | 230 | 126 | 133 | 142 |
| | *** | 2036 | 2629 | 4088 | 678 | 820 | 970 | 340 | 385 | 403 | 200 | 218 | 208 | 129 | 137 | 119 |
| 0.7 | *** | 1695 | 2027 | 3706 | 576 | 665 | 882 | 289 | 320 | 372 | 169 | 181 | 198 | 108 | 113 | 120 |
| | *** | 1825 | 2402 | 3714 | 614 | 742 | 865 | 303 | 342 | 351 | 175 | 189 | 176 | 110 | 116 | 97 |
| 0.75 | *** | 1477 | 1792 | 3253 | 504 | 581 | 757 | 247 | 272 | 311 | 140 | 149 | 161 | . | . | . |
| | *** | 1602 | 2137 | 3247 | 537 | 645 | 736 | 258 | 289 | 289 | 144 | 154 | 138 | . | . | . |
| 0.8 | *** | 1250 | 1531 | 2702 | 419 | 480 | 607 | 197 | 214 | 239 | . | . | . | . | . | . |
| | *** | 1363 | 1827 | 2687 | 446 | 529 | 584 | 205 | 225 | 216 | . | . | . | . | . | . |
| 0.85 | *** | 1005 | 1231 | 2053 | 319 | 359 | 432 | . | . | . | . | . | . | . | . | . |
| | *** | 1097 | 1459 | 2033 | 336 | 389 | 409 | . | . | . | . | . | . | . | . | . |
| 0.9 | *** | 720 | 870 | 1308 | . | . | . | . | . | . | . | . | . | . | . | . |
| | *** | 782 | 1009 | 1285 | . | . | . | . | . | . | . | . | . | . | . | . |

## TABLE 1: ALPHA= 0.005 POWER= 0.8    EXPECTED ACCRUAL THRU MINIMUM FOLLOW-UP= 425

| | | DEL=.05 | | | DEL=.10 | | | DEL=.15 | | | DEL=.20 | | | DEL=.25 | | |
|---|---|---|---|---|---|---|---|---|---|---|---|---|---|---|---|---|
| FACT= | | 1.0 .75 | .50 .25 | .00 BIN | 1.0 .75 | .50 .25 | .00 BIN | 1.0 .75 | .50 .25 | .00 BIN | 1.0 75 | .50 .25 | .00 BIN | 1.0 .75 | .50 .25 | .00 BIN |
| PCONT=*** | | | | | REQUIRED NUMBER OF PATIENTS | | | | | | | | | | | |
| 0.05 | *** | 706 | 715 | 746 | 255 | 259 | 265 | 150 | 152 | 155 | 106 | 107 | 109 | 83 | 84 | 84 |
| | *** | 709 | 725 | 1285 | 256 | 261 | 409 | 151 | 153 | 216 | 107 | 108 | 138 | 83 | 84 | 97 |
| 0.1 | *** | 1290 | 1312 | 1439 | 409 | 421 | 444 | 222 | 227 | 236 | 148 | 151 | 155 | 110 | 111 | 113 |
| | *** | 1298 | 1344 | 2033 | 414 | 430 | 584 | 224 | 231 | 289 | 149 | 153 | 176 | 110 | 112 | 119 |
| 0.15 | *** | 1789 | 1829 | 2109 | 537 | 559 | 609 | 281 | 291 | 307 | 181 | 186 | 193 | 130 | 133 | 137 |
| | *** | 1803 | 1890 | 2687 | 546 | 578 | 736 | 285 | 298 | 351 | 183 | 189 | 208 | 132 | 135 | 138 |
| 0.2 | *** | 2180 | 2241 | 2721 | 638 | 671 | 755 | 327 | 342 | 368 | 207 | 215 | 226 | 146 | 151 | 156 |
| | *** | 2201 | 2337 | 3247 | 651 | 701 | 865 | 334 | 353 | 403 | 210 | 220 | 234 | 149 | 154 | 153 |
| 0.25 | *** | 2459 | 2544 | 3256 | 712 | 758 | 879 | 362 | 382 | 419 | 226 | 237 | 252 | 158 | 164 | 172 |
| | *** | 2488 | 2680 | 3714 | 731 | 800 | 970 | 371 | 398 | 444 | 231 | 243 | 255 | 161 | 168 | 164 |
| 0.3 | *** | 2630 | 2745 | 3703 | 762 | 821 | 980 | 386 | 411 | 459 | 240 | 252 | 272 | 166 | 173 | 183 |
| | *** | 2670 | 2925 | 4088 | 786 | 875 | 1052 | 397 | 431 | 475 | 246 | 261 | 269 | 170 | 178 | 171 |
| 0.35 | *** | 2705 | 2854 | 4055 | 790 | 861 | 1056 | 400 | 431 | 488 | 248 | 262 | 285 | 170 | 178 | 189 |
| | *** | 2757 | 3079 | 4368 | 819 | 927 | 1110 | 414 | 454 | 496 | 254 | 272 | 278 | 174 | 183 | 175 |
| 0.4 | *** | 2696 | 2883 | 4309 | 800 | 882 | 1108 | 406 | 441 | 506 | 250 | 266 | 292 | 171 | 180 | 192 |
| | *** | 2762 | 3154 | 4555 | 834 | 958 | 1145 | 421 | 467 | 507 | 258 | 278 | 281 | 175 | 185 | 175 |
| 0.45 | *** | 2619 | 2846 | 4462 | 793 | 884 | 1133 | 404 | 441 | 512 | 248 | 265 | 292 | 169 | 178 | 190 |
| | *** | 2701 | 3159 | 4649 | 831 | 968 | 1157 | 420 | 470 | 507 | 256 | 277 | 278 | 173 | 183 | 171 |
| 0.5 | *** | 2490 | 2756 | 4514 | 773 | 870 | 1134 | 394 | 433 | 506 | 241 | 259 | 286 | 163 | 172 | 184 |
| | *** | 2588 | 3106 | 4649 | 814 | 960 | 1145 | 411 | 463 | 496 | 249 | 271 | 269 | 167 | 178 | 164 |
| 0.55 | *** | 2325 | 2626 | 4464 | 741 | 842 | 1109 | 379 | 418 | 490 | 230 | 247 | 274 | 154 | 163 | 174 |
| | *** | 2438 | 3002 | 4555 | 783 | 933 | 1110 | 396 | 447 | 475 | 238 | 259 | 255 | 158 | 168 | 153 |
| 0.6 | *** | 2135 | 2462 | 4312 | 698 | 799 | 1059 | 356 | 394 | 462 | 215 | 231 | 255 | 142 | 150 | 160 |
| | *** | 2261 | 2853 | 4368 | 741 | 888 | 1052 | 373 | 422 | 444 | 222 | 241 | 234 | 146 | 154 | 138 |
| 0.65 | *** | 1932 | 2272 | 4059 | 646 | 743 | 983 | 327 | 362 | 423 | 195 | 209 | 230 | 127 | 133 | 142 |
| | *** | 2065 | 2664 | 4088 | 687 | 827 | 970 | 343 | 387 | 403 | 201 | 218 | 208 | 130 | 137 | 119 |
| 0.7 | *** | 1721 | 2059 | 3706 | 584 | 672 | 882 | 292 | 322 | 372 | 170 | 182 | 198 | 108 | 113 | 120 |
| | *** | 1854 | 2436 | 3714 | 621 | 748 | 865 | 306 | 343 | 351 | 176 | 189 | 176 | 111 | 116 | 97 |
| 0.75 | *** | 1503 | 1822 | 3253 | 511 | 587 | 757 | 249 | 273 | 311 | 141 | 150 | 161 | . | . | . |
| | *** | 1630 | 2167 | 3247 | 544 | 650 | 736 | 260 | 290 | 289 | 145 | 155 | 138 | . | . | . |
| 0.8 | *** | 1274 | 1556 | 2702 | 425 | 485 | 606 | 198 | 215 | 239 | . | . | . | . | . | . |
| | *** | 1387 | 1852 | 2687 | 451 | 532 | 584 | 206 | 226 | 216 | . | . | . | . | . | . |
| 0.85 | *** | 1024 | 1251 | 2053 | 322 | 362 | 432 | . | . | . | . | . | . | . | . | . |
| | *** | 1117 | 1478 | 2033 | 340 | 391 | 409 | . | . | . | . | . | . | . | . | . |
| 0.9 | *** | 733 | 883 | 1308 | . | . | . | . | . | . | . | . | . | . | . | . |
| | *** | 796 | 1020 | 1285 | . | . | . | . | . | . | . | . | . | . | . | . |

**TABLE 1: ALPHA= 0.005 POWER= 0.8    EXPECTED ACCRUAL THRU MINIMUM FOLLOW-UP= 450**

| PCONT | FACT= | DEL=.05 1.0 .75 | .50 .25 | .00 BIN | DEL=.10 1.0 .75 | .50 .25 | .00 BIN | DEL=.15 1.0 .75 | .50 .25 | .00 BIN | DEL=.20 1.0 75 | .50 .25 | .00 BIN | DEL=.25 1.0 .75 | .50 .25 | .00 BIN |
|---|---|---|---|---|---|---|---|---|---|---|---|---|---|---|---|---|
| | | | | | REQUIRED NUMBER OF PATIENTS | | | | | | | | | | | |
| 0.05 | *** | 706 | 716 | 746 | 255 | 259 | 265 | 150 | 152 | 155 | 106 | 108 | 109 | 83 | 84 | 84 |
| | *** | 710 | 726 | 1285 | 257 | 262 | 409 | 151 | 153 | 216 | 107 | 108 | 138 | 83 | 84 | 97 |
| 0.1 | *** | 1291 | 1315 | 1439 | 410 | 422 | 444 | 222 | 228 | 236 | 148 | 151 | 154 | 110 | 111 | 113 |
| | *** | 1299 | 1347 | 2033 | 415 | 431 | 584 | 225 | 231 | 289 | 149 | 153 | 176 | 111 | 112 | 119 |
| 0.15 | *** | 1791 | 1833 | 2109 | 539 | 560 | 609 | 282 | 291 | 307 | 181 | 186 | 193 | 131 | 134 | 137 |
| | *** | 1806 | 1896 | 2687 | 548 | 579 | 736 | 286 | 298 | 351 | 184 | 190 | 208 | 132 | 135 | 138 |
| 0.2 | *** | 2184 | 2247 | 2721 | 640 | 674 | 755 | 328 | 343 | 369 | 208 | 215 | 226 | 147 | 151 | 157 |
| | *** | 2206 | 2346 | 3247 | 654 | 703 | 865 | 335 | 354 | 403 | 211 | 220 | 234 | 149 | 154 | 153 |
| 0.25 | *** | 2464 | 2554 | 3256 | 716 | 761 | 879 | 363 | 384 | 419 | 227 | 237 | 252 | 159 | 165 | 172 |
| | *** | 2495 | 2693 | 3714 | 734 | 803 | 970 | 372 | 399 | 444 | 232 | 244 | 255 | 162 | 168 | 164 |
| 0.3 | *** | 2637 | 2758 | 3703 | 766 | 825 | 980 | 388 | 414 | 459 | 241 | 253 | 272 | 167 | 174 | 183 |
| | *** | 2679 | 2942 | 4088 | 791 | 879 | 1052 | 399 | 432 | 475 | 247 | 262 | 269 | 170 | 178 | 171 |
| 0.35 | *** | 2714 | 2870 | 4055 | 796 | 867 | 1056 | 403 | 433 | 488 | 249 | 263 | 285 | 171 | 179 | 189 |
| | *** | 2769 | 3100 | 4368 | 825 | 932 | 1110 | 416 | 456 | 496 | 255 | 273 | 278 | 175 | 184 | 175 |
| 0.4 | *** | 2708 | 2903 | 4308 | 806 | 888 | 1108 | 409 | 443 | 506 | 252 | 268 | 292 | 172 | 180 | 192 |
| | *** | 2777 | 3178 | 4555 | 840 | 964 | 1145 | 424 | 469 | 507 | 259 | 279 | 281 | 176 | 185 | 175 |
| 0.45 | *** | 2634 | 2869 | 4462 | 801 | 892 | 1134 | 407 | 444 | 512 | 249 | 267 | 292 | 169 | 178 | 190 |
| | *** | 2719 | 3188 | 4649 | 838 | 974 | 1157 | 423 | 471 | 507 | 257 | 278 | 278 | 174 | 183 | 171 |
| 0.5 | *** | 2508 | 2783 | 4514 | 781 | 878 | 1134 | 398 | 436 | 507 | 243 | 260 | 286 | 164 | 172 | 184 |
| | *** | 2610 | 3137 | 4649 | 822 | 966 | 1145 | 415 | 465 | 496 | 251 | 272 | 269 | 168 | 178 | 164 |
| 0.55 | *** | 2346 | 2654 | 4464 | 749 | 850 | 1109 | 382 | 420 | 490 | 232 | 249 | 274 | 155 | 163 | 174 |
| | *** | 2462 | 3035 | 4555 | 792 | 939 | 1110 | 399 | 449 | 475 | 239 | 260 | 255 | 159 | 168 | 153 |
| 0.6 | *** | 2159 | 2493 | 4312 | 707 | 807 | 1059 | 360 | 396 | 462 | 216 | 232 | 255 | 143 | 150 | 160 |
| | *** | 2287 | 2887 | 4368 | 749 | 895 | 1052 | 376 | 423 | 444 | 223 | 242 | 234 | 146 | 155 | 138 |
| 0.65 | *** | 1958 | 2303 | 4059 | 654 | 750 | 983 | 330 | 365 | 423 | 196 | 210 | 230 | 127 | 134 | 142 |
| | *** | 2093 | 2697 | 4088 | 695 | 833 | 970 | 346 | 389 | 403 | 203 | 219 | 208 | 131 | 138 | 119 |
| 0.7 | *** | 1747 | 2089 | 3706 | 591 | 679 | 882 | 295 | 324 | 372 | 172 | 183 | 198 | 109 | 114 | 120 |
| | *** | 1882 | 2467 | 3714 | 629 | 753 | 865 | 308 | 345 | 351 | 177 | 190 | 176 | 111 | 117 | 97 |
| 0.75 | *** | 1527 | 1850 | 3253 | 517 | 593 | 757 | 252 | 275 | 311 | 142 | 150 | 161 | . | . | . |
| | *** | 1656 | 2196 | 3247 | 550 | 654 | 736 | 262 | 291 | 289 | 146 | 155 | 138 | . | . | . |
| 0.8 | *** | 1296 | 1581 | 2702 | 430 | 490 | 606 | 200 | 216 | 239 | . | . | . | . | . | . |
| | *** | 1411 | 1876 | 2687 | 456 | 536 | 584 | 207 | 226 | 216 | . | . | . | . | . | . |
| 0.85 | *** | 1042 | 1271 | 2053 | 326 | 365 | 432 | . | . | . | . | . | . | . | . | . |
| | *** | 1136 | 1496 | 2033 | 343 | 393 | 409 | . | . | . | . | . | . | . | . | . |
| 0.9 | *** | 745 | 895 | 1308 | . | . | . | . | . | . | . | . | . | . | . | . |
| | *** | 808 | 1031 | 1285 | . | . | . | . | . | . | . | . | . | . | . | . |

## TABLE 1: ALPHA= 0.005 POWER= 0.8     EXPECTED ACCRUAL THRU MINIMUM FOLLOW-UP= 475

| | | DEL=.05 | | | DEL=.10 | | | DEL=.15 | | | DEL=.20 | | | DEL=.25 | | |
|---|---|---|---|---|---|---|---|---|---|---|---|---|---|---|---|---|---|
| FACT= | | 1.0 .75 | .50 .25 | .00 BIN | 1.0 .75 | .50 .25 | .00 BIN | 1.0 .75 | .50 .25 | .00 BIN | 1.0 75 | .50 .25 | .00 BIN | 1.0 .75 | .50 .25 | .00 BIN |
| PCONT=*** | | | | | REQUIRED NUMBER OF PATIENTS | | | | | | | | | | | |
| 0.05 | *** | 707 | 716 | 746 | 255 | 259 | 265 | 150 | 152 | 155 | 107 | 108 | 109 | 83 | 83 | 84 |
| | *** | 710 | 726 | 1285 | 257 | 262 | 409 | 151 | 153 | 216 | 107 | 108 | 138 | 83 | 84 | 97 |
| 0.1 | *** | 1293 | 1317 | 1439 | 411 | 422 | 444 | 223 | 228 | 236 | 148 | 151 | 155 | 110 | 111 | 113 |
| | *** | 1301 | 1350 | 2033 | 416 | 431 | 584 | 225 | 232 | 289 | 150 | 153 | 176 | 110 | 112 | 119 |
| 0.15 | *** | 1794 | 1837 | 2109 | 541 | 562 | 609 | 282 | 292 | 307 | 182 | 187 | 193 | 131 | 134 | 137 |
| | *** | 1809 | 1901 | 2687 | 549 | 580 | 736 | 287 | 298 | 351 | 184 | 190 | 208 | 132 | 135 | 138 |
| 0.2 | *** | 2187 | 2254 | 2721 | 643 | 676 | 755 | 330 | 344 | 368 | 208 | 216 | 226 | 147 | 151 | 157 |
| | *** | 2211 | 2354 | 3247 | 657 | 705 | 865 | 336 | 355 | 403 | 212 | 220 | 234 | 149 | 154 | 153 |
| 0.25 | *** | 2469 | 2563 | 3256 | 719 | 765 | 879 | 365 | 385 | 419 | 228 | 238 | 252 | 159 | 165 | 172 |
| | *** | 2502 | 2705 | 3714 | 738 | 806 | 970 | 374 | 400 | 444 | 233 | 244 | 255 | 162 | 168 | 164 |
| 0.3 | *** | 2644 | 2770 | 3703 | 771 | 830 | 980 | 390 | 415 | 459 | 242 | 254 | 272 | 167 | 174 | 183 |
| | *** | 2688 | 2958 | 4088 | 795 | 883 | 1052 | 401 | 433 | 475 | 248 | 262 | 269 | 171 | 178 | 171 |
| 0.35 | *** | 2723 | 2885 | 4055 | 801 | 872 | 1056 | 406 | 435 | 488 | 250 | 264 | 285 | 172 | 179 | 189 |
| | *** | 2781 | 3120 | 4368 | 831 | 937 | 1110 | 419 | 457 | 496 | 257 | 273 | 278 | 175 | 184 | 175 |
| 0.4 | *** | 2720 | 2922 | 4309 | 813 | 895 | 1108 | 412 | 445 | 506 | 253 | 269 | 292 | 173 | 181 | 192 |
| | *** | 2792 | 3202 | 4555 | 847 | 969 | 1145 | 427 | 470 | 507 | 260 | 279 | 281 | 177 | 186 | 175 |
| 0.45 | *** | 2649 | 2892 | 4462 | 808 | 899 | 1134 | 410 | 447 | 512 | 251 | 267 | 292 | 170 | 179 | 190 |
| | *** | 2737 | 3215 | 4649 | 846 | 980 | 1157 | 426 | 473 | 507 | 259 | 279 | 278 | 174 | 184 | 171 |
| 0.5 | *** | 2526 | 2808 | 4513 | 789 | 886 | 1134 | 401 | 439 | 507 | 244 | 261 | 286 | 165 | 173 | 184 |
| | *** | 2631 | 3167 | 4649 | 830 | 972 | 1145 | 418 | 467 | 496 | 252 | 272 | 269 | 168 | 178 | 164 |
| 0.55 | *** | 2366 | 2682 | 4463 | 757 | 857 | 1109 | 385 | 423 | 490 | 233 | 250 | 274 | 156 | 164 | 174 |
| | *** | 2486 | 3066 | 4555 | 799 | 946 | 1110 | 402 | 450 | 475 | 241 | 260 | 255 | 159 | 168 | 153 |
| 0.6 | *** | 2182 | 2521 | 4312 | 715 | 815 | 1059 | 363 | 399 | 462 | 218 | 233 | 255 | 143 | 151 | 160 |
| | *** | 2313 | 2919 | 4368 | 757 | 901 | 1052 | 379 | 425 | 444 | 225 | 243 | 234 | 147 | 155 | 138 |
| 0.65 | *** | 1982 | 2333 | 4059 | 662 | 757 | 983 | 333 | 367 | 422 | 197 | 211 | 230 | 128 | 134 | 142 |
| | *** | 2119 | 2729 | 4088 | 702 | 839 | 970 | 348 | 390 | 403 | 204 | 219 | 208 | 131 | 138 | 119 |
| 0.7 | *** | 1771 | 2118 | 3706 | 598 | 686 | 882 | 298 | 326 | 372 | 172 | 184 | 198 | 110 | 114 | 120 |
| | *** | 1909 | 2497 | 3714 | 636 | 758 | 865 | 310 | 346 | 351 | 178 | 190 | 176 | 112 | 117 | 97 |
| 0.75 | *** | 1551 | 1876 | 3253 | 523 | 599 | 756 | 254 | 276 | 311 | 143 | 150 | 161 | . | . | . |
| | *** | 1681 | 2222 | 3247 | 556 | 659 | 736 | 264 | 292 | 289 | 146 | 155 | 138 | . | . | . |
| 0.8 | *** | 1317 | 1604 | 2702 | 435 | 494 | 606 | 202 | 217 | 239 | . | . | . | . | . | . |
| | *** | 1433 | 1898 | 2687 | 461 | 539 | 584 | 209 | 227 | 216 | . | . | . | . | . | . |
| 0.85 | *** | 1060 | 1289 | 2053 | 329 | 367 | 432 | . | . | . | . | . | . | . | . | . |
| | *** | 1153 | 1513 | 2033 | 346 | 395 | 409 | . | . | . | . | . | . | . | . | . |
| 0.9 | *** | 757 | 906 | 1308 | . | . | . | . | . | . | . | . | . | . | . | . |
| | *** | 820 | 1040 | 1285 | . | . | . | . | . | . | . | . | . | . | . | . |

TABLE 1: ALPHA= 0.005 POWER= 0.8     EXPECTED ACCRUAL THRU MINIMUM FOLLOW-UP= 500

| PCONT | | DEL=.05 1.0 / .75 | DEL=.05 .50 / .25 | DEL=.05 .00 / BIN | DEL=.10 1.0 / .75 | DEL=.10 .50 / .25 | DEL=.10 .00 / BIN | DEL=.15 1.0 / .75 | DEL=.15 .50 / .25 | DEL=.15 .00 / BIN | DEL=.20 1.0 / 75 | DEL=.20 .50 / .25 | DEL=.20 .00 / BIN | DEL=.25 1.0 / .75 | DEL=.25 .50 / .25 | DEL=.25 .00 / BIN |
|---|---|---|---|---|---|---|---|---|---|---|---|---|---|---|---|---|
| | | *REQUIRED NUMBER OF PATIENTS* | | | | | | | | | | | | | | |
| 0.05 | *** | 708 | 717 | 746 | 256 | 259 | 265 | 151 | 153 | 155 | 107 | 108 | 109 | 83 | 83 | 84 |
| | *** | 711 | 727 | 1285 | 258 | 262 | 409 | 152 | 153 | 216 | 107 | 108 | 138 | 83 | 84 | 97 |
| 0.1 | *** | 1294 | 1319 | 1439 | 412 | 423 | 444 | 223 | 228 | 236 | 149 | 151 | 155 | 110 | 112 | 113 |
| | *** | 1303 | 1353 | 2033 | 417 | 432 | 584 | 226 | 232 | 289 | 150 | 153 | 176 | 111 | 113 | 119 |
| 0.15 | *** | 1796 | 1842 | 2109 | 542 | 563 | 609 | 283 | 293 | 307 | 183 | 187 | 193 | 131 | 134 | 137 |
| | *** | 1812 | 1906 | 2687 | 551 | 581 | 736 | 288 | 299 | 351 | 185 | 190 | 208 | 133 | 136 | 138 |
| 0.2 | *** | 2191 | 2260 | 2721 | 645 | 678 | 755 | 331 | 345 | 368 | 209 | 216 | 226 | 148 | 152 | 157 |
| | *** | 2215 | 2363 | 3247 | 659 | 707 | 865 | 337 | 355 | 403 | 212 | 221 | 234 | 150 | 154 | 153 |
| 0.25 | *** | 2474 | 2572 | 3256 | 723 | 768 | 879 | 367 | 386 | 419 | 229 | 238 | 252 | 160 | 165 | 172 |
| | *** | 2508 | 2717 | 3714 | 742 | 809 | 970 | 376 | 400 | 444 | 233 | 245 | 255 | 163 | 168 | 164 |
| 0.3 | *** | 2651 | 2782 | 3703 | 775 | 834 | 980 | 392 | 417 | 459 | 243 | 255 | 272 | 168 | 174 | 183 |
| | *** | 2697 | 2973 | 4088 | 800 | 887 | 1052 | 403 | 435 | 475 | 248 | 263 | 269 | 171 | 178 | 171 |
| 0.35 | *** | 2733 | 2901 | 4055 | 807 | 878 | 1056 | 408 | 437 | 488 | 252 | 265 | 285 | 173 | 180 | 189 |
| | *** | 2792 | 3139 | 4368 | 836 | 941 | 1110 | 421 | 458 | 496 | 258 | 274 | 278 | 176 | 184 | 175 |
| 0.4 | *** | 2731 | 2940 | 4308 | 819 | 901 | 1108 | 415 | 448 | 506 | 254 | 270 | 292 | 173 | 181 | 192 |
| | *** | 2807 | 3225 | 4555 | 853 | 973 | 1145 | 429 | 472 | 507 | 262 | 280 | 281 | 177 | 186 | 175 |
| 0.45 | *** | 2663 | 2913 | 4462 | 814 | 905 | 1134 | 413 | 449 | 512 | 253 | 269 | 292 | 171 | 179 | 190 |
| | *** | 2755 | 3240 | 4649 | 853 | 985 | 1157 | 429 | 475 | 507 | 260 | 279 | 278 | 175 | 184 | 171 |
| 0.5 | *** | 2543 | 2833 | 4513 | 796 | 893 | 1134 | 404 | 441 | 507 | 246 | 262 | 286 | 165 | 173 | 184 |
| | *** | 2652 | 3195 | 4649 | 837 | 978 | 1145 | 421 | 468 | 496 | 253 | 273 | 269 | 169 | 178 | 164 |
| 0.55 | *** | 2386 | 2709 | 4463 | 765 | 865 | 1109 | 388 | 425 | 490 | 235 | 251 | 274 | 156 | 164 | 174 |
| | *** | 2509 | 3096 | 4555 | 807 | 951 | 1110 | 405 | 452 | 475 | 242 | 261 | 255 | 160 | 169 | 153 |
| 0.6 | *** | 2204 | 2549 | 4312 | 722 | 822 | 1058 | 366 | 401 | 462 | 219 | 234 | 255 | 144 | 151 | 160 |
| | *** | 2338 | 2949 | 4368 | 764 | 907 | 1052 | 382 | 427 | 444 | 226 | 243 | 234 | 148 | 155 | 138 |
| 0.65 | *** | 2005 | 2361 | 4059 | 669 | 764 | 983 | 336 | 369 | 423 | 199 | 212 | 230 | 129 | 135 | 142 |
| | *** | 2145 | 2758 | 4088 | 710 | 844 | 970 | 351 | 392 | 403 | 205 | 220 | 208 | 132 | 138 | 119 |
| 0.7 | *** | 1795 | 2145 | 3706 | 605 | 692 | 882 | 300 | 328 | 372 | 173 | 184 | 198 | 110 | 114 | 120 |
| | *** | 1934 | 2525 | 3714 | 642 | 763 | 865 | 313 | 347 | 351 | 178 | 191 | 176 | 112 | 117 | 97 |
| 0.75 | *** | 1573 | 1902 | 3253 | 529 | 603 | 757 | 256 | 278 | 311 | 143 | 151 | 161 | . | . | . |
| | *** | 1705 | 2248 | 3247 | 562 | 663 | 736 | 266 | 293 | 289 | 147 | 156 | 138 | . | . | . |
| 0.8 | *** | 1337 | 1626 | 2702 | 440 | 498 | 607 | 203 | 218 | 239 | . | . | . | . | . | . |
| | *** | 1454 | 1919 | 2687 | 465 | 541 | 584 | 210 | 228 | 216 | . | . | . | . | . | . |
| 0.85 | *** | 1076 | 1306 | 2053 | 333 | 370 | 432 | . | . | . | . | . | . | . | . | . |
| | *** | 1171 | 1528 | 2033 | 349 | 396 | 409 | . | . | . | . | . | . | . | . | . |
| 0.9 | *** | 768 | 917 | 1308 | . | . | . | . | . | . | . | . | . | . | . | . |
| | *** | 831 | 1049 | 1285 | . | . | . | . | . | . | . | . | . | . | . | . |

## TABLE 1: ALPHA= 0.005 POWER= 0.8    EXPECTED ACCRUAL THRU MINIMUM FOLLOW-UP= 550

| | DEL=.02 | | | DEL=.05 | | | DEL=.10 | | | DEL=.15 | | | DEL=.20 | | |
|---|---|---|---|---|---|---|---|---|---|---|---|---|---|---|---|
| FACT= | 1.0 .75 | .50 .25 | .00 BIN | 1.0 .75 | .50 .25 | .00 BIN | 1.0 .75 | .50 .25 | .00 BIN | 1.0 75 | .50 .25 | .00 BIN | 1.0 .75 | .50 .25 | .00 BIN |

PCONT=***  REQUIRED NUMBER OF PATIENTS

| PCONT | .02 1.0/.75 | .02 .50/.25 | .02 .00/BIN | .05 1.0/.75 | .05 .50/.25 | .05 .00/BIN | .10 1.0/.75 | .10 .50/.25 | .10 .00/BIN | .15 1.0/.75 | .15 .50/.25 | .15 .00/BIN | .20 1.0/.75 | .20 .50/.25 | .20 .00/BIN |
|---|---|---|---|---|---|---|---|---|---|---|---|---|---|---|---|
| 0.05 *** | 3323 | 3334 | 3518 | 709 | 718 | 746 | 256 | 260 | 265 | 151 | 153 | 155 | 107 | 107 | 109 |
| *** | 3326 | 3356 | 6576 | 712 | 728 | 1285 | 258 | 262 | 409 | 151 | 154 | 216 | 107 | 108 | 138 |
| 0.1 *** | 6912 | 6939 | 7730 | 1297 | 1324 | 1439 | 413 | 424 | 444 | 224 | 229 | 236 | 149 | 151 | 155 |
| *** | 6921 | 6993 | 11423 | 1306 | 1357 | 2033 | 418 | 433 | 584 | 226 | 232 | 289 | 150 | 153 | 176 |
| 0.15 *** | 10096 | 10144 | 11954 | 1801 | 1849 | 2109 | 545 | 566 | 609 | 285 | 294 | 307 | 183 | 188 | 193 |
| *** | 10112 | 10240 | 15685 | 1818 | 1916 | 2687 | 554 | 583 | 736 | 289 | 300 | 351 | 185 | 190 | 208 |
| 0.2 *** | 12630 | 12704 | 15884 | 2199 | 2273 | 2721 | 650 | 683 | 755 | 333 | 347 | 368 | 210 | 217 | 226 |
| *** | 12654 | 12851 | 19364 | 2225 | 2378 | 3247 | 664 | 710 | 865 | 339 | 356 | 403 | 213 | 221 | 234 |
| 0.25 *** | 14446 | 14552 | 19367 | 2485 | 2590 | 3256 | 729 | 774 | 879 | 370 | 389 | 419 | 231 | 239 | 252 |
| *** | 14481 | 14764 | 22459 | 2522 | 2739 | 3714 | 748 | 814 | 970 | 378 | 402 | 444 | 235 | 245 | 255 |
| 0.3 *** | 15555 | 15701 | 22320 | 2665 | 2805 | 3703 | 783 | 842 | 980 | 396 | 420 | 459 | 245 | 256 | 272 |
| *** | 15604 | 15991 | 24970 | 2715 | 3002 | 4088 | 808 | 893 | 1052 | 407 | 437 | 475 | 250 | 263 | 269 |
| 0.35 *** | 16008 | 16201 | 24695 | 2751 | 2930 | 4055 | 816 | 887 | 1056 | 412 | 440 | 488 | 254 | 267 | 285 |
| *** | 16072 | 16588 | 26897 | 2815 | 3175 | 4368 | 846 | 949 | 1110 | 425 | 461 | 496 | 259 | 275 | 278 |
| 0.4 *** | 15876 | 16128 | 26463 | 2754 | 2975 | 4309 | 830 | 912 | 1108 | 420 | 451 | 506 | 257 | 271 | 292 |
| *** | 15960 | 16632 | 28240 | 2835 | 3267 | 4555 | 864 | 982 | 1145 | 434 | 474 | 507 | 264 | 280 | 281 |
| 0.45 *** | 15243 | 15569 | 27607 | 2692 | 2955 | 4462 | 827 | 917 | 1134 | 419 | 453 | 512 | 255 | 270 | 292 |
| *** | 15352 | 16215 | 28999 | 2789 | 3288 | 4649 | 865 | 995 | 1157 | 434 | 478 | 507 | 262 | 280 | 278 |
| 0.5 *** | 14205 | 14621 | 28119 | 2577 | 2879 | 4513 | 809 | 905 | 1134 | 410 | 445 | 506 | 248 | 264 | 286 |
| *** | 14344 | 15438 | 28766 | 2692 | 3247 | 4649 | 850 | 988 | 1145 | 426 | 471 | 496 | 256 | 274 | 269 |
| 0.55 *** | 12860 | 13389 | 27996 | 2425 | 2759 | 4463 | 779 | 877 | 1109 | 394 | 430 | 490 | 237 | 252 | 274 |
| ***. | 13036 | 14403 | 28766 | 2554 | 3151 | 4555 | 821 | 961 | 1110 | 410 | 455 | 475 | 244 | 262 | 255 |
| 0.6 *** | 11311 | 11983 | 27237 | 2247 | 2602 | 4312 | 736 | 834 | 1059 | 371 | 405 | 462 | 221 | 235 | 255 |
| *** | 11537 | 13205 | 27773 | 2386 | 3005 | 4368 | 778 | 916 | 1052 | 386 | 429 | 444 | 228 | 244 | 234 |
| 0.65 *** | 9670 | 10510 | 25846 | 2050 | 2414 | 4059 | 683 | 776 | 983 | 341 | 373 | 423 | 201 | 213 | 230 |
| *** | 9958 | 11921 | 26196 | 2194 | 2814 | 4088 | 723 | 853 | 970 | 355 | 394 | 403 | 206 | 221 | 208 |
| 0.7 *** | 8051 | 9061 | 23826 | 1840 | 2197 | 3706 | 618 | 703 | 882 | 304 | 331 | 372 | 175 | 185 | 198 |
| *** | 8408 | 10599 | 24036 | 1982 | 2577 | 3714 | 654 | 771 | 865 | 316 | 349 | 351 | 180 | 191 | 176 |
| 0.75 *** | 6557 | 7688 | 21181 | 1616 | 1949 | 3253 | 540 | 613 | 756 | 259 | 280 | 311 | 145 | 152 | 161 |
| *** | 6972 | 9261 | 21291 | 1750 | 2294 | 3247 | 572 | 669 | 736 | 269 | 294 | 289 | 148 | 156 | 138 |
| 0.8 *** | 5241 | 6395 | 17920 | 1375 | 1667 | 2702 | 448 | 505 | 607 | 205 | 220 | 239 | . | . | . |
| *** | 5677 | 7894 | 17963 | 1494 | 1958 | 2687 | 473 | 546 | 584 | 212 | 228 | 216 | . | . | . |
| 0.85 *** | 4083 | 5143 | 14047 | 1107 | 1337 | 2053 | 338 | 374 | 432 | . | . | . | . | . | . |
| *** | 4491 | 6453 | 14050 | 1202 | 1557 | 2033 | 354 | 399 | 409 | . | . | . | . | . | . |
| 0.9 *** | 2994 | 3840 | 9570 | 789 | 936 | 1308 | . | . | . | . | . | . | . | . | . |
| *** | 3325 | 4839 | 9554 | 851 | 1065 | 1285 | . | . | . | . | . | . | . | . | . |
| 0.95 *** | 1787 | 2271 | 4496 | . | . | . | . | . | . | . | . | . | . | . | . |
| *** | 1981 | 2793 | 4474 | . | . | . | . | . | . | . | . | . | . | . | . |

TABLE 1: ALPHA= 0.005 POWER= 0.8    EXPECTED ACCRUAL THRU MINIMUM FOLLOW-UP= 600

| | | DEL=.02 | | | DEL=.05 | | | DEL=.10 | | | DEL=.15 | | | DEL=.20 | | |
|---|---|---|---|---|---|---|---|---|---|---|---|---|---|---|---|---|
| FACT= | | 1.0 .75 | .50 .25 | .00 BIN | 1.0 .75 | .50 .25 | .00 BIN | 1.0 .75 | .50 .25 | .00 BIN | 1.0 75 | .50 .25 | .00 BIN | 1.0 .75 | .50 .25 | .00 BIN |
| PCONT=*** | | | | REQUIRED NUMBER OF PATIENTS | | | | | | | | | | | | |
| 0.05 | *** *** | 3323 3328 | 3336 3360 | 3518 6576 | 710 713 | 719 729 | 746 1285 | 257 258 | 260 262 | 265 409 | 151 152 | 152 154 | 155 216 | 107 107 | 108 108 | 109 138 |
| 0.1 | *** *** | 6914 6925 | 6944 7003 | 7730 11423 | 1299 1310 | 1328 1361 | 1439 2033 | 415 420 | 426 433 | 444 584 | 225 227 | 229 232 | 236 289 | 149 151 | 152 153 | 154 176 |
| 0.15 | *** *** | 10100 10118 | 10153 10257 | 11954 15685 | 1806 1824 | 1857 1925 | 2109 2687 | 548 557 | 569 585 | 609 736 | 286 290 | 295 300 | 307 351 | 184 186 | 188 190 | 193 208 |
| 0.2 | *** *** | 12636 12663 | 12717 12878 | 15884 19364 | 2206 2234 | 2285 2393 | 2721 3247 | 654 668 | 687 713 | 755 865 | 335 341 | 348 357 | 368 403 | 211 214 | 217 221 | 226 234 |
| 0.25 | *** *** | 14455 14494 | 14571 14802 | 19367 22459 | 2495 2535 | 2606 2760 | 3256 3714 | 734 754 | 780 818 | 879 970 | 372 380 | 391 403 | 419 444 | 232 236 | 241 246 | 252 255 |
| 0.3 | *** *** | 15568 15621 | 15727 16044 | 22320 24970 | 2679 2732 | 2827 3029 | 3703 4088 | 791 815 | 849 898 | 980 1052 | 399 409 | 422 438 | 459 475 | 247 251 | 257 264 | 272 269 |
| 0.35 | *** *** | 16025 16096 | 16237 16658 | 24695 26897 | 2768 2837 | 2958 3208 | 4055 4368 | 825 855 | 895 955 | 1056 1110 | 416 428 | 443 463 | 488 496 | 256 261 | 268 275 | 285 278 |
| 0.4 | *** *** | 15898 15990 | 16174 16723 | 26462 28240 | 2777 2863 | 3009 3306 | 4308 4555 | 840 874 | 921 990 | 1108 1145 | 424 437 | 455 476 | 506 507 | 259 265 | 273 281 | 292 281 |
| 0.45 | *** *** | 15273 15391 | 15628 16330 | 27607 28999 | 2719 2822 | 2994 3332 | 4462 4649 | 838 876 | 928 1003 | 1133 1157 | 423 438 | 457 480 | 512 507 | 257 264 | 272 281 | 292 278 |
| 0.5 | *** *** | 14243 14394 | 14696 15581 | 28119 29175 | 2610 2729 | 2923 3295 | 4513 4649 | 822 862 | 917 997 | 1134 1145 | 415 430 | 449 473 | 506 496 | 251 257 | 265 275 | 286 269 |
| 0.55 | *** *** | 12908 13100 | 13485 14575 | 27996 28766 | 2462 2596 | 2806 3201 | 4463 4555 | 791 833 | 889 970 | 1109 1110 | 399 415 | 433 457 | 490 475 | 239 246 | 254 263 | 274 255 |
| 0.6 | *** *** | 11373 11619 | 12102 13404 | 27237 27773 | 2287 2430 | 2651 3056 | 4312 4368 | 749 790 | 846 925 | 1058 1052 | 376 391 | 409 431 | 462 444 | 223 230 | 237 245 | 255 234 |
| 0.65 | *** *** | 9749 10061 | 10654 12140 | 25846 26196 | 2092 2240 | 2463 2864 | 4059 4088 | 695 734 | 787 861 | 983 970 | 346 359 | 376 396 | 422 403 | 202 208 | 214 221 | 230 208 |
| 0.7 | *** *** | 8150 8533 | 9225 10829 | 23825 24036 | 1882 2027 | 2244 2624 | 3706 3714 | 629 665 | 712 778 | 882 865 | 308 320 | 334 350 | 372 351 | 177 181 | 186 192 | 198 176 |
| 0.75 | *** *** | 6674 7113 | 7862 9488 | 21181 21291 | 1656 1792 | 1993 2336 | 3253 3247 | 550 581 | 621 675 | 757 736 | 262 271 | 282 295 | 311 289 | 146 149 | 152 156 | 161 138 |
| 0.8 | *** *** | 5367 5821 | 6565 8104 | 17920 17963 | 1411 1531 | 1704 1993 | 2702 2687 | 456 480 | 511 550 | 607 584 | 207 214 | 221 229 | 239 216 | . . | . . | . . |
| 0.85 | *** *** | 4202 4624 | 5294 6633 | 14047 14050 | 1136 1231 | 1366 1582 | 2053 2033 | 343 359 | 378 401 | 432 409 | . . | . . | . . | . . | . . | . . |
| 0.9 | *** *** | 3091 3431 | 3958 4972 | 9570 9554 | 808 870 | 954 1079 | 1308 1285 | . . | . . | . . | . . | . . | . . | . . | . . | . . |
| 0.95 | *** *** | 1844 2041 | 2335 2859 | 4496 4474 | . . | . . | . . | . . | . . | . . | . . | . . | . . | . . | . . | . . |

# TABLE 1: ALPHA= 0.005 POWER= 0.8    EXPECTED ACCRUAL THRU MINIMUM FOLLOW-UP= 650

| | | DEL=.02 | | | DEL=.05 | | | DEL=.10 | | | DEL=.15 | | | DEL=.20 | | |
|---|---|---|---|---|---|---|---|---|---|---|---|---|---|---|---|---|
| FACT= | | 1.0 .75 | .50 .25 | .00 BIN | 1.0 .75 | .50 .25 | .00 BIN | 1.0 .75 | .50 .25 | .00 BIN | 1.0 75 | .50 .25 | .00 BIN | 1.0 .75 | .50 .25 | .00 BIN |
| PCONT=*** | | | | | REQUIRED NUMBER OF PATIENTS | | | | | | | | | | | |
| 0.05 | *** | 3325 3338 3518 | | | 711 721 746 | | | 257 261 265 | | | 151 153 155 | | | 107 108 109 | | |
| | *** | 3329 3364 6576 | | | 715 730 1285 | | | 259 263 409 | | | 152 154 216 | | | 107 108 138 | | |
| 0.1 | *** | 6917 6949 7730 | | | 1302 1332 1439 | | | 416 427 444 | | | 226 230 236 | | | 150 152 155 | | |
| | *** | 6928 7013 11423 | | | 1313 1365 2033 | | | 421 434 584 | | | 228 233 289 | | | 151 153 176 | | |
| 0.15 | *** | 10105 10161 11954 | | | 1810 1865 2109 | | | 550 571 609 | | | 287 295 307 | | | 184 188 193 | | |
| | *** | 10124 10274 15685 | | | 1830 1933 2687 | | | 559 587 736 | | | 291 301 351 | | | 186 191 208 | | |
| 0.2 | *** | 12643 12730 15884 | | | 2213 2296 2721 | | | 658 691 755 | | | 337 349 368 | | | 212 218 226 | | |
| | *** | 12672 12904 19364 | | | 2243 2406 3247 | | | 672 716 865 | | | 342 358 403 | | | 215 222 234 | | |
| 0.25 | *** | 14465 14590 19367 | | | 2505 2623 3256 | | | 740 785 879 | | | 375 392 419 | | | 233 241 252 | | |
| | *** | 14507 14841 22459 | | | 2547 2779 3714 | | | 759 821 970 | | | 383 404 444 | | | 237 246 255 | | |
| 0.3 | *** | 15582 15753 22320 | | | 2693 2849 3703 | | | 798 855 980 | | | 402 424 459 | | | 248 258 272 | | |
| | *** | 15639 16096 24970 | | | 2749 3054 4088 | | | 822 903 1052 | | | 412 439 475 | | | 253 264 269 | | |
| 0.35 | *** | 16043 16272 24695 | | | 2786 2985 4055 | | | 834 903 1056 | | | 419 446 488 | | | 257 269 285 | | |
| | *** | 16119 16728 26897 | | | 2859 3239 4368 | | | 863 961 1110 | | | 432 464 496 | | | 263 276 278 | | |
| 0.4 | *** | 15922 16220 26463 | | | 2799 3041 4309 | | | 850 930 1108 | | | 428 458 506 | | | 261 274 292 | | |
| | *** | 16021 16813 28240 | | | 2889 3343 4555 | | | 884 997 1145 | | | 441 478 507 | | | 267 282 281 | | |
| 0.45 | *** | 15303 15687 27607 | | | 2746 3031 4462 | | | 849 938 1134 | | | 428 460 512 | | | 259 273 292 | | |
| | *** | 15431 16445 28999 | | | 2854 3373 4649 | | | 887 1011 1157 | | | 442 482 507 | | | 266 282 278 | | |
| 0.5 | *** | 14281 14772 28119 | | | 2642 2964 4514 | | | 833 927 1134 | | | 419 453 506 | | | 253 267 286 | | |
| | *** | 14445 15722 29175 | | | 2766 3339 4649 | | | 873 1004 1145 | | | 435 476 496 | | | 259 276 269 | | |
| 0.55 | *** | 12956 13580 27996 | | | 2498 2850 4463 | | | 803 900 1109 | | | 403 437 490 | | | 242 255 274 | | |
| | *** | 13165 14743 28766 | | | 2635 3247 4555 | | | 844 978 1110 | | | 419 460 475 | | | 248 263 255 | | |
| 0.6 | *** | 11435 12220 27237 | | | 2326 2697 4312 | | | 761 856 1059 | | | 380 412 462 | | | 225 238 255 | | |
| | *** | 11700 13596 27773 | | | 2472 3104 4368 | | | 802 933 1052 | | | 395 434 444 | | | 231 246 234 | | |
| 0.65 | *** | 9828 10795 25846 | | | 2132 2509 4059 | | | 706 796 983 | | | 350 379 423 | | | 204 215 230 | | |
| | *** | 10163 12349 26196 | | | 2283 2910 4088 | | | 745 868 970 | | | 363 398 403 | | | 210 222 208 | | |
| 0.7 | *** | 8248 9384 23826 | | | 1921 2288 3706 | | | 639 721 882 | | | 311 336 372 | | | 178 187 198 | | |
| | *** | 8655 11046 24036 | | | 2069 2668 3714 | | | 675 784 865 | | | 323 352 351 | | | 182 192 176 | | |
| 0.75 | *** | 6789 8028 21181 | | | 1693 2033 3253 | | | 559 628 757 | | | 265 284 311 | | | 146 153 161 | | |
| | *** | 7249 9701 21291 | | | 1831 2375 3247 | | | 589 680 736 | | | 274 296 289 | | | 150 157 138 | | |
| 0.8 | *** | 5487 6726 17920 | | | 1444 1738 2702 | | | 463 516 606 | | | 209 222 239 | | | . . . | | |
| | *** | 5959 8302 17963 | | | 1565 2025 2687 | | | 487 554 584 | | | 215 230 216 | | | . . . | | |
| 0.85 | *** | 4315 5437 14047 | | | 1162 1393 2053 | | | 348 381 432 | | | . . . | | | . . . | | |
| | *** | 4749 6801 14050 | | | 1258 1605 2033 | | | 363 403 409 | | | . . . | | | . . . | | |
| 0.9 | *** | 3183 4068 9570 | | | 825 970 1308 | | | . . . | | | . . . | | | . . . | | |
| | *** | 3530 5096 9554 | | | 887 1091 1285 | | | . . . | | | . . . | | | . . . | | |
| 0.95 | *** | 1898 2395 4496 | | | . . . | | | . . . | | | . . . | | | . . . | | |
| | *** | 2098 2919 4474 | | | . . . | | | . . . | | | . . . | | | . . . | | |

TABLE 1: ALPHA= 0.005 POWER= 0.8    EXPECTED ACCRUAL THRU MINIMUM FOLLOW-UP= 700

| PCONT=*** | FACT= | DEL=.02 | | | DEL=.05 | | | DEL=.10 | | | DEL=.15 | | | DEL=.20 | | |
|---|---|---|---|---|---|---|---|---|---|---|---|---|---|---|---|---|
| | | 1.0 .75 | .50 .25 | .00 BIN | 1.0 .75 | .50 .25 | .00 BIN | 1.0 .75 | .50 .25 | .00 BIN | 1.0 75 | .50 .25 | .00 BIN | 1.0 .75 | .50 .25 | .00 BIN |
| | | REQUIRED NUMBER OF PATIENTS | | | | | | | | | | | | | | |
| 0.05 | *** | 3326 | 3340 | 3518 | 712 | 722 | 746 | 257 | 261 | 265 | 152 | 153 | 155 | 107 | 108 | 109 |
| | *** | 3330 | 3368 | 6576 | 716 | 731 | 1285 | 259 | 263 | 409 | 152 | 154 | 216 | 107 | 108 | 138 |
| 0.1 | *** | 6920 | 6954 | 7730 | 1305 | 1335 | 1439 | 418 | 428 | 444 | 226 | 230 | 236 | 150 | 152 | 155 |
| | *** | 6931 | 7023 | 11423 | 1316 | 1369 | 2033 | 422 | 435 | 584 | 228 | 233 | 289 | 151 | 153 | 176 |
| 0.15 | *** | 10109 | 10170 | 11954 | 1815 | 1871 | 2109 | 553 | 573 | 609 | 288 | 296 | 307 | 185 | 189 | 193 |
| | *** | 10129 | 10292 | 15685 | 1836 | 1940 | 2687 | 562 | 588 | 736 | 292 | 301 | 351 | 187 | 191 | 208 |
| 0.2 | *** | 12650 | 12744 | 15884 | 2220 | 2307 | 2721 | 662 | 693 | 754 | 338 | 351 | 369 | 213 | 219 | 226 |
| | *** | 12681 | 12931 | 19364 | 2252 | 2418 | 3247 | 675 | 718 | 865 | 344 | 359 | 403 | 215 | 222 | 234 |
| 0.25 | *** | 14475 | 14610 | 19367 | 2515 | 2638 | 3256 | 745 | 789 | 879 | 377 | 394 | 419 | 234 | 242 | 252 |
| | *** | 14520 | 14879 | 22459 | 2560 | 2796 | 3714 | 764 | 825 | 970 | 385 | 405 | 444 | 238 | 247 | 255 |
| 0.3 | *** | 15595 | 15780 | 22320 | 2706 | 2869 | 3703 | 804 | 861 | 980 | 405 | 426 | 459 | 249 | 259 | 272 |
| | *** | 15657 | 16149 | 24970 | 2766 | 3077 | 4088 | 828 | 907 | 1052 | 415 | 441 | 475 | 254 | 265 | 269 |
| 0.35 | *** | 16060 | 16307 | 24695 | 2804 | 3010 | 4055 | 841 | 910 | 1056 | 423 | 448 | 488 | 259 | 270 | 285 |
| | *** | 16143 | 16797 | 26897 | 2880 | 3267 | 4368 | 870 | 966 | 1110 | 434 | 466 | 496 | 264 | 277 | 278 |
| 0.4 | *** | 15944 | 16266 | 26462 | 2821 | 3071 | 4308 | 859 | 938 | 1108 | 432 | 460 | 506 | 262 | 275 | 292 |
| | *** | 16052 | 16903 | 28240 | 2915 | 3376 | 4555 | 893 | 1003 | 1145 | 445 | 480 | 507 | 268 | 283 | 281 |
| 0.45 | *** | 15332 | 15746 | 27607 | 2773 | 3065 | 4462 | 859 | 946 | 1134 | 432 | 463 | 512 | 261 | 275 | 292 |
| | *** | 15470 | 16557 | 28999 | 2884 | 3411 | 4649 | 896 | 1017 | 1157 | 446 | 484 | 507 | 267 | 282 | 278 |
| 0.5 | *** | 14318 | 14847 | 28119 | 2672 | 3002 | 4513 | 843 | 936 | 1134 | 423 | 456 | 506 | 254 | 268 | 286 |
| | *** | 14495 | 15860 | 29175 | 2800 | 3380 | 4649 | 884 | 1011 | 1145 | 438 | 478 | 496 | 261 | 276 | 269 |
| 0.55 | *** | 13004 | 13675 | 27996 | 2532 | 2892 | 4464 | 814 | 909 | 1109 | 408 | 439 | 490 | 243 | 256 | 274 |
| | *** | 13229 | 14906 | 28766 | 2673 | 3290 | 4555 | 855 | 985 | 1110 | 422 | 461 | 475 | 249 | 264 | 255 |
| 0.6 | *** | 11496 | 12337 | 27237 | 2362 | 2740 | 4312 | 772 | 865 | 1059 | 384 | 415 | 462 | 227 | 239 | 255 |
| | *** | 11782 | 13781 | 27773 | 2512 | 3147 | 4368 | 812 | 940 | 1052 | 398 | 436 | 444 | 233 | 246 | 234 |
| 0.65 | *** | 9906 | 10932 | 25846 | 2170 | 2551 | 4059 | 716 | 805 | 983 | 353 | 381 | 422 | 205 | 216 | 229 |
| | *** | 10264 | 12550 | 26196 | 2323 | 2952 | 4088 | 755 | 875 | 970 | 366 | 399 | 403 | 211 | 222 | 208 |
| 0.7 | *** | 8345 | 9537 | 23826 | 1958 | 2329 | 3706 | 649 | 729 | 882 | 314 | 338 | 372 | 179 | 188 | 198 |
| | *** | 8775 | 11253 | 24036 | 2108 | 2707 | 3714 | 684 | 790 | 865 | 325 | 353 | 351 | 183 | 193 | 176 |
| 0.75 | *** | 6900 | 8187 | 21181 | 1728 | 2070 | 3253 | 567 | 634 | 757 | 268 | 286 | 311 | 148 | 153 | 161 |
| | *** | 7380 | 9903 | 21291 | 1867 | 2410 | 3247 | 597 | 684 | 736 | 276 | 297 | 289 | 150 | 157 | 138 |
| 0.8 | *** | 5603 | 6879 | 17920 | 1475 | 1770 | 2702 | 469 | 520 | 607 | 211 | 223 | 239 | . | . | . |
| | *** | 6090 | 8488 | 17963 | 1596 | 2053 | 2687 | 492 | 557 | 584 | 217 | 230 | 216 | . | . | . |
| 0.85 | *** | 4422 | 5572 | 14047 | 1187 | 1416 | 2053 | 352 | 384 | 432 | . | . | . | . | . | . |
| | *** | 4868 | 6959 | 14050 | 1283 | 1626 | 2033 | 366 | 405 | 409 | . | . | . | . | . | . |
| 0.9 | *** | 3269 | 4172 | 9570 | 841 | 984 | 1308 | . | . | . | . | . | . | . | . | . |
| | *** | 3624 | 5212 | 9554 | 902 | 1103 | 1285 | . | . | . | . | . | . | . | . | . |
| 0.95 | *** | 1948 | 2451 | 4496 | . | . | . | . | . | . | . | . | . | . | . | . |
| | *** | 2151 | 2974 | 4474 | . | . | . | . | . | . | . | . | . | . | . | . |

## TABLE 1: ALPHA= 0.005 POWER= 0.8    EXPECTED ACCRUAL THRU MINIMUM FOLLOW-UP= 750

|  |  | DEL=.02 | | | DEL=.05 | | | DEL=.10 | | | DEL=.15 | | | DEL=.20 | | |
|---|---|---|---|---|---|---|---|---|---|---|---|---|---|---|---|---|
| FACT= | | 1.0 .75 | .50 .25 | .00 BIN | 1.0 .75 | .50 .25 | .00 BIN | 1.0 .75 | .50 .25 | .00 BIN | 1.0 75 | .50 .25 | .00 BIN | 1.0 .75 | .50 .25 | .00 BIN |

PCONT=***  REQUIRED NUMBER OF PATIENTS

| PCONT | | DEL=.02 | | | DEL=.05 | | | DEL=.10 | | | DEL=.15 | | | DEL=.20 | | |
|---|---|---|---|---|---|---|---|---|---|---|---|---|---|---|---|---|
| 0.05 | *** | 3327 | 3342 | 3518 | 713 | 723 | 746 | 258 | 261 | 265 | 152 | 153 | 154 | 107 | 108 | 109 |
|  | *** | 3332 | 3371 | 6576 | 717 | 732 | 1285 | 259 | 263 | 409 | 153 | 154 | 216 | 108 | 109 | 138 |
| 0.1 | *** | 6922 | 6959 | 7729 | 1308 | 1339 | 1439 | 419 | 429 | 444 | 227 | 230 | 235 | 150 | 152 | 154 |
|  | *** | 6934 | 7032 | 11423 | 1319 | 1372 | 2033 | 423 | 435 | 584 | 229 | 233 | 289 | 151 | 154 | 176 |
| 0.15 | *** | 10114 | 10179 | 11954 | 1820 | 1878 | 2109 | 555 | 574 | 609 | 289 | 296 | 307 | 185 | 189 | 193 |
|  | *** | 10135 | 10309 | 15685 | 1841 | 1947 | 2687 | 564 | 589 | 736 | 293 | 301 | 351 | 187 | 191 | 208 |
| 0.2 | *** | 12656 | 12757 | 15884 | 2227 | 2317 | 2721 | 665 | 696 | 755 | 340 | 351 | 368 | 214 | 219 | 226 |
|  | *** | 12690 | 12958 | 19364 | 2260 | 2429 | 3247 | 679 | 720 | 865 | 345 | 359 | 403 | 216 | 222 | 234 |
| 0.25 | *** | 14485 | 14629 | 19367 | 2525 | 2652 | 3256 | 749 | 793 | 879 | 379 | 395 | 419 | 235 | 243 | 252 |
|  | *** | 14532 | 14917 | 22459 | 2572 | 2813 | 3714 | 769 | 828 | 970 | 386 | 406 | 444 | 238 | 247 | 255 |
| 0.3 | *** | 15608 | 15806 | 22320 | 2719 | 2888 | 3703 | 810 | 866 | 980 | 407 | 428 | 460 | 250 | 260 | 272 |
|  | *** | 15674 | 16201 | 24970 | 2782 | 3098 | 4088 | 834 | 911 | 1052 | 417 | 442 | 475 | 255 | 265 | 269 |
| 0.35 | *** | 16078 | 16342 | 24695 | 2821 | 3034 | 4055 | 848 | 916 | 1056 | 426 | 450 | 488 | 260 | 271 | 285 |
|  | *** | 16166 | 16866 | 26897 | 2900 | 3294 | 4368 | 878 | 971 | 1110 | 437 | 467 | 496 | 265 | 277 | 278 |
| 0.4 | *** | 15967 | 16312 | 26463 | 2842 | 3100 | 4309 | 867 | 945 | 1107 | 435 | 463 | 505 | 264 | 276 | 292 |
|  | *** | 16082 | 16991 | 28240 | 2940 | 3407 | 4555 | 901 | 1008 | 1145 | 447 | 482 | 507 | 270 | 283 | 281 |
| 0.45 | *** | 15362 | 15805 | 27607 | 2798 | 3098 | 4462 | 868 | 954 | 1134 | 435 | 465 | 512 | 263 | 275 | 292 |
|  | *** | 15510 | 16669 | 28999 | 2914 | 3445 | 4649 | 905 | 1024 | 1157 | 449 | 485 | 507 | 269 | 283 | 278 |
| 0.5 | *** | 14356 | 14922 | 28119 | 2701 | 3039 | 4513 | 853 | 945 | 1134 | 427 | 458 | 506 | 256 | 269 | 286 |
|  | *** | 14545 | 15995 | 29175 | 2832 | 3417 | 4649 | 893 | 1018 | 1145 | 441 | 479 | 496 | 262 | 277 | 269 |
| 0.55 | *** | 13053 | 13769 | 27996 | 2564 | 2930 | 4464 | 824 | 918 | 1109 | 411 | 442 | 490 | 245 | 257 | 274 |
|  | *** | 13293 | 15065 | 28766 | 2709 | 3330 | 4555 | 865 | 992 | 1110 | 425 | 463 | 475 | 250 | 265 | 255 |
| 0.6 | *** | 11557 | 12452 | 27237 | 2397 | 2780 | 4312 | 781 | 874 | 1059 | 387 | 417 | 462 | 229 | 240 | 255 |
|  | *** | 11862 | 13960 | 27773 | 2549 | 3187 | 4368 | 821 | 946 | 1052 | 401 | 437 | 444 | 234 | 247 | 234 |
| 0.65 | *** | 9984 | 11066 | 25846 | 2206 | 2591 | 4059 | 726 | 813 | 983 | 356 | 383 | 423 | 207 | 217 | 230 |
|  | *** | 10363 | 12742 | 26196 | 2361 | 2991 | 4088 | 764 | 880 | 970 | 369 | 401 | 403 | 212 | 223 | 208 |
| 0.7 | *** | 8440 | 9685 | 23825 | 1994 | 2366 | 3706 | 657 | 736 | 882 | 317 | 340 | 372 | 180 | 188 | 199 |
|  | *** | 8891 | 11450 | 24036 | 2145 | 2743 | 3714 | 692 | 795 | 865 | 328 | 355 | 351 | 184 | 193 | 176 |
| 0.75 | *** | 7008 | 8339 | 21182 | 1761 | 2104 | 3253 | 574 | 640 | 757 | 270 | 287 | 311 | 148 | 154 | 161 |
|  | *** | 7506 | 10096 | 21291 | 1902 | 2441 | 3247 | 604 | 688 | 736 | 278 | 298 | 289 | 151 | 157 | 138 |
| 0.8 | *** | 5714 | 7025 | 17920 | 1504 | 1799 | 2702 | 475 | 525 | 606 | 213 | 224 | 239 | . | . | . |
|  | *** | 6216 | 8664 | 17963 | 1626 | 2079 | 2687 | 498 | 560 | 584 | 218 | 231 | 216 | . | . | . |
| 0.85 | *** | 4525 | 5700 | 14047 | 1210 | 1439 | 2053 | 355 | 386 | 432 | . | . | . | . | . | . |
|  | *** | 4982 | 7108 | 14050 | 1306 | 1644 | 2033 | 370 | 407 | 409 | . | . | . | . | . | . |
| 0.9 | *** | 3352 | 4270 | 9570 | 856 | 997 | 1308 | . | . | . | . | . | . | . | . | . |
|  | *** | 3714 | 5320 | 9554 | 917 | 1113 | 1285 | . | . | . | . | . | . | . | . | . |
| 0.95 | *** | 1996 | 2503 | 4496 | . | . | . | . | . | . | . | . | . | . | . | . |
|  | *** | 2201 | 3025 | 4474 | . | . | . | . | . | . | . | . | . | . | . | . |

## TABLE 1: ALPHA= 0.005 POWER= 0.8   EXPECTED ACCRUAL THRU MINIMUM FOLLOW-UP= 800

| | | DEL=.02 | | | DEL=.05 | | | DEL=.10 | | | DEL=.15 | | | DEL=.20 | | |
|---|---|---|---|---|---|---|---|---|---|---|---|---|---|---|---|---|---|
| FACT= | | 1.0 .75 | .50 .25 | .00 BIN | 1.0 .75 | .50 .25 | .00 BIN | 1.0 .75 | .50 .25 | .00 BIN | 1.0 75 | .50 .25 | .00 BIN | 1.0 .75 | .50 .25 | .00 BIN |
| PCONT=*** | | | | REQUIRED NUMBER OF PATIENTS | | | | | | | | | | | | |
| 0.05 | *** | 3328 | 3345 | 3518 | 714 | 724 | 746 | 258 | 261 | 265 | 152 | 153 | 155 | 107 | 108 | 109 |
| | *** | 3333 | 3375 | 6576 | 718 | 733 | 1285 | 260 | 263 | 409 | 153 | 154 | 216 | 108 | 108 | 138 |
| 0.1 | *** | 6925 | 6964 | 7730 | 1310 | 1342 | 1439 | 420 | 429 | 444 | 227 | 231 | 236 | 151 | 152 | 155 |
| | *** | 6938 | 7042 | 11423 | 1322 | 1375 | 2033 | 424 | 436 | 584 | 229 | 233 | 289 | 151 | 153 | 176 |
| 0.15 | *** | 10118 | 10187 | 11954 | 1824 | 1884 | 2109 | 557 | 576 | 609 | 290 | 297 | 307 | 186 | 189 | 193 |
| | *** | 10141 | 10326 | 15685 | 1847 | 1953 | 2687 | 565 | 590 | 736 | 293 | 302 | 351 | 187 | 191 | 208 |
| 0.2 | *** | 12663 | 12771 | 15884 | 2234 | 2327 | 2721 | 668 | 699 | 755 | 341 | 352 | 368 | 214 | 219 | 226 |
| | *** | 12699 | 12984 | 19364 | 2269 | 2440 | 3247 | 682 | 722 | 865 | 346 | 360 | 403 | 217 | 222 | 234 |
| 0.25 | *** | 14494 | 14648 | 19367 | 2535 | 2667 | 3256 | 754 | 797 | 879 | 381 | 397 | 419 | 236 | 243 | 252 |
| | *** | 14545 | 14955 | 22459 | 2584 | 2828 | 3714 | 773 | 830 | 970 | 388 | 407 | 444 | 239 | 247 | 255 |
| 0.3 | *** | 15621 | 15833 | 22320 | 2733 | 2907 | 3703 | 815 | 871 | 980 | 410 | 430 | 459 | 252 | 260 | 272 |
| | *** | 15692 | 16253 | 24970 | 2798 | 3118 | 4088 | 839 | 914 | 1052 | 419 | 443 | 475 | 256 | 266 | 269 |
| 0.35 | *** | 16096 | 16377 | 24695 | 2838 | 3057 | 4055 | 855 | 922 | 1056 | 428 | 452 | 488 | 261 | 272 | 285 |
| | *** | 16190 | 16935 | 26897 | 2920 | 3318 | 4368 | 884 | 975 | 1110 | 439 | 468 | 496 | 266 | 278 | 278 |
| 0.4 | *** | 15990 | 16358 | 26463 | 2863 | 3128 | 4308 | 875 | 952 | 1108 | 438 | 465 | 506 | 265 | 277 | 292 |
| | *** | 16113 | 17080 | 28240 | 2964 | 3435 | 4555 | 908 | 1013 | 1145 | 450 | 483 | 507 | 271 | 284 | 281 |
| 0.45 | *** | 15391 | 15864 | 27607 | 2822 | 3130 | 4462 | 876 | 962 | 1134 | 438 | 468 | 512 | 264 | 276 | 292 |
| | *** | 15549 | 16779 | 28999 | 2941 | 3478 | 4649 | 913 | 1029 | 1157 | 452 | 487 | 507 | 270 | 284 | 278 |
| 0.5 | *** | 14394 | 14997 | 28119 | 2729 | 3073 | 4514 | 862 | 952 | 1134 | 430 | 461 | 506 | 258 | 270 | 286 |
| | *** | 14596 | 16128 | 29175 | 2864 | 3453 | 4649 | 901 | 1023 | 1145 | 444 | 481 | 496 | 263 | 278 | 269 |
| 0.55 | *** | 13101 | 13862 | 27996 | 2596 | 2967 | 4464 | 833 | 925 | 1109 | 415 | 445 | 490 | 246 | 258 | 274 |
| | *** | 13357 | 15220 | 28766 | 2743 | 3366 | 4555 | 873 | 997 | 1110 | 428 | 465 | 475 | 252 | 265 | 255 |
| 0.6 | *** | 11619 | 12565 | 27237 | 2430 | 2818 | 4312 | 791 | 881 | 1059 | 391 | 420 | 462 | 230 | 241 | 255 |
| | *** | 11943 | 14133 | 27773 | 2585 | 3224 | 4368 | 830 | 951 | 1052 | 404 | 438 | 444 | 235 | 247 | 234 |
| 0.65 | *** | 10061 | 11198 | 25846 | 2240 | 2629 | 4059 | 735 | 820 | 983 | 359 | 385 | 423 | 208 | 218 | 230 |
| | *** | 10462 | 12927 | 26196 | 2397 | 3027 | 4088 | 772 | 885 | 970 | 371 | 402 | 403 | 213 | 223 | 208 |
| 0.7 | *** | 8533 | 9828 | 23826 | 2027 | 2402 | 3706 | 665 | 742 | 882 | 320 | 342 | 372 | 181 | 189 | 198 |
| | *** | 9005 | 11638 | 24036 | 2180 | 2777 | 3714 | 699 | 799 | 865 | 330 | 356 | 351 | 185 | 193 | 176 |
| 0.75 | *** | 7113 | 8486 | 21181 | 1792 | 2137 | 3253 | 581 | 645 | 757 | 272 | 289 | 311 | 149 | 154 | 161 |
| | *** | 7629 | 10278 | 21291 | 1934 | 2471 | 3247 | 610 | 692 | 736 | 280 | 299 | 289 | 152 | 158 | 138 |
| 0.8 | *** | 5821 | 7165 | 17920 | 1531 | 1827 | 2702 | 480 | 529 | 607 | 214 | 225 | 239 | . | . | . |
| | *** | 6337 | 8831 | 17963 | 1653 | 2103 | 2687 | 502 | 562 | 584 | 219 | 232 | 216 | . | . | . |
| 0.85 | *** | 4624 | 5822 | 14047 | 1231 | 1459 | 2053 | 359 | 389 | 432 | . | . | . | . | . | . |
| | *** | 5090 | 7248 | 14050 | 1327 | 1661 | 2033 | 373 | 408 | 409 | . | . | . | . | . | . |
| 0.9 | *** | 3431 | 4364 | 9570 | 870 | 1009 | 1308 | . | . | . | . | . | . | . | . | . |
| | *** | 3799 | 5422 | 9554 | 930 | 1122 | 1285 | . | . | . | . | . | . | . | . | . |
| 0.95 | *** | 2041 | 2552 | 4496 | . | . | . | . | . | . | . | . | . | . | . | . |
| | *** | 2248 | 3073 | 4474 | . | . | . | . | . | . | . | . | . | . | . | . |

TABLE 1: ALPHA= 0.005 POWER= 0.8    EXPECTED ACCRUAL THRU MINIMUM FOLLOW-UP= 850

|  |  | DEL=.02 | | | DEL=.05 | | | DEL=.10 | | | DEL=.15 | | | DEL=.20 | | |
|---|---|---|---|---|---|---|---|---|---|---|---|---|---|---|---|---|
| FACT= | | 1.0 .75 | .50 .25 | .00 BIN | 1.0 .75 | .50 .25 | .00 BIN | 1.0 .75 | .50 .25 | .00 BIN | 1.0 75 | .50 .25 | .00 BIN | 1.0 .75 | .50 .25 | .00 BIN |
| PCONT=*** | | | | | REQUIRED NUMBER OF PATIENTS | | | | | | | | | | | |
| 0.05 | *** | 3329 | 3347 | 3518 | 715 | 725 | 746 | 259 | 261 | 265 | 152 | 153 | 155 | 107 | 108 | 108 |
|  | *** | 3335 | 3378 | 6576 | 719 | 733 | 1285 | 260 | 263 | 409 | 153 | 154 | 216 | 107 | 108 | 138 |
| 0.1 | *** | 6927 | 6969 | 7730 | 1312 | 1344 | 1439 | 420 | 430 | 444 | 227 | 231 | 236 | 151 | 153 | 155 |
|  | *** | 6941 | 7052 | 11423 | 1325 | 1377 | 2033 | 425 | 436 | 584 | 229 | 233 | 289 | 152 | 154 | 176 |
| 0.15 | *** | 10122 | 10196 | 11954 | 1829 | 1890 | 2109 | 559 | 578 | 609 | 291 | 298 | 307 | 186 | 189 | 193 |
|  | *** | 10147 | 10342 | 15685 | 1852 | 1959 | 2687 | 567 | 591 | 736 | 294 | 302 | 351 | 188 | 191 | 208 |
| 0.2 | *** | 12670 | 12784 | 15883 | 2241 | 2337 | 2721 | 671 | 701 | 754 | 342 | 353 | 368 | 215 | 220 | 226 |
|  | *** | 12708 | 13011 | 19364 | 2277 | 2450 | 3247 | 684 | 724 | 865 | 347 | 360 | 403 | 217 | 223 | 234 |
| 0.25 | *** | 14504 | 14668 | 19367 | 2544 | 2680 | 3256 | 758 | 800 | 879 | 382 | 397 | 419 | 237 | 243 | 252 |
|  | *** | 14558 | 14993 | 22459 | 2595 | 2842 | 3714 | 776 | 833 | 970 | 389 | 408 | 444 | 240 | 248 | 255 |
| 0.3 | *** | 15634 | 15859 | 22320 | 2745 | 2925 | 3703 | 820 | 875 | 980 | 411 | 431 | 459 | 253 | 261 | 272 |
|  | *** | 15709 | 16305 | 24970 | 2813 | 3137 | 4088 | 844 | 918 | 1052 | 420 | 444 | 475 | 256 | 266 | 269 |
| 0.35 | *** | 16114 | 16412 | 24695 | 2854 | 3079 | 4055 | 861 | 927 | 1056 | 430 | 454 | 488 | 262 | 272 | 285 |
|  | *** | 16213 | 17003 | 26897 | 2940 | 3341 | 4368 | 890 | 979 | 1110 | 442 | 469 | 496 | 267 | 278 | 278 |
| 0.4 | *** | 16013 | 16404 | 26462 | 2883 | 3154 | 4309 | 882 | 958 | 1108 | 441 | 467 | 506 | 266 | 277 | 292 |
|  | *** | 16143 | 17167 | 28240 | 2987 | 3462 | 4555 | 915 | 1017 | 1145 | 452 | 484 | 507 | 272 | 284 | 281 |
| 0.45 | *** | 15421 | 15923 | 27607 | 2846 | 3160 | 4462 | 884 | 968 | 1133 | 441 | 470 | 512 | 265 | 277 | 292 |
|  | *** | 15589 | 16887 | 28999 | 2968 | 3508 | 4649 | 921 | 1034 | 1157 | 454 | 488 | 507 | 271 | 284 | 278 |
| 0.5 | *** | 14432 | 15072 | 28119 | 2756 | 3106 | 4514 | 870 | 960 | 1134 | 433 | 463 | 507 | 259 | 271 | 286 |
|  | *** | 14646 | 16258 | 29175 | 2894 | 3485 | 4649 | 909 | 1029 | 1145 | 447 | 482 | 496 | 265 | 278 | 269 |
| 0.55 | *** | 13149 | 13955 | 27996 | 2626 | 3002 | 4464 | 842 | 933 | 1109 | 418 | 447 | 490 | 247 | 259 | 274 |
|  | *** | 13421 | 15370 | 28766 | 2775 | 3401 | 4555 | 882 | 1003 | 1110 | 431 | 466 | 475 | 253 | 266 | 255 |
| 0.6 | *** | 11680 | 12676 | 27237 | 2462 | 2853 | 4312 | 799 | 888 | 1058 | 394 | 422 | 462 | 231 | 241 | 255 |
|  | *** | 12023 | 14300 | 27773 | 2619 | 3258 | 4368 | 838 | 956 | 1052 | 407 | 440 | 444 | 236 | 248 | 234 |
| 0.65 | *** | 10137 | 11325 | 25846 | 2272 | 2664 | 4059 | 743 | 827 | 983 | 362 | 387 | 423 | 209 | 219 | 230 |
|  | *** | 10559 | 13105 | 26196 | 2431 | 3060 | 4088 | 780 | 890 | 970 | 374 | 403 | 403 | 213 | 224 | 208 |
| 0.7 | *** | 8625 | 9966 | 23826 | 2059 | 2436 | 3706 | 672 | 748 | 882 | 322 | 343 | 372 | 182 | 189 | 198 |
|  | *** | 9116 | 11819 | 24036 | 2213 | 2808 | 3714 | 706 | 803 | 865 | 332 | 357 | 351 | 186 | 193 | 176 |
| 0.75 | *** | 7215 | 8627 | 21182 | 1822 | 2167 | 3253 | 587 | 650 | 757 | 273 | 290 | 311 | 150 | 155 | 161 |
|  | *** | 7747 | 10453 | 21291 | 1964 | 2498 | 3247 | 615 | 695 | 736 | 281 | 299 | 289 | 152 | 157 | 138 |
| 0.8 | *** | 5925 | 7298 | 17920 | 1556 | 1852 | 2702 | 485 | 532 | 606 | 215 | 225 | 239 | . | . | . |
|  | *** | 6453 | 8990 | 17963 | 1680 | 2125 | 2687 | 507 | 564 | 584 | 220 | 232 | 216 | . | . | . |
| 0.85 | *** | 4718 | 5938 | 14047 | 1251 | 1478 | 2053 | 362 | 391 | 432 | . | . | . | . | . | . |
|  | *** | 5194 | 7381 | 14050 | 1347 | 1677 | 2033 | 375 | 409 | 409 | . | . | . | . | . | . |
| 0.9 | *** | 3506 | 4452 | 9570 | 883 | 1020 | 1308 | . | . | . | . | . | . | . | . | . |
|  | *** | 3880 | 5517 | 9554 | 943 | 1130 | 1285 | . | . | . | . | . | . | . | . | . |
| 0.95 | *** | 2084 | 2598 | 4496 | . | . | . | . | . | . | . | . | . | . | . | . |
|  | *** | 2293 | 3117 | 4474 | . | . | . | . | . | . | . | . | . | . | . | . |

TABLE 1: ALPHA= 0.005 POWER= 0.8    EXPECTED ACCRUAL THRU MINIMUM FOLLOW-UP= 900

| | | DEL=.02 | | | DEL=.05 | | | DEL=.10 | | | DEL=.15 | | | DEL=.20 | | |
|---|---|---|---|---|---|---|---|---|---|---|---|---|---|---|---|---|---|
| FACT= | | 1.0 .75 | .50 .25 | .00 BIN | 1.0 .75 | .50 .25 | .00 BIN | 1.0 .75 | .50 .25 | .00 BIN | 1.0 75 | .50 .25 | .00 BIN | 1.0 .75 | .50 .25 | .00 BIN |
| PCONT=*** | | | | | REQUIRED | NUMBER | OF PATIENTS | | | | | | | | | |
| 0.05 | *** | 3330 | 3349 | 3518 | 716 | 726 | 746 | 259 | 262 | 265 | 152 | 153 | 155 | 108 | 108 | 109 |
| | *** | 3336 | 3381 | 6576 | 720 | 734 | 1285 | 260 | 263 | 409 | 153 | 154 | 216 | 108 | 108 | 138 |
| 0.1 | *** | 6930 | 6974 | 7730 | 1315 | 1347 | 1439 | 422 | 431 | 444 | 228 | 231 | 236 | 151 | 153 | 154 |
| | *** | 6944 | 7061 | 11423 | 1328 | 1380 | 2033 | 426 | 437 | 584 | 230 | 234 | 289 | 152 | 154 | 176 |
| 0.15 | *** | 10126 | 10205 | 11954 | 1833 | 1896 | 2109 | 560 | 579 | 609 | 291 | 298 | 307 | 186 | 190 | 193 |
| | *** | 10153 | 10360 | 15685 | 1857 | 1964 | 2687 | 569 | 592 | 736 | 294 | 302 | 351 | 188 | 191 | 208 |
| 0.2 | *** | 12677 | 12798 | 15884 | 2247 | 2346 | 2721 | 674 | 703 | 755 | 343 | 354 | 369 | 215 | 220 | 226 |
| | *** | 12717 | 13037 | 19364 | 2285 | 2459 | 3247 | 687 | 725 | 865 | 348 | 361 | 403 | 217 | 223 | 234 |
| 0.25 | *** | 14513 | 14687 | 19367 | 2554 | 2693 | 3256 | 761 | 803 | 879 | 384 | 398 | 419 | 237 | 244 | 252 |
| | *** | 14571 | 15031 | 22459 | 2606 | 2855 | 3714 | 780 | 835 | 970 | 390 | 408 | 444 | 240 | 248 | 255 |
| 0.3 | *** | 15648 | 15886 | 22320 | 2757 | 2942 | 3702 | 825 | 879 | 980 | 414 | 432 | 459 | 253 | 262 | 272 |
| | *** | 15727 | 16356 | 24970 | 2827 | 3155 | 4088 | 849 | 920 | 1052 | 422 | 444 | 475 | 257 | 266 | 269 |
| 0.35 | *** | 16131 | 16448 | 24695 | 2870 | 3100 | 4055 | 867 | 932 | 1056 | 433 | 456 | 488 | 263 | 273 | 285 |
| | *** | 16237 | 17071 | 26897 | 2958 | 3363 | 4368 | 896 | 982 | 1110 | 443 | 470 | 496 | 268 | 279 | 278 |
| 0.4 | *** | 16037 | 16449 | 26462 | 2903 | 3178 | 4308 | 888 | 964 | 1108 | 443 | 469 | 506 | 268 | 279 | 292 |
| | *** | 16174 | 17253 | 28240 | 3009 | 3488 | 4555 | 921 | 1021 | 1145 | 455 | 485 | 507 | 273 | 285 | 281 |
| 0.45 | *** | 15450 | 15982 | 27606 | 2870 | 3188 | 4462 | 892 | 974 | 1134 | 444 | 471 | 512 | 267 | 278 | 292 |
| | *** | 15628 | 16993 | 28999 | 2994 | 3537 | 4649 | 928 | 1038 | 1157 | 456 | 489 | 507 | 272 | 285 | 278 |
| 0.5 | *** | 14470 | 15146 | 28119 | 2783 | 3137 | 4514 | 878 | 966 | 1134 | 436 | 465 | 506 | 260 | 272 | 286 |
| | *** | 14697 | 16385 | 29175 | 2923 | 3516 | 4649 | 917 | 1033 | 1145 | 450 | 483 | 496 | 266 | 279 | 269 |
| 0.55 | *** | 13197 | 14046 | 27996 | 2654 | 3035 | 4464 | 850 | 939 | 1109 | 420 | 449 | 489 | 249 | 260 | 273 |
| | *** | 13485 | 15516 | 28766 | 2806 | 3432 | 4555 | 889 | 1007 | 1110 | 433 | 467 | 475 | 254 | 266 | 255 |
| 0.6 | *** | 11741 | 12785 | 27237 | 2493 | 2887 | 4312 | 807 | 895 | 1059 | 396 | 423 | 462 | 232 | 242 | 255 |
| | *** | 12102 | 14461 | 27773 | 2651 | 3290 | 4368 | 846 | 961 | 1052 | 409 | 441 | 444 | 237 | 248 | 234 |
| 0.65 | *** | 10214 | 11450 | 25846 | 2303 | 2697 | 4059 | 750 | 833 | 983 | 365 | 389 | 423 | 210 | 219 | 230 |
| | *** | 10654 | 13275 | 26196 | 2463 | 3092 | 4088 | 787 | 894 | 970 | 376 | 404 | 403 | 215 | 224 | 208 |
| 0.7 | *** | 8715 | 10100 | 23825 | 2089 | 2467 | 3706 | 679 | 753 | 882 | 324 | 344 | 372 | 183 | 190 | 198 |
| | *** | 9225 | 11991 | 24036 | 2244 | 2837 | 3714 | 712 | 807 | 865 | 334 | 357 | 351 | 186 | 194 | 176 |
| 0.75 | *** | 7314 | 8762 | 21182 | 1850 | 2196 | 3253 | 593 | 654 | 757 | 275 | 290 | 311 | 150 | 155 | 161 |
| | *** | 7862 | 10619 | 21291 | 1992 | 2523 | 3247 | 621 | 698 | 736 | 282 | 300 | 289 | 153 | 158 | 138 |
| 0.8 | *** | 6025 | 7426 | 17920 | 1581 | 1876 | 2702 | 489 | 536 | 606 | 216 | 226 | 239 | . | . | . |
| | *** | 6565 | 9141 | 17963 | 1704 | 2145 | 2687 | 510 | 567 | 584 | 221 | 233 | 216 | . | . | . |
| 0.85 | *** | 4809 | 6050 | 14047 | 1271 | 1496 | 2053 | 365 | 393 | 432 | . | . | . | . | . | . |
| | *** | 5294 | 7507 | 14050 | 1366 | 1691 | 2033 | 378 | 411 | 409 | . | . | . | . | . | . |
| 0.9 | *** | 3578 | 4537 | 9570 | 895 | 1031 | 1308 | . | . | . | . | . | . | . | . | . |
| | *** | 3958 | 5608 | 9554 | 954 | 1137 | 1285 | . | . | . | . | . | . | . | . | . |
| 0.95 | *** | 2125 | 2641 | 4496 | . | . | . | . | . | . | . | . | . | . | . | . |
| | *** | 2335 | 3158 | 4474 | . | . | . | . | . | . | . | . | . | . | . | . |

## TABLE 1: ALPHA= 0.005 POWER= 0.8    EXPECTED ACCRUAL THRU MINIMUM FOLLOW-UP= 950

| | DEL=.02 | | | DEL=.05 | | | DEL=.10 | | | DEL=.15 | | | DEL=.20 | | |
|---|---|---|---|---|---|---|---|---|---|---|---|---|---|---|---|
| FACT= | 1.0 .75 | .50 .25 | .00 BIN | 1.0 .75 | .50 .25 | .00 BIN | 1.0 .75 | .50 .25 | .00 BIN | 1.0 75 | .50 .25 | .00 BIN | 1.0 .75 | .50 .25 | .00 BIN |
| PCONT=*** | | | REQUIRED NUMBER OF PATIENTS | | | | | | | | | | | | |
| 0.05 *** | 3331 3338 | 3351 3384 | 3518 6576 | 716 720 | 726 735 | 746 1285 | 259 260 | 262 263 | 265 409 | 152 153 | 153 154 | 154 216 | 108 108 | 108 108 | 109 138 |
| 0.1 *** | 6932 6948 | 6979 7070 | 7729 11423 | 1317 1330 | 1350 1382 | 1439 2033 | 422 426 | 431 437 | 444 584 | 228 230 | 232 234 | 236 289 | 151 152 | 153 153 | 154 176 |
| 0.15 *** | 10131 10159 | 10213 10376 | 11954 15685 | 1837 1862 | 1901 1969 | 2109 2687 | 562 570 | 580 593 | 609 736 | 292 295 | 298 302 | 307 351 | 186 188 | 190 191 | 193 208 |
| 0.2 *** | 12683 12726 | 12811 13063 | 15884 19364 | 2254 2293 | 2354 2467 | 2721 3247 | 676 689 | 705 726 | 755 865 | 344 349 | 355 361 | 368 403 | 216 218 | 220 223 | 226 234 |
| 0.25 *** | 14523 14584 | 14706 15068 | 19367 22459 | 2563 2617 | 2705 2867 | 3256 3714 | 765 783 | 806 837 | 879 970 | 385 392 | 400 409 | 419 444 | 238 241 | 244 248 | 252 255 |
| 0.3 *** | 15661 15745 | 15912 16408 | 22320 24970 | 2770 2842 | 2958 3171 | 3703 4088 | 830 853 | 883 923 | 980 1052 | 415 424 | 433 445 | 459 475 | 254 258 | 262 267 | 272 269 |
| 0.35 *** | 16148 16260 | 16483 17138 | 24695 26897 | 2885 2976 | 3120 3383 | 4055 4368 | 872 901 | 937 985 | 1056 1110 | 435 445 | 457 471 | 488 496 | 264 268 | 273 279 | 285 278 |
| 0.4 *** | 16059 16205 | 16495 17338 | 26462 28240 | 2921 3031 | 3202 3511 | 4308 4555 | 895 927 | 969 1025 | 1108 1145 | 445 457 | 470 486 | 505 507 | 268 273 | 279 285 | 292 281 |
| 0.45 *** | 15480 15667 | 16040 17098 | 27607 28999 | 2892 3019 | 3215 3563 | 4461 4649 | 899 934 | 980 1042 | 1134 1157 | 447 458 | 473 490 | 512 507 | 267 273 | 279 285 | 292 278 |
| 0.5 *** | 14508 14746 | 15220 16509 | 28119 29175 | 2808 2951 | 3167 3545 | 4513 4649 | 886 923 | 972 1037 | 1134 1145 | 439 451 | 467 485 | 507 496 | 261 267 | 272 279 | 286 269 |
| 0.55 *** | 13245 13548 | 14137 15658 | 27996 28766 | 2682 2836 | 3066 3462 | 4463 4555 | 857 896 | 945 1011 | 1109 1110 | 423 436 | 450 468 | 490 475 | 249 255 | 260 267 | 274 255 |
| 0.6 *** | 11801 12181 | 12893 14617 | 27237 27773 | 2521 2682 | 2918 3320 | 4312 4368 | 815 853 | 901 965 | 1059 1052 | 399 411 | 425 442 | 462 444 | 233 238 | 242 248 | 255 234 |
| 0.65 *** | 10289 10748 | 11572 13440 | 25846 26196 | 2332 2494 | 2728 3121 | 4059 4088 | 757 793 | 838 898 | 983 970 | 367 378 | 390 405 | 422 403 | 211 215 | 219 224 | 230 208 |
| 0.7 *** | 8804 9331 | 10231 12157 | 23826 24036 | 2117 2274 | 2497 2864 | 3706 3714 | 686 718 | 758 810 | 882 865 | 326 335 | 346 358 | 372 351 | 184 186 | 190 194 | 198 176 |
| 0.75 *** | 7411 7974 | 8893 10778 | 21181 21291 | 1876 2020 | 2223 2547 | 3253 3247 | 599 625 | 659 700 | 756 736 | 276 283 | 292 300 | 311 289 | 150 153 | 155 158 | 161 138 |
| 0.8 *** | 6122 6673 | 7550 9285 | 17919 17963 | 1604 1727 | 1898 2165 | 2702 2687 | 494 514 | 539 568 | 606 584 | 217 222 | 227 232 | 239 216 | . . | . . | . . |
| 0.85 *** | 4897 5390 | 6157 7627 | 14047 14050 | 1288 1383 | 1512 1704 | 2053 2033 | 367 380 | 394 412 | 432 409 | . . | . . | . . | . . | . . | . . |
| 0.9 *** | 3647 4032 | 4617 5694 | 9570 9554 | 906 964 | 1040 1144 | 1308 1285 | . . | . . | . . | . . | . . | . . | . . | . . | . . |
| 0.95 *** | 2164 2376 | 2682 3197 | 4496 4474 | . . | . . | . . | . . | . . | . . | . . | . . | . . | . . | . . | . . |

## TABLE 1: ALPHA= 0.005 POWER= 0.8    EXPECTED ACCRUAL THRU MINIMUM FOLLOW-UP= 1000

| PCONT | | DEL=.02 | | | DEL=.05 | | | DEL=.10 | | | DEL=.15 | | | DEL=.20 | | |
|---|---|---|---|---|---|---|---|---|---|---|---|---|---|---|---|---|
| FACT= | | 1.0 .75 | .50 .25 | .00 BIN | 1.0 .75 | .50 .25 | .00 BIN | 1.0 .75 | .50 .25 | .00 BIN | 1.0 75 | .50 .25 | .00 BIN | 1.0 .75 | .50 .25 | .00 BIN |
| PCONT=*** | | | | REQUIRED NUMBER OF PATIENTS | | | | | | | | | | | | |
| 0.05 | *** | 3332 | 3353 | 3518 | 717 | 727 | 746 | 260 | 262 | 265 | 153 | 153 | 155 | 108 | 108 | 109 |
|  | *** | 3339 | 3387 | 6576 | 721 | 735 | 1285 | 261 | 263 | 409 | 153 | 154 | 216 | 108 | 108 | 138 |
| 0.1 | *** | 6935 | 6984 | 7730 | 1320 | 1353 | 1439 | 423 | 432 | 445 | 228 | 231 | 236 | 151 | 153 | 155 |
|  | *** | 6951 | 7079 | 11423 | 1333 | 1384 | 2033 | 427 | 438 | 584 | 230 | 233 | 289 | 152 | 154 | 176 |
| 0.15 | *** | 10135 | 10222 | 11954 | 1841 | 1906 | 2110 | 563 | 581 | 609 | 293 | 299 | 307 | 187 | 190 | 193 |
|  | *** | 10164 | 10393 | 15685 | 1866 | 1974 | 2687 | 571 | 593 | 736 | 296 | 303 | 351 | 188 | 191 | 208 |
| 0.2 | *** | 12690 | 12824 | 15884 | 2260 | 2363 | 2721 | 678 | 707 | 755 | 345 | 355 | 368 | 216 | 221 | 226 |
|  | *** | 12735 | 13090 | 19364 | 2300 | 2475 | 3247 | 691 | 728 | 865 | 350 | 361 | 403 | 218 | 223 | 234 |
| 0.25 | *** | 14533 | 14725 | 19367 | 2572 | 2717 | 3256 | 768 | 809 | 879 | 386 | 400 | 420 | 238 | 245 | 252 |
|  | *** | 14597 | 15106 | 22459 | 2628 | 2879 | 3714 | 786 | 838 | 970 | 393 | 409 | 444 | 241 | 248 | 255 |
| 0.3 | *** | 15674 | 15938 | 22320 | 2782 | 2973 | 3703 | 834 | 886 | 980 | 417 | 435 | 460 | 255 | 263 | 272 |
|  | *** | 15762 | 16458 | 24970 | 2856 | 3186 | 4088 | 857 | 925 | 1052 | 425 | 446 | 475 | 258 | 267 | 269 |
| 0.35 | *** | 16166 | 16518 | 24695 | 2901 | 3139 | 4055 | 878 | 941 | 1056 | 437 | 458 | 488 | 265 | 274 | 285 |
|  | *** | 16283 | 17204 | 26897 | 2993 | 3402 | 4368 | 906 | 988 | 1110 | 447 | 472 | 496 | 270 | 280 | 278 |
| 0.4 | *** | 16082 | 16541 | 26463 | 2940 | 3225 | 4308 | 901 | 973 | 1108 | 448 | 471 | 506 | 270 | 280 | 292 |
|  | *** | 16235 | 17422 | 28240 | 3051 | 3534 | 4555 | 933 | 1028 | 1145 | 458 | 487 | 507 | 275 | 285 | 281 |
| 0.45 | *** | 15510 | 16099 | 27607 | 2913 | 3240 | 4462 | 905 | 985 | 1134 | 449 | 475 | 512 | 269 | 279 | 292 |
|  | *** | 15707 | 17200 | 28999 | 3043 | 3588 | 4649 | 940 | 1046 | 1157 | 461 | 491 | 507 | 274 | 285 | 278 |
| 0.5 | *** | 14545 | 15293 | 28119 | 2833 | 3195 | 4513 | 893 | 978 | 1134 | 441 | 468 | 506 | 262 | 273 | 286 |
|  | *** | 14797 | 16630 | 29175 | 2977 | 3572 | 4649 | 930 | 1041 | 1145 | 454 | 485 | 496 | 267 | 279 | 269 |
| 0.55 | *** | 13293 | 14227 | 27996 | 2709 | 3096 | 4463 | 865 | 951 | 1109 | 425 | 452 | 490 | 251 | 261 | 274 |
|  | *** | 13611 | 15796 | 28766 | 2865 | 3491 | 4555 | 903 | 1016 | 1110 | 438 | 469 | 475 | 256 | 267 | 255 |
| 0.6 | *** | 11863 | 12999 | 27237 | 2550 | 2949 | 4312 | 821 | 906 | 1058 | 401 | 426 | 462 | 234 | 243 | 255 |
|  | *** | 12259 | 14768 | 27773 | 2711 | 3349 | 4368 | 859 | 969 | 1052 | 413 | 443 | 444 | 238 | 249 | 234 |
| 0.65 | *** | 10363 | 11691 | 25846 | 2361 | 2758 | 4059 | 764 | 844 | 983 | 369 | 391 | 423 | 211 | 220 | 230 |
|  | *** | 10841 | 13598 | 26196 | 2523 | 3148 | 4088 | 800 | 901 | 970 | 380 | 406 | 403 | 216 | 225 | 208 |
| 0.7 | *** | 8891 | 10358 | 23826 | 2145 | 2525 | 3706 | 691 | 763 | 882 | 328 | 347 | 372 | 184 | 191 | 198 |
|  | *** | 9435 | 12317 | 24036 | 2301 | 2889 | 3714 | 723 | 813 | 865 | 337 | 359 | 351 | 187 | 195 | 176 |
| 0.75 | *** | 7506 | 9020 | 21181 | 1902 | 2248 | 3253 | 603 | 663 | 756 | 278 | 293 | 311 | 151 | 156 | 161 |
|  | *** | 8081 | 10931 | 21291 | 2045 | 2570 | 3247 | 630 | 703 | 736 | 285 | 301 | 289 | 153 | 158 | 138 |
| 0.8 | *** | 6216 | 7669 | 17920 | 1626 | 1920 | 2702 | 498 | 541 | 606 | 218 | 228 | 239 | . | . | . |
|  | *** | 6778 | 9423 | 17963 | 1749 | 2183 | 2687 | 518 | 570 | 584 | 223 | 233 | 216 | . | . | . |
| 0.85 | *** | 4981 | 6260 | 14047 | 1306 | 1528 | 2053 | 370 | 396 | 432 | . | . | . | . | . | . |
|  | *** | 5483 | 7742 | 14050 | 1401 | 1717 | 2033 | 382 | 413 | 409 | . | . | . | . | . | . |
| 0.9 | *** | 3714 | 4694 | 9570 | 917 | 1049 | 1308 | . | . | . | . | . | . | . | . | . |
|  | *** | 4104 | 5775 | 9554 | 975 | 1151 | 1285 | . | . | . | . | . | . | . | . | . |
| 0.95 | *** | 2201 | 2721 | 4496 | . | . | . | . | . | . | . | . | . | . | . | . |
|  | *** | 2414 | 3233 | 4474 | . | . | . | . | . | . | . | . | . | . | . | . |

# TABLE 1: ALPHA= 0.005 POWER= 0.8    EXPECTED ACCRUAL THRU MINIMUM FOLLOW-UP= 1100

| | | DEL=.02 | | | DEL=.05 | | | DEL=.10 | | | DEL=.15 | | | DEL=.20 | | |
|---|---|---|---|---|---|---|---|---|---|---|---|---|---|---|---|---|
| FACT= | | 1.0 .75 | .50 .25 | .00 BIN | 1.0 .75 | .50 .25 | .00 BIN | 1.0 .75 | .50 .25 | .00 BIN | 1.0 75 | .50 .25 | .00 BIN | 1.0 .75 | .50 .25 | .00 BIN |
| PCONT=*** | | | | | REQUIRED NUMBER OF PATIENTS | | | | | | | | | | | |
| 0.05 | *** | 3334 | 3356 | 3518 | 719 | 728 | 746 | 260 | 262 | 265 | 153 | 153 | 155 | 107 | 108 | 109 |
| | *** | 3342 | 3393 | 6576 | 723 | 736 | 1285 | 261 | 263 | 409 | 153 | 154 | 216 | 108 | 109 | 138 |
| 0.1 | *** | 6939 | 6993 | 7730 | 1324 | 1357 | 1439 | 424 | 433 | 444 | 229 | 232 | 236 | 151 | 153 | 155 |
| | *** | 6957 | 7096 | 11423 | 1337 | 1387 | 2033 | 428 | 438 | 584 | 230 | 234 | 289 | 152 | 153 | 176 |
| 0.15 | *** | 10144 | 10240 | 11954 | 1849 | 1916 | 2109 | 566 | 583 | 609 | 294 | 300 | 307 | 188 | 191 | 193 |
| | *** | 10176 | 10426 | 15685 | 1875 | 1982 | 2687 | 574 | 595 | 736 | 296 | 303 | 351 | 189 | 192 | 208 |
| 0.2 | *** | 12704 | 12851 | 15883 | 2273 | 2378 | 2721 | 683 | 710 | 755 | 346 | 356 | 368 | 217 | 221 | 225 |
| | *** | 12753 | 13140 | 19364 | 2314 | 2490 | 3247 | 695 | 730 | 865 | 351 | 362 | 403 | 219 | 224 | 234 |
| 0.25 | *** | 14552 | 14763 | 19367 | 2590 | 2739 | 3256 | 774 | 813 | 879 | 389 | 401 | 419 | 239 | 246 | 252 |
| | *** | 14623 | 15179 | 22459 | 2648 | 2900 | 3714 | 792 | 841 | 970 | 395 | 410 | 444 | 242 | 248 | 255 |
| 0.3 | *** | 15701 | 15991 | 22320 | 2805 | 3002 | 3703 | 841 | 892 | 980 | 419 | 437 | 459 | 256 | 263 | 272 |
| | *** | 15797 | 16559 | 24970 | 2882 | 3214 | 4088 | 864 | 929 | 1052 | 428 | 447 | 475 | 259 | 268 | 269 |
| 0.35 | *** | 16201 | 16588 | 24695 | 2930 | 3175 | 4055 | 887 | 949 | 1056 | 440 | 461 | 488 | 267 | 275 | 285 |
| | *** | 16330 | 17335 | 26897 | 3026 | 3437 | 4368 | 914 | 994 | 1110 | 450 | 473 | 496 | 270 | 280 | 278 |
| 0.4 | *** | 16128 | 16632 | 26463 | 2975 | 3267 | 4309 | 912 | 983 | 1108 | 451 | 474 | 505 | 271 | 280 | 291 |
| | *** | 16296 | 17586 | 28240 | 3090 | 3574 | 4555 | 943 | 1034 | 1145 | 462 | 488 | 507 | 276 | 286 | 281 |
| 0.45 | *** | 15569 | 16215 | 27607 | 2955 | 3288 | 4462 | 917 | 995 | 1134 | 453 | 478 | 511 | 270 | 280 | 292 |
| | *** | 15786 | 17400 | 28999 | 3088 | 3634 | 4649 | 951 | 1052 | 1157 | 464 | 493 | 507 | 275 | 286 | 278 |
| 0.5 | *** | 14621 | 15438 | 28119 | 2879 | 3247 | 4514 | 906 | 988 | 1134 | 445 | 471 | 506 | 264 | 274 | 286 |
| | *** | 14897 | 16865 | 29175 | 3027 | 3621 | 4649 | 942 | 1048 | 1145 | 457 | 487 | 496 | 269 | 280 | 269 |
| 0.55 | *** | 13389 | 14403 | 27996 | 2759 | 3151 | 4463 | 877 | 961 | 1109 | 430 | 455 | 489 | 252 | 262 | 274 |
| | *** | 13738 | 16062 | 28766 | 2918 | 3542 | 4555 | 914 | 1022 | 1110 | 441 | 471 | 475 | 257 | 268 | 255 |
| 0.6 | *** | 11983 | 13205 | 27237 | 2602 | 3005 | 4312 | 834 | 917 | 1059 | 405 | 429 | 462 | 235 | 244 | 255 |
| | *** | 12413 | 15057 | 27773 | 2766 | 3400 | 4368 | 871 | 976 | 1052 | 417 | 444 | 444 | 239 | 249 | 234 |
| 0.65 | *** | 10510 | 11921 | 25846 | 2414 | 2814 | 4059 | 776 | 853 | 983 | 373 | 394 | 423 | 213 | 221 | 230 |
| | *** | 11022 | 13900 | 26196 | 2578 | 3198 | 4088 | 811 | 907 | 970 | 382 | 407 | 403 | 217 | 225 | 208 |
| 0.7 | *** | 9061 | 10599 | 23825 | 2197 | 2578 | 3706 | 703 | 771 | 882 | 331 | 349 | 372 | 185 | 191 | 198 |
| | *** | 9636 | 12618 | 24036 | 2354 | 2935 | 3714 | 733 | 818 | 865 | 340 | 360 | 351 | 188 | 195 | 176 |
| 0.75 | *** | 7688 | 9261 | 21181 | 1949 | 2294 | 3253 | 613 | 669 | 756 | 280 | 294 | 311 | 152 | 156 | 161 |
| | *** | 8289 | 11219 | 21291 | 2094 | 2609 | 3247 | 638 | 707 | 736 | 287 | 302 | 289 | 154 | 158 | 138 |
| 0.8 | *** | 6395 | 7894 | 17920 | 1666 | 1958 | 2702 | 505 | 546 | 606 | 219 | 228 | 239 | . | . | . |
| | *** | 6977 | 9682 | 17963 | 1790 | 2215 | 2687 | 523 | 573 | 584 | 224 | 233 | 216 | . | . | . |
| 0.85 | *** | 5142 | 6453 | 14047 | 1337 | 1556 | 2053 | 374 | 399 | 433 | . | . | . | . | . | . |
| | *** | 5658 | 7957 | 14050 | 1431 | 1739 | 2033 | 386 | 414 | 409 | . | . | . | . | . | . |
| 0.9 | *** | 3840 | 4839 | 9570 | 936 | 1065 | 1308 | . | . | . | . | . | . | . | . | . |
| | *** | 4239 | 5926 | 9554 | 993 | 1162 | 1285 | . | . | . | . | . | . | . | . | . |
| 0.95 | *** | 2271 | 2793 | 4496 | . | . | . | . | . | . | . | . | . | . | . | . |
| | *** | 2486 | 3299 | 4474 | . | . | . | . | . | . | . | . | . | . | . | . |

## TABLE 1: ALPHA= 0.005 POWER= 0.8    EXPECTED ACCRUAL THRU MINIMUM FOLLOW-UP= 1200

PCONT=***    REQUIRED NUMBER OF PATIENTS

| PCONT | DEL=.02 1.0/.75 | .50/.25 | .00/BIN | DEL=.05 1.0/.75 | .50/.25 | .00/BIN | DEL=.10 1.0/.75 | .50/.25 | .00/BIN | DEL=.15 1.0/.75 | .50/.25 | .00/BIN | DEL=.20 1.0/.75 | .50/.25 | .00/BIN |
|---|---|---|---|---|---|---|---|---|---|---|---|---|---|---|---|
| 0.05 | 3336 | 3360 | 3518 | 719 | 729 | 746 | 260 | 262 | 265 | 152 | 154 | 154 | 108 | 108 | 109 |
|  | 3344 | 3397 | 6576 | 724 | 736 | 1285 | 261 | 264 | 409 | 153 | 154 | 216 | 108 | 109 | 138 |
| 0.1 | 6944 | 7003 | 7729 | 1327 | 1361 | 1439 | 426 | 433 | 444 | 229 | 232 | 235 | 151 | 153 | 154 |
|  | 6964 | 7113 | 11423 | 1342 | 1391 | 2033 | 429 | 439 | 584 | 231 | 234 | 289 | 152 | 154 | 176 |
| 0.15 | 10153 | 10257 | 11954 | 1857 | 1924 | 2109 | 568 | 585 | 609 | 295 | 300 | 307 | 188 | 190 | 193 |
|  | 10187 | 10458 | 15685 | 1884 | 1990 | 2687 | 576 | 595 | 736 | 297 | 303 | 351 | 189 | 192 | 208 |
| 0.2 | 12717 | 12877 | 15883 | 2284 | 2392 | 2721 | 687 | 713 | 754 | 348 | 357 | 368 | 217 | 221 | 226 |
|  | 12770 | 13191 | 19364 | 2327 | 2503 | 3247 | 699 | 731 | 865 | 352 | 362 | 403 | 219 | 223 | 234 |
| 0.25 | 14571 | 14802 | 19366 | 2606 | 2760 | 3256 | 780 | 817 | 879 | 391 | 403 | 419 | 241 | 246 | 252 |
|  | 14648 | 15251 | 22459 | 2667 | 2919 | 3714 | 796 | 844 | 970 | 397 | 410 | 444 | 243 | 249 | 255 |
| 0.3 | 15727 | 16044 | 22320 | 2827 | 3029 | 3703 | 849 | 898 | 979 | 422 | 438 | 459 | 257 | 264 | 271 |
|  | 15832 | 16656 | 24970 | 2907 | 3239 | 4088 | 871 | 933 | 1052 | 430 | 448 | 475 | 260 | 268 | 269 |
| 0.35 | 16237 | 16657 | 24694 | 2958 | 3208 | 4054 | 895 | 955 | 1056 | 443 | 463 | 488 | 268 | 275 | 285 |
|  | 16377 | 17461 | 26897 | 3057 | 3468 | 4368 | 922 | 997 | 1110 | 452 | 474 | 496 | 271 | 280 | 278 |
| 0.4 | 16174 | 16723 | 26462 | 3009 | 3306 | 4308 | 921 | 990 | 1108 | 454 | 476 | 505 | 273 | 281 | 292 |
|  | 16357 | 17745 | 28240 | 3127 | 3611 | 4555 | 952 | 1039 | 1145 | 465 | 490 | 507 | 277 | 286 | 281 |
| 0.45 | 15628 | 16330 | 27607 | 2994 | 3332 | 4462 | 928 | 1003 | 1133 | 457 | 480 | 511 | 271 | 281 | 292 |
|  | 15864 | 17593 | 28999 | 3130 | 3675 | 4649 | 961 | 1057 | 1157 | 467 | 494 | 507 | 276 | 286 | 278 |
| 0.5 | 14696 | 15581 | 28119 | 2923 | 3295 | 4513 | 916 | 997 | 1134 | 449 | 473 | 506 | 265 | 274 | 286 |
|  | 14997 | 17089 | 29175 | 3073 | 3665 | 4649 | 952 | 1054 | 1145 | 460 | 488 | 496 | 270 | 280 | 269 |
| 0.55 | 13485 | 14575 | 27996 | 2806 | 3201 | 4463 | 889 | 970 | 1109 | 433 | 457 | 490 | 253 | 262 | 274 |
|  | 13862 | 16313 | 28766 | 2967 | 3588 | 4555 | 925 | 1028 | 1110 | 445 | 472 | 475 | 258 | 268 | 255 |
| 0.6 | 12102 | 13404 | 27237 | 2651 | 3056 | 4312 | 846 | 925 | 1058 | 409 | 431 | 462 | 237 | 245 | 255 |
|  | 12565 | 15329 | 27773 | 2818 | 3446 | 4368 | 881 | 982 | 1052 | 419 | 445 | 444 | 241 | 250 | 234 |
| 0.65 | 10654 | 12139 | 25846 | 2463 | 2864 | 4059 | 787 | 861 | 982 | 376 | 396 | 422 | 214 | 221 | 229 |
|  | 11197 | 14182 | 26196 | 2629 | 3242 | 4088 | 820 | 913 | 970 | 385 | 408 | 403 | 217 | 225 | 208 |
| 0.7 | 9225 | 10828 | 23825 | 2244 | 2624 | 3706 | 712 | 778 | 882 | 334 | 350 | 372 | 186 | 192 | 198 |
|  | 9828 | 12899 | 24036 | 2402 | 2976 | 3714 | 742 | 823 | 865 | 342 | 361 | 351 | 189 | 195 | 176 |
| 0.75 | 7861 | 9487 | 21181 | 1993 | 2336 | 3253 | 621 | 675 | 757 | 282 | 295 | 311 | 152 | 156 | 160 |
|  | 8485 | 11485 | 21291 | 2137 | 2644 | 3247 | 645 | 711 | 736 | 289 | 302 | 289 | 154 | 158 | 138 |
| 0.8 | 6565 | 8104 | 17920 | 1704 | 1993 | 2701 | 511 | 550 | 607 | 220 | 229 | 239 | . | . | . |
|  | 7165 | 9921 | 17963 | 1826 | 2242 | 2687 | 529 | 575 | 584 | 225 | 234 | 216 | . | . | . |
| 0.85 | 5294 | 6633 | 14047 | 1366 | 1582 | 2053 | 378 | 401 | 432 | . | . | . | . | . | . |
|  | 5822 | 8153 | 14050 | 1459 | 1758 | 2033 | 388 | 415 | 409 | . | . | . | . | . | . |
| 0.9 | 3958 | 4972 | 9570 | 954 | 1079 | 1308 | . | . | . | . | . | . | . | . | . |
|  | 4363 | 6064 | 9554 | 1009 | 1172 | 1285 | . | . | . | . | . | . | . | . | . |
| 0.95 | 2335 | 2859 | 4496 | . | . | . | . | . | . | . | . | . | . | . | . |
|  | 2551 | 3358 | 4474 | . | . | . | . | . | . | . | . | . | . | . | . |

# TABLE 1: ALPHA= 0.005 POWER= 0.8    EXPECTED ACCRUAL THRU MINIMUM FOLLOW-UP= 1300

|  |  | DEL=.02 | | | DEL=.05 | | | DEL=.10 | | | DEL=.15 | | | DEL=.20 | | |
|---|---|---|---|---|---|---|---|---|---|---|---|---|---|---|---|---|
| FACT= | | 1.0 .75 | .50 .25 | .00 BIN | 1.0 .75 | .50 .25 | .00 BIN | 1.0 .75 | .50 .25 | .00 BIN | 75 | .50 .25 | .00 BIN | 1.0 .75 | .50 .25 | .00 BIN |
| PCONT=*** | | | | | REQUIRED | NUMBER OF | PATIENTS | | | | | | | | | |
| 0.05 | *** | 3339 | 3364 | 3518 | 721 | 731 | 746 | 261 | 263 | 265 | 153 | 154 | 154 | 108 | 108 | 109 |
|  | *** | 3347 | 3403 | 6576 | 725 | 737 | 1285 | 262 | 264 | 409 | 154 | 154 | 216 | 108 | 108 | 138 |
| 0.1 | *** | 6949 | 7013 | 7729 | 1332 | 1365 | 1439 | 427 | 434 | 445 | 230 | 232 | 236 | 152 | 153 | 154 |
|  | *** | 6971 | 7130 | 11423 | 1345 | 1394 | 2033 | 431 | 439 | 584 | 231 | 234 | 289 | 153 | 154 | 176 |
| 0.15 | *** | 10161 | 10274 | 11954 | 1865 | 1933 | 2109 | 570 | 587 | 609 | 295 | 301 | 307 | 188 | 191 | 193 |
|  | *** | 10198 | 10489 | 15685 | 1892 | 1996 | 2687 | 578 | 596 | 736 | 297 | 304 | 351 | 189 | 192 | 208 |
| 0.2 | *** | 12730 | 12904 | 15884 | 2296 | 2406 | 2721 | 691 | 716 | 755 | 349 | 357 | 368 | 218 | 222 | 226 |
|  | *** | 12789 | 13240 | 19364 | 2340 | 2514 | 3247 | 702 | 733 | 865 | 354 | 362 | 403 | 219 | 224 | 234 |
| 0.25 | *** | 14590 | 14840 | 19367 | 2623 | 2779 | 3256 | 785 | 822 | 879 | 393 | 404 | 419 | 241 | 246 | 252 |
|  | *** | 14674 | 15322 | 22459 | 2684 | 2936 | 3714 | 801 | 847 | 970 | 398 | 411 | 444 | 244 | 249 | 255 |
| 0.3 | *** | 15754 | 16097 | 22320 | 2849 | 3054 | 3703 | 856 | 903 | 980 | 424 | 440 | 459 | 258 | 264 | 272 |
|  | *** | 15868 | 16752 | 24970 | 2931 | 3262 | 4088 | 877 | 936 | 1052 | 432 | 448 | 475 | 261 | 268 | 269 |
| 0.35 | *** | 16272 | 16728 | 24695 | 2984 | 3239 | 4054 | 903 | 961 | 1056 | 446 | 464 | 488 | 269 | 276 | 285 |
|  | *** | 16424 | 17586 | 26897 | 3086 | 3496 | 4368 | 929 | 1002 | 1110 | 454 | 475 | 496 | 272 | 280 | 278 |
| 0.4 | *** | 16220 | 16813 | 26462 | 3041 | 3343 | 4309 | 930 | 997 | 1108 | 458 | 479 | 505 | 274 | 282 | 292 |
|  | *** | 16419 | 17899 | 28240 | 3162 | 3644 | 4555 | 960 | 1044 | 1145 | 467 | 491 | 507 | 278 | 287 | 281 |
| 0.45 | *** | 15687 | 16445 | 27606 | 3031 | 3373 | 4462 | 938 | 1011 | 1134 | 460 | 482 | 512 | 273 | 282 | 292 |
|  | *** | 15943 | 17777 | 28999 | 3169 | 3712 | 4649 | 970 | 1063 | 1157 | 471 | 496 | 507 | 277 | 287 | 278 |
| 0.5 | *** | 14772 | 15722 | 28119 | 2964 | 3339 | 4514 | 927 | 1004 | 1134 | 453 | 476 | 506 | 266 | 276 | 286 |
|  | *** | 15096 | 17304 | 29175 | 3117 | 3706 | 4649 | 962 | 1059 | 1145 | 463 | 490 | 496 | 271 | 280 | 269 |
| 0.55 | *** | 13580 | 14743 | 27995 | 2850 | 3248 | 4463 | 900 | 978 | 1109 | 436 | 460 | 490 | 255 | 263 | 274 |
|  | *** | 13986 | 16553 | 28766 | 3013 | 3630 | 4555 | 935 | 1033 | 1110 | 448 | 474 | 475 | 259 | 268 | 255 |
| 0.6 | *** | 12220 | 13596 | 27238 | 2697 | 3104 | 4312 | 856 | 933 | 1059 | 412 | 434 | 461 | 238 | 245 | 255 |
|  | *** | 12712 | 15586 | 27773 | 2865 | 3488 | 4368 | 890 | 986 | 1052 | 422 | 447 | 444 | 241 | 250 | 234 |
| 0.65 | *** | 10795 | 12349 | 25846 | 2509 | 2910 | 4059 | 796 | 869 | 983 | 379 | 398 | 422 | 215 | 222 | 230 |
|  | *** | 11368 | 14447 | 26196 | 2676 | 3282 | 4088 | 829 | 917 | 970 | 388 | 409 | 403 | 219 | 226 | 208 |
| 0.7 | *** | 9384 | 11046 | 23826 | 2288 | 2668 | 3706 | 721 | 784 | 882 | 336 | 352 | 372 | 187 | 193 | 198 |
|  | *** | 10012 | 13162 | 24036 | 2447 | 3013 | 3714 | 750 | 827 | 865 | 344 | 362 | 351 | 189 | 195 | 176 |
| 0.75 | *** | 8027 | 9701 | 21181 | 2033 | 2375 | 3253 | 628 | 680 | 757 | 284 | 297 | 311 | 153 | 157 | 161 |
|  | *** | 8672 | 11734 | 21291 | 2177 | 2676 | 3247 | 652 | 714 | 736 | 290 | 303 | 289 | 155 | 159 | 138 |
| 0.8 | *** | 6726 | 8302 | 17920 | 1738 | 2025 | 2702 | 516 | 553 | 606 | 222 | 230 | 239 | . | . | . |
|  | *** | 7342 | 10143 | 17963 | 1860 | 2268 | 2687 | 533 | 578 | 584 | 226 | 234 | 216 | . | . | . |
| 0.85 | *** | 5437 | 6802 | 14047 | 1393 | 1605 | 2053 | 381 | 403 | 432 | . | . | . | . | . | . |
|  | *** | 5976 | 8335 | 14050 | 1485 | 1775 | 2033 | 392 | 417 | 409 | . | . | . | . | . | . |
| 0.9 | *** | 4068 | 5096 | 9571 | 969 | 1091 | 1308 | . | . | . | . | . | . | . | . | . |
|  | *** | 4481 | 6190 | 9554 | 1024 | 1181 | 1285 | . | . | . | . | . | . | . | . | . |
| 0.95 | *** | 2395 | 2919 | 4496 | . | . | . | . | . | . | . | . | . | . | . | . |
|  | *** | 2612 | 3412 | 4474 | . | . | . | . | . | . | . | . | . | . | . | . |

TABLE 1: ALPHA= 0.005 POWER= 0.8    EXPECTED ACCRUAL THRU MINIMUM FOLLOW-UP= 1400

|  | DEL=.02 | | | DEL=.05 | | | DEL=.10 | | | DEL=.15 | | | DEL=.20 | | |
|---|---|---|---|---|---|---|---|---|---|---|---|---|---|---|---|
| FACT= | 1.0 .75 | .50 .25 | .00 BIN | 1.0 .75 | .50 .25 | .00 BIN | 1.0 .75 | .50 .25 | .00 BIN | 1.0 75 | .50 .25 | .00 BIN | 1.0 .75 | .50 .25 | .00 BIN |
| PCONT=*** | REQUIRED NUMBER OF PATIENTS | | | | | | | | | | | | | | |
| 0.05 *** | 3340 | 3368 | 3518 | 722 | 731 | 746 | 261 | 262 | 265 | 153 | 154 | 155 | 108 | 108 | 108 |
| *** | 3349 | 3407 | 6576 | 726 | 738 | 1285 | 262 | 264 | 409 | 153 | 154 | 216 | 108 | 108 | 138 |
| 0.1 *** | 6954 | 7023 | 7730 | 1335 | 1368 | 1439 | 428 | 435 | 444 | 230 | 233 | 235 | 152 | 153 | 155 |
| *** | 6977 | 7145 | 11423 | 1349 | 1396 | 2033 | 431 | 439 | 584 | 231 | 234 | 289 | 152 | 154 | 176 |
| 0.15 *** | 10170 | 10292 | 11954 | 1872 | 1940 | 2110 | 573 | 588 | 609 | 296 | 301 | 307 | 189 | 191 | 193 |
| *** | 10210 | 10519 | 15685 | 1900 | 2003 | 2687 | 580 | 598 | 736 | 298 | 304 | 351 | 190 | 192 | 208 |
| 0.2 *** | 12743 | 12932 | 15884 | 2307 | 2418 | 2721 | 693 | 718 | 754 | 351 | 359 | 368 | 219 | 222 | 226 |
| *** | 12806 | 13289 | 19364 | 2352 | 2524 | 3247 | 704 | 734 | 865 | 354 | 363 | 403 | 220 | 224 | 234 |
| 0.25 *** | 14610 | 14878 | 19367 | 2638 | 2796 | 3256 | 789 | 825 | 878 | 394 | 405 | 419 | 241 | 247 | 252 |
| *** | 14699 | 15392 | 22459 | 2701 | 2951 | 3714 | 805 | 849 | 970 | 399 | 412 | 444 | 244 | 249 | 255 |
| 0.3 *** | 15780 | 16149 | 22320 | 2869 | 3077 | 3703 | 861 | 907 | 980 | 426 | 441 | 459 | 259 | 265 | 272 |
| *** | 15903 | 16845 | 24970 | 2952 | 3283 | 4088 | 882 | 939 | 1052 | 433 | 450 | 475 | 262 | 269 | 269 |
| 0.35 *** | 16306 | 16797 | 24695 | 3010 | 3267 | 4055 | 910 | 966 | 1056 | 448 | 465 | 488 | 270 | 276 | 285 |
| *** | 16471 | 17706 | 26897 | 3113 | 3522 | 4368 | 935 | 1005 | 1110 | 457 | 476 | 496 | 273 | 281 | 278 |
| 0.4 *** | 16265 | 16902 | 26463 | 3071 | 3376 | 4308 | 938 | 1003 | 1108 | 460 | 480 | 506 | 275 | 283 | 292 |
| *** | 16480 | 18049 | 28240 | 3195 | 3674 | 4555 | 967 | 1047 | 1145 | 470 | 492 | 507 | 279 | 287 | 281 |
| 0.45 *** | 15746 | 16558 | 27607 | 3065 | 3411 | 4462 | 946 | 1018 | 1134 | 463 | 484 | 512 | 275 | 283 | 292 |
| *** | 16021 | 17956 | 28999 | 3206 | 3746 | 4649 | 978 | 1067 | 1157 | 472 | 497 | 507 | 278 | 287 | 278 |
| 0.5 *** | 14847 | 15860 | 28119 | 3002 | 3380 | 4513 | 936 | 1011 | 1134 | 456 | 478 | 507 | 268 | 276 | 286 |
| *** | 15195 | 17509 | 29175 | 3157 | 3741 | 4649 | 970 | 1064 | 1145 | 466 | 491 | 496 | 272 | 281 | 269 |
| 0.55 *** | 13674 | 14906 | 27996 | 2892 | 3290 | 4463 | 909 | 985 | 1109 | 439 | 461 | 490 | 256 | 264 | 274 |
| *** | 14107 | 16780 | 28766 | 3055 | 3667 | 4555 | 943 | 1039 | 1110 | 450 | 474 | 475 | 260 | 269 | 255 |
| 0.6 *** | 12337 | 13781 | 27237 | 2740 | 3146 | 4312 | 865 | 940 | 1059 | 415 | 436 | 462 | 239 | 246 | 255 |
| *** | 12857 | 15829 | 27773 | 2908 | 3525 | 4368 | 899 | 990 | 1052 | 424 | 448 | 444 | 242 | 250 | 234 |
| 0.65 *** | 10932 | 12550 | 25846 | 2551 | 2952 | 4059 | 805 | 875 | 983 | 381 | 399 | 423 | 216 | 222 | 229 |
| *** | 11532 | 14697 | 26196 | 2719 | 3318 | 4088 | 836 | 921 | 970 | 389 | 410 | 403 | 220 | 226 | 208 |
| 0.7 *** | 9537 | 11253 | 23825 | 2328 | 2707 | 3706 | 729 | 790 | 882 | 338 | 353 | 372 | 188 | 192 | 199 |
| *** | 10188 | 13408 | 24036 | 2488 | 3045 | 3714 | 757 | 830 | 865 | 346 | 362 | 351 | 190 | 195 | 176 |
| 0.75 *** | 8186 | 9903 | 21181 | 2070 | 2410 | 3253 | 634 | 684 | 757 | 286 | 297 | 311 | 153 | 157 | 161 |
| *** | 8850 | 11966 | 21291 | 2214 | 2705 | 3247 | 657 | 717 | 736 | 291 | 304 | 289 | 155 | 159 | 138 |
| 0.8 *** | 6879 | 8488 | 17920 | 1770 | 2053 | 2702 | 521 | 556 | 606 | 223 | 230 | 239 | . | . | . |
| *** | 7509 | 10350 | 17963 | 1891 | 2290 | 2687 | 537 | 579 | 584 | 227 | 234 | 216 | . | . | . |
| 0.85 *** | 5572 | 6959 | 14047 | 1417 | 1626 | 2053 | 384 | 405 | 432 | . | . | . | . | . | . |
| *** | 6121 | 8503 | 14050 | 1508 | 1790 | 2033 | 394 | 417 | 409 | . | . | . | . | . | . |
| 0.9 *** | 4172 | 5211 | 9570 | 984 | 1102 | 1308 | . | . | . | . | . | . | . | . | . |
| *** | 4590 | 6306 | 9554 | 1037 | 1188 | 1285 | . | . | . | . | . | . | . | . | . |
| 0.95 *** | 2451 | 2974 | 4497 | . | . | . | . | . | . | . | . | . | . | . | . |
| *** | 2669 | 3460 | 4474 | . | . | . | . | . | . | . | . | . | . | . | . |

## TABLE 1: ALPHA= 0.005 POWER= 0.8    EXPECTED ACCRUAL THRU MINIMUM FOLLOW-UP= 1500

| | | DEL=.02 | | | DEL=.05 | | | DEL=.10 | | | DEL=.15 | | | DEL=.20 | | |
|---|---|---|---|---|---|---|---|---|---|---|---|---|---|---|---|---|---|
| FACT= | | 1.0 .75 | .50 .25 | .00 BIN | 1.0 .75 | .50 .25 | .00 BIN | 1.0 .75 | .50 .25 | .00 BIN | 1.0 75 | .50 .25 | .00 BIN | 1.0 .75 | .50 .25 | .00 BIN |
| PCONT=*** | | REQUIRED NUMBER OF PATIENTS | | | | | | | | | | | | | | |
| 0.05 | *** | 3342 | 3371 | 3518 | 723 | 732 | 746 | 260 | 262 | 265 | 153 | 154 | 155 | 108 | 109 | 109 |
| | *** | 3352 | 3412 | 6576 | 727 | 738 | 1285 | 262 | 264 | 409 | 154 | 154 | 216 | 108 | 109 | 138 |
| 0.1 | *** | 6959 | 7032 | 7730 | 1339 | 1372 | 1439 | 428 | 435 | 444 | 230 | 232 | 235 | 152 | 154 | 155 |
| | *** | 6983 | 7160 | 11423 | 1353 | 1399 | 2033 | 432 | 440 | 584 | 232 | 234 | 289 | 153 | 154 | 176 |
| 0.15 | *** | 10178 | 10309 | 11954 | 1878 | 1947 | 2109 | 575 | 589 | 608 | 296 | 301 | 307 | 189 | 191 | 193 |
| | *** | 10222 | 10549 | 15685 | 1906 | 2008 | 2687 | 581 | 598 | 736 | 299 | 304 | 351 | 190 | 192 | 208 |
| 0.2 | *** | 12757 | 12958 | 15884 | 2317 | 2429 | 2722 | 697 | 720 | 755 | 352 | 359 | 368 | 219 | 222 | 226 |
| | *** | 12824 | 13336 | 19364 | 2362 | 2534 | 3247 | 707 | 736 | 865 | 355 | 364 | 403 | 220 | 224 | 234 |
| 0.25 | *** | 14629 | 14917 | 19367 | 2652 | 2812 | 3256 | 793 | 828 | 879 | 395 | 406 | 419 | 243 | 247 | 252 |
| | *** | 14725 | 15459 | 22459 | 2717 | 2965 | 3714 | 809 | 850 | 970 | 400 | 412 | 444 | 245 | 249 | 255 |
| 0.3 | *** | 15806 | 16201 | 22320 | 2888 | 3098 | 3703 | 866 | 911 | 980 | 428 | 442 | 459 | 260 | 265 | 272 |
| | *** | 15938 | 16937 | 24970 | 2973 | 3302 | 4088 | 887 | 941 | 1052 | 435 | 450 | 475 | 262 | 268 | 269 |
| 0.35 | *** | 16342 | 16867 | 24695 | 3034 | 3293 | 4055 | 916 | 971 | 1057 | 450 | 467 | 488 | 271 | 277 | 285 |
| | *** | 16518 | 17824 | 26897 | 3139 | 3545 | 4368 | 941 | 1008 | 1110 | 458 | 477 | 496 | 274 | 281 | 278 |
| 0.4 | *** | 16312 | 16991 | 26463 | 3100 | 3407 | 4309 | 945 | 1008 | 1107 | 463 | 482 | 505 | 275 | 283 | 292 |
| | *** | 16540 | 18193 | 28240 | 3225 | 3701 | 4555 | 973 | 1051 | 1145 | 472 | 493 | 507 | 279 | 288 | 281 |
| 0.45 | *** | 15805 | 16669 | 27607 | 3098 | 3445 | 4462 | 954 | 1024 | 1133 | 465 | 485 | 512 | 275 | 283 | 292 |
| | *** | 16099 | 18127 | 28999 | 3240 | 3776 | 4649 | 985 | 1070 | 1157 | 474 | 498 | 507 | 279 | 288 | 278 |
| 0.5 | *** | 14922 | 15995 | 28119 | 3039 | 3417 | 4513 | 945 | 1018 | 1134 | 458 | 479 | 506 | 269 | 277 | 286 |
| | *** | 15292 | 17705 | 29175 | 3195 | 3774 | 4649 | 978 | 1068 | 1145 | 468 | 492 | 496 | 273 | 281 | 269 |
| 0.55 | *** | 13769 | 15065 | 27995 | 2930 | 3330 | 4463 | 918 | 992 | 1109 | 442 | 463 | 489 | 257 | 265 | 274 |
| | *** | 14227 | 16997 | 28766 | 3095 | 3701 | 4555 | 952 | 1042 | 1110 | 452 | 475 | 475 | 260 | 269 | 255 |
| 0.6 | *** | 12452 | 13960 | 27237 | 2780 | 3187 | 4312 | 874 | 946 | 1058 | 417 | 437 | 462 | 240 | 247 | 255 |
| | *** | 12999 | 16059 | 27773 | 2949 | 3560 | 4368 | 907 | 995 | 1052 | 427 | 448 | 444 | 243 | 250 | 234 |
| 0.65 | *** | 11066 | 12742 | 25846 | 2591 | 2990 | 4059 | 813 | 880 | 982 | 383 | 401 | 423 | 217 | 223 | 230 |
| | *** | 11690 | 14933 | 26196 | 2758 | 3350 | 4088 | 844 | 925 | 970 | 392 | 410 | 403 | 220 | 226 | 208 |
| 0.7 | *** | 9684 | 11450 | 23825 | 2366 | 2743 | 3706 | 736 | 795 | 882 | 340 | 354 | 372 | 188 | 193 | 199 |
| | *** | 10357 | 13640 | 24036 | 2525 | 3075 | 3714 | 763 | 833 | 865 | 347 | 363 | 351 | 190 | 196 | 176 |
| 0.75 | *** | 8339 | 10096 | 21182 | 2105 | 2441 | 3253 | 640 | 688 | 757 | 287 | 298 | 311 | 154 | 157 | 161 |
| | *** | 9020 | 12185 | 21291 | 2248 | 2730 | 3247 | 663 | 719 | 736 | 292 | 305 | 289 | 155 | 159 | 138 |
| 0.8 | *** | 7025 | 8664 | 17919 | 1799 | 2079 | 2702 | 525 | 560 | 607 | 224 | 230 | 239 | . | . | . |
| | *** | 7669 | 10544 | 17963 | 1919 | 2310 | 2687 | 541 | 581 | 584 | 228 | 235 | 216 | . | . | . |
| 0.85 | *** | 5700 | 7108 | 14047 | 1439 | 1644 | 2053 | 386 | 407 | 432 | . | . | . | . | . | . |
| | *** | 6260 | 8660 | 14050 | 1528 | 1804 | 2033 | 395 | 419 | 409 | . | . | . | . | . | . |
| 0.9 | *** | 4270 | 5320 | 9570 | 997 | 1113 | 1308 | . | . | . | . | . | . | . | . | . |
| | *** | 4694 | 6413 | 9554 | 1049 | 1195 | 1285 | . | . | . | . | . | . | . | . | . |
| 0.95 | *** | 2503 | 3025 | 4496 | . | . | . | . | . | . | . | . | . | . | . | . |
| | *** | 2722 | 3504 | 4474 | . | . | . | . | . | . | . | . | . | . | . | . |

TABLE 1: ALPHA= 0.005 POWER= 0.8    EXPECTED ACCRUAL THRU MINIMUM FOLLOW-UP= 1600

| | | DEL=.02 | | | DEL=.05 | | | DEL=.10 | | | DEL=.15 | | | DEL=.20 | | |
|---|---|---|---|---|---|---|---|---|---|---|---|---|---|---|---|---|---|
| FACT= | | 1.0 .75 | .50 .25 | .00 BIN | 1.0 .75 | .50 .25 | .00 BIN | 1.0 .75 | .50 .25 | .00 BIN | 1.0 75 | .50 .25 | .00 BIN | 1.0 .75 | .50 .25 | .00 BIN |
| PCONT=*** | | REQUIRED NUMBER OF PATIENTS | | | | | | | | | | | | | | |
| 0.05 | *** | 3345 | 3375 | 3518 | 724 | 733 | 746 | 261 | 263 | 265 | 153 | 154 | 155 | 108 | 108 | 109 |
| | *** | 3355 | 3415 | 6576 | 728 | 739 | 1285 | 262 | 264 | 409 | 154 | 154 | 216 | 108 | 109 | 138 |
| 0.1 | *** | 6964 | 7042 | 7730 | 1342 | 1375 | 1439 | 429 | 436 | 444 | 231 | 233 | 236 | 152 | 153 | 155 |
| | *** | 6990 | 7175 | 11423 | 1356 | 1401 | 2033 | 432 | 440 | 584 | 232 | 234 | 289 | 153 | 154 | 176 |
| 0.15 | *** | 10187 | 10326 | 11954 | 1884 | 1953 | 2109 | 576 | 590 | 609 | 297 | 302 | 307 | 189 | 191 | 193 |
| | *** | 10234 | 10578 | 15685 | 1913 | 2013 | 2687 | 583 | 599 | 736 | 299 | 304 | 351 | 190 | 192 | 208 |
| 0.2 | *** | 12771 | 12984 | 15884 | 2327 | 2440 | 2721 | 699 | 722 | 755 | 352 | 360 | 368 | 219 | 222 | 226 |
| | *** | 12842 | 13382 | 19364 | 2373 | 2542 | 3247 | 710 | 737 | 865 | 356 | 364 | 403 | 221 | 224 | 234 |
| 0.25 | *** | 14648 | 14955 | 19367 | 2667 | 2828 | 3256 | 797 | 830 | 879 | 397 | 407 | 419 | 243 | 247 | 252 |
| | *** | 14751 | 15526 | 22459 | 2732 | 2978 | 3714 | 812 | 852 | 970 | 401 | 413 | 444 | 245 | 250 | 255 |
| 0.3 | *** | 15833 | 16253 | 22320 | 2907 | 3118 | 3703 | 871 | 914 | 980 | 430 | 443 | 459 | 260 | 266 | 272 |
| | *** | 15974 | 17026 | 24970 | 2993 | 3319 | 4088 | 891 | 943 | 1052 | 436 | 451 | 475 | 263 | 269 | 269 |
| 0.35 | *** | 16377 | 16935 | 24695 | 3057 | 3318 | 4055 | 922 | 975 | 1056 | 452 | 468 | 488 | 272 | 278 | 285 |
| | *** | 16565 | 17937 | 26897 | 3164 | 3566 | 4368 | 946 | 1011 | 1110 | 460 | 478 | 496 | 275 | 281 | 278 |
| 0.4 | *** | 16358 | 17080 | 26463 | 3128 | 3435 | 4308 | 952 | 1013 | 1108 | 465 | 483 | 506 | 277 | 284 | 292 |
| | *** | 16602 | 18333 | 28240 | 3254 | 3726 | 4555 | 980 | 1054 | 1145 | 473 | 494 | 507 | 280 | 288 | 281 |
| 0.45 | *** | 15864 | 16779 | 27607 | 3130 | 3478 | 4462 | 962 | 1029 | 1134 | 468 | 487 | 512 | 276 | 284 | 292 |
| | *** | 16177 | 18293 | 28999 | 3273 | 3804 | 4649 | 992 | 1074 | 1157 | 477 | 499 | 507 | 280 | 288 | 278 |
| 0.5 | *** | 14997 | 16128 | 28119 | 3073 | 3453 | 4514 | 952 | 1023 | 1134 | 461 | 481 | 506 | 270 | 278 | 286 |
| | *** | 15390 | 17893 | 29175 | 3230 | 3805 | 4649 | 985 | 1072 | 1145 | 470 | 493 | 496 | 274 | 282 | 269 |
| 0.55 | *** | 13862 | 15220 | 27996 | 2967 | 3366 | 4464 | 925 | 997 | 1109 | 445 | 465 | 490 | 258 | 265 | 274 |
| | *** | 14345 | 17203 | 28766 | 3133 | 3732 | 4555 | 958 | 1046 | 1110 | 454 | 476 | 475 | 262 | 269 | 255 |
| 0.6 | *** | 12565 | 14133 | 27237 | 2818 | 3224 | 4312 | 881 | 951 | 1059 | 420 | 438 | 462 | 241 | 247 | 255 |
| | *** | 13137 | 16278 | 27773 | 2987 | 3591 | 4368 | 913 | 998 | 1052 | 428 | 449 | 444 | 244 | 251 | 234 |
| 0.65 | *** | 11198 | 12927 | 25846 | 2629 | 3027 | 4059 | 820 | 885 | 983 | 385 | 402 | 423 | 218 | 223 | 230 |
| | *** | 11845 | 15157 | 26196 | 2796 | 3381 | 4088 | 850 | 928 | 970 | 393 | 412 | 403 | 220 | 226 | 208 |
| 0.7 | *** | 9828 | 11638 | 23826 | 2402 | 2777 | 3706 | 742 | 799 | 882 | 342 | 356 | 372 | 189 | 193 | 198 |
| | *** | 10520 | 13860 | 24036 | 2561 | 3102 | 3714 | 768 | 836 | 865 | 348 | 364 | 351 | 191 | 196 | 176 |
| 0.75 | *** | 8486 | 10278 | 21181 | 2137 | 2471 | 3253 | 645 | 692 | 757 | 289 | 299 | 311 | 154 | 158 | 161 |
| | *** | 9182 | 12391 | 21291 | 2279 | 2753 | 3247 | 667 | 721 | 736 | 294 | 305 | 289 | 156 | 159 | 138 |
| 0.8 | *** | 7165 | 8831 | 17920 | 1827 | 2103 | 2702 | 529 | 562 | 607 | 225 | 232 | 239 | . | . | . |
| | *** | 7821 | 10725 | 17963 | 1946 | 2328 | 2687 | 544 | 583 | 584 | 228 | 235 | 216 | . | . | . |
| 0.85 | *** | 5822 | 7248 | 14047 | 1459 | 1661 | 2053 | 389 | 408 | 432 | . | . | . | . | . | . |
| | *** | 6390 | 8807 | 14050 | 1548 | 1816 | 2033 | 398 | 420 | 409 | . | . | . | . | . | . |
| 0.9 | *** | 4364 | 5422 | 9570 | 1009 | 1122 | 1308 | . | . | . | . | . | . | . | . | . |
| | *** | 4792 | 6513 | 9554 | 1060 | 1201 | 1285 | . | . | . | . | . | . | . | . | . |
| 0.95 | *** | 2552 | 3073 | 4496 | . | . | . | . | . | . | . | . | . | . | . | . |
| | *** | 2770 | 3544 | 4474 | . | . | . | . | . | . | . | . | . | . | . | . |

## TABLE 1: ALPHA= 0.005 POWER= 0.8     EXPECTED ACCRUAL THRU MINIMUM FOLLOW-UP= 1700

| | | DEL=.02 | | | DEL=.05 | | | DEL=.10 | | | DEL=.15 | | | DEL=.20 | | |
|---|---|---|---|---|---|---|---|---|---|---|---|---|---|---|---|---|---|
| FACT= | | 1.0 .75 | .50 .25 | .00 BIN | 1.0 .75 | .50 .25 | .00 BIN | 1.0 .75 | .50 .25 | .00 BIN | 1.0 75 | .50 .25 | .00 BIN | 1.0 .75 | .50 .25 | .00 BIN |
| PCONT=*** | | | | | REQUIRED NUMBER OF PATIENTS | | | | | | | | | | | |
| 0.05 | *** | 3347 | 3378 | 3518 | 724 | 733 | 746 | 261 | 263 | 265 | 153 | 154 | 155 | 108 | 108 | 108 |
| | *** | 3357 | 3419 | 6576 | 729 | 739 | 1285 | 262 | 265 | 409 | 154 | 154 | 216 | 108 | 108 | 138 |
| 0.1 | *** | 6969 | 7052 | 7730 | 1344 | 1377 | 1438 | 430 | 437 | 444 | 231 | 233 | 236 | 153 | 154 | 155 |
| | *** | 6997 | 7189 | 11423 | 1359 | 1402 | 2033 | 433 | 440 | 584 | 233 | 235 | 289 | 153 | 154 | 176 |
| 0.15 | *** | 10195 | 10342 | 11954 | 1890 | 1959 | 2109 | 578 | 590 | 609 | 297 | 301 | 307 | 189 | 191 | 193 |
| | *** | 10246 | 10606 | 15685 | 1919 | 2018 | 2687 | 584 | 599 | 736 | 299 | 305 | 351 | 190 | 192 | 208 |
| 0.2 | *** | 12784 | 13011 | 15883 | 2336 | 2450 | 2721 | 701 | 724 | 754 | 352 | 360 | 369 | 220 | 223 | 226 |
| | *** | 12860 | 13427 | 19364 | 2383 | 2550 | 3247 | 712 | 737 | 865 | 357 | 364 | 403 | 221 | 224 | 234 |
| 0.25 | *** | 14668 | 14993 | 19367 | 2681 | 2842 | 3257 | 800 | 833 | 879 | 397 | 408 | 420 | 243 | 248 | 252 |
| | *** | 14776 | 15590 | 22459 | 2747 | 2990 | 3714 | 815 | 853 | 970 | 403 | 413 | 444 | 245 | 250 | 255 |
| 0.3 | *** | 15859 | 16305 | 22320 | 2925 | 3138 | 3703 | 875 | 918 | 979 | 431 | 444 | 459 | 261 | 265 | 272 |
| | *** | 16009 | 17112 | 24970 | 3011 | 3334 | 4088 | 894 | 945 | 1052 | 437 | 452 | 475 | 263 | 269 | 269 |
| 0.35 | *** | 16412 | 17003 | 24694 | 3079 | 3342 | 4054 | 928 | 979 | 1056 | 454 | 469 | 488 | 272 | 278 | 284 |
| | *** | 16611 | 18047 | 26897 | 3186 | 3586 | 4368 | 951 | 1013 | 1110 | 461 | 478 | 496 | 275 | 282 | 278 |
| 0.4 | *** | 16404 | 17167 | 26462 | 3153 | 3463 | 4308 | 958 | 1017 | 1108 | 466 | 484 | 505 | 277 | 284 | 292 |
| | *** | 16662 | 18468 | 28240 | 3281 | 3750 | 4555 | 985 | 1057 | 1145 | 475 | 494 | 507 | 280 | 288 | 281 |
| 0.45 | *** | 15922 | 16887 | 27607 | 3160 | 3508 | 4461 | 968 | 1034 | 1134 | 469 | 488 | 512 | 277 | 284 | 292 |
| | *** | 16254 | 18451 | 28999 | 3303 | 3830 | 4649 | 998 | 1077 | 1157 | 478 | 499 | 507 | 280 | 288 | 278 |
| 0.5 | *** | 15072 | 16258 | 28119 | 3106 | 3485 | 4513 | 959 | 1028 | 1134 | 463 | 482 | 507 | 271 | 278 | 286 |
| | *** | 15486 | 18074 | 29175 | 3264 | 3832 | 4649 | 991 | 1075 | 1145 | 471 | 494 | 496 | 274 | 282 | 269 |
| 0.55 | *** | 13955 | 15370 | 27996 | 3002 | 3401 | 4464 | 933 | 1003 | 1109 | 447 | 466 | 490 | 259 | 265 | 274 |
| | *** | 14462 | 17401 | 28766 | 3168 | 3761 | 4555 | 964 | 1049 | 1110 | 456 | 477 | 475 | 262 | 270 | 255 |
| 0.6 | *** | 12675 | 14300 | 27237 | 2853 | 3257 | 4311 | 888 | 956 | 1058 | 422 | 440 | 462 | 241 | 248 | 255 |
| | *** | 13272 | 16487 | 27773 | 3023 | 3619 | 4368 | 919 | 1002 | 1052 | 430 | 450 | 444 | 244 | 250 | 234 |
| 0.65 | *** | 11325 | 13105 | 25846 | 2664 | 3060 | 4058 | 826 | 890 | 983 | 386 | 403 | 423 | 219 | 224 | 229 |
| | *** | 11995 | 15369 | 26196 | 2832 | 3407 | 4088 | 856 | 932 | 970 | 395 | 412 | 403 | 221 | 226 | 208 |
| 0.7 | *** | 9966 | 11819 | 23825 | 2436 | 2808 | 3706 | 748 | 803 | 882 | 343 | 357 | 372 | 189 | 193 | 199 |
| | *** | 10677 | 14069 | 24036 | 2594 | 3127 | 3714 | 773 | 838 | 865 | 350 | 364 | 351 | 191 | 195 | 176 |
| 0.75 | *** | 8626 | 10453 | 21182 | 2167 | 2498 | 3253 | 650 | 695 | 756 | 290 | 299 | 311 | 155 | 157 | 160 |
| | *** | 9338 | 12585 | 21291 | 2309 | 2774 | 3247 | 671 | 724 | 736 | 294 | 305 | 289 | 156 | 159 | 138 |
| 0.8 | *** | 7298 | 8990 | 17920 | 1852 | 2125 | 2702 | 532 | 564 | 607 | 225 | 231 | 239 | . | . | . |
| | *** | 7966 | 10897 | 17963 | 1970 | 2345 | 2687 | 547 | 584 | 584 | 228 | 236 | 216 | . | . | . |
| 0.85 | *** | 5938 | 7381 | 14047 | 1478 | 1676 | 2052 | 391 | 409 | 432 | . | . | . | . | . | . |
| | *** | 6514 | 8945 | 14050 | 1566 | 1827 | 2033 | .399 | 420 | 409 | . | . | . | . | . | . |
| 0.9 | *** | 4452 | 5518 | 9570 | 1020 | 1130 | 1308 | . | . | . | . | . | . | . | . | . |
| | *** | 4884 | 6606 | 9554 | 1070 | 1206 | 1285 | . | . | . | . | . | . | . | . | . |
| 0.95 | *** | 2598 | 3117 | 4496 | . | . | . | . | . | . | . | . | . | . | . | . |
| | *** | 2815 | 3580 | 4474 | . | . | . | . | . | . | . | . | . | . | . | . |

## TABLE 1: ALPHA= 0.005 POWER= 0.8    EXPECTED ACCRUAL THRU MINIMUM FOLLOW-UP= 1800

| | | DEL=.02 | | | DEL=.05 | | | DEL=.10 | | | DEL=.15 | | | DEL=.20 | | |
|---|---|---|---|---|---|---|---|---|---|---|---|---|---|---|---|---|
| FACT= | | 1.0<br>.75 | .50<br>.25 | .00<br>BIN | 1.0<br>.75 | .50<br>.25 | .00<br>BIN | 1.0<br>.75 | .50<br>.25 | .00<br>BIN | 1.0<br>75 | .50<br>.25 | .00<br>BIN | 1.0<br>.75 | .50<br>.25 | .00<br>BIN |
| PCONT=*** | | REQUIRED NUMBER OF PATIENTS | | | | | | | | | | | | | | |
| 0.05 | *** | 3349 | 3381 | 3518 | 726 | 733 | 746 | 262 | 263 | 265 | 153 | 154 | 155 | 108 | 108 | 109 |
| | *** | 3360 | 3422 | 6576 | 729 | 739 | 1285 | 262 | 264 | 409 | 154 | 154 | 216 | 108 | 109 | 138 |
| 0.1 | *** | 6974 | 7060 | 7730 | 1347 | 1380 | 1439 | 431 | 436 | 444 | 231 | 234 | 236 | 153 | 154 | 154 |
| | *** | 7003 | 7202 | 11423 | 1361 | 1404 | 2033 | 433 | 440 | 584 | 233 | 234 | 289 | 153 | 154 | 176 |
| 0.15 | *** | 10205 | 10360 | 11954 | 1896 | 1964 | 2109 | 579 | 591 | 609 | 298 | 303 | 307 | 190 | 191 | 193 |
| | *** | 10257 | 10632 | 15685 | 1925 | 2022 | 2687 | 585 | 600 | 736 | 300 | 305 | 351 | 190 | 192 | 208 |
| 0.2 | *** | 12798 | 13038 | 15884 | 2346 | 2459 | 2721 | 703 | 726 | 755 | 354 | 361 | 369 | 220 | 222 | 226 |
| | *** | 12878 | 13470 | 19364 | 2393 | 2557 | 3247 | 713 | 739 | 865 | 357 | 364 | 403 | 222 | 224 | 234 |
| 0.25 | *** | 14687 | 15031 | 19367 | 2693 | 2855 | 3255 | 803 | 834 | 879 | 398 | 408 | 420 | 244 | 247 | 252 |
| | *** | 14802 | 15652 | 22459 | 2760 | 3000 | 3714 | 818 | 855 | 970 | 402 | 414 | 444 | 246 | 249 | 255 |
| 0.3 | *** | 15886 | 16356 | 22320 | 2942 | 3154 | 3702 | 879 | 920 | 980 | 432 | 444 | 459 | 262 | 267 | 272 |
| | *** | 16044 | 17196 | 24970 | 3030 | 3349 | 4088 | 897 | 947 | 1052 | 438 | 451 | 475 | 264 | 269 | 269 |
| 0.35 | *** | 16447 | 17070 | 24695 | 3100 | 3363 | 4054 | 933 | 982 | 1056 | 456 | 470 | 488 | 273 | 279 | 285 |
| | *** | 16658 | 18155 | 26897 | 3208 | 3603 | 4368 | 955 | 1014 | 1110 | 462 | 479 | 496 | 276 | 282 | 278 |
| 0.4 | *** | 16449 | 17253 | 26462 | 3178 | 3487 | 4308 | 964 | 1021 | 1108 | 469 | 485 | 506 | 279 | 285 | 292 |
| | *** | 16723 | 18598 | 28240 | 3306 | 3771 | 4555 | 990 | 1059 | 1145 | 477 | 495 | 507 | 281 | 288 | 281 |
| 0.45 | *** | 15981 | 16993 | 27606 | 3188 | 3537 | 4461 | 974 | 1038 | 1134 | 471 | 489 | 512 | 278 | 285 | 292 |
| | *** | 16330 | 18605 | 28999 | 3332 | 3853 | 4649 | 1003 | 1080 | 1157 | 480 | 499 | 507 | 281 | 288 | 278 |
| 0.5 | *** | 15146 | 16384 | 28119 | 3138 | 3516 | 4513 | 966 | 1032 | 1134 | 465 | 483 | 506 | 272 | 279 | 285 |
| | *** | 15581 | 18247 | 29175 | 3295 | 3858 | 4649 | 996 | 1077 | 1145 | 474 | 494 | 496 | 274 | 282 | 269 |
| 0.55 | *** | 14046 | 15516 | 27996 | 3035 | 3432 | 4464 | 939 | 1007 | 1109 | 449 | 467 | 489 | 260 | 267 | 273 |
| | *** | 14575 | 17589 | 28766 | 3201 | 3788 | 4555 | 971 | 1052 | 1110 | 458 | 478 | 475 | 263 | 270 | 255 |
| 0.6 | *** | 12786 | 14460 | 27237 | 2886 | 3291 | 4312 | 895 | 960 | 1059 | 423 | 441 | 462 | 242 | 249 | 255 |
| | *** | 13404 | 16686 | 27773 | 3057 | 3645 | 4368 | 924 | 1005 | 1052 | 432 | 451 | 444 | 245 | 252 | 234 |
| 0.65 | *** | 11450 | 13275 | 25845 | 2697 | 3091 | 4059 | 832 | 894 | 983 | 389 | 404 | 423 | 219 | 224 | 229 |
| | *** | 12140 | 15571 | 26196 | 2864 | 3433 | 4088 | 861 | 933 | 970 | 396 | 413 | 403 | 222 | 227 | 208 |
| 0.7 | *** | 10100 | 11991 | 23825 | 2467 | 2837 | 3705 | 753 | 807 | 882 | 344 | 357 | 372 | 190 | 193 | 198 |
| | *** | 10829 | 14265 | 24036 | 2625 | 3150 | 3714 | 778 | 840 | 865 | 351 | 364 | 351 | 192 | 195 | 176 |
| 0.75 | *** | 8763 | 10619 | 21181 | 2196 | 2523 | 3253 | 654 | 697 | 757 | 290 | 300 | 312 | 155 | 157 | 161 |
| | *** | 9488 | 12768 | 21291 | 2337 | 2794 | 3247 | 675 | 724 | 736 | 296 | 306 | 289 | 156 | 159 | 138 |
| 0.8 | *** | 7426 | 9141 | 17920 | 1876 | 2145 | 2702 | 535 | 567 | 606 | 226 | 233 | 240 | . | . | . |
| | *** | 8104 | 11058 | 17963 | 1993 | 2360 | 2687 | 550 | 585 | 584 | 229 | 235 | 216 | . | . | . |
| 0.85 | *** | 6050 | 7507 | 14046 | 1496 | 1691 | 2053 | 393 | 411 | 432 | . | . | . | . | . | . |
| | *** | 6633 | 9074 | 14050 | 1581 | 1837 | 2033 | 402 | 420 | 409 | . | . | . | . | . | . |
| 0.9 | *** | 4537 | 5608 | 9570 | 1030 | 1137 | 1308 | . | . | . | . | . | . | . | . | . |
| | *** | 4972 | 6693 | 9554 | 1079 | 1212 | 1285 | . | . | . | . | . | . | . | . | . |
| 0.95 | *** | 2641 | 3158 | 4497 | . | . | . | . | . | . | . | . | . | . | . | . |
| | *** | 2859 | 3615 | 4474 | . | . | . | . | . | . | . | . | . | . | . | . |

TABLE 1: ALPHA= 0.005 POWER= 0.8     EXPECTED ACCRUAL THRU MINIMUM FOLLOW-UP= 1900

| | | DEL=.02 | | | DEL=.05 | | | DEL=.10 | | | DEL=.15 | | | DEL=.20 | |
|---|---|---|---|---|---|---|---|---|---|---|---|---|---|---|---|
| FACT= | 1.0 .75 | .50 .25 | .00 BIN | 1.0 .75 | .50 .25 | .00 BIN | 1.0 .75 | .50 .25 | .00 BIN | 1.0 75 | .50 .25 | .00 BIN | 1.0 .75 | .50 .25 | .00 BIN |
| PCONT=*** | | | | | | REQUIRED NUMBER OF PATIENTS | | | | | | | | | |
| 0.05 *** | 3351 | 3384 | 3518 | 726 | 735 | 745 | 262 | 263 | 265 | 153 | 154 | 154 | 108 | 108 | 109 |
| *** | 3363 | 3426 | 6576 | 730 | 740 | 1285 | 262 | 265 | 409 | 154 | 154 | 216 | 108 | 109 | 138 |
| 0.1 *** | 6979 | 7070 | 7729 | 1350 | 1382 | 1439 | 431 | 437 | 444 | 231 | 234 | 236 | 153 | 153 | 154 |
| *** | 7010 | 7215 | 11423 | 1364 | 1406 | 2033 | 434 | 440 | 584 | 232 | 235 | 289 | 153 | 154 | 176 |
| 0.15 *** | 10214 | 10376 | 11954 | 1901 | 1968 | 2109 | 581 | 592 | 609 | 298 | 303 | 307 | 190 | 191 | 193 |
| *** | 10268 | 10659 | 15685 | 1930 | 2025 | 2687 | 586 | 600 | 736 | 300 | 305 | 351 | 191 | 192 | 208 |
| 0.2 *** | 12810 | 13064 | 15884 | 2355 | 2467 | 2721 | 705 | 726 | 755 | 355 | 361 | 368 | 220 | 223 | 225 |
| *** | 12896 | 13512 | 19364 | 2402 | 2564 | 3247 | 714 | 740 | 865 | 357 | 364 | 403 | 222 | 224 | 234 |
| 0.25 *** | 14706 | 15068 | 19367 | 2705 | 2868 | 3256 | 806 | 837 | 878 | 400 | 408 | 419 | 244 | 248 | 251 |
| *** | 14828 | 15713 | 22459 | 2773 | 3010 | 3714 | 820 | 856 | 970 | 403 | 413 | 444 | 246 | 250 | 255 |
| 0.3 *** | 15912 | 16408 | 22320 | 2958 | 3170 | 3702 | 883 | 923 | 980 | 433 | 445 | 459 | 262 | 267 | 272 |
| *** | 16078 | 17278 | 24970 | 3046 | 3362 | 4088 | 901 | 949 | 1052 | 439 | 452 | 475 | 265 | 269 | 269 |
| 0.35 *** | 16482 | 17138 | 24695 | 3119 | 3383 | 4055 | 937 | 985 | 1056 | 457 | 471 | 488 | 273 | 279 | 285 |
| *** | 16704 | 18259 | 26897 | 3229 | 3621 | 4368 | 959 | 1018 | 1110 | 464 | 479 | 496 | 277 | 282 | 278 |
| 0.4 *** | 16495 | 17337 | 26462 | 3203 | 3511 | 4308 | 969 | 1025 | 1108 | 470 | 486 | 505 | 279 | 285 | 292 |
| *** | 16783 | 18724 | 28240 | 3331 | 3790 | 4555 | 995 | 1061 | 1145 | 477 | 495 | 507 | 282 | 288 | 281 |
| 0.45 *** | 16040 | 17097 | 27607 | 3214 | 3562 | 4461 | 980 | 1042 | 1134 | 474 | 490 | 512 | 279 | 285 | 292 |
| *** | 16406 | 18753 | 28999 | 3359 | 3876 | 4649 | 1008 | 1083 | 1157 | 482 | 501 | 507 | 281 | 288 | 278 |
| 0.5 *** | 15220 | 16508 | 28119 | 3167 | 3545 | 4514 | 972 | 1037 | 1134 | 467 | 484 | 507 | 272 | 279 | 286 |
| *** | 15675 | 18413 | 29175 | 3325 | 3882 | 4649 | 1002 | 1080 | 1145 | 475 | 495 | 496 | 275 | 282 | 269 |
| 0.55 *** | 14137 | 15658 | 27996 | 3066 | 3462 | 4464 | 945 | 1011 | 1109 | 450 | 467 | 490 | 260 | 267 | 274 |
| *** | 14688 | 17771 | 28766 | 3232 | 3811 | 4555 | 976 | 1054 | 1110 | 459 | 478 | 475 | 263 | 270 | 255 |
| 0.6 *** | 12893 | 14617 | 27238 | 2918 | 3320 | 4312 | 901 | 965 | 1059 | 425 | 441 | 462 | 242 | 248 | 255 |
| *** | 13532 | 16875 | 27773 | 3089 | 3669 | 4368 | 931 | 1007 | 1052 | 433 | 451 | 444 | 246 | 251 | 234 |
| 0.65 *** | 11572 | 13440 | 25846 | 2728 | 3120 | 4058 | 838 | 897 | 983 | 391 | 405 | 422 | 220 | 224 | 230 |
| *** | 12281 | 15764 | 26196 | 2895 | 3457 | 4088 | 866 | 935 | 970 | 398 | 413 | 403 | 222 | 227 | 208 |
| 0.7 *** | 10231 | 12157 | 23826 | 2497 | 2864 | 3706 | 759 | 809 | 882 | 345 | 358 | 372 | 190 | 194 | 198 |
| *** | 10974 | 14453 | 24036 | 2654 | 3170 | 3714 | 782 | 843 | 865 | 351 | 364 | 351 | 192 | 196 | 176 |
| 0.75 *** | 8893 | 10777 | 21181 | 2223 | 2547 | 3253 | 659 | 700 | 756 | 292 | 300 | 311 | 155 | 158 | 161 |
| *** | 9632 | 12943 | 21291 | 2362 | 2812 | 3247 | 678 | 726 | 736 | 296 | 306 | 289 | 156 | 159 | 138 |
| 0.8 *** | 7550 | 9285 | 17919 | 1899 | 2165 | 2701 | 539 | 569 | 607 | 227 | 232 | 239 | . | . | . |
| *** | 8238 | 11211 | 17963 | 2014 | 2374 | 2687 | 552 | 586 | 584 | 229 | 236 | 216 | . | . | . |
| 0.85 *** | 6157 | 7627 | 14047 | 1512 | 1704 | 2053 | 394 | 412 | 432 | . | . | . | . | . | . |
| *** | 6746 | 9197 | 14050 | 1597 | 1846 | 2033 | 402 | 421 | 409 | . | . | . | . | . | . |
| 0.9 *** | 4617 | 5694 | 9570 | 1040 | 1144 | 1308 | . | . | . | . | . | . | . | . | . |
| *** | 5056 | 6773 | 9554 | 1087 | 1216 | 1285 | . | . | . | . | . | . | . | . | . |
| 0.95 *** | 2682 | 3196 | 4495 | . | . | . | . | . | . | . | . | . | . | . | . |
| *** | 2899 | 3647 | 4474 | . | . | . | . | . | . | . | . | . | . | . | . |

## TABLE 1: ALPHA= 0.005 POWER= 0.8    EXPECTED ACCRUAL THRU MINIMUM FOLLOW-UP= 2000

| | | DEL=.02 | | | DEL=.05 | | | DEL=.10 | | | DEL=.15 | | | DEL=.20 | | |
|---|---|---|---|---|---|---|---|---|---|---|---|---|---|---|---|---|---|
| FACT= | | 1.0 .75 | .50 .25 | .00 BIN | 1.0 .75 | .50 .25 | .00 BIN | 1.0 .75 | .50 .25 | .00 BIN | 1.0 75 | .50 .25 | .00 BIN | 1.0 .75 | .50 .25 | .00 BIN |
| PCONT=*** | | | | REQUIRED | NUMBER | OF | PATIENTS | | | | | | | | | |
| 0.05 | *** | 3352 | 3387 | 3519 | 727 | 735 | 746 | 262 | 264 | 265 | 154 | 154 | 155 | 109 | 109 | 109 |
| | *** | 3365 | 3429 | 6576 | 731 | 740 | 1285 | 262 | 265 | 409 | 154 | 155 | 216 | 109 | 109 | 138 |
| 0.1 | *** | 6984 | 7079 | 7730 | 1352 | 1384 | 1439 | 432 | 437 | 445 | 231 | 234 | 236 | 152 | 154 | 155 |
| | *** | 7016 | 7227 | 11423 | 1366 | 1407 | 2033 | 435 | 441 | 584 | 232 | 235 | 289 | 154 | 154 | 176 |
| 0.15 | *** | 10222 | 10394 | 11954 | 1906 | 1974 | 2110 | 581 | 594 | 609 | 299 | 302 | 307 | 190 | 191 | 194 |
| | *** | 10280 | 10684 | 15685 | 1935 | 2029 | 2687 | 587 | 601 | 736 | 301 | 305 | 351 | 191 | 192 | 208 |
| 0.2 | *** | 12824 | 13090 | 15884 | 2362 | 2475 | 2721 | 707 | 727 | 755 | 355 | 361 | 369 | 221 | 224 | 226 |
| | *** | 12914 | 13552 | 19364 | 2410 | 2570 | 3247 | 717 | 740 | 865 | 359 | 365 | 403 | 222 | 225 | 234 |
| 0.25 | *** | 14725 | 15106 | 19367 | 2717 | 2879 | 3256 | 809 | 839 | 879 | 400 | 409 | 420 | 245 | 249 | 252 |
| | *** | 14854 | 15772 | 22459 | 2785 | 3020 | 3714 | 822 | 857 | 970 | 405 | 414 | 444 | 246 | 250 | 255 |
| 0.3 | *** | 15939 | 16459 | 22320 | 2974 | 3186 | 3702 | 886 | 925 | 980 | 435 | 446 | 460 | 262 | 267 | 272 |
| | *** | 16114 | 17357 | 24970 | 3062 | 3374 | 4088 | 905 | 950 | 1052 | 440 | 452 | 475 | 265 | 270 | 269 |
| 0.35 | *** | 16517 | 17204 | 24695 | 3139 | 3402 | 4055 | 941 | 989 | 1056 | 459 | 472 | 489 | 274 | 280 | 285 |
| | *** | 16751 | 18359 | 26897 | 3249 | 3636 | 4368 | 962 | 1019 | 1110 | 465 | 480 | 496 | 276 | 282 | 278 |
| 0.4 | *** | 16541 | 17422 | 26462 | 3225 | 3534 | 4309 | 974 | 1029 | 1107 | 471 | 487 | 506 | 280 | 285 | 292 |
| | *** | 16844 | 18847 | 28240 | 3354 | 3809 | 4555 | 999 | 1064 | 1145 | 479 | 496 | 507 | 282 | 289 | 281 |
| 0.45 | *** | 16099 | 17200 | 27607 | 3240 | 3589 | 4462 | 985 | 1046 | 1134 | 475 | 491 | 512 | 279 | 285 | 292 |
| | *** | 16482 | 18895 | 28999 | 3386 | 3896 | 4649 | 1014 | 1085 | 1157 | 482 | 501 | 507 | 282 | 289 | 278 |
| 0.5 | *** | 15292 | 16630 | 28119 | 3195 | 3572 | 4514 | 977 | 1041 | 1134 | 469 | 485 | 506 | 272 | 279 | 286 |
| | *** | 15769 | 18574 | 29175 | 3354 | 3904 | 4649 | 1007 | 1082 | 1145 | 476 | 495 | 496 | 276 | 282 | 269 |
| 0.55 | *** | 14227 | 15796 | 27996 | 3096 | 3491 | 4464 | 951 | 1016 | 1109 | 452 | 469 | 490 | 261 | 267 | 274 |
| | *** | 14799 | 17945 | 28766 | 3262 | 3835 | 4555 | 981 | 1057 | 1110 | 460 | 479 | 475 | 264 | 270 | 255 |
| 0.6 | *** | 12999 | 14769 | 27237 | 2949 | 3349 | 4312 | 906 | 969 | 1059 | 426 | 442 | 462 | 244 | 249 | 255 |
| | *** | 13659 | 17057 | 27773 | 3119 | 3692 | 4368 | 935 | 1009 | 1052 | 435 | 451 | 444 | 246 | 251 | 234 |
| 0.65 | *** | 11691 | 13599 | 25846 | 2759 | 3149 | 4059 | 844 | 901 | 982 | 391 | 406 | 422 | 220 | 225 | 230 |
| | *** | 12417 | 15947 | 26196 | 2925 | 3477 | 4088 | 871 | 939 | 970 | 399 | 414 | 403 | 222 | 227 | 208 |
| 0.7 | *** | 10357 | 12317 | 23826 | 2525 | 2889 | 3706 | 762 | 814 | 882 | 347 | 359 | 372 | 191 | 195 | 199 |
| | *** | 11116 | 14631 | 24036 | 2681 | 3191 | 3714 | 786 | 845 | 865 | 352 | 365 | 351 | 192 | 196 | 176 |
| 0.75 | *** | 9020 | 10931 | 21181 | 2247 | 2570 | 3254 | 662 | 702 | 756 | 292 | 301 | 311 | 156 | 159 | 161 |
| | *** | 9770 | 13110 | 21291 | 2386 | 2829 | 3247 | 681 | 727 | 736 | 296 | 306 | 289 | 157 | 160 | 138 |
| 0.8 | *** | 7669 | 9422 | 17920 | 1920 | 2182 | 2702 | 541 | 570 | 606 | 227 | 232 | 239 | . | . | . |
| | *** | 8365 | 11356 | 17963 | 2035 | 2386 | 2687 | 555 | 587 | 584 | 230 | 236 | 216 | . | . | . |
| 0.85 | *** | 6260 | 7742 | 14047 | 1529 | 1717 | 2054 | 396 | 412 | 432 | . | . | . | . | . | . |
| | *** | 6855 | 9312 | 14050 | 1612 | 1855 | 2033 | 404 | 422 | 409 | . | . | . | . | . | . |
| 0.9 | *** | 4694 | 5775 | 9570 | 1049 | 1151 | 1307 | . | . | . | . | . | . | . | . | . |
| | *** | 5136 | 6850 | 9554 | 1095 | 1220 | 1285 | . | . | . | . | . | . | . | . | . |
| 0.95 | *** | 2721 | 3234 | 4496 | . | . | . | . | . | . | . | . | . | . | . | . |
| | *** | 2939 | 3676 | 4474 | . | . | . | . | . | . | . | . | . | . | . | . |

## TABLE 1: ALPHA= 0.005 POWER= 0.8    EXPECTED ACCRUAL THRU MINIMUM FOLLOW-UP= 2250

|  |  | DEL=.02 | | | DEL=.05 | | | DEL=.10 | | | DEL=.15 | | | DEL=.20 | | |
|---|---|---|---|---|---|---|---|---|---|---|---|---|---|---|---|---|
| FACT= | | 1.0 .75 | .50 .25 | .00 BIN | 1.0 .75 | .50 .25 | .00 BIN | 1.0 .75 | .50 .25 | .00 BIN | 1.0 75 | .50 .25 | .00 BIN | 1.0 .75 | .50 .25 | .00 BIN |
| PCONT=*** | | REQUIRED NUMBER OF PATIENTS | | | | | | | | | | | | | | |
| 0.05 | *** | 3358 | 3394 | 3518 | 728 | 735 | 747 | 263 | 264 | 266 | 153 | 154 | 154 | 108 | 108 | 109 |
|  | *** | 3371 | 3435 | 6576 | 732 | 741 | 1285 | 263 | 264 | 409 | 154 | 154 | 216 | 108 | 108 | 138 |
| 0.1 | *** | 6996 | 7101 | 7730 | 1358 | 1389 | 1438 | 433 | 438 | 444 | 232 | 233 | 236 | 153 | 153 | 154 |
|  | *** | 7032 | 7255 | 11423 | 1372 | 1410 | 2033 | 435 | 441 | 584 | 233 | 235 | 289 | 153 | 154 | 176 |
| 0.15 | *** | 10244 | 10434 | 11954 | 1918 | 1984 | 2109 | 583 | 595 | 609 | 299 | 303 | 306 | 191 | 192 | 194 |
|  | *** | 10309 | 10743 | 15685 | 1947 | 2036 | 2687 | 589 | 601 | 736 | 300 | 305 | 351 | 191 | 192 | 208 |
| 0.2 | *** | 12857 | 13154 | 15883 | 2382 | 2493 | 2721 | 711 | 730 | 755 | 357 | 362 | 368 | 221 | 223 | 226 |
|  | *** | 12958 | 13650 | 19364 | 2429 | 2583 | 3247 | 719 | 742 | 865 | 359 | 365 | 403 | 222 | 224 | 234 |
| 0.25 | *** | 14774 | 15197 | 19366 | 2744 | 2905 | 3256 | 815 | 842 | 879 | 402 | 410 | 419 | 246 | 249 | 252 |
|  | *** | 14917 | 15913 | 22459 | 2812 | 3040 | 3714 | 828 | 859 | 970 | 406 | 415 | 444 | 247 | 250 | 255 |
| 0.3 | *** | 16004 | 16584 | 22319 | 3009 | 3222 | 3702 | 894 | 930 | 980 | 437 | 447 | 460 | 263 | 267 | 271 |
|  | *** | 16201 | 17546 | 24970 | 3098 | 3402 | 4088 | 911 | 953 | 1052 | 441 | 452 | 475 | 266 | 269 | 269 |
| 0.35 | *** | 16604 | 17367 | 24695 | 3183 | 3445 | 4055 | 950 | 994 | 1056 | 461 | 474 | 488 | 275 | 280 | 285 |
|  | *** | 16866 | 18597 | 26897 | 3293 | 3670 | 4368 | 972 | 1022 | 1110 | 466 | 480 | 496 | 277 | 282 | 278 |
| 0.4 | *** | 16654 | 17625 | 26462 | 3278 | 3584 | 4308 | 984 | 1036 | 1108 | 475 | 489 | 506 | 281 | 286 | 292 |
|  | *** | 16992 | 19135 | 28240 | 3407 | 3849 | 4555 | 1008 | 1068 | 1145 | 482 | 496 | 507 | 284 | 289 | 281 |
| 0.45 | *** | 16244 | 17448 | 27607 | 3300 | 3644 | 4462 | 997 | 1053 | 1133 | 478 | 493 | 511 | 281 | 286 | 292 |
|  | *** | 16669 | 19229 | 28999 | 3445 | 3942 | 4649 | 1023 | 1090 | 1157 | 485 | 502 | 507 | 284 | 289 | 278 |
| 0.5 | *** | 15474 | 16922 | 28119 | 3259 | 3633 | 4514 | 989 | 1050 | 1135 | 472 | 488 | 506 | 274 | 280 | 286 |
|  | *** | 15996 | 18947 | 29175 | 3417 | 3953 | 4649 | 1018 | 1088 | 1145 | 479 | 496 | 496 | 277 | 282 | 269 |
| 0.55 | *** | 14446 | 16126 | 27995 | 3164 | 3554 | 4463 | 964 | 1023 | 1109 | 455 | 471 | 489 | 263 | 268 | 274 |
|  | *** | 15065 | 18348 | 28766 | 3329 | 3885 | 4555 | 991 | 1063 | 1110 | 464 | 480 | 475 | 266 | 271 | 255 |
| 0.6 | *** | 13255 | 15127 | 27237 | 3019 | 3413 | 4311 | 919 | 977 | 1059 | 430 | 444 | 462 | 244 | 250 | 254 |
|  | *** | 13960 | 17479 | 27773 | 3186 | 3742 | 4368 | 946 | 1014 | 1052 | 437 | 452 | 444 | 247 | 252 | 234 |
| 0.65 | *** | 11977 | 13972 | 25845 | 2826 | 3209 | 4060 | 854 | 910 | 983 | 395 | 407 | 423 | 221 | 224 | 230 |
|  | *** | 12742 | 16373 | 26196 | 2991 | 3525 | 4088 | 880 | 943 | 970 | 401 | 415 | 403 | 223 | 227 | 208 |
| 0.7 | *** | 10658 | 12689 | 23826 | 2590 | 2946 | 3705 | 773 | 820 | 882 | 350 | 359 | 372 | 191 | 195 | 198 |
|  | *** | 11449 | 15044 | 24036 | 2743 | 3233 | 3714 | 794 | 848 | 865 | 354 | 365 | 351 | 192 | 196 | 176 |
| 0.75 | *** | 9319 | 11288 | 21182 | 2305 | 2618 | 3252 | 671 | 708 | 756 | 294 | 302 | 311 | 156 | 159 | 162 |
|  | *** | 10095 | 13491 | 21291 | 2441 | 2864 | 3247 | 689 | 731 | 736 | 298 | 306 | 289 | 157 | 160 | 138 |
| 0.8 | *** | 7948 | 9744 | 17920 | 1967 | 2221 | 2701 | 547 | 573 | 606 | 229 | 233 | 239 | . | . | . |
|  | *** | 8664 | 11688 | 17963 | 2080 | 2414 | 2687 | 559 | 589 | 584 | 230 | 236 | 216 | . | . | . |
| 0.85 | *** | 6499 | 8007 | 14047 | 1563 | 1743 | 2053 | 399 | 415 | 433 | . | . | . | . | . | . |
|  | *** | 7108 | 9575 | 14050 | 1644 | 1873 | 2033 | 406 | 423 | 409 | . | . | . | . | . | . |
| 0.9 | *** | 4872 | 5962 | 9570 | 1068 | 1166 | 1307 | . | . | . | . | . | . | . | . | . |
|  | *** | 5320 | 7022 | 9554 | 1112 | 1229 | 1285 | . | . | . | . | . | . | . | . | . |
| 0.95 | *** | 2811 | 3314 | 4497 | . | . | . | . | . | . | . | . | . | . | . | . |
|  | *** | 3026 | 3740 | 4474 | . | . | . | . | . | . | . | . | . | . | . | . |

TABLE 1: ALPHA= 0.005 POWER= 0.8    EXPECTED ACCRUAL THRU MINIMUM FOLLOW-UP= 2500

| | | DEL=.02 | | | DEL=.05 | | | DEL=.10 | | | DEL=.15 | | | DEL=.20 | | |
|---|---|---|---|---|---|---|---|---|---|---|---|---|---|---|---|---|---|
| FACT= | | 1.0 .75 | .50 .25 | .00 BIN | 1.0 .75 | .50 .25 | .00 BIN | 1.0 .75 | .50 .25 | .00 BIN | 1.0 75 | .50 .25 | .00 BIN | 1.0 .75 | .50 .25 | .00 BIN |
| PCONT=*** | | | | | REQUIRED NUMBER OF PATIENTS | | | | | | | | | | | |
| 0.05 | *** | 3362 | 3399 | 3518 | 729 | 737 | 746 | 262 | 264 | 265 | 154 | 154 | 154 | 108 | 109 | 109 |
| | *** | 3376 | 3440 | 6576 | 733 | 742 | 1285 | 264 | 264 | 409 | 154 | 154 | 216 | 109 | 109 | 138 |
| 0.1 | *** | 7009 | 7121 | 7729 | 1364 | 1392 | 1439 | 434 | 439 | 445 | 233 | 234 | 236 | 152 | 154 | 154 |
| | *** | 7048 | 7281 | 11423 | 1376 | 1412 | 2033 | 436 | 442 | 584 | 233 | 234 | 289 | 152 | 154 | 176 |
| 0.15 | *** | 10265 | 10473 | 11954 | 1929 | 1993 | 2109 | 586 | 596 | 609 | 299 | 302 | 308 | 190 | 192 | 193 |
| | *** | 10337 | 10798 | 15685 | 1958 | 2042 | 2687 | 590 | 602 | 736 | 301 | 306 | 351 | 192 | 193 | 208 |
| 0.2 | *** | 12892 | 13215 | 15884 | 2399 | 2509 | 2721 | 715 | 733 | 754 | 358 | 362 | 368 | 221 | 223 | 226 |
| | *** | 13002 | 13740 | 19364 | 2446 | 2595 | 3247 | 723 | 743 | 865 | 361 | 365 | 403 | 223 | 224 | 234 |
| 0.25 | *** | 14821 | 15287 | 19367 | 2770 | 2927 | 3256 | 820 | 845 | 879 | 404 | 411 | 420 | 246 | 249 | 252 |
| | *** | 14981 | 16043 | 22459 | 2837 | 3056 | 3714 | 833 | 861 | 970 | 408 | 415 | 444 | 248 | 251 | 255 |
| 0.3 | *** | 16070 | 16704 | 22320 | 3042 | 3251 | 3702 | 901 | 934 | 979 | 439 | 448 | 459 | 264 | 268 | 271 |
| | *** | 16287 | 17720 | 24970 | 3131 | 3424 | 4088 | 917 | 956 | 1052 | 443 | 454 | 475 | 265 | 270 | 269 |
| 0.35 | *** | 16693 | 17524 | 24695 | 3224 | 3483 | 4054 | 958 | 999 | 1056 | 464 | 474 | 489 | 276 | 281 | 286 |
| | *** | 16981 | 18818 | 26897 | 3334 | 3698 | 4368 | 977 | 1026 | 1110 | 468 | 481 | 496 | 277 | 283 | 278 |
| 0.4 | *** | 16768 | 17823 | 26462 | 3324 | 3627 | 4309 | 993 | 1042 | 1108 | 477 | 490 | 506 | 283 | 287 | 292 |
| | *** | 17137 | 19401 | 28240 | 3454 | 3883 | 4555 | 1015 | 1071 | 1145 | 484 | 498 | 507 | 284 | 289 | 281 |
| 0.45 | *** | 16387 | 17686 | 27608 | 3352 | 3693 | 4462 | 1008 | 1061 | 1134 | 481 | 495 | 512 | 281 | 287 | 292 |
| | *** | 16851 | 19537 | 28999 | 3498 | 3979 | 4649 | 1033 | 1093 | 1157 | 487 | 502 | 507 | 284 | 289 | 278 |
| 0.5 | *** | 15651 | 17198 | 28118 | 3317 | 3686 | 4514 | 1001 | 1058 | 1134 | 474 | 489 | 506 | 274 | 281 | 286 |
| | *** | 16215 | 19290 | 29175 | 3474 | 3993 | 4649 | 1026 | 1092 | 1145 | 483 | 498 | 496 | 277 | 284 | 269 |
| 0.55 | *** | 14659 | 16434 | 27996 | 3224 | 3609 | 4464 | 974 | 1031 | 1109 | 459 | 473 | 490 | 264 | 268 | 273 |
| | *** | 15320 | 18717 | 28766 | 3389 | 3927 | 4555 | 1001 | 1067 | 1110 | 465 | 481 | 475 | 265 | 271 | 255 |
| 0.6 | *** | 13501 | 15459 | 27237 | 3081 | 3467 | 4312 | 929 | 984 | 1059 | 433 | 446 | 462 | 245 | 249 | 254 |
| | *** | 14245 | 17862 | 27773 | 3246 | 3784 | 4368 | 954 | 1018 | 1052 | 439 | 454 | 444 | 248 | 252 | 234 |
| 0.65 | *** | 12245 | 14317 | 25846 | 2887 | 3262 | 4059 | 865 | 915 | 983 | 396 | 409 | 423 | 221 | 226 | 229 |
| | *** | 13046 | 16758 | 26196 | 3049 | 3565 | 4088 | 889 | 946 | 970 | 402 | 415 | 403 | 223 | 227 | 208 |
| 0.7 | *** | 10939 | 13033 | 23826 | 2646 | 2995 | 3706 | 781 | 824 | 883 | 351 | 361 | 371 | 192 | 195 | 198 |
| | *** | 11759 | 15414 | 24036 | 2798 | 3270 | 3714 | 801 | 851 | 865 | 356 | 367 | 351 | 193 | 196 | 176 |
| 0.75 | *** | 9596 | 11612 | 21181 | 2356 | 2661 | 3252 | 677 | 712 | 756 | 296 | 302 | 311 | 156 | 159 | 161 |
| | *** | 10395 | 13833 | 21291 | 2489 | 2895 | 3247 | 693 | 733 | 736 | 299 | 308 | 289 | 158 | 159 | 138 |
| 0.8 | *** | 8204 | 10034 | 17920 | 2009 | 2256 | 2701 | 551 | 576 | 606 | 229 | 234 | 239 | . | . | . |
| | *** | 8937 | 11984 | 17963 | 2118 | 2437 | 2687 | 564 | 590 | 584 | 233 | 237 | 216 | . | . | . |
| 0.85 | *** | 6718 | 8245 | 14046 | 1593 | 1767 | 2052 | 402 | 417 | 433 | . | . | . | . | . | . |
| | *** | 7337 | 9808 | 14050 | 1671 | 1889 | 2033 | 409 | 424 | 409 | . | . | . | . | . | . |
| 0.9 | *** | 5036 | 6127 | 9570 | 1086 | 1176 | 1308 | . | . | . | . | . | . | . | . | . |
| | *** | 5486 | 7173 | 9554 | 1127 | 1236 | 1285 | . | . | . | . | . | . | . | . | . |
| 0.95 | *** | 2890 | 3386 | 4496 | . | . | . | . | . | . | . | . | . | . | . | . |
| | *** | 3102 | 3795 | 4474 | . | . | . | . | . | . | . | . | . | . | . | . |

## TABLE 1: ALPHA= 0.005 POWER= 0.8    EXPECTED ACCRUAL THRU MINIMUM FOLLOW-UP= 2750

| | | DEL=.02 | | | DEL=.05 | | | DEL=.10 | | | DEL=.15 | | | DEL=.20 | | |
|---|---|---|---|---|---|---|---|---|---|---|---|---|---|---|---|---|
| FACT= | | 1.0 .75 | .50 .25 | .00 BIN | 1.0 .75 | .50 .25 | .00 BIN | 1.0 .75 | .50 .25 | .00 BIN | 1.0 75 | .50 .25 | .00 BIN | 1.0 .75 | .50 .25 | .00 BIN |
| PCONT=*** | | | | REQUIRED | NUMBER | OF | PATIENTS | | | | | | | | | |
| 0.05 | *** | 3367 | 3406 | 3518 | 731 | 737 | 745 | 263 | 264 | 266 | 154 | 154 | 154 | 108 | 108 | 109 |
| | *** | 3382 | 3446 | 6576 | 734 | 742 | 1285 | 263 | 264 | 409 | 154 | 154 | 216 | 108 | 108 | 138 |
| 0.1 | *** | 7021 | 7141 | 7729 | 1367 | 1395 | 1438 | 434 | 439 | 445 | 233 | 233 | 235 | 153 | 154 | 154 |
| | *** | 7063 | 7304 | 11423 | 1380 | 1414 | 2033 | 436 | 441 | 584 | 233 | 235 | 289 | 154 | 154 | 176 |
| 0.15 | *** | 10286 | 10511 | 11954 | 1938 | 2002 | 2109 | 587 | 597 | 608 | 300 | 304 | 307 | 190 | 192 | 194 |
| | *** | 10365 | 10848 | 15685 | 1965 | 2047 | 2687 | 593 | 603 | 736 | 302 | 305 | 351 | 192 | 192 | 208 |
| 0.2 | *** | 12924 | 13277 | 15884 | 2414 | 2522 | 2722 | 718 | 734 | 754 | 359 | 362 | 369 | 221 | 223 | 226 |
| | *** | 13047 | 13824 | 19364 | 2460 | 2604 | 3247 | 725 | 744 | 865 | 360 | 366 | 403 | 223 | 225 | 234 |
| 0.25 | *** | 14869 | 15374 | 19366 | 2793 | 2947 | 3257 | 824 | 848 | 879 | 405 | 412 | 419 | 247 | 249 | 252 |
| | *** | 15044 | 16166 | 22459 | 2859 | 3071 | 3714 | 835 | 862 | 970 | 408 | 415 | 444 | 247 | 250 | 255 |
| 0.3 | *** | 16135 | 16822 | 22319 | 3071 | 3277 | 3704 | 905 | 938 | 979 | 441 | 450 | 460 | 264 | 267 | 271 |
| | *** | 16374 | 17883 | 24970 | 3160 | 3444 | 4088 | 920 | 957 | 1052 | 445 | 453 | 475 | 266 | 269 | 269 |
| 0.35 | *** | 16780 | 17677 | 24694 | 3260 | 3516 | 4054 | 965 | 1005 | 1057 | 465 | 476 | 487 | 276 | 281 | 285 |
| | *** | 17093 | 19022 | 26897 | 3370 | 3724 | 4368 | 982 | 1027 | 1110 | 470 | 483 | 496 | 278 | 283 | 278 |
| 0.4 | *** | 16881 | 18012 | 26463 | 3368 | 3667 | 4309 | 1002 | 1046 | 1108 | 479 | 491 | 505 | 283 | 287 | 291 |
| | *** | 17282 | 19647 | 28240 | 3495 | 3911 | 4555 | 1022 | 1075 | 1145 | 486 | 498 | 507 | 285 | 290 | 281 |
| 0.45 | *** | 16529 | 17912 | 27606 | 3401 | 3738 | 4461 | 1015 | 1065 | 1134 | 484 | 496 | 511 | 283 | 287 | 291 |
| | *** | 17029 | 19820 | 28999 | 3545 | 4013 | 4649 | 1039 | 1098 | 1157 | 489 | 503 | 507 | 285 | 290 | 278 |
| 0.5 | *** | 15825 | 17458 | 28118 | 3370 | 3732 | 4513 | 1010 | 1064 | 1134 | 477 | 491 | 507 | 276 | 281 | 287 |
| | *** | 16427 | 19603 | 29175 | 3526 | 4028 | 4649 | 1034 | 1096 | 1145 | 484 | 498 | 496 | 278 | 283 | 269 |
| 0.55 | *** | 14866 | 16725 | 27996 | 3281 | 3659 | 4463 | 984 | 1037 | 1108 | 460 | 474 | 489 | 264 | 269 | 273 |
| | *** | 15564 | 19053 | 28766 | 3442 | 3965 | 4555 | 1009 | 1070 | 1110 | 467 | 483 | 475 | 266 | 271 | 255 |
| 0.6 | *** | 13735 | 15769 | 27237 | 3136 | 3516 | 4312 | 938 | 989 | 1058 | 434 | 448 | 462 | 245 | 250 | 256 |
| | *** | 14514 | 18211 | 27773 | 3301 | 3820 | 4368 | 962 | 1022 | 1052 | 441 | 455 | 444 | 249 | 252 | 234 |
| 0.65 | *** | 12500 | 14636 | 25846 | 2942 | 3310 | 4059 | 872 | 920 | 982 | 398 | 410 | 422 | 223 | 226 | 230 |
| | *** | 13330 | 17106 | 26196 | 3102 | 3600 | 4088 | 895 | 950 | 970 | 405 | 415 | 403 | 225 | 228 | 208 |
| 0.7 | *** | 11202 | 13349 | 23825 | 2698 | 3037 | 3705 | 789 | 830 | 881 | 353 | 362 | 373 | 192 | 195 | 199 |
| | *** | 12048 | 15750 | 24036 | 2845 | 3301 | 3714 | 807 | 854 | 865 | 357 | 367 | 351 | 194 | 197 | 176 |
| 0.75 | *** | 9855 | 11910 | 21181 | 2401 | 2698 | 3253 | 683 | 716 | 755 | 297 | 304 | 311 | 157 | 159 | 161 |
| | *** | 10673 | 14140 | 21291 | 2531 | 2921 | 3247 | 699 | 735 | 736 | 300 | 307 | 289 | 157 | 159 | 138 |
| 0.8 | *** | 8442 | 10300 | 17919 | 2047 | 2284 | 2701 | 556 | 579 | 606 | 230 | 235 | 239 | . | . | . |
| | *** | 9190 | 12249 | 17963 | 2151 | 2457 | 2687 | 566 | 593 | 584 | 232 | 236 | 216 | . | . | . |
| 0.85 | *** | 6921 | 8462 | 14047 | 1620 | 1787 | 2054 | 405 | 417 | 432 | . | . | . | . | . | . |
| | *** | 7548 | 10015 | 14050 | 1696 | 1900 | 2033 | 410 | 424 | 409 | . | . | . | . | . | . |
| 0.9 | *** | 5183 | 6278 | 9569 | 1099 | 1185 | 1308 | . | . | . | . | . | . | . | . | . |
| | *** | 5637 | 7306 | 9554 | 1140 | 1240 | 1285 | . | . | . | . | . | . | . | . | . |
| 0.95 | *** | 2961 | 3449 | 4495 | . | . | . | . | . | . | . | . | . | . | . | . |
| | *** | 3171 | 3842 | 4474 | . | . | . | . | . | . | . | . | . | . | . | . |

## TABLE 1: ALPHA= 0.005 POWER= 0.8    EXPECTED ACCRUAL THRU MINIMUM FOLLOW-UP= 3000

| | DEL=.01 | | | DEL=.02 | | | DEL=.05 | | | DEL=.10 | | | DEL=.15 | | |
|---|---|---|---|---|---|---|---|---|---|---|---|---|---|---|---|
| FACT= | 1.0 .75 | .50 .25 | .00 BIN | 1.0 .75 | .50 .25 | .00 BIN | 1.0 .75 | .50 .25 | .00 BIN | 1.0 75 | .50 .25 | .00 BIN | 1.0 .75 | .50 .25 | .00 BIN |
| PCONT=*** | | | | | | REQUIRED NUMBER OF PATIENTS | | | | | | | | | |
| 0.01 *** | 1783 | 1790 | 1802 | 655 | 658 | 658 | 215 | 215 | 215 | 110 | 110 | 110 | 77 | 77 | 77 |
| *** | 1787 | 1795 | 6891 | 658 | 658 | 2278 | 215 | 215 | 620 | 110 | 110 | 252 | 77 | 77 | 150 |
| 0.02 *** | 3940 | 3958 | 4018 | 1265 | 1273 | 1285 | 343 | 343 | 347 | 152 | 152 | 152 | 100 | 100 | 100 |
| *** | 3947 | 3977 | 11376 | 1270 | 1277 | 3387 | 343 | 347 | 792 | 152 | 152 | 293 | 100 | 100 | 167 |
| 0.05 *** | 11923 | 11980 | 12553 | 3370 | 3410 | 3520 | 733 | 737 | 745 | 260 | 265 | 265 | 152 | 152 | 155 |
| *** | 11942 | 12080 | 24269 | 3388 | 3448 | 6576 | 733 | 740 | 1285 | 265 | 265 | 409 | 152 | 155 | 216 |
| 0.1 *** | 26300 | 26440 | 29222 | 7033 | 7160 | 7730 | 1370 | 1397 | 1438 | 433 | 440 | 445 | 230 | 235 | 235 |
| *** | 26345 | 26713 | 43890 | 7078 | 7325 | 11423 | 1382 | 1415 | 2033 | 437 | 440 | 584 | 235 | 235 | 289 |
| 0.15 *** | 39265 | 39515 | 46165 | 10307 | 10547 | 11953 | 1948 | 2008 | 2110 | 587 | 598 | 610 | 302 | 302 | 305 |
| *** | 39347 | 40010 | 61175 | 10393 | 10892 | 15685 | 1975 | 2050 | 2687 | 595 | 602 | 736 | 302 | 305 | 351 |
| 0.2 *** | 49705 | 50090 | 62023 | 12958 | 13337 | 15883 | 2428 | 2533 | 2720 | 718 | 737 | 755 | 358 | 362 | 370 |
| *** | 49832 | 50863 | 76124 | 13090 | 13903 | 19364 | 2473 | 2612 | 3247 | 725 | 745 | 865 | 362 | 365 | 403 |
| 0.25 *** | 57295 | 57857 | 76145 | 14915 | 15460 | 19367 | 2810 | 2965 | 3257 | 827 | 850 | 880 | 407 | 410 | 418 |
| *** | 57482 | 58970 | 88737 | 15107 | 16280 | 22459 | 2878 | 3085 | 3714 | 838 | 865 | 970 | 407 | 415 | 444 |
| 0.3 *** | 62060 | 62830 | 88175 | 16202 | 16937 | 22318 | 3100 | 3302 | 3703 | 910 | 940 | 980 | 440 | 448 | 460 |
| *** | 62315 | 64367 | 99015 | 16457 | 18035 | 24970 | 3185 | 3460 | 4088 | 925 | 958 | 1052 | 445 | 455 | 475 |
| 0.35 *** | 64187 | 65215 | 97907 | 16865 | 17822 | 24695 | 3295 | 3545 | 4055 | 970 | 1007 | 1055 | 467 | 478 | 490 |
| *** | 64532 | 67258 | 106956 | 17203 | 19213 | 26897 | 3403 | 3745 | 4368 | 988 | 1030 | 1110 | 470 | 482 | 496 |
| 0.4 *** | 63962 | 65305 | 105223 | 16990 | 18193 | 26462 | 3407 | 3700 | 4307 | 1007 | 1052 | 1108 | 482 | 493 | 505 |
| *** | 64408 | 67960 | 112562 | 17420 | 19873 | 28240 | 3535 | 3935 | 4555 | 1030 | 1078 | 1145 | 485 | 497 | 507 |
| 0.45 *** | 61720 | 63452 | 110050 | 16667 | 18125 | 27605 | 3445 | 3775 | 4460 | 1022 | 1070 | 1135 | 485 | 497 | 512 |
| *** | 62297 | 66830 | 115833 | 17200 | 20083 | 28999 | 3587 | 4040 | 4649 | 1045 | 1100 | 1157 | 490 | 505 | 507 |
| 0.5 *** | 57842 | 60055 | 112352 | 15995 | 17705 | 28120 | 3418 | 3775 | 4513 | 1018 | 1067 | 1135 | 478 | 493 | 505 |
| *** | 58580 | 64262 | 116767 | 16630 | 19895 | 29175 | 3572 | 4060 | 4649 | 1040 | 1097 | 1145 | 485 | 497 | 496 |
| 0.55 *** | 52727 | 55528 | 112112 | 15065 | 16997 | 27995 | 3328 | 3700 | 4465 | 992 | 1040 | 1108 | 463 | 475 | 490 |
| *** | 53668 | 60632 | 115365 | 15797 | 19363 | 28766 | 3490 | 3995 | 4555 | 1015 | 1075 | 1110 | 467 | 482 | 475 |
| 0.6 *** | 46805 | 50312 | 109330 | 13960 | 16060 | 27238 | 3185 | 3560 | 4310 | 947 | 995 | 1060 | 437 | 448 | 463 |
| *** | 47998 | 56270 | 111628 | 14770 | 18530 | 27773 | 3347 | 3853 | 4368 | 970 | 1025 | 1052 | 440 | 455 | 444 |
| 0.65 *** | 40525 | 44788 | 104015 | 12740 | 14935 | 25847 | 2990 | 3350 | 4060 | 880 | 925 | 980 | 400 | 410 | 422 |
| *** | 42013 | 51437 | 105555 | 13600 | 17425 | 26196 | 3148 | 3628 | 4088 | 902 | 950 | 970 | 407 | 415 | 403 |
| 0.7 *** | 34322 | 39253 | 96185 | 11450 | 13640 | 23825 | 2743 | 3073 | 3707 | 793 | 835 | 883 | 355 | 362 | 373 |
| *** | 36107 | 46300 | 97146 | 12317 | 16055 | 24036 | 2890 | 3328 | 3714 | 812 | 857 | 865 | 358 | 365 | 351 |
| 0.75 *** | 28547 | 33857 | 85858 | 10097 | 12185 | 21182 | 2440 | 2728 | 3253 | 688 | 718 | 755 | 298 | 305 | 310 |
| *** | 30530 | 40907 | 86402 | 10930 | 14420 | 21291 | 2570 | 2942 | 3247 | 703 | 737 | 736 | 302 | 305 | 289 |
| 0.8 *** | 23323 | 28600 | 73055 | 8665 | 10543 | 17920 | 2080 | 2308 | 2702 | 560 | 580 | 605 | 230 | 235 | 238 |
| *** | 25337 | 35222 | 73321 | 9422 | 12490 | 17963 | 2180 | 2473 | 2687 | 568 | 595 | 584 | 230 | 238 | 216 |
| 0.85 *** | 18542 | 23315 | 57808 | 7108 | 8660 | 14045 | 1645 | 1802 | 2053 | 407 | 418 | 433 | . | . | . |
| *** | 20395 | 29060 | 57905 | 7742 | 10198 | 14050 | 1715 | 1910 | 2033 | 410 | 425 | 409 | . | . | . |
| 0.9 *** | 13870 | 17668 | 40142 | 5320 | 6415 | 9568 | 1112 | 1195 | 1307 | . | . | . | . | . | . |
| *** | 15365 | 22033 | 40153 | 5773 | 7423 | 9554 | 1150 | 1247 | 1285 | . | . | . | . | . | . |
| 0.95 *** | 8590 | 10817 | 20083 | 3025 | 3505 | 4495 | . | . | . | . | . | . | . | . | . |
| *** | 9490 | 13157 | 20065 | 3235 | 3883 | 4474 | . | . | . | . | . | . | . | . | . |
| 0.98 *** | 4123 | 4922 | 6913 | . | . | . | . | . | . | . | . | . | . | . | . |
| *** | 4460 | 5615 | 6891 | . | . | . | . | . | . | . | . | . | . | . | . |

# TABLE 1: ALPHA= 0.005 POWER= 0.8   EXPECTED ACCRUAL THRU MINIMUM FOLLOW-UP= 3250

| | | DEL=.01 | | | DEL=.02 | | | DEL=.05 | | | DEL=.10 | | | DEL=.15 | |
|---|---|---|---|---|---|---|---|---|---|---|---|---|---|---|---|---|
| FACT= | 1.0 .75 | .50 .25 | .00 BIN | 1.0 .75 | .50 .25 | .00 BIN | 1.0 .75 | .50 .25 | .00 BIN | 1.0 75 | .50 .25 | .00 BIN | 1.0 .75 | .50 .25 | .00 BIN |
| PCONT=*** | | | | | | REQUIRED NUMBER OF PATIENTS | | | | | | | | | |
| 0.01 *** | 1785 | 1790 | 1801 | 656 | 656 | 661 | 217 | 217 | 217 | 108 | 108 | 108 | 76 | 79 | 79 |
| *** | 1785 | 1793 | 6891 | 656 | 661 | 2278 | 217 | 217 | 620 | 108 | 108 | 252 | 76 | 79 | 150 |
| 0.02 *** | 3943 | 3959 | 4019 | 1265 | 1273 | 1286 | 344 | 344 | 347 | 152 | 152 | 152 | 100 | 100 | 100 |
| *** | 3951 | 3979 | 11376 | 1270 | 1278 | 3387 | 344 | 344 | 792 | 152 | 152 | 293 | 100 | 100 | 167 |
| 0.05 *** | 11930 | 11990 | 12556 | 3374 | 3415 | 3516 | 734 | 737 | 745 | 263 | 263 | 266 | 152 | 152 | 152 |
| *** | 11949 | 12096 | 24269 | 3391 | 3456 | 6576 | 734 | 742 | 1285 | 263 | 266 | 409 | 152 | 152 | 216 |
| 0.1 *** | 26311 | 26461 | 29223 | 7042 | 7177 | 7729 | 1376 | 1400 | 1441 | 436 | 441 | 444 | 233 | 233 | 233 |
| *** | 26363 | 26758 | 43890 | 7091 | 7342 | 11423 | 1387 | 1419 | 2033 | 436 | 441 | 584 | 233 | 233 | 289 |
| 0.15 *** | 39287 | 39555 | 46164 | 10329 | 10584 | 11954 | 1956 | 2012 | 2110 | 591 | 599 | 607 | 303 | 303 | 306 |
| *** | 39376 | 40091 | 61175 | 10419 | 10934 | 15685 | 1980 | 2053 | 2687 | 596 | 604 | 736 | 303 | 306 | 351 |
| 0.2 *** | 49736 | 50158 | 62024 | 12989 | 13393 | 15882 | 2443 | 2546 | 2719 | 721 | 737 | 753 | 360 | 363 | 368 |
| *** | 49877 | 50995 | 76124 | 13133 | 13972 | 19364 | 2489 | 2619 | 3247 | 729 | 745 | 865 | 360 | 368 | 403 |
| 0.25 *** | 57341 | 57950 | 76145 | 14964 | 15541 | 19367 | 2830 | 2979 | 3256 | 831 | 851 | 880 | 409 | 412 | 420 |
| *** | 57544 | 59156 | 88737 | 15167 | 16386 | 22459 | 2895 | 3093 | 3714 | 839 | 864 | 970 | 409 | 417 | 444 |
| 0.3 *** | 62126 | 62958 | 88175 | 16264 | 17049 | 22322 | 3123 | 3321 | 3702 | 916 | 945 | 981 | 441 | 449 | 458 |
| *** | 62403 | 64621 | 99015 | 16540 | 18178 | 24970 | 3212 | 3475 | 4088 | 929 | 961 | 1052 | 444 | 452 | 475 |
| 0.35 *** | 64274 | 65387 | 97909 | 16951 | 17967 | 24694 | 3326 | 3569 | 4052 | 978 | 1010 | 1054 | 469 | 477 | 490 |
| *** | 64645 | 67594 | 106956 | 17312 | 19392 | 26897 | 3431 | 3764 | 4368 | 994 | 1029 | 1110 | 474 | 482 | 496 |
| 0.4 *** | 64071 | 65531 | 105221 | 17101 | 18368 | 26461 | 3442 | 3732 | 4309 | 1013 | 1054 | 1108 | 482 | 493 | 506 |
| *** | 64559 | 68391 | 112562 | 17561 | 20088 | 28240 | 3569 | 3959 | 4555 | 1034 | 1078 | 1145 | 490 | 498 | 507 |
| 0.45 *** | 61866 | 63738 | 110051 | 16805 | 18333 | 27606 | 3483 | 3808 | 4463 | 1029 | 1075 | 1132 | 485 | 498 | 509 |
| *** | 62492 | 67370 | 115833 | 17366 | 20326 | 28999 | 3626 | 4065 | 4649 | 1051 | 1102 | 1157 | 493 | 506 | 507 |
| 0.5 *** | 58026 | 60420 | 112350 | 16158 | 17937 | 28118 | 3459 | 3813 | 4512 | 1026 | 1070 | 1135 | 482 | 493 | 506 |
| *** | 58828 | 64913 | 116767 | 16824 | 20164 | 29175 | 3613 | 4084 | 4649 | 1046 | 1099 | 1145 | 485 | 498 | 496 |
| 0.55 *** | 52961 | 55987 | 112111 | 15256 | 17252 | 27996 | 3374 | 3740 | 4463 | 997 | 1046 | 1108 | 466 | 477 | 490 |
| *** | 53980 | 61390 | 115365 | 16017 | 19649 | 28766 | 3532 | 4024 | 4555 | 1021 | 1075 | 1110 | 469 | 482 | 475 |
| 0.6 *** | 47106 | 50865 | 109333 | 14176 | 16329 | 27238 | 3231 | 3597 | 4312 | 953 | 997 | 1059 | 436 | 449 | 461 |
| *** | 48390 | 57121 | 111628 | 15009 | 18828 | 27773 | 3391 | 3878 | 4368 | 972 | 1026 | 1052 | 444 | 452 | 444 |
| 0.65 *** | 40904 | 45432 | 104019 | 12970 | 15213 | 25843 | 3036 | 3386 | 4060 | 888 | 929 | 981 | 401 | 412 | 420 |
| *** | 42496 | 52352 | 105555 | 13851 | 17718 | 26196 | 3191 | 3654 | 4088 | 907 | 953 | 970 | 409 | 417 | 403 |
| 0.7 *** | 34781 | 39961 | 96186 | 11686 | 13913 | 23825 | 2784 | 3109 | 3708 | 799 | 834 | 883 | 355 | 363 | 371 |
| *** | 36666 | 47236 | 97146 | 12567 | 16337 | 24036 | 2928 | 3350 | 3714 | 818 | 859 | 865 | 360 | 368 | 351 |
| 0.75 *** | 29066 | 34586 | 85859 | 10321 | 12442 | 21179 | 2476 | 2757 | 3253 | 693 | 721 | 758 | 298 | 303 | 311 |
| *** | 31138 | 41822 | 86402 | 11169 | 14676 | 21291 | 2603 | 2963 | 3247 | 704 | 737 | 736 | 303 | 306 | 289 |
| 0.8 *** | 23858 | 29296 | 73057 | 8870 | 10768 | 17918 | 2110 | 2329 | 2700 | 563 | 582 | 607 | 230 | 233 | 238 |
| *** | 25946 | 36061 | 73321 | 9639 | 12710 | 17963 | 2207 | 2489 | 2687 | 571 | 596 | 584 | 233 | 238 | 216 |
| 0.85 *** | 19039 | 23934 | 57812 | 7283 | 8843 | 14046 | 1663 | 1817 | 2053 | 409 | 420 | 433 | . | . | . |
| *** | 20944 | 29776 | 57905 | 7919 | 10370 | 14050 | 1736 | 1920 | 2033 | 412 | 425 | 409 | . | . | . |
| 0.9 *** | 14273 | 18149 | 40143 | 5446 | 6535 | 9569 | 1124 | 1200 | 1306 | . | . | . | . | . | . |
| *** | 15801 | 22561 | 40153 | 5901 | 7529 | 9554 | 1159 | 1249 | 1285 | . | . | . | . | . | . |
| 0.95 *** | 8834 | 11088 | 20082 | 3085 | 3553 | 4496 | . | . | . | . | . | . | . | . | . |
| *** | 9744 | 13425 | 20065 | 3288 | 3919 | 4474 | . | . | . | . | . | . | . | . | . |
| 0.98 *** | 4219 | 5008 | 6912 | . | . | . | . | . | . | . | . | . | . | . | . |
| *** | 4556 | 5685 | 6891 | . | . | . | . | . | . | . | . | . | . | . | . |

TABLE 1: ALPHA= 0.005 POWER= 0.8    EXPECTED ACCRUAL THRU MINIMUM FOLLOW-UP= 3500

| | | DEL=.01 | | | DEL=.02 | | | DEL=.05 | | | DEL=.10 | | | DEL=.15 | | |
|---|---|---|---|---|---|---|---|---|---|---|---|---|---|---|---|---|
| FACT= | | 1.0 .75 | .50 .25 | .00 BIN | 1.0 .75 | .50 .25 | .00 BIN | 1.0 .75 | .50 .25 | .00 BIN | 1.0 75 | .50 .25 | .00 BIN | 1.0 .75 | .50 .25 | .00 BIN |
| PCONT=*** | | | | | | | REQUIRED | NUMBER OF | PATIENTS | | | | | | | |
| 0.01 | *** | 1788 | 1791 | 1800 | 659 | 659 | 659 | 216 | 216 | 216 | 108 | 108 | 108 | 76 | 76 | 76 |
| | *** | 1788 | 1796 | 6891 | 659 | 659 | 2278 | 216 | 216 | 620 | 108 | 108 | 252 | 76 | 76 | 150 |
| 0.02 | *** | 3943 | 3961 | 4019 | 1266 | 1275 | 1283 | 344 | 344 | 344 | 151 | 151 | 151 | 99 | 99 | 99 |
| | *** | 3952 | 3984 | 11376 | 1271 | 1280 | 3387 | 344 | 344 | 792 | 151 | 151 | 293 | 99 | 99 | 167 |
| 0.05 | *** | 11932 | 11999 | 12553 | 3380 | 3418 | 3520 | 732 | 738 | 746 | 265 | 265 | 265 | 155 | 155 | 155 |
| | *** | 11955 | 12113 | 24269 | 3398 | 3459 | 6576 | 738 | 741 | 1285 | 265 | 265 | 409 | 155 | 155 | 216 |
| 0.1 | *** | 26323 | 26483 | 29222 | 7055 | 7195 | 7729 | 1376 | 1403 | 1438 | 435 | 440 | 443 | 233 | 233 | 233 |
| | *** | 26378 | 26804 | 43890 | 7108 | 7361 | 11423 | 1388 | 1420 | 2033 | 440 | 440 | 584 | 233 | 233 | 289 |
| 0.15 | *** | 39308 | 39596 | 46168 | 10348 | 10620 | 11955 | 1963 | 2018 | 2111 | 592 | 598 | 610 | 300 | 303 | 309 |
| | *** | 39404 | 40174 | 61175 | 10445 | 10975 | 15685 | 1989 | 2059 | 2687 | 592 | 601 | 736 | 303 | 303 | 351 |
| 0.2 | *** | 49767 | 50219 | 62023 | 13023 | 13446 | 15884 | 2453 | 2552 | 2718 | 723 | 738 | 755 | 361 | 365 | 370 |
| | *** | 49921 | 51120 | 76124 | 13175 | 14041 | 19364 | 2496 | 2622 | 3247 | 729 | 746 | 865 | 361 | 365 | 403 |
| 0.25 | *** | 57388 | 58041 | 76145 | 15012 | 15621 | 19366 | 2846 | 2995 | 3258 | 834 | 855 | 878 | 408 | 414 | 417 |
| | *** | 57607 | 59340 | 88737 | 15288 | 16482 | 22459 | 2911 | 3103 | 3714 | 843 | 863 | 970 | 408 | 417 | 444 |
| 0.3 | *** | 62189 | 63090 | 88176 | 16330 | 17153 | 22318 | 3144 | 3340 | 3704 | 916 | 948 | 977 | 443 | 452 | 458 |
| | *** | 62490 | 64870 | 99015 | 16622 | 18308 | 24970 | 3231 | 3488 | 4088 | 930 | 960 | 1052 | 449 | 452 | 475 |
| 0.35 | *** | 64359 | 65558 | 97906 | 17039 | 18101 | 24695 | 3354 | 3593 | 4054 | 983 | 1012 | 1056 | 470 | 478 | 487 |
| | *** | 64761 | 67923 | 106956 | 17418 | 19559 | 26897 | 3459 | 3783 | 4368 | 995 | 1035 | 1110 | 475 | 484 | 496 |
| 0.4 | *** | 64184 | 65753 | 105221 | 17208 | 18535 | 26463 | 3476 | 3760 | 4308 | 1018 | 1056 | 1108 | 484 | 493 | 505 |
| | *** | 64709 | 68813 | 112562 | 17690 | 20285 | 28240 | 3599 | 3978 | 4555 | 1038 | 1082 | 1145 | 487 | 501 | 507 |
| 0.45 | *** | 62008 | 64026 | 110051 | 16937 | 18530 | 27609 | 3523 | 3844 | 4460 | 1035 | 1079 | 1135 | 487 | 501 | 510 |
| | *** | 62682 | 67897 | 115833 | 17529 | 20551 | 28999 | 3660 | 4089 | 4649 | 1056 | 1105 | 1157 | 493 | 505 | 507 |
| 0.5 | *** | 58211 | 60783 | 112353 | 16321 | 18162 | 28120 | 3503 | 3844 | 4512 | 1030 | 1073 | 1135 | 484 | 493 | 505 |
| | *** | 59074 | 65549 | 116767 | 17016 | 20411 | 29175 | 3651 | 4110 | 4649 | 1053 | 1105 | 1145 | 487 | 501 | 496 |
| 0.55 | *** | 53197 | 56440 | 112111 | 15441 | 17497 | 27994 | 3415 | 3774 | 4465 | 1003 | 1053 | 1108 | 466 | 478 | 487 |
| | *** | 54291 | 62122 | 115365 | 16228 | 19918 | 28766 | 3573 | 4048 | 4555 | 1026 | 1079 | 1110 | 470 | 484 | 475 |
| 0.6 | *** | 47405 | 51409 | 109328 | 14379 | 16587 | 27236 | 3275 | 3634 | 4311 | 960 | 1003 | 1056 | 440 | 449 | 461 |
| | *** | 48784 | 57940 | 111628 | 15240 | 19098 | 27773 | 3433 | 3905 | 4368 | 977 | 1030 | 1052 | 443 | 458 | 444 |
| 0.65 | *** | 41276 | 46057 | 104017 | 13189 | 15473 | 25845 | 3077 | 3418 | 4057 | 890 | 933 | 983 | 405 | 414 | 423 |
| | *** | 42968 | 53223 | 105555 | 14090 | 17987 | 26196 | 3226 | 3678 | 4088 | 913 | 956 | 970 | 408 | 417 | 403 |
| 0.7 | *** | 35233 | 40641 | 96186 | 11906 | 14169 | 23823 | 2823 | 3138 | 3704 | 802 | 837 | 881 | 356 | 365 | 370 |
| | *** | 37216 | 48122 | 97146 | 12807 | 16596 | 24036 | 2963 | 3371 | 3714 | 820 | 860 | 865 | 361 | 370 | 351 |
| 0.75 | *** | 29569 | 35283 | 85858 | 10538 | 12676 | 21181 | 2508 | 2785 | 3252 | 697 | 723 | 755 | 300 | 303 | 309 |
| | *** | 31721 | 42680 | 86402 | 11398 | 14913 | 21291 | 2631 | 2981 | 3247 | 711 | 738 | 736 | 303 | 309 | 289 |
| 0.8 | *** | 24371 | 29963 | 73056 | 9068 | 10978 | 17917 | 2138 | 2351 | 2701 | 566 | 583 | 606 | 230 | 233 | 239 |
| | *** | 26518 | 36849 | 73321 | 9841 | 12909 | 17963 | 2234 | 2500 | 2687 | 575 | 592 | 584 | 233 | 239 | 216 |
| 0.85 | *** | 19510 | 24520 | 57808 | 7443 | 9010 | 14046 | 1683 | 1831 | 2053 | 408 | 423 | 431 | . | . | . |
| | *** | 21461 | 30444 | 57905 | 8088 | 10520 | 14050 | 1753 | 1931 | 2033 | 414 | 426 | 409 | . | . | . |
| 0.9 | *** | 14653 | 18600 | 40142 | 5562 | 6647 | 9570 | 1135 | 1210 | 1306 | . | . | . | . | . | . |
| | *** | 16216 | 23050 | 40153 | 6017 | 7624 | 9554 | 1170 | 1254 | 1285 | . | . | . | . | . | . |
| 0.95 | *** | 9068 | 11337 | 20084 | 3138 | 3599 | 4495 | . | . | . | . | . | . | . | . | . |
| | *** | 9986 | 13665 | 20065 | 3340 | 3952 | 4474 | . | . | . | . | . | . | . | . | . |
| 0.98 | *** | 4308 | 5086 | 6915 | . | . | . | . | . | . | . | . | . | . | . | . |
| | *** | 4640 | 5746 | 6891 | . | . | . | . | . | . | . | . | . | . | . | . |

## TABLE 1: ALPHA= 0.005 POWER= 0.8     EXPECTED ACCRUAL THRU MINIMUM FOLLOW-UP= 3750

|  | DEL=.01 | | | DEL=.02 | | | DEL=.05 | | | DEL=.10 | | | DEL=.15 | | |
|---|---|---|---|---|---|---|---|---|---|---|---|---|---|---|---|
| FACT= | 1.0 / .75 | .50 / .25 | .00 / BIN | 1.0 / .75 | .50 / .25 | .00 / BIN | 1.0 / .75 | .50 / .25 | .00 / BIN | 1.0 / 75 | .50 / .25 | .00 / BIN | 1.0 / .75 | .50 / .25 | .00 / BIN |

PCONT=***      REQUIRED NUMBER OF PATIENTS

| PCONT | DEL=.01 | | | DEL=.02 | | | DEL=.05 | | | DEL=.10 | | | DEL=.15 | | |
|---|---|---|---|---|---|---|---|---|---|---|---|---|---|---|---|
| 0.01 *** | 1788 | 1793 | 1803 | 659 | 659 | 659 | 218 | 218 | 218 | 109 | 109 | 109 | 78 | 78 | 78 |
| *** | 1788 | 1793 | 6891 | 659 | 659 | 2278 | 218 | 218 | 620 | 109 | 109 | 252 | 78 | 78 | 150 |
| 0.02 *** | 3944 | 3963 | 4019 | 1268 | 1272 | 1281 | 344 | 344 | 344 | 153 | 153 | 153 | 100 | 100 | 100 |
| *** | 3953 | 3981 | 11376 | 1272 | 1278 | 3387 | 344 | 344 | 792 | 153 | 153 | 293 | 100 | 100 | 167 |
| 0.05 *** | 11937 | 12006 | 12556 | 3381 | 3425 | 3518 | 734 | 738 | 747 | 265 | 265 | 265 | 153 | 153 | 153 |
| *** | 11959 | 12125 | 24269 | 3400 | 3462 | 6576 | 738 | 743 | 1285 | 265 | 265 | 409 | 153 | 153 | 216 |
| 0.1 *** | 26337 | 26509 | 29225 | 7066 | 7212 | 7728 | 1381 | 1403 | 1437 | 438 | 438 | 443 | 231 | 231 | 237 |
| *** | 26393 | 26847 | 43890 | 7122 | 7375 | 11423 | 1390 | 1422 | 2033 | 438 | 443 | 584 | 231 | 237 | 289 |
| 0.15 *** | 39325 | 39640 | 46165 | 10372 | 10653 | 11956 | 1966 | 2022 | 2106 | 593 | 597 | 606 | 303 | 303 | 303 |
| *** | 39434 | 40253 | 61175 | 10475 | 11013 | 15685 | 1994 | 2059 | 2687 | 597 | 603 | 736 | 303 | 306 | 351 |
| 0.2 *** | 49803 | 50284 | 62022 | 13056 | 13503 | 15884 | 2463 | 2562 | 2722 | 725 | 738 | 753 | 359 | 363 | 368 |
| *** | 49962 | 51247 | 76124 | 13216 | 14103 | 19364 | 2509 | 2631 | 3247 | 734 | 747 | 865 | 363 | 368 | 403 |
| 0.25 *** | 57434 | 58137 | 76147 | 15059 | 15697 | 19366 | 2862 | 3006 | 3256 | 837 | 856 | 878 | 409 | 415 | 419 |
| *** | 57668 | 59519 | 88737 | 15288 | 16578 | 22459 | 2928 | 3109 | 3714 | 847 | 865 | 970 | 409 | 415 | 444 |
| 0.3 *** | 62253 | 63218 | 88175 | 16394 | 17256 | 22319 | 3166 | 3359 | 3700 | 922 | 950 | 978 | 443 | 453 | 456 |
| *** | 62575 | 65122 | 99015 | 16703 | 18434 | 24970 | 3250 | 3500 | 4088 | 934 | 963 | 1052 | 447 | 456 | 475 |
| 0.35 *** | 64447 | 65731 | 97909 | 17122 | 18231 | 24697 | 3378 | 3616 | 4053 | 981 | 1015 | 1056 | 472 | 481 | 490 |
| *** | 64872 | 68253 | 106956 | 17525 | 19713 | 26897 | 3481 | 3794 | 4368 | 1000 | 1034 | 1110 | 475 | 484 | 496 |
| 0.4 *** | 64297 | 65975 | 105222 | 17318 | 18691 | 26463 | 3503 | 3784 | 4309 | 1025 | 1062 | 1109 | 484 | 494 | 503 |
| *** | 64859 | 69231 | 112562 | 17825 | 20472 | 28240 | 3625 | 3997 | 4555 | 1043 | 1081 | 1145 | 490 | 500 | 507 |
| 0.45 *** | 62153 | 64315 | 110050 | 17069 | 18715 | 27606 | 3556 | 3869 | 4459 | 1038 | 1081 | 1131 | 490 | 500 | 513 |
| *** | 62875 | 68412 | 115833 | 17684 | 20763 | 28999 | 3691 | 4109 | 4649 | 1062 | 1103 | 1157 | 494 | 503 | 507 |
| 0.5 *** | 58394 | 61147 | 112353 | 16478 | 18372 | 28118 | 3537 | 3875 | 4512 | 1034 | 1081 | 1131 | 484 | 494 | 503 |
| *** | 59318 | 66162 | 116767 | 17197 | 20647 | 29175 | 3687 | 4131 | 4649 | 1056 | 1103 | 1145 | 490 | 500 | 496 |
| 0.55 *** | 53434 | 56884 | 112113 | 15622 | 17725 | 27997 | 3456 | 3803 | 4465 | 1009 | 1053 | 1109 | 466 | 475 | 490 |
| *** | 54603 | 62834 | 115365 | 16431 | 20163 | 28766 | 3606 | 4072 | 4555 | 1028 | 1081 | 1110 | 472 | 484 | 475 |
| 0.6 *** | 47703 | 51944 | 109328 | 14581 | 16831 | 27237 | 3312 | 3663 | 4309 | 963 | 1006 | 1056 | 443 | 453 | 462 |
| *** | 49169 | 58722 | 111628 | 15456 | 19353 | 27773 | 3466 | 3925 | 4368 | 981 | 1028 | 1052 | 447 | 456 | 444 |
| 0.65 *** | 41647 | 46666 | 104018 | 13400 | 15715 | 25844 | 3115 | 3453 | 4056 | 897 | 934 | 981 | 406 | 415 | 425 |
| *** | 43437 | 54059 | 105555 | 14318 | 18241 | 26196 | 3259 | 3700 | 4088 | 916 | 959 | 970 | 409 | 419 | 403 |
| 0.7 *** | 35675 | 41300 | 96184 | 12115 | 14406 | 23825 | 2856 | 3166 | 3706 | 809 | 841 | 884 | 359 | 363 | 372 |
| *** | 37747 | 48968 | 97146 | 13034 | 16834 | 24036 | 2993 | 3391 | 3714 | 822 | 859 | 865 | 359 | 368 | 351 |
| 0.75 *** | 30059 | 35950 | 85859 | 10737 | 12903 | 21181 | 2543 | 2806 | 3250 | 700 | 725 | 756 | 303 | 306 | 312 |
| *** | 32284 | 43497 | 86402 | 11613 | 15128 | 21291 | 2659 | 2993 | 3247 | 709 | 738 | 736 | 303 | 306 | 289 |
| 0.8 *** | 24865 | 30593 | 73056 | 9250 | 11172 | 17918 | 2159 | 2369 | 2703 | 569 | 584 | 606 | 231 | 237 | 237 |
| *** | 27072 | 37591 | 73321 | 10034 | 13090 | 17963 | 2256 | 2515 | 2687 | 575 | 597 | 584 | 231 | 237 | 216 |
| 0.85 *** | 19962 | 25072 | 57809 | 7597 | 9166 | 14047 | 1700 | 1844 | 2050 | 409 | 419 | 434 | . | . | . |
| *** | 21959 | 31066 | 57905 | 8243 | 10662 | 14050 | 1765 | 1938 | 2033 | 415 | 425 | 409 | . | . | . |
| 0.9 *** | 15016 | 19025 | 40141 | 5675 | 6753 | 9569 | 1141 | 1212 | 1306 | . | . | . | . | . | . |
| *** | 16606 | 23509 | 40153 | 6128 | 7713 | 9554 | 1175 | 1259 | 1285 | . | . | . | . | . | . |
| 0.95 *** | 9284 | 11572 | 20084 | 3184 | 3640 | 4497 | . | . | . | . | . | . | . | . | . |
| *** | 10212 | 13891 | 20065 | 3387 | 3981 | 4474 | . | . | . | . | . | . | . | . | . |
| 0.98 *** | 4384 | 5159 | 6912 | . | . | . | . | . | . | . | . | . | . | . | . |
| *** | 4718 | 5806 | 6891 | . | . | . | . | . | . | . | . | . | . | . | . |

TABLE 1: ALPHA= 0.005 POWER= 0.8    EXPECTED ACCRUAL THRU MINIMUM FOLLOW-UP= 4000

| | | DEL=.01 | | | DEL=.02 | | | DEL=.05 | | | DEL=.10 | | | DEL=.15 | |
|---|---|---|---|---|---|---|---|---|---|---|---|---|---|---|---|---|
| FACT= | 1.0 .75 | .50 .25 | .00 BIN | 1.0 .75 | .50 .25 | .00 BIN | 1.0 .75 | .50 .25 | .00 BIN | 1.0 75 | .50 .25 | .00 BIN | 1.0 .75 | .50 .25 | .00 BIN |
| PCONT=*** | | | | REQUIRED NUMBER OF PATIENTS | | | | | | | | | | | |
| 0.01 *** | 1787 | 1793 | 1803 | 657 | 657 | 657 | 217 | 217 | 217 | 107 | 107 | 107 | 77 | 77 | 77 |
| *** | 1787 | 1797 | 6891 | 657 | 657 | 2278 | 217 | 217 | 620 | 107 | 107 | 252 | 77 | 77 | 150 |
| 0.02 *** | 3947 | 3967 | 4017 | 1267 | 1277 | 1283 | 343 | 343 | 347 | 153 | 153 | 153 | 97 | 97 | 97 |
| *** | 3953 | 3987 | 11376 | 1273 | 1277 | 3387 | 343 | 347 | 792 | 153 | 153 | 293 | 97 | 97 | 167 |
| 0.05 *** | 11943 | 12017 | 12553 | 3387 | 3427 | 3517 | 733 | 737 | 747 | 263 | 263 | 263 | 153 | 153 | 153 |
| *** | 11967 | 12137 | 24269 | 3403 | 3463 | 6576 | 737 | 743 | 1285 | 263 | 263 | 409 | 153 | 153 | 216 |
| 0.1 *** | 26347 | 26533 | 29223 | 7077 | 7227 | 7727 | 1383 | 1407 | 1437 | 437 | 443 | 443 | 233 | 233 | 237 |
| *** | 26407 | 26887 | 43890 | 7133 | 7393 | 11423 | 1393 | 1423 | 2033 | 437 | 443 | 584 | 233 | 233 | 289 |
| 0.15 *** | 39347 | 39683 | 46167 | 10393 | 10683 | 11953 | 1973 | 2027 | 2107 | 593 | 603 | 607 | 303 | 303 | 307 |
| *** | 39457 | 40333 | 61175 | 10497 | 11047 | 15685 | 1997 | 2063 | 2687 | 597 | 603 | 736 | 303 | 307 | 351 |
| 0.2 *** | 49833 | 50347 | 62023 | 13087 | 13553 | 15883 | 2473 | 2567 | 2723 | 727 | 737 | 753 | 363 | 363 | 367 |
| *** | 50007 | 51373 | 76124 | 13257 | 14163 | 19364 | 2517 | 2637 | 3247 | 733 | 747 | 865 | 363 | 367 | 403 |
| 0.25 *** | 57483 | 58227 | 76143 | 15107 | 15773 | 19367 | 2877 | 3017 | 3257 | 837 | 857 | 877 | 407 | 413 | 417 |
| *** | 57733 | 59703 | 88737 | 15347 | 16663 | 22459 | 2943 | 3117 | 3714 | 847 | 867 | 970 | 413 | 417 | 444 |
| 0.3 *** | 62317 | 63343 | 88173 | 16457 | 17357 | 22317 | 3187 | 3373 | 3703 | 923 | 947 | 977 | 447 | 453 | 457 |
| *** | 62657 | 65367 | 99015 | 16783 | 18547 | 24970 | 3267 | 3513 | 4088 | 937 | 963 | 1052 | 447 | 457 | 475 |
| 0.35 *** | 64533 | 65903 | 97907 | 17203 | 18357 | 24693 | 3403 | 3637 | 4053 | 987 | 1017 | 1057 | 473 | 477 | 487 |
| *** | 64987 | 68577 | 106956 | 17627 | 19857 | 26897 | 3503 | 3807 | 4368 | 1003 | 1037 | 1110 | 477 | 483 | 496 |
| 0.4 *** | 64407 | 66197 | 105223 | 17423 | 18847 | 26463 | 3533 | 3807 | 4307 | 1027 | 1063 | 1107 | 487 | 497 | 507 |
| *** | 65007 | 69643 | 112562 | 17947 | 20643 | 28240 | 3653 | 4013 | 4555 | 1043 | 1083 | 1145 | 493 | 503 | 507 |
| 0.45 *** | 62297 | 64597 | 110047 | 17197 | 18893 | 27607 | 3587 | 3897 | 4463 | 1047 | 1083 | 1133 | 493 | 503 | 513 |
| *** | 63067 | 68917 | 115833 | 17837 | 20963 | 28999 | 3723 | 4127 | 4649 | 1063 | 1107 | 1157 | 497 | 507 | 507 |
| 0.5 *** | 58577 | 61503 | 112353 | 16627 | 18573 | 28117 | 3573 | 3903 | 4513 | 1043 | 1083 | 1133 | 483 | 493 | 507 |
| *** | 59563 | 66763 | 116767 | 17373 | 20863 | 29175 | 3717 | 4153 | 4649 | 1063 | 1107 | 1145 | 487 | 503 | 496 |
| 0.55 *** | 53667 | 57327 | 112113 | 15797 | 17943 | 27997 | 3493 | 3833 | 4463 | 1017 | 1057 | 1107 | 467 | 477 | 487 |
| *** | 54913 | 63523 | 115365 | 16627 | 20393 | 28766 | 3643 | 4093 | 4555 | 1033 | 1083 | 1110 | 473 | 483 | 475 |
| 0.6 *** | 47997 | 52467 | 109333 | 14767 | 17057 | 27237 | 3347 | 3693 | 4313 | 967 | 1007 | 1057 | 443 | 453 | 463 |
| *** | 49553 | 59477 | 111628 | 15667 | 19587 | 27773 | 3503 | 3947 | 4368 | 987 | 1033 | 1052 | 447 | 457 | 444 |
| 0.65 *** | 42013 | 47257 | 104017 | 13597 | 15947 | 25847 | 3147 | 3477 | 4057 | 903 | 937 | 983 | 407 | 413 | 423 |
| *** | 43897 | 54853 | 105555 | 14533 | 18473 | 26196 | 3293 | 3717 | 4088 | 917 | 957 | 970 | 407 | 417 | 403 |
| 0.7 *** | 36107 | 41933 | 96187 | 12317 | 14633 | 23827 | 2887 | 3193 | 3707 | 813 | 843 | 883 | 357 | 363 | 373 |
| *** | 38263 | 49767 | 97146 | 13247 | 17057 | 24036 | 3023 | 3407 | 3714 | 827 | 863 | 865 | 363 | 367 | 351 |
| 0.75 *** | 30527 | 36587 | 85857 | 10933 | 13107 | 21183 | 2567 | 2827 | 3253 | 703 | 727 | 757 | 303 | 307 | 313 |
| *** | 32827 | 44273 | 86402 | 11813 | 15327 | 21291 | 2687 | 3007 | 3247 | 713 | 743 | 736 | 303 | 307 | 289 |
| 0.8 *** | 25337 | 31197 | 73057 | 9423 | 11357 | 17917 | 2183 | 2387 | 2703 | 567 | 587 | 607 | 233 | 237 | 237 |
| *** | 27603 | 38297 | 73321 | 10213 | 13263 | 17963 | 2273 | 2523 | 2687 | 577 | 597 | 584 | 233 | 237 | 216 |
| 0.85 *** | 20393 | 25597 | 57807 | 7743 | 9313 | 14047 | 1717 | 1853 | 2053 | 413 | 423 | 433 | . | . | . |
| *** | 22433 | 31657 | 57905 | 8393 | 10787 | 14050 | 1783 | 1943 | 2033 | 417 | 427 | 409 | . | . | . |
| 0.9 *** | 15363 | 19427 | 40143 | 5773 | 6847 | 9567 | 1153 | 1217 | 1307 | . | . | . | . | . | . |
| *** | 16977 | 23937 | 40153 | 6227 | 7793 | 9554 | 1183 | 1263 | 1285 | . | . | . | . | . | . |
| 0.95 *** | 9487 | 11787 | 20083 | 3233 | 3677 | 4497 | . | . | . | . | . | . | . | . | . |
| *** | 10427 | 14097 | 20065 | 3427 | 4007 | 4474 | . | . | . | . | . | . | . | . | . |
| 0.98 *** | 4463 | 5227 | 6913 | . | . | . | . | . | . | . | . | . | . | . | . |
| *** | 4793 | 5853 | 6891 | . | . | . | . | . | . | . | . | . | . | . | . |

## TABLE 1: ALPHA= 0.005 POWER= 0.8    EXPECTED ACCRUAL THRU MINIMUM FOLLOW-UP= 4250

| | | DEL=.01 | | | DEL=.02 | | | DEL=.05 | | | DEL=.10 | | | DEL=.15 | | |
|---|---|---|---|---|---|---|---|---|---|---|---|---|---|---|---|---|
| FACT= | | 1.0 | .50 | .00 | 1.0 | .50 | .00 | 1.0 | .50 | .00 | 1.0 | .50 | .00 | 1.0 | .50 | .00 |
| | | .75 | .25 | BIN | .75 | .25 | BIN | .75 | .25 | BIN | 75 | .25 | BIN | .75 | .25 | BIN |
| PCONT=*** | | | | | REQUIRED | NUMBER | OF | PATIENTS | | | | | | | | |
| 0.01 | *** | 1788 | 1792 | 1799 | 655 | 655 | 662 | 216 | 216 | 216 | 109 | 109 | 109 | 78 | 78 | 78 |
| | *** | 1788 | 1799 | 6891 | 655 | 662 | 2278 | 216 | 216 | 620 | 109 | 109 | 252 | 78 | 78 | 150 |
| 0.02 | *** | 3949 | 3966 | 4019 | 1272 | 1278 | 1282 | 343 | 343 | 347 | 152 | 152 | 152 | 99 | 99 | 99 |
| | *** | 3956 | 3988 | 11376 | 1272 | 1278 | 3387 | 343 | 343 | 792 | 152 | 152 | 293 | 99 | 99 | 167 |
| 0.05 | *** | 11950 | 12024 | 12555 | 3393 | 3428 | 3520 | 736 | 740 | 747 | 262 | 262 | 262 | 152 | 152 | 156 |
| | *** | 11978 | 12148 | 24269 | 3407 | 3467 | 6576 | 736 | 740 | 1285 | 262 | 262 | 409 | 152 | 152 | 216 |
| 0.1 | *** | 26357 | 26555 | 29222 | 7090 | 7239 | 7728 | 1384 | 1410 | 1438 | 439 | 439 | 443 | 230 | 237 | 237 |
| | *** | 26421 | 26927 | 43890 | 7147 | 7402 | 11423 | 1395 | 1420 | 2033 | 439 | 443 | 584 | 230 | 237 | 289 |
| 0.15 | *** | 39369 | 39723 | 46162 | 10416 | 10713 | 11956 | 1979 | 2033 | 2107 | 592 | 602 | 609 | 301 | 305 | 305 |
| | *** | 39486 | 40410 | 61175 | 10526 | 11078 | 15685 | 2005 | 2064 | 2687 | 598 | 602 | 736 | 305 | 305 | 351 |
| 0.2 | *** | 49866 | 50412 | 62021 | 13118 | 13603 | 15881 | 2483 | 2574 | 2723 | 730 | 740 | 751 | 358 | 364 | 368 |
| | *** | 50047 | 51496 | 76124 | 13295 | 14219 | 19364 | 2525 | 2638 | 3247 | 736 | 747 | 865 | 364 | 364 | 403 |
| 0.25 | *** | 57527 | 58324 | 76146 | 15154 | 15845 | 19366 | 2893 | 3031 | 3254 | 843 | 857 | 878 | 411 | 411 | 418 |
| | *** | 57793 | 59879 | 88737 | 15403 | 16748 | 22459 | 2950 | 3127 | 3714 | 847 | 868 | 970 | 411 | 418 | 444 |
| 0.3 | *** | 62383 | 63470 | 88173 | 16518 | 17453 | 22320 | 3205 | 3386 | 3701 | 928 | 953 | 981 | 443 | 453 | 460 |
| | *** | 62744 | 65613 | 99015 | 16858 | 18661 | 24970 | 3286 | 3520 | 4088 | 938 | 963 | 1052 | 449 | 453 | 475 |
| 0.35 | *** | 64618 | 66069 | 97906 | 17283 | 18480 | 24696 | 3424 | 3652 | 4055 | 991 | 1023 | 1055 | 471 | 481 | 485 |
| | *** | 65103 | 68896 | 106956 | 17726 | 19999 | 26897 | 3524 | 3822 | 4368 | 1006 | 1038 | 1110 | 475 | 485 | 496 |
| 0.4 | *** | 64522 | 66420 | 105223 | 17524 | 18994 | 26463 | 3556 | 3828 | 4306 | 1034 | 1066 | 1108 | 485 | 496 | 507 |
| | *** | 65156 | 70047 | 112562 | 18070 | 20807 | 28240 | 3679 | 4030 | 4555 | 1048 | 1087 | 1145 | 492 | 503 | 507 |
| 0.45 | *** | 62440 | 64883 | 110050 | 17326 | 19064 | 27607 | 3616 | 3917 | 4459 | 1048 | 1087 | 1133 | 492 | 503 | 513 |
| | *** | 63258 | 69410 | 115833 | 17985 | 21147 | 28999 | 3747 | 4140 | 4649 | 1066 | 1108 | 1157 | 496 | 507 | 507 |
| 0.5 | *** | 58763 | 61862 | 112352 | 16780 | 18767 | 28117 | 3605 | 3928 | 4512 | 1044 | 1087 | 1133 | 485 | 496 | 507 |
| | *** | 59811 | 67348 | 116767 | 17538 | 21066 | 29175 | 3747 | 4168 | 4649 | 1066 | 1108 | 1145 | 492 | 503 | 496 |
| 0.55 | *** | 53904 | 57765 | 112112 | 15962 | 18151 | 27993 | 3524 | 3860 | 4466 | 1017 | 1059 | 1108 | 471 | 481 | 492 |
| | *** | 55221 | 64182 | 115365 | 16816 | 20609 | 28766 | 3673 | 4108 | 4555 | 1038 | 1080 | 1110 | 475 | 485 | 475 |
| 0.6 | *** | 48294 | 52979 | 109328 | 14953 | 17273 | 27235 | 3382 | 3715 | 4310 | 974 | 1013 | 1059 | 443 | 453 | 460 |
| | *** | 49934 | 60204 | 111628 | 15866 | 19812 | 27773 | 3531 | 3966 | 4368 | 991 | 1034 | 1052 | 449 | 453 | 444 |
| 0.65 | *** | 42376 | 47837 | 104015 | 13788 | 16164 | 25847 | 3180 | 3503 | 4055 | 906 | 938 | 981 | 407 | 411 | 422 |
| | *** | 44345 | 55614 | 105555 | 14740 | 18693 | 26196 | 3322 | 3733 | 4088 | 921 | 959 | 970 | 411 | 418 | 403 |
| 0.7 | *** | 36525 | 42546 | 96185 | 12509 | 14840 | 23824 | 2918 | 3212 | 3705 | 815 | 847 | 878 | 358 | 364 | 368 |
| | *** | 38763 | 50536 | 97146 | 13448 | 17262 | 24036 | 3053 | 3418 | 3714 | 832 | 864 | 865 | 364 | 368 | 351 |
| 0.75 | *** | 30986 | 37201 | 85857 | 11110 | 13306 | 21183 | 2596 | 2844 | 3254 | 704 | 730 | 758 | 301 | 305 | 311 |
| | *** | 33348 | 45004 | 86402 | 12003 | 15516 | 21291 | 2706 | 3021 | 3247 | 715 | 740 | 736 | 305 | 311 | 289 |
| 0.8 | *** | 25794 | 31772 | 73054 | 9587 | 11525 | 17921 | 2203 | 2398 | 2702 | 570 | 588 | 609 | 230 | 237 | 237 |
| | *** | 28110 | 38965 | 73321 | 10384 | 13416 | 17963 | 2292 | 2532 | 2687 | 581 | 598 | 584 | 237 | 237 | 216 |
| 0.85 | *** | 20807 | 26098 | 57807 | 7876 | 9449 | 14049 | 1728 | 1863 | 2054 | 411 | 422 | 432 | . | . | . |
| | *** | 22883 | 32218 | 57905 | 8528 | 10908 | 14050 | 1792 | 1948 | 2033 | 418 | 428 | 409 | . | . | . |
| 0.9 | *** | 15696 | 19808 | 40144 | 5872 | 6941 | 9570 | 1155 | 1225 | 1310 | . | . | . | . | . | . |
| | *** | 17333 | 24338 | 40153 | 6325 | 7859 | 9554 | 1187 | 1261 | 1285 | . | . | . | . | . | . |
| 0.95 | *** | 9683 | 11992 | 20084 | 3276 | 3711 | 4498 | . | . | . | . | . | . | . | . | . |
| | *** | 10628 | 14294 | 20065 | 3467 | 4030 | 4474 | . | . | . | . | . | . | . | . | . |
| 0.98 | *** | 4533 | 5288 | 6913 | . | . | . | . | . | . | . | . | . | . | . | . |
| | *** | 4859 | 5900 | 6891 | . | . | . | . | . | . | . | . | . | . | . | . |

TABLE 1: ALPHA= 0.005 POWER= 0.8    EXPECTED ACCRUAL THRU MINIMUM FOLLOW-UP= 4500

| | | DEL=.01 | | | DEL=.02 | | | DEL=.05 | | | DEL=.10 | | | DEL=.15 | | |
|---|---|---|---|---|---|---|---|---|---|---|---|---|---|---|---|---|---|
| FACT= | | 1.0 .75 | .50 .25 | .00 BIN | 1.0 .75 | .50 .25 | .00 BIN | 1.0 .75 | .50 .25 | .00 BIN | 1.0 75 | .50 .25 | .00 BIN | 1.0 .75 | .50 .25 | .00 BIN |
| PCONT=*** | | | | | | REQUIRED NUMBER OF PATIENTS | | | | | | | | | | |
| 0.01 | *** | 1785 | 1792 | 1803 | 656 | 660 | 660 | 217 | 217 | 217 | 109 | 109 | 109 | 75 | 75 | 75 |
| | *** | 1792 | 1796 | 6891 | 656 | 660 | 2278 | 217 | 217 | 620 | 109 | 109 | 252 | 75 | 75 | 150 |
| 0.02 | *** | 3952 | 3968 | 4020 | 1268 | 1275 | 1286 | 345 | 345 | 345 | 150 | 150 | 150 | 98 | 98 | 98 |
| | *** | 3956 | 3986 | 11376 | 1275 | 1279 | 3387 | 345 | 345 | 792 | 150 | 150 | 293 | 98 | 98 | 167 |
| 0.05 | *** | 11951 | 12034 | 12551 | 3394 | 3435 | 3518 | 735 | 739 | 746 | 262 | 262 | 266 | 154 | 154 | 154 |
| | *** | 11978 | 12158 | 24269 | 3412 | 3468 | 6576 | 739 | 746 | 1285 | 262 | 262 | 409 | 154 | 154 | 216 |
| 0.1 | *** | 26366 | 26580 | 29224 | 7102 | 7253 | 7732 | 1387 | 1410 | 1436 | 435 | 442 | 442 | 233 | 233 | 233 |
| | *** | 26441 | 26970 | 43890 | 7158 | 7417 | 11423 | 1398 | 1425 | 2033 | 442 | 442 | 584 | 233 | 233 | 289 |
| 0.15 | *** | 39390 | 39765 | 46166 | 10432 | 10740 | 11955 | 1983 | 2033 | 2107 | 593 | 600 | 611 | 300 | 307 | 307 |
| | *** | 39513 | 40485 | 61175 | 10549 | 11107 | 15685 | 2006 | 2066 | 2687 | 600 | 604 | 736 | 300 | 307 | 351 |
| 0.2 | *** | 49897 | 50482 | 62025 | 13155 | 13650 | 15881 | 2494 | 2584 | 2719 | 728 | 739 | 757 | 363 | 363 | 368 |
| | *** | 50093 | 51618 | 76124 | 13335 | 14268 | 19364 | 2535 | 2640 | 3247 | 735 | 746 | 865 | 363 | 368 | 403 |
| 0.25 | *** | 57574 | 58413 | 76143 | 15195 | 15911 | 19365 | 2906 | 3041 | 3255 | 840 | 858 | 881 | 408 | 413 | 420 |
| | *** | 57855 | 60056 | 88737 | 15461 | 16822 | 22459 | 2966 | 3131 | 3714 | 851 | 870 | 970 | 413 | 420 | 444 |
| 0.3 | *** | 62445 | 63600 | 88174 | 16586 | 17546 | 22316 | 3221 | 3401 | 3705 | 930 | 953 | 982 | 446 | 453 | 458 |
| | *** | 62828 | 65850 | 99015 | 16935 | 18761 | 24970 | 3300 | 3529 | 4088 | 941 | 964 | 1052 | 446 | 458 | 475 |
| 0.35 | *** | 64702 | 66243 | 97905 | 17366 | 18600 | 24697 | 3446 | 3671 | 4053 | 993 | 1020 | 1054 | 476 | 480 | 487 |
| | *** | 65213 | 69213 | 106956 | 17823 | 20130 | 26897 | 3547 | 3833 | 4368 | 1009 | 1038 | 1110 | 476 | 487 | 496 |
| 0.4 | *** | 64635 | 66641 | 105225 | 17625 | 19133 | 26463 | 3585 | 3851 | 4305 | 1038 | 1065 | 1106 | 487 | 498 | 503 |
| | *** | 65303 | 70444 | 112562 | 18195 | 20962 | 28240 | 3698 | 4042 | 4555 | 1050 | 1088 | 1145 | 491 | 503 | 507 |
| 0.45 | *** | 62587 | 65168 | 110051 | 17445 | 19230 | 27604 | 3641 | 3941 | 4463 | 1054 | 1088 | 1133 | 491 | 503 | 510 |
| | *** | 63453 | 69893 | 115833 | 18127 | 21322 | 28999 | 3776 | 4155 | 4649 | 1072 | 1110 | 1157 | 498 | 510 | 507 |
| 0.5 | *** | 58946 | 62216 | 112350 | 16923 | 18948 | 28117 | 3630 | 3952 | 4515 | 1050 | 1088 | 1133 | 487 | 498 | 503 |
| | *** | 60056 | 67913 | 116767 | 17704 | 21259 | 29175 | 3772 | 4181 | 4649 | 1065 | 1110 | 1145 | 491 | 503 | 496 |
| 0.55 | *** | 54138 | 58193 | 112110 | 16125 | 18345 | 27993 | 3551 | 3885 | 4463 | 1020 | 1061 | 1110 | 469 | 480 | 487 |
| | *** | 55526 | 64826 | 115365 | 16995 | 20816 | 28766 | 3698 | 4125 | 4555 | 1043 | 1083 | 1110 | 476 | 487 | 475 |
| 0.6 | *** | 48585 | 53479 | 109331 | 15128 | 17479 | 27240 | 3412 | 3743 | 4312 | 975 | 1016 | 1061 | 442 | 453 | 465 |
| | *** | 50313 | 60904 | 111628 | 16057 | 20017 | 27773 | 3558 | 3979 | 4368 | 993 | 1031 | 1052 | 446 | 458 | 444 |
| 0.65 | *** | 42735 | 48394 | 104014 | 13969 | 16372 | 25845 | 3210 | 3525 | 4058 | 908 | 941 | 982 | 408 | 413 | 424 |
| | *** | 44790 | 56343 | 105555 | 14932 | 18896 | 26196 | 3349 | 3750 | 4088 | 926 | 960 | 970 | 408 | 420 | 403 |
| 0.7 | *** | 36941 | 43129 | 96184 | 12686 | 15045 | 23824 | 2944 | 3232 | 3705 | 818 | 847 | 881 | 356 | 363 | 375 |
| | *** | 39255 | 51270 | 97146 | 13638 | 17456 | 24036 | 3075 | 3435 | 3714 | 836 | 863 | 865 | 363 | 368 | 351 |
| 0.75 | *** | 31429 | 37785 | 85856 | 11287 | 13492 | 21180 | 2618 | 2865 | 3255 | 705 | 728 | 757 | 300 | 307 | 311 |
| | *** | 33859 | 45705 | 86402 | 12187 | 15690 | 21291 | 2730 | 3034 | 3247 | 716 | 746 | 736 | 307 | 307 | 289 |
| 0.8 | *** | 26238 | 32325 | 73054 | 9746 | 11685 | 17918 | 2220 | 2415 | 2703 | 570 | 588 | 604 | 233 | 233 | 240 |
| | *** | 28601 | 39596 | 73321 | 10545 | 13564 | 17963 | 2310 | 2539 | 2687 | 581 | 600 | 584 | 233 | 240 | 216 |
| 0.85 | *** | 21210 | 26576 | 57810 | 8006 | 9577 | 14048 | 1740 | 1871 | 2051 | 413 | 424 | 431 | . | . | . |
| | *** | 23318 | 32745 | 57905 | 8659 | 11017 | 14050 | 1803 | 1954 | 2033 | 420 | 424 | 409 | . | . | . |
| 0.9 | *** | 16012 | 20175 | 40143 | 5959 | 7023 | 9570 | 1166 | 1230 | 1308 | . | . | . | . | . | . |
| | *** | 17670 | 24720 | 40153 | 6416 | 7928 | 9554 | 1196 | 1263 | 1285 | . | . | . | . | . | . |
| 0.95 | *** | 9870 | 12187 | 20085 | 3315 | 3738 | 4496 | . | . | . | . | . | . | . | . | . |
| | *** | 10819 | 14471 | 20065 | 3502 | 4053 | 4474 | . | . | . | . | . | . | . | . | . |
| 0.98 | *** | 4598 | 5347 | 6915 | . | . | . | . | . | . | . | . | . | . | . | . |
| | *** | 4920 | 5943 | 6891 | . | . | . | . | . | . | . | . | . | . | . | . |

## TABLE 1: ALPHA= 0.005 POWER= 0.8    EXPECTED ACCRUAL THRU MINIMUM FOLLOW-UP= 4750

| | | DEL=.01 | | | DEL=.02 | | | DEL=.05 | | | DEL=.10 | | | DEL=.15 | | |
|---|---|---|---|---|---|---|---|---|---|---|---|---|---|---|---|---|---|
| FACT= | | 1.0 .75 | .50 .25 | .00 BIN | 1.0 .75 | .50 .25 | .00 BIN | 1.0 .75 | .50 .25 | .00 BIN | 1.0 75 | .50 .25 | .00 BIN | 1.0 .75 | .50 .25 | .00 BIN |

PCONT=***                            REQUIRED NUMBER OF PATIENTS

| PCONT | | DEL=.01 1.0/.75 | .50/.25 | .00/BIN | DEL=.02 1.0/.75 | .50/.25 | .00/BIN | DEL=.05 1.0/.75 | .50/.25 | .00/BIN | DEL=.10 1.0/75 | .50/.25 | .00/BIN | DEL=.15 1.0/.75 | .50/.25 | .00/BIN |
|---|---|---|---|---|---|---|---|---|---|---|---|---|---|---|---|---|
| 0.01 | *** | 1789 | 1789 | 1801 | 657 | 657 | 661 | 217 | 217 | 217 | 110 | 110 | 110 | 75 | 79 | 79 |
| | *** | 1789 | 1797 | 6891 | 657 | 661 | 2278 | 217 | 217 | 620 | 110 | 110 | 252 | 79 | 79 | 150 |
| 0.02 | *** | 3950 | 3970 | 4022 | 1274 | 1274 | 1286 | 340 | 348 | 348 | 150 | 150 | 150 | 98 | 98 | 98 |
| | *** | 3958 | 3986 | 11376 | 1274 | 1279 | 3387 | 348 | 348 | 792 | 150 | 150 | 293 | 98 | 98 | 167 |
| 0.05 | *** | 11954 | 12045 | 12555 | 3400 | 3435 | 3518 | 732 | 740 | 744 | 265 | 265 | 265 | 150 | 150 | 150 |
| | *** | 11985 | 12168 | 24269 | 3412 | 3471 | 6576 | 740 | 744 | 1285 | 265 | 265 | 409 | 150 | 150 | 216 |
| 0.1 | *** | 26382 | 26603 | 29220 | 7109 | 7271 | 7727 | 1393 | 1409 | 1440 | 435 | 443 | 443 | 234 | 234 | 234 |
| | *** | 26454 | 27007 | 43890 | 7169 | 7430 | 11423 | 1397 | 1421 | 2033 | 435 | 443 | 584 | 234 | 234 | 289 |
| 0.15 | *** | 39409 | 39801 | 46166 | 10453 | 10767 | 11954 | 1987 | 2039 | 2110 | 597 | 602 | 609 | 305 | 305 | 305 |
| | *** | 39540 | 40561 | 61175 | 10572 | 11135 | 15685 | 2010 | 2070 | 2687 | 597 | 602 | 736 | 305 | 305 | 351 |
| 0.2 | *** | 49930 | 50543 | 62019 | 13185 | 13695 | 15885 | 2502 | 2585 | 2723 | 732 | 740 | 756 | 360 | 364 | 364 |
| | *** | 50132 | 51735 | 76124 | 13375 | 14317 | 19364 | 2537 | 2644 | 3247 | 732 | 744 | 865 | 364 | 364 | 403 |
| 0.25 | *** | 57621 | 58504 | 76146 | 15244 | 15980 | 19364 | 2917 | 3048 | 3257 | 847 | 858 | 875 | 412 | 412 | 419 |
| | *** | 57918 | 60233 | 88737 | 15512 | 16894 | 22459 | 2977 | 3138 | 3714 | 851 | 870 | 970 | 412 | 419 | 444 |
| 0.3 | *** | 62506 | 63729 | 88175 | 16645 | 17630 | 22321 | 3238 | 3412 | 3701 | 930 | 953 | 977 | 447 | 455 | 459 |
| | *** | 62917 | 66088 | 99015 | 17008 | 18861 | 24970 | 3317 | 3535 | 4088 | 942 | 965 | 1052 | 447 | 455 | 475 |
| 0.35 | *** | 64786 | 66413 | 97905 | 17448 | 18711 | 24696 | 3464 | 3685 | 4053 | 994 | 1025 | 1053 | 471 | 478 | 490 |
| | *** | 65328 | 69524 | 106956 | 17915 | 20250 | 26897 | 3559 | 3839 | 4368 | 1013 | 1037 | 1110 | 478 | 483 | 496 |
| 0.4 | *** | 64746 | 66864 | 105220 | 17725 | 19269 | 26461 | 3606 | 3867 | 4307 | 1037 | 1072 | 1108 | 490 | 495 | 507 |
| | *** | 65451 | 70838 | 112562 | 18307 | 21110 | 28240 | 3720 | 4053 | 4555 | 1053 | 1089 | 1145 | 495 | 502 | 507 |
| 0.45 | *** | 62732 | 65451 | 110049 | 17567 | 19383 | 27605 | 3673 | 3962 | 4461 | 1053 | 1089 | 1132 | 495 | 502 | 514 |
| | *** | 63642 | 70367 | 115833 | 18267 | 21490 | 28999 | 3796 | 4172 | 4649 | 1072 | 1112 | 1157 | 495 | 507 | 507 |
| 0.5 | *** | 59134 | 62565 | 112353 | 17060 | 19122 | 28116 | 3661 | 3974 | 4516 | 1053 | 1089 | 1132 | 490 | 495 | 507 |
| | *** | 60297 | 68467 | 116767 | 17863 | 21438 | 29175 | 3796 | 4200 | 4649 | 1072 | 1112 | 1145 | 490 | 502 | 496 |
| 0.55 | *** | 54372 | 58618 | 112108 | 16284 | 18540 | 27997 | 3582 | 3903 | 4461 | 1029 | 1065 | 1108 | 471 | 478 | 490 |
| | *** | 55832 | 65447 | 115365 | 17167 | 21003 | 28766 | 3725 | 4140 | 4555 | 1048 | 1084 | 1110 | 478 | 483 | 475 |
| 0.6 | *** | 48881 | 53968 | 109329 | 15298 | 17673 | 27237 | 3440 | 3760 | 4314 | 982 | 1017 | 1060 | 443 | 455 | 459 |
| | *** | 50679 | 61575 | 111628 | 16241 | 20215 | 27773 | 3582 | 3993 | 4368 | 994 | 1037 | 1052 | 447 | 455 | 444 |
| 0.65 | *** | 43090 | 48933 | 104017 | 14147 | 16569 | 25843 | 3238 | 3547 | 4057 | 910 | 946 | 982 | 407 | 412 | 424 |
| | *** | 45216 | 57044 | 105555 | 15120 | 19087 | 26196 | 3376 | 3760 | 4088 | 930 | 965 | 970 | 412 | 419 | 403 |
| 0.7 | *** | 37350 | 43703 | 96184 | 12864 | 15232 | 23825 | 2972 | 3250 | 3708 | 823 | 851 | 882 | 360 | 364 | 372 |
| | *** | 39730 | 51968 | 97146 | 13826 | 17638 | 24036 | 3095 | 3447 | 3714 | 835 | 863 | 865 | 364 | 372 | 351 |
| 0.75 | *** | 31864 | 38352 | 85860 | 11451 | 13664 | 21181 | 2640 | 2882 | 3250 | 709 | 732 | 756 | 300 | 305 | 312 |
| | *** | 34350 | 46375 | 86402 | 12358 | 15849 | 21291 | 2751 | 3043 | 3247 | 720 | 744 | 736 | 305 | 305 | 289 |
| 0.8 | *** | 26663 | 32854 | 73058 | 9888 | 11843 | 17915 | 2240 | 2426 | 2699 | 573 | 590 | 609 | 234 | 234 | 241 |
| | *** | 29066 | 40200 | 73321 | 10695 | 13700 | 17963 | 2324 | 2549 | 2687 | 585 | 597 | 584 | 234 | 234 | 216 |
| 0.85 | *** | 21592 | 27031 | 57811 | 8130 | 9693 | 14044 | 1754 | 1880 | 2050 | 412 | 424 | 431 | . | . | . |
| | *** | 23734 | 33246 | 57905 | 8784 | 11118 | 14050 | 1813 | 1955 | 2033 | 419 | 424 | 409 | . | . | . |
| 0.9 | *** | 16312 | 20516 | 40141 | 6048 | 7097 | 9567 | 1172 | 1231 | 1310 | . | . | . | . | . | . |
| | *** | 17994 | 25076 | 40153 | 6499 | 7988 | 9554 | 1203 | 1267 | 1285 | . | . | . | . | . | . |
| 0.95 | *** | 10042 | 12370 | 20084 | 3352 | 3768 | 4497 | . | . | . | . | . | . | . | . | . |
| | *** | 11000 | 14638 | 20065 | 3535 | 4069 | 4474 | . | . | . | . | . | . | . | . | . |
| 0.98 | *** | 4658 | 5399 | 6915 | . | . | . | . | . | . | . | . | . | . | . | . |
| | *** | 4979 | 5981 | 6891 | . | . | . | . | . | . | . | . | . | . | . | . |

| TABLE 1: ALPHA= 0.005 POWER= 0.8 | | | | | EXPECTED ACCRUAL THRU MINIMUM FOLLOW-UP= 5000 | | | | | | | | | |

| | | DEL=.01 | | | DEL=.02 | | | DEL=.05 | | | DEL=.10 | | | DEL=.15 | | |
|---|---|---|---|---|---|---|---|---|---|---|---|---|---|---|---|---|
| FACT= | | 1.0 .75 | .50 .25 | .00 BIN | 1.0 .75 | .50 .25 | .00 BIN | 1.0 .75 | .50 .25 | .00 BIN | 1.0 75 | .50 .25 | .00 BIN | 1.0 .75 | .50 .25 | .00 BIN |
| PCONT=*** | | | | REQUIRED NUMBER OF PATIENTS | | | | | | | | | | | | |
| 0.01 | *** | 1791 | 1791 | 1804 | 658 | 658 | 658 | 216 | 216 | 216 | 108 | 108 | 108 | 79 | 79 | 79 |
| | *** | 1791 | 1796 | 6891 | 658 | 658 | 2278 | 216 | 216 | 620 | 108 | 108 | 252 | 79 | 79 | 150 |
| 0.02 | *** | 3954 | 3971 | 4021 | 1271 | 1279 | 1283 | 346 | 346 | 346 | 154 | 154 | 154 | 96 | 96 | 96 |
| | *** | 3958 | 3991 | 11376 | 1271 | 1279 | 3387 | 346 | 346 | 792 | 154 | 154 | 293 | 96 | 96 | 167 |
| 0.05 | *** | 11958 | 12054 | 12554 | 3396 | 3441 | 3516 | 733 | 741 | 746 | 266 | 266 | 266 | 154 | 154 | 154 |
| | *** | 11991 | 12179 | 24269 | 3416 | 3471 | 6576 | 741 | 741 | 1285 | 266 | 266 | 409 | 154 | 154 | 216 |
| 0.1 | *** | 26391 | 26621 | 29221 | 7121 | 7279 | 7729 | 1391 | 1408 | 1441 | 441 | 441 | 446 | 233 | 233 | 233 |
| | *** | 26471 | 27046 | 43890 | 7183 | 7441 | 11423 | 1404 | 1421 | 2033 | 441 | 441 | 584 | 233 | 233 | 289 |
| 0.15 | *** | 39433 | 39846 | 46166 | 10471 | 10796 | 11954 | 1991 | 2041 | 2108 | 596 | 604 | 608 | 304 | 304 | 308 |
| | *** | 39571 | 40641 | 61175 | 10596 | 11158 | 15685 | 2016 | 2071 | 2687 | 596 | 604 | 736 | 304 | 304 | 351 |
| 0.2 | *** | 49958 | 50608 | 62021 | 13216 | 13741 | 15883 | 2508 | 2596 | 2721 | 733 | 741 | 754 | 358 | 366 | 366 |
| | *** | 50179 | 51858 | 76124 | 13408 | 14366 | 19364 | 2546 | 2654 | 3247 | 733 | 746 | 865 | 366 | 366 | 403 |
| 0.25 | *** | 57666 | 58604 | 76146 | 15283 | 16041 | 19366 | 2929 | 3054 | 3254 | 846 | 858 | 879 | 408 | 416 | 421 |
| | *** | 57979 | 60404 | 88737 | 15566 | 16966 | 22459 | 2983 | 3141 | 3714 | 854 | 871 | 970 | 408 | 416 | 444 |
| 0.3 | *** | 62571 | 63858 | 88171 | 16704 | 17721 | 22321 | 3254 | 3421 | 3704 | 933 | 954 | 979 | 446 | 454 | 458 |
| | *** | 63004 | 66329 | 99015 | 17083 | 18954 | 24970 | 3329 | 3546 | 4088 | 946 | 966 | 1052 | 454 | 454 | 475 |
| 0.35 | *** | 64871 | 66583 | 97908 | 17521 | 18816 | 24696 | 3483 | 3696 | 4054 | 996 | 1029 | 1054 | 471 | 479 | 491 |
| | *** | 65446 | 69829 | 106956 | 18008 | 20366 | 26897 | 3579 | 3854 | 4368 | 1008 | 1041 | 1110 | 479 | 483 | 496 |
| 0.4 | *** | 64858 | 67083 | 105221 | 17821 | 19404 | 26458 | 3629 | 3883 | 4300 | 1041 | 1071 | 1108 | 491 | 496 | 504 |
| | *** | 65604 | 71216 | 112562 | 18421 | 21246 | 28240 | 3741 | 4066 | 4555 | 1054 | 1091 | 1145 | 491 | 504 | 507 |
| 0.45 | *** | 62871 | 65729 | 110046 | 17683 | 19533 | 27608 | 3691 | 3979 | 4458 | 1058 | 1091 | 1133 | 496 | 504 | 508 |
| | *** | 63833 | 70829 | 115833 | 18396 | 21646 | 28999 | 3821 | 4183 | 4649 | 1079 | 1108 | 1157 | 496 | 508 | 507 |
| 0.5 | *** | 59316 | 62916 | 112354 | 17196 | 19291 | 28116 | 3683 | 3991 | 4516 | 1058 | 1091 | 1133 | 491 | 496 | 504 |
| | *** | 60541 | 69004 | 116767 | 18016 | 21608 | 29175 | 3821 | 4208 | 4649 | 1071 | 1108 | 1145 | 491 | 504 | 496 |
| 0.55 | *** | 54604 | 59033 | 112108 | 16433 | 18716 | 27996 | 3608 | 3929 | 4466 | 1029 | 1066 | 1108 | 471 | 479 | 491 |
| | *** | 56141 | 66054 | 115365 | 17333 | 21183 | 28766 | 3754 | 4154 | 4555 | 1046 | 1083 | 1110 | 479 | 483 | 475 |
| 0.6 | *** | 49171 | 54454 | 109329 | 15458 | 17858 | 27233 | 3466 | 3783 | 4308 | 983 | 1016 | 1058 | 446 | 454 | 458 |
| | *** | 51046 | 62229 | 111628 | 16416 | 20396 | 27773 | 3608 | 4008 | 4368 | 996 | 1033 | 1052 | 446 | 458 | 444 |
| 0.65 | *** | 43441 | 49466 | 104016 | 14316 | 16758 | 25846 | 3258 | 3566 | 4058 | 916 | 946 | 983 | 408 | 416 | 421 |
| | *** | 45641 | 57721 | 105555 | 15296 | 19271 | 26196 | 3396 | 3779 | 4088 | 929 | 966 | 970 | 408 | 416 | 403 |
| 0.7 | *** | 37746 | 44254 | 96183 | 13033 | 15416 | 23829 | 2996 | 3271 | 3704 | 821 | 854 | 883 | 358 | 366 | 371 |
| | *** | 40191 | 52641 | 97146 | 13996 | 17808 | 24036 | 3116 | 3458 | 3714 | 833 | 866 | 865 | 366 | 371 | 351 |
| 0.75 | *** | 32283 | 38904 | 85858 | 11608 | 13833 | 21179 | 2658 | 2896 | 3254 | 708 | 733 | 754 | 304 | 308 | 308 |
| | *** | 34821 | 47016 | 86402 | 12521 | 16004 | 21291 | 2766 | 3054 | 3247 | 721 | 746 | 736 | 304 | 308 | 289 |
| 0.8 | *** | 27071 | 33358 | 73058 | 10033 | 11983 | 17921 | 2254 | 2433 | 2704 | 579 | 591 | 604 | 233 | 233 | 241 |
| | *** | 29521 | 40779 | 73321 | 10841 | 13829 | 17963 | 2341 | 2554 | 2687 | 583 | 596 | 584 | 233 | 233 | 216 |
| 0.85 | *** | 21958 | 27471 | 57808 | 8246 | 9808 | 14046 | 1766 | 1891 | 2054 | 416 | 421 | 433 | . | . | . |
| | *** | 24133 | 33721 | 57905 | 8896 | 11216 | 14050 | 1821 | 1966 | 2033 | 421 | 429 | 409 | . | . | . |
| 0.9 | *** | 16604 | 20846 | 40141 | 6129 | 7171 | 9571 | 1179 | 1233 | 1308 | . | . | . | . | . | . |
| | *** | 18304 | 25416 | 40153 | 6579 | 8046 | 9554 | 1204 | 1271 | 1285 | . | . | . | . | . | . |
| 0.95 | *** | 10208 | 12546 | 20083 | 3383 | 3796 | 4496 | . | . | . | . | . | . | . | . | . |
| | *** | 11171 | 14796 | 20065 | 3566 | 4091 | 4474 | . | . | . | . | . | . | . | . | . |
| 0.98 | *** | 4716 | 5446 | 6916 | . | . | . | . | . | . | . | . | . | . | . | . |
| | *** | 5033 | 6016 | 6891 | . | . | . | . | . | . | . | . | . | . | . | . |

# TABLE 1: ALPHA= 0.005 POWER= 0.8   EXPECTED ACCRUAL THRU MINIMUM FOLLOW-UP= 5500

|  |  | DEL=.01 | | | DEL=.02 | | | DEL=.05 | | | DEL=.10 | | | DEL=.15 | | |
|---|---|---|---|---|---|---|---|---|---|---|---|---|---|---|---|---|
| FACT= | | 1.0 .75 | .50 .25 | .00 BIN | 1.0 .75 | .50 .25 | .00 BIN | 1.0 .75 | .50 .25 | .00 BIN | 1.0 75 | .50 .25 | .00 BIN | 1.0 .75 | .50 .25 | .00 BIN |
| PCONT=*** | | | | | | REQUIRED NUMBER OF PATIENTS | | | | | | | | | | |
| 0.01 | *** | 1791 | 1791 | 1797 | 655 | 655 | 655 | 215 | 215 | 215 | 105 | 105 | 105 | 78 | 78 | 78 |
|  | *** | 1791 | 1797 | 6891 | 655 | 655 | 2278 | 215 | 215 | 620 | 105 | 105 | 252 | 78 | 78 | 150 |
| 0.02 | *** | 3955 | 3978 | 4019 | 1274 | 1274 | 1283 | 348 | 348 | 348 | 147 | 147 | 147 | 100 | 100 | 100 |
|  | *** | 3964 | 3991 | 11376 | 1274 | 1283 | 3387 | 348 | 348 | 792 | 147 | 147 | 293 | 100 | 100 | 167 |
| 0.05 | *** | 11972 | 12068 | 12558 | 3405 | 3447 | 3515 | 738 | 738 | 746 | 265 | 265 | 265 | 155 | 155 | 155 |
|  | *** | 12008 | 12200 | 24269 | 3419 | 3474 | 6576 | 738 | 746 | 1285 | 265 | 265 | 409 | 155 | 155 | 216 |
| 0.1 | *** | 26418 | 26670 | 29223 | 7140 | 7305 | 7731 | 1393 | 1412 | 1439 | 435 | 444 | 444 | 229 | 238 | 238 |
|  | *** | 26500 | 27119 | 43890 | 7209 | 7456 | 11423 | 1406 | 1425 | 2033 | 435 | 444 | 584 | 238 | 238 | 289 |
| 0.15 | *** | 39472 | 39925 | 46163 | 10509 | 10844 | 11953 | 2003 | 2044 | 2108 | 595 | 600 | 609 | 306 | 306 | 306 |
|  | *** | 39623 | 40786 | 61175 | 10638 | 11210 | 15685 | 2025 | 2072 | 2687 | 600 | 609 | 736 | 306 | 306 | 351 |
| 0.2 | *** | 50026 | 50733 | 62022 | 13278 | 13823 | 15885 | 2520 | 2603 | 2718 | 733 | 746 | 752 | 361 | 367 | 367 |
|  | *** | 50265 | 52094 | 76124 | 13484 | 14447 | 19364 | 2561 | 2658 | 3247 | 738 | 746 | 865 | 361 | 367 | 403 |
| 0.25 | *** | 57759 | 58785 | 76143 | 15376 | 16165 | 19364 | 2946 | 3070 | 3254 | 848 | 862 | 875 | 408 | 416 | 416 |
|  | *** | 58103 | 60743 | 88737 | 15670 | 17087 | 22459 | 3001 | 3153 | 3714 | 856 | 870 | 970 | 416 | 416 | 444 |
| 0.3 | *** | 62704 | 64112 | 88174 | 16820 | 17884 | 22320 | 3276 | 3441 | 3703 | 939 | 958 | 980 | 449 | 449 | 458 |
|  | *** | 63171 | 66788 | 99015 | 17224 | 19122 | 24970 | 3350 | 3557 | 4088 | 944 | 966 | 1052 | 449 | 458 | 475 |
| 0.35 | *** | 65047 | 66925 | 97909 | 17678 | 19020 | 24690 | 3515 | 3722 | 4052 | 1008 | 1027 | 1054 | 477 | 485 | 485 |
|  | *** | 65674 | 70423 | 106956 | 18187 | 20579 | 26897 | 3606 | 3868 | 4368 | 1013 | 1040 | 1110 | 477 | 485 | 496 |
| 0.4 | *** | 65083 | 67522 | 105224 | 18008 | 19644 | 26464 | 3667 | 3909 | 4308 | 1049 | 1076 | 1109 | 490 | 499 | 504 |
|  | *** | 65899 | 71958 | 112562 | 18640 | 21500 | 28240 | 3777 | 4079 | 4555 | 1063 | 1090 | 1145 | 490 | 499 | 507 |
| 0.45 | *** | 63163 | 66284 | 110050 | 17912 | 19818 | 27605 | 3735 | 4010 | 4459 | 1063 | 1095 | 1131 | 499 | 504 | 513 |
|  | *** | 64216 | 71715 | 115833 | 18654 | 21935 | 28999 | 3859 | 4203 | 4649 | 1082 | 1118 | 1157 | 499 | 504 | 507 |
| 0.5 | *** | 59684 | 63598 | 112347 | 17458 | 19603 | 28114 | 3730 | 4024 | 4514 | 1063 | 1095 | 1131 | 490 | 499 | 504 |
|  | *** | 61026 | 70033 | 116767 | 18305 | 21927 | 29175 | 3868 | 4239 | 4649 | 1076 | 1109 | 1145 | 490 | 499 | 496 |
| 0.55 | *** | 55064 | 59844 | 112113 | 16724 | 19053 | 27999 | 3661 | 3964 | 4464 | 1035 | 1068 | 1109 | 471 | 485 | 490 |
|  | *** | 56736 | 67200 | 115365 | 17650 | 21514 | 28766 | 3799 | 4175 | 4555 | 1054 | 1090 | 1110 | 477 | 485 | 475 |
| 0.6 | *** | 49743 | 55380 | 109330 | 15767 | 18209 | 27234 | 3515 | 3818 | 4313 | 985 | 1021 | 1054 | 449 | 458 | 463 |
|  | *** | 51764 | 63460 | 111628 | 16751 | 20730 | 27773 | 3653 | 4033 | 4368 | 1008 | 1040 | 1052 | 449 | 458 | 444 |
| 0.65 | *** | 44119 | 50480 | 104014 | 14634 | 17109 | 25845 | 3309 | 3598 | 4060 | 917 | 953 | 980 | 408 | 416 | 422 |
|  | *** | 46465 | 58997 | 105555 | 15638 | 19603 | 26196 | 3441 | 3799 | 4088 | 930 | 966 | 970 | 416 | 416 | 403 |
| 0.7 | *** | 38518 | 45310 | 96185 | 13347 | 15748 | 23824 | 3034 | 3304 | 3703 | 829 | 856 | 884 | 361 | 367 | 375 |
|  | *** | 41080 | 53904 | 97146 | 14331 | 18118 | 24036 | 3158 | 3474 | 3714 | 843 | 870 | 865 | 361 | 367 | 351 |
| 0.75 | *** | 33092 | 39939 | 85859 | 11911 | 14139 | 21179 | 2699 | 2919 | 3254 | 719 | 733 | 752 | 306 | 306 | 312 |
|  | *** | 35732 | 48217 | 86402 | 12824 | 16284 | 21291 | 2800 | 3070 | 3247 | 724 | 746 | 736 | 306 | 306 | 289 |
| 0.8 | *** | 27861 | 34324 | 73058 | 10303 | 12247 | 17920 | 2286 | 2457 | 2699 | 581 | 595 | 609 | 238 | 238 | 238 |
|  | *** | 30383 | 41850 | 73321 | 11105 | 14062 | 17963 | 2360 | 2567 | 2687 | 587 | 600 | 584 | 238 | 238 | 216 |
| 0.85 | *** | 22664 | 28293 | 57809 | 8460 | 10014 | 14048 | 1783 | 1901 | 2053 | 416 | 422 | 430 | . | . | . |
|  | *** | 24891 | 34613 | 57905 | 9112 | 11389 | 14050 | 1838 | 1970 | 2033 | 422 | 430 | 409 | . | . | . |
| 0.9 | *** | 17155 | 21468 | 40140 | 6279 | 7305 | 9565 | 1186 | 1241 | 1310 | . | . | . | . | . | . |
|  | *** | 18888 | 26046 | 40153 | 6719 | 8149 | 9554 | 1214 | 1274 | 1285 | . | . | . | . | . | . |
| 0.95 | *** | 10528 | 12865 | 20084 | 3447 | 3840 | 4492 | . | . | . | . | . | . | . | . | . |
|  | *** | 11490 | 15088 | 20065 | 3625 | 4120 | 4474 | . | . | . | . | . | . | . | . | . |
| 0.98 | *** | 4822 | 5537 | 6912 | . | . | . | . | . | . | . | . | . | . | . | . |
|  | *** | 5138 | 6081 | 6891 | . | . | . | . | . | . | . | . | . | . | . | . |

## TABLE 1: ALPHA= 0.005 POWER= 0.8    EXPECTED ACCRUAL THRU MINIMUM FOLLOW-UP= 6000

| FACT= | DEL=.01 1.0 / .75 | DEL=.01 .50 / .25 | DEL=.01 .00 BIN | DEL=.02 1.0 / .75 | DEL=.02 .50 / .25 | DEL=.02 .00 BIN | DEL=.05 1.0 / .75 | DEL=.05 .50 / .25 | DEL=.05 .00 BIN | DEL=.10 1.0 / 75 | DEL=.10 .50 / .25 | DEL=.10 .00 BIN | DEL=.15 1.0 / .75 | DEL=.15 .50 / .25 | DEL=.15 .00 BIN |
|---|---|---|---|---|---|---|---|---|---|---|---|---|---|---|---|

PCONT=***  REQUIRED NUMBER OF PATIENTS

| PCONT | 1.0/.75 | .50/.25 | .00/BIN | 1.0/.75 | .50/.25 | .00/BIN | 1.0/.75 | .50/.25 | .00/BIN | 1.0/75 | .50/.25 | .00/BIN | 1.0/.75 | .50/.25 | .00/BIN |
|---|---|---|---|---|---|---|---|---|---|---|---|---|---|---|---|
| 0.01 *** | 1789 | 1795 | 1804 | 655 | 655 | 655 | 214 | 214 | 214 | 109 | 109 | 109 | 79 | 79 | 79 |
| *** | 1789 | 1795 | 6891 | 655 | 655 | 2278 | 214 | 214 | 620 | 109 | 109 | 252 | 79 | 79 | 150 |
| 0.02 *** | 3955 | 3979 | 4015 | 1270 | 1279 | 1285 | 340 | 349 | 349 | 154 | 154 | 154 | 100 | 100 | 100 |
| *** | 3964 | 3994 | 11376 | 1279 | 1279 | 3387 | 340 | 349 | 792 | 154 | 154 | 293 | 100 | 100 | 167 |
| 0.05 *** | 11980 | 12079 | 12550 | 3409 | 3445 | 3520 | 739 | 739 | 745 | 265 | 265 | 265 | 154 | 154 | 154 |
| *** | 12019 | 12214 | 24269 | 3430 | 3475 | 6576 | 739 | 745 | 1285 | 265 | 265 | 409 | 154 | 154 | 216 |
| 0.1 *** | 26440 | 26710 | 29224 | 7159 | 7324 | 7729 | 1399 | 1414 | 1435 | 439 | 439 | 445 | 235 | 235 | 235 |
| *** | 26530 | 27190 | 43890 | 7225 | 7474 | 11423 | 1405 | 1429 | 2033 | 439 | 445 | 584 | 235 | 235 | 289 |
| 0.15 *** | 39514 | 40009 | 46165 | 10549 | 10894 | 11950 | 2005 | 2050 | 2110 | 595 | 604 | 610 | 304 | 304 | 304 |
| *** | 39679 | 40924 | 61175 | 10684 | 11254 | 15685 | 2029 | 2080 | 2687 | 604 | 604 | 736 | 304 | 304 | 351 |
| 0.2 *** | 50089 | 50860 | 62020 | 13339 | 13900 | 15880 | 2530 | 2614 | 2719 | 739 | 745 | 754 | 364 | 364 | 370 |
| *** | 50350 | 52315 | 76124 | 13549 | 14524 | 19364 | 2569 | 2659 | 3247 | 739 | 745 | 865 | 364 | 364 | 403 |
| 0.25 *** | 57859 | 58969 | 76144 | 15460 | 16279 | 19369 | 2965 | 3085 | 3259 | 850 | 865 | 880 | 409 | 415 | 415 |
| *** | 58225 | 61075 | 88737 | 15769 | 17200 | 22459 | 3019 | 3160 | 3714 | 859 | 874 | 970 | 415 | 415 | 444 |
| 0.3 *** | 62830 | 64369 | 88174 | 16939 | 18034 | 22315 | 3304 | 3460 | 3700 | 940 | 955 | 979 | 445 | 454 | 460 |
| *** | 63340 | 67234 | 99015 | 17359 | 19279 | 24970 | 3370 | 3565 | 4088 | 949 | 970 | 1052 | 454 | 454 | 475 |
| 0.35 *** | 65215 | 67255 | 97909 | 17824 | 19210 | 24694 | 3544 | 3745 | 4054 | 1009 | 1030 | 1054 | 475 | 484 | 490 |
| *** | 65899 | 70999 | 106956 | 18355 | 20770 | 26897 | 3634 | 3880 | 4368 | 1015 | 1039 | 1110 | 475 | 484 | 496 |
| 0.4 *** | 65305 | 67960 | 105220 | 18190 | 19870 | 26464 | 3700 | 3934 | 4309 | 1054 | 1075 | 1105 | 490 | 499 | 505 |
| *** | 66199 | 72670 | 112562 | 18844 | 21730 | 28240 | 3805 | 4099 | 4555 | 1060 | 1090 | 1145 | 499 | 499 | 507 |
| 0.45 *** | 63454 | 66829 | 110050 | 18124 | 20080 | 27604 | 3775 | 4039 | 4459 | 1069 | 1099 | 1135 | 499 | 505 | 514 |
| *** | 64600 | 72565 | 115833 | 18895 | 22195 | 28999 | 3895 | 4219 | 4649 | 1084 | 1114 | 1157 | 499 | 505 | 507 |
| 0.5 *** | 60055 | 64264 | 112354 | 17704 | 19894 | 28120 | 3775 | 4060 | 4510 | 1069 | 1099 | 1135 | 490 | 499 | 505 |
| *** | 61504 | 71005 | 116767 | 18574 | 22210 | 29175 | 3904 | 4255 | 4649 | 1084 | 1114 | 1145 | 490 | 499 | 496 |
| 0.55 *** | 55525 | 60634 | 112114 | 16999 | 19360 | 27994 | 3700 | 3994 | 4465 | 1039 | 1075 | 1105 | 475 | 484 | 490 |
| *** | 57325 | 68284 | 115365 | 17944 | 21814 | 28766 | 3835 | 4195 | 4555 | 1054 | 1090 | 1110 | 475 | 484 | 475 |
| 0.6 *** | 50314 | 56269 | 109330 | 16060 | 18529 | 27235 | 3559 | 3850 | 4309 | 994 | 1024 | 1060 | 445 | 454 | 460 |
| *** | 52465 | 64615 | 111628 | 17059 | 21040 | 27773 | 3694 | 4054 | 4368 | 1009 | 1039 | 1052 | 454 | 460 | 444 |
| 0.65 *** | 44785 | 51439 | 104014 | 14935 | 17425 | 25849 | 3349 | 3625 | 4060 | 925 | 949 | 979 | 409 | 415 | 424 |
| *** | 47260 | 60184 | 105555 | 15949 | 19900 | 26196 | 3475 | 3814 | 4088 | 940 | 964 | 970 | 415 | 415 | 403 |
| 0.7 *** | 39250 | 46300 | 96184 | 13639 | 16054 | 23824 | 3070 | 3325 | 3709 | 835 | 859 | 880 | 364 | 364 | 370 |
| *** | 41929 | 55084 | 97146 | 14629 | 18400 | 24036 | 3190 | 3490 | 3714 | 844 | 865 | 865 | 364 | 370 | 351 |
| 0.75 *** | 33859 | 40909 | 85855 | 12184 | 14419 | 21184 | 2725 | 2944 | 3250 | 715 | 739 | 754 | 304 | 304 | 310 |
| *** | 36589 | 49324 | 86402 | 13105 | 16534 | 21291 | 2830 | 3079 | 3247 | 724 | 745 | 736 | 304 | 310 | 289 |
| 0.8 *** | 28600 | 35224 | 73054 | 10540 | 12490 | 17920 | 2305 | 2470 | 2704 | 580 | 595 | 604 | 235 | 235 | 235 |
| *** | 31195 | 42844 | 73321 | 11359 | 14269 | 17963 | 2389 | 2575 | 2687 | 589 | 595 | 584 | 235 | 235 | 216 |
| 0.85 *** | 23314 | 29059 | 57805 | 8659 | 10195 | 14044 | 1804 | 1909 | 2050 | 415 | 424 | 430 | . | . | . |
| *** | 25594 | 35425 | 57905 | 9310 | 11539 | 14050 | 1855 | 1975 | 2033 | 424 | 430 | 409 | . | . | . |
| 0.9 *** | 17665 | 22030 | 40144 | 6415 | 7420 | 9565 | 1195 | 1249 | 1309 | . | . | . | . | . | . |
| *** | 19429 | 26614 | 40153 | 6850 | 8239 | 9554 | 1219 | 1279 | 1285 | . | . | . | . | . | . |
| 0.95 *** | 10819 | 13159 | 20080 | 3505 | 3880 | 4495 | . | . | . | . | . | . | . | . | . |
| *** | 11785 | 15340 | 20065 | 3679 | 4144 | 4474 | . | . | . | . | . | . | . | . | . |
| 0.98 *** | 4924 | 5614 | 6910 | . | . | . | . | . | . | . | . | . | . | . | . |
| *** | 5224 | 6139 | 6891 | . | . | . | . | . | . | . | . | . | . | . | . |

## TABLE 1: ALPHA= 0.005 POWER= 0.8    EXPECTED ACCRUAL THRU MINIMUM FOLLOW-UP= 6500

| | DEL=.01 | | | DEL=.02 | | | DEL=.05 | | | DEL=.10 | | | DEL=.15 | | |
|---|---|---|---|---|---|---|---|---|---|---|---|---|---|---|---|
| FACT= | 1.0 / .75 | .50 / .25 | .00 / BIN | 1.0 / .75 | .50 / .25 | .00 / BIN | 1.0 / .75 | .50 / .25 | .00 / BIN | 1.0 / 75 | .50 / .25 | .00 / BIN | 1.0 / .75 | .50 / .25 | .00 / BIN |

PCONT=***      REQUIRED NUMBER OF PATIENTS

| PCONT | | | | | | | | | | | | | | | |
|---|---|---|---|---|---|---|---|---|---|---|---|---|---|---|---|
| 0.01 *** | 1792 | 1792 | 1798 | 655 | 661 | 661 | 216 | 216 | 216 | 108 | 108 | 108 | 76 | 76 | 76 |
| *** | 1792 | 1798 | 6891 | 661 | 661 | 2278 | 216 | 216 | 620 | 108 | 108 | 252 | 76 | 76 | 150 |
| 0.02 *** | 3959 | 3976 | 4018 | 1272 | 1278 | 1288 | 346 | 346 | 346 | 151 | 151 | 151 | 102 | 102 | 102 |
| *** | 3970 | 3992 | 11376 | 1278 | 1278 | 3387 | 346 | 346 | 792 | 151 | 151 | 293 | 102 | 102 | 167 |
| 0.05 *** | 11987 | 12095 | 12556 | 3417 | 3456 | 3515 | 736 | 742 | 742 | 265 | 265 | 265 | 151 | 151 | 151 |
| *** | 12030 | 12231 | 24269 | 3433 | 3482 | 6576 | 742 | 742 | 1285 | 265 | 265 | 409 | 151 | 151 | 216 |
| 0.1 *** | 26460 | 26758 | 29222 | 7177 | 7339 | 7729 | 1402 | 1418 | 1441 | 443 | 443 | 443 | 232 | 232 | 232 |
| *** | 26563 | 27256 | 43890 | 7242 | 7486 | 11423 | 1408 | 1424 | 2033 | 443 | 443 | 584 | 232 | 232 | 289 |
| 0.15 *** | 39557 | 40093 | 46161 | 10583 | 10931 | 11954 | 2009 | 2052 | 2107 | 596 | 606 | 606 | 303 | 303 | 303 |
| *** | 39736 | 41058 | 61175 | 10719 | 11288 | 15685 | 2036 | 2074 | 2687 | 596 | 606 | 736 | 303 | 303 | 351 |
| 0.2 *** | 50158 | 50997 | 62021 | 13395 | 13969 | 15881 | 2546 | 2621 | 2718 | 736 | 742 | 752 | 362 | 368 | 368 |
| *** | 50434 | 52541 | 76124 | 13622 | 14587 | 19364 | 2578 | 2670 | 3247 | 742 | 752 | 865 | 362 | 368 | 403 |
| 0.25 *** | 57952 | 59155 | 76142 | 15540 | 16385 | 19364 | 2978 | 3092 | 3255 | 850 | 866 | 882 | 411 | 417 | 417 |
| *** | 58348 | 61397 | 88737 | 15865 | 17301 | 22459 | 3033 | 3163 | 3714 | 856 | 872 | 970 | 411 | 417 | 444 |
| 0.3 *** | 62957 | 64621 | 88177 | 17051 | 18178 | 22322 | 3320 | 3472 | 3699 | 947 | 963 | 980 | 449 | 449 | 460 |
| *** | 63516 | 67659 | 99015 | 17479 | 19413 | 24970 | 3391 | 3580 | 4088 | 953 | 969 | 1052 | 449 | 460 | 475 |
| 0.35 *** | 65384 | 67594 | 97911 | 17967 | 19391 | 24694 | 3569 | 3764 | 4051 | 1012 | 1028 | 1051 | 476 | 482 | 492 |
| *** | 66126 | 71553 | 106956 | 18519 | 20941 | 26897 | 3661 | 3888 | 4368 | 1018 | 1045 | 1110 | 482 | 482 | 496 |
| 0.4 *** | 65531 | 68391 | 105223 | 18367 | 20090 | 26460 | 3732 | 3959 | 4311 | 1051 | 1077 | 1110 | 492 | 498 | 508 |
| *** | 66500 | 73357 | 112562 | 19039 | 21932 | 28240 | 3840 | 4116 | 4555 | 1067 | 1093 | 1145 | 498 | 498 | 507 |
| 0.45 *** | 63737 | 67367 | 110050 | 18335 | 20323 | 27603 | 3807 | 4067 | 4463 | 1077 | 1099 | 1132 | 498 | 508 | 508 |
| *** | 64978 | 73379 | 115833 | 19121 | 22430 | 28999 | 3927 | 4236 | 4649 | 1083 | 1116 | 1157 | 498 | 508 | 507 |
| 0.5 *** | 60422 | 64913 | 112347 | 17934 | 20161 | 28117 | 3813 | 4083 | 4512 | 1067 | 1099 | 1132 | 492 | 498 | 508 |
| *** | 61982 | 71933 | 116767 | 18828 | 22468 | 29175 | 3937 | 4268 | 4649 | 1083 | 1116 | 1145 | 498 | 498 | 496 |
| 0.55 *** | 55986 | 61387 | 112113 | 17252 | 19651 | 27993 | 3742 | 4024 | 4463 | 1045 | 1077 | 1110 | 476 | 482 | 492 |
| *** | 57909 | 69301 | 115365 | 18221 | 22088 | 28766 | 3872 | 4213 | 4555 | 1061 | 1093 | 1110 | 476 | 482 | 475 |
| 0.6 *** | 50867 | 57123 | 109335 | 16326 | 18828 | 27240 | 3596 | 3878 | 4311 | 996 | 1028 | 1061 | 449 | 449 | 460 |
| *** | 53148 | 65703 | 111628 | 17343 | 21314 | 27773 | 3726 | 4067 | 4368 | 1012 | 1045 | 1052 | 449 | 460 | 444 |
| 0.65 *** | 45429 | 52352 | 104021 | 15215 | 17717 | 25842 | 3385 | 3651 | 4057 | 931 | 953 | 980 | 411 | 417 | 417 |
| *** | 48023 | 61289 | 105555 | 16238 | 20171 | 26196 | 3504 | 3829 | 4088 | 937 | 969 | 970 | 411 | 417 | 403 |
| 0.7 *** | 39963 | 47233 | 96188 | 13915 | 16336 | 23827 | 3108 | 3352 | 3710 | 833 | 856 | 882 | 362 | 368 | 368 |
| *** | 42742 | 56171 | 97146 | 14912 | 18649 | 24036 | 3222 | 3504 | 3714 | 850 | 866 | 865 | 362 | 368 | 351 |
| 0.75 *** | 34585 | 41822 | 85859 | 12442 | 14678 | 21178 | 2757 | 2962 | 3255 | 720 | 736 | 758 | 303 | 303 | 313 |
| *** | 37396 | 50353 | 86402 | 13368 | 16758 | 21291 | 2854 | 3092 | 3247 | 726 | 742 | 736 | 303 | 313 | 289 |
| 0.8 *** | 29293 | 36063 | 73054 | 10768 | 12712 | 17918 | 2328 | 2491 | 2702 | 579 | 596 | 606 | 232 | 238 | 238 |
| *** | 31958 | 43756 | 73321 | 11581 | 14451 | 17963 | 2399 | 2588 | 2687 | 590 | 596 | 584 | 238 | 238 | 216 |
| 0.85 *** | 23931 | 29775 | 57812 | 8845 | 10372 | 14045 | 1814 | 1922 | 2052 | 417 | 427 | 433 | . | . | . |
| *** | 26254 | 36167 | 57905 | 9495 | 11672 | 14050 | 1863 | 1977 | 2033 | 417 | 427 | 409 | . | . | . |
| 0.9 *** | 18146 | 22560 | 40142 | 6537 | 7528 | 9566 | 1197 | 1246 | 1305 | . | . | . | . | . | . |
| *** | 19933 | 27132 | 40153 | 6966 | 8314 | 9554 | 1223 | 1278 | 1285 | . | . | . | . | . | . |
| 0.95 *** | 11087 | 13427 | 20079 | 3553 | 3921 | 4496 | . | . | . | . | . | . | . | . | . |
| *** | 12062 | 15572 | 20065 | 3716 | 4171 | 4474 | . | . | . | . | . | . | . | . | . |
| 0.98 *** | 5010 | 5682 | 6911 | . | . | . | . | . | . | . | . | . | . | . | . |
| *** | 5308 | 6186 | 6891 | . | . | . | . | . | . | . | . | . | . | . | . |

TABLE 1: ALPHA= 0.005 POWER= 0.8    EXPECTED ACCRUAL THRU MINIMUM FOLLOW-UP= 7000

| | DEL=.01 | | | DEL=.02 | | | DEL=.05 | | | DEL=.10 | | | DEL=.15 | | |
|---|---|---|---|---|---|---|---|---|---|---|---|---|---|---|---|
| FACT= | 1.0 .75 | .50 .25 | .00 BIN | 1.0 .75 | .50 .25 | .00 BIN | 1.0 .75 | .50 .25 | .00 BIN | 1.0 75 | .50 .25 | .00 BIN | 1.0 .75 | .50 .25 | .00 BIN |
| PCONT=*** | | | REQUIRED NUMBER OF PATIENTS | | | | | | | | | | | | |
| 0.01 *** | 1790 | 1796 | 1796 | 659 | 659 | 659 | 215 | 215 | 215 | 110 | 110 | 110 | 75 | 75 | 75 |
| *** | 1790 | 1796 | 6891 | 659 | 659 | 2278 | 215 | 215 | 620 | 110 | 110 | 252 | 75 | 75 | 150 |
| 0.02 *** | 3960 | 3984 | 4019 | 1271 | 1282 | 1282 | 344 | 344 | 344 | 151 | 151 | 151 | 99 | 99 | 99 |
| *** | 3966 | 3995 | 11376 | 1271 | 1282 | 3387 | 344 | 344 | 792 | 151 | 151 | 293 | 99 | 99 | 167 |
| 0.05 *** | 11999 | 12115 | 12552 | 3417 | 3459 | 3522 | 740 | 740 | 746 | 267 | 267 | 267 | 151 | 151 | 151 |
| *** | 12034 | 12244 | 24269 | 3435 | 3487 | 6576 | 740 | 746 | 1285 | 267 | 267 | 409 | 151 | 151 | 216 |
| 0.1 *** | 26482 | 26804 | 29219 | 7197 | 7361 | 7729 | 1405 | 1422 | 1440 | 442 | 442 | 442 | 232 | 232 | 232 |
| *** | 26594 | 27322 | 43890 | 7267 | 7501 | 11423 | 1411 | 1429 | 2033 | 442 | 442 | 584 | 232 | 232 | 289 |
| 0.15 *** | 39596 | 40174 | 46170 | 10616 | 10977 | 11957 | 2017 | 2059 | 2111 | 600 | 600 | 606 | 302 | 302 | 309 |
| *** | 39789 | 41189 | 61175 | 10756 | 11316 | 15685 | 2035 | 2076 | 2687 | 600 | 606 | 736 | 302 | 302 | 351 |
| 0.2 *** | 50219 | 51122 | 62025 | 13445 | 14040 | 15884 | 2549 | 2619 | 2717 | 740 | 746 | 757 | 361 | 361 | 372 |
| *** | 50516 | 52750 | 76124 | 13679 | 14652 | 19364 | 2584 | 2671 | 3247 | 740 | 746 | 865 | 361 | 361 | 403 |
| 0.25 *** | 58041 | 59336 | 76147 | 15621 | 16479 | 19366 | 2997 | 3102 | 3260 | 851 | 862 | 880 | 414 | 414 | 414 |
| *** | 58479 | 61699 | 88737 | 15954 | 17400 | 22459 | 3050 | 3172 | 3714 | 862 | 869 | 970 | 414 | 414 | 444 |
| 0.3 *** | 63092 | 64866 | 88176 | 17155 | 18310 | 22317 | 3336 | 3487 | 3704 | 950 | 956 | 974 | 449 | 449 | 460 |
| *** | 63687 | 68080 | 99015 | 17599 | 19541 | 24970 | 3406 | 3581 | 4088 | 950 | 967 | 1052 | 449 | 460 | 475 |
| 0.35 *** | 65560 | 67922 | 97906 | 18100 | 19559 | 24697 | 3592 | 3785 | 4054 | 1009 | 1037 | 1055 | 477 | 484 | 484 |
| *** | 66534 | 72087 | 106956 | 18666 | 21110 | 26897 | 3680 | 3896 | 4368 | 1020 | 1044 | 1110 | 477 | 484 | 496 |
| 0.4 *** | 65752 | 68815 | 105221 | 18537 | 20287 | 26465 | 3756 | 3977 | 4310 | 1055 | 1079 | 1107 | 495 | 501 | 501 |
| *** | 66791 | 74012 | 112562 | 19226 | 22125 | 28240 | 3861 | 4124 | 4555 | 1072 | 1090 | 1145 | 495 | 501 | 507 |
| 0.45 *** | 64026 | 67894 | 110051 | 18526 | 20550 | 27609 | 3844 | 4089 | 4456 | 1079 | 1107 | 1131 | 501 | 501 | 512 |
| *** | 65356 | 74152 | 115833 | 19331 | 22639 | 28999 | 3949 | 4246 | 4649 | 1090 | 1114 | 1157 | 501 | 512 | 507 |
| 0.5 *** | 60782 | 65549 | 112355 | 18159 | 20410 | 28116 | 3844 | 4106 | 4509 | 1072 | 1107 | 1131 | 495 | 501 | 501 |
| *** | 62451 | 72811 | 116767 | 19062 | 22702 | 29175 | 3966 | 4281 | 4649 | 1090 | 1114 | 1145 | 495 | 501 | 496 |
| 0.55 *** | 56442 | 62119 | 112210 | 17494 | 19920 | 27994 | 3774 | 4047 | 4467 | 1055 | 1079 | 1107 | 477 | 484 | 484 |
| *** | 58472 | 70267 | 115365 | 18474 | 22335 | 28766 | 3896 | 4229 | 4555 | 1061 | 1090 | 1110 | 477 | 484 | 475 |
| 0.6 *** | 51409 | 57936 | 109327 | 16584 | 19097 | 27235 | 3634 | 3907 | 4310 | 1002 | 1026 | 1055 | 449 | 460 | 460 |
| *** | 53806 | 66721 | 111628 | 17610 | 21565 | 27773 | 3756 | 4082 | 4368 | 1020 | 1044 | 1052 | 449 | 460 | 444 |
| 0.65 *** | 46054 | 53222 | 104014 | 15475 | 17984 | 25841 | 3417 | 3680 | 4054 | 932 | 956 | 985 | 414 | 414 | 425 |
| *** | 48760 | 62340 | 105555 | 16507 | 20410 | 26196 | 3540 | 3844 | 4088 | 939 | 967 | 970 | 414 | 414 | 403 |
| 0.7 *** | 40640 | 48119 | 96185 | 14169 | 16595 | 23822 | 3137 | 3371 | 3704 | 834 | 862 | 880 | 361 | 372 | 372 |
| *** | 43516 | 57195 | 97146 | 15166 | 18876 | 24036 | 3242 | 3522 | 3714 | 851 | 869 | 865 | 361 | 372 | 351 |
| 0.75 *** | 35285 | 42676 | 85860 | 12675 | 14915 | 21180 | 2787 | 2980 | 3249 | 722 | 740 | 757 | 302 | 309 | 309 |
| *** | 38172 | 51315 | 86402 | 13609 | 16962 | 21291 | 2875 | 3102 | 3247 | 729 | 746 | 736 | 302 | 309 | 289 |
| 0.8 *** | 29965 | 36849 | 73056 | 10977 | 12909 | 17914 | 2350 | 2496 | 2700 | 582 | 589 | 606 | 232 | 239 | 239 |
| *** | 32677 | 44612 | 73321 | 11789 | 14617 | 17963 | 2420 | 2595 | 2687 | 589 | 600 | 584 | 232 | 239 | 216 |
| 0.85 *** | 24522 | 30444 | 57807 | 9006 | 10522 | 14046 | 1831 | 1930 | 2052 | 425 | 425 | 431 | . | . | . |
| *** | 26885 | 36860 | 57905 | 9654 | 11789 | 14050 | 1877 | 1989 | 2033 | 425 | 431 | 409 | . | . | . |
| 0.9 *** | 18596 | 23052 | 40139 | 6644 | 7624 | 9566 | 1212 | 1254 | 1306 | . | . | . | . | . | . |
| *** | 20399 | 27609 | 40153 | 7075 | 8387 | 9554 | 1230 | 1282 | 1285 | . | . | . | . | . | . |
| 0.95 *** | 11334 | 13661 | 20084 | 3599 | 3949 | 4491 | . | . | . | . | . | . | . | . | . |
| *** | 12314 | 15779 | 20065 | 3756 | 4187 | 4474 | . | . | . | . | . | . | . | . | . |
| 0.98 *** | 5086 | 5745 | 6917 | . | . | . | . | . | . | . | . | . | . | . | . |
| *** | 5377 | 6224 | 6891 | . | . | . | . | . | . | . | . | . | . | . | . |

## TABLE 1: ALPHA= 0.005 POWER= 0.8    EXPECTED ACCRUAL THRU MINIMUM FOLLOW-UP= 7500

|  |  | DEL=.01 | | | DEL=.02 | | | DEL=.05 | | | DEL=.10 | | | DEL=.15 | | |
|---|---|---|---|---|---|---|---|---|---|---|---|---|---|---|---|---|
| FACT= | | 1.0 .75 | .50 .25 | .00 BIN | 1.0 .75 | .50 .25 | .00 BIN | 1.0 .75 | .50 .25 | .00 BIN | 1.0 75 | .50 .25 | .00 BIN | 1.0 .75 | .50 .25 | .00 BIN |
| PCONT=*** | | | | | | | REQUIRED NUMBER OF PATIENTS | | | | | | | | | |
| 0.01 | *** | 1793 | 1793 | 1805 | 661 | 661 | 661 | 218 | 218 | 218 | 106 | 106 | 106 | 80 | 80 | 80 |
|  | *** | 1793 | 1793 | 6891 | 661 | 661 | 2278 | 218 | 218 | 620 | 106 | 106 | 252 | 80 | 80 | 150 |
| 0.02 | *** | 3961 | 3980 | 4018 | 1268 | 1280 | 1280 | 343 | 343 | 343 | 155 | 155 | 155 | 99 | 99 | 99 |
|  | *** | 3968 | 3999 | 11376 | 1280 | 1280 | 3387 | 343 | 343 | 792 | 155 | 155 | 293 | 99 | 99 | 167 |
| 0.05 | *** | 12005 | 12125 | 12556 | 3425 | 3462 | 3518 | 736 | 743 | 743 | 268 | 268 | 268 | 155 | 155 | 155 |
|  | *** | 12050 | 12256 | 24269 | 3436 | 3481 | 6576 | 743 | 743 | 1285 | 268 | 268 | 409 | 155 | 155 | 216 |
| 0.1 | *** | 26506 | 26843 | 29225 | 7212 | 7374 | 7730 | 1400 | 1418 | 1437 | 436 | 443 | 443 | 230 | 237 | 237 |
|  | *** | 26618 | 27380 | 43890 | 7280 | 7512 | 11423 | 1411 | 1430 | 2033 | 443 | 443 | 584 | 230 | 237 | 289 |
| 0.15 | *** | 39643 | 40250 | 46168 | 10655 | 11011 | 11956 | 2018 | 2056 | 2105 | 593 | 605 | 605 | 305 | 305 | 305 |
|  | *** | 39849 | 41318 | 61175 | 10793 | 11349 | 15685 | 2037 | 2086 | 2687 | 605 | 605 | 736 | 305 | 305 | 351 |
| 0.2 | *** | 50281 | 51249 | 62018 | 13505 | 14105 | 15886 | 2562 | 2630 | 2724 | 736 | 743 | 755 | 361 | 368 | 368 |
|  | *** | 50611 | 52955 | 76124 | 13737 | 14705 | 19364 | 2593 | 2675 | 3247 | 743 | 755 | 865 | 361 | 368 | 403 |
| 0.25 | *** | 58137 | 59518 | 76149 | 15699 | 16580 | 19362 | 3005 | 3106 | 3256 | 856 | 868 | 875 | 418 | 418 | 418 |
|  | *** | 58599 | 62000 | 88737 | 16043 | 17480 | 22459 | 3050 | 3174 | 3714 | 856 | 875 | 970 | 418 | 418 | 444 |
| 0.3 | *** | 63218 | 65124 | 88175 | 17255 | 18436 | 22318 | 3361 | 3500 | 3699 | 950 | 961 | 980 | 455 | 455 | 455 |
|  | *** | 63856 | 68480 | 99015 | 17724 | 19655 | 24970 | 3425 | 3593 | 4088 | 950 | 968 | 1052 | 455 | 455 | 475 |
| 0.35 | *** | 65731 | 68255 | 97906 | 18230 | 19711 | 24699 | 3612 | 3793 | 4055 | 1018 | 1036 | 1055 | 481 | 481 | 493 |
|  | *** | 66586 | 72605 | 106956 | 18818 | 21249 | 26897 | 3699 | 3912 | 4368 | 1025 | 1043 | 1110 | 481 | 481 | 496 |
| 0.4 | *** | 65975 | 69230 | 105218 | 18687 | 20468 | 26461 | 3781 | 3999 | 4306 | 1062 | 1081 | 1111 | 493 | 500 | 500 |
|  | *** | 67081 | 74637 | 112562 | 19400 | 22299 | 28240 | 3886 | 4137 | 4555 | 1074 | 1093 | 1145 | 500 | 500 | 507 |
| 0.45 | *** | 64318 | 68412 | 110049 | 18718 | 20761 | 27605 | 3868 | 4111 | 4456 | 1081 | 1100 | 1130 | 500 | 500 | 511 |
|  | *** | 65731 | 74893 | 115833 | 19531 | 22843 | 28999 | 3980 | 4261 | 4649 | 1093 | 1118 | 1157 | 500 | 511 | 507 |
| 0.5 | *** | 61149 | 66162 | 112355 | 18368 | 20649 | 28118 | 3875 | 4130 | 4512 | 1081 | 1100 | 1130 | 493 | 500 | 500 |
|  | *** | 62911 | 73643 | 116767 | 19287 | 22918 | 29175 | 3987 | 4299 | 4649 | 1093 | 1118 | 1145 | 500 | 500 | 496 |
| 0.55 | *** | 56881 | 62836 | 112111 | 17724 | 20161 | 27999 | 3800 | 4074 | 4468 | 1055 | 1081 | 1111 | 474 | 481 | 493 |
|  | *** | 59030 | 71180 | 115365 | 18718 | 22561 | 28766 | 3924 | 4243 | 4555 | 1062 | 1093 | 1110 | 481 | 481 | 475 |
| 0.6 | *** | 51943 | 58718 | 109325 | 16831 | 19355 | 27237 | 3661 | 3924 | 4306 | 1006 | 1025 | 1055 | 455 | 455 | 462 |
|  | *** | 54455 | 67681 | 111628 | 17862 | 21793 | 27773 | 3781 | 4100 | 4368 | 1018 | 1043 | 1052 | 455 | 455 | 444 |
| 0.65 | *** | 46662 | 54061 | 104018 | 15718 | 18237 | 25843 | 3455 | 3699 | 4055 | 931 | 961 | 980 | 418 | 418 | 425 |
|  | *** | 49468 | 63312 | 105555 | 16756 | 20630 | 26196 | 3568 | 3856 | 4088 | 943 | 968 | 970 | 418 | 418 | 403 |
| 0.7 | *** | 41300 | 48968 | 96181 | 14405 | 16831 | 23825 | 3162 | 3387 | 3706 | 837 | 856 | 886 | 361 | 368 | 368 |
|  | *** | 44255 | 58156 | 97146 | 15418 | 19081 | 24036 | 3268 | 3530 | 3714 | 849 | 868 | 865 | 368 | 368 | 351 |
| 0.75 | *** | 35949 | 43493 | 85861 | 12905 | 15125 | 21181 | 2806 | 2993 | 3249 | 725 | 736 | 755 | 305 | 305 | 312 |
|  | *** | 38900 | 52212 | 86402 | 13831 | 17143 | 21291 | 2893 | 3106 | 3247 | 736 | 743 | 736 | 305 | 305 | 289 |
| 0.8 | *** | 30593 | 37587 | 73055 | 11168 | 13093 | 17918 | 2368 | 2518 | 2705 | 586 | 593 | 605 | 237 | 237 | 237 |
|  | *** | 33361 | 45406 | 73321 | 11986 | 14768 | 17963 | 2431 | 2600 | 2687 | 586 | 605 | 584 | 237 | 237 | 216 |
| 0.85 | *** | 25074 | 31062 | 57811 | 9162 | 10662 | 14049 | 1843 | 1936 | 2049 | 418 | 425 | 436 | . | . | . |
|  | *** | 27474 | 37505 | 57905 | 9811 | 11900 | 14050 | 1887 | 1993 | 2033 | 425 | 425 | 409 | . | . | . |
| 0.9 | *** | 19025 | 23506 | 40137 | 6755 | 7711 | 9568 | 1212 | 1261 | 1306 | . | . | . | . | . | . |
|  | *** | 20843 | 28055 | 40153 | 7175 | 8443 | 9554 | 1231 | 1280 | 1285 | . | . | . | . | . | . |
| 0.95 | *** | 11574 | 13887 | 20086 | 3643 | 3980 | 4493 | . | . | . | . | . | . | . | . | . |
|  | *** | 12549 | 15968 | 20065 | 3793 | 4205 | 4474 | . | . | . | . | . | . | . | . | . |
| 0.98 | *** | 5161 | 5806 | 6912 | . | . | . | . | . | . | . | . | . | . | . | . |
|  | *** | 5450 | 6268 | 6891 | . | . | . | . | . | . | . | . | . | . | . | . |

## TABLE 1: ALPHA= 0.005 POWER= 0.8    EXPECTED ACCRUAL THRU MINIMUM FOLLOW-UP= 8000

| | | DEL=.01 | | | DEL=.02 | | | DEL=.05 | | | DEL=.10 | | | DEL=.15 | | |
|---|---|---|---|---|---|---|---|---|---|---|---|---|---|---|---|---|
| FACT= | | 1.0 .75 | .50 .25 | .00 BIN | 1.0 .75 | .50 .25 | .00 BIN | 1.0 .75 | .50 .25 | .00 BIN | 1.0 75 | .50 .25 | .00 BIN | 1.0 .75 | .50 .25 | .00 BIN |
| PCONT=*** | | | | | REQUIRED NUMBER OF PATIENTS | | | | | | | | | | | |
| 0.01 | *** | 1793 | 1793 | 1805 | 653 | 653 | 653 | 213 | 213 | 213 | 105 | 105 | 105 | 73 | 73 | 73 |
| | *** | 1793 | 1793 | 6891 | 653 | 653 | 2278 | 213 | 213 | 620 | 105 | 105 | 252 | 73 | 73 | 150 |
| 0.02 | *** | 3965 | 3985 | 4013 | 1273 | 1273 | 1285 | 345 | 345 | 345 | 153 | 153 | 153 | 93 | 93 | 93 |
| | *** | 3973 | 3993 | 11376 | 1273 | 1285 | 3387 | 345 | 345 | 792 | 153 | 153 | 293 | 93 | 93 | 167 |
| 0.05 | *** | 12013 | 12133 | 12553 | 3425 | 3465 | 3513 | 733 | 745 | 745 | 265 | 265 | 265 | 153 | 153 | 153 |
| | *** | 12065 | 12273 | 24269 | 3445 | 3485 | 6576 | 745 | 745 | 1285 | 265 | 265 | 409 | 153 | 153 | 216 |
| 0.1 | *** | 26533 | 26885 | 29225 | 7225 | 7393 | 7725 | 1405 | 1425 | 1433 | 445 | 445 | 445 | 233 | 233 | 233 |
| | *** | 26653 | 27433 | 43890 | 7293 | 7525 | 11423 | 1413 | 1425 | 2033 | 445 | 445 | 584 | 233 | 233 | 289 |
| 0.15 | *** | 39685 | 40333 | 46165 | 10685 | 11045 | 11953 | 2025 | 2065 | 2105 | 605 | 605 | 605 | 305 | 305 | 305 |
| | *** | 39905 | 41433 | 61175 | 10833 | 11385 | 15685 | 2045 | 2085 | 2687 | 605 | 605 | 736 | 305 | 305 | 351 |
| 0.2 | *** | 50345 | 51373 | 62025 | 13553 | 14165 | 15885 | 2565 | 2633 | 2725 | 733 | 745 | 753 | 365 | 365 | 365 |
| | *** | 50693 | 53153 | 76124 | 13793 | 14753 | 19364 | 2605 | 2673 | 3247 | 745 | 753 | 865 | 365 | 365 | 403 |
| 0.25 | *** | 58225 | 59705 | 76145 | 15773 | 16665 | 19365 | 3013 | 3113 | 3253 | 853 | 865 | 873 | 413 | 413 | 413 |
| | *** | 58725 | 62285 | 88737 | 16125 | 17565 | 22459 | 3065 | 3185 | 3714 | 865 | 873 | 970 | 413 | 413 | 444 |
| 0.3 | *** | 63345 | 65365 | 88173 | 17353 | 18545 | 22313 | 3373 | 3513 | 3705 | 945 | 965 | 973 | 453 | 453 | 453 |
| | *** | 64025 | 68865 | 99015 | 17825 | 19765 | 24970 | 3433 | 3593 | 4088 | 953 | 973 | 1052 | 453 | 453 | 475 |
| 0.35 | *** | 65905 | 68573 | 97905 | 18353 | 19853 | 24693 | 3633 | 3805 | 4053 | 1013 | 1033 | 1053 | 473 | 485 | 485 |
| | *** | 66805 | 73093 | 106956 | 18953 | 21385 | 26897 | 3713 | 3913 | 4368 | 1025 | 1045 | 1110 | 485 | 485 | 496 |
| 0.4 | *** | 66193 | 69645 | 105225 | 18845 | 20645 | 26465 | 3805 | 4013 | 4305 | 1065 | 1085 | 1105 | 493 | 505 | 505 |
| | *** | 67373 | 75233 | 112562 | 19565 | 22453 | 28240 | 3905 | 4145 | 4555 | 1073 | 1093 | 1145 | 493 | 505 | 507 |
| 0.45 | *** | 64593 | 68913 | 110045 | 18893 | 20965 | 27605 | 3893 | 4125 | 4465 | 1085 | 1105 | 1133 | 505 | 505 | 513 |
| | *** | 66105 | 75593 | 115833 | 19725 | 23025 | 28999 | 4005 | 4273 | 4649 | 1093 | 1113 | 1157 | 505 | 505 | 507 |
| 0.5 | *** | 61505 | 66765 | 112353 | 18573 | 20865 | 28113 | 3905 | 4153 | 4513 | 1085 | 1105 | 1133 | 493 | 505 | 505 |
| | *** | 63365 | 74445 | 116767 | 19505 | 23113 | 29175 | 4013 | 4313 | 4649 | 1093 | 1113 | 1145 | 493 | 505 | 496 |
| 0.55 | *** | 57325 | 63525 | 112113 | 17945 | 20393 | 27993 | 3833 | 4093 | 4465 | 1053 | 1085 | 1105 | 473 | 485 | 485 |
| | *** | 59573 | 72045 | 115365 | 18945 | 22765 | 28766 | 3953 | 4253 | 4555 | 1065 | 1093 | 1110 | 485 | 485 | 475 |
| 0.6 | *** | 52465 | 59473 | 109333 | 17053 | 19585 | 27233 | 3693 | 3945 | 4313 | 1005 | 1033 | 1053 | 453 | 453 | 465 |
| | *** | 55073 | 68593 | 111628 | 18093 | 22005 | 27773 | 3805 | 4105 | 4368 | 1025 | 1045 | 1052 | 453 | 453 | 444 |
| 0.65 | *** | 47253 | 54853 | 104013 | 15945 | 18473 | 25845 | 3473 | 3713 | 4053 | 933 | 953 | 985 | 413 | 413 | 425 |
| | *** | 50145 | 64245 | 105555 | 16993 | 20833 | 26196 | 3585 | 3873 | 4088 | 945 | 973 | 970 | 413 | 413 | 403 |
| 0.7 | *** | 41933 | 49765 | 96185 | 14633 | 17053 | 23825 | 3193 | 3405 | 3705 | 845 | 865 | 885 | 365 | 365 | 365 |
| | *** | 44965 | 59053 | 97146 | 15645 | 19273 | 24036 | 3293 | 3545 | 3714 | 853 | 873 | 865 | 365 | 373 | 351 |
| 0.75 | *** | 36585 | 44273 | 85853 | 13105 | 15325 | 21185 | 2825 | 3005 | 3253 | 725 | 745 | 753 | 305 | 305 | 313 |
| | *** | 39593 | 53053 | 86402 | 14045 | 17305 | 21291 | 2913 | 3125 | 3247 | 733 | 745 | 736 | 305 | 305 | 289 |
| 0.8 | *** | 31193 | 38293 | 73053 | 11353 | 13265 | 17913 | 2385 | 2525 | 2705 | 585 | 593 | 605 | 233 | 233 | 233 |
| | *** | 34013 | 46145 | 73321 | 12165 | 14905 | 17963 | 2453 | 2605 | 2687 | 593 | 605 | 584 | 233 | 233 | 216 |
| 0.85 | *** | 25593 | 31653 | 57805 | 9313 | 10785 | 14045 | 1853 | 1945 | 2053 | 425 | 425 | 433 | . | . | . |
| | *** | 28105 | 38105 | 57905 | 9945 | 12005 | 14050 | 1893 | 1993 | 2033 | 425 | 425 | 409 | . | . | . |
| 0.9 | *** | 19425 | 23933 | 40145 | 6845 | 7793 | 9565 | 1213 | 1265 | 1305 | . | . | . | . | . | . |
| | *** | 21265 | 28453 | 40153 | 7265 | 8505 | 9554 | 1233 | 1285 | 1285 | . | . | . | . | . | . |
| 0.95 | *** | 11785 | 14093 | 20085 | 3673 | 4005 | 4493 | . | . | . | . | . | . | . | . | . |
| | *** | 12765 | 16133 | 20065 | 3825 | 4225 | 4474 | . | . | . | . | . | . | . | . | . |
| 0.98 | *** | 5225 | 5853 | 6913 | . | . | . | . | . | . | . | . | . | . | . | . |
| | *** | 5505 | 6293 | 6891 | . | . | . | . | . | . | . | . | . | . | . | . |

# TABLE 1: ALPHA= 0.005 POWER= 0.8     EXPECTED ACCRUAL THRU MINIMUM FOLLOW-UP= 8500

| PCONT | FACT | DEL=.01 1.0 .75 | .50 .25 | .00 BIN | DEL=.02 1.0 .75 | .50 .25 | .00 BIN | DEL=.05 1.0 .75 | .50 .25 | .00 BIN | DEL=.10 1.0 75 | .50 .25 | .00 BIN | DEL=.15 1.0 .75 | .50 .25 | .00 BIN |
|---|---|---|---|---|---|---|---|---|---|---|---|---|---|---|---|---|
| PCONT=*** | | | | REQUIRED NUMBER OF PATIENTS | | | | | | | | | | | |
| 0.01 | *** | 1791 | 1799 | 1799 | 651 | 665 | 665 | 218 | 218 | 218 | 112 | 112 | 112 | 78 | 78 | 78 |
|  | *** | 1791 | 1799 | 6891 | 651 | 665 | 2278 | 218 | 218 | 620 | 112 | 112 | 252 | 78 | 78 | 150 |
| 0.02 | *** | 3966 | 3988 | 4022 | 1281 | 1281 | 1281 | 346 | 346 | 346 | 155 | 155 | 155 | 99 | 99 | 99 |
|  | *** | 3980 | 4001 | 11376 | 1281 | 1281 | 3387 | 346 | 346 | 792 | 155 | 155 | 293 | 99 | 99 | 167 |
| 0.05 | *** | 12020 | 12148 | 12551 | 3427 | 3470 | 3520 | 736 | 736 | 750 | 261 | 261 | 261 | 155 | 155 | 155 |
|  | *** | 12076 | 12288 | 24269 | 3448 | 3491 | 6576 | 736 | 750 | 1285 | 261 | 261 | 409 | 155 | 155 | 216 |
| 0.1 | *** | 26555 | 26930 | 29225 | 7239 | 7401 | 7728 | 1408 | 1416 | 1438 | 439 | 439 | 439 | 240 | 240 | 240 |
|  | *** | 26683 | 27482 | 43890 | 7316 | 7536 | 11423 | 1416 | 1430 | 2033 | 439 | 439 | 584 | 240 | 240 | 289 |
| 0.15 | *** | 39722 | 40410 | 46161 | 10716 | 11077 | 11956 | 2033 | 2067 | 2110 | 601 | 601 | 609 | 303 | 303 | 303 |
|  | *** | 39956 | 41550 | 61175 | 10865 | 11404 | 15685 | 2046 | 2088 | 2687 | 601 | 609 | 736 | 303 | 303 | 351 |
| 0.2 | *** | 50411 | 51495 | 62021 | 13606 | 14222 | 15880 | 2577 | 2641 | 2726 | 736 | 750 | 750 | 367 | 367 | 367 |
|  | *** | 50780 | 53343 | 76124 | 13848 | 14804 | 19364 | 2606 | 2670 | 3247 | 736 | 750 | 865 | 367 | 367 | 403 |
| 0.25 | *** | 58324 | 59875 | 76145 | 15845 | 16751 | 19365 | 3031 | 3130 | 3257 | 856 | 864 | 877 | 410 | 418 | 418 |
|  | *** | 58847 | 62566 | 88737 | 16206 | 17630 | 22459 | 3074 | 3180 | 3714 | 864 | 877 | 970 | 418 | 418 | 444 |
| 0.3 | *** | 63466 | 65613 | 88172 | 17452 | 18663 | 22318 | 3385 | 3520 | 3703 | 949 | 962 | 983 | 452 | 452 | 460 |
|  | *** | 64202 | 69238 | 99015 | 17928 | 19861 | 24970 | 3448 | 3605 | 4088 | 962 | 970 | 1052 | 452 | 460 | 475 |
| 0.35 | *** | 66072 | 68898 | 97905 | 18480 | 20002 | 24698 | 3648 | 3818 | 4051 | 1026 | 1034 | 1055 | 481 | 481 | 481 |
|  | *** | 67036 | 73573 | 106956 | 19088 | 21511 | 26897 | 3733 | 3924 | 4368 | 1026 | 1047 | 1110 | 481 | 481 | 496 |
| 0.4 | *** | 66420 | 70046 | 105223 | 18990 | 20810 | 26462 | 3831 | 4030 | 4306 | 1068 | 1090 | 1111 | 495 | 503 | 503 |
|  | *** | 67666 | 75813 | 112562 | 19726 | 22603 | 28240 | 3916 | 4150 | 4555 | 1076 | 1098 | 1145 | 495 | 503 | 507 |
| 0.45 | *** | 64882 | 69408 | 110046 | 19067 | 21150 | 27610 | 3916 | 4136 | 4455 | 1090 | 1111 | 1132 | 503 | 503 | 516 |
|  | *** | 66463 | 76272 | 115833 | 19904 | 23190 | 28999 | 4022 | 4285 | 4649 | 1098 | 1119 | 1157 | 503 | 503 | 507 |
| 0.5 | *** | 61865 | 67347 | 112355 | 18770 | 21065 | 28120 | 3924 | 4171 | 4511 | 1090 | 1111 | 1132 | 495 | 503 | 503 |
|  | *** | 63820 | 75210 | 116767 | 19705 | 23296 | 29175 | 4043 | 4320 | 4649 | 1098 | 1119 | 1145 | 495 | 503 | 496 |
| 0.55 | *** | 57763 | 64181 | 112108 | 18153 | 20605 | 27992 | 3860 | 4107 | 4468 | 1055 | 1076 | 1111 | 481 | 481 | 495 |
|  | *** | 60109 | 72872 | 115365 | 19160 | 22956 | 28766 | 3980 | 4264 | 4555 | 1068 | 1098 | 1110 | 481 | 481 | 475 |
| 0.6 | *** | 52982 | 60207 | 109324 | 17269 | 19811 | 27235 | 3711 | 3966 | 4306 | 1013 | 1034 | 1055 | 452 | 452 | 460 |
|  | *** | 55681 | 69459 | 111628 | 18323 | 22191 | 27773 | 3831 | 4115 | 4368 | 1026 | 1047 | 1052 | 452 | 460 | 444 |
| 0.65 | *** | 47840 | 55617 | 104011 | 16164 | 18693 | 25846 | 3499 | 3733 | 4051 | 941 | 962 | 983 | 410 | 418 | 418 |
|  | *** | 50801 | 65116 | 105555 | 17218 | 21022 | 26196 | 3605 | 3881 | 4088 | 949 | 970 | 970 | 418 | 418 | 403 |
| 0.7 | *** | 42548 | 50538 | 96183 | 14838 | 17261 | 23827 | 3215 | 3414 | 3703 | 843 | 864 | 877 | 367 | 367 | 367 |
|  | *** | 45638 | 59910 | 97146 | 15858 | 19450 | 24036 | 3308 | 3555 | 3714 | 856 | 877 | 865 | 367 | 367 | 351 |
| 0.75 | *** | 37201 | 45000 | 85856 | 13308 | 15518 | 21179 | 2840 | 3023 | 3257 | 728 | 736 | 758 | 303 | 311 | 311 |
|  | *** | 40261 | 53853 | 86402 | 14230 | 17460 | 21291 | 2925 | 3130 | 3247 | 736 | 750 | 736 | 303 | 311 | 289 |
| 0.8 | *** | 31775 | 38965 | 73050 | 11523 | 13415 | 17920 | 2394 | 2535 | 2705 | 588 | 601 | 609 | 240 | 240 | 240 |
|  | *** | 34630 | 46841 | 73321 | 12331 | 15030 | 17963 | 2458 | 2606 | 2687 | 588 | 601 | 584 | 240 | 240 | 216 |
| 0.85 | *** | 26101 | 32221 | 57806 | 9449 | 10907 | 14052 | 1863 | 1948 | 2054 | 418 | 431 | 431 | . | . | . |
|  | *** | 28553 | 38660 | 57905 | 10078 | 12084 | 14050 | 1905 | 2003 | 2033 | 418 | 431 | 409 | . | . | . |
| 0.9 | *** | 19811 | 24337 | 40147 | 6941 | 7855 | 9568 | 1225 | 1260 | 1310 | . | . | . | . | . | . |
|  | *** | 21660 | 28842 | 40153 | 7345 | 8548 | 9554 | 1238 | 1281 | 1285 | . | . | . | . | . | . |
| 0.95 | *** | 11991 | 14294 | 20087 | 3711 | 4030 | 4498 | . | . | . | . | . | . | . | . | . |
|  | *** | 12968 | 16291 | 20065 | 3860 | 4235 | 4474 | . | . | . | . | . | . | . | . | . |
| 0.98 | *** | 5284 | 5900 | 6912 | . | . | . | . | . | . | . | . | . | . | . | . |
|  | *** | 5560 | 6325 | 6891 | . | . | . | . | . | . | . | . | . | . | . | . |

TABLE 1: ALPHA= 0.005 POWER= 0.8    EXPECTED ACCRUAL THRU MINIMUM FOLLOW-UP= 9000

| | | DEL=.01 | | | DEL=.02 | | | DEL=.05 | | | DEL=.10 | | | DEL=.15 | | |
|---|---|---|---|---|---|---|---|---|---|---|---|---|---|---|---|---|---|
| FACT= | | 1.0 .75 | .50 .25 | .00 BIN | 1.0 .75 | .50 .25 | .00 BIN | 1.0 .75 | .50 .25 | .00 BIN | 1.0 75 | .50 .25 | .00 BIN | 1.0 .75 | .50 .25 | .00 BIN |
| PCONT=*** | | | REQUIRED NUMBER OF PATIENTS | | | | | | | | | | | | | | |
| 0.01 | *** | 1792 | 1792 | 1806 | 659 | 659 | 659 | 217 | 217 | 217 | 105 | 105 | 105 | 74 | 74 | 74 |
|  | *** | 1792 | 1792 | 6891 | 659 | 659 | 2278 | 217 | 217 | 620 | 105 | 105 | 252 | 74 | 74 | 150 |
| 0.02 | *** | 3966 | 3989 | 4020 | 1275 | 1275 | 1289 | 344 | 344 | 344 | 150 | 150 | 150 | 96 | 96 | 96 |
|  | *** | 3975 | 3997 | 11376 | 1275 | 1275 | 3387 | 344 | 344 | 792 | 150 | 150 | 293 | 96 | 96 | 167 |
| 0.05 | *** | 12030 | 12156 | 12547 | 3435 | 3471 | 3516 | 735 | 749 | 749 | 262 | 262 | 262 | 150 | 150 | 150 |
|  | *** | 12075 | 12291 | 24269 | 3449 | 3494 | 6576 | 735 | 749 | 1285 | 262 | 262 | 409 | 150 | 150 | 216 |
| 0.1 | *** | 26579 | 26970 | 29220 | 7251 | 7417 | 7732 | 1410 | 1424 | 1432 | 442 | 442 | 442 | 231 | 231 | 231 |
|  | *** | 26714 | 27532 | 43890 | 7327 | 7544 | 11423 | 1410 | 1432 | 2033 | 442 | 442 | 584 | 231 | 231 | 289 |
| 0.15 | *** | 39764 | 40484 | 46162 | 10739 | 11107 | 11954 | 2031 | 2062 | 2107 | 600 | 600 | 614 | 307 | 307 | 307 |
|  | *** | 40011 | 41662 | 61175 | 10896 | 11422 | 15685 | 2054 | 2085 | 2687 | 600 | 600 | 736 | 307 | 307 | 351 |
| 0.2 | *** | 50482 | 51621 | 62025 | 13650 | 14271 | 15877 | 2580 | 2639 | 2715 | 735 | 749 | 757 | 366 | 366 | 366 |
|  | *** | 50865 | 53534 | 76124 | 13897 | 14842 | 19364 | 2616 | 2684 | 3247 | 749 | 749 | 865 | 366 | 366 | 403 |
| 0.25 | *** | 58416 | 60059 | 76146 | 15914 | 16822 | 19365 | 3044 | 3134 | 3255 | 861 | 870 | 884 | 411 | 420 | 420 |
|  | *** | 58965 | 62835 | 88737 | 16282 | 17700 | 22459 | 3089 | 3187 | 3714 | 861 | 870 | 970 | 411 | 420 | 444 |
| 0.3 | *** | 63600 | 65850 | 88170 | 17542 | 18757 | 22312 | 3404 | 3525 | 3705 | 951 | 960 | 982 | 456 | 456 | 456 |
|  | *** | 64365 | 69599 | 99015 | 18037 | 19950 | 24970 | 3457 | 3606 | 4088 | 960 | 974 | 1052 | 456 | 456 | 475 |
| 0.35 | *** | 66246 | 69216 | 97904 | 18600 | 20130 | 24697 | 3674 | 3831 | 4056 | 1019 | 1041 | 1050 | 479 | 487 | 487 |
|  | *** | 67259 | 74031 | 106956 | 19207 | 21629 | 26897 | 3741 | 3930 | 4368 | 1027 | 1050 | 1110 | 479 | 487 | 496 |
| 0.4 | *** | 66637 | 70440 | 105225 | 19131 | 20962 | 26466 | 3854 | 4042 | 4304 | 1064 | 1086 | 1109 | 501 | 501 | 501 |
|  | *** | 67956 | 76371 | 112562 | 19874 | 22740 | 28240 | 3930 | 4155 | 4555 | 1072 | 1095 | 1145 | 501 | 501 | 507 |
| 0.45 | *** | 65166 | 69891 | 110054 | 19230 | 21322 | 27600 | 3944 | 4155 | 4461 | 1086 | 1109 | 1131 | 501 | 510 | 510 |
|  | *** | 66831 | 76911 | 115833 | 20085 | 23347 | 28999 | 4042 | 4290 | 4649 | 1095 | 1117 | 1157 | 501 | 510 | 507 |
| 0.5 | *** | 62219 | 67911 | 112349 | 18951 | 21255 | 28117 | 3952 | 4177 | 4515 | 1086 | 1109 | 1131 | 501 | 501 | 501 |
|  | *** | 64266 | 75930 | 116767 | 19896 | 23460 | 29175 | 4056 | 4335 | 4649 | 1095 | 1117 | 1145 | 501 | 501 | 496 |
| 0.55 | *** | 58191 | 64829 | 112110 | 18344 | 20819 | 27996 | 3885 | 4124 | 4461 | 1064 | 1086 | 1109 | 479 | 487 | 487 |
|  | *** | 60630 | 73657 | 115365 | 19365 | 23136 | 28766 | 3997 | 4281 | 4555 | 1072 | 1095 | 1110 | 479 | 487 | 475 |
| 0.6 | *** | 53475 | 60900 | 109334 | 17475 | 20017 | 27240 | 3741 | 3975 | 4312 | 1019 | 1027 | 1064 | 456 | 456 | 465 |
|  | *** | 56265 | 70282 | 111628 | 18532 | 22371 | 27773 | 3854 | 4132 | 4368 | 1027 | 1041 | 1052 | 456 | 456 | 444 |
| 0.65 | *** | 48390 | 56346 | 104010 | 16372 | 18892 | 25845 | 3525 | 3750 | 4056 | 937 | 960 | 982 | 411 | 420 | 420 |
|  | *** | 51441 | 65940 | 105555 | 17421 | 21201 | 26196 | 3629 | 3885 | 4088 | 951 | 974 | 970 | 411 | 420 | 403 |
| 0.7 | *** | 43125 | 51270 | 96180 | 15045 | 17452 | 23820 | 3232 | 3435 | 3705 | 847 | 861 | 884 | 366 | 366 | 375 |
|  | *** | 46297 | 60720 | 97146 | 16057 | 19612 | 24036 | 3322 | 3561 | 3714 | 861 | 870 | 865 | 366 | 366 | 351 |
| 0.75 | *** | 37784 | 45704 | 85852 | 13492 | 15689 | 21179 | 2864 | 3030 | 3255 | 726 | 749 | 757 | 307 | 307 | 307 |
|  | *** | 40911 | 54600 | 86402 | 14415 | 17601 | 21291 | 2940 | 3134 | 3247 | 735 | 749 | 736 | 307 | 307 | 289 |
| 0.8 | *** | 32325 | 39592 | 73050 | 11684 | 13560 | 17916 | 2414 | 2535 | 2706 | 591 | 600 | 600 | 231 | 240 | 240 |
|  | *** | 35219 | 47504 | 73321 | 12494 | 15149 | 17963 | 2467 | 2616 | 2687 | 591 | 600 | 584 | 240 | 240 | 216 |
| 0.85 | *** | 26579 | 32744 | 57809 | 9577 | 11017 | 14046 | 1874 | 1950 | 2054 | 420 | 420 | 434 | . | . | . |
|  | *** | 29062 | 39187 | 57905 | 10199 | 12179 | 14050 | 1905 | 1995 | 2033 | 420 | 434 | 409 | . | . | . |
| 0.9 | *** | 20175 | 24720 | 40146 | 7026 | 7926 | 9569 | 1230 | 1266 | 1311 | . | . | . | . | . | . |
|  | *** | 22034 | 29189 | 40153 | 7417 | 8601 | 9554 | 1244 | 1289 | 1285 | . | . | . | . | . | . |
| 0.95 | *** | 12187 | 14474 | 20085 | 3741 | 4056 | 4492 | . | . | . | . | . | . | . | . | . |
|  | *** | 13155 | 16440 | 20065 | 3885 | 4245 | 4474 | . | . | . | . | . | . | . | . | . |
| 0.98 | *** | 5347 | 5946 | 6914 | . | . | . | . | . | . | . | . | . | . | . | . |
|  | *** | 5617 | 6360 | 6891 | . | . | . | . | . | . | . | . | . | . | . | . |

# TABLE 1: ALPHA= 0.005 POWER= 0.8   EXPECTED ACCRUAL THRU MINIMUM FOLLOW-UP= 9500

| | | DEL=.01 | | | DEL=.02 | | | DEL=.05 | | | DEL=.10 | | | DEL=.15 | | |
|---|---|---|---|---|---|---|---|---|---|---|---|---|---|---|---|---|---|
| FACT= | | 1.0 .75 | .50 .25 | .00 BIN | 1.0 .75 | .50 .25 | .00 BIN | 1.0 .75 | .50 .25 | .00 BIN | 1.0 75 | .50 .25 | .00 BIN | 1.0 .75 | .50 .25 | .00 BIN |
| PCONT=*** | | | | | REQUIRED NUMBER OF PATIENTS | | | | | | | | | | | |
| 0.01 | *** | 1788 | 1797 | 1797 | 657 | 657 | 657 | 220 | 220 | 220 | 110 | 110 | 110 | 78 | 78 | 78 |
| | *** | 1797 | 1797 | 6891 | 657 | 657 | 2278 | 220 | 220 | 620 | 110 | 110 | 252 | 78 | 78 | 150 |
| 0.02 | *** | 3973 | 3982 | 4020 | 1274 | 1274 | 1289 | 348 | 348 | 348 | 149 | 149 | 149 | 101 | 101 | 101 |
| | *** | 3982 | 4005 | 11376 | 1274 | 1274 | 3387 | 348 | 348 | 792 | 149 | 149 | 293 | 101 | 101 | 167 |
| 0.05 | *** | 12048 | 12166 | 12555 | 3435 | 3474 | 3521 | 743 | 743 | 743 | 268 | 268 | 268 | 149 | 149 | 149 |
| | *** | 12095 | 12309 | 24269 | 3450 | 3498 | 6576 | 743 | 743 | 1285 | 268 | 268 | 409 | 149 | 149 | 216 |
| 0.1 | *** | 26606 | 27010 | 29219 | 7274 | 7425 | 7725 | 1408 | 1417 | 1440 | 443 | 443 | 443 | 229 | 229 | 229 |
| | *** | 26749 | 27580 | 43890 | 7330 | 7544 | 11423 | 1417 | 1431 | 2033 | 443 | 443 | 584 | 229 | 229 | 289 |
| 0.15 | *** | 39797 | 40557 | 46162 | 10765 | 11130 | 11953 | 2034 | 2073 | 2105 | 600 | 600 | 609 | 300 | 300 | 300 |
| | *** | 40058 | 41768 | 61175 | 10917 | 11454 | 15685 | 2049 | 2082 | 2687 | 600 | 609 | 736 | 300 | 300 | 351 |
| 0.2 | *** | 50546 | 51734 | 62018 | 13695 | 14313 | 15880 | 2580 | 2643 | 2723 | 743 | 743 | 752 | 363 | 363 | 363 |
| | *** | 50950 | 53705 | 76124 | 13948 | 14883 | 19364 | 2619 | 2675 | 3247 | 743 | 752 | 865 | 363 | 363 | 403 |
| 0.25 | *** | 58503 | 60236 | 76149 | 15975 | 16893 | 19363 | 3046 | 3141 | 3260 | 861 | 870 | 870 | 410 | 419 | 419 |
| | *** | 59096 | 63086 | 88737 | 16346 | 17757 | 22459 | 3094 | 3189 | 3714 | 861 | 870 | 970 | 410 | 419 | 444 |
| 0.3 | *** | 63728 | 66088 | 88175 | 17629 | 18864 | 22317 | 3412 | 3530 | 3697 | 956 | 965 | 980 | 458 | 458 | 458 |
| | *** | 64535 | 69950 | 99015 | 18128 | 20037 | 24970 | 3474 | 3616 | 4088 | 956 | 965 | 1052 | 458 | 458 | 475 |
| 0.35 | *** | 66411 | 69523 | 97904 | 18707 | 20250 | 24692 | 3688 | 3839 | 4053 | 1028 | 1037 | 1051 | 481 | 481 | 481 |
| | *** | 67480 | 74472 | 106956 | 19339 | 21723 | 26897 | 3759 | 3934 | 4368 | 1028 | 1051 | 1110 | 481 | 481 | 496 |
| 0.4 | *** | 66863 | 70838 | 105219 | 19268 | 21105 | 26464 | 3863 | 4053 | 4305 | 1075 | 1084 | 1108 | 490 | 505 | 505 |
| | *** | 68249 | 76909 | 112562 | 20013 | 22863 | 28240 | 3949 | 4172 | 4555 | 1075 | 1099 | 1145 | 505 | 505 | 507 |
| 0.45 | *** | 65447 | 70363 | 110049 | 19386 | 21485 | 27604 | 3958 | 4172 | 4457 | 1084 | 1108 | 1132 | 505 | 505 | 514 |
| | *** | 67195 | 77535 | 115833 | 20241 | 23495 | 28999 | 4053 | 4305 | 4649 | 1099 | 1123 | 1157 | 505 | 505 | 507 |
| 0.5 | *** | 62564 | 68463 | 112353 | 19125 | 21438 | 28112 | 3973 | 4195 | 4519 | 1084 | 1108 | 1132 | 490 | 505 | 505 |
| | *** | 64701 | 76624 | 116767 | 20075 | 23623 | 29175 | 4077 | 4338 | 4649 | 1099 | 1123 | 1145 | 505 | 505 | 496 |
| 0.55 | *** | 58621 | 65447 | 112106 | 18540 | 21001 | 27993 | 3901 | 4139 | 4457 | 1060 | 1084 | 1108 | 481 | 481 | 490 |
| | *** | 61139 | 74400 | 115365 | 19553 | 23305 | 28766 | 4020 | 4281 | 4555 | 1075 | 1099 | 1110 | 481 | 490 | 475 |
| 0.6 | *** | 53966 | 61575 | 109328 | 17676 | 20218 | 27233 | 3759 | 3996 | 4314 | 1013 | 1037 | 1060 | 458 | 458 | 458 |
| | *** | 56840 | 71066 | 111628 | 18730 | 22545 | 27773 | 3863 | 4139 | 4368 | 1028 | 1051 | 1052 | 458 | 458 | 444 |
| 0.65 | *** | 48931 | 57039 | 104017 | 16569 | 19087 | 25846 | 3545 | 3759 | 4053 | 942 | 965 | 980 | 410 | 419 | 419 |
| | *** | 52052 | 66729 | 105555 | 17614 | 21358 | 26196 | 3649 | 3901 | 4088 | 956 | 965 | 970 | 419 | 419 | 403 |
| 0.7 | *** | 43706 | 51971 | 96179 | 15230 | 17638 | 23828 | 3245 | 3450 | 3711 | 847 | 861 | 885 | 363 | 372 | 372 |
| | *** | 46922 | 61480 | 97146 | 16251 | 19766 | 24036 | 3340 | 3569 | 3714 | 861 | 870 | 865 | 363 | 372 | 351 |
| 0.75 | *** | 38348 | 46375 | 85863 | 13663 | 15848 | 21177 | 2880 | 3046 | 3245 | 728 | 743 | 752 | 300 | 300 | 315 |
| | *** | 41521 | 55305 | 86402 | 14589 | 17733 | 21291 | 2951 | 3141 | 3247 | 743 | 752 | 736 | 300 | 315 | 289 |
| 0.8 | *** | 32853 | 40200 | 73061 | 11843 | 13695 | 17914 | 2429 | 2548 | 2699 | 585 | 600 | 609 | 229 | 229 | 244 |
| | *** | 35783 | 48109 | 73321 | 12641 | 15254 | 17963 | 2485 | 2619 | 2687 | 585 | 600 | 584 | 229 | 244 | 216 |
| 0.85 | *** | 27034 | 33242 | 57814 | 9696 | 11121 | 14043 | 1883 | 1954 | 2049 | 419 | 419 | 434 | . | . | . |
| | *** | 29537 | 39678 | 57905 | 10314 | 12247 | 14050 | 1915 | 2001 | 2033 | 419 | 434 | 409 | . | . | . |
| 0.9 | *** | 20512 | 25072 | 40144 | 7093 | 7986 | 9563 | 1227 | 1265 | 1313 | . | . | . | . | . | . |
| | *** | 22388 | 29513 | 40153 | 7497 | 8637 | 9554 | 1250 | 1289 | 1285 | . | . | . | . | . | . |
| 0.95 | *** | 12365 | 14636 | 20084 | 3768 | 4068 | 4495 | . | . | . | . | . | . | . | . | . |
| | *** | 13339 | 16569 | 20065 | 3910 | 4258 | 4474 | . | . | . | . | . | . | . | . | . |
| 0.98 | *** | 5398 | 5977 | 6918 | . | . | . | . | . | . | . | . | . | . | . | . |
| | *** | 5659 | 6380 | 6891 | . | . | . | . | . | . | . | . | . | . | . | . |

TABLE 1: ALPHA= 0.005 POWER= 0.8    EXPECTED ACCRUAL THRU MINIMUM FOLLOW-UP= 10000

| | | DEL=.01 | | | DEL=.02 | | | DEL=.05 | | | DEL=.10 | | | DEL=.15 | | |
|---|---|---|---|---|---|---|---|---|---|---|---|---|---|---|---|---|
| FACT= | | 1.0 .75 | .50 .25 | .00 BIN | 1.0 .75 | .50 .25 | .00 BIN | 1.0 .75 | .50 .25 | .00 BIN | 1.0 75 | .50 .25 | .00 BIN | 1.0 .75 | .50 .25 | .00 BIN |
| PCONT=*** | | | | | REQUIRED | NUMBER OF | PATIENTS | | | | | | | | | |
| 0.01 | *** | 1791 | 1791 | 1807 | 657 | 657 | 657 | 216 | 216 | 216 | 107 | 107 | 107 | 82 | 82 | 82 |
| | *** | 1791 | 1791 | 6891 | 657 | 657 | 2278 | 216 | 216 | 620 | 107 | 107 | 252 | 82 | 82 | 150 |
| 0.02 | *** | 3966 | 3991 | 4016 | 1282 | 1282 | 1282 | 341 | 341 | 341 | 157 | 157 | 157 | 91 | 91 | 91 |
| | *** | 3982 | 4007 | 11376 | 1282 | 1282 | 3387 | 341 | 341 | 792 | 157 | 157 | 293 | 91 | 91 | 167 |
| 0.05 | *** | 12057 | 12182 | 12557 | 3441 | 3466 | 3516 | 741 | 741 | 741 | 266 | 266 | 266 | 157 | 157 | 157 |
| | *** | 12107 | 12316 | 24269 | 3457 | 3491 | 6576 | 741 | 741 | 1285 | 266 | 266 | 409 | 157 | 157 | 216 |
| 0.1 | *** | 26616 | 27041 | 29216 | 7282 | 7441 | 7732 | 1407 | 1416 | 1441 | 441 | 441 | 441 | 232 | 232 | 232 |
| | *** | 26766 | 27632 | 43890 | 7341 | 7557 | 11423 | 1416 | 1432 | 2033 | 441 | 441 | 584 | 232 | 232 | 289 |
| 0.15 | *** | 39841 | 40641 | 46166 | 10791 | 11157 | 11957 | 2041 | 2066 | 2107 | 607 | 607 | 607 | 307 | 307 | 307 |
| | *** | 40116 | 41866 | 61175 | 10941 | 11466 | 15685 | 2057 | 2091 | 2687 | 607 | 607 | 736 | 307 | 307 | 351 |
| 0.2 | *** | 50607 | 51857 | 62016 | 13741 | 14366 | 15882 | 2591 | 2657 | 2716 | 741 | 741 | 757 | 366 | 366 | 366 |
| | *** | 51032 | 53866 | 76124 | 13991 | 14932 | 19364 | 2616 | 2682 | 3247 | 741 | 757 | 865 | 366 | 366 | 403 |
| 0.25 | *** | 58607 | 60407 | 76141 | 16041 | 16966 | 19366 | 3057 | 3141 | 3257 | 857 | 866 | 882 | 416 | 416 | 416 |
| | *** | 59216 | 63341 | 88737 | 16416 | 17816 | 22459 | 3091 | 3191 | 3714 | 866 | 866 | 970 | 416 | 416 | 444 |
| 0.3 | *** | 63857 | 66332 | 88166 | 17716 | 18957 | 22316 | 3416 | 3541 | 3707 | 957 | 966 | 982 | 457 | 457 | 457 |
| | *** | 64707 | 70282 | 99015 | 18216 | 20116 | 24970 | 3482 | 3616 | 4088 | 957 | 966 | 1052 | 457 | 457 | 475 |
| 0.35 | *** | 66582 | 69832 | 97907 | 18816 | 20366 | 24691 | 3691 | 3857 | 4057 | 1032 | 1041 | 1057 | 482 | 482 | 491 |
| | *** | 67707 | 74891 | 106956 | 19441 | 21832 | 26897 | 3766 | 3941 | 4368 | 1032 | 1041 | 1110 | 482 | 482 | 496 |
| 0.4 | *** | 67082 | 71216 | 105216 | 19407 | 21241 | 26457 | 3882 | 4066 | 4307 | 1066 | 1091 | 1107 | 491 | 507 | 507 |
| | *** | 68532 | 77416 | 112562 | 20157 | 22991 | 28240 | 3966 | 4166 | 4555 | 1082 | 1091 | 1145 | 491 | 507 | 507 |
| 0.45 | *** | 65732 | 70832 | 110041 | 19532 | 21641 | 27607 | 3982 | 4182 | 4457 | 1091 | 1107 | 1132 | 507 | 507 | 507 |
| | *** | 67541 | 78132 | 115833 | 20407 | 23632 | 28999 | 4066 | 4307 | 4649 | 1107 | 1116 | 1157 | 507 | 507 | 507 |
| 0.5 | *** | 62916 | 69007 | 112357 | 19291 | 21607 | 28116 | 3991 | 4207 | 4516 | 1091 | 1107 | 1132 | 491 | 507 | 507 |
| | *** | 65132 | 77282 | 116767 | 20241 | 23766 | 29175 | 4091 | 4341 | 4649 | 1107 | 1116 | 1145 | 491 | 507 | 496 |
| 0.55 | *** | 59032 | 66057 | 112107 | 18716 | 21182 | 27991 | 3932 | 4157 | 4466 | 1066 | 1082 | 1107 | 482 | 482 | 491 |
| | *** | 61641 | 75116 | 115365 | 19741 | 23457 | 28766 | 4032 | 4291 | 4555 | 1082 | 1091 | 1110 | 482 | 482 | 475 |
| 0.6 | *** | 54457 | 62232 | 109332 | 17857 | 20391 | 27232 | 3782 | 4007 | 4307 | 1016 | 1032 | 1057 | 457 | 457 | 457 |
| | *** | 57391 | 71807 | 111628 | 18916 | 22691 | 27773 | 3891 | 4141 | 4368 | 1032 | 1041 | 1052 | 457 | 457 | 444 |
| 0.65 | *** | 49466 | 57716 | 104016 | 16757 | 19266 | 25841 | 3566 | 3782 | 4057 | 941 | 966 | 982 | 416 | 416 | 416 |
| | *** | 52641 | 67482 | 105555 | 17807 | 21507 | 26196 | 3666 | 3907 | 4088 | 957 | 966 | 970 | 416 | 416 | 403 |
| 0.7 | *** | 44257 | 52641 | 96182 | 15416 | 17807 | 23832 | 3266 | 3457 | 3707 | 857 | 866 | 882 | 366 | 366 | 366 |
| | *** | 47532 | 62207 | 97146 | 16416 | 19907 | 24036 | 3357 | 3566 | 3714 | 857 | 866 | 865 | 366 | 366 | 351 |
| 0.75 | *** | 38907 | 47016 | 85857 | 13832 | 16007 | 21182 | 2891 | 3057 | 3257 | 732 | 741 | 757 | 307 | 307 | 307 |
| | *** | 42116 | 55982 | 86402 | 14757 | 17857 | 21291 | 2966 | 3141 | 3247 | 741 | 741 | 736 | 307 | 307 | 289 |
| 0.8 | *** | 33357 | 40782 | 73057 | 11982 | 13832 | 17916 | 2432 | 2557 | 2707 | 591 | 591 | 607 | 232 | 232 | 241 |
| | *** | 36332 | 48707 | 73321 | 12782 | 15341 | 17963 | 2491 | 2616 | 2687 | 591 | 607 | 584 | 232 | 241 | 216 |
| 0.85 | *** | 27466 | 33716 | 57807 | 9807 | 11216 | 14041 | 1891 | 1966 | 2057 | 416 | 432 | 432 | . | . | . |
| | *** | 30007 | 40141 | 57905 | 10416 | 12316 | 14050 | 1916 | 2007 | 2033 | 432 | 432 | 409 | . | . | . |
| 0.9 | *** | 20841 | 25416 | 40141 | 7166 | 8041 | 9566 | 1232 | 1266 | 1307 | . | . | . | . | . | . |
| | *** | 22732 | 29832 | 40153 | 7566 | 8682 | 9554 | 1257 | 1291 | 1285 | . | . | . | . | . | . |
| 0.95 | *** | 12541 | 14791 | 20082 | 3791 | 4091 | 4491 | . | . | . | . | . | . | . | . | . |
| | *** | 13507 | 16707 | 20065 | 3932 | 4266 | 4474 | . | . | . | . | . | . | . | . | . |
| 0.98 | *** | 5441 | 6016 | 6916 | . | . | . | . | . | . | . | . | . | . | . | . |
| | *** | 5707 | 6407 | 6891 | . | . | . | . | . | . | . | . | . | . | . | . |

# TABLE 1: ALPHA= 0.005 POWER= 0.8    EXPECTED ACCRUAL THRU MINIMUM FOLLOW-UP= 11000

|  |  | DEL=.01 | | | DEL=.02 | | | DEL=.05 | | | DEL=.10 | | | DEL=.15 | | |
|---|---|---|---|---|---|---|---|---|---|---|---|---|---|---|---|---|
| FACT= | | 1.0 .75 | .50 .25 | .00 BIN | 1.0 .75 | .50 .25 | .00 BIN | 1.0 .75 | .50 .25 | .00 BIN | 1.0 75 | .50 .25 | .00 BIN | 1.0 .75 | .50 .25 | .00 BIN |
| PCONT=*** | | | | REQUIRED NUMBER OF PATIENTS | | | | | | | | | | | | |
| 0.01 | *** | 1795 1795 | 1795 1795 | 1795 6891 | 650 650 | 650 650 | 650 2278 | 210 210 | 210 210 | 210 620 | 100 100 | 100 100 | 100 252 | 73 73 | 73 73 | 73 150 |
| 0.02 | *** | 3978 3978 | 3995 4005 | 4022 11376 | 1272 1283 | 1283 1283 | 1283 3387 | 348 348 | 348 348 | 348 792 | 145 145 | 145 145 | 145 293 | 100 100 | 100 100 | 100 167 |
| 0.05 | *** | 12063 12118 | 12200 12327 | 12558 24269 | 3445 3455 | 3472 3500 | 3510 6576 | 733 733 | 750 750 | 750 1285 | 265 265 | 265 265 | 265 409 | 155 155 | 155 155 | 155 216 |
| 0.1 | *** | 26665 26830 | 27122 27710 | 29223 43890 | 7305 7377 | 7460 7570 | 7735 11423 | 1410 1420 | 1420 1437 | 1437 2033 | 447 447 | 447 447 | 447 584 | 238 238 | 238 238 | 238 289 |
| 0.15 | *** | 39920 40223 | 40790 42055 | 46163 61175 | 10842 11007 | 11210 11502 | 11953 15685 | 2042 2053 | 2070 2097 | 2108 2687 | 595 595 | 612 612 | 612 736 | 310 310 | 310 310 | 310 351 |
| 0.2 | *** | 50728 51195 | 52092 54193 | 62020 76124 | 13823 14087 | 14445 14995 | 15885 19364 | 2603 2630 | 2658 2685 | 2713 3247 | 750 750 | 750 750 | 750 865 | 365 365 | 365 365 | 365 403 |
| 0.25 | *** | 58785 59462 | 60738 63807 | 76138 88737 | 16160 16545 | 17085 17920 | 19367 22459 | 3070 3115 | 3153 3197 | 3252 3714 | 860 860 | 870 870 | 870 970 | 420 420 | 420 420 | 420 444 |
| 0.3 | *** | 64110 65028 | 66788 70913 | 88172 99015 | 17882 18388 | 19120 20258 | 22320 24970 | 3445 3500 | 3555 3620 | 3703 4088 | 953 953 | 970 970 | 980 1052 | 447 458 | 458 458 | 458 475 |
| 0.35 | *** | 66925 68135 | 70418 75698 | 97907 106956 | 19020 19670 | 20577 22007 | 24685 26897 | 3720 3785 | 3868 3950 | 4050 4368 | 1025 1035 | 1035 1052 | 1052 1110 | 485 485 | 485 485 | 485 496 |
| 0.4 | *** | 67520 69087 | 71958 78382 | 105222 112562 | 19642 20412 | 21495 23200 | 26462 28240 | 3912 3995 | 4077 4187 | 4308 4555 | 1080 1080 | 1090 1090 | 1107 1145 | 502 502 | 502 502 | 502 507 |
| 0.45 | *** | 66282 68245 | 71710 79245 | 110045 115833 | 19818 20698 | 21935 23860 | 27600 28999 | 4005 4105 | 4198 4325 | 4462 4649 | 1090 1107 | 1118 1118 | 1135 1157 | 502 502 | 502 513 | 513 507 |
| 0.5 | *** | 63598 65963 | 70033 78530 | 112345 116767 | 19598 20560 | 21925 24042 | 28112 29175 | 4022 4132 | 4242 4363 | 4517 4649 | 1090 1107 | 1107 1118 | 1135 1145 | 502 502 | 502 502 | 502 496 |
| 0.55 | *** | 59847 62597 | 67200 76457 | 112108 115365 | 19048 20082 | 21512 23723 | 28002 28766 | 3967 4060 | 4170 4308 | 4462 4555 | 1063 1080 | 1090 1090 | 1107 1110 | 485 485 | 485 485 | 485 475 |
| 0.6 | *** | 55375 58472 | 63460 73195 | 109330 111628 | 18212 19268 | 20725 22970 | 27232 27773 | 3813 3923 | 4033 4160 | 4308 4368 | 1025 1025 | 1035 1052 | 1052 1052 | 458 458 | 458 458 | 458 444 |
| 0.65 | *** | 50480 53780 | 58995 68878 | 104012 105555 | 17112 18157 | 19598 21787 | 25840 26196 | 3593 3692 | 3802 3912 | 4060 4088 | 953 953 | 970 970 | 980 970 | 420 420 | 420 420 | 420 403 |
| 0.7 | *** | 45310 48693 | 53907 63560 | 96185 97146 | 15748 16755 | 18113 20148 | 23822 24036 | 3307 3390 | 3472 3582 | 3703 3714 | 860 860 | 870 870 | 887 865 | 365 365 | 365 365 | 375 351 |
| 0.75 | *** | 39937 43237 | 48215 57218 | 85862 86402 | 14142 15060 | 16287 18075 | 21182 21291 | 2922 2988 | 3070 3153 | 3252 3247 | 733 733 | 750 750 | 750 736 | 310 310 | 310 310 | 310 289 |
| 0.8 | *** | 34327 37352 | 41845 49782 | 73058 73321 | 12245 13025 | 14060 15517 | 17920 17963 | 2455 2510 | 2565 2630 | 2702 2687 | 595 595 | 595 595 | 612 584 | 238 238 | 238 238 | 238 216 |
| 0.85 | *** | 28288 30862 | 34613 40993 | 57812 57905 | 10017 10622 | 11392 12437 | 14043 14050 | 1905 1932 | 1970 2015 | 2053 2033 | 420 420 | 430 430 | 430 409 | . . | . . | . . |
| 0.9 | *** | 21468 23355 | 26050 30395 | 40140 40153 | 7305 7680 | 8147 8752 | 9560 9554 | 1245 1255 | 1272 1283 | 1310 1285 | . . | . . | . . | . . | . . | . . |
| 0.95 | *** | 12860 13812 | 15088 16920 | 20082 20065 | 3840 3967 | 4115 4297 | 4490 4474 | . . | . . | . . | . . | . . | . . | . . | . . | . . |
| 0.98 | *** | 5535 5782 | 6085 6442 | 6910 6891 | . . | . . | . . | . . | . . | . . | . . | . . | . . | . . | . . | . . |

| TABLE 1: ALPHA= 0.005 POWER= 0.8 | | | EXPECTED ACCRUAL THRU MINIMUM FOLLOW-UP= 12000 | | | | | | | | | | | |

| | | DEL=.01 | | | DEL=.02 | | | DEL=.05 | | | DEL=.10 | | | DEL=.15 | | |
|---|---|---|---|---|---|---|---|---|---|---|---|---|---|---|---|---|
| FACT= | | 1.0 .75 | .50 .25 | .00 BIN | 1.0 .75 | .50 .25 | .00 BIN | 1.0 .75 | .50 .25 | .00 BIN | 1.0 75 | .50 .25 | .00 BIN | 1.0 .75 | .50 .25 | .00 BIN |
| PCONT=*** | | | | | REQUIRED NUMBER OF PATIENTS | | | | | | | | | | | |
| 0.01 | *** | 1789 | 1789 | 1808 | 649 | 649 | 649 | 218 | 218 | 218 | 109 | 109 | 109 | 79 | 79 | 79 |
|  | *** | 1789 | 1789 | 6891 | 649 | 649 | 2278 | 218 | 218 | 620 | 109 | 109 | 252 | 79 | 79 | 150 |
| 0.02 | *** | 3979 | 3998 | 4009 | 1279 | 1279 | 1279 | 349 | 349 | 349 | 158 | 158 | 158 | 98 | 98 | 98 |
|  | *** | 3979 | 4009 | 11376 | 1279 | 1279 | 3387 | 349 | 349 | 792 | 158 | 158 | 293 | 98 | 98 | 167 |
| 0.05 | *** | 12079 | 12218 | 12548 | 3439 | 3469 | 3518 | 739 | 739 | 739 | 259 | 259 | 259 | 158 | 158 | 158 |
|  | *** | 12139 | 12338 | 24269 | 3458 | 3499 | 6576 | 739 | 739 | 1285 | 259 | 259 | 409 | 158 | 158 | 216 |
| 0.1 | *** | 26708 | 27188 | 29228 | 7328 | 7478 | 7729 | 1418 | 1429 | 1429 | 439 | 439 | 439 | 229 | 229 | 229 |
|  | *** | 26888 | 27788 | 43890 | 7388 | 7579 | 11423 | 1418 | 1429 | 2033 | 439 | 439 | 584 | 229 | 229 | 289 |
| 0.15 | *** | 40009 | 40928 | 46159 | 10898 | 11258 | 11948 | 2048 | 2078 | 2108 | 608 | 608 | 608 | 308 | 308 | 308 |
|  | *** | 40328 | 42229 | 61175 | 11048 | 11528 | 15685 | 2059 | 2089 | 2687 | 608 | 608 | 736 | 308 | 308 | 351 |
| 0.2 | *** | 50858 | 52309 | 62018 | 13898 | 14528 | 15878 | 2618 | 2659 | 2719 | 739 | 739 | 758 | 368 | 368 | 368 |
|  | *** | 51368 | 54488 | 76124 | 14168 | 15049 | 19364 | 2629 | 2689 | 3247 | 739 | 758 | 865 | 368 | 368 | 403 |
| 0.25 | *** | 58969 | 61069 | 76148 | 16279 | 17198 | 19369 | 3079 | 3158 | 3259 | 859 | 878 | 878 | 409 | 409 | 409 |
|  | *** | 59708 | 64249 | 88737 | 16658 | 18008 | 22459 | 3109 | 3199 | 3714 | 859 | 878 | 970 | 409 | 409 | 444 |
| 0.3 | *** | 64369 | 67238 | 88178 | 18038 | 19279 | 22309 | 3458 | 3559 | 3698 | 949 | 968 | 979 | 458 | 458 | 458 |
|  | *** | 65359 | 71509 | 99015 | 18548 | 20378 | 24970 | 3518 | 3638 | 4088 | 968 | 968 | 1052 | 458 | 458 | 475 |
| 0.35 | *** | 67249 | 70999 | 97909 | 19208 | 20768 | 24698 | 3739 | 3878 | 4058 | 1028 | 1039 | 1058 | 488 | 488 | 488 |
|  | *** | 68569 | 76448 | 106956 | 19849 | 22159 | 26897 | 3799 | 3968 | 4368 | 1039 | 1039 | 1110 | 488 | 488 | 496 |
| 0.4 | *** | 67958 | 72668 | 105218 | 19868 | 21728 | 26468 | 3938 | 4099 | 4309 | 1069 | 1088 | 1099 | 499 | 499 | 499 |
|  | *** | 69638 | 79279 | 112562 | 20648 | 23389 | 28240 | 4009 | 4189 | 4555 | 1088 | 1099 | 1145 | 499 | 499 | 507 |
| 0.45 | *** | 66829 | 72559 | 110048 | 20078 | 22189 | 27608 | 4039 | 4219 | 4459 | 1099 | 1118 | 1129 | 499 | 499 | 518 |
|  | *** | 68918 | 80288 | 115833 | 20959 | 24079 | 28999 | 4129 | 4328 | 4649 | 1099 | 1118 | 1157 | 499 | 499 | 507 |
| 0.5 | *** | 64268 | 70999 | 112358 | 19898 | 22208 | 28118 | 4058 | 4249 | 4508 | 1099 | 1118 | 1129 | 499 | 499 | 499 |
|  | *** | 66758 | 79688 | 116767 | 20858 | 24259 | 29115 | 4148 | 4369 | 4649 | 1099 | 1118 | 1145 | 499 | 499 | 496 |
| 0.55 | *** | 60638 | 68288 | 112118 | 19358 | 21818 | 27998 | 3998 | 4189 | 4459 | 1069 | 1088 | 1099 | 488 | 488 | 488 |
|  | *** | 63518 | 77689 | 115365 | 20389 | 23978 | 28766 | 4088 | 4328 | 4555 | 1088 | 1099 | 1110 | 488 | 488 | 475 |
| 0.6 | *** | 56269 | 64609 | 109328 | 18529 | 21038 | 27229 | 3848 | 4058 | 4309 | 1028 | 1039 | 1058 | 458 | 458 | 458 |
|  | *** | 59479 | 74479 | 111628 | 19579 | 23228 | 27773 | 3949 | 4178 | 4368 | 1028 | 1039 | 1052 | 458 | 458 | 444 |
| 0.65 | *** | 51439 | 60188 | 104018 | 17419 | 19898 | 25849 | 3619 | 3818 | 4058 | 949 | 968 | 979 | 409 | 409 | 428 |
|  | *** | 54848 | 70159 | 105555 | 18469 | 22028 | 26196 | 3709 | 3919 | 4088 | 949 | 968 | 970 | 409 | 428 | 403 |
| 0.7 | *** | 46298 | 55088 | 96188 | 16058 | 18398 | 23828 | 3319 | 3488 | 3709 | 859 | 859 | 878 | 368 | 368 | 368 |
|  | *** | 49759 | 64789 | 97146 | 17059 | 20378 | 24036 | 3409 | 3589 | 3714 | 859 | 878 | 865 | 368 | 368 | 351 |
| 0.75 | *** | 40909 | 49328 | 85849 | 14419 | 16538 | 21188 | 2948 | 3079 | 3248 | 739 | 739 | 758 | 308 | 308 | 308 |
|  | *** | 44269 | 58358 | 86402 | 15319 | 18259 | 21291 | 3008 | 3158 | 3247 | 739 | 758 | 736 | 308 | 308 | 289 |
| 0.8 | *** | 35228 | 42848 | 73058 | 12488 | 14269 | 17918 | 2468 | 2569 | 2708 | 589 | 589 | 608 | 229 | 229 | 229 |
|  | *** | 38299 | 50768 | 73321 | 13268 | 15668 | 17963 | 2528 | 2629 | 2687 | 589 | 608 | 584 | 229 | 229 | 216 |
| 0.85 | *** | 29059 | 35419 | 57799 | 10189 | 11539 | 14048 | 1909 | 1969 | 2048 | 428 | 428 | 428 | . | . | . |
|  | *** | 31658 | 41768 | 57905 | 10789 | 12548 | 14050 | 1939 | 2018 | 2033 | 428 | 428 | 409 | . | . | . |
| 0.9 | *** | 22028 | 26618 | 40148 | 7418 | 8239 | 9559 | 1249 | 1279 | 1309 | . | . | . | . | . | . |
|  | *** | 23929 | 30889 | 40153 | 7789 | 8798 | 9554 | 1268 | 1298 | 1285 | . | . | . | . | . | . |
| 0.95 | *** | 13159 | 15338 | 20078 | 3878 | 4148 | 4489 | . | . | . | . | . | . | . | . | . |
|  | *** | 14089 | 17119 | 20065 | 4009 | 4309 | 4474 | . | . | . | . | . | . | . | . | . |
| 0.98 | *** | 5618 | 6139 | 6908 | . | . | . | . | . | . | . | . | . | . | . | . |
|  | *** | 5858 | 6488 | 6891 | . | . | . | . | . | . | . | . | . | . | . | . |

## TABLE 1: ALPHA= 0.005  POWER= 0.8   EXPECTED ACCRUAL THRU MINIMUM FOLLOW-UP= 13000

| | | DEL=.01 | | | DEL=.02 | | | DEL=.05 | | | DEL=.10 | | | DEL=.15 | | |
|---|---|---|---|---|---|---|---|---|---|---|---|---|---|---|---|---|
| FACT= | | 1.0 .75 | .50 .25 | .00 BIN | 1.0 .75 | .50 .25 | .00 BIN | 1.0 .75 | .50 .25 | .00 BIN | 1.0 75 | .50 .25 | .00 BIN | 1.0 .75 | .50 .25 | .00 BIN |
| PCONT=*** | | | | REQUIRED NUMBER OF PATIENTS | | | | | | | | | | | | |
| 0.01 | *** | 1796 | 1796 | 1796 | 659 | 659 | 659 | 216 | 216 | 216 | 106 | 106 | 106 | 74 | 74 | 74 |
|  | *** | 1796 | 1796 | 6891 | 659 | 659 | 2278 | 216 | 216 | 620 | 106 | 106 | 252 | 74 | 74 | 150 |
| 0.02 | *** | 3974 | 3986 | 4018 | 1276 | 1276 | 1288 | 346 | 346 | 346 | 151 | 151 | 151 | 106 | 106 | 106 |
|  | *** | 3986 | 4006 | 11376 | 1276 | 1276 | 3387 | 346 | 346 | 792 | 151 | 151 | 293 | 106 | 106 | 167 |
| 0.05 | *** | 12099 | 12229 | 12554 | 3454 | 3486 | 3519 | 736 | 736 | 736 | 269 | 269 | 269 | 151 | 151 | 151 |
|  | *** | 12143 | 12359 | 24269 | 3466 | 3498 | 6576 | 736 | 736 | 1285 | 269 | 269 | 409 | 151 | 151 | 216 |
| 0.1 | *** | 26756 | 27256 | 29226 | 7333 | 7484 | 7723 | 1418 | 1418 | 1439 | 443 | 443 | 443 | 236 | 236 | 236 |
|  | *** | 26931 | 27861 | 43890 | 7398 | 7593 | 11423 | 1418 | 1439 | 2033 | 443 | 443 | 584 | 236 | 236 | 289 |
| 0.15 | *** | 40093 | 41056 | 46159 | 10929 | 11286 | 11948 | 2056 | 2068 | 2101 | 606 | 606 | 606 | 301 | 301 | 301 |
|  | *** | 40439 | 42389 | 61175 | 11091 | 11558 | 15685 | 2068 | 2089 | 2687 | 606 | 606 | 736 | 301 | 301 | 351 |
| 0.2 | *** | 51001 | 52541 | 62019 | 13963 | 14581 | 15881 | 2621 | 2674 | 2718 | 736 | 756 | 756 | 366 | 366 | 366 |
|  | *** | 51533 | 54771 | 76124 | 14244 | 15101 | 19364 | 2641 | 2686 | 3247 | 736 | 756 | 865 | 366 | 366 | 403 |
| 0.25 | *** | 59159 | 61401 | 76136 | 16389 | 17299 | 19358 | 3096 | 3161 | 3259 | 866 | 866 | 886 | 411 | 411 | 411 |
|  | *** | 59939 | 64663 | 88737 | 16779 | 18091 | 22459 | 3129 | 3206 | 3714 | 866 | 866 | 970 | 411 | 411 | 444 |
| 0.3 | *** | 64619 | 67653 | 88181 | 18176 | 19411 | 22316 | 3466 | 3584 | 3693 | 963 | 963 | 984 | 443 | 464 | 464 |
|  | *** | 65691 | 72061 | 99015 | 18696 | 20484 | 24970 | 3519 | 3628 | 4088 | 963 | 963 | 1052 | 464 | 464 | 475 |
| 0.35 | *** | 67588 | 71553 | 97911 | 19391 | 20939 | 24688 | 3758 | 3888 | 4051 | 1028 | 1049 | 1049 | 476 | 476 | 496 |
|  | *** | 69006 | 77143 | 106956 | 20041 | 22304 | 26897 | 3823 | 3974 | 4368 | 1028 | 1049 | 1110 | 476 | 476 | 496 |
| 0.4 | *** | 68389 | 73361 | 105223 | 20094 | 21926 | 26464 | 3953 | 4116 | 4311 | 1081 | 1093 | 1114 | 496 | 496 | 508 |
|  | *** | 70176 | 80121 | 112562 | 20853 | 23551 | 28240 | 4039 | 4201 | 4555 | 1081 | 1093 | 1145 | 496 | 496 | 507 |
| 0.45 | *** | 67361 | 73373 | 110054 | 20321 | 22434 | 27601 | 4071 | 4234 | 4461 | 1093 | 1114 | 1126 | 508 | 508 | 508 |
|  | *** | 69571 | 81238 | 115833 | 21211 | 24266 | 28999 | 4148 | 4343 | 4649 | 1114 | 1126 | 1157 | 508 | 508 | 507 |
| 0.5 | *** | 64911 | 71931 | 112341 | 20159 | 22466 | 28121 | 4083 | 4266 | 4506 | 1093 | 1114 | 1126 | 496 | 496 | 508 |
|  | *** | 67544 | 80751 | 116767 | 21134 | 24481 | 29175 | 4169 | 4376 | 4649 | 1114 | 1126 | 1145 | 496 | 508 | 496 |
| 0.55 | *** | 61381 | 69299 | 112113 | 19651 | 22088 | 27991 | 4018 | 4213 | 4461 | 1081 | 1093 | 1114 | 476 | 476 | 496 |
|  | *** | 64403 | 78833 | 115365 | 20679 | 24189 | 28766 | 4116 | 4331 | 4555 | 1081 | 1093 | 1110 | 476 | 496 | 475 |
| 0.6 | *** | 57123 | 65703 | 109339 | 18826 | 21308 | 27244 | 3876 | 4071 | 4311 | 1028 | 1049 | 1061 | 443 | 464 | 464 |
|  | *** | 60438 | 75648 | 111628 | 19878 | 23441 | 27773 | 3974 | 4181 | 4368 | 1028 | 1049 | 1052 | 464 | 464 | 444 |
| 0.65 | *** | 52346 | 61283 | 104021 | 17721 | 20171 | 25846 | 3649 | 3823 | 4051 | 951 | 963 | 984 | 411 | 411 | 411 |
|  | *** | 55856 | 71326 | 105555 | 18761 | 22239 | 26196 | 3746 | 3941 | 4088 | 963 | 963 | 970 | 411 | 411 | 403 |
| 0.7 | *** | 47231 | 56169 | 96188 | 16336 | 18643 | 23831 | 3356 | 3498 | 3714 | 854 | 866 | 886 | 366 | 366 | 366 |
|  | *** | 50786 | 65919 | 97146 | 17331 | 20561 | 24036 | 3421 | 3596 | 3714 | 866 | 866 | 865 | 366 | 366 | 351 |
| 0.75 | *** | 41816 | 50351 | 85853 | 14678 | 16758 | 21178 | 2966 | 3096 | 3259 | 736 | 736 | 756 | 301 | 313 | 313 |
|  | *** | 45249 | 59386 | 86402 | 15576 | 18436 | 21291 | 3031 | 3161 | 3247 | 736 | 756 | 736 | 301 | 313 | 289 |
| 0.8 | *** | 36063 | 43754 | 73048 | 12716 | 14451 | 17916 | 2491 | 2588 | 2706 | 594 | 594 | 606 | 236 | 236 | 236 |
|  | *** | 39171 | 51651 | 73321 | 13464 | 15804 | 17963 | 2544 | 2641 | 2687 | 594 | 606 | 584 | 236 | 236 | 216 |
| 0.85 | *** | 29779 | 36161 | 57806 | 10376 | 11676 | 14049 | 1926 | 1971 | 2056 | 431 | 431 | 431 | . | . | . |
|  | *** | 32391 | 42454 | 57905 | 10941 | 12631 | 14050 | 1959 | 2024 | 2033 | 431 | 431 | 409 | . | . | . |
| 0.9 | *** | 22564 | 27126 | 40146 | 7528 | 8308 | 9564 | 1244 | 1276 | 1309 | . | . | . | . | . | . |
|  | *** | 24461 | 31339 | 40153 | 7886 | 8849 | 9554 | 1256 | 1288 | 1285 | . | . | . | . | . | . |
| 0.95 | *** | 13431 | 15576 | 20073 | 3921 | 4169 | 4494 | . | . | . | . | . | . | . | . | . |
|  | *** | 14353 | 17299 | 20065 | 4039 | 4311 | 4474 | . | . | . | . | . | . | . | . | . |
| 0.98 | *** | 5676 | 6184 | 6911 | . | . | . | . | . | . | . | . | . | . | . | . |
|  | *** | 5903 | 6509 | 6891 | . | . | . | . | . | . | . | . | . | . | . | . |

TABLE 1: ALPHA= 0.005 POWER= 0.8     EXPECTED ACCRUAL THRU MINIMUM FOLLOW-UP= 14000

| PCONT=*** | FACT= | DEL=.01 1.0 .75 | DEL=.01 .50 .25 | DEL=.01 .00 BIN | DEL=.02 1.0 .75 | DEL=.02 .50 .25 | DEL=.02 .00 BIN | DEL=.05 1.0 .75 | DEL=.05 .50 .25 | DEL=.05 .00 BIN | DEL=.10 1.0 75 | DEL=.10 .50 .25 | DEL=.10 .00 BIN | DEL=.15 1.0 .75 | DEL=.15 .50 .25 | DEL=.15 .00 BIN |
|---|---|---|---|---|---|---|---|---|---|---|---|---|---|---|---|---|
| | | | | | | | REQUIRED NUMBER OF PATIENTS | | | | | | | | | |
| 0.01 | *** | 1794 | 1794 | 1794 | 652 | 652 | 652 | 219 | 219 | 219 | 114 | 114 | 114 | 79 | 79 | 79 |
| | *** | 1794 | 1794 | 6891 | 652 | 652 | 2278 | 219 | 219 | 620 | 114 | 114 | 252 | 79 | 79 | 150 |
| 0.02 | *** | 3977 | 3999 | 4012 | 1282 | 1282 | 1282 | 337 | 337 | 337 | 149 | 149 | 149 | 92 | 92 | 92 |
| | *** | 3977 | 4012 | 11376 | 1282 | 1282 | 3387 | 337 | 337 | 792 | 149 | 149 | 293 | 92 | 92 | 167 |
| 0.05 | *** | 12119 | 12237 | 12552 | 3452 | 3487 | 3522 | 744 | 744 | 744 | 267 | 267 | 267 | 149 | 149 | 149 |
| | *** | 12167 | 12364 | 24269 | 3474 | 3487 | 6576 | 744 | 744 | 1285 | 267 | 267 | 409 | 149 | 149 | 216 |
| 0.1 | *** | 26797 | 27322 | 29212 | 7359 | 7499 | 7722 | 1422 | 1422 | 1444 | 442 | 442 | 442 | 232 | 232 | 232 |
| | *** | 26994 | 27917 | 43890 | 7429 | 7604 | 11423 | 1422 | 1422 | 2033 | 442 | 442 | 584 | 232 | 232 | 289 |
| 0.15 | *** | 40167 | 41182 | 46174 | 10977 | 11314 | 11957 | 2052 | 2074 | 2109 | 604 | 604 | 604 | 302 | 302 | 302 |
| | *** | 40539 | 42534 | 61175 | 11117 | 11572 | 15685 | 2074 | 2087 | 2687 | 604 | 604 | 736 | 302 | 302 | 351 |
| 0.2 | *** | 51122 | 52754 | 62029 | 14044 | 14652 | 15877 | 2612 | 2669 | 2717 | 744 | 744 | 757 | 359 | 359 | 372 |
| | *** | 51704 | 55029 | 76124 | 14302 | 15142 | 19364 | 2647 | 2682 | 3247 | 744 | 744 | 865 | 359 | 359 | 403 |
| 0.25 | *** | 59334 | 61692 | 76147 | 16472 | 17404 | 19364 | 3102 | 3172 | 3264 | 862 | 862 | 884 | 407 | 407 | 407 |
| | *** | 60174 | 65039 | 88737 | 16879 | 18152 | 22459 | 3137 | 3207 | 3714 | 862 | 884 | 970 | 407 | 407 | 444 |
| 0.3 | *** | 64864 | 68084 | 88174 | 18314 | 19539 | 22317 | 3487 | 3579 | 3697 | 954 | 967 | 967 | 442 | 464 | 464 |
| | *** | 66019 | 72577 | 99015 | 18817 | 20589 | 24970 | 3522 | 3649 | 4088 | 967 | 967 | 1052 | 464 | 464 | 475 |
| 0.35 | *** | 67922 | 72087 | 97904 | 19552 | 21114 | 24697 | 3789 | 3894 | 4047 | 1037 | 1037 | 1059 | 477 | 477 | 477 |
| | *** | 69414 | 77792 | 106956 | 20204 | 22422 | 26897 | 3837 | 3977 | 4368 | 1037 | 1037 | 1110 | 477 | 477 | 496 |
| 0.4 | *** | 68819 | 74012 | 105219 | 20287 | 22129 | 26469 | 3977 | 4117 | 4314 | 1072 | 1094 | 1107 | 499 | 499 | 499 |
| | *** | 70709 | 80907 | 112562 | 21057 | 23704 | 28240 | 4047 | 4209 | 4555 | 1094 | 1094 | 1145 | 499 | 499 | 507 |
| 0.45 | *** | 67887 | 74152 | 110049 | 20554 | 22632 | 27602 | 4082 | 4244 | 4454 | 1107 | 1107 | 1129 | 499 | 512 | 512 |
| | *** | 70219 | 82132 | 115833 | 21429 | 24439 | 28999 | 4174 | 4349 | 4649 | 1107 | 1129 | 1157 | 499 | 512 | 507 |
| 0.5 | *** | 65542 | 72809 | 112359 | 20414 | 22702 | 28114 | 4104 | 4279 | 4502 | 1107 | 1107 | 1129 | 499 | 499 | 499 |
| | *** | 68272 | 81734 | 116767 | 21372 | 24662 | 29175 | 4187 | 4397 | 4649 | 1107 | 1129 | 1145 | 499 | 499 | 496 |
| 0.55 | *** | 62112 | 70267 | 112114 | 19924 | 22339 | 27987 | 4047 | 4222 | 4467 | 1072 | 1094 | 1107 | 477 | 477 | 477 |
| | *** | 65249 | 79892 | 115365 | 20939 | 24382 | 28766 | 4139 | 4327 | 4555 | 1072 | 1094 | 1110 | 477 | 477 | 475 |
| 0.6 | *** | 57934 | 66719 | 109327 | 19097 | 21569 | 27239 | 3907 | 4082 | 4314 | 1024 | 1037 | 1059 | 464 | 464 | 464 |
| | *** | 61364 | 76742 | 111628 | 20147 | 23634 | 27773 | 3977 | 4187 | 4368 | 1037 | 1059 | 1052 | 464 | 464 | 444 |
| 0.65 | *** | 53222 | 62344 | 104007 | 17977 | 20414 | 25839 | 3684 | 3837 | 4047 | 954 | 967 | 989 | 407 | 407 | 429 |
| | *** | 56814 | 72424 | 105555 | 19027 | 22422 | 26196 | 3754 | 3942 | 4088 | 954 | 967 | 970 | 407 | 429 | 403 |
| 0.7 | *** | 48112 | 57199 | 96189 | 16599 | 18874 | 23822 | 3369 | 3522 | 3697 | 862 | 862 | 884 | 372 | 372 | 372 |
| | *** | 51739 | 66964 | 97146 | 17579 | 20742 | 24036 | 3439 | 3614 | 3714 | 862 | 884 | 865 | 372 | 372 | 351 |
| 0.75 | *** | 42674 | 51319 | 85864 | 14919 | 16962 | 21184 | 2984 | 3102 | 3242 | 744 | 744 | 757 | 302 | 302 | 302 |
| | *** | 46152 | 60349 | 86402 | 15794 | 18572 | 21291 | 3032 | 3172 | 3247 | 744 | 744 | 736 | 302 | 302 | 289 |
| 0.8 | *** | 36842 | 44612 | 73054 | 12902 | 14617 | 17907 | 2494 | 2599 | 2704 | 582 | 604 | 604 | 232 | 232 | 232 |
| | *** | 39992 | 52474 | 73321 | 13659 | 15934 | 17963 | 2542 | 2647 | 2687 | 604 | 604 | 584 | 232 | 232 | 216 |
| 0.85 | *** | 30437 | 36864 | 57807 | 10522 | 11782 | 14044 | 1934 | 1982 | 2052 | 429 | 429 | 429 | . | . | . |
| | *** | 33084 | 43094 | 57905 | 11082 | 12727 | 14050 | 1947 | 2017 | 2033 | 429 | 429 | 409 | . | . | . |
| 0.9 | *** | 23052 | 27602 | 40132 | 7617 | 8387 | 9564 | 1247 | 1282 | 1304 | . | . | . | . | . | . |
| | *** | 24964 | 31754 | 40153 | 7967 | 8899 | 9554 | 1269 | 1282 | 1285 | . | . | . | . | . | . |
| 0.95 | *** | 13659 | 15772 | 20077 | 3942 | 4187 | 4489 | . | . | . | . | . | . | . | . | . |
| | *** | 14582 | 17439 | 20065 | 4069 | 4327 | 4474 | . | . | . | . | . | . | . | . | . |
| 0.98 | *** | 5749 | 6217 | 6917 | . | . | . | . | . | . | . | . | . | . | . | . |
| | *** | 5972 | 6532 | 6891 | . | . | . | . | . | . | . | . | . | . | . | . |

## TABLE 1: ALPHA= 0.005 POWER= 0.8     EXPECTED ACCRUAL THRU MINIMUM FOLLOW-UP= 15000

| | FACT= | DEL=.01 | | | DEL=.02 | | | DEL=.05 | | | DEL=.10 | | | DEL=.15 | | |
|---|---|---|---|---|---|---|---|---|---|---|---|---|---|---|---|---|
| | | 1.0 .75 | .50 .25 | .00 BIN | 1.0 .75 | .50 .25 | .00 BIN | 1.0 .75 | .50 .25 | .00 BIN | 1.0 75 | .50 .25 | .00 BIN | 1.0 .75 | .50 .25 | .00 BIN |
| PCONT=*** | | | | | REQUIRED NUMBER OF PATIENTS | | | | | | | | | | | |
| 0.01 | *** | 1786 | 1786 | 1810 | 661 | 661 | 661 | 211 | 211 | 211 | 99 | 99 | 99 | 85 | 85 | 85 |
| | *** | 1786 | 1786 | 6891 | 661 | 661 | 2278 | 211 | 211 | 620 | 99 | 99 | 252 | 85 | 85 | 150 |
| 0.02 | *** | 3985 | 3999 | 4022 | 1285 | 1285 | 1285 | 347 | 347 | 347 | 160 | 160 | 160 | 99 | 99 | 99 |
| | *** | 3985 | 3999 | 11376 | 1285 | 1285 | 3387 | 347 | 347 | 792 | 160 | 160 | 293 | 99 | 99 | 167 |
| 0.05 | *** | 12122 | 12249 | 12549 | 3460 | 3474 | 3511 | 736 | 736 | 736 | 272 | 272 | 272 | 160 | 160 | 160 |
| | *** | 12174 | 12385 | 24269 | 3474 | 3497 | 6576 | 736 | 736 | 1285 | 272 | 272 | 409 | 160 | 160 | 216 |
| 0.1 | *** | 26836 | 27385 | 29222 | 7374 | 7510 | 7735 | 1411 | 1435 | 1435 | 436 | 436 | 436 | 235 | 235 | 235 |
| | *** | 27047 | 27961 | 43890 | 7435 | 7599 | 11423 | 1411 | 1435 | 2033 | 436 | 436 | 584 | 235 | 235 | 289 |
| 0.15 | *** | 40247 | 41311 | 46172 | 11011 | 11349 | 11949 | 2049 | 2086 | 2110 | 610 | 610 | 610 | 310 | 310 | 310 |
| | *** | 40636 | 42685 | 61175 | 11161 | 11597 | 15685 | 2072 | 2086 | 2687 | 610 | 610 | 736 | 310 | 310 | 351 |
| 0.2 | *** | 51249 | 52960 | 62011 | 14110 | 14710 | 15886 | 2635 | 2672 | 2724 | 736 | 760 | 760 | 361 | 361 | 361 |
| | *** | 51849 | 55261 | 76124 | 14372 | 15174 | 19364 | 2649 | 2686 | 3247 | 736 | 760 | 865 | 361 | 361 | 403 |
| 0.25 | *** | 59522 | 61997 | 76149 | 16585 | 17485 | 19360 | 3099 | 3174 | 3249 | 872 | 872 | 872 | 422 | 422 | 422 |
| | *** | 60399 | 65410 | 88737 | 16960 | 18211 | 22459 | 3136 | 3211 | 3714 | 872 | 872 | 970 | 422 | 422 | 444 |
| 0.3 | *** | 65124 | 68485 | 88172 | 18436 | 19660 | 22322 | 3497 | 3586 | 3699 | 961 | 961 | 985 | 460 | 460 | 460 |
| | *** | 66324 | 73060 | 99015 | 18947 | 20672 | 24970 | 3549 | 3647 | 4088 | 961 | 985 | 1052 | 460 | 460 | 475 |
| 0.35 | *** | 68260 | 72610 | 97899 | 19711 | 21249 | 24699 | 3797 | 3910 | 4060 | 1036 | 1036 | 1060 | 474 | 474 | 497 |
| | *** | 69835 | 78399 | 106956 | 20372 | 22547 | 26897 | 3849 | 3985 | 4368 | 1036 | 1060 | 1110 | 474 | 474 | 496 |
| 0.4 | *** | 69235 | 74635 | 105211 | 20461 | 22299 | 26461 | 3999 | 4135 | 4299 | 1074 | 1097 | 1111 | 497 | 497 | 497 |
| | *** | 71222 | 81624 | 112562 | 21249 | 23836 | 28240 | 4060 | 4210 | 4555 | 1097 | 1097 | 1145 | 497 | 497 | 507 |
| 0.45 | *** | 68410 | 74897 | 110049 | 20761 | 22847 | 27610 | 4111 | 4261 | 4449 | 1097 | 1111 | 1135 | 497 | 511 | 511 |
| | *** | 70824 | 82974 | 115833 | 21647 | 24586 | 28999 | 4186 | 4360 | 4649 | 1111 | 1135 | 1157 | 511 | 511 | 507 |
| 0.5 | *** | 66160 | 73636 | 112360 | 20649 | 22922 | 28111 | 4135 | 4299 | 4510 | 1097 | 1111 | 1135 | 497 | 497 | 497 |
| | *** | 69010 | 82660 | 116767 | 21610 | 24835 | 29175 | 4210 | 4397 | 4649 | 1111 | 1135 | 1145 | 497 | 497 | 496 |
| 0.55 | *** | 62836 | 71185 | 112111 | 20161 | 22561 | 27999 | 4074 | 4247 | 4472 | 1074 | 1097 | 1111 | 474 | 474 | 497 |
| | *** | 66047 | 80874 | 115365 | 21174 | 24572 | 28766 | 4149 | 4336 | 4555 | 1074 | 1097 | 1110 | 474 | 497 | 475 |
| 0.6 | *** | 58711 | 67674 | 109322 | 19360 | 21797 | 27235 | 3924 | 4097 | 4299 | 1022 | 1036 | 1060 | 460 | 460 | 460 |
| | *** | 62222 | 77761 | 111628 | 20386 | 23822 | 27773 | 3999 | 4186 | 4368 | 1036 | 1060 | 1052 | 460 | 460 | 444 |
| 0.65 | *** | 54061 | 63310 | 104011 | 18235 | 20635 | 25847 | 3699 | 3849 | 4060 | 961 | 961 | 985 | 422 | 422 | 422 |
| | *** | 57722 | 73435 | 105555 | 19261 | 22585 | 26196 | 3774 | 3947 | 4088 | 961 | 985 | 970 | 422 | 422 | 403 |
| 0.7 | *** | 48961 | 58149 | 96174 | 16824 | 19074 | 23822 | 3385 | 3535 | 3699 | 849 | 872 | 886 | 361 | 361 | 361 |
| | *** | 52636 | 67922 | 97146 | 17799 | 20897 | 24036 | 3460 | 3610 | 3714 | 872 | 872 | 865 | 361 | 361 | 351 |
| 0.75 | *** | 43486 | 52210 | 85861 | 15122 | 17147 | 21174 | 2986 | 3099 | 3249 | 736 | 736 | 760 | 310 | 310 | 310 |
| | *** | 47011 | 61224 | 86402 | 15999 | 18722 | 21291 | 3047 | 3174 | 3247 | 736 | 760 | 736 | 310 | 310 | 289 |
| 0.8 | *** | 37585 | 45399 | 73060 | 13097 | 14761 | 17911 | 2522 | 2597 | 2710 | 586 | 610 | 610 | 235 | 235 | 235 |
| | *** | 40772 | 53222 | 73321 | 13824 | 16036 | 17963 | 2560 | 2649 | 2687 | 586 | 610 | 584 | 235 | 235 | 216 |
| 0.85 | *** | 31060 | 37510 | 57811 | 10660 | 11897 | 14049 | 1936 | 1997 | 2049 | 422 | 422 | 436 | . | . | . |
| | *** | 33722 | 43674 | 57905 | 11222 | 12797 | 14050 | 1960 | 2011 | 2033 | 422 | 422 | 409 | . | . | . |
| 0.9 | *** | 23499 | 28060 | 40135 | 7711 | 8447 | 9572 | 1261 | 1285 | 1299 | . | . | . | . | . | . |
| | *** | 25411 | 32110 | 40153 | 8049 | 8935 | 9554 | 1261 | 1299 | 1285 | . | . | . | . | . | . |
| 0.95 | *** | 13885 | 15961 | 20086 | 3985 | 4210 | 4486 | . | . | . | . | . | . | . | . | . |
| | *** | 14799 | 17574 | 20065 | 4097 | 4336 | 4474 | . | . | . | . | . | . | . | . | . |
| 0.98 | *** | 5799 | 6272 | 6910 | . | . | . | . | . | . | . | . | . | . | . | . |
| | *** | 6010 | 6549 | 6891 | . | . | . | . | . | . | . | . | . | . | . | . |

## TABLE 1: ALPHA= 0.005 POWER= 0.8　　EXPECTED ACCRUAL THRU MINIMUM FOLLOW-UP= 17000

PCONT=***　REQUIRED NUMBER OF PATIENTS

| PCONT | FACT= | DEL=.01 1.0/.75 | DEL=.01 .50/.25 | DEL=.01 .00/BIN | DEL=.02 1.0/.75 | DEL=.02 .50/.25 | DEL=.02 .00/BIN | DEL=.05 1.0/.75 | DEL=.05 .50/.25 | DEL=.05 .00/BIN | DEL=.10 1.0/75 | DEL=.10 .50/.25 | DEL=.10 .00/BIN | DEL=.15 1.0/.75 | DEL=.15 .50/.25 | DEL=.15 .00/BIN |
|---|---|---|---|---|---|---|---|---|---|---|---|---|---|---|---|---|
| 0.01 | *** | 1796 | 1796 | 1796 | 665 | 665 | 665 | 224 | 224 | 224 | 112 | 112 | 112 | 70 | 70 | 70 |
|  | *** | 1796 | 1796 | 6891 | 665 | 665 | 2278 | 224 | 224 | 620 | 112 | 112 | 252 | 70 | 70 | 150 |
| 0.02 | *** | 3980 | 4006 | 4022 | 1286 | 1286 | 1286 | 351 | 351 | 351 | 155 | 155 | 155 | 96 | 96 | 96 |
|  | *** | 3980 | 4006 | 11376 | 1286 | 1286 | 3387 | 351 | 351 | 792 | 155 | 155 | 293 | 96 | 96 | 167 |
| 0.05 | *** | 12140 | 12294 | 12549 | 3470 | 3496 | 3512 | 734 | 750 | 750 | 266 | 266 | 266 | 155 | 155 | 155 |
|  | *** | 12209 | 12395 | 24269 | 3470 | 3496 | 6576 | 734 | 750 | 1285 | 266 | 266 | 409 | 155 | 155 | 216 |
| 0.1 | *** | 26930 | 27482 | 29225 | 7406 | 7534 | 7720 | 1414 | 1430 | 1430 | 436 | 436 | 436 | 240 | 240 | 240 |
|  | *** | 27142 | 28077 | 43890 | 7465 | 7619 | 11423 | 1430 | 1430 | 2033 | 436 | 436 | 584 | 240 | 240 | 289 |
| 0.15 | *** | 40402 | 41550 | 46166 | 11077 | 11401 | 11954 | 2067 | 2094 | 2110 | 606 | 606 | 606 | 309 | 309 | 309 |
|  | *** | 40827 | 42910 | 61175 | 11231 | 11630 | 15685 | 2067 | 2094 | 2687 | 606 | 606 | 736 | 309 | 309 | 351 |
| 0.2 | *** | 51495 | 53349 | 62019 | 14222 | 14801 | 15880 | 2646 | 2662 | 2731 | 750 | 750 | 750 | 367 | 367 | 367 |
|  | *** | 52175 | 55702 | 76124 | 14477 | 15242 | 19364 | 2662 | 2689 | 3247 | 750 | 750 | 865 | 367 | 367 | 403 |
| 0.25 | *** | 59867 | 62571 | 76145 | 16756 | 17622 | 19365 | 3130 | 3172 | 3257 | 861 | 877 | 877 | 410 | 410 | 410 |
|  | *** | 60845 | 66056 | 88737 | 17139 | 18329 | 22459 | 3156 | 3215 | 3714 | 861 | 877 | 970 | 410 | 410 | 444 |
| 0.3 | *** | 65605 | 69244 | 88172 | 18669 | 19859 | 22324 | 3512 | 3597 | 3709 | 962 | 962 | 989 | 452 | 452 | 452 |
|  | *** | 66922 | 73935 | 99015 | 19179 | 20836 | 24970 | 3555 | 3640 | 4088 | 962 | 962 | 1052 | 452 | 452 | 475 |
| 0.35 | *** | 68904 | 73579 | 97905 | 20002 | 21516 | 24704 | 3810 | 3921 | 4049 | 1031 | 1047 | 1047 | 479 | 479 | 479 |
|  | *** | 70620 | 79529 | 106956 | 20640 | 22749 | 26897 | 3879 | 3980 | 4368 | 1047 | 1047 | 1110 | 479 | 479 | 496 |
| 0.4 | *** | 70051 | 75805 | 105215 | 20810 | 22595 | 26462 | 4022 | 4150 | 4304 | 1090 | 1090 | 1116 | 495 | 495 | 495 |
|  | *** | 72192 | 82971 | 112562 | 21575 | 24082 | 28240 | 4091 | 4219 | 4555 | 1090 | 1090 | 1145 | 495 | 495 | 507 |
| 0.45 | *** | 69414 | 76272 | 110044 | 21150 | 23190 | 27610 | 4134 | 4277 | 4447 | 1116 | 1116 | 1132 | 495 | 495 | 521 |
|  | *** | 72006 | 84501 | 115833 | 22026 | 24874 | 28999 | 4219 | 4362 | 4649 | 1116 | 1132 | 1157 | 495 | 495 | 507 |
| 0.5 | *** | 67347 | 75210 | 112355 | 21065 | 23301 | 28120 | 4176 | 4320 | 4516 | 1116 | 1116 | 1132 | 495 | 495 | 495 |
|  | *** | 70365 | 84331 | 116767 | 22026 | 25129 | 29175 | 4235 | 4405 | 4649 | 1116 | 1132 | 1145 | 495 | 495 | 496 |
| 0.55 | *** | 64186 | 72872 | 112100 | 20597 | 22961 | 27992 | 4107 | 4261 | 4474 | 1074 | 1090 | 1116 | 479 | 479 | 495 |
|  | *** | 67560 | 82647 | 115365 | 21617 | 24874 | 28766 | 4176 | 4362 | 4555 | 1090 | 1090 | 1110 | 479 | 479 | 475 |
| 0.6 | *** | 60207 | 69456 | 109321 | 19816 | 22196 | 27227 | 3964 | 4107 | 4304 | 1031 | 1047 | 1047 | 452 | 452 | 452 |
|  | *** | 63846 | 79587 | 111628 | 20836 | 24109 | 27773 | 4049 | 4219 | 4368 | 1031 | 1047 | 1052 | 452 | 452 | 444 |
| 0.65 | *** | 55617 | 65121 | 104009 | 18685 | 21022 | 25851 | 3725 | 3879 | 4049 | 962 | 962 | 989 | 410 | 410 | 410 |
|  | *** | 59400 | 75236 | 105555 | 19705 | 22876 | 26196 | 3810 | 3964 | 4088 | 962 | 962 | 970 | 410 | 410 | 403 |
| 0.7 | *** | 50544 | 59910 | 96189 | 17266 | 19450 | 23827 | 3411 | 3555 | 3709 | 861 | 877 | 877 | 367 | 367 | 367 |
|  | *** | 54300 | 69642 | 97146 | 18217 | 21150 | 24036 | 3470 | 3624 | 3714 | 861 | 877 | 865 | 367 | 367 | 351 |
| 0.75 | *** | 44992 | 53859 | 85861 | 15524 | 17452 | 21176 | 3029 | 3130 | 3257 | 734 | 750 | 750 | 309 | 309 | 309 |
|  | *** | 48589 | 62784 | 86402 | 16374 | 18940 | 21291 | 3071 | 3172 | 3247 | 750 | 750 | 736 | 309 | 309 | 289 |
| 0.8 | *** | 38957 | 46846 | 73042 | 13415 | 15030 | 17920 | 2535 | 2604 | 2705 | 606 | 606 | 606 | 240 | 240 | 240 |
|  | *** | 42187 | 54555 | 73321 | 14137 | 16204 | 17963 | 2561 | 2646 | 2687 | 606 | 606 | 584 | 240 | 240 | 216 |
| 0.85 | *** | 32226 | 38660 | 57811 | 10907 | 12081 | 14052 | 1940 | 2009 | 2051 | 436 | 436 | 436 | . | . | . |
|  | *** | 34877 | 44695 | 57905 | 11444 | 12931 | 14050 | 1966 | 2025 | 2033 | 436 | 436 | 409 | . | . | . |
| 0.9 | *** | 24337 | 28842 | 40147 | 7847 | 8554 | 9574 | 1260 | 1286 | 1302 | . | . | . | . | . | . |
|  | *** | 26234 | 32752 | 40153 | 8171 | 8995 | 9554 | 1260 | 1286 | 1285 | . | . | . | . | . | . |
| 0.95 | *** | 14291 | 16289 | 20087 | 4022 | 4235 | 4490 | . | . | . | . | . | . | . | . | . |
|  | *** | 15184 | 17819 | 20065 | 4134 | 4362 | 4474 | . | . | . | . | . | . | . | . | . |
| 0.98 | *** | 5892 | 6317 | 6912 | . | . | . | . | . | . | . | . | . | . | . | . |
|  | *** | 6105 | 6599 | 6891 | . | . | . | . | . | . | . | . | . | . | . | . |

# TABLE 1: ALPHA= 0.005 POWER= 0.8 EXPECTED ACCRUAL THRU MINIMUM FOLLOW-UP= 20000

| | | DEL=.01 | | | DEL=.02 | | | DEL=.05 | | | DEL=.10 | | | DEL=.15 | |
|---|---|---|---|---|---|---|---|---|---|---|---|---|---|---|---|
| FACT= | 1.0 .75 | .50 .25 | .00 BIN | 1.0 .75 | .50 .25 | .00 BIN | 1.0 .75 | .50 .25 | .00 BIN | 1.0 75 | .50 .25 | .00 BIN | 1.0 .75 | .50 .25 | .00 BIN |
| PCONT=*** | | | | | | REQUIRED NUMBER OF PATIENTS | | | | | | | | | |
| 0.01 *** | 1782 | 1782 | 1813 | 663 | 663 | 663 | 213 | 213 | 213 | 113 | 113 | 113 | 82 | 82 | 82 |
| *** | 1782 | 1782 | 6891 | 663 | 663 | 2278 | 213 | 213 | 620 | 113 | 113 | 252 | 82 | 82 | 150 |
| 0.02 *** | 3982 | 4013 | 4013 | 1282 | 1282 | 1282 | 332 | 332 | 332 | 163 | 163 | 163 | 82 | 82 | 82 |
| *** | 3982 | 4013 | 11376 | 1282 | 1282 | 3387 | 332 | 332 | 792 | 163 | 163 | 293 | 82 | 82 | 167 |
| 0.05 *** | 12182 | 12313 | 12563 | 3463 | 3482 | 3513 | 732 | 732 | 732 | 263 | 263 | 263 | 163 | 163 | 163 |
| *** | 12232 | 12413 | 24269 | 3482 | 3513 | 6576 | 732 | 732 | 1285 | 263 | 263 | 409 | 163 | 163 | 216 |
| 0.1 *** | 27032 | 27632 | 29213 | 7432 | 7563 | 7732 | 1413 | 1432 | 1432 | 432 | 432 | 432 | 232 | 232 | 232 |
| *** | 27282 | 28182 | 43890 | 7482 | 7632 | 11423 | 1432 | 1432 | 2033 | 432 | 432 | 584 | 232 | 232 | 289 |
| 0.15 *** | 40632 | 41863 | 46163 | 11163 | 11463 | 11963 | 2063 | 2082 | 2113 | 613 | 613 | 613 | 313 | 313 | 313 |
| *** | 41113 | 43232 | 61175 | 11313 | 11682 | 15685 | 2082 | 2082 | 2687 | 613 | 613 | 736 | 313 | 313 | 351 |
| 0.2 *** | 51863 | 53863 | 62013 | 14363 | 14932 | 15882 | 2663 | 2682 | 2713 | 732 | 763 | 763 | 363 | 363 | 363 |
| *** | 52613 | 56263 | 76124 | 14613 | 15332 | 19364 | 2663 | 2713 | 3247 | 732 | 763 | 865 | 363 | 363 | 403 |
| 0.25 *** | 60413 | 63332 | 76132 | 16963 | 17813 | 19363 | 3132 | 3182 | 3263 | 863 | 863 | 882 | 413 | 413 | 413 |
| *** | 61482 | 66882 | 88737 | 17332 | 18463 | 22459 | 3163 | 3213 | 3714 | 863 | 882 | 970 | 413 | 413 | 444 |
| 0.3 *** | 66332 | 70282 | 88163 | 18963 | 20113 | 22313 | 3532 | 3613 | 3713 | 963 | 963 | 982 | 463 | 463 | 463 |
| *** | 67813 | 75082 | 99015 | 19463 | 21013 | 24970 | 3582 | 3663 | 4088 | 963 | 982 | 1052 | 463 | 463 | 475 |
| 0.35 *** | 69832 | 74882 | 97913 | 20363 | 21832 | 24682 | 3863 | 3932 | 4063 | 1032 | 1032 | 1063 | 482 | 482 | 482 |
| *** | 71732 | 80963 | 106956 | 21013 | 22963 | 26897 | 3882 | 3982 | 4368 | 1032 | 1063 | 1110 | 482 | 482 | 496 |
| 0.4 *** | 71213 | 77413 | 105213 | 21232 | 22982 | 26463 | 4063 | 4163 | 4313 | 1082 | 1082 | 1113 | 513 | 513 | 513 |
| *** | 73582 | 84682 | 112562 | 22013 | 24363 | 28240 | 4113 | 4232 | 4555 | 1082 | 1113 | 1145 | 513 | 513 | 507 |
| 0.45 *** | 70832 | 78132 | 110032 | 21632 | 23632 | 27613 | 4182 | 4313 | 4463 | 1113 | 1113 | 1132 | 513 | 513 | 513 |
| *** | 73632 | 86463 | 115833 | 22513 | 25182 | 28999 | 4232 | 4382 | 4649 | 1113 | 1132 | 1157 | 513 | 513 | 507 |
| 0.5 *** | 69013 | 77282 | 112363 | 21613 | 23763 | 28113 | 4213 | 4332 | 4513 | 1113 | 1113 | 1132 | 513 | 513 | 513 |
| *** | 72232 | 86482 | 116767 | 22532 | 25463 | 29175 | 4282 | 4432 | 4649 | 1113 | 1132 | 1145 | 513 | 513 | 496 |
| 0.55 *** | 66063 | 75113 | 112113 | 21182 | 23463 | 27982 | 4163 | 4282 | 4463 | 1082 | 1082 | 1113 | 482 | 482 | 482 |
| *** | 69632 | 84932 | 115365 | 22163 | 25232 | 28766 | 4213 | 4363 | 4555 | 1082 | 1113 | 1110 | 482 | 482 | 475 |
| 0.6 *** | 62232 | 71813 | 109332 | 20382 | 22682 | 27232 | 4013 | 4132 | 4313 | 1032 | 1032 | 1063 | 463 | 463 | 463 |
| *** | 66032 | 81932 | 111628 | 21382 | 24482 | 27773 | 4063 | 4213 | 4368 | 1032 | 1063 | 1052 | 463 | 463 | 444 |
| 0.65 *** | 57713 | 67482 | 104013 | 19263 | 21513 | 25832 | 3782 | 3913 | 4063 | 963 | 963 | 982 | 413 | 413 | 413 |
| *** | 61632 | 77563 | 105555 | 20263 | 23232 | 26196 | 3832 | 3982 | 4088 | 963 | 982 | 970 | 413 | 413 | 403 |
| 0.7 *** | 52632 | 62213 | 96182 | 17813 | 19913 | 23832 | 3463 | 3563 | 3713 | 863 | 863 | 882 | 363 | 363 | 363 |
| *** | 56513 | 71832 | 97146 | 18732 | 21482 | 24036 | 3513 | 3632 | 3714 | 863 | 882 | 865 | 363 | 363 | 351 |
| 0.75 *** | 47013 | 55982 | 85863 | 16013 | 17863 | 21182 | 3063 | 3132 | 3263 | 732 | 732 | 763 | 313 | 313 | 313 |
| *** | 50682 | 64782 | 86402 | 16832 | 19213 | 21291 | 3082 | 3182 | 3247 | 732 | 763 | 736 | 313 | 313 | 289 |
| 0.8 *** | 40782 | 48713 | 73063 | 13832 | 15332 | 17913 | 2563 | 2613 | 2713 | 582 | 613 | 613 | 232 | 232 | 232 |
| *** | 44063 | 56232 | 73321 | 14513 | 16432 | 17963 | 2582 | 2663 | 2687 | 582 | 613 | 584 | 232 | 232 | 216 |
| 0.85 *** | 33713 | 40132 | 57813 | 11213 | 12313 | 14032 | 1963 | 2013 | 2063 | 432 | 432 | 432 | . | . | . |
| *** | 36413 | 45963 | 57905 | 11713 | 13063 | 14050 | 1982 | 2032 | 2033 | 432 | 432 | 409 | . | . | . |
| 0.9 *** | 25413 | 29832 | 40132 | 8032 | 8682 | 9563 | 1263 | 1282 | 1313 | . | . | . | . | . | . |
| *** | 27282 | 33532 | 40153 | 8332 | 9082 | 9554 | 1282 | 1282 | 1285 | . | . | . | . | . | . |
| 0.95 *** | 14782 | 16713 | 20082 | 4082 | 4263 | 4482 | . | . | . | . | . | . | . | . | . |
| *** | 15632 | 18082 | 20065 | 4182 | 4382 | 4474 | . | . | . | . | . | . | . | . | . |
| 0.98 *** | 6013 | 6413 | 6913 | . | . | . | . | . | . | . | . | . | . | . | . |
| *** | 6213 | 6632 | 6891 | . | . | . | . | . | . | . | . | . | . | . | . |

TABLE 1: ALPHA= 0.005 POWER= 0.8    EXPECTED ACCRUAL THRU MINIMUM FOLLOW-UP= 25000

| | DEL=.01 | | | DEL=.02 | | | DEL=.05 | | | DEL=.10 | | | DEL=.15 | | |
|---|---|---|---|---|---|---|---|---|---|---|---|---|---|---|---|
| FACT= | 1.0 / .75 | .50 / .25 | .00 BIN | 1.0 / .75 | .50 / .25 | .00 BIN | 1.0 / .75 | .50 / .25 | .00 BIN | 1.0 / 75 | .50 / .25 | .00 BIN | 1.0 / .75 | .50 / .25 | .00 BIN |
| PCONT=*** | | | | REQUIRED NUMBER OF PATIENTS | | | | | | | | | | | |
| 0.01 *** | 1790 | 1790 | 1790 | 665 | 665 | 665 | 204 | 204 | 204 | 102 | 102 | 102 | 79 | 79 | 79 |
| *** | 1790 | 1790 | 6891 | 665 | 665 | 2278 | 204 | 204 | 620 | 102 | 102 | 252 | 79 | 79 | 150 |
| 0.02 *** | 3977 | 4016 | 4016 | 1266 | 1290 | 1290 | 352 | 352 | 352 | 141 | 141 | 141 | 102 | 102 | 102 |
| *** | 4016 | 4016 | 11376 | 1290 | 1290 | 3387 | 352 | 352 | 792 | 141 | 141 | 293 | 102 | 102 | 167 |
| 0.05 *** | 12227 | 12352 | 12540 | 3477 | 3477 | 3516 | 727 | 727 | 727 | 266 | 266 | 266 | 141 | 141 | 141 |
| *** | 12266 | 12454 | 24269 | 3477 | 3516 | 6576 | 727 | 727 | 1285 | 266 | 266 | 409 | 141 | 141 | 216 |
| 0.1 *** | 27227 | 27829 | 29227 | 7477 | 7579 | 7727 | 1415 | 1415 | 1454 | 454 | 454 | 454 | 227 | 227 | 227 |
| *** | 27454 | 28352 | 43890 | 7540 | 7641 | 11423 | 1415 | 1415 | 2033 | 454 | 454 | 584 | 227 | 227 | 289 |
| 0.15 *** | 40977 | 42290 | 46165 | 11266 | 11540 | 11954 | 2079 | 2079 | 2102 | 602 | 602 | 602 | 290 | 290 | 290 |
| *** | 41516 | 43641 | 61175 | 11391 | 11727 | 15685 | 2079 | 2102 | 2687 | 602 | 602 | 736 | 290 | 290 | 351 |
| 0.2 *** | 52415 | 54641 | 62016 | 14540 | 15079 | 15891 | 2665 | 2704 | 2727 | 727 | 766 | 766 | 352 | 352 | 352 |
| *** | 53290 | 57016 | 76124 | 14790 | 15415 | 19364 | 2665 | 2704 | 3247 | 766 | 766 | 865 | 352 | 352 | 403 |
| 0.25 *** | 61227 | 64454 | 76141 | 17266 | 18040 | 19352 | 3165 | 3204 | 3266 | 852 | 852 | 891 | 415 | 415 | 415 |
| *** | 62477 | 68016 | 88737 | 17602 | 18602 | 22459 | 3165 | 3227 | 3714 | 852 | 891 | 970 | 415 | 415 | 444 |
| 0.3 *** | 67454 | 71790 | 88165 | 19352 | 20415 | 22329 | 3579 | 3641 | 3704 | 977 | 977 | 977 | 454 | 454 | 454 |
| *** | 69102 | 76641 | 99015 | 19829 | 21227 | 24970 | 3602 | 3665 | 4088 | 977 | 977 | 1052 | 454 | 454 | 475 |
| 0.35 *** | 71266 | 76790 | 97915 | 20852 | 22227 | 24704 | 3891 | 3954 | 4040 | 1040 | 1040 | 1040 | 477 | 477 | 477 |
| *** | 73415 | 82891 | 106956 | 21477 | 23266 | 26897 | 3915 | 4016 | 4368 | 1040 | 1040 | 1110 | 477 | 477 | 496 |
| 0.4 *** | 73016 | 79704 | 105227 | 21829 | 23477 | 26454 | 4102 | 4204 | 4290 | 1079 | 1102 | 1102 | 516 | 516 | 516 |
| *** | 75641 | 87016 | 112562 | 22540 | 24704 | 28240 | 4141 | 4266 | 4555 | 1102 | 1102 | 1145 | 516 | 516 | 507 |
| 0.45 *** | 72977 | 80766 | 110040 | 22329 | 24165 | 27602 | 4227 | 4329 | 4454 | 1102 | 1102 | 1141 | 516 | 516 | 516 |
| *** | 76040 | 89102 | 115833 | 23141 | 25579 | 28999 | 4290 | 4391 | 4649 | 1102 | 1141 | 1157 | 516 | 516 | 507 |
| 0.5 *** | 71477 | 80227 | 112352 | 22329 | 24391 | 28102 | 4266 | 4391 | 4516 | 1102 | 1102 | 1141 | 516 | 516 | 516 |
| *** | 74954 | 89391 | 116767 | 23227 | 25891 | 29175 | 4329 | 4454 | 4649 | 1102 | 1141 | 1145 | 516 | 516 | 496 |
| 0.55 *** | 68790 | 78266 | 112102 | 21954 | 24079 | 27977 | 4204 | 4329 | 4454 | 1079 | 1102 | 1102 | 477 | 477 | 477 |
| *** | 72602 | 88016 | 115365 | 22891 | 25665 | 28766 | 4266 | 4391 | 4555 | 1102 | 1102 | 1110 | 477 | 477 | 475 |
| 0.6 *** | 65165 | 75079 | 109329 | 21165 | 23329 | 27227 | 4040 | 4165 | 4290 | 1040 | 1040 | 1040 | 454 | 454 | 454 |
| *** | 69165 | 85079 | 111628 | 22141 | 24915 | 27773 | 4102 | 4227 | 4368 | 1040 | 1040 | 1052 | 454 | 454 | 444 |
| 0.65 *** | 60727 | 70766 | 104016 | 20040 | 22141 | 25852 | 3829 | 3915 | 4040 | 954 | 977 | 977 | 415 | 415 | 415 |
| *** | 64829 | 80641 | 105555 | 20954 | 23665 | 26196 | 3891 | 3977 | 4088 | 977 | 977 | 970 | 415 | 415 | 403 |
| 0.7 *** | 55641 | 65352 | 96165 | 18516 | 20477 | 23829 | 3516 | 3602 | 3704 | 852 | 891 | 891 | 352 | 352 | 352 |
| *** | 59641 | 74766 | 97146 | 19391 | 21852 | 24036 | 3540 | 3641 | 3714 | 852 | 891 | 865 | 352 | 352 | 351 |
| 0.75 *** | 49852 | 58891 | 85852 | 16641 | 18352 | 21165 | 3079 | 3165 | 3266 | 727 | 766 | 766 | 290 | 290 | 290 |
| *** | 53579 | 67391 | 86402 | 17415 | 19540 | 21291 | 3141 | 3204 | 3247 | 727 | 766 | 736 | 290 | 290 | 289 |
| 0.8 *** | 43290 | 51204 | 73040 | 14352 | 15727 | 17915 | 2579 | 2641 | 2704 | 602 | 602 | 602 | 227 | 227 | 227 |
| *** | 46602 | 58415 | 73321 | 14977 | 16665 | 17963 | 2602 | 2665 | 2687 | 602 | 602 | 584 | 227 | 227 | 216 |
| 0.85 *** | 35790 | 42102 | 57790 | 11602 | 12602 | 14040 | 1977 | 2016 | 2040 | 415 | 415 | 415 | . | . | . |
| *** | 38477 | 47602 | 57905 | 12040 | 13227 | 14050 | 1977 | 2040 | 2033 | 415 | 415 | 409 | . | . | . |
| 0.9 *** | 26891 | 31102 | 40141 | 8266 | 8829 | 9579 | 1266 | 1290 | 1290 | . | . | . | . | . | . |
| *** | 28704 | 34540 | 40153 | 8540 | 9165 | 9554 | 1290 | 1290 | 1285 | . | . | . | . | . | . |
| 0.95 *** | 15454 | 17204 | 20079 | 4165 | 4329 | 4477 | . | . | . | . | . | . | . | . | . |
| *** | 16227 | 18415 | 20065 | 4227 | 4391 | 4474 | . | . | . | . | . | . | . | . | . |
| 0.98 *** | 6165 | 6477 | 6915 | . | . | . | . | . | . | . | . | . | . | . | . |
| *** | 6329 | 6704 | 6891 | . | . | . | . | . | . | . | . | . | . | . | . |

## TABLE 2: ALPHA= 0.005 POWER= 0.9    EXPECTED ACCRUAL THRU MINIMUM FOLLOW-UP= 30

| | | DEL=.10 | | | DEL=.15 | | | DEL=.20 | | | DEL=.25 | | | DEL=.30 | | |
|---|---|---|---|---|---|---|---|---|---|---|---|---|---|---|---|---|
| FACT= | | 1.0 .75 | .50 .25 | .00 BIN | 1.0 .75 | .50 .25 | .00 BIN | 1.0 .75 | .50 .25 | .00 BIN | 1.0 75 | .50 .25 | .00 BIN | 1.0 .75 | .50 .25 | .00 BIN |
| PCONT=*** | | | | | | REQUIRED NUMBER OF PATIENTS | | | | | | | | | | |
| 0.05 | *** | 312 | 313 | 338 | 181 | 182 | 197 | 127 | 128 | 138 | 99 | 100 | 107 | 81 | 83 | 88 |
| | *** | 312 | 315 | 521 | 181 | 184 | 275 | 128 | 131 | 175 | 99 | 102 | 123 | 82 | 84 | 91 |
| 0.1 | *** | 491 | 494 | 566 | 259 | 261 | 300 | 170 | 172 | 197 | 125 | 127 | 144 | 99 | 101 | 113 |
| | *** | 492 | 498 | 744 | 260 | 266 | 368 | 171 | 177 | 224 | 126 | 131 | 152 | 99 | 104 | 110 |
| 0.15 | *** | 634 | 637 | 776 | 317 | 321 | 391 | 200 | 204 | 246 | 142 | 146 | 175 | 110 | 113 | 133 |
| | *** | 635 | 644 | 938 | 318 | 328 | 447 | 201 | 211 | 265 | 144 | 153 | 175 | 111 | 119 | 124 |
| 0.2 | *** | 737 | 742 | 961 | 357 | 363 | 469 | 219 | 225 | 288 | 153 | 159 | 199 | 116 | 121 | 149 |
| | *** | 739 | 752 | 1102 | 359 | 374 | 513 | 221 | 235 | 298 | 155 | 167 | 195 | 118 | 128 | 136 |
| 0.25 | *** | 802 | 810 | 1120 | 380 | 388 | 534 | 229 | 238 | 321 | 158 | 166 | 219 | 119 | 126 | 161 |
| | *** | 805 | 824 | 1235 | 383 | 403 | 566 | 232 | 251 | 324 | 161 | 177 | 209 | 121 | 134 | 144 |
| 0.3 | *** | 833 | 843 | 1248 | 389 | 399 | 585 | 232 | 242 | 346 | 158 | 168 | 233 | 118 | 127 | 169 |
| | *** | 836 | 862 | 1340 | 392 | 419 | 606 | 235 | 260 | 343 | 162 | 182 | 218 | 121 | 137 | 149 |
| 0.35 | *** | 833 | 845 | 1346 | 384 | 398 | 622 | 228 | 241 | 363 | 155 | 167 | 241 | 115 | 125 | 173 |
| | *** | 837 | 870 | 1414 | 389 | 423 | 632 | 232 | 262 | 354 | 159 | 183 | 223 | 119 | 138 | 151 |
| 0.4 | *** | 806 | 822 | 1411 | 369 | 387 | 644 | 218 | 235 | 372 | 149 | 163 | 244 | 110 | 122 | 174 |
| | *** | 811 | 854 | 1459 | 375 | 417 | 645 | 224 | 259 | 358 | 154 | 181 | 223 | 115 | 135 | 149 |
| 0.45 | *** | 757 | 777 | 1444 | 346 | 368 | 652 | 205 | 225 | 372 | 140 | 156 | 242 | 104 | 117 | 170 |
| | *** | 764 | 818 | 1474 | 353 | 404 | 645 | 212 | 252 | 354 | 146 | 176 | 218 | 109 | 131 | 144 |
| 0.5 | *** | 691 | 717 | 1445 | 317 | 343 | 645 | 189 | 211 | 365 | 130 | 147 | 234 | 97 | 110 | 163 |
| | *** | 700 | 768 | 1459 | 326 | 384 | 632 | 198 | 241 | 343 | 137 | 168 | 209 | 102 | 125 | 136 |
| 0.55 | *** | 613 | 647 | 1413 | 284 | 315 | 624 | 172 | 196 | 349 | 119 | 137 | 222 | 89 | 102 | 153 |
| | *** | 625 | 708 | 1414 | 296 | 360 | 606 | 181 | 226 | 324 | 126 | 157 | 195 | 94 | 116 | 124 |
| 0.6 | *** | 530 | 572 | 1349 | 251 | 285 | 588 | 154 | 179 | 325 | 107 | 125 | 204 | 80 | 93 | 139 |
| | *** | 544 | 643 | 1340 | 264 | 333 | 566 | 164 | 209 | 298 | 114 | 145 | 175 | 85 | 106 | 110 |
| 0.65 | *** | 446 | 497 | 1252 | 217 | 254 | 538 | 136 | 161 | 293 | 95 | 112 | 181 | 71 | 82 | 121 |
| | *** | 464 | 575 | 1235 | 231 | 302 | 513 | 145 | 189 | 265 | 102 | 130 | 152 | 75 | 94 | 91 |
| 0.7 | *** | 367 | 425 | 1124 | 186 | 222 | 474 | 117 | 141 | 253 | 82 | 97 | 153 | . | . | . |
| | *** | 388 | 506 | 1102 | 200 | 268 | 447 | 126 | 167 | 224 | 88 | 112 | 123 | . | . | . |
| 0.75 | *** | 297 | 356 | 964 | 155 | 189 | 396 | 98 | 118 | 205 | . | . | . | . | . | . |
| | *** | 319 | 435 | 938 | 168 | 230 | 368 | 106 | 140 | 175 | . | . | . | . | . | . |
| 0.8 | *** | 234 | 291 | 773 | 124 | 153 | 304 | . | . | . | . | . | . | . | . | . |
| | *** | 256 | 361 | 744 | 136 | 186 | 275 | . | . | . | . | . | . | . | . | . |
| 0.85 | *** | 176 | 223 | 551 | . | . | . | . | . | . | . | . | . | . | . | . |
| | *** | 195 | 279 | 521 | . | . | . | . | . | . | . | . | . | . | . | . |

TABLE 2: ALPHA= 0.005 POWER= 0.9    EXPECTED ACCRUAL THRU MINIMUM FOLLOW-UP= 40

| | | DEL=.10 | | | DEL=.15 | | | DEL=.20 | | | DEL=.25 | | | DEL=.30 | | |
|---|---|---|---|---|---|---|---|---|---|---|---|---|---|---|---|---|
| FACT= | | 1.0 .75 | .50 .25 | .00 BIN | 1.0 .75 | .50 .25 | .00 BIN | 1.0 .75 | .50 .25 | .00 BIN | 1.0 75 | .50 .25 | .00 BIN | 1.0 .75 | .50 .25 | .00 BIN |
| PCONT=*** | | | | | REQUIRED NUMBER OF PATIENTS | | | | | | | | | | | |
| 0.05 | *** | 312 | 313 | 338 | 181 | 183 | 197 | 128 | 129 | 138 | 99 | 101 | 107 | 82 | 83 | 88 |
| | *** | 312 | 316 | 521 | 182 | 186 | 275 | 128 | 132 | 175 | 100 | 103 | 123 | 82 | 85 | 91 |
| 0.1 | *** | 492 | 495 | 566 | 260 | 263 | 300 | 171 | 174 | 197 | 126 | 129 | 144 | 100 | 102 | 113 |
| | *** | 493 | 501 | 744 | 261 | 269 | 368 | 172 | 179 | 224 | 127 | 133 | 152 | 101 | 106 | 110 |
| 0.15 | *** | 635 | 639 | 776 | 318 | 324 | 391 | 201 | 206 | 246 | 144 | 149 | 175 | 111 | 116 | 133 |
| | *** | 636 | 648 | 938 | 320 | 333 | 447 | 203 | 215 | 265 | 146 | 155 | 175 | 113 | 121 | 124 |
| 0.2 | *** | 739 | 745 | 961 | 359 | 366 | 469 | 221 | 229 | 288 | 155 | 162 | 199 | 118 | 124 | 149 |
| | *** | 741 | 759 | 1102 | 361 | 380 | 513 | 224 | 240 | 298 | 158 | 171 | 195 | 120 | 131 | 136 |
| 0.25 | *** | 805 | 814 | 1120 | 383 | 393 | 534 | 232 | 243 | 321 | 161 | 170 | 219 | 121 | 129 | 161 |
| | *** | 808 | 833 | 1235 | 386 | 412 | 566 | 236 | 258 | 324 | 164 | 182 | 209 | 124 | 138 | 144 |
| 0.3 | *** | 836 | 849 | 1248 | 392 | 406 | 585 | 235 | 249 | 346 | 162 | 174 | 233 | 121 | 131 | 169 |
| | *** | 841 | 875 | 1340 | 397 | 430 | 606 | 240 | 268 | 343 | 166 | 188 | 218 | 125 | 142 | 149 |
| 0.35 | *** | 837 | 854 | 1346 | 389 | 407 | 622 | 232 | 249 | 363 | 160 | 173 | 241 | 119 | 130 | 173 |
| | *** | 843 | 887 | 1414 | 395 | 437 | 632 | 238 | 272 | 354 | 165 | 190 | 223 | 124 | 143 | 151 |
| 0.4 | *** | 811 | 833 | 1411 | 375 | 398 | 644 | 224 | 244 | 372 | 154 | 170 | 244 | 115 | 128 | 174 |
| | *** | 818 | 875 | 1459 | 383 | 434 | 645 | 231 | 270 | 358 | 160 | 189 | 223 | 120 | 141 | 149 |
| 0.45 | *** | 764 | 791 | 1444 | 353 | 381 | 652 | 212 | 235 | 372 | 146 | 164 | 242 | 109 | 123 | 170 |
| | *** | 773 | 844 | 1474 | 363 | 423 | 645 | 221 | 264 | 354 | 153 | 184 | 218 | 115 | 137 | 144 |
| 0.5 | *** | 700 | 735 | 1445 | 326 | 359 | 645 | 198 | 223 | 365 | 137 | 156 | 234 | 102 | 116 | 163 |
| | *** | 711 | 799 | 1459 | 338 | 405 | 632 | 207 | 254 | 343 | 144 | 176 | 209 | 108 | 130 | 136 |
| 0.55 | *** | 625 | 669 | 1413 | 296 | 333 | 624 | 181 | 208 | 349 | 126 | 145 | 222 | 94 | 108 | 153 |
| | *** | 640 | 744 | 1414 | 309 | 382 | 606 | 192 | 240 | 324 | 134 | 166 | 195 | 100 | 122 | 124 |
| 0.6 | *** | 544 | 598 | 1349 | 264 | 304 | 588 | 164 | 191 | 325 | 114 | 133 | 204 | 85 | 99 | 139 |
| | *** | 563 | 682 | 1340 | 279 | 355 | 566 | 175 | 222 | 298 | 122 | 153 | 175 | 91 | 111 | 110 |
| 0.65 | *** | 464 | 526 | 1252 | 231 | 273 | 538 | 145 | 172 | 293 | 102 | 119 | 181 | 75 | 87 | 121 |
| | *** | 486 | 616 | 1235 | 247 | 323 | 513 | 156 | 202 | 265 | 109 | 137 | 152 | 80 | 98 | 91 |
| 0.7 | *** | 388 | 456 | 1124 | 200 | 240 | 474 | 126 | 151 | 253 | 88 | 103 | 153 | . | . | . |
| | *** | 413 | 546 | 1102 | 216 | 288 | 447 | 136 | 177 | 224 | 94 | 118 | 123 | . | . | . |
| 0.75 | *** | 319 | 387 | 964 | 168 | 205 | 396 | 106 | 127 | 205 | . | . | . | . | . | . |
| | *** | 345 | 473 | 938 | 183 | 247 | 368 | 115 | 149 | 175 | . | . | . | . | . | . |
| 0.8 | *** | 256 | 318 | 773 | 136 | 167 | 304 | . | . | . | . | . | . | . | . | . |
| | *** | 280 | 394 | 744 | 148 | 200 | 275 | . | . | . | . | . | . | . | . | . |
| 0.85 | *** | 195 | 245 | 551 | . | . | . | . | . | . | . | . | . | . | . | . |
| | *** | 214 | 304 | 521 | . | . | . | . | . | . | . | . | . | . | . | . |

TABLE 2: ALPHA= 0.005 POWER= 0.9    EXPECTED ACCRUAL THRU MINIMUM FOLLOW-UP= 50

| | | DEL=.10 | | | DEL=.15 | | | DEL=.20 | | | DEL=.25 | | | DEL=.30 | | |
|---|---|---|---|---|---|---|---|---|---|---|---|---|---|---|---|---|---|
| | FACT= | 1.0 .75 | .50 .25 | .00 BIN | 1.0 .75 | .50 .25 | .00 BIN | 1.0 .75 | .50 .25 | .00 BIN | 1.0 75 | .50 .25 | .00 BIN | 1.0 .75 | .50 .25 | .00 BIN |
| PCONT=*** | | | | | | REQUIRED NUMBER OF PATIENTS | | | | | | | | | | | |
| 0.05 | *** | 312 | 314 | 338 | 182 | 184 | 197 | 128 | 130 | 138 | 100 | 101 | 107 | 82 | 84 | 88 |
| | *** | 313 | 317 | 521 | 182 | 187 | 275 | 129 | 132 | 175 | 100 | 103 | 123 | 83 | 85 | 91 |
| 0.1 | *** | 493 | 496 | 566 | 261 | 265 | 300 | 171 | 175 | 197 | 127 | 130 | 144 | 100 | 103 | 113 |
| | *** | 494 | 503 | 744 | 262 | 271 | 368 | 173 | 181 | 224 | 128 | 134 | 152 | 102 | 107 | 110 |
| 0.15 | *** | 636 | 642 | 776 | 320 | 326 | 391 | 202 | 209 | 246 | 145 | 151 | 175 | 112 | 117 | 133 |
| | *** | 638 | 653 | 938 | 322 | 337 | 447 | 205 | 218 | 265 | 147 | 158 | 175 | 114 | 122 | 124 |
| 0.2 | *** | 740 | 749 | 961 | 361 | 370 | 469 | 223 | 232 | 288 | 157 | 165 | 199 | 120 | 126 | 149 |
| | *** | 743 | 766 | 1102 | 364 | 386 | 513 | 226 | 245 | 298 | 160 | 175 | 195 | 122 | 134 | 136 |
| 0.25 | *** | 807 | 819 | 1120 | 385 | 398 | 534 | 235 | 247 | 321 | 164 | 174 | 219 | 124 | 132 | 161 |
| | *** | 811 | 842 | 1235 | 390 | 420 | 566 | 239 | 264 | 324 | 167 | 186 | 209 | 127 | 141 | 144 |
| 0.3 | *** | 840 | 855 | 1248 | 396 | 413 | 585 | 239 | 255 | 346 | 165 | 178 | 233 | 124 | 135 | 169 |
| | *** | 845 | 887 | 1340 | 401 | 440 | 606 | 245 | 275 | 343 | 170 | 193 | 218 | 128 | 145 | 149 |
| 0.35 | *** | 841 | 862 | 1346 | 393 | 415 | 622 | 237 | 256 | 363 | 164 | 179 | 241 | 123 | 134 | 173 |
| | *** | 848 | 903 | 1414 | 401 | 449 | 632 | 244 | 280 | 354 | 169 | 196 | 223 | 127 | 146 | 151 |
| 0.4 | *** | 816 | 844 | 1411 | 381 | 408 | 644 | 230 | 252 | 372 | 159 | 176 | 244 | 119 | 132 | 174 |
| | *** | 826 | 895 | 1459 | 390 | 448 | 645 | 238 | 280 | 358 | 165 | 195 | 223 | 124 | 145 | 149 |
| 0.45 | *** | 771 | 805 | 1444 | 361 | 393 | 652 | 219 | 244 | 372 | 152 | 170 | 242 | 113 | 127 | 170 |
| | *** | 782 | 868 | 1474 | 372 | 439 | 645 | 228 | 274 | 354 | 159 | 190 | 218 | 119 | 141 | 144 |
| 0.5 | *** | 708 | 752 | 1445 | 335 | 372 | 645 | 205 | 232 | 365 | 143 | 162 | 234 | 107 | 121 | 163 |
| | *** | 723 | 827 | 1459 | 349 | 422 | 632 | 216 | 264 | 343 | 150 | 183 | 209 | 113 | 134 | 136 |
| 0.55 | *** | 636 | 689 | 1413 | 306 | 347 | 624 | 189 | 218 | 349 | 132 | 152 | 222 | 99 | 113 | 153 |
| | *** | 654 | 775 | 1414 | 321 | 400 | 606 | 200 | 250 | 324 | 140 | 172 | 195 | 105 | 126 | 124 |
| 0.6 | *** | 558 | 621 | 1349 | 275 | 319 | 588 | 172 | 201 | 325 | 120 | 140 | 204 | 90 | 103 | 139 |
| | *** | 581 | 715 | 1340 | 292 | 373 | 566 | 184 | 233 | 298 | 128 | 159 | 175 | 95 | 115 | 110 |
| 0.65 | *** | 481 | 552 | 1252 | 244 | 288 | 538 | 154 | 182 | 293 | 107 | 125 | 181 | 79 | 91 | 121 |
| | *** | 507 | 650 | 1235 | 261 | 341 | 513 | 165 | 211 | 265 | 115 | 143 | 152 | 84 | 101 | 91 |
| 0.7 | *** | 407 | 482 | 1124 | 212 | 255 | 474 | 134 | 160 | 253 | 93 | 108 | 153 | . | . | . |
| | *** | 436 | 580 | 1102 | 229 | 304 | 447 | 144 | 186 | 224 | 99 | 123 | 123 | . | . | . |
| 0.75 | *** | 339 | 413 | 964 | 180 | 219 | 396 | 113 | 134 | 205 | . | . | . | . | . | . |
| | *** | 367 | 504 | 938 | 195 | 261 | 368 | 122 | 155 | 175 | . | . | . | . | . | . |
| 0.8 | *** | 274 | 341 | 773 | 145 | 177 | 304 | . | . | . | . | . | . | . | . | . |
| | *** | 300 | 420 | 744 | 158 | 211 | 275 | . | . | . | . | . | . | . | . | . |
| 0.85 | *** | 210 | 263 | 551 | . | . | . | . | . | . | . | . | . | . | . | . |
| | *** | 231 | 324 | 521 | . | . | . | . | . | . | . | . | . | . | . | . |

TABLE 2: ALPHA= 0.005 POWER= 0.9    EXPECTED ACCRUAL THRU MINIMUM FOLLOW-UP= 60

|  |  | DEL=.10 | | | DEL=.15 | | | DEL=.20 | | | DEL=.25 | | | DEL=.30 | | |
|---|---|---|---|---|---|---|---|---|---|---|---|---|---|---|---|---|
| FACT= | | 1.0 .75 | .50 .25 | .00 BIN | 1.0 .75 | .50 .25 | .00 BIN | 1.0 .75 | .50 .25 | .00 BIN | 1.0 75 | .50 .25 | .00 BIN | 1.0 .75 | .50 .25 | .00 BIN |
| PCONT=*** | | | | REQUIRED | NUMBER | OF PATIENTS | | | | | | | | | | |
| 0.05 | *** | 313 | 315 | 338 | 182 | 184 | 197 | 128 | 131 | 138 | 100 | 102 | 107 | 83 | 84 | 88 |
|  | *** | 313 | 318 | 521 | 183 | 187 | 275 | 129 | 133 | 175 | 101 | 104 | 123 | 83 | 85 | 91 |
| 0.1 | *** | 494 | 498 | 566 | 261 | 266 | 300 | 172 | 177 | 197 | 127 | 131 | 144 | 101 | 104 | 113 |
|  | *** | 495 | 506 | 744 | 263 | 273 | 368 | 174 | 182 | 224 | 129 | 135 | 152 | 102 | 107 | 110 |
| 0.15 | *** | 637 | 644 | 776 | 321 | 328 | 391 | 204 | 211 | 246 | 146 | 153 | 175 | 113 | 119 | 133 |
|  | *** | 639 | 657 | 938 | 323 | 341 | 447 | 206 | 220 | 265 | 149 | 159 | 175 | 116 | 124 | 124 |
| 0.2 | *** | 742 | 752 | 961 | 363 | 374 | 469 | 225 | 235 | 288 | 159 | 167 | 199 | 121 | 128 | 149 |
|  | *** | 745 | 772 | 1102 | 366 | 391 | 513 | 229 | 248 | 298 | 162 | 177 | 195 | 124 | 135 | 136 |
| 0.25 | *** | 810 | 824 | 1120 | 388 | 403 | 534 | 238 | 251 | 321 | 166 | 177 | 219 | 126 | 134 | 161 |
|  | *** | 814 | 851 | 1235 | 393 | 427 | 566 | 242 | 268 | 324 | 170 | 189 | 209 | 129 | 143 | 144 |
| 0.3 | *** | 843 | 862 | 1248 | 399 | 419 | 585 | 242 | 260 | 346 | 168 | 182 | 233 | 127 | 137 | 169 |
|  | *** | 849 | 899 | 1340 | 406 | 449 | 606 | 249 | 281 | 343 | 174 | 197 | 218 | 131 | 148 | 149 |
| 0.35 | *** | 845 | 870 | 1346 | 398 | 423 | 622 | 241 | 262 | 363 | 167 | 183 | 241 | 125 | 138 | 173 |
|  | *** | 854 | 918 | 1414 | 407 | 460 | 632 | 249 | 287 | 354 | 173 | 200 | 223 | 130 | 149 | 151 |
| 0.4 | *** | 822 | 854 | 1411 | 387 | 417 | 644 | 235 | 259 | 372 | 163 | 181 | 244 | 122 | 135 | 174 |
|  | *** | 833 | 914 | 1459 | 398 | 460 | 645 | 244 | 287 | 358 | 170 | 199 | 223 | 128 | 148 | 149 |
| 0.45 | *** | 777 | 818 | 1444 | 368 | 404 | 652 | 225 | 252 | 372 | 156 | 176 | 242 | 117 | 131 | 170 |
|  | *** | 791 | 890 | 1474 | 381 | 452 | 645 | 235 | 282 | 354 | 164 | 195 | 218 | 123 | 144 | 144 |
| 0.5 | *** | 717 | 768 | 1445 | 343 | 384 | 645 | 211 | 241 | 365 | 147 | 168 | 234 | 110 | 125 | 163 |
|  | *** | 735 | 852 | 1459 | 359 | 437 | 632 | 223 | 273 | 343 | 156 | 188 | 209 | 116 | 138 | 136 |
| 0.55 | *** | 647 | 708 | 1413 | 315 | 360 | 624 | 196 | 226 | 349 | 137 | 157 | 222 | 102 | 116 | 153 |
|  | *** | 669 | 803 | 1414 | 333 | 415 | 606 | 208 | 259 | 324 | 145 | 177 | 195 | 108 | 129 | 124 |
| 0.6 | *** | 572 | 643 | 1349 | 286 | 333 | 588 | 179 | 209 | 325 | 125 | 145 | 204 | 93 | 106 | 139 |
|  | *** | 598 | 744 | 1340 | 304 | 388 | 566 | 191 | 241 | 298 | 133 | 164 | 175 | 99 | 118 | 110 |
| 0.65 | *** | 497 | 575 | 1252 | 254 | 302 | 538 | 161 | 189 | 293 | 112 | 130 | 181 | 82 | 94 | 121 |
|  | *** | 526 | 679 | 1235 | 273 | 355 | 513 | 172 | 219 | 265 | 119 | 147 | 152 | 87 | 104 | 91 |
| 0.7 | *** | 425 | 506 | 1124 | 223 | 268 | 474 | 141 | 167 | 253 | 97 | 112 | 153 | . | . | . |
|  | *** | 456 | 608 | 1102 | 240 | 317 | 447 | 151 | 192 | 224 | 103 | 126 | 123 | . | . | . |
| 0.75 | *** | 356 | 435 | 964 | 189 | 230 | 396 | 118 | 140 | 205 | . | . | . | . | . | . |
|  | *** | 387 | 530 | 938 | 205 | 272 | 368 | 127 | 160 | 175 | . | . | . | . | . | . |
| 0.8 | *** | 290 | 361 | 773 | 153 | 186 | 304 | . | . | . | . | . | . | . | . | . |
|  | *** | 318 | 442 | 744 | 167 | 219 | 275 | . | . | . | . | . | . | . | . | . |
| 0.85 | *** | 223 | 279 | 551 | . | . | . | . | . | . | . | . | . | . | . | . |
|  | *** | 245 | 340 | 521 | . | . | . | . | . | . | . | . | . | . | . | . |

## TABLE 2: ALPHA= 0.005 POWER= 0.9   EXPECTED ACCRUAL THRU MINIMUM FOLLOW-UP= 70

| | | DEL=.10 | | | DEL=.15 | | | DEL=.20 | | | DEL=.25 | | | DEL=.30 | | |
|---|---|---|---|---|---|---|---|---|---|---|---|---|---|---|---|---|
| FACT= | | 1.0 .75 | .50 .25 | .00 BIN | 1.0 .75 | .50 .25 | .00 BIN | 1.0 .75 | .50 .25 | .00 BIN | 1.0 75 | .50 .25 | .00 BIN | 1.0 .75 | .50 .25 | .00 BIN |
| PCONT=*** | | | | REQUIRED | NUMBER | OF | PATIENTS | | | | | | | | | |
| 0.05 | *** | 313 | 315 | 338 | 182 | 185 | 197 | 129 | 131 | 138 | 100 | 102 | 107 | 83 | 84 | 88 |
|  | *** | 314 | 319 | 521 | 183 | 188 | 275 | 130 | 133 | 175 | 101 | 104 | 123 | 83 | 86 | 91 |
| 0.1 | *** | 494 | 499 | 566 | 262 | 267 | 300 | 173 | 178 | 197 | 128 | 132 | 144 | 102 | 105 | 113 |
|  | *** | 496 | 508 | 744 | 264 | 275 | 368 | 175 | 183 | 224 | 130 | 136 | 152 | 103 | 108 | 110 |
| 0.15 | *** | 638 | 646 | 776 | 322 | 331 | 391 | 205 | 213 | 246 | 148 | 154 | 175 | 115 | 120 | 133 |
|  | *** | 641 | 662 | 938 | 325 | 344 | 447 | 208 | 222 | 265 | 150 | 161 | 175 | 117 | 125 | 124 |
| 0.2 | *** | 744 | 755 | 961 | 365 | 377 | 469 | 227 | 238 | 288 | 161 | 170 | 199 | 123 | 130 | 149 |
|  | *** | 748 | 778 | 1102 | 369 | 396 | 513 | 231 | 251 | 298 | 164 | 179 | 195 | 126 | 137 | 136 |
| 0.25 | *** | 812 | 828 | 1120 | 391 | 408 | 534 | 240 | 255 | 321 | 168 | 180 | 219 | 127 | 136 | 161 |
|  | *** | 817 | 860 | 1235 | 397 | 433 | 566 | 246 | 272 | 324 | 173 | 192 | 209 | 131 | 145 | 144 |
| 0.3 | *** | 846 | 868 | 1248 | 403 | 425 | 585 | 246 | 264 | 346 | 171 | 185 | 233 | 129 | 140 | 169 |
|  | *** | 853 | 910 | 1340 | 410 | 457 | 606 | 253 | 286 | 343 | 177 | 200 | 218 | 133 | 150 | 149 |
| 0.35 | *** | 850 | 879 | 1346 | 402 | 430 | 622 | 245 | 267 | 363 | 170 | 187 | 241 | 128 | 140 | 173 |
|  | *** | 859 | 932 | 1414 | 412 | 469 | 632 | 254 | 293 | 354 | 177 | 204 | 223 | 133 | 152 | 151 |
| 0.4 | *** | 827 | 865 | 1411 | 392 | 426 | 644 | 240 | 265 | 372 | 167 | 185 | 244 | 125 | 138 | 174 |
|  | *** | 840 | 931 | 1459 | 404 | 471 | 645 | 249 | 293 | 358 | 174 | 203 | 223 | 131 | 150 | 149 |
| 0.45 | *** | 784 | 832 | 1444 | 374 | 414 | 652 | 230 | 258 | 372 | 160 | 180 | 242 | 120 | 134 | 170 |
|  | *** | 800 | 910 | 1474 | 389 | 464 | 645 | 241 | 289 | 354 | 168 | 199 | 218 | 126 | 147 | 144 |
| 0.5 | *** | 726 | 784 | 1445 | 351 | 395 | 645 | 217 | 248 | 365 | 152 | 172 | 234 | 114 | 128 | 163 |
|  | *** | 746 | 875 | 1459 | 368 | 449 | 632 | 229 | 279 | 343 | 160 | 192 | 209 | 119 | 140 | 136 |
| 0.55 | *** | 658 | 727 | 1413 | 324 | 372 | 624 | 202 | 234 | 349 | 142 | 162 | 222 | 106 | 119 | 153 |
|  | *** | 682 | 827 | 1414 | 343 | 428 | 606 | 215 | 266 | 324 | 150 | 181 | 195 | 111 | 131 | 124 |
| 0.6 | *** | 585 | 663 | 1349 | 295 | 344 | 588 | 186 | 216 | 325 | 130 | 149 | 204 | 96 | 109 | 139 |
|  | *** | 614 | 770 | 1340 | 314 | 401 | 566 | 198 | 247 | 298 | 138 | 167 | 175 | 102 | 120 | 110 |
| 0.65 | *** | 512 | 596 | 1252 | 264 | 313 | 538 | 167 | 196 | 293 | 116 | 134 | 181 | 85 | 96 | 121 |
|  | *** | 544 | 705 | 1235 | 284 | 367 | 513 | 179 | 225 | 265 | 123 | 150 | 152 | 90 | 106 | 91 |
| 0.7 | *** | 441 | 527 | 1124 | 232 | 278 | 474 | 146 | 172 | 253 | 100 | 116 | 153 | . | . | . |
|  | *** | 474 | 633 | 1102 | 250 | 328 | 447 | 157 | 197 | 224 | 107 | 129 | 123 | . | . | . |
| 0.75 | *** | 372 | 455 | 964 | 198 | 239 | 396 | 123 | 145 | 205 | . | . | . | . | . | . |
|  | *** | 405 | 552 | 938 | 214 | 281 | 368 | 132 | 165 | 175 | . | . | . | . | . | . |
| 0.8 | *** | 305 | 378 | 773 | 160 | 194 | 304 | . | . | . | . | . | . | . | . | . |
|  | *** | 334 | 461 | 744 | 174 | 226 | 275 | . | . | . | . | . | . | . | . | . |
| 0.85 | *** | 235 | 292 | 551 | . | . | . | . | . | . | . | . | . | . | . | . |
|  | *** | 258 | 354 | 521 | . | . | . | . | . | . | . | . | . | . | . | . |

TABLE 2: ALPHA= 0.005 POWER= 0.9    EXPECTED ACCRUAL THRU MINIMUM FOLLOW-UP= 80

| | | DEL=.10 | | | DEL=.15 | | | DEL=.20 | | | DEL=.25 | | | DEL=.30 | | |
|---|---|---|---|---|---|---|---|---|---|---|---|---|---|---|---|---|---|
| FACT= | | 1.0 .75 | .50 .25 | .00 BIN | 1.0 .75 | .50 .25 | .00 BIN | 1.0 .75 | .50 .25 | .00 BIN | 1.0 75 | .50 .25 | .00 BIN | 1.0 .75 | .50 .25 | .00 BIN |
| PCONT=*** | | | | | REQUIRED NUMBER OF PATIENTS | | | | | | | | | | | |
| 0.05 | *** | 313 | 316 | 338 | 183 | 186 | 197 | 129 | 132 | 138 | 101 | 103 | 107 | 83 | 85 | 88 |
| | *** | 314 | 320 | 521 | 184 | 189 | 275 | 130 | 134 | 175 | 101 | 104 | 123 | 84 | 86 | 91 |
| 0.1 | *** | 495 | 501 | 566 | 263 | 269 | 300 | 174 | 179 | 197 | 129 | 133 | 144 | 102 | 106 | 113 |
| | *** | 497 | 511 | 744 | 265 | 277 | 368 | 176 | 185 | 224 | 131 | 137 | 152 | 104 | 109 | 110 |
| 0.15 | *** | 639 | 648 | 776 | 324 | 333 | 391 | 206 | 215 | 246 | 149 | 155 | 175 | 116 | 121 | 133 |
| | *** | 642 | 666 | 938 | 327 | 346 | 447 | 209 | 224 | 265 | 151 | 162 | 175 | 118 | 125 | 124 |
| 0.2 | *** | 745 | 759 | 961 | 366 | 380 | 469 | 229 | 240 | 288 | 162 | 171 | 199 | 124 | 131 | 149 |
| | *** | 750 | 784 | 1102 | 371 | 400 | 513 | 233 | 254 | 298 | 166 | 181 | 195 | 127 | 138 | 136 |
| 0.25 | *** | 814 | 833 | 1120 | 393 | 412 | 534 | 243 | 258 | 321 | 170 | 182 | 219 | 129 | 138 | 161 |
| | *** | 821 | 868 | 1235 | 400 | 439 | 566 | 248 | 276 | 324 | 175 | 194 | 209 | 133 | 146 | 144 |
| 0.3 | *** | 849 | 875 | 1248 | 406 | 430 | 585 | 249 | 268 | 346 | 174 | 188 | 233 | 131 | 142 | 169 |
| | *** | 858 | 921 | 1340 | 415 | 464 | 606 | 256 | 290 | 343 | 180 | 203 | 218 | 136 | 152 | 149 |
| 0.35 | *** | 854 | 887 | 1346 | 407 | 437 | 622 | 249 | 272 | 363 | 173 | 190 | 241 | 130 | 143 | 173 |
| | *** | 865 | 946 | 1414 | 418 | 477 | 632 | 258 | 297 | 354 | 180 | 207 | 223 | 136 | 154 | 151 |
| 0.4 | *** | 833 | 875 | 1411 | 398 | 434 | 644 | 244 | 270 | 372 | 170 | 189 | 244 | 128 | 141 | 174 |
| | *** | 847 | 947 | 1459 | 411 | 480 | 645 | 254 | 299 | 358 | 178 | 207 | 223 | 133 | 153 | 149 |
| 0.45 | *** | 791 | 844 | 1444 | 381 | 423 | 652 | 235 | 264 | 372 | 164 | 184 | 242 | 123 | 137 | 170 |
| | *** | 810 | 929 | 1474 | 397 | 474 | 645 | 247 | 295 | 354 | 172 | 203 | 218 | 129 | 149 | 144 |
| 0.5 | *** | 735 | 799 | 1445 | 359 | 405 | 645 | 223 | 254 | 365 | 156 | 176 | 234 | 116 | 130 | 163 |
| | *** | 757 | 896 | 1459 | 376 | 460 | 632 | 235 | 285 | 343 | 164 | 195 | 209 | 122 | 142 | 136 |
| 0.55 | *** | 669 | 744 | 1413 | 333 | 382 | 624 | 208 | 240 | 349 | 145 | 166 | 222 | 108 | 122 | 153 |
| | *** | 696 | 850 | 1414 | 352 | 439 | 606 | 221 | 272 | 324 | 154 | 185 | 195 | 114 | 133 | 124 |
| 0.6 | *** | 598 | 682 | 1349 | 304 | 355 | 588 | 191 | 222 | 325 | 133 | 153 | 204 | 99 | 111 | 139 |
| | *** | 629 | 794 | 1340 | 324 | 412 | 566 | 204 | 253 | 298 | 142 | 170 | 175 | 104 | 122 | 110 |
| 0.65 | *** | 526 | 616 | 1252 | 273 | 323 | 538 | 172 | 202 | 293 | 119 | 137 | 181 | 87 | 98 | 121 |
| | *** | 560 | 728 | 1235 | 293 | 378 | 513 | 184 | 230 | 265 | 127 | 153 | 152 | 92 | 107 | 91 |
| 0.7 | *** | 456 | 546 | 1124 | 240 | 288 | 474 | 151 | 177 | 253 | 103 | 118 | 153 | . | . | . |
| | *** | 491 | 655 | 1102 | 259 | 337 | 447 | 162 | 202 | 224 | 110 | 131 | 123 | . | . | . |
| 0.75 | *** | 387 | 473 | 964 | 205 | 247 | 396 | 127 | 149 | 205 | . | . | . | . | . | . |
| | *** | 421 | 572 | 938 | 222 | 289 | 368 | 136 | 168 | 175 | . | . | . | . | . | . |
| 0.8 | *** | 318 | 394 | 773 | 167 | 200 | 304 | . | . | . | . | . | . | . | . | . |
| | *** | 348 | 477 | 744 | 180 | 232 | 275 | . | . | . | . | . | . | . | . | . |
| 0.85 | *** | 245 | 304 | 551 | . | . | . | . | . | . | . | . | . | . | . | . |
| | *** | 269 | 366 | 521 | . | . | . | . | . | . | . | . | . | . | . | . |

TABLE 2: ALPHA= 0.005 POWER= 0.9    EXPECTED ACCRUAL THRU MINIMUM FOLLOW-UP= 90

|  |  | DEL=.10 | | | DEL=.15 | | | DEL=.20 | | | DEL=.25 | | | DEL=.30 | | |
|---|---|---|---|---|---|---|---|---|---|---|---|---|---|---|---|---|
| FACT= | | 1.0 .75 | .50 .25 | .00 BIN | 1.0 .75 | .50 .25 | .00 BIN | 1.0 .75 | .50 .25 | .00 BIN | 1.0 75 | .50 .25 | .00 BIN | 1.0 .75 | .50 .25 | .00 BIN |
| PCONT=*** | | | | | REQUIRED NUMBER OF PATIENTS | | | | | | | | | | | |
| 0.05 | *** | 314 | 317 | 338 | 183 | 186 | 197 | 130 | 132 | 138 | 101 | 103 | 107 | 83 | 85 | 88 |
|  | *** | 315 | 321 | 521 | 184 | 189 | 275 | 130 | 134 | 175 | 102 | 105 | 123 | 84 | 86 | 91 |
| 0.1 | *** | 496 | 502 | 566 | 264 | 270 | 300 | 175 | 180 | 197 | 130 | 134 | 144 | 103 | 106 | 113 |
|  | *** | 498 | 513 | 744 | 266 | 278 | 368 | 177 | 185 | 224 | 131 | 138 | 152 | 104 | 109 | 110 |
| 0.15 | *** | 640 | 651 | 776 | 325 | 335 | 391 | 208 | 216 | 246 | 150 | 157 | 175 | 116 | 122 | 133 |
|  | *** | 644 | 669 | 938 | 328 | 349 | 447 | 211 | 226 | 265 | 153 | 163 | 175 | 119 | 126 | 124 |
| 0.2 | *** | 747 | 762 | 961 | 368 | 383 | 469 | 230 | 243 | 288 | 164 | 173 | 199 | 125 | 133 | 149 |
|  | *** | 752 | 790 | 1102 | 374 | 404 | 513 | 235 | 256 | 298 | 167 | 182 | 195 | 128 | 139 | 136 |
| 0.25 | *** | 817 | 838 | 1120 | 396 | 416 | 534 | 245 | 261 | 321 | 172 | 184 | 219 | 131 | 140 | 161 |
|  | *** | 824 | 876 | 1235 | 403 | 443 | 566 | 251 | 279 | 324 | 177 | 196 | 209 | 134 | 148 | 144 |
| 0.3 | *** | 852 | 881 | 1248 | 409 | 435 | 585 | 252 | 272 | 346 | 176 | 191 | 233 | 133 | 144 | 169 |
|  | *** | 862 | 931 | 1340 | 419 | 470 | 606 | 260 | 294 | 343 | 182 | 205 | 218 | 137 | 153 | 149 |
| 0.35 | *** | 858 | 895 | 1346 | 411 | 443 | 622 | 252 | 276 | 363 | 176 | 193 | 241 | 132 | 145 | 173 |
|  | *** | 870 | 958 | 1414 | 423 | 484 | 632 | 262 | 302 | 354 | 183 | 209 | 223 | 138 | 155 | 151 |
| 0.4 | *** | 838 | 885 | 1411 | 403 | 441 | 644 | 248 | 275 | 372 | 173 | 192 | 244 | 130 | 143 | 174 |
|  | *** | 854 | 962 | 1459 | 417 | 488 | 645 | 259 | 303 | 358 | 181 | 209 | 223 | 135 | 154 | 149 |
| 0.45 | *** | 798 | 856 | 1444 | 387 | 431 | 652 | 240 | 269 | 372 | 167 | 187 | 242 | 125 | 139 | 170 |
|  | *** | 819 | 946 | 1474 | 404 | 483 | 645 | 252 | 300 | 354 | 176 | 206 | 218 | 131 | 150 | 144 |
| 0.5 | *** | 743 | 813 | 1445 | 366 | 414 | 645 | 228 | 259 | 364 | 159 | 180 | 234 | 119 | 133 | 163 |
|  | *** | 768 | 915 | 1459 | 384 | 470 | 632 | 241 | 291 | 343 | 168 | 198 | 209 | 125 | 144 | 136 |
| 0.55 | *** | 679 | 760 | 1413 | 340 | 392 | 624 | 213 | 245 | 349 | 149 | 169 | 222 | 111 | 124 | 153 |
|  | *** | 708 | 870 | 1414 | 360 | 449 | 606 | 226 | 277 | 324 | 157 | 187 | 195 | 116 | 135 | 124 |
| 0.6 | *** | 610 | 699 | 1349 | 312 | 364 | 588 | 196 | 228 | 325 | 137 | 156 | 204 | 101 | 113 | 139 |
|  | *** | 643 | 814 | 1340 | 333 | 421 | 566 | 209 | 258 | 298 | 145 | 173 | 175 | 106 | 123 | 110 |
| 0.65 | *** | 539 | 634 | 1252 | 281 | 333 | 538 | 177 | 207 | 293 | 123 | 140 | 181 | 89 | 100 | 121 |
|  | *** | 575 | 749 | 1235 | 302 | 387 | 513 | 189 | 234 | 265 | 130 | 155 | 152 | 94 | 108 | 91 |
| 0.7 | *** | 469 | 564 | 1124 | 248 | 296 | 474 | 156 | 182 | 253 | 106 | 121 | 153 | . | . | . |
|  | *** | 506 | 675 | 1102 | 268 | 345 | 447 | 167 | 205 | 224 | 112 | 133 | 123 | . | . | . |
| 0.75 | *** | 400 | 489 | 964 | 212 | 254 | 396 | 131 | 152 | 205 | . | . | . | . | . | . |
|  | *** | 435 | 590 | 938 | 229 | 296 | 368 | 140 | 171 | 175 | . | . | . | . | . | . |
| 0.8 | *** | 330 | 407 | 773 | 172 | 206 | 304 | . | . | . | . | . | . | . | . | . |
|  | *** | 361 | 492 | 744 | 186 | 237 | 275 | . | . | . | . | . | . | . | . | . |
| 0.85 | *** | 255 | 314 | 551 | . | . | . | . | . | . | . | . | . | . | . | . |
|  | *** | 279 | 376 | 521 | . | . | . | . | . | . | . | . | . | . | . | . |

TABLE 2: ALPHA= 0.005 POWER= 0.9    EXPECTED ACCRUAL THRU MINIMUM FOLLOW-UP= 100

| | | DEL=.10 | | | DEL=.15 | | | DEL=.20 | | | DEL=.25 | | | DEL=.30 | |
|---|---|---|---|---|---|---|---|---|---|---|---|---|---|---|---|---|
| FACT= | 1.0 .75 | .50 .25 | .00 BIN | 1.0 .75 | .50 .25 | .00 BIN | 1.0 .75 | .50 .25 | .00 BIN | 1.0 75 | .50 .25 | .00 BIN | 1.0 .75 | .50 .25 | .00 BIN |
| PCONT=*** | | | | REQUIRED | NUMBER OF | PATIENTS | | | | | | | | | |
| 0.05 *** | 314 | 317 | 338 | 184 | 187 | 197 | 130 | 132 | 138 | 101 | 103 | 107 | 84 | 85 | 88 |
| *** | 315 | 322 | 521 | 185 | 190 | 275 | 131 | 135 | 175 | 102 | 105 | 123 | 84 | 86 | 91 |
| 0.1 *** | 496 | 503 | 566 | 265 | 271 | 300 | 175 | 181 | 197 | 130 | 134 | 144 | 103 | 107 | 113 |
| *** | 499 | 515 | 744 | 267 | 279 | 368 | 177 | 186 | 224 | 132 | 138 | 152 | 105 | 109 | 110 |
| 0.15 *** | 642 | 653 | 776 | 326 | 337 | 391 | 209 | 218 | 246 | 151 | 158 | 175 | 117 | 122 | 133 |
| *** | 645 | 673 | 938 | 330 | 351 | 447 | 212 | 227 | 265 | 154 | 164 | 175 | 119 | 127 | 124 |
| 0.2 *** | 749 | 766 | 961 | 370 | 386 | 469 | 232 | 245 | 288 | 165 | 175 | 199 | 126 | 134 | 149 |
| *** | 754 | 795 | 1102 | 376 | 407 | 513 | 237 | 258 | 298 | 169 | 183 | 195 | 129 | 140 | 136 |
| 0.25 *** | 819 | 842 | 1120 | 398 | 420 | 534 | 247 | 264 | 321 | 174 | 186 | 219 | 132 | 141 | 161 |
| *** | 827 | 884 | 1235 | 406 | 448 | 566 | 254 | 281 | 324 | 179 | 198 | 209 | 136 | 149 | 144 |
| 0.3 *** | 855 | 887 | 1248 | 413 | 440 | 585 | 255 | 275 | 346 | 178 | 193 | 233 | 135 | 145 | 169 |
| *** | 866 | 941 | 1340 | 423 | 475 | 606 | 263 | 297 | 343 | 184 | 207 | 218 | 139 | 154 | 149 |
| 0.35 *** | 862 | 903 | 1346 | 415 | 449 | 622 | 256 | 280 | 363 | 179 | 196 | 241 | 134 | 146 | 173 |
| *** | 876 | 970 | 1414 | 428 | 491 | 632 | 265 | 305 | 354 | 186 | 211 | 223 | 139 | 156 | 151 |
| 0.4 *** | 844 | 895 | 1411 | 408 | 448 | 644 | 252 | 280 | 372 | 176 | 195 | 244 | 132 | 145 | 174 |
| *** | 861 | 976 | 1459 | 423 | 496 | 645 | 263 | 308 | 358 | 184 | 212 | 223 | 137 | 156 | 149 |
| 0.45 *** | 805 | 868 | 1444 | 393 | 439 | 652 | 244 | 274 | 372 | 170 | 190 | 242 | 127 | 141 | 170 |
| *** | 827 | 962 | 1474 | 410 | 491 | 645 | 256 | 304 | 354 | 179 | 208 | 218 | 133 | 152 | 144 |
| 0.5 *** | 752 | 827 | 1445 | 372 | 422 | 645 | 232 | 264 | 365 | 162 | 183 | 234 | 121 | 134 | 163 |
| *** | 779 | 932 | 1459 | 392 | 478 | 632 | 245 | 295 | 343 | 171 | 201 | 209 | 127 | 145 | 136 |
| 0.55 *** | 689 | 775 | 1413 | 347 | 400 | 624 | 218 | 250 | 349 | 152 | 172 | 222 | 113 | 126 | 153 |
| *** | 721 | 889 | 1414 | 368 | 458 | 606 | 231 | 281 | 324 | 161 | 190 | 195 | 118 | 136 | 124 |
| 0.6 *** | 621 | 715 | 1349 | 319 | 373 | 588 | 201 | 233 | 325 | 140 | 159 | 204 | 103 | 115 | 139 |
| *** | 657 | 834 | 1340 | 341 | 430 | 566 | 214 | 262 | 298 | 148 | 175 | 175 | 108 | 124 | 110 |
| 0.65 *** | 552 | 650 | 1252 | 288 | 341 | 538 | 182 | 211 | 293 | 125 | 143 | 181 | 91 | 101 | 121 |
| *** | 590 | 768 | 1235 | 310 | 395 | 513 | 194 | 238 | 265 | 133 | 157 | 152 | 96 | 109 | 91 |
| 0.7 *** | 482 | 580 | 1124 | 255 | 304 | 474 | 160 | 186 | 253 | 108 | 123 | 153 | . | . | . |
| *** | 520 | 692 | 1102 | 275 | 352 | 447 | 171 | 209 | 224 | 115 | 134 | 123 | . | . | . |
| 0.75 *** | 413 | 504 | 964 | 219 | 261 | 396 | 134 | 155 | 205 | . | . | . | . | . | . |
| *** | 449 | 605 | 938 | 236 | 302 | 368 | 143 | 173 | 175 | . | . | . | . | . | . |
| 0.8 *** | 341 | 420 | 773 | 177 | 211 | 304 | . | . | . | . | . | . | . | . | . |
| *** | 373 | 505 | 744 | 191 | 241 | 275 | . | . | . | . | . | . | . | . | . |
| 0.85 *** | 263 | 324 | 551 | . | . | . | . | . | . | . | . | . | . | . | . |
| *** | 288 | 385 | 521 | . | . | . | . | . | . | . | . | . | . | . | . |

# TABLE 2: ALPHA= 0.005 POWER= 0.9    EXPECTED ACCRUAL THRU MINIMUM FOLLOW-UP= 110

| PCONT=*** | FACT= | DEL=.05 1.0 .75 | .50 .25 | .00 BIN | DEL=.10 1.0 .75 | .50 .25 | .00 BIN | DEL=.15 1.0 .75 | .50 .25 | .00 BIN | DEL=.20 1.0 75 | .50 .25 | .00 BIN | DEL=.25 1.0 .75 | .50 .25 | .00 BIN |
|---|---|---|---|---|---|---|---|---|---|---|---|---|---|---|---|---|
| | | | | | REQUIRED NUMBER OF PATIENTS | | | | | | | | | | | |
| 0.05 | *** | 888 | 891 | 951 | 314 | 318 | 338 | 184 | 187 | 197 | 130 | 133 | 138 | 102 | 103 | 107 |
| | *** | 889 | 896 | 1637 | 316 | 323 | 521 | 185 | 190 | 275 | 131 | 135 | 175 | 102 | 105 | 123 |
| 0.1 | *** | 1618 | 1624 | 1833 | 497 | 505 | 566 | 265 | 272 | 300 | 176 | 181 | 197 | 131 | 135 | 144 |
| | *** | 1620 | 1637 | 2590 | 500 | 517 | 744 | 268 | 280 | 368 | 178 | 187 | 224 | 132 | 138 | 152 |
| 0.15 | *** | 2237 | 2248 | 2687 | 643 | 655 | 776 | 327 | 339 | 391 | 210 | 219 | 246 | 152 | 159 | 175 |
| | *** | 2240 | 2269 | 3423 | 647 | 676 | 938 | 331 | 353 | 447 | 213 | 228 | 265 | 155 | 164 | 175 |
| 0.2 | *** | 2713 | 2730 | 3467 | 750 | 769 | 961 | 372 | 389 | 469 | 234 | 247 | 288 | 166 | 176 | 199 |
| | *** | 2719 | 2762 | 4137 | 757 | 801 | 1102 | 378 | 410 | 513 | 239 | 260 | 298 | 170 | 184 | 195 |
| 0.25 | *** | 3042 | 3065 | 4148 | 821 | 847 | 1120 | 401 | 423 | 534 | 249 | 266 | 321 | 176 | 188 | 219 |
| | *** | 3049 | 3111 | 4732 | 830 | 891 | 1235 | 409 | 452 | 566 | 256 | 284 | 324 | 181 | 199 | 209 |
| 0.3 | *** | 3228 | 3259 | 4717 | 859 | 893 | 1248 | 416 | 445 | 585 | 257 | 278 | 346 | 180 | 195 | 233 |
| | *** | 3238 | 3322 | 5208 | 870 | 950 | 1340 | 427 | 480 | 606 | 265 | 300 | 343 | 186 | 208 | 218 |
| 0.35 | *** | 3283 | 3324 | 5166 | 866 | 911 | 1346 | 419 | 454 | 622 | 259 | 284 | 363 | 181 | 198 | 241 |
| | *** | 3297 | 3408 | 5565 | 881 | 981 | 1414 | 432 | 497 | 632 | 269 | 309 | 354 | 188 | 213 | 223 |
| 0.4 | *** | 3223 | 3277 | 5489 | 849 | 904 | 1411 | 413 | 454 | 644 | 256 | 283 | 372 | 178 | 197 | 244 |
| | *** | 3241 | 3385 | 5803 | 868 | 989 | 1459 | 428 | 503 | 645 | 267 | 311 | 358 | 186 | 214 | 223 |
| 0.45 | *** | 3067 | 3137 | 5684 | 812 | 879 | 1444 | 398 | 446 | 652 | 248 | 278 | 372 | 173 | 193 | 242 |
| | *** | 3090 | 3275 | 5922 | 836 | 977 | 1474 | 417 | 499 | 645 | 260 | 308 | 354 | 181 | 210 | 218 |
| 0.5 | *** | 2834 | 2923 | 5750 | 760 | 840 | 1445 | 379 | 430 | 645 | 237 | 269 | 365 | 165 | 185 | 234 |
| | *** | 2864 | 3097 | 5922 | 789 | 949 | 1459 | 399 | 486 | 632 | 250 | 299 | 343 | 174 | 203 | 209 |
| 0.55 | *** | 2544 | 2657 | 5687 | 699 | 789 | 1413 | 354 | 408 | 624 | 222 | 255 | 349 | 155 | 175 | 222 |
| | *** | 2582 | 2872 | 5803 | 732 | 906 | 1414 | 375 | 465 | 606 | 236 | 285 | 324 | 163 | 192 | 195 |
| 0.6 | *** | 2219 | 2362 | 5493 | 633 | 730 | 1348 | 326 | 381 | 588 | 205 | 237 | 325 | 142 | 161 | 204 |
| | *** | 2267 | 2618 | 5565 | 670 | 851 | 1340 | 348 | 437 | 566 | 218 | 266 | 298 | 151 | 177 | 175 |
| 0.65 | *** | 1882 | 2059 | 5171 | 564 | 665 | 1252 | 295 | 348 | 538 | 186 | 215 | 293 | 128 | 145 | 181 |
| | *** | 1943 | 2352 | 5208 | 603 | 785 | 1235 | 317 | 402 | 513 | 198 | 241 | 265 | 135 | 158 | 152 |
| 0.7 | *** | 1555 | 1766 | 4721 | 495 | 594 | 1124 | 262 | 311 | 474 | 163 | 189 | 253 | 111 | 125 | 153 |
| | *** | 1630 | 2080 | 4732 | 534 | 708 | 1102 | 282 | 359 | 447 | 174 | 211 | 224 | 117 | 136 | 123 |
| 0.75 | *** | 1258 | 1489 | 4144 | 424 | 517 | 964 | 224 | 267 | 396 | 137 | 158 | 205 | . | . | . |
| | *** | 1344 | 1805 | 4137 | 461 | 620 | 938 | 242 | 307 | 368 | 146 | 175 | 175 | . | . | . |
| 0.8 | *** | 999 | 1228 | 3442 | 351 | 431 | 773 | 182 | 215 | 304 | . | . | . | . | . | . |
| | *** | 1086 | 1523 | 3423 | 383 | 516 | 744 | 196 | 245 | 275 | . | . | . | . | . | . |
| 0.85 | *** | 768 | 972 | 2616 | 271 | 332 | 551 | . | . | . | . | . | . | . | . | . |
| | *** | 847 | 1222 | 2590 | 296 | 393 | 521 | . | . | . | . | . | . | . | . | . |
| 0.9 | *** | 545 | 699 | 1666 | . | . | . | . | . | . | . | . | . | . | . | . |
| | *** | 605 | 877 | 1637 | . | . | . | . | . | . | . | . | . | . | . | . |

TABLE 2: ALPHA= 0.005 POWER= 0.9    EXPECTED ACCRUAL THRU MINIMUM FOLLOW-UP= 120

| | | DEL=.05 | | | DEL=.10 | | | DEL=.15 | | | DEL=.20 | | | DEL=.25 | | |
|---|---|---|---|---|---|---|---|---|---|---|---|---|---|---|---|---|---|
| FACT= | | 1.0 .75 | .50 .25 | .00 BIN | 1.0 .75 | .50 .25 | .00 BIN | 1.0 .75 | .50 .25 | .00 BIN | 1.0 75 | .50 .25 | .00 BIN | 1.0 .75 | .50 .25 | .00 BIN |
| PCONT=*** | | | | | REQUIRED NUMBER OF PATIENTS | | | | | | | | | | | |
| 0.05 | *** | 888 | 891 | 950 | 315 | 318 | 338 | 184 | 187 | 197 | 130 | 133 | 138 | 102 | 104 | 107 |
| | *** | 889 | 897 | 1637 | 316 | 324 | 521 | 186 | 191 | 275 | 131 | 135 | 175 | 103 | 105 | 123 |
| 0.1 | *** | 1619 | 1626 | 1833 | 498 | 506 | 566 | 266 | 273 | 300 | 177 | 182 | 197 | 131 | 135 | 144 |
| | *** | 1621 | 1639 | 2590 | 501 | 519 | 744 | 269 | 282 | 368 | 179 | 187 | 224 | 133 | 139 | 152 |
| 0.15 | *** | 2238 | 2250 | 2687 | 644 | 657 | 776 | 328 | 340 | 391 | 211 | 220 | 246 | 153 | 159 | 175 |
| | *** | 2242 | 2273 | 3423 | 648 | 680 | 938 | 333 | 355 | 447 | 214 | 229 | 265 | 155 | 165 | 175 |
| 0.2 | *** | 2715 | 2733 | 3467 | 752 | 772 | 961 | 374 | 391 | 469 | 235 | 248 | 288 | 167 | 177 | 199 |
| | *** | 2721 | 2768 | 4137 | 759 | 805 | 1102 | 380 | 413 | 513 | 240 | 262 | 298 | 171 | 185 | 195 |
| 0.25 | *** | 3044 | 3069 | 4148 | 824 | 851 | 1120 | 403 | 427 | 534 | 251 | 268 | 321 | 177 | 189 | 219 |
| | *** | 3052 | 3119 | 4732 | 833 | 897 | 1235 | 412 | 456 | 566 | 258 | 286 | 324 | 182 | 200 | 209 |
| 0.3 | *** | 3230 | 3265 | 4717 | 862 | 899 | 1248 | 419 | 449 | 585 | 260 | 281 | 346 | 182 | 197 | 233 |
| | *** | 3242 | 3333 | 5208 | 874 | 958 | 1340 | 430 | 485 | 606 | 268 | 302 | 343 | 188 | 210 | 218 |
| 0.35 | *** | 3286 | 3332 | 5166 | 870 | 918 | 1346 | 423 | 460 | 622 | 262 | 287 | 363 | 183 | 200 | 241 |
| | *** | 3302 | 3423 | 5565 | 887 | 992 | 1414 | 437 | 502 | 632 | 272 | 311 | 354 | 190 | 215 | 223 |
| 0.4 | *** | 3228 | 3287 | 5489 | 854 | 914 | 1411 | 417 | 460 | 644 | 259 | 287 | 372 | 181 | 199 | 244 |
| | *** | 3248 | 3405 | 5803 | 875 | 1002 | 1459 | 434 | 509 | 645 | 270 | 314 | 358 | 189 | 216 | 223 |
| 0.45 | *** | 3074 | 3149 | 5684 | 818 | 890 | 1444 | 404 | 452 | 652 | 252 | 282 | 372 | 176 | 195 | 242 |
| | *** | 3099 | 3299 | 5922 | 844 | 991 | 1474 | 423 | 505 | 645 | 264 | 311 | 354 | 184 | 212 | 218 |
| 0.5 | *** | 2842 | 2939 | 5750 | 768 | 852 | 1445 | 384 | 437 | 645 | 241 | 273 | 364 | 168 | 188 | 234 |
| | *** | 2874 | 3127 | 5922 | 799 | 964 | 1459 | 405 | 493 | 632 | 254 | 302 | 343 | 176 | 205 | 209 |
| 0.55 | *** | 2554 | 2677 | 5687 | 708 | 802 | 1413 | 360 | 415 | 624 | 226 | 259 | 349 | 157 | 177 | 222 |
| | *** | 2596 | 2908 | 5803 | 744 | 922 | 1414 | 382 | 472 | 606 | 240 | 288 | 324 | 166 | 194 | 195 |
| 0.6 | *** | 2232 | 2387 | 5493 | 643 | 744 | 1348 | 333 | 388 | 588 | 209 | 241 | 325 | 145 | 163 | 204 |
| | *** | 2285 | 2660 | 5565 | 682 | 867 | 1340 | 355 | 444 | 566 | 222 | 269 | 298 | 153 | 179 | 175 |
| 0.65 | *** | 1899 | 2089 | 5171 | 575 | 679 | 1252 | 302 | 355 | 538 | 189 | 219 | 293 | 130 | 147 | 181 |
| | *** | 1965 | 2397 | 5208 | 616 | 801 | 1235 | 323 | 408 | 513 | 202 | 244 | 265 | 137 | 160 | 152 |
| 0.7 | *** | 1576 | 1799 | 4721 | 506 | 608 | 1124 | 268 | 317 | 474 | 167 | 192 | 253 | 112 | 126 | 153 |
| | *** | 1656 | 2126 | 4732 | 546 | 723 | 1102 | 288 | 364 | 447 | 177 | 214 | 224 | 118 | 137 | 123 |
| 0.75 | *** | 1283 | 1524 | 4144 | 435 | 530 | 964 | 229 | 272 | 396 | 140 | 160 | 205 | . | . | . |
| | *** | 1372 | 1850 | 4137 | 473 | 633 | 938 | 247 | 312 | 368 | 149 | 177 | 175 | . | . | . |
| 0.8 | *** | 1024 | 1262 | 3442 | 361 | 442 | 773 | 186 | 219 | 304 | . | . | . | . | . | . |
| | *** | 1115 | 1564 | 3423 | 394 | 527 | 744 | 200 | 248 | 275 | . | . | . | . | . | . |
| 0.85 | *** | 791 | 1001 | 2615 | 279 | 340 | 551 | . | . | . | . | . | . | . | . | . |
| | *** | 873 | 1256 | 2590 | 304 | 401 | 521 | . | . | . | . | . | . | . | . | . |
| 0.9 | *** | 563 | 720 | 1666 | . | . | . | . | . | . | . | . | . | . | . | . |
| | *** | 625 | 901 | 1637 | . | . | . | . | . | . | . | . | . | . | . | . |

# TABLE 2: ALPHA= 0.005 POWER= 0.9     EXPECTED ACCRUAL THRU MINIMUM FOLLOW-UP= 130

| | | DEL=.05 | | | DEL=.10 | | | DEL=.15 | | | DEL=.20 | | | DEL=.25 | | |
|---|---|---|---|---|---|---|---|---|---|---|---|---|---|---|---|---|---|
| FACT= | | 1.0 .75 | .50 .25 | .00 BIN | 1.0 .75 | .50 .25 | .00 BIN | 1.0 .75 | .50 .25 | .00 BIN | 1.0 75 | .50 .25 | .00 BIN | 1.0 .75 | .50 .25 | .00 BIN |
| PCONT=*** | | | | | REQUIRED | NUMBER | OF PATIENTS | | | | | | | | | |
| 0.05 | *** | 888 | 892 | 951 | 315 | 319 | 338 | 185 | 188 | 197 | 131 | 133 | 139 | 102 | 104 | 107 |
| | *** | 889 | 898 | 1637 | 316 | 324 | 521 | 186 | 191 | 275 | 132 | 135 | 175 | 103 | 105 | 123 |
| 0.1 | *** | 1619 | 1627 | 1833 | 498 | 507 | 566 | 267 | 274 | 300 | 177 | 183 | 197 | 132 | 136 | 144 |
| | *** | 1622 | 1642 | 2590 | 501 | 520 | 744 | 270 | 282 | 368 | 180 | 188 | 224 | 133 | 139 | 152 |
| 0.15 | *** | 2239 | 2251 | 2687 | 645 | 659 | 776 | 330 | 342 | 391 | 212 | 221 | 246 | 153 | 160 | 175 |
| | *** | 2243 | 2277 | 3423 | 650 | 683 | 938 | 334 | 357 | 447 | 216 | 230 | 265 | 156 | 166 | 175 |
| 0.2 | *** | 2716 | 2736 | 3467 | 754 | 775 | 961 | 375 | 394 | 469 | 237 | 250 | 288 | 169 | 178 | 200 |
| | *** | 2723 | 2774 | 4137 | 761 | 810 | 1102 | 382 | 415 | 513 | 242 | 263 | 298 | 173 | 186 | 195 |
| 0.25 | *** | 3046 | 3073 | 4148 | 826 | 856 | 1120 | 405 | 430 | 534 | 253 | 270 | 321 | 178 | 191 | 219 |
| | *** | 3055 | 3128 | 4732 | 836 | 904 | 1235 | 415 | 459 | 566 | 260 | 287 | 324 | 184 | 201 | 209 |
| 0.3 | *** | 3233 | 3270 | 4717 | 865 | 905 | 1248 | 422 | 453 | 585 | 262 | 283 | 346 | 184 | 198 | 233 |
| | *** | 3246 | 3345 | 5208 | 879 | 966 | 1340 | 434 | 489 | 606 | 271 | 304 | 343 | 190 | 211 | 218 |
| 0.35 | *** | 3290 | 3339 | 5166 | 875 | 925 | 1346 | 427 | 464 | 622 | 265 | 290 | 363 | 185 | 202 | 241 |
| | *** | 3307 | 3438 | 5565 | 892 | 1002 | 1414 | 441 | 507 | 632 | 275 | 314 | 354 | 192 | 216 | 223 |
| 0.4 | *** | 3233 | 3297 | 5489 | 860 | 922 | 1411 | 422 | 466 | 644 | 262 | 290 | 372 | 183 | 201 | 244 |
| | *** | 3254 | 3424 | 5803 | 882 | 1013 | 1459 | 439 | 514 | 645 | 274 | 317 | 358 | 191 | 217 | 223 |
| 0.45 | *** | 3080 | 3162 | 5684 | 825 | 901 | 1444 | 409 | 458 | 652 | 255 | 286 | 372 | 178 | 197 | 242 |
| | *** | 3107 | 3324 | 5922 | 852 | 1004 | 1474 | 428 | 511 | 645 | 268 | 314 | 358 | 186 | 214 | 218 |
| 0.5 | *** | 2850 | 2955 | 5750 | 776 | 864 | 1445 | 390 | 443 | 645 | 244 | 276 | 365 | 170 | 190 | 234 |
| | *** | 2885 | 3157 | 5922 | 809 | 978 | 1459 | 411 | 499 | 632 | 257 | 306 | 343 | 179 | 206 | 209 |
| 0.55 | *** | 2565 | 2698 | 5687 | 718 | 815 | 1413 | 366 | 422 | 624 | 230 | 262 | 349 | 160 | 179 | 222 |
| | *** | 2609 | 2943 | 5803 | 755 | 936 | 1414 | 389 | 479 | 606 | 244 | 291 | 324 | 168 | 195 | 195 |
| 0.6 | *** | 2245 | 2412 | 5493 | 653 | 758 | 1349 | 339 | 394 | 588 | 213 | 244 | 325 | 147 | 165 | 204 |
| | *** | 2302 | 2700 | 5565 | 694 | 882 | 1340 | 361 | 451 | 566 | 226 | 272 | 298 | 155 | 180 | 175 |
| 0.65 | *** | 1915 | 2119 | 5171 | 586 | 693 | 1252 | 308 | 361 | 538 | 193 | 222 | 293 | 132 | 148 | 181 |
| | *** | 1986 | 2440 | 5208 | 628 | 815 | 1235 | 330 | 414 | 513 | 205 | 247 | 265 | 139 | 161 | 152 |
| 0.7 | *** | 1597 | 1832 | 4721 | 517 | 621 | 1124 | 273 | 322 | 474 | 170 | 195 | 253 | 114 | 128 | 153 |
| | *** | 1682 | 2170 | 4732 | 558 | 737 | 1102 | 293 | 369 | 447 | 180 | 216 | 224 | 120 | 138 | 123 |
| 0.75 | *** | 1306 | 1558 | 4144 | 445 | 541 | 964 | 234 | 277 | 396 | 143 | 163 | 205 | . | . | . |
| | *** | 1400 | 1892 | 4137 | 484 | 645 | 938 | 252 | 316 | 368 | 151 | 179 | 175 | . | . | . |
| 0.8 | *** | 1048 | 1294 | 3442 | 370 | 452 | 773 | 190 | 223 | 304 | . | . | . | . | . | . |
| | *** | 1142 | 1603 | 3423 | 403 | 537 | 744 | 204 | 251 | 275 | . | . | . | . | . | . |
| 0.85 | *** | 813 | 1029 | 2615 | 286 | 347 | 551 | . | . | . | . | . | . | . | . | . |
| | *** | 897 | 1288 | 2590 | 311 | 407 | 521 | . | . | . | . | . | . | . | . | . |
| 0.9 | *** | 579 | 740 | 1666 | . | . | . | . | . | . | . | . | . | . | . | . |
| | *** | 643 | 923 | 1637 | . | . | . | . | . | . | . | . | . | . | . | . |

TABLE 2: ALPHA= 0.005 POWER= 0.9    EXPECTED ACCRUAL THRU MINIMUM FOLLOW-UP= 140

| | | DEL=.05 | | | DEL=.10 | | | DEL=.15 | | | DEL=.20 | | | DEL=.25 | | |
|---|---|---|---|---|---|---|---|---|---|---|---|---|---|---|---|---|---|
| FACT= | | 1.0 .75 | .50 .25 | .00 BIN | 1.0 .75 | .50 .25 | .00 BIN | 1.0 .75 | .50 .25 | .00 BIN | 1.0 75 | .50 .25 | .00 BIN | 1.0 .75 | .50 .25 | .00 BIN |
| PCONT=*** | | | | | REQUIRED | NUMBER | OF PATIENTS | | | | | | | | | |
| 0.05 | *** | 888 | 892 | 951 | 315 | 319 | 338 | 185 | 188 | 197 | 131 | 133 | 138 | 102 | 104 | 107 |
| | *** | 890 | 899 | 1637 | 317 | 325 | 521 | 186 | 191 | 275 | 132 | 135 | 175 | 103 | 105 | 123 |
| 0.1 | *** | 1620 | 1628 | 1833 | 499 | 508 | 566 | 267 | 275 | 300 | 178 | 183 | 197 | 132 | 136 | 144 |
| | *** | 1622 | 1644 | 2590 | 502 | 522 | 744 | 270 | 283 | 368 | 180 | 188 | 224 | 134 | 139 | 152 |
| 0.15 | *** | 2240 | 2253 | 2687 | 646 | 662 | 776 | 331 | 344 | 391 | 213 | 222 | 246 | 154 | 161 | 175 |
| | *** | 2244 | 2281 | 3423 | 651 | 685 | 938 | 336 | 358 | 447 | 217 | 231 | 265 | 157 | 166 | 175 |
| 0.2 | *** | 2718 | 2739 | 3467 | 755 | 778 | 961 | 377 | 396 | 469 | 238 | 251 | 288 | 170 | 179 | 200 |
| | *** | 2725 | 2780 | 4137 | 763 | 814 | 1102 | 384 | 417 | 513 | 243 | 264 | 298 | 174 | 187 | 195 |
| 0.25 | *** | 3048 | 3077 | 4148 | 828 | 860 | 1120 | 408 | 433 | 534 | 255 | 272 | 321 | 180 | 192 | 219 |
| | *** | 3058 | 3136 | 4732 | 839 | 910 | 1235 | 417 | 462 | 566 | 262 | 289 | 324 | 185 | 202 | 209 |
| 0.3 | *** | 3236 | 3276 | 4717 | 868 | 910 | 1248 | 425 | 457 | 585 | 264 | 286 | 346 | 185 | 200 | 233 |
| | *** | 3249 | 3356 | 5208 | 883 | 974 | 1340 | 437 | 493 | 606 | 273 | 306 | 343 | 192 | 212 | 218 |
| 0.35 | *** | 3294 | 3347 | 5166 | 879 | 932 | 1346 | 430 | 469 | 622 | 267 | 293 | 363 | 187 | 204 | 241 |
| | *** | 3312 | 3453 | 5565 | 898 | 1011 | 1414 | 445 | 512 | 632 | 278 | 316 | 354 | 194 | 218 | 223 |
| 0.4 | *** | 3238 | 3307 | 5489 | 865 | 931 | 1411 | 426 | 471 | 644 | 265 | 293 | 372 | 185 | 203 | 244 |
| | *** | 3261 | 3443 | 5803 | 888 | 1024 | 1459 | 443 | 519 | 645 | 277 | 320 | 358 | 193 | 219 | 223 |
| 0.45 | *** | 3086 | 3175 | 5684 | 832 | 910 | 1444 | 414 | 464 | 652 | 258 | 289 | 372 | 180 | 199 | 242 |
| | *** | 3116 | 3348 | 5922 | 860 | 1016 | 1474 | 433 | 517 | 645 | 271 | 317 | 354 | 188 | 215 | 218 |
| 0.5 | *** | 2858 | 2971 | 5750 | 784 | 875 | 1445 | 395 | 449 | 645 | 248 | 279 | 365 | 172 | 192 | 234 |
| | *** | 2896 | 3186 | 5922 | 818 | 991 | 1459 | 417 | 505 | 632 | 261 | 308 | 343 | 181 | 208 | 209 |
| 0.55 | *** | 2575 | 2718 | 5687 | 727 | 827 | 1413 | 372 | 428 | 624 | 234 | 266 | 349 | 162 | 181 | 222 |
| | *** | 2623 | 2977 | 5803 | 765 | 950 | 1414 | 395 | 485 | 606 | 247 | 294 | 324 | 170 | 197 | 195 |
| 0.6 | *** | 2259 | 2437 | 5493 | 663 | 770 | 1349 | 344 | 401 | 588 | 216 | 247 | 325 | 149 | 167 | 204 |
| | *** | 2319 | 2738 | 5565 | 705 | 896 | 1340 | 367 | 456 | 566 | 229 | 274 | 298 | 157 | 181 | 175 |
| 0.65 | *** | 1932 | 2147 | 5171 | 596 | 705 | 1252 | 313 | 367 | 538 | 196 | 225 | 293 | 134 | 150 | 181 |
| | *** | 2008 | 2481 | 5208 | 639 | 829 | 1235 | 335 | 419 | 513 | 208 | 249 | 265 | 141 | 162 | 152 |
| 0.7 | *** | 1617 | 1863 | 4721 | 527 | 633 | 1124 | 278 | 328 | 474 | 172 | 197 | 253 | 116 | 129 | 153 |
| | *** | 1706 | 2212 | 4732 | 569 | 749 | 1102 | 299 | 374 | 447 | 183 | 218 | 224 | 122 | 139 | 123 |
| 0.75 | *** | 1329 | 1590 | 4144 | 455 | 552 | 964 | 239 | 281 | 396 | 145 | 165 | 205 | . | . | . |
| | *** | 1427 | 1933 | 4137 | 494 | 655 | 938 | 257 | 319 | 368 | 153 | 180 | 175 | . | . | . |
| 0.8 | *** | 1071 | 1324 | 3442 | 378 | 461 | 773 | 194 | 226 | 304 | . | . | . | . | . | . |
| | *** | 1168 | 1639 | 3423 | 412 | 545 | 744 | 207 | 254 | 275 | . | . | . | . | . | . |
| 0.85 | *** | 834 | 1054 | 2615 | 292 | 354 | 551 | . | . | . | . | . | . | . | . | . |
| | *** | 920 | 1318 | 2590 | 318 | 413 | 521 | . | . | . | . | . | . | . | . | . |
| 0.9 | *** | 595 | 758 | 1666 | . | . | . | . | . | . | . | . | . | . | . | . |
| | *** | 660 | 943 | 1637 | . | . | . | . | . | . | . | . | . | . | . | . |

## TABLE 2: ALPHA= 0.005 POWER= 0.9    EXPECTED ACCRUAL THRU MINIMUM FOLLOW-UP= 150

| | | DEL=.05 | | | DEL=.10 | | | DEL=.15 | | | DEL=.20 | | | DEL=.25 | | |
|---|---|---|---|---|---|---|---|---|---|---|---|---|---|---|---|---|---|
| FACT= | | 1.0 .75 | .50 .25 | .00 BIN | 1.0 .75 | .50 .25 | .00 BIN | 1.0 .75 | .50 .25 | .00 BIN | 1.0 75 | .50 .25 | .00 BIN | 1.0 .75 | .50 .25 | .00 BIN |
| PCONT=*** | | | | | REQUIRED | NUMBER OF | PATIENTS | | | | | | | | | |
| 0.05 | *** | 889 | 893 | 950 | 316 | 320 | 338 | 185 | 189 | 197 | 131 | 134 | 138 | 102 | 104 | 107 |
| | *** | 890 | 900 | 1637 | 317 | 325 | 521 | 187 | 192 | 275 | 132 | 136 | 175 | 103 | 105 | 123 |
| 0.1 | *** | 1620 | 1629 | 1833 | 500 | 510 | 566 | 268 | 276 | 300 | 178 | 184 | 197 | 133 | 137 | 144 |
| | *** | 1623 | 1646 | 2590 | 503 | 523 | 744 | 271 | 284 | 368 | 181 | 189 | 224 | 134 | 140 | 152 |
| 0.15 | *** | 2241 | 2255 | 2687 | 647 | 664 | 776 | 332 | 345 | 391 | 214 | 223 | 246 | 155 | 161 | 175 |
| | *** | 2246 | 2285 | 3423 | 653 | 688 | 938 | 337 | 360 | 447 | 218 | 232 | 265 | 158 | 167 | 175 |
| 0.2 | *** | 2719 | 2742 | 3467 | 757 | 781 | 961 | 379 | 398 | 469 | 239 | 253 | 288 | 171 | 180 | 199 |
| | *** | 2727 | 2786 | 4137 | 766 | 818 | 1102 | 386 | 419 | 513 | 245 | 265 | 298 | 175 | 188 | 195 |
| 0.25 | *** | 3050 | 3082 | 4148 | 831 | 864 | 1120 | 410 | 436 | 534 | 256 | 274 | 321 | 181 | 193 | 219 |
| | *** | 3061 | 3145 | 4732 | 842 | 915 | 1235 | 420 | 465 | 566 | 264 | 290 | 324 | 186 | 203 | 209 |
| 0.3 | *** | 3239 | 3282 | 4717 | 871 | 916 | 1248 | 427 | 460 | 585 | 266 | 288 | 346 | 187 | 201 | 233 |
| | *** | 3253 | 3367 | 5208 | 887 | 981 | 1340 | 440 | 497 | 606 | 275 | 308 | 343 | 193 | 213 | 218 |
| 0.35 | *** | 3298 | 3355 | 5166 | 883 | 939 | 1346 | 433 | 473 | 622 | 270 | 295 | 363 | 189 | 205 | 241 |
| | *** | 3317 | 3467 | 5565 | 903 | 1020 | 1414 | 449 | 516 | 632 | 280 | 318 | 354 | 196 | 219 | 223 |
| 0.4 | *** | 3243 | 3317 | 5489 | 870 | 939 | 1411 | 430 | 475 | 644 | 268 | 296 | 372 | 187 | 205 | 244 |
| | *** | 3268 | 3462 | 5803 | 895 | 1034 | 1459 | 448 | 524 | 645 | 280 | 322 | 358 | 195 | 220 | 223 |
| 0.45 | *** | 3092 | 3187 | 5684 | 838 | 920 | 1444 | 418 | 469 | 652 | 261 | 292 | 372 | 182 | 201 | 242 |
| | *** | 3124 | 3371 | 5922 | 868 | 1028 | 1474 | 439 | 522 | 645 | 274 | 319 | 354 | 190 | 217 | 218 |
| 0.5 | *** | 2866 | 2987 | 5750 | 792 | 885 | 1445 | 400 | 455 | 645 | 251 | 283 | 365 | 174 | 194 | 234 |
| | *** | 2907 | 3214 | 5922 | 827 | 1003 | 1459 | 422 | 510 | 632 | 264 | 311 | 343 | 183 | 209 | 209 |
| 0.55 | *** | 2585 | 2738 | 5687 | 735 | 839 | 1413 | 377 | 434 | 624 | 237 | 269 | 349 | 164 | 183 | 222 |
| | *** | 2637 | 3010 | 5803 | 775 | 963 | 1414 | 400 | 490 | 606 | 250 | 297 | 324 | 172 | 198 | 195 |
| 0.6 | *** | 2272 | 2461 | 5493 | 673 | 782 | 1349 | 350 | 406 | 588 | 220 | 250 | 325 | 151 | 169 | 204 |
| | *** | 2336 | 2775 | 5565 | 715 | 909 | 1340 | 373 | 461 | 566 | 233 | 277 | 298 | 159 | 183 | 175 |
| 0.65 | *** | 1948 | 2175 | 5171 | 606 | 717 | 1252 | 319 | 373 | 538 | 199 | 227 | 293 | 136 | 151 | 181 |
| | *** | 2029 | 2520 | 5208 | 650 | 841 | 1235 | 341 | 424 | 513 | 211 | 251 | 265 | 142 | 163 | 152 |
| 0.7 | *** | 1637 | 1894 | 4721 | 537 | 644 | 1124 | 283 | 333 | 474 | 175 | 200 | 253 | 117 | 130 | 153 |
| | *** | 1731 | 2252 | 4732 | 580 | 761 | 1102 | 304 | 378 | 447 | 186 | 220 | 224 | 123 | 139 | 123 |
| 0.75 | *** | 1351 | 1620 | 4144 | 464 | 562 | 964 | 243 | 285 | 396 | 147 | 166 | 205 | . | . | . |
| | *** | 1452 | 1971 | 4137 | 504 | 666 | 938 | 261 | 323 | 368 | 155 | 181 | 175 | . | . | . |
| 0.8 | *** | 1093 | 1352 | 3442 | 386 | 469 | 773 | 197 | 229 | 304 | . | . | . | . | . | . |
| | *** | 1193 | 1673 | 3423 | 420 | 554 | 744 | 211 | 256 | 275 | . | . | . | . | . | . |
| 0.85 | *** | 854 | 1079 | 2615 | 298 | 360 | 551 | . | . | . | . | . | . | . | . | . |
| | *** | 941 | 1346 | 2590 | 324 | 419 | 521 | . | . | . | . | . | . | . | . | . |
| 0.9 | *** | 610 | 776 | 1666 | . | . | . | . | . | . | . | . | . | . | . | . |
| | *** | 676 | 962 | 1637 | . | . | . | . | . | . | . | . | . | . | . | . |

TABLE 2: ALPHA= 0.005 POWER= 0.9    EXPECTED ACCRUAL THRU MINIMUM FOLLOW-UP= 160

| | | DEL=.05 | | | DEL=.10 | | | DEL=.15 | | | DEL=.20 | | | DEL=.25 | | |
|---|---|---|---|---|---|---|---|---|---|---|---|---|---|---|---|---|---|
| FACT= | | 1.0 .75 | .50 .25 | .00 BIN | 1.0 .75 | .50 .25 | .00 BIN | 1.0 .75 | .50 .25 | .00 BIN | 1.0 75 | .50 .25 | .00 BIN | 1.0 .75 | .50 .25 | .00 BIN |
| PCONT=*** | | | | | REQUIRED NUMBER OF PATIENTS | | | | | | | | | | | |
| 0.05 | *** | 889 | 893 | 951 | 316 | 320 | 338 | 186 | 189 | 197 | 132 | 134 | 138 | 103 | 104 | 107 |
| | *** | 890 | 901 | 1637 | 318 | 326 | 521 | 187 | 192 | 275 | 133 | 136 | 175 | 103 | 106 | 123 |
| 0.1 | *** | 1621 | 1630 | 1833 | 501 | 511 | 566 | 269 | 277 | 300 | 179 | 185 | 197 | 133 | 137 | 144 |
| | *** | 1624 | 1649 | 2590 | 504 | 525 | 744 | 272 | 285 | 368 | 181 | 189 | 224 | 135 | 140 | 152 |
| 0.15 | *** | 2242 | 2257 | 2687 | 648 | 666 | 776 | 333 | 346 | 391 | 215 | 224 | 246 | 155 | 162 | 175 |
| | *** | 2247 | 2289 | 3423 | 654 | 691 | 938 | 338 | 361 | 447 | 218 | 232 | 265 | 158 | 167 | 175 |
| 0.2 | *** | 2721 | 2745 | 3467 | 759 | 784 | 961 | 380 | 400 | 469 | 240 | 254 | 288 | 171 | 181 | 199 |
| | *** | 2729 | 2792 | 4137 | 768 | 822 | 1102 | 388 | 421 | 513 | 246 | 266 | 298 | 175 | 188 | 195 |
| 0.25 | *** | 3052 | 3086 | 4148 | 833 | 868 | 1120 | 412 | 439 | 534 | 258 | 276 | 321 | 182 | 194 | 219 |
| | *** | 3063 | 3153 | 4732 | 846 | 921 | 1235 | 422 | 467 | 566 | 265 | 292 | 324 | 187 | 204 | 209 |
| 0.3 | *** | 3242 | 3288 | 4717 | 875 | 921 | 1248 | 430 | 464 | 585 | 268 | 290 | 346 | 188 | 203 | 233 |
| | *** | 3257 | 3379 | 5208 | 891 | 988 | 1340 | 443 | 500 | 606 | 277 | 310 | 343 | 194 | 214 | 218 |
| 0.35 | *** | 3302 | 3362 | 5166 | 887 | 946 | 1346 | 437 | 477 | 622 | 272 | 297 | 363 | 190 | 207 | 241 |
| | *** | 3322 | 3482 | 5565 | 908 | 1028 | 1414 | 453 | 520 | 632 | 283 | 320 | 354 | 197 | 220 | 223 |
| 0.4 | *** | 3248 | 3327 | 5489 | 875 | 947 | 1411 | 434 | 480 | 644 | 270 | 299 | 372 | 189 | 207 | 244 |
| | *** | 3274 | 3481 | 5803 | 901 | 1044 | 1459 | 452 | 528 | 645 | 282 | 324 | 358 | 196 | 221 | 223 |
| 0.45 | *** | 3099 | 3200 | 5684 | 844 | 929 | 1444 | 423 | 474 | 652 | 264 | 295 | 372 | 184 | 203 | 242 |
| | *** | 3133 | 3395 | 5922 | 876 | 1038 | 1474 | 443 | 527 | 645 | 277 | 322 | 354 | 192 | 218 | 218 |
| 0.5 | *** | 2874 | 3003 | 5750 | 799 | 896 | 1445 | 405 | 460 | 645 | 254 | 285 | 365 | 176 | 195 | 234 |
| | *** | 2917 | 3242 | 5922 | 835 | 1015 | 1459 | 427 | 515 | 632 | 267 | 313 | 343 | 185 | 211 | 209 |
| 0.55 | *** | 2596 | 2757 | 5687 | 744 | 850 | 1413 | 382 | 439 | 624 | 240 | 272 | 349 | 166 | 185 | 222 |
| | *** | 2650 | 3042 | 5803 | 784 | 975 | 1414 | 405 | 495 | 606 | 253 | 299 | 324 | 174 | 199 | 195 |
| 0.6 | *** | 2285 | 2485 | 5493 | 682 | 794 | 1349 | 355 | 412 | 588 | 222 | 253 | 325 | 153 | 170 | 204 |
| | *** | 2354 | 2811 | 5565 | 725 | 921 | 1340 | 378 | 466 | 566 | 235 | 279 | 298 | 161 | 184 | 175 |
| 0.65 | *** | 1965 | 2202 | 5171 | 616 | 728 | 1252 | 323 | 378 | 538 | 202 | 230 | 293 | 137 | 153 | 181 |
| | *** | 2049 | 2558 | 5208 | 660 | 853 | 1235 | 346 | 429 | 513 | 214 | 253 | 265 | 144 | 164 | 152 |
| 0.7 | *** | 1656 | 1923 | 4721 | 546 | 655 | 1124 | 288 | 337 | 474 | 177 | 202 | 253 | 118 | 131 | 153 |
| | *** | 1754 | 2290 | 4732 | 590 | 772 | 1102 | 308 | 382 | 447 | 188 | 221 | 224 | 124 | 140 | 123 |
| 0.75 | *** | 1372 | 1650 | 4144 | 473 | 572 | 964 | 247 | 289 | 396 | 149 | 168 | 205 | . | . | . |
| | *** | 1477 | 2007 | 4137 | 513 | 675 | 938 | 265 | 326 | 368 | 157 | 183 | 175 | . | . | . |
| 0.8 | *** | 1115 | 1380 | 3442 | 394 | 477 | 773 | 200 | 232 | 304 | . | . | . | . | . | . |
| | *** | 1217 | 1706 | 3423 | 428 | 561 | 744 | 214 | 258 | 275 | . | . | . | . | . | . |
| 0.85 | *** | 873 | 1102 | 2616 | 304 | 366 | 551 | . | . | . | . | . | . | . | . | . |
| | *** | 962 | 1373 | 2590 | 330 | 424 | 521 | . | . | . | . | . | . | . | . | . |
| 0.9 | *** | 625 | 793 | 1666 | . | . | . | . | . | . | . | . | . | . | . | . |
| | *** | 691 | 980 | 1637 | . | . | . | . | . | . | . | . | . | . | . | . |

TABLE 2: ALPHA= 0.005 POWER= 0.9    EXPECTED ACCRUAL THRU MINIMUM FOLLOW-UP= 170

|  |  | DEL=.05 | | | DEL=.10 | | | DEL=.15 | | | DEL=.20 | | | DEL=.25 | | |
|---|---|---|---|---|---|---|---|---|---|---|---|---|---|---|---|---|
| FACT= | | 1.0 .75 | .50 .25 | .00 BIN | 1.0 .75 | .50 .25 | .00 BIN | 1.0 .75 | .50 .25 | .00 BIN | 1.0 75 | .50 .25 | .00 BIN | 1.0 .75 | .50 .25 | .00 BIN |
| PCONT=*** | | | | | REQUIRED NUMBER OF PATIENTS | | | | | | | | | | | |
| 0.05 | *** | 889 | 894 | 951 | 316 | 321 | 338 | 186 | 189 | 197 | 132 | 134 | 138 | 103 | 104 | 107 |
|  | *** | 891 | 902 | 1637 | 318 | 326 | 521 | 187 | 192 | 275 | 133 | 136 | 175 | 103 | 106 | 123 |
| 0.1 | *** | 1622 | 1631 | 1833 | 501 | 512 | 566 | 269 | 277 | 300 | 179 | 185 | 197 | 133 | 137 | 144 |
|  | *** | 1625 | 1651 | 2590 | 505 | 526 | 744 | 273 | 285 | 368 | 182 | 190 | 224 | 135 | 140 | 152 |
| 0.15 | *** | 2243 | 2259 | 2687 | 650 | 667 | 776 | 334 | 348 | 391 | 215 | 225 | 246 | 156 | 162 | 175 |
|  | *** | 2248 | 2293 | 3423 | 656 | 693 | 938 | 339 | 362 | 447 | 219 | 233 | 265 | 159 | 167 | 175 |
| 0.2 | *** | 2722 | 2748 | 3467 | 761 | 787 | 961 | 382 | 402 | 469 | 242 | 255 | 288 | 172 | 181 | 199 |
|  | *** | 2731 | 2798 | 4137 | 770 | 826 | 1102 | 390 | 423 | 513 | 247 | 267 | 298 | 176 | 189 | 195 |
| 0.25 | *** | 3054 | 3090 | 4148 | 836 | 872 | 1120 | 414 | 441 | 534 | 259 | 277 | 321 | 183 | 195 | 219 |
|  | *** | 3066 | 3161 | 4732 | 849 | 926 | 1235 | 425 | 470 | 566 | 267 | 293 | 324 | 188 | 204 | 209 |
| 0.3 | *** | 3245 | 3293 | 4717 | 878 | 926 | 1248 | 433 | 467 | 585 | 270 | 292 | 346 | 190 | 204 | 233 |
|  | *** | 3261 | 3390 | 5208 | 895 | 995 | 1340 | 446 | 503 | 606 | 279 | 311 | 343 | 196 | 215 | 218 |
| 0.35 | *** | 3305 | 3370 | 5166 | 891 | 952 | 1346 | 440 | 481 | 622 | 274 | 300 | 363 | 192 | 208 | 241 |
|  | *** | 3327 | 3497 | 5565 | 913 | 1036 | 1414 | 456 | 523 | 632 | 285 | 322 | 354 | 199 | 221 | 223 |
| 0.4 | *** | 3253 | 3336 | 5489 | 880 | 955 | 1411 | 437 | 484 | 644 | 273 | 301 | 372 | 190 | 208 | 244 |
|  | *** | 3281 | 3500 | 5803 | 908 | 1053 | 1459 | 456 | 532 | 645 | 285 | 326 | 358 | 198 | 222 | 223 |
| 0.45 | *** | 3105 | 3212 | 5684 | 850 | 938 | 1444 | 427 | 479 | 652 | 267 | 297 | 372 | 186 | 204 | 242 |
|  | *** | 3141 | 3417 | 5922 | 883 | 1049 | 1474 | 448 | 531 | 645 | 280 | 324 | 354 | 194 | 219 | 218 |
| 0.5 | *** | 2882 | 3019 | 5750 | 806 | 905 | 1445 | 410 | 465 | 645 | 256 | 288 | 365 | 178 | 197 | 234 |
|  | *** | 2928 | 3270 | 5922 | 844 | 1026 | 1459 | 432 | 520 | 632 | 270 | 315 | 343 | 186 | 212 | 209 |
| 0.55 | *** | 2606 | 2777 | 5686 | 752 | 860 | 1413 | 387 | 444 | 624 | 243 | 274 | 349 | 168 | 186 | 222 |
|  | *** | 2664 | 3074 | 5803 | 794 | 986 | 1414 | 410 | 500 | 606 | 256 | 301 | 324 | 176 | 200 | 195 |
| 0.6 | *** | 2298 | 2508 | 5493 | 691 | 804 | 1349 | 360 | 416 | 588 | 225 | 256 | 325 | 155 | 172 | 204 |
|  | *** | 2371 | 2845 | 5565 | 735 | 932 | 1340 | 383 | 470 | 566 | 238 | 281 | 298 | 162 | 185 | 175 |
| 0.65 | *** | 1981 | 2229 | 5171 | 625 | 739 | 1252 | 328 | 382 | 538 | 204 | 232 | 293 | 139 | 154 | 181 |
|  | *** | 2069 | 2594 | 5208 | 670 | 864 | 1235 | 351 | 433 | 513 | 216 | 255 | 265 | 145 | 165 | 152 |
| 0.7 | *** | 1675 | 1951 | 4721 | 555 | 665 | 1124 | 292 | 341 | 474 | 180 | 204 | 253 | 120 | 132 | 153 |
|  | *** | 1777 | 2326 | 4732 | 599 | 782 | 1102 | 313 | 386 | 447 | 190 | 222 | 224 | 125 | 141 | 123 |
| 0.75 | *** | 1393 | 1678 | 4144 | 481 | 581 | 964 | 251 | 293 | 396 | 151 | 169 | 205 | . | . | . |
|  | *** | 1501 | 2042 | 4137 | 521 | 684 | 938 | 269 | 329 | 368 | 159 | 184 | 175 | . | . | . |
| 0.8 | *** | 1135 | 1406 | 3442 | 401 | 485 | 773 | 203 | 235 | 304 | . | . | . | . | . | . |
|  | *** | 1240 | 1737 | 3423 | 435 | 568 | 744 | 217 | 260 | 275 | . | . | . | . | . | . |
| 0.85 | *** | 891 | 1124 | 2615 | 309 | 371 | 551 | . | . | . | . | . | . | . | . | . |
|  | *** | 982 | 1398 | 2590 | 335 | 429 | 521 | . | . | . | . | . | . | . | . | . |
| 0.9 | *** | 638 | 808 | 1666 | . | . | . | . | . | . | . | . | . | . | . | . |
|  | *** | 706 | 997 | 1637 | . | . | . | . | . | . | . | . | . | . | . | . |

TABLE 2: ALPHA= 0.005 POWER= 0.9     EXPECTED ACCRUAL THRU MINIMUM FOLLOW-UP= 180

| | | DEL=.05 | | | DEL=.10 | | | DEL=.15 | | | DEL=.20 | | | DEL=.25 | | |
|---|---|---|---|---|---|---|---|---|---|---|---|---|---|---|---|---|---|
| FACT= | | 1.0 .75 | .50 .25 | .00 BIN | 1.0 .75 | .50 .25 | .00 BIN | 1.0 .75 | .50 .25 | .00 BIN | 1.0 75 | .50 .25 | .00 BIN | 1.0 .75 | .50 .25 | .00 BIN |
| PCONT=*** | | | | REQUIRED | NUMBER | OF | PATIENTS | | | | | | | | | |
| 0.05 | *** | 890 | 894 | 951 | 317 | 321 | 338 | 186 | 189 | 197 | 132 | 134 | 138 | 103 | 105 | 107 |
| | *** | 891 | 903 | 1637 | 318 | 327 | 521 | 188 | 192 | 275 | 133 | 136 | 175 | 104 | 106 | 123 |
| 0.1 | *** | 1622 | 1632 | 1833 | 502 | 513 | 566 | 270 | 278 | 300 | 180 | 185 | 197 | 134 | 138 | 144 |
| | *** | 1626 | 1653 | 2590 | 506 | 527 | 744 | 273 | 286 | 368 | 182 | 190 | 224 | 135 | 140 | 152 |
| 0.15 | *** | 2244 | 2261 | 2687 | 651 | 669 | 776 | 335 | 349 | 391 | 216 | 226 | 246 | 157 | 163 | 175 |
| | *** | 2250 | 2296 | 3423 | 657 | 695 | 938 | 341 | 363 | 447 | 220 | 233 | 265 | 159 | 168 | 175 |
| 0.2 | *** | 2724 | 2751 | 3467 | 762 | 790 | 961 | 383 | 404 | 469 | 243 | 256 | 288 | 173 | 182 | 199 |
| | *** | 2733 | 2804 | 4137 | 772 | 830 | 1102 | 391 | 425 | 513 | 248 | 268 | 298 | 177 | 189 | 195 |
| 0.25 | *** | 3057 | 3094 | 4148 | 838 | 876 | 1120 | 416 | 443 | 534 | 261 | 279 | 321 | 184 | 196 | 219 |
| | *** | 3069 | 3169 | 4732 | 852 | 930 | 1235 | 427 | 472 | 566 | 268 | 294 | 324 | 189 | 205 | 209 |
| 0.3 | *** | 3248 | 3299 | 4717 | 881 | 931 | 1248 | 435 | 470 | 585 | 272 | 294 | 346 | 191 | 205 | 233 |
| | *** | 3265 | 3401 | 5208 | 899 | 1001 | 1340 | 449 | 506 | 606 | 281 | 313 | 343 | 197 | 216 | 218 |
| 0.35 | *** | 3309 | 3377 | 5166 | 895 | 958 | 1346 | 443 | 484 | 622 | 276 | 302 | 363 | 193 | 209 | 241 |
| | *** | 3332 | 3511 | 5565 | 918 | 1043 | 1414 | 460 | 527 | 632 | 287 | 324 | 354 | 200 | 222 | 223 |
| 0.4 | *** | 3258 | 3346 | 5489 | 885 | 962 | 1411 | 441 | 488 | 644 | 275 | 303 | 372 | 192 | 209 | 244 |
| | *** | 3287 | 3518 | 5803 | 914 | 1061 | 1459 | 460 | 536 | 645 | 287 | 328 | 358 | 199 | 223 | 223 |
| 0.45 | *** | 3111 | 3225 | 5684 | 856 | 946 | 1444 | 431 | 483 | 652 | 269 | 300 | 372 | 187 | 206 | 242 |
| | *** | 3149 | 3440 | 5922 | 890 | 1058 | 1474 | 452 | 535 | 645 | 282 | 326 | 354 | 195 | 220 | 218 |
| 0.5 | *** | 2890 | 3035 | 5750 | 813 | 915 | 1445 | 414 | 470 | 645 | 259 | 291 | 364 | 180 | 198 | 234 |
| | *** | 2939 | 3296 | 5922 | 852 | 1036 | 1459 | 437 | 524 | 632 | 273 | 317 | 343 | 188 | 213 | 209 |
| 0.55 | *** | 2616 | 2796 | 5687 | 760 | 870 | 1413 | 392 | 449 | 624 | 245 | 277 | 349 | 169 | 187 | 222 |
| | *** | 2677 | 3104 | 5803 | 803 | 997 | 1414 | 415 | 504 | 606 | 259 | 303 | 324 | 177 | 201 | 195 |
| 0.6 | *** | 2311 | 2531 | 5493 | 699 | 814 | 1349 | 364 | 421 | 588 | 228 | 258 | 325 | 156 | 173 | 204 |
| | *** | 2387 | 2878 | 5565 | 744 | 943 | 1340 | 388 | 475 | 566 | 241 | 283 | 298 | 164 | 185 | 175 |
| 0.65 | *** | 1997 | 2255 | 5171 | 634 | 749 | 1252 | 333 | 387 | 538 | 207 | 234 | 293 | 140 | 155 | 181 |
| | *** | 2089 | 2629 | 5208 | 679 | 874 | 1235 | 355 | 436 | 513 | 219 | 256 | 265 | 147 | 165 | 152 |
| 0.7 | *** | 1694 | 1978 | 4721 | 564 | 675 | 1124 | 296 | 345 | 474 | 182 | 205 | 253 | 121 | 133 | 153 |
| | *** | 1799 | 2361 | 4732 | 608 | 791 | 1102 | 317 | 389 | 447 | 192 | 224 | 224 | 126 | 141 | 123 |
| 0.75 | *** | 1414 | 1705 | 4144 | 489 | 590 | 964 | 254 | 296 | 396 | 152 | 171 | 205 | . | . | . |
| | *** | 1524 | 2075 | 4137 | 530 | 692 | 938 | 272 | 331 | 368 | 161 | 185 | 175 | . | . | . |
| 0.8 | *** | 1155 | 1431 | 3442 | 407 | 492 | 773 | 206 | 237 | 304 | . | . | . | . | . | . |
| | *** | 1262 | 1766 | 3423 | 442 | 575 | 744 | 219 | 262 | 275 | . | . | . | . | . | . |
| 0.85 | *** | 908 | 1146 | 2616 | 314 | 376 | 551 | . | . | . | . | . | . | . | . | . |
| | *** | 1001 | 1422 | 2590 | 340 | 433 | 521 | . | . | . | . | . | . | . | . | . |
| 0.9 | *** | 651 | 823 | 1666 | . | . | . | . | . | . | . | . | . | . | . | . |
| | *** | 720 | 1013 | 1637 | . | . | . | . | . | . | . | . | . | . | . | . |

TABLE 2: ALPHA= 0.005 POWER= 0.9     EXPECTED ACCRUAL THRU MINIMUM FOLLOW-UP= 190

PCONT=*** : REQUIRED NUMBER OF PATIENTS

| PCONT | DEL=.05 1.0/.75 | .50/.25 | .00/BIN | DEL=.10 1.0/.75 | .50/.25 | .00/BIN | DEL=.15 1.0/.75 | .50/.25 | .00/BIN | DEL=.20 1.0/75 | .50/.25 | .00/BIN | DEL=.25 1.0/.75 | .50/.25 | .00/BIN |
|---|---|---|---|---|---|---|---|---|---|---|---|---|---|---|---|
| 0.05 | 890 | 895 | 951 | 317 | 322 | 338 | 186 | 190 | 197 | 132 | 134 | 138 | 103 | 105 | 107 |
|  | 892 | 904 | 1637 | 319 | 327 | 521 | 188 | 192 | 275 | 133 | 136 | 175 | 104 | 106 | 123 |
| 0.1 | 1623 | 1634 | 1833 | 503 | 514 | 566 | 271 | 279 | 300 | 180 | 186 | 197 | 134 | 138 | 144 |
|  | 1626 | 1655 | 2590 | 507 | 529 | 744 | 274 | 287 | 368 | 183 | 190 | 224 | 136 | 141 | 152 |
| 0.15 | 2245 | 2263 | 2687 | 652 | 671 | 776 | 336 | 350 | 391 | 217 | 226 | 246 | 157 | 163 | 175 |
|  | 2251 | 2300 | 3423 | 659 | 698 | 938 | 342 | 364 | 447 | 221 | 234 | 265 | 160 | 168 | 175 |
| 0.2 | 2725 | 2754 | 3467 | 764 | 793 | 961 | 385 | 405 | 469 | 244 | 257 | 288 | 174 | 183 | 199 |
|  | 2735 | 2809 | 4137 | 774 | 833 | 1102 | 393 | 426 | 513 | 249 | 269 | 298 | 178 | 190 | 195 |
| 0.25 | 3059 | 3099 | 4148 | 840 | 880 | 1120 | 418 | 446 | 534 | 262 | 280 | 321 | 185 | 197 | 219 |
|  | 3072 | 3178 | 4732 | 854 | 935 | 1235 | 429 | 474 | 566 | 270 | 295 | 324 | 190 | 206 | 209 |
| 0.3 | 3250 | 3305 | 4717 | 884 | 936 | 1248 | 438 | 473 | 585 | 273 | 295 | 346 | 192 | 206 | 233 |
|  | 3268 | 3412 | 5208 | 903 | 1007 | 1340 | 452 | 508 | 606 | 283 | 314 | 343 | 198 | 216 | 218 |
| 0.35 | 3313 | 3385 | 5166 | 899 | 964 | 1346 | 446 | 488 | 622 | 278 | 303 | 363 | 194 | 210 | 241 |
|  | 3337 | 3526 | 5565 | 923 | 1050 | 1414 | 463 | 530 | 632 | 289 | 325 | 354 | 201 | 222 | 223 |
| 0.4 | 3263 | 3356 | 5489 | 890 | 969 | 1411 | 445 | 492 | 644 | 277 | 306 | 372 | 193 | 211 | 244 |
|  | 3294 | 3536 | 5803 | 919 | 1070 | 1459 | 464 | 540 | 645 | 289 | 330 | 358 | 201 | 224 | 223 |
| 0.45 | 3118 | 3238 | 5684 | 862 | 955 | 1444 | 435 | 487 | 652 | 272 | 302 | 372 | 189 | 207 | 242 |
|  | 3158 | 3462 | 5922 | 897 | 1067 | 1474 | 456 | 539 | 645 | 284 | 328 | 354 | 197 | 221 | 218 |
| 0.5 | 2899 | 3050 | 5750 | 820 | 924 | 1445 | 418 | 474 | 645 | 262 | 293 | 364 | 181 | 200 | 234 |
|  | 2950 | 3322 | 5922 | 860 | 1046 | 1459 | 441 | 528 | 632 | 275 | 319 | 343 | 189 | 213 | 209 |
| 0.55 | 2626 | 2815 | 5687 | 767 | 880 | 1413 | 396 | 453 | 624 | 248 | 279 | 349 | 171 | 189 | 222 |
|  | 2691 | 3134 | 5803 | 811 | 1007 | 1414 | 420 | 508 | 606 | 261 | 305 | 324 | 179 | 202 | 195 |
| 0.6 | 2324 | 2553 | 5493 | 707 | 824 | 1348 | 369 | 426 | 588 | 230 | 260 | 325 | 158 | 174 | 204 |
|  | 2404 | 2910 | 5208 | 753 | 953 | 1340 | 392 | 478 | 566 | 243 | 284 | 298 | 165 | 186 | 175 |
| 0.65 | 2013 | 2280 | 5171 | 642 | 759 | 1252 | 337 | 391 | 538 | 209 | 236 | 293 | 141 | 156 | 181 |
|  | 2109 | 2662 | 5208 | 688 | 884 | 1235 | 359 | 440 | 513 | 221 | 258 | 265 | 148 | 166 | 152 |
| 0.7 | 1713 | 2005 | 4721 | 572 | 684 | 1124 | 300 | 349 | 474 | 184 | 207 | 253 | 122 | 134 | 153 |
|  | 1821 | 2394 | 4732 | 617 | 800 | 1102 | 321 | 392 | 447 | 194 | 225 | 224 | 127 | 142 | 123 |
| 0.75 | 1433 | 1731 | 4144 | 496 | 598 | 964 | 258 | 299 | 396 | 154 | 172 | 205 | . | . | . |
|  | 1547 | 2106 | 4137 | 538 | 700 | 938 | 275 | 334 | 368 | 162 | 185 | 175 | . | . | . |
| 0.8 | 1174 | 1455 | 3442 | 414 | 499 | 773 | 208 | 239 | 304 | . | . | . | . | . | . |
|  | 1283 | 1794 | 3423 | 449 | 581 | 744 | 222 | 264 | 275 | . | . | . | . | . | . |
| 0.85 | 925 | 1166 | 2616 | 319 | 381 | 551 | . | . | . | . | . | . | . | . | . |
|  | 1020 | 1444 | 2590 | 345 | 437 | 521 | . | . | . | . | . | . | . | . | . |
| 0.9 | 664 | 838 | 1666 | . | . | . | . | . | . | . | . | . | . | . | . |
|  | 733 | 1028 | 1637 | . | . | . | . | . | . | . | . | . | . | . | . |

TABLE 2: ALPHA= 0.005 POWER= 0.9     EXPECTED ACCRUAL THRU MINIMUM FOLLOW-UP= 200

| | | DEL=.05 | | | DEL=.10 | | | DEL=.15 | | | DEL=.20 | | | DEL=.25 | | |
|---|---|---|---|---|---|---|---|---|---|---|---|---|---|---|---|---|
| FACT= | | 1.0 .75 | .50 .25 | .00 BIN | 1.0 .75 | .50 .25 | .00 BIN | 1.0 .75 | .50 .25 | .00 BIN | 1.0 75 | .50 .25 | .00 BIN | 1.0 .75 | .50 .25 | .00 BIN |
| PCONT=*** | | | | | REQUIRED NUMBER OF PATIENTS | | | | | | | | | | | |
| 0.05 | *** | 890 | 895 | 951 | 317 | 322 | 338 | 187 | 190 | 197 | 132 | 135 | 138 | 103 | 105 | 107 |
| | *** | 892 | 905 | 1637 | 319 | 327 | 521 | 188 | 193 | 275 | 133 | 136 | 175 | 104 | 106 | 123 |
| 0.1 | *** | 1623 | 1635 | 1833 | 503 | 515 | 566 | 271 | 279 | 300 | 181 | 186 | 197 | 134 | 138 | 144 |
| | *** | 1627 | 1657 | 2590 | 508 | 530 | 744 | 274 | 287 | 368 | 183 | 190 | 224 | 136 | 141 | 152 |
| 0.15 | *** | 2246 | 2265 | 2687 | 653 | 673 | 776 | 337 | 351 | 391 | 218 | 227 | 246 | 158 | 164 | 175 |
| | *** | 2252 | 2304 | 3423 | 660 | 700 | 938 | 343 | 365 | 447 | 222 | 234 | 265 | 160 | 168 | 175 |
| 0.2 | *** | 2727 | 2756 | 3467 | 766 | 795 | 961 | 386 | 407 | 469 | 245 | 258 | 288 | 175 | 183 | 199 |
| | *** | 2737 | 2815 | 4137 | 776 | 836 | 1102 | 394 | 428 | 513 | 250 | 270 | 298 | 178 | 190 | 195 |
| 0.25 | *** | 3061 | 3103 | 4148 | 842 | 884 | 1120 | 420 | 448 | 534 | 264 | 281 | 321 | 186 | 198 | 219 |
| | *** | 3075 | 3186 | 4732 | 857 | 939 | 1235 | 431 | 476 | 566 | 271 | 296 | 324 | 191 | 206 | 209 |
| 0.3 | *** | 3253 | 3310 | 4717 | 887 | 941 | 1248 | 440 | 475 | 585 | 275 | 297 | 346 | 193 | 207 | 233 |
| | *** | 3272 | 3423 | 5208 | 906 | 1012 | 1340 | 454 | 511 | 606 | 284 | 315 | 343 | 199 | 217 | 218 |
| 0.35 | *** | 3317 | 3392 | 5166 | 903 | 970 | 1346 | 449 | 491 | 622 | 280 | 305 | 363 | 196 | 211 | 241 |
| | *** | 3342 | 3540 | 5565 | 928 | 1057 | 1414 | 466 | 533 | 632 | 291 | 327 | 354 | 203 | 223 | 223 |
| 0.4 | *** | 3268 | 3366 | 5489 | 895 | 976 | 1411 | 448 | 496 | 644 | 280 | 308 | 372 | 195 | 212 | 244 |
| | *** | 3300 | 3554 | 5803 | 925 | 1077 | 1459 | 467 | 543 | 645 | 291 | 331 | 358 | 202 | 225 | 223 |
| 0.45 | *** | 3124 | 3250 | 5684 | 868 | 962 | 1444 | 439 | 491 | 652 | 274 | 304 | 372 | 190 | 208 | 242 |
| | *** | 3166 | 3484 | 5922 | 904 | 1076 | 1474 | 460 | 542 | 645 | 287 | 329 | 354 | 198 | 222 | 218 |
| 0.5 | *** | 2907 | 3066 | 5750 | 827 | 932 | 1445 | 422 | 478 | 645 | 264 | 295 | 365 | 183 | 201 | 234 |
| | *** | 2960 | 3348 | 5922 | 867 | 1055 | 1459 | 445 | 532 | 632 | 277 | 321 | 343 | 191 | 214 | 209 |
| 0.55 | *** | 2637 | 2834 | 5687 | 775 | 889 | 1413 | 400 | 458 | 624 | 250 | 281 | 349 | 172 | 190 | 222 |
| | *** | 2704 | 3162 | 5803 | 819 | 1017 | 1414 | 424 | 511 | 606 | 263 | 306 | 324 | 180 | 203 | 195 |
| 0.6 | *** | 2337 | 2576 | 5493 | 715 | 834 | 1349 | 373 | 430 | 588 | 233 | 262 | 325 | 159 | 175 | 204 |
| | *** | 2420 | 2942 | 5565 | 762 | 963 | 1340 | 397 | 482 | 566 | 245 | 286 | 298 | 166 | 187 | 175 |
| 0.65 | *** | 2029 | 2304 | 5171 | 650 | 768 | 1252 | 341 | 395 | 538 | 211 | 238 | 293 | 143 | 157 | 181 |
| | *** | 2128 | 2694 | 5208 | 697 | 893 | 1235 | 363 | 443 | 513 | 223 | 259 | 265 | 149 | 167 | 152 |
| 0.7 | *** | 1731 | 2030 | 4721 | 580 | 692 | 1124 | 304 | 352 | 474 | 186 | 209 | 253 | 123 | 134 | 153 |
| | *** | 1842 | 2426 | 4732 | 625 | 808 | 1102 | 324 | 395 | 447 | 196 | 226 | 224 | 128 | 142 | 123 |
| 0.75 | *** | 1452 | 1757 | 4144 | 504 | 605 | 964 | 261 | 302 | 396 | 155 | 173 | 205 | . | . | . |
| | *** | 1568 | 2137 | 4137 | 545 | 707 | 938 | 278 | 336 | 368 | 163 | 186 | 175 | . | . | . |
| 0.8 | *** | 1193 | 1479 | 3442 | 420 | 505 | 773 | 211 | 241 | 304 | . | . | . | . | . | . |
| | *** | 1304 | 1821 | 3423 | 455 | 586 | 744 | 224 | 265 | 275 | . | . | . | . | . | . |
| 0.85 | *** | 942 | 1185 | 2616 | 324 | 385 | 551 | . | . | . | . | . | . | . | . | . |
| | *** | 1037 | 1466 | 2590 | 350 | 440 | 521 | . | . | . | . | . | . | . | . | . |
| 0.9 | *** | 676 | 852 | 1666 | . | . | . | . | . | . | . | . | . | . | . | . |
| | *** | 746 | 1042 | 1637 | . | . | . | . | . | . | . | . | . | . | . | . |

TABLE 2: ALPHA= 0.005 POWER= 0.9    EXPECTED ACCRUAL THRU MINIMUM FOLLOW-UP= 225

|  |  | DEL=.05 | | | DEL=.10 | | | DEL=.15 | | | DEL=.20 | | | DEL=.25 | | |
|---|---|---|---|---|---|---|---|---|---|---|---|---|---|---|---|---|
| FACT= | | 1.0 .75 | .50 .25 | .00 BIN | 1.0 .75 | .50 .25 | .00 BIN | 1.0 .75 | .50 .25 | .00 BIN | 1.0 75 | .50 .25 | .00 BIN | 1.0 .75 | .50 .25 | .00 BIN |
| PCONT=*** | | | | | REQUIRED NUMBER OF PATIENTS | | | | | | | | | | | |
| 0.05 | *** | 891 | 897 | 950 | 318 | 323 | 338 | 187 | 190 | 197 | 133 | 135 | 138 | 104 | 105 | 107 |
|  | *** | 893 | 907 | 1637 | 320 | 328 | 521 | 189 | 193 | 275 | 134 | 136 | 175 | 104 | 106 | 123 |
| 0.1 | *** | 1625 | 1638 | 1833 | 505 | 517 | 566 | 273 | 281 | 300 | 182 | 187 | 197 | 135 | 139 | 144 |
|  | *** | 1629 | 1663 | 2590 | 510 | 532 | 744 | 276 | 288 | 368 | 184 | 191 | 224 | 137 | 141 | 152 |
| 0.15 | *** | 2248 | 2270 | 2687 | 656 | 677 | 776 | 339 | 354 | 391 | 219 | 228 | 246 | 159 | 165 | 175 |
|  | *** | 2255 | 2313 | 3423 | 664 | 704 | 938 | 345 | 367 | 447 | 223 | 236 | 265 | 161 | 169 | 175 |
| 0.2 | *** | 2730 | 2764 | 3467 | 770 | 802 | 961 | 389 | 411 | 469 | 247 | 260 | 288 | 176 | 185 | 200 |
|  | *** | 2742 | 2829 | 4137 | 781 | 843 | 1102 | 398 | 431 | 513 | 253 | 271 | 298 | 180 | 191 | 195 |
| 0.25 | *** | 3066 | 3113 | 4148 | 848 | 892 | 1120 | 424 | 453 | 534 | 267 | 284 | 321 | 188 | 199 | 219 |
|  | *** | 3082 | 3206 | 4732 | 864 | 950 | 1235 | 436 | 480 | 566 | 274 | 298 | 324 | 193 | 207 | 209 |
| 0.3 | *** | 3260 | 3325 | 4717 | 894 | 952 | 1248 | 446 | 482 | 585 | 279 | 300 | 346 | 195 | 209 | 233 |
|  | *** | 3282 | 3450 | 5208 | 916 | 1025 | 1340 | 460 | 516 | 606 | 288 | 318 | 343 | 201 | 219 | 218 |
| 0.35 | *** | 3326 | 3411 | 5166 | 912 | 984 | 1346 | 456 | 498 | 622 | 284 | 309 | 363 | 199 | 214 | 241 |
|  | *** | 3355 | 3575 | 5565 | 939 | 1073 | 1414 | 473 | 539 | 632 | 295 | 330 | 354 | 205 | 225 | 223 |
| 0.4 | *** | 3280 | 3390 | 5489 | 907 | 992 | 1411 | 456 | 504 | 644 | 284 | 312 | 372 | 198 | 214 | 244 |
|  | *** | 3317 | 3598 | 5803 | 939 | 1095 | 1459 | 475 | 550 | 645 | 296 | 335 | 358 | 205 | 226 | 223 |
| 0.45 | *** | 3140 | 3281 | 5684 | 882 | 981 | 1444 | 447 | 500 | 652 | 279 | 309 | 372 | 194 | 211 | 242 |
|  | *** | 3187 | 3536 | 5922 | 920 | 1096 | 1474 | 469 | 550 | 645 | 292 | 333 | 354 | 201 | 223 | 218 |
| 0.5 | *** | 2927 | 3104 | 5750 | 843 | 952 | 1445 | 432 | 488 | 645 | 270 | 300 | 365 | 186 | 203 | 234 |
|  | *** | 2987 | 3409 | 5922 | 885 | 1076 | 1459 | 455 | 540 | 632 | 283 | 324 | 343 | 194 | 216 | 209 |
| 0.55 | *** | 2662 | 2881 | 5687 | 793 | 910 | 1413 | 410 | 467 | 624 | 256 | 286 | 349 | 176 | 192 | 222 |
|  | *** | 2738 | 3231 | 5803 | 839 | 1039 | 1414 | 434 | 520 | 606 | 269 | 310 | 324 | 183 | 204 | 195 |
| 0.6 | *** | 2368 | 2629 | 5493 | 734 | 855 | 1349 | 383 | 439 | 588 | 238 | 267 | 325 | 162 | 177 | 204 |
|  | *** | 2461 | 3015 | 5565 | 782 | 984 | 1340 | 406 | 490 | 566 | 250 | 289 | 298 | 169 | 188 | 175 |
| 0.65 | *** | 2067 | 2363 | 5171 | 669 | 789 | 1252 | 350 | 404 | 538 | 216 | 242 | 293 | 145 | 159 | 181 |
|  | *** | 2175 | 2770 | 5208 | 717 | 914 | 1235 | 373 | 450 | 513 | 227 | 262 | 265 | 151 | 168 | 152 |
| 0.7 | *** | 1774 | 2091 | 4721 | 598 | 712 | 1124 | 312 | 360 | 474 | 190 | 212 | 253 | 125 | 136 | 153 |
|  | *** | 1893 | 2501 | 4732 | 644 | 827 | 1102 | 333 | 401 | 447 | 200 | 228 | 224 | 130 | 143 | 123 |
| 0.75 | *** | 1498 | 1816 | 4144 | 520 | 623 | 964 | 268 | 308 | 396 | 159 | 176 | 205 | . | . | . |
|  | *** | 1620 | 2207 | 4137 | 562 | 723 | 938 | 285 | 341 | 368 | 166 | 188 | 175 | . | . | . |
| 0.8 | *** | 1237 | 1533 | 3442 | 434 | 519 | 773 | 216 | 246 | 304 | . | . | . | . | . | . |
|  | *** | 1352 | 1883 | 3423 | 469 | 599 | 744 | 229 | 269 | 275 | . | . | . | . | . | . |
| 0.85 | *** | 980 | 1231 | 2615 | 334 | 395 | 551 | . | . | . | . | . | . | . | . | . |
|  | *** | 1079 | 1516 | 2590 | 360 | 449 | 521 | . | . | . | . | . | . | . | . | . |
| 0.9 | *** | 704 | 883 | 1666 | . | . | . | . | . | . | . | . | . | . | . | . |
|  | *** | 776 | 1074 | 1637 | . | . | . | . | . | . | . | . | . | . | . | . |

TABLE 2: ALPHA= 0.005 POWER= 0.9    EXPECTED ACCRUAL THRU MINIMUM FOLLOW-UP= 250

| | | DEL=.05 | | | DEL=.10 | | | DEL=.15 | | | DEL=.20 | | | DEL=.25 | | |
|---|---|---|---|---|---|---|---|---|---|---|---|---|---|---|---|---|
| FACT= | | 1.0 .75 | .50 .25 | .00 BIN | 1.0 .75 | .50 .25 | .00 BIN | 1.0 .75 | .50 .25 | .00 BIN | 1.0 75 | .50 .25 | .00 BIN | 1.0 .75 | .50 .25 | .00 BIN |
| PCONT=*** | | | | | REQUIRED NUMBER OF PATIENTS | | | | | | | | | | | |
| 0.05 | *** | 891 | 898 | 951 | 319 | 324 | 338 | 188 | 191 | 197 | 133 | 135 | 138 | 104 | 105 | 107 |
| | *** | 894 | 909 | 1637 | 321 | 329 | 521 | 189 | 193 | 275 | 134 | 137 | 175 | 104 | 106 | 123 |
| 0.1 | *** | 1626 | 1641 | 1833 | 507 | 520 | 566 | 274 | 282 | 300 | 183 | 188 | 197 | 136 | 139 | 144 |
| | *** | 1631 | 1668 | 2590 | 512 | 534 | 744 | 277 | 289 | 368 | 185 | 192 | 224 | 137 | 141 | 152 |
| 0.15 | *** | 2251 | 2275 | 2687 | 658 | 681 | 776 | 341 | 356 | 391 | 221 | 230 | 246 | 160 | 165 | 175 |
| | *** | 2259 | 2322 | 3423 | 667 | 709 | 938 | 347 | 369 | 447 | 224 | 236 | 265 | 162 | 169 | 175 |
| 0.2 | *** | 2734 | 2771 | 3467 | 774 | 808 | 961 | 392 | 414 | 469 | 249 | 262 | 288 | 178 | 186 | 199 |
| | *** | 2747 | 2843 | 4137 | 786 | 850 | 1102 | 401 | 434 | 513 | 255 | 272 | 298 | 181 | 192 | 195 |
| 0.25 | *** | 3071 | 3124 | 4148 | 854 | 901 | 1120 | 428 | 457 | 534 | 269 | 287 | 321 | 190 | 201 | 219 |
| | *** | 3089 | 3226 | 4732 | 871 | 959 | 1235 | 440 | 484 | 566 | 277 | 300 | 324 | 195 | 208 | 209 |
| 0.3 | *** | 3267 | 3339 | 4717 | 902 | 962 | 1248 | 451 | 487 | 585 | 282 | 303 | 346 | 198 | 210 | 233 |
| | *** | 3291 | 3476 | 5208 | 924 | 1037 | 1340 | 466 | 521 | 606 | 291 | 320 | 343 | 203 | 220 | 218 |
| 0.35 | *** | 3336 | 3430 | 5166 | 922 | 997 | 1346 | 462 | 505 | 622 | 288 | 313 | 363 | 201 | 216 | 241 |
| | *** | 3367 | 3609 | 5565 | 950 | 1087 | 1414 | 480 | 545 | 632 | 299 | 332 | 354 | 207 | 226 | 223 |
| 0.4 | *** | 3292 | 3414 | 5489 | 918 | 1007 | 1411 | 463 | 512 | 644 | 289 | 316 | 372 | 200 | 216 | 244 |
| | *** | 3333 | 3639 | 5803 | 952 | 1111 | 1459 | 483 | 557 | 645 | 300 | 337 | 358 | 208 | 228 | 223 |
| 0.45 | *** | 3156 | 3312 | 5684 | 895 | 998 | 1444 | 455 | 508 | 652 | 284 | 313 | 372 | 196 | 213 | 242 |
| | *** | 3208 | 3586 | 5922 | 935 | 1113 | 1474 | 477 | 557 | 645 | 296 | 336 | 354 | 204 | 225 | 218 |
| 0.5 | *** | 2947 | 3142 | 5750 | 858 | 971 | 1445 | 440 | 496 | 645 | 274 | 304 | 364 | 189 | 206 | 234 |
| | *** | 3014 | 3467 | 5922 | 902 | 1095 | 1459 | 464 | 547 | 632 | 287 | 328 | 343 | 196 | 218 | 209 |
| 0.55 | *** | 2688 | 2925 | 5687 | 809 | 929 | 1413 | 419 | 476 | 624 | 261 | 290 | 349 | 178 | 194 | 222 |
| | *** | 2771 | 3295 | 5803 | 857 | 1058 | 1414 | 443 | 527 | 606 | 273 | 313 | 324 | 186 | 206 | 195 |
| 0.6 | *** | 2400 | 2680 | 5493 | 751 | 875 | 1349 | 391 | 447 | 588 | 242 | 270 | 325 | 164 | 179 | 204 |
| | *** | 2500 | 3084 | 5565 | 801 | 1004 | 1340 | 415 | 497 | 566 | 255 | 292 | 298 | 171 | 190 | 195 |
| 0.65 | *** | 2104 | 2418 | 5171 | 686 | 808 | 1252 | 358 | 411 | 538 | 220 | 246 | 293 | 147 | 160 | 181 |
| | *** | 2220 | 2840 | 5208 | 736 | 932 | 1235 | 381 | 457 | 513 | 231 | 264 | 265 | 153 | 169 | 152 |
| 0.7 | *** | 1816 | 2148 | 4721 | 615 | 730 | 1124 | 320 | 367 | 474 | 194 | 215 | 253 | 127 | 137 | 153 |
| | *** | 1942 | 2570 | 4732 | 662 | 844 | 1102 | 340 | 406 | 447 | 203 | 230 | 224 | 132 | 144 | 123 |
| 0.75 | *** | 1541 | 1872 | 4144 | 536 | 639 | 964 | 274 | 314 | 396 | 162 | 178 | 205 | . | . | . |
| | *** | 1669 | 2272 | 4137 | 578 | 738 | 938 | 291 | 345 | 368 | 169 | 189 | 175 | . | . | . |
| 0.8 | *** | 1278 | 1584 | 3442 | 447 | 532 | 773 | 221 | 250 | 304 | . | . | . | . | . | . |
| | *** | 1397 | 1940 | 3423 | 482 | 610 | 744 | 234 | 272 | 275 | . | . | . | . | . | . |
| 0.85 | *** | 1015 | 1273 | 2616 | 344 | 404 | 551 | . | . | . | . | . | . | . | . | . |
| | *** | 1117 | 1560 | 2590 | 369 | 456 | 521 | . | . | . | . | . | . | . | . | . |
| 0.9 | *** | 730 | 912 | 1666 | . | . | . | . | . | . | . | . | . | . | . | . |
| | *** | 803 | 1103 | 1637 | . | . | . | . | . | . | . | . | . | . | . | . |

## TABLE 2: ALPHA= 0.005 POWER= 0.9     EXPECTED ACCRUAL THRU MINIMUM FOLLOW-UP= 275

| | | DEL=.05 | | | DEL=.10 | | | DEL=.15 | | | DEL=.20 | | | DEL=.25 | | |
|---|---|---|---|---|---|---|---|---|---|---|---|---|---|---|---|---|---|
| FACT= | | 1.0 .75 | .50 .25 | .00 BIN | 1.0 .75 | .50 .25 | .00 BIN | 1.0 .75 | .50 .25 | .00 BIN | 1.0 75 | .50 .25 | .00 BIN | 1.0 .75 | .50 .25 | .00 BIN |
| PCONT=*** | | | | | | REQUIRED NUMBER OF PATIENTS | | | | | | | | | | |
| 0.05 | *** | 892 | 899 | 950 | 319 | 325 | 338 | 188 | 191 | 197 | 133 | 135 | 138 | 104 | 105 | 107 |
| | *** | 894 | 911 | 1637 | 321 | 330 | 521 | 189 | 194 | 275 | 134 | 137 | 175 | 105 | 106 | 123 |
| 0.1 | *** | 1628 | 1643 | 1833 | 508 | 521 | 566 | 275 | 283 | 300 | 183 | 188 | 197 | 136 | 139 | 144 |
| | *** | 1633 | 1673 | 2590 | 513 | 536 | 744 | 278 | 290 | 368 | 186 | 192 | 224 | 138 | 142 | 152 |
| 0.15 | *** | 2253 | 2280 | 2687 | 661 | 685 | 776 | 343 | 358 | 391 | 222 | 231 | 246 | 161 | 166 | 175 |
| | *** | 2262 | 2331 | 3423 | 670 | 712 | 938 | 349 | 370 | 447 | 226 | 237 | 265 | 163 | 170 | 175 |
| 0.2 | *** | 2738 | 2779 | 3467 | 777 | 813 | 961 | 395 | 417 | 469 | 251 | 264 | 288 | 179 | 187 | 199 |
| | *** | 2751 | 2857 | 4137 | 791 | 856 | 1102 | 404 | 436 | 513 | 257 | 274 | 298 | 182 | 192 | 195 |
| 0.25 | *** | 3076 | 3134 | 4148 | 859 | 908 | 1120 | 432 | 461 | 534 | 272 | 289 | 321 | 191 | 202 | 219 |
| | *** | 3096 | 3245 | 4732 | 877 | 967 | 1235 | 444 | 487 | 566 | 279 | 302 | 324 | 196 | 209 | 209 |
| 0.3 | *** | 3275 | 3353 | 4717 | 909 | 972 | 1248 | 456 | 492 | 585 | 285 | 306 | 346 | 200 | 212 | 233 |
| | *** | 3301 | 3502 | 5208 | 933 | 1047 | 1340 | 471 | 525 | 606 | 294 | 322 | 343 | 205 | 221 | 218 |
| 0.35 | *** | 3345 | 3449 | 5166 | 930 | 1009 | 1346 | 468 | 511 | 622 | 292 | 316 | 363 | 203 | 217 | 241 |
| | *** | 3380 | 3641 | 5565 | 960 | 1099 | 1414 | 486 | 550 | 632 | 302 | 334 | 354 | 210 | 227 | 223 |
| 0.4 | *** | 3304 | 3439 | 5489 | 929 | 1021 | 1411 | 469 | 518 | 644 | 293 | 319 | 372 | 203 | 218 | 244 |
| | *** | 3350 | 3680 | 5803 | 964 | 1126 | 1459 | 490 | 562 | 645 | 304 | 340 | 358 | 210 | 229 | 223 |
| 0.45 | *** | 3171 | 3342 | 5684 | 908 | 1013 | 1444 | 462 | 516 | 652 | 288 | 316 | 372 | 199 | 215 | 242 |
| | *** | 3229 | 3634 | 5922 | 949 | 1129 | 1474 | 485 | 563 | 645 | 300 | 338 | 354 | 206 | 226 | 218 |
| 0.5 | *** | 2967 | 3179 | 5750 | 872 | 988 | 1445 | 448 | 504 | 645 | 279 | 308 | 365 | 191 | 208 | 234 |
| | *** | 3040 | 3521 | 5922 | 918 | 1112 | 1459 | 471 | 553 | 632 | 291 | 330 | 343 | 199 | 219 | 209 |
| 0.55 | *** | 2713 | 2969 | 5687 | 824 | 947 | 1413 | 426 | 483 | 624 | 265 | 294 | 349 | 181 | 196 | 222 |
| | *** | 2803 | 3355 | 5803 | 873 | 1075 | 1414 | 450 | 533 | 606 | 277 | 315 | 324 | 188 | 207 | 195 |
| 0.6 | *** | 2431 | 2728 | 5493 | 767 | 893 | 1349 | 399 | 455 | 588 | 247 | 274 | 325 | 167 | 181 | 204 |
| | *** | 2538 | 3147 | 5565 | 818 | 1021 | 1340 | 423 | 502 | 566 | 259 | 294 | 298 | 173 | 191 | 175 |
| 0.65 | *** | 2140 | 2470 | 5171 | 702 | 826 | 1252 | 366 | 418 | 538 | 224 | 249 | 293 | 149 | 162 | 181 |
| | *** | 2263 | 2905 | 5208 | 752 | 949 | 1235 | 388 | 462 | 513 | 235 | 267 | 265 | 155 | 170 | 152 |
| 0.7 | *** | 1855 | 2201 | 4721 | 630 | 746 | 1124 | 326 | 373 | 474 | 197 | 217 | 253 | 128 | 138 | 153 |
| | *** | 1987 | 2633 | 4732 | 678 | 859 | 1102 | 346 | 411 | 447 | 206 | 232 | 224 | 133 | 145 | 123 |
| 0.75 | *** | 1582 | 1923 | 4144 | 550 | 653 | 964 | 280 | 319 | 396 | 164 | 180 | 205 | . | . | . |
| | *** | 1714 | 2331 | 4137 | 592 | 750 | 938 | 297 | 349 | 368 | 171 | 191 | 175 | . | . | . |
| 0.8 | *** | 1316 | 1630 | 3442 | 459 | 543 | 773 | 225 | 253 | 304 | . | . | . | . | . | . |
| | *** | 1439 | 1991 | 3423 | 494 | 619 | 744 | 238 | 274 | 275 | . | . | . | . | . | . |
| 0.85 | *** | 1048 | 1311 | 2615 | 352 | 412 | 551 | . | . | . | . | . | . | . | . | . |
| | *** | 1152 | 1601 | 2590 | 378 | 462 | 521 | . | . | . | . | . | . | . | . | . |
| 0.9 | *** | 754 | 938 | 1666 | . | . | . | . | . | . | . | . | . | . | . | . |
| | *** | 828 | 1129 | 1637 | . | . | . | . | . | . | . | . | . | . | . | . |

TABLE 2: ALPHA= 0.005 POWER= 0.9    EXPECTED ACCRUAL THRU MINIMUM FOLLOW-UP= 300

| PCONT | FACT | DEL=.05 1.0 / .75 | DEL=.05 .50 / .25 | DEL=.05 .00 / BIN | DEL=.10 1.0 / .75 | DEL=.10 .50 / .25 | DEL=.10 .00 / BIN | DEL=.15 1.0 / .75 | DEL=.15 .50 / .25 | DEL=.15 .00 / BIN | DEL=.20 1.0 / 75 | DEL=.20 .50 / .25 | DEL=.20 .00 / BIN | DEL=.25 1.0 / .75 | DEL=.25 .50 / .25 | DEL=.25 .00 / BIN |
|---|---|---|---|---|---|---|---|---|---|---|---|---|---|---|---|---|
| | | REQUIRED NUMBER OF PATIENTS | | | | | | | | | | | | | | |
| 0.05 | *** | 893 | 900 | 950 | 320 | 325 | 338 | 189 | 192 | 197 | 134 | 136 | 138 | 104 | 105 | 107 |
| | *** | 895 | 912 | 1637 | 322 | 330 | 521 | 190 | 194 | 275 | 134 | 137 | 175 | 105 | 106 | 123 |
| 0.1 | *** | 1629 | 1646 | 1833 | 510 | 523 | 566 | 276 | 284 | 300 | 184 | 189 | 197 | 137 | 140 | 144 |
| | *** | 1635 | 1677 | 2590 | 515 | 538 | 744 | 279 | 290 | 368 | 186 | 192 | 224 | 138 | 142 | 152 |
| 0.15 | *** | 2255 | 2285 | 2687 | 664 | 688 | 775 | 345 | 360 | 391 | 223 | 232 | 246 | 161 | 167 | 175 |
| | *** | 2265 | 2340 | 3423 | 673 | 715 | 938 | 351 | 372 | 447 | 227 | 238 | 265 | 164 | 170 | 175 |
| 0.2 | *** | 2742 | 2786 | 3467 | 781 | 818 | 961 | 398 | 419 | 469 | 253 | 265 | 288 | 180 | 187 | 199 |
| | *** | 2756 | 2870 | 4137 | 795 | 861 | 1102 | 407 | 438 | 513 | 258 | 274 | 298 | 183 | 193 | 195 |
| 0.25 | *** | 3082 | 3145 | 4148 | 864 | 915 | 1120 | 436 | 465 | 534 | 274 | 290 | 321 | 193 | 203 | 219 |
| | *** | 3103 | 3263 | 4732 | 884 | 974 | 1235 | 448 | 490 | 566 | 281 | 303 | 324 | 197 | 210 | 209 |
| 0.3 | *** | 3282 | 3367 | 4717 | 916 | 981 | 1248 | 460 | 496 | 585 | 288 | 308 | 346 | 201 | 213 | 232 |
| | *** | 3310 | 3526 | 5208 | 941 | 1056 | 1340 | 475 | 529 | 606 | 297 | 323 | 343 | 207 | 221 | 218 |
| 0.35 | *** | 3355 | 3467 | 5166 | 939 | 1020 | 1346 | 473 | 516 | 622 | 295 | 318 | 363 | 205 | 219 | 241 |
| | *** | 3392 | 3673 | 5565 | 970 | 1110 | 1414 | 491 | 554 | 632 | 305 | 336 | 354 | 211 | 228 | 223 |
| 0.4 | *** | 3317 | 3462 | 5489 | 939 | 1034 | 1411 | 475 | 524 | 644 | 296 | 322 | 372 | 205 | 220 | 244 |
| | *** | 3366 | 3718 | 5803 | 976 | 1138 | 1459 | 496 | 567 | 645 | 307 | 342 | 358 | 212 | 230 | 223 |
| 0.45 | *** | 3187 | 3371 | 5684 | 920 | 1028 | 1444 | 469 | 522 | 652 | 292 | 319 | 372 | 201 | 217 | 242 |
| | *** | 3250 | 3679 | 5922 | 962 | 1143 | 1474 | 491 | 568 | 645 | 304 | 341 | 354 | 208 | 227 | 218 |
| 0.5 | *** | 2987 | 3214 | 5750 | 885 | 1003 | 1445 | 455 | 510 | 645 | 283 | 311 | 364 | 194 | 209 | 234 |
| | *** | 3066 | 3572 | 5922 | 932 | 1127 | 1459 | 478 | 558 | 632 | 295 | 332 | 343 | 201 | 220 | 209 |
| 0.55 | *** | 2738 | 3010 | 5686 | 839 | 963 | 1413 | 434 | 490 | 624 | 269 | 297 | 349 | 183 | 198 | 222 |
| | *** | 2834 | 3411 | 5803 | 889 | 1091 | 1414 | 458 | 538 | 606 | 281 | 318 | 324 | 190 | 208 | 195 |
| 0.6 | *** | 2461 | 2775 | 5493 | 782 | 909 | 1348 | 406 | 461 | 588 | 250 | 277 | 325 | 169 | 183 | 204 |
| | *** | 2575 | 3206 | 5565 | 833 | 1036 | 1340 | 430 | 508 | 566 | 262 | 296 | 298 | 175 | 192 | 175 |
| 0.65 | *** | 2175 | 2520 | 5171 | 717 | 841 | 1252 | 373 | 424 | 538 | 227 | 251 | 292 | 151 | 163 | 181 |
| | *** | 2304 | 2965 | 5208 | 768 | 963 | 1235 | 395 | 466 | 513 | 238 | 268 | 265 | 157 | 171 | 152 |
| 0.7 | *** | 1894 | 2251 | 4721 | 644 | 761 | 1124 | 333 | 378 | 474 | 200 | 220 | 253 | 130 | 139 | 153 |
| | *** | 2030 | 2692 | 4732 | 692 | 872 | 1102 | 352 | 415 | 447 | 208 | 234 | 224 | 134 | 145 | 123 |
| 0.75 | *** | 1620 | 1971 | 4144 | 562 | 666 | 964 | 285 | 323 | 396 | 166 | 181 | 205 | . | . | . |
| | *** | 1756 | 2385 | 4137 | 605 | 761 | 938 | 302 | 352 | 368 | 173 | 192 | 175 | . | . | . |
| 0.8 | *** | 1352 | 1673 | 3442 | 469 | 553 | 773 | 229 | 256 | 304 | . | . | . | . | . | . |
| | *** | 1479 | 2038 | 3423 | 505 | 628 | 744 | 241 | 276 | 275 | . | . | . | . | . | . |
| 0.85 | *** | 1079 | 1346 | 2615 | 360 | 419 | 551 | . | . | . | . | . | . | . | . | . |
| | *** | 1185 | 1638 | 2590 | 385 | 467 | 521 | . | . | . | . | . | . | . | . | . |
| 0.9 | *** | 776 | 962 | 1666 | . | . | . | . | . | . | . | . | . | . | . | . |
| | *** | 852 | 1152 | 1637 | . | . | . | . | . | . | . | . | . | . | . | . |

# TABLE 2: ALPHA= 0.005 POWER= 0.9     EXPECTED ACCRUAL THRU MINIMUM FOLLOW-UP= 325

| | | DEL=.05 | | | DEL=.10 | | | DEL=.15 | | | DEL=.20 | | | DEL=.25 | |
|---|---|---|---|---|---|---|---|---|---|---|---|---|---|---|---|---|
| FACT= | | 1.0 .75 | .50 .25 | .00 BIN | 1.0 .75 | .50 .25 | .00 BIN | 1.0 .75 | .50 .25 | .00 BIN | 1.0 75 | .50 .25 | .00 BIN | 1.0 .75 | .50 .25 | .00 BIN |
| PCONT=*** | | | | | REQUIRED | NUMBER | OF | PATIENTS | | | | | | | | |
| 0.05 | *** | 893 | 902 | 950 | 320 | 326 | 338 | 189 | 192 | 197 | 134 | 136 | 138 | 104 | 106 | 107 |
| | *** | 896 | 914 | 1637 | 323 | 330 | 521 | 190 | 194 | 275 | 135 | 137 | 175 | 105 | 106 | 123 |
| 0.1 | *** | 1630 | 1649 | 1833 | 511 | 525 | 566 | 277 | 285 | 300 | 185 | 189 | 197 | 137 | 140 | 144 |
| | *** | 1637 | 1682 | 2590 | 517 | 539 | 744 | 280 | 291 | 368 | 187 | 193 | 224 | 138 | 142 | 152 |
| 0.15 | *** | 2258 | 2290 | 2687 | 666 | 691 | 775 | 347 | 361 | 391 | 224 | 232 | 246 | 162 | 167 | 175 |
| | *** | 2268 | 2348 | 3423 | 676 | 719 | 938 | 353 | 373 | 447 | 228 | 238 | 265 | 164 | 171 | 175 |
| 0.2 | *** | 2745 | 2793 | 3467 | 785 | 823 | 961 | 400 | 422 | 469 | 254 | 266 | 288 | 181 | 188 | 199 |
| | *** | 2761 | 2883 | 4137 | 800 | 866 | 1102 | 409 | 440 | 513 | 260 | 275 | 298 | 184 | 193 | 195 |
| 0.25 | *** | 3087 | 3155 | 4148 | 869 | 922 | 1120 | 439 | 468 | 534 | 276 | 292 | 321 | 194 | 204 | 219 |
| | *** | 3110 | 3281 | 4732 | 889 | 980 | 1235 | 451 | 493 | 566 | 283 | 304 | 324 | 199 | 210 | 209 |
| 0.3 | *** | 3289 | 3381 | 4717 | 922 | 990 | 1248 | 465 | 500 | 585 | 290 | 310 | 346 | 203 | 214 | 233 |
| | *** | 3320 | 3550 | 5208 | 948 | 1065 | 1340 | 480 | 532 | 606 | 299 | 325 | 343 | 208 | 222 | 218 |
| 0.35 | *** | 3364 | 3486 | 5166 | 947 | 1030 | 1346 | 478 | 521 | 622 | 298 | 321 | 363 | 207 | 220 | 241 |
| | *** | 3405 | 3703 | 5565 | 979 | 1120 | 1414 | 496 | 558 | 632 | 308 | 338 | 354 | 213 | 229 | 223 |
| 0.4 | *** | 3329 | 3486 | 5489 | 949 | 1046 | 1411 | 481 | 529 | 644 | 299 | 325 | 372 | 207 | 221 | 244 |
| | *** | 3382 | 3755 | 5803 | 987 | 1150 | 1459 | 502 | 571 | 645 | 311 | 344 | 358 | 213 | 231 | 223 |
| 0.45 | *** | 3203 | 3400 | 5684 | 931 | 1041 | 1444 | 475 | 528 | 652 | 295 | 322 | 372 | 203 | 218 | 242 |
| | *** | 3271 | 3723 | 5922 | 975 | 1156 | 1474 | 497 | 573 | 645 | 307 | 343 | 354 | 210 | 228 | 218 |
| 0.5 | *** | 3007 | 3249 | 5750 | 898 | 1018 | 1445 | 461 | 517 | 645 | 286 | 314 | 365 | 196 | 211 | 234 |
| | *** | 3092 | 3621 | 5922 | 946 | 1141 | 1459 | 485 | 563 | 632 | 298 | 335 | 343 | 203 | 221 | 209 |
| 0.55 | *** | 2762 | 3050 | 5686 | 852 | 978 | 1413 | 440 | 496 | 624 | 272 | 300 | 349 | 185 | 199 | 222 |
| | *** | 2865 | 3464 | 5803 | 903 | 1105 | 1414 | 464 | 543 | 606 | 284 | 320 | 324 | 192 | 209 | 195 |
| 0.6 | *** | 2491 | 2819 | 5493 | 796 | 924 | 1349 | 413 | 467 | 588 | 254 | 279 | 325 | 171 | 184 | 204 |
| | *** | 2611 | 3262 | 5565 | 848 | 1050 | 1340 | 436 | 512 | 566 | 265 | 298 | 298 | 177 | 193 | 175 |
| 0.65 | *** | 2209 | 2567 | 5171 | 731 | 856 | 1252 | 379 | 430 | 538 | 231 | 253 | 292 | 153 | 164 | 181 |
| | *** | 2344 | 3022 | 5208 | 782 | 977 | 1235 | 401 | 471 | 513 | 241 | 270 | 265 | 158 | 172 | 152 |
| 0.7 | *** | 1930 | 2299 | 4721 | 658 | 774 | 1124 | 338 | 383 | 474 | 202 | 222 | 253 | 131 | 140 | 153 |
| | *** | 2072 | 2747 | 4732 | 706 | 884 | 1102 | 358 | 418 | 447 | 211 | 235 | 224 | 135 | 146 | 123 |
| 0.75 | *** | 1657 | 2016 | 4144 | 574 | 677 | 964 | 290 | 327 | 396 | 168 | 183 | 205 | . | . | . |
| | *** | 1797 | 2435 | 4137 | 617 | 771 | 938 | 306 | 354 | 368 | 175 | 193 | 175 | . | . | . |
| 0.8 | *** | 1386 | 1714 | 3442 | 479 | 563 | 773 | 233 | 259 | 304 | . | . | . | . | . | . |
| | *** | 1516 | 2082 | 3423 | 515 | 636 | 744 | 244 | 278 | 275 | . | . | . | . | . | . |
| 0.85 | *** | 1108 | 1379 | 2615 | 367 | 425 | 551 | . | . | . | . | . | . | . | . | . |
| | *** | 1216 | 1672 | 2590 | 392 | 472 | 521 | . | . | . | . | . | . | . | . | . |
| 0.9 | *** | 797 | 984 | 1666 | . | . | . | . | . | . | . | . | . | . | . | . |
| | *** | 873 | 1173 | 1637 | . | . | . | . | . | . | . | . | . | . | . | . |

TABLE 2: ALPHA= 0.005 POWER= 0.9    EXPECTED ACCRUAL THRU MINIMUM FOLLOW-UP= 350

| | | DEL=.05 | | | DEL=.10 | | | DEL=.15 | | | DEL=.20 | | | DEL=.25 | | |
|---|---|---|---|---|---|---|---|---|---|---|---|---|---|---|---|---|
| FACT= | | 1.0 .75 | .50 .25 | .00 BIN | 1.0 .75 | .50 .25 | .00 BIN | 1.0 .75 | .50 .25 | .00 BIN | 1.0 75 | .50 .25 | .00 BIN | 1.0 .75 | .50 .25 | .00 BIN |
| PCONT=*** | | | | | REQUIRED | NUMBER OF | PATIENTS | | | | | | | | | |
| 0.05 | *** | 894 | 903 | 950 | 321 | 327 | 338 | 189 | 192 | 197 | 134 | 136 | 138 | 104 | 106 | 107 |
| | *** | 897 | 915 | 1637 | 323 | 331 | 521 | 191 | 194 | 275 | 135 | 137 | 175 | 105 | 106 | 123 |
| 0.1 | *** | 1632 | 1652 | 1833 | 512 | 527 | 566 | 278 | 286 | 300 | 185 | 190 | 197 | 138 | 140 | 144 |
| | *** | 1639 | 1686 | 2590 | 518 | 541 | 744 | 281 | 292 | 368 | 187 | 193 | 224 | 139 | 142 | 152 |
| 0.15 | *** | 2260 | 2294 | 2687 | 668 | 694 | 776 | 348 | 363 | 391 | 225 | 233 | 246 | 163 | 168 | 175 |
| | *** | 2272 | 2356 | 3423 | 678 | 721 | 938 | 355 | 374 | 447 | 229 | 239 | 265 | 165 | 171 | 175 |
| 0.2 | *** | 2749 | 2801 | 3467 | 789 | 828 | 961 | 403 | 424 | 469 | 256 | 268 | 288 | 182 | 189 | 199 |
| | *** | 2766 | 2895 | 4137 | 804 | 870 | 1102 | 412 | 442 | 513 | 261 | 276 | 298 | 185 | 194 | 195 |
| 0.25 | *** | 3092 | 3165 | 4148 | 874 | 928 | 1120 | 442 | 471 | 534 | 278 | 294 | 321 | 195 | 205 | 219 |
| | *** | 3117 | 3299 | 4732 | 895 | 986 | 1235 | 454 | 495 | 566 | 285 | 305 | 324 | 200 | 211 | 209 |
| 0.3 | *** | 3296 | 3395 | 4717 | 929 | 998 | 1248 | 468 | 504 | 585 | 293 | 312 | 346 | 204 | 215 | 232 |
| | *** | 3329 | 3574 | 5208 | 955 | 1072 | 1340 | 484 | 535 | 606 | 301 | 326 | 343 | 209 | 223 | 218 |
| 0.35 | *** | 3373 | 3504 | 5166 | 955 | 1040 | 1346 | 483 | 525 | 622 | 300 | 323 | 363 | 209 | 221 | 241 |
| | *** | 3417 | 3732 | 5565 | 988 | 1130 | 1414 | 501 | 561 | 632 | 311 | 339 | 354 | 214 | 230 | 223 |
| 0.4 | *** | 3341 | 3509 | 5489 | 958 | 1057 | 1411 | 486 | 534 | 644 | 302 | 327 | 372 | 209 | 223 | 244 |
| | *** | 3398 | 3790 | 5803 | 997 | 1161 | 1459 | 507 | 575 | 645 | 313 | 346 | 358 | 215 | 232 | 223 |
| 0.45 | *** | 3219 | 3429 | 5684 | 942 | 1053 | 1444 | 481 | 533 | 652 | 299 | 325 | 372 | 205 | 219 | 242 |
| | *** | 3291 | 3764 | 5922 | 986 | 1168 | 1474 | 503 | 577 | 645 | 310 | 344 | 354 | 211 | 229 | 218 |
| 0.5 | *** | 3027 | 3283 | 5750 | 910 | 1031 | 1445 | 467 | 522 | 645 | 289 | 316 | 365 | 198 | 212 | 234 |
| | *** | 3117 | 3667 | 5922 | 959 | 1153 | 1459 | 491 | 568 | 632 | 301 | 336 | 343 | 204 | 222 | 209 |
| 0.55 | *** | 2787 | 3089 | 5687 | 865 | 992 | 1413 | 447 | 502 | 624 | 275 | 302 | 349 | 187 | 201 | 222 |
| | *** | 2896 | 3514 | 5803 | 916 | 1118 | 1414 | 470 | 547 | 606 | 287 | 321 | 324 | 193 | 210 | 195 |
| 0.6 | *** | 2519 | 2862 | 5493 | 809 | 938 | 1349 | 419 | 473 | 588 | 257 | 282 | 325 | 172 | 185 | 204 |
| | *** | 2646 | 3315 | 5565 | 862 | 1063 | 1340 | 442 | 516 | 566 | 268 | 300 | 298 | 178 | 193 | 175 |
| 0.65 | *** | 2242 | 2611 | 5171 | 744 | 869 | 1252 | 384 | 435 | 538 | 233 | 256 | 293 | 154 | 165 | 181 |
| | *** | 2382 | 3075 | 5208 | 796 | 988 | 1235 | 406 | 474 | 513 | 243 | 271 | 265 | 159 | 172 | 152 |
| 0.7 | *** | 1965 | 2343 | 4721 | 670 | 787 | 1124 | 343 | 387 | 474 | 204 | 223 | 253 | 132 | 141 | 153 |
| | *** | 2111 | 2798 | 4732 | 718 | 895 | 1102 | 363 | 421 | 447 | 213 | 236 | 224 | 136 | 146 | 123 |
| 0.75 | *** | 1692 | 2058 | 4144 | 585 | 688 | 964 | 294 | 330 | 396 | 170 | 184 | 205 | . | . | . |
| | *** | 1835 | 2483 | 4137 | 628 | 780 | 938 | 310 | 357 | 368 | 176 | 193 | 175 | . | . | . |
| 0.8 | *** | 1419 | 1751 | 3442 | 488 | 571 | 773 | 236 | 261 | 304 | . | . | . | . | . | . |
| | *** | 1550 | 2123 | 3423 | 524 | 642 | 744 | 247 | 279 | 275 | . | . | . | . | . | . |
| 0.85 | *** | 1135 | 1410 | 2616 | 374 | 431 | 551 | . | . | . | . | . | . | . | . | . |
| | *** | 1245 | 1703 | 2590 | 398 | 476 | 521 | . | . | . | . | . | . | . | . | . |
| 0.9 | *** | 816 | 1005 | 1666 | . | . | . | . | . | . | . | . | . | . | . | . |
| | *** | 893 | 1193 | 1637 | . | . | . | . | . | . | . | . | . | . | . | . |

## TABLE 2: ALPHA= 0.005 POWER= 0.9    EXPECTED ACCRUAL THRU MINIMUM FOLLOW-UP= 375

| | | DEL=.05 | | | DEL=.10 | | | DEL=.15 | | | DEL=.20 | | | DEL=.25 | | |
|---|---|---|---|---|---|---|---|---|---|---|---|---|---|---|---|---|---|
| FACT= | | 1.0 .75 | .50 .25 | .00 BIN | 1.0 .75 | .50 .25 | .00 BIN | 1.0 .75 | .50 .25 | .00 BIN | 1.0 75 | .50 .25 | .00 BIN | 1.0 .75 | .50 .25 | .00 BIN |
| PCONT=*** | | | | | REQUIRED NUMBER OF PATIENTS | | | | | | | | | | | |
| 0.05 | *** | 895 | 904 | 950 | 322 | 327 | 338 | 190 | 193 | 197 | 134 | 136 | 138 | 105 | 106 | 107 |
| | *** | 898 | 917 | 1637 | 324 | 331 | 521 | 191 | 194 | 275 | 135 | 137 | 175 | 105 | 107 | 123 |
| 0.1 | *** | 1633 | 1655 | 1833 | 514 | 528 | 566 | 279 | 286 | 300 | 186 | 190 | 197 | 138 | 140 | 144 |
| | *** | 1640 | 1690 | 2590 | 520 | 542 | 744 | 282 | 292 | 368 | 188 | 193 | 224 | 139 | 142 | 152 |
| 0.15 | *** | 2263 | 2299 | 2687 | 671 | 697 | 776 | 350 | 364 | 391 | 226 | 234 | 246 | 163 | 168 | 175 |
| | *** | 2275 | 2364 | 3423 | 681 | 724 | 938 | 356 | 375 | 447 | 230 | 239 | 265 | 165 | 171 | 175 |
| 0.2 | *** | 2753 | 2808 | 3467 | 792 | 832 | 961 | 405 | 426 | 469 | 257 | 269 | 288 | 183 | 190 | 200 |
| | *** | 2771 | 2907 | 4137 | 808 | 874 | 1102 | 414 | 443 | 513 | 262 | 277 | 298 | 186 | 194 | 195 |
| 0.25 | *** | 3097 | 3176 | 4148 | 879 | 934 | 1120 | 445 | 474 | 534 | 280 | 295 | 321 | 197 | 205 | 219 |
| | *** | 3124 | 3316 | 4732 | 901 | 992 | 1235 | 457 | 497 | 566 | 287 | 306 | 324 | 200 | 211 | 209 |
| 0.3 | *** | 3303 | 3409 | 4717 | 935 | 1005 | 1248 | 472 | 508 | 585 | 295 | 314 | 346 | 205 | 216 | 233 |
| | *** | 3339 | 3596 | 5208 | 962 | 1079 | 1340 | 487 | 537 | 606 | 303 | 327 | 343 | 210 | 223 | 218 |
| 0.35 | *** | 3383 | 3522 | 5166 | 963 | 1049 | 1346 | 487 | 529 | 622 | 303 | 325 | 363 | 210 | 222 | 241 |
| | *** | 3430 | 3760 | 5565 | 997 | 1138 | 1414 | 505 | 564 | 632 | 313 | 341 | 354 | 215 | 230 | 223 |
| 0.4 | *** | 3354 | 3532 | 5489 | 967 | 1068 | 1411 | 491 | 539 | 644 | 305 | 329 | 372 | 210 | 224 | 244 |
| | *** | 3415 | 3824 | 5803 | 1007 | 1171 | 1459 | 512 | 578 | 645 | 316 | 347 | 358 | 216 | 233 | 223 |
| 0.45 | *** | 3234 | 3457 | 5684 | 953 | 1065 | 1444 | 486 | 538 | 652 | 301 | 327 | 372 | 207 | 221 | 242 |
| | *** | 3312 | 3803 | 5922 | 998 | 1179 | 1474 | 508 | 580 | 645 | 313 | 346 | 354 | 213 | 230 | 218 |
| 0.5 | *** | 3046 | 3316 | 5750 | 921 | 1043 | 1445 | 473 | 527 | 645 | 292 | 319 | 365 | 199 | 213 | 234 |
| | *** | 3142 | 3711 | 5922 | 971 | 1165 | 1459 | 496 | 571 | 632 | 304 | 338 | 343 | 206 | 223 | 209 |
| 0.55 | *** | 2811 | 3126 | 5687 | 877 | 1005 | 1413 | 452 | 507 | 624 | 278 | 304 | 349 | 188 | 202 | 222 |
| | *** | 2925 | 3562 | 5803 | 929 | 1129 | 1414 | 476 | 551 | 606 | 290 | 323 | 324 | 194 | 211 | 195 |
| 0.6 | *** | 2548 | 2902 | 5493 | 822 | 950 | 1348 | 425 | 478 | 588 | 260 | 284 | 325 | 174 | 186 | 204 |
| | *** | 2680 | 3364 | 5565 | 875 | 1074 | 1340 | 447 | 520 | 566 | 270 | 301 | 298 | 179 | 194 | 175 |
| 0.65 | *** | 2274 | 2654 | 5171 | 756 | 882 | 1252 | 390 | 439 | 538 | 236 | 257 | 293 | 155 | 166 | 181 |
| | *** | 2418 | 3124 | 5208 | 808 | 999 | 1235 | 411 | 478 | 513 | 245 | 272 | 265 | 160 | 173 | 152 |
| 0.7 | *** | 1998 | 2386 | 4721 | 681 | 798 | 1124 | 348 | 391 | 474 | 207 | 225 | 253 | 133 | 141 | 152 |
| | *** | 2148 | 2845 | 4732 | 730 | 905 | 1102 | 367 | 424 | 447 | 215 | 237 | 224 | 137 | 147 | 123 |
| 0.75 | *** | 1725 | 2099 | 4144 | 596 | 698 | 964 | 298 | 333 | 396 | 172 | 185 | 205 | . | . | . |
| | *** | 1871 | 2526 | 4137 | 639 | 789 | 938 | 314 | 359 | 368 | 178 | 194 | 175 | . | . | . |
| 0.8 | *** | 1450 | 1787 | 3442 | 497 | 579 | 773 | 238 | 264 | 304 | . | . | . | . | . | . |
| | *** | 1584 | 2160 | 3423 | 532 | 649 | 744 | 250 | 281 | 275 | . | . | . | . | . | . |
| 0.85 | *** | 1161 | 1439 | 2615 | 380 | 436 | 551 | . | . | . | . | . | . | . | . | . |
| | *** | 1273 | 1732 | 2590 | 404 | 480 | 521 | . | . | . | . | . | . | . | . | . |
| 0.9 | *** | 834 | 1024 | 1666 | . | . | . | . | . | . | . | . | . | . | . | . |
| | *** | 912 | 1210 | 1637 | . | . | . | . | . | . | . | . | . | . | . | . |

## TABLE 2: ALPHA= 0.005 POWER= 0.9    EXPECTED ACCRUAL THRU MINIMUM FOLLOW-UP= 400

|  |  | DEL=.05 | | | DEL=.10 | | | DEL=.15 | | | DEL=.20 | | | DEL=.25 | | |
|---|---|---|---|---|---|---|---|---|---|---|---|---|---|---|---|---|
| FACT= | | 1.0 .75 | .50 .25 | .00 BIN | 1.0 .75 | .50 .25 | .00 BIN | 1.0 .75 | .50 .25 | .00 BIN | 1.0 75 | .50 .25 | .00 BIN | 1.0 .75 | .50 .25 | .00 BIN |
| PCONT=*** | | | | | REQUIRED NUMBER OF PATIENTS | | | | | | | | | | | |
| 0.05 | *** | 895 | 905 | 951 | 322 | 327 | 338 | 190 | 193 | 197 | 135 | 136 | 138 | 105 | 106 | 107 |
|  | *** | 899 | 918 | 1637 | 324 | 332 | 521 | 191 | 195 | 275 | 135 | 137 | 175 | 105 | 107 | 123 |
| 0.1 | *** | 1635 | 1657 | 1833 | 515 | 530 | 566 | 279 | 287 | 300 | 186 | 190 | 197 | 138 | 141 | 144 |
|  | *** | 1643 | 1694 | 2590 | 521 | 543 | 744 | 283 | 293 | 368 | 188 | 193 | 224 | 139 | 142 | 152 |
| 0.15 | *** | 2265 | 2304 | 2687 | 673 | 700 | 776 | 351 | 365 | 391 | 227 | 234 | 246 | 164 | 168 | 175 |
|  | *** | 2278 | 2371 | 3423 | 684 | 726 | 938 | 357 | 376 | 447 | 230 | 240 | 265 | 166 | 171 | 175 |
| 0.2 | *** | 2756 | 2815 | 3467 | 795 | 836 | 961 | 407 | 428 | 469 | 258 | 270 | 288 | 183 | 190 | 199 |
|  | *** | 2776 | 2919 | 4137 | 811 | 877 | 1102 | 416 | 444 | 513 | 263 | 277 | 298 | 186 | 194 | 195 |
| 0.25 | *** | 3103 | 3186 | 4148 | 884 | 939 | 1120 | 448 | 476 | 534 | 281 | 296 | 321 | 198 | 206 | 219 |
|  | *** | 3131 | 3332 | 4732 | 906 | 997 | 1235 | 460 | 499 | 566 | 288 | 307 | 324 | 201 | 212 | 209 |
| 0.3 | *** | 3310 | 3423 | 4717 | 941 | 1012 | 1248 | 475 | 511 | 585 | 297 | 315 | 346 | 207 | 217 | 233 |
|  | *** | 3348 | 3618 | 5208 | 969 | 1086 | 1340 | 491 | 539 | 606 | 305 | 328 | 343 | 211 | 224 | 218 |
| 0.35 | *** | 3392 | 3540 | 5166 | 970 | 1057 | 1346 | 491 | 533 | 622 | 305 | 327 | 363 | 211 | 223 | 241 |
|  | *** | 3443 | 3787 | 5565 | 1005 | 1146 | 1414 | 509 | 567 | 632 | 315 | 342 | 354 | 217 | 231 | 223 |
| 0.4 | *** | 3366 | 3554 | 5489 | 976 | 1077 | 1411 | 496 | 543 | 644 | 308 | 331 | 372 | 212 | 225 | 244 |
|  | *** | 3431 | 3857 | 5803 | 1017 | 1180 | 1459 | 516 | 581 | 645 | 318 | 348 | 358 | 218 | 233 | 223 |
| 0.45 | *** | 3250 | 3484 | 5684 | 962 | 1076 | 1444 | 491 | 542 | 652 | 304 | 329 | 372 | 208 | 222 | 242 |
|  | *** | 3332 | 3841 | 5922 | 1008 | 1189 | 1474 | 513 | 584 | 645 | 315 | 347 | 354 | 214 | 231 | 218 |
| 0.5 | *** | 3066 | 3348 | 5750 | 932 | 1055 | 1445 | 478 | 532 | 645 | 295 | 321 | 365 | 201 | 214 | 234 |
|  | *** | 3166 | 3753 | 5922 | 982 | 1175 | 1459 | 501 | 575 | 632 | 307 | 339 | 343 | 207 | 223 | 209 |
| 0.55 | *** | 2834 | 3162 | 5687 | 889 | 1017 | 1413 | 458 | 511 | 624 | 281 | 306 | 349 | 190 | 203 | 222 |
|  | *** | 2954 | 3607 | 5803 | 941 | 1140 | 1414 | 481 | 555 | 606 | 292 | 324 | 324 | 196 | 211 | 195 |
| 0.6 | *** | 2576 | 2942 | 5493 | 834 | 963 | 1349 | 430 | 482 | 588 | 262 | 286 | 325 | 175 | 187 | 204 |
|  | *** | 2713 | 3411 | 5565 | 887 | 1085 | 1340 | 452 | 523 | 566 | 273 | 302 | 298 | 181 | 194 | 175 |
| 0.65 | *** | 2304 | 2694 | 5171 | 768 | 893 | 1252 | 395 | 443 | 538 | 238 | 259 | 293 | 157 | 167 | 181 |
|  | *** | 2453 | 3171 | 5208 | 820 | 1009 | 1235 | 416 | 481 | 513 | 248 | 274 | 265 | 161 | 173 | 152 |
| 0.7 | *** | 2030 | 2426 | 4721 | 692 | 808 | 1124 | 352 | 395 | 474 | 209 | 226 | 253 | 134 | 142 | 153 |
|  | *** | 2184 | 2890 | 4732 | 741 | 914 | 1102 | 371 | 427 | 447 | 217 | 238 | 224 | 138 | 147 | 123 |
| 0.75 | *** | 1757 | 2137 | 4144 | 605 | 707 | 964 | 302 | 336 | 396 | 173 | 186 | 205 | . | . | . |
|  | *** | 1906 | 2568 | 4137 | 648 | 796 | 938 | 317 | 361 | 368 | 179 | 195 | 175 | . | . | . |
| 0.8 | *** | 1479 | 1821 | 3442 | 505 | 586 | 773 | 241 | 265 | 304 | . | . | . | . | . | . |
|  | *** | 1615 | 2196 | 3423 | 540 | 654 | 744 | 252 | 282 | 275 | . | . | . | . | . | . |
| 0.85 | *** | 1185 | 1466 | 2616 | 385 | 440 | 551 | . | . | . | . | . | . | . | . | . |
|  | *** | 1298 | 1759 | 2590 | 409 | 484 | 521 | . | . | . | . | . | . | . | . | . |
| 0.9 | *** | 852 | 1042 | 1666 | . | . | . | . | . | . | . | . | . | . | . | . |
|  | *** | 930 | 1227 | 1637 | . | . | . | . | . | . | . | . | . | . | . | . |

TABLE 2: ALPHA= 0.005 POWER= 0.9    EXPECTED ACCRUAL THRU MINIMUM FOLLOW-UP= 425

| | | DEL=.05 | | | DEL=.10 | | | DEL=.15 | | | DEL=.20 | | | DEL=.25 | | |
|---|---|---|---|---|---|---|---|---|---|---|---|---|---|---|---|---|---|
| FACT= | | 1.0 .75 | .50 .25 | .00 BIN | 1.0 .75 | .50 .25 | .00 BIN | 1.0 .75 | .50 .25 | .00 BIN | 1.0 75 | .50 .25 | .00 BIN | 1.0 .75 | .50 .25 | .00 BIN |
| PCONT=*** | | | | | | REQUIRED NUMBER OF PATIENTS | | | | | | | | | | | |
| 0.05 | *** | 896 | 906 | 951 | 323 | 328 | 338 | 190 | 193 | 197 | 135 | 136 | 138 | 105 | 106 | 107 |
| | *** | 900 | 919 | 1637 | 325 | 332 | 521 | 191 | 195 | 275 | 136 | 137 | 175 | 105 | 107 | 123 |
| 0.1 | *** | 1636 | 1660 | 1833 | 516 | 531 | 566 | 280 | 288 | 300 | 187 | 191 | 197 | 138 | 141 | 144 |
| | *** | 1644 | 1698 | 2590 | 522 | 544 | 744 | 283 | 293 | 368 | 188 | 193 | 224 | 139 | 142 | 152 |
| 0.15 | *** | 2268 | 2309 | 2687 | 675 | 702 | 776 | 353 | 366 | 391 | 228 | 235 | 246 | 164 | 169 | 175 |
| | *** | 2281 | 2378 | 3423 | 686 | 728 | 938 | 358 | 376 | 447 | 231 | 240 | 265 | 166 | 171 | 175 |
| 0.2 | *** | 2760 | 2822 | 3467 | 799 | 840 | 961 | 409 | 430 | 469 | 259 | 271 | 288 | 184 | 190 | 200 |
| | *** | 2781 | 2930 | 4137 | 815 | 881 | 1102 | 418 | 445 | 513 | 264 | 278 | 298 | 187 | 195 | 195 |
| 0.25 | *** | 3108 | 3196 | 4148 | 888 | 945 | 1120 | 451 | 478 | 534 | 283 | 297 | 321 | 198 | 207 | 219 |
| | *** | 3138 | 3348 | 4732 | 911 | 1002 | 1235 | 462 | 501 | 566 | 289 | 308 | 324 | 202 | 212 | 209 |
| 0.3 | *** | 3317 | 3436 | 4717 | 946 | 1019 | 1248 | 479 | 513 | 585 | 298 | 316 | 346 | 208 | 218 | 232 |
| | *** | 3358 | 3638 | 5208 | 975 | 1092 | 1340 | 494 | 541 | 606 | 307 | 329 | 343 | 212 | 224 | 218 |
| 0.35 | *** | 3402 | 3558 | 5166 | 977 | 1065 | 1346 | 495 | 536 | 622 | 307 | 328 | 363 | 213 | 224 | 241 |
| | *** | 3455 | 3813 | 5565 | 1012 | 1154 | 1414 | 512 | 569 | 632 | 317 | 343 | 354 | 218 | 232 | 223 |
| 0.4 | *** | 3378 | 3576 | 5489 | 985 | 1087 | 1411 | 500 | 547 | 644 | 310 | 333 | 372 | 213 | 226 | 244 |
| | *** | 3447 | 3888 | 5803 | 1026 | 1188 | 1459 | 520 | 584 | 645 | 320 | 349 | 358 | 219 | 234 | 223 |
| 0.45 | *** | 3265 | 3510 | 5684 | 972 | 1086 | 1444 | 496 | 546 | 652 | 306 | 331 | 372 | 209 | 223 | 242 |
| | *** | 3351 | 3877 | 5922 | 1018 | 1198 | 1474 | 518 | 587 | 645 | 317 | 349 | 354 | 215 | 231 | 218 |
| 0.5 | *** | 3085 | 3379 | 5750 | 943 | 1066 | 1445 | 483 | 536 | 645 | 298 | 323 | 365 | 202 | 215 | 234 |
| | *** | 3190 | 3793 | 5922 | 993 | 1185 | 1459 | 506 | 578 | 632 | 309 | 340 | 343 | 208 | 224 | 209 |
| 0.55 | *** | 2858 | 3197 | 5687 | 900 | 1028 | 1413 | 462 | 516 | 624 | 283 | 308 | 349 | 191 | 204 | 222 |
| | *** | 2983 | 3650 | 5803 | 952 | 1150 | 1414 | 486 | 558 | 606 | 295 | 325 | 324 | 197 | 212 | 195 |
| 0.6 | *** | 2602 | 2979 | 5493 | 844 | 974 | 1348 | 435 | 486 | 588 | 264 | 288 | 325 | 176 | 188 | 204 |
| | *** | 2744 | 3455 | 5565 | 898 | 1095 | 1340 | 457 | 526 | 566 | 275 | 303 | 298 | 181 | 195 | 175 |
| 0.65 | *** | 2334 | 2733 | 5171 | 779 | 904 | 1252 | 399 | 447 | 538 | 240 | 261 | 292 | 158 | 167 | 181 |
| | *** | 2487 | 3215 | 5208 | 831 | 1019 | 1235 | 420 | 483 | 513 | 249 | 274 | 265 | 162 | 173 | 152 |
| 0.7 | *** | 2061 | 2465 | 4721 | 702 | 818 | 1124 | 356 | 398 | 474 | 210 | 227 | 253 | 135 | 143 | 153 |
| | *** | 2219 | 2933 | 4732 | 751 | 922 | 1102 | 375 | 429 | 447 | 218 | 239 | 224 | 139 | 147 | 123 |
| 0.75 | *** | 1787 | 2173 | 4144 | 614 | 715 | 964 | 305 | 339 | 396 | 175 | 187 | 205 | . | . | . |
| | *** | 1939 | 2606 | 4137 | 657 | 803 | 938 | 320 | 363 | 368 | 180 | 195 | 175 | . | . | . |
| 0.8 | *** | 1507 | 1853 | 3442 | 512 | 593 | 773 | 244 | 267 | 305 | . | . | . | . | . | . |
| | *** | 1645 | 2229 | 3423 | 547 | 659 | 744 | 254 | 283 | 275 | . | . | . | . | . | . |
| 0.85 | *** | 1209 | 1492 | 2615 | 391 | 445 | 551 | . | . | . | . | . | . | . | . | . |
| | *** | 1323 | 1785 | 2590 | 414 | 487 | 521 | . | . | . | . | . | . | . | . | . |
| 0.9 | *** | 868 | 1059 | 1666 | . | . | . | . | . | . | . | . | . | . | . | . |
| | *** | 946 | 1242 | 1637 | . | . | . | . | . | . | . | . | . | . | . | . |

## TABLE 2: ALPHA= 0.005 POWER= 0.9     EXPECTED ACCRUAL THRU MINIMUM FOLLOW-UP= 450

| | DEL=.05 | | | DEL=.10 | | | DEL=.15 | | | DEL=.20 | | | DEL=.25 | | |
|---|---|---|---|---|---|---|---|---|---|---|---|---|---|---|---|
| FACT= | 1.0 .75 | .50 .25 | .00 BIN | 1.0 .75 | .50 .25 | .00 BIN | 1.0 .75 | .50 .25 | .00 BIN | 1.0 75 | .50 .25 | .00 BIN | 1.0 .75 | .50 .25 | .00 BIN |

PCONT=***            REQUIRED NUMBER OF PATIENTS

| PCONT | 1.0/.75 | .50/.25 | .00/BIN | 1.0/.75 | .50/.25 | .00/BIN | 1.0/.75 | .50/.25 | .00/BIN | 1.0/75 | .50/.25 | .00/BIN | 1.0/.75 | .50/.25 | .00/BIN |
|---|---|---|---|---|---|---|---|---|---|---|---|---|---|---|---|
| 0.05 *** | 897 | 907 | 950 | 323 | 328 | 338 | 190 | 193 | 197 | 135 | 136 | 138 | 105 | 106 | 107 |
| *** | 900 | 920 | 1637 | 325 | 332 | 521 | 192 | 195 | 275 | 136 | 137 | 175 | 105 | 107 | 123 |
| 0.1 *** | 1638 | 1662 | 1833 | 517 | 532 | 566 | 281 | 288 | 300 | 187 | 191 | 197 | 139 | 141 | 144 |
| *** | 1646 | 1701 | 2590 | 523 | 545 | 744 | 284 | 293 | 368 | 189 | 194 | 224 | 140 | 143 | 152 |
| 0.15 *** | 2270 | 2313 | 2687 | 677 | 704 | 775 | 354 | 367 | 391 | 228 | 235 | 246 | 165 | 169 | 175 |
| *** | 2285 | 2385 | 3423 | 688 | 730 | 938 | 360 | 377 | 447 | 231 | 240 | 265 | 167 | 172 | 175 |
| 0.2 *** | 2764 | 2829 | 3467 | 802 | 843 | 961 | 411 | 431 | 469 | 261 | 271 | 288 | 185 | 191 | 199 |
| *** | 2786 | 2941 | 4137 | 819 | 884 | 1102 | 419 | 447 | 513 | 265 | 279 | 298 | 188 | 195 | 195 |
| 0.25 *** | 3113 | 3206 | 4148 | 892 | 950 | 1120 | 453 | 480 | 534 | 284 | 298 | 321 | 199 | 207 | 219 |
| *** | 3145 | 3363 | 4732 | 915 | 1006 | 1235 | 465 | 502 | 566 | 291 | 308 | 324 | 203 | 212 | 209 |
| 0.3 *** | 3325 | 3450 | 4717 | 952 | 1025 | 1248 | 482 | 516 | 585 | 300 | 318 | 346 | 209 | 219 | 233 |
| *** | 3367 | 3658 | 5208 | 981 | 1098 | 1340 | 496 | 543 | 606 | 308 | 330 | 343 | 213 | 225 | 218 |
| 0.35 *** | 3411 | 3575 | 5166 | 984 | 1073 | 1346 | 498 | 539 | 622 | 309 | 330 | 363 | 213 | 225 | 241 |
| *** | 3467 | 3839 | 5565 | 1020 | 1161 | 1414 | 516 | 572 | 632 | 318 | 344 | 354 | 219 | 232 | 223 |
| 0.4 *** | 3390 | 3597 | 5489 | 992 | 1095 | 1411 | 504 | 550 | 644 | 312 | 334 | 372 | 214 | 226 | 244 |
| *** | 3462 | 3918 | 5803 | 1034 | 1196 | 1459 | 524 | 587 | 645 | 322 | 351 | 358 | 220 | 234 | 223 |
| 0.45 *** | 3281 | 3536 | 5684 | 981 | 1096 | 1444 | 500 | 550 | 652 | 309 | 333 | 372 | 211 | 223 | 242 |
| *** | 3371 | 3911 | 5922 | 1028 | 1207 | 1474 | 522 | 590 | 645 | 320 | 350 | 354 | 217 | 232 | 218 |
| 0.5 *** | 3104 | 3409 | 5750 | 952 | 1076 | 1445 | 488 | 540 | 645 | 300 | 324 | 365 | 203 | 216 | 234 |
| *** | 3214 | 3831 | 5922 | 1003 | 1194 | 1459 | 510 | 581 | 632 | 311 | 342 | 343 | 209 | 224 | 209 |
| 0.55 *** | 2881 | 3231 | 5687 | 910 | 1039 | 1413 | 467 | 519 | 624 | 286 | 310 | 348 | 192 | 204 | 222 |
| *** | 3010 | 3690 | 5803 | 963 | 1159 | 1414 | 490 | 561 | 606 | 297 | 327 | 324 | 198 | 212 | 195 |
| 0.6 *** | 2629 | 3015 | 5493 | 855 | 984 | 1349 | 439 | 490 | 588 | 267 | 289 | 325 | 177 | 189 | 204 |
| *** | 2775 | 3497 | 5565 | 909 | 1104 | 1340 | 461 | 529 | 566 | 277 | 304 | 298 | 183 | 195 | 175 |
| 0.65 *** | 2363 | 2770 | 5171 | 789 | 914 | 1252 | 404 | 450 | 538 | 242 | 262 | 293 | 159 | 168 | 181 |
| *** | 2520 | 3257 | 5208 | 841 | 1027 | 1235 | 424 | 486 | 513 | 251 | 275 | 265 | 163 | 174 | 152 |
| 0.7 *** | 2091 | 2501 | 4721 | 712 | 828 | 1124 | 360 | 401 | 474 | 212 | 228 | 253 | 136 | 143 | 153 |
| *** | 2251 | 2973 | 4732 | 761 | 929 | 1102 | 378 | 431 | 447 | 219 | 239 | 224 | 139 | 147 | 123 |
| 0.75 *** | 1816 | 2207 | 4144 | 623 | 723 | 964 | 308 | 341 | 396 | 176 | 188 | 205 | . | . | . |
| *** | 1971 | 2643 | 4137 | 666 | 809 | 938 | 323 | 364 | 368 | 181 | 195 | 175 | . | . | . |
| 0.8 *** | 1533 | 1883 | 3442 | 519 | 599 | 773 | 246 | 269 | 304 | . | . | . | . | . | . |
| *** | 1673 | 2260 | 3423 | 554 | 664 | 744 | 256 | 284 | 275 | . | . | . | . | . | . |
| 0.85 *** | 1231 | 1516 | 2615 | 395 | 449 | 551 | . | . | . | . | . | . | . | . | . |
| *** | 1346 | 1808 | 2590 | 419 | 489 | 521 | . | . | . | . | . | . | . | . | . |
| 0.9 *** | 883 | 1074 | 1666 | . | . | . | . | . | . | . | . | . | . | . | . |
| *** | 962 | 1256 | 1637 | . | . | . | . | . | . | . | . | . | . | . | . |

# TABLE 2: ALPHA= 0.005 POWER= 0.9     EXPECTED ACCRUAL THRU MINIMUM FOLLOW-UP= 475

| PCONT | FACT= | DEL=.05 1.0 .75 | .50 .25 | .00 BIN | DEL=.10 1.0 .75 | .50 .25 | .00 BIN | DEL=.15 1.0 .75 | .50 .25 | .00 BIN | DEL=.20 1.0 75 | .50 .25 | .00 BIN | DEL=.25 1.0 .75 | .50 .25 | .00 BIN |
|---|---|---|---|---|---|---|---|---|---|---|---|---|---|---|---|---|
| | | | | | | REQUIRED NUMBER OF PATIENTS | | | | | | | | | | |
| 0.05 | *** | 897 | 908 | 951 | 324 | 329 | 338 | 191 | 193 | 197 | 135 | 137 | 138 | 105 | 106 | 107 |
| | *** | 901 | 921 | 1637 | 326 | 333 | 521 | 192 | 195 | 275 | 136 | 137 | 175 | 105 | 107 | 123 |
| 0.1 | *** | 1639 | 1665 | 1833 | 518 | 533 | 566 | 281 | 289 | 300 | 187 | 191 | 197 | 139 | 141 | 144 |
| | *** | 1648 | 1705 | 2590 | 525 | 546 | 744 | 285 | 294 | 368 | 189 | 194 | 224 | 140 | 143 | 152 |
| 0.15 | *** | 2273 | 2318 | 2687 | 679 | 707 | 775 | 355 | 368 | 391 | 229 | 236 | 246 | 165 | 169 | 175 |
| | *** | 2288 | 2392 | 3423 | 690 | 732 | 938 | 361 | 378 | 447 | 232 | 241 | 265 | 167 | 172 | 175 |
| 0.2 | *** | 2768 | 2836 | 3467 | 805 | 847 | 961 | 412 | 432 | 469 | 261 | 272 | 288 | 185 | 191 | 200 |
| | *** | 2791 | 2951 | 4137 | 822 | 887 | 1102 | 421 | 448 | 513 | 266 | 279 | 298 | 188 | 195 | 195 |
| 0.25 | *** | 3118 | 3216 | 4148 | 897 | 954 | 1120 | 455 | 482 | 534 | 285 | 299 | 321 | 200 | 208 | 219 |
| | *** | 3152 | 3378 | 4732 | 920 | 1010 | 1235 | 467 | 503 | 566 | 292 | 309 | 324 | 204 | 213 | 209 |
| 0.3 | *** | 3332 | 3463 | 4717 | 957 | 1031 | 1248 | 485 | 519 | 585 | 302 | 319 | 346 | 210 | 219 | 232 |
| | *** | 3377 | 3678 | 5208 | 987 | 1103 | 1340 | 499 | 545 | 606 | 309 | 331 | 343 | 214 | 225 | 218 |
| 0.35 | *** | 3421 | 3592 | 5166 | 990 | 1080 | 1346 | 502 | 542 | 622 | 311 | 331 | 363 | 215 | 226 | 241 |
| | *** | 3480 | 3863 | 5565 | 1027 | 1167 | 1414 | 519 | 574 | 632 | 320 | 345 | 354 | 220 | 232 | 223 |
| 0.4 | *** | 3402 | 3619 | 5489 | 1000 | 1103 | 1411 | 508 | 553 | 644 | 314 | 336 | 372 | 215 | 227 | 244 |
| | *** | 3478 | 3946 | 5803 | 1042 | 1203 | 1459 | 528 | 589 | 645 | 324 | 352 | 358 | 221 | 235 | 223 |
| 0.45 | *** | 3296 | 3562 | 5684 | 989 | 1105 | 1444 | 504 | 554 | 652 | 311 | 334 | 372 | 212 | 224 | 242 |
| | *** | 3391 | 3944 | 5922 | 1037 | 1214 | 1474 | 526 | 592 | 645 | 321 | 351 | 354 | 218 | 232 | 218 |
| 0.5 | *** | 3123 | 3438 | 5750 | 962 | 1086 | 1445 | 492 | 544 | 645 | 302 | 326 | 365 | 205 | 217 | 234 |
| | *** | 3238 | 3868 | 5922 | 1013 | 1202 | 1459 | 514 | 583 | 632 | 313 | 343 | 343 | 210 | 225 | 209 |
| 0.55 | *** | 2903 | 3263 | 5687 | 920 | 1049 | 1413 | 472 | 523 | 624 | 288 | 311 | 349 | 193 | 205 | 222 |
| | *** | 3037 | 3729 | 5803 | 973 | 1168 | 1414 | 494 | 563 | 606 | 299 | 327 | 324 | 199 | 213 | 195 |
| 0.6 | *** | 2655 | 3050 | 5493 | 865 | 994 | 1348 | 443 | 493 | 588 | 269 | 291 | 324 | 178 | 189 | 204 |
| | *** | 2805 | 3537 | 5565 | 919 | 1112 | 1340 | 465 | 531 | 566 | 279 | 305 | 298 | 184 | 196 | 175 |
| 0.65 | *** | 2391 | 2806 | 5171 | 799 | 924 | 1252 | 408 | 454 | 538 | 244 | 263 | 292 | 159 | 169 | 181 |
| | *** | 2551 | 3297 | 5208 | 851 | 1035 | 1235 | 428 | 488 | 513 | 253 | 276 | 265 | 164 | 174 | 152 |
| 0.7 | *** | 2120 | 2536 | 4721 | 721 | 836 | 1124 | 364 | 404 | 474 | 213 | 229 | 253 | 137 | 144 | 153 |
| | *** | 2283 | 3011 | 4732 | 770 | 936 | 1102 | 381 | 433 | 447 | 221 | 240 | 224 | 140 | 148 | 123 |
| 0.75 | *** | 1844 | 2240 | 4144 | 631 | 731 | 964 | 311 | 343 | 396 | 177 | 188 | 205 | . | . | . |
| | *** | 2001 | 2677 | 4137 | 674 | 815 | 938 | 325 | 366 | 368 | 182 | 196 | 175 | . | . | . |
| 0.8 | *** | 1559 | 1912 | 3442 | 526 | 604 | 773 | 248 | 270 | 304 | . | . | . | . | . | . |
| | *** | 1701 | 2289 | 3423 | 560 | 668 | 744 | 258 | 285 | 275 | . | . | . | . | . | . |
| 0.85 | *** | 1252 | 1539 | 2616 | 400 | 452 | 551 | . | . | . | . | . | . | . | . | . |
| | *** | 1368 | 1830 | 2590 | 423 | 492 | 521 | . | . | . | . | . | . | . | . | . |
| 0.9 | *** | 898 | 1089 | 1666 | . | . | . | . | . | . | . | . | . | . | . | . |
| | *** | 977 | 1269 | 1637 | . | . | . | . | . | . | . | . | . | . | . | . |

**TABLE 2: ALPHA= 0.005 POWER= 0.9    EXPECTED ACCRUAL THRU MINIMUM FOLLOW-UP= 500**

| | | DEL=.05 | | | DEL=.10 | | | DEL=.15 | | | DEL=.20 | | | DEL=.25 | | |
|---|---|---|---|---|---|---|---|---|---|---|---|---|---|---|---|---|---|
| FACT= | | 1.0 .75 | .50 .25 | .00 BIN | 1.0 .75 | .50 .25 | .00 BIN | 1.0 .75 | .50 .25 | .00 BIN | 1.0 75 | .50 .25 | .00 BIN | 1.0 .75 | .50 .25 | .00 BIN |
| PCONT=*** | | | | | | REQUIRED NUMBER OF PATIENTS | | | | | | | | | | |
| 0.05 | *** | 898 | 909 | 951 | 324 | 329 | 338 | 191 | 193 | 197 | 135 | 137 | 138 | 105 | 106 | 107 |
| | *** | 902 | 922 | 1637 | 326 | 333 | 521 | 192 | 195 | 275 | 136 | 138 | 175 | 106 | 107 | 123 |
| 0.1 | *** | 1641 | 1668 | 1833 | 520 | 534 | 566 | 282 | 289 | 300 | 188 | 192 | 197 | 139 | 141 | 144 |
| | *** | 1650 | 1708 | 2590 | 526 | 547 | 744 | 285 | 294 | 368 | 189 | 194 | 224 | 140 | 143 | 152 |
| 0.15 | *** | 2275 | 2323 | 2687 | 681 | 708 | 776 | 356 | 369 | 391 | 230 | 236 | 246 | 165 | 169 | 175 |
| | *** | 2291 | 2398 | 3423 | 693 | 733 | 938 | 362 | 378 | 447 | 233 | 241 | 265 | 167 | 172 | 175 |
| 0.2 | *** | 2771 | 2843 | 3467 | 808 | 850 | 961 | 414 | 434 | 469 | 262 | 273 | 288 | 186 | 192 | 199 |
| | *** | 2796 | 2961 | 4137 | 825 | 889 | 1102 | 423 | 448 | 513 | 267 | 279 | 298 | 188 | 195 | 195 |
| 0.25 | *** | 3124 | 3226 | 4148 | 901 | 958 | 1120 | 457 | 484 | 534 | 287 | 300 | 321 | 201 | 208 | 219 |
| | *** | 3158 | 3392 | 4732 | 924 | 1014 | 1235 | 469 | 505 | 566 | 293 | 309 | 324 | 204 | 213 | 209 |
| 0.3 | *** | 3339 | 3476 | 4717 | 963 | 1037 | 1248 | 487 | 521 | 585 | 303 | 320 | 346 | 210 | 220 | 233 |
| | *** | 3386 | 3696 | 5208 | 993 | 1108 | 1340 | 502 | 547 | 606 | 311 | 331 | 343 | 215 | 226 | 218 |
| 0.35 | *** | 3430 | 3609 | 5166 | 997 | 1087 | 1346 | 505 | 545 | 622 | 313 | 332 | 363 | 216 | 226 | 241 |
| | *** | 3492 | 3886 | 5565 | 1033 | 1173 | 1414 | 522 | 576 | 632 | 322 | 346 | 354 | 221 | 233 | 223 |
| 0.4 | *** | 3414 | 3639 | 5489 | 1008 | 1111 | 1411 | 512 | 557 | 644 | 316 | 338 | 372 | 216 | 228 | 244 |
| | *** | 3493 | 3974 | 5803 | 1050 | 1210 | 1459 | 531 | 591 | 645 | 326 | 352 | 358 | 222 | 235 | 223 |
| 0.45 | *** | 3312 | 3586 | 5684 | 998 | 1113 | 1444 | 508 | 557 | 652 | 313 | 336 | 372 | 213 | 225 | 242 |
| | *** | 3410 | 3975 | 5922 | 1045 | 1222 | 1474 | 529 | 595 | 645 | 323 | 352 | 354 | 218 | 233 | 218 |
| 0.5 | *** | 3142 | 3467 | 5750 | 971 | 1095 | 1445 | 496 | 547 | 645 | 304 | 328 | 364 | 206 | 218 | 234 |
| | *** | 3261 | 3903 | 5922 | 1022 | 1210 | 1459 | 518 | 586 | 632 | 315 | 343 | 343 | 211 | 225 | 209 |
| 0.55 | *** | 2925 | 3295 | 5687 | 929 | 1058 | 1413 | 476 | 527 | 624 | 290 | 313 | 348 | 194 | 206 | 222 |
| | *** | 3063 | 3766 | 5803 | 983 | 1176 | 1414 | 498 | 566 | 606 | 300 | 328 | 324 | 200 | 213 | 195 |
| 0.6 | *** | 2680 | 3083 | 5493 | 875 | 1003 | 1348 | 448 | 497 | 588 | 270 | 292 | 325 | 179 | 190 | 204 |
| | *** | 2834 | 3575 | 5565 | 928 | 1120 | 1340 | 469 | 533 | 566 | 280 | 306 | 298 | 184 | 196 | 175 |
| 0.65 | *** | 2418 | 2840 | 5171 | 808 | 933 | 1252 | 411 | 457 | 538 | 246 | 264 | 293 | 160 | 169 | 181 |
| | *** | 2582 | 3335 | 5208 | 860 | 1042 | 1235 | 431 | 490 | 513 | 254 | 277 | 265 | 164 | 174 | 152 |
| 0.7 | *** | 2148 | 2570 | 4721 | 730 | 844 | 1124 | 367 | 406 | 474 | 215 | 230 | 253 | 137 | 144 | 153 |
| | *** | 2314 | 3047 | 4732 | 778 | 943 | 1102 | 384 | 435 | 447 | 222 | 240 | 224 | 140 | 148 | 123 |
| 0.75 | *** | 1872 | 2272 | 4144 | 639 | 738 | 964 | 314 | 345 | 396 | 178 | 189 | 205 | . | . | . |
| | *** | 2030 | 2710 | 4137 | 681 | 820 | 938 | 328 | 367 | 368 | 183 | 197 | 175 | . | . | . |
| 0.8 | *** | 1583 | 1940 | 3442 | 532 | 610 | 773 | 250 | 272 | 304 | . | . | . | . | . | . |
| | *** | 1727 | 2317 | 3423 | 566 | 672 | 744 | 260 | 286 | 275 | . | . | . | . | . | . |
| 0.85 | *** | 1273 | 1560 | 2616 | 404 | 456 | 551 | . | . | . | . | . | . | . | . | . |
| | *** | 1390 | 1851 | 2590 | 427 | 494 | 521 | . | . | . | . | . | . | . | . | . |
| 0.9 | *** | 912 | 1103 | 1666 | . | . | . | . | . | . | . | . | . | . | . | . |
| | *** | 991 | 1281 | 1637 | . | . | . | . | . | . | . | . | . | . | . | . |

## TABLE 2: ALPHA= 0.005 POWER= 0.9   EXPECTED ACCRUAL THRU MINIMUM FOLLOW-UP= 550

|  | DEL=.02 | | | DEL=.05 | | | DEL=.10 | | | DEL=.15 | | | DEL=.20 | | |
|---|---|---|---|---|---|---|---|---|---|---|---|---|---|---|---|
| FACT= | 1.0 .75 | .50 .25 | .00 BIN | 1.0 .75 | .50 .25 | .00 BIN | 1.0 .75 | .50 .25 | .00 BIN | 1.0 75 | .50 .25 | .00 BIN | 1.0 .75 | .50 .25 | .00 BIN |
| PCONT=*** | REQUIRED NUMBER OF PATIENTS | | | | | | | | | | | | | | |
| 0.05 *** | 4230 | 4241 | 4482 | 899 | 910 | 950 | 324 | 330 | 338 | 191 | 193 | 197 | 135 | 137 | 138 |
| *** | 4234 | 4264 | 8378 | 903 | 924 | 1637 | 327 | 333 | 521 | 192 | 195 | 275 | 136 | 137 | 175 |
| 0.1 *** | 8799 | 8826 | 9848 | 1643 | 1673 | 1833 | 521 | 536 | 566 | 283 | 290 | 300 | 188 | 192 | 197 |
| *** | 8808 | 8880 | 14553 | 1654 | 1714 | 2590 | 528 | 548 | 744 | 286 | 294 | 368 | 190 | 194 | 224 |
| 0.15 *** | 12849 | 12897 | 15230 | 2280 | 2331 | 2687 | 685 | 712 | 775 | 358 | 371 | 391 | 231 | 237 | 246 |
| *** | 12865 | 12993 | 19984 | 2298 | 2410 | 3423 | 696 | 736 | 938 | 363 | 379 | 447 | 234 | 241 | 265 |
| 0.2 *** | 16070 | 16144 | 20236 | 2778 | 2857 | 3467 | 813 | 855 | 961 | 417 | 436 | 469 | 264 | 274 | 288 |
| *** | 16095 | 16292 | 24671 | 2806 | 2980 | 4137 | 831 | 894 | 1102 | 426 | 450 | 513 | 268 | 280 | 298 |
| 0.25 *** | 18375 | 18481 | 24674 | 3134 | 3245 | 4148 | 908 | 967 | 1119 | 461 | 487 | 534 | 289 | 302 | 321 |
| *** | 18411 | 18693 | 28614 | 3172 | 3419 | 4732 | 932 | 1020 | 1235 | 473 | 507 | 566 | 294 | 310 | 324 |
| 0.3 *** | 19778 | 19923 | 28436 | 3353 | 3502 | 4717 | 972 | 1047 | 1248 | 492 | 525 | 585 | 306 | 322 | 346 |
| *** | 19826 | 20214 | 31813 | 3404 | 3732 | 5208 | 1003 | 1116 | 1340 | 507 | 550 | 606 | 313 | 333 | 343 |
| 0.35 *** | 20341 | 20535 | 31462 | 3449 | 3641 | 5166 | 1009 | 1099 | 1346 | 511 | 550 | 622 | 316 | 334 | 363 |
| *** | 20406 | 20922 | 34268 | 3516 | 3930 | 5565 | 1046 | 1183 | 1414 | 528 | 579 | 632 | 324 | 347 | 354 |
| 0.4 *** | 20157 | 20409 | 33714 | 3438 | 3679 | 5489 | 1021 | 1126 | 1411 | 518 | 562 | 644 | 319 | 340 | 372 |
| *** | 20241 | 20914 | 35979 | 3524 | 4026 | 5803 | 1064 | 1222 | 1459 | 537 | 595 | 645 | 329 | 354 | 358 |
| 0.45 *** | 19331 | 19657 | 35172 | 3341 | 3634 | 5684 | 1013 | 1129 | 1444 | 516 | 563 | 652 | 316 | 338 | 372 |
| *** | 19440 | 20306 | 36946 | 3447 | 4035 | 5922 | 1061 | 1235 | 1474 | 536 | 599 | 645 | 327 | 353 | 354 |
| 0.5 *** | 17984 | 18400 | 35824 | 3179 | 3521 | 5750 | 987 | 1112 | 1445 | 503 | 553 | 645 | 308 | 330 | 365 |
| *** | 18122 | 19227 | 37169 | 3305 | 3968 | 5922 | 1039 | 1224 | 1459 | 525 | 590 | 632 | 318 | 345 | 343 |
| 0.55 *** | 16238 | 16768 | 35667 | 2969 | 3355 | 5687 | 947 | 1075 | 1413 | 483 | 533 | 624 | 294 | 316 | 349 |
| *** | 16415 | 17810 | 36648 | 3114 | 3836 | 5803 | 1001 | 1190 | 1414 | 505 | 570 | 606 | 303 | 330 | 324 |
| 0.6 *** | 14225 | 14902 | 34701 | 2728 | 3147 | 5493 | 893 | 1020 | 1348 | 455 | 503 | 588 | 274 | 294 | 324 |
| *** | 14451 | 16187 | 35384 | 2889 | 3646 | 5565 | 946 | 1134 | 1340 | 476 | 538 | 566 | 283 | 308 | 298 |
| 0.65 *** | 12082 | 12941 | 32928 | 2470 | 2905 | 5171 | 826 | 949 | 1252 | 418 | 462 | 538 | 248 | 267 | 292 |
| *** | 12372 | 14472 | 33375 | 2640 | 3405 | 5208 | 877 | 1056 | 1235 | 437 | 494 | 513 | 257 | 278 | 265 |
| 0.7 *** | 9953 | 11019 | 30354 | 2201 | 2633 | 4721 | 746 | 859 | 1124 | 373 | 411 | 474 | 217 | 232 | 253 |
| *** | 10322 | 12744 | 30622 | 2372 | 3114 | 4732 | 794 | 954 | 1102 | 390 | 437 | 447 | 224 | 241 | 224 |
| 0.75 *** | 7982 | 9226 | 26986 | 1923 | 2331 | 4144 | 653 | 750 | 964 | 319 | 349 | 396 | 180 | 191 | 205 |
| *** | 8431 | 11037 | 27126 | 2085 | 2771 | 4137 | 695 | 830 | 938 | 332 | 369 | 368 | 185 | 197 | 175 |
| 0.8 *** | 6269 | 7583 | 22830 | 1630 | 1991 | 3442 | 543 | 619 | 773 | 253 | 274 | 305 | . | . | . |
| *** | 6760 | 9342 | 22885 | 1776 | 2368 | 3423 | 576 | 679 | 744 | 263 | 288 | 275 | . | . | . |
| 0.85 *** | 4808 | 6042 | 17896 | 1311 | 1601 | 2615 | 412 | 462 | 551 | . | . | . | . | . | . |
| *** | 5280 | 7604 | 17900 | 1429 | 1889 | 2590 | 434 | 498 | 521 | . | . | . | . | . | . |
| 0.9 *** | 3490 | 4491 | 12193 | 938 | 1129 | 1666 | . | . | . | . | . | . | . | . | . |
| *** | 3879 | 5701 | 12172 | 1018 | 1303 | 1637 | . | . | . | . | . | . | . | . | . |
| 0.95 *** | 2081 | 2670 | 5728 | . | . | . | . | . | . | . | . | . | . | . | . |
| *** | 2314 | 3324 | 5699 | . | . | . | . | . | . | . | . | . | . | . | . |

TABLE 2: ALPHA= 0.005 POWER= 0.9     EXPECTED ACCRUAL THRU MINIMUM FOLLOW-UP= 600

| | | DEL=.02 | | | DEL=.05 | | | DEL=.10 | | | DEL=.15 | | | DEL=.20 | | |
|---|---|---|---|---|---|---|---|---|---|---|---|---|---|---|---|---|---|
| FACT= | | 1.0 .75 | .50 .25 | .00 BIN | 1.0 .75 | .50 .25 | .00 BIN | 1.0 .75 | .50 .25 | .00 BIN | 1.0 75 | .50 .25 | .00 BIN | 1.0 .75 | .50 .25 | .00 BIN |
| PCONT=*** | | REQUIRED NUMBER OF PATIENTS | | | | | | | | | | | | | | |
| 0.05 | *** | 4231 | 4243 | 4482 | 900 | 912 | 950 | 325 | 330 | 338 | 191 | 194 | 197 | 136 | 137 | 138 |
| | *** | 4235 | 4268 | 8378 | 905 | 925 | 1637 | 327 | 333 | 521 | 193 | 195 | 275 | 136 | 137 | 175 |
| 0.1 | *** | 8801 | 8831 | 9848 | 1646 | 1677 | 1833 | 523 | 538 | 566 | 284 | 290 | 300 | 189 | 192 | 197 |
| | *** | 8811 | 8890 | 14553 | 1657 | 1719 | 2590 | 530 | 549 | 744 | 287 | 295 | 368 | 190 | 194 | 224 |
| 0.15 | *** | 12854 | 12906 | 15230 | 2285 | 2340 | 2687 | 688 | 715 | 775 | 359 | 371 | 391 | 232 | 238 | 246 |
| | *** | 12871 | 13010 | 19984 | 2304 | 2421 | 3423 | 700 | 739 | 938 | 365 | 380 | 447 | 234 | 242 | 265 |
| 0.2 | *** | 16077 | 16157 | 20236 | 2786 | 2870 | 3467 | 818 | 861 | 961 | 419 | 438 | 469 | 265 | 274 | 287 |
| | *** | 16104 | 16318 | 24671 | 2815 | 2998 | 4137 | 836 | 898 | 1102 | 428 | 451 | 513 | 269 | 280 | 298 |
| 0.25 | *** | 18385 | 18500 | 24674 | 3145 | 3263 | 4148 | 915 | 974 | 1120 | 465 | 490 | 534 | 290 | 303 | 321 |
| | *** | 18424 | 18731 | 28614 | 3186 | 3444 | 4732 | 939 | 1027 | 1235 | 476 | 509 | 566 | 296 | 311 | 324 |
| 0.3 | *** | 19791 | 19950 | 28436 | 3367 | 3526 | 4717 | 981 | 1056 | 1248 | 496 | 529 | 585 | 308 | 323 | 346 |
| | *** | 19844 | 20267 | 31813 | 3423 | 3765 | 5208 | 1012 | 1124 | 1340 | 511 | 552 | 606 | 315 | 334 | 343 |
| 0.35 | *** | 20359 | 20570 | 31462 | 3467 | 3673 | 5166 | 1019 | 1110 | 1346 | 516 | 554 | 622 | 318 | 336 | 363 |
| | *** | 20429 | 20992 | 34268 | 3540 | 3971 | 5565 | 1057 | 1192 | 1414 | 532 | 582 | 632 | 326 | 348 | 354 |
| 0.4 | *** | 20179 | 20455 | 33714 | 3462 | 3718 | 5489 | 1034 | 1138 | 1411 | 524 | 566 | 644 | 322 | 342 | 372 |
| | *** | 20271 | 21005 | 35979 | 3554 | 4075 | 5803 | 1077 | 1233 | 1459 | 543 | 598 | 645 | 331 | 355 | 358 |
| 0.45 | *** | 19361 | 19716 | 35172 | 3371 | 3679 | 5683 | 1028 | 1143 | 1444 | 522 | 568 | 652 | 319 | 341 | 372 |
| | *** | 19479 | 20424 | 36946 | 3484 | 4090 | 5922 | 1076 | 1247 | 1474 | 542 | 602 | 645 | 329 | 355 | 354 |
| 0.5 | *** | 18021 | 18475 | 35824 | 3214 | 3572 | 5750 | 1003 | 1127 | 1445 | 510 | 558 | 645 | 311 | 332 | 364 |
| | *** | 18173 | 19375 | 37169 | 3347 | 4028 | 5922 | 1055 | 1237 | 1459 | 532 | 594 | 632 | 321 | 347 | 343 |
| 0.55 | *** | 16286 | 16865 | 35668 | 3010 | 3411 | 5686 | 963 | 1091 | 1413 | 490 | 538 | 624 | 296 | 317 | 349 |
| | *** | 16479 | 17992 | 36648 | 3162 | 3899 | 5803 | 1017 | 1203 | 1414 | 511 | 574 | 606 | 306 | 331 | 324 |
| 0.6 | *** | 14287 | 15023 | 34701 | 2775 | 3206 | 5493 | 909 | 1036 | 1348 | 461 | 508 | 588 | 277 | 296 | 325 |
| | *** | 14533 | 16404 | 35384 | 2941 | 3712 | 5565 | 962 | 1146 | 1340 | 482 | 541 | 566 | 286 | 309 | 298 |
| 0.65 | *** | 12161 | 13092 | 32928 | 2520 | 2965 | 5171 | 841 | 963 | 1252 | 424 | 466 | 538 | 251 | 268 | 292 |
| | *** | 12476 | 14718 | 33375 | 2694 | 3470 | 5208 | 893 | 1067 | 1235 | 443 | 497 | 513 | 259 | 279 | 265 |
| 0.7 | *** | 10055 | 11198 | 30354 | 2251 | 2692 | 4721 | 761 | 872 | 1124 | 378 | 415 | 474 | 220 | 233 | 253 |
| | *** | 10453 | 13008 | 30622 | 2426 | 3175 | 4732 | 808 | 965 | 1102 | 395 | 440 | 447 | 226 | 242 | 224 |
| 0.75 | *** | 8108 | 9422 | 26986 | 1971 | 2385 | 4144 | 665 | 761 | 964 | 323 | 352 | 396 | 181 | 191 | 205 |
| | *** | 8585 | 11303 | 27126 | 2137 | 2826 | 4137 | 707 | 838 | 938 | 336 | 371 | 368 | 186 | 198 | 175 |
| 0.8 | *** | 6410 | 7780 | 22830 | 1673 | 2038 | 3442 | 553 | 628 | 773 | 256 | 276 | 304 | . | . | . |
| | *** | 6924 | 9593 | 22885 | 1821 | 2414 | 3423 | 586 | 685 | 744 | 265 | 289 | 275 | . | . | . |
| 0.85 | *** | 4945 | 6221 | 17896 | 1346 | 1638 | 2615 | 419 | 467 | 551 | . | . | . | . | . | . |
| | *** | 5434 | 7822 | 17900 | 1466 | 1924 | 2590 | 440 | 502 | 521 | . | . | . | . | . | . |
| 0.9 | *** | 3604 | 4633 | 12193 | 962 | 1152 | 1666 | . | . | . | . | . | . | . | . | . |
| | *** | 4004 | 5866 | 12172 | 1042 | 1323 | 1637 | . | . | . | . | . | . | . | . | . |
| 0.95 | *** | 2150 | 2749 | 5728 | . | . | . | . | . | . | . | . | . | . | . | . |
| | *** | 2388 | 3409 | 5699 | . | . | . | . | . | . | . | . | . | . | . | . |

## TABLE 2: ALPHA= 0.005 POWER= 0.9  EXPECTED ACCRUAL THRU MINIMUM FOLLOW-UP= 650

| | | DEL=.02 | | | DEL=.05 | | | DEL=.10 | | | DEL=.15 | | | DEL=.20 | | |
|---|---|---|---|---|---|---|---|---|---|---|---|---|---|---|---|---|
| FACT= | | 1.0 .75 | .50 .25 | .00 BIN | 1.0 .75 | .50 .25 | .00 BIN | 1.0 .75 | .50 .25 | .00 BIN | 1.0 75 | .50 .25 | .00 BIN | 1.0 .75 | .50 .25 | .00 BIN |
| PCONT=*** | | REQUIRED NUMBER OF PATIENTS | | | | | | | | | | | | | | |
| 0.05 | *** | 4232 | 4246 | 4482 | 902 | 913 | 951 | 326 | 331 | 338 | 192 | 194 | 197 | 136 | 137 | 138 |
| | *** | 4236 | 4272 | 8378 | 906 | 926 | 1637 | 328 | 334 | 521 | 193 | 195 | 275 | 136 | 138 | 175 |
| 0.1 | *** | 8804 | 8836 | 9848 | 1649 | 1682 | 1833 | 525 | 539 | 566 | 285 | 291 | 300 | 189 | 192 | 197 |
| | *** | 8814 | 8900 | 14553 | 1661 | 1724 | 2590 | 531 | 550 | 744 | 288 | 295 | 368 | 191 | 194 | 224 |
| 0.15 | *** | 12858 | 12915 | 15230 | 2290 | 2348 | 2687 | 691 | 718 | 775 | 361 | 373 | 391 | 232 | 238 | 246 |
| | *** | 12877 | 13028 | 19984 | 2310 | 2431 | 3423 | 703 | 741 | 938 | 366 | 381 | 447 | 235 | 242 | 265 |
| 0.2 | *** | 16084 | 16171 | 20236 | 2793 | 2883 | 3467 | 823 | 866 | 961 | 422 | 440 | 469 | 266 | 275 | 288 |
| | *** | 16113 | 16345 | 24671 | 2824 | 3015 | 4137 | 841 | 902 | 1102 | 430 | 452 | 513 | 270 | 281 | 298 |
| 0.25 | *** | 18395 | 18520 | 24674 | 3155 | 3282 | 4149 | 922 | 981 | 1120 | 468 | 493 | 534 | 292 | 304 | 321 |
| | *** | 18436 | 18770 | 28614 | 3199 | 3468 | 4732 | 946 | 1032 | 1235 | 479 | 510 | 566 | 298 | 312 | 324 |
| 0.3 | *** | 19805 | 19976 | 28437 | 3382 | 3551 | 4717 | 990 | 1065 | 1248 | 500 | 532 | 585 | 310 | 325 | 346 |
| | *** | 19862 | 20320 | 31813 | 3441 | 3796 | 5208 | 1021 | 1131 | 1340 | 515 | 554 | 606 | 317 | 335 | 343 |
| 0.35 | *** | 20377 | 20605 | 31462 | 3486 | 3703 | 5166 | 1030 | 1120 | 1346 | 521 | 558 | 622 | 321 | 338 | 363 |
| | *** | 20453 | 21062 | 34268 | 3564 | 4009 | 5565 | 1068 | 1201 | 1414 | 537 | 584 | 632 | 329 | 349 | 354 |
| 0.4 | *** | 20203 | 20501 | 33714 | 3486 | 3755 | 5489 | 1046 | 1150 | 1411 | 529 | 571 | 644 | 325 | 344 | 372 |
| | *** | 20302 | 21097 | 35979 | 3583 | 4120 | 5803 | 1089 | 1243 | 1459 | 548 | 601 | 645 | 333 | 356 | 358 |
| 0.45 | *** | 19391 | 19775 | 35172 | 3400 | 3723 | 5684 | 1041 | 1156 | 1444 | 528 | 573 | 652 | 322 | 343 | 372 |
| | *** | 19519 | 20541 | 36946 | 3519 | 4141 | 5922 | 1089 | 1258 | 1474 | 548 | 606 | 645 | 332 | 356 | 354 |
| 0.5 | *** | 18059 | 18551 | 35825 | 3249 | 3621 | 5750 | 1017 | 1141 | 1445 | 517 | 563 | 645 | 314 | 335 | 365 |
| | *** | 18223 | 19521 | 37169 | 3389 | 4084 | 5922 | 1069 | 1248 | 1459 | 537 | 597 | 632 | 323 | 348 | 343 |
| 0.55 | *** | 16335 | 16961 | 35667 | 3050 | 3464 | 5687 | 978 | 1105 | 1413 | 496 | 543 | 624 | 300 | 320 | 348 |
| | *** | 16544 | 18171 | 36648 | 3208 | 3959 | 5803 | 1032 | 1215 | 1414 | 517 | 577 | 606 | 309 | 333 | 324 |
| 0.6 | *** | 14349 | 15144 | 34701 | 2819 | 3262 | 5493 | 924 | 1050 | 1349 | 467 | 512 | 588 | 279 | 298 | 324 |
| | *** | 14615 | 16615 | 35384 | 2991 | 3772 | 5565 | 977 | 1158 | 1340 | 487 | 544 | 566 | 288 | 310 | 298 |
| 0.65 | *** | 12240 | 13242 | 32928 | 2567 | 3022 | 5171 | 856 | 977 | 1252 | 430 | 471 | 538 | 253 | 270 | 292 |
| | *** | 12581 | 14956 | 33375 | 2746 | 3529 | 5208 | 907 | 1077 | 1235 | 448 | 500 | 513 | 261 | 280 | 265 |
| 0.7 | *** | 10156 | 11372 | 30354 | 2299 | 2746 | 4721 | 774 | 884 | 1124 | 383 | 418 | 474 | 222 | 235 | 253 |
| | *** | 10583 | 13260 | 30622 | 2477 | 3232 | 4732 | 821 | 974 | 1102 | 399 | 443 | 447 | 228 | 243 | 224 |
| 0.75 | *** | 8231 | 9611 | 26986 | 2016 | 2435 | 4144 | 678 | 771 | 964 | 327 | 354 | 396 | 183 | 192 | 205 |
| | *** | 8735 | 11556 | 27126 | 2185 | 2876 | 4137 | 718 | 846 | 938 | 340 | 373 | 368 | 188 | 198 | 175 |
| 0.8 | *** | 6545 | 7967 | 22830 | 1714 | 2082 | 3442 | 563 | 636 | 773 | 259 | 278 | 305 | . | . | . |
| | *** | 7080 | 9830 | 22885 | 1863 | 2456 | 3423 | 595 | 691 | 744 | 268 | 290 | 275 | . | . | . |
| 0.85 | *** | 5076 | 6389 | 17896 | 1379 | 1672 | 2615 | 425 | 472 | 551 | . | . | . | . | . | . |
| | *** | 5580 | 8026 | 17900 | 1500 | 1955 | 2590 | 446 | 505 | 521 | . | . | . | . | . | . |
| 0.9 | *** | 3711 | 4765 | 12193 | 984 | 1173 | 1666 | . | . | . | . | . | . | . | . | . |
| | *** | 4122 | 6019 | 12172 | 1064 | 1341 | 1637 | . | . | . | . | . | . | . | . | . |
| 0.95 | *** | 2215 | 2823 | 5728 | . | . | . | . | . | . | . | . | . | . | . | . |
| | *** | 2457 | 3486 | 5699 | . | . | . | . | . | . | . | . | . | . | . | . |

## TABLE 2: ALPHA= 0.005 POWER= 0.9    EXPECTED ACCRUAL THRU MINIMUM FOLLOW-UP= 700

| | DEL=.02 | | | DEL=.05 | | | DEL=.10 | | | DEL=.15 | | | DEL=.20 | | |
|---|---|---|---|---|---|---|---|---|---|---|---|---|---|---|---|
| FACT= | 1.0 .75 | .50 .25 | .00 BIN | 1.0 .75 | .50 .25 | .00 BIN | 1.0 .75 | .50 .25 | .00 BIN | 1.0 75 | .50 .25 | .00 BIN | 1.0 .75 | .50 .25 | .00 BIN |
| PCONT=*** | | | | REQUIRED NUMBER OF PATIENTS | | | | | | | | | | | |
| 0.05 *** | 4233 | 4247 | 4482 | 903 | 915 | 950 | 327 | 331 | 338 | 192 | 194 | 197 | 136 | 137 | 138 |
| *** | 4238 | 4276 | 8378 | 908 | 928 | 1637 | 328 | 334 | 521 | 193 | 195 | 275 | 136 | 138 | 175 |
| 0.1 *** | 8806 | 8841 | 9847 | 1652 | 1686 | 1833 | 527 | 541 | 566 | 285 | 292 | 300 | 190 | 193 | 197 |
| *** | 8818 | 8910 | 14553 | 1664 | 1729 | 2590 | 533 | 551 | 744 | 289 | 296 | 368 | 191 | 194 | 224 |
| 0.15 *** | 12862 | 12924 | 15230 | 2294 | 2356 | 2687 | 694 | 721 | 775 | 362 | 374 | 391 | 233 | 239 | 246 |
| *** | 12883 | 13045 | 19984 | 2316 | 2441 | 3423 | 706 | 743 | 938 | 368 | 381 | 447 | 236 | 242 | 265 |
| 0.2 *** | 16090 | 16184 | 20236 | 2801 | 2895 | 3467 | 828 | 870 | 961 | 424 | 442 | 469 | 268 | 276 | 288 |
| *** | 16122 | 16372 | 24671 | 2834 | 3030 | 4137 | 845 | 905 | 1102 | 432 | 453 | 513 | 271 | 282 | 298 |
| 0.25 *** | 18404 | 18539 | 24674 | 3165 | 3299 | 4148 | 928 | 986 | 1120 | 471 | 495 | 534 | 294 | 305 | 321 |
| *** | 18449 | 18809 | 28614 | 3212 | 3490 | 4732 | 953 | 1037 | 1235 | 481 | 512 | 566 | 299 | 312 | 324 |
| 0.3 *** | 19818 | 20003 | 28436 | 3395 | 3574 | 4717 | 998 | 1073 | 1248 | 504 | 534 | 585 | 312 | 326 | 346 |
| *** | 19879 | 20372 | 31813 | | 3824 | 5208 | 1029 | 1137 | 1340 | 518 | 556 | 606 | 318 | 335 | 343 |
| 0.35 *** | 20394 | 20640 | 31462 | 3504 | 3732 | 5166 | 1040 | 1130 | 1346 | 525 | 561 | 622 | 323 | 339 | 363 |
| *** | 20476 | 21132 | 34268 | 3586 | 4044 | 5565 | 1077 | 1208 | 1414 | 541 | 586 | 632 | 331 | 350 | 354 |
| 0.4 *** | 20225 | 20547 | 33714 | 3509 | 3790 | 5489 | 1057 | 1161 | 1411 | 534 | 575 | 644 | 327 | 345 | 372 |
| *** | 20333 | 21188 | 35979 | 3612 | 4162 | 5803 | 1101 | 1251 | 1459 | 552 | 604 | 645 | 335 | 357 | 358 |
| 0.45 *** | 19420 | 19834 | 35172 | 3429 | 3764 | 5684 | 1053 | 1168 | 1444 | 533 | 577 | 652 | 325 | 344 | 372 |
| *** | 19558 | 20657 | 36946 | 3553 | 4188 | 5922 | 1102 | 1267 | 1474 | 552 | 608 | 645 | 334 | 357 | 354 |
| 0.5 *** | 18097 | 18626 | 35824 | 3283 | 3667 | 5750 | 1031 | 1153 | 1445 | 522 | 568 | 645 | 317 | 336 | 365 |
| *** | 18274 | 19667 | 37169 | 3428 | 4136 | 5922 | 1083 | 1258 | 1459 | 542 | 600 | 632 | 326 | 349 | 343 |
| 0.55 *** | 16383 | 17057 | 35667 | 3089 | 3514 | 5686 | 992 | 1118 | 1413 | 502 | 547 | 624 | 302 | 321 | 348 |
| *** | 16608 | 18348 | 36648 | 3253 | 4013 | 5803 | 1045 | 1225 | 1414 | 522 | 579 | 606 | 311 | 334 | 324 |
| 0.6 *** | 14410 | 15265 | 34701 | 2862 | 3315 | 5493 | 938 | 1062 | 1349 | 473 | 516 | 588 | 282 | 299 | 324 |
| *** | 14697 | 16821 | 35384 | 3039 | 3828 | 5565 | 991 | 1167 | 1340 | 492 | 547 | 566 | 290 | 311 | 298 |
| 0.65 *** | 12319 | 13388 | 32928 | 2611 | 3075 | 5171 | 869 | 989 | 1252 | 435 | 474 | 538 | 256 | 271 | 292 |
| *** | 12685 | 15184 | 33375 | 2795 | 3584 | 5208 | 920 | 1087 | 1235 | 453 | 502 | 513 | 263 | 281 | 265 |
| 0.7 *** | 10256 | 11542 | 30354 | 2343 | 2798 | 4721 | 786 | 895 | 1124 | 387 | 422 | 474 | 223 | 236 | 253 |
| *** | 10710 | 13501 | 30622 | 2525 | 3283 | 4732 | 833 | 982 | 1102 | 403 | 444 | 447 | 229 | 243 | 224 |
| 0.75 *** | 8352 | 9792 | 26986 | 2058 | 2483 | 4144 | 688 | 780 | 964 | 330 | 357 | 396 | 184 | 193 | 205 |
| *** | 8881 | 11795 | 27126 | 2229 | 2922 | 4137 | 728 | 852 | 938 | 342 | 374 | 368 | 188 | 199 | 175 |
| 0.8 *** | 6676 | 8145 | 22830 | 1752 | 2123 | 3442 | 571 | 642 | 772 | 261 | 279 | 304 | . | . | . |
| *** | 7231 | 10054 | 22885 | 1903 | 2494 | 3423 | 603 | 695 | 744 | 270 | 291 | 275 | . | . | . |
| 0.85 *** | 5200 | 6550 | 17896 | 1410 | 1703 | 2616 | 431 | 476 | 551 | . | . | . | . | . | . |
| *** | 5720 | 8218 | 17900 | 1531 | 1983 | 2590 | 451 | 508 | 521 | . | . | . | . | . | . |
| 0.9 *** | 3813 | 4891 | 12192 | 1005 | 1192 | 1666 | . | . | . | . | . | . | . | . | . |
| *** | 4234 | 6162 | 12172 | 1084 | 1356 | 1637 | . | . | . | . | . | . | . | . | . |
| 0.95 *** | 2276 | 2892 | 5728 | . | . | . | . | . | . | . | . | . | . | . | . |
| *** | 2522 | 3558 | 5699 | . | . | . | . | . | . | . | . | . | . | . | . |

## TABLE 2: ALPHA= 0.005  POWER= 0.9  EXPECTED ACCRUAL THRU MINIMUM FOLLOW-UP= 750

| | | DEL=.02 | | | DEL=.05 | | | DEL=.10 | | | DEL=.15 | | | DEL=.20 | | |
|---|---|---|---|---|---|---|---|---|---|---|---|---|---|---|---|---|---|
| FACT= | | 1.0 | .50 | .00 | 1.0 | .50 | .00 | 1.0 | .50 | .00 | 1.0 | .50 | .00 | 1.0 | .50 | .00 |
| | | .75 | .25 | BIN | .75 | .25 | BIN | .75 | .25 | BIN | 75 | .25 | BIN | .75 | .25 | BIN |
| PCONT=*** | | | | | REQUIRED NUMBER OF PATIENTS | | | | | | | | | | | |
| 0.05 | *** | 4234 | 4249 | 4482 | 904 | 917 | 950 | 327 | 331 | 338 | 192 | 194 | 197 | 136 | 137 | 139 |
| | *** | 4239 | 4280 | 8378 | 909 | 929 | 1637 | 329 | 334 | 521 | 193 | 196 | 275 | 137 | 138 | 175 |
| 0.1 | *** | 8809 | 8845 | 9848 | 1654 | 1690 | 1833 | 528 | 542 | 566 | 286 | 292 | 300 | 190 | 193 | 197 |
| | *** | 8821 | 8920 | 14553 | 1668 | 1733 | 2590 | 534 | 552 | 744 | 289 | 295 | 368 | 191 | 195 | 224 |
| 0.15 | *** | 12867 | 12932 | 15230 | 2299 | 2364 | 2687 | 697 | 724 | 775 | 364 | 375 | 391 | 234 | 239 | 246 |
| | *** | 12889 | 13062 | 19984 | 2322 | 2449 | 3423 | 709 | 745 | 938 | 369 | 382 | 447 | 236 | 243 | 265 |
| 0.2 | *** | 16097 | 16198 | 20236 | 2808 | 2907 | 3467 | 832 | 874 | 961 | 426 | 443 | 469 | 269 | 277 | 288 |
| | *** | 16131 | 16399 | 24671 | 2843 | 3044 | 4137 | 850 | 908 | 1102 | 434 | 454 | 513 | 273 | 282 | 298 |
| 0.25 | *** | 18414 | 18559 | 24674 | 3175 | 3316 | 4148 | 934 | 992 | 1120 | 474 | 497 | 534 | 295 | 306 | 321 |
| | *** | 18462 | 18847 | 28614 | 3226 | 3510 | 4732 | 958 | 1041 | 1235 | 484 | 513 | 566 | 300 | 313 | 324 |
| 0.3 | *** | 19831 | 20029 | 28436 | 3409 | 3596 | 4717 | 1005 | 1079 | 1248 | 507 | 537 | 585 | 314 | 327 | 346 |
| | *** | 19897 | 20425 | 31813 | 3476 | 3851 | 5208 | 1037 | 1143 | 1340 | 521 | 558 | 606 | 320 | 336 | 343 |
| 0.35 | *** | 20412 | 20675 | 31462 | 3522 | 3760 | 5166 | 1049 | 1138 | 1345 | 529 | 564 | 622 | 325 | 341 | 363 |
| | *** | 20500 | 21202 | 34268 | 3609 | 4078 | 5565 | 1086 | 1215 | 1414 | 544 | 589 | 632 | 332 | 351 | 354 |
| 0.4 | *** | 20248 | 20593 | 33714 | 3532 | 3824 | 5489 | 1068 | 1171 | 1411 | 539 | 578 | 644 | 329 | 347 | 372 |
| | *** | 20363 | 21279 | 35979 | 3640 | 4201 | 5803 | 1111 | 1259 | 1459 | 557 | 606 | 645 | 337 | 358 | 358 |
| 0.45 | *** | 19450 | 19894 | 35172 | 3457 | 3803 | 5684 | 1065 | 1179 | 1444 | 538 | 580 | 652 | 327 | 346 | 372 |
| | *** | 19598 | 20772 | 36946 | 3586 | 4233 | 5922 | 1114 | 1276 | 1474 | 557 | 610 | 645 | 336 | 358 | 354 |
| 0.5 | *** | 18135 | 18702 | 35824 | 3316 | 3711 | 5750 | 1043 | 1165 | 1445 | 527 | 571 | 645 | 319 | 338 | 364 |
| | *** | 18324 | 19810 | 37169 | 3467 | 4184 | 5922 | 1095 | 1267 | 1459 | 547 | 603 | 632 | 327 | 350 | 343 |
| 0.55 | *** | 16431 | 17152 | 35667 | 3126 | 3562 | 5687 | 1005 | 1129 | 1413 | 507 | 551 | 624 | 304 | 323 | 349 |
| | *** | 16672 | 18520 | 36648 | 3295 | 4064 | 5803 | 1058 | 1234 | 1414 | 527 | 582 | 606 | 313 | 334 | 324 |
| 0.6 | *** | 14471 | 15384 | 34701 | 2902 | 3364 | 5494 | 950 | 1074 | 1348 | 477 | 520 | 588 | 284 | 301 | 325 |
| | *** | 14779 | 17020 | 35384 | 3084 | 3880 | 5565 | 1003 | 1176 | 1340 | 497 | 549 | 566 | 292 | 312 | 298 |
| 0.65 | *** | 12398 | 13533 | 32929 | 2654 | 3124 | 5171 | 881 | 999 | 1252 | 439 | 478 | 538 | 258 | 273 | 293 |
| | *** | 12788 | 15404 | 33375 | 2840 | 3635 | 5208 | 933 | 1095 | 1235 | 457 | 504 | 513 | 265 | 281 | 265 |
| 0.7 | *** | 10355 | 11707 | 30354 | 2386 | 2845 | 4721 | 798 | 904 | 1124 | 391 | 424 | 474 | 225 | 237 | 252 |
| | *** | 10836 | 13731 | 30622 | 2570 | 3331 | 4732 | 844 | 989 | 1102 | 406 | 446 | 447 | 230 | 244 | 224 |
| 0.75 | *** | 8470 | 9967 | 26986 | 2099 | 2526 | 4144 | 698 | 789 | 964 | 333 | 359 | 396 | 185 | 194 | 205 |
| | *** | 9022 | 12024 | 27126 | 2272 | 2965 | 4137 | 738 | 858 | 938 | 345 | 376 | 368 | 189 | 199 | 175 |
| 0.8 | *** | 6802 | 8316 | 22830 | 1787 | 2160 | 3442 | 579 | 649 | 773 | 264 | 281 | 304 | . | . | . |
| | *** | 7375 | 10266 | 22885 | 1940 | 2530 | 3423 | 610 | 700 | 744 | 272 | 292 | 275 | . | . | . |
| 0.85 | *** | 5320 | 6702 | 17896 | 1439 | 1732 | 2615 | 436 | 480 | 550 | . | . | . | . | . | . |
| | *** | 5853 | 8400 | 17900 | 1560 | 2008 | 2590 | 456 | 510 | 521 | . | . | . | . | . | . |
| 0.9 | *** | 3911 | 5009 | 12192 | 1024 | 1210 | 1666 | . | . | . | . | . | . | . | . | . |
| | *** | 4341 | 6297 | 12172 | 1103 | 1371 | 1637 | . | . | . | . | . | . | . | . | . |
| 0.95 | *** | 2333 | 2957 | 5728 | . | . | . | . | . | . | . | . | . | . | . | . |
| | *** | 2584 | 3624 | 5699 | . | . | . | . | . | . | . | . | . | . | . | . |

TABLE 2: ALPHA= 0.005 POWER= 0.9     EXPECTED ACCRUAL THRU MINIMUM FOLLOW-UP= 800

| | | DEL=.02 | | | DEL=.05 | | | DEL=.10 | | | DEL=.15 | | | DEL=.20 | | |
|---|---|---|---|---|---|---|---|---|---|---|---|---|---|---|---|---|---|
| FACT= | | 1.0 .75 | .50 .25 | .00 BIN | 1.0 .75 | .50 .25 | .00 BIN | 1.0 .75 | .50 .25 | .00 BIN | 1.0 75 | .50 .25 | .00 BIN | 1.0 .75 | .50 .25 | .00 BIN |
| PCONT=*** | | | | | | REQUIRED | NUMBER | OF PATIENTS | | | | | | | | | |
| 0.05 | *** | 4235 | 4252 | 4482 | 905 | 918 | 951 | 327 | 332 | 338 | 193 | 195 | 197 | 136 | 137 | 138 |
| | *** | 4241 | 4284 | 8378 | 910 | 930 | 1637 | 329 | 334 | 521 | 194 | 196 | 275 | 137 | 138 | 175 |
| 0.1 | *** | 8811 | 8851 | 9848 | 1657 | 1694 | 1833 | 530 | 543 | 566 | 287 | 293 | 300 | 190 | 193 | 197 |
| | *** | 8824 | 8930 | 14553 | 1671 | 1737 | 2590 | 536 | 553 | 744 | 290 | 296 | 368 | 192 | 195 | 224 |
| 0.15 | *** | 12871 | 12941 | 15230 | 2304 | 2371 | 2687 | 700 | 726 | 776 | 365 | 376 | 391 | 234 | 240 | 246 |
| | *** | 12894 | 13080 | 19984 | 2328 | 2458 | 3423 | 711 | 746 | 938 | 370 | 383 | 447 | 237 | 243 | 265 |
| 0.2 | *** | 16104 | 16211 | 20236 | 2815 | 2919 | 3467 | 836 | 877 | 961 | 428 | 444 | 469 | 270 | 277 | 288 |
| | *** | 16140 | 16426 | 24671 | 2852 | 3058 | 4137 | 854 | 911 | 1102 | 435 | 455 | 513 | 273 | 282 | 298 |
| 0.25 | *** | 18424 | 18578 | 24674 | 3186 | 3332 | 4148 | 939 | 997 | 1120 | 476 | 499 | 534 | 296 | 307 | 321 |
| | *** | 18475 | 18886 | 28614 | 3238 | 3530 | 4732 | 964 | 1045 | 1235 | 486 | 514 | 566 | 301 | 313 | 324 |
| 0.3 | *** | 19844 | 20055 | 28436 | 3423 | 3618 | 4717 | 1012 | 1086 | 1248 | 511 | 539 | 585 | 315 | 328 | 346 |
| | *** | 19915 | 20478 | 31813 | 3493 | 3877 | 5208 | 1044 | 1148 | 1340 | 524 | 559 | 606 | 321 | 337 | 343 |
| 0.35 | *** | 20429 | 20711 | 31462 | 3540 | 3787 | 5166 | 1057 | 1146 | 1346 | 533 | 567 | 622 | 327 | 342 | 363 |
| | *** | 20523 | 21272 | 34268 | 3631 | 4110 | 5565 | 1095 | 1221 | 1414 | 548 | 590 | 632 | 334 | 352 | 354 |
| 0.4 | *** | 20271 | 20639 | 33714 | 3554 | 3857 | 5489 | 1077 | 1180 | 1411 | 543 | 581 | 644 | 331 | 348 | 372 |
| | *** | 20394 | 21370 | 35979 | 3666 | 4238 | 5803 | 1121 | 1266 | 1459 | 560 | 608 | 645 | 339 | 359 | 358 |
| 0.45 | *** | 19479 | 19952 | 35172 | 3484 | 3841 | 5684 | 1076 | 1189 | 1444 | 542 | 584 | 652 | 329 | 347 | 372 |
| | *** | 19637 | 20887 | 36946 | 3618 | 4275 | 5922 | 1124 | 1284 | 1474 | 561 | 613 | 645 | 338 | 359 | 354 |
| 0.5 | *** | 18173 | 18777 | 35824 | 3348 | 3753 | 5750 | 1055 | 1175 | 1445 | 532 | 575 | 645 | 321 | 339 | 365 |
| | *** | 18374 | 19952 | 37169 | 3503 | 4230 | 5922 | 1106 | 1275 | 1459 | 551 | 605 | 632 | 329 | 351 | 343 |
| 0.55 | *** | 16479 | 17248 | 35668 | 3162 | 3607 | 5687 | 1017 | 1140 | 1413 | 511 | 555 | 624 | 306 | 324 | 349 |
| | *** | 16736 | 18689 | 36648 | 3335 | 4112 | 5803 | 1070 | 1242 | 1414 | 531 | 584 | 606 | 315 | 335 | 324 |
| 0.6 | *** | 14533 | 15503 | 34701 | 2942 | 3411 | 5493 | 963 | 1085 | 1349 | 482 | 523 | 588 | 286 | 302 | 325 |
| | *** | 14861 | 17215 | 35384 | 3126 | 3928 | 5565 | 1015 | 1184 | 1340 | 501 | 551 | 566 | 294 | 313 | 298 |
| 0.65 | *** | 12477 | 13674 | 32928 | 2694 | 3171 | 5171 | 893 | 1009 | 1252 | 443 | 481 | 538 | 259 | 274 | 293 |
| | *** | 12890 | 15617 | 33375 | 2884 | 3682 | 5208 | 944 | 1102 | 1235 | 460 | 506 | 513 | 266 | 282 | 265 |
| 0.7 | *** | 10454 | 11867 | 30354 | 2426 | 2890 | 4721 | 808 | 914 | 1124 | 395 | 427 | 474 | 226 | 238 | 253 |
| | *** | 10959 | 13953 | 30622 | 2613 | 3375 | 4732 | 854 | 996 | 1102 | 409 | 448 | 447 | 232 | 245 | 224 |
| 0.75 | *** | 8585 | 10136 | 26986 | 2137 | 2568 | 4144 | 707 | 796 | 964 | 336 | 361 | 396 | 186 | 195 | 205 |
| | *** | 9159 | 12241 | 27126 | 2312 | 3004 | 4137 | 746 | 863 | 938 | 348 | 377 | 368 | 190 | 199 | 175 |
| 0.8 | *** | 6924 | 8480 | 22830 | 1821 | 2196 | 3442 | 586 | 654 | 773 | 265 | 282 | 304 | . | . | . |
| | *** | 7515 | 10468 | 22885 | 1975 | 2562 | 3423 | 617 | 703 | 744 | 273 | 292 | 275 | . | . | . |
| 0.85 | *** | 5434 | 6847 | 17896 | 1466 | 1759 | 2616 | 440 | 484 | 551 | . | . | . | . | . | . |
| | *** | 5981 | 8572 | 17900 | 1588 | 2032 | 2590 | 460 | 513 | 521 | . | . | . | . | . | . |
| 0.9 | *** | 4004 | 5122 | 12193 | 1042 | 1227 | 1666 | . | . | . | . | . | . | . | . | . |
| | *** | 4442 | 6424 | 12172 | 1121 | 1384 | 1637 | . | . | . | . | . | . | . | . | . |
| 0.95 | *** | 2388 | 3018 | 5728 | . | . | . | . | . | . | . | . | . | . | . | . |
| | *** | 2642 | 3686 | 5699 | . | . | . | . | . | . | . | . | . | . | . | . |

TABLE 2: ALPHA= 0.005 POWER= 0.9      EXPECTED ACCRUAL THRU MINIMUM FOLLOW-UP= 850

| | | DEL=.02 | | | DEL=.05 | | | DEL=.10 | | | DEL=.15 | | | DEL=.20 | | |
|---|---|---|---|---|---|---|---|---|---|---|---|---|---|---|---|---|
| FACT= | | 1.0 .75 | .50 .25 | .00 BIN | 1.0 .75 | .50 .25 | .00 BIN | 1.0 .75 | .50 .25 | .00 BIN | 1.0 75 | .50 .25 | .00 BIN | 1.0 .75 | .50 .25 | .00 BIN |
| PCONT=*** | | | | | REQUIRED NUMBER OF PATIENTS | | | | | | | | | | | |
| 0.05 | *** | 4236 | 4254 | 4482 | 906 | 919 | 951 | 328 | 332 | 338 | 193 | 195 | 197 | 136 | 137 | 138 |
| | *** | 4242 | 4287 | 8378 | 911 | 930 | 1637 | 329 | 334 | 521 | 193 | 196 | 275 | 137 | 138 | 175 |
| 0.1 | *** | 8814 | 8856 | 9847 | 1660 | 1698 | 1833 | 531 | 544 | 566 | 288 | 293 | 300 | 191 | 193 | 197 |
| | *** | 8827 | 8939 | 14553 | 1674 | 1740 | 2590 | 537 | 553 | 744 | 290 | 296 | 368 | 192 | 195 | 224 |
| 0.15 | *** | 12875 | 12949 | 15230 | 2309 | 2378 | 2687 | 702 | 728 | 776 | 366 | 376 | 391 | 235 | 240 | 246 |
| | *** | 12900 | 13097 | 19984 | 2334 | 2466 | 3423 | 713 | 748 | 938 | 371 | 383 | 447 | 237 | 243 | 265 |
| 0.2 | *** | 16110 | 16224 | 20236 | 2822 | 2930 | 3467 | 839 | 881 | 961 | 429 | 445 | 469 | 271 | 278 | 288 |
| | *** | 16149 | 16453 | 24671 | 2861 | 3071 | 4137 | 858 | 913 | 1102 | 437 | 456 | 513 | 274 | 282 | 298 |
| 0.25 | *** | 18433 | 18597 | 24674 | 3196 | 3348 | 4148 | 945 | 1002 | 1120 | 478 | 501 | 534 | 297 | 308 | 321 |
| | *** | 18488 | 18924 | 28614 | 3251 | 3548 | 4732 | 969 | 1048 | 1235 | 488 | 515 | 566 | 302 | 314 | 324 |
| 0.3 | *** | 19857 | 20082 | 28436 | 3436 | 3638 | 4717 | 1019 | 1092 | 1248 | 513 | 542 | 585 | 316 | 329 | 346 |
| | *** | 19932 | 20530 | 31813 | 3510 | 3901 | 5208 | 1050 | 1152 | 1340 | 526 | 561 | 606 | 323 | 337 | 343 |
| 0.35 | *** | 20447 | 20746 | 31462 | 3557 | 3813 | 5166 | 1065 | 1154 | 1346 | 536 | 569 | 622 | 328 | 343 | 363 |
| | *** | 20547 | 21342 | 34268 | 3652 | 4139 | 5565 | 1103 | 1227 | 1414 | 551 | 592 | 632 | 335 | 352 | 354 |
| 0.4 | *** | 20295 | 20684 | 33714 | 3576 | 3888 | 5489 | 1087 | 1188 | 1411 | 547 | 584 | 644 | 333 | 349 | 372 |
| | *** | 20425 | 21459 | 35979 | 3692 | 4273 | 5803 | 1130 | 1273 | 1459 | 563 | 610 | 645 | 341 | 360 | 358 |
| 0.45 | *** | 19509 | 20011 | 35172 | 3510 | 3877 | 5684 | 1086 | 1198 | 1444 | 546 | 587 | 652 | 331 | 349 | 372 |
| | *** | 19677 | 21000 | 36946 | 3649 | 4314 | 5922 | 1134 | 1291 | 1474 | 565 | 615 | 645 | 339 | 359 | 354 |
| 0.5 | *** | 18210 | 18853 | 35824 | 3379 | 3793 | 5750 | 1066 | 1185 | 1445 | 536 | 578 | 645 | 323 | 340 | 365 |
| | *** | 18425 | 20091 | 37169 | 3538 | 4272 | 5922 | 1117 | 1283 | 1459 | 555 | 607 | 632 | 331 | 351 | 343 |
| 0.55 | *** | 16527 | 17343 | 35667 | 3197 | 3650 | 5687 | 1028 | 1150 | 1413 | 515 | 558 | 624 | 308 | 325 | 349 |
| | *** | 16800 | 18855 | 36648 | 3374 | 4157 | 5803 | 1081 | 1250 | 1414 | 535 | 586 | 606 | 316 | 336 | 324 |
| 0.6 | *** | 14595 | 15620 | 34701 | 2979 | 3455 | 5493 | 974 | 1094 | 1348 | 486 | 526 | 588 | 288 | 304 | 325 |
| | *** | 14942 | 17403 | 35384 | 3167 | 3973 | 5565 | 1026 | 1192 | 1340 | 504 | 553 | 566 | 295 | 313 | 298 |
| 0.65 | *** | 12555 | 13814 | 32928 | 2734 | 3215 | 5171 | 904 | 1019 | 1252 | 447 | 483 | 538 | 260 | 274 | 292 |
| | *** | 12992 | 15822 | 33375 | 2926 | 3726 | 5208 | 954 | 1109 | 1235 | 463 | 508 | 513 | 267 | 283 | 265 |
| 0.7 | *** | 10551 | 12023 | 30354 | 2465 | 2933 | 4721 | 818 | 922 | 1124 | 398 | 429 | 474 | 227 | 239 | 253 |
| | *** | 11080 | 14165 | 30622 | 2653 | 3416 | 4732 | 864 | 1002 | 1102 | 412 | 449 | 447 | 233 | 245 | 224 |
| 0.75 | *** | 8698 | 10298 | 26985 | 2173 | 2606 | 4145 | 715 | 803 | 964 | 339 | 362 | 396 | 187 | 195 | 205 |
| | *** | 9293 | 12450 | 27126 | 2349 | 3041 | 4137 | 754 | 868 | 938 | 350 | 378 | 368 | 191 | 200 | 175 |
| 0.8 | *** | 7042 | 8637 | 22830 | 1853 | 2229 | 3442 | 593 | 660 | 773 | 267 | 283 | 305 | . | . | . |
| | *** | 7650 | 10660 | 22885 | 2007 | 2592 | 3423 | 622 | 707 | 744 | 275 | 293 | 275 | . | . | . |
| 0.85 | *** | 5545 | 6987 | 17896 | 1491 | 1785 | 2616 | 445 | 487 | 550 | . | . | . | . | . | . |
| | *** | 6103 | 8736 | 17900 | 1614 | 2054 | 2590 | 464 | 514 | 521 | . | . | . | . | . | . |
| 0.9 | *** | 4094 | 5229 | 12192 | 1058 | 1242 | 1666 | . | . | . | . | . | . | . | . | . |
| | *** | 4540 | 6544 | 12172 | 1137 | 1396 | 1637 | . | . | . | . | . | . | . | . | . |
| 0.95 | *** | 2440 | 3076 | 5728 | . | . | . | . | . | . | . | . | . | . | . | . |
| | *** | 2696 | 3744 | 5699 | . | . | . | . | . | . | . | . | . | . | . | . |

TABLE 2: ALPHA= 0.005 POWER= 0.9    EXPECTED ACCRUAL THRU MINIMUM FOLLOW-UP= 900

| | DEL=.02 | | | DEL=.05 | | | DEL=.10 | | | DEL=.15 | | | DEL=.20 | | |
|---|---|---|---|---|---|---|---|---|---|---|---|---|---|---|---|
| FACT= | 1.0 .75 | .50 .25 | .00 BIN | 1.0 .75 | .50 .25 | .00 BIN | 1.0 .75 | .50 .25 | .00 BIN | 1.0 75 | .50 .25 | .00 BIN | 1.0 .75 | .50 .25 | .00 BIN |
| PCONT=*** | | | | REQUIRED NUMBER OF PATIENTS | | | | | | | | | | | |
| 0.05 *** | 4237 | 4256 | 4482 | 907 | 920 | 950 | 328 | 332 | 338 | 193 | 195 | 197 | 136 | 137 | 138 |
| *** | 4243 | 4291 | 8378 | 912 | 932 | 1637 | 330 | 335 | 521 | 194 | 196 | 275 | 137 | 138 | 175 |
| 0.1 *** | 8816 | 8861 | 9848 | 1662 | 1701 | 1833 | 532 | 545 | 566 | 288 | 293 | 300 | 191 | 194 | 197 |
| *** | 8831 | 8949 | 14553 | 1677 | 1744 | 2590 | 538 | 554 | 744 | 290 | 297 | 368 | 192 | 195 | 224 |
| 0.15 *** | 12880 | 12958 | 15230 | 2313 | 2385 | 2687 | 704 | 730 | 775 | 367 | 377 | 391 | 235 | 240 | 246 |
| *** | 12906 | 13114 | 19984 | 2340 | 2473 | 3423 | 716 | 749 | 938 | 371 | 383 | 447 | 237 | 243 | 265 |
| 0.2 *** | 16118 | 16238 | 20236 | 2829 | 2941 | 3467 | 843 | 884 | 962 | 431 | 447 | 469 | 271 | 279 | 288 |
| *** | 16157 | 16479 | 24671 | 2870 | 3083 | 4137 | 861 | 915 | 1102 | 438 | 457 | 513 | 275 | 282 | 298 |
| 0.25 *** | 18443 | 18616 | 24674 | 3206 | 3363 | 4148 | 950 | 1006 | 1119 | 480 | 502 | 534 | 298 | 308 | 321 |
| *** | 18501 | 18962 | 28614 | 3263 | 3565 | 4732 | 974 | 1051 | 1235 | 490 | 516 | 566 | 303 | 314 | 324 |
| 0.3 *** | 19871 | 20108 | 28436 | 3450 | 3658 | 4717 | 1025 | 1098 | 1248 | 516 | 543 | 585 | 318 | 330 | 346 |
| *** | 19950 | 20583 | 31813 | 3527 | 3924 | 5208 | 1056 | 1156 | 1340 | 528 | 561 | 606 | 324 | 338 | 343 |
| 0.35 *** | 20465 | 20781 | 31462 | 3575 | 3839 | 5166 | 1073 | 1161 | 1346 | 539 | 572 | 622 | 330 | 344 | 363 |
| *** | 20570 | 21411 | 34268 | 3673 | 4167 | 5565 | 1110 | 1232 | 1414 | 554 | 594 | 632 | 336 | 353 | 354 |
| 0.4 *** | 20317 | 20730 | 33714 | 3597 | 3918 | 5489 | 1095 | 1196 | 1411 | 550 | 587 | 644 | 334 | 351 | 372 |
| *** | 20455 | 21549 | 35979 | 3718 | 4305 | 5803 | 1139 | 1278 | 1459 | 567 | 612 | 645 | 342 | 360 | 358 |
| 0.45 *** | 19539 | 20071 | 35172 | 3536 | 3911 | 5684 | 1096 | 1207 | 1444 | 550 | 590 | 652 | 333 | 350 | 372 |
| *** | 19716 | 21113 | 36946 | 3680 | 4350 | 5922 | 1143 | 1297 | 1474 | 568 | 617 | 645 | 341 | 360 | 354 |
| 0.5 *** | 18248 | 18928 | 35825 | 3409 | 3831 | 5750 | 1076 | 1194 | 1445 | 540 | 581 | 645 | 324 | 342 | 365 |
| *** | 18475 | 20228 | 37169 | 3573 | 4312 | 5922 | 1127 | 1289 | 1459 | 558 | 609 | 632 | 333 | 352 | 343 |
| 0.55 *** | 16575 | 17437 | 35668 | 3231 | 3690 | 5687 | 1038 | 1160 | 1413 | 519 | 560 | 624 | 310 | 326 | 348 |
| *** | 16865 | 19017 | 36648 | 3411 | 4199 | 5803 | 1091 | 1256 | 1414 | 538 | 588 | 606 | 317 | 336 | 324 |
| 0.6 *** | 14656 | 15736 | 34701 | 3015 | 3497 | 5493 | 984 | 1104 | 1349 | 489 | 529 | 588 | 289 | 305 | 325 |
| *** | 15023 | 17587 | 35384 | 3206 | 4015 | 5565 | 1036 | 1198 | 1340 | 507 | 555 | 566 | 296 | 314 | 298 |
| 0.65 *** | 12633 | 13950 | 32928 | 2771 | 3257 | 5171 | 914 | 1027 | 1252 | 450 | 486 | 539 | 262 | 275 | 293 |
| *** | 13092 | 16021 | 33375 | 2966 | 3767 | 5208 | 963 | 1115 | 1235 | 467 | 509 | 513 | 269 | 283 | 265 |
| 0.7 *** | 10647 | 12174 | 30354 | 2501 | 2973 | 4721 | 828 | 929 | 1124 | 401 | 431 | 474 | 228 | 239 | 253 |
| *** | 11198 | 14369 | 30622 | 2692 | 3455 | 4732 | 872 | 1007 | 1102 | 415 | 450 | 447 | 234 | 245 | 224 |
| 0.75 *** | 8808 | 10455 | 26985 | 2207 | 2643 | 4144 | 723 | 809 | 964 | 341 | 364 | 396 | 188 | 195 | 205 |
| *** | 9423 | 12650 | 27126 | 2385 | 3075 | 4137 | 761 | 873 | 938 | 352 | 379 | 368 | 191 | 200 | 175 |
| 0.8 *** | 7156 | 8788 | 22830 | 1883 | 2260 | 3442 | 599 | 664 | 773 | 269 | 284 | 305 | . | . | . |
| *** | 7779 | 10844 | 22885 | 2039 | 2620 | 3423 | 628 | 710 | 744 | 276 | 294 | 275 | . | . | . |
| 0.85 *** | 5651 | 7120 | 17896 | 1515 | 1808 | 2615 | 449 | 489 | 551 | . | . | . | . | . | . |
| *** | 6221 | 8891 | 17900 | 1638 | 2074 | 2590 | 467 | 516 | 521 | . | . | . | . | . | . |
| 0.9 *** | 4179 | 5332 | 12192 | 1074 | 1256 | 1666 | . | . | . | . | . | . | . | . | . |
| *** | 4632 | 6658 | 12172 | 1152 | 1406 | 1637 | . | . | . | . | . | . | . | . | . |
| 0.95 *** | 2490 | 3131 | 5728 | . | . | . | . | . | . | . | . | . | . | . | . |
| *** | 2749 | 3798 | 5699 | . | . | . | . | . | . | . | . | . | . | . | . |

## TABLE 2: ALPHA= 0.005 POWER= 0.9   EXPECTED ACCRUAL THRU MINIMUM FOLLOW-UP= 950

| | | DEL=.02 | | | DEL=.05 | | | DEL=.10 | | | DEL=.15 | | | DEL=.20 | | |
|---|---|---|---|---|---|---|---|---|---|---|---|---|---|---|---|---|---|
| FACT= | | 1.0 .75 | .50 .25 | .00 BIN | 1.0 .75 | .50 .25 | .00 BIN | 1.0 .75 | .50 .25 | .00 BIN | 1.0 75 | .50 .25 | .00 BIN | 1.0 .75 | .50 .25 | .00 BIN |
| PCONT=*** | | REQUIRED NUMBER OF PATIENTS | | | | | | | | | | | | | | |
| 0.05 | *** | 4238 | 4258 | 4482 | 908 | 921 | 951 | 329 | 333 | 338 | 193 | 195 | 197 | 137 | 137 | 139 |
| | *** | 4245 | 4295 | 8378 | 913 | 932 | 1637 | 330 | 335 | 521 | 194 | 196 | 275 | 137 | 138 | 175 |
| 0.1 | *** | 8818 | 8865 | 9848 | 1665 | 1705 | 1833 | 533 | 546 | 566 | 289 | 293 | 300 | 191 | 194 | 197 |
| | *** | 8834 | 8959 | 14553 | 1680 | 1747 | 2590 | 539 | 555 | 744 | 291 | 296 | 368 | 192 | 195 | 224 |
| 0.15 | *** | 12884 | 12967 | 15230 | 2318 | 2392 | 2687 | 707 | 732 | 775 | 368 | 378 | 391 | 236 | 241 | 246 |
| | *** | 12912 | 13131 | 19984 | 2345 | 2480 | 3423 | 717 | 750 | 938 | 372 | 384 | 447 | 238 | 243 | 265 |
| 0.2 | *** | 16124 | 16251 | 20236 | 2837 | 2951 | 3467 | 847 | 887 | 961 | 432 | 448 | 469 | 272 | 279 | 287 |
| | *** | 16166 | 16506 | 24671 | 2879 | 3093 | 4137 | 864 | 918 | 1102 | 439 | 457 | 513 | 275 | 283 | 298 |
| 0.25 | *** | 18453 | 18635 | 24674 | 3216 | 3378 | 4148 | 954 | 1010 | 1120 | 482 | 503 | 534 | 299 | 309 | 321 |
| | *** | 18513 | 19000 | 28614 | 3275 | 3581 | 4732 | 978 | 1054 | 1235 | 492 | 517 | 566 | 304 | 314 | 324 |
| 0.3 | *** | 19884 | 20135 | 28437 | 3463 | 3678 | 4718 | 1031 | 1103 | 1248 | 519 | 545 | 585 | 319 | 331 | 346 |
| | *** | 19967 | 20635 | 31813 | 3542 | 3945 | 5208 | 1062 | 1160 | 1340 | 530 | 563 | 606 | 324 | 338 | 343 |
| 0.35 | *** | 20482 | 20816 | 31462 | 3592 | 3863 | 5166 | 1079 | 1167 | 1345 | 542 | 574 | 622 | 331 | 345 | 363 |
| | *** | 20593 | 21480 | 34268 | 3693 | 4193 | 5565 | 1117 | 1236 | 1414 | 557 | 595 | 632 | 337 | 353 | 354 |
| 0.4 | *** | 20340 | 20777 | 33714 | 3618 | 3946 | 5489 | 1103 | 1203 | 1411 | 553 | 589 | 644 | 336 | 352 | 372 |
| | *** | 20486 | 21638 | 35979 | 3743 | 4337 | 5803 | 1147 | 1283 | 1459 | 570 | 613 | 645 | 343 | 361 | 358 |
| 0.45 | *** | 19568 | 20129 | 35171 | 3561 | 3944 | 5684 | 1104 | 1214 | 1444 | 553 | 592 | 652 | 334 | 350 | 372 |
| | *** | 19755 | 21224 | 36946 | 3708 | 4385 | 5922 | 1152 | 1303 | 1474 | 571 | 618 | 645 | 342 | 361 | 354 |
| 0.5 | *** | 18286 | 19003 | 35825 | 3438 | 3868 | 5750 | 1085 | 1203 | 1445 | 543 | 583 | 645 | 326 | 343 | 365 |
| | *** | 18526 | 20364 | 37169 | 3605 | 4350 | 5922 | 1136 | 1296 | 1459 | 562 | 610 | 632 | 334 | 353 | 343 |
| 0.55 | *** | 16624 | 17531 | 35667 | 3263 | 3730 | 5687 | 1049 | 1168 | 1413 | 523 | 563 | 623 | 311 | 327 | 349 |
| | *** | 16929 | 19176 | 36648 | 3447 | 4238 | 5803 | 1100 | 1262 | 1414 | 542 | 590 | 606 | 319 | 337 | 324 |
| 0.6 | *** | 14717 | 15851 | 34701 | 3050 | 3537 | 5493 | 994 | 1112 | 1349 | 494 | 532 | 588 | 291 | 305 | 324 |
| | *** | 15104 | 17766 | 35384 | 3244 | 4055 | 5565 | 1046 | 1204 | 1340 | 511 | 557 | 566 | 298 | 314 | 298 |
| 0.65 | *** | 12711 | 14085 | 32928 | 2806 | 3297 | 5171 | 923 | 1035 | 1252 | 454 | 488 | 538 | 263 | 276 | 292 |
| | *** | 13192 | 16213 | 33375 | 3003 | 3806 | 5208 | 972 | 1121 | 1235 | 469 | 510 | 513 | 269 | 284 | 265 |
| 0.7 | *** | 10742 | 12322 | 30354 | 2536 | 3011 | 4721 | 836 | 937 | 1123 | 404 | 433 | 474 | 229 | 240 | 253 |
| | *** | 11315 | 14567 | 30622 | 2729 | 3491 | 4732 | 880 | 1012 | 1102 | 417 | 451 | 447 | 235 | 246 | 224 |
| 0.75 | *** | 8916 | 10608 | 26986 | 2240 | 2677 | 4144 | 730 | 815 | 964 | 343 | 366 | 396 | 188 | 196 | 205 |
| | *** | 9549 | 12841 | 27126 | 2419 | 3107 | 4137 | 768 | 876 | 938 | 353 | 380 | 368 | 192 | 200 | 175 |
| 0.8 | *** | 7268 | 8934 | 22830 | 1912 | 2289 | 3442 | 604 | 668 | 773 | 270 | 285 | 304 | . | . | . |
| | *** | 7905 | 11019 | 22885 | 2068 | 2646 | 3423 | 633 | 713 | 744 | 277 | 294 | 275 | . | . | . |
| 0.85 | *** | 5753 | 7248 | 17896 | 1539 | 1830 | 2616 | 452 | 492 | 551 | . | . | . | . | . | . |
| | *** | 6334 | 9039 | 17900 | 1661 | 2092 | 2590 | 470 | 518 | 521 | . | . | . | . | . | . |
| 0.9 | *** | 4262 | 5430 | 12193 | 1089 | 1269 | 1666 | . | . | . | . | . | . | . | . | . |
| | *** | 4722 | 6766 | 12172 | 1166 | 1416 | 1637 | . | . | . | . | . | . | . | . | . |
| 0.95 | *** | 2538 | 3183 | 5728 | . | . | . | . | . | . | . | . | . | . | . | . |
| | *** | 2799 | 3849 | 5699 | . | . | . | . | . | . | . | . | . | . | . | . |

## TABLE 2: ALPHA= 0.005 POWER= 0.9     EXPECTED ACCRUAL THRU MINIMUM FOLLOW-UP= 1000

| | | DEL=.02 | | | DEL=.05 | | | DEL=.10 | | | DEL=.15 | | | DEL=.20 | | |
|---|---|---|---|---|---|---|---|---|---|---|---|---|---|---|---|---|---|
| FACT= | | 1.0 / .75 | .50 / .25 | .00 / BIN | 1.0 / .75 | .50 / .25 | .00 / BIN | 1.0 / .75 | .50 / .25 | .00 / BIN | 1.0 / 75 | .50 / .25 | .00 / BIN | 1.0 / .75 | .50 / .25 | .00 / BIN |
| PCONT=*** | | | REQUIRED NUMBER OF PATIENTS | | | | | | | | | | | | | |
| 0.05 | *** | 4239 | 4260 | 4482 | 909 | 922 | 951 | 329 | 333 | 338 | 193 | 195 | 197 | 136 | 138 | 138 |
| | *** | 4246 | 4298 | 8378 | 914 | 933 | 1637 | 331 | 335 | 521 | 194 | 196 | 275 | 137 | 138 | 175 |
| 0.1 | *** | 8821 | 8870 | 9848 | 1668 | 1708 | 1833 | 535 | 546 | 566 | 289 | 294 | 300 | 191 | 194 | 197 |
| | *** | 8838 | 8968 | 14553 | 1683 | 1750 | 2590 | 540 | 555 | 744 | 291 | 297 | 368 | 193 | 195 | 224 |
| 0.15 | *** | 12889 | 12976 | 15230 | 2323 | 2398 | 2687 | 708 | 733 | 776 | 369 | 378 | 391 | 236 | 241 | 246 |
| | *** | 12918 | 13149 | 19984 | 2351 | 2486 | 3423 | 720 | 751 | 938 | 373 | 384 | 447 | 238 | 243 | 265 |
| 0.2 | *** | 16131 | 16265 | 20236 | 2843 | 2961 | 3467 | 850 | 890 | 961 | 434 | 448 | 470 | 273 | 279 | 288 |
| | *** | 16175 | 16532 | 24671 | 2887 | 3105 | 4137 | 867 | 919 | 1102 | 441 | 458 | 513 | 276 | 283 | 298 |
| 0.25 | *** | 18462 | 18655 | 24674 | 3226 | 3392 | 4148 | 958 | 1014 | 1120 | 484 | 505 | 534 | 300 | 310 | 321 |
| | *** | 18526 | 19038 | 28614 | 3287 | 3596 | 4732 | 983 | 1056 | 1235 | 493 | 518 | 566 | 305 | 315 | 324 |
| 0.3 | *** | 19897 | 20161 | 28436 | 3476 | 3696 | 4717 | 1036 | 1108 | 1248 | 521 | 547 | 585 | 320 | 331 | 346 |
| | *** | 19985 | 20687 | 31813 | 3558 | 3965 | 5208 | 1068 | 1164 | 1340 | 533 | 564 | 606 | 325 | 338 | 343 |
| 0.35 | *** | 20500 | 20851 | 31462 | 3609 | 3886 | 5166 | 1086 | 1173 | 1346 | 545 | 576 | 622 | 332 | 346 | 363 |
| | *** | 20617 | 21550 | 34268 | 3713 | 4218 | 5565 | 1124 | 1241 | 1414 | 559 | 596 | 632 | 338 | 354 | 354 |
| 0.4 | *** | 20363 | 20822 | 33714 | 3640 | 3974 | 5489 | 1111 | 1210 | 1411 | 556 | 591 | 644 | 338 | 352 | 372 |
| | *** | 20516 | 21726 | 35979 | 3767 | 4366 | 5803 | 1154 | 1288 | 1459 | 572 | 615 | 645 | 345 | 361 | 358 |
| 0.45 | *** | 19598 | 20189 | 35172 | 3586 | 3975 | 5685 | 1113 | 1222 | 1444 | 557 | 595 | 652 | 336 | 351 | 372 |
| | *** | 19795 | 21335 | 36946 | 3736 | 4418 | 5922 | 1160 | 1308 | 1474 | 574 | 620 | 645 | 343 | 361 | 354 |
| 0.5 | *** | 18324 | 19078 | 35825 | 3466 | 3903 | 5750 | 1095 | 1210 | 1445 | 547 | 586 | 645 | 328 | 343 | 365 |
| | *** | 18576 | 20497 | 37169 | 3637 | 4386 | 5922 | 1145 | 1301 | 1459 | 565 | 612 | 632 | 335 | 353 | 343 |
| 0.55 | *** | 16672 | 17625 | 35668 | 3295 | 3766 | 5686 | 1058 | 1176 | 1413 | 526 | 566 | 624 | 313 | 328 | 348 |
| | *** | 16993 | 19331 | 36648 | 3481 | 4275 | 5803 | 1110 | 1268 | 1414 | 545 | 591 | 606 | 320 | 338 | 324 |
| 0.6 | *** | 14779 | 15965 | 34701 | 3083 | 3575 | 5493 | 1003 | 1120 | 1348 | 496 | 533 | 588 | 292 | 306 | 325 |
| | *** | 15185 | 17940 | 35384 | 3280 | 4093 | 5565 | 1055 | 1210 | 1340 | 513 | 558 | 566 | 299 | 315 | 298 |
| 0.65 | *** | 12788 | 14216 | 32928 | 2840 | 3335 | 5171 | 933 | 1042 | 1252 | 456 | 490 | 538 | 265 | 277 | 293 |
| | *** | 13291 | 16400 | 33375 | 3040 | 3843 | 5208 | 981 | 1126 | 1235 | 472 | 511 | 513 | 270 | 285 | 265 |
| 0.7 | *** | 10836 | 12466 | 30355 | 2570 | 3047 | 4721 | 844 | 943 | 1124 | 406 | 435 | 475 | 230 | 240 | 253 |
| | *** | 11430 | 14756 | 30622 | 2764 | 3525 | 4732 | 888 | 1016 | 1102 | 420 | 453 | 447 | 235 | 246 | 224 |
| 0.75 | *** | 9022 | 10755 | 26986 | 2271 | 2710 | 4145 | 738 | 820 | 964 | 345 | 367 | 396 | 190 | 196 | 205 |
| | *** | 9672 | 13026 | 27126 | 2451 | 3137 | 4137 | 775 | 880 | 938 | 355 | 380 | 368 | 193 | 200 | 175 |
| 0.8 | *** | 7376 | 9075 | 22830 | 1940 | 2316 | 3442 | 610 | 672 | 773 | 271 | 286 | 305 | . | . | . |
| | *** | 8027 | 11188 | 22885 | 2096 | 2671 | 3423 | 638 | 715 | 744 | 278 | 295 | 275 | . | . | . |
| 0.85 | *** | 5853 | 7371 | 17896 | 1560 | 1851 | 2616 | 456 | 495 | 551 | . | . | . | . | . | . |
| | *** | 6444 | 9181 | 17900 | 1683 | 2110 | 2590 | 473 | 520 | 521 | . | . | . | . | . | . |
| 0.9 | *** | 4341 | 5524 | 12193 | 1103 | 1281 | 1666 | . | . | . | . | . | . | . | . | . |
| | *** | 4808 | 6869 | 12172 | 1180 | 1426 | 1637 | . | . | . | . | . | . | . | . | . |
| 0.95 | *** | 2583 | 3233 | 5728 | . | . | . | . | . | . | . | . | . | . | . | . |
| | *** | 2846 | 3897 | 5699 | . | . | . | . | . | . | . | . | . | . | . | . |

## TABLE 2: ALPHA= 0.005 POWER= 0.9 — EXPECTED ACCRUAL THRU MINIMUM FOLLOW-UP= 1100

|  |  | DEL=.02 | | | DEL=.05 | | | DEL=.10 | | | DEL=.15 | | | DEL=.20 | | |
|---|---|---|---|---|---|---|---|---|---|---|---|---|---|---|---|---|
| FACT= |  | 1.0 .75 | .50 .25 | .00 BIN | 1.0 .75 | .50 .25 | .00 BIN | 1.0 .75 | .50 .25 | .00 BIN | 1.0 75 | .50 .25 | .00 BIN | 1.0 .75 | .50 .25 | .00 BIN |
| PCONT=*** |  | REQUIRED NUMBER OF PATIENTS | | | | | | | | | | | | | | |
| 0.05 | *** | 4241 | 4264 | 4482 | 910 | 923 | 950 | 329 | 333 | 338 | 193 | 195 | 197 | 137 | 137 | 138 |
|  | *** | 4249 | 4305 | 8378 | 916 | 934 | 1637 | 331 | 335 | 521 | 195 | 196 | 275 | 137 | 138 | 175 |
| 0.1 | *** | 8826 | 8881 | 9848 | 1673 | 1714 | 1833 | 536 | 548 | 566 | 290 | 294 | 300 | 192 | 194 | 197 |
|  | *** | 8844 | 8987 | 14553 | 1688 | 1755 | 2590 | 541 | 555 | 744 | 291 | 297 | 368 | 193 | 195 | 224 |
| 0.15 | *** | 12897 | 12993 | 15229 | 2331 | 2410 | 2688 | 712 | 736 | 775 | 371 | 379 | 391 | 237 | 241 | 246 |
|  | *** | 12929 | 13183 | 19984 | 2361 | 2497 | 3423 | 723 | 753 | 938 | 375 | 384 | 447 | 239 | 243 | 265 |
| 0.2 | *** | 16144 | 16292 | 20236 | 2857 | 2980 | 3467 | 855 | 894 | 961 | 436 | 450 | 469 | 274 | 280 | 287 |
|  | *** | 16193 | 16585 | 24671 | 2903 | 3124 | 4137 | 873 | 922 | 1102 | 443 | 459 | 513 | 276 | 283 | 298 |
| 0.25 | *** | 18481 | 18693 | 24674 | 3244 | 3419 | 4148 | 967 | 1020 | 1119 | 488 | 507 | 534 | 302 | 310 | 321 |
|  | *** | 18551 | 19115 | 28614 | 3310 | 3624 | 4732 | 990 | 1061 | 1235 | 496 | 519 | 566 | 306 | 315 | 324 |
| 0.3 | *** | 19923 | 20214 | 28436 | 3502 | 3732 | 4717 | 1047 | 1116 | 1248 | 525 | 549 | 585 | 322 | 333 | 346 |
|  | *** | 20020 | 20791 | 31813 | 3589 | 4003 | 5208 | 1077 | 1170 | 1340 | 536 | 565 | 606 | 327 | 339 | 343 |
| 0.35 | *** | 20535 | 20921 | 31462 | 3641 | 3930 | 5166 | 1099 | 1183 | 1346 | 549 | 579 | 621 | 334 | 347 | 363 |
|  | *** | 20663 | 21686 | 34268 | 3751 | 4265 | 5565 | 1136 | 1248 | 1414 | 563 | 598 | 632 | 340 | 355 | 354 |
| 0.4 | *** | 20409 | 20914 | 33714 | 3679 | 4026 | 5489 | 1126 | 1222 | 1411 | 562 | 595 | 644 | 340 | 354 | 372 |
|  | *** | 20578 | 21900 | 35979 | 3813 | 4420 | 5803 | 1167 | 1297 | 1459 | 577 | 617 | 645 | 346 | 362 | 358 |
| 0.45 | *** | 19656 | 20306 | 35172 | 3634 | 4035 | 5684 | 1129 | 1236 | 1444 | 563 | 599 | 652 | 338 | 353 | 372 |
|  | *** | 19874 | 21550 | 36946 | 3790 | 4479 | 5922 | 1176 | 1318 | 1474 | 580 | 622 | 645 | 345 | 362 | 354 |
| 0.5 | *** | 18400 | 19227 | 35824 | 3521 | 3968 | 5750 | 1112 | 1225 | 1445 | 553 | 590 | 645 | 330 | 345 | 364 |
|  | *** | 18677 | 20756 | 37169 | 3697 | 4451 | 5922 | 1160 | 1312 | 1459 | 570 | 615 | 632 | 337 | 354 | 343 |
| 0.55 | *** | 16768 | 17810 | 35667 | 3355 | 3836 | 5686 | 1075 | 1190 | 1413 | 533 | 570 | 624 | 316 | 330 | 349 |
|  | *** | 17120 | 19632 | 36648 | 3546 | 4344 | 5803 | 1126 | 1279 | 1414 | 550 | 594 | 606 | 323 | 338 | 324 |
| 0.6 | *** | 14902 | 16187 | 34701 | 3147 | 3646 | 5493 | 1020 | 1134 | 1348 | 503 | 538 | 588 | 294 | 307 | 324 |
|  | *** | 15344 | 18274 | 35384 | 3348 | 4162 | 5565 | 1071 | 1220 | 1340 | 518 | 560 | 566 | 301 | 316 | 298 |
| 0.65 | *** | 12941 | 14472 | 32928 | 2905 | 3405 | 5171 | 949 | 1055 | 1252 | 462 | 494 | 538 | 267 | 278 | 292 |
|  | *** | 13485 | 16754 | 33375 | 3108 | 3910 | 5208 | 995 | 1135 | 1235 | 477 | 514 | 513 | 272 | 285 | 265 |
| 0.7 | *** | 11019 | 12743 | 30354 | 2633 | 3114 | 4721 | 859 | 954 | 1123 | 411 | 437 | 474 | 232 | 241 | 252 |
|  | *** | 11653 | 15117 | 30622 | 2830 | 3587 | 4732 | 901 | 1024 | 1102 | 423 | 455 | 447 | 236 | 247 | 224 |
| 0.75 | *** | 9226 | 11037 | 26986 | 2331 | 2771 | 4144 | 750 | 830 | 964 | 349 | 369 | 396 | 191 | 197 | 205 |
|  | *** | 9910 | 13374 | 27126 | 2512 | 3191 | 4137 | 786 | 886 | 938 | 358 | 382 | 368 | 194 | 201 | 175 |
| 0.8 | *** | 7583 | 9343 | 22830 | 1991 | 2368 | 3442 | 620 | 679 | 773 | 274 | 287 | 305 | . | . | . |
|  | *** | 8260 | 11505 | 22885 | 2148 | 2715 | 3423 | 646 | 720 | 744 | 280 | 296 | 275 | . | . | . |
| 0.85 | *** | 6043 | 7605 | 17896 | 1601 | 1889 | 2615 | 462 | 499 | 551 | . | . | . | . | . | . |
|  | *** | 6652 | 9448 | 17900 | 1723 | 2141 | 2590 | 478 | 522 | 521 | . | . | . | . | . | . |
| 0.9 | *** | 4492 | 5702 | 12193 | 1129 | 1303 | 1666 | . | . | . | . | . | . | . | . | . |
|  | *** | 4970 | 7061 | 12172 | 1204 | 1442 | 1637 | . | . | . | . | . | . | . | . | . |
| 0.95 | *** | 2670 | 3324 | 5728 | . | . | . | . | . | . | . | . | . | . | . | . |
|  | *** | 2936 | 3986 | 5699 | . | . | . | . | . | . | . | . | . | . | . | . |

TABLE 2: ALPHA= 0.005 POWER= 0.9    EXPECTED ACCRUAL THRU MINIMUM FOLLOW-UP= 1200

|  | | DEL=.02 | | | DEL=.05 | | | DEL=.10 | | | DEL=.15 | | | DEL=.20 | |
|---|---|---|---|---|---|---|---|---|---|---|---|---|---|---|---|
| FACT= | 1.0 .75 | .50 .25 | .00 BIN | 1.0 .75 | .50 .25 | .00 BIN | 1.0 .75 | .50 .25 | .00 BIN | 1.0 75 | .50 .25 | .00 BIN | 1.0 .75 | .50 .25 | .00 BIN |
| PCONT=*** | REQUIRED NUMBER OF PATIENTS | | | | | | | | | | | | | | |
| 0.05 *** | 4243 | 4268 | 4482 | 912 | 925 | 950 | 330 | 333 | 337 | 193 | 195 | 196 | 136 | 137 | 138 |
| *** | 4252 | 4310 | 8378 | 917 | 935 | 1637 | 331 | 335 | 521 | 194 | 196 | 275 | 137 | 138 | 175 |
| 0.1 *** | 8830 | 8890 | 9847 | 1677 | 1719 | 1833 | 538 | 549 | 565 | 290 | 295 | 300 | 192 | 194 | 196 |
| *** | 8851 | 9005 | 14553 | 1694 | 1760 | 2590 | 543 | 556 | 744 | 292 | 297 | 368 | 193 | 196 | 224 |
| 0.15 *** | 12906 | 13010 | 15229 | 2340 | 2421 | 2687 | 715 | 739 | 775 | 371 | 380 | 391 | 238 | 241 | 246 |
| *** | 12940 | 13216 | 19984 | 2371 | 2508 | 3423 | 726 | 754 | 938 | 376 | 385 | 447 | 239 | 244 | 265 |
| 0.2 *** | 16157 | 16318 | 20236 | 2870 | 2998 | 3467 | 861 | 898 | 961 | 438 | 451 | 469 | 274 | 280 | 287 |
| *** | 16211 | 16637 | 24671 | 2919 | 3141 | 4137 | 877 | 925 | 1102 | 444 | 460 | 513 | 277 | 283 | 298 |
| 0.25 *** | 18500 | 18731 | 24673 | 3263 | 3444 | 4148 | 973 | 1027 | 1120 | 490 | 508 | 534 | 303 | 311 | 321 |
| *** | 18577 | 19189 | 28614 | 3332 | 3650 | 4732 | 997 | 1065 | 1235 | 499 | 520 | 566 | 307 | 316 | 324 |
| 0.3 *** | 19950 | 20266 | 28436 | 3526 | 3765 | 4717 | 1056 | 1124 | 1248 | 529 | 552 | 585 | 323 | 334 | 346 |
| *** | 20055 | 20893 | 31813 | 3617 | 4036 | 5208 | 1086 | 1175 | 1340 | 539 | 567 | 606 | 328 | 340 | 343 |
| 0.35 *** | 20570 | 20992 | 31462 | 3673 | 3970 | 5166 | 1110 | 1192 | 1345 | 553 | 582 | 622 | 336 | 348 | 363 |
| *** | 20710 | 21820 | 34268 | 3787 | 4306 | 5565 | 1146 | 1255 | 1414 | 566 | 600 | 632 | 342 | 355 | 354 |
| 0.4 *** | 20455 | 21005 | 33714 | 3718 | 4075 | 5489 | 1138 | 1233 | 1411 | 566 | 598 | 644 | 342 | 355 | 372 |
| *** | 20638 | 22071 | 35979 | 3856 | 4468 | 5803 | 1180 | 1305 | 1459 | 581 | 619 | 645 | 348 | 363 | 358 |
| 0.45 *** | 19716 | 20424 | 35172 | 3679 | 4090 | 5684 | 1143 | 1247 | 1444 | 568 | 602 | 652 | 340 | 355 | 372 |
| *** | 19952 | 21761 | 36946 | 3841 | 4534 | 5922 | 1189 | 1327 | 1474 | 583 | 625 | 645 | 347 | 363 | 354 |
| 0.5 *** | 18475 | 19375 | 35824 | 3572 | 4028 | 5750 | 1126 | 1237 | 1444 | 558 | 594 | 645 | 332 | 346 | 364 |
| *** | 18777 | 21007 | 37169 | 3753 | 4510 | 5922 | 1175 | 1321 | 1459 | 574 | 616 | 632 | 339 | 355 | 343 |
| 0.55 *** | 16864 | 17992 | 35668 | 3411 | 3899 | 5686 | 1090 | 1203 | 1413 | 538 | 574 | 624 | 317 | 331 | 349 |
| *** | 17248 | 19920 | 36648 | 3607 | 4405 | 5803 | 1140 | 1288 | 1414 | 554 | 596 | 606 | 324 | 340 | 324 |
| 0.6 *** | 15023 | 16404 | 34701 | 3206 | 3712 | 5493 | 1036 | 1146 | 1348 | 508 | 541 | 588 | 296 | 309 | 325 |
| *** | 15502 | 18591 | 35384 | 3411 | 4224 | 5565 | 1084 | 1228 | 1340 | 523 | 562 | 566 | 302 | 316 | 298 |
| 0.65 *** | 13092 | 14718 | 32928 | 2965 | 3470 | 5171 | 963 | 1067 | 1252 | 466 | 496 | 538 | 268 | 279 | 292 |
| *** | 13674 | 17089 | 33375 | 3171 | 3970 | 5208 | 1009 | 1143 | 1235 | 481 | 515 | 513 | 274 | 286 | 265 |
| 0.7 *** | 11198 | 13008 | 30354 | 2692 | 3175 | 4721 | 872 | 964 | 1123 | 415 | 440 | 474 | 233 | 242 | 253 |
| *** | 11866 | 15454 | 30622 | 2890 | 3643 | 4732 | 913 | 1031 | 1102 | 427 | 456 | 447 | 238 | 247 | 224 |
| 0.75 *** | 9422 | 11303 | 26986 | 2385 | 2826 | 4144 | 761 | 838 | 964 | 352 | 371 | 396 | 191 | 198 | 205 |
| *** | 10135 | 13699 | 27126 | 2567 | 3240 | 4137 | 796 | 892 | 938 | 361 | 382 | 368 | 194 | 201 | 175 |
| 0.8 *** | 7780 | 9593 | 22830 | 2038 | 2413 | 3442 | 628 | 685 | 772 | 276 | 289 | 304 | . | . | . |
| *** | 8479 | 11800 | 22885 | 2195 | 2754 | 3423 | 654 | 724 | 744 | 282 | 296 | 275 | . | . | . |
| 0.85 *** | 6220 | 7822 | 17896 | 1638 | 1924 | 2615 | 467 | 502 | 550 | . | . | . | . | . | . |
| *** | 6847 | 9693 | 17900 | 1759 | 2169 | 2590 | 484 | 524 | 521 | . | . | . | . | . | . |
| 0.9 *** | 4633 | 5866 | 12193 | 1152 | 1323 | 1666 | . | . | . | . | . | . | . | . | . |
| *** | 5122 | 7236 | 12172 | 1226 | 1456 | 1637 | . | . | . | . | . | . | . | . | . |
| 0.95 *** | 2749 | 3409 | 5728 | . | . | . | . | . | . | . | . | . | . | . | . |
| *** | 3018 | 4065 | 5699 | . | . | . | . | . | . | . | . | . | . | . | . |

## TABLE 2: ALPHA= 0.005 POWER= 0.9   EXPECTED ACCRUAL THRU MINIMUM FOLLOW-UP= 1300

| | | DEL=.02 | | | DEL=.05 | | | DEL=.10 | | | DEL=.15 | | | DEL=.20 | | |
|---|---|---|---|---|---|---|---|---|---|---|---|---|---|---|---|---|---|
| FACT= | | 1.0 .75 | .50 .25 | .00 BIN | 1.0 .75 | .50 .25 | .00 BIN | 1.0 .75 | .50 .25 | .00 BIN | 1.0 75 | .50 .25 | .00 BIN | 1.0 .75 | .50 .25 | .00 BIN |
| PCONT=*** | | | | | REQUIRED NUMBER OF PATIENTS | | | | | | | | | | | |
| 0.05 | *** | 4245 | 4272 | 4483 | 913 | 926 | 951 | 331 | 334 | 338 | 194 | 195 | 197 | 136 | 137 | 138 |
| | *** | 4254 | 4317 | 8378 | 919 | 936 | 1637 | 332 | 336 | 521 | 195 | 196 | 275 | 137 | 138 | 175 |
| 0.1 | *** | 8836 | 8900 | 9847 | 1682 | 1724 | 1833 | 539 | 550 | 565 | 291 | 295 | 300 | 193 | 194 | 197 |
| | *** | 8857 | 9023 | 14553 | 1699 | 1764 | 2590 | 544 | 557 | 744 | 293 | 297 | 368 | 193 | 196 | 224 |
| 0.15 | *** | 12915 | 13028 | 15229 | 2348 | 2431 | 2687 | 718 | 741 | 775 | 373 | 381 | 391 | 238 | 242 | 246 |
| | *** | 12952 | 13250 | 19984 | 2381 | 2517 | 3423 | 729 | 757 | 938 | 376 | 385 | 447 | 240 | 244 | 265 |
| 0.2 | *** | 16171 | 16345 | 20236 | 2883 | 3014 | 3467 | 865 | 902 | 961 | 440 | 453 | 469 | 276 | 281 | 288 |
| | *** | 16229 | 16690 | 24671 | 2934 | 3157 | 4137 | 882 | 927 | 1102 | 446 | 460 | 513 | 278 | 284 | 298 |
| 0.25 | *** | 18520 | 18770 | 24674 | 3282 | 3468 | 4149 | 981 | 1032 | 1120 | 492 | 510 | 534 | 304 | 312 | 321 |
| | *** | 18603 | 19264 | 28614 | 3353 | 3673 | 4732 | 1004 | 1069 | 1235 | 500 | 521 | 566 | 308 | 316 | 324 |
| 0.3 | *** | 19976 | 20320 | 28437 | 3551 | 3796 | 4717 | 1064 | 1131 | 1248 | 531 | 554 | 585 | 325 | 335 | 346 |
| | *** | 20091 | 20994 | 31813 | 3645 | 4067 | 5208 | 1094 | 1180 | 1340 | 542 | 568 | 606 | 329 | 340 | 343 |
| 0.35 | *** | 20605 | 21063 | 31462 | 3703 | 4009 | 5166 | 1121 | 1201 | 1345 | 557 | 584 | 622 | 338 | 349 | 363 |
| | *** | 20758 | 21953 | 34268 | 3822 | 4344 | 5565 | 1156 | 1260 | 1414 | 570 | 601 | 632 | 344 | 356 | 354 |
| 0.4 | *** | 20501 | 21097 | 33714 | 3755 | 4119 | 5489 | 1150 | 1242 | 1411 | 571 | 601 | 644 | 344 | 356 | 372 |
| | *** | 20700 | 22239 | 35979 | 3898 | 4513 | 5803 | 1191 | 1311 | 1459 | 585 | 621 | 645 | 349 | 363 | 358 |
| 0.45 | *** | 19775 | 20541 | 35171 | 3723 | 4141 | 5684 | 1156 | 1258 | 1444 | 573 | 605 | 652 | 343 | 356 | 372 |
| | *** | 20031 | 21966 | 36946 | 3888 | 4583 | 5922 | 1201 | 1334 | 1474 | 588 | 627 | 645 | 349 | 363 | 354 |
| 0.5 | *** | 18551 | 19521 | 35825 | 3621 | 4084 | 5750 | 1141 | 1248 | 1445 | 563 | 597 | 645 | 335 | 348 | 365 |
| | *** | 18878 | 21249 | 37169 | 3806 | 4564 | 5922 | 1188 | 1329 | 1459 | 579 | 619 | 632 | 341 | 356 | 343 |
| 0.55 | *** | 16961 | 18172 | 35667 | 3464 | 3958 | 5687 | 1105 | 1215 | 1413 | 543 | 577 | 624 | 319 | 332 | 349 |
| | *** | 17374 | 20195 | 36648 | 3664 | 4461 | 5803 | 1153 | 1296 | 1414 | 558 | 598 | 606 | 326 | 341 | 324 |
| 0.6 | *** | 15144 | 16615 | 34701 | 3262 | 3773 | 5493 | 1050 | 1158 | 1349 | 512 | 544 | 588 | 298 | 310 | 324 |
| | *** | 15658 | 18892 | 35384 | 3469 | 4280 | 5565 | 1098 | 1236 | 1340 | 527 | 564 | 566 | 304 | 317 | 298 |
| 0.65 | *** | 13241 | 14956 | 32928 | 3022 | 3529 | 5172 | 977 | 1077 | 1252 | 471 | 500 | 538 | 270 | 280 | 292 |
| | *** | 13860 | 17405 | 33375 | 3230 | 4024 | 5208 | 1021 | 1150 | 1235 | 484 | 518 | 513 | 275 | 286 | 265 |
| 0.7 | *** | 11373 | 13260 | 30354 | 2746 | 3231 | 4722 | 884 | 973 | 1124 | 419 | 443 | 474 | 235 | 243 | 253 |
| | *** | 12074 | 15772 | 30622 | 2946 | 3693 | 4732 | 925 | 1037 | 1102 | 430 | 458 | 447 | 239 | 248 | 224 |
| 0.75 | *** | 9611 | 11555 | 26986 | 2435 | 2876 | 4145 | 771 | 846 | 964 | 354 | 373 | 396 | 193 | 198 | 205 |
| | *** | 10351 | 14003 | 27126 | 2619 | 3284 | 4137 | 805 | 896 | 938 | 363 | 383 | 368 | 195 | 201 | 175 |
| 0.8 | *** | 7967 | 9830 | 22831 | 2083 | 2456 | 3442 | 635 | 691 | 773 | 278 | 290 | 305 | . | . | . |
| | *** | 8688 | 12075 | 22885 | 2239 | 2789 | 3423 | 661 | 727 | 744 | 284 | 297 | 275 | . | . | . |
| 0.85 | *** | 6389 | 8026 | 17896 | 1672 | 1955 | 2616 | 472 | 505 | 551 | . | . | . | . | . | . |
| | *** | 7031 | 9922 | 17900 | 1792 | 2193 | 2590 | 487 | 526 | 521 | . | . | . | . | . | . |
| 0.9 | *** | 4765 | 6019 | 12192 | 1173 | 1341 | 1667 | . | . | . | . | . | . | . | . | . |
| | *** | 5264 | 7398 | 12172 | 1246 | 1469 | 1637 | . | . | . | . | . | . | . | . | . |
| 0.95 | *** | 2823 | 3487 | 5728 | . | . | . | . | . | . | . | . | . | . | . | . |
| | *** | 3095 | 4137 | 5699 | . | . | . | . | . | . | . | . | . | . | . | . |

TABLE 2: ALPHA= 0.005 POWER= 0.9    EXPECTED ACCRUAL THRU MINIMUM FOLLOW-UP= 1400

| | | DEL=.02 | | | DEL=.05 | | | DEL=.10 | | | DEL=.15 | | | DEL=.20 | | |
|---|---|---|---|---|---|---|---|---|---|---|---|---|---|---|---|---|---|
| FACT= | | 1.0 .75 | .50 .25 | .00 BIN | 1.0 .75 | .50 .25 | .00 BIN | 1.0 .75 | .50 .25 | .00 BIN | 1.0 75 | .50 .25 | .00 BIN | 1.0 .75 | .50 .25 | .00 BIN |
| PCONT=*** | | | | | REQUIRED NUMBER OF PATIENTS | | | | | | | | | | | |
| 0.05 | *** | 4247 | 4276 | 4483 | 915 | 927 | 950 | 331 | 334 | 338 | 194 | 195 | 197 | 137 | 137 | 138 |
| | *** | 4257 | 4322 | 8378 | 920 | 937 | 1637 | 332 | 336 | 521 | 195 | 196 | 275 | 137 | 138 | 175 |
| 0.1 | *** | 8841 | 8910 | 9847 | 1686 | 1729 | 1833 | 541 | 551 | 566 | 291 | 296 | 300 | 192 | 194 | 197 |
| | *** | 8864 | 9040 | 14553 | 1704 | 1767 | 2590 | 545 | 558 | 744 | 293 | 297 | 368 | 193 | 196 | 224 |
| 0.15 | *** | 12924 | 13045 | 15229 | 2356 | 2440 | 2687 | 721 | 743 | 775 | 374 | 381 | 391 | 239 | 242 | 246 |
| | *** | 12964 | 13282 | 19984 | 2390 | 2525 | 3423 | 731 | 758 | 938 | 377 | 386 | 447 | 241 | 244 | 265 |
| 0.2 | *** | 16184 | 16372 | 20236 | 2895 | 3030 | 3467 | 870 | 905 | 962 | 442 | 453 | 469 | 276 | 282 | 288 |
| | *** | 16247 | 16740 | 24671 | 2948 | 3172 | 4137 | 885 | 929 | 1102 | 447 | 461 | 513 | 278 | 284 | 298 |
| 0.25 | *** | 18539 | 18809 | 24674 | 3299 | 3489 | 4148 | 986 | 1037 | 1120 | 495 | 512 | 534 | 305 | 312 | 321 |
| | *** | 18629 | 19337 | 28614 | 3373 | 3694 | 4732 | 1009 | 1072 | 1235 | 503 | 522 | 566 | 309 | 317 | 324 |
| 0.3 | *** | 20002 | 20373 | 28437 | 3573 | 3825 | 4717 | 1073 | 1137 | 1249 | 535 | 556 | 585 | 326 | 335 | 346 |
| | *** | 20126 | 21094 | 31813 | 3671 | 4095 | 5208 | 1101 | 1184 | 1340 | 544 | 570 | 606 | 331 | 340 | 343 |
| 0.35 | *** | 20640 | 21132 | 31461 | 3732 | 4044 | 5166 | 1130 | 1208 | 1346 | 561 | 586 | 622 | 339 | 350 | 363 |
| | *** | 20805 | 22083 | 34268 | 3854 | 4378 | 5565 | 1165 | 1265 | 1414 | 573 | 603 | 632 | 345 | 356 | 354 |
| 0.4 | *** | 20547 | 21188 | 33714 | 3790 | 4161 | 5489 | 1161 | 1251 | 1411 | 575 | 604 | 644 | 346 | 357 | 372 |
| | *** | 20761 | 22403 | 35979 | 3937 | 4553 | 5803 | 1200 | 1318 | 1459 | 588 | 622 | 645 | 351 | 364 | 358 |
| 0.45 | *** | 19834 | 20657 | 35171 | 3763 | 4189 | 5684 | 1168 | 1267 | 1444 | 577 | 608 | 652 | 344 | 357 | 372 |
| | *** | 20110 | 22165 | 36946 | 3933 | 4629 | 5922 | 1212 | 1340 | 1474 | 591 | 628 | 645 | 350 | 364 | 354 |
| 0.5 | *** | 18626 | 19666 | 35824 | 3667 | 4136 | 5750 | 1153 | 1258 | 1445 | 568 | 600 | 645 | 336 | 349 | 365 |
| | *** | 18978 | 21483 | 37169 | 3855 | 4613 | 5922 | 1200 | 1335 | 1459 | 583 | 620 | 632 | 342 | 356 | 343 |
| 0.55 | *** | 17056 | 18348 | 35668 | 3514 | 4014 | 5687 | 1117 | 1225 | 1413 | 547 | 579 | 624 | 321 | 333 | 348 |
| | *** | 17500 | 20459 | 36648 | 3716 | 4512 | 5803 | 1165 | 1303 | 1414 | 563 | 599 | 606 | 327 | 340 | 324 |
| 0.6 | *** | 15264 | 16821 | 34701 | 3314 | 3828 | 5493 | 1062 | 1167 | 1348 | 516 | 547 | 588 | 299 | 311 | 325 |
| | *** | 15813 | 19179 | 35384 | 3524 | 4331 | 5565 | 1109 | 1242 | 1340 | 530 | 566 | 566 | 305 | 318 | 298 |
| 0.65 | *** | 13388 | 15184 | 32928 | 3075 | 3584 | 5171 | 989 | 1087 | 1252 | 474 | 501 | 538 | 271 | 281 | 292 |
| | *** | 14040 | 17705 | 33375 | 3284 | 4073 | 5208 | 1032 | 1156 | 1235 | 487 | 519 | 513 | 276 | 286 | 265 |
| 0.7 | *** | 11542 | 13500 | 30355 | 2797 | 3283 | 4721 | 895 | 982 | 1123 | 422 | 444 | 474 | 236 | 243 | 253 |
| | *** | 12274 | 16072 | 30622 | 2999 | 3739 | 4732 | 934 | 1042 | 1102 | 432 | 458 | 447 | 240 | 248 | 224 |
| 0.75 | *** | 9792 | 11795 | 26986 | 2482 | 2922 | 4144 | 780 | 852 | 963 | 357 | 374 | 396 | 193 | 199 | 205 |
| | *** | 10558 | 14289 | 27126 | 2666 | 3323 | 4137 | 813 | 900 | 938 | 365 | 385 | 368 | 196 | 201 | 175 |
| 0.8 | *** | 8145 | 10054 | 22830 | 2123 | 2495 | 3442 | 642 | 696 | 773 | 279 | 290 | 304 | . | . | . |
| | *** | 8886 | 12331 | 22885 | 2279 | 2821 | 3423 | 667 | 730 | 744 | 285 | 297 | 275 | . | . | . |
| 0.85 | *** | 6549 | 8218 | 17896 | 1704 | 1983 | 2615 | 476 | 508 | 550 | . | . | . | . | . | . |
| | *** | 7206 | 10133 | 17900 | 1823 | 2215 | 2590 | 491 | 528 | 521 | . | . | . | . | . | . |
| 0.9 | *** | 4890 | 6163 | 12192 | 1193 | 1356 | 1666 | . | . | . | . | . | . | . | . | . |
| | *** | 5398 | 7548 | 12172 | 1264 | 1480 | 1637 | . | . | . | . | . | . | . | . | . |
| 0.95 | *** | 2892 | 3558 | 5729 | . | . | . | . | . | . | . | . | . | . | . | . |
| | *** | 3166 | 4203 | 5699 | . | . | . | . | . | . | . | . | . | . | . | . |

TABLE 2: ALPHA= 0.005 POWER= 0.9      EXPECTED ACCRUAL THRU MINIMUM FOLLOW-UP= 1500

| | | DEL=.02 | | | DEL=.05 | | | DEL=.10 | | | DEL=.15 | | | DEL=.20 | | |
|---|---|---|---|---|---|---|---|---|---|---|---|---|---|---|---|---|
| FACT= | | 1.0 .75 | .50 .25 | .00 BIN | 1.0 .75 | .50 .25 | .00 BIN | 1.0 .75 | .50 .25 | .00 BIN | 1.0 75 | .50 .25 | .00 BIN | 1.0 .75 | .50 .25 | .00 BIN |
| PCONT=*** | | | | | | REQUIRED NUMBER OF PATIENTS | | | | | | | | | | |
| 0.05 | *** | 4250 | 4280 | 4482 | 917 | 929 | 950 | 331 | 334 | 337 | 194 | 196 | 197 | 137 | 138 | 139 |
| | *** | 4260 | 4327 | 8378 | 922 | 937 | 1637 | 333 | 335 | 521 | 195 | 196 | 275 | 138 | 138 | 175 |
| 0.1 | *** | 8845 | 8919 | 9847 | 1690 | 1733 | 1833 | 542 | 552 | 566 | 292 | 295 | 300 | 193 | 195 | 197 |
| | *** | 8870 | 9058 | 14553 | 1708 | 1771 | 2590 | 547 | 559 | 744 | 293 | 298 | 368 | 194 | 196 | 224 |
| 0.15 | *** | 12932 | 13062 | 15230 | 2363 | 2450 | 2687 | 724 | 744 | 775 | 375 | 382 | 391 | 239 | 243 | 247 |
| | *** | 12976 | 13314 | 19984 | 2398 | 2533 | 3423 | 733 | 758 | 938 | 378 | 386 | 447 | 241 | 245 | 265 |
| 0.2 | *** | 16198 | 16399 | 20236 | 2907 | 3044 | 3467 | 874 | 908 | 961 | 443 | 455 | 470 | 277 | 282 | 288 |
| | *** | 16265 | 16792 | 24671 | 2962 | 3185 | 4137 | 890 | 932 | 1102 | 448 | 461 | 513 | 279 | 285 | 298 |
| 0.25 | *** | 18559 | 18847 | 24674 | 3316 | 3510 | 4148 | 992 | 1040 | 1119 | 497 | 513 | 534 | 305 | 313 | 320 |
| | *** | 18654 | 19410 | 28614 | 3392 | 3713 | 4732 | 1013 | 1074 | 1235 | 504 | 523 | 566 | 309 | 317 | 324 |
| 0.3 | *** | 20029 | 20425 | 28436 | 3596 | 3851 | 4717 | 1079 | 1143 | 1248 | 537 | 558 | 585 | 327 | 335 | 346 |
| | *** | 20161 | 21192 | 31813 | 3697 | 4120 | 5208 | 1108 | 1188 | 1340 | 547 | 570 | 606 | 331 | 341 | 343 |
| 0.35 | *** | 20675 | 21202 | 31462 | 3760 | 4078 | 5165 | 1138 | 1215 | 1345 | 564 | 589 | 622 | 341 | 350 | 363 |
| | *** | 20852 | 22210 | 34268 | 3886 | 4410 | 5565 | 1173 | 1270 | 1414 | 575 | 604 | 632 | 346 | 357 | 354 |
| 0.4 | *** | 20593 | 21279 | 33714 | 3824 | 4201 | 5489 | 1171 | 1259 | 1411 | 578 | 607 | 644 | 347 | 358 | 372 |
| | *** | 20822 | 22563 | 35979 | 3974 | 4591 | 5803 | 1210 | 1323 | 1459 | 592 | 623 | 645 | 352 | 365 | 358 |
| 0.45 | *** | 19894 | 20772 | 35172 | 3803 | 4233 | 5684 | 1179 | 1276 | 1444 | 580 | 610 | 652 | 346 | 358 | 372 |
| | *** | 20189 | 22358 | 36946 | 3975 | 4670 | 5922 | 1222 | 1346 | 1474 | 594 | 630 | 645 | 352 | 365 | 354 |
| 0.5 | *** | 18702 | 19810 | 35825 | 3712 | 4184 | 5750 | 1164 | 1267 | 1445 | 571 | 603 | 645 | 337 | 350 | 365 |
| | *** | 19078 | 21709 | 37169 | 3903 | 4657 | 5922 | 1210 | 1342 | 1459 | 586 | 622 | 632 | 343 | 357 | 343 |
| 0.55 | *** | 17152 | 18520 | 35667 | 3562 | 4064 | 5687 | 1130 | 1234 | 1413 | 551 | 582 | 623 | 322 | 335 | 349 |
| | *** | 17625 | 20713 | 36648 | 3766 | 4558 | 5803 | 1175 | 1309 | 1414 | 565 | 601 | 606 | 328 | 341 | 324 |
| 0.6 | *** | 15384 | 17020 | 34702 | 3364 | 3879 | 5494 | 1074 | 1177 | 1348 | 519 | 549 | 588 | 301 | 312 | 324 |
| | *** | 15965 | 19453 | 35384 | 3575 | 4378 | 5565 | 1120 | 1249 | 1340 | 533 | 567 | 566 | 307 | 318 | 298 |
| 0.65 | *** | 13533 | 15404 | 32929 | 3125 | 3635 | 5171 | 999 | 1095 | 1252 | 478 | 504 | 538 | 273 | 281 | 292 |
| | *** | 14216 | 17989 | 33375 | 3335 | 4118 | 5208 | 1042 | 1162 | 1235 | 490 | 519 | 513 | 277 | 287 | 265 |
| 0.7 | *** | 11707 | 13732 | 30354 | 2845 | 3331 | 4721 | 905 | 989 | 1124 | 425 | 446 | 474 | 237 | 244 | 252 |
| | *** | 12466 | 16355 | 30622 | 3047 | 3780 | 4732 | 943 | 1047 | 1102 | 435 | 459 | 447 | 240 | 248 | 224 |
| 0.75 | *** | 9967 | 12023 | 26986 | 2527 | 2965 | 4145 | 788 | 858 | 964 | 359 | 376 | 397 | 194 | 199 | 204 |
| | *** | 10755 | 14557 | 27126 | 2710 | 3359 | 4137 | 820 | 905 | 938 | 367 | 385 | 368 | 197 | 202 | 175 |
| 0.8 | *** | 8317 | 10265 | 22830 | 2160 | 2529 | 3442 | 649 | 699 | 772 | 281 | 292 | 305 | . | . | . |
| | *** | 9075 | 12573 | 22885 | 2317 | 2849 | 3423 | 672 | 732 | 744 | 286 | 298 | 275 | . | . | . |
| 0.85 | *** | 6702 | 8400 | 17896 | 1732 | 2008 | 2615 | 480 | 510 | 550 | . | . | . | . | . | . |
| | *** | 7372 | 10332 | 17900 | 1852 | 2235 | 2590 | 494 | 529 | 521 | . | . | . | . | . | . |
| 0.9 | *** | 5009 | 6297 | 12192 | 1210 | 1370 | 1666 | . | . | . | . | . | . | . | . | . |
| | *** | 5524 | 7687 | 12172 | 1282 | 1490 | 1637 | . | . | . | . | . | . | . | . | . |
| 0.95 | *** | 2957 | 3624 | 5728 | . | . | . | . | . | . | . | . | . | . | . | . |
| | *** | 3232 | 4263 | 5699 | . | . | . | . | . | . | . | . | . | . | . | . |

TABLE 2: ALPHA= 0.005 POWER= 0.9    EXPECTED ACCRUAL THRU MINIMUM FOLLOW-UP= 1600

| | DEL=.02 | | | DEL=.05 | | | DEL=.10 | | | DEL=.15 | | | DEL=.20 | | |
|---|---|---|---|---|---|---|---|---|---|---|---|---|---|---|---|
| FACT= | 1.0 .75 | .50 .25 | .00 BIN | 1.0 .75 | .50 .25 | .00 BIN | 1.0 .75 | .50 .25 | .00 BIN | 1.0 75 | .50 .25 | .00 BIN | 1.0 .75 | .50 .25 | .00 BIN |
| PCONT=*** | | | | REQUIRED NUMBER OF PATIENTS | | | | | | | | | | | |
| 0.05 *** | 4252 | 4284 | 4482 | 918 | 930 | 951 | 332 | 334 | 338 | 195 | 196 | 197 | 137 | 138 | 138 |
| *** | 4263 | 4332 | 8378 | 923 | 939 | 1637 | 333 | 336 | 521 | 195 | 196 | 275 | 138 | 138 | 175 |
| 0.1 *** | 8851 | 8930 | 9848 | 1694 | 1737 | 1833 | 543 | 553 | 566 | 293 | 296 | 300 | 193 | 195 | 197 |
| *** | 8877 | 9074 | 14553 | 1712 | 1774 | 2590 | 548 | 559 | 744 | 294 | 298 | 368 | 194 | 196 | 224 |
| 0.15 *** | 12941 | 13080 | 15230 | 2371 | 2458 | 2687 | 726 | 746 | 776 | 376 | 383 | 391 | 240 | 243 | 246 |
| *** | 12987 | 13346 | 19984 | 2406 | 2540 | 3423 | 735 | 759 | 938 | 379 | 387 | 447 | 241 | 244 | 265 |
| 0.2 *** | 16211 | 16426 | 20236 | 2919 | 3058 | 3467 | 877 | 911 | 961 | 444 | 455 | 469 | 277 | 282 | 288 |
| *** | 16283 | 16841 | 24671 | 2974 | 3197 | 4137 | 893 | 933 | 1102 | 450 | 462 | 513 | 280 | 285 | 298 |
| 0.25 *** | 18578 | 18886 | 24674 | 3332 | 3530 | 4148 | 997 | 1045 | 1120 | 499 | 514 | 534 | 307 | 313 | 321 |
| *** | 18680 | 19482 | 28614 | 3410 | 3731 | 4732 | 1018 | 1077 | 1235 | 506 | 524 | 566 | 310 | 317 | 324 |
| 0.3 *** | 20055 | 20478 | 28436 | 3618 | 3877 | 4717 | 1086 | 1148 | 1248 | 539 | 559 | 585 | 328 | 337 | 346 |
| *** | 20196 | 21289 | 31813 | 3720 | 4144 | 5208 | 1114 | 1191 | 1340 | 549 | 571 | 606 | 332 | 341 | 343 |
| 0.35 *** | 20711 | 21272 | 31462 | 3787 | 4110 | 5166 | 1146 | 1221 | 1346 | 567 | 590 | 622 | 342 | 352 | 363 |
| *** | 20898 | 22336 | 34268 | 3916 | 4439 | 5565 | 1180 | 1274 | 1414 | 578 | 605 | 632 | 347 | 357 | 354 |
| 0.4 *** | 20639 | 21370 | 33714 | 3857 | 4238 | 5489 | 1180 | 1266 | 1411 | 581 | 608 | 644 | 348 | 359 | 372 |
| *** | 20883 | 22719 | 35979 | 4009 | 4625 | 5803 | 1218 | 1327 | 1459 | 594 | 625 | 645 | 353 | 365 | 358 |
| 0.45 *** | 19952 | 20887 | 35172 | 3841 | 4275 | 5684 | 1189 | 1284 | 1444 | 584 | 613 | 652 | 347 | 359 | 372 |
| *** | 20267 | 22546 | 36946 | 4016 | 4709 | 5922 | 1231 | 1351 | 1474 | 598 | 631 | 645 | 353 | 365 | 354 |
| 0.5 *** | 18777 | 19952 | 35824 | 3753 | 4230 | 5750 | 1175 | 1275 | 1445 | 575 | 605 | 645 | 339 | 351 | 365 |
| *** | 19177 | 21926 | 37169 | 3947 | 4699 | 5922 | 1220 | 1347 | 1459 | 589 | 623 | 632 | 345 | 357 | 343 |
| 0.55 *** | 17248 | 18689 | 35668 | 3607 | 4112 | 5687 | 1140 | 1242 | 1413 | 555 | 584 | 624 | 324 | 335 | 349 |
| *** | 17749 | 20956 | 36648 | 3813 | 4601 | 5803 | 1186 | 1314 | 1414 | 568 | 603 | 606 | 330 | 342 | 324 |
| 0.6 *** | 15503 | 17215 | 34701 | 3411 | 3928 | 5493 | 1085 | 1184 | 1349 | 523 | 551 | 588 | 302 | 313 | 325 |
| *** | 16113 | 19715 | 35384 | 3624 | 4421 | 5565 | 1130 | 1254 | 1340 | 536 | 568 | 566 | 307 | 318 | 298 |
| 0.65 *** | 13674 | 15617 | 32928 | 3171 | 3682 | 5171 | 1009 | 1102 | 1252 | 481 | 506 | 538 | 274 | 282 | 293 |
| *** | 14388 | 18260 | 33375 | 3383 | 4160 | 5208 | 1051 | 1167 | 1235 | 493 | 521 | 513 | 278 | 287 | 265 |
| 0.7 *** | 11867 | 13953 | 30354 | 2890 | 3375 | 4721 | 914 | 996 | 1124 | 427 | 448 | 474 | 238 | 245 | 253 |
| *** | 12653 | 16624 | 30622 | 3093 | 3818 | 4732 | 951 | 1051 | 1102 | 437 | 460 | 447 | 241 | 249 | 224 |
| 0.75 *** | 10136 | 12241 | 26986 | 2568 | 3004 | 4144 | 796 | 863 | 964 | 361 | 377 | 396 | 195 | 199 | 205 |
| *** | 10945 | 14812 | 27126 | 2751 | 3392 | 4137 | 827 | 908 | 938 | 369 | 386 | 368 | 197 | 202 | 175 |
| 0.8 *** | 8480 | 10468 | 22830 | 2196 | 2562 | 3442 | 654 | 703 | 773 | 282 | 292 | 304 | . | . | . |
| *** | 9255 | 12800 | 22885 | 2351 | 2875 | 3423 | 677 | 735 | 744 | 287 | 298 | 275 | . | . | . |
| 0.85 *** | 6847 | 8572 | 17896 | 1759 | 2032 | 2616 | 484 | 513 | 551 | . | . | . | . | . | . |
| *** | 7528 | 10519 | 17900 | 1877 | 2252 | 2590 | 497 | 530 | 521 | . | . | . | . | . | . |
| 0.9 *** | 5122 | 6424 | 12193 | 1227 | 1384 | 1666 | . | . | . | . | . | . | . | . | . |
| *** | 5644 | 7817 | 12172 | 1296 | 1499 | 1637 | . | . | . | . | . | . | . | . | . |
| 0.95 *** | 3018 | 3686 | 5728 | . | . | . | . | . | . | . | . | . | . | . | . |
| *** | 3295 | 4318 | 5699 | . | . | . | . | . | . | . | . | . | . | . | . |

## TABLE 2: ALPHA= 0.005 POWER= 0.9     EXPECTED ACCRUAL THRU MINIMUM FOLLOW-UP= 1700

| | DEL=.02 | | | DEL=.05 | | | DEL=.10 | | | DEL=.15 | | | DEL=.20 | | |
|---|---|---|---|---|---|---|---|---|---|---|---|---|---|---|---|
| **FACT=** | 1.0 | .50 | .00 | 1.0 | .50 | .00 | 1.0 | .50 | .00 | 1.0 | .50 | .00 | 1.0 | .50 | .00 |
| | .75 | .25 | BIN | .75 | .25 | BIN | .75 | .25 | BIN | 75 | .25 | BIN | .75 | .25 | BIN |

**PCONT=***     REQUIRED NUMBER OF PATIENTS

| PCONT | 1.0/.75 | .50/.25 | .00/BIN | 1.0/.75 | .50/.25 | .00/BIN | 1.0/.75 | .50/.25 | .00/BIN | 1.0/75 | .50/.25 | .00/BIN | 1.0/.75 | .50/.25 | .00/BIN |
|---|---|---|---|---|---|---|---|---|---|---|---|---|---|---|---|
| 0.05 | 4254 | 4287 | 4483 | 919 | 930 | 951 | 331 | 335 | 338 | 194 | 195 | 197 | 137 | 138 | 138 |
| | 4266 | 4337 | 8378 | 924 | 939 | 1637 | 333 | 335 | 521 | 195 | 197 | 275 | 138 | 138 | 175 |
| 0.1 | 8856 | 8939 | 9847 | 1698 | 1740 | 1833 | 544 | 554 | 566 | 293 | 296 | 301 | 193 | 195 | 197 |
| | 8884 | 9090 | 14553 | 1716 | 1778 | 2590 | 548 | 559 | 744 | 294 | 299 | 368 | 194 | 195 | 224 |
| 0.15 | 12949 | 13097 | 15230 | 2378 | 2466 | 2687 | 728 | 748 | 775 | 376 | 384 | 391 | 240 | 243 | 246 |
| | 12998 | 13377 | 19984 | 2414 | 2547 | 3423 | 737 | 760 | 938 | 379 | 386 | 447 | 241 | 244 | 265 |
| 0.2 | 16224 | 16453 | 20236 | 2930 | 3070 | 3467 | 881 | 913 | 962 | 445 | 456 | 469 | 278 | 282 | 288 |
| | 16301 | 16889 | 24671 | 2987 | 3208 | 4137 | 896 | 935 | 1102 | 450 | 462 | 513 | 280 | 284 | 298 |
| 0.25 | 18597 | 18924 | 24674 | 3348 | 3548 | 4148 | 1002 | 1047 | 1120 | 500 | 515 | 534 | 308 | 313 | 321 |
| | 18706 | 19552 | 28614 | 3427 | 3747 | 4732 | 1023 | 1079 | 1235 | 508 | 524 | 566 | 310 | 318 | 324 |
| 0.3 | 20082 | 20531 | 28436 | 3638 | 3901 | 4717 | 1092 | 1151 | 1248 | 542 | 561 | 585 | 329 | 337 | 346 |
| | 20232 | 21384 | 31813 | 3743 | 4165 | 5208 | 1119 | 1194 | 1340 | 550 | 571 | 606 | 333 | 341 | 343 |
| 0.35 | 20746 | 21342 | 31462 | 3813 | 4139 | 5166 | 1154 | 1227 | 1346 | 569 | 592 | 622 | 343 | 352 | 363 |
| | 20945 | 22458 | 34268 | 3944 | 4466 | 5565 | 1187 | 1278 | 1414 | 580 | 605 | 632 | 347 | 357 | 354 |
| 0.4 | 20684 | 21459 | 33714 | 3888 | 4273 | 5489 | 1188 | 1273 | 1411 | 584 | 610 | 644 | 350 | 360 | 372 |
| | 20945 | 22870 | 35979 | 4043 | 4656 | 5803 | 1226 | 1331 | 1459 | 596 | 626 | 645 | 355 | 365 | 358 |
| 0.45 | 20011 | 21000 | 35172 | 3877 | 4313 | 5684 | 1198 | 1291 | 1444 | 586 | 615 | 652 | 348 | 359 | 372 |
| | 20346 | 22729 | 36946 | 4053 | 4744 | 5922 | 1240 | 1355 | 1474 | 600 | 632 | 645 | 354 | 365 | 354 |
| 0.5 | 18853 | 20091 | 35824 | 3793 | 4272 | 5750 | 1185 | 1282 | 1445 | 578 | 607 | 645 | 340 | 352 | 364 |
| | 19277 | 22136 | 37169 | 3988 | 4738 | 5922 | 1229 | 1351 | 1459 | 592 | 624 | 632 | 345 | 358 | 343 |
| 0.55 | 17343 | 18855 | 35667 | 3650 | 4156 | 5686 | 1151 | 1249 | 1413 | 558 | 586 | 624 | 325 | 335 | 348 |
| | 17871 | 21189 | 36648 | 3858 | 4641 | 5803 | 1195 | 1319 | 1414 | 571 | 603 | 606 | 330 | 342 | 324 |
| 0.6 | 15620 | 17403 | 34701 | 3455 | 3973 | 5493 | 1094 | 1192 | 1348 | 526 | 554 | 588 | 304 | 313 | 325 |
| | 16260 | 19965 | 35384 | 3669 | 4460 | 5565 | 1138 | 1259 | 1340 | 539 | 569 | 566 | 308 | 318 | 298 |
| 0.65 | 13814 | 15822 | 32928 | 3215 | 3726 | 5171 | 1019 | 1109 | 1251 | 483 | 508 | 539 | 274 | 282 | 292 |
| | 14555 | 18518 | 33375 | 3427 | 4198 | 5268 | 1059 | 1171 | 1235 | 495 | 522 | 513 | 278 | 288 | 265 |
| 0.7 | 12023 | 14165 | 30355 | 2932 | 3416 | 4721 | 922 | 1002 | 1124 | 429 | 449 | 474 | 239 | 245 | 253 |
| | 12833 | 16879 | 30622 | 3135 | 3852 | 4732 | 958 | 1055 | 1102 | 439 | 461 | 447 | 242 | 248 | 224 |
| 0.75 | 10297 | 12450 | 26985 | 2606 | 3041 | 4145 | 803 | 868 | 964 | 362 | 378 | 396 | 195 | 199 | 205 |
| | 11128 | 15053 | 27126 | 2790 | 3422 | 4137 | 833 | 911 | 938 | 369 | 386 | 368 | 197 | 202 | 175 |
| 0.8 | 8637 | 10660 | 22830 | 2229 | 2592 | 3442 | 660 | 707 | 772 | 284 | 293 | 305 | . | . | . |
| | 9428 | 13015 | 22885 | 2384 | 2898 | 3423 | 681 | 736 | 744 | 288 | 299 | 275 | . | . | . |
| 0.85 | 6987 | 8736 | 17896 | 1785 | 2054 | 2616 | 486 | 514 | 550 | . | . | . | . | . | . |
| | 7679 | 10694 | 17900 | 1902 | 2268 | 2590 | 499 | 531 | 521 | . | . | . | . | . | . |
| 0.9 | 5229 | 6544 | 12192 | 1242 | 1396 | 1666 | . | . | . | . | . | . | . | . | . |
| | 5758 | 7938 | 12172 | 1310 | 1508 | 1637 | . | . | . | . | . | . | . | . | . |
| 0.95 | 3076 | 3744 | 5728 | . | . | . | . | . | . | . | . | . | . | . | . |
| | 3353 | 4369 | 5699 | . | . | . | . | . | . | . | . | . | . | . | . |

## TABLE 2: ALPHA= 0.005 POWER= 0.9     EXPECTED ACCRUAL THRU MINIMUM FOLLOW-UP= 1800

| | DEL=.02 | | | DEL=.05 | | | DEL=.10 | | | DEL=.15 | | | DEL=.20 | | |
|---|---|---|---|---|---|---|---|---|---|---|---|---|---|---|---|
| FACT= | 1.0 .75 | .50 .25 | .00 BIN | 1.0 .75 | .50 .25 | .00 BIN | 1.0 .75 | .50 .25 | .00 BIN | 1.0 75 | .50 .25 | .00 BIN | 1.0 .75 | .50 .25 | .00 BIN |

PCONT=***                                REQUIRED NUMBER OF PATIENTS

| PCONT | 1.0/.75 | .50/.25 | .00/BIN | 1.0/.75 | .50/.25 | .00/BIN | 1.0/.75 | .50/.25 | .00/BIN | 1.0/.75 | .50/.25 | .00/BIN | 1.0/.75 | .50/.25 | .00/BIN |
|---|---|---|---|---|---|---|---|---|---|---|---|---|---|---|---|
| 0.05 *** | 4256 | 4290 | 4482 | 920 | 931 | 951 | 332 | 335 | 337 | 195 | 195 | 197 | 137 | 138 | 138 |
| *** | 4268 | 4341 | 8378 | 924 | 939 | 1637 | 333 | 336 | 521 | 195 | 197 | 275 | 137 | 138 | 175 |
| 0.1 *** | 8860 | 8949 | 9848 | 1701 | 1743 | 1833 | 546 | 555 | 566 | 294 | 297 | 300 | 193 | 195 | 197 |
| *** | 8891 | 9105 | 14553 | 1719 | 1779 | 2590 | 549 | 559 | 744 | 294 | 298 | 368 | 195 | 195 | 224 |
| 0.15 *** | 12957 | 13114 | 15230 | 2385 | 2472 | 2688 | 730 | 749 | 775 | 377 | 384 | 391 | 240 | 243 | 246 |
| *** | 13011 | 13407 | 19984 | 2421 | 2553 | 3423 | 739 | 762 | 938 | 380 | 387 | 447 | 242 | 245 | 265 |
| 0.2 *** | 16238 | 16479 | 20236 | 2940 | 3082 | 3467 | 884 | 915 | 962 | 447 | 456 | 469 | 279 | 282 | 288 |
| *** | 16318 | 16938 | 24671 | 2998 | 3217 | 4137 | 897 | 936 | 1102 | 451 | 462 | 513 | 280 | 285 | 298 |
| 0.25 *** | 18616 | 18962 | 24673 | 3363 | 3565 | 4148 | 1005 | 1050 | 1119 | 501 | 516 | 534 | 308 | 314 | 321 |
| *** | 18731 | 19621 | 28614 | 3444 | 3763 | 4732 | 1027 | 1081 | 1235 | 508 | 524 | 566 | 312 | 317 | 324 |
| 0.3 *** | 20108 | 20583 | 28437 | 3658 | 3924 | 4717 | 1098 | 1156 | 1248 | 543 | 561 | 585 | 330 | 337 | 346 |
| *** | 20267 | 21477 | 31813 | 3765 | 4186 | 5208 | 1124 | 1196 | 1340 | 552 | 573 | 606 | 334 | 342 | 343 |
| 0.35 *** | 20781 | 21411 | 31461 | 3838 | 4167 | 5166 | 1161 | 1232 | 1345 | 571 | 594 | 622 | 344 | 353 | 363 |
| *** | 20992 | 22578 | 34268 | 3971 | 4491 | 5565 | 1192 | 1281 | 1414 | 582 | 606 | 632 | 348 | 357 | 354 |
| 0.4 *** | 20730 | 21549 | 33714 | 3918 | 4305 | 5489 | 1196 | 1278 | 1410 | 587 | 612 | 645 | 351 | 360 | 372 |
| *** | 21006 | 23019 | 35979 | 4074 | 4686 | 5803 | 1233 | 1335 | 1459 | 598 | 627 | 645 | 355 | 366 | 358 |
| 0.45 *** | 20071 | 21113 | 35172 | 3910 | 4350 | 5685 | 1207 | 1297 | 1444 | 589 | 616 | 652 | 350 | 360 | 372 |
| *** | 20424 | 22905 | 36946 | 4090 | 4776 | 5922 | 1248 | 1360 | 1474 | 603 | 633 | 645 | 354 | 366 | 354 |
| 0.5 *** | 18928 | 20229 | 35824 | 3831 | 4312 | 5750 | 1194 | 1289 | 1444 | 580 | 609 | 645 | 342 | 352 | 364 |
| *** | 19374 | 22339 | 37169 | 4029 | 4772 | 5922 | 1237 | 1356 | 1459 | 594 | 625 | 632 | 346 | 357 | 343 |
| 0.55 *** | 17437 | 19017 | 35668 | 3690 | 4198 | 5687 | 1160 | 1257 | 1413 | 560 | 588 | 624 | 326 | 336 | 348 |
| *** | 17992 | 21414 | 36648 | 3899 | 4677 | 5803 | 1203 | 1324 | 1414 | 573 | 605 | 606 | 332 | 342 | 324 |
| 0.6 *** | 15736 | 17587 | 34701 | 3498 | 4015 | 5493 | 1104 | 1198 | 1349 | 528 | 555 | 588 | 305 | 314 | 325 |
| *** | 16404 | 20205 | 35384 | 3712 | 4497 | 5565 | 1146 | 1263 | 1340 | 541 | 570 | 566 | 309 | 319 | 298 |
| 0.65 *** | 13950 | 16021 | 32928 | 3257 | 3768 | 5172 | 1027 | 1115 | 1252 | 486 | 510 | 539 | 276 | 283 | 292 |
| *** | 14718 | 18764 | 33375 | 3471 | 4233 | 5208 | 1068 | 1174 | 1235 | 497 | 523 | 513 | 279 | 288 | 265 |
| 0.7 *** | 12174 | 14370 | 30354 | 2973 | 3455 | 4722 | 929 | 1007 | 1124 | 431 | 450 | 474 | 240 | 245 | 253 |
| *** | 13008 | 17122 | 30622 | 3176 | 3885 | 4732 | 965 | 1059 | 1102 | 440 | 461 | 447 | 242 | 249 | 224 |
| 0.75 *** | 10455 | 12649 | 26985 | 2643 | 3075 | 4144 | 809 | 873 | 964 | 364 | 379 | 396 | 195 | 200 | 204 |
| *** | 11304 | 15282 | 27126 | 2826 | 3450 | 4137 | 838 | 913 | 938 | 371 | 387 | 368 | 198 | 202 | 175 |
| 0.8 *** | 8788 | 10844 | 22830 | 2260 | 2620 | 3442 | 663 | 710 | 773 | 285 | 294 | 305 | . | . | . |
| *** | 9594 | 13218 | 22885 | 2414 | 2920 | 3423 | 685 | 738 | 744 | 289 | 299 | 275 | . | . | . |
| 0.85 *** | 7120 | 8891 | 17896 | 1808 | 2074 | 2616 | 489 | 516 | 551 | . | . | . | . | . | . |
| *** | 7822 | 10860 | 17900 | 1923 | 2283 | 2590 | 501 | 532 | 521 | . | . | . | . | . | . |
| 0.9 *** | 5332 | 6657 | 12192 | 1255 | 1406 | 1666 | . | . | . | . | . | . | . | . | . |
| *** | 5865 | 8052 | 12172 | 1323 | 1515 | 1637 | . | . | . | . | . | . | . | . | . |
| 0.95 *** | 3131 | 3798 | 5728 | . | . | . | . | . | . | . | . | . | . | . | . |
| *** | 3408 | 4416 | 5699 | . | . | . | . | . | . | . | . | . | . | . | . |

TABLE 2: ALPHA= 0.005 POWER= 0.9     EXPECTED ACCRUAL THRU MINIMUM FOLLOW-UP= 1900

|  |  | DEL=.02 | | | DEL=.05 | | | DEL=.10 | | | DEL=.15 | | | DEL=.20 | | |
|---|---|---|---|---|---|---|---|---|---|---|---|---|---|---|---|---|
| FACT= | | 1.0 .75 | .50 .25 | .00 BIN | 1.0 .75 | .50 .25 | .00 BIN | 1.0 .75 | .50 .25 | .00 BIN | 1.0 75 | .50 .25 | .00 BIN | 1.0 .75 | .50 .25 | .00 BIN |
| PCONT=*** | | | | | REQUIRED NUMBER OF PATIENTS | | | | | | | | | | | |
| 0.05 | *** *** | 4258 4271 | 4295 4345 | 4483 8378 | 921 926 | 932 940 | 951 1637 | 332 334 | 334 336 | 338 521 | 194 196 | 196 196 | 197 275 | 137 137 | 137 137 | 139 175 |
| 0.1 | *** *** | 8865 8896 | 8958 9121 | 9848 14553 | 1705 1723 | 1747 1782 | 1833 2590 | 546 550 | 554 560 | 566 744 | 293 296 | 296 298 | 300 368 | 193 194 | 194 196 | 197 224 |
| 0.15 | *** *** | 12967 13022 | 13131 13436 | 15230 19984 | 2391 2428 | 2479 2557 | 2687 3423 | 731 740 | 750 762 | 775 938 | 377 381 | 383 387 | 391 447 | 241 242 | 243 244 | 246 265 |
| 0.2 | *** *** | 16251 16336 | 16506 16985 | 20236 24671 | 2951 3009 | 3093 3227 | 3467 4137 | 887 901 | 918 937 | 961 1102 | 448 452 | 457 463 | 469 513 | 279 281 | 282 285 | 287 298 |
| 0.25 | *** *** | 18635 18757 | 19000 19688 | 24673 28614 | 3378 3460 | 3581 3776 | 4148 4732 | 1010 1030 | 1054 1083 | 1120 1235 | 503 509 | 517 524 | 534 566 | 308 311 | 315 318 | 320 324 |
| 0.3 | *** *** | 20135 20301 | 20635 21568 | 28437 31813 | 3678 3785 | 3944 4203 | 4718 5208 | 1103 1129 | 1160 1199 | 1248 1340 | 545 553 | 562 573 | 585 606 | 331 334 | 338 342 | 346 343 |
| 0.35 | *** *** | 20816 21039 | 21481 22695 | 31461 34268 | 3863 3997 | 4193 4514 | 5165 5565 | 1167 1198 | 1236 1284 | 1345 1414 | 573 584 | 595 608 | 622 632 | 345 349 | 353 358 | 363 354 |
| 0.4 | *** *** | 20776 21066 | 21638 23163 | 33714 35979 | 3946 4105 | 4336 4713 | 5488 5803 | 1203 1239 | 1284 1338 | 1410 1459 | 589 600 | 612 628 | 645 645 | 351 356 | 361 365 | 372 358 |
| 0.45 | *** *** | 20129 20502 | 21224 23077 | 35171 36946 | 3944 4124 | 4385 4808 | 5684 5922 | 1215 1255 | 1303 1364 | 1444 1474 | 592 604 | 619 634 | 652 645 | 350 355 | 361 365 | 372 354 |
| 0.5 | *** *** | 19003 19472 | 20364 22536 | 35824 37169 | 3868 4066 | 4350 4806 | 5749 5922 | 1203 1244 | 1295 1360 | 1445 1459 | 583 596 | 610 627 | 645 632 | 343 348 | 353 358 | 364 343 |
| 0.55 | *** *** | 17531 18111 | 19175 21631 | 35667 36648 | 3730 3940 | 4238 4712 | 5687 5803 | 1168 1211 | 1262 1327 | 1413 1414 | 562 576 | 590 605 | 623 606 | 327 332 | 337 343 | 349 324 |
| 0.6 | *** *** | 15850 16545 | 17766 20436 | 34701 35205 | 3537 3752 | 4055 4531 | 5493 5565 | 1113 1154 | 1204 1267 | 1349 1340 | 532 543 | 557 571 | 588 566 | 305 310 | 315 319 | 324 298 |
| 0.65 | *** *** | 14085 14877 | 16213 19000 | 32928 33375 | 3806 3510 | 3806 4265 | 5171 5208 | 1035 1075 | 1121 1178 | 1251 1235 | 488 498 | 510 524 | 538 513 | 277 280 | 284 288 | 292 265 |
| 0.7 | *** *** | 12323 13178 | 14567 17354 | 30354 30622 | 3011 3213 | 3491 3915 | 4721 4732 | 937 971 | 1011 1061 | 1123 1102 | 433 441 | 451 462 | 474 447 | 239 243 | 246 249 | 253 224 |
| 0.75 | *** *** | 10608 11473 | 12841 15500 | 26986 27126 | 2678 2859 | 3108 3476 | 4144 4137 | 814 843 | 876 915 | 964 938 | 365 372 | 380 387 | 396 368 | 196 198 | 201 203 | 205 175 |
| 0.8 | *** *** | 8934 9753 | 11019 13411 | 22830 22885 | 2289 2443 | 2645 2940 | 3442 3423 | 668 688 | 712 740 | 773 744 | 285 289 | 294 299 | 304 275 | . . | . . | . . |
| 0.85 | *** *** | 7248 7960 | 9039 11016 | 17897 17900 | 1830 1945 | 2092 2296 | 2616 2590 | 491 505 | 517 533 | 551 521 | . . | . . | . . | . . | . . | . . |
| 0.9 | *** *** | 5430 5969 | 6766 8159 | 12193 12172 | 1269 1334 | 1417 1521 | 1666 1637 | . . | . . | . . | . . | . . | . . | . . | . . | . . |
| 0.95 | *** *** | 3182 3461 | 3849 4459 | 5728 5699 | . . | . . | . . | . . | . . | . . | . . | . . | . . | . . | . . | . . |

TABLE 2: ALPHA= 0.005 POWER= 0.9     EXPECTED ACCRUAL THRU MINIMUM FOLLOW-UP= 2000

| | DEL=.02 | | | DEL=.05 | | | DEL=.10 | | | DEL=.15 | | | DEL=.20 | | |
|---|---|---|---|---|---|---|---|---|---|---|---|---|---|---|---|
| FACT= | 1.0 .75 | .50 .25 | .00 BIN | 1.0 .75 | .50 .25 | .00 BIN | 1.0 .75 | .50 .25 | .00 BIN | 1.0 75 | .50 .25 | .00 BIN | 1.0 .75 | .50 .25 | .00 BIN |
| PCONT=*** | REQUIRED NUMBER OF PATIENTS | | | | | | | | | | | | | | |
| 0.05 *** | 4260 | 4297 | 4482 | 922 | 934 | 951 | 332 | 335 | 337 | 195 | 196 | 197 | 137 | 137 | 139 |
| *** | 4274 | 4350 | 8378 | 927 | 941 | 1637 | 334 | 336 | 521 | 195 | 196 | 275 | 137 | 139 | 175 |
| 0.1 *** | 8870 | 8969 | 9847 | 1707 | 1750 | 1834 | 546 | 555 | 566 | 294 | 297 | 300 | 194 | 195 | 197 |
| *** | 8904 | 9136 | 14553 | 1726 | 1784 | 2590 | 551 | 560 | 744 | 295 | 299 | 368 | 195 | 196 | 224 |
| 0.15 *** | 12976 | 13149 | 15230 | 2397 | 2486 | 2687 | 734 | 751 | 776 | 379 | 384 | 391 | 241 | 244 | 246 |
| *** | 13034 | 13465 | 19984 | 2435 | 2562 | 3423 | 741 | 762 | 938 | 381 | 387 | 447 | 242 | 245 | 265 |
| 0.2 *** | 16265 | 16532 | 20236 | 2961 | 3105 | 3467 | 890 | 919 | 961 | 449 | 457 | 470 | 279 | 284 | 287 |
| *** | 16355 | 17031 | 24671 | 3020 | 3236 | 4137 | 904 | 939 | 1102 | 454 | 464 | 513 | 281 | 285 | 298 |
| 0.25 *** | 18655 | 19039 | 24674 | 3392 | 3596 | 4149 | 1014 | 1056 | 1120 | 505 | 517 | 534 | 310 | 315 | 321 |
| *** | 18784 | 19755 | 28614 | 3475 | 3790 | 4732 | 1034 | 1085 | 1235 | 511 | 526 | 566 | 312 | 317 | 324 |
| 0.3 *** | 20161 | 20687 | 28436 | 3696 | 3965 | 4717 | 1107 | 1164 | 1249 | 547 | 564 | 585 | 331 | 339 | 346 |
| *** | 20337 | 21657 | 31813 | 3806 | 4221 | 5208 | 1134 | 1201 | 1340 | 555 | 574 | 606 | 335 | 342 | 343 |
| 0.35 *** | 20851 | 21241 | 31462 | 3886 | 4219 | 5166 | 1172 | 1241 | 1346 | 576 | 596 | 622 | 346 | 354 | 364 |
| *** | 21086 | 22810 | 34268 | 4021 | 4536 | 5565 | 1204 | 1286 | 1414 | 585 | 609 | 632 | 350 | 359 | 354 |
| 0.4 *** | 20822 | 21726 | 33714 | 3974 | 4366 | 5489 | 1210 | 1289 | 1411 | 591 | 615 | 644 | 352 | 361 | 372 |
| *** | 21127 | 23304 | 35979 | 4134 | 4739 | 5803 | 1246 | 1342 | 1459 | 602 | 629 | 645 | 356 | 366 | 358 |
| 0.45 *** | 20189 | 21335 | 35172 | 3975 | 4419 | 5685 | 1222 | 1309 | 1444 | 595 | 620 | 652 | 351 | 361 | 372 |
| *** | 20580 | 23242 | 36946 | 4157 | 4836 | 5922 | 1261 | 1367 | 1474 | 606 | 635 | 654 | 356 | 366 | 354 |
| 0.5 *** | 19077 | 20497 | 35825 | 3902 | 4386 | 5750 | 1210 | 1301 | 1445 | 586 | 612 | 645 | 344 | 354 | 365 |
| *** | 19570 | 22725 | 37169 | 4102 | 4836 | 5922 | 1251 | 1364 | 1459 | 599 | 627 | 632 | 349 | 359 | 343 |
| 0.55 *** | 17625 | 19331 | 35667 | 3766 | 4275 | 5686 | 1176 | 1269 | 1412 | 566 | 591 | 624 | 329 | 337 | 349 |
| *** | 18231 | 21840 | 36648 | 3977 | 4744 | 5803 | 1219 | 1331 | 1414 | 577 | 606 | 606 | 332 | 344 | 324 |
| 0.6 *** | 15965 | 17940 | 34701 | 3575 | 4094 | 5494 | 1120 | 1210 | 1349 | 534 | 557 | 589 | 306 | 315 | 325 |
| *** | 16685 | 20656 | 35384 | 3791 | 4562 | 5565 | 1161 | 1271 | 1340 | 545 | 572 | 566 | 310 | 320 | 298 |
| 0.65 *** | 14216 | 16400 | 32929 | 3335 | 3842 | 5171 | 1042 | 1126 | 1252 | 490 | 511 | 539 | 277 | 285 | 292 |
| *** | 15032 | 19226 | 33375 | 3549 | 4296 | 5208 | 1081 | 1181 | 1235 | 500 | 524 | 513 | 281 | 289 | 265 |
| 0.7 *** | 12466 | 14756 | 30355 | 3047 | 3525 | 4721 | 942 | 1016 | 1124 | 435 | 452 | 475 | 240 | 246 | 252 |
| *** | 13341 | 17576 | 30622 | 3249 | 3942 | 4732 | 976 | 1064 | 1102 | 444 | 462 | 447 | 244 | 250 | 224 |
| 0.75 *** | 10755 | 13026 | 26986 | 2710 | 3137 | 4145 | 820 | 880 | 964 | 367 | 380 | 396 | 196 | 200 | 205 |
| *** | 11637 | 15709 | 27126 | 2892 | 3499 | 4137 | 847 | 917 | 938 | 374 | 387 | 368 | 199 | 202 | 175 |
| 0.8 *** | 9075 | 11187 | 22830 | 2316 | 2671 | 3442 | 672 | 715 | 772 | 286 | 295 | 305 | . | . | . |
| *** | 9906 | 13596 | 22885 | 2469 | 2959 | 3423 | 692 | 741 | 744 | 290 | 300 | 275 | . | . | . |
| 0.85 *** | 7371 | 9181 | 17896 | 1851 | 2110 | 2616 | 495 | 520 | 551 | . | . | . | . | . | . |
| *** | 8091 | 11165 | 17900 | 1965 | 2310 | 2590 | 506 | 534 | 521 | . | . | . | . | . | . |
| 0.9 *** | 5524 | 6869 | 12192 | 1281 | 1426 | 1666 | . | . | . | . | . | . | . | . | . |
| *** | 6067 | 8260 | 12172 | 1346 | 1527 | 1637 | . | . | . | . | . | . | . | . | . |
| 0.95 *** | 3232 | 3897 | 5729 | . | . | . | . | . | . | . | . | . | . | . | . |
| *** | 3511 | 4500 | 5699 | . | . | . | . | . | . | . | . | . | . | . | . |

# TABLE 2: ALPHA= 0.005 POWER= 0.9 EXPECTED ACCRUAL THRU MINIMUM FOLLOW-UP= 2250

| | | DEL=.02 | | | DEL=.05 | | | DEL=.10 | | | DEL=.15 | | | DEL=.20 | | |
|---|---|---|---|---|---|---|---|---|---|---|---|---|---|---|---|---|
| FACT= | | 1.0 / .75 | .50 / .25 | .00 / BIN | 1.0 / .75 | .50 / .25 | .00 / BIN | 1.0 / .75 | .50 / .25 | .00 / BIN | 1.0 / 75 | .50 / .25 | .00 / BIN | 1.0 / .75 | .50 / .25 | .00 / BIN |
| PCONT=*** | | | | | | | REQUIRED NUMBER OF PATIENTS | | | | | | | | | |
| 0.05 | *** | 4265 | 4305 | 4483 | 924 | 935 | 950 | 333 | 336 | 337 | 195 | 196 | 196 | 137 | 137 | 139 |
| | *** | 4280 | 4358 | 8378 | 929 | 942 | 1637 | 334 | 336 | 521 | 195 | 196 | 275 | 137 | 137 | 175 |
| 0.1 | *** | 8883 | 8991 | 9848 | 1715 | 1756 | 1833 | 548 | 556 | 567 | 295 | 297 | 300 | 194 | 195 | 196 |
| | *** | 8920 | 9170 | 14553 | 1734 | 1788 | 2590 | 552 | 561 | 744 | 295 | 298 | 368 | 195 | 196 | 224 |
| 0.15 | *** | 12998 | 13192 | 15229 | 2413 | 2500 | 2687 | 736 | 753 | 776 | 379 | 385 | 390 | 241 | 243 | 246 |
| | *** | 13062 | 13535 | 19984 | 2449 | 2573 | 3423 | 745 | 763 | 938 | 382 | 388 | 447 | 243 | 244 | 265 |
| 0.2 | *** | 16298 | 16598 | 20235 | 2985 | 3129 | 3467 | 896 | 924 | 961 | 449 | 460 | 469 | 280 | 284 | 288 |
| | *** | 16399 | 17142 | 24671 | 3044 | 3255 | 4137 | 908 | 941 | 1102 | 454 | 464 | 513 | 282 | 285 | 298 |
| 0.25 | *** | 18703 | 19133 | 24674 | 3425 | 3632 | 4148 | 1022 | 1063 | 1119 | 507 | 520 | 534 | 311 | 314 | 320 |
| | *** | 18848 | 19915 | 28614 | 3509 | 3818 | 4732 | 1040 | 1088 | 1235 | 513 | 527 | 566 | 313 | 317 | 324 |
| 0.3 | *** | 20227 | 20817 | 28437 | 3740 | 4012 | 4718 | 1119 | 1171 | 1248 | 550 | 567 | 584 | 333 | 339 | 345 |
| | *** | 20426 | 21872 | 31813 | 3852 | 4259 | 5208 | 1143 | 1205 | 1340 | 558 | 575 | 606 | 336 | 343 | 343 |
| 0.35 | *** | 20939 | 21719 | 31462 | 3940 | 4274 | 5166 | 1185 | 1250 | 1346 | 579 | 599 | 621 | 347 | 354 | 362 |
| | *** | 21202 | 23083 | 34268 | 4078 | 4584 | 5565 | 1214 | 1292 | 1414 | 589 | 610 | 632 | 351 | 358 | 354 |
| 0.4 | *** | 20937 | 21943 | 33715 | 4038 | 4432 | 5488 | 1225 | 1299 | 1411 | 596 | 617 | 644 | 354 | 362 | 372 |
| | *** | 21279 | 23639 | 35979 | 4201 | 4795 | 5803 | 1258 | 1348 | 1459 | 606 | 629 | 645 | 358 | 367 | 358 |
| 0.45 | *** | 20336 | 21604 | 35172 | 4048 | 4493 | 5684 | 1239 | 1320 | 1444 | 600 | 623 | 652 | 354 | 362 | 372 |
| | *** | 20773 | 23637 | 36946 | 4232 | 4899 | 5922 | 1275 | 1375 | 1474 | 610 | 637 | 645 | 358 | 367 | 354 |
| 0.5 | *** | 19264 | 20820 | 35824 | 3984 | 4466 | 5750 | 1227 | 1315 | 1445 | 592 | 615 | 645 | 345 | 354 | 364 |
| | *** | 19810 | 23173 | 37169 | 4184 | 4904 | 5922 | 1267 | 1371 | 1459 | 603 | 629 | 632 | 350 | 359 | 343 |
| 0.55 | *** | 17856 | 19706 | 35668 | 3853 | 4359 | 5686 | 1194 | 1281 | 1413 | 570 | 595 | 624 | 330 | 339 | 348 |
| | *** | 18520 | 22330 | 36648 | 4064 | 4814 | 5803 | 1234 | 1340 | 1414 | 582 | 609 | 606 | 334 | 343 | 324 |
| 0.6 | *** | 16242 | 18354 | 34702 | 3663 | 4178 | 5494 | 1137 | 1222 | 1348 | 538 | 561 | 587 | 308 | 316 | 325 |
| | *** | 17021 | 21174 | 35384 | 3880 | 4633 | 5565 | 1177 | 1278 | 1340 | 550 | 573 | 566 | 312 | 320 | 298 |
| 0.65 | *** | 14534 | 16840 | 32928 | 3422 | 3926 | 5171 | 1059 | 1137 | 1253 | 494 | 514 | 538 | 278 | 285 | 292 |
| | *** | 15404 | 19752 | 33375 | 3635 | 4363 | 5208 | 1095 | 1188 | 1235 | 505 | 525 | 513 | 281 | 288 | 265 |
| 0.7 | *** | 12810 | 15204 | 30354 | 3130 | 3602 | 4721 | 957 | 1026 | 1123 | 438 | 455 | 474 | 241 | 247 | 253 |
| | *** | 13732 | 18089 | 30622 | 3331 | 4003 | 4732 | 989 | 1070 | 1102 | 446 | 464 | 447 | 244 | 250 | 224 |
| 0.75 | *** | 11105 | 13457 | 26985 | 2786 | 3205 | 4144 | 832 | 887 | 964 | 370 | 382 | 396 | 196 | 201 | 205 |
| | *** | 12023 | 16190 | 27126 | 2966 | 3552 | 4137 | 857 | 922 | 938 | 375 | 389 | 368 | 199 | 202 | 175 |
| 0.8 | *** | 9406 | 11581 | 22830 | 2379 | 2725 | 3442 | 680 | 721 | 773 | 288 | 295 | 305 | . | . | . |
| | *** | 10265 | 14020 | 22885 | 2530 | 2999 | 3423 | 700 | 745 | 744 | 292 | 299 | 275 | . | . | . |
| 0.85 | *** | 7660 | 9510 | 17895 | 1898 | 2148 | 2615 | 499 | 523 | 551 | . | . | . | . | . | . |
| | *** | 8399 | 11505 | 17900 | 2008 | 2337 | 2590 | 510 | 536 | 521 | . | . | . | . | . | . |
| 0.9 | *** | 5744 | 7106 | 12192 | 1309 | 1447 | 1666 | . | . | . | . | . | . | . | . | . |
| | *** | 6297 | 8489 | 12172 | 1371 | 1541 | 1637 | . | . | . | . | . | . | . | . | . |
| 0.95 | *** | 3346 | 4006 | 5729 | . | . | . | . | . | . | . | . | . | . | . | . |
| | *** | 3624 | 4591 | 5699 | . | . | . | . | . | . | . | . | . | . | . | . |

TABLE 2: ALPHA= 0.005 POWER= 0.9    EXPECTED ACCRUAL THRU MINIMUM FOLLOW-UP= 2500

| | | DEL=.02 | | | DEL=.05 | | | DEL=.10 | | | DEL=.15 | | | DEL=.20 | | |
|---|---|---|---|---|---|---|---|---|---|---|---|---|---|---|---|---|
| FACT= | | 1.0 .75 | .50 .25 | .00 BIN | 1.0 .75 | .50 .25 | .00 BIN | 1.0 .75 | .50 .25 | .00 BIN | 1.0 75 | .50 .25 | .00 BIN | 1.0 .75 | .50 .25 | .00 BIN |
| PCONT=*** | | | | | REQUIRED NUMBER OF PATIENTS | | | | | | | | | | | |
| 0.05 | *** | 4270 | 4314 | 4483 | 926 | 936 | 951 | 334 | 336 | 337 | 195 | 196 | 196 | 137 | 139 | 139 |
| | *** | 4286 | 4367 | 8378 | 931 | 942 | 1637 | 334 | 337 | 521 | 195 | 196 | 275 | 137 | 139 | 175 |
| 0.1 | *** | 8895 | 9014 | 9848 | 1721 | 1762 | 1833 | 549 | 558 | 565 | 295 | 298 | 299 | 195 | 195 | 196 |
| | *** | 8936 | 9201 | 14553 | 1739 | 1792 | 2590 | 552 | 561 | 744 | 296 | 298 | 368 | 195 | 196 | 224 |
| 0.15 | *** | 13018 | 13233 | 15229 | 2426 | 2512 | 2687 | 740 | 756 | 776 | 381 | 386 | 390 | 242 | 243 | 246 |
| | *** | 13092 | 13599 | 19984 | 2464 | 2583 | 3423 | 746 | 765 | 938 | 383 | 389 | 447 | 243 | 245 | 265 |
| 0.2 | *** | 16333 | 16664 | 20236 | 3006 | 3149 | 3467 | 899 | 926 | 961 | 452 | 461 | 470 | 281 | 284 | 287 |
| | *** | 16443 | 17246 | 24671 | 3067 | 3271 | 4137 | 912 | 942 | 1102 | 456 | 464 | 513 | 283 | 286 | 298 |
| 0.25 | *** | 18751 | 19226 | 24673 | 3456 | 3662 | 4148 | 1029 | 1067 | 1120 | 509 | 521 | 534 | 312 | 315 | 321 |
| | *** | 18911 | 20067 | 28614 | 3542 | 3842 | 4732 | 1046 | 1090 | 1235 | 515 | 527 | 566 | 314 | 318 | 324 |
| 0.3 | *** | 20293 | 20943 | 28436 | 3781 | 4051 | 4717 | 1127 | 1177 | 1248 | 552 | 568 | 586 | 334 | 340 | 346 |
| | *** | 20512 | 22076 | 31813 | 3893 | 4293 | 5208 | 1151 | 1209 | 1340 | 561 | 576 | 606 | 337 | 343 | 343 |
| 0.35 | *** | 21027 | 21887 | 31462 | 3990 | 4324 | 5165 | 1196 | 1258 | 1345 | 583 | 601 | 621 | 348 | 356 | 364 |
| | *** | 21318 | 23342 | 34268 | 4129 | 4624 | 5565 | 1224 | 1296 | 1414 | 592 | 611 | 632 | 352 | 359 | 354 |
| 0.4 | *** | 21051 | 22156 | 33714 | 4098 | 4492 | 5489 | 1237 | 1309 | 1411 | 599 | 620 | 643 | 356 | 364 | 371 |
| | *** | 21429 | 23952 | 35979 | 4262 | 4843 | 5803 | 1270 | 1354 | 1459 | 609 | 631 | 645 | 359 | 367 | 358 |
| 0.45 | *** | 20483 | 21865 | 35171 | 4115 | 4559 | 5684 | 1252 | 1331 | 1443 | 604 | 626 | 651 | 356 | 364 | 371 |
| | *** | 20962 | 24004 | 36946 | 4301 | 4954 | 5922 | 1289 | 1381 | 1474 | 614 | 639 | 645 | 359 | 367 | 354 |
| 0.5 | *** | 19448 | 21129 | 35824 | 4056 | 4537 | 5749 | 1243 | 1324 | 1445 | 595 | 618 | 645 | 346 | 356 | 364 |
| | *** | 20045 | 23587 | 37169 | 4259 | 4962 | 5922 | 1281 | 1377 | 1459 | 606 | 631 | 632 | 351 | 359 | 343 |
| 0.55 | *** | 18083 | 20059 | 35667 | 3929 | 4434 | 5687 | 1209 | 1292 | 1412 | 574 | 596 | 623 | 333 | 340 | 348 |
| | *** | 18799 | 22779 | 36648 | 4142 | 4874 | 5803 | 1246 | 1345 | 1414 | 586 | 609 | 606 | 336 | 343 | 324 |
| 0.6 | *** | 16511 | 18743 | 34701 | 3743 | 4252 | 5493 | 1152 | 1233 | 1348 | 543 | 564 | 589 | 309 | 317 | 324 |
| | *** | 17342 | 21645 | 35384 | 3959 | 4693 | 5565 | 1189 | 1284 | 1340 | 552 | 574 | 566 | 314 | 320 | 298 |
| 0.65 | *** | 14837 | 17249 | 32927 | 3499 | 3998 | 5171 | 1073 | 1146 | 1252 | 498 | 517 | 539 | 279 | 286 | 292 |
| | *** | 15754 | 20229 | 33375 | 3712 | 4420 | 5208 | 1108 | 1193 | 1235 | 508 | 526 | 513 | 283 | 289 | 265 |
| 0.7 | *** | 13136 | 15617 | 30354 | 3204 | 3668 | 4721 | 970 | 1034 | 1123 | 442 | 456 | 474 | 242 | 248 | 252 |
| | *** | 14095 | 18556 | 30622 | 3402 | 4056 | 4732 | 999 | 1074 | 1102 | 448 | 465 | 447 | 245 | 249 | 224 |
| 0.75 | *** | 11431 | 13852 | 26986 | 2851 | 3262 | 4145 | 842 | 895 | 964 | 371 | 384 | 396 | 198 | 201 | 204 |
| | *** | 12381 | 16623 | 27126 | 3029 | 3595 | 4137 | 867 | 926 | 938 | 377 | 390 | 368 | 199 | 202 | 175 |
| 0.8 | *** | 9714 | 11939 | 22831 | 2436 | 2771 | 3442 | 689 | 724 | 773 | 289 | 296 | 304 | . | . | . |
| | *** | 10596 | 14399 | 22885 | 2583 | 3034 | 3423 | 706 | 748 | 744 | 293 | 299 | 275 | . | . | . |
| 0.85 | *** | 7926 | 9809 | 17896 | 1940 | 2181 | 2615 | 504 | 524 | 551 | . | . | . | . | . | . |
| | *** | 8683 | 11809 | 17900 | 2046 | 2359 | 2590 | 514 | 537 | 521 | . | . | . | . | . | . |
| 0.9 | *** | 5943 | 7318 | 12192 | 1333 | 1464 | 1667 | . | . | . | . | . | . | . | . | . |
| | *** | 6504 | 8692 | 12172 | 1392 | 1551 | 1637 | . | . | . | . | . | . | . | . | . |
| 0.95 | *** | 3448 | 4101 | 5727 | . | . | . | . | . | . | . | . | . | . | . | . |
| | *** | 3724 | 4668 | 5699 | . | . | . | . | . | . | . | . | . | . | . | . |

## TABLE 2: ALPHA= 0.005 POWER= 0.9     EXPECTED ACCRUAL THRU MINIMUM FOLLOW-UP= 2750

|  |  | DEL=.02 | | | DEL=.05 | | | DEL=.10 | | | DEL=.15 | | | DEL=.20 | | |
|---|---|---|---|---|---|---|---|---|---|---|---|---|---|---|---|---|
| FACT= | | 1.0 / .75 | .50 / .25 | .00 / BIN | 1.0 / .75 | .50 / .25 | .00 / BIN | 1.0 / .75 | .50 / .25 | .00 / BIN | 1.0 / 75 | .50 / .25 | .00 / BIN | 1.0 / .75 | .50 / .25 | .00 / BIN |
| PCONT=*** | | REQUIRED NUMBER OF PATIENTS | | | | | | | | | | | | | | |
| 0.05 | *** | 4275 | 4320 | 4482 | 927 | 936 | 950 | 333 | 336 | 338 | 195 | 195 | 197 | 137 | 139 | 139 |
|  | *** | 4291 | 4374 | 8378 | 931 | 943 | 1637 | 335 | 336 | 521 | 195 | 197 | 275 | 137 | 139 | 175 |
| 0.1 | *** | 8908 | 9036 | 9848 | 1727 | 1766 | 1834 | 551 | 558 | 565 | 295 | 297 | 300 | 194 | 195 | 197 |
|  | *** | 8953 | 9231 | 14553 | 1745 | 1796 | 2590 | 555 | 562 | 744 | 297 | 298 | 368 | 195 | 195 | 224 |
| 0.15 | *** | 13041 | 13274 | 15229 | 2439 | 2522 | 2687 | 742 | 758 | 775 | 381 | 386 | 391 | 242 | 243 | 247 |
|  | *** | 13120 | 13660 | 19984 | 2474 | 2590 | 3423 | 749 | 766 | 938 | 383 | 388 | 447 | 243 | 245 | 265 |
| 0.2 | *** | 16365 | 16728 | 20236 | 3026 | 3169 | 3466 | 903 | 929 | 962 | 453 | 460 | 469 | 281 | 285 | 288 |
|  | *** | 16488 | 17347 | 24671 | 3086 | 3285 | 4137 | 916 | 943 | 1102 | 456 | 465 | 513 | 283 | 287 | 298 |
| 0.25 | *** | 18799 | 19320 | 24674 | 3484 | 3690 | 4148 | 1036 | 1070 | 1120 | 511 | 522 | 534 | 312 | 315 | 321 |
|  | *** | 18974 | 20210 | 28614 | 3571 | 3863 | 4732 | 1051 | 1092 | 1235 | 517 | 527 | 566 | 314 | 319 | 324 |
| 0.3 | *** | 20360 | 21070 | 28436 | 3817 | 4089 | 4718 | 1136 | 1182 | 1247 | 555 | 569 | 586 | 335 | 340 | 346 |
|  | *** | 20600 | 22267 | 31813 | 3930 | 4320 | 5208 | 1158 | 1213 | 1340 | 562 | 577 | 606 | 338 | 343 | 343 |
| 0.35 | *** | 21114 | 22051 | 31461 | 4035 | 4370 | 5166 | 1206 | 1264 | 1345 | 586 | 603 | 621 | 350 | 355 | 364 |
|  | *** | 21434 | 23584 | 34268 | 4176 | 4660 | 5565 | 1233 | 1301 | 1414 | 594 | 611 | 632 | 353 | 359 | 354 |
| 0.4 | *** | 21166 | 22362 | 33714 | 4152 | 4544 | 5489 | 1249 | 1316 | 1411 | 603 | 621 | 644 | 357 | 364 | 373 |
|  | *** | 21579 | 24247 | 35979 | 4315 | 4884 | 5803 | 1280 | 1359 | 1459 | 611 | 632 | 645 | 360 | 367 | 358 |
| 0.45 | *** | 20628 | 22116 | 35172 | 4178 | 4618 | 5684 | 1264 | 1339 | 1443 | 608 | 627 | 652 | 357 | 364 | 373 |
|  | *** | 21150 | 24347 | 36946 | 4361 | 5001 | 5922 | 1299 | 1387 | 1474 | 617 | 639 | 645 | 360 | 367 | 354 |
| 0.5 | *** | 19631 | 21425 | 35825 | 4123 | 4601 | 5750 | 1256 | 1333 | 1445 | 599 | 620 | 645 | 349 | 355 | 364 |
|  | *** | 20274 | 23971 | 37169 | 4326 | 5013 | 5922 | 1292 | 1383 | 1459 | 610 | 632 | 632 | 352 | 360 | 343 |
| 0.55 | *** | 18304 | 20394 | 35667 | 4000 | 4499 | 5687 | 1222 | 1301 | 1412 | 579 | 599 | 624 | 333 | 340 | 349 |
|  | *** | 19070 | 23194 | 36648 | 4212 | 4927 | 5803 | 1257 | 1350 | 1414 | 589 | 611 | 606 | 336 | 345 | 324 |
| 0.6 | *** | 16769 | 19108 | 34701 | 3815 | 4319 | 5492 | 1165 | 1240 | 1349 | 546 | 565 | 587 | 311 | 318 | 324 |
|  | *** | 17647 | 22078 | 35384 | 4028 | 4745 | 5565 | 1201 | 1290 | 1340 | 555 | 577 | 566 | 314 | 321 | 298 |
| 0.65 | *** | 15128 | 17632 | 32929 | 3571 | 4061 | 5171 | 1084 | 1154 | 1253 | 501 | 518 | 538 | 281 | 287 | 291 |
|  | *** | 16085 | 20668 | 33375 | 3780 | 4470 | 5208 | 1116 | 1199 | 1235 | 510 | 527 | 513 | 283 | 290 | 265 |
| 0.7 | *** | 13442 | 15999 | 30354 | 3270 | 3728 | 4721 | 979 | 1041 | 1123 | 445 | 459 | 474 | 243 | 247 | 252 |
|  | *** | 14435 | 18981 | 30622 | 3468 | 4100 | 4732 | 1009 | 1079 | 1102 | 452 | 465 | 447 | 245 | 250 | 224 |
| 0.75 | *** | 11737 | 14219 | 26986 | 2911 | 3313 | 4145 | 850 | 900 | 964 | 374 | 384 | 397 | 199 | 202 | 204 |
|  | *** | 12715 | 17017 | 27126 | 3086 | 3633 | 4137 | 874 | 929 | 938 | 379 | 390 | 368 | 201 | 202 | 175 |
| 0.8 | *** | 9999 | 12268 | 22830 | 2485 | 2813 | 3442 | 694 | 728 | 773 | 290 | 297 | 304 | . | . | . |
|  | *** | 10903 | 14743 | 22885 | 2629 | 3064 | 3423 | 711 | 749 | 744 | 294 | 300 | 275 | . | . | . |
| 0.85 | *** | 8172 | 10081 | 17897 | 1976 | 2210 | 2615 | 507 | 527 | 551 | . | . | . | . | . | . |
|  | *** | 8940 | 12081 | 17900 | 2081 | 2378 | 2590 | 517 | 538 | 521 | . | . | . | . | . | . |
| 0.9 | *** | 6127 | 7512 | 12192 | 1352 | 1477 | 1666 | . | . | . | . | . | . | . | . | . |
|  | *** | 6694 | 8870 | 12172 | 1411 | 1560 | 1637 | . | . | . | . | . | . | . | . | . |
| 0.95 | *** | 3540 | 4186 | 5728 | . | . | . | . | . | . | . | . | . | . | . | . |
|  | *** | 3815 | 4736 | 5699 | . | . | . | . | . | . | . | . | . | . | . | . |

TABLE 2: ALPHA= 0.005 POWER= 0.9    EXPECTED ACCRUAL THRU MINIMUM FOLLOW-UP= 3000

| | | DEL=.01 | | | DEL=.02 | | | DEL=.05 | | | DEL=.10 | | | DEL=.15 | | |
|---|---|---|---|---|---|---|---|---|---|---|---|---|---|---|---|---|
| FACT= | | 1.0 .75 | .50 .25 | .00 BIN | 1.0 .75 | .50 .25 | .00 BIN | 1.0 .75 | .50 .25 | .00 BIN | 1.0 75 | .50 .25 | .00 BIN | 1.0 .75 | .50 .25 | .00 BIN |
| PCONT=*** | | REQUIRED NUMBER OF PATIENTS | | | | | | | | | | | | | | |
| 0.01 | *** | 2270 2278 | | 2293 | 835 838 | | 842 | 275 275 | | 275 | 140 140 | | 140 | 100 100 | | 100 |
| | *** | 2275 2285 | | 8779 | 835 838 | | 2902 | 275 275 | | 790 | 140 140 | | 321 | 100 100 | | 191 |
| 0.02 | *** | 5015 5035 | | 5120 | 1610 1618 | | 1637 | 437 437 | | 440 | 193 193 | | 193 | 125 125 | | 125 |
| | *** | 5023 5057 | | 14493 | 1615 1625 | | 4316 | 437 440 | | 1009 | 193 193 | | 373 | 125 125 | | 213 |
| 0.05 | *** | 15178 15235 | | 15995 | 4280 4325 | | 4483 | 928 935 | | 950 | 332 335 | | 335 | 197 197 | | 197 |
| | *** | 15197 15340 | | 30920 | 4295 4378 | | 8378 | 932 943 | | 1637 | 335 335 | | 521 | 197 197 | | 275 |
| 0.1 | *** | 33470 33610 | | 37232 | 8920 9058 | | 9845 | 1735 1772 | | 1832 | 553 557 | | 565 | 295 298 | | 298 |
| | *** | 33515 33887 | | 55917 | 8968 9257 | | 14553 | 1750 1798 | | 2590 | 553 560 | | 744 | 298 298 | | 368 |
| 0.15 | *** | 49955 50207 | | 58817 | 13063 13315 | | 15230 | 2450 2533 | | 2687 | 745 760 | | 775 | 380 385 | | 392 |
| | *** | 50042 50705 | | 77939 | 13150 13715 | | 19984 | 2485 2597 | | 3423 | 752 767 | | 938 | 385 388 | | 447 |
| 0.2 | *** | 63220 63605 | | 79018 | 16397 16790 | | 20237 | 3043 3185 | | 3467 | 910 932 | | 962 | 455 460 | | 470 |
| | *** | 63347 64382 | | 96984 | 16532 17440 | | 24671 | 3103 3298 | | 4137 | 917 943 | | 1102 | 455 463 | | 513 |
| 0.25 | *** | 72842 73405 | | 97010 | 18845 19408 | | 24673 | 3508 3715 | | 4150 | 1040 1075 | | 1120 | 512 523 | | 535 |
| | *** | 73030 74522 | | 113054 | 19037 20345 | | 28614 | 3595 3883 | | 4732 | 1055 1097 | | 1235 | 515 527 | | 566 |
| 0.3 | *** | 78857 79625 | | 112337 | 20425 21193 | | 28435 | 3850 4120 | | 4715 | 1142 1187 | | 1247 | 557 568 | | 583 |
| | *** | 79112 81167 | | 126148 | 20687 22450 | | 31813 | 3965 4345 | | 5208 | 1165 1213 | | 1340 | 565 575 | | 606 |
| 0.35 | *** | 81497 82525 | | 124738 | 21200 22210 | | 31460 | 4078 4408 | | 5165 | 1213 1270 | | 1345 | 587 602 | | 620 |
| | *** | 81838 84575 | | 136266 | 21550 23815 | | 34268 | 4217 4690 | | 5565 | 1240 1303 | | 1414 | 595 613 | | 632 |
| 0.4 | *** | 81122 82465 | | 134057 | 21280 22562 | | 33715 | 4202 4592 | | 5488 | 1258 1322 | | 1412 | 605 625 | | 643 |
| | *** | 81568 85142 | | 143408 | 21725 24523 | | 35979 | 4367 4922 | | 5803 | 1288 1363 | | 1459 | 613 632 | | 645 |
| 0.45 | *** | 78160 79892 | | 140207 | 20773 22360 | | 35173 | 4232 4670 | | 5683 | 1277 1345 | | 1442 | 610 628 | | 650 |
| | *** | 78737 83327 | | 147574 | 21335 24665 | | 36946 | 4420 5042 | | 5922 | 1307 1390 | | 1474 | 620 640 | | 645 |
| 0.5 | *** | 73082 75298 | | 143140 | 19810 21707 | | 35825 | 4183 4655 | | 5750 | 1265 1340 | | 1445 | 602 620 | | 643 |
| | *** | 73825 79637 | | 148765 | 20495 24328 | | 37169 | 4385 5057 | | 5922 | 1300 1390 | | 1459 | 613 632 | | 632 |
| 0.55 | *** | 66403 69223 | | 142835 | 18520 20713 | | 35668 | 4063 4558 | | 5687 | 1232 1307 | | 1412 | 583 602 | | 625 |
| | *** | 67345 74590 | | 146979 | 19330 23578 | | 36648 | 4273 4975 | | 5803 | 1270 1355 | | 1414 | 590 613 | | 606 |
| 0.6 | *** | 58645 62215 | | 139292 | 17020 19453 | | 34700 | 3880 4378 | | 5492 | 1175 1247 | | 1348 | 550 568 | | 587 |
| | *** | 59845 68660 | | 142218 | 17938 22480 | | 35384 | 4093 4790 | | 5565 | 1210 1292 | | 1340 | 557 575 | | 566 |
| 0.65 | *** | 50372 54823 | | 132520 | 15403 17987 | | 32927 | 3635 4120 | | 5170 | 1093 1160 | | 1250 | 505 520 | | 538 |
| | *** | 51898 62233 | | 134480 | 16400 21070 | | 33375 | 3842 4513 | | 5208 | 1127 1202 | | 1235 | 512 527 | | 513 |
| 0.7 | *** | 42167 47500 | | 122545 | 13730 16355 | | 30355 | 3332 3778 | | 4720 | 988 1048 | | 1123 | 445 460 | | 475 |
| | *** | 44057 55562 | | 123767 | 14755 19370 | | 30622 | 3523 4138 | | 4732 | 1015 1082 | | 1102 | 452 467 | | 447 |
| 0.75 | *** | 34550 40510 | | 109385 | 12025 14555 | | 26987 | 2965 3358 | | 4145 | 857 905 | | 962 | 377 385 | | 395 |
| | *** | 36740 48748 | | 110078 | 13025 17375 | | 27126 | 3137 3665 | | 4137 | 880 932 | | 938 | 380 392 | | 368 |
| 0.8 | *** | 27800 33880 | | 93077 | 10265 12572 | | 22828 | 2530 2848 | | 3440 | 700 733 | | 770 | 290 298 | | 305 |
| | *** | 30100 41747 | | 93413 | 11188 15055 | | 22885 | 2672 3088 | | 3423 | 715 752 | | 744 | 295 302 | | 275 |
| 0.85 | *** | 21815 27430 | | 73652 | 8398 10333 | | 17897 | 2008 2233 | | 2615 | 508 527 | | 550 | . . | | . |
| | *** | 23980 34348 | | 73773 | 9182 12328 | | 17900 | 2110 2395 | | 2590 | 520 538 | | 521 | . . | | . |
| 0.9 | *** | 16187 20725 | | 51145 | 6298 7685 | | 12193 | 1370 1490 | | 1667 | . . | | . | . . | | . |
| | *** | 17960 26068 | | 51156 | 6868 9032 | | 12172 | 1427 1570 | | 1637 | . . | | . | . . | | . |
| 0.95 | *** | 10030 12760 | | 25588 | 3625 4262 | | 5728 | . . | | . | . . | | . | . . | | . |
| | *** | 11120 15725 | | 25563 | 3898 4795 | | 5699 | . . | | . | . . | | . | . . | | . |
| 0.98 | *** | 4892 5923 | | 8807 | . . | | . | . . | | . | . . | | . | . . | | . |
| | *** | 5323 6868 | | 8779 | . . | | . | . . | | . | . . | | . | . . | | . |

| TABLE 2: ALPHA= 0.005 POWER= 0.9 |  |  | EXPECTED ACCRUAL THRU MINIMUM FOLLOW-UP= 3250 |  |  |  |  |  |  |  |  |  |  |  |
|---|---|---|---|---|---|---|---|---|---|---|---|---|---|---|

| | | DEL=.01 | | | DEL=.02 | | | DEL=.05 | | | DEL=.10 | | | DEL=.15 | |
|---|---|---|---|---|---|---|---|---|---|---|---|---|---|---|---|
| FACT= | 1.0 .75 | .50 .25 | .00 BIN | 1.0 .75 | .50 .25 | .00 BIN | 1.0 .75 | .50 .25 | .00 BIN | 1.0 75 | .50 .25 | .00 BIN | 1.0 .75 | .50 .25 | .00 BIN |
| PCONT=*** | | | | REQUIRED NUMBER OF PATIENTS | | | | | | | | | | | |
| 0.01 *** | 2272 2272 | 2278 2286 | 2294 8779 | 834 834 | 839 839 | 839 2902 | 274 274 | 274 279 | 279 790 | 141 141 | 141 141 | 141 321 | 100 100 | 100 100 | 100 191 |
| 0.02 *** | 5019 5024 | 5035 5059 | 5121 14493 | 1611 1614 | 1619 1628 | 1636 4316 | 436 436 | 436 441 | 441 1009 | 192 192 | 192 192 | 192 373 | 124 124 | 124 127 | 127 213 |
| 0.05 *** | 15183 15204 | 15245 15359 | 15996 30920 | 4284 4304 | 4333 4385 | 4482 8378 | 929 932 | 937 945 | 948 1637 | 336 336 | 336 336 | 339 521 | 198 198 | 198 198 | 198 275 |
| 0.1 *** | 33481 33529 | 33632 33933 | 37231 55917 | 8932 8984 | 9078 9281 | 9845 14553 | 1736 1752 | 1774 1801 | 1834 2590 | 550 555 | 558 563 | 566 744 | 295 295 | 298 298 | 298 368 |
| 0.15 *** | 49979 50069 | 50248 50787 | 58814 77939 | 13084 13176 | 13352 13769 | 15229 19984 | 2459 2497 | 2541 2603 | 2687 3423 | 745 753 | 758 766 | 774 938 | 384 384 | 387 387 | 393 447 |
| 0.2 *** | 63251 63389 | 63670 64510 | 79018 96984 | 16431 16578 | 16854 17528 | 20237 24671 | 3061 3123 | 3199 3309 | 3467 4137 | 913 921 | 932 945 | 961 1102 | 458 458 | 461 466 | 469 513 |
| 0.25 *** | 72892 73090 | 73496 74707 | 97010 113054 | 18893 19099 | 19497 20472 | 24673 28614 | 3532 3621 | 3735 3897 | 4149 4732 | 1046 1059 | 1078 1094 | 1119 1235 | 514 517 | 523 531 | 534 566 |
| 0.3 *** | 78921 79200 | 79752 81423 | 112339 126148 | 20489 20773 | 21314 22617 | 28435 31813 | 3881 3995 | 4149 4369 | 4718 5208 | 1148 1167 | 1192 1216 | 1249 1340 | 558 566 | 571 579 | 582 606 |
| 0.35 *** | 81581 81951 | 82694 84917 | 124738 136266 | 21290 21664 | 22366 24028 | 31463 34268 | 4117 4255 | 4447 4718 | 5165 5565 | 1221 1246 | 1273 1306 | 1346 1414 | 591 599 | 604 612 | 620 632 |
| 0.4 *** | 81231 81719 | 82686 85583 | 134057 143408 | 21391 21870 | 22756 24784 | 33713 35979 | 4247 4409 | 4634 4954 | 5490 5803 | 1265 1294 | 1327 1368 | 1411 1459 | 607 615 | 623 631 | 644 645 |
| 0.45 *** | 78303 78929 | 80180 83888 | 140208 147574 | 20916 21512 | 22593 24966 | 35171 36946 | 4284 4471 | 4718 5081 | 5685 5922 | 1286 1314 | 1351 1395 | 1444 1474 | 612 620 | 631 639 | 653 645 |
| 0.5 *** | 73269 74070 | 75671 80329 | 143141 148765 | 19985 20713 | 21981 24662 | 35826 37169 | 4239 4439 | 4707 5097 | 5750 5922 | 1278 1311 | 1346 1392 | 1444 1459 | 604 615 | 623 631 | 644 632 |
| 0.55 *** | 66636 67659 | 69691 75422 | 142835 146979 | 18731 19584 | 21014 23939 | 35666 36648 | 4122 4333 | 4612 5016 | 5685 5803 | 1246 1278 | 1314 1359 | 1411 1414 | 582 591 | 604 612 | 623 606 |
| 0.6 *** | 58944 60244 | 62796 69618 | 139289 142218 | 17263 18219 | 19779 22850 | 34699 35384 | 3938 4149 | 4431 4832 | 5495 5565 | 1184 1216 | 1254 1297 | 1346 1340 | 550 558 | 566 579 | 588 566 |
| 0.65 *** | 50754 52401 | 55521 63288 | 132521 134480 | 15668 16694 | 18324 21444 | 32928 33375 | 3694 3897 | 4171 4553 | 5170 5208 | 1102 1132 | 1167 1205 | 1254 1235 | 506 514 | 523 531 | 539 513 |
| 0.7 *** | 42651 44661 | 48292 56661 | 122544 123767 | 14005 15058 | 16686 19730 | 30352 30622 | 3386 3578 | 3824 4174 | 4723 4732 | 997 1021 | 1051 1086 | 1124 1102 | 449 452 | 461 466 | 474 447 |
| 0.75 *** | 35122 37421 | 41346 49836 | 109384 110078 | 12296 13319 | 14874 17707 | 26986 27126 | 3012 3182 | 3399 3694 | 4146 4137 | 864 883 | 907 932 | 964 938 | 376 379 | 384 393 | 396 368 |
| 0.8 *** | 28408 30796 | 34699 42764 | 93077 93413 | 10516 11454 | 12856 15337 | 22829 22885 | 2570 2708 | 2882 3109 | 3442 3423 | 704 718 | 734 753 | 774 744 | 290 295 | 298 303 | 303 275 |
| 0.85 *** | 22395 24624 | 28164 35219 | 73651 73773 | 8615 9403 | 10565 12551 | 17897 17900 | 2037 2134 | 2256 2408 | 2614 2590 | 514 523 | 531 539 | 550 521 | . . | . . | . . |
| 0.9 *** | 16667 18482 | 21301 26726 | 51141 51156 | 6454 7031 | 7846 9176 | 12193 12172 | 1387 1441 | 1501 1574 | 1668 1637 | . . | . . | . . | . . | . . | . . |
| 0.95 *** | 10324 11434 | 13095 16069 | 25588 25563 | 3699 3971 | 4328 4848 | 5726 5699 | . . | . . | . . | . . | . . | . . | . . | . . | . . |
| 0.98 *** | 5011 5441 | 6039 6966 | 8810 8779 | . . | . . | . . | . . | . . | . . | . . | . . | . . | . . | . . | . . |

## TABLE 2: ALPHA= 0.005 POWER= 0.9    EXPECTED ACCRUAL THRU MINIMUM FOLLOW-UP= 3500

| | | DEL=.01 | | | DEL=.02 | | | DEL=.05 | | | DEL=.10 | | | DEL=.15 | | |
|---|---|---|---|---|---|---|---|---|---|---|---|---|---|---|---|---|---|
| FACT= | | 1.0 .75 | .50 .25 | .00 BIN | 1.0 .75 | .50 .25 | .00 BIN | 1.0 .75 | .50 .25 | .00 BIN | 1.0 75 | .50 .25 | .00 BIN | 1.0 .75 | .50 .25 | .00 BIN |
| PCONT=*** | | | | | REQUIRED NUMBER OF PATIENTS | | | | | | | | | | | |
| 0.01 | *** | 2272 2278 | 2278 2286 | 2295 8779 | 834 837 | 837 837 | 843 2902 | 277 277 | 277 277 | 277 790 | 137 137 | 137 137 | 137 321 | 99 99 | 99 99 | 99 191 |
| 0.02 | *** | 5020 5025 | 5037 5063 | 5121 14493 | 1613 1616 | 1621 1625 | 1633 4316 | 435 440 | 440 440 | 440 1009 | 190 190 | 190 190 | 190 373 | 125 125 | 125 125 | 125 213 |
| 0.05 | *** | 15187 15210 | 15254 15371 | 15998 30920 | 4290 4308 | 4337 4390 | 4483 8378 | 930 933 | 939 942 | 951 1637 | 335 335 | 335 335 | 338 521 | 195 195 | 195 195 | 195 275 |
| 0.1 | *** | 33492 33545 | 33655 33979 | 37234 55917 | 8945 8998 | 9097 9304 | 9846 14553 | 1744 1756 | 1779 1800 | 1831 2590 | 554 557 | 557 563 | 566 744 | 295 295 | 300 300 | 300 368 |
| 0.15 | *** | 50000 50096 | 50289 50870 | 58815 77939 | 13105 13206 | 13390 13819 | 15228 19984 | 2470 2505 | 2549 2605 | 2689 3423 | 746 755 | 758 767 | 776 938 | 382 382 | 388 388 | 391 447 |
| 0.2 | *** | 63283 63431 | 63732 64639 | 79018 96984 | 16465 16619 | 16911 17611 | 20236 24671 | 3077 3135 | 3214 3319 | 3468 4137 | 913 925 | 933 948 | 960 1102 | 458 458 | 461 466 | 470 513 |
| 0.25 | *** | 72937 73153 | 73590 74894 | 97008 113054 | 18941 19165 | 19585 20595 | 24672 28614 | 3555 3643 | 3756 3914 | 4150 4732 | 1047 1065 | 1079 1100 | 1117 1235 | 513 519 | 522 528 | 531 566 |
| 0.3 | *** | 78983 79286 | 79885 81675 | 112338 126148 | 20556 20857 | 21431 22782 | 28435 31813 | 3914 4022 | 4176 4386 | 4719 5208 | 1152 1175 | 1196 1219 | 1248 1340 | 563 566 | 571 580 | 583 606 |
| 0.35 | *** | 81666 82069 | 82865 85257 | 124737 136266 | 21379 21776 | 22516 24231 | 31462 34268 | 4153 4293 | 4477 4745 | 5165 5565 | 1228 1254 | 1280 1310 | 1345 1414 | 592 598 | 606 615 | 624 632 |
| 0.4 | *** | 81343 81868 | 82912 86024 | 134056 143408 | 21505 22012 | 22945 25028 | 33711 35979 | 4290 4451 | 4670 4981 | 5489 5803 | 1275 1301 | 1333 1368 | 1411 1459 | 610 618 | 627 636 | 645 645 |
| 0.45 | *** | 78446 79120 | 80468 84440 | 140207 147574 | 21055 21694 | 22817 25246 | 35172 36946 | 4334 4518 | 4763 5113 | 5685 5922 | 1292 1324 | 1359 1397 | 1441 1474 | 615 624 | 633 641 | 650 645 |
| 0.5 | *** | 73453 74316 | 76035 81013 | 143138 148765 | 20157 20924 | 22240 24970 | 35825 37169 | 4293 4491 | 4754 5130 | 5751 5922 | 1283 1318 | 1353 1394 | 1446 1459 | 606 615 | 624 633 | 645 632 |
| 0.55 | *** | 66873 67973 | 70151 76233 | 142832 146979 | 18938 19825 | 21303 24270 | 35668 36648 | 4176 4386 | 4658 5051 | 5685 5803 | 1254 1283 | 1318 1362 | 1411 1414 | 589 592 | 601 615 | 624 606 |
| 0.6 | *** | 59243 60640 | 63370 70545 | 139288 142218 | 17494 18486 | 20087 23199 | 34700 35384 | 3993 4203 | 4477 4868 | 5492 5565 | 1196 1228 | 1263 1301 | 1350 1340 | 554 563 | 571 580 | 589 566 |
| 0.65 | *** | 51138 52896 | 56204 64292 | 132521 134480 | 15922 16978 | 18640 21790 | 32929 33375 | 3748 3949 | 4215 4588 | 5168 5208 | 1114 1140 | 1170 1210 | 1254 1235 | 510 513 | 522 531 | 536 513 |
| 0.7 | *** | 43126 45252 | 49058 57709 | 122546 123767 | 14268 15345 | 17004 20061 | 30356 30622 | 3436 3625 | 3870 4203 | 4722 4732 | 1003 1030 | 1056 1088 | 1123 1102 | 449 452 | 461 466 | 475 447 |
| 0.75 | *** | 35676 38077 | 42151 50866 | 109386 110078 | 12550 13591 | 15170 18010 | 26988 27126 | 3056 3223 | 3436 3721 | 4145 4137 | 869 890 | 913 933 | 965 938 | 379 382 | 388 391 | 396 368 |
| 0.8 | *** | 28991 31462 | 35478 43718 | 93076 93413 | 10751 11705 | 13119 15604 | 22831 22885 | 2605 2741 | 2911 3130 | 3441 3423 | 706 720 | 738 755 | 773 744 | 291 295 | 300 300 | 303 275 |
| 0.85 | *** | 22945 25238 | 28860 36038 | 73651 73773 | 8814 9613 | 10777 12755 | 17896 17900 | 2062 2158 | 2278 2421 | 2613 2590 | 513 522 | 531 540 | 548 521 | . . | . . | . . |
| 0.9 | *** | 17118 18976 | 21851 27341 | 51141 51156 | 6600 7178 | 7995 9307 | 12191 12172 | 1403 1450 | 1511 1581 | 1665 1637 | . . | . . | . . | . . | . . | . . |
| 0.95 | *** | 10608 11731 | 13408 16386 | 25588 25563 | 3768 4040 | 4390 4894 | 5728 5699 | . . | . . | . . | . . | . . | . . | . . | . . | . . |
| 0.98 | *** | 5121 5553 | 6145 7050 | 8808 8779 | . . | . . | . . | . . | . . | . . | . . | . . | . . | . . | . . | . . |

## TABLE 2: ALPHA= 0.005 POWER= 0.9    EXPECTED ACCRUAL THRU MINIMUM FOLLOW-UP= 3750

PCONT=***  REQUIRED NUMBER OF PATIENTS

| | | DEL=.01 | | | DEL=.02 | | | DEL=.05 | | | DEL=.10 | | | DEL=.15 | | |
|---|---|---|---|---|---|---|---|---|---|---|---|---|---|---|---|---|
| FACT= | | 1.0 .75 | .50 .25 | .00 BIN | 1.0 .75 | .50 .25 | .00 BIN | 1.0 .75 | .50 .25 | .00 BIN | 1.0 75 | .50 .25 | .00 BIN | 1.0 .75 | .50 .25 | .00 BIN |
| 0.01 | *** | 2272 | 2281 | 2294 | 837 | 837 | 841 | 275 | 275 | 278 | 138 | 138 | 138 | 97 | 97 | 97 |
| | *** | 2275 | 2284 | 8779 | 837 | 841 | 2902 | 275 | 275 | 790 | 138 | 138 | 321 | 97 | 97 | 191 |
| 0.02 | *** | 5022 | 5041 | 5122 | 1615 | 1619 | 1634 | 438 | 438 | 438 | 190 | 190 | 190 | 125 | 125 | 125 |
| | *** | 5028 | 5065 | 14493 | 1615 | 1628 | 4316 | 438 | 438 | 1009 | 190 | 190 | 373 | 125 | 125 | 213 |
| 0.05 | *** | 15190 | 15259 | 15997 | 4291 | 4343 | 4484 | 931 | 940 | 950 | 334 | 334 | 334 | 194 | 194 | 194 |
| | *** | 15213 | 15387 | 30920 | 4315 | 4394 | 8378 | 934 | 944 | 1637 | 334 | 334 | 521 | 194 | 194 | 275 |
| 0.1 | *** | 33503 | 33678 | 37231 | 8956 | 9115 | 9847 | 1747 | 1778 | 1831 | 556 | 559 | 565 | 297 | 297 | 297 |
| | *** | 33559 | 34025 | 55917 | 9012 | 9325 | 14553 | 1759 | 1803 | 2590 | 556 | 559 | 744 | 297 | 297 | 368 |
| 0.15 | *** | 50018 | 50331 | 58816 | 13128 | 13428 | 15228 | 2478 | 2556 | 2688 | 747 | 762 | 775 | 381 | 387 | 391 |
| | *** | 50122 | 50950 | 77939 | 13231 | 13868 | 19984 | 2509 | 2613 | 3423 | 756 | 766 | 938 | 387 | 387 | 447 |
| 0.2 | *** | 63316 | 63800 | 79019 | 16497 | 16972 | 20234 | 3091 | 3222 | 3466 | 916 | 934 | 959 | 456 | 462 | 472 |
| | *** | 63475 | 64765 | 96984 | 16662 | 17688 | 24671 | 3147 | 3325 | 4137 | 925 | 950 | 1102 | 462 | 466 | 513 |
| 0.25 | *** | 72981 | 73681 | 97009 | 18991 | 19672 | 24672 | 3578 | 3772 | 4147 | 1053 | 1081 | 1118 | 518 | 522 | 531 |
| | *** | 73216 | 75078 | 113054 | 19225 | 20706 | 28614 | 3663 | 3925 | 4732 | 1066 | 1100 | 1235 | 522 | 528 | 566 |
| 0.3 | *** | 79047 | 80013 | 112338 | 20622 | 21547 | 28437 | 3940 | 4197 | 4718 | 1159 | 1197 | 1250 | 559 | 575 | 584 |
| | *** | 79372 | 81931 | 126148 | 20941 | 22934 | 31813 | 4053 | 4403 | 5208 | 1178 | 1222 | 1340 | 569 | 578 | 606 |
| 0.35 | *** | 81753 | 83037 | 124737 | 21462 | 22666 | 31459 | 4188 | 4506 | 5163 | 1234 | 1281 | 1343 | 593 | 606 | 622 |
| | *** | 82178 | 85591 | 136266 | 21888 | 24425 | 34268 | 4325 | 4765 | 5565 | 1259 | 1309 | 1414 | 603 | 612 | 632 |
| 0.4 | *** | 81456 | 83134 | 134056 | 21616 | 23125 | 33715 | 4328 | 4703 | 5487 | 1281 | 1338 | 1409 | 612 | 625 | 644 |
| | *** | 82015 | 86459 | 143408 | 22156 | 25259 | 35979 | 4493 | 5009 | 5803 | 1309 | 1372 | 1459 | 622 | 634 | 645 |
| 0.45 | *** | 78593 | 80759 | 140206 | 21194 | 23031 | 35172 | 4375 | 4797 | 5684 | 1300 | 1362 | 1441 | 616 | 634 | 650 |
| | *** | 79315 | 84991 | 147574 | 21865 | 25512 | 36946 | 4559 | 5140 | 5922 | 1328 | 1400 | 1474 | 625 | 640 | 645 |
| 0.5 | *** | 73638 | 76403 | 143140 | 20331 | 22488 | 35825 | 4338 | 4797 | 5750 | 1297 | 1356 | 1447 | 612 | 625 | 644 |
| | *** | 74562 | 81681 | 148765 | 21128 | 25263 | 37169 | 4534 | 5163 | 5922 | 1325 | 1400 | 1459 | 616 | 634 | 632 |
| 0.55 | *** | 67109 | 70615 | 142834 | 19137 | 21578 | 35665 | 4225 | 4703 | 5688 | 1259 | 1325 | 1413 | 588 | 606 | 622 |
| | *** | 68284 | 77022 | 146979 | 20059 | 24584 | 36648 | 4431 | 5084 | 5803 | 1291 | 1366 | 1414 | 597 | 612 | 606 |
| 0.6 | *** | 59543 | 63934 | 139291 | 17722 | 20378 | 34700 | 4043 | 4522 | 5491 | 1203 | 1263 | 1347 | 556 | 569 | 588 |
| | *** | 61038 | 71434 | 142218 | 18743 | 23519 | 35384 | 4253 | 4900 | 5565 | 1231 | 1306 | 1340 | 565 | 578 | 566 |
| 0.65 | *** | 51518 | 56872 | 132522 | 16165 | 18940 | 32928 | 3794 | 4259 | 5172 | 1118 | 1178 | 1253 | 509 | 522 | 537 |
| | *** | 53388 | 65262 | 134480 | 17247 | 22109 | 33375 | 3997 | 4615 | 5208 | 1147 | 1212 | 1235 | 518 | 531 | 513 |
| 0.7 | *** | 43597 | 49797 | 122543 | 14519 | 17294 | 30353 | 3481 | 3906 | 4722 | 1009 | 1062 | 1122 | 453 | 462 | 475 |
| | *** | 45837 | 58703 | 123767 | 15616 | 20369 | 30622 | 3668 | 4231 | 4732 | 1034 | 1090 | 1102 | 456 | 466 | 447 |
| 0.75 | *** | 36213 | 42922 | 109384 | 12794 | 15447 | 26984 | 3100 | 3472 | 4147 | 875 | 916 | 963 | 378 | 387 | 397 |
| | *** | 38716 | 51847 | 110078 | 13853 | 18293 | 27126 | 3259 | 3743 | 4137 | 893 | 940 | 938 | 381 | 391 | 368 |
| 0.8 | *** | 29556 | 36228 | 93078 | 10975 | 13366 | 22831 | 2641 | 2937 | 3443 | 709 | 738 | 772 | 293 | 297 | 303 |
| | *** | 32103 | 44622 | 93413 | 11937 | 15847 | 22885 | 2772 | 3147 | 3423 | 725 | 756 | 744 | 297 | 303 | 275 |
| 0.85 | *** | 23472 | 29519 | 73653 | 9003 | 10975 | 17894 | 2088 | 2294 | 2613 | 518 | 531 | 550 | . | . | . |
| | *** | 25822 | 36809 | 73773 | 9809 | 12944 | 17900 | 2181 | 2431 | 2590 | 522 | 541 | 521 | . | . | . |
| 0.9 | *** | 17547 | 22366 | 51143 | 6738 | 8131 | 12190 | 1413 | 1522 | 1666 | . | . | . | . | . | . |
| | *** | 19447 | 27912 | 51156 | 7319 | 9425 | 12172 | 1465 | 1587 | 1637 | . | . | . | . | . | . |
| 0.95 | *** | 10868 | 13703 | 25587 | 3837 | 4447 | 5725 | . | . | . | . | . | . | . | . | . |
| | *** | 12012 | 16681 | 25563 | 4100 | 4938 | 5699 | . | . | . | . | . | . | . | . | . |
| 0.98 | *** | 5225 | 6241 | 8809 | . | . | . | . | . | . | . | . | . | . | . | . |
| | *** | 5656 | 7131 | 8779 | . | . | . | . | . | . | . | . | . | . | . | . |

TABLE 2: ALPHA= 0.005 POWER= 0.9    EXPECTED ACCRUAL THRU MINIMUM FOLLOW-UP= 4000

| | DEL=.01 | | | DEL=.02 | | | DEL=.05 | | | DEL=.10 | | | DEL=.15 | | |
|---|---|---|---|---|---|---|---|---|---|---|---|---|---|---|---|
| FACT= | 1.0 .75 | .50 .25 | .00 BIN | 1.0 .75 | .50 .25 | .00 BIN | 1.0 .75 | .50 .25 | .00 BIN | 1.0 75 | .50 .25 | .00 BIN | 1.0 .75 | .50 .25 | .00 BIN |
| PCONT=*** | | | | | | REQUIRED NUMBER OF PATIENTS | | | | | | | | | |
| 0.01 *** | 2273 | 2283 | 2293 | 837 | 837 | 843 | 277 | 277 | 277 | 137 | 137 | 137 | 97 | 97 | 97 |
| *** | 2277 | 2287 | 8779 | 837 | 837 | 2902 | 277 | 277 | 790 | 137 | 137 | 321 | 97 | 97 | 191 |
| 0.02 *** | 5023 | 5043 | 5123 | 1613 | 1623 | 1637 | 437 | 437 | 443 | 193 | 193 | 193 | 127 | 127 | 127 |
| *** | 5033 | 5067 | 14493 | 1617 | 1627 | 4316 | 437 | 437 | 1009 | 193 | 193 | 373 | 127 | 127 | 213 |
| 0.05 *** | 15197 | 15273 | 15997 | 4297 | 4347 | 4483 | 933 | 943 | 953 | 333 | 337 | 337 | 197 | 197 | 197 |
| *** | 15223 | 15403 | 30920 | 4317 | 4397 | 8378 | 937 | 943 | 1637 | 337 | 337 | 521 | 197 | 197 | 275 |
| 0.1 *** | 33517 | 33703 | 37233 | 8967 | 9137 | 9847 | 1747 | 1783 | 1833 | 553 | 557 | 567 | 297 | 297 | 297 |
| *** | 33577 | 34067 | 55917 | 9027 | 9343 | 14553 | 1767 | 1807 | 2590 | 557 | 563 | 744 | 297 | 297 | 368 |
| 0.15 *** | 50043 | 50373 | 58817 | 13147 | 13463 | 15227 | 2487 | 2563 | 2687 | 753 | 763 | 777 | 383 | 387 | 393 |
| *** | 50153 | 51033 | 77939 | 13263 | 13907 | 19984 | 2517 | 2617 | 3423 | 757 | 767 | 938 | 387 | 387 | 447 |
| 0.2 *** | 63347 | 63863 | 79017 | 16533 | 17033 | 20237 | 3103 | 3237 | 3467 | 917 | 937 | 963 | 457 | 463 | 467 |
| *** | 63517 | 64893 | 96984 | 16707 | 17763 | 24671 | 3163 | 3333 | 4137 | 927 | 947 | 1102 | 463 | 467 | 513 |
| 0.25 *** | 73027 | 73777 | 97013 | 19037 | 19753 | 24673 | 3597 | 3787 | 4147 | 1057 | 1083 | 1117 | 517 | 527 | 533 |
| *** | 73277 | 75263 | 113054 | 19287 | 20817 | 28614 | 3683 | 3937 | 4732 | 1067 | 1103 | 1235 | 523 | 527 | 566 |
| 0.3 *** | 79113 | 80137 | 112337 | 20687 | 21657 | 28437 | 3963 | 4223 | 4717 | 1163 | 1203 | 1247 | 563 | 573 | 583 |
| *** | 79457 | 82183 | 126148 | 21027 | 23077 | 31813 | 4077 | 4417 | 5208 | 1183 | 1223 | 1340 | 567 | 577 | 606 |
| 0.35 *** | 81837 | 83207 | 124737 | 21547 | 22807 | 31463 | 4217 | 4537 | 5167 | 1243 | 1287 | 1347 | 597 | 607 | 623 |
| *** | 82297 | 85927 | 136266 | 21997 | 24607 | 34268 | 4357 | 4783 | 5565 | 1263 | 1313 | 1414 | 603 | 613 | 632 |
| 0.4 *** | 81567 | 83357 | 134057 | 21727 | 23303 | 33713 | 4367 | 4737 | 5387 | 1287 | 1343 | 1413 | 613 | 627 | 643 |
| *** | 82167 | 86893 | 143408 | 22293 | 25473 | 35979 | 4527 | 5033 | 5803 | 1313 | 1373 | 1459 | 623 | 637 | 645 |
| 0.45 *** | 78737 | 81043 | 140207 | 21333 | 23243 | 35173 | 4417 | 4837 | 5683 | 1307 | 1367 | 1443 | 617 | 633 | 653 |
| *** | 79507 | 85527 | 147574 | 22033 | 25763 | 36946 | 4597 | 5167 | 5922 | 1337 | 1403 | 1474 | 627 | 643 | 645 |
| 0.5 *** | 73823 | 76767 | 143137 | 20497 | 22723 | 35823 | 4387 | 4837 | 5747 | 1303 | 1363 | 1443 | 613 | 627 | 643 |
| *** | 74807 | 82337 | 148765 | 21327 | 25537 | 37169 | 4583 | 5193 | 5922 | 1333 | 1403 | 1459 | 617 | 637 | 632 |
| 0.55 *** | 67343 | 71073 | 142833 | 19333 | 21837 | 35667 | 4273 | 4743 | 5687 | 1267 | 1333 | 1413 | 593 | 607 | 623 |
| *** | 68597 | 77793 | 146979 | 20283 | 24877 | 36648 | 4477 | 5113 | 5803 | 1297 | 1367 | 1414 | 597 | 613 | 606 |
| 0.6 *** | 59843 | 64493 | 139293 | 17937 | 20657 | 34703 | 4093 | 4563 | 5493 | 1207 | 1273 | 1347 | 557 | 573 | 587 |
| *** | 61433 | 72303 | 142218 | 18987 | 23823 | 35384 | 4297 | 4927 | 5565 | 1237 | 1307 | 1340 | 563 | 577 | 566 |
| 0.65 *** | 51897 | 57523 | 132523 | 16397 | 19227 | 32927 | 3843 | 4297 | 5173 | 1127 | 1183 | 1253 | 513 | 523 | 537 |
| *** | 53873 | 66193 | 134480 | 17507 | 22413 | 33375 | 4043 | 4643 | 5208 | 1153 | 1213 | 1235 | 517 | 533 | 513 |
| 0.7 *** | 44057 | 50517 | 122543 | 14757 | 17577 | 30353 | 3523 | 3943 | 4723 | 1017 | 1063 | 1123 | 453 | 463 | 473 |
| *** | 46403 | 59663 | 123767 | 15873 | 20657 | 30622 | 3707 | 4257 | 4732 | 1037 | 1093 | 1102 | 457 | 467 | 447 |
| 0.75 *** | 36743 | 43663 | 109387 | 13027 | 15707 | 26987 | 3137 | 3497 | 4143 | 877 | 917 | 963 | 377 | 387 | 397 |
| *** | 39333 | 52777 | 110078 | 14097 | 18557 | 27126 | 3297 | 3763 | 4137 | 897 | 937 | 938 | 383 | 393 | 368 |
| 0.8 *** | 30097 | 36937 | 93077 | 11187 | 13597 | 22827 | 2673 | 2957 | 3443 | 713 | 743 | 773 | 293 | 297 | 303 |
| *** | 32717 | 45477 | 93413 | 12163 | 16073 | 22885 | 2797 | 3163 | 3423 | 727 | 757 | 744 | 297 | 303 | 275 |
| 0.85 *** | 23977 | 30153 | 73653 | 9183 | 11163 | 17897 | 2107 | 2307 | 2617 | 517 | 533 | 553 | . | . | . |
| *** | 26377 | 37543 | 73773 | 9993 | 13117 | 17900 | 2203 | 2443 | 2590 | 527 | 543 | 521 | . | . | . |
| 0.9 *** | 17963 | 22857 | 51143 | 6867 | 8257 | 12193 | 1427 | 1527 | 1667 | . | . | . | . | . | . |
| *** | 19887 | 28453 | 51156 | 7447 | 9537 | 12172 | 1473 | 1593 | 1637 | . | . | . | . | . | . |
| 0.95 *** | 11123 | 13977 | 25587 | 3897 | 4497 | 5727 | . | . | . | . | . | . | . | . | . |
| *** | 12273 | 16957 | 25563 | 4157 | 4973 | 5699 | . | . | . | . | . | . | . | . | . |
| 0.98 *** | 5323 | 6333 | 8807 | . | . | . | . | . | . | . | . | . | . | . | . |
| *** | 5753 | 7203 | 8779 | . | . | . | . | . | . | . | . | . | . | . | . |

# TABLE 2: ALPHA= 0.005 POWER= 0.9     EXPECTED ACCRUAL THRU MINIMUM FOLLOW-UP= 4250

|  |  | DEL=.01 | | | DEL=.02 | | | DEL=.05 | | | DEL=.10 | | | DEL=.15 | | |
|---|---|---|---|---|---|---|---|---|---|---|---|---|---|---|---|---|
| FACT= | | 1.0 .75 | .50 .25 | .00 BIN | 1.0 .75 | .50 .25 | .00 BIN | 1.0 .75 | .50 .25 | .00 BIN | 1.0 75 | .50 .25 | .00 BIN | 1.0 .75 | .50 .25 | .00 BIN |
| PCONT=*** | | REQUIRED NUMBER OF PATIENTS | | | | | | | | | | | | | | |
| 0.01 | *** | 2277 2281 | 2292 | | 836 836 | 843 | | 273 279 | 279 | | 141 141 | 141 | | 99 99 | 99 | |
|  | *** | 2277 2288 | 8779 | | 836 843 | 2902 | | 273 279 | 790 | | 141 141 | 321 | | 99 99 | 191 | |
| 0.02 | *** | 5022 5043 | 5124 | | 1612 1622 | 1633 | | 439 439 | 439 | | 194 194 | 194 | | 124 124 | 124 | |
|  | *** | 5033 5071 | 14493 | | 1618 1629 | 4316 | | 439 439 | 1009 | | 194 194 | 373 | | 124 124 | 213 | |
| 0.05 | *** | 15201 15282 | 15994 | | 4300 4353 | 4480 | | 932 942 | 949 | | 337 337 | 337 | | 194 194 | 194 | |
|  | *** | 15229 15420 | 30920 | | 4321 4402 | 8378 | | 938 942 | 1637 | | 337 337 | 521 | | 194 194 | 275 | |
| 0.1 | *** | 33525 33727 | 37233 | | 8981 9151 | 9846 | | 1750 1788 | 1831 | | 556 560 | 566 | | 294 301 | 301 | |
|  | *** | 33593 34109 | 55917 | | 9045 9364 | 14553 | | 1767 1809 | 2590 | | 556 560 | 744 | | 294 301 | 368 | |
| 0.15 | *** | 50062 50412 | 58817 | | 13168 13501 | 15229 | | 2493 2568 | 2685 | | 751 762 | 772 | | 386 386 | 390 | |
|  | *** | 50178 51113 | 77939 | | 13288 13954 | 19984 | | 2525 2621 | 3423 | | 758 768 | 938 | | 386 390 | 447 | |
| 0.2 | *** | 63381 63927 | 79021 | | 16568 17088 | 20237 | | 3116 3244 | 3467 | | 921 938 | 959 | | 460 464 | 471 | |
|  | *** | 63562 65022 | 96984 | | 16748 17832 | 24671 | | 3173 3339 | 4137 | | 928 949 | 1102 | | 460 464 | 513 | |
| 0.25 | *** | 73075 73868 | 97009 | | 19086 19833 | 24674 | | 3616 3807 | 4147 | | 1059 1087 | 1119 | | 517 524 | 534 | |
|  | *** | 73341 75445 | 113054 | | 19351 20917 | 28614 | | 3694 3945 | 4732 | | 1070 1102 | 1235 | | 524 528 | 566 | |
| 0.3 | *** | 79174 80268 | 112335 | | 20754 21767 | 28436 | | 3988 4243 | 4714 | | 1165 1204 | 1246 | | 566 577 | 588 | |
|  | *** | 79542 82436 | 126148 | | 21108 23219 | 31813 | | 4098 4434 | 5208 | | 1183 1225 | 1340 | | 570 581 | 606 | |
| 0.35 | *** | 81926 83382 | 124741 | | 21636 22947 | 31464 | | 4247 4561 | 5167 | | 1246 1289 | 1346 | | 598 609 | 619 | |
|  | *** | 82411 86261 | 136266 | | 22103 24781 | 34268 | | 4385 4799 | 5565 | | 1268 1314 | 1414 | | 602 613 | 632 | |
| 0.4 | *** | 81682 83583 | 134059 | | 21838 23474 | 33716 | | 4402 4767 | 5490 | | 1293 1346 | 1410 | | 613 630 | 645 | |
|  | *** | 82315 87319 | 143408 | | 22426 25677 | 35979 | | 4561 5054 | 5803 | | 1321 1374 | 1459 | | 623 634 | 645 | |
| 0.45 | *** | 78883 81331 | 140204 | | 21470 23442 | 35172 | | 4455 4869 | 5681 | | 1314 1374 | 1442 | | 619 634 | 651 | |
|  | *** | 79701 86059 | 147574 | | 22199 25996 | 36946 | | 4636 5188 | 5922 | | 1342 1406 | 1474 | | 630 645 | 645 | |
| 0.5 | *** | 74006 77134 | 143137 | | 20658 22953 | 35824 | | 4427 4869 | 5751 | | 1310 1367 | 1442 | | 613 630 | 645 | |
|  | *** | 75052 82978 | 148765 | | 21523 25801 | 37169 | | 4618 5220 | 5922 | | 1335 1406 | 1459 | | 619 634 | 632 | |
| 0.55 | *** | 67578 71531 | 142835 | | 19521 22086 | 35665 | | 4317 4778 | 5688 | | 1272 1335 | 1410 | | 592 609 | 623 | |
|  | *** | 68910 78537 | 146979 | | 20503 25153 | 36648 | | 4519 5139 | 5803 | | 1303 1374 | 1414 | | 598 613 | 606 | |
| 0.6 | *** | 60145 65043 | 139290 | | 18151 20917 | 34698 | | 4136 4597 | 5490 | | 1214 1272 | 1346 | | 560 570 | 588 | |
|  | *** | 61823 73139 | 142218 | | 19224 24105 | 35384 | | 4338 4954 | 5565 | | 1246 1310 | 1340 | | 566 581 | 566 | |
| 0.65 | *** | 52272 58158 | 132522 | | 16625 19493 | 32930 | | 3885 4332 | 5171 | | 1129 1187 | 1250 | | 513 524 | 538 | |
|  | *** | 54350 67089 | 134480 | | 17751 22692 | 33375 | | 4083 4668 | 5208 | | 1155 1214 | 1235 | | 517 528 | 513 | |
| 0.7 | *** | 44511 51216 | 122545 | | 14984 17836 | 30352 | | 3563 3970 | 4721 | | 1023 1066 | 1123 | | 453 464 | 475 | |
|  | *** | 46959 60576 | 123767 | | 16121 20928 | 30622 | | 3747 4278 | 4732 | | 1044 1091 | 1102 | | 460 471 | 447 | |
| 0.75 | *** | 37254 44373 | 109388 | | 13246 15955 | 26984 | | 3169 3524 | 4147 | | 885 921 | 963 | | 379 390 | 396 | |
|  | *** | 39932 53663 | 110078 | | 14336 18803 | 27126 | | 3329 3779 | 4137 | | 900 942 | 938 | | 386 390 | 368 | |
| 0.8 | *** | 30624 37620 | 93078 | | 11387 13816 | 22830 | | 2695 2978 | 3439 | | 719 740 | 772 | | 294 301 | 305 | |
|  | *** | 33306 46296 | 93413 | | 12371 16281 | 22885 | | 2823 3173 | 3423 | | 730 758 | 744 | | 294 301 | 275 | |
| 0.85 | *** | 24466 30752 | 73649 | | 9347 11340 | 17896 | | 2128 2323 | 2617 | | 517 534 | 549 | | . . | . | |
|  | *** | 26916 38232 | 73773 | | 10165 13278 | 17900 | | 2217 2451 | 2590 | | 528 545 | 521 | | . . | . | |
| 0.9 | *** | 18353 23325 | 51141 | | 6988 8380 | 12190 | | 1438 1533 | 1665 | | . . | . | | . . | . | |
|  | *** | 20318 28960 | 51156 | | 7572 9633 | 12172 | | 1480 1597 | 1637 | | . . | . | | . . | . | |
| 0.95 | *** | 11361 14241 | 25588 | | 3956 4544 | 5730 | | . . | . | | . . | . | | . . | . | |
|  | *** | 12523 17209 | 25563 | | 4211 5008 | 5699 | | . . | . | | . . | . | | . . | . | |
| 0.98 | *** | 5415 6414 | 8811 | | . . | . | | . . | . | | . . | . | | . . | . | |
|  | *** | 5840 7271 | 8779 | | . . | . | | . . | . | | . . | . | | . . | . | |

## TABLE 2: ALPHA= 0.005 POWER= 0.9    EXPECTED ACCRUAL THRU MINIMUM FOLLOW-UP= 4500

| | | DEL=.01 | | | DEL=.02 | | | DEL=.05 | | | DEL=.10 | | | DEL=.15 | | |
|---|---|---|---|---|---|---|---|---|---|---|---|---|---|---|---|---|
| FACT= | | 1.0 .75 | .50 .25 | .00 BIN | 1.0 .75 | .50 .25 | .00 BIN | 1.0 .75 | .50 .25 | .00 BIN | 1.0 75 | .50 .25 | .00 BIN | 1.0 .75 | .50 .25 | .00 BIN |
| PCONT=*** | | | | REQUIRED NUMBER OF PATIENTS | | | | | | | | | | | | |
| 0.01 | *** | 2276 2276 | 2280 2287 | 2291 8779 | 836 836 | 840 840 | 840 2902 | 278 278 | 278 278 | 278 790 | 138 138 | 138 138 | 138 321 | 98 98 | 98 98 | 98 191 |
| 0.02 | *** | 5025 5032 | 5048 5070 | 5122 14493 | 1616 1616 | 1623 1628 | 1635 4316 | 435 435 | 442 442 | 442 1009 | 195 195 | 195 195 | 195 373 | 127 127 | 127 127 | 127 213 |
| 0.05 | *** | 15206 15236 | 15292 15431 | 15994 30920 | 4305 4328 | 4357 4406 | 4481 8378 | 937 937 | 941 948 | 948 1637 | 334 334 | 334 334 | 334 521 | 195 195 | 195 195 | 195 275 |
| 0.1 | *** | 33540 33607 | 33746 34151 | 37230 55917 | 8992 9060 | 9172 9379 | 9847 14553 | 1758 1770 | 1785 1808 | 1830 2590 | 555 559 | 559 566 | 566 744 | 296 296 | 296 300 | 300 368 |
| 0.15 | *** | 50081 50205 | 50453 51195 | 58818 77939 | 13193 13312 | 13537 13991 | 15229 19984 | 2501 2535 | 2573 2625 | 2685 3423 | 750 757 | 761 768 | 773 938 | 386 386 | 386 390 | 390 447 |
| 0.2 | *** | 63413 63604 | 63993 65152 | 79016 96984 | 16597 16793 | 17141 17902 | 20235 24671 | 3131 3187 | 3255 3345 | 3468 4137 | 926 930 | 941 948 | 960 1102 | 458 458 | 465 465 | 469 513 |
| 0.25 | *** | 73121 73403 | 73961 75630 | 97012 113054 | 19133 19410 | 19916 21018 | 24675 28614 | 3630 3716 | 3817 3956 | 4148 4732 | 1061 1072 | 1088 1106 | 1117 1235 | 521 521 | 525 532 | 532 566 |
| 0.3 | *** | 79241 79624 | 80396 82684 | 112339 126148 | 20816 21191 | 21873 23347 | 28436 31813 | 4013 4121 | 4260 4447 | 4717 5208 | 1173 1189 | 1207 1223 | 1245 1340 | 566 570 | 577 581 | 581 606 |
| 0.35 | *** | 82009 82522 | 83550 86595 | 124736 136266 | 21720 22211 | 23081 24945 | 31463 34268 | 4271 4406 | 4582 4818 | 5167 5565 | 1252 1268 | 1290 1320 | 1346 1414 | 600 604 | 611 615 | 622 632 |
| 0.4 | *** | 81791 82466 | 83805 87742 | 134058 143408 | 21941 22564 | 23640 25878 | 33713 35979 | 4429 4593 | 4796 5070 | 5486 5803 | 1297 1324 | 1346 1376 | 1410 1459 | 615 622 | 626 638 | 645 645 |
| 0.45 | *** | 79023 79890 | 81622 86588 | 140205 147574 | 21603 22357 | 23640 26220 | 35171 36946 | 4492 4672 | 4897 5212 | 5685 5922 | 1320 1346 | 1376 1410 | 1443 1474 | 622 626 | 638 645 | 649 645 |
| 0.5 | *** | 74190 75300 | 77498 83613 | 143137 148765 | 20820 21709 | 23171 26047 | 35823 37169 | 4463 4654 | 4901 5239 | 5752 5922 | 1313 1342 | 1369 1403 | 1443 1459 | 615 622 | 626 638 | 645 632 |
| 0.55 | *** | 67811 69225 | 71981 79264 | 142833 146979 | 19706 20715 | 22328 25417 | 35666 36648 | 4357 4560 | 4811 5160 | 5685 5803 | 1279 1308 | 1342 1376 | 1414 1414 | 593 600 | 611 615 | 622 606 |
| 0.6 | *** | 60443 62216 | 65584 73950 | 139290 142218 | 18352 19455 | 21176 24375 | 34703 35384 | 4177 4380 | 4631 4976 | 5493 5565 | 1223 1245 | 1279 1313 | 1346 1340 | 559 566 | 570 581 | 588 566 |
| 0.65 | *** | 52646 54825 | 58785 67946 | 132521 134480 | 16838 17985 | 19751 22958 | 32925 33375 | 3923 4121 | 4361 4688 | 5171 5208 | 1140 1162 | 1189 1218 | 1252 1235 | 514 521 | 525 532 | 536 513 |
| 0.7 | *** | 44958 47501 | 51888 61451 | 122543 123767 | 15202 16354 | 18086 21180 | 30356 30622 | 3603 3776 | 4001 4301 | 4721 4732 | 1027 1050 | 1072 1095 | 1121 1102 | 453 458 | 465 469 | 476 447 |
| 0.75 | *** | 37751 40508 | 45064 54514 | 109387 110078 | 13458 14554 | 16192 19031 | 26985 27126 | 3203 3360 | 3551 3799 | 4143 4137 | 885 903 | 919 941 | 964 938 | 379 386 | 390 390 | 397 368 |
| 0.8 | *** | 31132 33881 | 38276 47073 | 93079 93413 | 11580 12574 | 14021 16478 | 22830 22885 | 2726 2850 | 3000 3187 | 3439 3423 | 723 735 | 746 757 | 773 744 | 296 296 | 300 300 | 307 275 |
| 0.85 | *** | 24933 27431 | 31328 38888 | 73650 73773 | 9510 10331 | 11505 13429 | 17895 17900 | 2145 2235 | 2336 2460 | 2613 2590 | 521 525 | 536 543 | 548 521 | . . | . . | . . |
| 0.9 | *** | 18735 20726 | 23768 29445 | 51146 51156 | 7106 7687 | 8490 9728 | 12191 12172 | 1448 1488 | 1538 1601 | 1668 1637 | . . | . . | . . | . . | . . | . . |
| 0.95 | *** | 11584 12761 | 14482 17452 | 25586 25563 | 4008 4260 | 4593 5043 | 5730 5699 | . . | . . | . . | . . | . . | . . | . . | . . | . . |
| 0.98 | *** | 5498 5925 | 6495 7331 | 8805 8779 | . . | . . | . . | . . | . . | . . | . . | . . | . . | . . | . . | . . |

TABLE 2: ALPHA= 0.005 POWER= 0.9    EXPECTED ACCRUAL THRU MINIMUM FOLLOW-UP= 4750

| | | DEL=.01 | | | DEL=.02 | | | DEL=.05 | | | DEL=.10 | | | DEL=.15 | | |
|---|---|---|---|---|---|---|---|---|---|---|---|---|---|---|---|---|---|
| FACT= | | 1.0 .75 | .50 .25 | .00 BIN | 1.0 .75 | .50 .25 | .00 BIN | 1.0 .75 | .50 .25 | .00 BIN | 1.0 75 | .50 .25 | .00 BIN | 1.0 .75 | .50 .25 | .00 BIN |
| PCONT=*** | | | | | REQUIRED NUMBER OF PATIENTS | | | | | | | | | | | |
| 0.01 | *** | 2276 | 2283 | 2295 | 835 | 839 | 839 | 277 | 277 | 277 | 139 | 139 | 139 | 98 | 98 | 98 |
| | *** | 2276 | 2288 | 8779 | 839 | 839 | 2902 | 277 | 277 | 790 | 139 | 139 | 321 | 98 | 98 | 191 |
| 0.02 | *** | 5027 | 5050 | 5122 | 1618 | 1623 | 1635 | 435 | 435 | 443 | 193 | 193 | 193 | 127 | 127 | 127 |
| | *** | 5038 | 5074 | 14493 | 1618 | 1630 | 4316 | 435 | 443 | 1009 | 193 | 193 | 373 | 127 | 127 | 213 |
| 0.05 | *** | 15208 | 15298 | 15992 | 4307 | 4362 | 4480 | 934 | 942 | 953 | 336 | 336 | 336 | 193 | 198 | 198 |
| | *** | 15239 | 15445 | 30920 | 4330 | 4409 | 8378 | 934 | 946 | 1637 | 336 | 336 | 521 | 193 | 198 | 275 |
| 0.1 | *** | 33550 | 33769 | 37232 | 9005 | 9187 | 9848 | 1761 | 1789 | 1832 | 554 | 562 | 566 | 293 | 300 | 300 |
| | *** | 33622 | 34196 | 55917 | 9069 | 9397 | 14553 | 1773 | 1808 | 2590 | 562 | 562 | 744 | 300 | 300 | 368 |
| 0.15 | *** | 50104 | 50496 | 58813 | 13213 | 13565 | 15227 | 2509 | 2580 | 2687 | 756 | 763 | 775 | 383 | 388 | 388 |
| | *** | 50235 | 51272 | 77939 | 13339 | 14028 | 19984 | 2537 | 2628 | 3423 | 756 | 768 | 938 | 388 | 388 | 447 |
| 0.2 | *** | 63444 | 64057 | 79020 | 16628 | 17198 | 20238 | 3138 | 3262 | 3464 | 922 | 942 | 958 | 459 | 467 | 467 |
| | *** | 63646 | 65273 | 96984 | 16830 | 17963 | 24671 | 3190 | 3352 | 4137 | 934 | 953 | 1102 | 459 | 467 | 513 |
| 0.25 | *** | 73170 | 74056 | 97010 | 19182 | 19989 | 24672 | 3649 | 3832 | 4148 | 1065 | 1089 | 1120 | 519 | 526 | 530 |
| | *** | 73467 | 75813 | 113054 | 19471 | 21110 | 28614 | 3725 | 3962 | 4732 | 1077 | 1100 | 1235 | 526 | 530 | 566 |
| 0.3 | *** | 79305 | 80528 | 112341 | 20880 | 21977 | 28437 | 4034 | 4278 | 4718 | 1172 | 1207 | 1250 | 566 | 573 | 585 |
| | *** | 79713 | 82938 | 126148 | 21272 | 23473 | 31813 | 4140 | 4457 | 5208 | 1191 | 1227 | 1340 | 573 | 578 | 606 |
| 0.35 | *** | 82095 | 83722 | 124738 | 21806 | 23212 | 31460 | 4302 | 4604 | 5162 | 1255 | 1290 | 1345 | 597 | 609 | 621 |
| | *** | 82634 | 86921 | 136266 | 22317 | 25100 | 34268 | 4433 | 4837 | 5565 | 1274 | 1322 | 1414 | 602 | 614 | 632 |
| 0.4 | *** | 81905 | 84031 | 134060 | 22048 | 23801 | 33717 | 4461 | 4817 | 5490 | 1302 | 1350 | 1409 | 621 | 633 | 645 |
| | *** | 82610 | 88156 | 143408 | 22689 | 26062 | 35979 | 4615 | 5090 | 5803 | 1326 | 1381 | 1459 | 625 | 637 | 645 |
| 0.45 | *** | 79167 | 81905 | 140204 | 21735 | 23825 | 35170 | 4528 | 4924 | 5684 | 1326 | 1381 | 1445 | 625 | 637 | 649 |
| | *** | 80081 | 87099 | 147574 | 22518 | 26430 | 36946 | 4699 | 5233 | 5922 | 1350 | 1409 | 1474 | 633 | 645 | 645 |
| 0.5 | *** | 74377 | 77860 | 143137 | 20975 | 23385 | 35823 | 4504 | 4936 | 5751 | 1322 | 1374 | 1445 | 614 | 633 | 645 |
| | *** | 75545 | 84225 | 148765 | 21889 | 26275 | 37169 | 4694 | 5264 | 5922 | 1345 | 1405 | 1459 | 621 | 637 | 632 |
| 0.55 | *** | 68047 | 72429 | 142836 | 19882 | 22559 | 35669 | 4397 | 4848 | 5684 | 1286 | 1345 | 1409 | 597 | 609 | 621 |
| | *** | 69532 | 79974 | 146979 | 20915 | 25658 | 36648 | 4592 | 5185 | 5803 | 1314 | 1374 | 1414 | 602 | 614 | 606 |
| 0.6 | *** | 60744 | 66123 | 139290 | 18552 | 21414 | 34702 | 4219 | 4663 | 5494 | 1227 | 1279 | 1350 | 562 | 573 | 585 |
| | *** | 62601 | 74733 | 142218 | 19673 | 24632 | 35384 | 4414 | 5003 | 5565 | 1250 | 1314 | 1340 | 566 | 578 | 566 |
| 0.65 | *** | 53018 | 59390 | 132521 | 17049 | 19994 | 32925 | 3962 | 4390 | 5169 | 1143 | 1191 | 1250 | 514 | 526 | 538 |
| | *** | 55293 | 68776 | 134480 | 18212 | 23212 | 33375 | 4152 | 4710 | 5208 | 1167 | 1219 | 1235 | 519 | 530 | 513 |
| 0.7 | *** | 45402 | 52543 | 122542 | 15410 | 18327 | 30356 | 3637 | 4029 | 4722 | 1029 | 1072 | 1124 | 455 | 467 | 471 |
| | *** | 48030 | 62292 | 123767 | 16581 | 21419 | 30622 | 3808 | 4314 | 4732 | 1048 | 1096 | 1102 | 459 | 467 | 447 |
| 0.75 | *** | 38241 | 45727 | 109384 | 13660 | 16407 | 26983 | 3233 | 3570 | 4140 | 894 | 922 | 965 | 383 | 388 | 395 |
| | *** | 41072 | 55329 | 110078 | 14769 | 19253 | 27126 | 3388 | 3815 | 4137 | 906 | 942 | 938 | 383 | 395 | 368 |
| 0.8 | *** | 31627 | 38910 | 93080 | 11764 | 14210 | 22832 | 2747 | 3020 | 3440 | 720 | 744 | 775 | 293 | 300 | 305 |
| | *** | 34429 | 47812 | 93413 | 12762 | 16657 | 22885 | 2870 | 3202 | 3423 | 732 | 756 | 744 | 300 | 300 | 275 |
| 0.85 | *** | 25385 | 31880 | 73652 | 9662 | 11665 | 17899 | 2165 | 2347 | 2616 | 526 | 538 | 550 | . | . | . |
| | *** | 27922 | 39512 | 73773 | 10489 | 13569 | 17900 | 2248 | 2466 | 2590 | 530 | 542 | 521 | . | . | . |
| 0.9 | *** | 19091 | 24193 | 51142 | 7216 | 8594 | 12192 | 1452 | 1547 | 1666 | . | . | . | . | . | . |
| | *** | 21117 | 29905 | 51156 | 7793 | 9817 | 12172 | 1500 | 1599 | 1637 | . | . | . | . | . | . |
| 0.95 | *** | 11800 | 14717 | 25587 | 4053 | 4627 | 5727 | . | . | . | . | . | . | . | . | . |
| | *** | 12987 | 17673 | 25563 | 4307 | 5067 | 5699 | . | . | . | . | . | . | . | . | . |
| 0.98 | *** | 5577 | 6563 | 8807 | . | . | . | . | . | . | . | . | . | . | . | . |
| | *** | 6000 | 7390 | 8779 | . | . | . | . | . | . | . | . | . | . | . | . |

TABLE 2: ALPHA= 0.005 POWER= 0.9     EXPECTED ACCRUAL THRU MINIMUM FOLLOW-UP= 5000

| | | DEL=.01 | | | DEL=.02 | | | DEL=.05 | | | DEL=.10 | | | DEL=.15 | | |
|---|---|---|---|---|---|---|---|---|---|---|---|---|---|---|---|---|
| FACT= | | 1.0 .75 | .50 .25 | .00 BIN | 1.0 .75 | .50 .25 | .00 BIN | 1.0 .75 | .50 .25 | .00 BIN | 1.0 75 | .50 .25 | .00 BIN | 1.0 .75 | .50 .25 | .00 BIN |
| PCONT=*** | | | | | REQUIRED | NUMBER | OF PATIENTS | | | | | | | | | |
| 0.01 | *** | 2279 | 2283 | 2296 | 833 | 841 | 841 | 279 | 279 | 279 | 141 | 141 | 141 | 96 | 96 | 96 |
| | *** | 2279 | 2283 | 8779 | 841 | 841 | 2902 | 279 | 279 | 790 | 141 | 141 | 321 | 96 | 96 | 191 |
| 0.02 | *** | 5029 | 5054 | 5121 | 1616 | 1621 | 1633 | 441 | 441 | 441 | 191 | 191 | 191 | 129 | 129 | 129 |
| | *** | 5033 | 5079 | 14493 | 1621 | 1629 | 4316 | 441 | 441 | 1009 | 191 | 191 | 373 | 129 | 129 | 213 |
| 0.05 | *** | 15216 | 15308 | 15996 | 4316 | 4366 | 4483 | 933 | 941 | 954 | 333 | 333 | 333 | 196 | 196 | 196 |
| | *** | 15246 | 15458 | 30920 | 4333 | 4408 | 8378 | 941 | 946 | 1637 | 333 | 333 | 521 | 196 | 196 | 275 |
| 0.1 | *** | 33558 | 33796 | 37233 | 9016 | 9204 | 9846 | 1758 | 1791 | 1833 | 558 | 558 | 566 | 296 | 296 | 296 |
| | *** | 33641 | 34241 | 55917 | 9083 | 9408 | 14553 | 1779 | 1808 | 2590 | 558 | 566 | 744 | 296 | 296 | 368 |
| 0.15 | *** | 50121 | 50541 | 58816 | 13233 | 13596 | 15229 | 2508 | 2583 | 2683 | 754 | 766 | 779 | 383 | 391 | 391 |
| | *** | 50258 | 51354 | 77939 | 13366 | 14058 | 19984 | 2546 | 2629 | 3423 | 758 | 771 | 938 | 383 | 391 | 447 |
| 0.2 | *** | 63479 | 64121 | 79021 | 16666 | 17246 | 20233 | 3146 | 3271 | 3466 | 929 | 941 | 958 | 458 | 466 | 471 |
| | *** | 63691 | 65404 | 96984 | 16871 | 18021 | 24671 | 3204 | 3354 | 4137 | 933 | 954 | 1102 | 458 | 466 | 513 |
| 0.25 | *** | 73216 | 74146 | 97008 | 19229 | 20066 | 24671 | 3658 | 3841 | 4146 | 1066 | 1091 | 1121 | 521 | 529 | 533 |
| | *** | 73529 | 75991 | 113054 | 19529 | 21196 | 28614 | 3741 | 3971 | 4732 | 1079 | 1104 | 1235 | 521 | 529 | 566 |
| 0.3 | *** | 79371 | 80654 | 112341 | 20941 | 22079 | 28433 | 4054 | 4291 | 4716 | 1179 | 1208 | 1246 | 566 | 579 | 583 |
| | *** | 79796 | 83183 | 126148 | 21354 | 23591 | 31813 | 4158 | 4471 | 5208 | 1191 | 1229 | 1340 | 571 | 579 | 606 |
| 0.35 | *** | 82179 | 83896 | 124741 | 21883 | 23341 | 31458 | 4321 | 4621 | 5166 | 1258 | 1296 | 1346 | 604 | 608 | 621 |
| | *** | 82754 | 87246 | 136266 | 22416 | 25246 | 34268 | 4796 | 4846 | 5565 | 1279 | 1321 | 1414 | 604 | 616 | 632 |
| 0.4 | *** | 82016 | 84254 | 134058 | 22154 | 23954 | 33716 | 4491 | 4841 | 5491 | 1308 | 1354 | 1408 | 621 | 629 | 641 |
| | *** | 82758 | 88571 | 143408 | 22821 | 26233 | 35979 | 4646 | 5108 | 5803 | 1329 | 1379 | 1459 | 621 | 633 | 645 |
| 0.45 | *** | 79316 | 82191 | 140208 | 21866 | 24004 | 35171 | 4558 | 4954 | 5683 | 1329 | 1379 | 1441 | 629 | 641 | 654 |
| | *** | 80279 | 87608 | 147574 | 22666 | 26633 | 36946 | 4733 | 5254 | 5922 | 1354 | 1408 | 1474 | 629 | 646 | 645 |
| 0.5 | *** | 74558 | 78221 | 143141 | 21129 | 23583 | 35821 | 4533 | 4958 | 5746 | 1321 | 1379 | 1446 | 616 | 629 | 646 |
| | *** | 75791 | 84829 | 148765 | 22066 | 26496 | 37169 | 4721 | 5283 | 5922 | 1346 | 1408 | 1459 | 621 | 633 | 632 |
| 0.55 | *** | 68283 | 72866 | 142833 | 20058 | 22779 | 35666 | 4433 | 4871 | 5683 | 1291 | 1346 | 1408 | 596 | 608 | 621 |
| | *** | 69841 | 80666 | 146979 | 21108 | 25896 | 36648 | 4629 | 5204 | 5803 | 1316 | 1379 | 1414 | 604 | 616 | 606 |
| 0.6 | *** | 61041 | 66646 | 139291 | 18741 | 21646 | 34704 | 4254 | 4691 | 5491 | 1233 | 1283 | 1346 | 566 | 571 | 591 |
| | *** | 62983 | 75491 | 142218 | 19883 | 24866 | 35384 | 4446 | 5021 | 5565 | 1258 | 1316 | 1340 | 566 | 579 | 566 |
| 0.65 | *** | 53383 | 59983 | 132521 | 17246 | 20229 | 32929 | 3996 | 4421 | 5171 | 1146 | 1191 | 1254 | 516 | 529 | 541 |
| | *** | 55746 | 69583 | 134480 | 18433 | 23446 | 33375 | 4183 | 4729 | 5208 | 1171 | 1221 | 1235 | 521 | 533 | 513 |
| 0.7 | *** | 45833 | 53183 | 122546 | 15616 | 18554 | 30354 | 3666 | 4054 | 4721 | 1033 | 1071 | 1121 | 454 | 466 | 471 |
| | *** | 48554 | 63104 | 123767 | 16796 | 21646 | 30622 | 3841 | 4333 | 4732 | 1054 | 1096 | 1102 | 458 | 471 | 447 |
| 0.75 | *** | 38716 | 46371 | 109383 | 13854 | 16621 | 26983 | 3258 | 3596 | 4146 | 896 | 929 | 966 | 383 | 391 | 396 |
| | *** | 41616 | 56108 | 110078 | 14971 | 19454 | 27126 | 3408 | 3829 | 4137 | 908 | 941 | 938 | 383 | 391 | 368 |
| 0.8 | *** | 32104 | 39516 | 93079 | 11941 | 14396 | 22829 | 2771 | 3033 | 3441 | 721 | 746 | 771 | 296 | 296 | 304 |
| | *** | 34966 | 48521 | 93413 | 12946 | 16833 | 22885 | 2891 | 3208 | 3423 | 733 | 758 | 744 | 296 | 304 | 275 |
| 0.85 | *** | 25821 | 32416 | 73654 | 9808 | 11808 | 17896 | 2179 | 2358 | 2616 | 521 | 533 | 554 | . | . | . |
| | *** | 28396 | 40108 | 73773 | 10633 | 13696 | 17900 | 2266 | 2471 | 2590 | 529 | 541 | 521 | . | . | . |
| 0.9 | *** | 19446 | 24596 | 51141 | 7316 | 8691 | 12191 | 1466 | 1554 | 1666 | . | . | . | . | . | . |
| | *** | 21491 | 30333 | 51156 | 7896 | 9896 | 12172 | 1504 | 1604 | 1637 | . | . | . | . | . | . |
| 0.95 | *** | 12008 | 14941 | 25591 | 4104 | 4666 | 5729 | . | . | . | . | . | . | . | . | . |
| | *** | 13204 | 17883 | 25563 | 4354 | 5096 | 5699 | . | . | . | . | . | . | . | . | . |
| 0.98 | *** | 5654 | 6633 | 8808 | . | . | . | . | . | . | . | . | . | . | . | . |
| | *** | 6079 | 7441 | 8779 | . | . | . | . | . | . | . | . | . | . | . | . |

# TABLE 2: ALPHA= 0.005 POWER= 0.9     EXPECTED ACCRUAL THRU MINIMUM FOLLOW-UP= 5500

| | DEL=.01 | | | DEL=.02 | | | DEL=.05 | | | DEL=.10 | | | DEL=.15 | | |
|---|---|---|---|---|---|---|---|---|---|---|---|---|---|---|---|
| FACT= | 1.0 .75 | .50 .25 | .00 BIN | 1.0 .75 | .50 .25 | .00 BIN | 1.0 .75 | .50 .25 | .00 BIN | 1.0 75 | .50 .25 | .00 BIN | 1.0 .75 | .50 .25 | .00 BIN |

PCONT=***          REQUIRED NUMBER OF PATIENTS

| PCONT | .01a | .01b | .01c | .02a | .02b | .02c | .05a | .05b | .05c | .10a | .10b | .10c | .15a | .15b | .15c |
|---|---|---|---|---|---|---|---|---|---|---|---|---|---|---|---|
| 0.01 *** | 2278 | 2286 | 2292 | 834 | 834 | 843 | 279 | 279 | 279 | 141 | 141 | 141 | 100 | 100 | 100 |
| *** | 2278 | 2286 | 8779 | 834 | 843 | 2902 | 279 | 279 | 790 | 141 | 141 | 321 | 100 | 100 | 191 |
| 0.02 *** | 5028 | 5055 | 5119 | 1618 | 1626 | 1632 | 435 | 435 | 444 | 188 | 188 | 188 | 128 | 128 | 128 |
| *** | 5042 | 5078 | 14493 | 1618 | 1632 | 4316 | 435 | 435 | 1009 | 188 | 188 | 373 | 128 | 128 | 213 |
| 0.05 *** | 15225 | 15321 | 15995 | 4321 | 4376 | 4478 | 939 | 944 | 953 | 334 | 334 | 339 | 196 | 196 | 196 |
| *** | 15258 | 15478 | 30920 | 4340 | 4418 | 8378 | 939 | 944 | 1637 | 334 | 334 | 521 | 196 | 196 | 275 |
| 0.1 *** | 33587 | 33843 | 37230 | 9038 | 9230 | 9849 | 1764 | 1797 | 1833 | 559 | 559 | 568 | 298 | 298 | 298 |
| *** | 33669 | 34324 | 55917 | 9112 | 9436 | 14553 | 1778 | 1810 | 2590 | 559 | 559 | 744 | 298 | 298 | 368 |
| 0.15 *** | 50164 | 50623 | 58818 | 13273 | 13658 | 15230 | 2520 | 2589 | 2685 | 760 | 765 | 774 | 389 | 389 | 389 |
| *** | 50315 | 51511 | 77939 | 13415 | 14125 | 19984 | 2553 | 2635 | 3423 | 760 | 774 | 938 | 389 | 389 | 447 |
| 0.2 *** | 63543 | 64249 | 79017 | 16729 | 17348 | 20235 | 3166 | 3282 | 3469 | 930 | 944 | 958 | 458 | 463 | 471 |
| *** | 63776 | 65646 | 96984 | 16949 | 18132 | 24671 | 3221 | 3364 | 4137 | 939 | 953 | 1102 | 463 | 463 | 513 |
| 0.25 *** | 73310 | 74336 | 97010 | 19323 | 20208 | 24671 | 3689 | 3859 | 4148 | 1068 | 1090 | 1118 | 518 | 526 | 532 |
| *** | 73649 | 76349 | 113054 | 19644 | 21363 | 28614 | 3763 | 3983 | 4732 | 1082 | 1104 | 1235 | 526 | 532 | 566 |
| 0.3 *** | 79498 | 80909 | 112341 | 21069 | 22265 | 28439 | 4088 | 4321 | 4720 | 1178 | 1214 | 1247 | 568 | 573 | 587 |
| *** | 79965 | 83673 | 126148 | 21509 | 23810 | 31813 | 4189 | 4486 | 5208 | 1200 | 1228 | 1340 | 573 | 581 | 606 |
| 0.35 *** | 82353 | 84236 | 124735 | 22050 | 23585 | 31464 | 4368 | 4657 | 5165 | 1260 | 1302 | 1343 | 600 | 609 | 623 |
| *** | 82977 | 87885 | 136266 | 22614 | 25524 | 34268 | 4500 | 4871 | 5565 | 1283 | 1324 | 1414 | 609 | 614 | 632 |
| 0.4 *** | 82243 | 84695 | 134058 | 22361 | 24245 | 33710 | 4541 | 4885 | 5490 | 1315 | 1357 | 1412 | 623 | 628 | 642 |
| *** | 83059 | 89379 | 143408 | 23068 | 26560 | 35979 | 4693 | 5133 | 5803 | 1338 | 1384 | 1459 | 628 | 636 | 645 |
| 0.45 *** | 79603 | 82765 | 140204 | 22114 | 24347 | 35168 | 4615 | 5000 | 5683 | 1338 | 1384 | 1439 | 628 | 636 | 650 |
| *** | 80661 | 88600 | 147574 | 22958 | 27000 | 36946 | 4789 | 5284 | 5922 | 1357 | 1412 | 1474 | 636 | 642 | 645 |
| 0.5 *** | 74928 | 78934 | 143141 | 21426 | 23970 | 35823 | 4602 | 5014 | 5751 | 1329 | 1384 | 1448 | 623 | 628 | 642 |
| *** | 76280 | 85996 | 148765 | 22403 | 26904 | 37169 | 4780 | 5317 | 5922 | 1357 | 1412 | 1459 | 623 | 636 | 632 |
| 0.55 *** | 68754 | 73737 | 142830 | 20395 | 23192 | 35663 | 4500 | 4926 | 5688 | 1302 | 1351 | 1412 | 600 | 609 | 623 |
| *** | 70459 | 81995 | 146979 | 21487 | 26327 | 36648 | 4693 | 5243 | 5803 | 1324 | 1379 | 1414 | 600 | 614 | 606 |
| 0.6 *** | 61631 | 67668 | 139291 | 19108 | 22078 | 34700 | 4321 | 4748 | 5490 | 1241 | 1288 | 1351 | 568 | 573 | 587 |
| *** | 63749 | 76940 | 142218 | 20285 | 25309 | 35384 | 4505 | 5055 | 5565 | 1260 | 1315 | 1340 | 568 | 581 | 566 |
| 0.65 *** | 54110 | 61136 | 132518 | 17631 | 20670 | 32927 | 4060 | 4473 | 5174 | 1150 | 1200 | 1255 | 518 | 526 | 540 |
| *** | 56645 | 71105 | 134480 | 18841 | 23888 | 33375 | 4244 | 4761 | 5208 | 1173 | 1219 | 1235 | 526 | 532 | 513 |
| 0.7 *** | 46685 | 54404 | 122544 | 16000 | 18979 | 30355 | 3730 | 4101 | 4720 | 1040 | 1076 | 1123 | 458 | 463 | 471 |
| *** | 49559 | 64634 | 123767 | 17197 | 22059 | 30622 | 3895 | 4363 | 4732 | 1063 | 1095 | 1102 | 463 | 471 | 447 |
| 0.75 *** | 39631 | 47598 | 109385 | 14221 | 17018 | 26987 | 3309 | 3634 | 4143 | 898 | 930 | 966 | 380 | 389 | 394 |
| *** | 42670 | 57580 | 110078 | 15354 | 19823 | 27126 | 3460 | 3854 | 4137 | 911 | 944 | 938 | 389 | 394 | 368 |
| 0.8 *** | 33018 | 40668 | 93078 | 12269 | 14744 | 22829 | 2814 | 3062 | 3441 | 724 | 746 | 774 | 298 | 298 | 306 |
| *** | 35979 | 49861 | 93413 | 13286 | 17150 | 22885 | 2924 | 3227 | 3423 | 738 | 760 | 744 | 298 | 298 | 275 |
| 0.85 *** | 26651 | 33416 | 73649 | 10083 | 12082 | 17898 | 2209 | 2374 | 2616 | 526 | 540 | 554 | . | . | . |
| *** | 29305 | 41226 | 73773 | 10913 | 13938 | 17900 | 2286 | 2484 | 2590 | 532 | 545 | 521 | . | . | . |
| 0.9 *** | 20106 | 25364 | 51140 | 7511 | 8873 | 12192 | 1475 | 1558 | 1668 | . | . | . | . | . | . |
| *** | 22196 | 31139 | 51156 | 8089 | 10041 | 12172 | 1516 | 1613 | 1637 | . | . | . | . | . | . |
| 0.95 *** | 12398 | 15349 | 25584 | 4184 | 4734 | 5729 | . | . | . | . | . | . | . | . | . |
| *** | 13608 | 18269 | 25563 | 4431 | 5138 | 5699 | . | . | . | . | . | . | . | . | . |
| 0.98 *** | 5798 | 6755 | 8809 | . | . | . | . | . | . | . | . | . | . | . | . |
| *** | 6210 | 7530 | 8779 | . | . | . | . | . | . | . | . | . | . | . | . |

TABLE 2: ALPHA= 0.005 POWER= 0.9     EXPECTED ACCRUAL THRU MINIMUM FOLLOW-UP= 6000

| | | DEL=.01 | | | DEL=.02 | | | DEL=.05 | | | DEL=.10 | | | DEL=.15 | | |
|---|---|---|---|---|---|---|---|---|---|---|---|---|---|---|---|---|---|
| FACT= | | 1.0 .75 | .50 .25 | .00 BIN | 1.0 .75 | .50 .25 | .00 BIN | 1.0 .75 | .50 .25 | .00 BIN | 1.0 75 | .50 .25 | .00 BIN | 1.0 .75 | .50 .25 | .00 BIN |
| PCONT=*** | | | | | | REQUIRED NUMBER OF PATIENTS | | | | | | | | | | |
| 0.01 | *** | 2275 2284 | 2284 2290 | 2290 8779 | 835 835 | 835 835 | 844 2902 | 274 274 | 274 274 | 274 790 | 139 139 | 139 139 | 139 321 | 100 100 | 100 100 | 100 191 |
| 0.02 | *** | 5035 5044 | 5059 5080 | 5119 14493 | 1615 1624 | 1624 1630 | 1639 4316 | 439 439 | 439 439 | 439 1009 | 190 190 | 190 190 | 190 373 | 124 124 | 124 124 | 124 213 |
| 0.05 | *** | 15235 15274 | 15340 15505 | 15994 30920 | 4324 4345 | 4375 4420 | 4480 8378 | 934 940 | 940 949 | 949 1637 | 334 334 | 334 334 | 334 521 | 199 199 | 199 199 | 199 275 |
| 0.1 | *** | 33610 33700 | 33889 34399 | 37234 55917 | 9055 9139 | 9259 9460 | 9844 14553 | 1774 1780 | 1795 1810 | 1834 2399 | 559 559 | 559 565 | 565 744 | 295 295 | 295 295 | 295 368 |
| 0.15 | *** | 50209 50374 | 50704 51664 | 58819 77939 | 13315 13465 | 13714 14179 | 15229 19984 | 2530 2560 | 2599 2635 | 2689 3423 | 760 760 | 769 769 | 775 938 | 385 385 | 385 385 | 394 447 |
| 0.2 | *** | 63604 63865 | 64384 65890 | 79015 96984 | 16789 17029 | 17440 18229 | 20239 24671 | 3184 3235 | 3295 3370 | 3469 4137 | 934 940 | 940 955 | 964 1102 | 460 460 | 460 469 | 469 513 |
| 0.25 | *** | 73405 73774 | 74524 76705 | 97009 113054 | 19405 19750 | 20344 21505 | 24670 28614 | 3715 3790 | 3880 3994 | 4150 4732 | 1075 1084 | 1099 1105 | 1120 1235 | 520 529 | 529 529 | 535 566 |
| 0.3 | *** | 79624 80140 | 81169 84154 | 112339 126148 | 21190 21655 | 22450 24010 | 28435 31813 | 4120 4219 | 4345 4504 | 4714 5208 | 1189 1204 | 1210 1234 | 1249 1340 | 565 574 | 574 580 | 580 606 |
| 0.35 | *** | 82525 83209 | 84574 88510 | 124735 136266 | 22210 22810 | 23815 25774 | 31459 34268 | 4405 4534 | 4690 4894 | 5164 5565 | 1270 1285 | 1300 1324 | 1345 1414 | 604 610 | 610 619 | 619 632 |
| 0.4 | *** | 82465 83359 | 85144 90169 | 134059 143408 | 22564 23305 | 24520 26860 | 33715 35979 | 4594 4735 | 4924 5155 | 5485 5803 | 1324 1339 | 1360 1384 | 1414 1459 | 625 625 | 634 640 | 640 645 |
| 0.45 | *** | 79894 81040 | 83329 89554 | 140209 147574 | 22360 23239 | 24664 27340 | 35170 36946 | 4669 4834 | 5044 5314 | 5680 5922 | 1345 1369 | 1390 1414 | 1444 1474 | 625 634 | 640 649 | 649 645 |
| 0.5 | *** | 75295 76765 | 79639 87115 | 143140 148765 | 21709 22720 | 24325 27280 | 35824 37169 | 4654 4834 | 5059 5344 | 5749 5922 | 1339 1360 | 1390 1414 | 1444 1459 | 619 625 | 634 640 | 640 632 |
| 0.55 | *** | 69220 71074 | 74590 83254 | 142834 146979 | 20710 21835 | 23575 26719 | 35665 36648 | 4555 4744 | 4975 5269 | 5689 5803 | 1309 1330 | 1354 1384 | 1414 1414 | 604 604 | 610 619 | 625 606 |
| 0.6 | *** | 62215 64495 | 68659 78310 | 139294 142218 | 19450 20659 | 22480 25714 | 34699 35384 | 4375 4564 | 4789 5089 | 5494 5565 | 1249 1270 | 1294 1315 | 1345 1340 | 565 574 | 574 580 | 589 566 |
| 0.65 | *** | 54820 57520 | 62230 72535 | 132520 134480 | 17989 19225 | 21070 24280 | 32929 33375 | 4120 4294 | 4510 4789 | 5170 5208 | 1159 1180 | 1204 1225 | 1249 1235 | 520 520 | 529 535 | 535 513 |
| 0.7 | *** | 47500 50515 | 55564 66064 | 122545 123767 | 16354 17575 | 19369 22435 | 30355 30622 | 3775 3940 | 4135 4390 | 4720 4732 | 1045 1060 | 1084 1099 | 1120 1102 | 460 460 | 469 469 | 475 447 |
| 0.75 | *** | 40510 43660 | 48745 58945 | 109384 110078 | 14554 15709 | 17374 20164 | 26989 27126 | 3355 3499 | 3664 3874 | 4144 4137 | 904 919 | 934 949 | 964 938 | 385 385 | 394 394 | 394 368 |
| 0.8 | *** | 33880 36940 | 41749 51094 | 93079 93413 | 12574 13594 | 15055 17425 | 22825 22885 | 2845 2959 | 3085 3244 | 3439 3423 | 730 739 | 754 760 | 769 744 | 295 295 | 304 304 | 304 275 |
| 0.85 | *** | 27430 30154 | 34345 42250 | 73654 73773 | 10330 11164 | 12325 14149 | 17899 17900 | 2230 2305 | 2395 2494 | 2614 2590 | 529 535 | 535 544 | 550 521 | . . | . . | . . |
| 0.9 | *** | 20725 22855 | 26065 31879 | 51145 51156 | 7684 8260 | 9034 10165 | 12190 12172 | 1489 1525 | 1570 1615 | 1669 1637 | . . | . . | . . | . . | . . | . . |
| 0.95 | *** | 12760 13975 | 15724 18619 | 25585 25563 | 4264 4495 | 4795 5179 | 5725 5699 | . . | . . | . . | . . | . . | . . | . . | . . | . . |
| 0.98 | *** | 5920 6334 | 6865 7615 | 8809 8779 | . . | . . | . . | . . | . . | . . | . . | . . | . . | . . | . . | . . |

# TABLE 2: ALPHA= 0.005 POWER= 0.9    EXPECTED ACCRUAL THRU MINIMUM FOLLOW-UP= 6500

| | DEL=.01 | | | DEL=.02 | | | DEL=.05 | | | DEL=.10 | | | DEL=.15 | | |
|---|---|---|---|---|---|---|---|---|---|---|---|---|---|---|---|
| FACT= | 1.0 .75 | .50 .25 | .00 BIN | 1.0 .75 | .50 .25 | .00 BIN | 1.0 .75 | .50 .25 | .00 BIN | 1.0 75 | .50 .25 | .00 BIN | 1.0 .75 | .50 .25 | .00 BIN |

PCONT=***                    REQUIRED NUMBER OF PATIENTS

| PCONT | 1.0 .75 | .50 .25 | .00 BIN | 1.0 .75 | .50 .25 | .00 BIN | 1.0 .75 | .50 .25 | .00 BIN | 1.0 75 | .50 .25 | .00 BIN | 1.0 .75 | .50 .25 | .00 BIN |
|---|---|---|---|---|---|---|---|---|---|---|---|---|---|---|---|
| 0.01 *** | 2280 | 2286 | 2296 | 839 | 839 | 839 | 271 | 281 | 281 | 141 | 141 | 141 | 102 | 102 | 102 |
| *** | 2280 | 2286 | 8779 | 839 | 839 | 2902 | 281 | 281 | 790 | 141 | 141 | 321 | 102 | 102 | 191 |
| 0.02 *** | 5032 | 5058 | 5123 | 1619 | 1630 | 1636 | 433 | 443 | 443 | 189 | 189 | 189 | 124 | 124 | 124 |
| *** | 5048 | 5081 | 14493 | 1619 | 1630 | 4316 | 443 | 443 | 1009 | 189 | 189 | 373 | 124 | 124 | 213 |
| 0.05 *** | 15247 | 15361 | 15995 | 4333 | 4382 | 4479 | 937 | 947 | 947 | 336 | 336 | 336 | 200 | 200 | 200 |
| *** | 15280 | 15523 | 30920 | 4360 | 4425 | 8378 | 937 | 947 | 1637 | 336 | 336 | 521 | 200 | 200 | 275 |
| 0.1 *** | 33632 | 33935 | 37233 | 9078 | 9283 | 9842 | 1776 | 1798 | 1831 | 557 | 563 | 563 | 297 | 297 | 297 |
| *** | 33729 | 34477 | 55917 | 9159 | 9484 | 14553 | 1782 | 1814 | 2590 | 557 | 563 | 744 | 297 | 297 | 368 |
| 0.15 *** | 50250 | 50786 | 58813 | 13352 | 13768 | 15231 | 2540 | 2605 | 2686 | 758 | 768 | 774 | 384 | 384 | 395 |
| *** | 50428 | 51816 | 77939 | 13508 | 14229 | 19984 | 2572 | 2643 | 3423 | 758 | 768 | 938 | 384 | 384 | 447 |
| 0.2 *** | 63672 | 64507 | 79018 | 16856 | 17528 | 20236 | 3196 | 3309 | 3466 | 931 | 947 | 963 | 460 | 466 | 466 |
| *** | 63948 | 66132 | 96984 | 17106 | 18324 | 24671 | 3244 | 3374 | 4137 | 937 | 953 | 1102 | 466 | 466 | 513 |
| 0.25 *** | 73493 | 74706 | 97007 | 19494 | 20469 | 24672 | 3732 | 3894 | 4148 | 1077 | 1093 | 1116 | 525 | 531 | 531 |
| *** | 73899 | 77046 | 113054 | 19862 | 21650 | 28614 | 3807 | 4008 | 4732 | 1083 | 1110 | 1235 | 525 | 531 | 566 |
| 0.3 *** | 79749 | 81423 | 112341 | 21314 | 22614 | 28432 | 4148 | 4366 | 4717 | 1191 | 1213 | 1246 | 573 | 579 | 579 |
| *** | 80312 | 84618 | 126148 | 21802 | 24191 | 31813 | 4246 | 4522 | 5208 | 1207 | 1229 | 1340 | 573 | 579 | 606 |
| 0.35 *** | 82691 | 84917 | 124740 | 22365 | 24028 | 31465 | 4447 | 4717 | 5162 | 1272 | 1305 | 1343 | 606 | 612 | 622 |
| *** | 83438 | 89120 | 136266 | 22988 | 26005 | 34268 | 4571 | 4912 | 5565 | 1288 | 1327 | 1414 | 606 | 612 | 632 |
| 0.4 *** | 82685 | 85583 | 134057 | 22755 | 24786 | 33713 | 4636 | 4951 | 5487 | 1327 | 1370 | 1408 | 622 | 628 | 644 |
| *** | 83660 | 90929 | 143408 | 23524 | 27132 | 35979 | 4772 | 5178 | 5803 | 1343 | 1386 | 1459 | 628 | 638 | 645 |
| 0.45 *** | 80182 | 83887 | 140210 | 22592 | 24965 | 35170 | 4717 | 5081 | 5682 | 1353 | 1392 | 1441 | 628 | 638 | 655 |
| *** | 81423 | 90474 | 147574 | 23508 | 27652 | 36946 | 4880 | 5335 | 5922 | 1370 | 1418 | 1474 | 638 | 644 | 645 |
| 0.5 *** | 75671 | 80328 | 143141 | 21981 | 24662 | 35826 | 4707 | 5097 | 5747 | 1343 | 1392 | 1441 | 622 | 628 | 644 |
| *** | 77257 | 88183 | 148765 | 23031 | 27619 | 37169 | 4880 | 5373 | 5922 | 1370 | 1418 | 1459 | 628 | 638 | 632 |
| 0.55 *** | 69691 | 75421 | 142832 | 21016 | 23941 | 35663 | 4609 | 5016 | 5682 | 1311 | 1359 | 1408 | 606 | 612 | 622 |
| *** | 71673 | 84456 | 146979 | 22170 | 27077 | 36648 | 4788 | 5302 | 5803 | 1337 | 1386 | 1414 | 606 | 622 | 606 |
| 0.6 *** | 62795 | 69620 | 139289 | 19781 | 22852 | 34698 | 4431 | 4831 | 5497 | 1256 | 1294 | 1343 | 563 | 579 | 590 |
| *** | 65222 | 79603 | 142218 | 21006 | 26076 | 35384 | 4609 | 5113 | 5565 | 1272 | 1321 | 1340 | 573 | 579 | 566 |
| 0.65 *** | 55521 | 63288 | 132523 | 18324 | 21444 | 32927 | 4171 | 4555 | 5172 | 1164 | 1207 | 1256 | 525 | 531 | 541 |
| *** | 58364 | 73877 | 134480 | 19586 | 24640 | 33375 | 4343 | 4815 | 5208 | 1181 | 1229 | 1235 | 525 | 531 | 513 |
| 0.7 *** | 48289 | 56658 | 122546 | 16683 | 19732 | 30349 | 3823 | 4171 | 4723 | 1051 | 1083 | 1126 | 460 | 466 | 476 |
| *** | 51442 | 67399 | 123767 | 17928 | 22771 | 30622 | 3986 | 4408 | 4732 | 1067 | 1099 | 1102 | 466 | 466 | 447 |
| 0.75 *** | 41345 | 49833 | 109383 | 14873 | 17707 | 26986 | 3401 | 3693 | 4148 | 904 | 931 | 963 | 384 | 395 | 395 |
| *** | 44611 | 60217 | 110078 | 16033 | 20463 | 27126 | 3537 | 3894 | 4137 | 921 | 947 | 938 | 384 | 395 | 368 |
| 0.8 *** | 34698 | 42764 | 93074 | 12858 | 15334 | 22826 | 2881 | 3108 | 3439 | 736 | 752 | 774 | 297 | 303 | 303 |
| *** | 37841 | 52238 | 93413 | 13882 | 17685 | 22885 | 2984 | 3261 | 3423 | 742 | 758 | 744 | 297 | 303 | 275 |
| 0.85 *** | 28166 | 35218 | 73650 | 10567 | 12550 | 17896 | 2253 | 2410 | 2611 | 531 | 541 | 547 | . | . | . |
| *** | 30951 | 43203 | 73773 | 11396 | 14337 | 17900 | 2328 | 2507 | 2590 | 531 | 547 | 521 | . | . | . |
| 0.9 *** | 21298 | 26726 | 51143 | 7843 | 9176 | 12192 | 1500 | 1571 | 1668 | . | . | . | . | . | . |
| *** | 23476 | 32553 | 51156 | 8412 | 10281 | 12172 | 1538 | 1619 | 1637 | . | . | . | . | . | . |
| 0.95 *** | 13092 | 16066 | 25588 | 4327 | 4847 | 5725 | . | . | . | . | . | . | . | . | . |
| *** | 14321 | 18926 | 25563 | 4561 | 5221 | 5699 | . | . | . | . | . | . | . | . | . |
| 0.98 *** | 6039 | 6966 | 8812 | . | . | . | . | . | . | . | . | . | . | . | . |
| *** | 6446 | 7681 | 8779 | . | . | . | . | . | . | . | . | . | . | . | . |

## TABLE 2: ALPHA= 0.005 POWER= 0.9     EXPECTED ACCRUAL THRU MINIMUM FOLLOW-UP= 7000

| | | DEL=.01 | | | DEL=.02 | | | DEL=.05 | | | DEL=.10 | | | DEL=.15 | | |
|---|---|---|---|---|---|---|---|---|---|---|---|---|---|---|---|---|---|
| FACT= | | 1.0 .75 | .50 .25 | .00 BIN | 1.0 .75 | .50 .25 | .00 BIN | 1.0 .75 | .50 .25 | .00 BIN | 1.0 75 | .50 .25 | .00 BIN | 1.0 .75 | .50 .25 | .00 BIN |
| PCONT=*** | | | | REQUIRED NUMBER OF PATIENTS | | | | | | | | | | | | |
| 0.01 | *** | 2280 | 2286 | 2297 | 834 | 834 | 845 | 274 | 274 | 274 | 134 | 134 | 134 | 99 | 99 | 99 |
| | *** | 2280 | 2286 | 8779 | 834 | 834 | 2902 | 274 | 274 | 790 | 134 | 134 | 321 | 99 | 99 | 191 |
| 0.02 | *** | 5034 | 5062 | 5121 | 1621 | 1621 | 1632 | 442 | 442 | 442 | 186 | 186 | 186 | 127 | 127 | 127 |
| | *** | 5051 | 5086 | 14493 | 1621 | 1632 | 4316 | 442 | 442 | 1009 | 186 | 186 | 373 | 127 | 127 | 213 |
| 0.05 | *** | 15254 | 15370 | 16000 | 4334 | 4386 | 4485 | 939 | 939 | 950 | 337 | 337 | 337 | 197 | 197 | 197 |
| | *** | 15289 | 15545 | 30920 | 4362 | 4432 | 8378 | 939 | 950 | 1637 | 337 | 337 | 521 | 197 | 197 | 275 |
| 0.1 | *** | 33657 | 33979 | 37234 | 9094 | 9304 | 9846 | 1779 | 1796 | 1831 | 554 | 565 | 565 | 302 | 302 | 302 |
| | *** | 33762 | 34550 | 55917 | 9181 | 9496 | 14553 | 1790 | 1814 | 2590 | 565 | 565 | 744 | 302 | 302 | 368 |
| 0.15 | *** | 50289 | 50866 | 58811 | 13392 | 13819 | 15230 | 2549 | 2601 | 2689 | 757 | 764 | 775 | 390 | 390 | 390 |
| | *** | 50481 | 51962 | 77939 | 13556 | 14274 | 19984 | 2577 | 2647 | 3423 | 764 | 775 | 938 | 390 | 390 | 447 |
| 0.2 | *** | 63729 | 64639 | 79017 | 16910 | 17610 | 20235 | 3214 | 3319 | 3470 | 932 | 950 | 956 | 460 | 466 | 466 |
| | *** | 64037 | 66365 | 96984 | 17179 | 18404 | 24671 | 3260 | 3382 | 4137 | 939 | 956 | 1102 | 460 | 466 | 513 |
| 0.25 | *** | 73592 | 74894 | 97007 | 19587 | 20591 | 24669 | 3756 | 3914 | 4152 | 1079 | 1096 | 1114 | 519 | 530 | 530 |
| | *** | 74019 | 77390 | 113054 | 19961 | 21764 | 28614 | 3826 | 4012 | 4732 | 1090 | 1107 | 1235 | 530 | 530 | 566 |
| 0.3 | *** | 79881 | 81677 | 112337 | 21431 | 22779 | 28431 | 4176 | 4386 | 4719 | 1195 | 1219 | 1247 | 571 | 582 | 582 |
| | *** | 80476 | 85079 | 126148 | 21939 | 24365 | 31813 | 4275 | 4526 | 5208 | 1201 | 1230 | 1340 | 571 | 582 | 606 |
| 0.35 | *** | 82867 | 85254 | 124734 | 22516 | 24231 | 31459 | 4474 | 4747 | 5167 | 1282 | 1306 | 1341 | 606 | 617 | 624 |
| | *** | 83661 | 89716 | 136266 | 23175 | 26209 | 34268 | 4596 | 4922 | 5565 | 1289 | 1324 | 1414 | 606 | 617 | 632 |
| 0.4 | *** | 82909 | 86024 | 134055 | 22947 | 25030 | 33710 | 4666 | 4981 | 5489 | 1335 | 1370 | 1411 | 624 | 635 | 641 |
| | *** | 83952 | 91670 | 143408 | 23741 | 27381 | 35979 | 4806 | 5202 | 5803 | 1352 | 1387 | 1459 | 635 | 641 | 645 |
| 0.45 | *** | 80470 | 84442 | 140204 | 22814 | 25246 | 35169 | 4765 | 5115 | 5681 | 1359 | 1394 | 1440 | 635 | 641 | 652 |
| | *** | 81806 | 91361 | 147574 | 23759 | 27941 | 36946 | 4922 | 5360 | 5922 | 1376 | 1422 | 1474 | 635 | 641 | 645 |
| 0.5 | *** | 76031 | 81012 | 143137 | 22236 | 24966 | 35827 | 4754 | 5132 | 5751 | 1352 | 1394 | 1446 | 624 | 635 | 641 |
| | *** | 77740 | 89209 | 148765 | 23315 | 27935 | 37169 | 4922 | 5395 | 5922 | 1370 | 1422 | 1459 | 624 | 641 | 632 |
| 0.55 | *** | 70151 | 76235 | 142829 | 21302 | 24266 | 35670 | 4660 | 5051 | 5681 | 1317 | 1359 | 1411 | 600 | 617 | 624 |
| | *** | 72280 | 85597 | 146979 | 22481 | 27410 | 36648 | 4835 | 5325 | 5803 | 1341 | 1387 | 1414 | 606 | 617 | 606 |
| 0.6 | *** | 63372 | 70547 | 139287 | 20084 | 23199 | 34696 | 4474 | 4870 | 5489 | 1265 | 1300 | 1352 | 571 | 582 | 589 |
| | *** | 65945 | 80837 | 142218 | 21337 | 26412 | 35384 | 4649 | 5132 | 5565 | 1282 | 1324 | 1340 | 571 | 582 | 566 |
| 0.65 | *** | 56204 | 64289 | 132521 | 18642 | 21792 | 32929 | 4211 | 4590 | 5167 | 1166 | 1212 | 1254 | 519 | 530 | 536 |
| | *** | 59190 | 75139 | 134480 | 19920 | 24966 | 33375 | 4380 | 4835 | 5208 | 1195 | 1230 | 1235 | 530 | 530 | 513 |
| 0.7 | *** | 49057 | 57709 | 122546 | 17004 | 20060 | 30356 | 3872 | 4205 | 4719 | 1055 | 1090 | 1125 | 460 | 466 | 477 |
| | *** | 52330 | 68664 | 123767 | 18246 | 23076 | 30622 | 4019 | 4432 | 4732 | 1072 | 1107 | 1102 | 466 | 466 | 447 |
| 0.75 | *** | 42151 | 50866 | 109386 | 15166 | 18012 | 26990 | 3435 | 3721 | 4141 | 915 | 932 | 967 | 390 | 390 | 396 |
| | *** | 45511 | 61412 | 110078 | 16339 | 20742 | 27126 | 3564 | 3907 | 4137 | 921 | 950 | 938 | 390 | 390 | 368 |
| 0.8 | *** | 35477 | 43720 | 93076 | 13119 | 15604 | 22831 | 2910 | 3126 | 3441 | 740 | 757 | 775 | 302 | 302 | 302 |
| | *** | 38697 | 53310 | 93413 | 14151 | 17907 | 22885 | 3015 | 3266 | 3423 | 746 | 764 | 744 | 302 | 302 | 275 |
| 0.85 | *** | 28862 | 36037 | 73651 | 10774 | 12751 | 17896 | 2280 | 2420 | 2612 | 530 | 536 | 547 | . | . | . |
| | *** | 31697 | 44087 | 73773 | 11607 | 14501 | 17900 | 2339 | 2507 | 2590 | 536 | 547 | 521 | . | . | . |
| 0.9 | *** | 21851 | 27340 | 51140 | 7991 | 9304 | 12191 | 1510 | 1580 | 1667 | . | . | . | . | . | . |
| | *** | 24050 | 33174 | 51156 | 8562 | 10382 | 12172 | 1545 | 1621 | 1637 | . | . | . | . | . | . |
| 0.95 | *** | 13410 | 16385 | 25590 | 4386 | 4894 | 5727 | . | . | . | . | . | . | . | . | . |
| | *** | 14641 | 19220 | 25563 | 4614 | 5244 | 5699 | . | . | . | . | . | . | . | . | . |
| 0.98 | *** | 6147 | 7046 | 8807 | . | . | . | . | . | . | . | . | . | . | . | . |
| | *** | 6539 | 7746 | 8779 | . | . | . | . | . | . | . | . | . | . | . | . |

# TABLE 2: ALPHA= 0.005 POWER= 0.9     EXPECTED ACCRUAL THRU MINIMUM FOLLOW-UP= 7500

| | | DEL=.01 | | | DEL=.02 | | | DEL=.05 | | | DEL=.10 | | | DEL=.15 | | |
|---|---|---|---|---|---|---|---|---|---|---|---|---|---|---|---|---|---|
| FACT= | | 1.0 .75 | .50 .25 | .00 BIN | 1.0 .75 | .50 .25 | .00 BIN | 1.0 .75 | .50 .25 | .00 BIN | 1.0 75 | .50 .25 | .00 BIN | 1.0 .75 | .50 .25 | .00 BIN |
| PCONT=*** | | | | | REQUIRED NUMBER OF PATIENTS | | | | | | | | | | | |
| 0.01 | *** | 2281 | 2281 | 2293 | 837 | 837 | 837 | 275 | 275 | 275 | 136 | 136 | 136 | 99 | 99 | 99 |
| | *** | 2281 | 2293 | 8779 | 837 | 837 | 2902 | 275 | 275 | 790 | 136 | 136 | 321 | 99 | 99 | 191 |
| 0.02 | *** | 5037 | 5068 | 5124 | 1618 | 1625 | 1636 | 436 | 436 | 436 | 193 | 193 | 193 | 125 | 125 | 125 |
| | *** | 5049 | 5086 | 14493 | 1625 | 1636 | 4316 | 436 | 436 | 1009 | 193 | 193 | 373 | 125 | 125 | 213 |
| 0.05 | *** | 15256 | 15387 | 15999 | 4343 | 4393 | 4486 | 943 | 943 | 950 | 331 | 331 | 331 | 193 | 193 | 193 |
| | *** | 15305 | 15556 | 30920 | 4362 | 4430 | 8378 | 943 | 950 | 1637 | 331 | 331 | 521 | 193 | 193 | 275 |
| 0.1 | *** | 33680 | 34025 | 37231 | 9118 | 9324 | 9849 | 1775 | 1805 | 1831 | 556 | 556 | 568 | 293 | 293 | 293 |
| | *** | 33793 | 34618 | 55917 | 9200 | 9518 | 14553 | 1793 | 1812 | 2590 | 556 | 568 | 744 | 293 | 293 | 368 |
| 0.15 | *** | 50330 | 50949 | 58812 | 13430 | 13868 | 15230 | 2555 | 2611 | 2686 | 762 | 762 | 774 | 387 | 387 | 387 |
| | *** | 50536 | 52100 | 77939 | 13599 | 14318 | 19984 | 2581 | 2649 | 3423 | 762 | 774 | 938 | 387 | 387 | 447 |
| 0.2 | *** | 63800 | 64768 | 79018 | 16974 | 17686 | 20236 | 3218 | 3324 | 3462 | 931 | 950 | 961 | 462 | 462 | 474 |
| | *** | 64118 | 66593 | 96984 | 17243 | 18481 | 24671 | 3268 | 3387 | 4137 | 943 | 950 | 1102 | 462 | 462 | 513 |
| 0.25 | *** | 73681 | 75080 | 97006 | 19674 | 20705 | 24668 | 3774 | 3924 | 4149 | 1081 | 1100 | 1118 | 518 | 530 | 530 |
| | *** | 74150 | 77712 | 113054 | 20068 | 21886 | 28614 | 3837 | 4025 | 4732 | 1093 | 1111 | 1235 | 530 | 530 | 566 |
| 0.3 | *** | 80011 | 81931 | 112336 | 21549 | 22936 | 28437 | 4193 | 4400 | 4718 | 1193 | 1224 | 1250 | 575 | 575 | 586 |
| | *** | 80656 | 85524 | 126148 | 22074 | 24511 | 31813 | 4287 | 4543 | 5208 | 1205 | 1231 | 1340 | 575 | 586 | 606 |
| 0.35 | *** | 83037 | 85587 | 124737 | 22662 | 24425 | 31456 | 4505 | 4768 | 5161 | 1280 | 1306 | 1343 | 605 | 612 | 624 |
| | *** | 83893 | 90293 | 136266 | 23337 | 26405 | 34268 | 4625 | 4936 | 5565 | 1299 | 1325 | 1414 | 612 | 612 | 632 |
| 0.4 | *** | 83131 | 86461 | 134056 | 23124 | 25261 | 33718 | 4700 | 5011 | 5487 | 1336 | 1374 | 1411 | 624 | 631 | 643 |
| | *** | 84256 | 92386 | 143408 | 23949 | 27612 | 35979 | 4843 | 5218 | 5803 | 1355 | 1393 | 1459 | 631 | 643 | 645 |
| 0.45 | *** | 80761 | 84987 | 140206 | 23030 | 25512 | 35168 | 4793 | 5143 | 5686 | 1362 | 1400 | 1437 | 631 | 643 | 650 |
| | *** | 82193 | 92218 | 147574 | 24005 | 28205 | 36946 | 4955 | 5375 | 5922 | 1381 | 1418 | 1474 | 643 | 643 | 645 |
| 0.5 | *** | 76400 | 81680 | 143143 | 22486 | 25261 | 35825 | 4793 | 5161 | 5750 | 1355 | 1400 | 1449 | 624 | 631 | 643 |
| | *** | 78218 | 90193 | 148765 | 23581 | 28212 | 37169 | 4962 | 5412 | 5922 | 1374 | 1418 | 1459 | 631 | 643 | 632 |
| 0.55 | *** | 70618 | 77018 | 142831 | 21575 | 24586 | 35668 | 4700 | 5086 | 5686 | 1325 | 1362 | 1411 | 605 | 612 | 624 |
| | *** | 72868 | 86686 | 146979 | 22775 | 27706 | 36648 | 4868 | 5337 | 5803 | 1343 | 1393 | 1414 | 605 | 612 | 606 |
| 0.6 | *** | 63931 | 71431 | 139287 | 20375 | 23518 | 34700 | 4524 | 4899 | 5487 | 1261 | 1306 | 1343 | 568 | 575 | 586 |
| | *** | 66643 | 81999 | 142218 | 21643 | 26724 | 35384 | 4693 | 5150 | 5565 | 1280 | 1325 | 1340 | 575 | 586 | 566 |
| 0.65 | *** | 56874 | 65262 | 132518 | 18943 | 22111 | 32930 | 4261 | 4618 | 5168 | 1175 | 1212 | 1250 | 518 | 530 | 537 |
| | *** | 59986 | 76343 | 134480 | 20225 | 25268 | 33375 | 4418 | 4861 | 5208 | 1193 | 1231 | 1235 | 530 | 530 | 513 |
| 0.7 | *** | 49793 | 58700 | 122543 | 17293 | 20368 | 30350 | 3905 | 4231 | 4718 | 1062 | 1093 | 1118 | 462 | 462 | 474 |
| | *** | 53180 | 69849 | 123767 | 18556 | 23368 | 30622 | 4055 | 4449 | 4732 | 1074 | 1100 | 1102 | 462 | 474 | 447 |
| 0.75 | *** | 42924 | 51849 | 109381 | 15443 | 18293 | 26986 | 3474 | 3743 | 4149 | 912 | 943 | 961 | 387 | 387 | 399 |
| | *** | 46374 | 62536 | 110078 | 16625 | 20993 | 27126 | 3593 | 3924 | 4137 | 924 | 950 | 938 | 387 | 387 | 368 |
| 0.8 | *** | 36230 | 44618 | 93080 | 13362 | 15849 | 22831 | 2937 | 3143 | 3443 | 736 | 755 | 774 | 293 | 305 | 305 |
| | *** | 39518 | 54305 | 93413 | 14393 | 18118 | 22885 | 3031 | 3275 | 3423 | 743 | 762 | 744 | 293 | 305 | 275 |
| 0.85 | *** | 29518 | 36811 | 73655 | 10974 | 12943 | 17893 | 2293 | 2431 | 2611 | 530 | 537 | 549 | . | . | . |
| | *** | 32412 | 44900 | 73773 | 11806 | 14656 | 17900 | 2356 | 2518 | 2590 | 537 | 549 | 521 | . | . | . |
| 0.9 | *** | 22362 | 27912 | 51143 | 8131 | 9425 | 12193 | 1524 | 1587 | 1662 | . | . | . | . | . | . |
| | *** | 24593 | 33755 | 51156 | 8693 | 10468 | 12172 | 1550 | 1625 | 1637 | . | . | . | . | . | . |
| 0.95 | *** | 13700 | 16681 | 25587 | 4449 | 4936 | 5724 | . | . | . | . | . | . | . | . | . |
| | *** | 14937 | 19475 | 25563 | 4662 | 5274 | 5699 | . | . | . | . | . | . | . | . | . |
| 0.98 | *** | 6237 | 7130 | 8806 | . | . | . | . | . | . | . | . | . | . | . | . |
| | *** | 6631 | 7805 | 8779 | . | . | . | . | . | . | . | . | . | . | . | . |

TABLE 2: ALPHA= 0.005 POWER= 0.9    EXPECTED ACCRUAL THRU MINIMUM FOLLOW-UP= 8000

| | DEL=.01 | | | DEL=.02 | | | DEL=.05 | | | DEL=.10 | | | DEL=.15 | | |
|---|---|---|---|---|---|---|---|---|---|---|---|---|---|---|---|
| FACT= | 1.0 .75 | .50 .25 | .00 BIN | 1.0 .75 | .50 .25 | .00 BIN | 1.0 .75 | .50 .25 | .00 BIN | 1.0 75 | .50 .25 | .00 BIN | 1.0 .75 | .50 .25 | .00 BIN |
| PCONT=*** | | | | REQUIRED NUMBER OF PATIENTS | | | | | | | | | | | |
| 0.01 *** | 2285 2285 | 2285 2285 | 2293 8779 | 833 833 | 833 833 | 845 2902 | 273 273 | 273 273 | 273 790 | 133 133 | 133 133 | 133 321 | 93 93 | 93 93 | 93 191 |
| 0.02 *** | 5045 5053 | 5065 5093 | 5125 14493 | 1625 1625 | 1625 1633 | 1633 4316 | 433 433 | 433 433 | 445 1009 | 193 193 | 193 193 | 193 373 | 125 125 | 125 125 | 125 213 |
| 0.05 *** | 15273 15313 | 15405 15573 | 15993 30920 | 4345 4373 | 4393 4433 | 4485 8378 | 945 945 | 945 945 | 953 1637 | 333 333 | 333 333 | 333 521 | 193 193 | 193 193 | 193 275 |
| 0.1 *** | 33705 33825 | 34065 34685 | 37233 55917 | 9133 9225 | 9345 9533 | 9845 14553 | 1785 1793 | 1805 1813 | 1833 2590 | 553 565 | 565 565 | 565 744 | 293 293 | 293 293 | 293 368 |
| 0.15 *** | 50373 50593 | 51033 52233 | 58813 77939 | 13465 13633 | 13905 14365 | 15225 19984 | 2565 2585 | 2613 2645 | 2685 3423 | 765 765 | 765 773 | 773 938 | 385 385 | 385 385 | 393 447 |
| 0.2 *** | 63865 64205 | 64893 66813 | 79013 96984 | 17033 17313 | 17765 18553 | 20233 24671 | 3233 3285 | 3333 3393 | 3465 4137 | 933 945 | 945 953 | 965 1102 | 465 465 | 465 465 | 465 513 |
| 0.25 *** | 73773 74273 | 75265 78033 | 97013 113054 | 19753 20165 | 20813 21993 | 24673 28614 | 3785 3853 | 3933 4033 | 4145 4732 | 1085 1093 | 1105 1105 | 1113 1235 | 525 525 | 525 533 | 533 566 |
| 0.3 *** | 80133 80825 | 82185 85965 | 112333 126148 | 21653 22205 | 23073 24653 | 28433 31813 | 4225 4313 | 4413 4553 | 4713 5208 | 1205 1213 | 1225 1233 | 1245 1340 | 573 573 | 573 585 | 585 606 |
| 0.35 *** | 83205 84125 | 85925 90853 | 124733 136266 | 22805 23505 | 24605 26585 | 31465 34268 | 4533 4645 | 4785 4953 | 5165 5565 | 1285 1293 | 1313 1325 | 1345 1414 | 605 613 | 613 613 | 625 632 |
| 0.4 *** | 83353 84553 | 86893 93073 | 134053 143408 | 23305 24153 | 25473 27833 | 33713 35979 | 4733 4873 | 5033 5233 | 5485 5803 | 1345 1353 | 1373 1393 | 1413 1459 | 625 633 | 633 633 | 645 645 |
| 0.45 *** | 81045 82573 | 85525 93033 | 140205 147574 | 23245 24233 | 25765 28445 | 35173 36946 | 4833 4985 | 5165 5393 | 5685 5922 | 1365 1385 | 1405 1425 | 1445 1474 | 633 633 | 645 645 | 653 645 |
| 0.5 *** | 76765 78693 | 82333 91133 | 143133 148765 | 22725 23845 | 25533 28485 | 35825 37169 | 4833 4993 | 5193 5433 | 5745 5922 | 1365 1385 | 1405 1425 | 1445 1459 | 625 633 | 633 633 | 645 632 |
| 0.55 *** | 71073 73453 | 77793 87725 | 142833 146979 | 21833 23053 | 24873 27993 | 35665 36648 | 4745 4913 | 5113 5365 | 5685 5803 | 1333 1345 | 1365 1385 | 1413 1414 | 605 613 | 613 613 | 625 606 |
| 0.6 *** | 64493 67333 | 72305 83105 | 139293 142218 | 20653 21933 | 23825 27005 | 34705 35384 | 4565 4725 | 4925 5173 | 5493 5565 | 1273 1285 | 1305 1325 | 1345 1340 | 573 573 | 573 585 | 585 566 |
| 0.65 *** | 57525 60753 | 66193 77473 | 132525 134480 | 19225 20525 | 22413 25545 | 32925 33375 | 4293 4453 | 4645 4873 | 5173 5208 | 1185 1193 | 1213 1233 | 1253 1235 | 525 525 | 533 533 | 533 513 |
| 0.7 *** | 50513 54005 | 59665 70965 | 122545 123767 | 17573 18845 | 20653 23625 | 30353 30622 | 3945 4085 | 4253 4465 | 4725 4732 | 1065 1073 | 1093 1105 | 1125 1102 | 465 465 | 465 473 | 473 447 |
| 0.75 *** | 43665 47193 | 52773 63585 | 109385 110078 | 15705 16885 | 18553 21225 | 26985 27126 | 3493 3625 | 3765 3933 | 4145 4137 | 913 925 | 933 953 | 965 938 | 385 385 | 393 393 | 393 368 |
| 0.8 *** | 36933 40293 | 45473 55245 | 93073 93413 | 13593 14633 | 16073 18313 | 22825 22885 | 2953 3053 | 3165 3285 | 3445 3423 | 745 745 | 753 765 | 773 744 | 293 305 | 305 305 | 305 275 |
| 0.85 *** | 30153 33085 | 37545 45673 | 73653 73773 | 11165 11993 | 13113 14793 | 17893 17900 | 2305 2373 | 2445 2525 | 2613 2590 | 533 533 | 545 545 | 553 521 | . . | . . | . . |
| 0.9 *** | 22853 25113 | 28453 34285 | 51145 51156 | 8253 8813 | 9533 10553 | 12193 12172 | 1525 1553 | 1593 1625 | 1665 1637 | . . | . . | . . | . . | . . | . . |
| 0.95 *** | 13973 15213 | 16953 19713 | 25585 25563 | 4493 4713 | 4973 5293 | 5725 5699 | . . | . . | . . | . . | . . | . . | . . | . . | . . |
| 0.98 *** | 6333 6713 | 7205 7853 | 8805 8779 | . . | . . | . . | . . | . . | . . | . . | . . | . . | . . | . . | . . |

# TABLE 2: ALPHA= 0.005 POWER= 0.9    EXPECTED ACCRUAL THRU MINIMUM FOLLOW-UP= 8500

| | | DEL=.01 | | | DEL=.02 | | | DEL=.05 | | | DEL=.10 | | | DEL=.15 | | |
|---|---|---|---|---|---|---|---|---|---|---|---|---|---|---|---|---|---|
| FACT= | | 1.0 .75 | .50 .25 | .00 BIN | 1.0 .75 | .50 .25 | .00 BIN | 1.0 .75 | .50 .25 | .00 BIN | 1.0 75 | .50 .25 | .00 BIN | 1.0 .75 | .50 .25 | .00 BIN |
| PCONT=*** | | REQUIRED NUMBER OF PATIENTS | | | | | | | | | | | | | | |
| 0.01 | *** | 2280 | 2288 | 2288 | 835 | 843 | 843 | 282 | 282 | 282 | 141 | 141 | 141 | 99 | 99 | 99 |
| | *** | 2280 | 2288 | 8779 | 835 | 843 | 2902 | 282 | 282 | 790 | 141 | 141 | 321 | 99 | 99 | 191 |
| 0.02 | *** | 5042 | 5071 | 5127 | 1621 | 1629 | 1629 | 439 | 439 | 439 | 197 | 197 | 197 | 120 | 120 | 120 |
| | *** | 5050 | 5093 | 14493 | 1629 | 1629 | 4316 | 439 | 439 | 1009 | 197 | 197 | 373 | 120 | 120 | 213 |
| 0.05 | *** | 15285 | 15420 | 15994 | 4349 | 4405 | 4476 | 941 | 941 | 949 | 333 | 333 | 333 | 197 | 197 | 197 |
| | *** | 15327 | 15590 | 30920 | 4370 | 4434 | 8378 | 941 | 949 | 1637 | 333 | 333 | 521 | 197 | 197 | 275 |
| 0.1 | *** | 33730 | 34112 | 37236 | 9151 | 9364 | 9845 | 1791 | 1812 | 1833 | 558 | 558 | 566 | 303 | 303 | 303 |
| | *** | 33857 | 34750 | 55917 | 9236 | 9547 | 14553 | 1799 | 1820 | 2590 | 558 | 566 | 744 | 303 | 303 | 368 |
| 0.15 | *** | 50411 | 51112 | 58813 | 13500 | 13954 | 15229 | 2564 | 2620 | 2683 | 758 | 771 | 771 | 388 | 388 | 388 |
| | *** | 50645 | 52374 | 77939 | 13678 | 14400 | 19984 | 2585 | 2649 | 3423 | 771 | 771 | 938 | 388 | 388 | 447 |
| 0.2 | *** | 63926 | 65018 | 79021 | 17091 | 17835 | 20236 | 3244 | 3342 | 3470 | 941 | 949 | 962 | 460 | 460 | 473 |
| | *** | 64295 | 67028 | 96984 | 17375 | 18621 | 24671 | 3286 | 3393 | 4137 | 941 | 949 | 1102 | 460 | 460 | 513 |
| 0.25 | *** | 73871 | 75443 | 97012 | 19832 | 20916 | 24677 | 3810 | 3945 | 4150 | 1090 | 1098 | 1119 | 524 | 524 | 537 |
| | *** | 74402 | 78355 | 113054 | 20257 | 22085 | 28614 | 3873 | 4030 | 4732 | 1090 | 1111 | 1235 | 524 | 537 | 566 |
| 0.3 | *** | 80267 | 82435 | 112333 | 21766 | 23219 | 28438 | 4243 | 4434 | 4710 | 1204 | 1225 | 1246 | 580 | 580 | 588 |
| | *** | 80998 | 86387 | 126148 | 22326 | 24791 | 31813 | 4328 | 4561 | 5208 | 1217 | 1238 | 1340 | 580 | 580 | 606 |
| 0.35 | *** | 83378 | 86260 | 124743 | 22943 | 24783 | 31464 | 4561 | 4795 | 5170 | 1289 | 1310 | 1345 | 609 | 609 | 622 |
| | *** | 84347 | 91402 | 136266 | 23665 | 26760 | 34268 | 4668 | 4965 | 5565 | 1302 | 1331 | 1414 | 609 | 622 | 632 |
| 0.4 | *** | 83582 | 87322 | 134059 | 23474 | 25676 | 33716 | 4766 | 5050 | 5488 | 1345 | 1374 | 1408 | 630 | 630 | 643 |
| | *** | 84844 | 93748 | 143408 | 24337 | 28035 | 35979 | 4893 | 5241 | 5803 | 1353 | 1395 | 1459 | 630 | 643 | 645 |
| 0.45 | *** | 81330 | 86055 | 140200 | 23445 | 25995 | 35175 | 4872 | 5191 | 5680 | 1374 | 1408 | 1438 | 630 | 643 | 651 |
| | *** | 82953 | 93825 | 147574 | 24451 | 28672 | 36946 | 5008 | 5403 | 5922 | 1387 | 1416 | 1474 | 643 | 643 | 645 |
| 0.5 | *** | 77130 | 82974 | 143133 | 22956 | 25803 | 35820 | 4872 | 5220 | 5751 | 1366 | 1408 | 1438 | 630 | 630 | 643 |
| | *** | 79170 | 92040 | 148765 | 24090 | 28723 | 37169 | 5029 | 5446 | 5922 | 1387 | 1416 | 1459 | 630 | 643 | 632 |
| 0.55 | *** | 71533 | 78533 | 142835 | 22085 | 25153 | 35663 | 4774 | 5135 | 5688 | 1331 | 1374 | 1408 | 609 | 609 | 622 |
| | *** | 74028 | 88725 | 146979 | 23325 | 28247 | 36648 | 4944 | 5382 | 5803 | 1353 | 1387 | 1414 | 609 | 622 | 606 |
| 0.6 | *** | 65039 | 73135 | 139286 | 20916 | 24103 | 34694 | 4596 | 4957 | 5488 | 1268 | 1310 | 1345 | 566 | 580 | 588 |
| | *** | 68006 | 84156 | 142218 | 22212 | 27270 | 35384 | 4766 | 5191 | 5565 | 1289 | 1323 | 1340 | 580 | 580 | 566 |
| 0.65 | *** | 58154 | 67092 | 132521 | 19492 | 22688 | 32930 | 4328 | 4668 | 5170 | 1183 | 1217 | 1246 | 524 | 524 | 537 |
| | *** | 61503 | 78554 | 134480 | 20810 | 25803 | 33375 | 4490 | 4893 | 5208 | 1196 | 1238 | 1235 | 524 | 537 | 513 |
| 0.7 | *** | 51218 | 60576 | 122541 | 17835 | 20924 | 30351 | 3966 | 4277 | 4723 | 1068 | 1090 | 1119 | 460 | 473 | 473 |
| | *** | 54796 | 72022 | 123767 | 19110 | 23870 | 30622 | 4115 | 4476 | 4732 | 1076 | 1111 | 1102 | 460 | 473 | 447 |
| 0.75 | *** | 44376 | 53662 | 109388 | 15951 | 18799 | 26980 | 3520 | 3775 | 4150 | 920 | 941 | 962 | 388 | 388 | 396 |
| | *** | 47988 | 64585 | 110078 | 17141 | 21434 | 27126 | 3648 | 3945 | 4137 | 928 | 949 | 938 | 388 | 396 | 368 |
| 0.8 | *** | 37618 | 46296 | 93081 | 13818 | 16283 | 22828 | 2981 | 3172 | 3435 | 736 | 758 | 771 | 303 | 303 | 303 |
| | *** | 41040 | 56135 | 93413 | 14846 | 18480 | 22885 | 3074 | 3300 | 3423 | 750 | 758 | 744 | 303 | 303 | 275 |
| 0.85 | *** | 30755 | 38235 | 73645 | 11340 | 13274 | 17898 | 2322 | 2450 | 2620 | 537 | 545 | 545 | . | . | . |
| | *** | 33730 | 46395 | 73773 | 12161 | 14923 | 17900 | 2386 | 2521 | 2590 | 537 | 545 | 521 | . | . | . |
| 0.9 | *** | 23325 | 28956 | 51141 | 8378 | 9632 | 12190 | 1536 | 1600 | 1663 | . | . | . | . | . | . |
| | *** | 25599 | 34792 | 51156 | 8931 | 10631 | 12172 | 1565 | 1629 | 1637 | . | . | . | . | . | . |
| 0.95 | *** | 14243 | 17205 | 25591 | 4540 | 5008 | 5730 | . | . | . | . | . | . | . | . | . |
| | *** | 15476 | 19925 | 25563 | 4753 | 5318 | 5699 | . | . | . | . | . | . | . | . | . |
| 0.98 | *** | 6410 | 7273 | 8811 | . | . | . | . | . | . | . | . | . | . | . | . |
| | *** | 6793 | 7898 | 8779 | . | . | . | . | . | . | . | . | . | . | . | . |

## TABLE 2: ALPHA= 0.005 POWER= 0.9    EXPECTED ACCRUAL THRU MINIMUM FOLLOW-UP= 9000

| | DEL=.01 | | | DEL=.02 | | | DEL=.05 | | | DEL=.10 | | | DEL=.15 | | |
|---|---|---|---|---|---|---|---|---|---|---|---|---|---|---|---|
| FACT= | 1.0 / .75 | .50 / .25 | .00 BIN | 1.0 / .75 | .50 / .25 | .00 BIN | 1.0 / .75 | .50 / .25 | .00 BIN | 1.0 / 75 | .50 / .25 | .00 BIN | 1.0 / .75 | .50 / .25 | .00 BIN |
| PCONT=*** | REQUIRED NUMBER OF PATIENTS | | | | | | | | | | | | | | |
| 0.01 *** | 2279 2287 | 2287 | 839 839 | 839 | 276 276 | 276 | 141 141 | 141 | 96 96 | 96 |
| *** | 2287 2287 | 8779 | 839 839 | 2902 | 276 276 | 790 | 141 141 | 321 | 96 96 | 191 |
| 0.02 *** | 5046 5069 | 5122 | 1626 1626 | 1635 | 442 442 | 442 | 195 195 | 195 | 127 127 | 127 |
| *** | 5055 5091 | 14493 | 1626 1635 | 4316 | 442 442 | 1009 | 195 195 | 373 | 127 127 | 213 |
| 0.05 *** | 15292 15427 | 15990 | 4357 4402 | 4484 | 937 951 | 951 | 330 330 | 330 | 195 195 | 195 |
| *** | 15337 15607 | 30920 | 4380 4439 | 8378 | 937 951 | 1637 | 330 330 | 521 | 195 195 | 275 |
| 0.1 *** | 33742 34147 | 37230 | 9172 9375 | 9847 | 1784 1806 | 1829 | 555 569 | 569 | 299 299 | 299 |
| *** | 33891 34814 | 55917 | 9254 9555 | 14553 | 1792 1815 | 2590 | 555 569 | 744 | 299 299 | 368 |
| 0.15 *** | 50451 51194 | 58821 | 13537 13987 | 15225 | 2571 2625 | 2684 | 757 771 | 771 | 389 389 | 389 |
| *** | 50707 52499 | 77939 | 13717 14429 | 19984 | 2594 2647 | 3423 | 771 771 | 938 | 389 389 | 447 |
| 0.2 *** | 63996 65152 | 79012 | 17137 17902 | 20234 | 3255 3345 | 3471 | 937 951 | 960 | 465 465 | 465 |
| *** | 64379 67245 | 96984 | 17444 18681 | 24671 | 3300 3404 | 4137 | 937 951 | 1102 | 465 465 | 513 |
| 0.25 *** | 73964 75629 | 97012 | 19919 21021 | 24675 | 3817 3952 | 4146 | 1086 1109 | 1117 | 524 532 | 532 |
| *** | 74526 78652 | 113054 | 20346 22177 | 28614 | 3885 4042 | 4732 | 1095 1109 | 1235 | 524 532 | 566 |
| 0.3 *** | 80399 82680 | 112335 | 21876 23347 | 28432 | 4259 4447 | 4717 | 1207 1221 | 1244 | 577 577 | 577 |
| *** | 81164 86797 | 126148 | 22447 24914 | 31813 | 4349 4574 | 5208 | 1207 1230 | 1340 | 577 577 | 606 |
| 0.35 *** | 83549 86595 | 124732 | 23077 24945 | 31461 | 4582 4821 | 5167 | 1289 1320 | 1342 | 614 614 | 622 |
| *** | 84570 91927 | 136266 | 23811 26916 | 34268 | 4686 4979 | 5565 | 1297 1334 | 1414 | 614 614 | 632 |
| 0.4 *** | 83805 87742 | 134061 | 23640 25881 | 33711 | 4799 5069 | 5482 | 1342 1379 | 1410 | 622 636 | 645 |
| *** | 85146 94394 | 143408 | 24517 28221 | 35979 | 4920 5257 | 5803 | 1365 1387 | 1459 | 636 636 | 645 |
| 0.45 *** | 81622 86586 | 140204 | 23640 26219 | 35174 | 4897 5212 | 5685 | 1379 1410 | 1446 | 636 645 | 645 |
| *** | 83324 94596 | 147574 | 24666 28882 | 36946 | 5046 5415 | 5922 | 1387 1424 | 1474 | 636 645 | 645 |
| 0.5 *** | 77496 83616 | 143137 | 23167 26047 | 35826 | 4897 5235 | 5752 | 1365 1401 | 1446 | 622 636 | 645 |
| *** | 79634 92909 | 148765 | 24329 28964 | 37169 | 5055 5460 | 5922 | 1387 1424 | 1459 | 636 636 | 632 |
| 0.55 *** | 71984 79260 | 142836 | 22326 25417 | 35669 | 4807 5159 | 5685 | 1342 1379 | 1410 | 614 614 | 622 |
| *** | 74594 89669 | 146979 | 23572 28491 | 36648 | 4979 5392 | 5803 | 1356 1387 | 1414 | 614 622 | 606 |
| 0.6 *** | 65580 73950 | 139290 | 21179 24374 | 34701 | 4627 4979 | 5496 | 1275 1311 | 1342 | 569 577 | 591 |
| *** | 68662 85169 | 142218 | 22484 27510 | 35384 | 4785 5204 | 5565 | 1289 1334 | 1340 | 577 577 | 566 |
| 0.65 *** | 58785 67942 | 132517 | 19747 22956 | 32924 | 4357 4686 | 5167 | 1185 1221 | 1252 | 524 532 | 532 |
| *** | 62227 79575 | 134480 | 21066 26039 | 33375 | 4515 4897 | 5208 | 1199 1230 | 1235 | 524 532 | 513 |
| 0.7 *** | 51891 61454 | 122541 | 18082 21179 | 30359 | 3997 4304 | 4717 | 1072 1095 | 1117 | 465 465 | 479 |
| *** | 55559 73027 | 123767 | 19365 24090 | 30622 | 4132 4484 | 4732 | 1086 1109 | 1102 | 465 465 | 447 |
| 0.75 *** | 45060 54510 | 109387 | 16192 19027 | 26984 | 3547 3795 | 4146 | 915 937 | 960 | 389 389 | 397 |
| *** | 48750 65526 | 110078 | 17376 21637 | 27126 | 3660 3952 | 4137 | 929 951 | 938 | 389 397 | 368 |
| 0.8 *** | 38279 47076 | 93075 | 14024 16476 | 22830 | 2999 3187 | 3435 | 749 757 | 771 | 299 299 | 307 |
| *** | 41744 56962 | 93413 | 15059 18645 | 22885 | 3089 3300 | 3423 | 749 757 | 744 | 299 299 | 275 |
| 0.85 *** | 31326 38886 | 73649 | 11504 13425 | 17894 | 2332 2459 | 2616 | 532 546 | 546 | . . | . |
| *** | 34350 47076 | 73773 | 12322 15045 | 17900 | 2391 2535 | 2590 | 532 546 | 521 | . . | . |
| 0.9 *** | 23766 29445 | 51149 | 8489 9726 | 12187 | 1536 1604 | 1671 | . . | . | . . | . |
| *** | 26070 35250 | 51156 | 9029 10694 | 12172 | 1567 1626 | 1637 | . . | . | . . | . |
| 0.95 *** | 14482 17452 | 25589 | 4596 5046 | 5730 | . . | . | . . | . | . . | . |
| *** | 15720 20130 | 25563 | 4799 5339 | 5699 | . . | . | . . | . | . . | . |
| 0.98 *** | 6495 7327 | 8804 | . . | . | . . | . | . . | . | . . | . |
| *** | 6869 7935 | 8779 | . . | . | . . | . | . . | . | . . | . |

## TABLE 2: ALPHA= 0.005 POWER= 0.9    EXPECTED ACCRUAL THRU MINIMUM FOLLOW-UP= 9500

| | | DEL=.01 | | | DEL=.02 | | | DEL=.05 | | | DEL=.10 | | | DEL=.15 | |
|---|---|---|---|---|---|---|---|---|---|---|---|---|---|---|---|---|
| FACT= | 1.0 .75 | .50 .25 | .00 BIN | 1.0 .75 | .50 .25 | .00 BIN | 1.0 .75 | .50 .25 | .00 BIN | 1.0 75 | .50 .25 | .00 BIN | 1.0 .75 | .50 .25 | .00 BIN |
| PCONT=*** | | | | REQUIRED NUMBER OF PATIENTS | | | | | | | | | | | | |
| 0.01 *** | 2286 | 2286 | 2295 | 838 | 838 | 838 | 277 | 277 | 277 | 134 | 134 | 134 | 101 | 101 | 101 |
| *** | 2286 | 2286 | 8779 | 838 | 838 | 2902 | 277 | 277 | 790 | 134 | 134 | 321 | 101 | 101 | 191 |
| 0.02 *** | 5050 | 5074 | 5122 | 1621 | 1630 | 1630 | 434 | 443 | 443 | 196 | 196 | 196 | 125 | 125 | 125 |
| *** | 5065 | 5089 | 14493 | 1621 | 1630 | 4316 | 443 | 443 | 1009 | 196 | 196 | 373 | 125 | 125 | 213 |
| 0.05 *** | 15301 | 15444 | 15990 | 4362 | 4409 | 4480 | 942 | 942 | 956 | 339 | 339 | 339 | 196 | 196 | 196 |
| *** | 15349 | 15619 | 30920 | 4385 | 4433 | 8378 | 942 | 942 | 1637 | 339 | 339 | 521 | 196 | 196 | 275 |
| 0.1 *** | 33764 | 34192 | 37232 | 9183 | 9397 | 9848 | 1788 | 1811 | 1835 | 562 | 562 | 562 | 300 | 300 | 300 |
| *** | 33921 | 34871 | 55917 | 9269 | 9578 | 14553 | 1797 | 1820 | 2590 | 562 | 562 | 744 | 300 | 300 | 368 |
| 0.15 *** | 50499 | 51268 | 58811 | 13568 | 14028 | 15230 | 2580 | 2628 | 2690 | 766 | 766 | 775 | 386 | 386 | 386 |
| *** | 50760 | 52622 | 77939 | 13758 | 14455 | 19984 | 2595 | 2652 | 3423 | 766 | 775 | 938 | 386 | 386 | 447 |
| 0.2 *** | 64060 | 65271 | 79023 | 17201 | 17961 | 20241 | 3260 | 3355 | 3459 | 942 | 956 | 956 | 467 | 467 | 467 |
| *** | 64464 | 67442 | 96984 | 17495 | 18730 | 24671 | 3308 | 3403 | 4137 | 942 | 956 | 1102 | 467 | 467 | 513 |
| 0.25 *** | 74059 | 75816 | 97010 | 19989 | 21105 | 24668 | 3830 | 3958 | 4148 | 1084 | 1099 | 1123 | 529 | 529 | 529 |
| *** | 74638 | 78951 | 113054 | 20431 | 22260 | 28614 | 3887 | 4044 | 4732 | 1099 | 1108 | 1235 | 529 | 529 | 566 |
| 0.3 *** | 80528 | 82941 | 112344 | 21975 | 23471 | 28435 | 4281 | 4457 | 4718 | 1203 | 1227 | 1250 | 576 | 576 | 585 |
| *** | 81335 | 87202 | 126148 | 22569 | 25024 | 31813 | 4362 | 4575 | 5208 | 1218 | 1241 | 1340 | 576 | 585 | 606 |
| 0.35 *** | 83725 | 86917 | 124741 | 23210 | 25095 | 31460 | 4599 | 4837 | 5160 | 1289 | 1322 | 1345 | 609 | 609 | 624 |
| *** | 84803 | 92441 | 136266 | 23955 | 27058 | 34268 | 4709 | 4979 | 5565 | 1298 | 1336 | 1414 | 609 | 624 | 632 |
| 0.4 *** | 84034 | 88152 | 134060 | 23804 | 26060 | 33717 | 4813 | 5089 | 5493 | 1345 | 1384 | 1408 | 633 | 633 | 648 |
| *** | 85435 | 95015 | 143408 | 24692 | 28388 | 35979 | 4946 | 5264 | 5803 | 1360 | 1393 | 1459 | 633 | 633 | 645 |
| 0.45 *** | 81905 | 87098 | 140203 | 23828 | 26425 | 35165 | 4923 | 5231 | 5683 | 1384 | 1408 | 1440 | 633 | 648 | 648 |
| *** | 83701 | 95324 | 147574 | 24873 | 29076 | 36946 | 5065 | 5430 | 5922 | 1393 | 1431 | 1474 | 633 | 648 | 645 |
| 0.5 *** | 77859 | 84224 | 143133 | 23385 | 26274 | 35821 | 4932 | 5264 | 5754 | 1369 | 1408 | 1440 | 633 | 633 | 648 |
| *** | 80100 | 93733 | 148765 | 24549 | 29171 | 37169 | 5089 | 5478 | 5922 | 1393 | 1431 | 1459 | 633 | 633 | 632 |
| 0.55 *** | 72429 | 79973 | 142839 | 22554 | 25656 | 35664 | 4851 | 5184 | 5683 | 1345 | 1369 | 1408 | 609 | 609 | 624 |
| *** | 75151 | 90589 | 146979 | 23813 | 28720 | 36648 | 5003 | 5407 | 5803 | 1360 | 1393 | 1414 | 609 | 624 | 606 |
| 0.6 *** | 66126 | 74733 | 139285 | 21414 | 24635 | 34705 | 4661 | 5003 | 5493 | 1274 | 1313 | 1345 | 576 | 576 | 585 |
| *** | 69309 | 86124 | 142218 | 22735 | 27732 | 35384 | 4813 | 5217 | 5565 | 1298 | 1322 | 1340 | 576 | 585 | 566 |
| 0.65 *** | 59390 | 68772 | 132517 | 19989 | 23210 | 32924 | 4385 | 4709 | 5169 | 1194 | 1218 | 1250 | 529 | 529 | 538 |
| *** | 62944 | 80566 | 134480 | 21319 | 26259 | 33375 | 4543 | 4908 | 5208 | 1203 | 1241 | 1235 | 529 | 538 | 513 |
| 0.7 *** | 52541 | 62288 | 122542 | 18327 | 21414 | 30359 | 4029 | 4314 | 4718 | 1075 | 1099 | 1123 | 467 | 467 | 467 |
| *** | 56303 | 73988 | 123767 | 19609 | 24288 | 30622 | 4163 | 4495 | 4732 | 1084 | 1108 | 1102 | 467 | 467 | 447 |
| 0.75 *** | 45725 | 55329 | 109384 | 16403 | 19253 | 26986 | 3569 | 3815 | 4139 | 918 | 942 | 965 | 386 | 395 | 395 |
| *** | 49478 | 66420 | 110078 | 17590 | 21818 | 27126 | 3688 | 3958 | 4137 | 933 | 956 | 938 | 386 | 395 | 368 |
| 0.8 *** | 38909 | 47815 | 93083 | 14209 | 16655 | 22830 | 3023 | 3198 | 3435 | 743 | 752 | 775 | 300 | 300 | 300 |
| *** | 42433 | 57766 | 93413 | 15239 | 18793 | 22885 | 3103 | 3308 | 3423 | 752 | 766 | 744 | 300 | 300 | 275 |
| 0.85 *** | 31879 | 39512 | 73655 | 11668 | 13568 | 17899 | 2343 | 2462 | 2619 | 538 | 538 | 553 | . | . | . |
| *** | 34928 | 47720 | 73773 | 12475 | 15159 | 17900 | 2405 | 2533 | 2590 | 538 | 553 | 521 | . | . | . |
| 0.9 *** | 24193 | 29908 | 51140 | 8589 | 9815 | 12190 | 1550 | 1598 | 1669 | . | . | . | . | . | . |
| *** | 26511 | 35688 | 51156 | 9126 | 10750 | 12172 | 1574 | 1630 | 1637 | . | . | . | . | . | . |
| 0.95 *** | 14717 | 17676 | 25585 | 4623 | 5065 | 5730 | . | . | . | . | . | . | . | . | . |
| *** | 15952 | 20322 | 25563 | 4828 | 5359 | 5699 | . | . | . | . | . | . | . | . | . |
| 0.98 *** | 6561 | 7393 | 8803 | . | . | . | . | . | . | . | . | . | . | . | . |
| *** | 6927 | 7972 | 8779 | . | . | . | . | . | . | . | . | . | . | . | . |

TABLE 2: ALPHA= 0.005 POWER= 0.9    EXPECTED ACCRUAL THRU MINIMUM FOLLOW-UP= 10000

| PCONT | FACT | DEL=.01 1.0/.75 | DEL=.01 .50/.25 | DEL=.01 .00/BIN | DEL=.02 1.0/.75 | DEL=.02 .50/.25 | DEL=.02 .00/BIN | DEL=.05 1.0/.75 | DEL=.05 .50/.25 | DEL=.05 .00/BIN | DEL=.10 1.0/75 | DEL=.10 .50/.25 | DEL=.10 .00/BIN | DEL=.15 1.0/.75 | DEL=.15 .50/.25 | DEL=.15 .00/BIN |
|---|---|---|---|---|---|---|---|---|---|---|---|---|---|---|---|---|
| | | REQUIRED NUMBER OF PATIENTS | | | | | | | | | | | | | | |
| 0.01 | *** | 2282 | 2282 | 2291 | 841 | 841 | 841 | 282 | 282 | 282 | 141 | 141 | 141 | 91 | 91 | 91 |
| | *** | 2282 | 2291 | 8779 | 841 | 841 | 2902 | 282 | 282 | 790 | 141 | 141 | 321 | 91 | 91 | 191 |
| 0.02 | *** | 5057 | 5082 | 5116 | 1616 | 1632 | 1632 | 441 | 441 | 441 | 191 | 191 | 191 | 132 | 132 | 132 |
| | *** | 5066 | 5091 | 14493 | 1632 | 1632 | 4316 | 441 | 441 | 1009 | 191 | 191 | 373 | 132 | 132 | 213 |
| 0.05 | *** | 15307 | 15457 | 15991 | 4366 | 4407 | 4482 | 941 | 941 | 957 | 332 | 332 | 332 | 191 | 191 | 191 |
| | *** | 15366 | 15632 | 30920 | 4382 | 4441 | 8378 | 941 | 941 | 1637 | 332 | 332 | 521 | 191 | 191 | 275 |
| 0.1 | *** | 33791 | 34241 | 37232 | 9207 | 9407 | 9841 | 1791 | 1807 | 1832 | 557 | 566 | 566 | 291 | 291 | 291 |
| | *** | 33941 | 34932 | 55917 | 9291 | 9582 | 14553 | 1807 | 1816 | 2590 | 557 | 566 | 744 | 291 | 291 | 368 |
| 0.15 | *** | 50541 | 51357 | 58816 | 13591 | 14057 | 15232 | 2582 | 2632 | 2682 | 766 | 766 | 782 | 391 | 391 | 391 |
| | *** | 50816 | 52741 | 77939 | 13782 | 14491 | 19984 | 2607 | 2657 | 3423 | 766 | 766 | 938 | 391 | 391 | 447 |
| 0.2 | *** | 64116 | 65407 | 79016 | 17241 | 18016 | 20232 | 3266 | 3357 | 3466 | 941 | 957 | 957 | 466 | 466 | 466 |
| | *** | 64557 | 67641 | 96984 | 17557 | 18782 | 24671 | 3307 | 3407 | 4137 | 941 | 957 | 1102 | 466 | 466 | 513 |
| 0.25 | *** | 74141 | 75991 | 97007 | 20066 | 21191 | 24666 | 3841 | 3966 | 4141 | 1091 | 1107 | 1116 | 532 | 532 | 532 |
| | *** | 74766 | 79241 | 113054 | 20516 | 22341 | 28614 | 3907 | 4057 | 4732 | 1091 | 1107 | 1235 | 532 | 532 | 566 |
| 0.3 | *** | 80657 | 83182 | 112341 | 22082 | 23591 | 28432 | 4291 | 4466 | 4716 | 1207 | 1232 | 1241 | 582 | 582 | 582 |
| | *** | 81507 | 87591 | 126148 | 22666 | 25141 | 31813 | 4366 | 4582 | 5208 | 1216 | 1232 | 1340 | 582 | 582 | 606 |
| 0.35 | *** | 83891 | 87241 | 124741 | 23341 | 25241 | 31457 | 4616 | 4841 | 5166 | 1291 | 1316 | 1341 | 607 | 616 | 616 |
| | *** | 85032 | 92941 | 136266 | 24091 | 27191 | 34268 | 4732 | 4991 | 5565 | 1307 | 1332 | 1414 | 616 | 616 | 632 |
| 0.4 | *** | 84257 | 88566 | 134057 | 23957 | 26232 | 33716 | 4841 | 5107 | 5491 | 1357 | 1382 | 1407 | 632 | 632 | 641 |
| | *** | 85732 | 95632 | 143408 | 24866 | 28557 | 35979 | 4966 | 5282 | 5803 | 1366 | 1391 | 1459 | 632 | 641 | 645 |
| 0.45 | *** | 82191 | 87607 | 140207 | 24007 | 26632 | 35166 | 4957 | 5257 | 5682 | 1382 | 1407 | 1441 | 641 | 641 | 657 |
| | *** | 84066 | 96041 | 147574 | 25057 | 29266 | 36946 | 5091 | 5441 | 5922 | 1391 | 1432 | 1474 | 641 | 641 | 645 |
| 0.5 | *** | 78216 | 84832 | 143141 | 23582 | 26491 | 35816 | 4957 | 5282 | 5741 | 1382 | 1407 | 1441 | 632 | 632 | 641 |
| | *** | 80557 | 94541 | 148765 | 24766 | 29382 | 37169 | 5107 | 5491 | 5922 | 1391 | 1432 | 1459 | 632 | 641 | 632 |
| 0.55 | *** | 72866 | 80666 | 142832 | 22782 | 25891 | 35666 | 4866 | 5207 | 5682 | 1341 | 1382 | 1407 | 607 | 616 | 616 |
| | *** | 75691 | 91457 | 146979 | 24057 | 28932 | 36648 | 5032 | 5416 | 5803 | 1357 | 1391 | 1414 | 616 | 616 | 606 |
| 0.6 | *** | 66641 | 75491 | 139291 | 21641 | 24866 | 34707 | 4691 | 5016 | 5491 | 1282 | 1316 | 1341 | 566 | 582 | 591 |
| | *** | 69932 | 87041 | 142218 | 22966 | 27957 | 35384 | 4841 | 5232 | 5565 | 1291 | 1332 | 1340 | 582 | 582 | 566 |
| 0.65 | *** | 59982 | 69582 | 132516 | 20232 | 23441 | 32932 | 4416 | 4732 | 5166 | 1191 | 1216 | 1257 | 532 | 532 | 541 |
| | *** | 63632 | 81491 | 134480 | 21557 | 26466 | 33375 | 4566 | 4932 | 5208 | 1207 | 1232 | 1235 | 532 | 532 | 513 |
| 0.7 | *** | 53182 | 63107 | 122541 | 18557 | 21641 | 30357 | 4057 | 4332 | 4716 | 1066 | 1091 | 1116 | 466 | 466 | 466 |
| | *** | 57016 | 74907 | 123767 | 19841 | 24491 | 30622 | 4182 | 4507 | 4732 | 1082 | 1107 | 1102 | 466 | 466 | 447 |
| 0.75 | *** | 46366 | 56107 | 109382 | 16616 | 19457 | 26982 | 3591 | 3832 | 4141 | 932 | 941 | 966 | 391 | 391 | 391 |
| | *** | 50182 | 67282 | 110078 | 17807 | 21991 | 27126 | 3707 | 3966 | 4137 | 932 | 957 | 938 | 391 | 391 | 368 |
| 0.8 | *** | 39516 | 48516 | 93082 | 14391 | 16832 | 22832 | 3032 | 3207 | 3441 | 741 | 757 | 766 | 291 | 307 | 307 |
| | *** | 43082 | 58516 | 93413 | 15432 | 18932 | 22885 | 3116 | 3316 | 3423 | 757 | 766 | 744 | 307 | 307 | 275 |
| 0.85 | *** | 32416 | 40107 | 73657 | 11807 | 13691 | 17891 | 2357 | 2466 | 2616 | 532 | 541 | 557 | . | . | . |
| | *** | 35491 | 48316 | 73773 | 12616 | 15257 | 17900 | 2416 | 2541 | 2590 | 541 | 541 | 521 | . | . | . |
| 0.9 | *** | 24591 | 30332 | 51141 | 8691 | 9891 | 12191 | 1557 | 1607 | 1666 | . | . | . | . | . | . |
| | *** | 26932 | 36107 | 51156 | 9216 | 10807 | 12172 | 1582 | 1632 | 1637 | . | . | . | . | . | . |
| 0.95 | *** | 14941 | 17882 | 25591 | 4666 | 5091 | 5732 | . | . | . | . | . | . | . | . | . |
| | *** | 16182 | 20491 | 25563 | 4866 | 5382 | 5699 | . | . | . | . | . | . | . | . | . |
| 0.98 | *** | 6632 | 7441 | 8807 | . | . | . | . | . | . | . | . | . | . | . | . |
| | *** | 6991 | 8016 | 8779 | . | . | . | . | . | . | . | . | . | . | . | . |

# TABLE 2: ALPHA= 0.005 POWER= 0.9    EXPECTED ACCRUAL THRU MINIMUM FOLLOW-UP= 11000

| | | DEL=.01 | | | DEL=.02 | | | DEL=.05 | | | DEL=.10 | | | DEL=.15 | | |
|---|---|---|---|---|---|---|---|---|---|---|---|---|---|---|---|---|---|
| FACT= | | 1.0 .75 | .50 .25 | .00 BIN | 1.0 .75 | .50 .25 | .00 BIN | 1.0 .75 | .50 .25 | .00 BIN | 1.0 75 | .50 .25 | .00 BIN | 1.0 .75 | .50 .25 | .00 BIN |
| PCONT=*** | | | | | REQUIRED NUMBER OF PATIENTS | | | | | | | | | | | |
| 0.01 | *** | 2290 | 2290 | 2290 | 832 | 843 | 843 | 282 | 282 | 282 | 145 | 145 | 145 | 100 | 100 | 100 |
| | *** | 2290 | 2290 | 8779 | 843 | 843 | 2902 | 282 | 282 | 790 | 145 | 145 | 321 | 100 | 100 | 191 |
| 0.02 | *** | 5050 | 5078 | 5122 | 1630 | 1630 | 1630 | 430 | 430 | 447 | 183 | 183 | 183 | 128 | 128 | 128 |
| | *** | 5067 | 5095 | 14493 | 1630 | 1630 | 4316 | 430 | 447 | 1009 | 183 | 183 | 373 | 128 | 128 | 213 |
| 0.05 | *** | 15325 | 15473 | 15995 | 4380 | 4418 | 4473 | 942 | 942 | 953 | 337 | 337 | 337 | 200 | 200 | 200 |
| | *** | 15380 | 15655 | 30920 | 4390 | 4445 | 8378 | 942 | 942 | 1637 | 337 | 337 | 521 | 200 | 200 | 275 |
| 0.1 | *** | 33843 | 34327 | 37225 | 9230 | 9440 | 9852 | 1795 | 1805 | 1833 | 557 | 557 | 568 | 293 | 293 | 293 |
| | *** | 34008 | 35042 | 55917 | 9313 | 9605 | 14553 | 1805 | 1822 | 2590 | 557 | 568 | 744 | 293 | 293 | 368 |
| 0.15 | *** | 50618 | 51515 | 58813 | 13658 | 14125 | 15225 | 2592 | 2630 | 2685 | 760 | 777 | 777 | 392 | 392 | 392 |
| | *** | 50920 | 52972 | 77939 | 13850 | 14538 | 19984 | 2603 | 2658 | 3423 | 760 | 777 | 938 | 392 | 392 | 447 |
| 0.2 | *** | 64247 | 65650 | 79015 | 17343 | 18130 | 20230 | 3280 | 3362 | 3472 | 942 | 953 | 953 | 458 | 458 | 475 |
| | *** | 64725 | 68025 | 96984 | 17662 | 18872 | 24671 | 3318 | 3417 | 4137 | 942 | 953 | 1102 | 458 | 475 | 513 |
| 0.25 | *** | 74340 | 76347 | 97010 | 20203 | 21358 | 24675 | 3857 | 3978 | 4143 | 1090 | 1107 | 1118 | 530 | 530 | 530 |
| | *** | 75010 | 79795 | 113054 | 20670 | 22485 | 28614 | 3923 | 4060 | 4732 | 1090 | 1107 | 1235 | 530 | 530 | 566 |
| 0.3 | *** | 80912 | 83673 | 112345 | 22265 | 23805 | 28442 | 4325 | 4490 | 4720 | 1217 | 1228 | 1245 | 568 | 585 | 585 |
| | *** | 81847 | 88337 | 126148 | 22887 | 25335 | 31813 | 4390 | 4600 | 5208 | 1217 | 1245 | 1340 | 585 | 585 | 606 |
| 0.35 | *** | 84240 | 87880 | 124730 | 23585 | 25527 | 31467 | 4655 | 4875 | 5160 | 1300 | 1327 | 1338 | 612 | 612 | 623 |
| | *** | 85477 | 93892 | 136266 | 24355 | 27435 | 34268 | 4765 | 4995 | 5565 | 1310 | 1327 | 1414 | 612 | 623 | 632 |
| 0.4 | *** | 84690 | 89382 | 134053 | 24245 | 26555 | 33705 | 4885 | 5133 | 5490 | 1355 | 1382 | 1410 | 623 | 640 | 640 |
| | *** | 86313 | 96780 | 143408 | 25180 | 28855 | 35979 | 4995 | 5298 | 5803 | 1365 | 1393 | 1459 | 640 | 640 | 645 |
| 0.45 | *** | 82765 | 88595 | 140202 | 24345 | 26995 | 35163 | 4995 | 5287 | 5683 | 1382 | 1410 | 1437 | 640 | 640 | 650 |
| | *** | 84800 | 97395 | 147574 | 25428 | 29597 | 36946 | 5133 | 5463 | 5922 | 1393 | 1420 | 1474 | 640 | 650 | 645 |
| 0.5 | *** | 78932 | 86000 | 143145 | 23970 | 26902 | 35823 | 5012 | 5315 | 5755 | 1382 | 1410 | 1448 | 623 | 640 | 640 |
| | *** | 81462 | 96065 | 148765 | 25170 | 29735 | 37169 | 5150 | 5507 | 5922 | 1393 | 1420 | 1459 | 640 | 640 | 632 |
| 0.55 | *** | 73735 | 81995 | 142825 | 23190 | 26325 | 35658 | 4930 | 5243 | 5683 | 1355 | 1382 | 1410 | 612 | 612 | 623 |
| | *** | 76760 | 93105 | 146979 | 24482 | 29305 | 36648 | 5067 | 5435 | 5803 | 1365 | 1393 | 1414 | 612 | 623 | 606 |
| 0.6 | *** | 67668 | 76935 | 139295 | 22073 | 25307 | 34695 | 4748 | 5050 | 5490 | 1283 | 1310 | 1355 | 568 | 585 | 585 |
| | *** | 71150 | 88777 | 142218 | 23410 | 28343 | 35384 | 4885 | 5243 | 5565 | 1300 | 1327 | 1340 | 585 | 585 | 566 |
| 0.65 | *** | 61140 | 71105 | 132513 | 20670 | 23888 | 32925 | 4473 | 4765 | 5177 | 1200 | 1217 | 1255 | 530 | 530 | 540 |
| | *** | 64945 | 83250 | 134480 | 22007 | 26847 | 33375 | 4600 | 4940 | 5208 | 1217 | 1228 | 1235 | 530 | 530 | 513 |
| 0.7 | *** | 54402 | 64632 | 122547 | 18982 | 22062 | 30350 | 4105 | 4363 | 4720 | 1080 | 1090 | 1118 | 458 | 475 | 475 |
| | *** | 58373 | 76605 | 123767 | 20275 | 24840 | 30622 | 4225 | 4528 | 4732 | 1090 | 1107 | 1102 | 458 | 475 | 447 |
| 0.75 | *** | 47593 | 57575 | 109385 | 17013 | 19818 | 26985 | 3637 | 3857 | 4143 | 925 | 942 | 970 | 392 | 392 | 392 |
| | *** | 51525 | 68867 | 110078 | 18195 | 22293 | 27126 | 3730 | 3978 | 4137 | 942 | 953 | 938 | 392 | 392 | 368 |
| 0.8 | *** | 40663 | 49865 | 93078 | 14747 | 17150 | 22832 | 3060 | 3225 | 3445 | 750 | 760 | 777 | 293 | 293 | 310 |
| | *** | 44320 | 59902 | 93413 | 15765 | 19185 | 22885 | 3142 | 3335 | 3423 | 750 | 760 | 744 | 293 | 310 | 275 |
| 0.85 | *** | 33420 | 41230 | 73652 | 12080 | 13933 | 17893 | 2372 | 2482 | 2620 | 540 | 540 | 557 | . | . | . |
| | *** | 36555 | 49435 | 73773 | 12877 | 15435 | 17900 | 2427 | 2548 | 2590 | 540 | 540 | 521 | . | . | . |
| 0.9 | *** | 25362 | 31137 | 51140 | 8873 | 10045 | 12190 | 1558 | 1613 | 1668 | . | . | . | . | . | . |
| | *** | 27727 | 36857 | 51156 | 9385 | 10908 | 12172 | 1585 | 1640 | 1637 | . | . | . | . | . | . |
| 0.95 | *** | 15352 | 18267 | 25582 | 4737 | 5133 | 5727 | . | . | . | . | . | . | . | . | . |
| | *** | 16590 | 20808 | 25563 | 4930 | 5397 | 5699 | . | . | . | . | . | . | . | . | . |
| 0.98 | *** | 6755 | 7525 | 8807 | . | . | . | . | . | . | . | . | . | . | . | . |
| | *** | 7102 | 8075 | 8779 | . | . | . | . | . | . | . | . | . | . | . | . |

## TABLE 2: ALPHA= 0.005 POWER= 0.9    EXPECTED ACCRUAL THRU MINIMUM FOLLOW-UP= 12000

| | | DEL=.01 | | | DEL=.02 | | | DEL=.05 | | | DEL=.10 | | | DEL=.15 | | |
|---|---|---|---|---|---|---|---|---|---|---|---|---|---|---|---|---|
| FACT= | | 1.0 .75 | .50 .25 | .00 BIN | 1.0 .75 | .50 .25 | .00 BIN | 1.0 .75 | .50 .25 | .00 BIN | 1.0 75 | .50 .25 | .00 BIN | 1.0 .75 | .50 .25 | .00 BIN |
| PCONT=*** | | | | REQUIRED NUMBER OF PATIENTS | | | | | | | | | | | | |
| 0.01 | *** | 2288 | 2288 | 2288 | 829 | 829 | 848 | 278 | 278 | 278 | 139 | 139 | 139 | 98 | 98 | 98 |
| | *** | 2288 | 2288 | 8779 | 829 | 848 | 2902 | 278 | 278 | 790 | 139 | 139 | 321 | 98 | 98 | 191 |
| 0.02 | *** | 5059 | 5078 | 5119 | 1628 | 1628 | 1639 | 439 | 439 | 439 | 188 | 188 | 188 | 128 | 128 | 128 |
| | *** | 5059 | 5089 | 14493 | 1628 | 1628 | 4316 | 439 | 439 | 1009 | 188 | 188 | 373 | 128 | 128 | 213 |
| 0.05 | *** | 15338 | 15499 | 15998 | 4369 | 4418 | 4478 | 938 | 949 | 949 | 338 | 338 | 338 | 199 | 199 | 199 |
| | *** | 15398 | 15668 | 30920 | 4399 | 4448 | 8378 | 938 | 949 | 1637 | 338 | 338 | 521 | 199 | 199 | 275 |
| 0.1 | *** | 33889 | 34399 | 37238 | 9259 | 9458 | 9848 | 1789 | 1808 | 1838 | 559 | 559 | 559 | 289 | 289 | 289 |
| | *** | 34069 | 35138 | 55917 | 9338 | 9619 | 14553 | 1808 | 1819 | 2590 | 559 | 559 | 744 | 289 | 289 | 368 |
| 0.15 | *** | 50708 | 51668 | 58819 | 13718 | 14179 | 15229 | 2599 | 2629 | 2689 | 769 | 769 | 769 | 379 | 379 | 398 |
| | *** | 51038 | 53179 | 77939 | 13909 | 14588 | 19984 | 2618 | 2659 | 3423 | 769 | 769 | 938 | 379 | 379 | 447 |
| 0.2 | *** | 64388 | 65888 | 79009 | 17438 | 18229 | 20239 | 3289 | 3368 | 3469 | 938 | 949 | 968 | 458 | 469 | 469 |
| | *** | 64898 | 68389 | 96984 | 17768 | 18968 | 24671 | 3338 | 3409 | 4137 | 949 | 949 | 1102 | 469 | 469 | 513 |
| 0.25 | *** | 74528 | 76699 | 97009 | 20348 | 21499 | 24668 | 3878 | 3998 | 4148 | 1099 | 1099 | 1118 | 529 | 529 | 529 |
| | *** | 75259 | 80329 | 113054 | 20809 | 22609 | 28614 | 3938 | 4069 | 4732 | 1099 | 1118 | 1235 | 529 | 529 | 566 |
| 0.3 | *** | 81169 | 84158 | 112339 | 22448 | 24008 | 28429 | 4339 | 4508 | 4718 | 1208 | 1238 | 1249 | 578 | 578 | 578 |
| | *** | 82178 | 89048 | 126148 | 23078 | 25508 | 31813 | 4418 | 4598 | 5208 | 1219 | 1238 | 1340 | 578 | 578 | 606 |
| 0.35 | *** | 84578 | 88508 | 124729 | 23809 | 25778 | 31459 | 4688 | 4898 | 5168 | 1298 | 1328 | 1339 | 608 | 619 | 619 |
| | *** | 85928 | 94789 | 136266 | 24608 | 27668 | 34268 | 4778 | 5018 | 5565 | 1309 | 1328 | 1414 | 608 | 619 | 632 |
| 0.4 | *** | 85148 | 90169 | 134059 | 24518 | 26858 | 33709 | 4928 | 5149 | 5479 | 1358 | 1388 | 1418 | 638 | 638 | 638 |
| | *** | 86888 | 97868 | 143408 | 25478 | 29108 | 35979 | 5029 | 5299 | 5803 | 1369 | 1399 | 1459 | 638 | 638 | 645 |
| 0.45 | *** | 83329 | 89558 | 140209 | 24668 | 27338 | 35168 | 5048 | 5318 | 5678 | 1388 | 1418 | 1448 | 638 | 649 | 649 |
| | *** | 85519 | 98659 | 147574 | 25759 | 29899 | 36946 | 5168 | 5479 | 5922 | 1399 | 1429 | 1474 | 638 | 649 | 645 |
| 0.5 | *** | 79639 | 87109 | 143138 | 24319 | 27278 | 35828 | 5059 | 5348 | 5749 | 1388 | 1418 | 1448 | 638 | 638 | 638 |
| | *** | 82339 | 97478 | 148765 | 25538 | 30068 | 37169 | 5198 | 5528 | 5922 | 1399 | 1429 | 1459 | 638 | 638 | 632 |
| 0.55 | *** | 74588 | 83258 | 142838 | 23569 | 26719 | 35659 | 4969 | 5269 | 5689 | 1358 | 1388 | 1418 | 608 | 619 | 619 |
| | *** | 77798 | 94678 | 146979 | 24878 | 29648 | 36648 | 5108 | 5449 | 5803 | 1369 | 1399 | 1414 | 608 | 619 | 606 |
| 0.6 | *** | 68659 | 78308 | 139298 | 22478 | 25718 | 34699 | 4789 | 5089 | 5498 | 1298 | 1309 | 1339 | 578 | 578 | 589 |
| | *** | 72308 | 90379 | 142218 | 23828 | 28688 | 35384 | 4928 | 5269 | 5565 | 1309 | 1328 | 1340 | 578 | 578 | 566 |
| 0.65 | *** | 62228 | 72529 | 132518 | 21068 | 24278 | 32929 | 4508 | 4789 | 5168 | 1208 | 1219 | 1249 | 529 | 529 | 529 |
| | *** | 66188 | 84859 | 134480 | 22418 | 27188 | 33375 | 4639 | 4958 | 5208 | 1208 | 1238 | 1235 | 529 | 529 | 513 |
| 0.7 | *** | 55568 | 66068 | 122539 | 19369 | 22429 | 30349 | 4129 | 4388 | 4718 | 1088 | 1099 | 1118 | 469 | 469 | 469 |
| | *** | 59659 | 78169 | 123767 | 20659 | 25148 | 30622 | 4249 | 4538 | 4732 | 1088 | 1118 | 1102 | 469 | 469 | 447 |
| 0.75 | *** | 48739 | 58939 | 109388 | 17378 | 20168 | 26989 | 3668 | 3878 | 4148 | 938 | 949 | 968 | 398 | 398 | 398 |
| | *** | 52778 | 70328 | 110078 | 18559 | 22568 | 27126 | 3758 | 3998 | 4137 | 938 | 949 | 938 | 398 | 398 | 368 |
| 0.8 | *** | 41749 | 51098 | 93079 | 15049 | 17419 | 22819 | 3079 | 3248 | 3439 | 758 | 758 | 769 | 308 | 308 | 308 |
| | *** | 45469 | 61178 | 93413 | 16069 | 19399 | 22885 | 3158 | 3338 | 3423 | 758 | 769 | 744 | 308 | 308 | 275 |
| 0.85 | *** | 34339 | 42248 | 73658 | 12319 | 14149 | 17899 | 2389 | 2498 | 2618 | 529 | 548 | 548 | . | . | . |
| | *** | 37538 | 50449 | 73773 | 13118 | 15589 | 17900 | 2438 | 2558 | 2590 | 548 | 548 | 521 | . | . | . |
| 0.9 | *** | 26059 | 31879 | 51139 | 9038 | 10159 | 12188 | 1568 | 1609 | 1669 | . | . | . | . | . | . |
| | *** | 28448 | 37538 | 51156 | 9529 | 10999 | 12172 | 1598 | 1639 | 1637 | . | . | . | . | . | . |
| 0.95 | *** | 15728 | 18619 | 25579 | 4789 | 5179 | 5719 | . | . | . | . | . | . | . | . | . |
| | *** | 16958 | 21098 | 25563 | 4969 | 5419 | 5699 | . | . | . | . | . | . | . | . | . |
| 0.98 | *** | 6859 | 7609 | 8809 | . | . | . | . | . | . | . | . | . | . | . | . |
| | *** | 7208 | 8119 | 8779 | . | . | . | . | . | . | . | . | . | . | . | . |

# TABLE 2: ALPHA= 0.005 POWER= 0.9    EXPECTED ACCRUAL THRU MINIMUM FOLLOW-UP= 13000

|  |  | DEL=.01 | | | DEL=.02 | | | DEL=.05 | | | DEL=.10 | | | DEL=.15 | | |
|---|---|---|---|---|---|---|---|---|---|---|---|---|---|---|---|---|
| FACT= | | 1.0 .75 | .50 .25 | .00 BIN | 1.0 .75 | .50 .25 | .00 BIN | 1.0 .75 | .50 .25 | .00 BIN | 1.0 75 | .50 .25 | .00 BIN | 1.0 .75 | .50 .25 | .00 BIN |
| PCONT=*** | | REQUIRED NUMBER OF PATIENTS | | | | | | | | | | | | | | |
| 0.01 | *** | 2284 | 2284 | 2296 | 833 | 833 | 833 | 281 | 281 | 281 | 139 | 139 | 139 | 106 | 106 | 106 |
|  | *** | 2284 | 2284 | 8779 | 833 | 833 | 2902 | 281 | 281 | 790 | 139 | 139 | 321 | 106 | 106 | 191 |
| 0.02 | *** | 5058 | 5079 | 5123 | 1634 | 1634 | 1634 | 443 | 443 | 443 | 183 | 183 | 183 | 118 | 118 | 118 |
|  | *** | 5079 | 5091 | 14493 | 1634 | 1634 | 4316 | 443 | 443 | 1009 | 183 | 183 | 373 | 118 | 118 | 213 |
| 0.05 | *** | 15361 | 15523 | 15999 | 4376 | 4429 | 4473 | 951 | 951 | 951 | 334 | 334 | 334 | 204 | 204 | 204 |
|  | *** | 15426 | 15686 | 30920 | 4396 | 4441 | 8378 | 951 | 951 | 1637 | 334 | 334 | 521 | 204 | 204 | 275 |
| 0.1 | *** | 33939 | 34471 | 37233 | 9283 | 9478 | 9836 | 1796 | 1808 | 1829 | 561 | 561 | 561 | 301 | 301 | 301 |
|  | *** | 34134 | 35218 | 55917 | 9369 | 9629 | 14553 | 1808 | 1829 | 2590 | 561 | 561 | 744 | 301 | 301 | 368 |
| 0.15 | *** | 50786 | 51814 | 58813 | 13768 | 14223 | 15231 | 2609 | 2641 | 2686 | 768 | 768 | 768 | 378 | 378 | 399 |
|  | *** | 51143 | 53386 | 77939 | 13963 | 14613 | 19984 | 2621 | 2653 | 3423 | 768 | 768 | 938 | 378 | 378 | 447 |
| 0.2 | *** | 64501 | 66126 | 79016 | 17526 | 18318 | 20236 | 3303 | 3368 | 3466 | 951 | 951 | 963 | 464 | 464 | 464 |
|  | *** | 65053 | 68726 | 96984 | 17851 | 19033 | 24671 | 3336 | 3421 | 4137 | 951 | 951 | 1102 | 464 | 464 | 513 |
| 0.25 | *** | 74706 | 77046 | 97001 | 20463 | 21654 | 24676 | 3888 | 4006 | 4148 | 1093 | 1114 | 1114 | 529 | 529 | 529 |
|  | *** | 75506 | 80816 | 113054 | 20951 | 22726 | 28614 | 3953 | 4071 | 4732 | 1093 | 1114 | 1235 | 529 | 529 | 566 |
| 0.3 | *** | 81421 | 84618 | 112341 | 22608 | 24189 | 28426 | 4364 | 4526 | 4721 | 1211 | 1223 | 1244 | 573 | 573 | 573 |
|  | *** | 82526 | 89709 | 126148 | 23258 | 25663 | 31813 | 4441 | 4603 | 5208 | 1223 | 1244 | 1340 | 573 | 573 | 606 |
| 0.35 | *** | 84911 | 89124 | 124744 | 24026 | 26009 | 31469 | 4721 | 4916 | 5156 | 1309 | 1321 | 1341 | 606 | 606 | 626 |
|  | *** | 86373 | 95636 | 136266 | 24839 | 27861 | 34268 | 4798 | 5026 | 5565 | 1309 | 1341 | 1414 | 606 | 626 | 632 |
| 0.4 | *** | 85581 | 90923 | 134051 | 24786 | 27126 | 33711 | 4949 | 5176 | 5481 | 1374 | 1386 | 1406 | 626 | 638 | 638 |
|  | *** | 87466 | 98886 | 143408 | 25749 | 29356 | 35979 | 5058 | 5318 | 5803 | 1374 | 1406 | 1459 | 638 | 638 | 645 |
| 0.45 | *** | 83891 | 90468 | 140214 | 24969 | 27646 | 35174 | 5079 | 5339 | 5676 | 1386 | 1418 | 1439 | 638 | 638 | 659 |
|  | *** | 86231 | 99828 | 147574 | 26074 | 30169 | 36946 | 5188 | 5501 | 5922 | 1406 | 1439 | 1474 | 638 | 638 | 645 |
| 0.5 | *** | 80328 | 88181 | 143139 | 24656 | 27613 | 35824 | 5091 | 5371 | 5741 | 1386 | 1418 | 1439 | 626 | 638 | 638 |
|  | *** | 83188 | 98809 | 148765 | 25879 | 30364 | 37169 | 5221 | 5546 | 5922 | 1406 | 1439 | 1459 | 638 | 638 | 632 |
| 0.55 | *** | 75421 | 84456 | 142826 | 23941 | 27081 | 35661 | 5014 | 5306 | 5676 | 1353 | 1386 | 1406 | 606 | 626 | 626 |
|  | *** | 78789 | 96058 | 146979 | 25241 | 29953 | 36648 | 5144 | 5469 | 5803 | 1374 | 1406 | 1414 | 606 | 626 | 606 |
| 0.6 | *** | 69624 | 79601 | 139283 | 22856 | 26074 | 34698 | 4831 | 5111 | 5501 | 1288 | 1321 | 1341 | 573 | 573 | 594 |
|  | *** | 73406 | 91854 | 142218 | 24201 | 28999 | 35384 | 4961 | 5286 | 5565 | 1309 | 1341 | 1340 | 573 | 594 | 566 |
| 0.65 | *** | 63286 | 73881 | 132523 | 21438 | 24644 | 32931 | 4559 | 4819 | 5176 | 1211 | 1223 | 1256 | 529 | 529 | 541 |
|  | *** | 67381 | 86341 | 134480 | 22791 | 27483 | 33375 | 4668 | 4981 | 5208 | 1211 | 1244 | 1235 | 529 | 529 | 513 |
| 0.7 | *** | 56656 | 67393 | 122546 | 19736 | 22771 | 30343 | 4169 | 4408 | 4721 | 1081 | 1093 | 1126 | 464 | 464 | 476 |
|  | *** | 60861 | 79613 | 123767 | 21016 | 25424 | 30622 | 4278 | 4559 | 4732 | 1093 | 1114 | 1102 | 464 | 476 | 447 |
| 0.75 | *** | 49831 | 60211 | 109383 | 17701 | 20463 | 26984 | 3693 | 3888 | 4148 | 931 | 951 | 963 | 399 | 399 | 399 |
|  | *** | 53959 | 71651 | 110078 | 18871 | 22803 | 27126 | 3791 | 4006 | 4137 | 931 | 951 | 938 | 399 | 399 | 368 |
| 0.8 | *** | 42758 | 52236 | 93068 | 15328 | 17689 | 22824 | 3108 | 3259 | 3433 | 756 | 756 | 768 | 301 | 301 | 301 |
|  | *** | 46561 | 62344 | 93413 | 16336 | 19606 | 22885 | 3173 | 3336 | 3423 | 756 | 768 | 744 | 301 | 301 | 275 |
| 0.85 | *** | 35218 | 43201 | 73654 | 12554 | 14341 | 17896 | 2414 | 2511 | 2609 | 541 | 541 | 541 | . | . | . |
|  | *** | 38456 | 51371 | 73773 | 13334 | 15718 | 17900 | 2458 | 2556 | 2590 | 541 | 541 | 521 | . | . | . |
| 0.9 | *** | 26724 | 32553 | 51143 | 9174 | 10279 | 12196 | 1569 | 1613 | 1666 | . | . | . | . | . | . |
|  | *** | 29129 | 38143 | 51156 | 9661 | 11071 | 12172 | 1601 | 1634 | 1637 | . | . | . | . | . | . |
| 0.95 | *** | 16064 | 18924 | 25586 | 4851 | 5221 | 5729 | . | . | . | . | . | . | . | . | . |
|  | *** | 17299 | 21341 | 25563 | 5014 | 5448 | 5699 | . | . | . | . | . | . | . | . | . |
| 0.98 | *** | 6964 | 7679 | 8816 | . | . | . | . | . | . | . | . | . | . | . | . |
|  | *** | 7289 | 8166 | 8779 | . | . | . | . | . | . | . | . | . | . | . | . |

TABLE 2: ALPHA= 0.005 POWER= 0.9    EXPECTED ACCRUAL THRU MINIMUM FOLLOW-UP= 14000

| | | DEL=.01 | | | DEL=.02 | | | DEL=.05 | | | DEL=.10 | | | DEL=.15 | | |
|---|---|---|---|---|---|---|---|---|---|---|---|---|---|---|---|---|---|
| FACT= | | 1.0 .75 | .50 .25 | .00 BIN | 1.0 .75 | .50 .25 | .00 BIN | 1.0 .75 | .50 .25 | .00 BIN | 1.0 75 | .50 .25 | .00 BIN | 1.0 .75 | .50 .25 | .00 BIN |
| PCONT=*** | | | | | REQUIRED NUMBER OF PATIENTS | | | | | | | | | | | |
| 0.01 | *** | 2284 | 2284 | 2297 | 827 | 827 | 849 | 267 | 267 | 267 | 127 | 127 | 127 | 92 | 92 | 92 |
| | *** | 2284 | 2284 | 8779 | 827 | 849 | 2902 | 267 | 267 | 790 | 127 | 127 | 321 | 92 | 92 | 191 |
| 0.02 | *** | 5062 | 5084 | 5119 | 1619 | 1632 | 1632 | 442 | 442 | 442 | 184 | 184 | 184 | 127 | 127 | 127 |
| | *** | 5062 | 5097 | 14493 | 1632 | 1632 | 4316 | 442 | 442 | 1009 | 184 | 184 | 373 | 127 | 127 | 213 |
| 0.05 | *** | 15374 | 15549 | 16004 | 4384 | 4432 | 4489 | 932 | 954 | 954 | 337 | 337 | 337 | 197 | 197 | 197 |
| | *** | 15444 | 15702 | 30920 | 4397 | 4454 | 8378 | 954 | 954 | 1637 | 337 | 337 | 521 | 197 | 197 | 275 |
| 0.1 | *** | 33972 | 34554 | 37227 | 9297 | 9494 | 9844 | 1794 | 1807 | 1829 | 569 | 569 | 569 | 302 | 302 | 302 |
| | *** | 34182 | 35302 | 55917 | 9389 | 9647 | 14553 | 1807 | 1829 | 2590 | 569 | 569 | 744 | 302 | 302 | 368 |
| 0.15 | *** | 50864 | 51962 | 58809 | 13812 | 14267 | 15234 | 2599 | 2647 | 2682 | 757 | 779 | 779 | 394 | 394 | 394 |
| | *** | 51249 | 53572 | 77939 | 14009 | 14652 | 19984 | 2612 | 2669 | 3423 | 757 | 779 | 938 | 394 | 394 | 447 |
| 0.2 | *** | 64632 | 66369 | 79017 | 17614 | 18397 | 20239 | 3312 | 3382 | 3474 | 954 | 954 | 954 | 464 | 464 | 464 |
| | *** | 65227 | 69042 | 96984 | 17942 | 19097 | 24671 | 3347 | 3417 | 4137 | 954 | 954 | 1102 | 464 | 464 | 513 |
| 0.25 | *** | 74887 | 77394 | 97007 | 20589 | 21757 | 24662 | 3907 | 4012 | 4152 | 1094 | 1107 | 1107 | 534 | 534 | 534 |
| | *** | 75749 | 81292 | 113054 | 21079 | 22829 | 28614 | 3964 | 4082 | 4732 | 1107 | 1107 | 1235 | 534 | 534 | 566 |
| 0.3 | *** | 81677 | 85072 | 112337 | 22772 | 24369 | 28429 | 4384 | 4524 | 4712 | 1212 | 1234 | 1247 | 582 | 582 | 582 |
| | *** | 82854 | 90344 | 126148 | 23424 | 25804 | 31813 | 4454 | 4607 | 5208 | 1234 | 1234 | 1340 | 582 | 582 | 606 |
| 0.35 | *** | 85247 | 89714 | 124727 | 24229 | 26202 | 31452 | 4747 | 4922 | 5167 | 1304 | 1317 | 1339 | 617 | 617 | 617 |
| | *** | 86809 | 96434 | 136266 | 25047 | 28044 | 34268 | 4817 | 5027 | 5565 | 1317 | 1339 | 1414 | 617 | 617 | 632 |
| 0.4 | *** | 86017 | 91674 | 134059 | 25034 | 27379 | 33714 | 4979 | 5202 | 5482 | 1374 | 1387 | 1409 | 639 | 639 | 639 |
| | *** | 88012 | 99842 | 143408 | 25992 | 29562 | 35979 | 5084 | 5329 | 5803 | 1374 | 1387 | 1459 | 639 | 639 | 645 |
| 0.45 | *** | 84442 | 91359 | 140197 | 25244 | 27939 | 35162 | 5119 | 5364 | 5679 | 1387 | 1422 | 1444 | 639 | 639 | 652 |
| | *** | 86927 | 100949 | 147574 | 26364 | 30402 | 36946 | 5224 | 5504 | 5922 | 1409 | 1422 | 1474 | 639 | 652 | 645 |
| 0.5 | *** | 81012 | 89202 | 143137 | 24964 | 27939 | 35827 | 5132 | 5399 | 5749 | 1387 | 1422 | 1444 | 639 | 639 | 639 |
| | *** | 84022 | 100039 | 148765 | 26202 | 30612 | 37169 | 5259 | 5552 | 5922 | 1409 | 1422 | 1459 | 639 | 639 | 632 |
| 0.55 | *** | 76239 | 85597 | 142822 | 22464 | 27414 | 35674 | 5049 | 5329 | 5679 | 1352 | 1387 | 1409 | 617 | 617 | 617 |
| | *** | 79739 | 97392 | 146979 | 25572 | 30227 | 36648 | 5167 | 5482 | 5803 | 1374 | 1387 | 1414 | 617 | 617 | 606 |
| 0.6 | *** | 70547 | 80837 | 139287 | 23192 | 26412 | 34694 | 4874 | 5132 | 5482 | 1304 | 1317 | 1352 | 582 | 582 | 582 |
| | *** | 74467 | 93249 | 142218 | 24544 | 29269 | 35384 | 4992 | 5294 | 5565 | 1304 | 1339 | 1340 | 582 | 582 | 566 |
| 0.65 | *** | 64282 | 75132 | 132519 | 21792 | 24964 | 32922 | 4594 | 4839 | 5167 | 1212 | 1234 | 1247 | 534 | 534 | 534 |
| | *** | 68504 | 87732 | 134480 | 23122 | 27742 | 33375 | 4699 | 4992 | 5208 | 1212 | 1234 | 1235 | 534 | 534 | 513 |
| 0.7 | *** | 57702 | 68657 | 122544 | 20064 | 23074 | 30354 | 4209 | 4432 | 4712 | 1094 | 1107 | 1129 | 464 | 464 | 477 |
| | *** | 62007 | 80964 | 123767 | 21337 | 25664 | 30622 | 4314 | 4559 | 4732 | 1094 | 1107 | 1102 | 464 | 464 | 447 |
| 0.75 | *** | 50864 | 61412 | 109384 | 18012 | 20742 | 26994 | 3719 | 3907 | 4139 | 932 | 954 | 967 | 394 | 394 | 394 |
| | *** | 55064 | 72892 | 110078 | 19167 | 23017 | 27126 | 3802 | 4012 | 4137 | 932 | 954 | 938 | 394 | 394 | 368 |
| 0.8 | *** | 43724 | 53314 | 93074 | 15597 | 17907 | 22829 | 3124 | 3264 | 3439 | 757 | 757 | 779 | 302 | 302 | 302 |
| | *** | 47574 | 63407 | 93413 | 16599 | 19762 | 22885 | 3194 | 3347 | 3423 | 757 | 757 | 744 | 302 | 302 | 275 |
| 0.85 | *** | 36037 | 44087 | 73649 | 12749 | 14499 | 17894 | 2424 | 2507 | 2612 | 534 | 547 | 547 | . | . | . |
| | *** | 39314 | 52229 | 73773 | 13519 | 15842 | 17900 | 2459 | 2564 | 2590 | 547 | 547 | 521 | . | . | . |
| 0.9 | *** | 27344 | 33167 | 51144 | 9297 | 10382 | 12189 | 1584 | 1619 | 1667 | . | . | . | . | . | . |
| | *** | 29759 | 38719 | 51156 | 9787 | 11139 | 12172 | 1597 | 1632 | 1637 | . | . | . | . | . | . |
| 0.95 | *** | 16389 | 19224 | 25594 | 4887 | 5237 | 5727 | . | . | . | . | . | . | . | . | . |
| | *** | 17592 | 21547 | 25563 | 5062 | 5469 | 5699 | . | . | . | . | . | . | . | . | . |
| 0.98 | *** | 7044 | 7744 | 8807 | . | . | . | . | . | . | . | . | . | . | . | . |
| | *** | 7372 | 8212 | 8779 | . | . | . | . | . | . | . | . | . | . | . | . |

## TABLE 2: ALPHA= 0.005 POWER= 0.9    EXPECTED ACCRUAL THRU MINIMUM FOLLOW-UP= 15000

| | | DEL=.01 | | | DEL=.02 | | | DEL=.05 | | | DEL=.10 | | | DEL=.15 | | |
|---|---|---|---|---|---|---|---|---|---|---|---|---|---|---|---|---|---|
| FACT= | | 1.0 .75 | .50 .25 | .00 BIN | 1.0 .75 | .50 .25 | .00 BIN | 1.0 .75 | .50 .25 | .00 BIN | 1.0 75 | .50 .25 | .00 BIN | 1.0 .75 | .50 .25 | .00 BIN |
| PCONT=*** | | | | | REQUIRED NUMBER OF PATIENTS | | | | | | | | | | | |
| 0.01 | *** | 2274 2297 | 2297 | 835 835 | 835 | 272 272 | 272 | 136 136 | 136 | 99 99 | 99 |
| | *** | 2274 2297 | 8779 | 835 835 | 2902 | 272 272 | 790 | 136 136 | 321 | 99 99 | 191 |
| 0.02 | *** | 5072 5086 | 5124 | 1622 1636 | 1636 | 436 436 | 436 | 197 197 | 197 | 122 122 | 122 |
| | *** | 5072 5110 | 14493 | 1622 1636 | 4316 | 436 436 | 1009 | 197 197 | 373 | 122 122 | 213 |
| 0.05 | *** | 15385 15549 | 15999 | 4397 4435 | 4486 | 947 947 | 947 | 324 324 | 324 | 197 197 | 197 |
| | *** | 15460 15722 | 30920 | 4411 4449 | 8378 | 947 947 | 1637 | 324 324 | 521 | 197 197 | 275 |
| 0.1 | *** | 34022 34622 | 37224 | 9324 9511 | 9849 | 1810 1810 | 1824 | 549 572 | 572 | 286 286 | 286 |
| | *** | 34247 35372 | 55917 | 9399 9661 | 14553 | 1810 1824 | 2590 | 572 572 | 744 | 286 286 | 368 |
| 0.15 | *** | 50949 52097 | 58810 | 13861 14311 | 15235 | 2611 2649 | 2686 | 760 774 | 774 | 385 385 | 385 |
| | *** | 51347 53747 | 77939 | 14049 14686 | 19984 | 2635 2672 | 3423 | 774 774 | 938 | 385 385 | 447 |
| 0.2 | *** | 64772 66586 | 79022 | 17686 18474 | 20236 | 3324 3385 | 3460 | 947 947 | 961 | 460 460 | 474 |
| | *** | 65410 69347 | 96984 | 18024 19149 | 24671 | 3347 3422 | 4137 | 947 961 | 1102 | 460 460 | 513 |
| 0.25 | *** | 75085 77710 | 96999 | 20710 21886 | 24661 | 3924 4022 | 4149 | 1097 1111 | 1111 | 535 535 | 535 |
| | *** | 75985 81736 | 113054 | 21197 22922 | 28614 | 3961 4074 | 4732 | 1097 1111 | 1235 | 535 535 | 566 |
| 0.3 | *** | 81924 85524 | 112336 | 22936 24511 | 28435 | 4397 4547 | 4711 | 1224 1224 | 1247 | 572 586 | 586 |
| | *** | 83185 90947 | 126148 | 23597 25922 | 31813 | 4472 4622 | 5208 | 1224 1247 | 1340 | 572 586 | 606 |
| 0.35 | *** | 85585 90286 | 124735 | 24422 26410 | 31449 | 4772 4936 | 5161 | 1299 1322 | 1336 | 610 610 | 624 |
| | *** | 87249 97186 | 136266 | 25247 28186 | 34268 | 4847 5049 | 5565 | 1322 1336 | 1414 | 610 624 | 632 |
| 0.4 | *** | 86461 92386 | 134049 | 25261 27610 | 33722 | 5011 5222 | 5485 | 1374 1397 | 1411 | 624 647 | 647 |
| | *** | 88561 100749 | 143408 | 26236 29747 | 35979 | 5110 5335 | 5803 | 1374 1397 | 1459 | 624 647 | 645 |
| 0.45 | *** | 84985 92222 | 140199 | 25510 28210 | 35161 | 5147 5372 | 5686 | 1397 1411 | 1435 | 647 647 | 647 |
| | *** | 87610 101986 | 147574 | 26635 30624 | 36946 | 5260 5522 | 5922 | 1411 1435 | 1474 | 647 647 | 645 |
| 0.5 | *** | 81685 90197 | 143147 | 25261 28210 | 35822 | 5161 5410 | 5747 | 1397 1411 | 1449 | 624 647 | 647 |
| | *** | 84835 101199 | 148765 | 26499 30849 | 37169 | 5274 5574 | 5922 | 1411 1435 | 1459 | 624 647 | 632 |
| 0.55 | *** | 77011 86686 | 142824 | 24586 27699 | 35672 | 5086 5335 | 5686 | 1360 1397 | 1411 | 610 610 | 624 |
| | *** | 80672 98635 | 146979 | 25899 30474 | 36648 | 5199 5499 | 5803 | 1374 1397 | 1414 | 610 624 | 606 |
| 0.6 | *** | 71424 81999 | 139285 | 23522 26724 | 34697 | 4899 5147 | 5485 | 1299 1322 | 1336 | 572 586 | 586 |
| | *** | 75497 94524 | 142218 | 24872 29522 | 35384 | 5011 5311 | 5565 | 1322 1336 | 1340 | 572 586 | 566 |
| 0.65 | *** | 65260 76336 | 132511 | 22111 25261 | 32935 | 4622 4861 | 5161 | 1210 1224 | 1247 | 535 535 | 535 |
| | *** | 69586 89035 | 134480 | 23447 27985 | 33375 | 4735 4997 | 5208 | 1224 1247 | 1235 | 535 535 | 513 |
| 0.7 | *** | 58697 69849 | 122536 | 20372 23372 | 30347 | 4224 4449 | 4711 | 1097 1097 | 1111 | 460 474 | 474 |
| | *** | 63099 82210 | 123767 | 21647 25885 | 30622 | 4336 4561 | 4732 | 1097 1111 | 1102 | 474 474 | 447 |
| 0.75 | *** | 51849 62536 | 109374 | 18286 20986 | 26986 | 3736 3924 | 4149 | 947 947 | 961 | 385 385 | 399 |
| | *** | 56110 74035 | 110078 | 19449 23222 | 27126 | 3835 4022 | 4137 | 947 961 | 938 | 385 399 | 368 |
| 0.8 | *** | 44611 54310 | 93085 | 15849 18122 | 22824 | 3136 3272 | 3436 | 760 760 | 774 | 310 310 | 310 |
| | *** | 48511 64397 | 93413 | 16824 19922 | 22885 | 3211 3361 | 3423 | 760 760 | 744 | 310 310 | 275 |
| 0.85 | *** | 36811 44897 | 73660 | 12947 14649 | 17897 | 2424 2522 | 2611 | 535 549 | 549 | . . | . |
| | *** | 40111 52997 | 73773 | 13697 15961 | 17900 | 2461 2560 | 2590 | 535 549 | 521 | . . | . |
| 0.9 | *** | 27910 33760 | 51136 | 9422 10472 | 12197 | 1585 1622 | 1660 | . . | . | . . | . |
| | *** | 30324 39211 | 51156 | 9886 11199 | 12172 | 1599 1636 | 1637 | . . | . | . . | . |
| 0.95 | *** | 16674 19472 | 25585 | 4936 5274 | 5724 | . . | . | . . | . | . . | . |
| | *** | 17874 21760 | 25563 | 5086 5485 | 5699 | . . | . | . . | . | . . | . |
| 0.98 | *** | 7135 7810 | 8799 | . . | . | . . | . | . . | . | . . | . |
| | *** | 7435 8236 | 8779 | . . | . | . . | . | . . | . | . . | . |

TABLE 2: ALPHA= 0.005 POWER= 0.9    EXPECTED ACCRUAL THRU MINIMUM FOLLOW-UP= 17000

| | | DEL=.01 | | | DEL=.02 | | | DEL=.05 | | | DEL=.10 | | | DEL=.15 | | |
|---|---|---|---|---|---|---|---|---|---|---|---|---|---|---|---|---|
| FACT= | | 1.0 .75 | .50 .25 | .00 BIN | 1.0 .75 | .50 .25 | .00 BIN | 1.0 .75 | .50 .25 | .00 BIN | 1.0 75 | .50 .25 | .00 BIN | 1.0 .75 | .50 .25 | .00 BIN |
| PCONT=*** | | | | | | | REQUIRED NUMBER OF PATIENTS | | | | | | | | |
| 0.01 | *** | 2280 | 2280 | 2280 | 835 | 835 | 835 | 282 | 282 | 282 | 139 | 139 | 139 | 96 | 96 | 96 |
| | *** | 2280 | 2280 | 8779 | 835 | 835 | 2902 | 282 | 282 | 790 | 139 | 139 | 321 | 96 | 96 | 191 |
| 0.02 | *** | 5069 | 5085 | 5127 | 1626 | 1626 | 1626 | 436 | 436 | 436 | 197 | 197 | 197 | 112 | 112 | 112 |
| | *** | 5085 | 5111 | 14493 | 1626 | 1626 | 4316 | 436 | 436 | 1009 | 197 | 197 | 373 | 112 | 112 | 213 |
| 0.05 | *** | 15412 | 15582 | 15991 | 4405 | 4431 | 4474 | 946 | 946 | 946 | 325 | 325 | 325 | 197 | 197 | 197 |
| | *** | 15481 | 15752 | 30920 | 4405 | 4447 | 8378 | 946 | 946 | 1637 | 325 | 325 | 521 | 197 | 197 | 275 |
| 0.1 | *** | 34112 | 34750 | 37241 | 9361 | 9547 | 9845 | 1812 | 1812 | 1839 | 564 | 564 | 564 | 309 | 309 | 309 |
| | *** | 34351 | 35515 | 55917 | 9446 | 9675 | 14553 | 1812 | 1812 | 2590 | 564 | 564 | 744 | 309 | 309 | 368 |
| 0.15 | *** | 51112 | 52371 | 58805 | 13951 | 14392 | 15226 | 2620 | 2646 | 2689 | 776 | 776 | 776 | 394 | 394 | 394 |
| | *** | 51564 | 54071 | 77939 | 14137 | 14732 | 19984 | 2620 | 2662 | 3423 | 776 | 776 | 938 | 394 | 394 | 447 |
| 0.2 | *** | 65010 | 67034 | 79019 | 17835 | 18626 | 20241 | 3342 | 3385 | 3470 | 946 | 946 | 962 | 452 | 452 | 479 |
| | *** | 65732 | 69897 | 96984 | 18159 | 19264 | 24671 | 3369 | 3427 | 4137 | 946 | 962 | 1102 | 452 | 479 | 513 |
| 0.25 | *** | 75449 | 78355 | 97012 | 20921 | 22085 | 24677 | 3937 | 4022 | 4150 | 1090 | 1116 | 1116 | 521 | 537 | 537 |
| | *** | 76469 | 82546 | 113054 | 21405 | 23062 | 28614 | 3980 | 4091 | 4732 | 1116 | 1116 | 1235 | 521 | 537 | 566 |
| 0.3 | *** | 82435 | 86387 | 112339 | 23216 | 24789 | 28444 | 4431 | 4559 | 4702 | 1217 | 1244 | 1244 | 580 | 580 | 580 |
| | *** | 83837 | 92040 | 126148 | 23870 | 26149 | 31813 | 4490 | 4644 | 5208 | 1217 | 1244 | 1340 | 580 | 580 | 606 |
| 0.35 | *** | 86260 | 91402 | 124749 | 24789 | 26760 | 31461 | 4787 | 4957 | 5170 | 1302 | 1329 | 1345 | 606 | 622 | 622 |
| | *** | 88087 | 98569 | 136266 | 25612 | 28486 | 34268 | 4872 | 5069 | 5565 | 1329 | 1329 | 1414 | 622 | 622 | 632 |
| 0.4 | *** | 87322 | 93740 | 134056 | 25681 | 28035 | 33714 | 5042 | 5239 | 5494 | 1371 | 1387 | 1414 | 622 | 649 | 649 |
| | *** | 89644 | 102436 | 143408 | 26659 | 30075 | 35979 | 5154 | 5366 | 5803 | 1387 | 1387 | 1459 | 649 | 649 | 645 |
| 0.45 | *** | 86047 | 93825 | 140192 | 25995 | 28672 | 35175 | 5196 | 5409 | 5680 | 1414 | 1414 | 1430 | 649 | 649 | 649 |
| | *** | 88921 | 103924 | 147574 | 27126 | 31010 | 36946 | 5297 | 5536 | 5922 | 1414 | 1430 | 1474 | 649 | 649 | 645 |
| 0.5 | *** | 82971 | 92040 | 143125 | 25809 | 28715 | 35812 | 5212 | 5451 | 5749 | 1414 | 1414 | 1430 | 622 | 649 | 649 |
| | *** | 86371 | 103329 | 148765 | 27041 | 31265 | 37169 | 5324 | 5595 | 5922 | 1414 | 1430 | 1459 | 649 | 649 | 632 |
| 0.55 | *** | 78525 | 88725 | 142827 | 25145 | 28247 | 35669 | 5127 | 5382 | 5680 | 1371 | 1387 | 1414 | 606 | 622 | 622 |
| | *** | 82419 | 100906 | 146979 | 26462 | 30909 | 36648 | 5255 | 5510 | 5803 | 1371 | 1387 | 1414 | 622 | 622 | 606 |
| 0.6 | *** | 73127 | 84161 | 139284 | 24109 | 27270 | 34691 | 4957 | 5196 | 5494 | 1302 | 1329 | 1345 | 580 | 580 | 580 |
| | *** | 77404 | 96869 | 142218 | 25442 | 29947 | 35384 | 5069 | 5324 | 5565 | 1329 | 1329 | 1340 | 580 | 580 | 566 |
| 0.65 | *** | 67092 | 78551 | 132526 | 22680 | 25809 | 32922 | 4660 | 4899 | 5170 | 1217 | 1244 | 1244 | 521 | 537 | 537 |
| | *** | 71597 | 91360 | 134480 | 24024 | 28401 | 33375 | 4771 | 5026 | 5208 | 1217 | 1244 | 1235 | 537 | 537 | 513 |
| 0.7 | *** | 60574 | 72022 | 122539 | 20921 | 23870 | 30356 | 4277 | 4474 | 4729 | 1090 | 1116 | 1116 | 479 | 479 | 479 |
| | *** | 65121 | 84459 | 123767 | 22196 | 26276 | 30622 | 4362 | 4601 | 4732 | 1090 | 1116 | 1102 | 479 | 479 | 447 |
| 0.75 | *** | 53662 | 64585 | 109380 | 18796 | 21431 | 26972 | 3767 | 3937 | 4150 | 946 | 946 | 962 | 394 | 394 | 394 |
| | *** | 58040 | 76102 | 110078 | 19944 | 23556 | 27126 | 3852 | 4049 | 4137 | 946 | 962 | 938 | 394 | 394 | 368 |
| 0.8 | *** | 46294 | 56127 | 93086 | 16289 | 18472 | 22834 | 3172 | 3300 | 3427 | 750 | 750 | 776 | 309 | 309 | 309 |
| | *** | 50289 | 66184 | 93413 | 17240 | 20199 | 22885 | 3241 | 3369 | 3423 | 750 | 776 | 744 | 309 | 309 | 275 |
| 0.85 | *** | 38235 | 46395 | 73637 | 13271 | 14929 | 17904 | 2450 | 2519 | 2620 | 537 | 537 | 537 | . | . | . |
| | *** | 41576 | 54385 | 73773 | 14010 | 16135 | 17900 | 2492 | 2561 | 2590 | 537 | 537 | 521 | . | . | . |
| 0.9 | *** | 28954 | 34792 | 51139 | 9632 | 10636 | 12182 | 1600 | 1626 | 1669 | . | . | . | . | . | . |
| | *** | 31392 | 40105 | 51156 | 10084 | 11290 | 12172 | 1600 | 1642 | 1637 | . | . | . | . | . | . |
| 0.95 | *** | 17197 | 19917 | 25596 | 5000 | 5324 | 5722 | . | . | . | . | . | . | . | . | . |
| | *** | 18387 | 22085 | 25563 | 5154 | 5510 | 5699 | . | . | . | . | . | . | . | . | . |
| 0.98 | *** | 7279 | 7890 | 8809 | . | . | . | . | . | . | . | . | . | . | . | . |
| | *** | 7550 | 8299 | 8779 | . | . | . | . | . | . | . | . | . | . | . | . |

## TABLE 2: ALPHA= 0.005 POWER= 0.9 EXPECTED ACCRUAL THRU MINIMUM FOLLOW-UP= 20000

| | | DEL=.01 | | | DEL=.02 | | | DEL=.05 | | | DEL=.10 | | | DEL=.15 | | |
|---|---|---|---|---|---|---|---|---|---|---|---|---|---|---|---|---|
| FACT= | | 1.0 .75 | .50 .25 | .00 BIN | 1.0 .75 | .50 .25 | .00 BIN | 1.0 .75 | .50 .25 | .00 BIN | 1.0 75 | .50 .25 | .00 BIN | 1.0 .75 | .50 .25 | .00 BIN |
| PCONT=*** | | | | | REQUIRED NUMBER OF PATIENTS | | | | | | | | | | | |
| 0.01 | *** | 2282 | 2282 | 2282 | 832 | 832 | 832 | 282 | 282 | 282 | 132 | 132 | 132 | 82 | 82 | 82 |
| | *** | 2282 | 2282 | 8779 | 832 | 832 | 2902 | 282 | 282 | 790 | 132 | 132 | 321 | 82 | 82 | 191 |
| 0.02 | *** | 5082 | 5082 | 5113 | 1632 | 1632 | 1632 | 432 | 432 | 432 | 182 | 182 | 182 | 132 | 132 | 132 |
| | *** | 5082 | 5113 | 14493 | 1632 | 1632 | 4316 | 432 | 432 | 1009 | 182 | 182 | 373 | 132 | 132 | 213 |
| 0.05 | *** | 15463 | 15632 | 15982 | 4413 | 4432 | 4482 | 932 | 932 | 963 | 332 | 332 | 332 | 182 | 182 | 182 |
| | *** | 15532 | 15782 | 30920 | 4432 | 4463 | 8378 | 932 | 932 | 1637 | 332 | 332 | 521 | 182 | 182 | 275 |
| 0.1 | *** | 34232 | 34932 | 37232 | 9413 | 9582 | 9832 | 1813 | 1813 | 1832 | 563 | 563 | 563 | 282 | 282 | 282 |
| | *** | 34513 | 35682 | 55917 | 9482 | 9713 | 14553 | 1813 | 1832 | 2590 | 563 | 563 | 744 | 282 | 282 | 368 |
| 0.15 | *** | 51363 | 52732 | 58813 | 14063 | 14482 | 15232 | 2632 | 2663 | 2682 | 763 | 763 | 782 | 382 | 382 | 382 |
| | *** | 51863 | 54482 | 77939 | 14232 | 14813 | 19984 | 2632 | 2663 | 3423 | 763 | 763 | 938 | 382 | 382 | 447 |
| 0.2 | *** | 65413 | 67632 | 79013 | 18013 | 18782 | 20232 | 3363 | 3413 | 3463 | 963 | 963 | 963 | 463 | 463 | 463 |
| | *** | 66213 | 70613 | 96984 | 18363 | 19382 | 24671 | 3382 | 3432 | 4137 | 963 | 963 | 1102 | 463 | 463 | 513 |
| 0.25 | *** | 75982 | 79232 | 97013 | 21182 | 22332 | 24663 | 3963 | 4063 | 4132 | 1113 | 1113 | 1113 | 532 | 532 | 532 |
| | *** | 77163 | 83632 | 113054 | 21682 | 23263 | 28614 | 4013 | 4082 | 4732 | 1113 | 1113 | 1235 | 532 | 532 | 566 |
| 0.3 | *** | 83182 | 87582 | 112332 | 23582 | 25132 | 28432 | 4463 | 4582 | 4713 | 1232 | 1232 | 1232 | 582 | 582 | 582 |
| | *** | 84782 | 93482 | 126148 | 24232 | 26413 | 31813 | 4513 | 4632 | 5208 | 1232 | 1232 | 1340 | 582 | 582 | 606 |
| 0.35 | *** | 87232 | 92932 | 124732 | 25232 | 27182 | 31463 | 4832 | 4982 | 5163 | 1313 | 1332 | 1332 | 613 | 613 | 613 |
| | *** | 89313 | 100413 | 136266 | 26082 | 28813 | 34268 | 4913 | 5063 | 5565 | 1332 | 1332 | 1414 | 613 | 613 | 632 |
| 0.4 | *** | 88563 | 95632 | 134063 | 26232 | 28563 | 33713 | 5113 | 5282 | 5482 | 1382 | 1382 | 1413 | 632 | 632 | 632 |
| | *** | 91182 | 104613 | 143408 | 27213 | 30482 | 35979 | 5182 | 5382 | 5803 | 1382 | 1413 | 1459 | 632 | 632 | 645 |
| 0.45 | *** | 87613 | 96032 | 140213 | 26632 | 29263 | 35163 | 5263 | 5432 | 5682 | 1413 | 1432 | 1432 | 632 | 632 | 663 |
| | *** | 90763 | 106432 | 147574 | 27763 | 31463 | 36946 | 5332 | 5563 | 5922 | 1413 | 1432 | 1474 | 632 | 632 | 645 |
| 0.5 | *** | 84832 | 94532 | 143132 | 26482 | 29382 | 35813 | 5282 | 5482 | 5732 | 1413 | 1432 | 1432 | 632 | 632 | 632 |
| | *** | 88532 | 106082 | 148765 | 27732 | 31763 | 37169 | 5382 | 5613 | 5922 | 1413 | 1432 | 1459 | 632 | 632 | 632 |
| 0.55 | *** | 80663 | 91463 | 142832 | 25882 | 28932 | 35663 | 5213 | 5413 | 5682 | 1382 | 1382 | 1413 | 613 | 613 | 613 |
| | *** | 84832 | 103863 | 146979 | 27182 | 31432 | 36648 | 5313 | 5532 | 5803 | 1382 | 1413 | 1414 | 613 | 613 | 606 |
| 0.6 | *** | 75482 | 87032 | 139282 | 24863 | 27963 | 34713 | 5013 | 5232 | 5482 | 1313 | 1332 | 1332 | 582 | 582 | 582 |
| | *** | 80013 | 99913 | 142218 | 26182 | 30482 | 35384 | 5113 | 5363 | 5565 | 1313 | 1332 | 1340 | 582 | 582 | 566 |
| 0.65 | *** | 69582 | 81482 | 132513 | 23432 | 26463 | 32932 | 4732 | 4932 | 5163 | 1213 | 1232 | 1263 | 532 | 532 | 532 |
| | *** | 74313 | 94382 | 134480 | 24763 | 28913 | 33375 | 4813 | 5032 | 5208 | 1232 | 1232 | 1235 | 532 | 532 | 513 |
| 0.7 | *** | 63113 | 74913 | 122532 | 21632 | 24482 | 30363 | 4332 | 4513 | 4713 | 1082 | 1113 | 1113 | 463 | 463 | 463 |
| | *** | 67832 | 87332 | 123767 | 22882 | 26732 | 30622 | 4413 | 4613 | 4732 | 1113 | 1113 | 1102 | 463 | 463 | 447 |
| 0.75 | *** | 56113 | 67282 | 109382 | 19463 | 21982 | 26982 | 3832 | 3963 | 4132 | 932 | 963 | 963 | 382 | 382 | 382 |
| | *** | 60632 | 78732 | 110078 | 20563 | 23963 | 27126 | 3882 | 4063 | 4137 | 932 | 963 | 938 | 382 | 382 | 368 |
| 0.8 | *** | 48513 | 58513 | 93082 | 16832 | 18932 | 22832 | 3213 | 3313 | 3432 | 763 | 763 | 763 | 313 | 313 | 313 |
| | *** | 52613 | 68432 | 93413 | 17763 | 20513 | 22885 | 3263 | 3382 | 3423 | 763 | 763 | 744 | 313 | 313 | 275 |
| 0.85 | *** | 40113 | 48313 | 73663 | 13682 | 15263 | 17882 | 2463 | 2532 | 2613 | 532 | 532 | 563 | . | . | . |
| | *** | 43513 | 56113 | 73773 | 14382 | 16363 | 17900 | 2513 | 2582 | 2590 | 532 | 532 | 521 | . | . | . |
| 0.9 | *** | 30332 | 36113 | 51132 | 9882 | 10813 | 12182 | 1613 | 1632 | 1663 | . | . | . | . | . | . |
| | *** | 32763 | 41213 | 51156 | 10313 | 11413 | 12172 | 1613 | 1632 | 1637 | . | . | . | . | . | . |
| 0.95 | *** | 17882 | 20482 | 25582 | 5082 | 5382 | 5732 | . | . | . | . | . | . | . | . | . |
| | *** | 19032 | 22513 | 25563 | 5232 | 5532 | 5699 | . | . | . | . | . | . | . | . | . |
| 0.98 | *** | 7432 | 8013 | 8813 | . | . | . | . | . | . | . | . | . | . | . | . |
| | *** | 7713 | 8363 | 8779 | . | . | . | . | . | . | . | . | . | . | . | . |

TABLE 2: ALPHA= 0.005 POWER= 0.9    EXPECTED ACCRUAL THRU MINIMUM FOLLOW-UP= 25000

| PCONT | FACT | DEL=.01 1.0 .75 | DEL=.01 .50 .25 | DEL=.01 .00 BIN | DEL=.02 1.0 .75 | DEL=.02 .50 .25 | DEL=.02 .00 BIN | DEL=.05 1.0 .75 | DEL=.05 .50 .25 | DEL=.05 .00 BIN | DEL=.10 1.0 75 | DEL=.10 .50 .25 | DEL=.10 .00 BIN | DEL=.15 1.0 .75 | DEL=.15 .50 .25 | DEL=.15 .00 BIN |
|---|---|---|---|---|---|---|---|---|---|---|---|---|---|---|---|---|
| PCONT=*** | | | | | REQUIRED NUMBER OF PATIENTS | | | | | | | | | | | |
| 0.01 | *** | 2290 | 2290 | 2290 | 829 | 829 | 829 | 266 | 266 | 266 | 141 | 141 | 141 | 102 | 102 | 102 |
|  | *** | 2290 | 2290 | 8779 | 829 | 829 | 2902 | 266 | 266 | 790 | 141 | 141 | 321 | 102 | 102 | 191 |
| 0.02 | *** | 5079 | 5102 | 5102 | 1641 | 1641 | 1641 | 454 | 454 | 454 | 204 | 204 | 204 | 141 | 141 | 141 |
|  | *** | 5079 | 5102 | 14493 | 1641 | 1641 | 4316 | 454 | 454 | 1009 | 204 | 204 | 373 | 141 | 141 | 213 |
| 0.05 | *** | 15516 | 15665 | 15977 | 4415 | 4454 | 4477 | 954 | 954 | 954 | 329 | 329 | 329 | 204 | 204 | 204 |
|  | *** | 15579 | 15829 | 30920 | 4415 | 4454 | 8378 | 954 | 954 | 1637 | 329 | 329 | 521 | 204 | 204 | 275 |
| 0.1 | *** | 34454 | 35165 | 37227 | 9477 | 9641 | 9852 | 1829 | 1829 | 1829 | 579 | 579 | 579 | 290 | 290 | 290 |
|  | *** | 34727 | 35915 | 55917 | 9540 | 9727 | 14553 | 1829 | 1829 | 2590 | 579 | 579 | 744 | 290 | 290 | 368 |
| 0.15 | *** | 51727 | 53290 | 58829 | 14204 | 14602 | 15227 | 2641 | 2665 | 2665 | 766 | 766 | 766 | 391 | 391 | 391 |
|  | *** | 52329 | 55040 | 77939 | 14391 | 14891 | 19984 | 2641 | 2665 | 3423 | 766 | 766 | 938 | 391 | 391 | 447 |
| 0.2 | *** | 66016 | 68540 | 79016 | 18266 | 18977 | 20227 | 3391 | 3415 | 3454 | 954 | 954 | 954 | 454 | 454 | 477 |
|  | *** | 66954 | 71602 | 96984 | 18602 | 19516 | 24671 | 3391 | 3454 | 4137 | 954 | 954 | 1102 | 454 | 454 | 513 |
| 0.25 | *** | 76891 | 80579 | 97016 | 21579 | 22665 | 24665 | 4016 | 4079 | 4141 | 1102 | 1102 | 1102 | 516 | 540 | 540 |
|  | *** | 78227 | 85102 | 113054 | 22040 | 23477 | 28614 | 4040 | 4102 | 4732 | 1102 | 1102 | 1235 | 540 | 540 | 566 |
| 0.3 | *** | 84391 | 89391 | 112329 | 24102 | 25579 | 28415 | 4516 | 4602 | 4704 | 1227 | 1227 | 1227 | 579 | 579 | 579 |
|  | *** | 86227 | 95477 | 126148 | 24727 | 26727 | 31813 | 4540 | 4665 | 5208 | 1227 | 1227 | 1340 | 579 | 579 | 606 |
| 0.35 | *** | 88829 | 95204 | 124727 | 25891 | 27766 | 31454 | 4891 | 5016 | 5165 | 1329 | 1329 | 1352 | 602 | 602 | 602 |
|  | *** | 91204 | 102915 | 136266 | 26704 | 29227 | 34268 | 4954 | 5079 | 5565 | 1329 | 1329 | 1414 | 602 | 602 | 632 |
| 0.4 | *** | 90540 | 98391 | 134040 | 27016 | 29227 | 33704 | 5165 | 5329 | 5477 | 1391 | 1391 | 1415 | 641 | 641 | 641 |
|  | *** | 93516 | 107641 | 143408 | 27954 | 30977 | 35979 | 5227 | 5391 | 5803 | 1391 | 1391 | 1459 | 641 | 641 | 645 |
| 0.45 | *** | 90016 | 99266 | 140204 | 27516 | 30040 | 35165 | 5329 | 5477 | 5665 | 1415 | 1415 | 1454 | 641 | 641 | 641 |
|  | *** | 93579 | 109852 | 147574 | 28602 | 32040 | 36946 | 5391 | 5579 | 5922 | 1415 | 1415 | 1474 | 641 | 641 | 645 |
| 0.5 | *** | 87665 | 98141 | 143141 | 27454 | 30204 | 35829 | 5352 | 5540 | 5727 | 1415 | 1415 | 1454 | 641 | 641 | 641 |
|  | *** | 91727 | 109891 | 148765 | 28641 | 32391 | 37169 | 5454 | 5641 | 5922 | 1415 | 1415 | 1459 | 641 | 641 | 632 |
| 0.55 | *** | 83852 | 95352 | 142829 | 26891 | 29790 | 35665 | 5290 | 5454 | 5665 | 1391 | 1391 | 1415 | 602 | 602 | 602 |
|  | *** | 88391 | 107891 | 146979 | 28165 | 32079 | 36648 | 5352 | 5579 | 5803 | 1391 | 1391 | 1414 | 602 | 602 | 606 |
| 0.6 | *** | 78977 | 91141 | 139290 | 25891 | 28829 | 34704 | 5102 | 5266 | 5477 | 1329 | 1329 | 1352 | 579 | 579 | 579 |
|  | *** | 83790 | 104040 | 142218 | 27165 | 31141 | 35384 | 5165 | 5391 | 5565 | 1329 | 1329 | 1340 | 579 | 579 | 566 |
| 0.65 | *** | 73204 | 85602 | 132516 | 24454 | 27329 | 32915 | 4790 | 4977 | 5165 | 1227 | 1227 | 1266 | 540 | 540 | 540 |
|  | *** | 78204 | 98477 | 134480 | 25727 | 29540 | 33375 | 4891 | 5079 | 5208 | 1227 | 1227 | 1235 | 540 | 540 | 513 |
| 0.7 | *** | 66727 | 78915 | 122540 | 22602 | 25290 | 30352 | 4391 | 4540 | 4727 | 1102 | 1102 | 1102 | 477 | 477 | 477 |
|  | *** | 71665 | 91204 | 123767 | 23790 | 27329 | 30622 | 4477 | 4641 | 4732 | 1102 | 1102 | 1102 | 477 | 477 | 447 |
| 0.75 | *** | 59602 | 71016 | 109391 | 20329 | 22704 | 26977 | 3891 | 4016 | 4141 | 954 | 954 | 954 | 391 | 391 | 391 |
|  | *** | 64266 | 82227 | 110078 | 21352 | 24454 | 27126 | 3954 | 4079 | 4137 | 954 | 954 | 938 | 391 | 391 | 368 |
| 0.8 | *** | 51665 | 61766 | 93079 | 17540 | 19516 | 22829 | 3266 | 3329 | 3454 | 766 | 766 | 766 | 290 | 290 | 290 |
|  | *** | 55829 | 71391 | 93413 | 18415 | 20891 | 22885 | 3290 | 3391 | 3423 | 766 | 766 | 744 | 290 | 290 | 275 |
| 0.85 | *** | 42727 | 50915 | 73641 | 14227 | 15665 | 17891 | 2477 | 2540 | 2602 | 540 | 540 | 540 | . | . | . |
|  | *** | 46165 | 58391 | 73773 | 14891 | 16641 | 17900 | 2516 | 2579 | 2590 | 540 | 540 | 521 | . | . | . |
| 0.9 | *** | 32227 | 37852 | 51141 | 10227 | 11040 | 12204 | 1602 | 1641 | 1665 | . | . | . | . | . | . |
|  | *** | 34602 | 42641 | 51156 | 10602 | 11540 | 12172 | 1641 | 1641 | 1637 | . | . | . | . | . | . |
| 0.95 | *** | 18766 | 21227 | 25579 | 5204 | 5454 | 5727 | . | . | . | . | . | . | . | . | . |
|  | *** | 19852 | 23016 | 25563 | 5329 | 5579 | 5699 | . | . | . | . | . | . | . | . | . |
| 0.98 | *** | 7641 | 8141 | 8790 | . | . | . | . | . | . | . | . | . | . | . | . |
|  | *** | 7891 | 8454 | 8779 | . | . | . | . | . | . | . | . | . | . | . | . |

## TABLE 3: ALPHA= 0.01  POWER= 0.8    EXPECTED ACCRUAL THRU MINIMUM FOLLOW-UP= 30

| | | DEL=.10 | | | DEL=.15 | | | DEL=.20 | | | DEL=.25 | | | DEL=.30 | | |
|---|---|---|---|---|---|---|---|---|---|---|---|---|---|---|---|---|
| FACT= | | 1.0 .75 | .50 .25 | .00 BIN | 1.0 .75 | .50 .25 | .00 BIN | 1.0 .75 | .50 .25 | .00 BIN | 1.0 75 | .50 .25 | .00 BIN | 1.0 .75 | .50 .25 | .00 BIN |
| PCONT=*** | | | | | REQUIRED NUMBER OF PATIENTS | | | | | | | | | | | |
| 0.05 | *** | 211 | 212 | 228 | 123 | 124 | 133 | 86 | 88 | 94 | 67 | 68 | 72 | 55 | 56 | 60 |
| | *** | 211 | 214 | 352 | 123 | 126 | 186 | 87 | 89 | 118 | 68 | 70 | 83 | 56 | 57 | 62 |
| 0.1 | *** | 332 | 334 | 382 | 176 | 178 | 203 | 115 | 118 | 133 | 85 | 87 | 98 | 68 | 70 | 77 |
| | *** | 333 | 339 | 502 | 176 | 182 | 248 | 116 | 121 | 151 | 86 | 90 | 102 | 68 | 72 | 74 |
| 0.15 | *** | 429 | 432 | 523 | 215 | 219 | 264 | 136 | 140 | 166 | 98 | 101 | 118 | 75 | 79 | 90 |
| | *** | 430 | 439 | 633 | 217 | 226 | 302 | 138 | 146 | 179 | 99 | 106 | 119 | 77 | 82 | 84 |
| 0.2 | *** | 499 | 504 | 649 | 243 | 248 | 317 | 150 | 156 | 194 | 105 | 110 | 135 | 80 | 85 | 101 |
| | *** | 500 | 514 | 743 | 245 | 258 | 346 | 152 | 164 | 201 | 107 | 117 | 131 | 82 | 89 | 92 |
| 0.25 | *** | 544 | 551 | 755 | 259 | 267 | 360 | 158 | 165 | 217 | 109 | 116 | 148 | 83 | 88 | 109 |
| | *** | 546 | 565 | 833 | 262 | 280 | 382 | 160 | 176 | 219 | 112 | 124 | 141 | 85 | 94 | 98 |
| 0.3 | *** | 565 | 575 | 842 | 266 | 276 | 395 | 160 | 170 | 234 | 111 | 119 | 157 | 83 | 90 | 114 |
| | *** | 568 | 594 | 904 | 269 | 293 | 409 | 164 | 183 | 231 | 114 | 129 | 147 | 86 | 97 | 101 |
| 0.35 | *** | 566 | 579 | 908 | 264 | 277 | 420 | 158 | 170 | 245 | 109 | 119 | 163 | 82 | 89 | 117 |
| | *** | 570 | 603 | 954 | 268 | 299 | 426 | 163 | 186 | 239 | 113 | 130 | 151 | 85 | 98 | 102 |
| 0.4 | *** | 549 | 565 | 952 | 255 | 271 | 435 | 153 | 167 | 251 | 105 | 117 | 165 | 79 | 88 | 117 |
| | *** | 554 | 597 | 984 | 261 | 297 | 435 | 158 | 185 | 241 | 110 | 129 | 151 | 82 | 96 | 101 |
| 0.45 | *** | 517 | 538 | 974 | 241 | 261 | 440 | 145 | 161 | 251 | 100 | 113 | 163 | 75 | 84 | 115 |
| | *** | 524 | 577 | 994 | 248 | 290 | 435 | 151 | 181 | 239 | 105 | 126 | 147 | 79 | 94 | 98 |
| 0.5 | *** | 475 | 501 | 975 | 223 | 246 | 435 | 136 | 154 | 246 | 94 | 107 | 158 | 71 | 80 | 110 |
| | *** | 484 | 548 | 984 | 231 | 279 | 426 | 143 | 175 | 231 | 99 | 121 | 141 | 74 | 89 | 92 |
| 0.55 | *** | 425 | 457 | 953 | 203 | 229 | 421 | 125 | 144 | 235 | 87 | 100 | 150 | 65 | 75 | 103 |
| | *** | 436 | 512 | 954 | 212 | 264 | 409 | 132 | 165 | 219 | 92 | 114 | 131 | 69 | 84 | 84 |
| 0.6 | *** | 371 | 411 | 910 | 181 | 210 | 397 | 113 | 132 | 219 | 79 | 92 | 138 | 59 | 68 | 94 |
| | *** | 385 | 471 | 904 | 192 | 245 | 382 | 121 | 153 | 201 | 84 | 105 | 119 | 63 | 76 | 74 |
| 0.65 | *** | 318 | 363 | 845 | 160 | 189 | 363 | 101 | 119 | 197 | 71 | 83 | 122 | 52 | 60 | 82 |
| | *** | 334 | 426 | 833 | 171 | 224 | 346 | 108 | 139 | 179 | 75 | 94 | 102 | 56 | 68 | 62 |
| 0.7 | *** | 268 | 316 | 758 | 139 | 167 | 320 | 88 | 105 | 171 | 61 | 72 | 103 | . | . | . |
| | *** | 286 | 379 | 743 | 150 | 199 | 302 | 95 | 122 | 151 | 65 | 81 | 83 | . | . | . |
| 0.75 | *** | 222 | 269 | 650 | 117 | 143 | 267 | 74 | 88 | 138 | . | . | . | . | . | . |
| | *** | 240 | 329 | 633 | 127 | 171 | 248 | 80 | 103 | 118 | . | . | . | . | . | . |
| 0.8 | *** | 178 | 222 | 521 | 95 | 116 | 205 | . | . | . | . | . | . | . | . | . |
| | *** | 195 | 274 | 502 | 103 | 139 | 186 | . | . | . | . | . | . | . | . | . |
| 0.85 | *** | 136 | 171 | 372 | . | . | . | . | . | . | . | . | . | . | . | . |
| | *** | 150 | 211 | 352 | . | . | . | . | . | . | . | . | . | . | . | . |

## TABLE 3: ALPHA= 0.01  POWER= 0.8    EXPECTED ACCRUAL THRU MINIMUM FOLLOW-UP= 40

| | DEL=.10 | | | DEL=.15 | | | DEL=.20 | | | DEL=.25 | | | DEL=.30 | | |
|---|---|---|---|---|---|---|---|---|---|---|---|---|---|---|---|
| FACT= | 1.0 .75 | .50 .25 | .00 BIN | 1.0 .75 | .50 .25 | .00 BIN | 1.0 .75 | .50 .25 | .00 BIN | 1.0 75 | .50 .25 | .00 BIN | 1.0 .75 | .50 .25 | .00 BIN |
| PCONT=*** | REQUIRED NUMBER OF PATIENTS | | | | | | | | | | | | | | |
| 0.05 *** | 211 | 212 | 228 | 123 | 124 | 133 | 87 | 88 | 94 | 68 | 69 | 73 | 56 | 57 | 60 |
| *** | 211 | 215 | 352 | 123 | 127 | 186 | 87 | 90 | 118 | 68 | 70 | 83 | 56 | 58 | 62 |
| 0.1 *** | 333 | 336 | 382 | 176 | 180 | 203 | 116 | 119 | 133 | 86 | 89 | 98 | 68 | 70 | 77 |
| *** | 334 | 341 | 502 | 177 | 184 | 248 | 117 | 123 | 151 | 87 | 91 | 102 | 69 | 73 | 74 |
| 0.15 *** | 430 | 434 | 523 | 217 | 222 | 264 | 138 | 142 | 166 | 99 | 103 | 118 | 77 | 80 | 90 |
| *** | 431 | 443 | 633 | 218 | 230 | 302 | 139 | 148 | 179 | 100 | 108 | 119 | 78 | 83 | 84 |
| 0.2 *** | 501 | 507 | 649 | 245 | 252 | 317 | 152 | 159 | 194 | 107 | 113 | 135 | 82 | 87 | 101 |
| *** | 503 | 521 | 743 | 247 | 264 | 346 | 154 | 168 | 201 | 109 | 119 | 131 | 84 | 91 | 92 |
| 0.25 *** | 546 | 556 | 755 | 262 | 272 | 360 | 160 | 169 | 217 | 112 | 119 | 148 | 85 | 91 | 109 |
| *** | 549 | 574 | 833 | 265 | 288 | 382 | 164 | 181 | 219 | 115 | 128 | 141 | 87 | 97 | 98 |
| 0.3 *** | 568 | 581 | 842 | 269 | 282 | 395 | 164 | 175 | 234 | 114 | 123 | 157 | 86 | 93 | 114 |
| *** | 573 | 606 | 904 | 274 | 303 | 409 | 168 | 189 | 231 | 117 | 133 | 147 | 88 | 100 | 101 |
| 0.35 *** | 570 | 587 | 908 | 268 | 285 | 420 | 163 | 176 | 245 | 113 | 124 | 163 | 85 | 93 | 117 |
| *** | 576 | 619 | 954 | 274 | 310 | 426 | 168 | 193 | 239 | 117 | 135 | 151 | 88 | 101 | 102 |
| 0.4 *** | 554 | 576 | 952 | 261 | 281 | 435 | 158 | 174 | 251 | 110 | 122 | 165 | 82 | 91 | 117 |
| *** | 562 | 616 | 984 | 268 | 310 | 435 | 164 | 193 | 241 | 115 | 134 | 151 | 86 | 100 | 101 |
| 0.45 *** | 524 | 552 | 974 | 248 | 272 | 440 | 151 | 169 | 251 | 105 | 118 | 163 | 79 | 88 | 115 |
| *** | 533 | 600 | 994 | 257 | 304 | 435 | 158 | 190 | 239 | 111 | 132 | 147 | 83 | 97 | 98 |
| 0.5 *** | 484 | 518 | 975 | 231 | 259 | 435 | 143 | 162 | 246 | 99 | 113 | 158 | 74 | 84 | 110 |
| *** | 495 | 574 | 984 | 242 | 294 | 426 | 150 | 184 | 231 | 105 | 127 | 141 | 78 | 93 | 92 |
| 0.55 *** | 436 | 477 | 953 | 212 | 243 | 421 | 132 | 152 | 235 | 92 | 106 | 150 | 69 | 78 | 103 |
| *** | 450 | 540 | 954 | 224 | 280 | 409 | 140 | 174 | 219 | 98 | 119 | 131 | 73 | 87 | 84 |
| 0.6 *** | 385 | 433 | 910 | 192 | 224 | 397 | 121 | 141 | 219 | 84 | 98 | 138 | 63 | 72 | 94 |
| *** | 402 | 501 | 904 | 205 | 261 | 382 | 129 | 162 | 201 | 90 | 110 | 119 | 67 | 79 | 74 |
| 0.65 *** | 334 | 387 | 845 | 171 | 203 | 363 | 108 | 128 | 197 | 75 | 88 | 122 | 56 | 63 | 82 |
| *** | 354 | 457 | 833 | 184 | 239 | 346 | 116 | 147 | 179 | 81 | 99 | 102 | 59 | 70 | 62 |
| 0.7 *** | 286 | 340 | 758 | 150 | 180 | 320 | 95 | 112 | 171 | 65 | 76 | 103 | . | . | . |
| *** | 307 | 409 | 743 | 162 | 213 | 302 | 102 | 129 | 151 | 70 | 85 | 83 | . | . | . |
| 0.75 *** | 240 | 293 | 650 | 127 | 154 | 267 | 80 | 94 | 138 | . | . | . | . | . | . |
| *** | 260 | 356 | 633 | 138 | 183 | 248 | 86 | 108 | 118 | . | . | . | . | . | . |
| 0.8 *** | 195 | 243 | 521 | 103 | 125 | 205 | . | . | . | . | . | . | . | . | . |
| *** | 214 | 297 | 502 | 112 | 148 | 186 | . | . | . | . | . | . | . | . | . |
| 0.85 *** | 150 | 188 | 372 | . | . | . | . | . | . | . | . | . | . | . | . |
| *** | 165 | 229 | 352 | . | . | . | . | . | . | . | . | . | . | . | . |

## TABLE 3: ALPHA= 0.01 POWER= 0.8     EXPECTED ACCRUAL THRU MINIMUM FOLLOW-UP= 50

| PCONT=*** | FACT= | DEL=.10 1.0/.75 | .50/.25 | .00/BIN | DEL=.15 1.0/.75 | .50/.25 | .00/BIN | DEL=.20 1.0/.75 | .50/.25 | .00/BIN | DEL=.25 1.0/75 | .50/.25 | .00/BIN | DEL=.30 1.0/.75 | .50/.25 | .00/BIN |
|---|---|---|---|---|---|---|---|---|---|---|---|---|---|---|---|---|
| | | REQUIRED NUMBER OF PATIENTS | | | | | | | | | | | | | | |
| 0.05 | *** | 211 | 213 | 228 | 123 | 125 | 133 | 87 | 89 | 94 | 68 | 69 | 73 | 56 | 57 | 60 |
| | *** | 212 | 216 | 352 | 124 | 127 | 186 | 88 | 90 | 118 | 68 | 70 | 83 | 57 | 58 | 62 |
| 0.1 | *** | 334 | 337 | 382 | 177 | 181 | 203 | 117 | 120 | 133 | 87 | 90 | 98 | 69 | 71 | 77 |
| | *** | 335 | 344 | 502 | 179 | 186 | 248 | 118 | 124 | 151 | 88 | 92 | 102 | 70 | 73 | 74 |
| 0.15 | *** | 431 | 437 | 523 | 218 | 224 | 264 | 139 | 144 | 166 | 100 | 104 | 118 | 78 | 81 | 90 |
| | *** | 433 | 448 | 633 | 220 | 233 | 302 | 141 | 151 | 179 | 102 | 109 | 119 | 79 | 84 | 84 |
| 0.2 | *** | 502 | 511 | 649 | 247 | 255 | 317 | 154 | 161 | 194 | 109 | 115 | 135 | 83 | 88 | 101 |
| | *** | 505 | 527 | 743 | 250 | 268 | 346 | 157 | 171 | 201 | 111 | 121 | 131 | 85 | 93 | 92 |
| 0.25 | *** | 548 | 560 | 755 | 264 | 276 | 360 | 163 | 173 | 217 | 114 | 122 | 148 | 87 | 93 | 109 |
| | *** | 552 | 583 | 833 | 269 | 294 | 382 | 167 | 185 | 219 | 117 | 130 | 141 | 89 | 98 | 98 |
| 0.3 | *** | 572 | 588 | 842 | 273 | 288 | 395 | 167 | 179 | 234 | 116 | 126 | 157 | 88 | 95 | 114 |
| | *** | 577 | 617 | 904 | 278 | 310 | 409 | 172 | 194 | 231 | 120 | 136 | 147 | 91 | 102 | 101 |
| 0.35 | *** | 574 | 595 | 908 | 273 | 292 | 420 | 167 | 182 | 245 | 116 | 127 | 163 | 87 | 95 | 117 |
| | *** | 581 | 633 | 954 | 280 | 319 | 426 | 172 | 199 | 239 | 121 | 138 | 151 | 91 | 103 | 102 |
| 0.4 | *** | 560 | 586 | 952 | 266 | 290 | 435 | 163 | 180 | 251 | 114 | 126 | 165 | 85 | 94 | 117 |
| | *** | 569 | 633 | 984 | 275 | 320 | 435 | 170 | 200 | 241 | 119 | 138 | 151 | 89 | 102 | 101 |
| 0.45 | *** | 531 | 565 | 974 | 255 | 282 | 440 | 157 | 176 | 251 | 109 | 123 | 163 | 82 | 91 | 115 |
| | *** | 543 | 620 | 994 | 265 | 316 | 435 | 164 | 197 | 239 | 115 | 136 | 147 | 86 | 100 | 98 |
| 0.5 | *** | 492 | 533 | 975 | 239 | 270 | 435 | 148 | 169 | 246 | 104 | 118 | 158 | 78 | 87 | 110 |
| | *** | 507 | 596 | 984 | 251 | 306 | 426 | 157 | 190 | 231 | 109 | 131 | 141 | 82 | 95 | 92 |
| 0.55 | *** | 447 | 495 | 953 | 221 | 254 | 421 | 138 | 159 | 235 | 97 | 111 | 150 | 72 | 81 | 103 |
| | *** | 464 | 565 | 954 | 234 | 292 | 409 | 147 | 181 | 219 | 102 | 123 | 131 | 76 | 89 | 84 |
| 0.6 | *** | 398 | 453 | 910 | 202 | 236 | 397 | 127 | 148 | 219 | 89 | 102 | 138 | 66 | 74 | 94 |
| | *** | 418 | 526 | 904 | 215 | 274 | 382 | 135 | 169 | 201 | 94 | 114 | 119 | 69 | 81 | 74 |
| 0.65 | *** | 349 | 408 | 845 | 181 | 214 | 363 | 114 | 134 | 197 | 79 | 91 | 122 | 58 | 66 | 82 |
| | *** | 371 | 483 | 833 | 194 | 251 | 346 | 122 | 153 | 179 | 84 | 102 | 102 | 61 | 72 | 62 |
| 0.7 | *** | 302 | 361 | 758 | 159 | 191 | 320 | 100 | 118 | 171 | 69 | 79 | 103 | . | . | . |
| | *** | 325 | 433 | 743 | 172 | 224 | 302 | 108 | 135 | 151 | 73 | 88 | 83 | . | . | . |
| 0.75 | *** | 255 | 312 | 650 | 136 | 164 | 267 | 84 | 99 | 138 | . | . | . | . | . | . |
| | *** | 278 | 378 | 633 | 147 | 192 | 248 | 91 | 112 | 118 | . | . | . | . | . | . |
| 0.8 | *** | 210 | 260 | 521 | 110 | 133 | 205 | . | . | . | . | . | . | . | . | . |
| | *** | 229 | 316 | 502 | 119 | 154 | 186 | . | . | . | . | . | . | . | . | . |
| 0.85 | *** | 162 | 201 | 372 | . | . | . | . | . | . | . | . | . | . | . | . |
| | *** | 177 | 242 | 352 | . | . | . | . | . | . | . | . | . | . | . | . |

## TABLE 3: ALPHA= 0.01 POWER= 0.8    EXPECTED ACCRUAL THRU MINIMUM FOLLOW-UP= 60

| | DEL=.10 | | | DEL=.15 | | | DEL=.20 | | | DEL=.25 | | | DEL=.30 | | |
|---|---|---|---|---|---|---|---|---|---|---|---|---|---|---|---|
| FACT= | 1.0 .75 | .50 .25 | .00 BIN | 1.0 .75 | .50 .25 | .00 BIN | 1.0 .75 | .50 .25 | .00 BIN | 1.0 75 | .50 .25 | .00 BIN | 1.0 .75 | .50 .25 | .00 BIN |
| PCONT=*** | | | | | REQUIRED NUMBER OF PATIENTS | | | | | | | | | | |
| 0.05 *** | 212 | 214 | 228 | 124 | 126 | 133 | 88 | 89 | 94 | 68 | 70 | 73 | 56 | 57 | 60 |
| *** | 212 | 217 | 352 | 124 | 128 | 186 | 88 | 91 | 118 | 69 | 71 | 83 | 57 | 58 | 62 |
| 0.1 *** | 334 | 339 | 382 | 178 | 182 | 203 | 118 | 121 | 133 | 88 | 90 | 98 | 70 | 72 | 77 |
| *** | 336 | 346 | 502 | 179 | 188 | 248 | 119 | 125 | 151 | 89 | 93 | 102 | 70 | 74 | 74 |
| 0.15 *** | 432 | 439 | 523 | 219 | 226 | 264 | 140 | 146 | 166 | 101 | 106 | 118 | 79 | 82 | 90 |
| *** | 434 | 451 | 633 | 222 | 235 | 302 | 142 | 152 | 179 | 103 | 110 | 119 | 80 | 85 | 84 |
| 0.2 *** | 504 | 514 | 649 | 248 | 258 | 317 | 155 | 164 | 194 | 110 | 117 | 135 | 85 | 89 | 101 |
| *** | 507 | 533 | 743 | 252 | 272 | 346 | 159 | 173 | 201 | 113 | 123 | 131 | 87 | 94 | 92 |
| 0.25 *** | 551 | 565 | 755 | 267 | 280 | 360 | 165 | 176 | 217 | 116 | 124 | 148 | 88 | 94 | 109 |
| *** | 556 | 591 | 833 | 272 | 299 | 382 | 169 | 188 | 219 | 119 | 132 | 141 | 91 | 100 | 98 |
| 0.3 *** | 575 | 594 | 842 | 276 | 293 | 395 | 170 | 183 | 234 | 119 | 129 | 157 | 90 | 97 | 114 |
| *** | 581 | 627 | 904 | 282 | 317 | 409 | 175 | 198 | 231 | 123 | 138 | 147 | 93 | 103 | 101 |
| 0.35 *** | 579 | 603 | 908 | 277 | 299 | 420 | 170 | 186 | 245 | 119 | 130 | 163 | 89 | 98 | 117 |
| *** | 587 | 646 | 954 | 285 | 326 | 426 | 176 | 203 | 239 | 124 | 141 | 151 | 93 | 105 | 102 |
| 0.4 *** | 565 | 597 | 952 | 271 | 297 | 435 | 167 | 185 | 251 | 117 | 129 | 165 | 88 | 96 | 117 |
| *** | 576 | 648 | 984 | 281 | 329 | 435 | 174 | 205 | 241 | 122 | 141 | 151 | 91 | 104 | 101 |
| 0.45 *** | 538 | 577 | 974 | 261 | 290 | 440 | 161 | 181 | 251 | 113 | 126 | 163 | 84 | 94 | 115 |
| *** | 552 | 637 | 994 | 272 | 325 | 435 | 169 | 202 | 239 | 118 | 139 | 147 | 88 | 102 | 98 |
| 0.5 *** | 501 | 548 | 975 | 246 | 279 | 435 | 154 | 175 | 246 | 107 | 121 | 158 | 80 | 89 | 110 |
| *** | 518 | 616 | 984 | 259 | 316 | 426 | 162 | 196 | 231 | 113 | 134 | 141 | 84 | 97 | 92 |
| 0.55 *** | 457 | 512 | 953 | 229 | 264 | 421 | 144 | 165 | 235 | 100 | 114 | 150 | 75 | 84 | 103 |
| *** | 477 | 586 | 954 | 243 | 302 | 409 | 152 | 186 | 219 | 106 | 126 | 131 | 78 | 91 | 84 |
| 0.6 *** | 411 | 471 | 910 | 210 | 245 | 397 | 132 | 153 | 219 | 92 | 105 | 138 | 68 | 76 | 94 |
| *** | 433 | 548 | 904 | 224 | 284 | 382 | 141 | 174 | 201 | 98 | 117 | 119 | 72 | 83 | 74 |
| 0.65 *** | 363 | 426 | 845 | 189 | 224 | 363 | 119 | 139 | 197 | 83 | 94 | 122 | 60 | 68 | 82 |
| *** | 387 | 504 | 833 | 203 | 260 | 346 | 128 | 158 | 179 | 88 | 104 | 102 | 63 | 73 | 62 |
| 0.7 *** | 316 | 379 | 758 | 167 | 199 | 320 | 105 | 122 | 171 | 72 | 82 | 103 | . | . | . |
| *** | 340 | 454 | 743 | 180 | 232 | 302 | 112 | 138 | 151 | 76 | 90 | 83 | . | . | . |
| 0.75 *** | 269 | 329 | 650 | 143 | 171 | 267 | 88 | 103 | 138 | . | . | . | . | . | . |
| *** | 293 | 397 | 633 | 154 | 199 | 248 | 94 | 115 | 118 | . | . | . | . | . | . |
| 0.8 *** | 222 | 274 | 521 | 116 | 139 | 205 | . | . | . | . | . | . | . | . | . |
| *** | 243 | 331 | 502 | 125 | 160 | 186 | . | . | . | . | . | . | . | . | . |
| 0.85 *** | 171 | 211 | 372 | . | . | . | . | . | . | . | . | . | . | . | . |
| *** | 188 | 253 | 352 | . | . | . | . | . | . | . | . | . | . | . | . |

# TABLE 3: ALPHA= 0.01 POWER= 0.8    EXPECTED ACCRUAL THRU MINIMUM FOLLOW-UP= 70

| | | DEL=.10 | | | DEL=.15 | | | DEL=.20 | | | DEL=.25 | | | DEL=.30 | | |
|---|---|---|---|---|---|---|---|---|---|---|---|---|---|---|---|---|
| FACT= | | 1.0 .75 | .50 .25 | .00 BIN | 1.0 .75 | .50 .25 | .00 BIN | 1.0 .75 | .50 .25 | .00 BIN | 1.0 75 | .50 .25 | .00 BIN | 1.0 .75 | .50 .25 | .00 BIN |
| PCONT=*** | | REQUIRED NUMBER OF PATIENTS | | | | | | | | | | | | | | |
| 0.05 | *** | 212 | 214 | 228 | 124 | 126 | 133 | 88 | 89 | 94 | 69 | 70 | 72 | 57 | 58 | 60 |
| | *** | 213 | 218 | 352 | 125 | 128 | 186 | 89 | 91 | 118 | 69 | 71 | 83 | 57 | 58 | 62 |
| 0.1 | *** | 335 | 340 | 382 | 179 | 183 | 203 | 119 | 122 | 133 | 88 | 91 | 97 | 70 | 72 | 77 |
| | *** | 337 | 348 | 502 | 180 | 189 | 248 | 120 | 126 | 151 | 89 | 93 | 102 | 71 | 74 | 74 |
| 0.15 | *** | 433 | 441 | 523 | 220 | 228 | 264 | 141 | 147 | 166 | 102 | 107 | 118 | 79 | 83 | 90 |
| | *** | 436 | 455 | 633 | 223 | 238 | 302 | 144 | 153 | 179 | 104 | 111 | 119 | 81 | 86 | 84 |
| 0.2 | *** | 506 | 517 | 649 | 250 | 261 | 317 | 157 | 166 | 194 | 112 | 118 | 135 | 86 | 90 | 101 |
| | *** | 510 | 538 | 743 | 254 | 275 | 346 | 160 | 175 | 201 | 114 | 124 | 131 | 88 | 94 | 92 |
| 0.25 | *** | 553 | 570 | 755 | 269 | 284 | 360 | 167 | 179 | 217 | 118 | 126 | 148 | 90 | 96 | 109 |
| | *** | 559 | 598 | 833 | 275 | 303 | 382 | 172 | 190 | 219 | 121 | 134 | 141 | 92 | 101 | 98 |
| 0.3 | *** | 578 | 600 | 842 | 279 | 298 | 395 | 172 | 186 | 234 | 121 | 131 | 157 | 91 | 98 | 114 |
| | *** | 585 | 637 | 904 | 286 | 322 | 409 | 178 | 201 | 231 | 125 | 140 | 147 | 94 | 104 | 101 |
| 0.35 | *** | 583 | 611 | 908 | 281 | 304 | 420 | 173 | 190 | 245 | 121 | 133 | 163 | 91 | 99 | 117 |
| | *** | 592 | 657 | 954 | 290 | 333 | 426 | 180 | 207 | 239 | 126 | 143 | 151 | 95 | 106 | 102 |
| 0.4 | *** | 571 | 606 | 952 | 276 | 304 | 435 | 171 | 190 | 251 | 119 | 132 | 165 | 90 | 98 | 117 |
| | *** | 583 | 662 | 984 | 287 | 336 | 435 | 179 | 208 | 241 | 125 | 143 | 151 | 93 | 105 | 101 |
| 0.45 | *** | 545 | 589 | 974 | 267 | 298 | 440 | 166 | 186 | 251 | 116 | 129 | 163 | 87 | 96 | 115 |
| | *** | 560 | 653 | 994 | 279 | 333 | 435 | 174 | 206 | 239 | 121 | 141 | 147 | 90 | 103 | 98 |
| 0.5 | *** | 509 | 561 | 975 | 253 | 287 | 435 | 158 | 179 | 246 | 110 | 124 | 158 | 82 | 91 | 110 |
| | *** | 528 | 633 | 984 | 266 | 325 | 426 | 167 | 200 | 231 | 116 | 136 | 141 | 86 | 99 | 92 |
| 0.55 | *** | 467 | 526 | 953 | 236 | 272 | 421 | 148 | 170 | 235 | 103 | 117 | 150 | 77 | 85 | 103 |
| | *** | 489 | 604 | 954 | 250 | 311 | 409 | 157 | 191 | 219 | 109 | 129 | 131 | 80 | 92 | 84 |
| 0.6 | *** | 422 | 487 | 910 | 217 | 254 | 397 | 137 | 158 | 219 | 95 | 108 | 138 | 70 | 78 | 94 |
| | *** | 446 | 567 | 904 | 232 | 292 | 382 | 146 | 178 | 201 | 101 | 119 | 119 | 73 | 84 | 74 |
| 0.65 | *** | 376 | 443 | 845 | 197 | 232 | 363 | 124 | 144 | 197 | 85 | 97 | 122 | 62 | 69 | 82 |
| | *** | 401 | 523 | 833 | 211 | 268 | 346 | 132 | 162 | 179 | 90 | 106 | 102 | 65 | 74 | 62 |
| 0.7 | *** | 329 | 395 | 758 | 174 | 207 | 320 | 109 | 126 | 171 | 74 | 83 | 103 | . | . | . |
| | *** | 355 | 471 | 743 | 187 | 239 | 302 | 116 | 142 | 151 | 78 | 91 | 83 | . | . | . |
| 0.75 | *** | 282 | 343 | 650 | 149 | 178 | 267 | 92 | 106 | 138 | . | . | . | . | . | . |
| | *** | 306 | 412 | 633 | 161 | 205 | 248 | 98 | 118 | 118 | . | . | . | . | . | . |
| 0.8 | *** | 233 | 286 | 521 | 121 | 143 | 205 | . | . | . | . | . | . | . | . | . |
| | *** | 254 | 344 | 502 | 130 | 164 | 186 | . | . | . | . | . | . | . | . | . |
| 0.85 | *** | 180 | 221 | 372 | . | . | . | . | . | . | . | . | . | . | . | . |
| | *** | 197 | 262 | 352 | . | . | . | . | . | . | . | . | . | . | . | . |

TABLE 3: ALPHA= 0.01  POWER= 0.8     EXPECTED ACCRUAL THRU MINIMUM FOLLOW-UP= 80

| | | DEL=.10 | | | DEL=.15 | | | DEL=.20 | | | DEL=.25 | | | DEL=.30 | | |
|---|---|---|---|---|---|---|---|---|---|---|---|---|---|---|---|---|
| FACT= | | 1.0 | .50 | .00 | 1.0 | .50 | .00 | 1.0 | .50 | .00 | 1.0 | .50 | .00 | 1.0 | .50 | .00 |
| | | .75 | .25 | BIN | .75 | .25 | BIN | .75 | .25 | BIN | 75 | .25 | BIN | .75 | .25 | BIN |
| PCONT=*** | | | | | REQUIRED NUMBER OF PATIENTS | | | | | | | | | | | |
| 0.05 | *** | 212 | 215 | 228 | 124 | 127 | 133 | 88 | 90 | 94 | 69 | 70 | 73 | 57 | 58 | 60 |
| | *** | 213 | 218 | 352 | 125 | 129 | 186 | 89 | 91 | 118 | 69 | 71 | 83 | 57 | 59 | 62 |
| 0.1 | *** | 336 | 341 | 382 | 180 | 184 | 203 | 119 | 123 | 133 | 89 | 91 | 98 | 70 | 73 | 77 |
| | *** | 338 | 350 | 502 | 181 | 190 | 248 | 121 | 127 | 151 | 90 | 94 | 102 | 71 | 74 | 74 |
| 0.15 | *** | 434 | 443 | 523 | 222 | 230 | 264 | 142 | 148 | 166 | 103 | 108 | 118 | 80 | 83 | 90 |
| | *** | 437 | 458 | 633 | 225 | 239 | 302 | 145 | 155 | 179 | 105 | 112 | 119 | 82 | 86 | 84 |
| 0.2 | *** | 507 | 521 | 649 | 252 | 264 | 317 | 159 | 168 | 194 | 113 | 119 | 135 | 87 | 91 | 101 |
| | *** | 512 | 543 | 743 | 256 | 278 | 346 | 162 | 176 | 201 | 116 | 125 | 131 | 89 | 95 | 92 |
| 0.25 | *** | 556 | 574 | 755 | 272 | 288 | 360 | 169 | 181 | 217 | 119 | 128 | 148 | 91 | 97 | 109 |
| | *** | 562 | 605 | 833 | 278 | 307 | 382 | 174 | 193 | 219 | 123 | 135 | 141 | 93 | 101 | 98 |
| 0.3 | *** | 581 | 606 | 842 | 282 | 303 | 395 | 175 | 189 | 234 | 123 | 133 | 157 | 93 | 100 | 114 |
| | *** | 590 | 646 | 904 | 290 | 327 | 409 | 181 | 204 | 231 | 127 | 142 | 147 | 96 | 105 | 101 |
| 0.35 | *** | 587 | 619 | 908 | 285 | 310 | 420 | 176 | 193 | 245 | 124 | 135 | 163 | 93 | 101 | 117 |
| | *** | 598 | 668 | 954 | 294 | 338 | 426 | 183 | 210 | 239 | 128 | 145 | 151 | 96 | 107 | 102 |
| 0.4 | *** | 576 | 616 | 952 | 281 | 310 | 435 | 174 | 193 | 251 | 122 | 134 | 165 | 91 | 100 | 117 |
| | *** | 590 | 675 | 984 | 292 | 343 | 435 | 182 | 212 | 241 | 127 | 145 | 151 | 95 | 107 | 101 |
| 0.45 | *** | 552 | 600 | 974 | 272 | 304 | 440 | 169 | 190 | 251 | 118 | 132 | 163 | 88 | 97 | 115 |
| | *** | 569 | 667 | 994 | 285 | 340 | 435 | 178 | 210 | 239 | 124 | 143 | 147 | 92 | 104 | 98 |
| 0.5 | *** | 518 | 574 | 975 | 259 | 294 | 435 | 162 | 184 | 246 | 113 | 127 | 158 | 84 | 93 | 110 |
| | *** | 538 | 649 | 984 | 273 | 332 | 426 | 171 | 204 | 231 | 119 | 138 | 141 | 88 | 100 | 92 |
| 0.55 | *** | 477 | 540 | 953 | 243 | 280 | 421 | 152 | 174 | 235 | 106 | 119 | 150 | 78 | 87 | 103 |
| | *** | 501 | 620 | 954 | 257 | 318 | 409 | 162 | 194 | 219 | 112 | 131 | 131 | 82 | 93 | 84 |
| 0.6 | *** | 433 | 501 | 910 | 224 | 261 | 397 | 141 | 162 | 219 | 98 | 110 | 138 | 72 | 79 | 94 |
| | *** | 459 | 584 | 904 | 239 | 299 | 382 | 150 | 181 | 201 | 103 | 121 | 119 | 75 | 85 | 74 |
| 0.65 | *** | 387 | 457 | 845 | 203 | 239 | 363 | 128 | 147 | 197 | 88 | 99 | 122 | 63 | 70 | 82 |
| | *** | 414 | 539 | 833 | 218 | 275 | 346 | 136 | 165 | 179 | 93 | 108 | 102 | 66 | 75 | 62 |
| 0.7 | *** | 340 | 409 | 758 | 180 | 213 | 320 | 112 | 129 | 171 | 76 | 85 | 103 | . | . | . |
| | *** | 367 | 487 | 743 | 194 | 245 | 302 | 120 | 144 | 151 | 80 | 92 | 83 | . | . | . |
| 0.75 | *** | 293 | 356 | 650 | 154 | 183 | 267 | 94 | 108 | 138 | . | . | . | . | . | . |
| | *** | 318 | 426 | 633 | 166 | 210 | 248 | 100 | 119 | 118 | . | . | . | . | . | . |
| 0.8 | *** | 243 | 297 | 521 | 125 | 148 | 205 | . | . | . | . | . | . | . | . | . |
| | *** | 265 | 355 | 502 | 135 | 167 | 186 | . | . | . | . | . | . | . | . | . |
| 0.85 | *** | 188 | 229 | 372 | . | . | . | . | . | . | . | . | . | . | . | . |
| | *** | 204 | 270 | 352 | . | . | . | . | . | . | . | . | . | . | . | . |

## TABLE 3: ALPHA= 0.01  POWER= 0.8     EXPECTED ACCRUAL THRU MINIMUM FOLLOW-UP= 90

| | | DEL=.10 | | | DEL=.15 | | | DEL=.20 | | | DEL=.25 | | | DEL=.30 | | |
|---|---|---|---|---|---|---|---|---|---|---|---|---|---|---|---|---|---|
| FACT= | | 1.0 .75 | .50 .25 | .00 BIN | 1.0 .75 | .50 .25 | .00 BIN | 1.0 .75 | .50 .25 | .00 BIN | 1.0 75 | .50 .25 | .00 BIN | 1.0 .75 | .50 .25 | .00 BIN |
| PCONT=*** | | | | | REQUIRED | NUMBER | OF PATIENTS | | | | | | | | | |
| 0.05 | *** | 213 | 215 | 228 | 125 | 127 | 133 | 88 | 90 | 94 | 69 | 70 | 73 | 57 | 58 | 60 |
| | *** | 214 | 219 | 352 | 126 | 129 | 186 | 89 | 91 | 118 | 70 | 71 | 83 | 57 | 59 | 62 |
| 0.1 | *** | 336 | 343 | 382 | 180 | 185 | 203 | 120 | 124 | 133 | 89 | 92 | 97 | 71 | 73 | 77 |
| | *** | 339 | 352 | 502 | 182 | 191 | 248 | 121 | 127 | 151 | 90 | 94 | 102 | 72 | 74 | 74 |
| 0.15 | *** | 435 | 445 | 523 | 223 | 231 | 264 | 143 | 150 | 166 | 104 | 108 | 118 | 81 | 84 | 90 |
| | *** | 439 | 461 | 633 | 226 | 241 | 302 | 146 | 155 | 179 | 106 | 112 | 119 | 82 | 87 | 84 |
| 0.2 | *** | 509 | 524 | 649 | 254 | 266 | 317 | 160 | 169 | 194 | 114 | 120 | 135 | 87 | 92 | 101 |
| | *** | 514 | 547 | 743 | 258 | 281 | 346 | 164 | 178 | 201 | 117 | 126 | 131 | 89 | 96 | 92 |
| 0.25 | *** | 558 | 578 | 755 | 274 | 291 | 360 | 171 | 183 | 217 | 121 | 129 | 148 | 92 | 98 | 109 |
| | *** | 565 | 611 | 833 | 280 | 310 | 382 | 176 | 194 | 219 | 124 | 136 | 141 | 94 | 102 | 98 |
| 0.3 | *** | 584 | 612 | 842 | 285 | 307 | 395 | 177 | 192 | 234 | 124 | 134 | 157 | 94 | 101 | 114 |
| | *** | 594 | 654 | 904 | 293 | 331 | 409 | 183 | 206 | 231 | 129 | 143 | 147 | 97 | 106 | 101 |
| 0.35 | *** | 591 | 626 | 908 | 289 | 314 | 420 | 179 | 196 | 245 | 125 | 137 | 163 | 94 | 102 | 117 |
| | *** | 603 | 678 | 954 | 299 | 343 | 426 | 186 | 213 | 239 | 130 | 146 | 151 | 98 | 108 | 102 |
| 0.4 | *** | 581 | 624 | 952 | 285 | 315 | 435 | 178 | 197 | 251 | 124 | 136 | 165 | 93 | 101 | 117 |
| | *** | 597 | 686 | 984 | 297 | 348 | 435 | 185 | 215 | 241 | 129 | 147 | 151 | 96 | 108 | 101 |
| 0.45 | *** | 558 | 610 | 974 | 277 | 310 | 440 | 173 | 194 | 251 | 121 | 134 | 163 | 90 | 99 | 115 |
| | *** | 577 | 680 | 994 | 290 | 346 | 435 | 181 | 213 | 239 | 126 | 145 | 147 | 94 | 105 | 98 |
| 0.5 | *** | 525 | 585 | 975 | 264 | 301 | 435 | 166 | 187 | 246 | 115 | 129 | 158 | 86 | 94 | 110 |
| | *** | 548 | 663 | 984 | 279 | 338 | 426 | 175 | 207 | 231 | 121 | 140 | 141 | 89 | 101 | 92 |
| 0.55 | *** | 486 | 553 | 953 | 249 | 286 | 421 | 156 | 178 | 235 | 108 | 122 | 150 | 80 | 88 | 103 |
| | *** | 511 | 635 | 954 | 264 | 325 | 409 | 165 | 197 | 219 | 114 | 132 | 131 | 84 | 94 | 84 |
| 0.6 | *** | 443 | 514 | 910 | 230 | 268 | 397 | 145 | 166 | 219 | 100 | 112 | 138 | 73 | 81 | 94 |
| | *** | 471 | 598 | 904 | 245 | 305 | 382 | 153 | 184 | 201 | 105 | 122 | 119 | 76 | 86 | 74 |
| 0.65 | *** | 398 | 470 | 845 | 209 | 245 | 363 | 131 | 150 | 198 | 90 | 101 | 122 | 65 | 71 | 82 |
| | *** | 426 | 553 | 833 | 224 | 281 | 346 | 139 | 167 | 179 | 94 | 109 | 102 | 67 | 75 | 62 |
| 0.7 | *** | 351 | 422 | 758 | 186 | 219 | 320 | 115 | 132 | 171 | 78 | 87 | 103 | . | . | . |
| | *** | 379 | 500 | 743 | 199 | 250 | 302 | 122 | 146 | 151 | 82 | 93 | 83 | . | . | . |
| 0.75 | *** | 303 | 368 | 650 | 159 | 188 | 267 | 97 | 110 | 138 | . | . | . | . | . | . |
| | *** | 329 | 438 | 633 | 171 | 214 | 248 | 103 | 121 | 118 | . | . | . | . | . | . |
| 0.8 | *** | 252 | 307 | 521 | 129 | 151 | 205 | . | . | . | . | . | . | . | . | . |
| | *** | 274 | 364 | 502 | 138 | 170 | 186 | . | . | . | . | . | . | . | . | . |
| 0.85 | *** | 194 | 236 | 372 | . | . | . | . | . | . | . | . | . | . | . | . |
| | *** | 211 | 276 | 352 | . | . | . | . | . | . | . | . | . | . | . | . |

TABLE 3: ALPHA= 0.01　POWER= 0.8　　EXPECTED ACCRUAL THRU MINIMUM FOLLOW-UP= 100

| | | DEL=.10 | | | DEL=.15 | | | DEL=.20 | | | DEL=.25 | | | DEL=.30 | | |
|---|---|---|---|---|---|---|---|---|---|---|---|---|---|---|---|---|
| FACT= | | 1.0 .75 | .50 .25 | .00 BIN | 1.0 .75 | .50 .25 | .00 BIN | 1.0 .75 | .50 .25 | .00 BIN | 1.0 75 | .50 .25 | .00 BIN | 1.0 .75 | .50 .25 | .00 BIN |
| PCONT=*** | | | | | REQUIRED NUMBER OF PATIENTS | | | | | | | | | | | |
| 0.05 | *** *** | 213 214 | 216 220 | 228 352 | 125 126 | 127 129 | 133 186 | 89 89 | 90 92 | 94 118 | 69 70 | 70 71 | 73 83 | 57 58 | 58 59 | 60 62 |
| 0.1 | *** *** | 337 340 | 344 353 | 382 502 | 181 183 | 186 192 | 203 248 | 120 122 | 124 128 | 133 151 | 90 91 | 92 94 | 98 102 | 71 72 | 73 75 | 77 74 |
| 0.15 | *** *** | 437 440 | 448 464 | 523 633 | 224 227 | 233 243 | 264 302 | 144 147 | 151 156 | 166 179 | 104 106 | 109 113 | 118 119 | 81 83 | 84 87 | 90 84 |
| 0.2 | *** *** | 511 516 | 527 552 | 649 743 | 255 260 | 268 283 | 317 346 | 161 165 | 171 179 | 194 201 | 115 118 | 121 127 | 135 131 | 88 90 | 93 96 | 101 92 |
| 0.25 | *** *** | 560 568 | 583 617 | 755 833 | 276 283 | 294 313 | 360 382 | 173 178 | 185 196 | 217 219 | 122 126 | 130 137 | 148 141 | 93 95 | 98 103 | 109 98 |
| 0.3 | *** *** | 588 598 | 617 661 | 842 904 | 288 297 | 310 335 | 395 409 | 179 185 | 194 208 | 234 231 | 126 130 | 136 144 | 157 147 | 95 98 | 102 107 | 114 101 |
| 0.35 | *** *** | 595 608 | 633 687 | 908 954 | 292 303 | 319 348 | 420 426 | 182 189 | 199 215 | 245 239 | 127 132 | 138 148 | 163 151 | 95 99 | 103 109 | 117 102 |
| 0.4 | *** *** | 586 603 | 633 696 | 952 984 | 290 302 | 320 353 | 435 435 | 180 188 | 200 217 | 251 241 | 126 131 | 138 148 | 165 151 | 94 98 | 102 108 | 117 101 |
| 0.45 | *** *** | 565 585 | 620 692 | 974 994 | 282 295 | 316 352 | 440 435 | 176 185 | 197 215 | 251 239 | 123 128 | 136 146 | 163 147 | 91 95 | 100 106 | 115 98 |
| 0.5 | *** *** | 533 557 | 596 675 | 975 984 | 270 284 | 306 344 | 435 426 | 169 178 | 190 210 | 246 231 | 118 123 | 131 141 | 158 141 | 87 91 | 95 102 | 110 92 |
| 0.55 | *** *** | 495 522 | 565 648 | 953 954 | 254 269 | 292 330 | 421 409 | 159 169 | 181 200 | 235 219 | 111 116 | 123 134 | 150 131 | 81 85 | 89 95 | 103 84 |
| 0.6 | *** *** | 453 481 | 526 612 | 910 904 | 236 251 | 274 311 | 397 382 | 148 157 | 169 187 | 219 201 | 102 107 | 114 123 | 138 119 | 74 78 | 81 87 | 94 74 |
| 0.65 | *** *** | 408 437 | 483 566 | 845 833 | 214 229 | 251 286 | 363 346 | 134 142 | 153 169 | 197 179 | 91 96 | 102 110 | 122 102 | 66 68 | 72 76 | 82 62 |
| 0.7 | *** *** | 361 390 | 433 512 | 758 743 | 191 204 | 224 255 | 320 302 | 118 125 | 135 148 | 171 151 | 79 83 | 88 94 | 103 83 | . . | . . | . . |
| 0.75 | *** *** | 312 339 | 378 448 | 650 633 | 164 176 | 192 218 | 267 248 | 99 105 | 112 122 | 138 118 | . . | . . | . . | . . | . . | . . |
| 0.8 | *** *** | 260 282 | 316 373 | 521 502 | 133 142 | 154 173 | 205 186 | . . | . . | . . | . . | . . | . . | . . | . . | . . |
| 0.85 | *** *** | 201 218 | 242 282 | 372 352 | . . | . . | . . | . . | . . | . . | . . | . . | . . | . . | . . | . . |

TABLE 3: ALPHA= 0.01  POWER= 0.8     EXPECTED ACCRUAL THRU MINIMUM FOLLOW-UP= 110

| | | DEL=.05 | | | DEL=.10 | | | DEL=.15 | | | DEL=.20 | | | DEL=.25 | | |
|---|---|---|---|---|---|---|---|---|---|---|---|---|---|---|---|---|---|
| FACT= | | 1.0 .75 | .50 .25 | .00 BIN | 1.0 .75 | .50 .25 | .00 BIN | 1.0 .75 | .50 .25 | .00 BIN | 1.0 75 | .50 .25 | .00 BIN | 1.0 .75 | .50 .25 | .00 BIN |
| PCONT=*** | | | | | REQUIRED NUMBER OF PATIENTS | | | | | | | | | | | |
| 0.05 | *** | 600 | 603 | 641 | 213 | 216 | 228 | 125 | 128 | 133 | 89 | 91 | 94 | 69 | 71 | 72 |
| | *** | 601 | 608 | 1104 | 214 | 220 | 352 | 126 | 130 | 186 | 90 | 92 | 118 | 70 | 71 | 83 |
| 0.1 | *** | 1094 | 1100 | 1237 | 338 | 345 | 382 | 182 | 187 | 203 | 121 | 125 | 133 | 90 | 93 | 98 |
| | *** | 1096 | 1113 | 1747 | 340 | 354 | 502 | 184 | 192 | 248 | 122 | 128 | 151 | 91 | 95 | 102 |
| 0.15 | *** | 1512 | 1523 | 1813 | 438 | 449 | 523 | 225 | 234 | 264 | 145 | 151 | 166 | 105 | 109 | 118 |
| | *** | 1516 | 1545 | 2309 | 442 | 467 | 633 | 229 | 244 | 302 | 148 | 157 | 179 | 107 | 113 | 119 |
| 0.2 | *** | 1836 | 1852 | 2339 | 512 | 530 | 649 | 257 | 270 | 317 | 163 | 172 | 194 | 116 | 122 | 135 |
| | *** | 1841 | 1884 | 2791 | 518 | 556 | 743 | 262 | 285 | 346 | 166 | 180 | 201 | 119 | 127 | 131 |
| 0.25 | *** | 2059 | 2082 | 2798 | 563 | 587 | 755 | 278 | 296 | 361 | 174 | 186 | 217 | 123 | 131 | 148 |
| | *** | 2067 | 2129 | 3192 | 571 | 622 | 833 | 285 | 316 | 382 | 179 | 197 | 219 | 127 | 138 | 141 |
| 0.3 | *** | 2187 | 2219 | 3182 | 591 | 622 | 842 | 291 | 314 | 395 | 181 | 196 | 234 | 127 | 137 | 157 |
| | *** | 2198 | 2281 | 3513 | 602 | 668 | 904 | 300 | 338 | 409 | 188 | 209 | 231 | 132 | 145 | 147 |
| 0.35 | *** | 2228 | 2269 | 3484 | 599 | 639 | 908 | 295 | 323 | 420 | 184 | 201 | 245 | 129 | 140 | 163 |
| | *** | 2242 | 2352 | 3754 | 614 | 695 | 954 | 306 | 351 | 426 | 191 | 217 | 239 | 133 | 149 | 151 |
| 0.4 | *** | 2192 | 2246 | 3702 | 592 | 641 | 952 | 293 | 325 | 435 | 183 | 202 | 251 | 128 | 140 | 165 |
| | *** | 2210 | 2352 | 3915 | 609 | 706 | 984 | 306 | 357 | 435 | 191 | 219 | 241 | 133 | 149 | 151 |
| 0.45 | *** | 2092 | 2161 | 3834 | 571 | 629 | 974 | 286 | 321 | 440 | 179 | 199 | 251 | 125 | 137 | 163 |
| | *** | 2115 | 2295 | 3995 | 592 | 703 | 994 | 300 | 356 | 435 | 187 | 218 | 239 | 130 | 147 | 147 |
| 0.5 | *** | 1941 | 2029 | 3879 | 541 | 606 | 975 | 274 | 312 | 435 | 172 | 193 | 246 | 119 | 132 | 158 |
| | *** | 1970 | 2193 | 3995 | 565 | 687 | 984 | 289 | 349 | 426 | 181 | 212 | 231 | 125 | 142 | 141 |
| 0.55 | *** | 1753 | 1864 | 3836 | 504 | 575 | 953 | 259 | 297 | 421 | 163 | 184 | 235 | 112 | 125 | 150 |
| | *** | 1791 | 2059 | 3915 | 531 | 660 | 954 | 275 | 335 | 409 | 172 | 202 | 219 | 118 | 135 | 131 |
| 0.6 | *** | 1544 | 1681 | 3705 | 462 | 538 | 910 | 241 | 279 | 397 | 151 | 171 | 219 | 104 | 115 | 138 |
| | *** | 1591 | 1903 | 3754 | 492 | 624 | 904 | 256 | 315 | 382 | 160 | 189 | 201 | 109 | 124 | 119 |
| 0.65 | *** | 1329 | 1491 | 3488 | 417 | 494 | 845 | 219 | 256 | 363 | 137 | 156 | 197 | 93 | 103 | 122 |
| | *** | 1387 | 1733 | 3513 | 448 | 578 | 833 | 234 | 290 | 346 | 145 | 171 | 179 | 98 | 111 | 102 |
| 0.7 | *** | 1121 | 1303 | 3185 | 370 | 444 | 758 | 195 | 228 | 320 | 120 | 137 | 171 | 80 | 89 | 103 |
| | *** | 1188 | 1552 | 3192 | 400 | 523 | 743 | 209 | 259 | 302 | 127 | 150 | 151 | 84 | 95 | 83 |
| 0.75 | *** | 930 | 1119 | 2796 | 321 | 388 | 650 | 168 | 196 | 267 | 101 | 114 | 138 | . | . | . |
| | *** | 1002 | 1361 | 2791 | 348 | 457 | 633 | 180 | 221 | 248 | 107 | 124 | 118 | . | . | . |
| 0.8 | *** | 756 | 936 | 2322 | 267 | 324 | 521 | 136 | 157 | 205 | . | . | . | . | . | . |
| | *** | 826 | 1157 | 2309 | 290 | 380 | 502 | 145 | 175 | 186 | . | . | . | . | . | . |
| 0.85 | *** | 593 | 748 | 1764 | 206 | 248 | 372 | . | . | . | . | . | . | . | . | . |
| | *** | 653 | 931 | 1747 | 224 | 287 | 352 | . | . | . | . | . | . | . | . | . |
| 0.9 | *** | 424 | 538 | 1124 | . | . | . | . | . | . | . | . | . | . | . | . |
| | *** | 469 | 665 | 1104 | . | . | . | . | . | . | . | . | . | . | . | . |

## TABLE 3: ALPHA= 0.01  POWER= 0.8     EXPECTED ACCRUAL THRU MINIMUM FOLLOW-UP= 120

| | | DEL=.05 | | | DEL=.10 | | | DEL=.15 | | | DEL=.20 | | | DEL=.25 | | |
|---|---|---|---|---|---|---|---|---|---|---|---|---|---|---|---|---|
| FACT= | | 1.0 .75 | .50 .25 | .00 BIN | 1.0 .75 | .50 .25 | .00 BIN | 1.0 .75 | .50 .25 | .00 BIN | 1.0 75 | .50 .25 | .00 BIN | 1.0 .75 | .50 .25 | .00 BIN |
| PCONT=*** | | | | | REQUIRED NUMBER OF PATIENTS | | | | | | | | | | | |
| 0.05 | *** | 600 | 603 | 641 | 214 | 217 | 228 | 126 | 128 | 133 | 89 | 91 | 94 | 70 | 71 | 73 |
| | *** | 601 | 609 | 1104 | 215 | 220 | 352 | 127 | 130 | 186 | 90 | 92 | 118 | 70 | 71 | 83 |
| 0.1 | *** | 1094 | 1101 | 1237 | 339 | 346 | 382 | 182 | 188 | 203 | 121 | 125 | 133 | 90 | 93 | 97 |
| | *** | 1096 | 1115 | 1747 | 341 | 356 | 502 | 184 | 193 | 248 | 123 | 128 | 151 | 91 | 95 | 102 |
| 0.15 | *** | 1513 | 1525 | 1813 | 439 | 451 | 523 | 226 | 235 | 264 | 146 | 152 | 166 | 106 | 110 | 118 |
| | *** | 1517 | 1549 | 2309 | 443 | 469 | 633 | 230 | 245 | 302 | 148 | 158 | 179 | 108 | 113 | 119 |
| 0.2 | *** | 1837 | 1855 | 2339 | 514 | 533 | 649 | 258 | 272 | 317 | 164 | 173 | 194 | 117 | 123 | 135 |
| | *** | 1843 | 1890 | 2791 | 521 | 559 | 743 | 264 | 286 | 346 | 168 | 181 | 201 | 119 | 128 | 131 |
| 0.25 | *** | 2061 | 2087 | 2798 | 565 | 591 | 755 | 280 | 299 | 360 | 176 | 188 | 217 | 124 | 132 | 148 |
| | *** | 2070 | 2137 | 3192 | 574 | 627 | 833 | 288 | 318 | 382 | 181 | 198 | 219 | 128 | 138 | 141 |
| 0.3 | *** | 2190 | 2224 | 3182 | 594 | 627 | 842 | 293 | 317 | 395 | 183 | 198 | 234 | 129 | 138 | 157 |
| | *** | 2202 | 2292 | 3513 | 606 | 674 | 904 | 303 | 341 | 409 | 189 | 211 | 231 | 133 | 146 | 147 |
| 0.35 | *** | 2232 | 2277 | 3484 | 603 | 646 | 908 | 299 | 326 | 420 | 186 | 203 | 245 | 130 | 141 | 163 |
| | *** | 2247 | 2366 | 3754 | 619 | 703 | 954 | 310 | 355 | 426 | 193 | 218 | 239 | 135 | 150 | 151 |
| 0.4 | *** | 2197 | 2256 | 3702 | 597 | 648 | 952 | 297 | 329 | 435 | 185 | 205 | 251 | 129 | 141 | 165 |
| | *** | 2216 | 2370 | 3915 | 616 | 715 | 984 | 310 | 361 | 435 | 193 | 221 | 241 | 134 | 150 | 151 |
| 0.45 | *** | 2098 | 2174 | 3834 | 577 | 637 | 974 | 290 | 325 | 440 | 181 | 202 | 251 | 126 | 139 | 163 |
| | *** | 2123 | 2317 | 3995 | 600 | 713 | 994 | 304 | 360 | 435 | 190 | 220 | 239 | 132 | 148 | 147 |
| 0.5 | *** | 1949 | 2045 | 3879 | 548 | 616 | 975 | 279 | 316 | 435 | 175 | 196 | 246 | 121 | 134 | 158 |
| | *** | 1981 | 2220 | 3995 | 574 | 697 | 984 | 294 | 353 | 426 | 184 | 214 | 231 | 127 | 143 | 141 |
| 0.55 | *** | 1763 | 1884 | 3836 | 511 | 586 | 953 | 264 | 302 | 421 | 165 | 186 | 235 | 114 | 126 | 150 |
| | *** | 1804 | 2090 | 3915 | 540 | 671 | 954 | 280 | 339 | 409 | 174 | 204 | 219 | 119 | 136 | 131 |
| 0.6 | *** | 1557 | 1704 | 3705 | 471 | 548 | 910 | 245 | 284 | 397 | 153 | 174 | 219 | 105 | 117 | 138 |
| | *** | 1608 | 1937 | 3754 | 501 | 635 | 904 | 261 | 320 | 382 | 162 | 191 | 201 | 110 | 125 | 119 |
| 0.65 | *** | 1345 | 1517 | 3488 | 426 | 504 | 845 | 224 | 260 | 363 | 139 | 158 | 197 | 94 | 104 | 122 |
| | *** | 1407 | 1768 | 3513 | 457 | 589 | 833 | 239 | 294 | 346 | 147 | 173 | 179 | 99 | 112 | 102 |
| 0.7 | *** | 1140 | 1331 | 3185 | 379 | 454 | 758 | 199 | 232 | 320 | 122 | 138 | 171 | 82 | 90 | 103 |
| | *** | 1211 | 1588 | 3192 | 409 | 532 | 743 | 213 | 262 | 302 | 129 | 151 | 151 | 85 | 95 | 83 |
| 0.75 | *** | 951 | 1146 | 2796 | 329 | 397 | 650 | 171 | 199 | 267 | 103 | 115 | 138 | . | . | . |
| | *** | 1025 | 1395 | 2791 | 356 | 466 | 633 | 183 | 223 | 248 | 108 | 124 | 118 | . | . | . |
| 0.8 | *** | 776 | 962 | 2322 | 274 | 331 | 521 | 139 | 160 | 205 | . | . | . | . | . | . |
| | *** | 848 | 1187 | 2309 | 297 | 387 | 502 | 148 | 177 | 186 | . | . | . | . | . | . |
| 0.85 | *** | 610 | 770 | 1764 | 211 | 253 | 372 | . | . | . | . | . | . | . | . | . |
| | *** | 673 | 956 | 1747 | 229 | 291 | 352 | . | . | . | . | . | . | . | . | . |
| 0.9 | *** | 438 | 554 | 1124 | . | . | . | . | . | . | . | . | . | . | . | . |
| | *** | 484 | 681 | 1104 | . | . | . | . | . | . | . | . | . | . | . | . |

## TABLE 3: ALPHA= 0.01  POWER= 0.8    EXPECTED ACCRUAL THRU MINIMUM FOLLOW-UP= 130

| | | DEL=.05 | | | DEL=.10 | | | DEL=.15 | | | DEL=.20 | | | DEL=.25 | | |
|---|---|---|---|---|---|---|---|---|---|---|---|---|---|---|---|---|---|
| FACT= | | 1.0<br>.75 | .50<br>.25 | .00<br>BIN | 1.0<br>.75 | .50<br>.25 | .00<br>BIN | 1.0<br>.75 | .50<br>.25 | .00<br>BIN | 1.0<br>75 | .50<br>.25 | .00<br>BIN | 1.0<br>.75 | .50<br>.25 | .00<br>BIN |
| PCONT=*** | | REQUIRED NUMBER OF PATIENTS | | | | | | | | | | | | | | |
| 0.05 | *** | 600 | 604 | 641 | 214 | 217 | 228 | 126 | 128 | 133 | 89 | 91 | 94 | 70 | 71 | 73 |
| | *** | 602 | 610 | 1104 | 215 | 221 | 352 | 127 | 130 | 186 | 90 | 92 | 118 | 70 | 72 | 83 |
| 0.1 | *** | 1095 | 1102 | 1237 | 339 | 347 | 382 | 183 | 188 | 203 | 122 | 126 | 133 | 91 | 93 | 98 |
| | *** | 1097 | 1117 | 1747 | 342 | 357 | 502 | 185 | 193 | 248 | 123 | 128 | 151 | 92 | 95 | 102 |
| 0.15 | *** | 1514 | 1527 | 1813 | 440 | 453 | 523 | 227 | 236 | 264 | 147 | 153 | 166 | 106 | 110 | 118 |
| | *** | 1519 | 1552 | 2309 | 445 | 471 | 633 | 231 | 246 | 302 | 149 | 158 | 179 | 108 | 114 | 119 |
| 0.2 | *** | 1839 | 1858 | 2339 | 516 | 535 | 649 | 260 | 274 | 317 | 165 | 174 | 194 | 118 | 124 | 135 |
| | *** | 1845 | 1896 | 2791 | 523 | 563 | 743 | 265 | 288 | 346 | 169 | 182 | 201 | 120 | 128 | 131 |
| 0.25 | *** | 2064 | 2091 | 2798 | 567 | 594 | 755 | 282 | 301 | 360 | 177 | 189 | 217 | 125 | 133 | 148 |
| | *** | 2073 | 2145 | 3192 | 577 | 632 | 833 | 290 | 320 | 382 | 182 | 200 | 219 | 129 | 139 | 141 |
| 0.3 | *** | 2193 | 2230 | 3182 | 597 | 632 | 842 | 296 | 320 | 395 | 185 | 200 | 234 | 130 | 139 | 157 |
| | *** | 2205 | 2303 | 3513 | 610 | 680 | 904 | 305 | 343 | 409 | 191 | 212 | 231 | 134 | 146 | 147 |
| 0.35 | *** | 2235 | 2285 | 3484 | 607 | 652 | 908 | 302 | 330 | 420 | 188 | 205 | 245 | 132 | 142 | 163 |
| | *** | 2252 | 2381 | 3754 | 623 | 710 | 954 | 313 | 358 | 426 | 195 | 220 | 239 | 136 | 150 | 151 |
| 0.4 | *** | 2202 | 2266 | 3702 | 601 | 655 | 952 | 301 | 333 | 435 | 188 | 207 | 251 | 131 | 142 | 165 |
| | *** | 2223 | 2389 | 3705 | 621 | 723 | 984 | 314 | 365 | 435 | 196 | 223 | 241 | 136 | 151 | 151 |
| 0.45 | *** | 2104 | 2186 | 3834 | 583 | 646 | 974 | 294 | 330 | 440 | 184 | 204 | 251 | 128 | 140 | 163 |
| | *** | 2132 | 2339 | 3995 | 607 | 722 | 994 | 309 | 364 | 435 | 192 | 221 | 239 | 133 | 149 | 147 |
| 0.5 | *** | 1957 | 2060 | 3879 | 555 | 625 | 975 | 283 | 321 | 435 | 177 | 198 | 246 | 123 | 135 | 158 |
| | *** | 1992 | 2246 | 3995 | 582 | 707 | 984 | 298 | 357 | 426 | 186 | 216 | 231 | 128 | 144 | 141 |
| 0.55 | *** | 1773 | 1903 | 3836 | 519 | 595 | 953 | 268 | 307 | 421 | 168 | 189 | 235 | 116 | 128 | 150 |
| | *** | 1818 | 2119 | 3915 | 549 | 681 | 954 | 284 | 343 | 409 | 177 | 206 | 219 | 121 | 137 | 131 |
| 0.6 | *** | 1570 | 1727 | 3705 | 479 | 558 | 910 | 250 | 288 | 397 | 156 | 176 | 219 | 107 | 118 | 138 |
| | *** | 1625 | 1969 | 3754 | 510 | 645 | 904 | 266 | 323 | 382 | 165 | 192 | 201 | 112 | 126 | 119 |
| 0.65 | *** | 1361 | 1543 | 3488 | 435 | 514 | 845 | 228 | 265 | 363 | 141 | 160 | 197 | 96 | 105 | 122 |
| | *** | 1426 | 1802 | 3513 | 466 | 598 | 833 | 243 | 297 | 346 | 149 | 174 | 179 | 100 | 112 | 102 |
| 0.7 | *** | 1159 | 1357 | 3185 | 387 | 463 | 758 | 203 | 236 | 320 | 124 | 140 | 171 | 83 | 90 | 103 |
| | *** | 1233 | 1621 | 3192 | 418 | 541 | 743 | 217 | 265 | 302 | 131 | 152 | 151 | 86 | 96 | 83 |
| 0.75 | *** | 970 | 1173 | 2796 | 336 | 405 | 650 | 175 | 202 | 267 | 104 | 116 | 138 | . | . | . |
| | *** | 1047 | 1427 | 2791 | 364 | 474 | 633 | 186 | 226 | 248 | 110 | 125 | 118 | . | . | . |
| 0.8 | *** | 796 | 986 | 2322 | 280 | 338 | 521 | 141 | 162 | 205 | . | . | . | . | . | . |
| | *** | 869 | 1215 | 2309 | 304 | 393 | 502 | 150 | 178 | 186 | . | . | . | . | . | . |
| 0.85 | *** | 627 | 790 | 1764 | 216 | 258 | 372 | . | . | . | . | . | . | . | . | . |
| | *** | 691 | 978 | 1747 | 234 | 295 | 352 | . | . | . | . | . | . | . | . | . |
| 0.9 | *** | 450 | 568 | 1124 | . | . | . | . | . | . | . | . | . | . | . | . |
| | *** | 497 | 696 | 1104 | . | . | . | . | . | . | . | . | . | . | . | . |

## TABLE 3: ALPHA= 0.01　POWER= 0.8　EXPECTED ACCRUAL THRU MINIMUM FOLLOW-UP= 140

REQUIRED NUMBER OF PATIENTS

| PCONT | FACT= | DEL=.05 1.0/.75 | .50/.25 | .00/BIN | DEL=.10 1.0/.75 | .50/.25 | .00/BIN | DEL=.15 1.0/.75 | .50/.25 | .00/BIN | DEL=.20 1.0/75 | .50/.25 | .00/BIN | DEL=.25 1.0/.75 | .50/.25 | .00/BIN |
|---|---|---|---|---|---|---|---|---|---|---|---|---|---|---|---|---|
| 0.05 | *** | 601 | 604 | 641 | 214 | 218 | 228 | 126 | 128 | 133 | 90 | 91 | 94 | 70 | 71 | 72 |
|  | *** | 602 | 611 | 1104 | 216 | 221 | 352 | 127 | 130 | 186 | 90 | 92 | 118 | 70 | 72 | 83 |
| 0.1 | *** | 1095 | 1103 | 1237 | 340 | 348 | 382 | 183 | 189 | 203 | 122 | 126 | 133 | 91 | 93 | 97 |
|  | *** | 1098 | 1119 | 1747 | 343 | 358 | 502 | 186 | 194 | 248 | 124 | 129 | 151 | 92 | 95 | 102 |
| 0.15 | *** | 1515 | 1529 | 1813 | 441 | 455 | 523 | 228 | 238 | 264 | 147 | 153 | 166 | 107 | 111 | 118 |
|  | *** | 1520 | 1556 | 2309 | 446 | 473 | 633 | 232 | 247 | 302 | 150 | 159 | 179 | 109 | 114 | 119 |
| 0.2 | *** | 1840 | 1861 | 2339 | 517 | 538 | 649 | 261 | 275 | 317 | 166 | 175 | 194 | 118 | 124 | 135 |
|  | *** | 1847 | 1902 | 2791 | 525 | 566 | 743 | 267 | 289 | 346 | 170 | 182 | 201 | 121 | 128 | 131 |
| 0.25 | *** | 2066 | 2095 | 2798 | 570 | 598 | 755 | 284 | 303 | 361 | 179 | 190 | 217 | 126 | 134 | 148 |
|  | *** | 2075 | 2153 | 3192 | 580 | 636 | 833 | 292 | 322 | 382 | 184 | 200 | 219 | 130 | 139 | 141 |
| 0.3 | *** | 2196 | 2236 | 3182 | 600 | 637 | 842 | 298 | 322 | 395 | 186 | 201 | 234 | 131 | 140 | 157 |
|  | *** | 2209 | 2314 | 3513 | 613 | 686 | 904 | 308 | 346 | 409 | 193 | 213 | 231 | 135 | 147 | 147 |
| 0.35 | *** | 2239 | 2292 | 3484 | 611 | 657 | 908 | 304 | 333 | 420 | 190 | 207 | 245 | 133 | 143 | 163 |
|  | *** | 2257 | 2395 | 3754 | 628 | 717 | 954 | 316 | 361 | 426 | 197 | 221 | 239 | 137 | 151 | 151 |
| 0.4 | *** | 2207 | 2275 | 3702 | 606 | 662 | 952 | 304 | 336 | 435 | 190 | 209 | 251 | 132 | 144 | 165 |
|  | *** | 2230 | 2406 | 3915 | 627 | 731 | 984 | 317 | 368 | 435 | 198 | 224 | 241 | 137 | 152 | 151 |
| 0.45 | *** | 2111 | 2199 | 3834 | 589 | 653 | 974 | 298 | 333 | 440 | 186 | 206 | 251 | 129 | 141 | 163 |
|  | *** | 2140 | 2361 | 3995 | 613 | 730 | 994 | 312 | 368 | 435 | 195 | 223 | 239 | 134 | 150 | 147 |
| 0.5 | *** | 1965 | 2076 | 3879 | 561 | 633 | 975 | 287 | 325 | 435 | 179 | 200 | 246 | 124 | 136 | 158 |
|  | *** | 2002 | 2271 | 3995 | 589 | 716 | 984 | 302 | 361 | 426 | 188 | 217 | 231 | 129 | 145 | 141 |
| 0.55 | *** | 1784 | 1922 | 3836 | 526 | 604 | 953 | 272 | 311 | 421 | 170 | 191 | 235 | 117 | 129 | 150 |
|  | *** | 1831 | 2148 | 3915 | 557 | 691 | 954 | 288 | 347 | 409 | 179 | 208 | 219 | 122 | 137 | 131 |
| 0.6 | *** | 1583 | 1748 | 3705 | 487 | 567 | 910 | 254 | 292 | 397 | 158 | 178 | 219 | 108 | 119 | 138 |
|  | *** | 1641 | 2000 | 3754 | 518 | 654 | 904 | 270 | 327 | 382 | 167 | 194 | 201 | 113 | 127 | 119 |
| 0.65 | *** | 1376 | 1567 | 3488 | 442 | 523 | 845 | 232 | 268 | 363 | 144 | 162 | 197 | 97 | 106 | 122 |
|  | *** | 1446 | 1833 | 3513 | 475 | 607 | 833 | 247 | 301 | 346 | 151 | 176 | 179 | 101 | 113 | 102 |
| 0.7 | *** | 1176 | 1382 | 3185 | 395 | 471 | 758 | 207 | 239 | 320 | 126 | 142 | 171 | 83 | 91 | 103 |
|  | *** | 1254 | 1652 | 3192 | 426 | 550 | 743 | 221 | 268 | 302 | 133 | 153 | 151 | 87 | 96 | 83 |
| 0.75 | *** | 989 | 1197 | 2796 | 343 | 412 | 650 | 178 | 205 | 267 | 106 | 118 | 138 | . | . | . |
|  | *** | 1069 | 1456 | 2791 | 371 | 481 | 633 | 189 | 228 | 248 | 111 | 126 | 118 | . | . | . |
| 0.8 | *** | 814 | 1009 | 2322 | 286 | 344 | 521 | 143 | 164 | 205 | . | . | . | . | . | . |
|  | *** | 890 | 1242 | 2309 | 310 | 398 | 502 | 152 | 180 | 186 | . | . | . | . | . | . |
| 0.85 | *** | 643 | 809 | 1764 | 221 | 262 | 372 | . | . | . | . | . | . | . | . | . |
|  | *** | 709 | 999 | 1747 | 238 | 299 | 352 | . | . | . | . | . | . | . | . | . |
| 0.9 | *** | 462 | 581 | 1124 | . | . | . | . | . | . | . | . | . | . | . | . |
|  | *** | 510 | 710 | 1104 | . | . | . | . | . | . | . | . | . | . | . | . |

## TABLE 3: ALPHA= 0.01  POWER= 0.8     EXPECTED ACCRUAL THRU MINIMUM FOLLOW-UP= 150

|  |  | DEL=.05 | | | DEL=.10 | | | DEL=.15 | | | DEL=.20 | | | DEL=.25 | | |
|---|---|---|---|---|---|---|---|---|---|---|---|---|---|---|---|---|
| FACT= | | 1.0 | .50 | .00 | 1.0 | .50 | .00 | 1.0 | .50 | .00 | 1.0 | .50 | .00 | 1.0 | .50 | .00 |
| | | .75 | .25 | BIN | .75 | .25 | BIN | .75 | .25 | BIN | 75 | .25 | BIN | .75 | .25 | BIN |

PCONT=*** | REQUIRED NUMBER OF PATIENTS

| PCONT | | .05a | .05b | .05c | .10a | .10b | .10c | .15a | .15b | .15c | .20a | .20b | .20c | .25a | .25b | .25c |
|---|---|---|---|---|---|---|---|---|---|---|---|---|---|---|---|---|
| 0.05 | *** | 601 | 605 | 641 | 215 | 218 | 228 | 126 | 129 | 133 | 90 | 91 | 94 | 70 | 71 | 73 |
| | *** | 602 | 612 | 1104 | 216 | 221 | 352 | 127 | 130 | 186 | 90 | 92 | 118 | 70 | 72 | 83 |
| 0.1 | *** | 1096 | 1105 | 1237 | 341 | 349 | 382 | 184 | 189 | 203 | 123 | 126 | 133 | 91 | 94 | 97 |
| | *** | 1099 | 1121 | 1747 | 344 | 359 | 502 | 186 | 194 | 248 | 124 | 129 | 151 | 92 | 95 | 102 |
| 0.15 | *** | 1516 | 1531 | 1813 | 442 | 457 | 523 | 229 | 239 | 264 | 148 | 154 | 166 | 107 | 111 | 118 |
| | *** | 1521 | 1560 | 2309 | 448 | 475 | 633 | 233 | 248 | 302 | 151 | 159 | 179 | 109 | 114 | 119 |
| 0.2 | *** | 1842 | 1864 | 2339 | 519 | 541 | 649 | 263 | 277 | 317 | 167 | 176 | 194 | 119 | 125 | 135 |
| | *** | 1849 | 1908 | 2791 | 527 | 568 | 743 | 268 | 291 | 346 | 170 | 183 | 201 | 121 | 129 | 131 |
| 0.25 | *** | 2068 | 2099 | 2798 | 572 | 601 | 755 | 286 | 305 | 360 | 180 | 192 | 217 | 127 | 134 | 148 |
| | *** | 2078 | 2161 | 3192 | 583 | 640 | 833 | 294 | 324 | 382 | 185 | 201 | 219 | 130 | 140 | 141 |
| 0.3 | *** | 2199 | 2242 | 3182 | 603 | 641 | 842 | 301 | 325 | 395 | 188 | 202 | 234 | 132 | 141 | 157 |
| | *** | 2213 | 2325 | 3513 | 617 | 691 | 904 | 310 | 348 | 409 | 194 | 214 | 231 | 136 | 147 | 147 |
| 0.35 | *** | 2243 | 2300 | 3484 | 615 | 663 | 908 | 307 | 336 | 420 | 192 | 208 | 245 | 134 | 144 | 163 |
| | *** | 2262 | 2409 | 3754 | 633 | 723 | 954 | 319 | 363 | 426 | 199 | 222 | 239 | 138 | 152 | 151 |
| 0.4 | *** | 2212 | 2285 | 3702 | 611 | 668 | 952 | 307 | 340 | 435 | 192 | 210 | 251 | 133 | 144 | 165 |
| | *** | 2236 | 2424 | 3915 | 633 | 738 | 984 | 320 | 371 | 435 | 200 | 226 | 241 | 138 | 153 | 151 |
| 0.45 | *** | 2117 | 2211 | 3834 | 594 | 660 | 974 | 301 | 337 | 440 | 188 | 208 | 251 | 130 | 142 | 163 |
| | *** | 2148 | 2382 | 3995 | 620 | 738 | 994 | 316 | 371 | 435 | 197 | 224 | 239 | 136 | 151 | 147 |
| 0.5 | *** | 1973 | 2091 | 3879 | 568 | 641 | 975 | 291 | 329 | 435 | 182 | 202 | 246 | 125 | 137 | 158 |
| | *** | 2013 | 2295 | 3995 | 596 | 725 | 984 | 306 | 364 | 426 | 190 | 219 | 231 | 131 | 146 | 141 |
| 0.55 | *** | 1794 | 1940 | 3836 | 533 | 612 | 953 | 276 | 315 | 421 | 172 | 193 | 235 | 118 | 130 | 150 |
| | *** | 1844 | 2175 | 3915 | 565 | 699 | 954 | 292 | 350 | 409 | 181 | 209 | 219 | 123 | 138 | 131 |
| 0.6 | *** | 1595 | 1770 | 3705 | 494 | 575 | 910 | 257 | 296 | 397 | 160 | 180 | 219 | 109 | 120 | 138 |
| | *** | 1657 | 2029 | 3754 | 526 | 663 | 904 | 274 | 330 | 382 | 169 | 195 | 201 | 114 | 127 | 119 |
| 0.65 | *** | 1392 | 1590 | 3488 | 450 | 531 | 845 | 236 | 272 | 363 | 145 | 163 | 197 | 98 | 107 | 122 |
| | *** | 1464 | 1864 | 3513 | 483 | 615 | 833 | 251 | 303 | 346 | 153 | 177 | 179 | 102 | 113 | 102 |
| 0.7 | *** | 1194 | 1407 | 3185 | 402 | 479 | 758 | 210 | 243 | 320 | 128 | 143 | 170 | 84 | 92 | 103 |
| | *** | 1274 | 1682 | 3192 | 433 | 557 | 743 | 224 | 270 | 302 | 134 | 154 | 151 | 88 | 97 | 83 |
| 0.75 | *** | 1007 | 1221 | 2795 | 350 | 419 | 650 | 180 | 208 | 267 | 107 | 119 | 138 | . | . | . |
| | *** | 1089 | 1484 | 2791 | 378 | 487 | 633 | 192 | 230 | 248 | 112 | 127 | 118 | . | . | . |
| 0.8 | *** | 831 | 1031 | 2322 | 292 | 349 | 521 | 146 | 166 | 205 | . | . | . | . | . | . |
| | *** | 909 | 1266 | 2309 | 316 | 403 | 502 | 154 | 181 | 186 | . | . | . | . | . | . |
| 0.85 | *** | 658 | 827 | 1764 | 225 | 266 | 372 | . | . | . | . | . | . | . | . | . |
| | *** | 725 | 1019 | 1747 | 242 | 302 | 352 | . | . | . | . | . | . | . | . | . |
| 0.9 | *** | 473 | 594 | 1124 | . | . | . | . | . | . | . | . | . | . | . | . |
| | *** | 521 | 723 | 1104 | . | . | . | . | . | . | . | . | . | . | . | . |

TABLE 3: ALPHA= 0.01 POWER= 0.8     EXPECTED ACCRUAL THRU MINIMUM FOLLOW-UP= 160

| | | DEL=.05 | | | DEL=.10 | | | DEL=.15 | | | DEL=.20 | | | DEL=.25 | |
|---|---|---|---|---|---|---|---|---|---|---|---|---|---|---|---|
| FACT= | 1.0 .75 | .50 .25 | .00 BIN | 1.0 .75 | .50 .25 | .00 BIN | 1.0 .75 | .50 .25 | .00 BIN | 1.0 75 | .50 .25 | .00 BIN | 1.0 .75 | .50 .25 | .00 BIN |
| PCONT=*** | | | | | REQUIRED | NUMBER | OF | PATIENTS | | | | | | | |
| 0.05 *** | 601 | 605 | 641 | 215 | 218 | 228 | 127 | 129 | 133 | 90 | 91 | 94 | 70 | 71 | 73 |
| *** | 603 | 613 | 1104 | 216 | 222 | 352 | 128 | 130 | 186 | 90 | 92 | 118 | 71 | 72 | 83 |
| 0.1 *** | 1096 | 1106 | 1237 | 341 | 350 | 382 | 184 | 190 | 203 | 123 | 127 | 133 | 91 | 94 | 98 |
| *** | 1100 | 1123 | 1747 | 345 | 360 | 502 | 187 | 195 | 248 | 125 | 129 | 151 | 93 | 95 | 102 |
| 0.15 *** | 1517 | 1533 | 1813 | 443 | 458 | 523 | 230 | 239 | 264 | 148 | 155 | 166 | 108 | 112 | 118 |
| *** | 1523 | 1564 | 2309 | 449 | 477 | 633 | 234 | 248 | 302 | 151 | 159 | 179 | 109 | 114 | 119 |
| 0.2 *** | 1843 | 1867 | 2339 | 521 | 543 | 649 | 264 | 278 | 317 | 168 | 176 | 194 | 119 | 125 | 135 |
| *** | 1851 | 1913 | 2791 | 529 | 571 | 743 | 270 | 292 | 346 | 171 | 183 | 201 | 122 | 129 | 131 |
| 0.25 *** | 2070 | 2103 | 2798 | 574 | 605 | 755 | 288 | 307 | 360 | 181 | 193 | 217 | 128 | 135 | 148 |
| *** | 2081 | 2169 | 3192 | 585 | 644 | 833 | 296 | 325 | 382 | 186 | 202 | 219 | 131 | 140 | 141 |
| 0.3 *** | 2202 | 2247 | 3182 | 606 | 646 | 842 | 303 | 327 | 395 | 189 | 204 | 234 | 133 | 142 | 157 |
| *** | 2217 | 2336 | 3513 | 621 | 695 | 904 | 313 | 350 | 409 | 195 | 215 | 231 | 137 | 148 | 147 |
| 0.35 *** | 2247 | 2307 | 3484 | 619 | 668 | 908 | 310 | 338 | 420 | 193 | 210 | 245 | 135 | 145 | 163 |
| *** | 2267 | 2423 | 3754 | 637 | 728 | 954 | 321 | 366 | 426 | 200 | 223 | 239 | 139 | 152 | 151 |
| 0.4 *** | 2216 | 2295 | 3702 | 616 | 675 | 952 | 310 | 343 | 435 | 193 | 212 | 251 | 134 | 145 | 165 |
| *** | 2243 | 2441 | 3915 | 638 | 744 | 984 | 323 | 373 | 435 | 201 | 227 | 241 | 139 | 153 | 151 |
| 0.45 *** | 2123 | 2223 | 3834 | 600 | 667 | 974 | 304 | 340 | 440 | 190 | 210 | 251 | 132 | 143 | 163 |
| *** | 2157 | 2402 | 3995 | 626 | 745 | 994 | 319 | 374 | 435 | 199 | 226 | 239 | 137 | 151 | 147 |
| 0.5 *** | 1981 | 2106 | 3879 | 574 | 649 | 975 | 294 | 332 | 435 | 184 | 204 | 246 | 127 | 138 | 158 |
| *** | 2024 | 2319 | 3995 | 603 | 732 | 984 | 310 | 367 | 426 | 192 | 220 | 231 | 132 | 146 | 141 |
| 0.55 *** | 1804 | 1958 | 3836 | 540 | 620 | 953 | 280 | 318 | 421 | 174 | 194 | 235 | 119 | 131 | 150 |
| *** | 1858 | 2201 | 3915 | 572 | 707 | 954 | 296 | 353 | 409 | 183 | 210 | 219 | 124 | 139 | 131 |
| 0.6 *** | 1608 | 1790 | 3705 | 501 | 584 | 910 | 261 | 299 | 397 | 162 | 181 | 219 | 110 | 121 | 138 |
| *** | 1673 | 2057 | 3754 | 534 | 671 | 904 | 277 | 333 | 382 | 171 | 196 | 201 | 115 | 128 | 119 |
| 0.65 *** | 1407 | 1612 | 3488 | 457 | 539 | 845 | 239 | 275 | 363 | 147 | 165 | 197 | 99 | 108 | 122 |
| *** | 1482 | 1892 | 3513 | 490 | 623 | 833 | 254 | 306 | 346 | 155 | 178 | 179 | 103 | 114 | 102 |
| 0.7 *** | 1211 | 1430 | 3185 | 409 | 487 | 758 | 213 | 245 | 320 | 129 | 144 | 171 | 85 | 92 | 103 |
| *** | 1293 | 1710 | 3192 | 441 | 564 | 743 | 227 | 272 | 302 | 136 | 155 | 151 | 88 | 97 | 83 |
| 0.75 *** | 1025 | 1244 | 2796 | 356 | 426 | 650 | 183 | 210 | 267 | 108 | 119 | 138 | . | . | . |
| *** | 1109 | 1511 | 2791 | 385 | 493 | 633 | 195 | 232 | 248 | 113 | 127 | 118 | . | . | . |
| 0.8 *** | 848 | 1051 | 2322 | 297 | 355 | 521 | 148 | 167 | 205 | . | . | . | . | . | . |
| *** | 927 | 1290 | 2309 | 321 | 408 | 502 | 156 | 182 | 186 | . | . | . | . | . | . |
| 0.85 *** | 673 | 844 | 1764 | 229 | 270 | 372 | . | . | . | . | . | . | . | . | . |
| *** | 741 | 1038 | 1747 | 246 | 305 | 352 | . | . | . | . | . | . | . | . | . |
| 0.9 *** | 484 | 606 | 1124 | . | . | . | . | . | . | . | . | . | . | . | . |
| *** | 533 | 735 | 1104 | . | . | . | . | . | . | . | . | . | . | . | . |

TABLE 3: ALPHA= 0.01  POWER= 0.8    EXPECTED ACCRUAL THRU MINIMUM FOLLOW-UP= 170

|  |  | DEL=.05 | | | DEL=.10 | | | DEL=.15 | | | DEL=.20 | | | DEL=.25 | | |
|---|---|---|---|---|---|---|---|---|---|---|---|---|---|---|---|---|
| FACT= | | 1.0 .75 | .50 .25 | .00 BIN | 1.0 .75 | .50 .25 | .00 BIN | 1.0 .75 | .50 .25 | .00 BIN | 1.0 75 | .50 .25 | .00 BIN | 1.0 .75 | .50 .25 | .00 BIN |
| PCONT=*** | | | | | REQUIRED NUMBER OF PATIENTS | | | | | | | | | | | |
| 0.05 | *** | 602 | 606 | 641 | 215 | 219 | 228 | 127 | 129 | 133 | 90 | 91 | 93 | 70 | 71 | 72 |
|  | *** | 603 | 613 | 1104 | 217 | 222 | 352 | 128 | 131 | 186 | 91 | 92 | 118 | 71 | 72 | 83 |
| 0.1 | *** | 1097 | 1107 | 1237 | 342 | 351 | 382 | 185 | 190 | 203 | 123 | 127 | 133 | 92 | 94 | 98 |
|  | *** | 1100 | 1125 | 1747 | 345 | 361 | 502 | 187 | 195 | 248 | 125 | 129 | 151 | 93 | 96 | 102 |
| 0.15 | *** | 1518 | 1535 | 1813 | 444 | 460 | 523 | 230 | 240 | 264 | 149 | 155 | 166 | 108 | 112 | 118 |
|  | *** | 1524 | 1567 | 2309 | 450 | 478 | 633 | 235 | 249 | 302 | 152 | 160 | 179 | 110 | 114 | 119 |
| 0.2 | *** | 1844 | 1870 | 2339 | 522 | 545 | 649 | 265 | 280 | 317 | 168 | 177 | 194 | 120 | 126 | 135 |
|  | *** | 1853 | 1919 | 2791 | 531 | 574 | 743 | 271 | 293 | 346 | 172 | 184 | 201 | 122 | 129 | 131 |
| 0.25 | *** | 2072 | 2108 | 2798 | 576 | 608 | 755 | 289 | 309 | 361 | 182 | 194 | 217 | 128 | 136 | 148 |
|  | *** | 2084 | 2177 | 3192 | 588 | 647 | 833 | 297 | 327 | 382 | 187 | 203 | 219 | 132 | 141 | 141 |
| 0.3 | *** | 2204 | 2253 | 3182 | 609 | 650 | 842 | 305 | 329 | 395 | 191 | 205 | 234 | 134 | 142 | 157 |
|  | *** | 2221 | 2346 | 3513 | 624 | 700 | 904 | 315 | 352 | 409 | 197 | 216 | 231 | 137 | 148 | 147 |
| 0.35 | *** | 2251 | 2315 | 3484 | 622 | 673 | 908 | 312 | 341 | 420 | 195 | 211 | 245 | 136 | 146 | 163 |
|  | *** | 2272 | 2436 | 3754 | 642 | 734 | 954 | 324 | 368 | 426 | 202 | 224 | 239 | 140 | 153 | 151 |
| 0.4 | *** | 2221 | 2305 | 3702 | 620 | 680 | 952 | 313 | 346 | 435 | 195 | 213 | 251 | 135 | 146 | 165 |
|  | *** | 2249 | 2457 | 3915 | 643 | 751 | 984 | 326 | 376 | 435 | 203 | 228 | 241 | 140 | 154 | 151 |
| 0.45 | *** | 2130 | 2235 | 3834 | 605 | 674 | 974 | 308 | 343 | 440 | 192 | 211 | 251 | 133 | 144 | 163 |
|  | *** | 2165 | 2422 | 3995 | 632 | 752 | 994 | 322 | 376 | 435 | 200 | 227 | 239 | 138 | 152 | 147 |
| 0.5 | *** | 1989 | 2121 | 3879 | 580 | 656 | 975 | 297 | 335 | 435 | 186 | 205 | 246 | 128 | 139 | 158 |
|  | *** | 2034 | 2341 | 3995 | 610 | 740 | 984 | 313 | 369 | 426 | 194 | 221 | 231 | 133 | 147 | 141 |
| 0.55 | *** | 1814 | 1976 | 3836 | 547 | 628 | 953 | 283 | 322 | 421 | 176 | 196 | 235 | 121 | 131 | 150 |
|  | *** | 1871 | 2226 | 3915 | 579 | 715 | 954 | 299 | 356 | 409 | 185 | 211 | 219 | 125 | 139 | 131 |
| 0.6 | *** | 1621 | 1810 | 3705 | 508 | 591 | 910 | 264 | 302 | 397 | 164 | 183 | 219 | 111 | 121 | 138 |
|  | *** | 1689 | 2084 | 3754 | 541 | 678 | 904 | 280 | 335 | 382 | 172 | 197 | 201 | 116 | 128 | 119 |
| 0.65 | *** | 1422 | 1634 | 3488 | 464 | 546 | 845 | 242 | 278 | 363 | 149 | 166 | 198 | 100 | 108 | 122 |
|  | *** | 1500 | 1920 | 3513 | 497 | 630 | 833 | 257 | 308 | 346 | 156 | 179 | 179 | 104 | 114 | 102 |
| 0.7 | *** | 1227 | 1452 | 3185 | 416 | 493 | 758 | 216 | 248 | 320 | 131 | 145 | 171 | 86 | 93 | 103 |
|  | *** | 1312 | 1737 | 3192 | 447 | 570 | 743 | 230 | 274 | 302 | 137 | 156 | 151 | 89 | 97 | 83 |
| 0.75 | *** | 1042 | 1265 | 2796 | 362 | 432 | 650 | 186 | 212 | 267 | 109 | 120 | 138 | . | . | . |
|  | *** | 1128 | 1536 | 2791 | 391 | 498 | 633 | 197 | 233 | 248 | 114 | 128 | 118 | . | . | . |
| 0.8 | *** | 864 | 1071 | 2322 | 302 | 360 | 521 | 150 | 169 | 205 | . | . | . | . | . | . |
|  | *** | 945 | 1311 | 2309 | 326 | 412 | 502 | 158 | 184 | 186 | . | . | . | . | . | . |
| 0.85 | *** | 687 | 861 | 1764 | 232 | 273 | 372 | . | . | . | . | . | . | . | . | . |
|  | *** | 756 | 1055 | 1747 | 250 | 308 | 352 | . | . | . | . | . | . | . | . | . |
| 0.9 | *** | 494 | 617 | 1124 | . | . | . | . | . | . | . | . | . | . | . | . |
|  | *** | 543 | 746 | 1104 | . | . | . | . | . | . | . | . | . | . | . | . |

TABLE 3: ALPHA= 0.01  POWER= 0.8    EXPECTED ACCRUAL THRU MINIMUM FOLLOW-UP= 180

| | | DEL=.05 | | | DEL=.10 | | | DEL=.15 | | | DEL=.20 | | | DEL=.25 | | |
|---|---|---|---|---|---|---|---|---|---|---|---|---|---|---|---|---|---|
| FACT= | | 1.0 .75 | .50 .25 | .00 BIN | 1.0 .75 | .50 .25 | .00 BIN | 1.0 .75 | .50 .25 | .00 BIN | 1.0 75 | .50 .25 | .00 BIN | 1.0 .75 | .50 .25 | .00 BIN |
| PCONT=*** | | | | | REQUIRED NUMBER OF PATIENTS | | | | | | | | | | | |
| 0.05 | *** | 602 | 606 | 641 | 215 | 219 | 228 | 127 | 129 | 133 | 90 | 91 | 94 | 70 | 71 | 73 |
| | *** | 603 | 614 | 1104 | 217 | 222 | 352 | 128 | 131 | 186 | 91 | 92 | 118 | 71 | 72 | 83 |
| 0.1 | *** | 1098 | 1108 | 1237 | 343 | 352 | 382 | 185 | 191 | 203 | 124 | 127 | 133 | 92 | 94 | 98 |
| | *** | 1101 | 1127 | 1747 | 346 | 361 | 502 | 188 | 195 | 248 | 125 | 130 | 151 | 93 | 96 | 102 |
| 0.15 | *** | 1519 | 1537 | 1813 | 445 | 461 | 523 | 231 | 241 | 264 | 150 | 155 | 166 | 108 | 112 | 118 |
| | *** | 1525 | 1571 | 2309 | 451 | 480 | 633 | 235 | 250 | 302 | 152 | 160 | 179 | 110 | 115 | 119 |
| 0.2 | *** | 1846 | 1873 | 2339 | 524 | 548 | 649 | 266 | 281 | 317 | 169 | 178 | 194 | 120 | 126 | 135 |
| | *** | 1855 | 1924 | 2791 | 533 | 576 | 743 | 272 | 294 | 346 | 173 | 184 | 201 | 123 | 130 | 131 |
| 0.25 | *** | 2074 | 2112 | 2798 | 578 | 611 | 755 | 291 | 310 | 360 | 183 | 194 | 217 | 129 | 136 | 148 |
| | *** | 2087 | 2184 | 3192 | 591 | 650 | 833 | 299 | 328 | 382 | 188 | 203 | 219 | 132 | 141 | 141 |
| 0.3 | *** | 2207 | 2259 | 3182 | 612 | 654 | 842 | 307 | 331 | 395 | 192 | 206 | 234 | 134 | 143 | 157 |
| | *** | 2224 | 2357 | 3513 | 627 | 704 | 904 | 317 | 353 | 409 | 198 | 217 | 231 | 138 | 149 | 147 |
| 0.35 | *** | 2254 | 2322 | 3484 | 626 | 678 | 908 | 314 | 343 | 420 | 196 | 213 | 245 | 137 | 146 | 163 |
| | *** | 2277 | 2449 | 3754 | 646 | 739 | 954 | 326 | 370 | 426 | 203 | 225 | 239 | 141 | 153 | 151 |
| 0.4 | *** | 2226 | 2314 | 3702 | 624 | 686 | 952 | 315 | 348 | 435 | 197 | 215 | 251 | 136 | 147 | 165 |
| | *** | 2256 | 2473 | 3915 | 648 | 756 | 984 | 329 | 378 | 435 | 204 | 229 | 241 | 141 | 154 | 151 |
| 0.45 | *** | 2136 | 2247 | 3834 | 610 | 680 | 974 | 310 | 346 | 440 | 194 | 213 | 251 | 134 | 145 | 163 |
| | *** | 2174 | 2441 | 3995 | 637 | 758 | 995 | 325 | 379 | 435 | 202 | 228 | 239 | 139 | 153 | 147 |
| 0.5 | *** | 1997 | 2136 | 3879 | 585 | 663 | 975 | 301 | 338 | 435 | 187 | 207 | 246 | 129 | 140 | 158 |
| | *** | 2045 | 2363 | 3995 | 616 | 746 | 984 | 316 | 372 | 426 | 196 | 222 | 231 | 134 | 148 | 141 |
| 0.55 | *** | 1824 | 1993 | 3836 | 553 | 635 | 953 | 286 | 325 | 421 | 178 | 197 | 235 | 122 | 132 | 150 |
| | *** | 1884 | 2250 | 3915 | 586 | 722 | 954 | 302 | 358 | 409 | 186 | 212 | 219 | 126 | 140 | 131 |
| 0.6 | *** | 1633 | 1830 | 3705 | 514 | 598 | 910 | 268 | 305 | 397 | 166 | 184 | 219 | 112 | 122 | 138 |
| | *** | 1704 | 2109 | 3754 | 548 | 685 | 904 | 284 | 338 | 382 | 174 | 198 | 201 | 117 | 129 | 119 |
| 0.65 | *** | 1436 | 1655 | 3488 | 470 | 553 | 845 | 245 | 281 | 363 | 150 | 167 | 198 | 101 | 109 | 122 |
| | *** | 1517 | 1946 | 3513 | 504 | 637 | 833 | 260 | 311 | 346 | 158 | 180 | 179 | 104 | 115 | 102 |
| 0.7 | *** | 1243 | 1474 | 3185 | 422 | 500 | 758 | 219 | 250 | 320 | 132 | 146 | 171 | 87 | 93 | 103 |
| | *** | 1331 | 1763 | 3192 | 454 | 576 | 743 | 232 | 276 | 302 | 138 | 156 | 151 | 90 | 98 | 83 |
| 0.75 | *** | 1058 | 1286 | 2796 | 368 | 438 | 650 | 188 | 214 | 267 | 110 | 121 | 138 | . | . | . |
| | *** | 1146 | 1560 | 2791 | 397 | 504 | 633 | 199 | 235 | 248 | 115 | 128 | 118 | . | . | . |
| 0.8 | *** | 880 | 1090 | 2322 | 307 | 364 | 521 | 151 | 170 | 206 | . | . | . | . | . | . |
| | *** | 962 | 1332 | 2309 | 331 | 416 | 502 | 160 | 184 | 186 | . | . | . | . | . | . |
| 0.85 | *** | 700 | 876 | 1764 | 236 | 276 | 372 | . | . | . | . | . | . | . | . | . |
| | *** | 770 | 1071 | 1747 | 253 | 310 | 352 | . | . | . | . | . | . | . | . | . |
| 0.9 | *** | 504 | 627 | 1124 | . | . | . | . | . | . | . | . | . | . | . | . |
| | *** | 554 | 756 | 1104 | . | . | . | . | . | . | . | . | . | . | . | . |

## TABLE 3: ALPHA= 0.01  POWER= 0.8     EXPECTED ACCRUAL THRU MINIMUM FOLLOW-UP= 190

| | DEL=.05 | | | DEL=.10 | | | DEL=.15 | | | DEL=.20 | | | DEL=.25 | | |
|---|---|---|---|---|---|---|---|---|---|---|---|---|---|---|---|
| FACT= | 1.0 .75 | .50 .25 | .00 BIN | 1.0 .75 | .50 .25 | .00 BIN | 1.0 .75 | .50 .25 | .00 BIN | 1.0 75 | .50 .25 | .00 BIN | 1.0 .75 | .50 .25 | .00 BIN |
| PCONT=*** | | | | | | REQUIRED NUMBER OF PATIENTS | | | | | | | | | |
| 0.05 *** | 602 | 607 | 641 | 216 | 219 | 228 | 127 | 129 | 133 | 90 | 92 | 94 | 70 | 71 | 73 |
| *** | 604 | 615 | 1104 | 217 | 222 | 352 | 128 | 131 | 186 | 91 | 92 | 118 | 71 | 72 | 83 |
| 0.1 *** | 1098 | 1109 | 1237 | 343 | 352 | 382 | 186 | 191 | 203 | 124 | 127 | 133 | 92 | 94 | 98 |
| *** | 1102 | 1129 | 1747 | 347 | 362 | 502 | 188 | 196 | 248 | 125 | 130 | 151 | 93 | 96 | 102 |
| 0.15 *** | 1520 | 1539 | 1813 | 446 | 463 | 523 | 232 | 242 | 264 | 150 | 156 | 166 | 109 | 112 | 118 |
| *** | 1526 | 1574 | 2309 | 453 | 481 | 633 | 236 | 250 | 302 | 153 | 160 | 179 | 110 | 115 | 119 |
| 0.2 *** | 1847 | 1876 | 2339 | 525 | 550 | 649 | 267 | 282 | 317 | 170 | 178 | 194 | 121 | 126 | 135 |
| *** | 1857 | 1930 | 2791 | 534 | 578 | 743 | 273 | 295 | 346 | 174 | 185 | 201 | 123 | 130 | 131 |
| 0.25 *** | 2076 | 2116 | 2798 | 581 | 614 | 755 | 292 | 312 | 360 | 184 | 195 | 217 | 130 | 136 | 148 |
| *** | 2089 | 2192 | 3192 | 593 | 653 | 833 | 301 | 329 | 382 | 189 | 204 | 219 | 133 | 141 | 141 |
| 0.3 *** | 2210 | 2264 | 3182 | 614 | 658 | 842 | 308 | 333 | 395 | 193 | 207 | 234 | 135 | 143 | 157 |
| *** | 2228 | 2367 | 3513 | 631 | 708 | 904 | 319 | 355 | 409 | 199 | 218 | 231 | 139 | 149 | 147 |
| 0.35 *** | 2258 | 2330 | 3484 | 629 | 683 | 908 | 317 | 345 | 420 | 198 | 214 | 245 | 138 | 147 | 163 |
| *** | 2282 | 2462 | 3754 | 650 | 744 | 954 | 329 | 372 | 426 | 205 | 226 | 239 | 142 | 154 | 151 |
| 0.4 *** | 2231 | 2324 | 3702 | 629 | 691 | 952 | 318 | 351 | 435 | 198 | 216 | 251 | 137 | 148 | 165 |
| *** | 2262 | 2489 | 3915 | 653 | 762 | 984 | 332 | 380 | 435 | 206 | 230 | 241 | 142 | 155 | 151 |
| 0.45 *** | 2142 | 2260 | 3834 | 615 | 686 | 974 | 313 | 349 | 440 | 195 | 214 | 251 | 135 | 145 | 163 |
| *** | 2182 | 2460 | 3995 | 643 | 764 | 994 | 328 | 381 | 435 | 203 | 229 | 239 | 139 | 153 | 147 |
| 0.5 *** | 2005 | 2151 | 3879 | 591 | 669 | 975 | 303 | 341 | 435 | 189 | 208 | 246 | 130 | 141 | 158 |
| *** | 2055 | 2384 | 3995 | 622 | 753 | 984 | 319 | 374 | 426 | 197 | 223 | 231 | 135 | 148 | 141 |
| 0.55 *** | 1834 | 2010 | 3836 | 559 | 642 | 953 | 289 | 327 | 421 | 179 | 199 | 235 | 122 | 133 | 150 |
| *** | 1896 | 2273 | 3915 | 592 | 728 | 954 | 305 | 361 | 409 | 188 | 213 | 219 | 127 | 140 | 131 |
| 0.6 *** | 1645 | 1849 | 3705 | 520 | 605 | 910 | 271 | 308 | 397 | 167 | 185 | 219 | 113 | 123 | 138 |
| *** | 1719 | 2134 | 3754 | 555 | 692 | 904 | 287 | 340 | 382 | 175 | 199 | 201 | 117 | 129 | 119 |
| 0.65 *** | 1450 | 1675 | 3488 | 477 | 560 | 845 | 248 | 283 | 363 | 152 | 168 | 197 | 101 | 110 | 122 |
| *** | 1534 | 1971 | 3513 | 511 | 643 | 833 | 263 | 313 | 346 | 159 | 180 | 179 | 105 | 115 | 102 |
| 0.7 *** | 1259 | 1494 | 3185 | 428 | 506 | 758 | 221 | 253 | 320 | 133 | 147 | 170 | 87 | 94 | 103 |
| *** | 1348 | 1787 | 3192 | 460 | 582 | 743 | 235 | 278 | 302 | 140 | 157 | 151 | 90 | 98 | 83 |
| 0.75 *** | 1074 | 1306 | 2796 | 373 | 443 | 650 | 190 | 216 | 267 | 111 | 122 | 138 | . | . | . |
| *** | 1164 | 1582 | 2791 | 402 | 508 | 633 | 201 | 236 | 248 | 116 | 129 | 118 | . | . | . |
| 0.8 *** | 895 | 1108 | 2322 | 312 | 369 | 521 | 153 | 172 | 206 | . | . | . | . | . | . |
| *** | 978 | 1352 | 2309 | 335 | 420 | 502 | 161 | 185 | 186 | . | . | . | . | . | . |
| 0.85 *** | 713 | 891 | 1764 | 239 | 279 | 372 | . | . | . | . | . | . | . | . | . |
| *** | 784 | 1087 | 1747 | 256 | 313 | 352 | . | . | . | . | . | . | . | . | . |
| 0.9 *** | 513 | 637 | 1124 | . | . | . | . | . | . | . | . | . | . | . | . |
| *** | 563 | 766 | 1104 | . | . | . | . | . | . | . | . | . | . | . | . |

TABLE 3: ALPHA= 0.01  POWER= 0.8     EXPECTED ACCRUAL THRU MINIMUM FOLLOW-UP= 200

| | | DEL=.05 | | | DEL=.10 | | | DEL=.15 | | | DEL=.20 | | | DEL=.25 | | |
|---|---|---|---|---|---|---|---|---|---|---|---|---|---|---|---|---|---|
| FACT= | | 1.0 .75 | .50 .25 | .00 BIN | 1.0 .75 | .50 .25 | .00 BIN | 1.0 .75 | .50 .25 | .00 BIN | 1.0 75 | .50 .25 | .00 BIN | 1.0 .75 | .50 .25 | .00 BIN |
| PCONT=*** | | | | | | | REQUIRED | NUMBER | OF | PATIENTS | | | | | | |
| 0.05 | *** | 602 | 607 | 641 | 216 | 220 | 228 | 127 | 129 | 133 | 90 | 92 | 94 | 70 | 71 | 73 |
| | *** | 604 | 615 | 1104 | 217 | 223 | 352 | 128 | 131 | 186 | 91 | 92 | 118 | 71 | 72 | 83 |
| 0.1 | *** | 1099 | 1110 | 1237 | 344 | 353 | 382 | 186 | 192 | 203 | 124 | 128 | 133 | 92 | 94 | 98 |
| | *** | 1103 | 1131 | 1747 | 347 | 363 | 502 | 189 | 196 | 248 | 126 | 130 | 151 | 93 | 96 | 102 |
| 0.15 | *** | 1521 | 1541 | 1813 | 448 | 464 | 523 | 233 | 243 | 264 | 151 | 156 | 166 | 109 | 113 | 118 |
| | *** | 1528 | 1578 | 2309 | 454 | 483 | 633 | 237 | 251 | 302 | 153 | 161 | 179 | 111 | 115 | 119 |
| 0.2 | *** | 1849 | 1879 | 2339 | 527 | 552 | 649 | 268 | 283 | 317 | 171 | 179 | 194 | 121 | 127 | 135 |
| | *** | 1859 | 1935 | 2791 | 536 | 580 | 743 | 274 | 296 | 346 | 174 | 185 | 201 | 124 | 130 | 131 |
| 0.25 | *** | 2078 | 2120 | 2798 | 583 | 617 | 755 | 294 | 313 | 360 | 185 | 196 | 217 | 130 | 137 | 148 |
| | *** | 2092 | 2200 | 3192 | 596 | 656 | 833 | 302 | 331 | 382 | 190 | 204 | 219 | 133 | 142 | 141 |
| 0.3 | *** | 2213 | 2270 | 3182 | 617 | 661 | 842 | 310 | 335 | 395 | 194 | 208 | 234 | 136 | 144 | 157 |
| | *** | 2232 | 2376 | 3513 | 634 | 712 | 904 | 320 | 356 | 409 | 200 | 218 | 231 | 139 | 150 | 147 |
| 0.35 | *** | 2262 | 2337 | 3484 | 633 | 687 | 908 | 319 | 348 | 420 | 199 | 215 | 245 | 138 | 148 | 163 |
| | *** | 2287 | 2475 | 3754 | 654 | 748 | 954 | 331 | 373 | 426 | 206 | 227 | 239 | 143 | 154 | 151 |
| 0.4 | *** | 2236 | 2333 | 3702 | 633 | 696 | 952 | 320 | 353 | 435 | 200 | 217 | 251 | 138 | 148 | 165 |
| | *** | 2269 | 2504 | 3915 | 658 | 767 | 984 | 334 | 382 | 435 | 207 | 231 | 241 | 143 | 155 | 151 |
| 0.45 | *** | 2148 | 2271 | 3834 | 620 | 692 | 974 | 316 | 352 | 440 | 197 | 215 | 251 | 136 | 146 | 163 |
| | *** | 2190 | 2478 | 3995 | 648 | 770 | 994 | 331 | 383 | 435 | 205 | 230 | 239 | 140 | 153 | 147 |
| 0.5 | *** | 2013 | 2165 | 3879 | 596 | 675 | 975 | 306 | 344 | 435 | 190 | 210 | 246 | 131 | 141 | 158 |
| | *** | 2066 | 2405 | 3995 | 628 | 759 | 984 | 322 | 376 | 426 | 199 | 224 | 231 | 135 | 149 | 141 |
| 0.55 | *** | 1844 | 2027 | 3836 | 565 | 648 | 953 | 292 | 330 | 421 | 181 | 200 | 235 | 123 | 134 | 150 |
| | *** | 1909 | 2296 | 3915 | 598 | 735 | 954 | 308 | 363 | 409 | 189 | 214 | 219 | 128 | 140 | 131 |
| 0.6 | *** | 1657 | 1868 | 3705 | 526 | 612 | 910 | 274 | 311 | 397 | 169 | 187 | 219 | 114 | 123 | 138 |
| | *** | 1734 | 2157 | 3754 | 561 | 698 | 904 | 289 | 342 | 382 | 177 | 200 | 201 | 118 | 129 | 119 |
| 0.65 | *** | 1464 | 1695 | 3488 | 483 | 566 | 845 | 251 | 286 | 363 | 153 | 169 | 197 | 102 | 110 | 122 |
| | *** | 1551 | 1995 | 3513 | 517 | 649 | 833 | 266 | 314 | 346 | 160 | 181 | 179 | 106 | 115 | 102 |
| 0.7 | *** | 1274 | 1514 | 3185 | 433 | 512 | 758 | 224 | 255 | 320 | 135 | 148 | 171 | 88 | 94 | 103 |
| | *** | 1366 | 1811 | 3192 | 466 | 587 | 743 | 237 | 280 | 302 | 141 | 158 | 151 | 91 | 98 | 83 |
| 0.75 | *** | 1089 | 1325 | 2796 | 378 | 448 | 650 | 192 | 218 | 267 | 112 | 122 | 138 | . | . | . |
| | *** | 1181 | 1604 | 2791 | 407 | 513 | 633 | 203 | 237 | 248 | 117 | 129 | 118 | . | . | . |
| 0.8 | *** | 909 | 1125 | 2322 | 316 | 373 | 521 | 154 | 173 | 205 | . | . | . | . | . | . |
| | *** | 994 | 1371 | 2309 | 340 | 423 | 502 | 163 | 186 | 186 | . | . | . | . | . | . |
| 0.85 | *** | 725 | 905 | 1764 | 242 | 282 | 372 | . | . | . | . | . | . | . | . | . |
| | *** | 797 | 1102 | 1747 | 259 | 315 | 352 | . | . | . | . | . | . | . | . | . |
| 0.9 | *** | 522 | 647 | 1124 | . | . | . | . | . | . | . | . | . | . | . | . |
| | *** | 572 | 775 | 1104 | . | . | . | . | . | . | . | . | . | . | . | . |

## TABLE 3: ALPHA= 0.01  POWER= 0.8     EXPECTED ACCRUAL THRU MINIMUM FOLLOW-UP= 225

| | | DEL=.05 | | | DEL=.10 | | | DEL=.15 | | | DEL=.20 | | | DEL=.25 | | |
|---|---|---|---|---|---|---|---|---|---|---|---|---|---|---|---|---|---|
| FACT= | | 1.0 .75 | .50 .25 | .00 BIN | 1.0 .75 | .50 .25 | .00 BIN | 1.0 .75 | .50 .25 | .00 BIN | 1.0 75 | .50 .25 | .00 BIN | 1.0 .75 | .50 .25 | .00 BIN |
| PCONT=*** | | | | | | | | REQUIRED NUMBER OF PATIENTS | | | | | | | | |
| 0.05 | *** | 603 | 608 | 641 | 217 | 220 | 228 | 128 | 130 | 133 | 91 | 92 | 93 | 71 | 71 | 73 |
| | *** | 605 | 617 | 1104 | 218 | 223 | 352 | 129 | 131 | 186 | 91 | 93 | 118 | 71 | 72 | 83 |
| 0.1 | *** | 1100 | 1113 | 1237 | 345 | 355 | 382 | 187 | 192 | 203 | 125 | 128 | 133 | 93 | 95 | 97 |
| | *** | 1105 | 1136 | 1747 | 349 | 364 | 502 | 189 | 197 | 248 | 126 | 130 | 151 | 94 | 96 | 102 |
| 0.15 | *** | 1524 | 1546 | 1813 | 450 | 467 | 523 | 234 | 244 | 264 | 152 | 157 | 166 | 110 | 113 | 118 |
| | *** | 1531 | 1586 | 2309 | 457 | 485 | 633 | 239 | 252 | 302 | 154 | 161 | 179 | 111 | 115 | 119 |
| 0.2 | *** | 1853 | 1886 | 2339 | 530 | 556 | 649 | 271 | 285 | 317 | 172 | 180 | 194 | 122 | 127 | 135 |
| | *** | 1864 | 1947 | 2791 | 541 | 585 | 743 | 277 | 297 | 346 | 176 | 186 | 201 | 125 | 131 | 131 |
| 0.25 | *** | 2084 | 2131 | 2798 | 588 | 623 | 755 | 297 | 317 | 360 | 187 | 198 | 217 | 131 | 138 | 148 |
| | *** | 2099 | 2217 | 3192 | 601 | 663 | 833 | 305 | 333 | 382 | 192 | 206 | 219 | 134 | 142 | 141 |
| 0.3 | *** | 2220 | 2284 | 3182 | 624 | 670 | 842 | 314 | 339 | 395 | 197 | 210 | 234 | 137 | 145 | 157 |
| | *** | 2242 | 2400 | 3513 | 641 | 720 | 904 | 325 | 359 | 409 | 202 | 220 | 231 | 141 | 150 | 147 |
| 0.35 | *** | 2271 | 2356 | 3484 | 641 | 697 | 908 | 324 | 352 | 420 | 202 | 217 | 245 | 140 | 149 | 163 |
| | *** | 2300 | 2505 | 3754 | 663 | 758 | 954 | 336 | 377 | 426 | 209 | 228 | 239 | 144 | 155 | 151 |
| 0.4 | *** | 2248 | 2357 | 3702 | 642 | 708 | 952 | 326 | 358 | 435 | 203 | 220 | 251 | 140 | 150 | 165 |
| | *** | 2285 | 2541 | 3915 | 668 | 779 | 984 | 340 | 386 | 435 | 210 | 232 | 241 | 144 | 156 | 151 |
| 0.45 | *** | 2164 | 2300 | 3834 | 631 | 705 | 974 | 322 | 357 | 440 | 200 | 218 | 251 | 138 | 148 | 163 |
| | *** | 2211 | 2521 | 3995 | 660 | 783 | 994 | 337 | 387 | 435 | 208 | 232 | 239 | 142 | 154 | 147 |
| 0.5 | *** | 2033 | 2199 | 3879 | 609 | 690 | 975 | 313 | 350 | 435 | 194 | 212 | 246 | 133 | 143 | 158 |
| | *** | 2091 | 2453 | 3995 | 641 | 773 | 984 | 329 | 381 | 426 | 202 | 226 | 231 | 137 | 149 | 141 |
| 0.55 | *** | 1869 | 2067 | 3836 | 578 | 663 | 953 | 299 | 336 | 421 | 185 | 203 | 235 | 125 | 135 | 150 |
| | *** | 1940 | 2349 | 3915 | 612 | 748 | 954 | 315 | 367 | 409 | 193 | 216 | 219 | 130 | 141 | 131 |
| 0.6 | *** | 1687 | 1912 | 3705 | 540 | 627 | 910 | 280 | 317 | 397 | 172 | 189 | 219 | 116 | 124 | 138 |
| | *** | 1770 | 2213 | 3754 | 576 | 711 | 904 | 296 | 347 | 382 | 180 | 202 | 201 | 120 | 130 | 119 |
| 0.65 | *** | 1498 | 1742 | 3488 | 496 | 581 | 845 | 257 | 291 | 363 | 156 | 172 | 197 | 104 | 111 | 122 |
| | *** | 1590 | 2051 | 3513 | 531 | 662 | 833 | 272 | 318 | 346 | 163 | 183 | 179 | 107 | 116 | 102 |
| 0.7 | *** | 1310 | 1561 | 3185 | 446 | 525 | 758 | 230 | 260 | 320 | 137 | 150 | 171 | 89 | 95 | 103 |
| | *** | 1407 | 1865 | 3192 | 479 | 599 | 743 | 243 | 283 | 302 | 143 | 159 | 151 | 92 | 99 | 83 |
| 0.75 | *** | 1126 | 1370 | 2795 | 390 | 460 | 650 | 197 | 221 | 267 | 114 | 124 | 138 | . | . | . |
| | *** | 1221 | 1654 | 2791 | 419 | 523 | 633 | 208 | 240 | 248 | 119 | 130 | 118 | . | . | . |
| 0.8 | *** | 943 | 1165 | 2322 | 326 | 382 | 521 | 158 | 175 | 205 | . | . | . | . | . | . |
| | *** | 1031 | 1414 | 2309 | 349 | 431 | 502 | 166 | 188 | 186 | . | . | . | . | . | . |
| 0.85 | *** | 754 | 938 | 1764 | 249 | 288 | 372 | . | . | . | . | . | . | . | . | . |
| | *** | 827 | 1135 | 1747 | 266 | 320 | 352 | . | . | . | . | . | . | . | . | . |
| 0.9 | *** | 542 | 669 | 1124 | . | . | . | . | . | . | . | . | . | . | . | . |
| | *** | 594 | 796 | 1104 | . | . | . | . | . | . | . | . | . | . | . | . |

TABLE 3: ALPHA= 0.01  POWER= 0.8   EXPECTED ACCRUAL THRU MINIMUM FOLLOW-UP= 250

| | | DEL=.05 | | | DEL=.10 | | | DEL=.15 | | | DEL=.20 | | | DEL=.25 | | |
|---|---|---|---|---|---|---|---|---|---|---|---|---|---|---|---|---|
| FACT= | | 1.0 .75 | .50 .25 | .00 BIN | 1.0 .75 | .50 .25 | .00 BIN | 1.0 .75 | .50 .25 | .00 BIN | 1.0 75 | .50 .25 | .00 BIN | 1.0 .75 | .50 .25 | .00 BIN |
| PCONT=*** | | | | | REQUIRED NUMBER OF PATIENTS | | | | | | | | | | | |
| 0.05 | *** | 604 | 610 | 641 | 217 | 221 | 228 | 128 | 130 | 133 | 91 | 92 | 94 | 71 | 72 | 72 |
| | *** | 606 | 618 | 1104 | 219 | 224 | 352 | 129 | 131 | 186 | 91 | 93 | 118 | 71 | 72 | 83 |
| 0.1 | *** | 1102 | 1116 | 1237 | 347 | 356 | 382 | 188 | 193 | 203 | 125 | 128 | 133 | 93 | 95 | 97 |
| | *** | 1107 | 1140 | 1747 | 350 | 366 | 502 | 190 | 197 | 248 | 127 | 130 | 151 | 94 | 96 | 102 |
| 0.15 | *** | 1526 | 1550 | 1813 | 452 | 470 | 523 | 236 | 245 | 264 | 152 | 158 | 166 | 110 | 113 | 118 |
| | *** | 1534 | 1594 | 2309 | 459 | 488 | 633 | 240 | 253 | 302 | 155 | 162 | 179 | 112 | 116 | 119 |
| 0.2 | *** | 1856 | 1893 | 2339 | 534 | 561 | 649 | 273 | 287 | 317 | 173 | 181 | 194 | 123 | 128 | 135 |
| | *** | 1869 | 1960 | 2791 | 544 | 589 | 743 | 279 | 299 | 346 | 177 | 187 | 201 | 125 | 131 | 131 |
| 0.25 | *** | 2089 | 2141 | 2798 | 592 | 629 | 755 | 300 | 319 | 360 | 189 | 199 | 217 | 133 | 139 | 148 |
| | *** | 2106 | 2235 | 3192 | 607 | 669 | 833 | 308 | 335 | 382 | 193 | 207 | 219 | 135 | 143 | 141 |
| 0.3 | *** | 2227 | 2298 | 3182 | 630 | 677 | 842 | 318 | 342 | 395 | 199 | 212 | 234 | 139 | 146 | 157 |
| | *** | 2251 | 2423 | 3513 | 649 | 727 | 904 | 328 | 362 | 409 | 204 | 221 | 231 | 142 | 151 | 147 |
| 0.35 | *** | 2281 | 2374 | 3484 | 649 | 707 | 908 | 328 | 357 | 420 | 204 | 219 | 245 | 142 | 150 | 163 |
| | *** | 2312 | 2533 | 3754 | 672 | 767 | 954 | 340 | 380 | 426 | 211 | 230 | 239 | 145 | 156 | 151 |
| 0.4 | *** | 2261 | 2380 | 3702 | 652 | 719 | 952 | 331 | 363 | 435 | 206 | 222 | 251 | 142 | 151 | 165 |
| | *** | 2301 | 2576 | 3915 | 679 | 789 | 984 | 345 | 390 | 435 | 213 | 234 | 241 | 146 | 157 | 151 |
| 0.45 | *** | 2180 | 2328 | 3834 | 642 | 717 | 974 | 328 | 362 | 440 | 203 | 221 | 251 | 139 | 149 | 163 |
| | *** | 2231 | 2561 | 3995 | 672 | 794 | 994 | 342 | 391 | 435 | 211 | 233 | 239 | 144 | 155 | 147 |
| 0.5 | *** | 2053 | 2233 | 3879 | 620 | 702 | 975 | 319 | 355 | 435 | 197 | 215 | 246 | 134 | 144 | 158 |
| | *** | 2116 | 2498 | 3995 | 654 | 784 | 984 | 334 | 385 | 426 | 205 | 228 | 231 | 139 | 150 | 141 |
| 0.55 | *** | 1893 | 2105 | 3836 | 590 | 676 | 953 | 305 | 341 | 421 | 188 | 205 | 235 | 127 | 136 | 150 |
| | *** | 1970 | 2397 | 3915 | 625 | 761 | 954 | 320 | 372 | 409 | 195 | 218 | 219 | 131 | 142 | 131 |
| 0.6 | *** | 1715 | 1953 | 3705 | 553 | 640 | 910 | 286 | 322 | 397 | 175 | 191 | 219 | 117 | 126 | 138 |
| | *** | 1804 | 2264 | 3754 | 589 | 723 | 904 | 301 | 350 | 382 | 182 | 203 | 201 | 121 | 131 | 119 |
| 0.65 | *** | 1530 | 1785 | 3488 | 509 | 593 | 845 | 262 | 296 | 363 | 159 | 174 | 197 | 105 | 112 | 122 |
| | *** | 1627 | 2102 | 3513 | 544 | 673 | 833 | 277 | 322 | 346 | 166 | 184 | 179 | 108 | 117 | 102 |
| 0.7 | *** | 1344 | 1604 | 3185 | 458 | 537 | 758 | 234 | 264 | 320 | 139 | 152 | 171 | 90 | 96 | 103 |
| | *** | 1445 | 1914 | 3192 | 491 | 609 | 743 | 247 | 286 | 302 | 145 | 160 | 151 | 93 | 99 | 83 |
| 0.75 | *** | 1160 | 1411 | 2796 | 401 | 470 | 650 | 201 | 225 | 267 | 116 | 125 | 138 | . | . | . |
| | *** | 1258 | 1699 | 2791 | 430 | 531 | 633 | 211 | 242 | 248 | 120 | 131 | 118 | . | . | . |
| 0.8 | *** | 974 | 1202 | 2322 | 334 | 390 | 521 | 161 | 178 | 205 | . | . | . | . | . | . |
| | *** | 1064 | 1453 | 2309 | 358 | 437 | 502 | 168 | 189 | 186 | . | . | . | . | . | . |
| 0.85 | *** | 780 | 967 | 1764 | 256 | 294 | 372 | . | . | . | . | . | . | . | . | . |
| | *** | 855 | 1165 | 1747 | 272 | 324 | 352 | . | . | . | . | . | . | . | . | . |
| 0.9 | *** | 561 | 689 | 1124 | . | . | . | . | . | . | . | . | . | . | . | . |
| | *** | 613 | 814 | 1104 | . | . | . | . | . | . | . | . | . | . | . | . |

TABLE 3: ALPHA= 0.01  POWER= 0.8     EXPECTED ACCRUAL THRU MINIMUM FOLLOW-UP= 275

|  |  | DEL=.05 | | | DEL=.10 | | | DEL=.15 | | | DEL=.20 | | | DEL=.25 | | |
|---|---|---|---|---|---|---|---|---|---|---|---|---|---|---|---|---|
| FACT= | | 1.0 .75 | .50 .25 | .00 BIN | 1.0 .75 | .50 .25 | .00 BIN | 1.0 .75 | .50 .25 | .00 BIN | 1.0 75 | .50 .25 | .00 BIN | 1.0 .75 | .50 .25 | .00 BIN |
| PCONT=*** | | | | | REQUIRED NUMBER OF PATIENTS | | | | | | | | | | | |
| 0.05 | *** | 604 | 611 | 641 | 217 | 221 | 228 | 128 | 130 | 133 | 91 | 92 | 94 | 71 | 72 | 72 |
|  | *** | 607 | 619 | 1104 | 219 | 224 | 352 | 129 | 131 | 186 | 91 | 93 | 118 | 71 | 72 | 83 |
| 0.1 | *** | 1103 | 1119 | 1237 | 348 | 358 | 382 | 189 | 194 | 202 | 126 | 129 | 133 | 93 | 95 | 98 |
|  | *** | 1108 | 1144 | 1747 | 352 | 367 | 502 | 191 | 198 | 248 | 127 | 131 | 151 | 94 | 96 | 102 |
| 0.15 | *** | 1529 | 1555 | 1813 | 454 | 473 | 523 | 237 | 246 | 264 | 153 | 158 | 166 | 111 | 114 | 118 |
|  | *** | 1537 | 1601 | 2309 | 462 | 490 | 633 | 241 | 254 | 302 | 156 | 162 | 179 | 112 | 116 | 119 |
| 0.2 | *** | 1860 | 1900 | 2339 | 537 | 565 | 649 | 275 | 289 | 317 | 175 | 182 | 194 | 124 | 128 | 135 |
|  | *** | 1874 | 1971 | 2791 | 548 | 593 | 743 | 281 | 300 | 346 | 178 | 187 | 201 | 126 | 131 | 131 |
| 0.25 | *** | 2094 | 2151 | 2798 | 597 | 635 | 755 | 303 | 322 | 360 | 190 | 200 | 217 | 134 | 139 | 148 |
|  | *** | 2113 | 2251 | 3192 | 612 | 674 | 833 | 311 | 337 | 382 | 195 | 207 | 219 | 136 | 143 | 141 |
| 0.3 | *** | 2234 | 2312 | 3182 | 636 | 684 | 842 | 321 | 345 | 395 | 201 | 213 | 234 | 140 | 147 | 157 |
|  | *** | 2261 | 2444 | 3513 | 655 | 734 | 904 | 332 | 364 | 409 | 206 | 222 | 231 | 143 | 151 | 147 |
| 0.35 | *** | 2290 | 2391 | 3484 | 656 | 715 | 908 | 332 | 360 | 420 | 206 | 221 | 245 | 143 | 151 | 163 |
|  | *** | 2325 | 2560 | 3754 | 679 | 775 | 954 | 344 | 383 | 426 | 213 | 231 | 239 | 146 | 156 | 151 |
| 0.4 | *** | 2273 | 2402 | 3702 | 660 | 729 | 952 | 336 | 367 | 435 | 208 | 224 | 251 | 143 | 152 | 165 |
|  | *** | 2317 | 2608 | 3915 | 688 | 798 | 984 | 349 | 393 | 435 | 215 | 235 | 241 | 147 | 158 | 151 |
| 0.45 | *** | 2195 | 2356 | 3834 | 651 | 728 | 974 | 332 | 367 | 440 | 206 | 223 | 251 | 141 | 150 | 163 |
|  | *** | 2251 | 2598 | 3995 | 682 | 804 | 994 | 347 | 395 | 435 | 213 | 235 | 239 | 145 | 156 | 147 |
| 0.5 | *** | 2072 | 2265 | 3879 | 631 | 714 | 975 | 324 | 360 | 435 | 200 | 217 | 246 | 136 | 145 | 158 |
|  | *** | 2141 | 2540 | 3995 | 665 | 795 | 984 | 339 | 388 | 426 | 208 | 229 | 231 | 140 | 151 | 141 |
| 0.55 | *** | 1917 | 2141 | 3836 | 602 | 688 | 953 | 310 | 346 | 421 | 190 | 207 | 235 | 128 | 137 | 150 |
|  | *** | 1999 | 2442 | 3915 | 637 | 771 | 954 | 326 | 375 | 409 | 198 | 219 | 219 | 132 | 143 | 131 |
| 0.6 | *** | 1743 | 1992 | 3705 | 565 | 652 | 910 | 291 | 326 | 397 | 177 | 193 | 219 | 118 | 126 | 138 |
|  | *** | 1836 | 2310 | 3754 | 601 | 734 | 904 | 306 | 354 | 382 | 185 | 204 | 201 | 122 | 131 | 119 |
| 0.65 | *** | 1561 | 1826 | 3488 | 520 | 605 | 845 | 267 | 300 | 363 | 161 | 175 | 198 | 106 | 113 | 122 |
|  | *** | 1662 | 2148 | 3513 | 556 | 683 | 833 | 282 | 325 | 346 | 168 | 185 | 179 | 109 | 117 | 102 |
| 0.7 | *** | 1376 | 1645 | 3185 | 469 | 547 | 758 | 239 | 267 | 320 | 141 | 153 | 171 | 91 | 96 | 103 |
|  | *** | 1481 | 1959 | 3192 | 502 | 618 | 743 | 251 | 288 | 302 | 147 | 161 | 151 | 93 | 99 | 83 |
| 0.75 | *** | 1191 | 1449 | 2796 | 410 | 479 | 650 | 204 | 227 | 267 | 117 | 126 | 138 | . | . | . |
|  | *** | 1293 | 1740 | 2791 | 439 | 539 | 633 | 215 | 244 | 248 | 121 | 132 | 118 | . | . | . |
| 0.8 | *** | 1003 | 1235 | 2322 | 342 | 397 | 521 | 163 | 179 | 205 | . | . | . | . | . | . |
|  | *** | 1096 | 1488 | 2309 | 366 | 442 | 502 | 171 | 191 | 186 | . | . | . | . | . | . |
| 0.85 | *** | 805 | 994 | 1764 | 261 | 298 | 371 | . | . | . | . | . | . | . | . | . |
|  | *** | 881 | 1192 | 1747 | 277 | 327 | 352 | . | . | . | . | . | . | . | . | . |
| 0.9 | *** | 578 | 706 | 1124 | . | . | . | . | . | . | . | . | . | . | . | . |
|  | *** | 631 | 831 | 1104 | . | . | . | . | . | . | . | . | . | . | . | . |

## TABLE 3: ALPHA= 0.01  POWER= 0.8    EXPECTED ACCRUAL THRU MINIMUM FOLLOW-UP= 300

| | DEL=.05 | | | DEL=.10 | | | DEL=.15 | | | DEL=.20 | | | DEL=.25 | | |
|---|---|---|---|---|---|---|---|---|---|---|---|---|---|---|---|
| FACT= | 1.0 .75 | .50 .25 | .00 BIN | 1.0 .75 | .50 .25 | .00 BIN | 1.0 .75 | .50 .25 | .00 BIN | 1.0 75 | .50 .25 | .00 BIN | 1.0 .75 | .50 .25 | .00 BIN |
| PCONT=*** | | | | | | REQUIRED NUMBER OF PATIENTS | | | | | | | | | |
| 0.05 *** | 605 | 612 | 641 | 218 | 221 | 228 | 129 | 130 | 133 | 91 | 92 | 94 | 71 | 72 | 73 |
| *** | 607 | 620 | 1104 | 220 | 224 | 352 | 129 | 131 | 186 | 91 | 93 | 118 | 71 | 72 | 83 |
| 0.1 *** | 1105 | 1121 | 1237 | 349 | 359 | 382 | 189 | 194 | 202 | 126 | 129 | 133 | 94 | 95 | 97 |
| *** | 1110 | 1147 | 1747 | 353 | 368 | 502 | 192 | 198 | 248 | 127 | 131 | 151 | 94 | 96 | 102 |
| 0.15 *** | 1531 | 1560 | 1813 | 457 | 475 | 523 | 238 | 248 | 264 | 154 | 159 | 166 | 111 | 114 | 118 |
| *** | 1541 | 1608 | 2309 | 464 | 492 | 633 | 242 | 254 | 302 | 156 | 162 | 179 | 112 | 116 | 119 |
| 0.2 *** | 1864 | 1908 | 2339 | 541 | 568 | 649 | 277 | 291 | 317 | 176 | 183 | 194 | 125 | 129 | 135 |
| *** | 1879 | 1982 | 2791 | 552 | 596 | 743 | 283 | 301 | 346 | 179 | 188 | 201 | 127 | 131 | 131 |
| 0.25 *** | 2099 | 2161 | 2798 | 601 | 640 | 755 | 305 | 324 | 360 | 192 | 201 | 217 | 134 | 140 | 148 |
| *** | 2120 | 2266 | 3192 | 617 | 678 | 833 | 313 | 338 | 382 | 196 | 208 | 219 | 137 | 143 | 141 |
| 0.3 *** | 2242 | 2325 | 3182 | 641 | 691 | 842 | 325 | 348 | 395 | 202 | 214 | 234 | 141 | 147 | 157 |
| *** | 2270 | 2465 | 3513 | 661 | 740 | 904 | 335 | 366 | 409 | 208 | 223 | 231 | 144 | 152 | 147 |
| 0.35 *** | 2300 | 2409 | 3484 | 663 | 723 | 908 | 336 | 363 | 420 | 208 | 222 | 245 | 144 | 152 | 163 |
| *** | 2337 | 2586 | 3754 | 687 | 782 | 954 | 348 | 385 | 426 | 215 | 232 | 239 | 148 | 157 | 151 |
| 0.4 *** | 2285 | 2424 | 3702 | 668 | 738 | 952 | 340 | 371 | 435 | 210 | 226 | 251 | 144 | 153 | 165 |
| *** | 2333 | 2638 | 3915 | 696 | 806 | 984 | 353 | 396 | 435 | 217 | 236 | 241 | 148 | 158 | 151 |
| 0.45 *** | 2211 | 2382 | 3834 | 660 | 738 | 974 | 337 | 371 | 440 | 208 | 224 | 251 | 142 | 151 | 163 |
| *** | 2271 | 2633 | 3995 | 692 | 813 | 994 | 352 | 397 | 435 | 215 | 236 | 239 | 146 | 156 | 147 |
| 0.5 *** | 2091 | 2295 | 3879 | 641 | 724 | 975 | 328 | 364 | 435 | 202 | 219 | 246 | 137 | 146 | 158 |
| *** | 2165 | 2579 | 3995 | 675 | 804 | 984 | 344 | 391 | 426 | 210 | 230 | 231 | 141 | 151 | 141 |
| 0.55 *** | 1940 | 2175 | 3836 | 612 | 699 | 953 | 315 | 350 | 421 | 193 | 209 | 235 | 130 | 138 | 150 |
| *** | 2027 | 2484 | 3915 | 648 | 781 | 954 | 330 | 378 | 409 | 200 | 220 | 219 | 133 | 143 | 131 |
| 0.6 *** | 1770 | 2029 | 3705 | 575 | 663 | 910 | 296 | 330 | 397 | 180 | 195 | 219 | 120 | 127 | 138 |
| *** | 1867 | 2353 | 3754 | 612 | 743 | 904 | 311 | 356 | 382 | 187 | 205 | 201 | 123 | 132 | 119 |
| 0.65 *** | 1590 | 1864 | 3488 | 531 | 615 | 845 | 272 | 303 | 363 | 163 | 177 | 197 | 107 | 113 | 122 |
| *** | 1695 | 2191 | 3513 | 566 | 692 | 833 | 286 | 327 | 346 | 169 | 186 | 179 | 110 | 117 | 102 |
| 0.7 *** | 1407 | 1682 | 3184 | 479 | 557 | 758 | 243 | 270 | 320 | 143 | 154 | 170 | 92 | 97 | 103 |
| *** | 1514 | 2000 | 3192 | 512 | 626 | 743 | 255 | 291 | 302 | 148 | 161 | 151 | 94 | 100 | 83 |
| 0.75 *** | 1221 | 1484 | 2795 | 419 | 487 | 650 | 208 | 230 | 267 | 118 | 127 | 138 | . | . | . |
| *** | 1325 | 1778 | 2791 | 448 | 545 | 633 | 217 | 246 | 248 | 122 | 132 | 118 | . | . | . |
| 0.8 *** | 1031 | 1266 | 2322 | 349 | 403 | 521 | 166 | 181 | 205 | . | . | . | . | . | . |
| *** | 1125 | 1520 | 2309 | 373 | 447 | 502 | 173 | 192 | 186 | . | . | . | . | . | . |
| 0.85 *** | 827 | 1019 | 1764 | 266 | 302 | 372 | . | . | . | . | . | . | . | . | . |
| *** | 905 | 1216 | 1747 | 282 | 330 | 352 | . | . | . | . | . | . | . | . | . |
| 0.9 *** | 594 | 723 | 1124 | . | . | . | . | . | . | . | . | . | . | . | . |
| *** | 647 | 845 | 1104 | . | . | . | . | . | . | . | . | . | . | . | . |

# TABLE 3: ALPHA= 0.01  POWER= 0.8    EXPECTED ACCRUAL THRU MINIMUM FOLLOW-UP= 325

| | | DEL=.05 | | | DEL=.10 | | | DEL=.15 | | | DEL=.20 | | | DEL=.25 | | |
|---|---|---|---|---|---|---|---|---|---|---|---|---|---|---|---|---|---|
| FACT= | | 1.0 .75 | .50 .25 | .00 BIN | 1.0 .75 | .50 .25 | .00 BIN | 1.0 .75 | .50 .25 | .00 BIN | 1.0 75 | .50 .25 | .00 BIN | 1.0 .75 | .50 .25 | .00 BIN |
| PCONT=*** | | | | | REQUIRED NUMBER OF PATIENTS | | | | | | | | | | | |
| 0.05 | *** | 606 | 613 | 641 | 218 | 222 | 228 | 129 | 131 | 133 | 91 | 92 | 94 | 71 | 72 | 73 |
| | *** | 608 | 622 | 1104 | 220 | 224 | 352 | 130 | 132 | 186 | 92 | 93 | 118 | 71 | 72 | 83 |
| 0.1 | *** | 1106 | 1124 | 1237 | 350 | 360 | 382 | 190 | 195 | 203 | 127 | 129 | 133 | 94 | 95 | 97 |
| | *** | 1112 | 1150 | 1747 | 354 | 368 | 502 | 192 | 198 | 248 | 128 | 131 | 151 | 95 | 96 | 102 |
| 0.15 | *** | 1533 | 1564 | 1813 | 459 | 477 | 523 | 240 | 249 | 264 | 155 | 159 | 166 | 112 | 114 | 118 |
| | *** | 1544 | 1614 | 2309 | 466 | 494 | 633 | 244 | 255 | 302 | 157 | 162 | 179 | 113 | 116 | 119 |
| 0.2 | *** | 1867 | 1915 | 2339 | 544 | 572 | 649 | 279 | 292 | 317 | 177 | 184 | 194 | 125 | 129 | 135 |
| | *** | 1884 | 1993 | 2791 | 555 | 599 | 743 | 285 | 302 | 346 | 180 | 188 | 201 | 127 | 132 | 131 |
| 0.25 | *** | 2105 | 2171 | 2798 | 606 | 645 | 755 | 307 | 326 | 361 | 193 | 202 | 217 | 135 | 140 | 148 |
| | *** | 2127 | 2281 | 3192 | 621 | 682 | 833 | 315 | 340 | 382 | 197 | 209 | 219 | 138 | 144 | 141 |
| 0.3 | *** | 2249 | 2338 | 3182 | 647 | 697 | 842 | 327 | 350 | 395 | 204 | 216 | 234 | 142 | 148 | 157 |
| | *** | 2279 | 2484 | 3513 | 667 | 745 | 904 | 337 | 368 | 409 | 209 | 223 | 231 | 145 | 152 | 147 |
| 0.35 | *** | 2309 | 2426 | 3484 | 669 | 730 | 908 | 339 | 366 | 420 | 210 | 224 | 245 | 145 | 152 | 163 |
| | *** | 2350 | 2610 | 3754 | 694 | 788 | 954 | 351 | 387 | 426 | 216 | 233 | 239 | 148 | 157 | 151 |
| 0.4 | *** | 2297 | 2445 | 3703 | 676 | 746 | 952 | 343 | 374 | 435 | 212 | 227 | 251 | 146 | 154 | 165 |
| | *** | 2349 | 2667 | 3915 | 705 | 813 | 984 | 357 | 398 | 435 | 219 | 237 | 241 | 149 | 159 | 151 |
| 0.45 | *** | 2226 | 2407 | 3834 | 669 | 747 | 974 | 341 | 374 | 440 | 210 | 226 | 251 | 143 | 151 | 163 |
| | *** | 2291 | 2666 | 3995 | 701 | 821 | 994 | 355 | 400 | 435 | 217 | 237 | 239 | 147 | 157 | 147 |
| 0.5 | *** | 2110 | 2324 | 3879 | 651 | 734 | 975 | 333 | 367 | 435 | 204 | 220 | 246 | 138 | 147 | 158 |
| | *** | 2188 | 2615 | 3995 | 685 | 813 | 984 | 348 | 394 | 426 | 212 | 232 | 231 | 142 | 152 | 141 |
| 0.55 | *** | 1963 | 2207 | 3836 | 622 | 709 | 953 | 319 | 354 | 421 | 195 | 211 | 235 | 131 | 139 | 150 |
| | *** | 2054 | 2522 | 3915 | 658 | 790 | 954 | 334 | 380 | 409 | 202 | 221 | 219 | 134 | 144 | 131 |
| 0.6 | *** | 1795 | 2064 | 3705 | 586 | 673 | 910 | 300 | 333 | 397 | 182 | 196 | 219 | 121 | 128 | 138 |
| | *** | 1897 | 2393 | 3754 | 622 | 752 | 904 | 315 | 359 | 382 | 188 | 206 | 201 | 124 | 132 | 119 |
| 0.65 | *** | 1618 | 1899 | 3488 | 541 | 625 | 845 | 276 | 307 | 363 | 165 | 178 | 197 | 108 | 114 | 122 |
| | *** | 1727 | 2231 | 3513 | 576 | 700 | 833 | 289 | 330 | 346 | 171 | 187 | 179 | 111 | 118 | 102 |
| 0.7 | *** | 1435 | 1717 | 3185 | 488 | 566 | 758 | 246 | 273 | 320 | 144 | 155 | 171 | 92 | 97 | 103 |
| | *** | 1546 | 2038 | 3192 | 521 | 633 | 743 | 258 | 292 | 302 | 149 | 162 | 151 | 95 | 100 | 83 |
| 0.75 | *** | 1249 | 1517 | 2796 | 427 | 494 | 650 | 210 | 232 | 268 | 120 | 128 | 138 | . | . | . |
| | *** | 1355 | 1812 | 2791 | 456 | 551 | 633 | 220 | 247 | 248 | 123 | 132 | 118 | . | . | . |
| 0.8 | *** | 1056 | 1295 | 2322 | 356 | 409 | 521 | 168 | 183 | 206 | . | . | . | . | . | . |
| | *** | 1152 | 1549 | 2309 | 379 | 452 | 502 | 174 | 193 | 186 | . | . | . | . | . | . |
| 0.85 | *** | 849 | 1042 | 1764 | 271 | 306 | 372 | . | . | . | . | . | . | . | . | . |
| | *** | 927 | 1239 | 1747 | 286 | 333 | 352 | . | . | . | . | . | . | . | . | . |
| 0.9 | *** | 609 | 737 | 1124 | . | . | . | . | . | . | . | . | . | . | . | . |
| | *** | 662 | 858 | 1104 | . | . | . | . | . | . | . | . | . | . | . | . |

TABLE 3: ALPHA= 0.01  POWER= 0.8     EXPECTED ACCRUAL THRU MINIMUM FOLLOW-UP= 350

| | | DEL=.05 | | | DEL=.10 | | | DEL=.15 | | | DEL=.20 | | | DEL=.25 | | |
|---|---|---|---|---|---|---|---|---|---|---|---|---|---|---|---|---|---|
| FACT= | | 1.0 .75 | .50 .25 | .00 BIN | 1.0 .75 | .50 .25 | .00 BIN | 1.0 .75 | .50 .25 | .00 BIN | 1.0 75 | .50 .25 | .00 BIN | 1.0 .75 | .50 .25 | .00 BIN |
| PCONT=*** | | | | | REQUIRED | NUMBER OF | PATIENTS | | | | | | | | | |
| 0.05 | *** | 606 | 614 | 641 | 219 | 222 | 228 | 129 | 131 | 133 | 91 | 92 | 94 | 71 | 72 | 73 |
| | *** | 609 | 622 | 1104 | 220 | 225 | 352 | 130 | 132 | 186 | 92 | 93 | 118 | 71 | 72 | 83 |
| 0.1 | *** | 1107 | 1126 | 1237 | 351 | 361 | 382 | 191 | 195 | 202 | 127 | 129 | 133 | 94 | 96 | 97 |
| | *** | 1114 | 1154 | 1747 | 355 | 369 | 502 | 193 | 199 | 248 | 128 | 131 | 151 | 95 | 96 | 102 |
| 0.15 | *** | 1536 | 1569 | 1813 | 461 | 479 | 523 | 241 | 249 | 264 | 155 | 160 | 166 | 112 | 115 | 118 |
| | *** | 1547 | 1621 | 2309 | 468 | 496 | 633 | 244 | 256 | 302 | 157 | 163 | 179 | 113 | 116 | 119 |
| 0.2 | *** | 1871 | 1921 | 2339 | 546 | 575 | 649 | 280 | 293 | 317 | 177 | 184 | 194 | 126 | 130 | 135 |
| | *** | 1888 | 2002 | 2791 | 558 | 601 | 743 | 286 | 303 | 346 | 181 | 189 | 201 | 127 | 132 | 131 |
| 0.25 | *** | 2110 | 2181 | 2798 | 610 | 649 | 755 | 310 | 328 | 360 | 194 | 203 | 217 | 136 | 141 | 148 |
| | *** | 2134 | 2295 | 3192 | 626 | 686 | 833 | 318 | 341 | 382 | 198 | 209 | 219 | 138 | 144 | 141 |
| 0.3 | *** | 2256 | 2351 | 3182 | 652 | 702 | 842 | 330 | 353 | 395 | 205 | 216 | 234 | 143 | 149 | 157 |
| | *** | 2289 | 2503 | 3513 | 672 | 750 | 904 | 340 | 370 | 409 | 210 | 224 | 231 | 145 | 152 | 147 |
| 0.35 | *** | 2318 | 2442 | 3484 | 676 | 736 | 908 | 342 | 369 | 420 | 212 | 225 | 245 | 146 | 153 | 163 |
| | *** | 2362 | 2633 | 3754 | 700 | 794 | 954 | 354 | 389 | 426 | 218 | 234 | 239 | 149 | 157 | 151 |
| 0.4 | *** | 2309 | 2465 | 3702 | 683 | 754 | 952 | 347 | 377 | 435 | 214 | 228 | 251 | 146 | 154 | 165 |
| | *** | 2364 | 2694 | 3915 | 712 | 820 | 984 | 360 | 400 | 435 | 221 | 238 | 241 | 150 | 159 | 151 |
| 0.45 | *** | 2241 | 2432 | 3834 | 677 | 755 | 974 | 345 | 377 | 440 | 212 | 227 | 251 | 144 | 152 | 163 |
| | *** | 2310 | 2697 | 3995 | 709 | 828 | 994 | 359 | 402 | 435 | 219 | 238 | 239 | 148 | 157 | 147 |
| 0.5 | *** | 2129 | 2352 | 3879 | 659 | 743 | 975 | 337 | 371 | 435 | 206 | 222 | 246 | 139 | 147 | 158 |
| | *** | 2211 | 2649 | 3995 | 694 | 820 | 984 | 352 | 397 | 426 | 213 | 232 | 231 | 143 | 152 | 141 |
| 0.55 | *** | 1984 | 2238 | 3836 | 631 | 718 | 953 | 323 | 357 | 421 | 197 | 212 | 235 | 132 | 139 | 150 |
| | *** | 2080 | 2559 | 3915 | 668 | 797 | 954 | 338 | 383 | 409 | 204 | 222 | 219 | 135 | 144 | 131 |
| 0.6 | *** | 1820 | 2096 | 3705 | 595 | 682 | 910 | 304 | 337 | 397 | 183 | 198 | 219 | 122 | 128 | 138 |
| | *** | 1926 | 2430 | 3754 | 631 | 759 | 904 | 318 | 361 | 382 | 190 | 207 | 201 | 125 | 133 | 119 |
| 0.65 | *** | 1645 | 1933 | 3488 | 550 | 633 | 845 | 279 | 309 | 363 | 167 | 179 | 197 | 109 | 115 | 122 |
| | *** | 1757 | 2268 | 3513 | 585 | 707 | 833 | 293 | 332 | 346 | 172 | 187 | 179 | 111 | 118 | 102 |
| 0.7 | *** | 1463 | 1750 | 3184 | 497 | 573 | 758 | 249 | 275 | 320 | 146 | 156 | 171 | 93 | 97 | 103 |
| | *** | 1576 | 2073 | 3192 | 529 | 639 | 743 | 261 | 294 | 302 | 150 | 163 | 151 | 95 | 100 | 83 |
| 0.75 | *** | 1276 | 1548 | 2796 | 435 | 501 | 650 | 213 | 234 | 267 | 121 | 128 | 138 | . | . | . |
| | *** | 1384 | 1844 | 2791 | 463 | 556 | 633 | 222 | 248 | 248 | 124 | 133 | 118 | . | . | . |
| 0.8 | *** | 1080 | 1322 | 2322 | 362 | 414 | 521 | 169 | 184 | 206 | . | . | . | . | . | . |
| | *** | 1177 | 1576 | 2309 | 384 | 455 | 502 | 176 | 194 | 186 | . | . | . | . | . | . |
| 0.85 | *** | 869 | 1063 | 1764 | 275 | 309 | 372 | . | . | . | . | . | . | . | . | . |
| | *** | 948 | 1259 | 1747 | 290 | 335 | 352 | . | . | . | . | . | . | . | . | . |
| 0.9 | *** | 622 | 751 | 1124 | . | . | . | . | . | . | . | . | . | . | . | . |
| | *** | 676 | 870 | 1104 | . | . | . | . | . | . | . | . | . | . | . | . |

## TABLE 3: ALPHA= 0.01  POWER= 0.8    EXPECTED ACCRUAL THRU MINIMUM FOLLOW-UP= 375

| | | DEL=.05 | | | DEL=.10 | | | DEL=.15 | | | DEL=.20 | | | DEL=.25 | | |
|---|---|---|---|---|---|---|---|---|---|---|---|---|---|---|---|---|
| FACT= | | 1.0 .75 | .50 .25 | .00 BIN | 1.0 .75 | .50 .25 | .00 BIN | 1.0 .75 | .50 .25 | .00 BIN | 1.0 75 | .50 .25 | .00 BIN | 1.0 .75 | .50 .25 | .00 BIN |
| PCONT=*** | | | | | REQUIRED NUMBER OF PATIENTS | | | | | | | | | | | |
| 0.05 | *** | 607 | 614 | 641 | 219 | 223 | 228 | 129 | 131 | 133 | 92 | 92 | 94 | 71 | 72 | 73 |
| | *** | 610 | 623 | 1104 | 221 | 225 | 352 | 130 | 132 | 186 | 92 | 93 | 118 | 71 | 72 | 83 |
| 0.1 | *** | 1109 | 1129 | 1237 | 352 | 362 | 382 | 191 | 196 | 203 | 127 | 130 | 133 | 94 | 96 | 97 |
| | *** | 1116 | 1157 | 1747 | 356 | 370 | 502 | 193 | 199 | 248 | 128 | 131 | 151 | 95 | 96 | 102 |
| 0.15 | *** | 1538 | 1573 | 1813 | 462 | 481 | 523 | 242 | 250 | 264 | 156 | 160 | 166 | 112 | 115 | 118 |
| | *** | 1550 | 1626 | 2309 | 470 | 497 | 633 | 245 | 256 | 302 | 158 | 163 | 179 | 113 | 116 | 119 |
| 0.2 | *** | 1875 | 1928 | 2339 | 549 | 578 | 649 | 282 | 295 | 317 | 178 | 185 | 194 | 126 | 130 | 135 |
| | *** | 1893 | 2012 | 2791 | 561 | 604 | 743 | 287 | 304 | 346 | 181 | 189 | 201 | 128 | 132 | 131 |
| 0.25 | *** | 2115 | 2190 | 2798 | 613 | 653 | 755 | 312 | 329 | 360 | 195 | 204 | 217 | 136 | 141 | 148 |
| | *** | 2141 | 2308 | 3192 | 629 | 689 | 833 | 319 | 342 | 382 | 199 | 209 | 219 | 139 | 144 | 141 |
| 0.3 | *** | 2263 | 2364 | 3182 | 657 | 707 | 842 | 332 | 355 | 395 | 207 | 217 | 234 | 143 | 149 | 157 |
| | *** | 2298 | 2520 | 3513 | 677 | 754 | 904 | 342 | 371 | 409 | 212 | 225 | 231 | 146 | 153 | 147 |
| 0.35 | *** | 2328 | 2459 | 3484 | 681 | 742 | 908 | 345 | 371 | 420 | 213 | 226 | 245 | 147 | 154 | 163 |
| | *** | 2374 | 2654 | 3754 | 707 | 799 | 954 | 356 | 391 | 426 | 219 | 234 | 239 | 150 | 158 | 151 |
| 0.4 | *** | 2321 | 2485 | 3703 | 690 | 760 | 952 | 350 | 380 | 435 | 216 | 230 | 251 | 148 | 155 | 165 |
| | *** | 2380 | 2720 | 3915 | 719 | 825 | 984 | 363 | 402 | 435 | 222 | 239 | 241 | 151 | 159 | 151 |
| 0.45 | *** | 2256 | 2455 | 3834 | 685 | 763 | 974 | 348 | 380 | 440 | 214 | 229 | 251 | 145 | 153 | 163 |
| | *** | 2328 | 2726 | 3995 | 717 | 835 | 994 | 362 | 404 | 435 | 220 | 238 | 239 | 149 | 158 | 147 |
| 0.5 | *** | 2147 | 2379 | 3879 | 668 | 751 | 975 | 340 | 374 | 435 | 208 | 223 | 246 | 140 | 148 | 158 |
| | *** | 2233 | 2682 | 3995 | 703 | 827 | 984 | 355 | 399 | 426 | 215 | 233 | 231 | 144 | 153 | 141 |
| 0.55 | *** | 2006 | 2268 | 3836 | 640 | 727 | 953 | 327 | 360 | 421 | 198 | 213 | 235 | 133 | 140 | 150 |
| | *** | 2105 | 2593 | 3915 | 676 | 804 | 954 | 341 | 385 | 409 | 205 | 223 | 219 | 136 | 145 | 131 |
| 0.6 | *** | 1844 | 2128 | 3705 | 603 | 690 | 910 | 307 | 340 | 397 | 185 | 199 | 219 | 122 | 129 | 137 |
| | *** | 1953 | 2465 | 3754 | 640 | 766 | 904 | 322 | 363 | 382 | 191 | 208 | 201 | 125 | 133 | 119 |
| 0.65 | *** | 1670 | 1965 | 3488 | 558 | 641 | 845 | 283 | 312 | 363 | 168 | 180 | 197 | 109 | 115 | 122 |
| | *** | 1785 | 2303 | 3513 | 593 | 713 | 833 | 296 | 333 | 346 | 174 | 188 | 179 | 112 | 118 | 102 |
| 0.7 | *** | 1489 | 1781 | 3185 | 505 | 581 | 758 | 252 | 278 | 320 | 147 | 157 | 170 | 94 | 98 | 103 |
| | *** | 1604 | 2106 | 3192 | 537 | 645 | 743 | 264 | 296 | 302 | 152 | 163 | 151 | 95 | 100 | 83 |
| 0.75 | *** | 1301 | 1577 | 2795 | 441 | 507 | 650 | 215 | 236 | 267 | 122 | 129 | 138 | . | . | . |
| | *** | 1411 | 1874 | 2791 | 470 | 560 | 633 | 225 | 249 | 248 | 125 | 133 | 118 | . | . | . |
| 0.8 | *** | 1103 | 1347 | 2322 | 367 | 419 | 521 | 171 | 185 | 205 | . | . | . | . | . | . |
| | *** | 1202 | 1601 | 2309 | 390 | 459 | 502 | 178 | 194 | 186 | . | . | . | . | . | . |
| 0.85 | *** | 887 | 1083 | 1764 | 279 | 312 | 372 | . | . | . | . | . | . | . | . | . |
| | *** | 967 | 1277 | 1747 | 294 | 337 | 352 | . | . | . | . | . | . | . | . | . |
| 0.9 | *** | 635 | 763 | 1124 | . | . | . | . | . | . | . | . | . | . | . | . |
| | *** | 689 | 881 | 1104 | . | . | . | . | . | . | . | . | . | . | . | . |

TABLE 3: ALPHA= 0.01  POWER= 0.8     EXPECTED ACCRUAL THRU MINIMUM FOLLOW-UP= 400

| | | DEL=.05 | | | DEL=.10 | | | DEL=.15 | | | DEL=.20 | | | DEL=.25 | |
|---|---|---|---|---|---|---|---|---|---|---|---|---|---|---|---|---|
| FACT= | 1.0 .75 | .50 .25 | .00 BIN | 1.0 .75 | .50 .25 | .00 BIN | 1.0 .75 | .50 .25 | .00 BIN | 1.0 75 | .50 .25 | .00 BIN | 1.0 .75 | .50 .25 | .00 BIN |
| PCONT=*** | | | | REQUIRED NUMBER OF PATIENTS | | | | | | | | | | | |
| 0.05 *** | 607 | 615 | 641 | 220 | 223 | 228 | 129 | 131 | 133 | 92 | 92 | 94 | 71 | 72 | 73 |
| *** | 610 | 624 | 1104 | 221 | 225 | 352 | 130 | 132 | 186 | 92 | 93 | 118 | 72 | 72 | 83 |
| 0.1 *** | 1110 | 1131 | 1237 | 353 | 363 | 382 | 192 | 196 | 203 | 128 | 130 | 133 | 94 | 96 | 98 |
| *** | 1118 | 1159 | 1747 | 357 | 371 | 502 | 194 | 199 | 248 | 129 | 131 | 151 | 95 | 97 | 102 |
| 0.15 *** | 1541 | 1578 | 1813 | 464 | 483 | 523 | 243 | 251 | 264 | 156 | 161 | 166 | 113 | 115 | 118 |
| *** | 1554 | 1632 | 2309 | 472 | 498 | 633 | 246 | 256 | 302 | 158 | 163 | 179 | 114 | 116 | 119 |
| 0.2 *** | 1879 | 1935 | 2339 | 552 | 580 | 649 | 283 | 296 | 317 | 179 | 185 | 194 | 127 | 130 | 135 |
| *** | 1898 | 2021 | 2791 | 564 | 606 | 743 | 289 | 305 | 346 | 182 | 189 | 201 | 128 | 132 | 131 |
| 0.25 *** | 2120 | 2200 | 2798 | 617 | 656 | 755 | 313 | 331 | 360 | 196 | 204 | 217 | 137 | 142 | 148 |
| *** | 2148 | 2321 | 3192 | 633 | 692 | 833 | 321 | 343 | 382 | 200 | 210 | 219 | 139 | 144 | 141 |
| 0.3 *** | 2270 | 2376 | 3182 | 661 | 712 | 842 | 335 | 356 | 395 | 208 | 218 | 234 | 144 | 150 | 157 |
| *** | 2307 | 2537 | 3513 | 682 | 758 | 904 | 344 | 372 | 409 | 213 | 225 | 231 | 147 | 153 | 147 |
| 0.35 *** | 2337 | 2475 | 3484 | 687 | 748 | 908 | 348 | 373 | 420 | 215 | 227 | 245 | 148 | 154 | 163 |
| *** | 2386 | 2675 | 3754 | 712 | 804 | 954 | 359 | 392 | 426 | 220 | 235 | 239 | 151 | 158 | 151 |
| 0.4 *** | 2333 | 2504 | 3702 | 696 | 767 | 952 | 353 | 382 | 435 | 217 | 231 | 251 | 148 | 155 | 165 |
| *** | 2395 | 2744 | 3915 | 726 | 831 | 984 | 366 | 404 | 435 | 223 | 240 | 241 | 152 | 160 | 151 |
| 0.45 *** | 2271 | 2478 | 3834 | 692 | 770 | 974 | 352 | 383 | 440 | 215 | 230 | 251 | 146 | 153 | 163 |
| *** | 2347 | 2754 | 3995 | 725 | 840 | 994 | 365 | 406 | 435 | 222 | 239 | 239 | 150 | 158 | 147 |
| 0.5 *** | 2165 | 2405 | 3879 | 675 | 759 | 975 | 344 | 376 | 435 | 210 | 224 | 246 | 141 | 149 | 158 |
| *** | 2254 | 2712 | 3995 | 710 | 833 | 984 | 358 | 400 | 426 | 216 | 234 | 231 | 145 | 153 | 141 |
| 0.55 *** | 2027 | 2296 | 3836 | 648 | 735 | 953 | 330 | 363 | 421 | 200 | 214 | 235 | 134 | 140 | 150 |
| *** | 2129 | 2625 | 3915 | 685 | 811 | 954 | 345 | 387 | 409 | 207 | 224 | 219 | 137 | 145 | 131 |
| 0.6 *** | 1868 | 2157 | 3705 | 612 | 698 | 910 | 311 | 342 | 397 | 187 | 200 | 219 | 123 | 129 | 138 |
| *** | 1979 | 2498 | 3754 | 648 | 772 | 904 | 325 | 365 | 382 | 193 | 208 | 201 | 126 | 133 | 119 |
| 0.65 *** | 1695 | 1995 | 3488 | 566 | 649 | 845 | 286 | 314 | 363 | 169 | 181 | 197 | 110 | 115 | 122 |
| *** | 1813 | 2335 | 3513 | 601 | 719 | 833 | 299 | 335 | 346 | 175 | 188 | 179 | 113 | 118 | 102 |
| 0.7 *** | 1514 | 1811 | 3185 | 512 | 587 | 758 | 255 | 280 | 320 | 148 | 158 | 171 | 94 | 98 | 103 |
| *** | 1632 | 2136 | 3192 | 544 | 650 | 743 | 266 | 297 | 302 | 153 | 164 | 151 | 96 | 100 | 83 |
| 0.75 *** | 1325 | 1604 | 2796 | 448 | 513 | 650 | 218 | 237 | 267 | 122 | 129 | 138 | . | . | . |
| *** | 1437 | 1901 | 2791 | 476 | 565 | 633 | 226 | 250 | 248 | 126 | 133 | 118 | . | . | . |
| 0.8 *** | 1125 | 1371 | 2322 | 373 | 423 | 521 | 173 | 186 | 205 | . | . | . | . | . | . |
| *** | 1224 | 1624 | 2309 | 395 | 462 | 502 | 179 | 195 | 186 | . | . | . | . | . | . |
| 0.85 *** | 905 | 1102 | 1764 | 282 | 315 | 372 | . | . | . | . | . | . | . | . | . |
| *** | 986 | 1295 | 1747 | 297 | 339 | 352 | . | . | . | . | . | . | . | . | . |
| 0.9 *** | 647 | 775 | 1124 | . | . | . | . | . | . | . | . | . | . | . | . |
| *** | 701 | 891 | 1104 | . | . | . | . | . | . | . | . | . | . | . | . |

## TABLE 3: ALPHA= 0.01  POWER= 0.8      EXPECTED ACCRUAL THRU MINIMUM FOLLOW-UP= 425

| | | DEL=.05 | | | DEL=.10 | | | DEL=.15 | | | DEL=.20 | | | DEL=.25 | |
|---|---|---|---|---|---|---|---|---|---|---|---|---|---|---|---|
| FACT= | 1.0 .75 | .50 .25 | .00 BIN | 1.0 .75 | .50 .25 | .00 BIN | 1.0 .75 | .50 .25 | .00 BIN | 1.0 75 | .50 .25 | .00 BIN | 1.0 .75 | .50 .25 | .00 BIN |
| PCONT=*** | | | | | REQUIRED NUMBER OF PATIENTS | | | | | | | | | | |
| 0.05 *** | 608 | 616 | 641 | 220 | 223 | 228 | 129 | 131 | 133 | 92 | 93 | 94 | 71 | 72 | 73 |
| *** | 611 | 625 | 1104 | 221 | 225 | 352 | 130 | 132 | 186 | 92 | 93 | 118 | 71 | 72 | 83 |
| 0.1 *** | 1112 | 1133 | 1237 | 354 | 363 | 382 | 192 | 196 | 203 | 128 | 130 | 133 | 95 | 96 | 98 |
| *** | 1119 | 1162 | 1747 | 358 | 371 | 502 | 194 | 199 | 248 | 129 | 131 | 151 | 95 | 97 | 102 |
| 0.15 *** | 1543 | 1582 | 1813 | 466 | 484 | 523 | 243 | 251 | 264 | 157 | 161 | 166 | 113 | 115 | 118 |
| *** | 1557 | 1637 | 2309 | 473 | 499 | 633 | 247 | 257 | 302 | 159 | 163 | 179 | 114 | 116 | 119 |
| 0.2 *** | 1882 | 1941 | 2339 | 554 | 583 | 649 | 284 | 297 | 317 | 180 | 186 | 194 | 127 | 130 | 135 |
| *** | 1903 | 2029 | 2791 | 566 | 608 | 743 | 290 | 305 | 346 | 182 | 189 | 201 | 129 | 132 | 131 |
| 0.25 *** | 2125 | 2209 | 2798 | 620 | 660 | 756 | 315 | 332 | 360 | 197 | 205 | 217 | 137 | 142 | 148 |
| *** | 2154 | 2333 | 3192 | 637 | 695 | 833 | 323 | 344 | 382 | 201 | 210 | 219 | 139 | 145 | 141 |
| 0.3 *** | 2277 | 2389 | 3182 | 665 | 716 | 842 | 337 | 358 | 395 | 209 | 219 | 234 | 144 | 150 | 157 |
| *** | 2316 | 2552 | 3513 | 686 | 761 | 904 | 346 | 373 | 409 | 213 | 226 | 231 | 147 | 153 | 147 |
| 0.35 *** | 2346 | 2490 | 3485 | 692 | 753 | 908 | 350 | 375 | 419 | 216 | 228 | 245 | 148 | 154 | 163 |
| *** | 2397 | 2694 | 3754 | 717 | 808 | 954 | 361 | 394 | 426 | 221 | 235 | 239 | 151 | 158 | 151 |
| 0.4 *** | 2345 | 2523 | 3702 | 703 | 773 | 952 | 356 | 384 | 435 | 218 | 232 | 251 | 149 | 156 | 165 |
| *** | 2409 | 2767 | 3915 | 732 | 836 | 984 | 368 | 405 | 435 | 224 | 240 | 241 | 152 | 160 | 151 |
| 0.45 *** | 2286 | 2500 | 3834 | 699 | 777 | 974 | 355 | 385 | 440 | 217 | 231 | 251 | 147 | 154 | 163 |
| *** | 2364 | 2780 | 3995 | 731 | 846 | 994 | 368 | 408 | 435 | 223 | 240 | 239 | 150 | 158 | 147 |
| 0.5 *** | 2182 | 2430 | 3879 | 683 | 766 | 975 | 347 | 379 | 435 | 211 | 225 | 246 | 142 | 149 | 158 |
| *** | 2275 | 2740 | 3995 | 718 | 839 | 984 | 361 | 402 | 426 | 218 | 234 | 231 | 145 | 153 | 141 |
| 0.55 *** | 2047 | 2323 | 3836 | 656 | 742 | 953 | 333 | 365 | 421 | 201 | 215 | 235 | 134 | 141 | 150 |
| *** | 2152 | 2655 | 3915 | 692 | 816 | 954 | 348 | 388 | 409 | 208 | 224 | 219 | 137 | 145 | 131 |
| 0.6 *** | 1890 | 2186 | 3705 | 619 | 705 | 910 | 314 | 344 | 397 | 188 | 201 | 219 | 124 | 130 | 138 |
| *** | 2005 | 2529 | 3754 | 656 | 778 | 904 | 327 | 366 | 382 | 194 | 209 | 201 | 127 | 133 | 119 |
| 0.65 *** | 1719 | 2024 | 3488 | 574 | 655 | 845 | 289 | 317 | 363 | 171 | 182 | 197 | 111 | 116 | 122 |
| *** | 1839 | 2365 | 3513 | 609 | 724 | 833 | 301 | 336 | 346 | 176 | 189 | 179 | 113 | 119 | 102 |
| 0.7 *** | 1538 | 1838 | 3185 | 519 | 594 | 758 | 257 | 281 | 320 | 149 | 158 | 171 | 94 | 98 | 103 |
| *** | 1657 | 2165 | 3192 | 551 | 655 | 743 | 268 | 298 | 302 | 153 | 164 | 151 | 96 | 101 | 83 |
| 0.75 *** | 1348 | 1630 | 2796 | 454 | 518 | 650 | 220 | 239 | 267 | 123 | 130 | 138 | . | . | . |
| *** | 1461 | 1927 | 2791 | 482 | 569 | 633 | 228 | 251 | 248 | 126 | 134 | 118 | . | . | . |
| 0.8 *** | 1145 | 1393 | 2322 | 377 | 427 | 521 | 174 | 187 | 205 | . | . | . | . | . | . |
| *** | 1246 | 1646 | 2309 | 399 | 465 | 502 | 180 | 195 | 186 | . | . | . | . | . | . |
| 0.85 *** | 922 | 1119 | 1764 | 285 | 317 | 371 | . | . | . | . | . | . | . | . | . |
| *** | 1003 | 1311 | 1747 | 300 | 340 | 352 | . | . | . | . | . | . | . | . | . |
| 0.9 *** | 658 | 786 | 1124 | . | . | . | . | . | . | . | . | . | . | . | . |
| *** | 712 | 900 | 1104 | . | . | . | . | . | . | . | . | . | . | . | . |

TABLE 3: ALPHA= 0.01  POWER= 0.8     EXPECTED ACCRUAL THRU MINIMUM FOLLOW-UP= 450

| | DEL=.05 | | | DEL=.10 | | | DEL=.15 | | | DEL=.20 | | | DEL=.25 | | |
|---|---|---|---|---|---|---|---|---|---|---|---|---|---|---|---|
| FACT= | 1.0 .75 | .50 .25 | .00 BIN | 1.0 .75 | .50 .25 | .00 BIN | 1.0 .75 | .50 .25 | .00 BIN | 1.0 75 | .50 .25 | .00 BIN | 1.0 .75 | .50 .25 | .00 BIN |
| PCONT=*** | REQUIRED NUMBER OF PATIENTS | | | | | | | | | | | | | | |
| 0.05 *** | 608 | 617 | 641 | 220 | 223 | 228 | 130 | 131 | 133 | 92 | 93 | 93 | 72 | 72 | 73 |
| *** | 612 | 625 | 1104 | 221 | 225 | 352 | 130 | 132 | 186 | 92 | 93 | 118 | 72 | 72 | 83 |
| 0.1 *** | 1113 | 1135 | 1237 | 355 | 364 | 382 | 192 | 197 | 203 | 128 | 130 | 133 | 95 | 96 | 97 |
| *** | 1121 | 1164 | 1747 | 359 | 372 | 502 | 194 | 199 | 248 | 129 | 131 | 151 | 95 | 97 | 102 |
| 0.15 *** | 1545 | 1586 | 1813 | 467 | 486 | 523 | 244 | 252 | 264 | 157 | 161 | 166 | 113 | 115 | 118 |
| *** | 1560 | 1642 | 2309 | 475 | 500 | 633 | 248 | 257 | 302 | 159 | 163 | 179 | 114 | 117 | 119 |
| 0.2 *** | 1886 | 1947 | 2339 | 556 | 585 | 649 | 285 | 297 | 317 | 180 | 186 | 194 | 127 | 131 | 135 |
| *** | 1908 | 2037 | 2791 | 568 | 609 | 743 | 291 | 306 | 346 | 183 | 190 | 201 | 129 | 132 | 131 |
| 0.25 *** | 2130 | 2217 | 2798 | 623 | 663 | 756 | 316 | 333 | 360 | 198 | 206 | 217 | 138 | 142 | 148 |
| *** | 2161 | 2344 | 3192 | 640 | 697 | 833 | 324 | 345 | 382 | 201 | 211 | 219 | 140 | 145 | 141 |
| 0.3 *** | 2284 | 2400 | 3182 | 670 | 720 | 842 | 339 | 360 | 395 | 210 | 220 | 234 | 145 | 150 | 157 |
| *** | 2325 | 2567 | 3513 | 691 | 765 | 904 | 348 | 374 | 409 | 214 | 226 | 231 | 147 | 153 | 147 |
| 0.35 *** | 2355 | 2505 | 3484 | 697 | 758 | 908 | 352 | 377 | 420 | 217 | 228 | 245 | 149 | 155 | 163 |
| *** | 2409 | 2713 | 3754 | 723 | 812 | 954 | 363 | 395 | 426 | 222 | 236 | 239 | 152 | 158 | 151 |
| 0.4 *** | 2357 | 2541 | 3702 | 708 | 779 | 952 | 358 | 386 | 435 | 220 | 232 | 251 | 150 | 156 | 165 |
| *** | 2424 | 2789 | 3915 | 738 | 840 | 984 | 371 | 406 | 435 | 226 | 241 | 241 | 153 | 160 | 151 |
| 0.45 *** | 2300 | 2521 | 3834 | 705 | 783 | 974 | 357 | 387 | 440 | 218 | 231 | 251 | 148 | 154 | 163 |
| *** | 2382 | 2804 | 3995 | 738 | 851 | 994 | 371 | 409 | 435 | 225 | 240 | 239 | 151 | 158 | 147 |
| 0.5 *** | 2199 | 2453 | 3879 | 690 | 773 | 975 | 350 | 381 | 435 | 212 | 226 | 246 | 143 | 149 | 158 |
| *** | 2295 | 2767 | 3995 | 725 | 844 | 984 | 364 | 404 | 426 | 219 | 235 | 231 | 146 | 154 | 141 |
| 0.55 *** | 2067 | 2349 | 3836 | 663 | 748 | 953 | 336 | 367 | 421 | 203 | 216 | 235 | 135 | 141 | 150 |
| *** | 2175 | 2683 | 3915 | 699 | 822 | 954 | 350 | 390 | 409 | 209 | 225 | 219 | 138 | 145 | 131 |
| 0.6 *** | 1912 | 2213 | 3705 | 627 | 711 | 910 | 316 | 347 | 397 | 189 | 202 | 219 | 124 | 130 | 138 |
| *** | 2029 | 2558 | 3754 | 663 | 783 | 904 | 330 | 368 | 382 | 195 | 210 | 201 | 127 | 134 | 119 |
| 0.65 *** | 1742 | 2051 | 3488 | 581 | 662 | 845 | 291 | 318 | 363 | 172 | 183 | 198 | 111 | 116 | 122 |
| *** | 1864 | 2394 | 3513 | 615 | 729 | 833 | 303 | 338 | 346 | 177 | 189 | 179 | 113 | 119 | 102 |
| 0.7 *** | 1561 | 1865 | 3185 | 525 | 599 | 758 | 260 | 283 | 320 | 150 | 159 | 171 | 95 | 99 | 103 |
| *** | 1682 | 2192 | 3192 | 557 | 659 | 743 | 270 | 299 | 302 | 154 | 164 | 151 | 96 | 101 | 83 |
| 0.75 *** | 1370 | 1654 | 2795 | 460 | 523 | 650 | 221 | 240 | 267 | 124 | 130 | 138 | . | . | . |
| *** | 1484 | 1951 | 2791 | 487 | 572 | 633 | 230 | 252 | 248 | 127 | 134 | 118 | . | . | . |
| 0.8 *** | 1165 | 1414 | 2322 | 382 | 431 | 521 | 175 | 188 | 205 | . | . | . | . | . | . |
| *** | 1266 | 1666 | 2309 | 403 | 467 | 502 | 181 | 196 | 186 | . | . | . | . | . | . |
| 0.85 *** | 938 | 1135 | 1764 | 288 | 320 | 372 | . | . | . | . | . | . | . | . | . |
| *** | 1019 | 1325 | 1747 | 302 | 342 | 352 | . | . | . | . | . | . | . | . | . |
| 0.9 *** | 669 | 796 | 1124 | . | . | . | . | . | . | . | . | . | . | . | . |
| *** | 723 | 908 | 1104 | . | . | . | . | . | . | . | . | . | . | . | . |

## TABLE 3: ALPHA= 0.01  POWER= 0.8    EXPECTED ACCRUAL THRU MINIMUM FOLLOW-UP= 475

|  | | DEL=.05 | | | DEL=.10 | | | DEL=.15 | | | DEL=.20 | | | DEL=.25 | |
|---|---|---|---|---|---|---|---|---|---|---|---|---|---|---|---|---|
| FACT= | | 1.0 .75 | .50 .25 | .00 BIN | 1.0 .75 | .50 .25 | .00 BIN | 1.0 .75 | .50 .25 | .00 BIN | 1.0 75 | .50 .25 | .00 BIN | 1.0 .75 | .50 .25 | .00 BIN |
| PCONT=*** | | | | | REQUIRED NUMBER OF PATIENTS | | | | | | | | | | | |
| 0.05 | *** | 609 | 618 | 641 | 220 | 223 | 228 | 130 | 131 | 133 | 92 | 93 | 93 | 72 | 72 | 72 |
|  | *** | 612 | 626 | 1104 | 222 | 225 | 352 | 130 | 132 | 186 | 92 | 93 | 118 | 72 | 72 | 83 |
| 0.1 | *** | 1115 | 1138 | 1237 | 355 | 365 | 382 | 193 | 197 | 203 | 128 | 130 | 133 | 95 | 96 | 97 |
|  | *** | 1123 | 1166 | 1747 | 359 | 372 | 502 | 195 | 200 | 248 | 129 | 131 | 151 | 95 | 97 | 102 |
| 0.15 | *** | 1548 | 1590 | 1813 | 469 | 487 | 523 | 245 | 252 | 264 | 157 | 161 | 166 | 113 | 115 | 118 |
|  | *** | 1563 | 1647 | 2309 | 476 | 501 | 633 | 248 | 257 | 302 | 159 | 164 | 179 | 114 | 117 | 119 |
| 0.2 | *** | 1890 | 1954 | 2338 | 559 | 587 | 649 | 286 | 298 | 317 | 181 | 186 | 194 | 128 | 131 | 135 |
|  | *** | 1912 | 2045 | 2791 | 571 | 611 | 743 | 292 | 306 | 346 | 184 | 190 | 201 | 129 | 133 | 131 |
| 0.25 | *** | 2136 | 2226 | 2798 | 626 | 666 | 755 | 318 | 334 | 360 | 198 | 206 | 217 | 138 | 143 | 148 |
|  | *** | 2168 | 2355 | 3192 | 643 | 699 | 833 | 325 | 346 | 382 | 202 | 211 | 219 | 140 | 145 | 141 |
| 0.3 | *** | 2291 | 2412 | 3182 | 674 | 724 | 842 | 340 | 361 | 395 | 211 | 220 | 234 | 146 | 150 | 157 |
|  | *** | 2334 | 2581 | 3513 | 695 | 767 | 904 | 349 | 375 | 409 | 215 | 226 | 231 | 148 | 153 | 147 |
| 0.35 | *** | 2365 | 2519 | 3484 | 702 | 763 | 908 | 355 | 378 | 419 | 218 | 229 | 245 | 149 | 155 | 163 |
|  | *** | 2420 | 2730 | 3754 | 727 | 815 | 954 | 365 | 396 | 426 | 223 | 236 | 239 | 152 | 159 | 151 |
| 0.4 | *** | 2368 | 2559 | 3702 | 714 | 784 | 952 | 361 | 388 | 435 | 221 | 233 | 251 | 150 | 156 | 165 |
|  | *** | 2438 | 2810 | 3915 | 743 | 845 | 984 | 373 | 408 | 435 | 226 | 241 | 241 | 153 | 160 | 151 |
| 0.45 | *** | 2314 | 2541 | 3834 | 711 | 789 | 974 | 360 | 390 | 440 | 219 | 232 | 251 | 148 | 155 | 163 |
|  | *** | 2399 | 2828 | 3995 | 744 | 856 | 994 | 373 | 411 | 435 | 225 | 241 | 239 | 151 | 159 | 147 |
| 0.5 | *** | 2217 | 2476 | 3879 | 696 | 779 | 975 | 352 | 383 | 435 | 214 | 227 | 246 | 143 | 150 | 158 |
|  | *** | 2315 | 2793 | 3995 | 731 | 849 | 984 | 366 | 405 | 426 | 220 | 235 | 231 | 146 | 154 | 141 |
| 0.55 | *** | 2086 | 2373 | 3836 | 670 | 755 | 953 | 339 | 370 | 421 | 204 | 217 | 235 | 135 | 142 | 150 |
|  | *** | 2197 | 2710 | 3915 | 706 | 827 | 954 | 353 | 391 | 409 | 210 | 225 | 219 | 138 | 146 | 131 |
| 0.6 | *** | 1933 | 2239 | 3705 | 633 | 718 | 910 | 319 | 349 | 397 | 190 | 203 | 219 | 125 | 131 | 137 |
|  | *** | 2052 | 2585 | 3754 | 669 | 788 | 904 | 333 | 369 | 382 | 196 | 210 | 201 | 128 | 134 | 119 |
| 0.65 | *** | 1764 | 2077 | 3488 | 587 | 667 | 845 | 294 | 320 | 363 | 172 | 183 | 197 | 112 | 116 | 122 |
|  | *** | 1888 | 2420 | 3513 | 622 | 734 | 833 | 305 | 339 | 346 | 178 | 190 | 179 | 114 | 119 | 102 |
| 0.7 | *** | 1583 | 1890 | 3185 | 531 | 604 | 758 | 262 | 285 | 320 | 151 | 159 | 170 | 95 | 99 | 103 |
|  | *** | 1706 | 2217 | 3192 | 563 | 663 | 743 | 272 | 300 | 302 | 155 | 165 | 151 | 97 | 101 | 83 |
| 0.75 | *** | 1391 | 1677 | 2795 | 465 | 527 | 650 | 223 | 241 | 267 | 124 | 131 | 138 | . | . | . |
|  | *** | 1506 | 1974 | 2791 | 492 | 575 | 633 | 231 | 253 | 248 | 127 | 134 | 118 | . | . | . |
| 0.8 | *** | 1184 | 1434 | 2322 | 386 | 434 | 521 | 177 | 189 | 205 | . | . | . | . | . | . |
|  | *** | 1286 | 1685 | 2309 | 407 | 469 | 502 | 182 | 196 | 186 | . | . | . | . | . | . |
| 0.85 | *** | 953 | 1151 | 1764 | 291 | 321 | 371 | . | . | . | . | . | . | . | . | . |
|  | *** | 1035 | 1339 | 1747 | 305 | 343 | 352 | . | . | . | . | . | . | . | . | . |
| 0.9 | *** | 679 | 805 | 1124 | . | . | . | . | . | . | . | . | . | . | . | . |
|  | *** | 732 | 916 | 1104 | . | . | . | . | . | . | . | . | . | . | . | . |

TABLE 3: ALPHA= 0.01  POWER= 0.8    EXPECTED ACCRUAL THRU MINIMUM FOLLOW-UP= 500

| | | DEL=.05 | | | DEL=.10 | | | DEL=.15 | | | DEL=.20 | | | DEL=.25 | |
|---|---|---|---|---|---|---|---|---|---|---|---|---|---|---|---|---|
| FACT= | 1.0 .75 | .50 .25 | .00 BIN | 1.0 .75 | .50 .25 | .00 BIN | 1.0 .75 | .50 .25 | .00 BIN | 1.0 75 | .50 .25 | .00 BIN | 1.0 .75 | .50 .25 | .00 BIN |
| PCONT=*** | | | REQUIRED NUMBER OF PATIENTS | | | | | | | | | | | | | |
| 0.05 *** | 610 | 618 | 641 | 221 | 223 | 228 | 130 | 131 | 133 | 92 | 93 | 93 | 72 | 72 | 73 |
| *** | 613 | 627 | 1104 | 222 | 226 | 352 | 131 | 132 | 186 | 92 | 93 | 118 | 72 | 72 | 83 |
| 0.1 *** | 1116 | 1140 | 1237 | 356 | 366 | 382 | 193 | 197 | 203 | 128 | 130 | 133 | 95 | 96 | 98 |
| *** | 1125 | 1169 | 1747 | 360 | 373 | 502 | 195 | 200 | 248 | 129 | 132 | 151 | 96 | 97 | 102 |
| 0.15 *** | 1550 | 1593 | 1813 | 470 | 488 | 523 | 245 | 253 | 264 | 158 | 162 | 166 | 113 | 116 | 118 |
| *** | 1566 | 1651 | 2309 | 478 | 502 | 633 | 249 | 258 | 302 | 160 | 164 | 179 | 114 | 117 | 119 |
| 0.2 *** | 1893 | 1960 | 2339 | 561 | 589 | 649 | 287 | 299 | 317 | 181 | 187 | 194 | 128 | 131 | 135 |
| *** | 1917 | 2052 | 2791 | 573 | 612 | 743 | 293 | 307 | 346 | 184 | 190 | 201 | 129 | 133 | 131 |
| 0.25 *** | 2141 | 2235 | 2798 | 629 | 669 | 755 | 319 | 335 | 360 | 199 | 207 | 217 | 139 | 143 | 148 |
| *** | 2174 | 2366 | 3192 | 646 | 702 | 833 | 327 | 346 | 382 | 203 | 211 | 219 | 141 | 145 | 141 |
| 0.3 *** | 2298 | 2423 | 3182 | 677 | 728 | 842 | 342 | 362 | 395 | 212 | 221 | 234 | 146 | 151 | 157 |
| *** | 2343 | 2595 | 3513 | 698 | 770 | 904 | 351 | 376 | 409 | 216 | 227 | 231 | 148 | 154 | 147 |
| 0.35 *** | 2374 | 2533 | 3484 | 707 | 767 | 908 | 357 | 380 | 420 | 219 | 230 | 245 | 150 | 156 | 163 |
| *** | 2432 | 2747 | 3754 | 732 | 819 | 954 | 367 | 397 | 426 | 224 | 237 | 239 | 153 | 159 | 151 |
| 0.4 *** | 2380 | 2576 | 3703 | 719 | 789 | 952 | 363 | 390 | 435 | 222 | 234 | 251 | 151 | 157 | 165 |
| *** | 2452 | 2829 | 3915 | 748 | 848 | 984 | 375 | 409 | 435 | 228 | 242 | 241 | 154 | 161 | 151 |
| 0.45 *** | 2328 | 2561 | 3834 | 717 | 794 | 974 | 363 | 391 | 440 | 221 | 233 | 251 | 149 | 155 | 163 |
| *** | 2415 | 2850 | 3995 | 750 | 860 | 994 | 375 | 412 | 435 | 227 | 241 | 239 | 152 | 159 | 147 |
| 0.5 *** | 2233 | 2498 | 3879 | 703 | 784 | 975 | 355 | 385 | 435 | 215 | 228 | 246 | 144 | 150 | 158 |
| *** | 2334 | 2817 | 3995 | 737 | 854 | 984 | 368 | 406 | 426 | 221 | 236 | 231 | 147 | 154 | 141 |
| 0.55 *** | 2105 | 2397 | 3836 | 676 | 761 | 953 | 341 | 372 | 421 | 205 | 218 | 235 | 136 | 142 | 150 |
| *** | 2218 | 2736 | 3915 | 712 | 831 | 954 | 355 | 393 | 409 | 211 | 226 | 219 | 139 | 146 | 131 |
| 0.6 *** | 1953 | 2263 | 3705 | 640 | 723 | 910 | 322 | 350 | 397 | 191 | 203 | 219 | 126 | 131 | 138 |
| *** | 2075 | 2611 | 3754 | 676 | 793 | 904 | 335 | 370 | 382 | 197 | 210 | 201 | 128 | 134 | 119 |
| 0.65 *** | 1785 | 2102 | 3488 | 593 | 673 | 845 | 296 | 322 | 363 | 173 | 184 | 198 | 112 | 117 | 122 |
| *** | 1911 | 2446 | 3513 | 628 | 738 | 833 | 308 | 340 | 346 | 178 | 190 | 179 | 114 | 119 | 102 |
| 0.7 *** | 1604 | 1914 | 3185 | 537 | 609 | 758 | 263 | 286 | 320 | 152 | 160 | 171 | 96 | 99 | 103 |
| *** | 1728 | 2241 | 3192 | 568 | 667 | 743 | 274 | 301 | 302 | 155 | 165 | 151 | 97 | 101 | 83 |
| 0.75 *** | 1411 | 1699 | 2796 | 470 | 531 | 650 | 225 | 242 | 268 | 125 | 131 | 138 | . | . | . |
| *** | 1528 | 1995 | 2791 | 497 | 578 | 633 | 233 | 253 | 248 | 128 | 134 | 118 | . | . | . |
| 0.8 *** | 1202 | 1453 | 2322 | 390 | 437 | 521 | 178 | 189 | 205 | . | . | . | . | . | . |
| *** | 1304 | 1702 | 2309 | 411 | 472 | 502 | 183 | 197 | 186 | . | . | . | . | . | . |
| 0.85 *** | 967 | 1165 | 1764 | 293 | 323 | 372 | . | . | . | . | . | . | . | . | . |
| *** | 1049 | 1352 | 1747 | 307 | 344 | 352 | . | . | . | . | . | . | . | . | . |
| 0.9 *** | 689 | 814 | 1124 | . | . | . | . | . | . | . | . | . | . | . | . |
| *** | 742 | 923 | 1104 | . | . | . | . | . | . | . | . | . | . | . | . |

## TABLE 3: ALPHA= 0.01 POWER= 0.8 EXPECTED ACCRUAL THRU MINIMUM FOLLOW-UP= 550

| | | DEL=.02 | | | DEL=.05 | | | DEL=.10 | | | DEL=.15 | | | DEL=.20 | | |
|---|---|---|---|---|---|---|---|---|---|---|---|---|---|---|---|---|
| FACT= | | 1.0 .75 | .50 .25 | .00 BIN | 1.0 .75 | .50 .25 | .00 BIN | 1.0 .75 | .50 .25 | .00 BIN | 1.0 75 | .50 .25 | .00 BIN | 1.0 .75 | .50 .25 | .00 BIN |
| PCONT=*** | | REQUIRED NUMBER OF PATIENTS | | | | | | | | | | | | | | |
| 0.05 | *** | 2857 | 2868 | 3024 | 611 | 619 | 641 | 221 | 224 | 228 | 130 | 131 | 133 | 92 | 93 | 93 |
| | *** | 2861 | 2890 | 5651 | 614 | 627 | 1104 | 222 | 226 | 352 | 131 | 132 | 186 | 92 | 93 | 118 |
| 0.1 | *** | 5944 | 5971 | 6642 | 1119 | 1144 | 1237 | 358 | 367 | 382 | 194 | 198 | 202 | 129 | 131 | 133 |
| | *** | 5953 | 6025 | 9816 | 1128 | 1172 | 1747 | 362 | 373 | 502 | 195 | 200 | 248 | 129 | 132 | 151 |
| 0.15 | *** | 8683 | 8731 | 10273 | 1555 | 1601 | 1812 | 473 | 490 | 523 | 246 | 254 | 264 | 158 | 162 | 166 |
| | *** | 8698 | 8826 | 13479 | 1572 | 1660 | 2309 | 480 | 504 | 633 | 250 | 258 | 302 | 160 | 164 | 179 |
| 0.2 | *** | 10863 | 10937 | 13649 | 1900 | 1971 | 2338 | 565 | 593 | 649 | 289 | 300 | 316 | 182 | 187 | 194 |
| | *** | 10888 | 11085 | 16640 | 1926 | 2065 | 2791 | 577 | 615 | 743 | 294 | 308 | 346 | 184 | 190 | 201 |
| 0.25 | *** | 12429 | 12535 | 16643 | 2151 | 2251 | 2798 | 635 | 674 | 756 | 322 | 337 | 360 | 200 | 207 | 217 |
| | *** | 12464 | 12746 | 19300 | 2187 | 2385 | 3192 | 651 | 705 | 833 | 329 | 347 | 382 | 203 | 212 | 219 |
| 0.3 | *** | 13388 | 13533 | 19180 | 2312 | 2444 | 3182 | 684 | 734 | 842 | 345 | 364 | 395 | 213 | 222 | 234 |
| | *** | 13436 | 13823 | 21458 | 2360 | 2620 | 3513 | 705 | 775 | 904 | 354 | 378 | 409 | 217 | 227 | 231 |
| 0.35 | *** | 13783 | 13977 | 21221 | 2391 | 2560 | 3484 | 715 | 775 | 908 | 360 | 383 | 420 | 221 | 231 | 245 |
| | *** | 13848 | 14363 | 23113 | 2453 | 2778 | 3754 | 740 | 825 | 954 | 371 | 399 | 426 | 225 | 237 | 239 |
| 0.4 | *** | 13678 | 13930 | 22740 | 2402 | 2608 | 3702 | 729 | 798 | 952 | 367 | 393 | 435 | 224 | 235 | 251 |
| | *** | 13762 | 14433 | 24268 | 2479 | 2866 | 3915 | 758 | 855 | 984 | 379 | 411 | 435 | 229 | 242 | 241 |
| 0.45 | *** | 13145 | 13470 | 23723 | 2356 | 2598 | 3834 | 728 | 804 | 974 | 367 | 395 | 440 | 223 | 235 | 251 |
| | *** | 13253 | 14112 | 24920 | 2447 | 2892 | 3995 | 760 | 868 | 994 | 379 | 414 | 435 | 228 | 242 | 239 |
| 0.5 | *** | 12265 | 12681 | 24164 | 2265 | 2540 | 3878 | 714 | 795 | 974 | 360 | 388 | 435 | 217 | 229 | 246 |
| | *** | 12404 | 13487 | 25070 | 2370 | 2862 | 3995 | 749 | 862 | 984 | 373 | 409 | 426 | 223 | 237 | 231 |
| 0.55 | *** | 11125 | 11653 | 24058 | 2140 | 2442 | 3836 | 688 | 771 | 953 | 346 | 375 | 421 | 207 | 219 | 235 |
| | *** | 11302 | 12641 | 24719 | 2258 | 2783 | 3915 | 724 | 839 | 954 | 359 | 395 | 409 | 213 | 226 | 219 |
| 0.6 | *** | 9815 | 10481 | 23406 | 1992 | 2310 | 3705 | 652 | 734 | 910 | 326 | 354 | 397 | 193 | 204 | 219 |
| | *** | 10040 | 11651 | 23866 | 2117 | 2659 | 3754 | 687 | 800 | 904 | 338 | 372 | 382 | 198 | 211 | 201 |
| 0.65 | *** | 8432 | 9253 | 22210 | 1826 | 2148 | 3488 | 605 | 683 | 844 | 300 | 325 | 363 | 175 | 185 | 198 |
| | *** | 8716 | 10577 | 22511 | 1954 | 2493 | 3513 | 639 | 745 | 833 | 311 | 342 | 346 | 180 | 191 | 179 |
| 0.7 | *** | 7071 | 8037 | 20474 | 1645 | 1959 | 3184 | 547 | 618 | 758 | 267 | 288 | 320 | 153 | 161 | 170 |
| | *** | 7417 | 9456 | 20655 | 1771 | 2285 | 3192 | 578 | 673 | 743 | 277 | 302 | 302 | 157 | 165 | 151 |
| 0.75 | *** | 5814 | 6871 | 18202 | 1449 | 1740 | 2796 | 479 | 539 | 650 | 228 | 244 | 267 | 126 | 132 | 138 |
| | *** | 6206 | 8301 | 18296 | 1567 | 2034 | 2791 | 505 | 583 | 633 | 235 | 255 | 248 | 129 | 135 | 118 |
| 0.8 | *** | 4695 | 5753 | 15399 | 1235 | 1488 | 2322 | 397 | 442 | 521 | 179 | 191 | 206 | . | . | . |
| | *** | 5097 | 7101 | 15436 | 1339 | 1735 | 2309 | 417 | 475 | 502 | 185 | 198 | 186 | . | . | . |
| 0.85 | *** | 3689 | 4648 | 12071 | 994 | 1192 | 1764 | 298 | 327 | 371 | . | . | . | . | . | . |
| | *** | 4060 | 5816 | 12074 | 1077 | 1376 | 1747 | 311 | 346 | 352 | . | . | . | . | . | . |
| 0.9 | *** | 2720 | 3478 | 8224 | 706 | 831 | 1124 | . | . | . | . | . | . | . | . | . |
| | *** | 3017 | 4359 | 8210 | 759 | 936 | 1104 | . | . | . | . | . | . | . | . | . |
| 0.95 | *** | 1622 | 2048 | 3864 | . | . | . | . | . | . | . | . | . | . | . | . |
| | *** | 1794 | 2499 | 3844 | . | . | . | . | . | . | . | . | . | . | . | . |

TABLE 3: ALPHA= 0.01  POWER= 0.8    EXPECTED ACCRUAL THRU MINIMUM FOLLOW-UP= 600

| | | DEL=.02 | | | DEL=.05 | | | DEL=.10 | | | DEL=.15 | | | DEL=.20 | | |
|---|---|---|---|---|---|---|---|---|---|---|---|---|---|---|---|---|
| FACT= | | 1.0 .75 | .50 .25 | .00 BIN | 1.0 .75 | .50 .25 | .00 BIN | 1.0 .75 | .50 .25 | .00 BIN | 1.0 75 | .50 .25 | .00 BIN | 1.0 .75 | .50 .25 | .00 BIN |
| PCONT=*** | | | | | REQUIRED NUMBER OF PATIENTS | | | | | | | | | | | |
| 0.05 | *** | 2858 | 2870 | 3023 | 612 | 620 | 641 | 221 | 224 | 228 | 130 | 131 | 133 | 92 | 93 | 94 |
| | *** | 2862 | 2894 | 5651 | 615 | 628 | 1104 | 223 | 226 | 352 | 131 | 132 | 186 | 92 | 93 | 118 |
| 0.1 | *** | 5946 | 5976 | 6642 | 1121 | 1147 | 1237 | 359 | 368 | 382 | 194 | 198 | 202 | 129 | 131 | 133 |
| | *** | 5956 | 6035 | 9816 | 1131 | 1176 | 1747 | 363 | 374 | 502 | 196 | 200 | 248 | 130 | 132 | 151 |
| 0.15 | *** | 8687 | 8739 | 10273 | 1560 | 1608 | 1813 | 475 | 492 | 523 | 248 | 254 | 264 | 159 | 162 | 166 |
| | *** | 8704 | 8843 | 13479 | 1577 | 1667 | 2309 | 482 | 505 | 633 | 251 | 259 | 302 | 160 | 164 | 179 |
| 0.2 | *** | 10870 | 10951 | 13649 | 1907 | 1982 | 2339 | 568 | 596 | 649 | 290 | 301 | 317 | 183 | 188 | 194 |
| | *** | 10897 | 11111 | 16640 | 1935 | 2078 | 2791 | 580 | 617 | 743 | 295 | 308 | 346 | 185 | 191 | 201 |
| 0.25 | *** | 12438 | 12554 | 16642 | 2161 | 2266 | 2798 | 640 | 678 | 755 | 324 | 338 | 360 | 201 | 208 | 217 |
| | *** | 12477 | 12785 | 19300 | 2200 | 2402 | 3192 | 656 | 709 | 833 | 331 | 348 | 382 | 204 | 212 | 219 |
| 0.3 | *** | 13401 | 13559 | 19180 | 2325 | 2465 | 3182 | 691 | 740 | 842 | 348 | 366 | 395 | 214 | 223 | 233 |
| | *** | 13454 | 13876 | 21458 | 2376 | 2644 | 3513 | 712 | 779 | 904 | 356 | 379 | 409 | 218 | 227 | 231 |
| 0.35 | *** | 13801 | 14012 | 21221 | 2409 | 2585 | 3484 | 722 | 782 | 908 | 363 | 385 | 419 | 222 | 232 | 245 |
| | *** | 13871 | 14432 | 23113 | 2474 | 2807 | 3754 | 748 | 830 | 954 | 373 | 400 | 426 | 227 | 238 | 239 |
| 0.4 | *** | 13701 | 13976 | 22740 | 2423 | 2638 | 3702 | 738 | 806 | 952 | 371 | 395 | 434 | 226 | 236 | 251 |
| | *** | 13793 | 14522 | 24268 | 2504 | 2900 | 3915 | 767 | 862 | 984 | 382 | 412 | 435 | 230 | 243 | 241 |
| 0.45 | *** | 13174 | 13529 | 23723 | 2382 | 2633 | 3834 | 738 | 813 | 974 | 371 | 397 | 440 | 224 | 236 | 251 |
| | *** | 13293 | 14225 | 24920 | 2477 | 2930 | 3995 | 770 | 874 | 994 | 383 | 416 | 435 | 230 | 243 | 231 |
| 0.5 | *** | 12303 | 12756 | 24163 | 2295 | 2579 | 3878 | 724 | 804 | 974 | 364 | 391 | 435 | 219 | 230 | 246 |
| | *** | 12454 | 13625 | 25070 | 2405 | 2903 | 3995 | 759 | 869 | 984 | 376 | 410 | 426 | 224 | 238 | 231 |
| 0.55 | *** | 11173 | 11748 | 24058 | 2174 | 2483 | 3836 | 699 | 781 | 953 | 350 | 378 | 421 | 209 | 220 | 235 |
| | *** | 11366 | 12805 | 24719 | 2296 | 2826 | 3915 | 734 | 847 | 954 | 362 | 397 | 409 | 214 | 227 | 219 |
| 0.6 | *** | 9877 | 10598 | 23406 | 2029 | 2353 | 3705 | 662 | 743 | 910 | 330 | 356 | 397 | 195 | 205 | 219 |
| | *** | 10122 | 11837 | 23866 | 2157 | 2703 | 3754 | 698 | 807 | 904 | 342 | 374 | 382 | 200 | 212 | 201 |
| 0.65 | *** | 8510 | 9390 | 22210 | 1864 | 2191 | 3488 | 615 | 692 | 845 | 303 | 327 | 363 | 176 | 186 | 197 |
| | *** | 8817 | 10778 | 22511 | 1995 | 2536 | 3513 | 649 | 751 | 833 | 314 | 343 | 346 | 181 | 191 | 179 |
| 0.7 | *** | 7168 | 8191 | 20474 | 1682 | 2000 | 3184 | 557 | 626 | 758 | 270 | 290 | 320 | 154 | 161 | 170 |
| | *** | 7537 | 9664 | 20655 | 1810 | 2325 | 3192 | 587 | 679 | 743 | 280 | 304 | 302 | 157 | 166 | 151 |
| 0.75 | *** | 5926 | 7030 | 18202 | 1484 | 1778 | 2795 | 487 | 545 | 650 | 230 | 245 | 267 | 127 | 132 | 138 |
| | *** | 6337 | 8504 | 18296 | 1604 | 2069 | 2791 | 512 | 588 | 633 | 237 | 256 | 248 | 129 | 135 | 118 |
| 0.8 | *** | 4811 | 5907 | 15399 | 1266 | 1520 | 2322 | 403 | 447 | 521 | 181 | 192 | 205 | . | . | . |
| | *** | 5229 | 7288 | 15436 | 1371 | 1763 | 2309 | 423 | 478 | 502 | 186 | 198 | 186 | . | . | . |
| 0.85 | *** | 3797 | 4784 | 12071 | 1019 | 1216 | 1764 | 302 | 330 | 371 | . | . | . | . | . | . |
| | *** | 4180 | 5975 | 12074 | 1102 | 1396 | 1747 | 315 | 348 | 352 | . | . | . | . | . | . |
| 0.9 | *** | 2807 | 3582 | 8224 | 722 | 845 | 1124 | . | . | . | . | . | . | . | . | . |
| | *** | 3112 | 4475 | 8210 | 775 | 947 | 1104 | . | . | . | . | . | . | . | . | . |
| 0.95 | *** | 1673 | 2104 | 3864 | . | . | . | . | . | . | . | . | . | . | . | . |
| | *** | 1847 | 2554 | 3844 | . | . | . | . | . | . | . | . | . | . | . | . |

TABLE 3: ALPHA= 0.01  POWER= 0.8    EXPECTED ACCRUAL THRU MINIMUM FOLLOW-UP= 650

| | DEL=.02 | | | DEL=.05 | | | DEL=.10 | | | DEL=.15 | | | DEL=.20 | | |
|---|---|---|---|---|---|---|---|---|---|---|---|---|---|---|---|
| FACT= | 1.0 .75 | .50 .25 | .00 BIN | 1.0 .75 | .50 .25 | .00 BIN | 1.0 .75 | .50 .25 | .00 BIN | 1.0 75 | .50 .25 | .00 BIN | 1.0 .75 | .50 .25 | .00 BIN |
| PCONT=*** | REQUIRED NUMBER OF PATIENTS | | | | | | | | | | | | | | |
| 0.05 *** | 2859 2872 | | 3024 | 613 621 | | 641 | 222 224 | | 228 | 131 132 | | 133 | 92 93 | | 94 |
| *** | 2863 2897 | | 5651 | 616 629 | | 1104 | 223 226 | | 352 | 131 132 | | 186 | 93 93 | | 118 |
| 0.1 *** | 5949 5981 | | 6642 | 1124 1150 | | 1237 | 360 368 | | 382 | 195 198 | | 203 | 129 131 | | 133 |
| *** | 5959 6044 | | 9816 | 1134 1179 | | 1747 | 364 374 | | 502 | 197 200 | | 248 | 130 132 | | 151 |
| 0.15 *** | 8691 8748 | | 10273 | 1564 1614 | | 1813 | 477 494 | | 523 | 249 255 | | 264 | 159 162 | | 166 |
| *** | 8710 8861 | | 13479 | 1583 1674 | | 2309 | 484 506 | | 633 | 252 259 | | 302 | 161 164 | | 179 |
| 0.2 *** | 10877 10964 | | 13649 | 1914 1992 | | 2339 | 572 599 | | 649 | 292 302 | | 317 | 184 188 | | 194 |
| *** | 10906 11138 | | 16640 | 1943 2089 | | 2791 | 584 619 | | 743 | 297 309 | | 346 | 186 191 | | 201 |
| 0.25 *** | 12448 12573 | | 16642 | 2171 2281 | | 2798 | 645 682 | | 756 | 326 340 | | 361 | 202 209 | | 217 |
| *** | 12490 12823 | | 19300 | 2212 2419 | | 3192 | 661 712 | | 833 | 332 349 | | 382 | 205 212 | | 219 |
| 0.3 *** | 13414 13586 | | 19180 | 2338 2484 | | 3182 | 697 745 | | 842 | 350 368 | | 395 | 216 223 | | 234 |
| *** | 13471 13928 | | 21458 | 2393 2665 | | 3513 | 717 783 | | 904 | 359 380 | | 409 | 219 228 | | 231 |
| 0.35 *** | 13818 14047 | | 21221 | 2426 2610 | | 3484 | 730 788 | | 908 | 366 387 | | 419 | 224 233 | | 245 |
| *** | 13894 14501 | | 23113 | 2495 2833 | | 3754 | 755 835 | | 954 | 376 402 | | 426 | 228 239 | | 239 |
| 0.4 *** | 13724 14022 | | 22740 | 2445 2667 | | 3702 | 746 813 | | 952 | 374 398 | | 435 | 227 237 | | 251 |
| *** | 13823 14611 | | 24268 | 2529 2931 | | 3915 | 775 867 | | 984 | 385 414 | | 435 | 232 244 | | 241 |
| 0.45 *** | 13204 13588 | | 23723 | 2407 2666 | | 3834 | 747 821 | | 974 | 374 400 | | 440 | 226 237 | | 251 |
| *** | 13332 14336 | | 24920 | 2507 2964 | | 3995 | 779 880 | | 994 | 386 418 | | 435 | 231 244 | | 239 |
| 0.5 *** | 12341 12831 | | 24164 | 2324 2615 | | 3879 | 734 813 | | 974 | 367 394 | | 435 | 220 231 | | 246 |
| *** | 12505 13760 | | 25070 | 2438 2941 | | 3995 | 768 875 | | 984 | 380 412 | | 426 | 226 238 | | 231 |
| 0.55 *** | 11222 11842 | | 24058 | 2207 2522 | | 3836 | 709 790 | | 953 | 354 380 | | 421 | 211 221 | | 235 |
| *** | 11430 12963 | | 24719 | 2331 2866 | | 3915 | 744 853 | | 954 | 366 398 | | 409 | 216 228 | | 219 |
| 0.6 *** | 9938 10713 | | 23406 | 2064 2393 | | 3705 | 673 752 | | 910 | 333 359 | | 397 | 197 206 | | 219 |
| *** | 10203 12015 | | 23866 | 2195 2742 | | 3754 | 707 814 | | 904 | 345 376 | | 382 | 201 212 | | 201 |
| 0.65 *** | 8588 9524 | | 22210 | 1900 2231 | | 3488 | 625 699 | | 845 | 307 330 | | 363 | 178 187 | | 197 |
| *** | 8916 10971 | | 22511 | 2033 2574 | | 3513 | 658 757 | | 833 | 317 345 | | 346 | 182 192 | | 179 |
| 0.7 *** | 7263 8338 | | 20474 | 1717 2038 | | 3184 | 566 633 | | 758 | 273 292 | | 320 | 155 162 | | 171 |
| *** | 7653 9861 | | 20655 | 1848 2361 | | 3192 | 595 684 | | 743 | 282 305 | | 302 | 158 166 | | 151 |
| 0.75 *** | 6034 7182 | | 18202 | 1517 1812 | | 2796 | 494 551 | | 650 | 232 247 | | 268 | 127 132 | | 138 |
| *** | 6464 8696 | | 18296 | 1638 2101 | | 2791 | 519 592 | | 633 | 239 256 | | 248 | 130 135 | | 118 |
| 0.8 *** | 4922 6053 | | 15399 | 1295 1549 | | 2322 | 409 452 | | 522 | 183 193 | | 205 | . . | | . |
| *** | 5355 7464 | | 15436 | 1400 1789 | | 2309 | 428 481 | | 502 | 188 198 | | 186 | . . | | . |
| 0.85 *** | 3899 4912 | | 12071 | 1042 1238 | | 1764 | 306 333 | | 372 | . . | | . | . . | | . |
| *** | 4293 6124 | | 12074 | 1125 1415 | | 1747 | 318 350 | | 352 | . . | | . | . . | | . |
| 0.9 *** | 2889 3681 | | 8224 | 737 858 | | 1124 | . . | | . | . . | | . | . . | | . |
| *** | 3201 4583 | | 8210 | 790 957 | | 1104 | . . | | . | . . | | . | . . | | . |
| 0.95 *** | 1720 2156 | | 3864 | . . | | . | . . | | . | . . | | . | . . | | . |
| *** | 1897 2606 | | 3844 | . . | | . | . . | | . | . . | | . | . . | | . |

TABLE 3: ALPHA= 0.01  POWER= 0.8    EXPECTED ACCRUAL THRU MINIMUM FOLLOW-UP= 700

| | | DEL=.02 | | | DEL=.05 | | | DEL=.10 | | | DEL=.15 | | | DEL=.20 | | |
|---|---|---|---|---|---|---|---|---|---|---|---|---|---|---|---|---|---|
| FACT= | | 1.0 .75 | .50 .25 | .00 BIN | 1.0 .75 | .50 .25 | .00 BIN | 1.0 .75 | .50 .25 | .00 BIN | 1.0 75 | .50 .25 | .00 BIN | 1.0 .75 | .50 .25 | .00 BIN |
| PCONT=*** | | | | | REQUIRED NUMBER OF PATIENTS | | | | | | | | | | | |
| 0.05 | *** | 2860 2865 | 2875 2901 | 3023 5651 | 614 617 | 622 630 | 641 1104 | 222 223 | 225 226 | 228 352 | 131 131 | 131 132 | 133 186 | 92 93 | 93 93 | 93 118 |
| 0.1 | *** | 5951 5962 | 5986 6054 | 6642 9816 | 1126 1137 | 1153 1182 | 1237 1747 | 361 365 | 369 375 | 382 502 | 195 197 | 198 200 | 202 248 | 129 130 | 131 132 | 133 151 |
| 0.15 | *** | 8696 8716 | 8756 8878 | 10272 13479 | 1569 1588 | 1621 1680 | 1813 2309 | 479 486 | 495 507 | 523 633 | 249 252 | 256 259 | 264 302 | 160 161 | 163 164 | 166 179 |
| 0.2 | *** | 10883 10915 | 10978 11164 | 13649 16640 | 1921 1951 | 2002 2099 | 2339 2791 | 575 586 | 601 621 | 649 743 | 293 298 | 303 309 | 317 346 | 184 186 | 189 191 | 194 201 |
| 0.25 | *** | 12458 12503 | 12592 12861 | 16642 19300 | 2181 2223 | 2295 2434 | 2798 3192 | 649 665 | 686 714 | 755 833 | 327 334 | 341 350 | 360 382 | 203 206 | 209 212 | 217 219 |
| 0.3 | *** | 13427 13489 | 13612 13980 | 19180 21458 | 2351 2408 | 2503 2685 | 3182 3513 | 702 723 | 750 786 | 842 904 | 352 360 | 369 381 | 395 409 | 216 220 | 224 229 | 234 231 |
| 0.35 | *** | 13836 13918 | 14082 14570 | 21221 23113 | 2442 2515 | 2633 2858 | 3484 3754 | 736 761 | 794 839 | 908 954 | 369 378 | 389 403 | 420 426 | 225 229 | 234 239 | 245 239 |
| 0.4 | *** | 13746 13854 | 14068 14699 | 22740 24268 | 2465 2553 | 2694 2959 | 3702 3915 | 754 782 | 820 872 | 952 984 | 377 387 | 400 415 | 435 435 | 228 233 | 238 244 | 251 241 |
| 0.45 | *** | 13234 13372 | 13647 14446 | 23723 24920 | 2431 2534 | 2697 2996 | 3834 3995 | 755 787 | 828 885 | 974 994 | 377 389 | 402 419 | 440 435 | 227 232 | 238 244 | 251 239 |
| 0.5 | *** | 12379 12555 | 12906 13892 | 24163 25070 | 2352 2469 | 2649 2975 | 3879 3995 | 743 777 | 820 881 | 975 984 | 371 383 | 397 414 | 435 426 | 222 227 | 232 239 | 246 231 |
| 0.55 | *** | 11270 11494 | 11935 13117 | 24057 24719 | 2238 2365 | 2559 2902 | 3836 3915 | 718 753 | 797 859 | 953 954 | 357 369 | 383 400 | 421 409 | 212 217 | 222 228 | 235 219 |
| 0.6 | *** | 10000 10283 | 10825 12187 | 23406 23866 | 2096 2230 | 2431 2779 | 3705 3754 | 681 716 | 759 819 | 910 904 | 337 348 | 361 377 | 397 382 | 198 202 | 207 213 | 219 201 |
| 0.65 | *** | 8664 9014 | 9655 11153 | 22210 22511 | 1933 2068 | 2268 2610 | 3488 3513 | 633 666 | 707 762 | 845 833 | 310 320 | 331 346 | 363 346 | 179 183 | 187 192 | 198 179 |
| 0.7 | *** | 7356 7767 | 8480 10047 | 20474 20655 | 1750 1881 | 2073 2394 | 3184 3192 | 573 603 | 639 688 | 758 743 | 275 284 | 294 306 | 320 302 | 156 159 | 163 166 | 170 151 |
| 0.75 | *** | 6138 6585 | 7328 8877 | 18202 18296 | 1548 1670 | 1844 2130 | 2795 2791 | 501 526 | 556 595 | 650 633 | 234 240 | 248 257 | 268 248 | 128 131 | 133 135 | 138 118 |
| 0.8 | *** | 5029 5475 | 6191 7629 | 15399 15436 | 1322 1427 | 1576 1813 | 2322 2309 | 414 433 | 455 484 | 521 502 | 184 188 | 194 199 | 205 186 | . . | . . | . . |
| 0.85 | *** | 3997 4401 | 5033 6263 | 12071 12074 | 1063 1146 | 1259 1432 | 1764 1747 | 309 321 | 334 351 | 372 352 | . . | . . | . . | . . | . . | . . |
| 0.9 | *** | 2967 3285 | 3772 4684 | 8224 8210 | 751 803 | 870 966 | 1124 1104 | . . | . . | . . | . . | . . | . . | . . | . . | . . |
| 0.95 | *** | 1765 1944 | 2204 2652 | 3864 3844 | . . | . . | . . | . . | . . | . . | . . | . . | . . | . . | . . | . . |

TABLE 3: ALPHA= 0.01  POWER= 0.8    EXPECTED ACCRUAL THRU MINIMUM FOLLOW-UP= 750

| | | DEL=.02 | | | DEL=.05 | | | DEL=.10 | | | DEL=.15 | | | DEL=.20 | | |
|---|---|---|---|---|---|---|---|---|---|---|---|---|---|---|---|---|---|
| FACT= | | 1.0 | .50 | .00 | 1.0 | .50 | .00 | 1.0 | .50 | .00 | 1.0 | .50 | .00 | 1.0 | .50 | .00 |
| | | .75 | .25 | BIN | .75 | .25 | BIN | .75 | .25 | BIN | 75 | .25 | BIN | .75 | .25 | BIN |
| PCONT=*** | | | | | REQUIRED NUMBER OF PATIENTS | | | | | | | | | | | |
| 0.05 | *** | 2861 | 2876 | 3024 | 614 | 623 | 641 | 222 | 225 | 228 | 130 | 132 | 133 | 93 | 93 | 94 |
| | *** | 2866 | 2904 | 5651 | 618 | 630 | 1104 | 223 | 226 | 352 | 131 | 132 | 186 | 93 | 93 | 118 |
| 0.1 | *** | 5953 | 5991 | 6642 | 1129 | 1157 | 1237 | 362 | 370 | 382 | 196 | 199 | 203 | 130 | 131 | 133 |
| | *** | 5966 | 6063 | 9816 | 1140 | 1185 | 1747 | 365 | 375 | 502 | 197 | 200 | 248 | 130 | 132 | 151 |
| 0.15 | *** | 8700 | 8765 | 10272 | 1573 | 1626 | 1813 | 481 | 497 | 523 | 250 | 256 | 264 | 160 | 163 | 166 |
| | *** | 8722 | 8894 | 13479 | 1594 | 1685 | 2309 | 488 | 508 | 633 | 253 | 259 | 302 | 161 | 164 | 179 |
| 0.2 | *** | 10890 | 10991 | 13649 | 1928 | 2012 | 2339 | 578 | 604 | 649 | 295 | 304 | 317 | 185 | 189 | 194 |
| | *** | 10924 | 11191 | 16640 | 1960 | 2109 | 2791 | 589 | 622 | 743 | 299 | 310 | 346 | 187 | 191 | 201 |
| 0.25 | *** | 12467 | 12611 | 16642 | 2190 | 2308 | 2798 | 653 | 689 | 755 | 329 | 342 | 360 | 204 | 209 | 217 |
| | *** | 12515 | 12899 | 19300 | 2235 | 2447 | 3192 | 669 | 716 | 833 | 335 | 350 | 382 | 206 | 213 | 219 |
| 0.3 | *** | 13440 | 13639 | 19180 | 2364 | 2520 | 3182 | 707 | 754 | 842 | 355 | 371 | 395 | 217 | 225 | 234 |
| | *** | 13506 | 14031 | 21458 | 2423 | 2703 | 3513 | 727 | 790 | 904 | 362 | 382 | 409 | 220 | 229 | 231 |
| 0.35 | *** | 13854 | 14118 | 21221 | 2459 | 2654 | 3484 | 742 | 799 | 908 | 371 | 391 | 420 | 226 | 234 | 245 |
| | *** | 13941 | 14638 | 23113 | 2533 | 2880 | 3754 | 767 | 843 | 954 | 380 | 404 | 426 | 230 | 239 | 239 |
| 0.4 | *** | 13770 | 14114 | 22740 | 2485 | 2720 | 3702 | 760 | 825 | 952 | 379 | 402 | 435 | 229 | 239 | 251 |
| | *** | 13885 | 14785 | 24268 | 2575 | 2985 | 3915 | 789 | 876 | 984 | 390 | 416 | 435 | 234 | 244 | 241 |
| 0.45 | *** | 13263 | 13706 | 23723 | 2455 | 2726 | 3834 | 763 | 835 | 974 | 380 | 404 | 440 | 229 | 238 | 251 |
| | *** | 13411 | 14553 | 24920 | 2560 | 3026 | 3995 | 794 | 890 | 994 | 391 | 420 | 435 | 233 | 244 | 239 |
| 0.5 | *** | 12416 | 12980 | 24163 | 2379 | 2681 | 3879 | 751 | 827 | 975 | 374 | 399 | 435 | 223 | 233 | 246 |
| | *** | 12605 | 14021 | 25070 | 2498 | 3007 | 3995 | 784 | 886 | 984 | 385 | 415 | 426 | 228 | 239 | 231 |
| 0.55 | *** | 11318 | 12027 | 24057 | 2268 | 2593 | 3835 | 727 | 804 | 953 | 360 | 385 | 421 | 213 | 223 | 235 |
| | *** | 11558 | 13265 | 24719 | 2397 | 2935 | 3915 | 760 | 864 | 954 | 371 | 401 | 409 | 218 | 229 | 219 |
| 0.6 | *** | 10061 | 10936 | 23406 | 2128 | 2465 | 3705 | 690 | 766 | 910 | 340 | 363 | 397 | 199 | 208 | 219 |
| | *** | 10363 | 12352 | 23866 | 2263 | 2813 | 3754 | 724 | 824 | 904 | 350 | 378 | 382 | 203 | 213 | 201 |
| 0.65 | *** | 8741 | 9782 | 22210 | 1965 | 2303 | 3488 | 641 | 713 | 844 | 312 | 334 | 363 | 180 | 188 | 198 |
| | *** | 9111 | 11329 | 22511 | 2102 | 2643 | 3513 | 673 | 767 | 833 | 322 | 347 | 346 | 184 | 192 | 179 |
| 0.7 | *** | 7447 | 8617 | 20474 | 1781 | 2106 | 3184 | 580 | 645 | 758 | 278 | 295 | 320 | 157 | 163 | 170 |
| | *** | 7877 | 10225 | 20655 | 1914 | 2425 | 3192 | 609 | 692 | 743 | 286 | 307 | 302 | 160 | 167 | 151 |
| 0.75 | *** | 6239 | 7466 | 18202 | 1577 | 1874 | 2795 | 507 | 560 | 650 | 235 | 249 | 267 | 129 | 133 | 139 |
| | *** | 6702 | 9048 | 18296 | 1699 | 2157 | 2791 | 531 | 598 | 633 | 242 | 258 | 248 | 131 | 136 | 118 |
| 0.8 | *** | 5131 | 6322 | 15399 | 1347 | 1601 | 2322 | 419 | 459 | 521 | 185 | 194 | 205 | . | . | . |
| | *** | 5590 | 7785 | 15436 | 1453 | 1834 | 2309 | 437 | 486 | 502 | 190 | 199 | 186 | . | . | . |
| 0.85 | *** | 4090 | 5147 | 12071 | 1083 | 1278 | 1764 | 312 | 337 | 371 | . | . | . | . | . | . |
| | *** | 4503 | 6393 | 12074 | 1165 | 1447 | 1747 | 324 | 352 | 352 | . | . | . | . | . | . |
| 0.9 | *** | 3041 | 3859 | 8224 | 763 | 881 | 1124 | . | . | . | . | . | . | . | . | . |
| | *** | 3365 | 4777 | 8210 | 814 | 974 | 1104 | . | . | . | . | . | . | . | . | . |
| 0.95 | *** | 1807 | 2250 | 3864 | . | . | . | . | . | . | . | . | . | . | . | . |
| | *** | 1987 | 2695 | 3844 | . | . | . | . | . | . | . | . | . | . | . | . |

TABLE 3: ALPHA= 0.01  POWER= 0.8     EXPECTED ACCRUAL THRU MINIMUM FOLLOW-UP= 800

| | | DEL=.02 | | | DEL=.05 | | | DEL=.10 | | | DEL=.15 | | | DEL=.20 | | |
|---|---|---|---|---|---|---|---|---|---|---|---|---|---|---|---|---|---|
| FACT= | | 1.0 .75 | .50 .25 | .00 BIN | 1.0 .75 | .50 .25 | .00 BIN | 1.0 .75 | .50 .25 | .00 BIN | 1.0 75 | .50 .25 | .00 BIN | 1.0 .75 | .50 .25 | .00 BIN |
| PCONT=*** | | | | | REQUIRED | NUMBER OF | PATIENTS | | | | | | | | | |
| 0.05 | *** | 2862 | 2879 | 3023 | 615 | 624 | 641 | 223 | 225 | 228 | 131 | 132 | 133 | 92 | 93 | 94 |
| | *** | 2868 | 2907 | 5651 | 619 | 631 | 1104 | 224 | 226 | 352 | 131 | 132 | 186 | 93 | 93 | 118 |
| 0.1 | *** | 5956 | 5996 | 6642 | 1131 | 1159 | 1237 | 363 | 371 | 382 | 196 | 199 | 203 | 130 | 131 | 133 |
| | *** | 5969 | 6072 | 9816 | 1142 | 1187 | 1747 | 366 | 376 | 502 | 197 | 201 | 248 | 131 | 132 | 151 |
| 0.15 | *** | 8704 | 8774 | 10273 | 1578 | 1632 | 1813 | 483 | 498 | 523 | 251 | 256 | 264 | 161 | 163 | 166 |
| | *** | 8728 | 8911 | 13479 | 1599 | 1691 | 2309 | 490 | 509 | 633 | 253 | 260 | 302 | 162 | 165 | 179 |
| 0.2 | *** | 10897 | 11004 | 13649 | 1935 | 2021 | 2339 | 580 | 606 | 649 | 296 | 305 | 317 | 185 | 189 | 194 |
| | *** | 10933 | 11217 | 16640 | 1967 | 2117 | 2791 | 592 | 624 | 743 | 300 | 310 | 346 | 187 | 192 | 201 |
| 0.25 | *** | 12477 | 12631 | 16643 | 2200 | 2321 | 2798 | 656 | 692 | 755 | 331 | 343 | 360 | 204 | 210 | 217 |
| | *** | 12528 | 12936 | 19300 | 2246 | 2460 | 3192 | 672 | 718 | 833 | 336 | 351 | 382 | 207 | 213 | 219 |
| 0.3 | *** | 13454 | 13665 | 19180 | 2376 | 2537 | 3182 | 712 | 758 | 842 | 356 | 372 | 395 | 218 | 225 | 234 |
| | *** | 13524 | 14083 | 21458 | 2438 | 2720 | 3513 | 732 | 792 | 904 | 364 | 382 | 409 | 221 | 229 | 231 |
| 0.35 | *** | 13871 | 14153 | 21221 | 2475 | 2675 | 3484 | 748 | 804 | 908 | 373 | 392 | 420 | 227 | 235 | 245 |
| | *** | 13965 | 14705 | 23113 | 2551 | 2901 | 3754 | 772 | 846 | 954 | 382 | 405 | 426 | 231 | 240 | 239 |
| 0.4 | *** | 13793 | 14160 | 22740 | 2504 | 2744 | 3702 | 767 | 831 | 952 | 382 | 404 | 435 | 231 | 240 | 251 |
| | *** | 13915 | 14871 | 24268 | 2598 | 3010 | 3915 | 795 | 880 | 984 | 392 | 417 | 435 | 235 | 245 | 241 |
| 0.45 | *** | 13293 | 13765 | 23723 | 2478 | 2754 | 3834 | 770 | 840 | 974 | 383 | 406 | 440 | 230 | 239 | 251 |
| | *** | 13451 | 14659 | 24920 | 2586 | 3053 | 3995 | 801 | 894 | 994 | 394 | 421 | 435 | 234 | 245 | 239 |
| 0.5 | *** | 12454 | 13055 | 24163 | 2405 | 2712 | 3879 | 759 | 833 | 975 | 376 | 400 | 435 | 224 | 234 | 246 |
| | *** | 12656 | 14146 | 25070 | 2527 | 3037 | 3995 | 792 | 890 | 984 | 387 | 416 | 426 | 229 | 240 | 231 |
| 0.55 | *** | 11366 | 12119 | 24058 | 2296 | 2625 | 3836 | 735 | 811 | 953 | 363 | 387 | 421 | 214 | 224 | 235 |
| | *** | 11622 | 13409 | 24719 | 2427 | 2966 | 3915 | 768 | 868 | 954 | 374 | 402 | 409 | 219 | 229 | 219 |
| 0.6 | *** | 10122 | 11044 | 23406 | 2157 | 2498 | 3705 | 698 | 772 | 910 | 342 | 365 | 397 | 200 | 208 | 219 |
| | *** | 10442 | 12510 | 23866 | 2295 | 2844 | 3866 | 731 | 828 | 904 | 353 | 379 | 382 | 204 | 213 | 201 |
| 0.65 | *** | 8817 | 9905 | 22210 | 1995 | 2335 | 3488 | 649 | 719 | 845 | 314 | 335 | 363 | 181 | 188 | 197 |
| | *** | 9206 | 11496 | 22511 | 2133 | 2672 | 3513 | 680 | 771 | 833 | 324 | 348 | 346 | 185 | 193 | 179 |
| 0.7 | *** | 7537 | 8750 | 20474 | 1811 | 2136 | 3185 | 587 | 650 | 758 | 280 | 297 | 320 | 158 | 164 | 171 |
| | *** | 7984 | 10394 | 20655 | 1944 | 2452 | 3192 | 615 | 695 | 743 | 288 | 308 | 302 | 160 | 167 | 151 |
| 0.75 | *** | 6338 | 7600 | 18202 | 1604 | 1901 | 2796 | 513 | 565 | 650 | 237 | 250 | 267 | 129 | 133 | 138 |
| | *** | 6816 | 9210 | 18296 | 1727 | 2181 | 2791 | 536 | 601 | 633 | 243 | 258 | 248 | 131 | 136 | 118 |
| 0.8 | *** | 5229 | 6448 | 15399 | 1371 | 1624 | 2322 | 423 | 462 | 521 | 186 | 195 | 205 | . | . | . |
| | *** | 5700 | 7932 | 15436 | 1477 | 1854 | 2309 | 441 | 488 | 502 | 190 | 200 | 186 | . | . | . |
| 0.85 | *** | 4180 | 5256 | 12071 | 1102 | 1295 | 1764 | 315 | 339 | 372 | . | . | . | . | . | . |
| | *** | 4601 | 6516 | 12074 | 1184 | 1461 | 1747 | 326 | 353 | 352 | . | . | . | . | . | . |
| 0.9 | *** | 3112 | 3942 | 8224 | 775 | 891 | 1124 | . | . | . | . | . | . | . | . | . |
| | *** | 3441 | 4865 | 8210 | 826 | 981 | 1104 | . | . | . | . | . | . | . | . | . |
| 0.95 | *** | 1847 | 2292 | 3864 | . | . | . | . | . | . | . | . | . | . | . | . |
| | *** | 2029 | 2735 | 3844 | . | . | . | . | . | . | . | . | . | . | . | . |

## TABLE 3: ALPHA= 0.01  POWER= 0.8     EXPECTED ACCRUAL THRU MINIMUM FOLLOW-UP= 850

|  |  | DEL=.02 | | | DEL=.05 | | | DEL=.10 | | | DEL=.15 | | | DEL=.20 | | |
|---|---|---|---|---|---|---|---|---|---|---|---|---|---|---|---|---|
| FACT= | | 1.0<br>.75 | .50<br>.25 | .00<br>BIN | 1.0<br>.75 | .50<br>.25 | .00<br>BIN | 1.0<br>.75 | .50<br>.25 | .00<br>BIN | 1.0<br>75 | .50<br>.25 | .00<br>BIN | 1.0<br>.75 | .50<br>.25 | .00<br>BIN |
| PCONT=*** | | REQUIRED NUMBER OF PATIENTS | | | | | | | | | | | | | | |
| 0.05 | *** | 2863 | 2881 | 3024 | 616 | 624 | 641 | 223 | 225 | 228 | 131 | 132 | 133 | 93 | 93 | 94 |
|  | *** | 2869 | 2910 | 5651 | 620 | 631 | 1104 | 224 | 226 | 352 | 131 | 133 | 186 | 93 | 93 | 118 |
| 0.1 | *** | 5959 | 6001 | 6642 | 1133 | 1162 | 1236 | 363 | 371 | 382 | 196 | 199 | 203 | 130 | 131 | 133 |
|  | *** | 5972 | 6081 | 9816 | 1144 | 1189 | 1747 | 367 | 376 | 502 | 198 | 201 | 248 | 131 | 132 | 151 |
| 0.15 | *** | 8708 | 8783 | 10272 | 1582 | 1637 | 1813 | 484 | 499 | 524 | 252 | 257 | 264 | 161 | 163 | 167 |
|  | *** | 8733 | 8928 | 13479 | 1603 | 1695 | 2309 | 491 | 510 | 633 | 254 | 260 | 302 | 162 | 165 | 179 |
| 0.2 | *** | 10903 | 11018 | 13649 | 1941 | 2029 | 2339 | 583 | 607 | 649 | 297 | 305 | 317 | 186 | 189 | 194 |
|  | *** | 10942 | 11243 | 16640 | 1975 | 2126 | 2791 | 594 | 625 | 743 | 300 | 310 | 346 | 188 | 192 | 201 |
| 0.25 | *** | 12487 | 12650 | 16643 | 2209 | 2333 | 2798 | 660 | 695 | 756 | 332 | 344 | 360 | 205 | 210 | 217 |
|  | *** | 12541 | 12974 | 19300 | 2256 | 2472 | 3192 | 675 | 720 | 833 | 338 | 351 | 382 | 207 | 213 | 219 |
| 0.3 | *** | 13467 | 13691 | 19180 | 2389 | 2552 | 3182 | 716 | 762 | 842 | 358 | 373 | 395 | 219 | 225 | 233 |
|  | *** | 13542 | 14133 | 21458 | 2451 | 2735 | 3513 | 736 | 795 | 904 | 365 | 383 | 409 | 222 | 229 | 231 |
| 0.35 | *** | 13889 | 14188 | 21221 | 2490 | 2694 | 3485 | 753 | 808 | 907 | 375 | 394 | 419 | 227 | 236 | 245 |
|  | *** | 13989 | 14772 | 23113 | 2569 | 2920 | 3754 | 777 | 849 | 954 | 384 | 406 | 426 | 231 | 240 | 239 |
| 0.4 | *** | 13815 | 14205 | 22740 | 2523 | 2767 | 3703 | 773 | 836 | 952 | 384 | 405 | 435 | 232 | 240 | 251 |
|  | *** | 13945 | 14955 | 24268 | 2618 | 3032 | 3915 | 801 | 883 | 984 | 394 | 418 | 435 | 236 | 245 | 241 |
| 0.45 | *** | 13322 | 13823 | 23723 | 2500 | 2780 | 3834 | 777 | 846 | 974 | 385 | 408 | 440 | 231 | 240 | 252 |
|  | *** | 13490 | 14761 | 24920 | 2610 | 3079 | 3995 | 807 | 898 | 994 | 395 | 422 | 435 | 235 | 245 | 239 |
| 0.5 | *** | 12492 | 13128 | 24163 | 2430 | 2740 | 3879 | 766 | 839 | 974 | 379 | 402 | 435 | 225 | 235 | 246 |
|  | *** | 12706 | 14268 | 25070 | 2553 | 3064 | 3995 | 798 | 894 | 984 | 390 | 417 | 426 | 230 | 240 | 231 |
| 0.55 | *** | 11414 | 12209 | 24058 | 2323 | 2655 | 3836 | 742 | 816 | 953 | 365 | 389 | 421 | 215 | 224 | 235 |
|  | *** | 11685 | 13549 | 24719 | 2456 | 2994 | 3915 | 775 | 872 | 954 | 376 | 403 | 409 | 220 | 229 | 219 |
| 0.6 | *** | 10183 | 11151 | 23406 | 2186 | 2529 | 3705 | 705 | 778 | 910 | 344 | 366 | 397 | 201 | 209 | 219 |
|  | *** | 10520 | 12663 | 23866 | 2325 | 2873 | 3754 | 737 | 832 | 904 | 355 | 380 | 382 | 205 | 214 | 201 |
| 0.65 | *** | 8892 | 10024 | 22210 | 2024 | 2365 | 3488 | 655 | 724 | 845 | 317 | 337 | 363 | 182 | 189 | 197 |
|  | *** | 9299 | 11656 | 22511 | 2163 | 2700 | 3513 | 686 | 774 | 833 | 326 | 349 | 346 | 185 | 193 | 179 |
| 0.7 | *** | 7625 | 8877 | 20474 | 1838 | 2165 | 3184 | 594 | 655 | 758 | 281 | 298 | 320 | 158 | 164 | 171 |
|  | *** | 8089 | 10555 | 20655 | 1973 | 2478 | 3192 | 621 | 698 | 743 | 289 | 308 | 302 | 161 | 167 | 151 |
| 0.75 | *** | 6432 | 7728 | 18202 | 1630 | 1927 | 2796 | 518 | 569 | 650 | 239 | 252 | 267 | 130 | 134 | 138 |
|  | *** | 6925 | 9365 | 18296 | 1753 | 2204 | 2791 | 541 | 604 | 633 | 244 | 259 | 248 | 131 | 136 | 118 |
| 0.8 | *** | 5324 | 6568 | 15399 | 1393 | 1646 | 2322 | 427 | 464 | 521 | 187 | 195 | 205 | . | . | . |
|  | *** | 5805 | 8072 | 15436 | 1499 | 1872 | 2309 | 444 | 490 | 502 | 191 | 200 | 186 | . | . | . |
| 0.85 | *** | 4265 | 5360 | 12071 | 1119 | 1311 | 1765 | 317 | 340 | 372 | . | . | . | . | . | . |
|  | *** | 4694 | 6632 | 12074 | 1201 | 1473 | 1747 | 328 | 355 | 352 | . | . | . | . | . | . |
| 0.9 | *** | 3179 | 4020 | 8224 | 786 | 900 | 1124 | . | . | . | . | . | . | . | . | . |
|  | *** | 3513 | 4948 | 8210 | 836 | 988 | 1104 | . | . | . | . | . | . | . | . | . |
| 0.95 | *** | 1885 | 2331 | 3864 | . | . | . | . | . | . | . | . | . | . | . | . |
|  | *** | 2067 | 2772 | 3844 | . | . | . | . | . | . | . | . | . | . | . | . |

TABLE 3: ALPHA= 0.01  POWER= 0.8    EXPECTED ACCRUAL THRU MINIMUM FOLLOW-UP= 900

| | | DEL=.02 | | | DEL=.05 | | | DEL=.10 | | | DEL=.15 | | | DEL=.20 | | |
|---|---|---|---|---|---|---|---|---|---|---|---|---|---|---|---|---|
| FACT= | | 1.0 .75 | .50 .25 | .00 BIN | 1.0 .75 | .50 .25 | .00 BIN | 1.0 .75 | .50 .25 | .00 BIN | 1.0 75 | .50 .25 | .00 BIN | 1.0 .75 | .50 .25 | .00 BIN |
| PCONT=*** | | | | | REQUIRED NUMBER OF PATIENTS | | | | | | | | | | | |
| 0.05 | *** | 2864 | 2882 | 3024 | 617 | 625 | 641 | 223 | 225 | 228 | 131 | 132 | 133 | 92 | 93 | 93 |
| | *** | 2871 | 2913 | 5651 | 621 | 632 | 1104 | 224 | 226 | 352 | 131 | 132 | 186 | 93 | 93 | 118 |
| 0.1 | *** | 5961 | 6005 | 6642 | 1135 | 1164 | 1236 | 364 | 371 | 382 | 197 | 199 | 203 | 130 | 131 | 133 |
| | *** | 5976 | 6090 | 9816 | 1147 | 1191 | 1747 | 368 | 376 | 502 | 198 | 201 | 248 | 131 | 132 | 151 |
| 0.15 | *** | 8713 | 8792 | 10272 | 1586 | 1642 | 1812 | 486 | 500 | 523 | 252 | 257 | 264 | 161 | 163 | 166 |
| | *** | 8739 | 8945 | 13479 | 1608 | 1700 | 2309 | 492 | 510 | 633 | 254 | 260 | 302 | 162 | 165 | 179 |
| 0.2 | *** | 10910 | 11031 | 13649 | 1947 | 2037 | 2339 | 585 | 609 | 649 | 297 | 306 | 317 | 186 | 190 | 194 |
| | *** | 10950 | 11269 | 16640 | 1982 | 2133 | 2791 | 596 | 626 | 743 | 301 | 311 | 346 | 188 | 192 | 201 |
| 0.25 | *** | 12496 | 12669 | 16642 | 2217 | 2344 | 2798 | 663 | 697 | 756 | 333 | 345 | 360 | 206 | 210 | 217 |
| | *** | 12554 | 13011 | 19300 | 2267 | 2483 | 3192 | 678 | 722 | 833 | 338 | 352 | 382 | 208 | 213 | 219 |
| 0.3 | *** | 13480 | 13718 | 19180 | 2400 | 2567 | 3182 | 720 | 765 | 842 | 360 | 374 | 395 | 219 | 226 | 234 |
| | *** | 13559 | 14184 | 21458 | 2465 | 2750 | 3513 | 740 | 797 | 904 | 366 | 384 | 409 | 222 | 230 | 231 |
| 0.35 | *** | 13906 | 14223 | 21221 | 2504 | 2712 | 3484 | 758 | 812 | 908 | 377 | 395 | 420 | 228 | 236 | 245 |
| | *** | 14012 | 14837 | 23113 | 2585 | 2938 | 3754 | 782 | 852 | 954 | 386 | 406 | 426 | 232 | 240 | 239 |
| 0.4 | *** | 13838 | 14251 | 22740 | 2541 | 2789 | 3702 | 779 | 840 | 952 | 386 | 406 | 434 | 233 | 241 | 251 |
| | *** | 13976 | 15039 | 24268 | 2638 | 3054 | 3915 | 806 | 886 | 984 | 396 | 419 | 435 | 236 | 245 | 241 |
| 0.45 | *** | 13352 | 13881 | 23723 | 2521 | 2804 | 3834 | 783 | 851 | 974 | 387 | 409 | 440 | 231 | 240 | 251 |
| | *** | 13529 | 14862 | 24920 | 2633 | 3102 | 3995 | 813 | 901 | 994 | 397 | 423 | 435 | 236 | 245 | 239 |
| 0.5 | *** | 12530 | 13201 | 24164 | 2453 | 2767 | 3879 | 773 | 845 | 974 | 381 | 404 | 435 | 226 | 235 | 246 |
| | *** | 12756 | 14388 | 25070 | 2579 | 3090 | 3995 | 804 | 898 | 984 | 392 | 418 | 426 | 230 | 240 | 231 |
| 0.55 | *** | 11462 | 12297 | 24058 | 2349 | 2683 | 3836 | 748 | 822 | 953 | 368 | 390 | 421 | 216 | 225 | 235 |
| | *** | 11748 | 13683 | 24719 | 2484 | 3021 | 3915 | 781 | 876 | 954 | 378 | 404 | 409 | 220 | 230 | 219 |
| 0.6 | *** | 10243 | 11255 | 23406 | 2213 | 2558 | 3705 | 711 | 783 | 910 | 347 | 368 | 397 | 201 | 209 | 219 |
| | *** | 10598 | 12810 | 23866 | 2353 | 2899 | 3754 | 743 | 836 | 904 | 356 | 381 | 382 | 206 | 214 | 201 |
| 0.65 | *** | 8965 | 10141 | 22210 | 2051 | 2394 | 3488 | 662 | 729 | 845 | 318 | 338 | 363 | 182 | 189 | 198 |
| | *** | 9390 | 11810 | 22511 | 2191 | 2726 | 3513 | 692 | 777 | 833 | 327 | 350 | 346 | 186 | 193 | 179 |
| 0.7 | *** | 7710 | 9000 | 20474 | 1865 | 2192 | 3185 | 599 | 659 | 758 | 283 | 299 | 320 | 159 | 164 | 171 |
| | *** | 8191 | 10709 | 20655 | 2000 | 2502 | 3192 | 626 | 701 | 743 | 290 | 309 | 302 | 162 | 167 | 151 |
| 0.75 | *** | 6525 | 7851 | 18201 | 1654 | 1951 | 2795 | 523 | 572 | 650 | 240 | 252 | 267 | 130 | 134 | 138 |
| | *** | 7030 | 9513 | 18296 | 1778 | 2225 | 2791 | 545 | 606 | 633 | 245 | 259 | 248 | 132 | 136 | 118 |
| 0.8 | *** | 5415 | 6683 | 15399 | 1414 | 1666 | 2322 | 431 | 467 | 521 | 188 | 196 | 206 | . | . | . |
| | *** | 5907 | 8205 | 15436 | 1520 | 1889 | 2309 | 447 | 491 | 502 | 192 | 200 | 186 | . | . | . |
| 0.85 | *** | 4348 | 5459 | 12071 | 1135 | 1325 | 1764 | 320 | 342 | 371 | . | . | . | . | . | . |
| | *** | 4784 | 6742 | 12074 | 1216 | 1485 | 1747 | 330 | 355 | 352 | . | . | . | . | . | . |
| 0.9 | *** | 3243 | 4094 | 8224 | 796 | 908 | 1124 | . | . | . | . | . | . | . | . | . |
| | *** | 3582 | 5025 | 8210 | 845 | 994 | 1104 | . | . | . | . | . | . | . | . | . |
| 0.95 | *** | 1920 | 2368 | 3864 | . | . | . | . | . | . | . | . | . | . | . | . |
| | *** | 2105 | 2806 | 3844 | . | . | . | . | . | . | . | . | . | . | . | . |

## TABLE 3: ALPHA= 0.01  POWER= 0.8    EXPECTED ACCRUAL THRU MINIMUM FOLLOW-UP= 950

| | | DEL=.02 | | | DEL=.05 | | | DEL=.10 | | | DEL=.15 | | | DEL=.20 | | |
|---|---|---|---|---|---|---|---|---|---|---|---|---|---|---|---|---|---|
| FACT= | | 1.0 .75 | .50 .25 | .00 BIN | 1.0 .75 | .50 .25 | .00 BIN | 1.0 .75 | .50 .25 | .00 BIN | 1.0 75 | .50 .25 | .00 BIN | 1.0 .75 | .50 .25 | .00 BIN |
| PCONT=*** | | | | REQUIRED NUMBER OF PATIENTS | | | | | | | | | | | |
| 0.05 | *** | 2865 | 2884 | 3023 | 618 | 626 | 641 | 223 | 225 | 228 | 131 | 132 | 133 | 93 | 93 | 93 |
| | *** | 2871 | 2915 | 5651 | 621 | 633 | 1104 | 224 | 226 | 352 | 131 | 133 | 186 | 93 | 93 | 118 |
| 0.1 | *** | 5963 | 6010 | 6642 | 1138 | 1166 | 1237 | 365 | 372 | 382 | 197 | 200 | 203 | 130 | 131 | 133 |
| | *** | 5979 | 6099 | 9816 | 1150 | 1193 | 1747 | 368 | 376 | 502 | 198 | 201 | 248 | 131 | 132 | 151 |
| 0.15 | *** | 8717 | 8800 | 10273 | 1590 | 1647 | 1813 | 487 | 501 | 523 | 253 | 257 | 264 | 161 | 163 | 166 |
| | *** | 8745 | 8961 | 13479 | 1612 | 1704 | 2309 | 494 | 511 | 633 | 255 | 260 | 302 | 162 | 165 | 179 |
| 0.2 | *** | 10917 | 11045 | 13649 | 1953 | 2044 | 2338 | 587 | 610 | 648 | 298 | 306 | 317 | 186 | 190 | 194 |
| | *** | 10959 | 11294 | 16640 | 1989 | 2140 | 2791 | 598 | 627 | 743 | 302 | 311 | 346 | 188 | 192 | 201 |
| 0.25 | *** | 12506 | 12688 | 16642 | 2226 | 2355 | 2798 | 666 | 699 | 755 | 334 | 346 | 361 | 206 | 211 | 217 |
| | *** | 12567 | 13047 | 19300 | 2276 | 2493 | 3192 | 680 | 723 | 833 | 339 | 352 | 382 | 209 | 214 | 219 |
| 0.3 | *** | 13493 | 13744 | 19180 | 2412 | 2581 | 3182 | 724 | 767 | 842 | 361 | 375 | 395 | 220 | 226 | 234 |
| | *** | 13577 | 14233 | 21458 | 2478 | 2763 | 3513 | 743 | 799 | 904 | 368 | 384 | 409 | 223 | 230 | 231 |
| 0.35 | *** | 13924 | 14258 | 21221 | 2519 | 2730 | 3484 | 762 | 815 | 908 | 378 | 396 | 419 | 229 | 236 | 245 |
| | *** | 14035 | 14902 | 23113 | 2602 | 2955 | 3754 | 786 | 854 | 954 | 387 | 407 | 426 | 233 | 241 | 239 |
| 0.4 | *** | 13861 | 14296 | 22740 | 2559 | 2810 | 3702 | 784 | 844 | 952 | 388 | 407 | 435 | 234 | 241 | 251 |
| | *** | 14007 | 15120 | 24268 | 2658 | 3073 | 3915 | 811 | 889 | 984 | 397 | 420 | 435 | 237 | 246 | 241 |
| 0.45 | *** | 13382 | 13940 | 23723 | 2541 | 2828 | 3834 | 789 | 856 | 974 | 390 | 410 | 440 | 232 | 241 | 251 |
| | *** | 13568 | 14961 | 24920 | 2655 | 3125 | 3995 | 818 | 904 | 994 | 399 | 424 | 435 | 236 | 246 | 239 |
| 0.5 | *** | 12568 | 13273 | 24163 | 2476 | 2793 | 3878 | 779 | 849 | 975 | 383 | 405 | 435 | 227 | 235 | 246 |
| | *** | 12806 | 14504 | 25070 | 2604 | 3114 | 3995 | 810 | 901 | 984 | 393 | 419 | 426 | 231 | 241 | 231 |
| 0.55 | *** | 11510 | 12385 | 24058 | 2373 | 2710 | 3836 | 755 | 827 | 953 | 369 | 391 | 421 | 217 | 225 | 235 |
| | *** | 11811 | 13815 | 24719 | 2510 | 3046 | 3915 | 787 | 879 | 954 | 380 | 405 | 409 | 221 | 230 | 219 |
| 0.6 | *** | 10303 | 11357 | 23406 | 2238 | 2585 | 3705 | 717 | 788 | 910 | 349 | 369 | 397 | 203 | 210 | 219 |
| | *** | 10674 | 12952 | 23866 | 2380 | 2924 | 3754 | 749 | 838 | 904 | 358 | 382 | 382 | 206 | 215 | 201 |
| 0.65 | *** | 9039 | 10254 | 22210 | 2077 | 2420 | 3488 | 667 | 733 | 844 | 320 | 338 | 363 | 183 | 190 | 197 |
| | *** | 9480 | 11958 | 22511 | 2218 | 2750 | 3513 | 697 | 780 | 833 | 329 | 350 | 346 | 186 | 193 | 179 |
| 0.7 | *** | 7794 | 9120 | 20474 | 1890 | 2217 | 3184 | 604 | 663 | 758 | 285 | 300 | 320 | 159 | 165 | 171 |
| | *** | 8290 | 10857 | 20655 | 2025 | 2524 | 3192 | 631 | 704 | 743 | 292 | 310 | 302 | 162 | 167 | 151 |
| 0.75 | *** | 6615 | 7969 | 18202 | 1677 | 1974 | 2795 | 527 | 576 | 650 | 241 | 253 | 267 | 131 | 134 | 139 |
| | *** | 7133 | 9653 | 18296 | 1801 | 2244 | 2791 | 549 | 608 | 633 | 247 | 260 | 248 | 133 | 136 | 118 |
| 0.8 | *** | 5504 | 6794 | 15399 | 1434 | 1685 | 2322 | 433 | 469 | 521 | 189 | 196 | 205 | . | . | . |
| | *** | 6005 | 8332 | 15436 | 1540 | 1904 | 2309 | 450 | 492 | 502 | 192 | 201 | 186 | . | . | . |
| 0.85 | *** | 4427 | 5554 | 12071 | 1151 | 1339 | 1764 | 321 | 343 | 371 | . | . | . | . | . | . |
| | *** | 4870 | 6847 | 12074 | 1231 | 1495 | 1747 | 331 | 356 | 352 | . | . | . | . | . | . |
| 0.9 | *** | 3306 | 4165 | 8224 | 805 | 916 | 1124 | . | . | . | . | . | . | . | . | . |
| | *** | 3648 | 5099 | 8210 | 854 | 999 | 1104 | . | . | . | . | . | . | . | . | . |
| 0.95 | *** | 1955 | 2404 | 3864 | . | . | . | . | . | . | . | . | . | . | . | . |
| | *** | 2139 | 2838 | 3844 | . | . | . | . | . | . | . | . | . | . | . | . |

TABLE 3: ALPHA= 0.01  POWER= 0.8    EXPECTED ACCRUAL THRU MINIMUM FOLLOW-UP= 1000

| | | DEL=.02 | | | DEL=.05 | | | DEL=.10 | | | DEL=.15 | | | DEL=.20 | | |
|---|---|---|---|---|---|---|---|---|---|---|---|---|---|---|---|---|
| FACT= | | 1.0 .75 | .50 .25 | .00 BIN | 1.0 .75 | .50 .25 | .00 BIN | 1.0 .75 | .50 .25 | .00 BIN | 1.0 75 | .50 .25 | .00 BIN | 1.0 .75 | .50 .25 | .00 BIN |
| PCONT=*** | | | | | REQUIRED NUMBER OF PATIENTS | | | | | | | | | | | |
| 0.05 | *** | 2866 | 2886 | 3023 | 618 | 626 | 641 | 223 | 226 | 228 | 131 | 132 | 133 | 93 | 93 | 93 |
| | *** | 2873 | 2918 | 5651 | 622 | 633 | 1104 | 225 | 226 | 352 | 131 | 133 | 186 | 93 | 93 | 118 |
| 0.1 | *** | 5966 | 6015 | 6642 | 1140 | 1169 | 1236 | 366 | 373 | 382 | 197 | 200 | 203 | 130 | 131 | 133 |
| | *** | 5983 | 6108 | 9816 | 1151 | 1195 | 1747 | 369 | 377 | 502 | 198 | 201 | 248 | 131 | 132 | 151 |
| 0.15 | *** | 8721 | 8809 | 10273 | 1593 | 1651 | 1813 | 488 | 502 | 523 | 253 | 258 | 264 | 161 | 164 | 166 |
| | *** | 8751 | 8977 | 13479 | 1616 | 1708 | 2309 | 495 | 511 | 633 | 255 | 261 | 302 | 163 | 165 | 179 |
| 0.2 | *** | 10924 | 11058 | 13650 | 1960 | 2052 | 2339 | 589 | 612 | 649 | 299 | 306 | 316 | 187 | 190 | 194 |
| | *** | 10968 | 11320 | 16640 | 1996 | 2146 | 2791 | 600 | 628 | 743 | 303 | 311 | 346 | 188 | 192 | 201 |
| 0.25 | *** | 12515 | 12708 | 16643 | 2235 | 2366 | 2798 | 669 | 701 | 755 | 335 | 346 | 360 | 206 | 211 | 216 |
| | *** | 12580 | 13084 | 19300 | 2286 | 2503 | 3192 | 683 | 725 | 833 | 340 | 353 | 382 | 209 | 214 | 219 |
| 0.3 | *** | 13506 | 13771 | 19180 | 2423 | 2595 | 3182 | 728 | 770 | 842 | 362 | 376 | 395 | 221 | 226 | 234 |
| | *** | 13595 | 14283 | 21458 | 2490 | 2776 | 3513 | 746 | 801 | 904 | 369 | 385 | 409 | 223 | 230 | 231 |
| 0.35 | *** | 13941 | 14293 | 21221 | 2533 | 2747 | 3485 | 767 | 819 | 908 | 380 | 397 | 420 | 230 | 237 | 245 |
| | *** | 14059 | 14966 | 23113 | 2618 | 2971 | 3754 | 790 | 856 | 954 | 388 | 407 | 426 | 233 | 241 | 239 |
| 0.4 | *** | 13885 | 14342 | 22740 | 2576 | 2830 | 3703 | 789 | 848 | 952 | 390 | 409 | 435 | 234 | 241 | 251 |
| | *** | 14038 | 15200 | 24268 | 2676 | 3092 | 3915 | 815 | 891 | 984 | 399 | 421 | 435 | 238 | 246 | 241 |
| 0.45 | *** | 13411 | 13998 | 23723 | 2561 | 2850 | 3834 | 794 | 860 | 974 | 391 | 412 | 440 | 233 | 241 | 251 |
| | *** | 13608 | 15058 | 24920 | 2676 | 3146 | 3995 | 823 | 908 | 994 | 401 | 425 | 435 | 237 | 246 | 239 |
| 0.5 | *** | 12606 | 13345 | 24163 | 2498 | 2817 | 3879 | 785 | 854 | 975 | 385 | 406 | 435 | 228 | 236 | 246 |
| | *** | 12856 | 14616 | 25070 | 2627 | 3136 | 3995 | 815 | 904 | 984 | 395 | 420 | 426 | 232 | 241 | 231 |
| 0.55 | *** | 11558 | 12472 | 24058 | 2397 | 2736 | 3836 | 761 | 831 | 953 | 371 | 393 | 421 | 218 | 226 | 235 |
| | *** | 11873 | 13941 | 24719 | 2535 | 3070 | 3915 | 792 | 882 | 954 | 381 | 406 | 409 | 221 | 230 | 219 |
| 0.6 | *** | 10363 | 11457 | 23406 | 2263 | 2611 | 3705 | 723 | 793 | 910 | 350 | 370 | 397 | 203 | 210 | 219 |
| | *** | 10750 | 13090 | 23866 | 2406 | 2948 | 3754 | 755 | 842 | 904 | 360 | 383 | 382 | 206 | 215 | 201 |
| 0.65 | *** | 9111 | 10365 | 22210 | 2102 | 2446 | 3488 | 673 | 738 | 845 | 322 | 340 | 363 | 184 | 190 | 198 |
| | *** | 9568 | 12101 | 22511 | 2244 | 2773 | 3513 | 702 | 783 | 833 | 330 | 351 | 346 | 187 | 194 | 179 |
| 0.7 | *** | 7877 | 9235 | 20474 | 1914 | 2241 | 3185 | 609 | 666 | 758 | 286 | 301 | 320 | 160 | 165 | 171 |
| | *** | 8386 | 10999 | 20655 | 2050 | 2545 | 3192 | 635 | 706 | 743 | 293 | 310 | 302 | 162 | 168 | 151 |
| 0.75 | *** | 6703 | 8084 | 18202 | 1699 | 1995 | 2796 | 531 | 578 | 650 | 242 | 253 | 268 | 131 | 135 | 138 |
| | *** | 7231 | 9788 | 18296 | 1823 | 2262 | 2791 | 553 | 610 | 633 | 248 | 260 | 248 | 133 | 136 | 118 |
| 0.8 | *** | 5590 | 6900 | 15399 | 1453 | 1702 | 2322 | 437 | 471 | 521 | 190 | 197 | 205 | . | . | . |
| | *** | 6100 | 8453 | 15436 | 1558 | 1919 | 2309 | 453 | 494 | 502 | 193 | 201 | 186 | . | . | . |
| 0.85 | *** | 4503 | 5645 | 12071 | 1165 | 1352 | 1765 | 323 | 344 | 371 | . | . | . | . | . | . |
| | *** | 4953 | 6946 | 12074 | 1246 | 1505 | 1747 | 333 | 357 | 352 | . | . | . | . | . | . |
| 0.9 | *** | 3365 | 4232 | 8224 | 815 | 923 | 1124 | . | . | . | . | . | . | . | . | . |
| | *** | 3711 | 5169 | 8210 | 863 | 1005 | 1104 | . | . | . | . | . | . | . | . | . |
| 0.95 | *** | 1987 | 2437 | 3864 | . | . | . | . | . | . | . | . | . | . | . | . |
| | *** | 2173 | 2868 | 3844 | . | . | . | . | . | . | . | . | . | . | . | . |

# TABLE 3: ALPHA= 0.01  POWER= 0.8    EXPECTED ACCRUAL THRU MINIMUM FOLLOW-UP= 1100

| | | DEL=.02 | | | DEL=.05 | | | DEL=.10 | | | DEL=.15 | | | DEL=.20 | | |
|---|---|---|---|---|---|---|---|---|---|---|---|---|---|---|---|---|---|
| FACT= | | 1.0 .75 | .50 .25 | .00 BIN | 1.0 .75 | .50 .25 | .00 BIN | 1.0 .75 | .50 .25 | .00 BIN | 1.0 75 | .50 .25 | .00 BIN | 1.0 .75 | .50 .25 | .00 BIN |
| PCONT=*** | | REQUIRED NUMBER OF PATIENTS | | | | | | | | | | | | | | |
| 0.05 | *** | 2868 | 2890 | 3024 | 620 | 627 | 642 | 224 | 225 | 228 | 131 | 132 | 133 | 93 | 93 | 93 |
| | *** | 2876 | 2923 | 5651 | 623 | 633 | 1104 | 225 | 227 | 352 | 131 | 133 | 186 | 93 | 93 | 118 |
| 0.1 | *** | 5971 | 6025 | 6642 | 1143 | 1172 | 1237 | 367 | 373 | 382 | 197 | 200 | 202 | 131 | 131 | 133 |
| | *** | 5989 | 6124 | 9816 | 1156 | 1198 | 1747 | 370 | 377 | 502 | 199 | 201 | 248 | 131 | 132 | 151 |
| 0.15 | *** | 8731 | 8826 | 10273 | 1600 | 1660 | 1812 | 490 | 504 | 523 | 254 | 258 | 264 | 162 | 164 | 166 |
| | *** | 8762 | 9008 | 13479 | 1625 | 1715 | 2309 | 496 | 512 | 633 | 256 | 261 | 302 | 163 | 165 | 179 |
| 0.2 | *** | 10938 | 11085 | 13649 | 1971 | 2065 | 2338 | 593 | 615 | 648 | 300 | 307 | 316 | 187 | 191 | 194 |
| | *** | 10986 | 11369 | 16640 | 2009 | 2159 | 2791 | 603 | 630 | 743 | 303 | 312 | 346 | 189 | 192 | 201 |
| 0.25 | *** | 12534 | 12746 | 16642 | 2251 | 2385 | 2798 | 674 | 705 | 756 | 337 | 347 | 360 | 207 | 212 | 217 |
| | *** | 12605 | 13155 | 19300 | 2304 | 2520 | 3192 | 688 | 727 | 833 | 342 | 353 | 382 | 209 | 214 | 219 |
| 0.3 | *** | 13533 | 13823 | 19180 | 2444 | 2620 | 3182 | 734 | 775 | 842 | 364 | 378 | 395 | 221 | 227 | 234 |
| | *** | 13630 | 14379 | 21458 | 2514 | 2799 | 3513 | 752 | 804 | 904 | 371 | 386 | 409 | 224 | 230 | 231 |
| 0.35 | *** | 13977 | 14363 | 21221 | 2560 | 2778 | 3484 | 775 | 825 | 907 | 383 | 399 | 419 | 231 | 237 | 245 |
| | *** | 14106 | 15091 | 23113 | 2647 | 3000 | 3754 | 797 | 860 | 954 | 390 | 408 | 426 | 234 | 241 | 239 |
| 0.4 | *** | 13930 | 14433 | 22740 | 2608 | 2866 | 3702 | 797 | 855 | 951 | 393 | 411 | 434 | 235 | 242 | 251 |
| | *** | 14099 | 15355 | 24268 | 2711 | 3126 | 3915 | 824 | 896 | 984 | 401 | 422 | 435 | 239 | 246 | 241 |
| 0.45 | *** | 13470 | 14112 | 23723 | 2598 | 2892 | 3834 | 804 | 868 | 974 | 395 | 414 | 440 | 235 | 242 | 251 |
| | *** | 13686 | 15246 | 24920 | 2716 | 3184 | 3995 | 833 | 912 | 994 | 404 | 426 | 435 | 238 | 246 | 239 |
| 0.5 | *** | 12681 | 13487 | 24164 | 2540 | 2862 | 3878 | 795 | 862 | 974 | 389 | 408 | 435 | 229 | 236 | 246 |
| | *** | 12956 | 14833 | 25070 | 2671 | 3178 | 3995 | 825 | 910 | 984 | 398 | 421 | 426 | 233 | 241 | 231 |
| 0.55 | *** | 11653 | 12640 | 24058 | 2442 | 2783 | 3836 | 771 | 840 | 953 | 375 | 395 | 421 | 219 | 226 | 235 |
| | *** | 11997 | 14184 | 24719 | 2582 | 3112 | 3915 | 802 | 888 | 954 | 384 | 407 | 409 | 223 | 230 | 219 |
| 0.6 | *** | 10481 | 11651 | 23406 | 2310 | 2659 | 3705 | 734 | 800 | 910 | 353 | 372 | 397 | 204 | 211 | 219 |
| | *** | 10899 | 13351 | 23866 | 2454 | 2991 | 3754 | 764 | 847 | 904 | 362 | 384 | 382 | 208 | 214 | 201 |
| 0.65 | *** | 9252 | 10576 | 22210 | 2149 | 2493 | 3488 | 683 | 745 | 844 | 324 | 342 | 363 | 185 | 191 | 197 |
| | *** | 9740 | 12371 | 22511 | 2292 | 2814 | 3513 | 711 | 788 | 833 | 333 | 351 | 346 | 188 | 194 | 179 |
| 0.7 | *** | 8037 | 9456 | 20474 | 1959 | 2285 | 3184 | 618 | 673 | 758 | 288 | 302 | 320 | 161 | 165 | 170 |
| | *** | 8573 | 11267 | 20655 | 2095 | 2583 | 3192 | 643 | 710 | 743 | 295 | 311 | 302 | 163 | 168 | 151 |
| 0.75 | *** | 6871 | 8301 | 18202 | 1740 | 2034 | 2795 | 538 | 583 | 650 | 244 | 254 | 268 | 131 | 135 | 138 |
| | *** | 7421 | 10042 | 18296 | 1864 | 2294 | 2791 | 559 | 613 | 633 | 249 | 261 | 248 | 133 | 136 | 118 |
| 0.8 | *** | 5753 | 7101 | 15399 | 1488 | 1735 | 2322 | 442 | 475 | 521 | 191 | 197 | 206 | . | . | . |
| | *** | 6279 | 8679 | 15436 | 1593 | 1944 | 2309 | 458 | 496 | 502 | 194 | 202 | 186 | . | . | . |
| 0.85 | *** | 4648 | 5816 | 12071 | 1192 | 1376 | 1764 | 327 | 346 | 371 | . | . | . | . | . | . |
| | *** | 5109 | 7132 | 12074 | 1271 | 1523 | 1747 | 336 | 358 | 352 | . | . | . | . | . | . |
| 0.9 | *** | 3477 | 4359 | 8224 | 830 | 936 | 1124 | . | . | . | . | . | . | . | . | . |
| | *** | 3831 | 5298 | 8210 | 877 | 1013 | 1104 | . | . | . | . | . | . | . | . | . |
| 0.95 | *** | 2048 | 2498 | 3864 | . | . | . | . | . | . | . | . | . | . | . | . |
| | *** | 2235 | 2923 | 3844 | . | . | . | . | . | . | . | . | . | . | . | . |

TABLE 3: ALPHA= 0.01  POWER= 0.8    EXPECTED ACCRUAL THRU MINIMUM FOLLOW-UP= 1200

| | | DEL=.02 | | | DEL=.05 | | | DEL=.10 | | | DEL=.15 | | | DEL=.20 | | |
|---|---|---|---|---|---|---|---|---|---|---|---|---|---|---|---|---|---|
| FACT= | | 1.0 .75 | .50 .25 | .00 BIN | 1.0 .75 | .50 .25 | .00 BIN | 1.0 .75 | .50 .25 | .00 BIN | 1.0 75 | .50 .25 | .00 BIN | 1.0 .75 | .50 .25 | .00 BIN |
| PCONT=*** | | | | REQUIRED NUMBER OF PATIENTS | | | | | | | | | | | | |
| 0.05 | *** | 2870 | 2893 | 3023 | 620 | 628 | 641 | 224 | 226 | 228 | 131 | 132 | 133 | 93 | 93 | 94 |
| | *** | 2878 | 2928 | 5651 | 624 | 634 | 1104 | 225 | 226 | 352 | 132 | 133 | 186 | 93 | 93 | 118 |
| 0.1 | *** | 5976 | 6034 | 6642 | 1147 | 1176 | 1237 | 367 | 373 | 382 | 198 | 200 | 202 | 130 | 132 | 133 |
| | *** | 5995 | 6139 | 9816 | 1159 | 1200 | 1747 | 370 | 377 | 502 | 199 | 201 | 248 | 131 | 132 | 151 |
| 0.15 | *** | 8739 | 8843 | 10273 | 1608 | 1667 | 1813 | 492 | 505 | 523 | 254 | 259 | 264 | 162 | 164 | 166 |
| | *** | 8773 | 9039 | 13479 | 1632 | 1720 | 2309 | 498 | 513 | 633 | 256 | 261 | 302 | 163 | 165 | 179 |
| 0.2 | *** | 10951 | 11111 | 13649 | 1982 | 2077 | 2338 | 595 | 617 | 649 | 301 | 308 | 316 | 187 | 190 | 194 |
| | *** | 11004 | 11418 | 16640 | 2020 | 2169 | 2791 | 605 | 631 | 743 | 304 | 312 | 346 | 189 | 192 | 201 |
| 0.25 | *** | 12553 | 12784 | 16642 | 2266 | 2402 | 2798 | 678 | 709 | 755 | 338 | 348 | 360 | 208 | 212 | 217 |
| | *** | 12631 | 13225 | 19300 | 2320 | 2536 | 3192 | 692 | 729 | 833 | 343 | 354 | 382 | 210 | 214 | 219 |
| 0.3 | *** | 13559 | 13876 | 19180 | 2464 | 2644 | 3181 | 739 | 779 | 842 | 366 | 379 | 394 | 223 | 227 | 233 |
| | *** | 13665 | 14473 | 21458 | 2536 | 2821 | 3513 | 757 | 806 | 904 | 372 | 386 | 409 | 225 | 230 | 231 |
| 0.35 | *** | 14011 | 14432 | 21220 | 2585 | 2806 | 3484 | 781 | 830 | 907 | 385 | 400 | 419 | 232 | 238 | 245 |
| | *** | 14152 | 15212 | 23113 | 2674 | 3025 | 3754 | 803 | 863 | 954 | 392 | 409 | 426 | 235 | 241 | 239 |
| 0.4 | *** | 13976 | 14522 | 22740 | 2638 | 2899 | 3702 | 805 | 862 | 952 | 395 | 412 | 434 | 236 | 243 | 250 |
| | *** | 14159 | 15505 | 24268 | 2744 | 3157 | 3915 | 831 | 900 | 984 | 403 | 423 | 435 | 239 | 247 | 241 |
| 0.45 | *** | 13529 | 14225 | 23723 | 2633 | 2929 | 3834 | 813 | 874 | 974 | 397 | 415 | 439 | 235 | 243 | 251 |
| | *** | 13765 | 15424 | 24920 | 2754 | 3217 | 3995 | 840 | 916 | 994 | 406 | 427 | 435 | 239 | 247 | 239 |
| 0.5 | *** | 12756 | 13624 | 24163 | 2579 | 2903 | 3878 | 804 | 869 | 974 | 391 | 410 | 435 | 230 | 238 | 246 |
| | *** | 13054 | 15040 | 25070 | 2711 | 3214 | 3995 | 833 | 914 | 984 | 400 | 422 | 426 | 234 | 241 | 231 |
| 0.55 | *** | 11748 | 12805 | 24058 | 2483 | 2826 | 3835 | 781 | 847 | 953 | 378 | 397 | 421 | 220 | 227 | 235 |
| | *** | 12118 | 14413 | 24719 | 2624 | 3150 | 3915 | 811 | 892 | 954 | 386 | 408 | 409 | 223 | 231 | 219 |
| 0.6 | *** | 10597 | 11837 | 23406 | 2353 | 2703 | 3705 | 743 | 807 | 910 | 356 | 374 | 397 | 205 | 211 | 219 |
| | *** | 11044 | 13594 | 23866 | 2497 | 3028 | 3754 | 772 | 851 | 904 | 364 | 385 | 382 | 208 | 215 | 201 |
| 0.65 | *** | 9390 | 10778 | 22210 | 2191 | 2536 | 3488 | 691 | 751 | 844 | 327 | 343 | 363 | 186 | 191 | 197 |
| | *** | 9904 | 12622 | 22511 | 2335 | 2850 | 3513 | 718 | 792 | 833 | 334 | 352 | 346 | 188 | 194 | 179 |
| 0.7 | *** | 8191 | 9664 | 20473 | 1999 | 2325 | 3184 | 625 | 679 | 758 | 290 | 304 | 320 | 161 | 166 | 170 |
| | *** | 8749 | 11515 | 20655 | 2136 | 2616 | 3192 | 650 | 713 | 743 | 297 | 311 | 302 | 163 | 168 | 151 |
| 0.75 | *** | 7030 | 8504 | 18202 | 1777 | 2069 | 2795 | 545 | 588 | 650 | 245 | 256 | 267 | 132 | 135 | 138 |
| | *** | 7600 | 10276 | 18296 | 1901 | 2323 | 2791 | 565 | 616 | 633 | 250 | 261 | 248 | 133 | 136 | 118 |
| 0.8 | *** | 5907 | 7288 | 15399 | 1520 | 1763 | 2322 | 447 | 478 | 521 | 192 | 198 | 205 | . | . | . |
| | *** | 6448 | 8888 | 15436 | 1624 | 1967 | 2309 | 462 | 498 | 502 | 195 | 202 | 186 | . | . | . |
| 0.85 | *** | 4783 | 5975 | 12071 | 1216 | 1396 | 1764 | 330 | 348 | 371 | . | . | . | . | . | . |
| | *** | 5256 | 7302 | 12074 | 1294 | 1538 | 1747 | 338 | 359 | 352 | . | . | . | . | . | . |
| 0.9 | *** | 3582 | 4475 | 8224 | 845 | 947 | 1124 | . | . | . | . | . | . | . | . | . |
| | *** | 3941 | 5415 | 8210 | 891 | 1021 | 1104 | . | . | . | . | . | . | . | . | . |
| 0.95 | *** | 2104 | 2554 | 3864 | . | . | . | . | . | . | . | . | . | . | . | . |
| | *** | 2291 | 2972 | 3844 | . | . | . | . | . | . | . | . | . | . | . | . |

## TABLE 3: ALPHA= 0.01  POWER= 0.8    EXPECTED ACCRUAL THRU MINIMUM FOLLOW-UP= 1300

| | | DEL=.02 | | | DEL=.05 | | | DEL=.10 | | | DEL=.15 | | | DEL=.20 | |
|---|---|---|---|---|---|---|---|---|---|---|---|---|---|---|---|---|
| FACT= | 1.0 .75 | .50 .25 | .00 BIN | 1.0 .75 | .50 .25 | .00 BIN | 1.0 .75 | .50 .25 | .00 BIN | 1.0 75 | .50 .25 | .00 BIN | 1.0 .75 | .50 .25 | .00 BIN |

PCONT=***          REQUIRED NUMBER OF PATIENTS

| PCONT | | 1.0/.75 | .50/.25 | .00/BIN | 1.0/.75 | .50/.25 | .00/BIN | 1.0/.75 | .50/.25 | .00/BIN | 1.0/75 | .50/.25 | .00/BIN | 1.0/.75 | .50/.25 | .00/BIN |
|---|---|---|---|---|---|---|---|---|---|---|---|---|---|---|---|---|
| 0.05 | *** | 2872 | 2897 | 3023 | 622 | 629 | 641 | 224 | 226 | 228 | 132 | 133 | 133 | 93 | 94 | 94 |
| | *** | 2881 | 2931 | 5651 | 625 | 635 | 1104 | 225 | 227 | 352 | 132 | 133 | 186 | 93 | 94 | 118 |
| 0.1 | *** | 5981 | 6044 | 6642 | 1150 | 1179 | 1237 | 368 | 375 | 382 | 198 | 200 | 202 | 131 | 132 | 133 |
| | *** | 6002 | 6155 | 9816 | 1163 | 1202 | 1747 | 371 | 378 | 502 | 199 | 201 | 248 | 132 | 133 | 151 |
| 0.15 | *** | 8747 | 8860 | 10273 | 1615 | 1674 | 1813 | 494 | 506 | 523 | 255 | 259 | 264 | 162 | 164 | 167 |
| | *** | 8786 | 9068 | 13479 | 1639 | 1726 | 2309 | 500 | 514 | 633 | 257 | 262 | 302 | 163 | 165 | 179 |
| 0.2 | *** | 10964 | 11138 | 13649 | 1992 | 2089 | 2338 | 599 | 619 | 648 | 302 | 309 | 317 | 188 | 191 | 194 |
| | *** | 11022 | 11465 | 16640 | 2032 | 2178 | 2791 | 608 | 632 | 743 | 305 | 313 | 346 | 189 | 193 | 201 |
| 0.25 | *** | 12574 | 12823 | 16643 | 2281 | 2419 | 2798 | 682 | 712 | 756 | 340 | 349 | 361 | 209 | 212 | 217 |
| | *** | 12656 | 13292 | 19300 | 2337 | 2550 | 3192 | 695 | 731 | 833 | 344 | 354 | 382 | 211 | 214 | 219 |
| 0.3 | *** | 13586 | 13928 | 19180 | 2484 | 2665 | 3182 | 745 | 783 | 842 | 368 | 380 | 395 | 224 | 228 | 234 |
| | *** | 13700 | 14564 | 21458 | 2557 | 2839 | 3513 | 762 | 809 | 904 | 374 | 387 | 409 | 226 | 231 | 231 |
| 0.35 | *** | 14047 | 14501 | 21221 | 2610 | 2833 | 3484 | 788 | 835 | 908 | 388 | 401 | 419 | 233 | 239 | 245 |
| | *** | 14199 | 15329 | 23113 | 2700 | 3048 | 3754 | 809 | 866 | 954 | 394 | 410 | 426 | 236 | 241 | 239 |
| 0.4 | *** | 14022 | 14611 | 22740 | 2668 | 2931 | 3703 | 813 | 867 | 952 | 398 | 414 | 435 | 237 | 244 | 251 |
| | *** | 14220 | 15650 | 24268 | 2775 | 3183 | 3915 | 838 | 903 | 984 | 406 | 423 | 435 | 240 | 247 | 241 |
| 0.45 | *** | 13588 | 14337 | 23723 | 2666 | 2964 | 3834 | 821 | 880 | 974 | 400 | 418 | 440 | 237 | 244 | 251 |
| | *** | 13843 | 15596 | 24920 | 2788 | 3248 | 3995 | 848 | 921 | 994 | 408 | 428 | 435 | 240 | 247 | 239 |
| 0.5 | *** | 12831 | 13760 | 24164 | 2616 | 2941 | 3879 | 812 | 875 | 974 | 394 | 412 | 435 | 232 | 238 | 246 |
| | *** | 13153 | 15236 | 25070 | 2749 | 3247 | 3995 | 841 | 918 | 984 | 403 | 422 | 426 | 235 | 242 | 231 |
| 0.55 | *** | 11842 | 12964 | 24057 | 2522 | 2866 | 3836 | 790 | 853 | 953 | 380 | 398 | 421 | 221 | 227 | 235 |
| | *** | 12239 | 14629 | 24719 | 2664 | 3184 | 3915 | 818 | 896 | 954 | 388 | 409 | 409 | 224 | 232 | 219 |
| 0.6 | *** | 10713 | 12015 | 23406 | 2393 | 2742 | 3705 | 752 | 813 | 910 | 359 | 375 | 396 | 206 | 212 | 219 |
| | *** | 11186 | 13825 | 23866 | 2538 | 3062 | 3754 | 780 | 856 | 904 | 367 | 386 | 382 | 209 | 215 | 201 |
| 0.65 | *** | 9524 | 10970 | 22210 | 2231 | 2574 | 3488 | 700 | 757 | 845 | 330 | 344 | 363 | 187 | 192 | 198 |
| | *** | 10064 | 12858 | 22511 | 2375 | 2883 | 3513 | 726 | 796 | 833 | 336 | 354 | 346 | 189 | 194 | 179 |
| 0.7 | *** | 8338 | 9860 | 20474 | 2038 | 2361 | 3184 | 633 | 683 | 758 | 292 | 305 | 320 | 162 | 166 | 171 |
| | *** | 8919 | 11747 | 20655 | 2174 | 2645 | 3192 | 656 | 717 | 743 | 298 | 312 | 302 | 164 | 168 | 151 |
| 0.75 | *** | 7182 | 8696 | 18202 | 1812 | 2101 | 2796 | 551 | 591 | 650 | 247 | 256 | 267 | 133 | 135 | 138 |
| | *** | 7769 | 10494 | 18296 | 1935 | 2349 | 2791 | 570 | 618 | 633 | 251 | 262 | 248 | 134 | 136 | 118 |
| 0.8 | *** | 6052 | 7464 | 15399 | 1550 | 1789 | 2321 | 452 | 481 | 522 | 193 | 198 | 206 | . | . | . |
| | *** | 6607 | 9081 | 15436 | 1653 | 1987 | 2309 | 466 | 500 | 502 | 196 | 201 | 186 | . | . | . |
| 0.85 | *** | 4912 | 6124 | 12071 | 1238 | 1415 | 1764 | 332 | 349 | 371 | . | . | . | . | . | . |
| | *** | 5393 | 7459 | 12074 | 1316 | 1552 | 1747 | 341 | 360 | 352 | . | . | . | . | . | . |
| 0.9 | *** | 3681 | 4583 | 8224 | 858 | 957 | 1124 | . | . | . | . | . | . | . | . | . |
| | *** | 4045 | 5523 | 8210 | 903 | 1028 | 1104 | . | . | . | . | . | . | . | . | . |
| 0.95 | *** | 2156 | 2606 | 3864 | . | . | . | . | . | . | . | . | . | . | . | . |
| | *** | 2344 | 3016 | 3844 | . | . | . | . | . | . | . | . | . | . | . | . |

TABLE 3: ALPHA= 0.01  POWER= 0.8    EXPECTED ACCRUAL THRU MINIMUM FOLLOW-UP= 1400

| | | DEL=.02 | | | DEL=.05 | | | DEL=.10 | | | DEL=.15 | | | DEL=.20 | | |
|---|---|---|---|---|---|---|---|---|---|---|---|---|---|---|---|---|
| FACT= | | 1.0 .75 | .50 .25 | .00 BIN | 1.0 .75 | .50 .25 | .00 BIN | 1.0 .75 | .50 .25 | .00 BIN | 1.0 75 | .50 .25 | .00 BIN | 1.0 .75 | .50 .25 | .00 BIN |
| PCONT=*** | | REQUIRED NUMBER OF PATIENTS | | | | | | | | | | | | | | |
| 0.05 | *** | 2874 | 2901 | 3023 | 622 | 630 | 641 | 225 | 226 | 228 | 131 | 132 | 133 | 93 | 93 | 94 |
| | *** | 2884 | 2936 | 5651 | 626 | 635 | 1104 | 226 | 227 | 352 | 132 | 133 | 186 | 93 | 94 | 118 |
| 0.1 | *** | 5986 | 6054 | 6642 | 1153 | 1182 | 1236 | 369 | 374 | 381 | 199 | 200 | 202 | 131 | 132 | 133 |
| | *** | 6009 | 6169 | 9816 | 1165 | 1204 | 1747 | 372 | 378 | 502 | 199 | 201 | 248 | 131 | 132 | 151 |
| 0.15 | *** | 8756 | 8878 | 10272 | 1620 | 1680 | 1813 | 495 | 507 | 523 | 255 | 259 | 264 | 163 | 164 | 166 |
| | *** | 8797 | 9096 | 13479 | 1645 | 1731 | 2309 | 501 | 514 | 633 | 257 | 262 | 302 | 164 | 165 | 179 |
| 0.2 | *** | 10978 | 11164 | 13649 | 2002 | 2099 | 2339 | 601 | 621 | 648 | 303 | 309 | 317 | 189 | 192 | 194 |
| | *** | 11040 | 11511 | 16640 | 2042 | 2187 | 2791 | 610 | 633 | 743 | 306 | 312 | 346 | 190 | 192 | 201 |
| 0.25 | *** | 12592 | 12861 | 16642 | 2295 | 2433 | 2798 | 686 | 714 | 755 | 341 | 350 | 360 | 209 | 213 | 217 |
| | *** | 12682 | 13358 | 19300 | 2351 | 2562 | 3192 | 699 | 732 | 833 | 345 | 354 | 382 | 211 | 214 | 219 |
| 0.3 | *** | 13612 | 13980 | 19180 | 2502 | 2684 | 3181 | 750 | 787 | 842 | 369 | 381 | 395 | 224 | 228 | 234 |
| | *** | 13736 | 14653 | 21458 | 2577 | 2856 | 3513 | 766 | 811 | 904 | 375 | 388 | 409 | 226 | 231 | 231 |
| 0.35 | *** | 14082 | 14570 | 21220 | 2633 | 2858 | 3484 | 794 | 839 | 907 | 389 | 402 | 420 | 234 | 239 | 245 |
| | *** | 14246 | 15442 | 23113 | 2725 | 3069 | 3754 | 815 | 869 | 954 | 395 | 410 | 426 | 236 | 241 | 239 |
| 0.4 | *** | 14068 | 14699 | 22739 | 2694 | 2959 | 3702 | 820 | 871 | 952 | 400 | 416 | 435 | 238 | 244 | 251 |
| | *** | 14282 | 15788 | 24268 | 2803 | 3208 | 3915 | 843 | 906 | 984 | 407 | 424 | 435 | 241 | 248 | 241 |
| 0.45 | *** | 13647 | 14445 | 23723 | 2697 | 2996 | 3834 | 828 | 885 | 974 | 402 | 419 | 440 | 238 | 244 | 251 |
| | *** | 13920 | 15760 | 24920 | 2820 | 3276 | 3995 | 854 | 924 | 994 | 410 | 429 | 435 | 241 | 248 | 239 |
| 0.5 | *** | 12906 | 13892 | 24163 | 2649 | 2975 | 3879 | 820 | 881 | 975 | 396 | 414 | 435 | 232 | 239 | 246 |
| | *** | 13249 | 15422 | 25070 | 2784 | 3277 | 3995 | 848 | 921 | 984 | 404 | 423 | 426 | 235 | 242 | 231 |
| 0.55 | *** | 11935 | 13117 | 24057 | 2558 | 2901 | 3836 | 797 | 858 | 953 | 382 | 400 | 421 | 222 | 228 | 235 |
| | *** | 12356 | 14834 | 24719 | 2701 | 3215 | 3915 | 825 | 899 | 954 | 391 | 409 | 409 | 225 | 232 | 219 |
| 0.6 | *** | 10825 | 12187 | 23405 | 2431 | 2779 | 3706 | 759 | 819 | 910 | 361 | 377 | 397 | 207 | 213 | 219 |
| | *** | 11323 | 14041 | 23866 | 2576 | 3093 | 3754 | 787 | 858 | 904 | 368 | 387 | 382 | 210 | 216 | 201 |
| 0.65 | *** | 9655 | 11154 | 22210 | 2268 | 2610 | 3488 | 707 | 762 | 844 | 332 | 346 | 363 | 187 | 192 | 198 |
| | *** | 10216 | 13079 | 22511 | 2411 | 2912 | 3513 | 732 | 799 | 833 | 339 | 354 | 346 | 190 | 194 | 179 |
| 0.7 | *** | 8480 | 10047 | 20474 | 2073 | 2394 | 3184 | 639 | 688 | 758 | 294 | 306 | 320 | 163 | 166 | 171 |
| | *** | 9080 | 11964 | 20655 | 2209 | 2672 | 3192 | 661 | 719 | 743 | 300 | 312 | 302 | 164 | 168 | 151 |
| 0.75 | *** | 7328 | 8877 | 18202 | 1844 | 2131 | 2796 | 556 | 595 | 650 | 248 | 257 | 268 | 133 | 136 | 138 |
| | *** | 7930 | 10698 | 18296 | 1966 | 2371 | 2791 | 574 | 620 | 633 | 253 | 262 | 248 | 134 | 136 | 118 |
| 0.8 | *** | 6191 | 7629 | 15399 | 1576 | 1813 | 2321 | 455 | 484 | 521 | 193 | 199 | 206 | . | . | . |
| | *** | 6758 | 9260 | 15436 | 1678 | 2005 | 2309 | 469 | 501 | 502 | 196 | 202 | 186 | . | . | . |
| 0.85 | *** | 5033 | 6262 | 12071 | 1259 | 1431 | 1764 | 334 | 351 | 372 | . | . | . | . | . | . |
| | *** | 5523 | 7604 | 12074 | 1334 | 1564 | 1747 | 342 | 360 | 352 | . | . | . | . | . | . |
| 0.9 | *** | 3772 | 4684 | 8224 | 870 | 966 | 1124 | . | . | . | . | . | . | . | . | . |
| | *** | 4141 | 5621 | 8210 | 913 | 1033 | 1104 | . | . | . | . | . | . | . | . | . |
| 0.95 | *** | 2204 | 2652 | 3864 | . | . | . | . | . | . | . | . | . | . | . | . |
| | *** | 2392 | 3055 | 3844 | . | . | . | . | . | . | . | . | . | . | . | . |

## TABLE 3: ALPHA= 0.01  POWER= 0.8    EXPECTED ACCRUAL THRU MINIMUM FOLLOW-UP= 1500

| | | DEL=.02 | | | DEL=.05 | | | DEL=.10 | | | DEL=.15 | | | DEL=.20 | | |
|---|---|---|---|---|---|---|---|---|---|---|---|---|---|---|---|---|---|
| FACT= | | 1.0 .75 | .50 .25 | .00 BIN | 1.0 .75 | .50 .25 | .00 BIN | 1.0 .75 | .50 .25 | .00 BIN | 1.0 75 | .50 .25 | .00 BIN | 1.0 .75 | .50 .25 | .00 BIN |
| PCONT=*** | | REQUIRED NUMBER OF PATIENTS | | | | | | | | | | | | | | |
| 0.05 | *** | 2876 2904 3023 | | | 623 630 641 | | | 225 226 228 | | | 132 132 133 | | | 93 93 94 | | |
| | *** | 2887 2939 5651 | | | 626 635 1104 | | | 226 227 352 | | | 132 132 186 | | | 93 94 118 | | |
| 0.1 | *** | 5990 6063 6642 | | | 1157 1185 1237 | | | 370 375 382 | | | 199 200 202 | | | 131 132 133 | | |
| | *** | 6015 6183 9816 | | | 1169 1207 1747 | | | 372 379 502 | | | 200 202 248 | | | 131 132 151 | | |
| 0.15 | *** | 8765 8894 10272 | | | 1627 1685 1813 | | | 497 508 523 | | | 256 260 263 | | | 163 164 166 | | |
| | *** | 8809 9125 13479 | | | 1651 1735 2309 | | | 502 515 633 | | | 258 262 302 | | | 164 165 179 | | |
| 0.2 | *** | 10991 11191 13649 | | | 2012 2108 2339 | | | 604 622 649 | | | 304 309 317 | | | 189 191 194 | | |
| | *** | 11058 11555 16640 | | | 2052 2195 2791 | | | 612 635 743 | | | 307 313 346 | | | 190 193 201 | | |
| 0.25 | *** | 12611 12899 16642 | | | 2308 2447 2798 | | | 689 716 755 | | | 342 350 360 | | | 209 213 217 | | |
| | *** | 12708 13421 19300 | | | 2365 2573 3192 | | | 701 734 833 | | | 346 355 382 | | | 211 215 219 | | |
| 0.3 | *** | 13639 14032 19180 | | | 2520 2703 3182 | | | 754 789 842 | | | 371 382 395 | | | 225 229 233 | | |
| | *** | 13771 14738 21458 | | | 2595 2870 3513 | | | 770 813 904 | | | 376 388 409 | | | 227 232 231 | | |
| 0.35 | *** | 14118 14638 21221 | | | 2654 2880 3485 | | | 799 843 907 | | | 391 404 420 | | | 234 239 245 | | |
| | *** | 14293 15551 23113 | | | 2747 3089 3754 | | | 818 872 954 | | | 397 412 426 | | | 237 242 239 | | |
| 0.4 | *** | 14114 14785 22740 | | | 2720 2985 3702 | | | 825 875 952 | | | 402 416 435 | | | 239 245 251 | | |
| | *** | 14342 15922 24268 | | | 2829 3230 3915 | | | 848 909 984 | | | 409 425 435 | | | 242 247 241 | | |
| 0.45 | *** | 13706 14553 23723 | | | 2726 3026 3834 | | | 834 890 974 | | | 404 420 440 | | | 238 245 251 | | |
| | *** | 13998 15917 24920 | | | 2850 3301 3995 | | | 860 927 994 | | | 412 429 435 | | | 241 247 239 | | |
| 0.5 | *** | 12980 14021 24163 | | | 2681 3007 3878 | | | 827 886 975 | | | 398 415 435 | | | 233 239 245 | | |
| | *** | 13345 15600 25070 | | | 2817 3304 3995 | | | 854 924 984 | | | 406 425 426 | | | 236 243 231 | | |
| 0.55 | *** | 12027 13265 24057 | | | 2593 2935 3835 | | | 804 863 953 | | | 384 401 421 | | | 223 229 235 | | |
| | *** | 12472 15028 24719 | | | 2735 3243 3915 | | | 832 903 954 | | | 393 410 409 | | | 226 232 219 | | |
| 0.6 | *** | 10936 12352 23405 | | | 2465 2812 3705 | | | 766 824 909 | | | 363 378 397 | | | 208 213 219 | | |
| | *** | 11457 14246 23866 | | | 2611 3121 3754 | | | 792 862 904 | | | 370 387 382 | | | 210 215 201 | | |
| 0.65 | *** | 9782 11329 22210 | | | 2302 2643 3488 | | | 713 767 845 | | | 334 347 363 | | | 187 192 198 | | |
| | *** | 10365 13287 22511 | | | 2446 2938 3513 | | | 738 802 833 | | | 339 354 346 | | | 190 195 179 | | |
| 0.7 | *** | 8617 10224 20474 | | | 2105 2424 3185 | | | 645 692 758 | | | 295 307 320 | | | 163 167 170 | | |
| | *** | 9235 12168 20655 | | | 2242 2696 3192 | | | 667 722 743 | | | 301 313 302 | | | 165 169 151 | | |
| 0.75 | *** | 7466 9048 18202 | | | 1874 2157 2795 | | | 560 598 650 | | | 249 258 267 | | | 133 136 139 | | |
| | *** | 8084 10887 18296 | | | 1995 2392 2791 | | | 578 622 633 | | | 253 262 248 | | | 134 137 118 | | |
| 0.8 | *** | 6322 7785 15399 | | | 1601 1835 2322 | | | 458 485 521 | | | 194 200 205 | | | . . . | | |
| | *** | 6900 9428 15436 | | | 1702 2021 2309 | | | 472 502 502 | | | 197 202 186 | | | . . . | | |
| 0.85 | *** | 5147 6393 12071 | | | 1278 1447 1764 | | | 337 352 371 | | | . . . | | | . . . | | |
| | *** | 5645 7738 12074 | | | 1352 1574 1747 | | | 344 362 352 | | | . . . | | | . . . | | |
| 0.9 | *** | 3860 4777 8224 | | | 881 974 1124 | | | . . . | | | . . . | | | . . . | | |
| | *** | 4232 5711 8210 | | | 923 1039 1104 | | | . . . | | | . . . | | | . . . | | |
| 0.95 | *** | 2250 2695 3863 | | | . . . | | | . . . | | | . . . | | | . . . | | |
| | *** | 2437 3091 3844 | | | . . . | | | . . . | | | . . . | | | . . . | | |

TABLE 3: ALPHA= 0.01  POWER= 0.8     EXPECTED ACCRUAL THRU MINIMUM FOLLOW-UP= 1600

PCONT=***          REQUIRED NUMBER OF PATIENTS

| PCONT | FACT | DEL=.02 1.0/.75 | .50/.25 | .00/BIN | DEL=.05 1.0/.75 | .50/.25 | .00/BIN | DEL=.10 1.0/.75 | .50/.25 | .00/BIN | DEL=.15 1.0/.75 | .50/.25 | .00/BIN | DEL=.20 1.0/.75 | .50/.25 | .00/BIN |
|---|---|---|---|---|---|---|---|---|---|---|---|---|---|---|---|---|
| 0.05 | *** | 2879 | 2907 | 3023 | 624 | 631 | 641 | 225 | 226 | 228 | 132 | 132 | 133 | 93 | 93 | 94 |
|  | *** | 2889 | 2943 | 5651 | 627 | 636 | 1104 | 226 | 227 | 352 | 132 | 133 | 186 | 93 | 93 | 118 |
| 0.1 | *** | 5996 | 6072 | 6642 | 1159 | 1187 | 1237 | 371 | 376 | 382 | 199 | 201 | 203 | 131 | 132 | 133 |
|  | *** | 6022 | 6196 | 9816 | 1171 | 1208 | 1747 | 373 | 379 | 502 | 200 | 202 | 248 | 132 | 132 | 151 |
| 0.15 | *** | 8774 | 8911 | 10273 | 1632 | 1691 | 1813 | 498 | 509 | 523 | 256 | 260 | 264 | 163 | 165 | 166 |
|  | *** | 8820 | 9151 | 13479 | 1657 | 1739 | 2309 | 503 | 516 | 633 | 258 | 262 | 302 | 164 | 165 | 179 |
| 0.2 | *** | 11004 | 11217 | 13649 | 2021 | 2117 | 2339 | 606 | 624 | 649 | 305 | 310 | 317 | 189 | 192 | 194 |
|  | *** | 11076 | 11598 | 16640 | 2061 | 2201 | 2791 | 614 | 635 | 743 | 307 | 313 | 346 | 190 | 193 | 201 |
| 0.25 | *** | 12631 | 12936 | 16643 | 2321 | 2460 | 2798 | 692 | 718 | 755 | 343 | 351 | 360 | 210 | 213 | 217 |
|  | *** | 12734 | 13483 | 19300 | 2379 | 2584 | 3192 | 704 | 735 | 833 | 347 | 356 | 382 | 211 | 215 | 219 |
| 0.3 | *** | 13665 | 14083 | 19180 | 2537 | 2720 | 3182 | 758 | 792 | 842 | 372 | 382 | 395 | 225 | 229 | 234 |
|  | *** | 13806 | 14821 | 21458 | 2612 | 2885 | 3513 | 774 | 815 | 904 | 377 | 388 | 409 | 227 | 231 | 231 |
| 0.35 | *** | 14153 | 14705 | 21221 | 2675 | 2901 | 3484 | 804 | 846 | 908 | 392 | 405 | 420 | 235 | 240 | 245 |
|  | *** | 14339 | 15656 | 23113 | 2768 | 3106 | 3754 | 823 | 873 | 954 | 398 | 412 | 426 | 237 | 242 | 239 |
| 0.4 | *** | 14160 | 14871 | 22740 | 2744 | 3010 | 3702 | 831 | 880 | 952 | 404 | 417 | 435 | 240 | 245 | 251 |
|  | *** | 14402 | 16050 | 24268 | 2854 | 3251 | 3915 | 853 | 912 | 984 | 410 | 426 | 435 | 242 | 248 | 241 |
| 0.45 | *** | 13765 | 14659 | 23723 | 2754 | 3053 | 3834 | 840 | 894 | 974 | 406 | 421 | 440 | 239 | 245 | 251 |
|  | *** | 14074 | 16067 | 24920 | 2878 | 3323 | 3995 | 865 | 930 | 994 | 413 | 430 | 435 | 242 | 248 | 239 |
| 0.5 | *** | 13055 | 14146 | 24163 | 2712 | 3037 | 3879 | 833 | 890 | 975 | 400 | 416 | 435 | 234 | 240 | 246 |
|  | *** | 13440 | 15769 | 25070 | 2848 | 3328 | 3995 | 859 | 928 | 984 | 408 | 425 | 426 | 237 | 243 | 231 |
| 0.55 | *** | 12119 | 13409 | 24058 | 2625 | 2966 | 3836 | 811 | 868 | 953 | 387 | 402 | 421 | 224 | 229 | 235 |
|  | *** | 12585 | 15213 | 24719 | 2768 | 3268 | 3915 | 837 | 906 | 954 | 394 | 411 | 409 | 226 | 232 | 219 |
| 0.6 | *** | 11044 | 12510 | 23406 | 2498 | 2844 | 3705 | 772 | 828 | 910 | 365 | 379 | 397 | 208 | 213 | 219 |
|  | *** | 11587 | 14440 | 23866 | 2644 | 3146 | 3754 | 798 | 864 | 904 | 372 | 388 | 382 | 211 | 216 | 201 |
| 0.65 | *** | 9905 | 11496 | 22210 | 2335 | 2672 | 3488 | 719 | 771 | 845 | 335 | 348 | 363 | 188 | 193 | 197 |
|  | *** | 10507 | 13484 | 22511 | 2478 | 2963 | 3513 | 743 | 804 | 833 | 341 | 355 | 346 | 191 | 195 | 179 |
| 0.7 | *** | 8750 | 10394 | 20474 | 2136 | 2452 | 3185 | 650 | 695 | 758 | 297 | 308 | 320 | 164 | 167 | 171 |
|  | *** | 9384 | 12359 | 20655 | 2271 | 2718 | 3192 | 671 | 724 | 743 | 302 | 314 | 302 | 165 | 169 | 151 |
| 0.75 | *** | 7600 | 9210 | 18202 | 1901 | 2181 | 2796 | 565 | 601 | 650 | 250 | 258 | 267 | 133 | 136 | 138 |
|  | *** | 8230 | 11066 | 18296 | 2022 | 2411 | 2791 | 582 | 624 | 633 | 254 | 263 | 248 | 135 | 137 | 118 |
| 0.8 | *** | 6448 | 7932 | 15399 | 1624 | 1854 | 2322 | 462 | 488 | 521 | 195 | 200 | 205 | . | . | . |
|  | *** | 7036 | 9585 | 15436 | 1724 | 2035 | 2309 | 474 | 503 | 502 | 197 | 203 | 186 | . | . | . |
| 0.85 | *** | 5256 | 6516 | 12071 | 1295 | 1461 | 1764 | 339 | 353 | 372 | . | . | . | . | . | . |
|  | *** | 5761 | 7864 | 12074 | 1368 | 1584 | 1747 | 346 | 362 | 352 | . | . | . | . | . | . |
| 0.9 | *** | 3942 | 4865 | 8224 | 891 | 981 | 1124 | . | . | . | . | . | . | . | . | . |
|  | *** | 4318 | 5795 | 8210 | 932 | 1043 | 1104 | . | . | . | . | . | . | . | . | . |
| 0.95 | *** | 2292 | 2735 | 3864 | . | . | . | . | . | . | . | . | . | . | . | . |
|  | *** | 2479 | 3124 | 3844 | . | . | . | . | . | . | . | . | . | . | . | . |

## TABLE 3: ALPHA= 0.01  POWER= 0.8     EXPECTED ACCRUAL THRU MINIMUM FOLLOW-UP= 1700

|  |  | DEL=.02 | | | DEL=.05 | | | DEL=.10 | | | DEL=.15 | | | DEL=.20 | | |
|---|---|---|---|---|---|---|---|---|---|---|---|---|---|---|---|---|
| FACT= | | 1.0 .75 | .50 .25 | .00 BIN | 1.0 .75 | .50 .25 | .00 BIN | 1.0 .75 | .50 .25 | .00 BIN | 1.0 75 | .50 .25 | .00 BIN | 1.0 .75 | .50 .25 | .00 BIN |
| PCONT=*** | | REQUIRED NUMBER OF PATIENTS | | | | | | | | | | | | | | |
| 0.05 | *** | 2880 | 2910 | 3024 | 624 | 631 | 641 | 225 | 226 | 228 | 131 | 133 | 133 | 93 | 93 | 93 |
|  | *** | 2891 | 2945 | 5651 | 628 | 636 | 1104 | 226 | 227 | 352 | 131 | 133 | 186 | 93 | 93 | 118 |
| 0.1 | *** | 6001 | 6081 | 6642 | 1162 | 1189 | 1236 | 371 | 376 | 381 | 199 | 201 | 203 | 131 | 131 | 133 |
|  | *** | 6028 | 6208 | 9816 | 1174 | 1209 | 1747 | 373 | 379 | 502 | 199 | 202 | 248 | 131 | 133 | 151 |
| 0.15 | *** | 8782 | 8928 | 10272 | 1637 | 1695 | 1812 | 499 | 510 | 524 | 257 | 260 | 263 | 163 | 165 | 167 |
|  | *** | 8831 | 9175 | 13479 | 1661 | 1742 | 2309 | 505 | 516 | 633 | 258 | 262 | 302 | 163 | 165 | 179 |
| 0.2 | *** | 11018 | 11243 | 13649 | 2029 | 2126 | 2339 | 607 | 624 | 649 | 305 | 310 | 316 | 189 | 192 | 194 |
|  | *** | 11094 | 11638 | 16640 | 2069 | 2208 | 2791 | 616 | 636 | 743 | 308 | 313 | 346 | 190 | 193 | 201 |
| 0.25 | *** | 12650 | 12974 | 16643 | 2333 | 2472 | 2798 | 695 | 720 | 755 | 344 | 352 | 360 | 210 | 214 | 216 |
|  | *** | 12760 | 13542 | 19300 | 2390 | 2594 | 3192 | 707 | 736 | 833 | 347 | 356 | 382 | 211 | 214 | 219 |
| 0.3 | *** | 13691 | 14133 | 19180 | 2552 | 2735 | 3182 | 762 | 794 | 843 | 373 | 384 | 395 | 225 | 229 | 233 |
|  | *** | 13841 | 14900 | 21458 | 2628 | 2897 | 3513 | 777 | 816 | 904 | 378 | 389 | 409 | 227 | 231 | 231 |
| 0.35 | *** | 14188 | 14772 | 21221 | 2694 | 2919 | 3485 | 807 | 849 | 907 | 394 | 406 | 420 | 236 | 240 | 245 |
|  | *** | 14386 | 15758 | 23113 | 2788 | 3121 | 3754 | 826 | 875 | 954 | 399 | 412 | 426 | 238 | 242 | 239 |
| 0.4 | *** | 14205 | 14955 | 22739 | 2766 | 3032 | 3703 | 836 | 883 | 952 | 405 | 418 | 435 | 240 | 245 | 250 |
|  | *** | 14462 | 16173 | 24268 | 2878 | 3269 | 3915 | 857 | 913 | 984 | 411 | 426 | 435 | 242 | 248 | 241 |
| 0.45 | *** | 13823 | 14761 | 23723 | 2779 | 3079 | 3835 | 845 | 898 | 974 | 408 | 422 | 440 | 240 | 245 | 252 |
|  | *** | 14150 | 16211 | 24920 | 2905 | 3344 | 3995 | 870 | 932 | 994 | 414 | 430 | 435 | 242 | 248 | 239 |
| 0.5 | *** | 13128 | 14268 | 24163 | 2740 | 3064 | 3879 | 839 | 894 | 974 | 403 | 418 | 435 | 235 | 240 | 246 |
|  | *** | 13533 | 15931 | 25070 | 2876 | 3350 | 3995 | 865 | 930 | 984 | 409 | 426 | 426 | 237 | 243 | 231 |
| 0.55 | *** | 12209 | 13549 | 24058 | 2655 | 2994 | 3835 | 816 | 872 | 953 | 389 | 403 | 420 | 224 | 229 | 235 |
|  | *** | 12696 | 15388 | 24719 | 2798 | 3291 | 3915 | 843 | 908 | 954 | 395 | 411 | 409 | 226 | 233 | 219 |
| 0.6 | *** | 11151 | 12663 | 23406 | 2528 | 2873 | 3705 | 777 | 832 | 909 | 367 | 380 | 397 | 209 | 214 | 219 |
|  | *** | 11714 | 14624 | 23866 | 2674 | 3169 | 3754 | 803 | 867 | 904 | 373 | 388 | 382 | 211 | 216 | 201 |
| 0.65 | *** | 10025 | 11657 | 22210 | 2365 | 2700 | 3488 | 724 | 775 | 845 | 337 | 348 | 363 | 189 | 193 | 197 |
|  | *** | 10645 | 13670 | 22511 | 2507 | 2985 | 3513 | 747 | 806 | 833 | 342 | 356 | 346 | 191 | 195 | 179 |
| 0.7 | *** | 8877 | 10555 | 20474 | 2165 | 2477 | 3184 | 654 | 698 | 758 | 299 | 308 | 320 | 163 | 167 | 171 |
|  | *** | 9526 | 12541 | 20655 | 2299 | 2738 | 3192 | 675 | 726 | 743 | 303 | 313 | 302 | 165 | 169 | 151 |
| 0.75 | *** | 7728 | 9365 | 18202 | 1927 | 2203 | 2795 | 568 | 603 | 650 | 252 | 259 | 267 | 134 | 136 | 138 |
|  | *** | 8370 | 11235 | 18296 | 2046 | 2428 | 2791 | 585 | 624 | 633 | 255 | 263 | 248 | 135 | 137 | 118 |
| 0.8 | *** | 6568 | 8072 | 15399 | 1646 | 1872 | 2322 | 464 | 490 | 522 | 195 | 199 | 205 | . | . | . |
|  | *** | 7165 | 9732 | 15436 | 1744 | 2048 | 2309 | 476 | 505 | 502 | 197 | 203 | 186 | . | . | . |
| 0.85 | *** | 5360 | 6632 | 12071 | 1311 | 1474 | 1765 | 340 | 355 | 372 | . | . | . | . | . | . |
|  | *** | 5870 | 7981 | 12074 | 1382 | 1593 | 1747 | 347 | 362 | 352 | . | . | . | . | . | . |
| 0.9 | *** | 4019 | 4948 | 8223 | 900 | 988 | 1124 | . | . | . | . | . | . | . | . | . |
|  | *** | 4398 | 5872 | 8210 | 940 | 1047 | 1104 | . | . | . | . | . | . | . | . | . |
| 0.95 | *** | 2331 | 2772 | 3864 | . | . | . | . | . | . | . | . | . | . | . | . |
|  | *** | 2518 | 3153 | 3844 | . | . | . | . | . | . | . | . | . | . | . | . |

TABLE 3: ALPHA= 0.01  POWER= 0.8     EXPECTED ACCRUAL THRU MINIMUM FOLLOW-UP= 1800

| | DEL=.02 | | | DEL=.05 | | | DEL=.10 | | | DEL=.15 | | | DEL=.20 | | |
|---|---|---|---|---|---|---|---|---|---|---|---|---|---|---|---|
| FACT= | 1.0 .75 | .50 .25 | .00 BIN | 1.0 .75 | .50 .25 | .00 BIN | 1.0 .75 | .50 .25 | .00 BIN | 1.0 75 | .50 .25 | .00 BIN | 1.0 .75 | .50 .25 | .00 BIN |
| PCONT=*** | REQUIRED NUMBER OF PATIENTS | | | | | | | | | | | | | | |
| 0.05 *** | 2882 | 2913 | 3024 | 625 | 632 | 641 | 225 | 226 | 228 | 132 | 132 | 132 | 93 | 93 | 93 |
| *** | 2893 | 2949 | 5651 | 629 | 636 | 1104 | 226 | 227 | 352 | 132 | 132 | 186 | 93 | 93 | 118 |
| 0.1 *** | 6005 | 6090 | 6642 | 1164 | 1191 | 1236 | 371 | 375 | 382 | 199 | 201 | 202 | 132 | 132 | 132 |
| *** | 6034 | 6220 | 9816 | 1176 | 1210 | 1747 | 373 | 379 | 502 | 200 | 201 | 248 | 132 | 132 | 151 |
| 0.15 *** | 8792 | 8945 | 10272 | 1642 | 1700 | 1812 | 501 | 510 | 523 | 258 | 260 | 264 | 163 | 165 | 166 |
| *** | 8844 | 9200 | 13479 | 1667 | 1746 | 2309 | 505 | 516 | 633 | 258 | 262 | 302 | 164 | 165 | 179 |
| 0.2 *** | 11031 | 11269 | 13650 | 2037 | 2133 | 2339 | 609 | 627 | 649 | 306 | 310 | 317 | 190 | 192 | 195 |
| *** | 11112 | 11679 | 16640 | 2078 | 2213 | 2791 | 618 | 636 | 743 | 308 | 314 | 346 | 191 | 193 | 201 |
| 0.25 *** | 12669 | 13011 | 16642 | 2344 | 2483 | 2798 | 697 | 722 | 756 | 345 | 352 | 360 | 210 | 213 | 217 |
| *** | 12784 | 13600 | 19300 | 2403 | 2602 | 3192 | 708 | 737 | 833 | 348 | 357 | 382 | 213 | 215 | 219 |
| 0.3 *** | 13718 | 14184 | 19180 | 2567 | 2749 | 3181 | 765 | 796 | 843 | 375 | 384 | 395 | 226 | 229 | 234 |
| *** | 13875 | 14978 | 21458 | 2643 | 2909 | 3513 | 780 | 818 | 904 | 379 | 389 | 409 | 227 | 231 | 231 |
| 0.35 *** | 14223 | 14838 | 21221 | 2712 | 2938 | 3484 | 812 | 852 | 908 | 395 | 406 | 420 | 236 | 240 | 245 |
| *** | 14433 | 15855 | 23113 | 2807 | 3136 | 3754 | 830 | 877 | 954 | 400 | 413 | 426 | 238 | 243 | 239 |
| 0.4 *** | 14251 | 15039 | 22740 | 2789 | 3054 | 3702 | 840 | 886 | 951 | 406 | 420 | 434 | 240 | 245 | 251 |
| *** | 14523 | 16292 | 24268 | 2900 | 3286 | 3915 | 861 | 915 | 984 | 413 | 426 | 435 | 243 | 249 | 241 |
| 0.45 *** | 13881 | 14862 | 23723 | 2805 | 3102 | 3834 | 850 | 901 | 974 | 409 | 423 | 440 | 240 | 245 | 251 |
| *** | 14226 | 16348 | 24920 | 2929 | 3363 | 3995 | 874 | 933 | 994 | 416 | 431 | 435 | 243 | 249 | 239 |
| 0.5 *** | 13200 | 14388 | 24164 | 2767 | 3090 | 3879 | 845 | 897 | 974 | 404 | 418 | 435 | 235 | 240 | 246 |
| *** | 13625 | 16086 | 25070 | 2904 | 3372 | 3995 | 870 | 933 | 984 | 411 | 426 | 426 | 237 | 243 | 231 |
| 0.55 *** | 12297 | 13683 | 24058 | 2683 | 3021 | 3836 | 822 | 876 | 953 | 390 | 404 | 420 | 225 | 229 | 235 |
| *** | 12804 | 15555 | 24719 | 2826 | 3313 | 3915 | 847 | 910 | 954 | 397 | 411 | 409 | 227 | 233 | 219 |
| 0.6 *** | 11256 | 12810 | 23406 | 2558 | 2899 | 3705 | 783 | 836 | 910 | 368 | 381 | 397 | 209 | 213 | 219 |
| *** | 11837 | 14800 | 23866 | 2703 | 3190 | 3754 | 807 | 868 | 904 | 375 | 389 | 382 | 211 | 217 | 201 |
| 0.65 *** | 10140 | 11810 | 22209 | 2394 | 2726 | 3489 | 729 | 777 | 845 | 337 | 350 | 363 | 189 | 193 | 198 |
| *** | 10779 | 13848 | 22511 | 2535 | 3005 | 3513 | 751 | 807 | 833 | 343 | 357 | 346 | 191 | 195 | 179 |
| 0.7 *** | 9000 | 10709 | 20474 | 2191 | 2502 | 3185 | 659 | 701 | 758 | 299 | 309 | 321 | 164 | 168 | 171 |
| *** | 9663 | 12712 | 20655 | 2325 | 2756 | 3192 | 678 | 726 | 743 | 303 | 314 | 302 | 165 | 168 | 151 |
| 0.75 *** | 7851 | 9513 | 18201 | 1950 | 2225 | 2796 | 573 | 606 | 650 | 252 | 258 | 267 | 134 | 136 | 138 |
| *** | 8505 | 11394 | 18296 | 2070 | 2443 | 2791 | 588 | 627 | 633 | 255 | 263 | 248 | 135 | 137 | 118 |
| 0.8 *** | 6684 | 8205 | 15399 | 1666 | 1889 | 2322 | 467 | 492 | 521 | 195 | 200 | 206 | . | . | . |
| *** | 7289 | 9870 | 15436 | 1764 | 2060 | 2309 | 478 | 505 | 502 | 198 | 202 | 186 | . | . | . |
| 0.85 *** | 5460 | 6742 | 12071 | 1325 | 1485 | 1764 | 342 | 355 | 371 | . | . | . | . | . | . |
| *** | 5976 | 8091 | 12074 | 1396 | 1601 | 1747 | 348 | 363 | 352 | . | . | . | . | . | . |
| 0.9 *** | 4094 | 5025 | 8223 | 908 | 994 | 1124 | . | . | . | . | . | . | . | . | . |
| *** | 4475 | 5946 | 8210 | 947 | 1050 | 1104 | . | . | . | . | . | . | . | . | . |
| 0.95 *** | 2368 | 2805 | 3864 | . | . | . | . | . | . | . | . | . | . | . | . |
| *** | 2555 | 3181 | 3844 | . | . | . | . | . | . | . | . | . | . | . | . |

## TABLE 3: ALPHA= 0.01  POWER= 0.8    EXPECTED ACCRUAL THRU MINIMUM FOLLOW-UP= 1900

| | | DEL=.02 | | | DEL=.05 | | | DEL=.10 | | | DEL=.15 | | | DEL=.20 | | |
|---|---|---|---|---|---|---|---|---|---|---|---|---|---|---|---|---|---|
| FACT= | | 1.0 .75 | .50 .25 | .00 BIN | 1.0 .75 | .50 .25 | .00 BIN | 1.0 .75 | .50 .25 | .00 BIN | 1.0 75 | .50 .25 | .00 BIN | 1.0 .75 | .50 .25 | .00 BIN |
| PCONT=*** | | REQUIRED NUMBER OF PATIENTS | | | | | | | | | | | | | | |
| 0.05 | *** | 2884 | 2915 | 3023 | 626 | 633 | 641 | 225 | 227 | 228 | 132 | 133 | 133 | 92 | 94 | 94 |
| | *** | 2896 | 2951 | 5651 | 629 | 636 | 1104 | 225 | 228 | 352 | 132 | 133 | 186 | 94 | 94 | 118 |
| 0.1 | *** | 6010 | 6099 | 6642 | 1166 | 1193 | 1237 | 372 | 376 | 382 | 199 | 201 | 203 | 132 | 132 | 133 |
| | *** | 6041 | 6231 | 9816 | 1178 | 1211 | 1747 | 374 | 379 | 502 | 201 | 201 | 248 | 132 | 133 | 151 |
| 0.15 | *** | 8800 | 8960 | 10273 | 1647 | 1704 | 1813 | 501 | 510 | 524 | 258 | 260 | 263 | 163 | 165 | 166 |
| | *** | 8855 | 9224 | 13479 | 1672 | 1748 | 2309 | 505 | 516 | 633 | 258 | 262 | 302 | 163 | 166 | 179 |
| 0.2 | *** | 11045 | 11294 | 13649 | 2044 | 2139 | 2338 | 610 | 627 | 648 | 306 | 311 | 317 | 190 | 192 | 194 |
| | *** | 11129 | 11717 | 16640 | 2085 | 2218 | 2791 | 619 | 638 | 743 | 308 | 313 | 346 | 191 | 193 | 201 |
| 0.25 | *** | 12688 | 13047 | 16643 | 2355 | 2493 | 2797 | 699 | 723 | 755 | 345 | 353 | 361 | 211 | 213 | 217 |
| | *** | 12810 | 13656 | 19300 | 2413 | 2610 | 3192 | 711 | 738 | 833 | 349 | 356 | 382 | 212 | 215 | 219 |
| 0.3 | *** | 13744 | 14233 | 19180 | 2581 | 2763 | 3182 | 767 | 799 | 842 | 375 | 384 | 395 | 227 | 230 | 234 |
| | *** | 13910 | 15052 | 21458 | 2657 | 2920 | 3513 | 782 | 818 | 904 | 380 | 389 | 409 | 228 | 231 | 231 |
| 0.35 | *** | 14258 | 14902 | 21220 | 2730 | 2956 | 3484 | 816 | 854 | 908 | 396 | 407 | 419 | 236 | 241 | 246 |
| | *** | 14478 | 15950 | 23113 | 2825 | 3149 | 3754 | 833 | 878 | 954 | 401 | 413 | 426 | 239 | 243 | 239 |
| 0.4 | *** | 14296 | 15120 | 22740 | 2809 | 3073 | 3702 | 844 | 889 | 952 | 407 | 420 | 434 | 241 | 246 | 250 |
| | *** | 14581 | 16406 | 24268 | 2921 | 3302 | 3915 | 866 | 918 | 984 | 413 | 427 | 435 | 243 | 248 | 241 |
| 0.45 | *** | 13940 | 14961 | 23723 | 2828 | 3125 | 3834 | 856 | 904 | 973 | 410 | 424 | 440 | 241 | 246 | 251 |
| | *** | 14299 | 16481 | 24920 | 2953 | 3381 | 3995 | 878 | 935 | 994 | 417 | 431 | 435 | 243 | 248 | 239 |
| 0.5 | *** | 13273 | 14504 | 24163 | 2793 | 3115 | 3878 | 849 | 901 | 975 | 405 | 419 | 436 | 235 | 241 | 246 |
| | *** | 13715 | 16234 | 25070 | 2928 | 3390 | 3995 | 873 | 934 | 984 | 412 | 426 | 426 | 239 | 243 | 231 |
| 0.55 | *** | 12385 | 13815 | 24057 | 2709 | 3046 | 3835 | 826 | 878 | 953 | 391 | 405 | 421 | 225 | 230 | 235 |
| | *** | 12910 | 15716 | 24719 | 2852 | 3332 | 3915 | 851 | 912 | 954 | 398 | 412 | 409 | 228 | 232 | 219 |
| 0.6 | *** | 11357 | 12952 | 23405 | 2585 | 2925 | 3705 | 788 | 838 | 909 | 369 | 382 | 396 | 210 | 215 | 220 |
| | *** | 11957 | 14967 | 23866 | 2730 | 3210 | 3754 | 812 | 870 | 904 | 375 | 389 | 382 | 212 | 217 | 201 |
| 0.65 | *** | 10254 | 11958 | 22210 | 2420 | 2750 | 3488 | 733 | 780 | 844 | 338 | 350 | 363 | 190 | 193 | 197 |
| | *** | 10907 | 14014 | 22511 | 2561 | 3023 | 3513 | 755 | 809 | 833 | 344 | 356 | 346 | 191 | 196 | 179 |
| 0.7 | *** | 9120 | 10857 | 20474 | 2217 | 2524 | 3184 | 662 | 704 | 759 | 300 | 310 | 320 | 165 | 167 | 171 |
| | *** | 9796 | 12874 | 20655 | 2350 | 2773 | 3192 | 681 | 729 | 743 | 305 | 315 | 302 | 166 | 168 | 151 |
| 0.75 | *** | 7969 | 9653 | 18202 | 1973 | 2244 | 2795 | 576 | 608 | 650 | 253 | 260 | 267 | 134 | 136 | 139 |
| | *** | 8633 | 11544 | 18296 | 2091 | 2457 | 2791 | 590 | 628 | 633 | 256 | 263 | 248 | 135 | 137 | 118 |
| 0.8 | *** | 6794 | 8331 | 15399 | 1685 | 1904 | 2321 | 469 | 493 | 521 | 196 | 201 | 205 | . | . | . |
| | *** | 7406 | 10002 | 15436 | 1781 | 2071 | 2309 | 481 | 505 | 502 | 198 | 203 | 186 | . | . | . |
| 0.85 | *** | 5554 | 6847 | 12071 | 1339 | 1495 | 1764 | 343 | 356 | 372 | . | . | . | . | . | . |
| | *** | 6075 | 8195 | 12074 | 1409 | 1607 | 1747 | 349 | 363 | 352 | . | . | . | . | . | . |
| 0.9 | *** | 4164 | 5099 | 8224 | 915 | 999 | 1124 | . | . | . | . | . | . | . | . | . |
| | *** | 4548 | 6013 | 8210 | 954 | 1054 | 1104 | . | . | . | . | . | . | . | . | . |
| 0.95 | *** | 2403 | 2838 | 3864 | . | . | . | . | . | . | . | . | . | . | . | . |
| | *** | 2588 | 3206 | 3844 | . | . | . | . | . | . | . | . | . | . | . | . |

TABLE 3: ALPHA= 0.01  POWER= 0.8     EXPECTED ACCRUAL THRU MINIMUM FOLLOW-UP= 2000

| | | DEL=.02 | | | DEL=.05 | | | DEL=.10 | | | DEL=.15 | | | DEL=.20 | | |
|---|---|---|---|---|---|---|---|---|---|---|---|---|---|---|---|---|---|
| FACT= | | 1.0 .75 | .50 .25 | .00 BIN | 1.0 .75 | .50 .25 | .00 BIN | 1.0 .75 | .50 .25 | .00 BIN | 1.0 75 | .50 .25 | .00 BIN | 1.0 .75 | .50 .25 | .00 BIN |
| PCONT=*** | | | | | REQUIRED | NUMBER OF | PATIENTS | | | | | | | | | |
| 0.05 | *** | 2886 | 2919 | 3024 | 626 | 632 | 641 | 226 | 226 | 229 | 132 | 132 | 132 | 94 | 94 | 94 |
| | *** | 2899 | 2954 | 5651 | 630 | 636 | 1104 | 226 | 227 | 352 | 132 | 132 | 186 | 94 | 94 | 118 |
| 0.1 | *** | 6015 | 6107 | 6642 | 1169 | 1195 | 1236 | 372 | 377 | 382 | 200 | 201 | 202 | 131 | 132 | 132 |
| | *** | 6047 | 6241 | 9816 | 1180 | 1212 | 1747 | 375 | 379 | 502 | 200 | 202 | 248 | 132 | 132 | 151 |
| 0.15 | *** | 8809 | 8977 | 10272 | 1651 | 1707 | 1812 | 502 | 511 | 524 | 257 | 261 | 264 | 164 | 165 | 166 |
| | *** | 8866 | 9246 | 13479 | 1676 | 1751 | 2309 | 506 | 517 | 633 | 259 | 262 | 302 | 165 | 166 | 179 |
| 0.2 | *** | 11057 | 11320 | 13650 | 2052 | 2146 | 2339 | 612 | 629 | 649 | 306 | 311 | 316 | 190 | 192 | 194 |
| | *** | 11147 | 11755 | 16640 | 2092 | 2222 | 2791 | 620 | 637 | 743 | 309 | 314 | 346 | 191 | 194 | 201 |
| 0.25 | *** | 12707 | 13084 | 16642 | 2366 | 2502 | 2799 | 701 | 725 | 755 | 346 | 352 | 360 | 211 | 214 | 216 |
| | *** | 12836 | 13710 | 19300 | 2424 | 2617 | 3192 | 712 | 739 | 833 | 350 | 356 | 382 | 212 | 215 | 219 |
| 0.3 | *** | 13771 | 14282 | 19180 | 2595 | 2776 | 3182 | 770 | 801 | 842 | 376 | 385 | 395 | 226 | 230 | 234 |
| | *** | 13945 | 15125 | 21458 | 2671 | 2930 | 3513 | 785 | 820 | 904 | 380 | 390 | 409 | 229 | 232 | 231 |
| 0.35 | *** | 14292 | 14966 | 21221 | 2747 | 2971 | 3485 | 819 | 856 | 907 | 397 | 407 | 420 | 237 | 241 | 245 |
| | *** | 14525 | 16041 | 23113 | 2841 | 3162 | 3754 | 836 | 880 | 954 | 402 | 414 | 426 | 239 | 242 | 239 |
| 0.4 | *** | 14342 | 15200 | 22740 | 2830 | 3092 | 3702 | 849 | 891 | 952 | 409 | 421 | 435 | 241 | 246 | 251 |
| | *** | 14641 | 16516 | 24268 | 2940 | 3316 | 3915 | 869 | 919 | 984 | 415 | 427 | 435 | 244 | 249 | 241 |
| 0.45 | *** | 13997 | 15059 | 23724 | 2850 | 3146 | 3834 | 860 | 907 | 974 | 412 | 425 | 440 | 241 | 246 | 251 |
| | *** | 14372 | 16609 | 24920 | 2975 | 3397 | 3995 | 882 | 937 | 994 | 417 | 432 | 435 | 244 | 249 | 239 |
| 0.5 | *** | 13345 | 14616 | 24164 | 2817 | 3136 | 3879 | 854 | 904 | 975 | 406 | 420 | 435 | 236 | 241 | 246 |
| | *** | 13805 | 16376 | 25070 | 2952 | 3407 | 3995 | 877 | 936 | 984 | 412 | 427 | 426 | 239 | 244 | 231 |
| 0.55 | *** | 12472 | 13941 | 24057 | 2736 | 3070 | 3836 | 831 | 882 | 954 | 392 | 406 | 421 | 226 | 230 | 235 |
| | *** | 13015 | 15869 | 24719 | 2877 | 3350 | 3915 | 855 | 915 | 954 | 399 | 412 | 409 | 227 | 232 | 219 |
| 0.6 | *** | 11457 | 13090 | 23406 | 2611 | 2947 | 3705 | 792 | 842 | 910 | 370 | 382 | 397 | 210 | 215 | 219 |
| | *** | 12074 | 15126 | 23866 | 2755 | 3227 | 3754 | 815 | 872 | 904 | 376 | 390 | 382 | 212 | 217 | 201 |
| 0.65 | *** | 10365 | 12101 | 22210 | 2446 | 2772 | 3489 | 737 | 784 | 845 | 340 | 351 | 364 | 190 | 194 | 197 |
| | *** | 11032 | 14175 | 22511 | 2586 | 3041 | 3513 | 759 | 811 | 833 | 345 | 356 | 346 | 192 | 196 | 179 |
| 0.7 | *** | 9235 | 10999 | 20474 | 2241 | 2545 | 3185 | 666 | 706 | 759 | 301 | 310 | 320 | 165 | 167 | 171 |
| | *** | 9924 | 13030 | 20655 | 2372 | 2789 | 3192 | 685 | 730 | 743 | 305 | 315 | 302 | 166 | 169 | 151 |
| 0.75 | *** | 8084 | 9789 | 18202 | 1995 | 2262 | 2796 | 579 | 610 | 650 | 254 | 260 | 267 | 135 | 136 | 139 |
| | *** | 8757 | 11687 | 18296 | 2111 | 2470 | 2791 | 594 | 629 | 633 | 256 | 264 | 248 | 135 | 137 | 118 |
| 0.8 | *** | 6900 | 8452 | 15399 | 1702 | 1919 | 2322 | 471 | 494 | 521 | 197 | 201 | 205 | . | . | . |
| | *** | 7520 | 10126 | 15436 | 1797 | 2081 | 2309 | 482 | 507 | 502 | 199 | 204 | 186 | . | . | . |
| 0.85 | *** | 5645 | 6946 | 12071 | 1352 | 1505 | 1765 | 344 | 357 | 371 | . | . | . | . | . | . |
| | *** | 6171 | 8292 | 12074 | 1421 | 1614 | 1747 | 350 | 364 | 352 | . | . | . | . | . | . |
| 0.9 | *** | 4232 | 5169 | 8224 | 924 | 1005 | 1124 | . | . | . | . | . | . | . | . | . |
| | *** | 4617 | 6077 | 8210 | 960 | 1057 | 1104 | . | . | . | . | . | . | . | . | . |
| 0.95 | *** | 2437 | 2869 | 3864 | . | . | . | . | . | . | . | . | . | . | . | . |
| | *** | 2621 | 3230 | 3844 | . | . | . | . | . | . | . | . | . | . | . | . |

## TABLE 3: ALPHA= 0.01  POWER= 0.8     EXPECTED ACCRUAL THRU MINIMUM FOLLOW-UP= 2250

|  |  | DEL=.02 | | | DEL=.05 | | | DEL=.10 | | | DEL=.15 | | | DEL=.20 | | |
|---|---|---|---|---|---|---|---|---|---|---|---|---|---|---|---|---|
| FACT= | | 1.0 .75 | .50 .25 | .00 BIN | 1.0 .75 | .50 .25 | .00 BIN | 1.0 .75 | .50 .25 | .00 BIN | 1.0 75 | .50 .25 | .00 BIN | 1.0 .75 | .50 .25 | .00 BIN |
| PCONT=*** | | REQUIRED NUMBER OF PATIENTS | | | | | | | | | | | | | | |
| 0.05 | *** | 2891 | 2924 | 3023 | 628 | 634 | 641 | 226 | 226 | 227 | 132 | 132 | 133 | 92 | 94 | 94 |
|  | *** | 2904 | 2958 | 5651 | 629 | 637 | 1104 | 226 | 227 | 352 | 132 | 133 | 186 | 92 | 94 | 118 |
| 0.1 | *** | 6027 | 6128 | 6643 | 1174 | 1198 | 1237 | 374 | 376 | 382 | 199 | 201 | 202 | 132 | 132 | 133 |
|  | *** | 6063 | 6266 | 9816 | 1185 | 1214 | 1747 | 375 | 379 | 502 | 201 | 202 | 248 | 132 | 132 | 151 |
| 0.15 | *** | 8830 | 9016 | 10272 | 1662 | 1717 | 1812 | 505 | 513 | 523 | 258 | 261 | 264 | 164 | 165 | 165 |
|  | *** | 8894 | 9299 | 13479 | 1686 | 1756 | 2309 | 509 | 517 | 633 | 260 | 263 | 302 | 164 | 165 | 179 |
| 0.2 | *** | 11091 | 11382 | 13649 | 2068 | 2161 | 2338 | 615 | 629 | 648 | 308 | 312 | 316 | 191 | 192 | 194 |
|  | *** | 11190 | 11842 | 16640 | 2109 | 2233 | 2791 | 623 | 638 | 743 | 309 | 314 | 346 | 191 | 194 | 201 |
| 0.25 | *** | 12756 | 13172 | 16643 | 2389 | 2524 | 2798 | 705 | 728 | 755 | 347 | 354 | 359 | 212 | 213 | 216 |
|  | *** | 12899 | 13837 | 19300 | 2446 | 2632 | 3192 | 717 | 741 | 833 | 350 | 357 | 382 | 213 | 215 | 219 |
| 0.3 | *** | 13836 | 14402 | 19180 | 2626 | 2805 | 3182 | 776 | 804 | 842 | 378 | 387 | 395 | 227 | 230 | 233 |
|  | *** | 14031 | 15296 | 21458 | 2702 | 2952 | 3513 | 790 | 822 | 904 | 382 | 390 | 409 | 229 | 232 | 231 |
| 0.35 | *** | 14380 | 15121 | 21222 | 2786 | 3006 | 3484 | 826 | 862 | 908 | 399 | 409 | 420 | 237 | 241 | 244 |
|  | *** | 14637 | 16256 | 23113 | 2879 | 3189 | 3754 | 842 | 883 | 954 | 403 | 413 | 426 | 239 | 243 | 239 |
| 0.4 | *** | 14455 | 15394 | 22740 | 2876 | 3134 | 3702 | 857 | 897 | 952 | 412 | 421 | 434 | 243 | 247 | 252 |
|  | *** | 14785 | 16773 | 24268 | 2985 | 3349 | 3915 | 876 | 922 | 984 | 416 | 429 | 435 | 244 | 249 | 241 |
| 0.45 | *** | 14141 | 15291 | 23723 | 2902 | 3192 | 3835 | 869 | 914 | 974 | 415 | 426 | 440 | 243 | 247 | 252 |
|  | *** | 14553 | 16905 | 24920 | 3026 | 3434 | 3995 | 890 | 942 | 994 | 420 | 433 | 435 | 244 | 249 | 239 |
| 0.5 | *** | 13521 | 14886 | 24163 | 2873 | 3188 | 3878 | 863 | 911 | 974 | 409 | 421 | 435 | 237 | 241 | 246 |
|  | *** | 14022 | 16707 | 25070 | 3008 | 3447 | 3995 | 885 | 941 | 984 | 415 | 427 | 426 | 239 | 243 | 231 |
| 0.55 | *** | 12683 | 14242 | 24058 | 2794 | 3121 | 3836 | 840 | 888 | 953 | 395 | 407 | 420 | 226 | 230 | 235 |
|  | *** | 13265 | 16225 | 24719 | 2935 | 3390 | 3915 | 863 | 918 | 954 | 401 | 413 | 409 | 229 | 233 | 219 |
| 0.6 | *** | 11698 | 13412 | 23405 | 2670 | 3000 | 3705 | 803 | 848 | 910 | 372 | 384 | 396 | 210 | 215 | 219 |
|  | *** | 12352 | 15495 | 23866 | 2812 | 3268 | 3754 | 824 | 876 | 904 | 378 | 390 | 382 | 213 | 216 | 201 |
| 0.65 | *** | 10628 | 12435 | 22210 | 2504 | 2823 | 3489 | 747 | 789 | 845 | 342 | 351 | 362 | 191 | 194 | 198 |
|  | *** | 11328 | 14545 | 22511 | 2642 | 3078 | 3513 | 766 | 814 | 833 | 347 | 357 | 346 | 192 | 195 | 179 |
| 0.7 | *** | 9509 | 11330 | 20473 | 2296 | 2592 | 3185 | 674 | 711 | 758 | 303 | 311 | 320 | 165 | 168 | 170 |
|  | *** | 10225 | 13386 | 20655 | 2424 | 2822 | 3192 | 691 | 732 | 743 | 306 | 314 | 302 | 167 | 168 | 151 |
| 0.75 | *** | 8353 | 10102 | 18202 | 2043 | 2302 | 2795 | 584 | 614 | 651 | 254 | 261 | 267 | 134 | 136 | 139 |
|  | *** | 9047 | 12014 | 18296 | 2157 | 2499 | 2791 | 599 | 631 | 633 | 257 | 264 | 248 | 136 | 137 | 118 |
| 0.8 | *** | 7149 | 8732 | 15400 | 1742 | 1950 | 2322 | 477 | 496 | 522 | 198 | 201 | 205 | . | . | . |
|  | *** | 7784 | 10409 | 15436 | 1835 | 2103 | 2309 | 486 | 509 | 502 | 199 | 204 | 186 | . | . | . |
| 0.85 | *** | 5857 | 7176 | 12071 | 1380 | 1527 | 1765 | 347 | 358 | 371 | . | . | . | . | . | . |
|  | *** | 6392 | 8515 | 12074 | 1447 | 1628 | 1747 | 353 | 364 | 352 | . | . | . | . | . | . |
| 0.9 | *** | 4389 | 5328 | 8223 | 939 | 1015 | 1123 | . | . | . | . | . | . | . | . | . |
|  | *** | 4777 | 6221 | 8210 | 974 | 1064 | 1104 | . | . | . | . | . | . | . | . | . |
| 0.95 | *** | 2513 | 2936 | 3864 | . | . | . | . | . | . | . | . | . | . | . | . |
|  | *** | 2696 | 3282 | 3844 | . | . | . | . | . | . | . | . | . | . | . | . |

TABLE 3: ALPHA= 0.01  POWER= 0.8    EXPECTED ACCRUAL THRU MINIMUM FOLLOW-UP= 2500

| | DEL=.02 | | | DEL=.05 | | | DEL=.10 | | | DEL=.15 | | | DEL=.20 | | |
|---|---|---|---|---|---|---|---|---|---|---|---|---|---|---|---|
| FACT= | 1.0 .75 | .50 .25 | .00 BIN | 1.0 .75 | .50 .25 | .00 BIN | 1.0 .75 | .50 .25 | .00 BIN | 1.0 75 | .50 .25 | .00 BIN | 1.0 .75 | .50 .25 | .00 BIN |
| PCONT=*** | | | | REQUIRED NUMBER OF PATIENTS | | | | | | | | | | | |
| 0.05 *** | 2895 | 2929 | 3023 | 629 | 634 | 642 | 226 | 226 | 227 | 133 | 133 | 133 | 93 | 93 | 93 |
| *** | 2909 | 2964 | 5651 | 631 | 637 | 1104 | 226 | 227 | 352 | 133 | 133 | 186 | 93 | 93 | 118 |
| 0.1 *** | 6040 | 6148 | 6642 | 1177 | 1201 | 1237 | 374 | 377 | 383 | 199 | 201 | 202 | 133 | 133 | 133 |
| *** | 6077 | 6287 | 9816 | 1189 | 1217 | 1747 | 376 | 379 | 502 | 201 | 201 | 248 | 133 | 133 | 151 |
| 0.15 *** | 8851 | 9054 | 10273 | 1670 | 1723 | 1812 | 506 | 514 | 523 | 259 | 261 | 264 | 164 | 165 | 167 |
| *** | 8923 | 9348 | 13479 | 1693 | 1762 | 2309 | 509 | 518 | 633 | 261 | 262 | 302 | 165 | 165 | 179 |
| 0.2 *** | 11124 | 11442 | 13649 | 2084 | 2173 | 2339 | 618 | 633 | 648 | 309 | 312 | 317 | 190 | 192 | 193 |
| *** | 11234 | 11923 | 16640 | 2123 | 2242 | 2791 | 624 | 640 | 743 | 311 | 314 | 346 | 192 | 193 | 201 |
| 0.25 *** | 12804 | 13259 | 16642 | 2411 | 2543 | 2798 | 711 | 729 | 756 | 348 | 354 | 361 | 212 | 214 | 217 |
| *** | 12961 | 13954 | 19300 | 2468 | 2646 | 3192 | 720 | 742 | 833 | 351 | 358 | 382 | 214 | 215 | 219 |
| 0.3 *** | 13901 | 14518 | 19181 | 2654 | 2829 | 3183 | 781 | 808 | 842 | 379 | 387 | 395 | 227 | 231 | 234 |
| *** | 14117 | 15451 | 21458 | 2729 | 2970 | 3513 | 793 | 823 | 904 | 383 | 390 | 409 | 229 | 233 | 231 |
| 0.35 *** | 14467 | 15271 | 21221 | 2820 | 3037 | 3484 | 833 | 865 | 908 | 401 | 409 | 420 | 239 | 242 | 245 |
| *** | 14749 | 16452 | 23113 | 2914 | 3212 | 3754 | 848 | 886 | 954 | 404 | 414 | 426 | 240 | 243 | 239 |
| 0.4 *** | 14567 | 15577 | 22740 | 2915 | 3170 | 3702 | 864 | 901 | 951 | 414 | 423 | 434 | 243 | 246 | 251 |
| *** | 14927 | 17009 | 24268 | 3024 | 3376 | 3915 | 883 | 924 | 984 | 418 | 429 | 435 | 245 | 249 | 241 |
| 0.45 *** | 14281 | 15512 | 23723 | 2948 | 3234 | 3834 | 877 | 918 | 974 | 417 | 427 | 440 | 243 | 246 | 251 |
| *** | 14727 | 17177 | 24920 | 3070 | 3464 | 3995 | 896 | 945 | 994 | 421 | 434 | 435 | 245 | 249 | 239 |
| 0.5 *** | 13693 | 15139 | 24164 | 2923 | 3231 | 3879 | 871 | 917 | 974 | 411 | 423 | 436 | 237 | 242 | 246 |
| *** | 14227 | 17008 | 25070 | 3056 | 3479 | 3995 | 893 | 943 | 984 | 417 | 429 | 426 | 240 | 243 | 231 |
| 0.55 *** | 12884 | 14523 | 24058 | 2846 | 3167 | 3836 | 849 | 895 | 952 | 398 | 409 | 421 | 227 | 231 | 236 |
| *** | 13502 | 16546 | 24719 | 2986 | 3424 | 3915 | 870 | 921 | 954 | 402 | 414 | 409 | 229 | 233 | 219 |
| 0.6 *** | 11927 | 13712 | 23406 | 2723 | 3045 | 3706 | 811 | 852 | 909 | 374 | 386 | 396 | 212 | 215 | 218 |
| *** | 12612 | 15827 | 23866 | 2864 | 3301 | 3915 | 831 | 879 | 904 | 379 | 390 | 382 | 214 | 217 | 201 |
| 0.65 *** | 10876 | 12742 | 22211 | 2556 | 2867 | 3489 | 754 | 793 | 845 | 343 | 352 | 364 | 192 | 195 | 198 |
| *** | 11604 | 14876 | 22511 | 2692 | 3111 | 3513 | 773 | 817 | 833 | 348 | 358 | 346 | 193 | 196 | 179 |
| 0.7 *** | 9764 | 11633 | 20473 | 2343 | 2631 | 3184 | 681 | 715 | 758 | 304 | 312 | 320 | 165 | 168 | 170 |
| *** | 10501 | 13704 | 20655 | 2470 | 2851 | 3192 | 696 | 736 | 743 | 308 | 315 | 302 | 167 | 170 | 151 |
| 0.75 *** | 8601 | 10387 | 18201 | 2086 | 2337 | 2795 | 590 | 617 | 649 | 256 | 261 | 267 | 136 | 137 | 139 |
| *** | 9314 | 12308 | 18296 | 2196 | 2523 | 2791 | 602 | 633 | 633 | 259 | 264 | 248 | 136 | 137 | 118 |
| 0.8 *** | 7377 | 8986 | 15399 | 1776 | 1977 | 2321 | 479 | 498 | 521 | 198 | 201 | 206 | . | . | . |
| *** | 8026 | 10661 | 15436 | 1867 | 2121 | 2309 | 489 | 509 | 502 | 199 | 202 | 186 | . | . | . |
| 0.85 *** | 6051 | 7383 | 12071 | 1406 | 1545 | 1764 | 349 | 359 | 371 | . | . | . | . | . | . |
| *** | 6593 | 8709 | 12074 | 1468 | 1640 | 1747 | 354 | 365 | 352 | . | . | . | . | . | . |
| 0.9 *** | 4529 | 5470 | 8224 | 952 | 1024 | 1124 | . | . | . | . | . | . | . | . | . |
| *** | 4921 | 6345 | 8210 | 986 | 1070 | 1104 | . | . | . | . | . | . | . | . | . |
| 0.95 *** | 2581 | 2995 | 3864 | . | . | . | . | . | . | . | . | . | . | . | . |
| *** | 2759 | 3326 | 3844 | . | . | . | . | . | . | . | . | . | . | . | . |

## TABLE 3: ALPHA= 0.01  POWER= 0.8    EXPECTED ACCRUAL THRU MINIMUM FOLLOW-UP= 2750

| | | DEL=.02 | | | DEL=.05 | | | DEL=.10 | | | DEL=.15 | | | DEL=.20 | | |
|---|---|---|---|---|---|---|---|---|---|---|---|---|---|---|---|---|---|
| FACT= | | 1.0 .75 | .50 .25 | .00 BIN | 1.0 .75 | .50 .25 | .00 BIN | 1.0 .75 | .50 .25 | .00 BIN | 1.0 75 | .50 .25 | .00 BIN | 1.0 .75 | .50 .25 | .00 BIN |
| PCONT=*** | | | | | REQUIRED NUMBER OF PATIENTS | | | | | | | | | | | |
| 0.05 | *** | 2899 | 2935 | 3023 | 630 | 635 | 641 | 226 | 226 | 228 | 132 | 132 | 133 | 92 | 94 | 94 |
| | *** | 2914 | 2968 | 5651 | 632 | 637 | 1104 | 226 | 228 | 352 | 132 | 132 | 186 | 92 | 94 | 118 |
| 0.1 | *** | 6051 | 6166 | 6643 | 1182 | 1204 | 1237 | 374 | 377 | 381 | 201 | 201 | 202 | 132 | 132 | 133 |
| | *** | 6093 | 6307 | 9816 | 1192 | 1218 | 1747 | 376 | 379 | 502 | 201 | 202 | 248 | 132 | 132 | 151 |
| 0.15 | *** | 8874 | 9090 | 10273 | 1679 | 1730 | 1813 | 507 | 515 | 524 | 259 | 260 | 264 | 164 | 164 | 166 |
| | *** | 8949 | 9390 | 13479 | 1701 | 1766 | 2309 | 510 | 518 | 633 | 260 | 263 | 302 | 164 | 166 | 179 |
| 0.2 | *** | 11157 | 11500 | 13650 | 2096 | 2184 | 2339 | 620 | 634 | 649 | 309 | 312 | 315 | 190 | 192 | 194 |
| | *** | 11278 | 11996 | 16640 | 2136 | 2249 | 2791 | 627 | 641 | 743 | 311 | 314 | 346 | 192 | 194 | 201 |
| 0.25 | *** | 12851 | 13342 | 16642 | 2430 | 2559 | 2797 | 713 | 731 | 755 | 350 | 355 | 360 | 212 | 214 | 216 |
| | *** | 13023 | 14062 | 19300 | 2487 | 2656 | 3192 | 723 | 744 | 833 | 352 | 357 | 382 | 212 | 216 | 219 |
| 0.3 | *** | 13966 | 14631 | 19180 | 2679 | 2851 | 3182 | 785 | 810 | 841 | 381 | 388 | 395 | 228 | 232 | 233 |
| | *** | 14200 | 15595 | 21458 | 2755 | 2985 | 3513 | 797 | 824 | 904 | 384 | 391 | 409 | 230 | 232 | 231 |
| 0.35 | *** | 14552 | 15413 | 21221 | 2851 | 3064 | 3485 | 838 | 869 | 907 | 401 | 410 | 419 | 239 | 242 | 245 |
| | *** | 14860 | 16633 | 23113 | 2944 | 3230 | 3754 | 852 | 886 | 954 | 407 | 415 | 426 | 240 | 243 | 239 |
| 0.4 | *** | 14677 | 15753 | 22740 | 2952 | 3202 | 3701 | 871 | 905 | 951 | 415 | 424 | 434 | 243 | 247 | 250 |
| | *** | 15066 | 17227 | 24268 | 3061 | 3399 | 3915 | 886 | 927 | 984 | 419 | 429 | 435 | 245 | 249 | 241 |
| 0.45 | *** | 14418 | 15719 | 23724 | 2989 | 3268 | 3834 | 885 | 923 | 974 | 419 | 429 | 439 | 243 | 247 | 250 |
| | *** | 14896 | 17426 | 24920 | 3110 | 3490 | 3995 | 902 | 947 | 994 | 424 | 434 | 435 | 245 | 249 | 239 |
| 0.5 | *** | 13859 | 15377 | 24164 | 2968 | 3270 | 3879 | 879 | 920 | 974 | 414 | 424 | 434 | 239 | 242 | 245 |
| | *** | 14426 | 17282 | 25070 | 3099 | 3508 | 3995 | 899 | 945 | 984 | 419 | 429 | 426 | 240 | 243 | 231 |
| 0.55 | *** | 13079 | 14784 | 24057 | 2892 | 3206 | 3835 | 857 | 899 | 954 | 400 | 408 | 421 | 228 | 232 | 235 |
| | *** | 13727 | 16838 | 24719 | 3030 | 3454 | 3915 | 876 | 924 | 954 | 404 | 415 | 409 | 230 | 233 | 219 |
| 0.6 | *** | 12144 | 13989 | 23405 | 2770 | 3085 | 3705 | 817 | 857 | 910 | 376 | 386 | 397 | 212 | 216 | 219 |
| | *** | 12858 | 16130 | 23866 | 2907 | 3330 | 3754 | 837 | 881 | 904 | 381 | 391 | 382 | 214 | 218 | 201 |
| 0.65 | *** | 11108 | 13024 | 22209 | 2601 | 2904 | 3488 | 761 | 797 | 845 | 345 | 353 | 364 | 192 | 194 | 197 |
| | *** | 11861 | 15176 | 22511 | 2734 | 3138 | 3513 | 778 | 819 | 833 | 350 | 359 | 346 | 194 | 195 | 179 |
| 0.7 | *** | 10001 | 11910 | 20473 | 2387 | 2665 | 3184 | 687 | 718 | 758 | 305 | 312 | 319 | 166 | 168 | 170 |
| | *** | 10759 | 13992 | 20655 | 2509 | 2875 | 3192 | 703 | 737 | 743 | 309 | 315 | 302 | 168 | 170 | 151 |
| 0.75 | *** | 8832 | 10647 | 18201 | 2124 | 2366 | 2796 | 594 | 620 | 651 | 257 | 263 | 267 | 135 | 137 | 139 |
| | *** | 9561 | 12569 | 18296 | 2230 | 2543 | 2791 | 606 | 634 | 633 | 259 | 264 | 248 | 135 | 137 | 118 |
| 0.8 | *** | 7589 | 9217 | 15399 | 1807 | 2000 | 2322 | 483 | 501 | 522 | 199 | 202 | 205 | . | . | . |
| | *** | 8248 | 10884 | 15436 | 1893 | 2136 | 2309 | 491 | 510 | 502 | 201 | 204 | 186 | . | . | . |
| 0.85 | *** | 6228 | 7569 | 12070 | 1428 | 1560 | 1765 | 350 | 360 | 370 | . | . | . | . | . | . |
| | *** | 6778 | 8882 | 12074 | 1488 | 1649 | 1747 | 355 | 366 | 352 | . | . | . | . | . | . |
| 0.9 | *** | 4659 | 5598 | 8224 | 964 | 1033 | 1123 | . | . | . | . | . | . | . | . | . |
| | *** | 5051 | 6454 | 8210 | 996 | 1074 | 1104 | . | . | . | . | . | . | . | . | . |
| 0.95 | *** | 2641 | 3045 | 3863 | . | . | . | . | . | . | . | . | . | . | . | . |
| | *** | 2817 | 3363 | 3844 | . | . | . | . | . | . | . | . | . | . | . | . |

TABLE 3: ALPHA= 0.01  POWER= 0.8    EXPECTED ACCRUAL THRU MINIMUM FOLLOW-UP= 3000

| | | DEL=.01 | | | DEL=.02 | | | DEL=.05 | | | DEL=.10 | | | DEL=.15 | | |
|---|---|---|---|---|---|---|---|---|---|---|---|---|---|---|---|---|---|---|
| FACT= | | 1.0 .75 | .50 .25 | .00 BIN | 1.0 .75 | .50 .25 | .00 BIN | 1.0 .75 | .50 .25 | .00 BIN | 1.0 75 | .50 .25 | .00 BIN | 1.0 .75 | .50 .25 | .00 BIN |
| PCONT=*** | | | | | REQUIRED NUMBER OF PATIENTS | | | | | | | | | | | | |
| 0.01 | *** | 1535 | 1540 | 1547 | 565 | 565 | 568 | 185 | 185 | 185 | 95 | 95 | 95 | 65 | 65 | 65 |
| | *** | 1535 | 1543 | 5922 | 565 | 565 | 1958 | 185 | 185 | 533 | 95 | 95 | 217 | 65 | 65 | 129 |
| 0.02 | *** | 3388 | 3403 | 3455 | 1090 | 1093 | 1105 | 295 | 295 | 298 | 130 | 130 | 130 | 85 | 85 | 85 |
| | *** | 3395 | 3422 | 9776 | 1093 | 1097 | 2911 | 295 | 298 | 681 | 130 | 130 | 252 | 85 | 85 | 144 |
| 0.05 | *** | 10255 | 10310 | 10790 | 2905 | 2938 | 3025 | 628 | 635 | 640 | 227 | 227 | 227 | 133 | 133 | 133 |
| | *** | 10273 | 10408 | 20855 | 2920 | 2972 | 5651 | 632 | 640 | 1104 | 227 | 227 | 352 | 133 | 133 | 186 |
| 0.1 | *** | 22618 | 22760 | 25112 | 6062 | 6182 | 6643 | 1183 | 1205 | 1235 | 373 | 377 | 380 | 200 | 200 | 200 |
| | *** | 22667 | 23030 | 37716 | 6107 | 6325 | 9816 | 1195 | 1220 | 1747 | 377 | 380 | 502 | 200 | 200 | 248 |
| 0.15 | *** | 33778 | 34025 | 39670 | 8893 | 9125 | 10273 | 1685 | 1735 | 1813 | 508 | 515 | 523 | 260 | 260 | 265 |
| | *** | 33860 | 34520 | 52569 | 8975 | 9430 | 13479 | 1708 | 1768 | 2309 | 512 | 520 | 633 | 260 | 260 | 302 |
| 0.2 | *** | 42767 | 43153 | 53297 | 11192 | 11555 | 13648 | 2110 | 2195 | 2338 | 620 | 635 | 647 | 310 | 313 | 317 |
| | *** | 42895 | 43925 | 65415 | 11320 | 12065 | 16640 | 2147 | 2255 | 2791 | 628 | 640 | 743 | 310 | 313 | 346 |
| 0.25 | *** | 49315 | 49873 | 65432 | 12898 | 13420 | 16640 | 2447 | 2575 | 2800 | 715 | 733 | 755 | 350 | 355 | 358 |
| | *** | 49502 | 50987 | 76254 | 13082 | 14162 | 19300 | 2503 | 2668 | 3192 | 725 | 745 | 833 | 350 | 358 | 382 |
| 0.3 | *** | 53440 | 54208 | 75770 | 14030 | 14740 | 19180 | 2702 | 2870 | 3182 | 790 | 812 | 842 | 380 | 388 | 395 |
| | *** | 53695 | 55738 | 85086 | 14282 | 15730 | 21458 | 2777 | 2998 | 3513 | 800 | 827 | 904 | 385 | 392 | 409 |
| 0.35 | *** | 55303 | 56330 | 84133 | 14638 | 15550 | 21220 | 2878 | 3088 | 3485 | 842 | 872 | 905 | 403 | 410 | 418 |
| | *** | 55645 | 58360 | 91910 | 14965 | 16802 | 23113 | 2972 | 3250 | 3754 | 857 | 887 | 954 | 407 | 415 | 426 |
| 0.4 | *** | 55153 | 56495 | 90422 | 14785 | 15920 | 22738 | 2983 | 3230 | 3703 | 875 | 910 | 950 | 415 | 425 | 433 |
| | *** | 55600 | 59120 | 96728 | 15200 | 17425 | 24268 | 3092 | 3418 | 3915 | 890 | 928 | 984 | 422 | 430 | 435 |
| 0.45 | *** | 53282 | 55010 | 94570 | 14552 | 15917 | 23725 | 3025 | 3302 | 3835 | 890 | 928 | 973 | 418 | 430 | 440 |
| | *** | 53860 | 58330 | 99538 | 15058 | 17653 | 24920 | 3145 | 3512 | 3995 | 905 | 947 | 994 | 425 | 433 | 435 |
| 0.5 | *** | 50015 | 52220 | 96545 | 14020 | 15598 | 24163 | 3005 | 3302 | 3880 | 887 | 925 | 973 | 415 | 425 | 433 |
| | *** | 50755 | 56308 | 100341 | 14615 | 17533 | 25070 | 3137 | 3530 | 3995 | 902 | 947 | 984 | 418 | 430 | 426 |
| 0.55 | *** | 45707 | 48485 | 96340 | 13265 | 15028 | 24058 | 2935 | 3242 | 3835 | 865 | 902 | 955 | 400 | 410 | 422 |
| | *** | 46645 | 53365 | 99136 | 13940 | 17105 | 24719 | 3070 | 3478 | 3915 | 883 | 925 | 954 | 407 | 415 | 409 |
| 0.6 | *** | 40727 | 44162 | 93950 | 12350 | 14245 | 23405 | 2810 | 3122 | 3703 | 823 | 860 | 910 | 377 | 388 | 395 |
| | *** | 41908 | 49765 | 95925 | 13090 | 16405 | 23866 | 2945 | 3355 | 3754 | 842 | 883 | 904 | 380 | 392 | 382 |
| 0.65 | *** | 35458 | 39560 | 89383 | 11327 | 13288 | 22210 | 2642 | 2938 | 3490 | 767 | 800 | 845 | 347 | 355 | 362 |
| | *** | 36913 | 45710 | 90706 | 12100 | 15448 | 22511 | 2773 | 3160 | 3513 | 782 | 820 | 833 | 350 | 358 | 346 |
| 0.7 | *** | 30260 | 34907 | 82655 | 10225 | 12167 | 20473 | 2425 | 2695 | 3185 | 692 | 722 | 760 | 305 | 313 | 320 |
| | *** | 31963 | 41327 | 83480 | 10997 | 14252 | 20655 | 2545 | 2897 | 3192 | 707 | 737 | 743 | 310 | 317 | 302 |
| 0.75 | *** | 25393 | 30298 | 73780 | 9047 | 10888 | 18200 | 2158 | 2390 | 2795 | 598 | 620 | 650 | 257 | 260 | 268 |
| | *** | 27242 | 36655 | 74247 | 9790 | 12805 | 18296 | 2263 | 2560 | 2791 | 610 | 635 | 633 | 260 | 265 | 248 |
| 0.8 | *** | 20927 | 25727 | 62780 | 7783 | 9430 | 15400 | 1835 | 2020 | 2323 | 485 | 500 | 520 | 200 | 200 | 205 |
| | *** | 22772 | 31640 | 63007 | 8450 | 11087 | 15436 | 1918 | 2150 | 2309 | 493 | 512 | 502 | 200 | 205 | 186 |
| 0.85 | *** | 16753 | 21050 | 49678 | 6392 | 7738 | 12070 | 1445 | 1573 | 1765 | 350 | 362 | 370 | . | . | . |
| | *** | 18430 | 26140 | 49759 | 6947 | 9035 | 12074 | 1505 | 1660 | 1747 | 358 | 365 | 352 | . | . | . |
| 0.9 | *** | 12583 | 15970 | 34495 | 4775 | 5710 | 8222 | 973 | 1037 | 1123 | . | . | . | . | . | . |
| | *** | 13922 | 19795 | 34504 | 5170 | 6550 | 8210 | 1003 | 1078 | 1104 | . | . | . | . | . | . |
| 0.95 | *** | 7783 | 9737 | 17260 | 2695 | 3092 | 3865 | . | . | . | . | . | . | . | . | . |
| | *** | 8575 | 11735 | 17242 | 2867 | 3395 | 3844 | . | . | . | . | . | . | . | . | . |
| 0.98 | *** | 3695 | 4370 | 5942 | . | . | . | . | . | . | . | . | . | . | . | . |
| | *** | 3985 | 4937 | 5922 | . | . | . | . | . | . | . | . | . | . | . | . |

## TABLE 3: ALPHA= 0.01  POWER= 0.8    EXPECTED ACCRUAL THRU MINIMUM FOLLOW-UP= 3250

PCONT=***                    REQUIRED NUMBER OF PATIENTS

| | | DEL=.01 | | | DEL=.02 | | | DEL=.05 | | | DEL=.10 | | | DEL=.15 | | |
|---|---|---|---|---|---|---|---|---|---|---|---|---|---|---|---|---|---|
| | FACT= | 1.0 .75 | .50 .25 | .00 BIN | 1.0 .75 | .50 .25 | .00 BIN | 1.0 .75 | .50 .25 | .00 BIN | 1.0 75 | .50 .25 | .00 BIN | 1.0 .75 | .50 .25 | .00 BIN |
| 0.01 | *** | 1533 1538 | 1538 1541 | 1546 5922 | 563 566 | 566 566 | 566 1958 | 184 184 | 184 184 | 184 533 | 95 95 | 95 95 | 95 217 | 68 68 | 68 68 | 68 129 |
| 0.02 | *** | 3391 3399 | 3407 3423 | 3456 9776 | 1091 1091 | 1094 1099 | 1102 2911 | 295 295 | 295 298 | 298 681 | 127 127 | 127 127 | 127 252 | 84 84 | 84 84 | 84 144 |
| 0.05 | *** | 10259 10281 | 10321 10419 | 10787 20855 | 2906 2922 | 2944 2976 | 3025 5651 | 631 631 | 636 639 | 639 1104 | 225 225 | 225 225 | 230 352 | 133 133 | 133 133 | 133 186 |
| 0.1 | *** | 22631 22682 | 22785 23072 | 25112 37716 | 6075 6121 | 6197 6340 | 6641 9816 | 1189 1197 | 1208 1221 | 1238 1747 | 376 376 | 379 379 | 379 502 | 201 201 | 201 201 | 201 248 |
| 0.15 | *** | 33797 33887 | 34066 34599 | 39672 52569 | 8916 9005 | 9154 9468 | 10273 13479 | 1693 1712 | 1741 1774 | 1814 2309 | 509 514 | 514 517 | 523 633 | 257 263 | 263 263 | 263 302 |
| 0.2 | *** | 42797 42938 | 43219 44051 | 53297 65415 | 11223 11361 | 11608 12128 | 13647 16640 | 2118 2156 | 2204 2261 | 2337 2791 | 623 628 | 636 639 | 647 743 | 311 311 | 314 314 | 314 346 |
| 0.25 | *** | 49362 49565 | 49966 51169 | 65433 76254 | 12946 13144 | 13498 14254 | 16643 19300 | 2464 2516 | 2586 2676 | 2798 3192 | 718 726 | 734 745 | 753 833 | 352 352 | 355 355 | 360 382 |
| 0.3 | *** | 53501 53782 | 54337 55987 | 75771 85086 | 14094 14362 | 14842 15854 | 19181 21458 | 2724 2798 | 2887 3009 | 3182 3513 | 794 802 | 815 826 | 842 904 | 384 384 | 387 393 | 396 409 |
| 0.35 | *** | 55391 55759 | 56504 58689 | 84137 91910 | 14720 15069 | 15684 16954 | 21220 23113 | 2906 2996 | 3109 3264 | 3483 3754 | 848 859 | 875 888 | 907 954 | 404 409 | 412 417 | 420 426 |
| 0.4 | *** | 55264 55748 | 56718 59537 | 90421 96728 | 14891 15329 | 16082 17609 | 22739 24268 | 3017 3123 | 3256 3434 | 3702 3915 | 880 896 | 913 932 | 953 984 | 417 420 | 425 428 | 433 435 |
| 0.45 | *** | 53424 54050 | 55296 58844 | 94569 99538 | 14684 15216 | 16101 17864 | 23722 24920 | 3061 3179 | 3329 3532 | 3832 3995 | 896 913 | 929 948 | 972 994 | 420 425 | 428 433 | 441 435 |
| 0.5 | *** | 50202 50998 | 52582 56921 | 96547 100341 | 14176 14798 | 15809 17767 | 24161 25070 | 3044 3171 | 3334 3553 | 3878 3995 | 891 907 | 929 948 | 972 984 | 417 420 | 425 428 | 436 426 |
| 0.55 | *** | 45941 46957 | 48931 54074 | 96341 99136 | 13444 14143 | 15256 17352 | 24056 24719 | 2971 3106 | 3272 3499 | 3838 3915 | 867 888 | 904 929 | 953 954 | 401 404 | 412 417 | 420 409 |
| 0.6 | *** | 41026 42296 | 44693 50548 | 93952 95925 | 12548 13306 | 14489 16659 | 23406 23866 | 2849 2984 | 3150 3377 | 3702 3754 | 826 848 | 864 883 | 907 904 | 379 384 | 387 393 | 396 382 |
| 0.65 | *** | 35829 37378 | 40167 46543 | 89386 90706 | 11535 12328 | 13531 15700 | 22208 22511 | 2679 2806 | 2968 3179 | 3488 3513 | 769 786 | 802 823 | 842 833 | 347 352 | 355 360 | 363 346 |
| 0.7 | *** | 30702 32494 | 35561 42166 | 82653 83480 | 10435 11223 | 12404 14489 | 20472 20655 | 2459 2578 | 2724 2914 | 3182 3192 | 696 709 | 726 742 | 758 743 | 306 311 | 314 314 | 319 302 |
| 0.75 | *** | 25881 27806 | 30962 37467 | 73781 74247 | 9249 9999 | 11109 13022 | 18203 18296 | 2188 2289 | 2416 2573 | 2798 2791 | 604 612 | 623 636 | 647 633 | 257 263 | 263 266 | 266 248 |
| 0.8 | *** | 21420 23324 | 26355 32384 | 62779 63007 | 7968 8642 | 9623 11267 | 15399 15436 | 1858 1939 | 2037 2159 | 2321 2309 | 490 493 | 501 509 | 523 502 | 201 201 | 201 206 | 206 186 |
| 0.85 | *** | 17203 18921 | 21602 26766 | 49679 49759 | 6546 7104 | 7892 9176 | 12071 12074 | 1465 1522 | 1587 1663 | 1766 1747 | 352 355 | 363 368 | 371 352 | . . | . . | . . |
| 0.9 | *** | 12946 14311 | 16394 20250 | 34496 34504 | 4886 5276 | 5815 6636 | 8225 8210 | 981 1010 | 1043 1083 | 1124 1104 | . . | . . | . . | . . | . . | . . |
| 0.95 | *** | 8001 8802 | 9967 11963 | 17260 17242 | 2744 2914 | 3131 3423 | 3862 3844 | . . | . . | . . | . . | . . | . . | . . | . . | . . |
| 0.98 | *** | 3776 4065 | 4442 4991 | 5942 5922 | . . | . . | . . | . . | . . | . . | . . | . . | . . | . . | . . | . . |

TABLE 3: ALPHA= 0.01  POWER= 0.8    EXPECTED ACCRUAL THRU MINIMUM FOLLOW-UP= 3500

| | | DEL=.01 | | | DEL=.02 | | | DEL=.05 | | | DEL=.10 | | | DEL=.15 | | |
|---|---|---|---|---|---|---|---|---|---|---|---|---|---|---|---|---|---|
| FACT= | | 1.0 .75 | .50 .25 | .00 BIN | 1.0 .75 | .50 .25 | .00 BIN | 1.0 .75 | .50 .25 | .00 BIN | 1.0 75 | .50 .25 | .00 BIN | 1.0 .75 | .50 .25 | .00 BIN |
| PCONT=*** | | | | | | | REQUIRED NUMBER OF PATIENTS | | | | | | | | |
| 0.01 | *** | 1534 | 1537 | 1546 | 566 | 566 | 566 | 186 | 186 | 186 | 93 | 93 | 93 | 67 | 67 | 67 |
| | *** | 1537 | 1543 | 5922 | 566 | 566 | 1958 | 186 | 186 | 533 | 93 | 93 | 217 | 67 | 67 | 129 |
| 0.02 | *** | 3392 | 3410 | 3453 | 1091 | 1096 | 1105 | 295 | 295 | 295 | 128 | 128 | 128 | 85 | 85 | 85 |
| | *** | 3398 | 3424 | 9776 | 1091 | 1100 | 2911 | 295 | 295 | 681 | 128 | 128 | 252 | 85 | 85 | 144 |
| 0.05 | *** | 10266 | 10328 | 10791 | 2911 | 2946 | 3021 | 633 | 636 | 641 | 225 | 225 | 230 | 134 | 134 | 134 |
| | *** | 10287 | 10433 | 20855 | 2925 | 2978 | 5651 | 633 | 636 | 1104 | 225 | 225 | 352 | 134 | 134 | 186 |
| 0.1 | *** | 22642 | 22805 | 25115 | 6084 | 6215 | 6644 | 1187 | 1210 | 1236 | 373 | 379 | 382 | 198 | 198 | 204 |
| | *** | 22695 | 23115 | 37716 | 6136 | 6355 | 9816 | 1201 | 1222 | 1747 | 379 | 379 | 502 | 198 | 204 | 248 |
| 0.15 | *** | 33816 | 34110 | 39670 | 8936 | 9190 | 10270 | 1695 | 1744 | 1814 | 510 | 513 | 522 | 260 | 260 | 265 |
| | *** | 33918 | 34679 | 52569 | 9027 | 9500 | 13479 | 1718 | 1773 | 2309 | 513 | 519 | 633 | 260 | 260 | 302 |
| 0.2 | *** | 42828 | 43283 | 53299 | 11255 | 11658 | 13647 | 2129 | 2211 | 2339 | 624 | 636 | 650 | 309 | 312 | 318 |
| | *** | 42983 | 44176 | 65415 | 11404 | 12186 | 16640 | 2164 | 2263 | 2791 | 633 | 641 | 743 | 312 | 312 | 346 |
| 0.25 | *** | 49408 | 50061 | 65435 | 12991 | 13574 | 16640 | 2479 | 2596 | 2797 | 720 | 738 | 755 | 353 | 356 | 361 |
| | *** | 49624 | 51348 | 76254 | 13201 | 14338 | 19300 | 2531 | 2683 | 3192 | 729 | 746 | 833 | 353 | 356 | 382 |
| 0.3 | *** | 53565 | 54466 | 75772 | 14160 | 14939 | 19177 | 2741 | 2902 | 3182 | 793 | 816 | 843 | 382 | 388 | 396 |
| | *** | 53868 | 56233 | 85086 | 14440 | 15966 | 21458 | 2815 | 3021 | 3513 | 808 | 828 | 904 | 388 | 391 | 409 |
| 0.35 | *** | 55472 | 56671 | 84134 | 14802 | 15805 | 21221 | 2928 | 3130 | 3485 | 851 | 878 | 907 | 405 | 414 | 417 |
| | *** | 55875 | 59013 | 91910 | 15170 | 17100 | 23113 | 3016 | 3275 | 3754 | 863 | 890 | 954 | 408 | 414 | 426 |
| 0.4 | *** | 55376 | 56942 | 90420 | 14995 | 16234 | 22738 | 3042 | 3278 | 3704 | 886 | 913 | 951 | 417 | 426 | 435 |
| | *** | 55898 | 59949 | 96728 | 15455 | 17783 | 24268 | 3147 | 3450 | 3915 | 898 | 930 | 984 | 423 | 431 | 435 |
| 0.45 | *** | 53570 | 55583 | 94567 | 14811 | 16281 | 23724 | 3091 | 3354 | 3835 | 898 | 933 | 974 | 423 | 431 | 440 |
| | *** | 54244 | 59348 | 99538 | 15368 | 18063 | 24920 | 3205 | 3550 | 3995 | 916 | 951 | 994 | 426 | 435 | 435 |
| 0.5 | *** | 50385 | 52943 | 96545 | 14326 | 16010 | 24161 | 3077 | 3363 | 3879 | 895 | 930 | 974 | 417 | 426 | 435 |
| | *** | 51246 | 57520 | 100341 | 14974 | 17978 | 25070 | 3200 | 3573 | 3995 | 913 | 951 | 984 | 423 | 431 | 426 |
| 0.55 | *** | 46176 | 49373 | 96340 | 13618 | 15473 | 24056 | 3007 | 3301 | 3835 | 872 | 907 | 951 | 405 | 414 | 423 |
| | *** | 47265 | 54755 | 99136 | 14338 | 17581 | 24719 | 3138 | 3520 | 3915 | 890 | 930 | 954 | 408 | 417 | 409 |
| 0.6 | *** | 41320 | 45217 | 93951 | 12737 | 14711 | 23403 | 2885 | 3179 | 3704 | 834 | 869 | 907 | 379 | 388 | 396 |
| | *** | 42680 | 51295 | 95925 | 13516 | 16890 | 23866 | 3016 | 3398 | 3754 | 851 | 886 | 904 | 382 | 391 | 382 |
| 0.65 | *** | 36196 | 40755 | 89384 | 11736 | 13758 | 22210 | 2715 | 2995 | 3488 | 776 | 808 | 843 | 347 | 356 | 361 |
| | *** | 37832 | 47331 | 90706 | 12541 | 15931 | 22511 | 2838 | 3200 | 3513 | 790 | 825 | 833 | 353 | 361 | 346 |
| 0.7 | *** | 31135 | 36187 | 82655 | 10634 | 12629 | 20472 | 2491 | 2745 | 3182 | 697 | 723 | 758 | 309 | 312 | 321 |
| | *** | 33008 | 42965 | 83480 | 11433 | 14711 | 20655 | 2605 | 2928 | 3192 | 711 | 741 | 743 | 312 | 318 | 302 |
| 0.75 | *** | 26349 | 31593 | 73777 | 9438 | 11316 | 18203 | 2216 | 2435 | 2794 | 606 | 624 | 650 | 260 | 265 | 268 |
| | *** | 28344 | 38231 | 74247 | 10200 | 13218 | 18296 | 2313 | 2587 | 2791 | 615 | 636 | 633 | 260 | 265 | 248 |
| 0.8 | *** | 21890 | 26953 | 62778 | 8140 | 9803 | 15397 | 1878 | 2053 | 2321 | 487 | 505 | 522 | 198 | 204 | 204 |
| | *** | 23846 | 33078 | 63007 | 8817 | 11433 | 15436 | 1957 | 2173 | 2309 | 496 | 513 | 502 | 198 | 204 | 186 |
| 0.85 | *** | 17628 | 22123 | 49676 | 6688 | 8035 | 12069 | 1476 | 1595 | 1765 | 356 | 361 | 370 | . | . | . |
| | *** | 19393 | 27346 | 49759 | 7248 | 9304 | 12074 | 1534 | 1674 | 1747 | 356 | 365 | 352 | . | . | . |
| 0.9 | *** | 13288 | 16794 | 34495 | 4985 | 5909 | 8222 | 991 | 1047 | 1123 | . | . | . | . | . | . |
| | *** | 14680 | 20673 | 34504 | 5378 | 6714 | 8210 | 1018 | 1082 | 1104 | . | . | . | . | . | . |
| 0.95 | *** | 8201 | 10182 | 17258 | 2788 | 3165 | 3865 | . | . | . | . | . | . | . | . | . |
| | *** | 9010 | 12165 | 17242 | 2955 | 3450 | 3844 | . | . | . | . | . | . | . | . | . |
| 0.98 | *** | 3853 | 4509 | 5938 | . | . | . | . | . | . | . | . | . | . | . | . |
| | *** | 4133 | 5043 | 5922 | . | . | . | . | . | . | . | . | . | . | . | . |

## TABLE 3: ALPHA= 0.01  POWER= 0.8    EXPECTED ACCRUAL THRU MINIMUM FOLLOW-UP= 3750

| | | DEL=.01 | | | DEL=.02 | | | DEL=.05 | | | DEL=.10 | | | DEL=.15 | | |
|---|---|---|---|---|---|---|---|---|---|---|---|---|---|---|---|---|
| FACT= | | 1.0 / .75 | .50 / .25 | .00 / BIN | 1.0 / .75 | .50 / .25 | .00 / BIN | 1.0 / .75 | .50 / .25 | .00 / BIN | 1.0 / 75 | .50 / .25 | .00 / BIN | 1.0 / .75 | .50 / .25 | .00 / BIN |
| PCONT=*** | | REQUIRED NUMBER OF PATIENTS | | | | | | | | | | | | | | |
| 0.01 | *** | 1534 | 1540 | 1550 | 565 | 565 | 565 | 184 | 184 | 184 | 97 | 97 | 97 | 68 | 68 | 68 |
| | *** | 1540 | 1544 | 5922 | 565 | 565 | 1958 | 184 | 184 | 533 | 97 | 97 | 217 | 68 | 68 | 129 |
| 0.02 | *** | 3391 | 3409 | 3453 | 1090 | 1094 | 1103 | 297 | 297 | 297 | 128 | 128 | 128 | 87 | 87 | 87 |
| | *** | 3400 | 3425 | 9776 | 1094 | 1100 | 2911 | 297 | 297 | 681 | 128 | 128 | 252 | 87 | 87 | 144 |
| 0.05 | *** | 10268 | 10338 | 10788 | 2913 | 2950 | 3022 | 631 | 634 | 640 | 228 | 228 | 228 | 134 | 134 | 134 |
| | *** | 10291 | 10447 | 20855 | 2928 | 2978 | 5651 | 634 | 640 | 1104 | 228 | 228 | 352 | 134 | 134 | 186 |
| 0.1 | *** | 22656 | 22831 | 25113 | 6097 | 6228 | 6640 | 1193 | 1212 | 1234 | 378 | 378 | 381 | 200 | 200 | 203 |
| | *** | 22713 | 23159 | 37716 | 6147 | 6368 | 9816 | 1203 | 1222 | 1747 | 378 | 381 | 502 | 200 | 203 | 248 |
| 0.15 | *** | 33837 | 34150 | 39672 | 8956 | 9218 | 10272 | 1703 | 1747 | 1812 | 509 | 518 | 522 | 259 | 259 | 265 |
| | *** | 33944 | 34756 | 52569 | 9053 | 9531 | 13479 | 1722 | 1775 | 2309 | 513 | 518 | 633 | 259 | 265 | 302 |
| 0.2 | *** | 42865 | 43347 | 53300 | 11290 | 11706 | 13647 | 2140 | 2215 | 2337 | 625 | 634 | 650 | 312 | 312 | 316 |
| | *** | 43025 | 44300 | 65415 | 11440 | 12237 | 16640 | 2172 | 2272 | 2791 | 631 | 640 | 743 | 312 | 316 | 346 |
| 0.25 | *** | 49456 | 50153 | 65434 | 13038 | 13643 | 16643 | 2491 | 2609 | 2797 | 725 | 738 | 756 | 353 | 353 | 359 |
| | *** | 49684 | 51528 | 76254 | 13259 | 14422 | 19300 | 2543 | 2688 | 3192 | 728 | 747 | 833 | 353 | 359 | 382 |
| 0.3 | *** | 53631 | 54593 | 75772 | 14219 | 15034 | 19178 | 2759 | 2918 | 3181 | 800 | 818 | 841 | 381 | 387 | 397 |
| | *** | 53950 | 56478 | 85086 | 14519 | 16075 | 21458 | 2828 | 3031 | 3513 | 809 | 828 | 904 | 387 | 391 | 409 |
| 0.35 | *** | 55559 | 56843 | 84134 | 14884 | 15925 | 21222 | 2950 | 3147 | 3484 | 850 | 878 | 906 | 406 | 409 | 419 |
| | *** | 55990 | 59328 | 91910 | 15269 | 17234 | 23113 | 3034 | 3288 | 3754 | 865 | 893 | 954 | 409 | 415 | 426 |
| 0.4 | *** | 55488 | 57166 | 90419 | 15100 | 16375 | 22741 | 3068 | 3297 | 3700 | 888 | 916 | 950 | 419 | 425 | 434 |
| | *** | 56047 | 60350 | 96728 | 15578 | 17941 | 24268 | 3172 | 3466 | 3915 | 903 | 934 | 984 | 425 | 428 | 435 |
| 0.45 | *** | 53716 | 55868 | 94568 | 14937 | 16447 | 23722 | 3119 | 3378 | 3831 | 903 | 934 | 972 | 425 | 428 | 438 |
| | *** | 54434 | 59838 | 99538 | 15513 | 18241 | 24920 | 3231 | 3565 | 3995 | 916 | 953 | 994 | 428 | 434 | 435 |
| 0.5 | *** | 50572 | 53300 | 96547 | 14472 | 16197 | 24162 | 3109 | 3387 | 3878 | 897 | 934 | 972 | 419 | 425 | 434 |
| | *** | 51490 | 58094 | 100341 | 15138 | 18181 | 25070 | 3231 | 3588 | 3995 | 916 | 953 | 984 | 425 | 428 | 426 |
| 0.55 | *** | 46413 | 49806 | 96340 | 13784 | 15678 | 24059 | 3040 | 3325 | 3837 | 878 | 912 | 953 | 406 | 409 | 419 |
| | *** | 47575 | 55409 | 99136 | 14525 | 17791 | 24719 | 3166 | 3537 | 3915 | 893 | 931 | 954 | 409 | 415 | 409 |
| 0.6 | *** | 41618 | 45725 | 93950 | 12916 | 14928 | 23406 | 2918 | 3203 | 3706 | 837 | 869 | 906 | 381 | 387 | 397 |
| | *** | 43056 | 52009 | 95925 | 13713 | 17106 | 23866 | 3044 | 3409 | 3754 | 850 | 888 | 904 | 387 | 391 | 382 |
| 0.65 | *** | 36556 | 41328 | 89384 | 11922 | 13972 | 22212 | 2744 | 3016 | 3490 | 781 | 809 | 847 | 350 | 353 | 363 |
| | *** | 38281 | 48078 | 90706 | 12743 | 16147 | 22511 | 2866 | 3213 | 3513 | 794 | 828 | 833 | 353 | 359 | 346 |
| 0.7 | *** | 31553 | 36790 | 82656 | 10822 | 12837 | 20472 | 2519 | 2768 | 3184 | 700 | 728 | 756 | 306 | 312 | 322 |
| | *** | 33503 | 43718 | 83480 | 11631 | 14913 | 20655 | 2631 | 2947 | 3192 | 715 | 743 | 743 | 312 | 316 | 302 |
| 0.75 | *** | 26806 | 32200 | 73778 | 9616 | 11506 | 18200 | 2238 | 2453 | 2797 | 606 | 625 | 650 | 259 | 265 | 265 |
| | *** | 28859 | 38950 | 74247 | 10384 | 13403 | 18296 | 2337 | 2600 | 2791 | 616 | 640 | 633 | 259 | 265 | 248 |
| 0.8 | *** | 22338 | 27522 | 62781 | 8300 | 9968 | 15400 | 1900 | 2069 | 2322 | 490 | 503 | 522 | 200 | 203 | 203 |
| | *** | 24350 | 33734 | 63007 | 8984 | 11590 | 15436 | 1975 | 2178 | 2309 | 500 | 513 | 502 | 200 | 203 | 186 |
| 0.85 | *** | 18040 | 22615 | 49675 | 6822 | 8168 | 12072 | 1493 | 1606 | 1765 | 353 | 363 | 372 | . | . | . |
| | *** | 19834 | 27893 | 49759 | 7381 | 9419 | 12074 | 1544 | 1675 | 1747 | 359 | 368 | 352 | . | . | . |
| 0.9 | *** | 13609 | 17168 | 34497 | 5078 | 5997 | 8225 | 997 | 1053 | 1122 | . | . | . | . | . | . |
| | *** | 15025 | 21068 | 34504 | 5468 | 6784 | 8210 | 1025 | 1084 | 1104 | . | . | . | . | . | . |
| 0.95 | *** | 8393 | 10384 | 17256 | 2828 | 3200 | 3865 | . | . | . | . | . | . | . | . | . |
| | *** | 9209 | 12353 | 17242 | 2993 | 3472 | 3844 | . | . | . | . | . | . | . | . | . |
| 0.98 | *** | 3922 | 4568 | 5941 | . | . | . | . | . | . | . | . | . | . | . | . |
| | *** | 4203 | 5088 | 5922 | . | . | . | . | . | . | . | . | . | . | . | . |

**TABLE 3: ALPHA= 0.01  POWER= 0.8     EXPECTED ACCRUAL THRU MINIMUM FOLLOW-UP= 4000**

| | DEL=.01 | | | DEL=.02 | | | DEL=.05 | | | DEL=.10 | | | DEL=.15 | | |
|---|---|---|---|---|---|---|---|---|---|---|---|---|---|---|---|
| FACT= | 1.0 .75 | .50 .25 | .00 BIN | 1.0 .75 | .50 .25 | .00 BIN | 1.0 .75 | .50 .25 | .00 BIN | 1.0 75 | .50 .25 | .00 BIN | 1.0 .75 | .50 .25 | .00 BIN |
| PCONT=*** | | | | | REQUIRED NUMBER OF PATIENTS | | | | | | | | | | |
| 0.01 *** | 1537 | 1543 | 1547 | 563 | 567 | 567 | 187 | 187 | 187 | 93 | 93 | 93 | 67 | 67 | 67 |
| *** | 1537 | 1543 | 5922 | 567 | 567 | 1958 | 187 | 187 | 533 | 93 | 93 | 217 | 67 | 67 | 129 |
| 0.02 *** | 3397 | 3413 | 3453 | 1093 | 1097 | 1103 | 297 | 297 | 297 | 127 | 127 | 127 | 83 | 83 | 87 |
| *** | 3403 | 3427 | 9776 | 1093 | 1097 | 2911 | 297 | 297 | 681 | 127 | 127 | 252 | 83 | 83 | 144 |
| 0.05 *** | 10273 | 10347 | 10787 | 2917 | 2953 | 3023 | 633 | 637 | 643 | 227 | 227 | 227 | 133 | 133 | 133 |
| *** | 10297 | 10453 | 20855 | 2933 | 2983 | 5651 | 633 | 637 | 1104 | 227 | 227 | 352 | 133 | 133 | 186 |
| 0.1 *** | 22667 | 22853 | 25113 | 6107 | 6243 | 6643 | 1193 | 1213 | 1237 | 377 | 377 | 383 | 203 | 203 | 203 |
| *** | 22727 | 23197 | 37716 | 6157 | 6377 | 9816 | 1203 | 1223 | 1747 | 377 | 383 | 502 | 203 | 203 | 248 |
| 0.15 *** | 33857 | 34193 | 39673 | 8977 | 9247 | 10273 | 1707 | 1753 | 1813 | 513 | 517 | 523 | 263 | 263 | 263 |
| *** | 33973 | 34833 | 52569 | 9077 | 9563 | 13479 | 1727 | 1777 | 2309 | 513 | 517 | 633 | 263 | 263 | 302 |
| 0.2 *** | 42897 | 43413 | 53297 | 11317 | 11753 | 13647 | 2147 | 2223 | 2337 | 627 | 637 | 647 | 313 | 313 | 317 |
| *** | 43067 | 44423 | 65415 | 11477 | 12287 | 16640 | 2183 | 2273 | 2791 | 633 | 643 | 743 | 313 | 313 | 346 |
| 0.25 *** | 49503 | 50247 | 65433 | 13083 | 13707 | 16643 | 2503 | 2617 | 2797 | 723 | 737 | 753 | 353 | 357 | 357 |
| *** | 49747 | 51703 | 76254 | 13313 | 14493 | 19300 | 2553 | 2693 | 3192 | 733 | 747 | 833 | 353 | 357 | 382 |
| 0.3 *** | 53697 | 54723 | 75773 | 14283 | 15123 | 19177 | 2777 | 2927 | 3183 | 803 | 817 | 843 | 383 | 387 | 393 |
| *** | 54037 | 56717 | 85086 | 14593 | 16177 | 21458 | 2843 | 3037 | 3513 | 807 | 827 | 904 | 387 | 393 | 409 |
| 0.35 *** | 55647 | 57013 | 84133 | 14967 | 16043 | 21223 | 2973 | 3163 | 3483 | 857 | 877 | 907 | 407 | 413 | 417 |
| *** | 56103 | 59643 | 91910 | 15367 | 17363 | 23113 | 3057 | 3297 | 3754 | 867 | 893 | 954 | 407 | 417 | 426 |
| 0.4 *** | 55603 | 57387 | 90423 | 15197 | 16517 | 22737 | 3093 | 3317 | 3703 | 893 | 917 | 953 | 423 | 427 | 433 |
| *** | 56197 | 60743 | 96728 | 15697 | 18093 | 24268 | 3193 | 3477 | 3915 | 903 | 933 | 984 | 423 | 433 | 435 |
| 0.45 *** | 53857 | 56153 | 94567 | 15057 | 16607 | 23723 | 3147 | 3397 | 3833 | 907 | 937 | 973 | 423 | 433 | 437 |
| *** | 54627 | 60317 | 99538 | 15653 | 18413 | 24920 | 3257 | 3577 | 3995 | 923 | 953 | 994 | 427 | 437 | 435 |
| 0.5 *** | 50753 | 53647 | 96547 | 14617 | 16377 | 24163 | 3137 | 3407 | 3877 | 903 | 937 | 973 | 417 | 427 | 433 |
| *** | 51733 | 58657 | 100341 | 15297 | 18367 | 25070 | 3257 | 3603 | 3995 | 917 | 953 | 984 | 423 | 433 | 426 |
| 0.55 *** | 46647 | 50233 | 96343 | 13943 | 15867 | 24057 | 3067 | 3347 | 3837 | 883 | 913 | 953 | 407 | 413 | 423 |
| *** | 47883 | 56043 | 99136 | 14697 | 17987 | 24719 | 3193 | 3553 | 3915 | 897 | 933 | 954 | 407 | 417 | 409 |
| 0.6 *** | 41907 | 46217 | 93953 | 13087 | 15127 | 23407 | 2947 | 3227 | 3703 | 843 | 873 | 907 | 383 | 387 | 397 |
| *** | 43433 | 52697 | 95925 | 13897 | 17307 | 23866 | 3073 | 3427 | 3754 | 857 | 887 | 904 | 387 | 393 | 382 |
| 0.65 *** | 36913 | 41873 | 89383 | 12103 | 14173 | 22207 | 2773 | 3043 | 3487 | 783 | 813 | 843 | 353 | 357 | 363 |
| *** | 38717 | 48793 | 90706 | 12933 | 16343 | 22511 | 2893 | 3227 | 3513 | 797 | 827 | 833 | 353 | 357 | 346 |
| 0.7 *** | 31963 | 37367 | 82653 | 10997 | 13027 | 20473 | 2543 | 2787 | 3183 | 707 | 727 | 757 | 307 | 313 | 317 |
| *** | 33987 | 44433 | 83480 | 11823 | 15097 | 20655 | 2653 | 2957 | 3192 | 717 | 743 | 743 | 313 | 317 | 302 |
| 0.75 *** | 27243 | 32777 | 73777 | 9787 | 11687 | 18203 | 2263 | 2467 | 2797 | 607 | 627 | 647 | 257 | 263 | 267 |
| *** | 29357 | 39637 | 74247 | 10563 | 13567 | 18296 | 2357 | 2613 | 2791 | 617 | 637 | 633 | 263 | 263 | 248 |
| 0.8 *** | 22773 | 28063 | 62777 | 8453 | 10127 | 15397 | 1917 | 2083 | 2323 | 493 | 507 | 523 | 203 | 203 | 203 |
| *** | 24827 | 34347 | 63007 | 9143 | 11727 | 15436 | 1993 | 2187 | 2309 | 497 | 513 | 502 | 203 | 203 | 186 |
| 0.85 *** | 18427 | 23083 | 49677 | 6947 | 8293 | 12073 | 1503 | 1613 | 1763 | 357 | 363 | 373 | . | . | . |
| *** | 20257 | 28407 | 49759 | 7507 | 9523 | 12074 | 1557 | 1683 | 1747 | 357 | 367 | 352 | . | . | . |
| 0.9 *** | 13923 | 17517 | 34497 | 5167 | 6077 | 8223 | 1003 | 1057 | 1123 | . | . | . | . | . | . |
| *** | 15357 | 21433 | 34504 | 5557 | 6847 | 8210 | 1027 | 1087 | 1104 | . | . | . | . | . | . |
| 0.95 *** | 8573 | 10573 | 17257 | 2867 | 3227 | 3863 | . | . | . | . | . | . | . | . | . |
| *** | 9393 | 12527 | 17242 | 3027 | 3493 | 3844 | . | . | . | . | . | . | . | . | . |
| 0.98 *** | 3983 | 4623 | 5943 | . | . | . | . | . | . | . | . | . | . | . | . |
| *** | 4263 | 5127 | 5922 | . | . | . | . | . | . | . | . | . | . | . | . |

## TABLE 3: ALPHA= 0.01  POWER= 0.8    EXPECTED ACCRUAL THRU MINIMUM FOLLOW-UP= 4250

| | | DEL=.01 | | | DEL=.02 | | | DEL=.05 | | | DEL=.10 | | | DEL=.15 | |
|---|---|---|---|---|---|---|---|---|---|---|---|---|---|---|---|---|
| FACT= | 1.0 .75 | .50 .25 | .00 BIN | 1.0 .75 | .50 .25 | .00 BIN | 1.0 .75 | .50 .25 | .00 BIN | 1.0 75 | .50 .25 | .00 BIN | 1.0 .75 | .50 .25 | .00 BIN |
| PCONT=*** | | | | | | REQUIRED NUMBER OF PATIENTS | | | | | | | | | |
| 0.01 *** | 1537 | 1544 | 1548 | 566 | 566 | 566 | 188 | 188 | 188 | 92 | 92 | 92 | 67 | 67 | 67 |
| *** | 1537 | 1544 | 5922 | 566 | 566 | 1958 | 188 | 188 | 533 | 92 | 92 | 217 | 67 | 67 | 129 |
| 0.02 *** | 3397 | 3414 | 3456 | 1091 | 1098 | 1102 | 294 | 294 | 294 | 131 | 131 | 131 | 82 | 82 | 88 |
| *** | 3403 | 3428 | 9776 | 1098 | 1102 | 2911 | 294 | 294 | 681 | 131 | 131 | 252 | 82 | 82 | 144 |
| 0.05 *** | 10278 | 10356 | 10788 | 2918 | 2957 | 3025 | 634 | 634 | 641 | 226 | 226 | 226 | 131 | 131 | 131 |
| *** | 10303 | 10462 | 20855 | 2936 | 2982 | 5651 | 634 | 641 | 1104 | 226 | 226 | 352 | 131 | 131 | 186 |
| 0.1 *** | 22677 | 22872 | 25114 | 6117 | 6255 | 6644 | 1197 | 1214 | 1236 | 375 | 379 | 379 | 198 | 198 | 205 |
| *** | 22745 | 23233 | 37716 | 6170 | 6389 | 9816 | 1204 | 1225 | 1747 | 379 | 379 | 502 | 198 | 198 | 248 |
| 0.15 *** | 33880 | 34230 | 39670 | 8996 | 9272 | 10271 | 1714 | 1756 | 1813 | 513 | 517 | 524 | 262 | 262 | 262 |
| *** | 33997 | 34910 | 52569 | 9102 | 9587 | 13479 | 1728 | 1782 | 2309 | 513 | 517 | 633 | 262 | 262 | 302 |
| 0.2 *** | 42928 | 43474 | 53298 | 11351 | 11797 | 13650 | 2153 | 2228 | 2341 | 630 | 641 | 651 | 311 | 315 | 315 |
| *** | 43109 | 44543 | 65415 | 11521 | 12332 | 16640 | 2185 | 2277 | 2791 | 634 | 641 | 743 | 311 | 315 | 346 |
| 0.25 *** | 49548 | 50338 | 65432 | 13129 | 13773 | 16642 | 2515 | 2628 | 2798 | 726 | 740 | 758 | 354 | 358 | 358 |
| *** | 49813 | 51874 | 76254 | 13369 | 14563 | 19300 | 2564 | 2702 | 3192 | 730 | 747 | 833 | 354 | 358 | 382 |
| 0.3 *** | 53759 | 54849 | 75770 | 14340 | 15212 | 19181 | 2791 | 2940 | 3180 | 804 | 821 | 843 | 386 | 390 | 396 |
| *** | 54120 | 56953 | 85086 | 14666 | 16270 | 21458 | 2855 | 3046 | 3513 | 811 | 832 | 904 | 386 | 390 | 409 |
| 0.35 *** | 55731 | 57187 | 84136 | 15042 | 16153 | 21221 | 2989 | 3173 | 3482 | 857 | 878 | 906 | 407 | 411 | 418 |
| *** | 56213 | 59949 | 91910 | 15463 | 17481 | 23113 | 3074 | 3308 | 3754 | 868 | 896 | 954 | 411 | 418 | 426 |
| 0.4 *** | 55710 | 57605 | 90422 | 15297 | 16646 | 22741 | 3116 | 3333 | 3701 | 896 | 921 | 953 | 422 | 428 | 432 |
| *** | 56348 | 61129 | 96728 | 15813 | 18229 | 24268 | 3212 | 3488 | 3915 | 906 | 938 | 984 | 422 | 432 | 435 |
| 0.45 *** | 54003 | 56433 | 94570 | 15176 | 16759 | 23722 | 3169 | 3414 | 3832 | 910 | 938 | 974 | 422 | 432 | 439 |
| *** | 54822 | 60778 | 99538 | 15785 | 18569 | 24920 | 3280 | 3594 | 3995 | 921 | 953 | 994 | 428 | 432 | 435 |
| 0.5 *** | 50939 | 53999 | 96546 | 14755 | 16546 | 24164 | 3163 | 3428 | 3881 | 906 | 938 | 974 | 422 | 428 | 432 |
| *** | 51981 | 59195 | 100341 | 15452 | 18537 | 25070 | 3280 | 3616 | 3995 | 921 | 953 | 984 | 422 | 432 | 426 |
| 0.55 *** | 46881 | 50653 | 96340 | 14096 | 16051 | 24058 | 3095 | 3371 | 3832 | 885 | 917 | 953 | 407 | 411 | 422 |
| *** | 48188 | 56649 | 99136 | 14868 | 18172 | 24719 | 3216 | 3567 | 3915 | 900 | 932 | 954 | 411 | 418 | 409 |
| 0.6 *** | 42199 | 46704 | 93949 | 13253 | 15314 | 23403 | 2972 | 3248 | 3705 | 843 | 874 | 910 | 386 | 390 | 396 |
| *** | 43799 | 53351 | 95925 | 14075 | 17492 | 23866 | 3095 | 3439 | 3754 | 857 | 889 | 904 | 386 | 390 | 382 |
| 0.65 *** | 37265 | 42408 | 89385 | 12268 | 14362 | 22209 | 2798 | 3057 | 3488 | 783 | 811 | 843 | 354 | 358 | 364 |
| *** | 39146 | 49477 | 90706 | 13114 | 16525 | 22511 | 2914 | 3244 | 3513 | 800 | 825 | 833 | 354 | 358 | 346 |
| 0.7 *** | 32360 | 37928 | 82655 | 11170 | 13214 | 20471 | 2568 | 2808 | 3184 | 708 | 730 | 758 | 311 | 315 | 322 |
| *** | 34453 | 45110 | 83480 | 11999 | 15271 | 20655 | 2674 | 2968 | 3192 | 719 | 747 | 743 | 311 | 315 | 302 |
| 0.75 *** | 27664 | 33327 | 73777 | 9948 | 11854 | 18204 | 2281 | 2483 | 2798 | 613 | 630 | 651 | 258 | 262 | 269 |
| *** | 29838 | 40283 | 74247 | 10728 | 13724 | 18296 | 2377 | 2621 | 2791 | 619 | 641 | 633 | 262 | 262 | 248 |
| 0.8 *** | 23187 | 28574 | 62780 | 8599 | 10271 | 15399 | 1937 | 2090 | 2319 | 496 | 507 | 524 | 198 | 205 | 205 |
| *** | 25284 | 34932 | 63007 | 9289 | 11861 | 15436 | 2005 | 2196 | 2309 | 503 | 513 | 502 | 198 | 205 | 186 |
| 0.85 *** | 18803 | 23527 | 49675 | 7062 | 8408 | 12073 | 1516 | 1622 | 1767 | 358 | 364 | 368 | . | . | . |
| *** | 20662 | 28893 | 49759 | 7625 | 9619 | 12074 | 1565 | 1686 | 1747 | 358 | 368 | 352 | . | . | . |
| 0.9 *** | 14213 | 17853 | 34496 | 5252 | 6148 | 8220 | 1013 | 1059 | 1123 | . | . | . | . | . | . |
| *** | 15668 | 21778 | 34504 | 5634 | 6903 | 8210 | 1034 | 1091 | 1104 | . | . | . | . | . | . |
| 0.95 *** | 8748 | 10749 | 17258 | 2904 | 3254 | 3864 | . | . | . | . | . | . | . | . | . |
| *** | 9570 | 12689 | 17242 | 3063 | 3509 | 3844 | . | . | . | . | . | . | . | . | . |
| 0.98 *** | 4045 | 4672 | 5943 | . | . | . | . | . | . | . | . | . | . | . | . |
| *** | 4317 | 5167 | 5922 | . | . | . | . | . | . | . | . | . | . | . | . |

| TABLE 3: ALPHA= 0.01 POWER= 0.8 | | EXPECTED ACCRUAL THRU MINIMUM FOLLOW-UP= 4500 | | | | | | | | | | | | |

| | | DEL=.01 | | | DEL=.02 | | | DEL=.05 | | | DEL=.10 | | | DEL=.15 | |
|---|---|---|---|---|---|---|---|---|---|---|---|---|---|---|---|
| FACT= | | 1.0 .75 | .50 .25 | .00 BIN | 1.0 .75 | .50 .25 | .00 BIN | 1.0 .75 | .50 .25 | .00 BIN | 1.0 75 | .50 .25 | .00 BIN | 1.0 .75 | .50 .25 | .00 BIN |
| PCONT=*** | | | | | REQUIRED NUMBER OF PATIENTS | | | | | | | | | | |
| 0.01 | *** | 1538 | 1538 | 1549 | 566 | 566 | 566 | 188 | 188 | 188 | 93 | 93 | 93 | 64 | 64 | 64 |
| | *** | 1538 | 1545 | 5922 | 566 | 566 | 1958 | 188 | 188 | 533 | 93 | 93 | 217 | 64 | 64 | 129 |
| 0.02 | *** | 3401 | 3416 | 3457 | 1095 | 1099 | 1106 | 296 | 296 | 296 | 127 | 131 | 131 | 86 | 86 | 86 |
| | *** | 3405 | 3428 | 9776 | 1095 | 1099 | 2911 | 296 | 296 | 681 | 131 | 131 | 252 | 86 | 86 | 144 |
| 0.05 | *** | 10286 | 10365 | 10792 | 2921 | 2955 | 3023 | 633 | 638 | 638 | 228 | 228 | 228 | 131 | 131 | 131 |
| | *** | 10313 | 10477 | 20855 | 2940 | 2985 | 5651 | 633 | 638 | 1104 | 228 | 228 | 352 | 131 | 131 | 186 |
| 0.1 | *** | 22688 | 22897 | 25113 | 6128 | 6263 | 6641 | 1196 | 1211 | 1234 | 375 | 379 | 379 | 199 | 199 | 199 |
| | *** | 22762 | 23273 | 37716 | 6184 | 6398 | 9816 | 1207 | 1223 | 1747 | 379 | 379 | 502 | 199 | 199 | 248 |
| 0.15 | *** | 33900 | 34275 | 39671 | 9015 | 9300 | 10275 | 1718 | 1758 | 1815 | 514 | 514 | 521 | 262 | 262 | 262 |
| | *** | 34028 | 34984 | 52569 | 9127 | 9611 | 13479 | 1736 | 1781 | 2309 | 514 | 521 | 633 | 262 | 262 | 302 |
| 0.2 | *** | 42960 | 43541 | 53299 | 11381 | 11843 | 13650 | 2163 | 2231 | 2336 | 626 | 638 | 649 | 311 | 311 | 318 |
| | *** | 43151 | 44659 | 65415 | 11557 | 12378 | 16640 | 2197 | 2280 | 2791 | 633 | 645 | 743 | 311 | 311 | 346 |
| 0.25 | *** | 49593 | 50430 | 65433 | 13170 | 13834 | 16642 | 2523 | 2629 | 2798 | 728 | 739 | 757 | 352 | 356 | 356 |
| | *** | 49875 | 52046 | 76254 | 13418 | 14628 | 19300 | 2573 | 2703 | 3192 | 735 | 746 | 833 | 356 | 356 | 382 |
| 0.3 | *** | 53823 | 54975 | 75772 | 14403 | 15296 | 19178 | 2805 | 2951 | 3180 | 802 | 825 | 840 | 386 | 390 | 397 |
| | *** | 54210 | 57180 | 85086 | 14741 | 16354 | 21458 | 2872 | 3052 | 3513 | 813 | 829 | 904 | 386 | 390 | 409 |
| 0.35 | *** | 55815 | 57356 | 84135 | 15123 | 16253 | 21221 | 3007 | 3187 | 3484 | 863 | 881 | 908 | 408 | 413 | 420 |
| | *** | 56332 | 60251 | 91910 | 15551 | 17587 | 23113 | 3090 | 3315 | 3754 | 870 | 892 | 954 | 413 | 413 | 426 |
| 0.4 | *** | 55826 | 57828 | 90420 | 15393 | 16770 | 22740 | 3135 | 3349 | 3705 | 896 | 919 | 953 | 420 | 431 | 435 |
| | *** | 56494 | 61500 | 96728 | 15922 | 18363 | 24268 | 3232 | 3502 | 3915 | 908 | 937 | 984 | 424 | 431 | 435 |
| 0.45 | *** | 54150 | 56708 | 94571 | 15292 | 16905 | 23723 | 3191 | 3435 | 3833 | 915 | 941 | 975 | 424 | 431 | 442 |
| | *** | 55009 | 61230 | 99538 | 15915 | 18723 | 24920 | 3300 | 3603 | 3995 | 926 | 960 | 994 | 431 | 435 | 435 |
| 0.5 | *** | 51123 | 54341 | 96544 | 14887 | 16710 | 24161 | 3187 | 3446 | 3878 | 908 | 941 | 975 | 420 | 424 | 435 |
| | *** | 52219 | 59723 | 100341 | 15600 | 18701 | 25070 | 3304 | 3630 | 3995 | 926 | 953 | 984 | 424 | 431 | 426 |
| 0.55 | *** | 47111 | 51060 | 96341 | 14239 | 16226 | 24056 | 3120 | 3390 | 3833 | 885 | 919 | 953 | 408 | 413 | 420 |
| | *** | 48484 | 57232 | 99136 | 15026 | 18345 | 24719 | 3243 | 3581 | 3915 | 903 | 937 | 954 | 408 | 420 | 409 |
| 0.6 | *** | 42488 | 47175 | 93952 | 13413 | 15495 | 23403 | 3000 | 3266 | 3705 | 847 | 874 | 908 | 386 | 390 | 397 |
| | *** | 44160 | 53985 | 95925 | 14246 | 17670 | 23866 | 3120 | 3450 | 3754 | 863 | 892 | 904 | 386 | 390 | 382 |
| 0.65 | *** | 37605 | 42922 | 89385 | 12435 | 14543 | 22211 | 2820 | 3079 | 3491 | 791 | 813 | 847 | 352 | 356 | 363 |
| | *** | 39563 | 50126 | 90706 | 13290 | 16698 | 22511 | 2940 | 3255 | 3513 | 802 | 829 | 833 | 352 | 356 | 346 |
| 0.7 | *** | 32752 | 38467 | 82657 | 11332 | 13384 | 20471 | 2591 | 2820 | 3187 | 712 | 735 | 757 | 311 | 311 | 318 |
| | *** | 34905 | 45761 | 83480 | 12169 | 15431 | 20655 | 2696 | 2978 | 3192 | 723 | 746 | 743 | 311 | 318 | 302 |
| 0.75 | *** | 28076 | 33859 | 73781 | 10099 | 12011 | 18199 | 2303 | 2501 | 2793 | 615 | 633 | 649 | 262 | 262 | 266 |
| | *** | 30300 | 40901 | 74247 | 10886 | 13868 | 18296 | 2393 | 2629 | 2791 | 622 | 638 | 633 | 262 | 266 | 248 |
| 0.8 | *** | 23588 | 29066 | 62778 | 8733 | 10410 | 15398 | 1950 | 2100 | 2321 | 498 | 510 | 521 | 199 | 206 | 206 |
| | *** | 25725 | 35486 | 63007 | 9431 | 11978 | 15436 | 2021 | 2201 | 2309 | 503 | 514 | 502 | 199 | 206 | 186 |
| 0.85 | *** | 19162 | 23948 | 49676 | 7174 | 8513 | 12068 | 1526 | 1628 | 1763 | 356 | 363 | 368 | . | . | . |
| | *** | 21052 | 29348 | 49759 | 7736 | 9712 | 12074 | 1571 | 1691 | 1747 | 363 | 368 | 352 | . | . | . |
| 0.9 | *** | 14498 | 18172 | 34496 | 5329 | 6218 | 8220 | 1016 | 1065 | 1121 | . | . | . | . | . | . |
| | *** | 15971 | 22103 | 34504 | 5711 | 6956 | 8210 | 1038 | 1095 | 1104 | . | . | . | . | . | . |
| 0.95 | *** | 8906 | 10916 | 17261 | 2933 | 3281 | 3862 | . | . | . | . | . | . | . | . | . |
| | *** | 9735 | 12840 | 17242 | 3090 | 3525 | 3844 | . | . | . | . | . | . | . | . | . |
| 0.98 | *** | 4098 | 4717 | 5943 | . | . | . | . | . | . | . | . | . | . | . | . |
| | *** | 4368 | 5201 | 5922 | . | . | . | . | . | . | . | . | . | . | . | . |

## TABLE 3: ALPHA= 0.01  POWER= 0.8     EXPECTED ACCRUAL THRU MINIMUM FOLLOW-UP= 4750

| | | DEL=.01 | | | DEL=.02 | | | DEL=.05 | | | DEL=.10 | | | DEL=.15 | | |
|---|---|---|---|---|---|---|---|---|---|---|---|---|---|---|---|---|
| FACT= | | 1.0 .75 | .50 .25 | .00 BIN | 1.0 .75 | .50 .25 | .00 BIN | 1.0 .75 | .50 .25 | .00 BIN | 1.0 75 | .50 .25 | .00 BIN | 1.0 .75 | .50 .25 | .00 BIN |
| PCONT=*** | | | | | REQUIRED | NUMBER OF | PATIENTS | | | | | | | | | |
| 0.01 | *** | 1535 | 1540 | 1547 | 566 | 566 | 566 | 186 | 186 | 186 | 91 | 91 | 91 | 67 | 67 | 67 |
| | *** | 1540 | 1547 | 5922 | 566 | 566 | 1958 | 186 | 186 | 533 | 91 | 91 | 217 | 67 | 67 | 129 |
| 0.02 | *** | 3400 | 3416 | 3452 | 1096 | 1096 | 1100 | 293 | 293 | 300 | 127 | 127 | 127 | 87 | 87 | 87 |
| | *** | 3404 | 3428 | 9776 | 1096 | 1100 | 2911 | 293 | 293 | 681 | 127 | 127 | 252 | 87 | 87 | 144 |
| 0.05 | *** | 10287 | 10370 | 10790 | 2925 | 2960 | 3024 | 633 | 637 | 637 | 229 | 229 | 229 | 134 | 134 | 134 |
| | *** | 10315 | 10482 | 20855 | 2941 | 2989 | 5651 | 633 | 637 | 1104 | 229 | 229 | 352 | 134 | 134 | 186 |
| 0.1 | *** | 22701 | 22922 | 25112 | 6135 | 6278 | 6642 | 1195 | 1215 | 1238 | 376 | 376 | 383 | 198 | 198 | 205 |
| | *** | 22772 | 23307 | 37716 | 6195 | 6409 | 9816 | 1207 | 1227 | 1747 | 376 | 383 | 502 | 198 | 198 | 248 |
| 0.15 | *** | 33923 | 34315 | 39670 | 9033 | 9325 | 10275 | 1718 | 1761 | 1813 | 514 | 519 | 526 | 257 | 265 | 265 |
| | *** | 34054 | 35051 | 52569 | 9147 | 9634 | 13479 | 1737 | 1785 | 2309 | 514 | 519 | 633 | 265 | 265 | 302 |
| 0.2 | *** | 42991 | 43608 | 53298 | 11408 | 11883 | 13648 | 2169 | 2236 | 2335 | 633 | 637 | 649 | 312 | 312 | 317 |
| | *** | 43197 | 44777 | 65415 | 11593 | 12417 | 16640 | 2200 | 2283 | 2791 | 633 | 645 | 743 | 312 | 317 | 346 |
| 0.25 | *** | 49641 | 50524 | 65435 | 13213 | 13897 | 16640 | 2533 | 2640 | 2799 | 728 | 740 | 756 | 352 | 360 | 360 |
| | *** | 49938 | 52218 | 76254 | 13474 | 14693 | 19300 | 2580 | 2711 | 3192 | 732 | 744 | 833 | 352 | 360 | 382 |
| 0.3 | *** | 53885 | 55103 | 75770 | 14460 | 15374 | 19182 | 2818 | 2960 | 3179 | 804 | 823 | 839 | 383 | 388 | 395 |
| | *** | 54296 | 57412 | 85086 | 14804 | 16438 | 21458 | 2882 | 3055 | 3513 | 815 | 835 | 904 | 388 | 395 | 409 |
| 0.35 | *** | 55904 | 57526 | 84138 | 15196 | 16355 | 21217 | 3024 | 3202 | 3483 | 863 | 882 | 906 | 407 | 412 | 419 |
| | *** | 56445 | 60547 | 91910 | 15635 | 17690 | 23113 | 3103 | 3321 | 3754 | 870 | 894 | 954 | 412 | 419 | 426 |
| 0.4 | *** | 55935 | 58048 | 90420 | 15488 | 16894 | 22737 | 3150 | 3364 | 3701 | 899 | 922 | 953 | 424 | 431 | 435 |
| | *** | 56647 | 61872 | 96728 | 16027 | 18485 | 24268 | 3245 | 3507 | 3915 | 910 | 934 | 984 | 424 | 431 | 435 |
| 0.45 | *** | 54289 | 56984 | 94569 | 15405 | 17044 | 23722 | 3214 | 3447 | 3832 | 918 | 942 | 970 | 424 | 431 | 443 |
| | *** | 55203 | 61670 | 99538 | 16039 | 18861 | 24920 | 3321 | 3613 | 3995 | 930 | 958 | 994 | 431 | 435 | 435 |
| 0.5 | *** | 51308 | 54680 | 96547 | 15013 | 16859 | 24162 | 3210 | 3464 | 3879 | 910 | 942 | 977 | 419 | 431 | 435 |
| | *** | 52460 | 60226 | 100341 | 15742 | 18854 | 25070 | 3321 | 3642 | 3995 | 930 | 958 | 984 | 424 | 431 | 426 |
| 0.55 | *** | 47342 | 51462 | 96338 | 14384 | 16391 | 24055 | 3143 | 3404 | 3832 | 894 | 918 | 953 | 407 | 412 | 419 |
| | *** | 48786 | 57799 | 99136 | 15180 | 18505 | 24719 | 3262 | 3590 | 3915 | 906 | 934 | 954 | 412 | 419 | 409 |
| 0.6 | *** | 42777 | 47634 | 93951 | 13565 | 15667 | 23402 | 3024 | 3285 | 3701 | 851 | 875 | 910 | 383 | 388 | 395 |
| | *** | 44515 | 54593 | 95925 | 14408 | 17832 | 23866 | 3143 | 3464 | 3754 | 863 | 894 | 904 | 388 | 395 | 382 |
| 0.65 | *** | 37949 | 43423 | 89387 | 12591 | 14717 | 22210 | 2846 | 3095 | 3487 | 792 | 815 | 847 | 352 | 360 | 364 |
| | *** | 39967 | 50757 | 90706 | 13450 | 16859 | 22511 | 2960 | 3262 | 3513 | 804 | 827 | 833 | 352 | 360 | 346 |
| 0.7 | *** | 33135 | 38982 | 82653 | 11487 | 13545 | 20476 | 2609 | 2834 | 3186 | 716 | 732 | 756 | 312 | 317 | 317 |
| | *** | 35343 | 46380 | 83480 | 12330 | 15583 | 20655 | 2715 | 2989 | 3192 | 720 | 744 | 743 | 312 | 317 | 302 |
| 0.75 | *** | 28472 | 34370 | 73783 | 10244 | 12163 | 18200 | 2319 | 2509 | 2794 | 614 | 633 | 649 | 257 | 265 | 265 |
| | *** | 30748 | 41487 | 74247 | 11035 | 14004 | 18296 | 2407 | 2640 | 2791 | 621 | 637 | 633 | 265 | 265 | 248 |
| 0.8 | *** | 23972 | 29541 | 62779 | 8862 | 10537 | 15398 | 1963 | 2110 | 2319 | 495 | 507 | 519 | 198 | 205 | 205 |
| | *** | 26152 | 36013 | 63007 | 9555 | 12092 | 15436 | 2034 | 2205 | 2309 | 502 | 514 | 502 | 205 | 205 | 186 |
| 0.85 | *** | 19502 | 24352 | 49677 | 7283 | 8613 | 12068 | 1535 | 1635 | 1765 | 360 | 364 | 372 | . | . | . |
| | *** | 21426 | 29779 | 49759 | 7841 | 9793 | 12074 | 1583 | 1694 | 1747 | 360 | 364 | 352 | . | . | . |
| 0.9 | *** | 14769 | 18474 | 34493 | 5399 | 6285 | 8225 | 1017 | 1065 | 1124 | . | . | . | . | . | . |
| | *** | 16253 | 22412 | 34504 | 5779 | 7010 | 8210 | 1041 | 1096 | 1104 | . | . | . | . | . | . |
| 0.95 | *** | 9064 | 11071 | 17258 | 2965 | 3305 | 3863 | . | . | . | . | . | . | . | . | . |
| | *** | 9895 | 12975 | 17242 | 3119 | 3542 | 3844 | . | . | . | . | . | . | . | . | . |
| 0.98 | *** | 4152 | 4758 | 5941 | . | . | . | . | . | . | . | . | . | . | . | . |
| | *** | 4421 | 5228 | 5922 | . | . | . | . | . | . | . | . | . | . | . | . |

## TABLE 3: ALPHA= 0.01 POWER= 0.8    EXPECTED ACCRUAL THRU MINIMUM FOLLOW-UP= 5000

| | DEL=.01 | | | DEL=.02 | | | DEL=.05 | | | DEL=.10 | | | DEL=.15 | | |
|---|---|---|---|---|---|---|---|---|---|---|---|---|---|---|---|
| FACT= | 1.0 .75 | .50 .25 | .00 BIN | 1.0 .75 | .50 .25 | .00 BIN | 1.0 .75 | .50 .25 | .00 BIN | 1.0 75 | .50 .25 | .00 BIN | 1.0 .75 | .50 .25 | .00 BIN |
| PCONT=*** | | | | REQUIRED NUMBER OF PATIENTS | | | | | | | | | | | |
| 0.01 *** | 1541 1541 | 1541 1546 | 1546 5922 | 566 566 | 566 566 | 566 1958 | 183 183 | 183 183 | 183 533 | 96 96 | 96 96 | 96 217 | 66 66 | 66 66 | 66 129 |
| 0.02 *** | 3404 3408 | 3416 3433 | 3454 9776 | 1091 1096 | 1096 1104 | 1104 2911 | 296 296 | 296 296 | 296 681 | 129 129 | 129 129 | 129 252 | 83 83 | 83 83 | 83 144 |
| 0.05 *** | 10291 10321 | 10379 10491 | 10791 20855 | 2929 2946 | 2966 2991 | 3021 5651 | 633 633 | 633 641 | 641 1104 | 229 229 | 229 229 | 229 352 | 133 133 | 133 133 | 133 186 |
| 0.1 *** | 22716 22791 | 22941 23341 | 25116 37716 | 6146 6204 | 6283 6416 | 6641 9816 | 1204 1208 | 1216 1229 | 1233 1747 | 379 379 | 379 379 | 383 502 | 204 204 | 204 204 | 204 248 |
| 0.15 *** | 33941 34079 | 34358 35129 | 39671 52569 | 9054 9166 | 9346 9654 | 10271 13479 | 1721 1741 | 1758 1783 | 1808 2309 | 516 516 | 516 521 | 521 633 | 258 258 | 258 266 | 266 302 |
| 0.2 *** | 43021 43241 | 43671 44891 | 53296 65415 | 11441 11621 | 11921 12458 | 13646 16640 | 2171 2204 | 2241 2283 | 2341 2791 | 633 633 | 641 641 | 646 743 | 308 316 | 316 316 | 316 346 |
| 0.25 *** | 49683 49996 | 50616 52379 | 65433 76254 | 13258 13521 | 13954 14746 | 16641 19300 | 2541 2591 | 2646 2716 | 2796 3192 | 729 733 | 741 746 | 754 833 | 354 354 | 358 358 | 358 382 |
| 0.3 *** | 53954 54379 | 55233 57633 | 75771 85086 | 14516 14871 | 15454 16516 | 19179 21458 | 2829 2891 | 2971 3058 | 3183 3513 | 808 816 | 821 833 | 841 904 | 383 391 | 391 391 | 396 409 |
| 0.35 *** | 55991 56558 | 57691 60833 | 84133 91910 | 15271 15721 | 16454 17791 | 21221 23113 | 3033 3116 | 3208 3329 | 3483 3754 | 866 871 | 883 896 | 908 954 | 408 408 | 416 416 | 421 426 |
| 0.4 *** | 56046 56791 | 58266 62229 | 90421 96728 | 15579 16133 | 17008 18604 | 22741 24268 | 3171 3266 | 3379 3516 | 3704 3915 | 904 916 | 921 933 | 954 984 | 421 429 | 429 429 | 433 435 |
| 0.45 *** | 54433 55391 | 57258 62096 | 94566 99538 | 15508 16166 | 17179 18991 | 23721 24920 | 3233 3333 | 3466 3621 | 3833 3995 | 916 929 | 946 958 | 971 994 | 429 429 | 433 433 | 441 435 |
| 0.5 *** | 51491 52704 | 55016 60721 | 96546 100341 | 15141 15879 | 17008 18996 | 24166 25070 | 3229 3341 | 3479 3654 | 3879 3995 | 916 929 | 941 958 | 971 984 | 421 429 | 429 433 | 433 426 |
| 0.55 *** | 47571 49079 | 51858 58346 | 96341 99136 | 14521 15329 | 16546 18654 | 24058 24719 | 3166 3283 | 3421 3604 | 3833 3915 | 896 908 | 921 933 | 954 954 | 408 408 | 416 416 | 421 409 |
| 0.6 *** | 43058 44871 | 48079 55171 | 93954 95925 | 13708 14566 | 15829 17983 | 23404 23866 | 3046 3158 | 3304 3479 | 3704 3754 | 854 866 | 879 891 | 908 904 | 383 383 | 391 391 | 396 382 |
| 0.65 *** | 38279 40366 | 43908 51354 | 89383 90706 | 12741 13608 | 14879 17008 | 22208 22511 | 2866 2979 | 3108 3271 | 3491 3513 | 791 804 | 816 829 | 846 833 | 354 354 | 358 358 | 366 346 |
| 0.7 *** | 33504 35771 | 39483 46971 | 82654 83480 | 11633 12479 | 13704 15729 | 20471 20655 | 2629 2733 | 2854 2996 | 3183 3192 | 716 721 | 733 746 | 758 743 | 308 316 | 316 316 | 321 302 |
| 0.75 *** | 28858 31179 | 34858 42046 | 73779 74247 | 10383 11179 | 12308 14133 | 18204 18296 | 2333 2421 | 2521 2646 | 2796 2791 | 616 621 | 633 641 | 646 633 | 258 258 | 266 266 | 266 248 |
| 0.8 *** | 24346 26558 | 29991 36516 | 62779 63007 | 8983 9683 | 10658 12196 | 15396 15436 | 1979 2041 | 2121 2208 | 2321 2309 | 496 504 | 508 516 | 521 502 | 204 204 | 204 204 | 204 186 |
| 0.85 *** | 19833 21779 | 24741 30196 | 49679 49759 | 7383 7941 | 8708 9871 | 12071 12074 | 1546 1591 | 1641 1696 | 1766 1747 | 358 358 | 366 366 | 371 352 | . . | . . | . . |
| 0.9 *** | 15029 16529 | 18758 22696 | 34496 34504 | 5471 5846 | 6346 7054 | 8221 8210 | 1021 1046 | 1071 1096 | 1121 1104 | . . | . . | . . | . . | . . | . . |
| 0.95 *** | 9208 10041 | 11216 13108 | 17258 17242 | 2996 3141 | 3329 3554 | 3866 3844 | . . | . . | . . | . . | . . | . . | . . | . . | . . |
| 0.98 *** | 4204 4466 | 4804 5258 | 5941 5922 | . . | . . | . . | . . | . . | . . | . . | . . | . . | . . | . . | . . |

## TABLE 3: ALPHA= 0.01  POWER= 0.8     EXPECTED ACCRUAL THRU MINIMUM FOLLOW-UP= 5500

| | FACT= | DEL=.01 | | | DEL=.02 | | | DEL=.05 | | | DEL=.10 | | | DEL=.15 | | |
|---|---|---|---|---|---|---|---|---|---|---|---|---|---|---|---|---|
| | | 1.0 .75 | .50 .25 | .00 BIN | 1.0 .75 | .50 .25 | .00 BIN | 1.0 .75 | .50 .25 | .00 BIN | 1.0 75 | .50 .25 | .00 BIN | 1.0 .75 | .50 .25 | .00 BIN |
| PCONT=*** | | REQUIRED NUMBER OF PATIENTS | | | | | | | | | | | | | | |
| 0.01 | *** | 1535 1544 | 1549 | | 568 568 | 568 | | 188 188 | 188 | | 92 92 | 92 | | 64 64 | 64 | |
| | *** | 1535 1544 | 5922 | | 568 568 | 1958 | | 188 188 | 533 | | 92 92 | 217 | | 64 64 | 129 | |
| 0.02 | *** | 3400 3419 | 3455 | | 1095 1095 | 1104 | | 298 298 | 298 | | 128 128 | 128 | | 86 86 | 86 | |
| | *** | 3405 3433 | 9776 | | 1095 1104 | 2911 | | 298 298 | 681 | | 128 128 | 252 | | 86 86 | 144 | |
| 0.05 | *** | 10303 10390 | 10789 | | 2933 2965 | 3020 | | 636 636 | 642 | | 224 229 | 229 | | 133 133 | 133 | |
| | *** | 10335 10509 | 20855 | | 2946 2993 | 5651 | | 636 636 | 1104 | | 224 229 | 352 | | 133 133 | 186 | |
| 0.1 | *** | 22738 22985 | 25111 | | 6164 6307 | 6645 | | 1205 1219 | 1233 | | 375 380 | 380 | | 202 202 | 202 | |
| | *** | 22820 23412 | 37716 | | 6224 6430 | 9816 | | 1214 1228 | 1747 | | 380 380 | 502 | | 202 202 | 248 | |
| 0.15 | *** | 33985 34439 | 39673 | | 9093 9387 | 10275 | | 1728 1764 | 1810 | | 513 518 | 526 | | 257 265 | 265 | |
| | *** | 34137 35264 | 52569 | | 9208 9698 | 13479 | | 1742 1783 | 2309 | | 518 518 | 633 | | 265 265 | 302 | |
| 0.2 | *** | 43088 43798 | 53299 | | 11499 11994 | 13649 | | 2182 2250 | 2341 | | 636 642 | 650 | | 312 312 | 312 | |
| | *** | 43322 45109 | 65415 | | 11691 12530 | 16640 | | 2218 2292 | 2791 | | 636 642 | 743 | | 312 312 | 346 | |
| 0.25 | *** | 49779 50802 | 65432 | | 13341 14062 | 16641 | | 2561 2658 | 2795 | | 733 746 | 752 | | 353 353 | 361 | |
| | *** | 50123 52699 | 76254 | | 13616 14854 | 19300 | | 2603 2718 | 3192 | | 738 746 | 833 | | 353 361 | 382 | |
| 0.3 | *** | 54083 55485 | 75772 | | 14634 15596 | 19177 | | 2850 2988 | 3180 | | 807 820 | 843 | | 389 389 | 394 | |
| | *** | 54550 58070 | 85086 | | 15005 16660 | 21458 | | 2910 3070 | 3513 | | 815 834 | 904 | | 389 394 | 409 | |
| 0.35 | *** | 56159 58029 | 84132 | | 15409 16633 | 21220 | | 3062 3227 | 3483 | | 870 884 | 903 | | 408 416 | 416 | |
| | *** | 56783 61398 | 91910 | | 15885 17967 | 23113 | | 3139 3345 | 3754 | | 875 898 | 954 | | 408 416 | 426 | |
| 0.4 | *** | 56269 58694 | 90424 | | 15753 17224 | 22738 | | 3199 3400 | 3703 | | 903 925 | 953 | | 422 430 | 435 | |
| | *** | 57094 62915 | 96728 | | 16330 18814 | 24268 | | 3290 3529 | 3915 | | 917 939 | 984 | | 422 430 | 435 | |
| 0.45 | *** | 54720 57800 | 94568 | | 15720 17425 | 23723 | | 3268 3488 | 3832 | | 925 944 | 972 | | 430 435 | 435 | |
| | *** | 55774 62915 | 99538 | | 16394 19232 | 24920 | | 3373 3639 | 3995 | | 930 958 | 994 | | 430 435 | 435 | |
| 0.5 | *** | 51855 55669 | 96548 | | 15376 17279 | 24163 | | 3268 3510 | 3881 | | 917 944 | 972 | | 422 430 | 435 | |
| | *** | 53180 61659 | 100341 | | 16133 19268 | 25070 | | 3378 3667 | 3995 | | 930 958 | 984 | | 422 430 | 426 | |
| 0.55 | *** | 48033 52625 | 96342 | | 14785 16839 | 24058 | | 3208 3455 | 3832 | | 898 925 | 953 | | 408 416 | 422 | |
| | *** | 49660 59382 | 99136 | | 15610 18938 | 24719 | | 3318 3620 | 3915 | | 911 939 | 954 | | 408 416 | 409 | |
| 0.6 | *** | 43619 48940 | 93949 | | 13988 16133 | 23406 | | 3084 3331 | 3703 | | 856 884 | 911 | | 389 389 | 394 | |
| | *** | 45558 56274 | 95925 | | 14854 18269 | 23866 | | 3194 3496 | 3754 | | 870 898 | 904 | | 389 394 | 382 | |
| 0.65 | *** | 38930 44834 | 89384 | | 13025 15175 | 22210 | | 2905 3139 | 3488 | | 793 820 | 843 | | 353 361 | 361 | |
| | *** | 41135 52488 | 90706 | | 13905 17288 | 22511 | | 3007 3290 | 3513 | | 807 829 | 833 | | 353 361 | 346 | |
| 0.7 | *** | 34219 40434 | 82655 | | 11911 13993 | 20469 | | 2663 2878 | 3185 | | 719 738 | 760 | | 312 312 | 320 | |
| | *** | 36593 48088 | 83480 | | 12764 15987 | 20655 | | 2759 3015 | 3192 | | 724 746 | 743 | | 312 320 | 302 | |
| 0.75 | *** | 29599 35787 | 73778 | | 10646 12571 | 18200 | | 2369 2539 | 2795 | | 623 636 | 650 | | 265 265 | 265 | |
| | *** | 32000 43102 | 74247 | | 11444 14364 | 18296 | | 2443 2658 | 2791 | | 628 642 | 633 | | 265 265 | 248 | |
| 0.8 | *** | 25056 30845 | 62778 | | 9216 10885 | 15395 | | 1998 2135 | 2319 | | 499 513 | 518 | | 202 202 | 202 | |
| | *** | 27339 37450 | 63007 | | 9918 12384 | 15436 | | 2066 2218 | 2309 | | 504 513 | 502 | | 202 202 | 186 | |
| 0.85 | *** | 20464 25469 | 49674 | | 7566 8878 | 12068 | | 1558 1645 | 1764 | | 361 367 | 367 | | . | . | . |
| | *** | 22458 30960 | 49759 | | 8122 10005 | 12074 | | 1604 1700 | 1747 | | 361 367 | 352 | | . | . | . |
| 0.9 | *** | 15514 19300 | 34494 | | 5600 6453 | 8226 | | 1035 1076 | 1123 | | . | . | . | . | . | . |
| | *** | 17045 23233 | 34504 | | 5971 7132 | 8210 | | 1049 1095 | 1104 | | . | . | . | . | . | . |
| 0.95 | *** | 9483 11490 | 17260 | | 3043 3364 | 3859 | | . | . | . | . | . | . | . | . | . |
| | *** | 10316 13341 | 17242 | | 3185 3579 | 3844 | | . | . | . | . | . | . | . | . | . |
| 0.98 | *** | 4285 4871 | 5944 | | . | . | . | . | . | . | . | . | . | . | . | . |
| | *** | 4547 5303 | 5922 | | . | . | . | . | . | . | . | . | . | . | . | . |

TABLE 3: ALPHA= 0.01  POWER= 0.8    EXPECTED ACCRUAL THRU MINIMUM FOLLOW-UP= 6000

| | | DEL=.01 | | | DEL=.02 | | | DEL=.05 | | | DEL=.10 | | | DEL=.15 | | |
|---|---|---|---|---|---|---|---|---|---|---|---|---|---|---|---|---|---|
| FACT= | | 1.0 .75 | .50 .25 | .00 BIN | 1.0 .75 | .50 .25 | .00 BIN | 1.0 .75 | .50 .25 | .00 BIN | 1.0 75 | .50 .25 | .00 BIN | 1.0 .75 | .50 .25 | .00 BIN |
| PCONT=*** | | | | | REQUIRED NUMBER OF PATIENTS | | | | | | | | | | | | |
| 0.01 | *** | 1540 | 1540 | 1549 | 565 | 565 | 565 | 184 | 184 | 184 | 94 | 94 | 94 | 64 | 64 | 64 |
| | *** | 1540 | 1540 | 5922 | 565 | 565 | 1958 | 184 | 184 | 533 | 94 | 94 | 217 | 64 | 64 | 129 |
| 0.02 | *** | 3400 | 3424 | 3454 | 1090 | 1099 | 1105 | 295 | 295 | 295 | 130 | 130 | 130 | 85 | 85 | 85 |
| | *** | 3409 | 3439 | 9776 | 1099 | 1099 | 2911 | 295 | 295 | 681 | 130 | 130 | 252 | 85 | 85 | 144 |
| 0.05 | *** | 10309 | 10405 | 10789 | 2935 | 2974 | 3025 | 634 | 640 | 640 | 229 | 229 | 229 | 130 | 130 | 130 |
| | *** | 10345 | 10525 | 20855 | 2950 | 2995 | 5651 | 634 | 640 | 1104 | 229 | 229 | 352 | 130 | 130 | 186 |
| 0.1 | *** | 22759 | 23029 | 25114 | 6184 | 6325 | 6640 | 1204 | 1219 | 1234 | 379 | 379 | 379 | 199 | 199 | 199 |
| | *** | 22849 | 23470 | 37716 | 6244 | 6445 | 9816 | 1210 | 1225 | 1747 | 379 | 379 | 502 | 199 | 199 | 248 |
| 0.15 | *** | 34024 | 34519 | 39670 | 9124 | 9430 | 10270 | 1735 | 1765 | 1810 | 514 | 520 | 520 | 259 | 259 | 265 |
| | *** | 34189 | 35395 | 52569 | 9244 | 9730 | 13479 | 1750 | 1789 | 2309 | 514 | 520 | 633 | 259 | 265 | 302 |
| 0.2 | *** | 43150 | 43924 | 53299 | 11554 | 12064 | 13645 | 2194 | 2254 | 2335 | 634 | 640 | 649 | 310 | 310 | 319 |
| | *** | 43414 | 45325 | 65415 | 11755 | 12589 | 16640 | 2224 | 2290 | 2791 | 634 | 640 | 743 | 310 | 319 | 346 |
| 0.25 | *** | 49870 | 50989 | 65434 | 13420 | 14164 | 16639 | 2575 | 2665 | 2800 | 730 | 745 | 754 | 355 | 355 | 355 |
| | *** | 50245 | 53014 | 76254 | 13705 | 14950 | 19300 | 2614 | 2725 | 3192 | 739 | 745 | 833 | 355 | 355 | 382 |
| 0.3 | *** | 54205 | 55735 | 75769 | 14740 | 15730 | 19180 | 2869 | 2995 | 3184 | 814 | 829 | 844 | 385 | 394 | 394 |
| | *** | 54724 | 58489 | 85086 | 15124 | 16789 | 21458 | 2929 | 3079 | 3513 | 820 | 835 | 904 | 385 | 394 | 409 |
| 0.35 | *** | 56329 | 58360 | 84130 | 15550 | 16804 | 21220 | 3085 | 3250 | 3484 | 874 | 889 | 904 | 409 | 415 | 415 |
| | *** | 57010 | 61930 | 91910 | 16039 | 18130 | 23113 | 3160 | 3355 | 3754 | 880 | 895 | 954 | 415 | 415 | 426 |
| 0.4 | *** | 56494 | 59119 | 90424 | 15919 | 17425 | 22735 | 3229 | 3415 | 3700 | 910 | 925 | 949 | 424 | 430 | 430 |
| | *** | 57385 | 63580 | 96728 | 16519 | 19009 | 24268 | 3319 | 3544 | 3915 | 919 | 940 | 984 | 424 | 430 | 435 |
| 0.45 | *** | 55009 | 58330 | 94570 | 15919 | 17650 | 23725 | 3304 | 3514 | 3835 | 925 | 949 | 970 | 430 | 430 | 439 |
| | *** | 56149 | 63694 | 99538 | 16609 | 19450 | 24920 | 3394 | 3655 | 3915 | 934 | 964 | 994 | 430 | 439 | 435 |
| 0.5 | *** | 52219 | 56305 | 96544 | 15595 | 17530 | 24160 | 3304 | 3529 | 3880 | 925 | 949 | 970 | 424 | 430 | 430 |
| | *** | 53650 | 62545 | 100341 | 16375 | 19504 | 25070 | 3409 | 3685 | 3995 | 934 | 964 | 984 | 424 | 430 | 426 |
| 0.55 | *** | 48484 | 53365 | 96340 | 15025 | 17104 | 24055 | 3244 | 3475 | 3835 | 904 | 925 | 955 | 409 | 415 | 424 |
| | *** | 50230 | 60349 | 99136 | 15865 | 19180 | 24719 | 3349 | 3634 | 3915 | 910 | 940 | 954 | 409 | 415 | 409 |
| 0.6 | *** | 44164 | 49765 | 93949 | 14245 | 16405 | 23404 | 3124 | 3355 | 3700 | 859 | 880 | 910 | 385 | 394 | 394 |
| | *** | 46219 | 57304 | 95925 | 15124 | 18520 | 23866 | 3229 | 3505 | 3754 | 874 | 895 | 904 | 385 | 394 | 382 |
| 0.65 | *** | 39559 | 45709 | 89380 | 13285 | 15445 | 22210 | 2935 | 3160 | 3490 | 799 | 820 | 844 | 355 | 355 | 364 |
| | *** | 41875 | 53539 | 90706 | 14170 | 17530 | 22511 | 3040 | 3304 | 3513 | 814 | 829 | 833 | 355 | 364 | 346 |
| 0.7 | *** | 34909 | 41329 | 82654 | 12169 | 14254 | 20470 | 2695 | 2899 | 3184 | 724 | 739 | 760 | 310 | 319 | 319 |
| | *** | 37369 | 49120 | 83480 | 13030 | 16219 | 20655 | 2785 | 3025 | 3192 | 730 | 745 | 743 | 310 | 319 | 302 |
| 0.75 | *** | 30295 | 36655 | 73780 | 10885 | 12805 | 18199 | 2389 | 2560 | 2794 | 619 | 634 | 649 | 259 | 265 | 265 |
| | *** | 32779 | 44065 | 74247 | 11689 | 14569 | 18296 | 2470 | 2665 | 2791 | 625 | 640 | 633 | 265 | 265 | 248 |
| 0.8 | *** | 25729 | 31639 | 62779 | 9430 | 11089 | 15400 | 2020 | 2149 | 2320 | 499 | 514 | 520 | 199 | 205 | 205 |
| | *** | 28060 | 38305 | 63007 | 10129 | 12559 | 15436 | 2080 | 2230 | 2309 | 505 | 514 | 502 | 205 | 205 | 186 |
| 0.85 | *** | 21049 | 26140 | 49675 | 7735 | 9034 | 12070 | 1570 | 1660 | 1765 | 364 | 364 | 370 | . | . | . |
| | *** | 23080 | 31654 | 49759 | 8290 | 10129 | 12074 | 1615 | 1705 | 1747 | 364 | 370 | 352 | . | . | . |
| 0.9 | *** | 15970 | 19795 | 34495 | 5710 | 6550 | 8224 | 1039 | 1075 | 1120 | . | . | . | . | . | . |
| | *** | 17515 | 23710 | 34504 | 6079 | 7204 | 8210 | 1054 | 1099 | 1104 | . | . | . | . | . | . |
| 0.95 | *** | 9739 | 11734 | 17260 | 3094 | 3394 | 3865 | . | . | . | . | . | . | . | . | . |
| | *** | :0570 | 13555 | 17242 | 3229 | 3595 | 3844 | . | . | . | . | . | . | . | . | . |
| 0.98 | *** | 4369 | 4939 | 5944 | . | . | . | . | . | . | . | . | . | . | . | . |
| | *** | 4624 | 5350 | 5922 | . | . | . | . | . | . | . | . | . | . | . | . |

## TABLE 3: ALPHA= 0.01  POWER= 0.8    EXPECTED ACCRUAL THRU MINIMUM FOLLOW-UP= 6500

| | | DEL=.01 | | | DEL=.02 | | | DEL=.05 | | | DEL=.10 | | | DEL=.15 | | |
|---|---|---|---|---|---|---|---|---|---|---|---|---|---|---|---|---|---|
| FACT= | | 1.0 .75 | .50 .25 | .00 BIN | 1.0 .75 | .50 .25 | .00 BIN | 1.0 .75 | .50 .25 | .00 BIN | 1.0 75 | .50 .25 | .00 BIN | 1.0 .75 | .50 .25 | .00 BIN |
| PCONT=*** | | | | REQUIRED NUMBER OF PATIENTS | | | | | | | | | | | | |
| 0.01 | *** | 1538 | 1538 | 1548 | 563 | 563 | 563 | 183 | 183 | 183 | 92 | 92 | 92 | 70 | 70 | 70 |
| | *** | 1538 | 1548 | 5922 | 563 | 563 | 1958 | 183 | 183 | 533 | 92 | 92 | 217 | 70 | 70 | 129 |
| 0.02 | *** | 3407 | 3423 | 3456 | 1093 | 1099 | 1099 | 297 | 297 | 297 | 124 | 124 | 124 | 86 | 86 | 86 |
| | *** | 3417 | 3433 | 9776 | 1099 | 1099 | 2911 | 297 | 297 | 681 | 124 | 124 | 252 | 86 | 86 | 144 |
| 0.05 | *** | 10323 | 10421 | 10784 | 2946 | 2978 | 3027 | 638 | 638 | 638 | 222 | 222 | 232 | 135 | 135 | 135 |
| | *** | 10356 | 10535 | 20855 | 2952 | 2995 | 5651 | 638 | 638 | 1104 | 222 | 222 | 352 | 135 | 135 | 186 |
| 0.1 | *** | 22787 | 23069 | 25111 | 6196 | 6342 | 6641 | 1207 | 1223 | 1240 | 378 | 378 | 378 | 200 | 200 | 200 |
| | *** | 22885 | 23535 | 37716 | 6261 | 6456 | 9816 | 1213 | 1229 | 1747 | 378 | 378 | 502 | 200 | 200 | 248 |
| 0.15 | *** | 34065 | 34601 | 39671 | 9153 | 9468 | 10275 | 1743 | 1776 | 1814 | 514 | 514 | 525 | 265 | 265 | 265 |
| | *** | 34243 | 35517 | 52569 | 9283 | 9761 | 13479 | 1749 | 1792 | 2309 | 514 | 525 | 633 | 265 | 265 | 302 |
| 0.2 | *** | 43219 | 44048 | 53294 | 11607 | 12127 | 13644 | 2204 | 2263 | 2334 | 638 | 638 | 644 | 313 | 313 | 313 |
| | *** | 43496 | 45527 | 65415 | 11808 | 12647 | 16640 | 2231 | 2296 | 2791 | 638 | 644 | 743 | 313 | 313 | 346 |
| 0.25 | *** | 49963 | 51166 | 65433 | 13498 | 14256 | 16645 | 2588 | 2676 | 2800 | 736 | 742 | 752 | 352 | 352 | 362 |
| | *** | 50369 | 53311 | 76254 | 13791 | 15036 | 19300 | 2627 | 2735 | 3192 | 742 | 752 | 833 | 352 | 362 | 382 |
| 0.3 | *** | 54334 | 55986 | 75768 | 14841 | 15854 | 19180 | 2887 | 3011 | 3179 | 817 | 823 | 839 | 384 | 395 | 395 |
| | *** | 54887 | 58895 | 85086 | 15237 | 16905 | 21458 | 2946 | 3082 | 3513 | 823 | 833 | 904 | 384 | 395 | 409 |
| 0.35 | *** | 56506 | 58689 | 84137 | 15686 | 16953 | 21217 | 3108 | 3261 | 3482 | 872 | 888 | 904 | 411 | 417 | 417 |
| | *** | 57243 | 62443 | 91910 | 16190 | 18276 | 23113 | 3179 | 3358 | 3754 | 882 | 898 | 954 | 411 | 417 | 426 |
| 0.4 | *** | 56717 | 59534 | 90420 | 16082 | 17609 | 22738 | 3255 | 3433 | 3699 | 915 | 931 | 953 | 427 | 427 | 433 |
| | *** | 57682 | 64208 | 96728 | 16693 | 19180 | 24268 | 3336 | 3553 | 3915 | 921 | 937 | 984 | 427 | 433 | 435 |
| 0.45 | *** | 55293 | 58846 | 94569 | 16098 | 17863 | 23719 | 3326 | 3531 | 3829 | 931 | 947 | 969 | 427 | 433 | 443 |
| | *** | 56522 | 64436 | 99538 | 16807 | 19651 | 24920 | 3423 | 3667 | 3995 | 937 | 963 | 994 | 433 | 433 | 435 |
| 0.5 | *** | 52579 | 56918 | 96546 | 15806 | 17766 | 24158 | 3336 | 3553 | 3878 | 931 | 947 | 969 | 427 | 427 | 433 |
| | *** | 54117 | 63380 | 100341 | 16602 | 19716 | 25070 | 3433 | 3699 | 3995 | 937 | 963 | 984 | 427 | 433 | 426 |
| 0.55 | *** | 48933 | 54074 | 96341 | 15253 | 17349 | 24055 | 3271 | 3498 | 3840 | 904 | 931 | 953 | 411 | 417 | 417 |
| | *** | 50786 | 61257 | 99136 | 16108 | 19407 | 24719 | 3374 | 3651 | 3915 | 915 | 937 | 954 | 411 | 417 | 409 |
| 0.6 | *** | 44692 | 50548 | 93952 | 14489 | 16661 | 23405 | 3147 | 3374 | 3699 | 866 | 882 | 904 | 384 | 395 | 395 |
| | *** | 46859 | 58267 | 95925 | 15377 | 18747 | 23866 | 3255 | 3521 | 3754 | 872 | 898 | 904 | 384 | 395 | 382 |
| 0.65 | *** | 40164 | 46545 | 89386 | 13531 | 15702 | 22208 | 2968 | 3179 | 3488 | 801 | 823 | 839 | 352 | 362 | 362 |
| | *** | 42580 | 54513 | 90706 | 14424 | 17756 | 22511 | 3066 | 3320 | 3513 | 817 | 833 | 833 | 352 | 362 | 346 |
| 0.7 | *** | 35560 | 42163 | 82652 | 12403 | 14489 | 20469 | 2724 | 2913 | 3179 | 726 | 742 | 758 | 313 | 313 | 319 |
| | *** | 38111 | 50077 | 83480 | 13271 | 16423 | 20655 | 2816 | 3033 | 3192 | 736 | 752 | 743 | 313 | 319 | 302 |
| 0.75 | *** | 30961 | 37467 | 73780 | 11109 | 13021 | 18205 | 2416 | 2572 | 2800 | 622 | 638 | 644 | 265 | 265 | 265 |
| | *** | 33502 | 44968 | 74247 | 11906 | 14749 | 18296 | 2491 | 2676 | 2791 | 628 | 644 | 633 | 265 | 265 | 248 |
| 0.8 | *** | 26352 | 32381 | 62778 | 9625 | 11266 | 15399 | 2036 | 2156 | 2318 | 498 | 508 | 525 | 200 | 206 | 206 |
| | *** | 28741 | 39102 | 63007 | 10313 | 12702 | 15436 | 2091 | 2237 | 2309 | 508 | 514 | 502 | 200 | 206 | 186 |
| 0.85 | *** | 21601 | 26768 | 49681 | 7892 | 9176 | 12068 | 1587 | 1662 | 1766 | 362 | 368 | 368 | . | . | . |
| | *** | 23671 | 32299 | 49759 | 8444 | 10242 | 12074 | 1619 | 1711 | 1747 | 362 | 368 | 352 | . | . | . |
| 0.9 | *** | 16391 | 20252 | 34493 | 5812 | 6635 | 8227 | 1045 | 1083 | 1126 | . | . | . | . | . | . |
| | *** | 17961 | 24152 | 34504 | 6169 | 7268 | 8210 | 1061 | 1099 | 1104 | . | . | . | . | . | . |
| 0.95 | *** | 9966 | 11965 | 17262 | 3131 | 3423 | 3862 | . | . | . | . | . | . | . | . | . |
| | *** | 10801 | 13742 | 17242 | 3261 | 3618 | 3844 | . | . | . | . | . | . | . | . | . |
| 0.98 | *** | 4441 | 4993 | 5942 | . | . | . | . | . | . | . | . | . | . | . | . |
| | *** | 4685 | 5389 | 5922 | . | . | . | . | . | . | . | . | . | . | . | . |

TABLE 3: ALPHA= 0.01  POWER= 0.8     EXPECTED ACCRUAL THRU MINIMUM FOLLOW-UP= 7000

|  |  | DEL=.01 | | | DEL=.02 | | | DEL=.05 | | | DEL=.10 | | | DEL=.15 | | |
|---|---|---|---|---|---|---|---|---|---|---|---|---|---|---|---|---|
| FACT= | | 1.0 .75 | .50 .25 | .00 BIN | 1.0 .75 | .50 .25 | .00 BIN | 1.0 .75 | .50 .25 | .00 BIN | 1.0 75 | .50 .25 | .00 BIN | 1.0 .75 | .50 .25 | .00 BIN |
| PCONT=*** | | | | | REQUIRED NUMBER OF PATIENTS | | | | | | | | | | | |
| 0.01 | *** | 1534 | 1545 | 1545 | 565 | 565 | 565 | 186 | 186 | 186 | 92 | 92 | 92 | 64 | 64 | 64 |
|  | *** | 1545 | 1545 | 5922 | 565 | 565 | 1958 | 186 | 186 | 533 | 92 | 92 | 217 | 64 | 64 | 129 |
| 0.02 | *** | 3406 | 3424 | 3452 | 1096 | 1096 | 1107 | 291 | 291 | 291 | 127 | 127 | 127 | 81 | 81 | 81 |
|  | *** | 3417 | 3435 | 9776 | 1096 | 1096 | 2911 | 291 | 291 | 681 | 127 | 127 | 252 | 81 | 81 | 144 |
| 0.05 | *** | 10330 | 10435 | 10791 | 2945 | 2980 | 3021 | 635 | 635 | 641 | 221 | 221 | 232 | 134 | 134 | 134 |
|  | *** | 10365 | 10546 | 20855 | 2962 | 2997 | 5651 | 635 | 641 | 1104 | 221 | 221 | 352 | 134 | 134 | 186 |
| 0.1 | *** | 22807 | 23111 | 25117 | 6217 | 6357 | 6644 | 1212 | 1219 | 1236 | 379 | 379 | 379 | 197 | 204 | 204 |
|  | *** | 22912 | 23584 | 37716 | 6270 | 6469 | 9816 | 1212 | 1230 | 1747 | 379 | 379 | 502 | 204 | 204 | 248 |
| 0.15 | *** | 34112 | 34679 | 39666 | 9192 | 9496 | 10266 | 1744 | 1772 | 1814 | 512 | 519 | 519 | 256 | 256 | 267 |
|  | *** | 34305 | 35635 | 52569 | 9315 | 9787 | 13479 | 1755 | 1790 | 2309 | 519 | 519 | 633 | 256 | 267 | 302 |
| 0.2 | *** | 43282 | 44175 | 53299 | 11660 | 12185 | 13644 | 2210 | 2262 | 2339 | 635 | 641 | 652 | 309 | 309 | 320 |
|  | *** | 43586 | 45721 | 65415 | 11870 | 12692 | 16640 | 2234 | 2297 | 2791 | 635 | 641 | 743 | 309 | 320 | 346 |
| 0.25 | *** | 50061 | 51350 | 65437 | 13574 | 14337 | 16636 | 2595 | 2682 | 2794 | 740 | 746 | 757 | 355 | 355 | 361 |
|  | *** | 50492 | 53596 | 76254 | 13871 | 15107 | 19300 | 2636 | 2735 | 3192 | 740 | 746 | 833 | 355 | 361 | 382 |
| 0.3 | *** | 54465 | 56232 | 75769 | 14939 | 15965 | 19174 | 2899 | 3021 | 3179 | 816 | 827 | 845 | 390 | 390 | 396 |
|  | *** | 55060 | 59277 | 85086 | 15352 | 17004 | 21458 | 2951 | 3091 | 3513 | 816 | 834 | 904 | 390 | 390 | 409 |
| 0.35 | *** | 56670 | 59015 | 84134 | 15807 | 17102 | 21221 | 3126 | 3277 | 3487 | 880 | 886 | 904 | 414 | 414 | 414 |
|  | *** | 57464 | 62935 | 91910 | 16321 | 18404 | 23113 | 3196 | 3371 | 3754 | 880 | 897 | 954 | 414 | 414 | 426 |
| 0.4 | *** | 56939 | 59949 | 90416 | 16234 | 17785 | 22737 | 3277 | 3452 | 3704 | 915 | 932 | 950 | 425 | 431 | 431 |
|  | *** | 57971 | 64796 | 96728 | 16857 | 19342 | 24268 | 3354 | 3564 | 3915 | 921 | 939 | 984 | 425 | 431 | 435 |
| 0.45 | *** | 55585 | 59347 | 94564 | 16280 | 18065 | 23724 | 3354 | 3546 | 3837 | 932 | 950 | 974 | 431 | 431 | 442 |
|  | *** | 56897 | 65129 | 99538 | 16997 | 19832 | 24920 | 3441 | 3680 | 3995 | 939 | 967 | 994 | 431 | 431 | 435 |
| 0.5 | *** | 52942 | 57516 | 96541 | 16006 | 17977 | 24161 | 3365 | 3575 | 3879 | 932 | 950 | 974 | 425 | 431 | 431 |
|  | *** | 54570 | 64166 | 100341 | 16811 | 19909 | 25070 | 3459 | 3704 | 3995 | 939 | 956 | 984 | 425 | 431 | 426 |
| 0.55 | *** | 49372 | 54751 | 96342 | 15475 | 17581 | 24056 | 3301 | 3522 | 3837 | 904 | 932 | 950 | 414 | 414 | 425 |
|  | *** | 51332 | 62119 | 99136 | 16332 | 19611 | 24719 | 3400 | 3662 | 3915 | 921 | 939 | 954 | 414 | 414 | 409 |
| 0.6 | *** | 45214 | 51297 | 93951 | 14711 | 16892 | 23402 | 3179 | 3400 | 3704 | 869 | 886 | 904 | 390 | 390 | 396 |
|  | *** | 47482 | 59161 | 95925 | 15604 | 18957 | 23866 | 3277 | 3529 | 3754 | 880 | 897 | 904 | 390 | 396 | 382 |
| 0.65 | *** | 40751 | 47331 | 89384 | 13760 | 15930 | 22212 | 2997 | 3196 | 3487 | 810 | 827 | 845 | 355 | 361 | 361 |
|  | *** | 43254 | 55427 | 90706 | 14659 | 17949 | 22511 | 3091 | 3330 | 3513 | 816 | 834 | 833 | 355 | 361 | 346 |
| 0.7 | *** | 36184 | 42967 | 82657 | 12629 | 14711 | 20469 | 2741 | 2927 | 3179 | 722 | 740 | 757 | 309 | 320 | 320 |
|  | *** | 38809 | 50971 | 83480 | 13497 | 16612 | 20655 | 2829 | 3050 | 3192 | 729 | 746 | 743 | 320 | 320 | 302 |
| 0.75 | *** | 31592 | 38231 | 73774 | 11316 | 13217 | 18205 | 2437 | 2584 | 2794 | 624 | 635 | 652 | 267 | 267 | 267 |
|  | *** | 34200 | 45791 | 74247 | 12115 | 14915 | 18296 | 2507 | 2682 | 2791 | 635 | 641 | 633 | 267 | 267 | 248 |
| 0.8 | *** | 26955 | 33080 | 62777 | 9805 | 11432 | 15394 | 2052 | 2175 | 2321 | 501 | 512 | 519 | 204 | 204 | 204 |
|  | *** | 29387 | 39835 | 63007 | 10494 | 12839 | 15436 | 2111 | 2245 | 2309 | 512 | 519 | 502 | 204 | 204 | 186 |
| 0.85 | *** | 22125 | 27346 | 49676 | 8037 | 9304 | 12069 | 1597 | 1674 | 1761 | 361 | 361 | 372 | . | . | . |
|  | *** | 24225 | 32887 | 49759 | 8580 | 10336 | 12074 | 1632 | 1720 | 1747 | 361 | 372 | 352 | . | . | . |
| 0.9 | *** | 16794 | 20672 | 34497 | 5909 | 6714 | 8219 | 1044 | 1079 | 1125 | . | . | . | . | . | . |
|  | *** | 18369 | 24557 | 34504 | 6259 | 7320 | 8210 | 1061 | 1107 | 1104 | . | . | . | . | . | . |
| 0.95 | *** | 10179 | 12167 | 17260 | 3161 | 3452 | 3861 | . | . | . | . | . | . | . | . | . |
|  | *** | 11019 | 13906 | 17242 | 3295 | 3634 | 3844 | . | . | . | . | . | . | . | . | . |
| 0.98 | *** | 4509 | 5045 | 5937 | . | . | . | . | . | . | . | . | . | . | . | . |
|  | *** | 4747 | 5419 | 5922 | . | . | . | . | . | . | . | . | . | . | . | . |

## TABLE 3: ALPHA= 0.01  POWER= 0.8     EXPECTED ACCRUAL THRU MINIMUM FOLLOW-UP= 7500

| | | DEL=.01 | | | DEL=.02 | | | DEL=.05 | | | DEL=.10 | | | DEL=.15 | | |
|---|---|---|---|---|---|---|---|---|---|---|---|---|---|---|---|---|
| FACT= | | 1.0 .75 | .50 .25 | .00 BIN | 1.0 .75 | .50 .25 | .00 BIN | 1.0 .75 | .50 .25 | .00 BIN | 1.0 75 | .50 .25 | .00 BIN | 1.0 .75 | .50 .25 | .00 BIN |
| PCONT=*** | | | | REQUIRED NUMBER OF PATIENTS | | | | | | | | | | | | |
| 0.01 | *** | 1543 | 1543 | 1550 | 568 | 568 | 568 | 181 | 181 | 181 | 99 | 99 | 99 | 68 | 68 | 68 |
| | *** | 1543 | 1543 | 5922 | 568 | 568 | 1958 | 181 | 181 | 533 | 99 | 99 | 217 | 68 | 68 | 129 |
| 0.02 | *** | 3406 | 3425 | 3455 | 1093 | 1100 | 1100 | 293 | 293 | 293 | 125 | 125 | 125 | 87 | 87 | 87 |
| | *** | 3418 | 3436 | 9776 | 1100 | 1100 | 2911 | 293 | 293 | 681 | 125 | 125 | 252 | 87 | 87 | 144 |
| 0.05 | *** | 10336 | 10449 | 10786 | 2949 | 2975 | 3024 | 631 | 643 | 643 | 230 | 230 | 230 | 136 | 136 | 136 |
| | *** | 10374 | 10561 | 20855 | 2968 | 2993 | 5651 | 631 | 643 | 1104 | 230 | 230 | 352 | 136 | 136 | 186 |
| 0.1 | *** | 22831 | 23161 | 25111 | 6230 | 6368 | 6643 | 1212 | 1224 | 1231 | 380 | 380 | 380 | 200 | 200 | 200 |
| | *** | 22943 | 23637 | 37716 | 6286 | 6481 | 9816 | 1212 | 1231 | 1747 | 380 | 380 | 502 | 200 | 200 | 248 |
| 0.15 | *** | 34149 | 34756 | 39668 | 9218 | 9530 | 10268 | 1749 | 1775 | 1812 | 518 | 518 | 518 | 256 | 268 | 268 |
| | *** | 34355 | 35750 | 52569 | 9350 | 9811 | 13479 | 1756 | 1793 | 2309 | 518 | 518 | 633 | 256 | 268 | 302 |
| 0.2 | *** | 43343 | 44300 | 53300 | 11705 | 12237 | 13643 | 2218 | 2274 | 2337 | 631 | 643 | 650 | 312 | 312 | 312 |
| | *** | 43674 | 45912 | 65415 | 11918 | 12736 | 16640 | 2243 | 2300 | 2791 | 643 | 643 | 743 | 312 | 312 | 346 |
| 0.25 | *** | 50150 | 51530 | 65431 | 13643 | 14424 | 16643 | 2611 | 2686 | 2799 | 736 | 743 | 755 | 350 | 361 | 361 |
| | *** | 50618 | 53862 | 76254 | 13955 | 15174 | 19300 | 2649 | 2743 | 3192 | 743 | 755 | 833 | 361 | 361 | 382 |
| 0.3 | *** | 54593 | 56480 | 75774 | 15031 | 16074 | 19175 | 2918 | 3031 | 3181 | 818 | 830 | 837 | 387 | 387 | 399 |
| | *** | 55231 | 59649 | 85086 | 15455 | 17105 | 21458 | 2968 | 3099 | 3513 | 818 | 837 | 904 | 387 | 387 | 409 |
| 0.35 | *** | 56843 | 59330 | 84136 | 15924 | 17236 | 21218 | 3143 | 3286 | 3481 | 875 | 893 | 905 | 406 | 418 | 418 |
| | *** | 57687 | 63399 | 91910 | 16449 | 18530 | 23113 | 3211 | 3380 | 3754 | 886 | 893 | 954 | 418 | 418 | 426 |
| 0.4 | *** | 57162 | 60350 | 90418 | 16374 | 17937 | 22737 | 3293 | 3462 | 3699 | 912 | 931 | 950 | 425 | 425 | 436 |
| | *** | 58261 | 65368 | 96728 | 17011 | 19486 | 24268 | 3380 | 3575 | 3915 | 924 | 943 | 984 | 425 | 436 | 435 |
| 0.45 | *** | 55868 | 59836 | 94568 | 16449 | 18237 | 23724 | 3380 | 3568 | 3830 | 931 | 950 | 968 | 425 | 436 | 436 |
| | *** | 57256 | 65799 | 99538 | 17180 | 19993 | 24920 | 3462 | 3687 | 3995 | 943 | 961 | 994 | 436 | 436 | 435 |
| 0.5 | *** | 53300 | 58093 | 96549 | 16193 | 18181 | 24162 | 3387 | 3586 | 3875 | 931 | 950 | 968 | 425 | 425 | 436 |
| | *** | 55018 | 64906 | 100341 | 17011 | 20086 | 25070 | 3481 | 3718 | 3995 | 943 | 961 | 984 | 425 | 436 | 426 |
| 0.55 | *** | 49805 | 55411 | 96343 | 15680 | 17787 | 24061 | 3324 | 3537 | 3837 | 912 | 931 | 950 | 406 | 418 | 418 |
| | *** | 51856 | 62930 | 99136 | 16543 | 19793 | 24719 | 3425 | 3668 | 3915 | 924 | 943 | 954 | 418 | 418 | 409 |
| 0.6 | *** | 45725 | 52006 | 93950 | 14930 | 17105 | 23405 | 3200 | 3406 | 3706 | 868 | 886 | 905 | 387 | 387 | 399 |
| | *** | 48080 | 60012 | 95925 | 15830 | 19149 | 23866 | 3305 | 3549 | 3754 | 875 | 893 | 904 | 387 | 399 | 382 |
| 0.65 | *** | 41330 | 48080 | 89386 | 13974 | 16149 | 22212 | 3012 | 3211 | 3493 | 811 | 830 | 849 | 350 | 361 | 361 |
| | *** | 43906 | 56281 | 90706 | 14874 | 18136 | 22511 | 3106 | 3343 | 3513 | 818 | 837 | 833 | 361 | 361 | 346 |
| 0.7 | *** | 36793 | 43718 | 82655 | 12837 | 14911 | 20468 | 2768 | 2949 | 3181 | 725 | 743 | 755 | 312 | 312 | 324 |
| | *** | 39481 | 51800 | 83480 | 13700 | 16775 | 20655 | 2855 | 3050 | 3192 | 736 | 743 | 743 | 312 | 312 | 302 |
| 0.75 | *** | 32199 | 38949 | 73775 | 11506 | 13400 | 18200 | 2450 | 2600 | 2799 | 624 | 643 | 650 | 268 | 268 | 268 |
| | *** | 34861 | 46568 | 74247 | 12305 | 15061 | 18296 | 2525 | 2686 | 2791 | 631 | 643 | 633 | 268 | 268 | 248 |
| 0.8 | *** | 27518 | 33736 | 62780 | 9968 | 11593 | 15399 | 2068 | 2180 | 2318 | 500 | 511 | 518 | 200 | 200 | 200 |
| | *** | 29993 | 40512 | 63007 | 10662 | 12961 | 15436 | 2124 | 2243 | 2309 | 511 | 518 | 502 | 200 | 200 | 186 |
| 0.85 | *** | 22618 | 27893 | 49674 | 8168 | 9418 | 12068 | 1606 | 1674 | 1768 | 361 | 368 | 368 | . | . | . |
| | *** | 24736 | 33436 | 49759 | 8705 | 10418 | 12074 | 1636 | 1718 | 1747 | 361 | 368 | 352 | . | . | . |
| 0.9 | *** | 17168 | 21068 | 34493 | 5993 | 6781 | 8225 | 1055 | 1081 | 1118 | . | . | . | . | . | . |
| | *** | 18762 | 24924 | 34504 | 6343 | 7362 | 8210 | 1074 | 1100 | 1104 | . | . | . | . | . | . |
| 0.95 | *** | 10381 | 12350 | 17255 | 3200 | 3474 | 3868 | . | . | . | . | . | . | . | . | . |
| | *** | 11218 | 14068 | 17242 | 3324 | 3650 | 3844 | . | . | . | . | . | . | . | . | . |
| 0.98 | *** | 4568 | 5086 | 5937 | . | . | . | . | . | . | . | . | . | . | . | . |
| | *** | 4805 | 5450 | 5922 | . | . | . | . | . | . | . | . | . | . | . | . |

TABLE 3: ALPHA= 0.01  POWER= 0.8    EXPECTED ACCRUAL THRU MINIMUM FOLLOW-UP= 8000

| | | DEL=.01 | | | DEL=.02 | | | DEL=.05 | | | DEL=.10 | | | DEL=.15 | | |
|---|---|---|---|---|---|---|---|---|---|---|---|---|---|---|---|---|---|
| FACT= | | 1.0<br>.75 | .50<br>.25 | .00<br>BIN | 1.0<br>.75 | .50<br>.25 | .00<br>BIN | 1.0<br>.75 | .50<br>.25 | .00<br>BIN | 1.0<br>75 | .50<br>.25 | .00<br>BIN | 1.0<br>.75 | .50<br>.25 | .00<br>BIN |
| PCONT=*** | | | | | REQUIRED NUMBER OF PATIENTS | | | | | | | | | | | |
| 0.01 | *** | 1545 | 1545 | 1545 | 565 | 565 | 565 | 185 | 185 | 185 | 93 | 93 | 93 | 65 | 65 | 65 |
| | *** | 1545 | 1545 | 5922 | 565 | 565 | 1958 | 185 | 185 | 533 | 93 | 93 | 217 | 65 | 65 | 129 |
| 0.02 | *** | 3413 | 3425 | 3453 | 1093 | 1093 | 1105 | 293 | 293 | 293 | 125 | 125 | 125 | 85 | 85 | 85 |
| | *** | 3413 | 3433 | 9776 | 1093 | 1105 | 2911 | 293 | 293 | 681 | 125 | 125 | 252 | 85 | 85 | 144 |
| 0.05 | *** | 10345 | 10453 | 10785 | 2953 | 2985 | 3025 | 633 | 633 | 645 | 225 | 225 | 225 | 133 | 133 | 133 |
| | *** | 10385 | 10573 | 20855 | 2965 | 3005 | 5651 | 633 | 633 | 1104 | 225 | 225 | 352 | 133 | 133 | 186 |
| 0.1 | *** | 22853 | 23193 | 25113 | 6245 | 6373 | 6645 | 1213 | 1225 | 1233 | 373 | 385 | 385 | 205 | 205 | 205 |
| | *** | 22973 | 23685 | 37716 | 6305 | 6485 | 9816 | 1213 | 1225 | 1747 | 373 | 385 | 502 | 205 | 205 | 248 |
| 0.15 | *** | 34193 | 34833 | 39673 | 9245 | 9565 | 10273 | 1753 | 1773 | 1813 | 513 | 513 | 525 | 265 | 265 | 265 |
| | *** | 34413 | 35853 | 52569 | 9373 | 9833 | 13479 | 1765 | 1793 | 2309 | 513 | 525 | 633 | 265 | 265 | 302 |
| 0.2 | *** | 43413 | 44425 | 53293 | 11753 | 12285 | 13645 | 2225 | 2273 | 2333 | 633 | 645 | 645 | 313 | 313 | 313 |
| | *** | 43753 | 46093 | 65415 | 11973 | 12785 | 16640 | 2245 | 2305 | 2791 | 633 | 645 | 743 | 313 | 313 | 346 |
| 0.25 | *** | 50245 | 51705 | 65433 | 13705 | 14493 | 16645 | 2613 | 2693 | 2793 | 733 | 745 | 753 | 353 | 353 | 353 |
| | *** | 50745 | 54133 | 76254 | 14025 | 15245 | 19300 | 2653 | 2745 | 3192 | 745 | 753 | 833 | 353 | 353 | 382 |
| 0.3 | *** | 54725 | 56713 | 75773 | 15125 | 16173 | 19173 | 2925 | 3033 | 3185 | 813 | 825 | 845 | 385 | 393 | 393 |
| | *** | 55405 | 59993 | 85086 | 15545 | 17193 | 21458 | 2973 | 3105 | 3513 | 825 | 833 | 904 | 393 | 393 | 409 |
| 0.35 | *** | 57013 | 59645 | 84133 | 16045 | 17365 | 21225 | 3165 | 3293 | 3485 | 873 | 893 | 905 | 413 | 413 | 413 |
| | *** | 57913 | 63853 | 91910 | 16573 | 18633 | 23113 | 3225 | 3385 | 3754 | 885 | 893 | 954 | 413 | 413 | 426 |
| 0.4 | *** | 57385 | 60745 | 90425 | 16513 | 18093 | 22733 | 3313 | 3473 | 3705 | 913 | 933 | 953 | 425 | 433 | 433 |
| | *** | 58553 | 65913 | 96728 | 17153 | 19613 | 24268 | 3393 | 3573 | 3915 | 925 | 945 | 984 | 425 | 433 | 435 |
| 0.45 | *** | 56153 | 60313 | 94565 | 16605 | 18413 | 23725 | 3393 | 3573 | 3833 | 933 | 953 | 973 | 433 | 433 | 433 |
| | *** | 57625 | 66425 | 99538 | 17345 | 20145 | 24920 | 3485 | 3693 | 3995 | 945 | 965 | 994 | 433 | 433 | 435 |
| 0.5 | *** | 53645 | 58653 | 96545 | 16373 | 18365 | 24165 | 3405 | 3605 | 3873 | 933 | 953 | 973 | 425 | 433 | 433 |
| | *** | 55453 | 65625 | 100341 | 17193 | 20253 | 25070 | 3493 | 3725 | 3995 | 945 | 965 | 984 | 425 | 433 | 426 |
| 0.55 | *** | 50233 | 56045 | 96345 | 15865 | 17985 | 24053 | 3345 | 3553 | 3833 | 913 | 933 | 953 | 413 | 413 | 425 |
| | *** | 52373 | 63693 | 99136 | 16745 | 19965 | 24719 | 3445 | 3685 | 3915 | 925 | 945 | 954 | 413 | 413 | 409 |
| 0.6 | *** | 46213 | 52693 | 93953 | 15125 | 17305 | 23405 | 3225 | 3425 | 3705 | 873 | 885 | 905 | 385 | 393 | 393 |
| | *** | 48665 | 60813 | 95925 | 16033 | 19313 | 23866 | 3325 | 3553 | 3754 | 885 | 893 | 904 | 393 | 393 | 382 |
| 0.65 | *** | 41873 | 48793 | 89385 | 14173 | 16345 | 22205 | 3045 | 3225 | 3485 | 813 | 825 | 845 | 353 | 353 | 365 |
| | *** | 44533 | 57093 | 90706 | 15073 | 18305 | 22511 | 3125 | 3345 | 3513 | 813 | 833 | 833 | 353 | 365 | 346 |
| 0.7 | *** | 37365 | 44433 | 82653 | 13025 | 15093 | 20473 | 2785 | 2953 | 3185 | 725 | 745 | 753 | 313 | 313 | 313 |
| | *** | 40125 | 52585 | 83480 | 13893 | 16933 | 20655 | 2865 | 3065 | 3192 | 733 | 753 | 743 | 313 | 313 | 302 |
| 0.75 | *** | 32773 | 39633 | 73773 | 11685 | 13565 | 18205 | 2465 | 2613 | 2793 | 625 | 633 | 645 | 265 | 265 | 265 |
| | *** | 35485 | 47305 | 74247 | 12485 | 15193 | 18296 | 2533 | 2693 | 2791 | 633 | 645 | 633 | 265 | 265 | 248 |
| 0.8 | *** | 28065 | 34345 | 62773 | 10125 | 11725 | 15393 | 2085 | 2185 | 2325 | 505 | 513 | 525 | 205 | 205 | 205 |
| | *** | 30573 | 41145 | 62773 | 10813 | 13065 | 15436 | 2133 | 2253 | 2309 | 505 | 513 | 502 | 205 | 205 | 186 |
| 0.85 | *** | 23085 | 28405 | 49673 | 8293 | 9525 | 12073 | 1613 | 1685 | 1765 | 365 | 365 | 373 | . | . | . |
| | *** | 25233 | 33933 | 49759 | 8825 | 10505 | 12074 | 1645 | 1725 | 1747 | 365 | 365 | 352 | . | . | . |
| 0.9 | *** | 17513 | 21433 | 34493 | 6073 | 6845 | 8225 | 1053 | 1085 | 1125 | . | . | . | . | . | . |
| | *** | 19125 | 25265 | 34504 | 6413 | 7413 | 8210 | 1073 | 1105 | 1104 | . | . | . | . | . | . |
| 0.95 | *** | 10573 | 12525 | 17253 | 3225 | 3493 | 3865 | . | . | . | . | . | . | . | . | . |
| | *** | 11405 | 14205 | 17242 | 3353 | 3653 | 3844 | . | . | . | . | . | . | . | . | . |
| 0.98 | *** | 4625 | 5125 | 5945 | . | . | . | . | . | . | . | . | . | . | . | . |
| | *** | 4853 | 5473 | 5922 | . | . | . | . | . | . | . | . | . | . | . | . |

TABLE 3: ALPHA= 0.01  POWER= 0.8    EXPECTED ACCRUAL THRU MINIMUM FOLLOW-UP= 8500

| | | DEL=.01 | | | DEL=.02 | | | DEL=.05 | | | DEL=.10 | | | DEL=.15 | | |
|---|---|---|---|---|---|---|---|---|---|---|---|---|---|---|---|---|---|
| FACT= | | 1.0 .75 | .50 .25 | .00 BIN | 1.0 .75 | .50 .25 | .00 BIN | 1.0 .75 | .50 .25 | .00 BIN | 1.0 75 | .50 .25 | .00 BIN | 1.0 .75 | .50 .25 | .00 BIN |
| PCONT=*** | | | | | | REQUIRED NUMBER OF PATIENTS | | | | | | | | | | |
| 0.01 | *** | 1544 | 1544 | 1544 | 566 | 566 | 566 | 184 | 184 | 184 | 91 | 91 | 91 | 70 | 70 | 70 |
| | *** | 1544 | 1544 | 5922 | 566 | 566 | 1958 | 184 | 184 | 533 | 91 | 91 | 217 | 70 | 70 | 129 |
| 0.02 | *** | 3414 | 3427 | 3456 | 1098 | 1098 | 1098 | 290 | 290 | 290 | 133 | 133 | 133 | 78 | 78 | 91 |
| | *** | 3414 | 3435 | 9776 | 1098 | 1098 | 2911 | 290 | 290 | 681 | 133 | 133 | 252 | 78 | 91 | 144 |
| 0.05 | *** | 10355 | 10461 | 10788 | 2960 | 2981 | 3023 | 630 | 643 | 643 | 226 | 226 | 226 | 133 | 133 | 133 |
| | *** | 10397 | 10575 | 20855 | 2968 | 3002 | 5651 | 630 | 643 | 1104 | 226 | 226 | 352 | 133 | 133 | 186 |
| 0.1 | *** | 22871 | 23232 | 25110 | 6253 | 6389 | 6644 | 1217 | 1225 | 1238 | 375 | 375 | 375 | 197 | 197 | 205 |
| | *** | 22998 | 23729 | 37716 | 6317 | 6495 | 9816 | 1217 | 1225 | 1747 | 375 | 375 | 502 | 197 | 205 | 248 |
| 0.15 | *** | 34226 | 34906 | 39666 | 9271 | 9590 | 10270 | 1756 | 1778 | 1812 | 516 | 516 | 524 | 261 | 261 | 261 |
| | *** | 34460 | 35961 | 52569 | 9406 | 9853 | 13479 | 1770 | 1791 | 2309 | 516 | 524 | 633 | 261 | 261 | 302 |
| 0.2 | *** | 43470 | 44546 | 53301 | 11800 | 12331 | 13648 | 2224 | 2280 | 2343 | 643 | 643 | 651 | 311 | 311 | 311 |
| | *** | 43845 | 46267 | 65415 | 12020 | 12820 | 16640 | 2245 | 2309 | 2791 | 643 | 643 | 743 | 311 | 311 | 346 |
| 0.25 | *** | 50334 | 51877 | 65435 | 13776 | 14562 | 16645 | 2628 | 2705 | 2798 | 736 | 750 | 758 | 354 | 354 | 354 |
| | *** | 50865 | 54385 | 76254 | 14095 | 15293 | 19300 | 2662 | 2747 | 3192 | 736 | 750 | 833 | 354 | 354 | 382 |
| 0.3 | *** | 54852 | 56956 | 75770 | 15208 | 16270 | 19181 | 2938 | 3045 | 3180 | 821 | 835 | 843 | 388 | 388 | 396 |
| | *** | 55575 | 60335 | 85086 | 15646 | 17269 | 21458 | 2989 | 3108 | 3513 | 821 | 835 | 904 | 388 | 388 | 409 |
| 0.35 | *** | 57190 | 59952 | 84135 | 16156 | 17481 | 21221 | 3172 | 3308 | 3478 | 877 | 898 | 906 | 410 | 418 | 418 |
| | *** | 58133 | 64274 | 91910 | 16687 | 18735 | 23113 | 3236 | 3385 | 3754 | 885 | 898 | 954 | 418 | 418 | 426 |
| 0.4 | *** | 57601 | 61129 | 90425 | 16645 | 18225 | 22743 | 3329 | 3491 | 3703 | 920 | 941 | 949 | 431 | 431 | 431 |
| | *** | 58834 | 66433 | 96728 | 17290 | 19734 | 24268 | 3406 | 3584 | 3915 | 928 | 941 | 984 | 431 | 431 | 435 |
| 0.45 | *** | 56433 | 60781 | 94568 | 16759 | 18565 | 23721 | 3414 | 3597 | 3831 | 941 | 949 | 970 | 431 | 431 | 439 |
| | *** | 57976 | 67028 | 99538 | 17503 | 20278 | 24920 | 3499 | 3703 | 3995 | 949 | 962 | 994 | 431 | 439 | 435 |
| 0.5 | *** | 54002 | 59195 | 96545 | 16546 | 18536 | 24167 | 3427 | 3618 | 3881 | 941 | 949 | 970 | 431 | 431 | 431 |
| | *** | 55880 | 66293 | 100341 | 17367 | 20393 | 25070 | 3512 | 3733 | 3995 | 949 | 962 | 984 | 431 | 431 | 426 |
| 0.55 | *** | 50653 | 56645 | 96340 | 16050 | 18175 | 24061 | 3371 | 3563 | 3831 | 920 | 928 | 949 | 410 | 418 | 418 |
| | *** | 52876 | 64423 | 99136 | 16929 | 20130 | 24719 | 3456 | 3690 | 3915 | 928 | 941 | 954 | 418 | 418 | 409 |
| 0.6 | *** | 46700 | 53351 | 93952 | 15314 | 17495 | 23402 | 3244 | 3435 | 3703 | 877 | 885 | 906 | 388 | 388 | 396 |
| | *** | 49221 | 61567 | 95925 | 16220 | 19471 | 23866 | 3342 | 3563 | 3754 | 885 | 898 | 904 | 388 | 396 | 382 |
| 0.65 | *** | 42408 | 49476 | 89383 | 14358 | 16525 | 22212 | 3053 | 3244 | 3491 | 813 | 821 | 843 | 354 | 354 | 367 |
| | *** | 45128 | 57848 | 90706 | 15271 | 18459 | 22511 | 3151 | 3350 | 3513 | 821 | 835 | 833 | 354 | 354 | 346 |
| 0.7 | *** | 37924 | 45106 | 82655 | 13210 | 15271 | 20470 | 2811 | 2968 | 3180 | 728 | 750 | 758 | 311 | 311 | 325 |
| | *** | 40742 | 53322 | 83480 | 14081 | 17078 | 20655 | 2883 | 3066 | 3192 | 736 | 750 | 743 | 311 | 311 | 302 |
| 0.75 | *** | 33326 | 40283 | 73773 | 11850 | 13720 | 18204 | 2479 | 2620 | 2798 | 630 | 643 | 651 | 261 | 261 | 269 |
| | *** | 36075 | 47988 | 74247 | 12650 | 15327 | 18296 | 2543 | 2705 | 2791 | 630 | 643 | 633 | 261 | 269 | 248 |
| 0.8 | *** | 28574 | 34928 | 62778 | 10270 | 11863 | 15399 | 2088 | 2195 | 2322 | 503 | 516 | 524 | 205 | 205 | 205 |
| | *** | 31116 | 41741 | 63007 | 10950 | 13168 | 15436 | 2139 | 2258 | 2309 | 516 | 516 | 502 | 205 | 205 | 186 |
| 0.85 | *** | 23530 | 28893 | 49675 | 8408 | 9619 | 12076 | 1621 | 1685 | 1770 | 367 | 367 | 367 | . | . | . |
| | *** | 25697 | 34410 | 49759 | 8931 | 10575 | 12074 | 1650 | 1727 | 1747 | 367 | 367 | 352 | . | . | . |
| 0.9 | *** | 17856 | 21774 | 34495 | 6147 | 6899 | 8216 | 1055 | 1090 | 1119 | . | . | . | . | . | . |
| | *** | 19471 | 25578 | 34504 | 6487 | 7451 | 8210 | 1076 | 1111 | 1104 | . | . | . | . | . | . |
| 0.95 | *** | 10745 | 12692 | 17261 | 3257 | 3512 | 3860 | . | . | . | . | . | . | . | . | . |
| | *** | 11574 | 14328 | 17242 | 3371 | 3669 | 3844 | . | . | . | . | . | . | . | . | . |
| 0.98 | *** | 4668 | 5170 | 5943 | . | . | . | . | . | . | . | . | . | . | . | . |
| | *** | 4893 | 5496 | 5922 | . | . | . | . | . | . | . | . | . | . | . | . |

TABLE 3: ALPHA= 0.01  POWER= 0.8    EXPECTED ACCRUAL THRU MINIMUM FOLLOW-UP= 9000

| | | DEL=.01 | | | DEL=.02 | | | DEL=.05 | | | DEL=.10 | | | DEL=.15 | | |
|---|---|---|---|---|---|---|---|---|---|---|---|---|---|---|---|---|---|
| FACT= | | 1.0 .75 | .50 .25 | .00 BIN | 1.0 .75 | .50 .25 | .00 BIN | 1.0 .75 | .50 .25 | .00 BIN | 1.0 75 | .50 .25 | .00 BIN | 1.0 .75 | .50 .25 | .00 BIN |
| PCONT=*** | | | | | REQUIRED NUMBER OF PATIENTS | | | | | | | | | | | |
| 0.01 | *** | 1536 | 1545 | 1545 | 569 | 569 | 569 | 186 | 186 | 186 | 96 | 96 | 96 | 60 | 60 | 60 |
| | *** | 1545 | 1545 | 5922 | 569 | 569 | 1958 | 186 | 186 | 533 | 96 | 96 | 217 | 60 | 60 | 129 |
| 0.02 | *** | 3412 | 3426 | 3457 | 1095 | 1095 | 1109 | 299 | 299 | 299 | 127 | 127 | 127 | 82 | 82 | 82 |
| | *** | 3426 | 3435 | 9776 | 1095 | 1095 | 2911 | 299 | 299 | 681 | 127 | 127 | 252 | 82 | 82 | 144 |
| 0.05 | *** | 10365 | 10477 | 10792 | 2954 | 2985 | 3021 | 636 | 636 | 636 | 231 | 231 | 231 | 127 | 127 | 127 |
| | *** | 10410 | 10590 | 20855 | 2976 | 2999 | 5651 | 636 | 636 | 1104 | 231 | 231 | 352 | 127 | 127 | 186 |
| 0.1 | *** | 22897 | 23271 | 25116 | 6261 | 6396 | 6644 | 1207 | 1221 | 1230 | 375 | 375 | 375 | 195 | 195 | 195 |
| | *** | 23032 | 23775 | 37716 | 6329 | 6495 | 9816 | 1221 | 1230 | 1747 | 375 | 375 | 502 | 195 | 195 | 248 |
| 0.15 | *** | 34274 | 34980 | 39674 | 9299 | 9614 | 10275 | 1761 | 1784 | 1815 | 510 | 524 | 524 | 262 | 262 | 262 |
| | *** | 34521 | 36051 | 52569 | 9434 | 9870 | 13479 | 1770 | 1792 | 2309 | 524 | 524 | 633 | 262 | 262 | 302 |
| 0.2 | *** | 43544 | 44655 | 53295 | 11841 | 12381 | 13650 | 2234 | 2279 | 2332 | 636 | 645 | 645 | 307 | 307 | 321 |
| | *** | 43926 | 46432 | 65415 | 12066 | 12854 | 16640 | 2256 | 2310 | 2791 | 636 | 645 | 743 | 307 | 321 | 346 |
| 0.25 | *** | 50429 | 52049 | 65436 | 13830 | 14631 | 16642 | 2625 | 2706 | 2796 | 735 | 749 | 757 | 352 | 352 | 352 |
| | *** | 50991 | 54622 | 76254 | 14159 | 15351 | 19300 | 2670 | 2751 | 3192 | 749 | 749 | 833 | 352 | 352 | 382 |
| 0.3 | *** | 54974 | 57179 | 75772 | 15292 | 16350 | 19176 | 2954 | 3052 | 3179 | 825 | 825 | 839 | 389 | 389 | 397 |
| | *** | 55739 | 60666 | 85086 | 15734 | 17340 | 21458 | 2999 | 3111 | 3513 | 825 | 839 | 904 | 389 | 389 | 409 |
| 0.35 | *** | 57359 | 60247 | 84134 | 16251 | 17587 | 21224 | 3187 | 3314 | 3480 | 884 | 892 | 906 | 411 | 411 | 420 |
| | *** | 58357 | 64694 | 91910 | 16800 | 18839 | 23113 | 3246 | 3390 | 3754 | 884 | 906 | 954 | 411 | 420 | 426 |
| 0.4 | *** | 57831 | 61499 | 90420 | 16769 | 18366 | 22740 | 3345 | 3502 | 3705 | 915 | 937 | 951 | 434 | 434 | 434 |
| | *** | 59122 | 66930 | 96728 | 17421 | 19851 | 24268 | 3412 | 3592 | 3915 | 929 | 937 | 984 | 434 | 434 | 435 |
| 0.45 | *** | 56706 | 61229 | 94574 | 16904 | 18726 | 23721 | 3435 | 3606 | 3831 | 937 | 960 | 974 | 434 | 434 | 442 |
| | *** | 58326 | 67605 | 99538 | 17655 | 20400 | 24920 | 3516 | 3705 | 3995 | 951 | 960 | 994 | 434 | 434 | 435 |
| 0.5 | *** | 54344 | 59721 | 96540 | 16710 | 18704 | 24157 | 3449 | 3629 | 3876 | 937 | 951 | 974 | 420 | 434 | 434 |
| | *** | 56310 | 66930 | 100341 | 17534 | 20535 | 25070 | 3525 | 3741 | 3995 | 951 | 960 | 984 | 434 | 434 | 426 |
| 0.55 | *** | 51059 | 57232 | 96337 | 16229 | 18344 | 24059 | 3390 | 3584 | 3831 | 915 | 937 | 951 | 411 | 420 | 420 |
| | *** | 53362 | 65107 | 99136 | 17106 | 20265 | 24719 | 3480 | 3696 | 3915 | 929 | 937 | 954 | 411 | 420 | 409 |
| 0.6 | *** | 47175 | 53984 | 93952 | 15495 | 17669 | 23406 | 3269 | 3449 | 3705 | 870 | 892 | 906 | 389 | 389 | 397 |
| | *** | 49762 | 62286 | 95925 | 16409 | 19626 | 23866 | 3359 | 3570 | 3754 | 884 | 906 | 904 | 389 | 397 | 382 |
| 0.65 | *** | 42922 | 50122 | 89385 | 14541 | 16701 | 22214 | 3075 | 3255 | 3494 | 816 | 825 | 847 | 352 | 352 | 366 |
| | *** | 45712 | 58574 | 90706 | 15450 | 18600 | 22511 | 3156 | 3359 | 3513 | 816 | 839 | 833 | 352 | 366 | 346 |
| 0.7 | *** | 38467 | 45757 | 82657 | 13380 | 15427 | 20467 | 2819 | 2976 | 3187 | 735 | 749 | 757 | 307 | 321 | 321 |
| | *** | 41325 | 54015 | 83480 | 14249 | 17205 | 20655 | 2895 | 3075 | 3192 | 735 | 749 | 743 | 321 | 321 | 302 |
| 0.75 | *** | 33855 | 40897 | 73784 | 12007 | 13866 | 18195 | 2504 | 2625 | 2796 | 636 | 636 | 645 | 262 | 262 | 262 |
| | *** | 36659 | 48629 | 74247 | 12809 | 15441 | 18296 | 2557 | 2706 | 2791 | 636 | 645 | 633 | 262 | 262 | 248 |
| 0.8 | *** | 29062 | 35489 | 62781 | 10410 | 11976 | 15396 | 2099 | 2197 | 2324 | 510 | 510 | 524 | 209 | 209 | 209 |
| | *** | 31641 | 42306 | 63007 | 11085 | 13259 | 15436 | 2152 | 2256 | 2309 | 510 | 510 | 502 | 209 | 209 | 186 |
| 0.85 | *** | 23946 | 29346 | 49672 | 8511 | 9712 | 12066 | 1626 | 1694 | 1761 | 366 | 366 | 366 | . | . | . |
| | *** | 26137 | 34859 | 49759 | 9037 | 10635 | 12074 | 1657 | 1725 | 1747 | 366 | 366 | 352 | . | . | . |
| 0.9 | *** | 18172 | 22101 | 34499 | 6216 | 6959 | 8219 | 1064 | 1095 | 1117 | . | . | . | . | . | . |
| | *** | 19792 | 25867 | 34504 | 6554 | 7485 | 8210 | 1072 | 1109 | 1104 | . | . | . | . | . | . |
| 0.95 | *** | 10919 | 12840 | 17264 | 3277 | 3525 | 3862 | . | . | . | . | . | . | . | . | . |
| | *** | 11737 | 14451 | 17242 | 3390 | 3682 | 3844 | . | . | . | . | . | . | . | . | . |
| 0.98 | *** | 4717 | 5204 | 5946 | . | . | . | . | . | . | . | . | . | . | . | . |
| | *** | 4934 | 5519 | 5922 | . | . | . | . | . | . | . | . | . | . | . | . |

## TABLE 3: ALPHA= 0.01  POWER= 0.8    EXPECTED ACCRUAL THRU MINIMUM FOLLOW-UP= 9500

|  |  | DEL=.01 | | | DEL=.02 | | | DEL=.05 | | | DEL=.10 | | | DEL=.15 | | |
|---|---|---|---|---|---|---|---|---|---|---|---|---|---|---|---|---|
| FACT= | | 1.0 / .75 | .50 / .25 | .00 / BIN | 1.0 / .75 | .50 / .25 | .00 / BIN | 1.0 / .75 | .50 / .25 | .00 / BIN | 1.0 / 75 | .50 / .25 | .00 / BIN | 1.0 / .75 | .50 / .25 | .00 / BIN |
| PCONT=*** | | | | | REQUIRED NUMBER OF PATIENTS | | | | | | | | | | | |
| 0.01 | *** | 1535 | 1550 | 1550 | 562 | 562 | 562 | 182 | 182 | 182 | 87 | 87 | 87 | 63 | 63 | 63 |
|  | *** | 1535 | 1550 | 5922 | 562 | 562 | 1958 | 182 | 182 | 533 | 87 | 87 | 217 | 63 | 63 | 129 |
| 0.02 | *** | 3412 | 3426 | 3450 | 1099 | 1099 | 1099 | 291 | 291 | 300 | 125 | 125 | 125 | 87 | 87 | 87 |
|  | *** | 3426 | 3435 | 9776 | 1099 | 1099 | 2911 | 291 | 291 | 681 | 125 | 125 | 252 | 87 | 87 | 144 |
| 0.05 | *** | 10370 | 10480 | 10789 | 2960 | 2984 | 3023 | 633 | 633 | 633 | 229 | 229 | 229 | 134 | 134 | 134 |
|  | *** | 10418 | 10599 | 20855 | 2975 | 2999 | 5651 | 633 | 633 | 1104 | 229 | 229 | 352 | 134 | 134 | 186 |
| 0.1 | *** | 22925 | 23305 | 25110 | 6276 | 6404 | 6642 | 1218 | 1227 | 1241 | 372 | 386 | 386 | 196 | 196 | 205 |
|  | *** | 23053 | 23813 | 37716 | 6333 | 6514 | 9816 | 1218 | 1227 | 1747 | 372 | 386 | 502 | 196 | 205 | 248 |
| 0.15 | *** | 34310 | 35047 | 39669 | 9325 | 9634 | 10275 | 1764 | 1788 | 1811 | 514 | 514 | 529 | 268 | 268 | 268 |
|  | *** | 34572 | 36154 | 52569 | 9459 | 9886 | 13479 | 1773 | 1797 | 2309 | 514 | 514 | 633 | 268 | 268 | 302 |
| 0.2 | *** | 43611 | 44775 | 53301 | 11881 | 12413 | 13648 | 2239 | 2286 | 2334 | 633 | 648 | 648 | 315 | 315 | 315 |
|  | *** | 44015 | 46589 | 65415 | 12104 | 12888 | 16640 | 2263 | 2310 | 2791 | 633 | 648 | 743 | 315 | 315 | 346 |
| 0.25 | *** | 50523 | 52218 | 65438 | 13900 | 14693 | 16640 | 2643 | 2714 | 2794 | 743 | 743 | 752 | 363 | 363 | 363 |
|  | *** | 51102 | 54854 | 76254 | 14218 | 15405 | 19300 | 2675 | 2747 | 3192 | 743 | 752 | 833 | 363 | 363 | 382 |
| 0.3 | *** | 55106 | 57410 | 75769 | 15373 | 16441 | 19182 | 2960 | 3055 | 3174 | 823 | 838 | 838 | 386 | 395 | 395 |
|  | *** | 55899 | 60973 | 85086 | 15809 | 17415 | 21458 | 3008 | 3118 | 3513 | 823 | 838 | 904 | 386 | 395 | 409 |
| 0.35 | *** | 57529 | 60545 | 84138 | 16355 | 17685 | 21215 | 3198 | 3317 | 3483 | 885 | 894 | 909 | 410 | 419 | 419 |
|  | *** | 58574 | 65081 | 91910 | 16902 | 18920 | 23113 | 3260 | 3403 | 3754 | 885 | 894 | 954 | 410 | 419 | 426 |
| 0.4 | *** | 58051 | 61875 | 90423 | 16893 | 18484 | 22735 | 3364 | 3507 | 3697 | 918 | 933 | 956 | 434 | 434 | 434 |
|  | *** | 59405 | 67409 | 96728 | 17543 | 19942 | 24268 | 3426 | 3593 | 3915 | 933 | 942 | 984 | 434 | 434 | 435 |
| 0.45 | *** | 56983 | 61670 | 94564 | 17044 | 18864 | 23718 | 3450 | 3616 | 3830 | 942 | 956 | 965 | 434 | 434 | 443 |
|  | *** | 58669 | 68154 | 99538 | 17795 | 20526 | 24920 | 3521 | 3711 | 3995 | 942 | 965 | 994 | 434 | 434 | 435 |
| 0.5 | *** | 54679 | 60222 | 96550 | 16854 | 18849 | 24160 | 3459 | 3640 | 3878 | 942 | 956 | 980 | 434 | 434 | 434 |
|  | *** | 56721 | 67537 | 100341 | 17685 | 20669 | 25070 | 3545 | 3744 | 3995 | 942 | 965 | 984 | 434 | 434 | 426 |
| 0.55 | *** | 51458 | 57799 | 96336 | 16394 | 18508 | 24050 | 3403 | 3593 | 3830 | 918 | 933 | 956 | 410 | 419 | 419 |
|  | *** | 53833 | 65770 | 99136 | 17273 | 20408 | 24719 | 3498 | 3697 | 3915 | 933 | 942 | 954 | 410 | 419 | 409 |
| 0.6 | *** | 47634 | 54593 | 93947 | 15667 | 17828 | 23400 | 3284 | 3459 | 3697 | 870 | 894 | 909 | 386 | 395 | 395 |
|  | *** | 50294 | 62968 | 95925 | 16569 | 19752 | 23866 | 3364 | 3578 | 3754 | 885 | 894 | 904 | 386 | 395 | 382 |
| 0.65 | *** | 43421 | 50760 | 89387 | 14717 | 16854 | 22213 | 3094 | 3260 | 3483 | 814 | 823 | 847 | 363 | 363 | 363 |
|  | *** | 46271 | 59248 | 90706 | 15619 | 18730 | 22511 | 3174 | 3364 | 3513 | 823 | 838 | 833 | 363 | 363 | 346 |
| 0.7 | *** | 38980 | 46375 | 82656 | 13544 | 15586 | 20479 | 2833 | 2984 | 3189 | 728 | 743 | 752 | 315 | 315 | 315 |
|  | *** | 41887 | 54679 | 83480 | 14408 | 17329 | 20655 | 2904 | 3079 | 3192 | 743 | 752 | 743 | 315 | 315 | 302 |
| 0.75 | *** | 34373 | 41483 | 73783 | 12166 | 14004 | 18199 | 2509 | 2643 | 2794 | 633 | 633 | 648 | 268 | 268 | 268 |
|  | *** | 37199 | 49225 | 74247 | 12950 | 15539 | 18296 | 2571 | 2714 | 2791 | 633 | 648 | 633 | 268 | 268 | 248 |
| 0.8 | *** | 29537 | 36011 | 62778 | 10537 | 12095 | 15396 | 2105 | 2200 | 2319 | 505 | 514 | 514 | 205 | 205 | 205 |
|  | *** | 32140 | 42828 | 63007 | 11202 | 13339 | 15436 | 2153 | 2263 | 2309 | 514 | 514 | 502 | 205 | 205 | 186 |
| 0.85 | *** | 24350 | 29774 | 49677 | 8613 | 9791 | 12071 | 1630 | 1693 | 1764 | 363 | 363 | 372 | . | . | . |
|  | *** | 26559 | 35260 | 49759 | 9126 | 10694 | 12074 | 1669 | 1725 | 1747 | 363 | 372 | 352 | . | . | . |
| 0.9 | *** | 18469 | 22412 | 34491 | 6285 | 7013 | 8224 | 1060 | 1099 | 1123 | . | . | . | . | . | . |
|  | *** | 20099 | 26140 | 34504 | 6609 | 7520 | 8210 | 1075 | 1108 | 1104 | . | . | . | . | . | . |
| 0.95 | *** | 11074 | 12974 | 17258 | 3308 | 3545 | 3863 | . | . | . | . | . | . | . | . | . |
|  | *** | 11890 | 14550 | 17242 | 3412 | 3688 | 3844 | . | . | . | . | . | . | . | . | . |
| 0.98 | *** | 4756 | 5231 | 5944 | . | . | . | . | . | . | . | . | . | . | . | . |
|  | *** | 4970 | 5540 | 5922 | . | . | . | . | . | . | . | . | . | . | . | . |

TABLE 3: ALPHA= 0.01  POWER= 0.8    EXPECTED ACCRUAL THRU MINIMUM FOLLOW-UP= 10000

| | DEL=.01 | | | DEL=.02 | | | DEL=.05 | | | DEL=.10 | | | DEL=.15 | | |
|---|---|---|---|---|---|---|---|---|---|---|---|---|---|---|---|
| FACT= | 1.0 .75 | .50 .25 | .00 BIN | 1.0 .75 | .50 .25 | .00 BIN | 1.0 .75 | .50 .25 | .00 BIN | 1.0 75 | .50 .25 | .00 BIN | 1.0 .75 | .50 .25 | .00 BIN |
| PCONT=*** | | | | | REQUIRED NUMBER OF PATIENTS | | | | | | | | | | |
| 0.01 *** | 1541 | 1541 | 1541 | 566 | 566 | 566 | 182 | 182 | 182 | 91 | 91 | 91 | 66 | 66 | 66 |
| *** | 1541 | 1541 | 5922 | 566 | 566 | 1958 | 182 | 182 | 533 | 91 | 91 | 217 | 66 | 66 | 129 |
| 0.02 *** | 3416 | 3432 | 3457 | 1091 | 1107 | 1107 | 291 | 291 | 291 | 132 | 132 | 132 | 82 | 82 | 82 |
| *** | 3416 | 3441 | 9776 | 1091 | 1107 | 2911 | 291 | 291 | 681 | 132 | 132 | 252 | 82 | 82 | 144 |
| 0.05 *** | 10382 | 10491 | 10791 | 2966 | 2991 | 3016 | 632 | 641 | 641 | 232 | 232 | 232 | 132 | 132 | 132 |
| *** | 10416 | 10607 | 20855 | 2966 | 3007 | 5651 | 641 | 641 | 1104 | 232 | 232 | 352 | 132 | 132 | 186 |
| 0.1 *** | 22941 | 23341 | 25116 | 6282 | 6416 | 6641 | 1216 | 1232 | 1232 | 382 | 382 | 382 | 207 | 207 | 207 |
| *** | 23091 | 23857 | 37716 | 6341 | 6516 | 9816 | 1216 | 1232 | 1747 | 382 | 382 | 502 | 207 | 207 | 248 |
| 0.15 *** | 34357 | 35132 | 39666 | 9341 | 9657 | 10266 | 1757 | 1782 | 1807 | 516 | 516 | 516 | 257 | 266 | 266 |
| *** | 34632 | 36232 | 52569 | 9482 | 9907 | 13479 | 1766 | 1791 | 2309 | 516 | 516 | 633 | 257 | 266 | 302 |
| 0.2 *** | 43666 | 44891 | 53291 | 11916 | 12457 | 13641 | 2241 | 2282 | 2341 | 641 | 641 | 641 | 316 | 316 | 316 |
| *** | 44091 | 46732 | 65415 | 12141 | 12916 | 16640 | 2257 | 2307 | 2791 | 641 | 641 | 743 | 316 | 316 | 346 |
| 0.25 *** | 50616 | 52382 | 65432 | 13957 | 14741 | 16641 | 2641 | 2716 | 2791 | 741 | 741 | 757 | 357 | 357 | 357 |
| *** | 51232 | 55082 | 76254 | 14282 | 15441 | 19300 | 2682 | 2757 | 3192 | 741 | 757 | 833 | 357 | 357 | 382 |
| 0.3 *** | 55232 | 57632 | 75766 | 15457 | 16516 | 19182 | 2966 | 3057 | 3182 | 816 | 832 | 841 | 391 | 391 | 391 |
| *** | 56066 | 61266 | 85086 | 15891 | 17482 | 21458 | 3016 | 3116 | 3513 | 832 | 832 | 904 | 391 | 391 | 409 |
| 0.35 *** | 57691 | 60832 | 84132 | 16457 | 17791 | 21216 | 3207 | 3332 | 3482 | 882 | 891 | 907 | 416 | 416 | 416 |
| *** | 58791 | 65466 | 91910 | 17007 | 19007 | 23113 | 3266 | 3407 | 3754 | 891 | 907 | 954 | 416 | 416 | 426 |
| 0.4 *** | 58266 | 62232 | 90416 | 17007 | 18607 | 22741 | 3382 | 3516 | 3707 | 916 | 932 | 957 | 432 | 432 | 432 |
| *** | 59682 | 67857 | 96728 | 17666 | 20041 | 24268 | 3441 | 3607 | 3915 | 932 | 941 | 984 | 432 | 432 | 435 |
| 0.45 *** | 57257 | 62091 | 94566 | 17182 | 18991 | 23716 | 3466 | 3616 | 3832 | 941 | 957 | 966 | 432 | 432 | 441 |
| *** | 59016 | 68682 | 99538 | 17932 | 20632 | 24920 | 3541 | 3716 | 3995 | 957 | 966 | 994 | 432 | 441 | 435 |
| 0.5 *** | 55016 | 60716 | 96541 | 17007 | 18991 | 24166 | 3482 | 3657 | 3882 | 941 | 957 | 966 | 432 | 432 | 432 |
| *** | 57116 | 68116 | 100341 | 17841 | 20782 | 25070 | 3557 | 3757 | 3995 | 957 | 966 | 984 | 432 | 432 | 426 |
| 0.55 *** | 51857 | 58341 | 96341 | 16541 | 18657 | 24057 | 3416 | 3607 | 3832 | 916 | 932 | 957 | 416 | 416 | 416 |
| *** | 54307 | 66391 | 99136 | 17432 | 20532 | 24719 | 3507 | 3707 | 3915 | 932 | 941 | 954 | 416 | 416 | 409 |
| 0.6 *** | 48082 | 55166 | 93957 | 15832 | 17982 | 23407 | 3307 | 3482 | 3707 | 882 | 891 | 907 | 391 | 391 | 391 |
| *** | 50807 | 63616 | 95925 | 16732 | 19882 | 23866 | 3382 | 3582 | 3754 | 882 | 907 | 904 | 391 | 391 | 382 |
| 0.65 *** | 43907 | 51357 | 89382 | 14882 | 17007 | 22207 | 3107 | 3266 | 3491 | 816 | 832 | 841 | 357 | 357 | 366 |
| *** | 46807 | 59907 | 90706 | 15782 | 18857 | 22511 | 3182 | 3366 | 3513 | 816 | 832 | 833 | 357 | 357 | 346 |
| 0.7 *** | 39482 | 46966 | 82657 | 13707 | 15732 | 20466 | 2857 | 2991 | 3182 | 732 | 741 | 757 | 316 | 316 | 316 |
| *** | 42441 | 55307 | 83480 | 14566 | 17441 | 20655 | 2916 | 3082 | 3192 | 741 | 757 | 743 | 316 | 316 | 302 |
| 0.75 *** | 34857 | 42041 | 73782 | 12307 | 14132 | 18207 | 2516 | 2641 | 2791 | 632 | 641 | 641 | 266 | 266 | 266 |
| *** | 37732 | 49807 | 74247 | 13091 | 15641 | 18296 | 2582 | 2716 | 2791 | 632 | 641 | 633 | 266 | 266 | 248 |
| 0.8 *** | 29991 | 36516 | 62782 | 10657 | 12191 | 15391 | 2116 | 2207 | 2316 | 507 | 516 | 516 | 207 | 207 | 207 |
| *** | 32616 | 43332 | 63007 | 11332 | 13416 | 15436 | 2166 | 2266 | 2309 | 507 | 516 | 502 | 207 | 207 | 186 |
| 0.85 *** | 24741 | 30191 | 49682 | 8707 | 9866 | 12066 | 1641 | 1691 | 1766 | 366 | 366 | 366 | . | . | . |
| *** | 26966 | 35657 | 49759 | 9216 | 10757 | 12074 | 1666 | 1732 | 1747 | 366 | 366 | 352 | . | . | . |
| 0.9 *** | 18757 | 22691 | 34491 | 6341 | 7057 | 8216 | 1066 | 1091 | 1116 | . | . | . | . | . | . |
| *** | 20391 | 26391 | 34504 | 6657 | 7541 | 8210 | 1082 | 1107 | 1104 | . | . | . | . | . | . |
| 0.95 *** | 11216 | 13107 | 17257 | 3332 | 3557 | 3866 | . | . | . | . | . | . | . | . | . |
| *** | 12032 | 14657 | 17242 | 3432 | 3691 | 3844 | . | . | . | . | . | . | . | . | . |
| 0.98 *** | 4807 | 5257 | 5941 | . | . | . | . | . | . | . | . | . | . | . | . |
| *** | 5007 | 5557 | 5922 | . | . | . | . | . | . | . | . | . | . | . | . |

TABLE 3: ALPHA= 0.01  POWER= 0.8    EXPECTED ACCRUAL THRU MINIMUM FOLLOW-UP= 11000

| | | DEL=.01 | | | DEL=.02 | | | DEL=.05 | | | DEL=.10 | | | DEL=.15 | | |
|---|---|---|---|---|---|---|---|---|---|---|---|---|---|---|---|---|---|
| FACT= | | 1.0 .75 | .50 .25 | .00 BIN | 1.0 .75 | .50 .25 | .00 BIN | 1.0 .75 | .50 .25 | .00 BIN | 1.0 75 | .50 .25 | .00 BIN | 1.0 .75 | .50 .25 | .00 BIN |
| PCONT=*** | | | | | REQUIRED NUMBER OF PATIENTS | | | | | | | | | | | | |
| 0.01 | *** | 1547 | 1547 | 1547 | 568 | 568 | 568 | 183 | 183 | 183 | 90 | 90 | 90 | 62 | 62 | 62 |
|  | *** | 1547 | 1547 | 5922 | 568 | 568 | 1958 | 183 | 183 | 533 | 90 | 90 | 217 | 62 | 62 | 129 |
| 0.02 | *** | 3417 | 3428 | 3455 | 1090 | 1107 | 1107 | 293 | 293 | 293 | 128 | 128 | 128 | 90 | 90 | 90 |
|  | *** | 3428 | 3445 | 9776 | 1090 | 1107 | 2911 | 293 | 293 | 681 | 128 | 128 | 252 | 90 | 90 | 144 |
| 0.05 | *** | 10385 | 10512 | 10787 | 2960 | 2988 | 3015 | 640 | 640 | 640 | 227 | 227 | 227 | 128 | 128 | 128 |
|  | *** | 10440 | 10622 | 20855 | 2977 | 3005 | 5651 | 640 | 640 | 1104 | 227 | 227 | 352 | 128 | 128 | 186 |
| 0.1 | *** | 22980 | 23410 | 25115 | 6305 | 6425 | 6645 | 1217 | 1228 | 1228 | 375 | 375 | 375 | 200 | 200 | 200 |
|  | *** | 23145 | 23932 | 37716 | 6360 | 6525 | 9816 | 1217 | 1228 | 1747 | 375 | 375 | 502 | 200 | 200 | 248 |
| 0.15 | *** | 34437 | 35262 | 39673 | 9385 | 9698 | 10275 | 1767 | 1778 | 1805 | 513 | 513 | 530 | 265 | 265 | 265 |
|  | *** | 34723 | 36400 | 52569 | 9522 | 9935 | 13479 | 1778 | 1795 | 2309 | 513 | 513 | 633 | 265 | 265 | 302 |
| 0.2 | *** | 43798 | 45107 | 53302 | 11997 | 12530 | 13647 | 2245 | 2290 | 2345 | 640 | 640 | 650 | 310 | 310 | 310 |
|  | *** | 44255 | 47015 | 65415 | 12217 | 12970 | 16640 | 2262 | 2317 | 2791 | 640 | 640 | 743 | 310 | 310 | 346 |
| 0.25 | *** | 50800 | 52697 | 65430 | 14060 | 14857 | 16645 | 2658 | 2713 | 2795 | 750 | 750 | 750 | 348 | 365 | 365 |
|  | *** | 51470 | 55502 | 76254 | 14390 | 15528 | 19300 | 2685 | 2757 | 3192 | 750 | 750 | 833 | 365 | 365 | 382 |
| 0.3 | *** | 55485 | 58070 | 75770 | 15600 | 16655 | 19175 | 2988 | 3070 | 3180 | 815 | 832 | 843 | 392 | 392 | 392 |
|  | *** | 56393 | 61838 | 85086 | 16040 | 17590 | 21458 | 3032 | 3125 | 3513 | 832 | 832 | 904 | 392 | 392 | 409 |
| 0.35 | *** | 58032 | 61398 | 84130 | 16628 | 17965 | 21220 | 3225 | 3345 | 3483 | 887 | 898 | 898 | 420 | 420 | 420 |
|  | *** | 59225 | 66172 | 91910 | 17195 | 19147 | 23113 | 3280 | 3400 | 3754 | 887 | 898 | 954 | 420 | 420 | 426 |
| 0.4 | *** | 58692 | 62910 | 90427 | 17222 | 18817 | 22733 | 3400 | 3527 | 3703 | 925 | 942 | 953 | 430 | 430 | 430 |
|  | *** | 60215 | 68713 | 96728 | 17893 | 20220 | 24268 | 3455 | 3610 | 3915 | 925 | 942 | 984 | 430 | 430 | 435 |
| 0.45 | *** | 57795 | 62910 | 94563 | 17425 | 19230 | 23723 | 3483 | 3637 | 3830 | 942 | 953 | 970 | 430 | 430 | 430 |
|  | *** | 59682 | 69665 | 99538 | 18185 | 20825 | 24920 | 3555 | 3730 | 3995 | 953 | 970 | 994 | 430 | 430 | 435 |
| 0.5 | *** | 55667 | 61662 | 96543 | 17277 | 19268 | 24163 | 3510 | 3665 | 3885 | 942 | 953 | 970 | 430 | 430 | 430 |
|  | *** | 57905 | 69208 | 100341 | 18113 | 21000 | 25070 | 3582 | 3758 | 3995 | 953 | 970 | 984 | 430 | 430 | 426 |
| 0.55 | *** | 52625 | 59380 | 96340 | 16837 | 18938 | 24053 | 3455 | 3620 | 3830 | 925 | 942 | 953 | 420 | 420 | 420 |
|  | *** | 55200 | 67547 | 99136 | 17717 | 20753 | 24719 | 3527 | 3720 | 3915 | 925 | 942 | 954 | 420 | 420 | 409 |
| 0.6 | *** | 48940 | 56272 | 93947 | 16133 | 18267 | 23410 | 3335 | 3500 | 3703 | 887 | 898 | 915 | 392 | 392 | 392 |
|  | *** | 51773 | 64825 | 95925 | 17030 | 20110 | 23866 | 3400 | 3593 | 3754 | 887 | 898 | 904 | 392 | 392 | 382 |
| 0.65 | *** | 44832 | 52488 | 89382 | 15170 | 17288 | 22210 | 3142 | 3290 | 3483 | 815 | 832 | 843 | 365 | 365 | 365 |
|  | *** | 47830 | 61095 | 90706 | 16078 | 19065 | 22511 | 3208 | 3390 | 3513 | 832 | 832 | 833 | 365 | 365 | 346 |
| 0.7 | *** | 40432 | 48088 | 82655 | 13988 | 15985 | 20467 | 2878 | 3015 | 3180 | 733 | 750 | 760 | 310 | 320 | 320 |
|  | *** | 43468 | 56465 | 83480 | 14840 | 17635 | 20655 | 2933 | 3087 | 3192 | 733 | 750 | 743 | 320 | 320 | 302 |
| 0.75 | *** | 35785 | 43100 | 73773 | 12575 | 14362 | 18195 | 2537 | 2658 | 2795 | 640 | 640 | 650 | 265 | 265 | 265 |
|  | *** | 38710 | 50865 | 74247 | 13345 | 15820 | 18296 | 2592 | 2713 | 2791 | 640 | 640 | 633 | 265 | 265 | 248 |
| 0.8 | *** | 30845 | 37445 | 62773 | 10880 | 12382 | 15390 | 2135 | 2218 | 2317 | 513 | 513 | 513 | 200 | 200 | 200 |
|  | *** | 33513 | 44238 | 63007 | 11540 | 13565 | 15436 | 2180 | 2262 | 2309 | 513 | 513 | 502 | 200 | 200 | 186 |
| 0.85 | *** | 25472 | 30955 | 49672 | 8873 | 10000 | 12063 | 1640 | 1695 | 1767 | 365 | 365 | 365 | . | . | . |
|  | *** | 27710 | 36373 | 49759 | 9385 | 10842 | 12074 | 1668 | 1723 | 1747 | 365 | 365 | 352 | . | . | . |
| 0.9 | *** | 19295 | 23228 | 34492 | 6453 | 7130 | 8230 | 1080 | 1090 | 1118 | . | . | . | . | . | . |
|  | *** | 20935 | 26858 | 34504 | 6755 | 7597 | 8210 | 1080 | 1107 | 1104 | . | . | . | . | . | . |
| 0.95 | *** | 11485 | 13345 | 17260 | 3362 | 3582 | 3857 | . | . | . | . | . | . | . | . | . |
|  | *** | 12283 | 14830 | 17242 | 3455 | 3703 | 3844 | . | . | . | . | . | . | . | . | . |
| 0.98 | *** | 4875 | 5298 | 5947 | . | . | . | . | . | . | . | . | . | . | . | . |
|  | *** | 5067 | 5590 | 5922 | . | . | . | . | . | . | . | . | . | . | . | . |

## TABLE 3: ALPHA= 0.01  POWER= 0.8    EXPECTED ACCRUAL THRU MINIMUM FOLLOW-UP= 12000

| | | DEL=.01 | | | DEL=.02 | | | DEL=.05 | | | DEL=.10 | | | DEL=.15 | | |
|---|---|---|---|---|---|---|---|---|---|---|---|---|---|---|---|---|---|
| FACT= | | 1.0 .75 | .50 .25 | .00 BIN | 1.0 .75 | .50 .25 | .00 BIN | 1.0 .75 | .50 .25 | .00 BIN | 1.0 75 | .50 .25 | .00 BIN | 1.0 .75 | .50 .25 | .00 BIN |

PCONT=***    REQUIRED NUMBER OF PATIENTS

| PCONT | | DEL=.01 1.0/.75 | .50/.25 | .00/BIN | DEL=.02 1.0/.75 | .50/.25 | .00/BIN | DEL=.05 1.0/.75 | .50/.25 | .00/BIN | DEL=.10 1.0/.75 | .50/.25 | .00/BIN | DEL=.15 1.0/.75 | .50/.25 | .00/BIN |
|---|---|---|---|---|---|---|---|---|---|---|---|---|---|---|---|---|
| 0.01 | *** | 1538 | 1538 | 1549 | 559 | 559 | 559 | 188 | 188 | 188 | 98 | 98 | 98 | 68 | 68 | 68 |
| | *** | 1538 | 1549 | 5922 | 559 | 559 | 1958 | 188 | 188 | 533 | 98 | 98 | 217 | 68 | 68 | 129 |
| 0.02 | *** | 3428 | 3439 | 3458 | 1099 | 1099 | 1099 | 289 | 289 | 289 | 128 | 128 | 128 | 79 | 79 | 79 |
| | *** | 3428 | 3439 | 9776 | 1099 | 1099 | 2911 | 289 | 289 | 681 | 128 | 128 | 252 | 79 | 79 | 144 |
| 0.05 | *** | 10399 | 10519 | 10789 | 2978 | 2989 | 3019 | 638 | 638 | 638 | 229 | 229 | 229 | 128 | 128 | 128 |
| | *** | 10448 | 10628 | 20855 | 2978 | 3008 | 5651 | 638 | 638 | 1104 | 229 | 229 | 352 | 128 | 128 | 186 |
| 0.1 | *** | 23029 | 23468 | 25118 | 6319 | 6439 | 6638 | 1219 | 1219 | 1238 | 379 | 379 | 379 | 199 | 199 | 199 |
| | *** | 23198 | 23989 | 37716 | 6379 | 6529 | 9816 | 1219 | 1238 | 1747 | 379 | 379 | 502 | 199 | 199 | 248 |
| 0.15 | *** | 34519 | 35389 | 39668 | 9428 | 9728 | 10268 | 1759 | 1789 | 1808 | 518 | 518 | 518 | 259 | 259 | 259 |
| | *** | 34838 | 36548 | 52569 | 9559 | 9949 | 13479 | 1778 | 1808 | 2309 | 518 | 518 | 633 | 259 | 259 | 302 |
| 0.2 | *** | 43928 | 45319 | 53299 | 12068 | 12589 | 13639 | 2258 | 2288 | 2329 | 638 | 638 | 649 | 308 | 319 | 319 |
| | *** | 44419 | 47288 | 65415 | 12289 | 13009 | 16640 | 2269 | 2318 | 2791 | 638 | 649 | 743 | 308 | 319 | 346 |
| 0.25 | *** | 50989 | 53018 | 65438 | 14168 | 14948 | 16639 | 2659 | 2719 | 2798 | 739 | 739 | 758 | 349 | 349 | 349 |
| | *** | 51698 | 55879 | 76254 | 14498 | 15608 | 19300 | 2689 | 2768 | 3192 | 739 | 758 | 833 | 349 | 349 | 382 |
| 0.3 | *** | 55729 | 58489 | 75769 | 15728 | 16789 | 19178 | 2989 | 3079 | 3188 | 829 | 829 | 848 | 398 | 398 | 398 |
| | *** | 56719 | 62359 | 85086 | 16178 | 17689 | 21458 | 3038 | 3128 | 3513 | 829 | 829 | 904 | 398 | 398 | 409 |
| 0.35 | *** | 58358 | 61928 | 84128 | 16808 | 18128 | 21218 | 3248 | 3349 | 3488 | 889 | 889 | 908 | 409 | 409 | 409 |
| | *** | 59648 | 66829 | 91910 | 17359 | 19268 | 23113 | 3289 | 3409 | 3754 | 889 | 908 | 954 | 409 | 409 | 426 |
| 0.4 | *** | 59119 | 63578 | 90428 | 17419 | 19009 | 22729 | 3409 | 3548 | 3698 | 919 | 938 | 949 | 428 | 428 | 428 |
| | *** | 60739 | 69499 | 96728 | 18098 | 20378 | 24268 | 3469 | 3619 | 3915 | 938 | 949 | 984 | 428 | 428 | 435 |
| 0.45 | *** | 58328 | 63698 | 94568 | 17648 | 19448 | 23719 | 3518 | 3649 | 3829 | 949 | 968 | 968 | 428 | 439 | 439 |
| | *** | 60319 | 70568 | 99538 | 18409 | 21008 | 24920 | 3578 | 3739 | 3995 | 949 | 968 | 994 | 439 | 439 | 435 |
| 0.5 | *** | 56299 | 62539 | 96548 | 17528 | 19508 | 24158 | 3529 | 3679 | 3878 | 949 | 968 | 968 | 428 | 428 | 428 |
| | *** | 58658 | 70208 | 100341 | 18388 | 21188 | 25070 | 3608 | 3769 | 3995 | 949 | 968 | 984 | 428 | 428 | 426 |
| 0.55 | *** | 53359 | 60349 | 96338 | 17108 | 19178 | 24049 | 3469 | 3638 | 3829 | 919 | 938 | 949 | 409 | 409 | 428 |
| | *** | 56048 | 68618 | 99136 | 17989 | 20948 | 24719 | 3548 | 3728 | 3915 | 938 | 949 | 954 | 409 | 409 | 409 |
| 0.6 | *** | 49759 | 57308 | 93949 | 16399 | 18518 | 23408 | 3349 | 3499 | 3698 | 878 | 889 | 908 | 398 | 398 | 398 |
| | *** | 52699 | 65918 | 95925 | 17299 | 20299 | 23866 | 3428 | 3608 | 3754 | 889 | 908 | 904 | 398 | 398 | 382 |
| 0.65 | *** | 45709 | 53539 | 89378 | 15439 | 17528 | 22208 | 3158 | 3308 | 3488 | 818 | 829 | 848 | 349 | 368 | 368 |
| | *** | 48788 | 62198 | 90706 | 16339 | 19268 | 22511 | 3229 | 3398 | 3513 | 829 | 829 | 833 | 349 | 368 | 346 |
| 0.7 | *** | 41329 | 49118 | 82658 | 14258 | 16219 | 20468 | 2899 | 3019 | 3188 | 739 | 739 | 758 | 319 | 319 | 319 |
| | *** | 44438 | 57499 | 83480 | 15098 | 17809 | 20655 | 2959 | 3098 | 3192 | 739 | 758 | 743 | 319 | 319 | 302 |
| 0.75 | *** | 36649 | 44059 | 73778 | 12799 | 14569 | 18199 | 2558 | 2659 | 2798 | 638 | 638 | 649 | 259 | 259 | 259 |
| | *** | 39638 | 51829 | 74247 | 13568 | 15968 | 18296 | 2618 | 2719 | 2791 | 638 | 649 | 633 | 259 | 259 | 248 |
| 0.8 | *** | 31639 | 38299 | 62779 | 11089 | 12559 | 15398 | 2149 | 2228 | 2318 | 518 | 518 | 518 | 199 | 199 | 199 |
| | *** | 34339 | 45068 | 63007 | 11719 | 13688 | 15436 | 2179 | 2269 | 2309 | 518 | 518 | 502 | 199 | 199 | 186 |
| 0.85 | *** | 26138 | 31658 | 49669 | 9038 | 10129 | 12068 | 1658 | 1699 | 1759 | 368 | 368 | 368 | . | . | . |
| | *** | 28399 | 37009 | 49759 | 9518 | 10928 | 12074 | 1688 | 1729 | 1747 | 368 | 368 | 352 | . | . | . |
| 0.9 | *** | 19789 | 23708 | 34489 | 6548 | 7208 | 8228 | 1069 | 1099 | 1118 | . | . | . | . | . | . |
| | *** | 21428 | 27259 | 34504 | 6848 | 7639 | 8210 | 1088 | 1118 | 1104 | . | . | . | . | . | . |
| 0.95 | *** | 11738 | 13549 | 17258 | 3398 | 3589 | 3859 | . | . | . | . | . | . | . | . | . |
| | *** | 12529 | 14989 | 17242 | 3488 | 3728 | 3844 | . | . | . | . | . | . | . | . | . |
| 0.98 | *** | 4939 | 5348 | 5948 | . | . | . | . | . | . | . | . | . | . | . | . |
| | *** | 5119 | 5618 | 5922 | . | . | . | . | . | . | . | . | . | . | . | . |

## TABLE 3: ALPHA= 0.01  POWER= 0.8    EXPECTED ACCRUAL THRU MINIMUM FOLLOW-UP= 13000

| | | DEL=.01 | | | DEL=.02 | | | DEL=.05 | | | DEL=.10 | | | DEL=.15 | | |
|---|---|---|---|---|---|---|---|---|---|---|---|---|---|---|---|---|---|
| FACT= | | 1.0 .75 | .50 .25 | .00 BIN | 1.0 .75 | .50 .25 | .00 BIN | 1.0 .75 | .50 .25 | .00 BIN | 1.0 75 | .50 .25 | .00 BIN | 1.0 .75 | .50 .25 | .00 BIN |
| PCONT=*** | | | | | REQUIRED | NUMBER OF | PATIENTS | | | | | | | | | |
| 0.01 | *** | 1536 1548 | 1548 | 561 561 | 561 | 183 183 | 183 | 86 86 | 86 | 74 74 | 74 |
| | *** | 1536 1548 | 5922 | 561 561 | 1958 | 183 183 | 533 | 86 86 | 217 | 74 74 | 129 |
| 0.02 | *** | 3421 3433 | 3454 | 1093 1093 | 1093 | 301 301 | 301 | 118 118 | 118 | 86 86 | 86 |
| | *** | 3433 3433 | 9776 | 1093 1093 | 2911 | 301 301 | 681 | 118 118 | 252 | 86 86 | 144 |
| 0.05 | *** | 10421 10539 | 10778 | 2978 2999 | 3031 | 638 638 | 638 | 216 216 | 236 | 139 139 | 139 |
| | *** | 10474 10636 | 20855 | 2978 3011 | 5651 | 638 638 | 1104 | 216 216 | 352 | 139 139 | 186 |
| 0.1 | *** | 23063 23539 | 25111 | 6346 6456 | 6639 | 1223 1223 | 1244 | 378 378 | 378 | 204 204 | 204 |
| | *** | 23246 24038 | 37716 | 6391 6541 | 9816 | 1223 1223 | 1747 | 378 378 | 502 | 204 204 | 248 |
| 0.15 | *** | 34601 35511 | 39671 | 9466 9759 | 10279 | 1776 1796 | 1808 | 508 529 | 529 | 269 269 | 269 |
| | *** | 34926 36681 | 52569 | 9596 9966 | 13479 | 1776 1796 | 2309 | 508 529 | 633 | 269 269 | 302 |
| 0.2 | *** | 44046 45521 | 53288 | 12131 12651 | 13638 | 2263 2296 | 2328 | 638 638 | 638 | 313 313 | 313 |
| | *** | 44578 47524 | 65415 | 12359 13053 | 16640 | 2284 2316 | 2791 | 638 638 | 743 | 313 313 | 346 |
| 0.25 | *** | 51164 53309 | 65431 | 14256 15036 | 16649 | 2674 2739 | 2804 | 736 756 | 756 | 346 366 | 366 |
| | *** | 51923 56234 | 76254 | 14581 15653 | 19300 | 2706 2771 | 3192 | 736 756 | 833 | 366 366 | 382 |
| 0.3 | *** | 55986 58899 | 75766 | 15848 16909 | 19184 | 3011 3076 | 3173 | 821 833 | 833 | 399 399 | 399 |
| | *** | 57026 62843 | 85086 | 16303 17766 | 21458 | 3043 3129 | 3513 | 833 833 | 904 | 399 399 | 409 |
| 0.35 | *** | 58683 62441 | 84131 | 16953 18274 | 21211 | 3259 3356 | 3486 | 886 898 | 898 | 411 411 | 411 |
| | *** | 60048 67446 | 91910 | 17506 19379 | 23113 | 3303 3421 | 3754 | 886 898 | 954 | 411 411 | 426 |
| 0.4 | *** | 59528 64208 | 90424 | 17603 19184 | 22738 | 3433 3551 | 3693 | 931 931 | 951 | 431 431 | 431 |
| | *** | 61251 70221 | 96728 | 18274 20496 | 24268 | 3486 3628 | 3915 | 931 951 | 984 | 431 431 | 435 |
| 0.45 | *** | 58846 64436 | 94563 | 17863 19651 | 23713 | 3531 3661 | 3823 | 951 963 | 963 | 431 431 | 443 |
| | *** | 60926 71391 | 99538 | 18611 21146 | 24920 | 3596 3746 | 3995 | 951 963 | 994 | 431 431 | 435 |
| 0.5 | *** | 56916 63384 | 96546 | 17766 19716 | 24156 | 3551 3693 | 3876 | 951 963 | 963 | 431 431 | 431 |
| | *** | 59366 71131 | 100341 | 18599 21361 | 25070 | 3616 3779 | 3995 | 951 963 | 984 | 431 431 | 426 |
| 0.55 | *** | 54068 61251 | 96339 | 17343 19411 | 24059 | 3498 3649 | 3844 | 931 931 | 951 | 411 411 | 411 |
| | *** | 56851 69603 | 99136 | 18221 21134 | 24719 | 3563 3726 | 3915 | 931 951 | 954 | 411 411 | 409 |
| 0.6 | *** | 50546 58261 | 93946 | 16661 18741 | 23409 | 3368 3519 | 3693 | 886 898 | 898 | 399 399 | 399 |
| | *** | 53569 66926 | 95925 | 17559 20484 | 23866 | 3454 3616 | 3754 | 886 898 | 904 | 399 399 | 382 |
| 0.65 | *** | 46549 54511 | 89384 | 15706 17754 | 22206 | 3173 3324 | 3486 | 821 833 | 833 | 366 366 | 366 |
| | *** | 49701 63201 | 90706 | 16584 19423 | 22511 | 3238 3401 | 3513 | 821 833 | 833 | 366 366 | 346 |
| 0.7 | *** | 42161 50071 | 82656 | 14483 16421 | 20463 | 2913 3031 | 3173 | 736 756 | 756 | 313 313 | 313 |
| | *** | 45326 58476 | 83480 | 15328 17961 | 20655 | 2966 3108 | 3192 | 736 756 | 743 | 313 313 | 302 |
| 0.75 | *** | 37461 44968 | 73784 | 13021 14743 | 18209 | 2576 2674 | 2804 | 638 638 | 638 | 269 269 | 269 |
| | *** | 40483 52703 | 74247 | 13768 16096 | 18296 | 2621 2739 | 2791 | 638 638 | 633 | 269 269 | 248 |
| 0.8 | *** | 32379 39106 | 62778 | 11266 12696 | 15393 | 2154 2231 | 2316 | 508 508 | 529 | 204 204 | 204 |
| | *** | 35121 45813 | 63007 | 11904 13789 | 15436 | 2198 2284 | 2309 | 508 508 | 502 | 204 204 | 186 |
| 0.85 | *** | 26768 32293 | 49681 | 9174 10246 | 12066 | 1666 1711 | 1764 | 366 366 | 366 | . . | . |
| | *** | 29043 37591 | 49759 | 9641 11006 | 12074 | 1678 1731 | 1747 | 366 366 | 352 | . . | . |
| 0.9 | *** | 20256 24156 | 34491 | 6639 7268 | 8231 | 1081 1093 | 1126 | . . | . | . . | . |
| | *** | 21893 27634 | 34504 | 6931 7679 | 8210 | 1093 1114 | 1104 | . . | . | . . | . |
| 0.95 | *** | 11969 13736 | 17266 | 3421 3616 | 3856 | . . | . | . . | . | . . | . |
| | *** | 12728 15121 | 17242 | 3519 3726 | 3844 | . . | . | . . | . | . . | . |
| 0.98 | *** | 4993 5383 | 5936 | . . | . | . . | . | . . | . | . . | . |
| | *** | 5176 5631 | 5922 | . . | . | . . | . | . . | . | . . | . |

TABLE 3: ALPHA= 0.01  POWER= 0.8    EXPECTED ACCRUAL THRU MINIMUM FOLLOW-UP= 14000

| | | DEL=.01 | | | DEL=.02 | | | DEL=.05 | | | DEL=.10 | | | DEL=.15 | |
|---|---|---|---|---|---|---|---|---|---|---|---|---|---|---|---|---|
| FACT= | 1.0 / .75 | .50 / .25 | .00 BIN | 1.0 / .75 | .50 / .25 | .00 BIN | 1.0 / .75 | .50 / .25 | .00 BIN | 1.0 / 75 | .50 / .25 | .00 BIN | 1.0 / .75 | .50 / .25 | .00 BIN |

PCONT=***                REQUIRED NUMBER OF PATIENTS

| PCONT | | .01 (1.0/.75) | .01 (.50/.25) | .01 (.00/BIN) | .02 (1.0/.75) | .02 (.50/.25) | .02 (.00/BIN) | .05 (1.0/.75) | .05 (.50/.25) | .05 (.00/BIN) | .10 (1.0/75) | .10 (.50/.25) | .10 (.00/BIN) | .15 (1.0/.75) | .15 (.50/.25) | .15 (.00/BIN) |
|---|---|---|---|---|---|---|---|---|---|---|---|---|---|---|---|---|
| 0.01 | *** | 1549 | 1549 | 1549 | 569 | 569 | 569 | 184 | 184 | 184 | 92 | 92 | 92 | 57 | 57 | 57 |
| | *** | 1549 | 1549 | 5922 | 569 | 569 | 1958 | 184 | 184 | 533 | 92 | 92 | 217 | 57 | 57 | 129 |
| 0.02 | *** | 3417 | 3439 | 3452 | 1094 | 1094 | 1107 | 289 | 289 | 289 | 127 | 127 | 127 | 79 | 79 | 79 |
| | *** | 3439 | 3439 | 9776 | 1094 | 1094 | 2911 | 289 | 289 | 681 | 127 | 127 | 252 | 79 | 79 | 144 |
| 0.05 | *** | 10439 | 10544 | 10789 | 2984 | 2997 | 3019 | 639 | 639 | 639 | 219 | 219 | 232 | 127 | 127 | 127 |
| | *** | 10474 | 10649 | 20855 | 2984 | 2997 | 5651 | 639 | 639 | 1104 | 219 | 219 | 352 | 127 | 127 | 186 |
| 0.1 | *** | 23109 | 23577 | 25117 | 6357 | 6462 | 6637 | 1212 | 1234 | 1234 | 372 | 372 | 372 | 197 | 197 | 197 |
| | *** | 23297 | 24089 | 37716 | 6414 | 6554 | 9816 | 1234 | 1234 | 1747 | 372 | 372 | 502 | 197 | 197 | 248 |
| 0.15 | *** | 34672 | 35639 | 39664 | 9494 | 9787 | 10264 | 1772 | 1794 | 1807 | 512 | 512 | 512 | 254 | 267 | 267 |
| | *** | 35022 | 36807 | 52569 | 9634 | 9997 | 13479 | 1772 | 1794 | 2309 | 512 | 512 | 633 | 267 | 267 | 302 |
| 0.2 | *** | 44179 | 45719 | 53292 | 12189 | 12692 | 13637 | 2262 | 2297 | 2332 | 639 | 639 | 652 | 302 | 324 | 324 |
| | *** | 44739 | 47749 | 65415 | 12399 | 13077 | 16640 | 2284 | 2319 | 2791 | 639 | 639 | 743 | 302 | 324 | 346 |
| 0.25 | *** | 51354 | 53594 | 65437 | 14337 | 15107 | 16634 | 2682 | 2739 | 2787 | 744 | 744 | 757 | 359 | 359 | 359 |
| | *** | 52159 | 56569 | 76254 | 14674 | 15724 | 19300 | 2704 | 2774 | 3192 | 744 | 744 | 833 | 359 | 359 | 382 |
| 0.3 | *** | 56232 | 59277 | 75762 | 15969 | 16997 | 19167 | 3019 | 3089 | 3172 | 827 | 827 | 849 | 394 | 394 | 394 |
| | *** | 57339 | 63289 | 85086 | 16402 | 17859 | 21458 | 3054 | 3137 | 3513 | 827 | 827 | 904 | 394 | 394 | 409 |
| 0.35 | *** | 59019 | 62939 | 84127 | 17102 | 18397 | 21219 | 3277 | 3369 | 3487 | 884 | 897 | 897 | 407 | 407 | 407 |
| | *** | 60454 | 68014 | 91910 | 17662 | 19482 | 23113 | 3312 | 3417 | 3754 | 897 | 897 | 954 | 407 | 407 | 426 |
| 0.4 | *** | 59942 | 64794 | 90414 | 17789 | 19342 | 22737 | 3452 | 3557 | 3697 | 932 | 932 | 954 | 429 | 429 | 429 |
| | *** | 61749 | 70897 | 96728 | 18454 | 20624 | 24268 | 3509 | 3627 | 3915 | 932 | 954 | 984 | 429 | 429 | 435 |
| 0.45 | *** | 59347 | 65122 | 94557 | 18069 | 19832 | 23717 | 3544 | 3684 | 3837 | 954 | 967 | 967 | 429 | 429 | 442 |
| | *** | 61517 | 72179 | 99538 | 18817 | 21289 | 24920 | 3614 | 3754 | 3995 | 954 | 967 | 994 | 429 | 442 | 435 |
| 0.5 | *** | 57514 | 64164 | 96539 | 17977 | 19902 | 24159 | 3579 | 3697 | 3872 | 954 | 954 | 967 | 429 | 429 | 429 |
| | *** | 60069 | 71982 | 100341 | 18804 | 21499 | 25070 | 3627 | 3789 | 3995 | 954 | 967 | 984 | 429 | 429 | 426 |
| 0.55 | *** | 54749 | 62112 | 96342 | 17579 | 19609 | 24054 | 3522 | 3662 | 3837 | 932 | 932 | 954 | 407 | 407 | 429 |
| | *** | 57619 | 70512 | 99136 | 18454 | 21289 | 24719 | 3579 | 3732 | 3915 | 932 | 954 | 954 | 407 | 407 | 409 |
| 0.6 | *** | 51297 | 59159 | 93949 | 16892 | 18957 | 23402 | 3404 | 3522 | 3697 | 884 | 897 | 897 | 394 | 394 | 394 |
| | *** | 54399 | 67852 | 95925 | 17767 | 20637 | 23866 | 3452 | 3614 | 3754 | 884 | 897 | 904 | 394 | 394 | 382 |
| 0.65 | *** | 47329 | 55427 | 89377 | 15934 | 17942 | 22212 | 3194 | 3334 | 3487 | 827 | 827 | 849 | 359 | 359 | 359 |
| | *** | 50549 | 64129 | 90706 | 16809 | 19574 | 22511 | 3264 | 3404 | 3513 | 827 | 827 | 833 | 359 | 359 | 346 |
| 0.7 | *** | 42967 | 50969 | 82657 | 14709 | 16612 | 20462 | 2927 | 3054 | 3172 | 744 | 744 | 757 | 324 | 324 | 324 |
| | *** | 46174 | 59347 | 83480 | 15527 | 18104 | 20655 | 2984 | 3102 | 3192 | 744 | 757 | 743 | 324 | 324 | 302 |
| 0.75 | *** | 38229 | 45789 | 73767 | 13217 | 14919 | 18209 | 2577 | 2682 | 2787 | 639 | 639 | 652 | 267 | 267 | 267 |
| | *** | 41287 | 53502 | 74247 | 13952 | 16214 | 18296 | 2634 | 2739 | 2791 | 639 | 639 | 633 | 267 | 267 | 248 |
| 0.8 | *** | 33084 | 39839 | 62777 | 11432 | 12832 | 15387 | 2179 | 2249 | 2319 | 512 | 512 | 512 | 197 | 197 | 197 |
| | *** | 35849 | 46489 | 63007 | 12049 | 13882 | 15436 | 2192 | 2284 | 2309 | 512 | 512 | 502 | 197 | 197 | 186 |
| 0.85 | *** | 27344 | 32887 | 49674 | 9297 | 10334 | 12062 | 1667 | 1724 | 1759 | 359 | 372 | 372 | . | . | . |
| | *** | 29632 | 38102 | 49759 | 9774 | 11069 | 12074 | 1689 | 1737 | 1747 | 372 | 372 | 352 | . | . | . |
| 0.9 | *** | 20672 | 24557 | 34497 | 6707 | 7324 | 8212 | 1072 | 1107 | 1129 | . | . | . | . | . | . |
| | *** | 22304 | 27974 | 34504 | 6987 | 7722 | 8210 | 1094 | 1107 | 1104 | . | . | . | . | . | . |
| 0.95 | *** | 12167 | 13904 | 17264 | 3452 | 3627 | 3859 | . | . | . | . | . | . | . | . | . |
| | *** | 12924 | 15234 | 17242 | 3544 | 3732 | 3844 | . | . | . | . | . | . | . | . | . |
| 0.98 | *** | 5049 | 5412 | 5937 | . | . | . | . | . | . | . | . | . | . | . | . |
| | *** | 5224 | 5657 | 5922 | . | . | . | . | . | . | . | . | . | . | . | . |

TABLE 3: ALPHA= 0.01  POWER= 0.8    EXPECTED ACCRUAL THRU MINIMUM FOLLOW-UP= 15000

| | | DEL=.01 | | | DEL=.02 | | | DEL=.05 | | | DEL=.10 | | | DEL=.15 | |
|---|---|---|---|---|---|---|---|---|---|---|---|---|---|---|---|---|
| FACT= | 1.0 .75 | .50 .25 | .00 BIN | 1.0 .75 | .50 .25 | .00 BIN | 1.0 .75 | .50 .25 | .00 BIN | 1.0 75 | .50 .25 | .00 BIN | 1.0 .75 | .50 .25 | .00 BIN |

PCONT=***                    REQUIRED NUMBER OF PATIENTS

| PCONT | | 1.0/.75 | .50/.25 | .00 BIN | 1.0/.75 | .50/.25 | .00 BIN | 1.0/.75 | .50/.25 | .00 BIN | 1.0/75 | .50/.25 | .00 BIN | 1.0/.75 | .50/.25 | .00 BIN |
|---|---|---|---|---|---|---|---|---|---|---|---|---|---|---|---|---|
| 0.01 | *** | 1547 | 1547 | 1547 | 572 | 572 | 572 | 174 | 174 | 174 | 99 | 99 | 99 | 61 | 61 | 61 |
| | *** | 1547 | 1547 | 5922 | 572 | 572 | 1958 | 174 | 174 | 533 | 99 | 99 | 217 | 61 | 61 | 129 |
| 0.02 | *** | 3422 | 3436 | 3460 | 1097 | 1097 | 1097 | 286 | 286 | 286 | 122 | 122 | 122 | 85 | 85 | 85 |
| | *** | 3436 | 3436 | 9776 | 1097 | 1097 | 2911 | 286 | 286 | 681 | 122 | 122 | 252 | 85 | 85 | 144 |
| 0.05 | *** | 10449 | 10561 | 10786 | 2972 | 2986 | 3024 | 647 | 647 | 647 | 235 | 235 | 235 | 136 | 136 | 136 |
| | *** | 10486 | 10660 | 20855 | 2986 | 3010 | 5651 | 647 | 647 | 1104 | 235 | 235 | 352 | 136 | 136 | 186 |
| 0.1 | *** | 23161 | 23635 | 25111 | 6361 | 6474 | 6647 | 1224 | 1224 | 1224 | 385 | 385 | 385 | 197 | 197 | 197 |
| | *** | 23335 | 24136 | 37716 | 6422 | 6549 | 9816 | 1224 | 1224 | 1747 | 385 | 385 | 502 | 197 | 197 | 248 |
| 0.15 | *** | 34749 | 35747 | 39661 | 9535 | 9811 | 10261 | 1772 | 1786 | 1810 | 511 | 511 | 511 | 272 | 272 | 272 |
| | *** | 35124 | 36924 | 52569 | 9647 | 9999 | 13479 | 1786 | 1810 | 2309 | 511 | 511 | 633 | 272 | 272 | 302 |
| 0.2 | *** | 44297 | 45910 | 53297 | 12235 | 12736 | 13636 | 2274 | 2297 | 2335 | 647 | 647 | 647 | 310 | 310 | 310 |
| | *** | 44897 | 47949 | 65415 | 12460 | 13111 | 16640 | 2274 | 2311 | 2791 | 647 | 647 | 743 | 310 | 310 | 346 |
| 0.25 | *** | 51535 | 53860 | 65424 | 14424 | 15174 | 16636 | 2686 | 2747 | 2799 | 736 | 760 | 760 | 361 | 361 | 361 |
| | *** | 52374 | 56874 | 76254 | 14747 | 15760 | 19300 | 2710 | 2761 | 3192 | 736 | 760 | 833 | 361 | 361 | 382 |
| 0.3 | *** | 56485 | 59649 | 75774 | 16074 | 17110 | 19172 | 3024 | 3099 | 3174 | 835 | 835 | 835 | 385 | 385 | 399 |
| | *** | 57624 | 63699 | 85086 | 16510 | 17911 | 21458 | 3061 | 3136 | 3513 | 835 | 835 | 904 | 385 | 385 | 409 |
| 0.35 | *** | 59335 | 63399 | 84136 | 17236 | 18535 | 21211 | 3286 | 3385 | 3474 | 886 | 886 | 910 | 422 | 422 | 422 |
| | *** | 60835 | 68536 | 91910 | 17785 | 19561 | 23113 | 3324 | 3422 | 3754 | 886 | 910 | 954 | 422 | 422 | 426 |
| 0.4 | *** | 60347 | 65372 | 90422 | 17935 | 19486 | 22735 | 3460 | 3572 | 3699 | 924 | 947 | 947 | 422 | 436 | 436 |
| | *** | 62222 | 71536 | 96728 | 18610 | 20724 | 24268 | 3511 | 3624 | 3915 | 924 | 947 | 984 | 422 | 436 | 435 |
| 0.45 | *** | 59836 | 65799 | 94561 | 18235 | 19997 | 23724 | 3572 | 3685 | 3835 | 947 | 961 | 961 | 436 | 436 | 436 |
| | *** | 62086 | 72886 | 99538 | 18985 | 21422 | 24920 | 3624 | 3760 | 3995 | 961 | 961 | 994 | 436 | 436 | 435 |
| 0.5 | *** | 58097 | 64899 | 96549 | 18174 | 20086 | 24160 | 3586 | 3722 | 3872 | 947 | 961 | 961 | 422 | 436 | 436 |
| | *** | 60722 | 72774 | 100341 | 18999 | 21647 | 25070 | 3647 | 3797 | 3995 | 961 | 961 | 984 | 436 | 436 | 436 |
| 0.55 | *** | 55411 | 62935 | 96347 | 17785 | 19786 | 24061 | 3535 | 3661 | 3835 | 924 | 947 | 947 | 422 | 422 | 422 |
| | *** | 58336 | 71349 | 99136 | 18647 | 21422 | 24719 | 3610 | 3736 | 3915 | 924 | 947 | 954 | 422 | 422 | 409 |
| 0.6 | *** | 51999 | 60010 | 93947 | 17110 | 19149 | 23410 | 3399 | 3549 | 3699 | 886 | 886 | 910 | 385 | 399 | 399 |
| | *** | 55172 | 68724 | 95925 | 17986 | 20785 | 23866 | 3474 | 3624 | 3754 | 886 | 910 | 904 | 385 | 399 | 382 |
| 0.65 | *** | 48085 | 56274 | 89386 | 16149 | 18136 | 22210 | 3211 | 3347 | 3497 | 835 | 835 | 849 | 361 | 361 | 361 |
| | *** | 51347 | 64974 | 90706 | 17011 | 19711 | 22511 | 3272 | 3399 | 3513 | 835 | 835 | 833 | 361 | 361 | 346 |
| 0.7 | *** | 43711 | 51797 | 82660 | 14911 | 16772 | 20461 | 2949 | 3047 | 3174 | 736 | 736 | 760 | 310 | 310 | 324 |
| | *** | 46974 | 60160 | 83480 | 15722 | 18235 | 20655 | 2986 | 3122 | 3192 | 736 | 760 | 743 | 310 | 324 | 302 |
| 0.75 | *** | 38949 | 46561 | 73772 | 13397 | 15061 | 18197 | 2597 | 2686 | 2799 | 647 | 647 | 647 | 272 | 272 | 272 |
| | *** | 42047 | 54235 | 74247 | 14124 | 16322 | 18296 | 2649 | 2747 | 2791 | 647 | 647 | 633 | 272 | 272 | 248 |
| 0.8 | *** | 33736 | 40510 | 62785 | 11597 | 12961 | 15399 | 2185 | 2236 | 2311 | 511 | 511 | 511 | 197 | 197 | 197 |
| | *** | 36511 | 47110 | 63007 | 12197 | 13960 | 15436 | 2199 | 2274 | 2309 | 511 | 511 | 502 | 197 | 197 | 186 |
| 0.85 | *** | 27886 | 33436 | 49674 | 9422 | 10411 | 12061 | 1674 | 1711 | 1772 | 361 | 361 | 361 | . | . | . |
| | *** | 30197 | 38597 | 49759 | 9872 | 11124 | 12074 | 1697 | 1735 | 1747 | 361 | 361 | 352 | . | . | . |
| 0.9 | *** | 21061 | 24924 | 34486 | 6774 | 7360 | 8222 | 1074 | 1097 | 1111 | . | . | . | . | . | . |
| | *** | 22697 | 28261 | 34504 | 7060 | 7749 | 8210 | 1097 | 1111 | 1104 | . | . | . | . | . | . |
| 0.95 | *** | 12347 | 14072 | 17260 | 3474 | 3647 | 3872 | . | . | . | . | . | . | . | . | . |
| | *** | 13111 | 15347 | 17242 | 3549 | 3736 | 3844 | . | . | . | . | . | . | . | . | . |
| 0.98 | *** | 5086 | 5447 | 5935 | . | . | . | . | . | . | . | . | . | . | . | . |
| | *** | 5260 | 5672 | 5922 | . | . | . | . | . | . | . | . | . | . | . | . |

TABLE 3: ALPHA= 0.01  POWER= 0.8    EXPECTED ACCRUAL THRU MINIMUM FOLLOW-UP= 17000

| | | DEL=.01 | | | DEL=.02 | | | DEL=.05 | | | DEL=.10 | | | DEL=.15 | | |
|---|---|---|---|---|---|---|---|---|---|---|---|---|---|---|---|---|---|
| FACT= | | 1.0 .75 | .50 .25 | .00 BIN | 1.0 .75 | .50 .25 | .00 BIN | 1.0 .75 | .50 .25 | .00 BIN | 1.0 75 | .50 .25 | .00 BIN | 1.0 .75 | .50 .25 | .00 BIN |
| PCONT=*** | | | | | REQUIRED NUMBER OF PATIENTS | | | | | | | | | | | |
| 0.01 | *** | 1541 | 1541 | 1541 | 564 | 564 | 564 | 181 | 181 | 181 | 96 | 96 | 96 | 70 | 70 | 70 |
| | *** | 1541 | 1541 | 5922 | 564 | 564 | 1958 | 181 | 181 | 533 | 96 | 96 | 217 | 70 | 70 | 129 |
| 0.02 | *** | 3427 | 3427 | 3454 | 1090 | 1090 | 1090 | 282 | 282 | 282 | 139 | 139 | 139 | 70 | 96 | 96 |
| | *** | 3427 | 3454 | 9776 | 1090 | 1090 | 2911 | 282 | 282 | 681 | 139 | 139 | 252 | 70 | 96 | 144 |
| 0.05 | *** | 10466 | 10567 | 10780 | 2986 | 3002 | 3029 | 649 | 649 | 649 | 224 | 224 | 224 | 139 | 139 | 139 |
| | *** | 10509 | 10652 | 20855 | 2986 | 3002 | 5651 | 649 | 649 | 1104 | 224 | 224 | 352 | 139 | 139 | 186 |
| 0.1 | *** | 23232 | 23726 | 25102 | 6386 | 6487 | 6641 | 1217 | 1217 | 1244 | 367 | 367 | 367 | 197 | 197 | 197 |
| | *** | 23429 | 24236 | 37716 | 6429 | 6556 | 9816 | 1217 | 1244 | 1747 | 367 | 367 | 502 | 197 | 197 | 248 |
| 0.15 | *** | 34904 | 35966 | 39664 | 9590 | 9845 | 10270 | 1770 | 1796 | 1812 | 521 | 521 | 521 | 266 | 266 | 266 |
| | *** | 35302 | 37130 | 52569 | 9701 | 10041 | 13479 | 1796 | 1796 | 2309 | 521 | 521 | 633 | 266 | 266 | 302 |
| 0.2 | *** | 44551 | 46267 | 53306 | 12336 | 12820 | 13654 | 2280 | 2306 | 2349 | 649 | 649 | 649 | 309 | 309 | 309 |
| | *** | 45189 | 48307 | 65415 | 12549 | 13160 | 16640 | 2280 | 2322 | 2791 | 649 | 649 | 743 | 309 | 309 | 346 |
| 0.25 | *** | 51877 | 54385 | 65435 | 14562 | 15285 | 16645 | 2705 | 2747 | 2790 | 750 | 750 | 750 | 351 | 351 | 351 |
| | *** | 52812 | 57429 | 76254 | 14886 | 15864 | 19300 | 2731 | 2774 | 3192 | 750 | 750 | 833 | 351 | 351 | 382 |
| 0.3 | *** | 56961 | 60335 | 75762 | 16262 | 17266 | 19179 | 3045 | 3114 | 3172 | 835 | 835 | 835 | 394 | 394 | 394 |
| | *** | 58210 | 64457 | 85086 | 16714 | 18047 | 21458 | 3071 | 3130 | 3513 | 835 | 835 | 904 | 394 | 394 | 409 |
| 0.35 | *** | 59952 | 64271 | 84135 | 17479 | 18727 | 21219 | 3300 | 3385 | 3470 | 904 | 904 | 904 | 410 | 410 | 410 |
| | *** | 61567 | 69499 | 91910 | 18031 | 19731 | 23113 | 3342 | 3427 | 3754 | 904 | 904 | 954 | 410 | 410 | 426 |
| 0.4 | *** | 61126 | 66439 | 90425 | 18217 | 19731 | 22749 | 3496 | 3581 | 3709 | 946 | 946 | 946 | 436 | 436 | 436 |
| | *** | 63140 | 72686 | 96728 | 18881 | 20921 | 24268 | 3539 | 3640 | 3915 | 946 | 946 | 984 | 436 | 436 | 435 |
| 0.45 | *** | 60786 | 67034 | 94574 | 18557 | 20284 | 23726 | 3597 | 3709 | 3836 | 946 | 962 | 962 | 436 | 436 | 436 |
| | *** | 63182 | 74190 | 99538 | 19306 | 21617 | 24920 | 3640 | 3767 | 3995 | 962 | 962 | 994 | 436 | 436 | 435 |
| 0.5 | *** | 59187 | 66285 | 96545 | 18541 | 20385 | 24167 | 3624 | 3725 | 3879 | 946 | 962 | 962 | 436 | 436 | 436 |
| | *** | 61950 | 74216 | 100341 | 19349 | 21872 | 25070 | 3666 | 3794 | 3995 | 962 | 962 | 984 | 436 | 436 | 426 |
| 0.55 | *** | 56637 | 64415 | 96332 | 18175 | 20130 | 24066 | 3555 | 3682 | 3836 | 920 | 946 | 946 | 410 | 410 | 410 |
| | *** | 59697 | 72856 | 99136 | 19025 | 21660 | 24719 | 3624 | 3751 | 3915 | 946 | 946 | 954 | 410 | 410 | 409 |
| 0.6 | *** | 53349 | 61567 | 93952 | 17495 | 19476 | 23402 | 3427 | 3555 | 3709 | 877 | 904 | 904 | 394 | 394 | 394 |
| | *** | 56621 | 70280 | 95925 | 18345 | 21022 | 23866 | 3496 | 3624 | 3754 | 904 | 904 | 904 | 394 | 394 | 382 |
| 0.65 | *** | 49481 | 57854 | 89389 | 16517 | 18456 | 22212 | 3241 | 3342 | 3496 | 819 | 835 | 835 | 351 | 351 | 367 |
| | *** | 52839 | 66524 | 90706 | 17367 | 19944 | 22511 | 3300 | 3411 | 3513 | 835 | 835 | 833 | 351 | 367 | 346 |
| 0.7 | *** | 45104 | 53322 | 82647 | 15269 | 17070 | 20470 | 2960 | 3071 | 3172 | 750 | 750 | 750 | 309 | 309 | 325 |
| | *** | 48435 | 61610 | 83480 | 16076 | 18430 | 20655 | 3002 | 3114 | 3192 | 750 | 750 | 743 | 309 | 325 | 302 |
| 0.75 | *** | 40275 | 47994 | 73765 | 13712 | 15327 | 18201 | 2620 | 2705 | 2790 | 649 | 649 | 649 | 266 | 266 | 266 |
| | *** | 43420 | 55559 | 74247 | 14435 | 16501 | 18296 | 2662 | 2747 | 2791 | 649 | 649 | 633 | 266 | 266 | 248 |
| 0.8 | *** | 34920 | 41746 | 62784 | 11869 | 13160 | 15396 | 2195 | 2264 | 2322 | 521 | 521 | 521 | 197 | 197 | 197 |
| | *** | 37751 | 48222 | 63007 | 12437 | 14095 | 15436 | 2221 | 2280 | 2309 | 521 | 521 | 502 | 197 | 197 | 186 |
| 0.85 | *** | 28885 | 34410 | 49667 | 9616 | 10567 | 12081 | 1685 | 1727 | 1770 | 367 | 367 | 367 | . | . | . |
| | *** | 31206 | 39425 | 49759 | 10057 | 11231 | 12074 | 1711 | 1754 | 1747 | 367 | 367 | 352 | . | . | . |
| 0.9 | *** | 21771 | 25570 | 34495 | 6896 | 7449 | 8214 | 1090 | 1116 | 1116 | . | . | . | . | . | . |
| | *** | 23402 | 28784 | 34504 | 7151 | 7805 | 8210 | 1090 | 1116 | 1104 | . | . | . | . | . | . |
| 0.95 | *** | 12692 | 14334 | 17266 | 3512 | 3666 | 3852 | . | . | . | . | . | . | . | . | . |
| | *** | 13415 | 15524 | 17242 | 3581 | 3767 | 3844 | . | . | . | . | . | . | . | . | . |
| 0.98 | *** | 5170 | 5494 | 5935 | . | . | . | . | . | . | . | . | . | . | . | . |
| | *** | 5324 | 5706 | 5922 | . | . | . | . | . | . | . | . | . | . | . | . |

## TABLE 3: ALPHA= 0.01  POWER= 0.8    EXPECTED ACCRUAL THRU MINIMUM FOLLOW-UP= 20000

| | | DEL=.01 | | | DEL=.02 | | | DEL=.05 | | | DEL=.10 | | | DEL=.15 | | |
|---|---|---|---|---|---|---|---|---|---|---|---|---|---|---|---|---|---|
| FACT= | | 1.0 .75 | .50 .25 | .00 BIN | 1.0 .75 | .50 .25 | .00 BIN | 1.0 .75 | .50 .25 | .00 BIN | 1.0 75 | .50 .25 | .00 BIN | 1.0 .75 | .50 .25 | .00 BIN |
| PCONT=*** | | | | | REQUIRED NUMBER OF PATIENTS | | | | | | | | | | | |
| 0.01 | *** | 1532 | 1532 | 1532 | 563 | 563 | 563 | 182 | 182 | 182 | 82 | 82 | 82 | 63 | 63 | 63 |
| | *** | 1532 | 1532 | 5922 | 563 | 563 | 1958 | 182 | 182 | 533 | 82 | 82 | 217 | 63 | 63 | 129 |
| 0.02 | *** | 3432 | 3432 | 3463 | 1113 | 1113 | 1113 | 282 | 282 | 282 | 132 | 132 | 132 | 82 | 82 | 82 |
| | *** | 3432 | 3432 | 9776 | 1113 | 1113 | 2911 | 282 | 282 | 681 | 132 | 132 | 252 | 82 | 82 | 144 |
| 0.05 | *** | 10482 | 10613 | 10782 | 2982 | 3013 | 3013 | 632 | 632 | 632 | 232 | 232 | 232 | 132 | 132 | 132 |
| | *** | 10532 | 10682 | 20855 | 2982 | 3013 | 5651 | 632 | 632 | 1104 | 232 | 232 | 352 | 132 | 132 | 186 |
| 0.1 | *** | 23332 | 23863 | 25113 | 6413 | 6513 | 6632 | 1232 | 1232 | 1232 | 382 | 382 | 382 | 213 | 213 | 213 |
| | *** | 23563 | 24332 | 37716 | 6463 | 6563 | 9816 | 1232 | 1232 | 1747 | 382 | 382 | 502 | 213 | 213 | 248 |
| 0.15 | *** | 35132 | 36232 | 39663 | 9663 | 9913 | 10263 | 1782 | 1782 | 1813 | 513 | 513 | 513 | 263 | 263 | 263 |
| | *** | 35563 | 37382 | 52569 | 9763 | 10063 | 13479 | 1782 | 1813 | 2309 | 513 | 513 | 633 | 263 | 263 | 302 |
| 0.2 | *** | 44882 | 46732 | 53282 | 12463 | 12913 | 13632 | 2282 | 2313 | 2332 | 632 | 632 | 632 | 313 | 313 | 313 |
| | *** | 45582 | 48782 | 65415 | 12663 | 13232 | 16640 | 2282 | 2313 | 2791 | 632 | 632 | 743 | 313 | 313 | 346 |
| 0.25 | *** | 52382 | 55082 | 65432 | 14732 | 15432 | 16632 | 2713 | 2763 | 2782 | 732 | 763 | 763 | 363 | 363 | 363 |
| | *** | 53413 | 58132 | 76254 | 15063 | 15963 | 19300 | 2732 | 2763 | 3192 | 732 | 763 | 833 | 363 | 363 | 382 |
| 0.3 | *** | 57632 | 61263 | 75763 | 16513 | 17482 | 19182 | 3063 | 3113 | 3182 | 832 | 832 | 832 | 382 | 382 | 382 |
| | *** | 59013 | 65432 | 85086 | 16932 | 18182 | 21458 | 3082 | 3132 | 3513 | 832 | 832 | 904 | 382 | 382 | 409 |
| 0.35 | *** | 60832 | 65463 | 84132 | 17782 | 19013 | 21213 | 3332 | 3413 | 3482 | 882 | 913 | 913 | 413 | 413 | 413 |
| | *** | 62613 | 70713 | 91910 | 18313 | 19913 | 23113 | 3363 | 3432 | 3754 | 882 | 913 | 954 | 413 | 413 | 426 |
| 0.4 | *** | 62232 | 67863 | 90413 | 18613 | 20032 | 22732 | 3513 | 3613 | 3713 | 932 | 932 | 963 | 432 | 432 | 432 |
| | *** | 64413 | 74132 | 96728 | 19232 | 21132 | 24268 | 3563 | 3663 | 3915 | 932 | 932 | 984 | 432 | 432 | 435 |
| 0.45 | *** | 62082 | 68682 | 94563 | 18982 | 20632 | 23713 | 3613 | 3713 | 3832 | 963 | 963 | 963 | 432 | 432 | 432 |
| | *** | 64663 | 75863 | 99538 | 19713 | 21882 | 24920 | 3663 | 3763 | 3995 | 963 | 963 | 994 | 432 | 432 | 435 |
| 0.5 | *** | 60713 | 68113 | 96532 | 18982 | 20782 | 24163 | 3663 | 3763 | 3882 | 963 | 963 | 963 | 432 | 432 | 432 |
| | *** | 63632 | 76032 | 100341 | 19782 | 22132 | 25070 | 3713 | 3813 | 3995 | 963 | 963 | 984 | 432 | 432 | 426 |
| 0.55 | *** | 58332 | 66382 | 96332 | 18663 | 20532 | 24063 | 3613 | 3713 | 3832 | 932 | 932 | 963 | 413 | 413 | 413 |
| | *** | 61563 | 74782 | 99136 | 19482 | 21932 | 24719 | 3663 | 3763 | 3915 | 932 | 932 | 954 | 413 | 413 | 409 |
| 0.6 | *** | 55163 | 63613 | 93963 | 17982 | 19882 | 23413 | 3482 | 3582 | 3713 | 882 | 913 | 913 | 382 | 382 | 382 |
| | *** | 58563 | 72232 | 95925 | 18813 | 21313 | 23866 | 3532 | 3632 | 3754 | 882 | 913 | 904 | 382 | 382 | 382 |
| 0.65 | *** | 51363 | 59913 | 89382 | 17013 | 18863 | 22213 | 3263 | 3363 | 3482 | 832 | 832 | 832 | 363 | 363 | 363 |
| | *** | 54813 | 68463 | 90706 | 17813 | 20213 | 22511 | 3313 | 3432 | 3513 | 832 | 832 | 833 | 363 | 363 | 346 |
| 0.7 | *** | 46963 | 55313 | 82663 | 15732 | 17432 | 20463 | 2982 | 3082 | 3182 | 732 | 763 | 763 | 313 | 313 | 313 |
| | *** | 50382 | 63463 | 83480 | 16482 | 18682 | 20655 | 3032 | 3132 | 3192 | 732 | 763 | 743 | 313 | 313 | 302 |
| 0.75 | *** | 42032 | 49813 | 73782 | 14132 | 15632 | 18213 | 2632 | 2713 | 2782 | 632 | 632 | 632 | 263 | 263 | 263 |
| | *** | 45232 | 57213 | 74247 | 14813 | 16713 | 18296 | 2682 | 2763 | 2791 | 632 | 632 | 633 | 263 | 263 | 248 |
| 0.8 | *** | 36513 | 43332 | 62782 | 12182 | 13413 | 15382 | 2213 | 2263 | 2313 | 513 | 513 | 513 | 213 | 213 | 213 |
| | *** | 39363 | 49613 | 63007 | 12763 | 14263 | 15436 | 2232 | 2282 | 2309 | 513 | 513 | 502 | 213 | 213 | 186 |
| 0.85 | *** | 30182 | 35663 | 49682 | 9863 | 10763 | 12063 | 1682 | 1732 | 1763 | 363 | 363 | 363 | . | . | . |
| | *** | 32482 | 40463 | 49759 | 10263 | 11332 | 12074 | 1713 | 1732 | 1747 | 363 | 363 | 352 | . | . | . |
| 0.9 | *** | 22682 | 26382 | 34482 | 7063 | 7532 | 8213 | 1082 | 1113 | 1113 | . | . | . | . | . | . |
| | *** | 24282 | 29413 | 34504 | 7282 | 7863 | 8210 | 1113 | 1113 | 1104 | . | . | . | . | . | . |
| 0.95 | *** | 13113 | 14663 | 17263 | 3563 | 3682 | 3863 | . | . | . | . | . | . | . | . | . |
| | *** | 13782 | 15732 | 17242 | 3613 | 3782 | 3844 | . | . | . | . | . | . | . | . | . |
| 0.98 | *** | 5263 | 5563 | 5932 | . | . | . | . | . | . | . | . | . | . | . | . |
| | *** | 5382 | 5732 | 5922 | . | . | . | . | . | . | . | . | . | . | . | . |

TABLE 3: ALPHA= 0.01  POWER= 0.8    EXPECTED ACCRUAL THRU MINIMUM FOLLOW-UP= 25000

| | | DEL=.01 | | | DEL=.02 | | | DEL=.05 | | | DEL=.10 | | | DEL=.15 | | |
|---|---|---|---|---|---|---|---|---|---|---|---|---|---|---|---|---|---|
| FACT= | | 1.0 .75 | .50 .25 | .00 BIN | 1.0 .75 | .50 .25 | .00 BIN | 1.0 .75 | .50 .25 | .00 BIN | 1.0 75 | .50 .25 | .00 BIN | 1.0 .75 | .50 .25 | .00 BIN |
| PCONT=*** | | REQUIRED NUMBER OF PATIENTS | | | | | | | | | | | | | | | |
| 0.01 | *** | 1540 | 1540 | 1540 | 579 | 579 | 579 | 165 | 165 | 165 | 102 | 102 | 102 | 79 | 79 | 79 |
| | *** | 1540 | 1540 | 5922 | 579 | 579 | 1958 | 165 | 165 | 533 | 102 | 102 | 217 | 79 | 79 | 129 |
| 0.02 | *** | 3415 | 3454 | 3454 | 1102 | 1102 | 1102 | 290 | 290 | 290 | 141 | 141 | 141 | 79 | 79 | 79 |
| | *** | 3454 | 3454 | 9776 | 1102 | 1102 | 2911 | 290 | 290 | 681 | 141 | 141 | 252 | 79 | 79 | 144 |
| 0.05 | *** | 10516 | 10641 | 10790 | 2977 | 3016 | 3016 | 641 | 641 | 641 | 227 | 227 | 227 | 141 | 141 | 141 |
| | *** | 10579 | 10704 | 20855 | 3016 | 3016 | 5651 | 641 | 641 | 1104 | 227 | 227 | 352 | 141 | 141 | 186 |
| 0.1 | *** | 23516 | 24016 | 25102 | 6454 | 6540 | 6641 | 1227 | 1227 | 1227 | 391 | 391 | 391 | 204 | 204 | 204 |
| | *** | 23704 | 24454 | 37716 | 6477 | 6579 | 9816 | 1227 | 1227 | 1747 | 391 | 391 | 502 | 204 | 204 | 248 |
| 0.15 | *** | 35454 | 36602 | 39665 | 9727 | 9954 | 10266 | 1790 | 1790 | 1790 | 516 | 516 | 516 | 266 | 266 | 266 |
| | *** | 35915 | 37727 | 52569 | 9852 | 10102 | 13479 | 1790 | 1790 | 2309 | 516 | 516 | 633 | 266 | 266 | 302 |
| 0.2 | *** | 45415 | 47391 | 53290 | 12602 | 13040 | 13641 | 2290 | 2329 | 2329 | 641 | 641 | 641 | 329 | 329 | 329 |
| | *** | 46204 | 49391 | 65415 | 12790 | 13290 | 16640 | 2290 | 2329 | 2791 | 641 | 641 | 743 | 329 | 329 | 346 |
| 0.25 | *** | 53165 | 56079 | 65415 | 14977 | 15641 | 16641 | 2727 | 2766 | 2790 | 727 | 766 | 766 | 352 | 352 | 352 |
| | *** | 54290 | 59079 | 76254 | 15266 | 16079 | 19300 | 2727 | 2766 | 3192 | 766 | 766 | 833 | 352 | 352 | 382 |
| 0.3 | *** | 58704 | 62602 | 75766 | 16852 | 17727 | 19165 | 3079 | 3141 | 3165 | 829 | 829 | 829 | 391 | 391 | 391 |
| | *** | 60227 | 66704 | 85086 | 17227 | 18352 | 21458 | 3102 | 3141 | 3513 | 829 | 829 | 904 | 391 | 391 | 409 |
| 0.35 | *** | 62204 | 67141 | 84141 | 18204 | 19329 | 21227 | 3352 | 3415 | 3477 | 891 | 891 | 915 | 415 | 415 | 415 |
| | *** | 64141 | 72329 | 91910 | 18704 | 20141 | 23113 | 3391 | 3454 | 3754 | 891 | 891 | 954 | 415 | 415 | 426 |
| 0.4 | *** | 63891 | 69852 | 90415 | 19102 | 20454 | 22727 | 3540 | 3602 | 3704 | 954 | 954 | 954 | 415 | 415 | 415 |
| | *** | 66266 | 76079 | 96728 | 19704 | 21415 | 24268 | 3579 | 3665 | 3915 | 954 | 954 | 984 | 415 | 415 | 435 |
| 0.45 | *** | 64079 | 70977 | 94579 | 19540 | 21079 | 23727 | 3665 | 3727 | 3829 | 954 | 954 | 977 | 415 | 454 | 454 |
| | *** | 66829 | 78079 | 99538 | 20227 | 22165 | 24920 | 3704 | 3790 | 3995 | 954 | 977 | 994 | 415 | 454 | 435 |
| 0.5 | *** | 62954 | 70665 | 96540 | 19602 | 21266 | 24165 | 3704 | 3766 | 3891 | 954 | 954 | 977 | 415 | 415 | 415 |
| | *** | 66079 | 78454 | 100341 | 20352 | 22477 | 25070 | 3727 | 3829 | 3995 | 954 | 977 | 984 | 415 | 415 | 426 |
| 0.55 | *** | 60829 | 69102 | 96329 | 19290 | 21040 | 24040 | 3641 | 3727 | 3829 | 954 | 954 | 954 | 415 | 415 | 415 |
| | *** | 64165 | 77352 | 99136 | 20079 | 22290 | 24719 | 3665 | 3790 | 3915 | 954 | 954 | 954 | 415 | 415 | 409 |
| 0.6 | *** | 57790 | 66415 | 93954 | 18641 | 20391 | 23391 | 3516 | 3602 | 3704 | 891 | 891 | 915 | 391 | 391 | 391 |
| | *** | 61329 | 74852 | 95925 | 19415 | 21641 | 23866 | 3540 | 3641 | 3754 | 891 | 891 | 904 | 391 | 391 | 382 |
| 0.65 | *** | 54040 | 62704 | 89391 | 17641 | 19352 | 22204 | 3290 | 3391 | 3477 | 829 | 829 | 852 | 352 | 352 | 352 |
| | *** | 57602 | 71016 | 90706 | 18415 | 20540 | 22511 | 3352 | 3454 | 3513 | 829 | 829 | 833 | 352 | 352 | 346 |
| 0.7 | *** | 49602 | 57977 | 82641 | 16329 | 17891 | 20477 | 3016 | 3102 | 3165 | 727 | 766 | 766 | 329 | 329 | 329 |
| | *** | 53079 | 65852 | 83480 | 17016 | 18977 | 20655 | 3079 | 3141 | 3192 | 766 | 766 | 743 | 329 | 329 | 302 |
| 0.75 | *** | 44516 | 52266 | 73766 | 14665 | 16040 | 18204 | 2665 | 2727 | 2790 | 641 | 641 | 641 | 266 | 266 | 266 |
| | *** | 47766 | 59352 | 74247 | 15290 | 16977 | 18296 | 2704 | 2766 | 2791 | 641 | 641 | 633 | 266 | 266 | 248 |
| 0.8 | *** | 38704 | 45454 | 62766 | 12641 | 13727 | 15391 | 2227 | 2266 | 2329 | 516 | 516 | 516 | 204 | 204 | 204 |
| | *** | 41540 | 51391 | 63007 | 13141 | 14454 | 15436 | 2266 | 2290 | 2309 | 516 | 516 | 502 | 204 | 204 | 186 |
| 0.85 | *** | 31977 | 37290 | 49665 | 10204 | 10977 | 12079 | 1704 | 1727 | 1766 | 352 | 352 | 352 | . | . | . |
| | *** | 34266 | 41790 | 49759 | 10540 | 11454 | 12074 | 1727 | 1727 | 1747 | 352 | 352 | 352 | . | . | . |
| 0.9 | *** | 23954 | 27454 | 34477 | 7227 | 7665 | 8227 | 1102 | 1102 | 1102 | . | . | . | . | . | . |
| | *** | 25477 | 30204 | 34504 | 7454 | 7915 | 8210 | 1102 | 1102 | 1104 | . | . | . | . | . | . |
| 0.95 | *** | 13641 | 15040 | 17266 | 3602 | 3727 | 3852 | . | . | . | . | . | . | . | . | . |
| | *** | 14290 | 16016 | 17242 | 3665 | 3790 | 3844 | . | . | . | . | . | . | . | . | . |
| 0.98 | *** | 5352 | 5641 | 5954 | . | . | . | . | . | . | . | . | . | . | . | . |
| | *** | 5477 | 5766 | 5922 | . | . | . | . | . | . | . | . | . | . | . | . |

## TABLE 4: ALPHA= 0.01  POWER= 0.9    EXPECTED ACCRUAL THRU MINIMUM FOLLOW-UP= 30

| | | DEL=.10 | | | DEL=.15 | | | DEL=.20 | | | DEL=.25 | | | DEL=.30 | | |
|---|---|---|---|---|---|---|---|---|---|---|---|---|---|---|---|---|
| FACT= | | 1.0 .75 | .50 .25 | .00 BIN | 1.0 .75 | .50 .25 | .00 BIN | 1.0 .75 | .50 .25 | .00 BIN | 1.0 75 | .50 .25 | .00 BIN | 1.0 .75 | .50 .25 | .00 BIN |
| PCONT=*** | | | | | | | REQUIRED NUMBER OF PATIENTS | | | | | | | | |
| 0.05 | *** | 273 | 274 | 296 | 158 | 160 | 172 | 111 | 113 | 121 | 87 | 88 | 94 | 71 | 72 | 77 |
| | *** | 273 | 276 | 456 | 159 | 162 | 241 | 112 | 115 | 153 | 87 | 89 | 108 | 72 | 74 | 80 |
| 0.1 | *** | 430 | 432 | 495 | 227 | 229 | 263 | 149 | 151 | 172 | 110 | 112 | 126 | 87 | 89 | 99 |
| | *** | 431 | 437 | 651 | 228 | 234 | 322 | 150 | 156 | 196 | 110 | 116 | 133 | 88 | 92 | 96 |
| 0.15 | *** | 555 | 558 | 679 | 278 | 282 | 342 | 175 | 179 | 216 | 125 | 129 | 153 | 96 | 100 | 117 |
| | *** | 556 | 565 | 821 | 279 | 289 | 391 | 177 | 186 | 232 | 127 | 135 | 154 | 98 | 105 | 109 |
| 0.2 | *** | 645 | 650 | 841 | 313 | 319 | 411 | 192 | 198 | 252 | 135 | 140 | 175 | 102 | 107 | 131 |
| | *** | 647 | 661 | 964 | 315 | 329 | 449 | 194 | 208 | 261 | 137 | 148 | 170 | 104 | 114 | 119 |
| 0.25 | *** | 703 | 710 | 980 | 334 | 342 | 467 | 202 | 210 | 281 | 139 | 147 | 191 | 105 | 111 | 141 |
| | *** | 705 | 724 | 1081 | 336 | 356 | 495 | 204 | 222 | 284 | 142 | 157 | 183 | 107 | 119 | 126 |
| 0.3 | *** | 730 | 740 | 1092 | 341 | 352 | 512 | 204 | 215 | 303 | 140 | 150 | 204 | 105 | 113 | 148 |
| | *** | 733 | 759 | 1172 | 345 | 371 | 530 | 208 | 231 | 300 | 144 | 162 | 191 | 108 | 122 | 131 |
| 0.35 | *** | 730 | 743 | 1177 | 338 | 351 | 544 | 201 | 214 | 318 | 137 | 149 | 211 | 102 | 112 | 152 |
| | *** | 734 | 768 | 1237 | 343 | 375 | 553 | 206 | 233 | 310 | 142 | 163 | 195 | 106 | 123 | 132 |
| 0.4 | *** | 707 | 723 | 1235 | 325 | 343 | 564 | 193 | 209 | 325 | 132 | 145 | 214 | 98 | 109 | 152 |
| | *** | 712 | 755 | 1276 | 331 | 372 | 565 | 199 | 231 | 313 | 137 | 161 | 195 | 103 | 121 | 131 |
| 0.45 | *** | 665 | 685 | 1263 | 306 | 327 | 570 | 182 | 201 | 326 | 125 | 140 | 212 | 93 | 105 | 149 |
| | *** | 672 | 726 | 1289 | 313 | 361 | 565 | 189 | 225 | 310 | 131 | 157 | 191 | 98 | 117 | 126 |
| 0.5 | *** | 608 | 634 | 1264 | 281 | 306 | 564 | 169 | 190 | 319 | 117 | 132 | 205 | 87 | 99 | 143 |
| | *** | 616 | 684 | 1276 | 290 | 345 | 553 | 177 | 216 | 300 | 123 | 150 | 183 | 92 | 111 | 119 |
| 0.55 | *** | 541 | 574 | 1236 | 253 | 283 | 546 | 154 | 176 | 305 | 107 | 123 | 194 | 80 | 92 | 134 |
| | *** | 552 | 634 | 1237 | 264 | 324 | 530 | 163 | 204 | 284 | 113 | 141 | 170 | 85 | 104 | 109 |
| 0.6 | *** | 469 | 510 | 1180 | 224 | 257 | 515 | 139 | 162 | 284 | 97 | 113 | 178 | 72 | 84 | 121 |
| | *** | 483 | 578 | 1172 | 236 | 300 | 495 | 148 | 189 | 261 | 103 | 130 | 154 | 77 | 95 | 96 |
| 0.65 | *** | 397 | 446 | 1095 | 196 | 230 | 471 | 123 | 145 | 256 | 86 | 101 | 158 | 64 | 74 | 106 |
| | *** | 414 | 519 | 1081 | 209 | 273 | 449 | 132 | 171 | 232 | 92 | 117 | 133 | 68 | 84 | 80 |
| 0.7 | *** | 329 | 384 | 983 | 168 | 202 | 415 | 106 | 127 | 221 | 74 | 87 | 134 | . | . | . |
| | *** | 349 | 459 | 964 | 181 | 242 | 391 | 115 | 150 | 196 | 79 | 101 | 108 | . | . | . |
| 0.75 | *** | 268 | 324 | 843 | 141 | 172 | 347 | 89 | 107 | 179 | . | . | . | . | . | . |
| | *** | 289 | 396 | 821 | 153 | 208 | 322 | 96 | 126 | 153 | . | . | . | . | . | . |
| 0.8 | *** | 213 | 265 | 676 | 113 | 140 | 266 | . | . | . | . | . | . | . | . | . |
| | *** | 233 | 329 | 651 | 124 | 169 | 241 | . | . | . | . | . | . | . | . | . |
| 0.85 | *** | 162 | 204 | 482 | . | . | . | . | . | . | . | . | . | . | . | . |
| | *** | 178 | 254 | 456 | . | . | . | . | . | . | . | . | . | . | . | . |

## TABLE 4: ALPHA= 0.01  POWER= 0.9    EXPECTED ACCRUAL THRU MINIMUM FOLLOW-UP= 40

| | | DEL=.10 | | | DEL=.15 | | | DEL=.20 | | | DEL=.25 | | | DEL=.30 | | |
|---|---|---|---|---|---|---|---|---|---|---|---|---|---|---|---|---|
| FACT= | | 1.0 .75 | .50 .25 | .00 BIN | 1.0 .75 | .50 .25 | .00 BIN | 1.0 .75 | .50 .25 | .00 BIN | 1.0 75 | .50 .25 | .00 BIN | 1.0 .75 | .50 .25 | .00 BIN |
| PCONT=*** | | | | | REQUIRED NUMBER OF PATIENTS | | | | | | | | | | | |
| 0.05 | *** | 273 | 274 | 296 | 159 | 160 | 172 | 112 | 113 | 121 | 87 | 88 | 94 | 72 | 73 | 77 |
| | *** | 274 | 277 | 456 | 159 | 163 | 241 | 112 | 116 | 153 | 88 | 90 | 108 | 72 | 74 | 80 |
| 0.1 | *** | 431 | 434 | 495 | 228 | 231 | 263 | 150 | 153 | 172 | 111 | 113 | 126 | 88 | 90 | 99 |
| | *** | 432 | 439 | 651 | 229 | 236 | 322 | 151 | 158 | 196 | 112 | 117 | 133 | 89 | 93 | 96 |
| 0.15 | *** | 556 | 560 | 679 | 279 | 284 | 342 | 177 | 182 | 216 | 127 | 131 | 153 | 98 | 102 | 117 |
| | *** | 557 | 570 | 821 | 281 | 293 | 391 | 178 | 189 | 232 | 128 | 137 | 154 | 99 | 107 | 109 |
| 0.2 | *** | 647 | 654 | 841 | 315 | 322 | 411 | 194 | 202 | 252 | 137 | 143 | 175 | 104 | 110 | 131 |
| | *** | 649 | 667 | 964 | 317 | 336 | 449 | 197 | 213 | 261 | 139 | 152 | 170 | 106 | 116 | 119 |
| 0.25 | *** | 705 | 715 | 980 | 336 | 347 | 467 | 205 | 215 | 281 | 142 | 151 | 191 | 107 | 115 | 141 |
| | *** | 708 | 734 | 1081 | 340 | 365 | 495 | 208 | 229 | 284 | 145 | 162 | 183 | 110 | 122 | 126 |
| 0.3 | *** | 733 | 746 | 1092 | 345 | 359 | 512 | 208 | 221 | 303 | 144 | 154 | 204 | 108 | 117 | 148 |
| | *** | 738 | 771 | 1172 | 350 | 382 | 530 | 212 | 238 | 300 | 148 | 167 | 191 | 111 | 126 | 131 |
| 0.35 | *** | 734 | 751 | 1177 | 343 | 360 | 544 | 206 | 221 | 318 | 142 | 155 | 211 | 106 | 116 | 152 |
| | *** | 740 | 784 | 1237 | 349 | 388 | 553 | 211 | 242 | 310 | 147 | 169 | 195 | 110 | 127 | 132 |
| 0.4 | *** | 712 | 734 | 1235 | 331 | 353 | 564 | 199 | 218 | 325 | 137 | 152 | 214 | 103 | 114 | 152 |
| | *** | 720 | 776 | 1276 | 339 | 387 | 565 | 206 | 241 | 313 | 143 | 168 | 195 | 107 | 125 | 131 |
| 0.45 | *** | 672 | 699 | 1263 | 313 | 339 | 570 | 189 | 210 | 326 | 131 | 147 | 212 | 98 | 110 | 149 |
| | *** | 681 | 751 | 1289 | 322 | 378 | 565 | 197 | 236 | 310 | 137 | 164 | 191 | 103 | 122 | 126 |
| 0.5 | *** | 617 | 651 | 1264 | 290 | 321 | 564 | 177 | 200 | 319 | 123 | 140 | 205 | 92 | 104 | 143 |
| | *** | 628 | 713 | 1276 | 301 | 363 | 553 | 186 | 227 | 300 | 129 | 158 | 183 | 97 | 116 | 119 |
| 0.55 | *** | 552 | 595 | 1236 | 264 | 299 | 546 | 163 | 187 | 305 | 113 | 131 | 194 | 85 | 97 | 134 |
| | *** | 567 | 667 | 1237 | 277 | 344 | 530 | 172 | 215 | 284 | 120 | 149 | 170 | 90 | 109 | 109 |
| 0.6 | *** | 483 | 535 | 1180 | 236 | 274 | 515 | 148 | 173 | 284 | 103 | 120 | 178 | 77 | 89 | 121 |
| | *** | 501 | 614 | 1172 | 251 | 320 | 495 | 157 | 200 | 261 | 110 | 137 | 154 | 82 | 99 | 96 |
| 0.65 | *** | 414 | 474 | 1095 | 209 | 247 | 471 | 132 | 156 | 256 | 92 | 108 | 158 | 68 | 78 | 106 |
| | *** | 436 | 556 | 1081 | 224 | 292 | 449 | 141 | 182 | 232 | 98 | 123 | 133 | 72 | 88 | 80 |
| 0.7 | *** | 349 | 412 | 983 | 181 | 218 | 415 | 115 | 137 | 221 | 79 | 93 | 134 | . | . | . |
| | *** | 373 | 495 | 964 | 196 | 260 | 391 | 124 | 160 | 196 | 85 | 106 | 108 | . | . | . |
| 0.75 | *** | 289 | 352 | 843 | 153 | 187 | 347 | 96 | 115 | 179 | . | . | . | . | . | . |
| | *** | 313 | 430 | 821 | 166 | 223 | 322 | 104 | 134 | 153 | . | . | . | . | . | . |
| 0.8 | *** | 233 | 290 | 676 | 124 | 151 | 266 | . | . | . | . | . | . | . | . | . |
| | *** | 255 | 358 | 651 | 135 | 181 | 241 | . | . | . | . | . | . | . | . | . |
| 0.85 | *** | 178 | 224 | 482 | . | . | . | . | . | . | . | . | . | . | . | . |
| | *** | 196 | 276 | 456 | . | . | . | . | . | . | . | . | . | . | . | . |

# TABLE 4: ALPHA= 0.01  POWER= 0.9    EXPECTED ACCRUAL THRU MINIMUM FOLLOW-UP= 50

|  | FACT= | DEL=.10 | | | DEL=.15 | | | DEL=.20 | | | DEL=.25 | | | DEL=.30 | | |
|---|---|---|---|---|---|---|---|---|---|---|---|---|---|---|---|---|
|  |  | 1.0 / .75 | .50 / .25 | .00 / BIN | 1.0 / .75 | .50 / .25 | .00 / BIN | 1.0 / .75 | .50 / .25 | .00 / BIN | 1.0 / 75 | .50 / .25 | .00 / BIN | 1.0 / .75 | .50 / .25 | .00 / BIN |
| PCONT=*** |  | REQUIRED NUMBER OF PATIENTS | | | | | | | | | | | | | | |
| 0.05 | *** | 273 | 275 | 296 | 159 | 161 | 172 | 112 | 114 | 121 | 87 | 89 | 94 | 72 | 74 | 77 |
|  | *** | 274 | 278 | 456 | 160 | 164 | 241 | 113 | 116 | 153 | 88 | 91 | 108 | 73 | 75 | 80 |
| 0.1 | *** | 432 | 435 | 495 | 229 | 232 | 263 | 151 | 154 | 172 | 111 | 115 | 126 | 88 | 91 | 99 |
|  | *** | 433 | 442 | 651 | 230 | 239 | 322 | 152 | 159 | 196 | 113 | 118 | 133 | 89 | 94 | 96 |
| 0.15 | *** | 557 | 563 | 679 | 281 | 287 | 342 | 178 | 184 | 216 | 128 | 133 | 153 | 99 | 103 | 117 |
|  | *** | 559 | 574 | 821 | 283 | 297 | 391 | 180 | 192 | 232 | 130 | 139 | 154 | 101 | 108 | 109 |
| 0.2 | *** | 649 | 657 | 841 | 317 | 326 | 411 | 196 | 205 | 252 | 139 | 146 | 175 | 106 | 112 | 131 |
|  | *** | 652 | 674 | 964 | 320 | 341 | 449 | 200 | 217 | 261 | 141 | 154 | 170 | 108 | 118 | 119 |
| 0.25 | *** | 708 | 720 | 980 | 339 | 352 | 467 | 207 | 219 | 281 | 145 | 154 | 191 | 109 | 117 | 141 |
|  | *** | 712 | 743 | 1081 | 343 | 372 | 495 | 211 | 234 | 284 | 148 | 165 | 183 | 113 | 125 | 126 |
| 0.3 | *** | 737 | 752 | 1092 | 348 | 365 | 512 | 211 | 226 | 303 | 147 | 158 | 204 | 110 | 120 | 148 |
|  | *** | 742 | 783 | 1172 | 354 | 391 | 530 | 217 | 244 | 300 | 151 | 171 | 191 | 114 | 129 | 131 |
| 0.35 | *** | 739 | 760 | 1177 | 347 | 368 | 544 | 210 | 228 | 318 | 145 | 159 | 211 | 109 | 120 | 152 |
|  | *** | 746 | 799 | 1237 | 354 | 400 | 553 | 217 | 249 | 310 | 151 | 174 | 195 | 113 | 130 | 132 |
| 0.4 | *** | 718 | 745 | 1235 | 337 | 363 | 564 | 204 | 225 | 325 | 142 | 157 | 214 | 106 | 118 | 152 |
|  | *** | 727 | 795 | 1276 | 346 | 400 | 565 | 212 | 249 | 313 | 148 | 173 | 195 | 111 | 129 | 131 |
| 0.45 | *** | 678 | 713 | 1263 | 320 | 351 | 570 | 195 | 218 | 326 | 136 | 152 | 212 | 102 | 114 | 149 |
|  | *** | 690 | 773 | 1289 | 331 | 392 | 565 | 204 | 245 | 310 | 142 | 170 | 191 | 107 | 125 | 126 |
| 0.5 | *** | 625 | 668 | 1264 | 298 | 333 | 564 | 184 | 209 | 319 | 128 | 146 | 205 | 96 | 108 | 143 |
|  | *** | 640 | 739 | 1276 | 311 | 379 | 553 | 193 | 237 | 300 | 135 | 163 | 183 | 101 | 120 | 119 |
| 0.55 | *** | 563 | 615 | 1236 | 274 | 312 | 546 | 170 | 196 | 305 | 119 | 137 | 194 | 89 | 101 | 134 |
|  | *** | 581 | 696 | 1237 | 288 | 360 | 530 | 180 | 224 | 284 | 126 | 154 | 170 | 94 | 112 | 109 |
| 0.6 | *** | 497 | 558 | 1180 | 247 | 288 | 515 | 155 | 181 | 284 | 108 | 126 | 178 | 81 | 92 | 121 |
|  | *** | 519 | 644 | 1172 | 263 | 336 | 495 | 166 | 209 | 261 | 116 | 142 | 154 | 86 | 102 | 96 |
| 0.65 | *** | 431 | 498 | 1095 | 220 | 261 | 471 | 139 | 164 | 256 | 97 | 113 | 158 | 71 | 82 | 106 |
|  | *** | 456 | 588 | 1081 | 236 | 307 | 449 | 149 | 190 | 232 | 103 | 127 | 133 | 76 | 90 | 80 |
| 0.7 | *** | 367 | 437 | 983 | 192 | 231 | 415 | 121 | 144 | 221 | 84 | 98 | 134 | . | . | . |
|  | *** | 394 | 525 | 964 | 208 | 274 | 391 | 131 | 167 | 196 | 90 | 110 | 108 | . | . | . |
| 0.75 | *** | 308 | 375 | 843 | 163 | 198 | 347 | 102 | 121 | 179 | . | . | . | . | . | . |
|  | *** | 334 | 457 | 821 | 177 | 235 | 322 | 110 | 139 | 153 | . | . | . | . | . | . |
| 0.8 | *** | 250 | 311 | 676 | 132 | 161 | 266 | . | . | . | . | . | . | . | . | . |
|  | *** | 274 | 382 | 651 | 144 | 190 | 241 | . | . | . | . | . | . | . | . | . |
| 0.85 | *** | 192 | 240 | 482 | . | . | . | . | . | . | . | . | . | . | . | . |
|  | *** | 211 | 294 | 456 | . | . | . | . | . | . | . | . | . | . | . | . |

TABLE 4: ALPHA= 0.01  POWER= 0.9    EXPECTED ACCRUAL THRU MINIMUM FOLLOW-UP= 60

| | | DEL=.10 | | | DEL=.15 | | | DEL=.20 | | | DEL=.25 | | | DEL=.30 | |
|---|---|---|---|---|---|---|---|---|---|---|---|---|---|---|---|---|
| FACT= | 1.0 .75 | .50 .25 | .00 BIN | 1.0 .75 | .50 .25 | .00 BIN | 1.0 .75 | .50 .25 | .00 BIN | 1.0 75 | .50 .25 | .00 BIN | 1.0 .75 | .50 .25 | .00 BIN |
| PCONT=*** | | | | REQUIRED NUMBER OF PATIENTS | | | | | | | | | | | |
| 0.05 *** | 274 | 276 | 296 | 160 | 162 | 172 | 113 | 115 | 121 | 88 | 89 | 94 | 73 | 74 | 77 |
| *** | 274 | 279 | 456 | 160 | 165 | 241 | 113 | 117 | 153 | 88 | 91 | 108 | 73 | 75 | 80 |
| 0.1 *** | 432 | 437 | 495 | 229 | 234 | 263 | 151 | 155 | 172 | 112 | 116 | 126 | 89 | 92 | 99 |
| *** | 434 | 445 | 651 | 231 | 240 | 322 | 153 | 160 | 196 | 113 | 119 | 133 | 90 | 95 | 96 |
| 0.15 *** | 558 | 565 | 679 | 282 | 289 | 342 | 179 | 186 | 216 | 129 | 135 | 153 | 100 | 105 | 117 |
| *** | 560 | 578 | 821 | 284 | 300 | 391 | 182 | 194 | 232 | 131 | 141 | 154 | 102 | 109 | 109 |
| 0.2 *** | 650 | 661 | 841 | 319 | 329 | 411 | 198 | 208 | 252 | 140 | 148 | 175 | 107 | 114 | 131 |
| *** | 654 | 680 | 964 | 322 | 346 | 449 | 202 | 220 | 261 | 143 | 156 | 170 | 110 | 119 | 119 |
| 0.25 *** | 710 | 724 | 980 | 342 | 356 | 467 | 210 | 222 | 281 | 147 | 157 | 191 | 111 | 119 | 141 |
| *** | 715 | 751 | 1081 | 347 | 378 | 495 | 215 | 238 | 284 | 151 | 168 | 183 | 115 | 127 | 126 |
| 0.3 *** | 740 | 759 | 1092 | 352 | 371 | 512 | 215 | 231 | 303 | 150 | 162 | 203 | 113 | 122 | 148 |
| *** | 746 | 795 | 1172 | 359 | 399 | 530 | 221 | 250 | 300 | 154 | 175 | 191 | 117 | 131 | 131 |
| 0.35 *** | 743 | 768 | 1177 | 352 | 375 | 544 | 214 | 233 | 318 | 149 | 163 | 211 | 112 | 122 | 152 |
| *** | 751 | 814 | 1237 | 360 | 409 | 553 | 221 | 255 | 310 | 155 | 178 | 195 | 116 | 132 | 132 |
| 0.4 *** | 723 | 755 | 1235 | 343 | 371 | 564 | 209 | 231 | 325 | 145 | 161 | 214 | 109 | 121 | 152 |
| *** | 734 | 812 | 1276 | 353 | 411 | 565 | 218 | 256 | 313 | 152 | 177 | 195 | 114 | 131 | 131 |
| 0.45 *** | 685 | 726 | 1263 | 327 | 361 | 570 | 201 | 225 | 326 | 140 | 157 | 212 | 105 | 117 | 149 |
| *** | 699 | 794 | 1289 | 339 | 404 | 565 | 210 | 252 | 310 | 147 | 174 | 191 | 110 | 128 | 126 |
| 0.5 *** | 634 | 684 | 1264 | 306 | 345 | 564 | 190 | 216 | 319 | 132 | 150 | 205 | 99 | 111 | 143 |
| *** | 651 | 763 | 1276 | 321 | 392 | 553 | 200 | 244 | 300 | 140 | 167 | 183 | 104 | 122 | 119 |
| 0.55 *** | 574 | 634 | 1236 | 283 | 324 | 546 | 176 | 204 | 305 | 123 | 141 | 194 | 92 | 104 | 134 |
| *** | 595 | 721 | 1237 | 299 | 373 | 530 | 187 | 232 | 284 | 131 | 158 | 170 | 97 | 115 | 109 |
| 0.6 *** | 510 | 578 | 1180 | 257 | 300 | 515 | 162 | 189 | 284 | 113 | 130 | 178 | 84 | 95 | 121 |
| *** | 535 | 671 | 1172 | 274 | 349 | 495 | 173 | 216 | 261 | 120 | 146 | 154 | 89 | 105 | 96 |
| 0.65 *** | 446 | 519 | 1095 | 230 | 273 | 471 | 145 | 171 | 256 | 101 | 117 | 158 | 74 | 84 | 106 |
| *** | 473 | 614 | 1081 | 247 | 320 | 449 | 156 | 196 | 232 | 108 | 131 | 133 | 78 | 92 | 80 |
| 0.7 *** | 384 | 459 | 983 | 202 | 242 | 415 | 127 | 150 | 221 | 88 | 101 | 134 | . | . | . |
| *** | 412 | 551 | 964 | 218 | 285 | 391 | 137 | 172 | 196 | 93 | 112 | 108 | . | . | . |
| 0.75 *** | 324 | 396 | 843 | 172 | 208 | 347 | 107 | 126 | 179 | . | . | . | . | . | . |
| *** | 352 | 481 | 821 | 187 | 245 | 322 | 115 | 144 | 153 | . | . | . | . | . | . |
| 0.8 *** | 265 | 329 | 676 | 140 | 169 | 266 | . | . | . | . | . | . | . | . | . |
| *** | 290 | 401 | 651 | 151 | 197 | 241 | . | . | . | . | . | . | . | . | . |
| 0.85 *** | 204 | 254 | 482 | . | . | . | . | . | . | . | . | . | . | . | . |
| *** | 224 | 308 | 456 | . | . | . | . | . | . | . | . | . | . | . | . |

## TABLE 4: ALPHA= 0.01  POWER= 0.9   EXPECTED ACCRUAL THRU MINIMUM FOLLOW-UP= 70

|  | | DEL=.10 | | | DEL=.15 | | | DEL=.20 | | | DEL=.25 | | | DEL=.30 | | |
|---|---|---|---|---|---|---|---|---|---|---|---|---|---|---|---|---|
| FACT= | | 1.0 .75 | .50 .25 | .00 BIN | 1.0 .75 | .50 .25 | .00 BIN | 1.0 .75 | .50 .25 | .00 BIN | 1.0 75 | .50 .25 | .00 BIN | 1.0 .75 | .50 .25 | .00 BIN |
| PCONT=*** | | REQUIRED NUMBER OF PATIENTS | | | | | | | | | | | | | | |
| 0.05 | *** | 274 | 277 | 296 | 160 | 162 | 172 | 113 | 115 | 121 | 88 | 90 | 94 | 73 | 74 | 77 |
|  | *** | 275 | 280 | 456 | 161 | 165 | 241 | 114 | 117 | 153 | 89 | 91 | 108 | 73 | 75 | 80 |
| 0.1 | *** | 433 | 438 | 495 | 230 | 235 | 263 | 152 | 157 | 172 | 113 | 116 | 126 | 90 | 92 | 99 |
|  | *** | 435 | 447 | 651 | 232 | 242 | 322 | 154 | 161 | 196 | 114 | 120 | 133 | 91 | 95 | 96 |
| 0.15 | *** | 559 | 567 | 679 | 283 | 291 | 342 | 181 | 188 | 216 | 130 | 136 | 153 | 101 | 106 | 117 |
|  | *** | 562 | 582 | 821 | 286 | 303 | 391 | 183 | 196 | 232 | 132 | 142 | 154 | 103 | 110 | 109 |
| 0.2 | *** | 652 | 664 | 841 | 321 | 333 | 411 | 200 | 210 | 252 | 142 | 150 | 175 | 109 | 115 | 131 |
|  | *** | 656 | 686 | 964 | 325 | 350 | 449 | 204 | 222 | 261 | 145 | 158 | 170 | 111 | 121 | 119 |
| 0.25 | *** | 712 | 729 | 980 | 344 | 360 | 467 | 212 | 226 | 281 | 149 | 159 | 191 | 113 | 121 | 141 |
|  | *** | 718 | 760 | 1081 | 350 | 384 | 495 | 217 | 241 | 284 | 153 | 170 | 183 | 116 | 128 | 126 |
| 0.3 | *** | 743 | 765 | 1092 | 355 | 376 | 512 | 218 | 235 | 303 | 152 | 165 | 204 | 115 | 124 | 148 |
|  | *** | 750 | 806 | 1172 | 363 | 406 | 530 | 224 | 254 | 300 | 157 | 177 | 191 | 119 | 133 | 131 |
| 0.35 | *** | 747 | 776 | 1177 | 356 | 382 | 544 | 218 | 238 | 318 | 152 | 166 | 211 | 114 | 125 | 152 |
|  | *** | 757 | 827 | 1237 | 365 | 417 | 553 | 226 | 260 | 310 | 158 | 181 | 195 | 119 | 134 | 132 |
| 0.4 | *** | 729 | 766 | 1235 | 348 | 380 | 564 | 214 | 237 | 325 | 149 | 165 | 214 | 112 | 123 | 152 |
|  | *** | 741 | 829 | 1276 | 360 | 420 | 565 | 223 | 261 | 313 | 155 | 181 | 195 | 116 | 133 | 131 |
| 0.45 | *** | 692 | 739 | 1263 | 333 | 370 | 570 | 206 | 231 | 326 | 143 | 161 | 212 | 107 | 120 | 149 |
|  | *** | 708 | 813 | 1289 | 347 | 415 | 565 | 216 | 258 | 310 | 151 | 177 | 191 | 113 | 130 | 126 |
| 0.5 | *** | 643 | 699 | 1264 | 314 | 354 | 564 | 195 | 222 | 319 | 136 | 154 | 205 | 102 | 114 | 143 |
|  | *** | 663 | 784 | 1276 | 329 | 403 | 553 | 206 | 250 | 300 | 144 | 171 | 183 | 107 | 125 | 119 |
| 0.55 | *** | 585 | 651 | 1236 | 291 | 334 | 546 | 182 | 210 | 305 | 127 | 145 | 194 | 95 | 107 | 134 |
|  | *** | 609 | 743 | 1237 | 308 | 384 | 530 | 193 | 238 | 284 | 135 | 162 | 170 | 100 | 117 | 109 |
| 0.6 | *** | 523 | 597 | 1180 | 266 | 311 | 515 | 167 | 195 | 284 | 117 | 134 | 178 | 86 | 97 | 121 |
|  | *** | 550 | 694 | 1172 | 283 | 360 | 495 | 179 | 221 | 261 | 124 | 149 | 154 | 91 | 106 | 96 |
| 0.65 | *** | 460 | 539 | 1095 | 239 | 283 | 471 | 151 | 177 | 256 | 105 | 120 | 158 | 76 | 86 | 106 |
|  | *** | 490 | 637 | 1081 | 256 | 330 | 449 | 161 | 201 | 232 | 111 | 134 | 133 | 81 | 94 | 80 |
| 0.7 | *** | 399 | 478 | 983 | 210 | 252 | 415 | 132 | 155 | 221 | 91 | 104 | 134 | . | . | . |
|  | *** | 429 | 573 | 964 | 227 | 295 | 391 | 142 | 177 | 196 | 96 | 115 | 108 | . | . | . |
| 0.75 | *** | 339 | 414 | 843 | 180 | 216 | 347 | 111 | 130 | 179 | . | . | . | . | . | . |
|  | *** | 368 | 500 | 821 | 195 | 253 | 322 | 119 | 147 | 153 | . | . | . | . | . | . |
| 0.8 | *** | 278 | 344 | 676 | 146 | 175 | 266 | . | . | . | . | . | . | . | . | . |
|  | *** | 305 | 418 | 651 | 158 | 203 | 241 | . | . | . | . | . | . | . | . | . |
| 0.85 | *** | 215 | 266 | 482 | . | . | . | . | . | . | . | . | . | . | . | . |
|  | *** | 235 | 320 | 456 | . | . | . | . | . | . | . | . | . | . | . | . |

TABLE 4: ALPHA= 0.01   POWER= 0.9    EXPECTED ACCRUAL THRU MINIMUM FOLLOW-UP= 80

| | | DEL=.10 | | | DEL=.15 | | | DEL=.20 | | | DEL=.25 | | | DEL=.30 | |
|---|---|---|---|---|---|---|---|---|---|---|---|---|---|---|---|
| FACT= | 1.0 .75 | .50 .25 | .00 BIN | 1.0 .75 | .50 .25 | .00 BIN | 1.0 .75 | .50 .25 | .00 BIN | 1.0 75 | .50 .25 | .00 BIN | 1.0 .75 | .50 .25 | .00 BIN |
| PCONT=*** | | | REQUIRED NUMBER OF PATIENTS | | | | | | | | | | | | |
| 0.05 *** | 274 275 | 277 281 | 296 456 | 160 161 | 163 166 | 172 241 | 113 114 | 116 118 | 121 153 | 88 89 | 90 92 | 94 108 | 73 74 | 74 75 | 77 80 |
| 0.1 *** | 434 436 | 439 449 | 495 651 | 231 233 | 236 244 | 263 322 | 153 155 | 158 162 | 172 196 | 113 115 | 117 120 | 126 133 | 90 91 | 93 95 | 99 96 |
| 0.15 *** | 560 564 | 570 586 | 679 821 | 284 288 | 293 306 | 342 391 | 182 185 | 189 198 | 216 232 | 131 134 | 137 143 | 153 154 | 102 104 | 107 110 | 117 109 |
| 0.2 *** | 654 658 | 667 692 | 841 964 | 322 327 | 336 354 | 411 449 | 202 206 | 213 225 | 252 261 | 143 147 | 152 160 | 175 170 | 110 113 | 116 122 | 131 119 |
| 0.25 *** | 715 721 | 734 768 | 980 1081 | 347 353 | 365 389 | 467 495 | 215 220 | 229 244 | 281 284 | 151 155 | 162 172 | 191 183 | 115 118 | 122 129 | 141 126 |
| 0.3 *** | 746 755 | 771 816 | 1092 1172 | 359 367 | 382 412 | 512 530 | 221 228 | 238 257 | 303 300 | 154 160 | 167 179 | 204 191 | 117 121 | 126 134 | 148 131 |
| 0.35 *** | 751 762 | 784 840 | 1177 1237 | 360 371 | 388 425 | 544 553 | 221 230 | 242 264 | 318 310 | 155 161 | 169 183 | 211 195 | 116 121 | 127 136 | 152 132 |
| 0.4 *** | 734 748 | 776 844 | 1235 1276 | 353 366 | 387 428 | 564 565 | 218 227 | 241 266 | 325 313 | 152 159 | 168 184 | 214 195 | 114 119 | 125 135 | 152 131 |
| 0.45 *** | 699 717 | 751 830 | 1263 1289 | 339 354 | 378 424 | 570 565 | 210 221 | 236 263 | 326 310 | 147 154 | 164 180 | 212 191 | 110 115 | 122 132 | 149 126 |
| 0.5 *** | 651 674 | 713 803 | 1264 1276 | 321 337 | 363 412 | 564 553 | 200 211 | 227 255 | 319 300 | 140 147 | 158 174 | 205 183 | 104 109 | 116 126 | 143 119 |
| 0.55 *** | 595 621 | 667 764 | 1236 1237 | 299 316 | 344 394 | 546 530 | 187 199 | 215 243 | 305 284 | 131 138 | 149 164 | 194 170 | 97 102 | 109 118 | 134 109 |
| 0.6 *** | 535 565 | 614 715 | 1180 1172 | 274 292 | 320 370 | 515 495 | 173 184 | 200 226 | 284 261 | 120 127 | 137 152 | 178 154 | 89 93 | 99 108 | 121 96 |
| 0.65 *** | 474 505 | 556 658 | 1095 1081 | 247 265 | 292 339 | 471 449 | 156 166 | 182 205 | 256 232 | 108 114 | 123 136 | 158 133 | 78 83 | 88 95 | 106 80 |
| 0.7 *** | 412 445 | 495 592 | 983 964 | 218 235 | 260 303 | 415 391 | 137 146 | 160 180 | 221 196 | 93 99 | 106 116 | 134 108 | . . | . . | . . |
| 0.75 *** | 352 383 | 430 518 | 843 821 | 187 202 | 223 260 | 347 322 | 115 123 | 134 150 | 179 153 | . . | . . | . . | . . | . . | . . |
| 0.8 *** | 290 317 | 358 432 | 676 651 | 151 164 | 181 208 | 266 241 | . . | . . | . . | . . | . . | . . | . . | . . | . . |
| 0.85 *** | 224 245 | 276 330 | 482 456 | . . | . . | . . | . . | . . | . . | . . | . . | . . | . . | . . | . . |

## TABLE 4: ALPHA= 0.01  POWER= 0.9    EXPECTED ACCRUAL THRU MINIMUM FOLLOW-UP= 90

| | | DEL=.10 | | | DEL=.15 | | | DEL=.20 | | | DEL=.25 | | | DEL=.30 | | |
|---|---|---|---|---|---|---|---|---|---|---|---|---|---|---|---|---|
| FACT= | | 1.0 .75 | .50 .25 | .00 BIN | 1.0 .75 | .50 .25 | .00 BIN | 1.0 .75 | .50 .25 | .00 BIN | 1.0 75 | .50 .25 | .00 BIN | 1.0 .75 | .50 .25 | .00 BIN |
| PCONT=*** | | | | | REQUIRED NUMBER OF PATIENTS | | | | | | | | | | | |
| 0.05 | *** | 275 | 278 | 296 | 161 | 163 | 172 | 114 | 116 | 121 | 89 | 90 | 94 | 73 | 75 | 77 |
| | *** | 276 | 282 | 456 | 162 | 166 | 241 | 115 | 118 | 153 | 89 | 92 | 108 | 74 | 76 | 80 |
| 0.1 | *** | 434 | 441 | 495 | 232 | 238 | 263 | 154 | 158 | 172 | 114 | 118 | 126 | 91 | 93 | 99 |
| | *** | 437 | 451 | 651 | 234 | 245 | 322 | 155 | 163 | 196 | 116 | 121 | 133 | 92 | 96 | 96 |
| 0.15 | *** | 562 | 572 | 679 | 286 | 295 | 342 | 183 | 191 | 216 | 132 | 138 | 153 | 103 | 107 | 117 |
| | *** | 565 | 590 | 821 | 289 | 308 | 391 | 186 | 199 | 232 | 135 | 144 | 154 | 105 | 111 | 109 |
| 0.2 | *** | 655 | 671 | 841 | 324 | 338 | 411 | 204 | 215 | 252 | 145 | 153 | 175 | 111 | 117 | 131 |
| | *** | 661 | 697 | 964 | 329 | 357 | 449 | 208 | 226 | 261 | 148 | 161 | 170 | 114 | 122 | 119 |
| 0.25 | *** | 717 | 738 | 980 | 349 | 368 | 467 | 217 | 231 | 281 | 153 | 163 | 191 | 116 | 124 | 141 |
| | *** | 724 | 775 | 1081 | 356 | 393 | 495 | 222 | 247 | 284 | 157 | 173 | 183 | 119 | 130 | 126 |
| 0.3 | *** | 749 | 777 | 1092 | 362 | 386 | 512 | 223 | 241 | 303 | 156 | 169 | 204 | 118 | 127 | 148 |
| | *** | 759 | 825 | 1172 | 371 | 417 | 530 | 231 | 260 | 300 | 162 | 181 | 191 | 122 | 135 | 131 |
| 0.35 | *** | 755 | 792 | 1177 | 364 | 394 | 544 | 225 | 246 | 318 | 157 | 172 | 211 | 118 | 128 | 152 |
| | *** | 768 | 852 | 1237 | 375 | 431 | 553 | 233 | 268 | 310 | 163 | 185 | 195 | 123 | 137 | 132 |
| 0.4 | *** | 739 | 785 | 1235 | 358 | 393 | 564 | 221 | 246 | 325 | 155 | 171 | 214 | 116 | 127 | 152 |
| | *** | 755 | 857 | 1276 | 371 | 436 | 565 | 231 | 270 | 313 | 161 | 186 | 195 | 121 | 137 | 131 |
| 0.45 | *** | 706 | 762 | 1263 | 345 | 385 | 570 | 214 | 241 | 326 | 150 | 167 | 212 | 112 | 124 | 149 |
| | *** | 726 | 846 | 1289 | 361 | 432 | 565 | 225 | 267 | 310 | 157 | 183 | 191 | 117 | 133 | 126 |
| 0.5 | *** | 660 | 727 | 1264 | 327 | 371 | 564 | 204 | 232 | 319 | 143 | 161 | 205 | 106 | 118 | 143 |
| | *** | 684 | 820 | 1276 | 345 | 421 | 553 | 216 | 259 | 300 | 150 | 176 | 183 | 111 | 128 | 119 |
| 0.55 | *** | 605 | 682 | 1236 | 306 | 352 | 546 | 192 | 220 | 305 | 134 | 151 | 194 | 99 | 111 | 134 |
| | *** | 634 | 782 | 1237 | 324 | 402 | 530 | 204 | 247 | 284 | 141 | 167 | 170 | 104 | 120 | 109 |
| 0.6 | *** | 547 | 630 | 1180 | 281 | 328 | 515 | 177 | 205 | 284 | 123 | 140 | 178 | 90 | 101 | 121 |
| | *** | 578 | 734 | 1172 | 300 | 378 | 495 | 189 | 230 | 261 | 130 | 154 | 154 | 95 | 109 | 96 |
| 0.65 | *** | 486 | 573 | 1095 | 254 | 300 | 471 | 160 | 186 | 256 | 110 | 125 | 158 | 80 | 89 | 106 |
| | *** | 519 | 676 | 1081 | 273 | 347 | 449 | 171 | 209 | 232 | 117 | 138 | 133 | 84 | 96 | 80 |
| 0.7 | *** | 425 | 511 | 983 | 225 | 268 | 415 | 141 | 163 | 221 | 95 | 108 | 134 | . | . | . |
| | *** | 459 | 610 | 964 | 242 | 310 | 391 | 150 | 183 | 196 | 101 | 118 | 108 | . | . | . |
| 0.75 | *** | 364 | 444 | 843 | 193 | 230 | 347 | 118 | 137 | 179 | . | . | . | . | . | . |
| | *** | 396 | 533 | 821 | 208 | 265 | 322 | 126 | 152 | 153 | . | . | . | . | . | . |
| 0.8 | *** | 301 | 370 | 676 | 156 | 186 | 266 | . | . | . | . | . | . | . | . | . |
| | *** | 329 | 445 | 651 | 169 | 212 | 241 | . | . | . | . | . | . | . | . | . |
| 0.85 | *** | 233 | 286 | 482 | . | . | . | . | . | . | . | . | . | . | . | . |
| | *** | 254 | 339 | 456 | . | . | . | . | . | . | . | . | . | . | . | . |

## TABLE 4: ALPHA= 0.01 POWER= 0.9    EXPECTED ACCRUAL THRU MINIMUM FOLLOW-UP= 100

| | | DEL=.10 | | | DEL=.15 | | | DEL=.20 | | | DEL=.25 | | | DEL=.30 | | |
|---|---|---|---|---|---|---|---|---|---|---|---|---|---|---|---|---|
| FACT= | | 1.0 .75 | .50 .25 | .00 BIN | 1.0 .75 | .50 .25 | .00 BIN | 1.0 .75 | .50 .25 | .00 BIN | 1.0 75 | .50 .25 | .00 BIN | 1.0 .75 | .50 .25 | .00 BIN |
| PCONT=*** | | REQUIRED NUMBER OF PATIENTS | | | | | | | | | | | | | | |
| 0.05 | *** | 275 | 278 | 296 | 161 | 164 | 172 | 114 | 116 | 121 | 89 | 91 | 94 | 74 | 75 | 77 |
| | *** | 276 | 283 | 456 | 162 | 167 | 241 | 115 | 118 | 153 | 90 | 92 | 108 | 74 | 76 | 80 |
| 0.1 | *** | 435 | 442 | 495 | 232 | 239 | 263 | 154 | 159 | 172 | 115 | 118 | 126 | 91 | 94 | 99 |
| | *** | 438 | 453 | 651 | 235 | 246 | 322 | 156 | 164 | 196 | 116 | 121 | 133 | 92 | 96 | 96 |
| 0.15 | *** | 563 | 574 | 679 | 287 | 297 | 342 | 184 | 192 | 216 | 133 | 139 | 153 | 103 | 108 | 117 |
| | *** | 567 | 593 | 821 | 291 | 310 | 391 | 187 | 200 | 232 | 136 | 144 | 154 | 105 | 111 | 109 |
| 0.2 | *** | 657 | 674 | 841 | 326 | 341 | 411 | 205 | 217 | 252 | 146 | 154 | 175 | 112 | 118 | 131 |
| | *** | 663 | 702 | 964 | 332 | 360 | 449 | 210 | 228 | 261 | 149 | 162 | 170 | 115 | 123 | 119 |
| 0.25 | *** | 720 | 743 | 980 | 352 | 372 | 467 | 219 | 234 | 281 | 154 | 165 | 191 | 117 | 125 | 141 |
| | *** | 727 | 782 | 1081 | 359 | 397 | 495 | 225 | 249 | 284 | 159 | 175 | 183 | 120 | 131 | 126 |
| 0.3 | *** | 752 | 783 | 1092 | 365 | 391 | 512 | 226 | 244 | 303 | 158 | 171 | 204 | 120 | 129 | 148 |
| | *** | 763 | 834 | 1172 | 375 | 422 | 530 | 233 | 263 | 300 | 164 | 183 | 191 | 124 | 136 | 131 |
| 0.35 | *** | 760 | 799 | 1177 | 368 | 400 | 544 | 228 | 249 | 318 | 159 | 174 | 211 | 120 | 130 | 152 |
| | *** | 773 | 863 | 1237 | 380 | 437 | 553 | 236 | 271 | 310 | 165 | 187 | 195 | 124 | 138 | 132 |
| 0.4 | *** | 745 | 795 | 1235 | 363 | 400 | 564 | 225 | 249 | 325 | 157 | 173 | 214 | 118 | 129 | 152 |
| | *** | 762 | 870 | 1276 | 377 | 442 | 565 | 235 | 273 | 313 | 164 | 188 | 195 | 122 | 138 | 131 |
| 0.45 | *** | 713 | 773 | 1263 | 351 | 392 | 570 | 218 | 245 | 326 | 152 | 170 | 212 | 114 | 125 | 149 |
| | *** | 734 | 860 | 1289 | 367 | 439 | 565 | 229 | 271 | 310 | 160 | 185 | 191 | 119 | 135 | 126 |
| 0.5 | *** | 668 | 739 | 1264 | 333 | 379 | 564 | 209 | 237 | 319 | 146 | 163 | 205 | 108 | 120 | 143 |
| | *** | 694 | 836 | 1276 | 351 | 428 | 553 | 220 | 263 | 300 | 153 | 178 | 183 | 113 | 129 | 119 |
| 0.55 | *** | 615 | 696 | 1236 | 312 | 360 | 546 | 196 | 224 | 305 | 137 | 154 | 194 | 101 | 112 | 134 |
| | *** | 645 | 799 | 1237 | 331 | 410 | 530 | 208 | 251 | 284 | 144 | 169 | 170 | 106 | 121 | 109 |
| 0.6 | *** | 558 | 644 | 1180 | 288 | 336 | 515 | 181 | 209 | 284 | 126 | 142 | 178 | 92 | 102 | 121 |
| | *** | 591 | 751 | 1172 | 307 | 385 | 495 | 193 | 234 | 261 | 133 | 156 | 154 | 97 | 110 | 96 |
| 0.65 | *** | 498 | 588 | 1095 | 261 | 307 | 471 | 164 | 190 | 256 | 113 | 127 | 158 | 82 | 90 | 106 |
| | *** | 533 | 693 | 1081 | 280 | 354 | 449 | 175 | 212 | 232 | 119 | 139 | 133 | 86 | 97 | 80 |
| 0.7 | *** | 437 | 525 | 983 | 231 | 274 | 415 | 144 | 167 | 221 | 98 | 110 | 134 | . | . | . |
| | *** | 472 | 625 | 964 | 249 | 316 | 391 | 154 | 186 | 196 | 103 | 119 | 108 | . | . | . |
| 0.75 | *** | 375 | 457 | 843 | 198 | 235 | 347 | 121 | 139 | 179 | . | . | . | . | . | . |
| | *** | 408 | 547 | 821 | 214 | 270 | 322 | 129 | 154 | 153 | . | . | . | . | . | . |
| 0.8 | *** | 311 | 382 | 676 | 161 | 190 | 266 | . | . | . | . | . | . | . | . | . |
| | *** | 339 | 456 | 651 | 173 | 216 | 241 | . | . | . | . | . | . | . | . | . |
| 0.85 | *** | 240 | 294 | 482 | . | . | . | . | . | . | . | . | . | . | . | . |
| | *** | 262 | 347 | 456 | . | . | . | . | . | . | . | . | . | . | . | . |

## TABLE 4: ALPHA= 0.01 POWER= 0.9  EXPECTED ACCRUAL THRU MINIMUM FOLLOW-UP= 110

| | | DEL=.05 | | | DEL=.10 | | | DEL=.15 | | | DEL=.20 | | | DEL=.25 | | |
|---|---|---|---|---|---|---|---|---|---|---|---|---|---|---|---|---|---|
| FACT= | | 1.0 .75 | .50 .25 | .00 BIN | 1.0 .75 | .50 .25 | .00 BIN | 1.0 .75 | .50 .25 | .00 BIN | 1.0 75 | .50 .25 | .00 BIN | 1.0 .75 | .50 .25 | .00 BIN |
| PCONT=*** | | | | | | | | REQUIRED NUMBER OF PATIENTS | | | | | | | | |
| 0.05 | *** | 777 | 780 | 832 | 276 | 279 | 296 | 161 | 164 | 172 | 114 | 116 | 121 | 89 | 91 | 94 |
| | *** | 778 | 786 | 1432 | 277 | 283 | 456 | 163 | 167 | 241 | 115 | 118 | 153 | 90 | 92 | 108 |
| 0.1 | *** | 1416 | 1423 | 1604 | 436 | 443 | 495 | 233 | 240 | 263 | 155 | 160 | 172 | 115 | 119 | 126 |
| | *** | 1418 | 1435 | 2265 | 438 | 455 | 651 | 236 | 247 | 322 | 157 | 164 | 196 | 117 | 122 | 133 |
| 0.15 | *** | 1958 | 1969 | 2351 | 564 | 576 | 679 | 288 | 299 | 342 | 185 | 193 | 215 | 134 | 140 | 153 |
| | *** | 1962 | 1991 | 2994 | 568 | 596 | 821 | 292 | 311 | 391 | 188 | 201 | 232 | 136 | 145 | 154 |
| 0.2 | *** | 2376 | 2392 | 3033 | 659 | 677 | 841 | 328 | 344 | 411 | 207 | 218 | 252 | 147 | 155 | 175 |
| | *** | 2381 | 2425 | 3619 | 665 | 707 | 964 | 334 | 362 | 449 | 211 | 230 | 261 | 151 | 163 | 170 |
| 0.25 | *** | 2664 | 2687 | 3629 | 722 | 747 | 980 | 354 | 375 | 467 | 221 | 236 | 281 | 156 | 166 | 191 |
| | *** | 2672 | 2733 | 4140 | 731 | 788 | 1081 | 362 | 400 | 495 | 227 | 251 | 284 | 160 | 176 | 183 |
| 0.3 | *** | 2828 | 2859 | 4127 | 756 | 789 | 1092 | 368 | 395 | 512 | 228 | 247 | 303 | 160 | 173 | 203 |
| | *** | 2838 | 2922 | 4556 | 767 | 842 | 1172 | 378 | 427 | 530 | 236 | 265 | 300 | 166 | 184 | 191 |
| 0.35 | *** | 2877 | 2919 | 4519 | 764 | 807 | 1177 | 372 | 405 | 544 | 230 | 253 | 318 | 161 | 176 | 211 |
| | *** | 2891 | 3002 | 4869 | 779 | 873 | 1237 | 384 | 442 | 553 | 239 | 274 | 310 | 168 | 189 | 195 |
| 0.4 | *** | 2827 | 2881 | 4802 | 750 | 804 | 1235 | 367 | 405 | 564 | 228 | 253 | 325 | 159 | 176 | 214 |
| | *** | 2845 | 2988 | 5077 | 769 | 882 | 1276 | 382 | 448 | 565 | 238 | 276 | 313 | 166 | 189 | 195 |
| 0.45 | *** | 2692 | 2762 | 4973 | 719 | 784 | 1263 | 356 | 399 | 570 | 222 | 249 | 326 | 155 | 172 | 212 |
| | *** | 2715 | 2899 | 5181 | 743 | 874 | 1289 | 373 | 445 | 565 | 233 | 274 | 310 | 162 | 186 | 191 |
| 0.5 | *** | 2490 | 2579 | 5031 | 676 | 751 | 1264 | 339 | 385 | 564 | 212 | 240 | 319 | 148 | 165 | 205 |
| | *** | 2520 | 2751 | 5181 | 704 | 850 | 1276 | 358 | 435 | 553 | 224 | 266 | 300 | 155 | 180 | 183 |
| 0.55 | *** | 2240 | 2353 | 4975 | 625 | 709 | 1236 | 318 | 367 | 546 | 200 | 228 | 305 | 139 | 156 | 194 |
| | *** | 2278 | 2562 | 5077 | 656 | 814 | 1237 | 338 | 417 | 530 | 212 | 254 | 284 | 146 | 170 | 170 |
| 0.6 | *** | 1959 | 2101 | 4806 | 568 | 658 | 1180 | 294 | 343 | 515 | 185 | 212 | 284 | 128 | 144 | 178 |
| | *** | 2008 | 2347 | 4869 | 603 | 766 | 1172 | 314 | 392 | 495 | 197 | 237 | 261 | 135 | 157 | 154 |
| 0.65 | *** | 1669 | 1843 | 4524 | 509 | 601 | 1095 | 267 | 314 | 471 | 168 | 193 | 256 | 115 | 129 | 158 |
| | *** | 1730 | 2118 | 4556 | 545 | 708 | 1081 | 286 | 360 | 449 | 178 | 215 | 232 | 121 | 140 | 133 |
| 0.7 | *** | 1389 | 1591 | 4130 | 448 | 539 | 983 | 237 | 280 | 415 | 147 | 170 | 221 | 99 | 111 | 134 |
| | *** | 1462 | 1882 | 4140 | 484 | 639 | 964 | 255 | 321 | 391 | 157 | 188 | 196 | 105 | 120 | 108 |
| 0.75 | *** | 1134 | 1350 | 3626 | 386 | 469 | 843 | 203 | 240 | 347 | 124 | 142 | 179 | . | . | . |
| | *** | 1215 | 1640 | 3619 | 419 | 560 | 821 | 219 | 275 | 322 | 131 | 156 | 153 | . | . | . |
| 0.8 | *** | 908 | 1120 | 3011 | 320 | 392 | 676 | 165 | 194 | 266 | . | . | . | . | . | . |
| | *** | 989 | 1388 | 2994 | 349 | 466 | 651 | 177 | 219 | 241 | . | . | . | . | . | . |
| 0.85 | *** | 703 | 890 | 2288 | 248 | 301 | 482 | . | . | . | . | . | . | . | . | . |
| | *** | 776 | 1115 | 2265 | 270 | 354 | 456 | . | . | . | . | . | . | . | . | . |
| 0.9 | *** | 501 | 640 | 1458 | . | . | . | . | . | . | . | . | . | . | . | . |
| | *** | 556 | 799 | 1432 | . | . | . | . | . | . | . | . | . | . | . | . |

## TABLE 4: ALPHA= 0.01  POWER= 0.9    EXPECTED ACCRUAL THRU MINIMUM FOLLOW-UP= 120

| | | DEL=.05 | | | DEL=.10 | | | DEL=.15 | | | DEL=.20 | | | DEL=.25 | | |
|---|---|---|---|---|---|---|---|---|---|---|---|---|---|---|---|---|---|
| FACT= | | 1.0 .75 | .50 .25 | .00 BIN | 1.0 .75 | .50 .25 | .00 BIN | 1.0 .75 | .50 .25 | .00 BIN | 1.0 75 | .50 .25 | .00 BIN | 1.0 .75 | .50 .25 | .00 BIN |
| PCONT=*** | | \multicolumn{16}{REQUIRED NUMBER OF PATIENTS} | | | | | | | | | | | | | | |
| 0.05 | *** | 777 | 780 | 832 | 276 | 279 | 296 | 162 | 165 | 172 | 115 | 117 | 121 | 89 | 91 | 94 |
| | *** | 778 | 787 | 1432 | 277 | 284 | 456 | 163 | 167 | 241 | 115 | 118 | 153 | 90 | 92 | 108 |
| 0.1 | *** | 1417 | 1424 | 1604 | 437 | 445 | 495 | 234 | 240 | 263 | 155 | 160 | 172 | 116 | 119 | 126 |
| | *** | 1419 | 1438 | 2265 | 439 | 456 | 651 | 236 | 248 | 322 | 157 | 165 | 196 | 117 | 122 | 133 |
| 0.15 | *** | 1959 | 1971 | 2351 | 565 | 578 | 679 | 289 | 300 | 342 | 186 | 194 | 216 | 135 | 141 | 153 |
| | *** | 1963 | 1994 | 2994 | 570 | 599 | 821 | 293 | 313 | 391 | 189 | 202 | 232 | 137 | 145 | 154 |
| 0.2 | *** | 2377 | 2395 | 3033 | 661 | 680 | 841 | 329 | 346 | 411 | 208 | 220 | 252 | 148 | 156 | 175 |
| | *** | 2383 | 2431 | 3619 | 667 | 711 | 964 | 336 | 365 | 449 | 213 | 231 | 261 | 152 | 163 | 170 |
| 0.25 | *** | 2666 | 2691 | 3629 | 724 | 751 | 980 | 356 | 378 | 467 | 222 | 238 | 281 | 157 | 168 | 191 |
| | *** | 2674 | 2742 | 4140 | 734 | 794 | 1081 | 364 | 403 | 495 | 229 | 253 | 284 | 162 | 177 | 183 |
| 0.3 | *** | 2830 | 2865 | 4127 | 759 | 795 | 1092 | 371 | 399 | 512 | 231 | 250 | 303 | 162 | 175 | 203 |
| | *** | 2842 | 2933 | 4556 | 771 | 850 | 1172 | 382 | 430 | 530 | 238 | 268 | 300 | 167 | 185 | 191 |
| 0.35 | *** | 2881 | 2926 | 4519 | 768 | 814 | 1177 | 375 | 409 | 544 | 233 | 255 | 318 | 163 | 178 | 211 |
| | *** | 2896 | 3017 | 4869 | 784 | 882 | 1237 | 388 | 447 | 553 | 242 | 276 | 310 | 169 | 190 | 195 |
| 0.4 | *** | 2832 | 2891 | 4802 | 755 | 812 | 1234 | 371 | 411 | 564 | 231 | 256 | 325 | 161 | 177 | 214 |
| | *** | 2851 | 3008 | 5077 | 776 | 893 | 1276 | 387 | 453 | 565 | 241 | 279 | 313 | 168 | 191 | 195 |
| 0.45 | *** | 2698 | 2774 | 4973 | 726 | 794 | 1263 | 361 | 404 | 570 | 225 | 252 | 326 | 157 | 174 | 212 |
| | *** | 2724 | 2923 | 5181 | 751 | 886 | 1289 | 378 | 451 | 565 | 236 | 277 | 310 | 164 | 188 | 191 |
| 0.5 | *** | 2498 | 2595 | 5031 | 684 | 763 | 1264 | 345 | 392 | 564 | 216 | 244 | 319 | 150 | 167 | 205 |
| | *** | 2531 | 2780 | 5181 | 713 | 864 | 1276 | 363 | 441 | 553 | 227 | 269 | 300 | 158 | 182 | 183 |
| 0.55 | *** | 2250 | 2373 | 4975 | 634 | 721 | 1236 | 324 | 373 | 546 | 204 | 232 | 305 | 141 | 158 | 194 |
| | *** | 2291 | 2596 | 5077 | 667 | 828 | 1237 | 344 | 423 | 530 | 215 | 257 | 284 | 149 | 172 | 170 |
| 0.6 | *** | 1973 | 2126 | 4806 | 578 | 671 | 1180 | 300 | 349 | 515 | 189 | 216 | 284 | 130 | 146 | 178 |
| | *** | 2025 | 2386 | 4869 | 614 | 780 | 1172 | 320 | 398 | 495 | 200 | 240 | 261 | 137 | 158 | 154 |
| 0.65 | *** | 1686 | 1872 | 4524 | 519 | 614 | 1095 | 273 | 320 | 471 | 171 | 196 | 256 | 117 | 131 | 158 |
| | *** | 1751 | 2160 | 4556 | 556 | 722 | 1081 | 292 | 366 | 449 | 181 | 217 | 232 | 123 | 142 | 133 |
| 0.7 | *** | 1410 | 1622 | 4130 | 459 | 551 | 983 | 242 | 285 | 415 | 150 | 172 | 221 | 101 | 112 | 134 |
| | *** | 1487 | 1925 | 4140 | 495 | 652 | 964 | 260 | 326 | 391 | 160 | 190 | 196 | 106 | 121 | 108 |
| 0.75 | *** | 1157 | 1383 | 3626 | 396 | 481 | 843 | 208 | 245 | 347 | 126 | 144 | 179 | . | . | . |
| | *** | 1242 | 1681 | 3619 | 430 | 571 | 821 | 223 | 279 | 322 | 134 | 157 | 153 | . | . | . |
| 0.8 | *** | 931 | 1151 | 3011 | 329 | 401 | 676 | 169 | 197 | 266 | . | . | . | . | . | . |
| | *** | 1015 | 1425 | 2994 | 358 | 475 | 651 | 181 | 222 | 241 | . | . | . | . | . | . |
| 0.85 | *** | 725 | 916 | 2288 | 254 | 308 | 482 | . | . | . | . | . | . | . | . | . |
| | *** | 799 | 1146 | 2265 | 276 | 360 | 456 | . | . | . | . | . | . | . | . | . |
| 0.9 | *** | 517 | 659 | 1458 | . | . | . | . | . | . | . | . | . | . | . | . |
| | *** | 573 | 820 | 1432 | . | . | . | . | . | . | . | . | . | . | . | . |

# TABLE 4: ALPHA= 0.01 POWER= 0.9 EXPECTED ACCRUAL THRU MINIMUM FOLLOW-UP= 130

| | | DEL=.05 | | | DEL=.10 | | | DEL=.15 | | | DEL=.20 | | | DEL=.25 | | |
|---|---|---|---|---|---|---|---|---|---|---|---|---|---|---|---|---|---|
| FACT= | | 1.0 .75 | .50 .25 | .00 BIN | 1.0 .75 | .50 .25 | .00 BIN | 1.0 .75 | .50 .25 | .00 BIN | 1.0 75 | .50 .25 | .00 BIN | 1.0 .75 | .50 .25 | .00 BIN |
| PCONT=*** | | | | | | REQUIRED NUMBER OF PATIENTS | | | | | | | | | | |
| 0.05 | *** | 778 | 781 | 832 | 276 | 280 | 296 | 162 | 165 | 172 | 115 | 117 | 121 | 90 | 91 | 94 |
| | *** | 779 | 788 | 1432 | 278 | 285 | 456 | 163 | 168 | 241 | 116 | 119 | 153 | 90 | 92 | 108 |
| 0.1 | *** | 1418 | 1425 | 1604 | 437 | 446 | 495 | 235 | 241 | 263 | 156 | 161 | 172 | 116 | 120 | 126 |
| | *** | 1420 | 1440 | 2265 | 440 | 458 | 651 | 237 | 248 | 322 | 158 | 165 | 196 | 118 | 122 | 133 |
| 0.15 | *** | 1960 | 1973 | 2351 | 566 | 580 | 679 | 290 | 302 | 342 | 187 | 195 | 216 | 135 | 141 | 153 |
| | *** | 1964 | 1998 | 2994 | 571 | 602 | 821 | 295 | 314 | 391 | 190 | 203 | 232 | 138 | 146 | 154 |
| 0.2 | *** | 2379 | 2398 | 3033 | 662 | 683 | 841 | 331 | 348 | 411 | 209 | 221 | 252 | 149 | 157 | 175 |
| | *** | 2385 | 2437 | 3619 | 670 | 716 | 964 | 338 | 367 | 449 | 214 | 232 | 261 | 153 | 164 | 170 |
| 0.25 | *** | 2668 | 2696 | 3629 | 727 | 756 | 980 | 358 | 381 | 467 | 224 | 240 | 281 | 158 | 169 | 191 |
| | *** | 2677 | 2750 | 4140 | 737 | 800 | 1081 | 367 | 406 | 495 | 230 | 254 | 284 | 163 | 178 | 183 |
| 0.3 | *** | 2833 | 2870 | 4127 | 762 | 800 | 1092 | 374 | 402 | 512 | 233 | 252 | 303 | 163 | 176 | 204 |
| | *** | 2846 | 2944 | 4556 | 775 | 858 | 1172 | 385 | 434 | 530 | 240 | 269 | 300 | 169 | 187 | 191 |
| 0.35 | *** | 2885 | 2934 | 4519 | 772 | 821 | 1177 | 379 | 413 | 544 | 236 | 258 | 318 | 165 | 179 | 211 |
| | *** | 2901 | 3032 | 4869 | 789 | 891 | 1237 | 392 | 451 | 553 | 245 | 278 | 310 | 171 | 191 | 195 |
| 0.4 | *** | 2837 | 2900 | 4802 | 761 | 821 | 1234 | 376 | 415 | 564 | 234 | 259 | 325 | 163 | 179 | 214 |
| | *** | 2858 | 3027 | 5077 | 782 | 903 | 1276 | 391 | 458 | 565 | 244 | 282 | 313 | 170 | 192 | 195 |
| 0.45 | *** | 2705 | 2787 | 4973 | 732 | 804 | 1263 | 365 | 410 | 570 | 228 | 255 | 326 | 159 | 176 | 212 |
| | *** | 2732 | 2947 | 5181 | 759 | 898 | 1289 | 383 | 456 | 565 | 239 | 279 | 310 | 166 | 189 | 191 |
| 0.5 | *** | 2507 | 2611 | 5031 | 692 | 773 | 1264 | 350 | 397 | 564 | 219 | 247 | 319 | 152 | 169 | 205 |
| | *** | 2542 | 2809 | 5181 | 722 | 876 | 1276 | 369 | 446 | 553 | 231 | 272 | 300 | 160 | 183 | 183 |
| 0.55 | *** | 2260 | 2393 | 4975 | 642 | 732 | 1236 | 329 | 379 | 546 | 207 | 235 | 305 | 143 | 160 | 194 |
| | *** | 2305 | 2629 | 5077 | 677 | 841 | 1237 | 349 | 428 | 530 | 219 | 259 | 284 | 151 | 173 | 170 |
| 0.6 | *** | 1986 | 2150 | 4806 | 587 | 683 | 1180 | 305 | 355 | 515 | 192 | 219 | 284 | 132 | 148 | 178 |
| | *** | 2042 | 2423 | 4869 | 625 | 794 | 1172 | 326 | 403 | 495 | 203 | 242 | 261 | 139 | 160 | 154 |
| 0.65 | *** | 1703 | 1900 | 4524 | 529 | 626 | 1095 | 278 | 325 | 471 | 174 | 199 | 256 | 119 | 132 | 158 |
| | *** | 1772 | 2200 | 4556 | 567 | 735 | 1081 | 298 | 371 | 449 | 184 | 220 | 232 | 125 | 143 | 133 |
| 0.7 | *** | 1430 | 1653 | 4130 | 469 | 562 | 983 | 247 | 290 | 415 | 153 | 174 | 221 | 102 | 114 | 134 |
| | *** | 1511 | 1965 | 4140 | 506 | 664 | 964 | 265 | 330 | 391 | 162 | 192 | 196 | 107 | 122 | 108 |
| 0.75 | *** | 1179 | 1414 | 3626 | 405 | 491 | 843 | 212 | 249 | 347 | 128 | 145 | 179 | . | . | . |
| | *** | 1268 | 1720 | 3619 | 440 | 581 | 821 | 228 | 282 | 322 | 136 | 159 | 153 | . | . | . |
| 0.8 | *** | 954 | 1180 | 3011 | 337 | 410 | 676 | 172 | 200 | 266 | . | . | . | . | . | . |
| | *** | 1041 | 1460 | 2994 | 366 | 483 | 651 | 184 | 224 | 241 | . | . | . | . | . | . |
| 0.85 | *** | 745 | 941 | 2288 | 260 | 314 | 482 | . | . | . | . | . | . | . | . | . |
| | *** | 821 | 1174 | 2265 | 283 | 366 | 456 | . | . | . | . | . | . | . | . | . |
| 0.9 | *** | 532 | 677 | 1458 | . | . | . | . | . | . | . | . | . | . | . | . |
| | *** | 589 | 840 | 1432 | . | . | . | . | . | . | . | . | . | . | . | . |

TABLE 4: ALPHA= 0.01  POWER= 0.9     EXPECTED ACCRUAL THRU MINIMUM FOLLOW-UP= 140

| | | DEL=.05 | | | DEL=.10 | | | DEL=.15 | | | DEL=.20 | | | DEL=.25 | | |
|---|---|---|---|---|---|---|---|---|---|---|---|---|---|---|---|---|---|
| FACT= | | 1.0 .75 | .50 .25 | .00 BIN | 1.0 .75 | .50 .25 | .00 BIN | 1.0 .75 | .50 .25 | .00 BIN | 1.0 75 | .50 .25 | .00 BIN | 1.0 .75 | .50 .25 | .00 BIN |
| PCONT=*** | | | | | | REQUIRED NUMBER OF PATIENTS | | | | | | | | | | |
| 0.05 | *** | 778 | 782 | 832 | 277 | 280 | 296 | 162 | 165 | 172 | 115 | 117 | 121 | 90 | 91 | 94 |
| | *** | 779 | 789 | 1432 | 278 | 285 | 456 | 164 | 168 | 241 | 116 | 119 | 153 | 90 | 92 | 108 |
| 0.1 | *** | 1418 | 1426 | 1604 | 438 | 447 | 495 | 235 | 242 | 263 | 157 | 161 | 172 | 116 | 120 | 126 |
| | *** | 1421 | 1442 | 2265 | 441 | 459 | 651 | 238 | 249 | 322 | 159 | 166 | 196 | 118 | 123 | 133 |
| 0.15 | *** | 1961 | 1975 | 2351 | 567 | 582 | 679 | 291 | 303 | 342 | 188 | 196 | 216 | 136 | 142 | 153 |
| | *** | 1966 | 2002 | 2994 | 573 | 604 | 821 | 296 | 316 | 391 | 191 | 203 | 232 | 138 | 146 | 154 |
| 0.2 | *** | 2380 | 2401 | 3033 | 664 | 686 | 841 | 333 | 350 | 411 | 210 | 222 | 252 | 150 | 158 | 175 |
| | *** | 2387 | 2443 | 3619 | 672 | 719 | 964 | 339 | 369 | 449 | 215 | 233 | 261 | 154 | 165 | 170 |
| 0.25 | *** | 2670 | 2700 | 3629 | 729 | 760 | 980 | 360 | 384 | 467 | 226 | 241 | 281 | 159 | 170 | 191 |
| | *** | 2680 | 2758 | 4140 | 740 | 805 | 1081 | 370 | 409 | 495 | 232 | 255 | 284 | 164 | 178 | 183 |
| 0.3 | *** | 2836 | 2876 | 4127 | 765 | 806 | 1092 | 376 | 406 | 512 | 235 | 254 | 303 | 165 | 177 | 204 |
| | *** | 2849 | 2956 | 4556 | 779 | 865 | 1172 | 388 | 437 | 530 | 243 | 271 | 300 | 170 | 187 | 191 |
| 0.35 | *** | 2888 | 2941 | 4519 | 776 | 827 | 1177 | 382 | 417 | 544 | 238 | 260 | 318 | 167 | 181 | 211 |
| | *** | 2906 | 3046 | 4869 | 794 | 899 | 1237 | 396 | 455 | 553 | 247 | 280 | 310 | 173 | 192 | 195 |
| 0.4 | *** | 2841 | 2910 | 4802 | 766 | 829 | 1235 | 379 | 420 | 564 | 237 | 261 | 325 | 165 | 181 | 214 |
| | *** | 2864 | 3045 | 5077 | 789 | 913 | 1276 | 396 | 462 | 565 | 247 | 284 | 313 | 172 | 193 | 195 |
| 0.45 | *** | 2711 | 2799 | 4973 | 739 | 813 | 1263 | 370 | 415 | 570 | 231 | 258 | 326 | 161 | 177 | 212 |
| | *** | 2741 | 2970 | 5181 | 766 | 909 | 1289 | 388 | 461 | 565 | 242 | 282 | 310 | 168 | 191 | 191 |
| 0.5 | *** | 2515 | 2627 | 5031 | 699 | 784 | 1264 | 354 | 403 | 564 | 222 | 250 | 319 | 154 | 171 | 205 |
| | *** | 2552 | 2837 | 5181 | 731 | 888 | 1276 | 374 | 451 | 553 | 234 | 274 | 300 | 162 | 184 | 183 |
| 0.55 | *** | 2271 | 2412 | 4975 | 651 | 743 | 1236 | 335 | 384 | 546 | 210 | 238 | 305 | 145 | 162 | 194 |
| | *** | 2319 | 2662 | 5077 | 686 | 853 | 1237 | 355 | 433 | 530 | 222 | 262 | 284 | 152 | 174 | 170 |
| 0.6 | *** | 1999 | 2174 | 4806 | 597 | 694 | 1180 | 311 | 360 | 515 | 195 | 221 | 284 | 134 | 149 | 178 |
| | *** | 2059 | 2459 | 4869 | 635 | 806 | 1172 | 331 | 408 | 495 | 206 | 244 | 261 | 141 | 161 | 154 |
| 0.65 | *** | 1719 | 1927 | 4524 | 539 | 637 | 1095 | 283 | 330 | 471 | 177 | 201 | 256 | 120 | 134 | 158 |
| | *** | 1793 | 2238 | 4556 | 578 | 746 | 1081 | 303 | 375 | 449 | 187 | 221 | 232 | 126 | 144 | 133 |
| 0.7 | *** | 1449 | 1682 | 4130 | 478 | 573 | 983 | 252 | 295 | 415 | 155 | 176 | 221 | 104 | 115 | 134 |
| | *** | 1535 | 2003 | 4140 | 516 | 675 | 964 | 270 | 334 | 391 | 165 | 194 | 196 | 109 | 123 | 108 |
| 0.75 | *** | 1201 | 1443 | 3626 | 414 | 501 | 843 | 216 | 253 | 347 | 130 | 147 | 179 | . | . | . |
| | *** | 1292 | 1756 | 3619 | 449 | 591 | 821 | 232 | 285 | 322 | 138 | 160 | 153 | . | . | . |
| 0.8 | *** | 975 | 1207 | 3011 | 344 | 418 | 676 | 175 | 203 | 266 | . | . | . | . | . | . |
| | *** | 1065 | 1492 | 2994 | 374 | 491 | 651 | 187 | 226 | 241 | . | . | . | . | . | . |
| 0.85 | *** | 764 | 964 | 2288 | 266 | 320 | 482 | . | . | . | . | . | . | . | . | . |
| | *** | 842 | 1201 | 2265 | 288 | 371 | 456 | . | . | . | . | . | . | . | . | . |
| 0.9 | *** | 546 | 694 | 1458 | . | . | . | . | . | . | . | . | . | . | . | . |
| | *** | 605 | 858 | 1432 | . | . | . | . | . | . | . | . | . | . | . | . |

## TABLE 4: ALPHA= 0.01  POWER= 0.9    EXPECTED ACCRUAL THRU MINIMUM FOLLOW-UP= 150

| | | DEL=.05 | | | DEL=.10 | | | DEL=.15 | | | DEL=.20 | | | DEL=.25 | | |
|---|---|---|---|---|---|---|---|---|---|---|---|---|---|---|---|---|---|
| FACT= | | 1.0 .75 | .50 .25 | .00 BIN | 1.0 .75 | .50 .25 | .00 BIN | 1.0 .75 | .50 .25 | .00 BIN | 1.0 75 | .50 .25 | .00 BIN | 1.0 .75 | .50 .25 | .00 BIN |
| PCONT=*** | | | | | | | REQUIRED NUMBER OF PATIENTS | | | | | | | | | |
| 0.05 | *** | 778 | 782 | 832 | 277 | 281 | 296 | 163 | 166 | 172 | 115 | 117 | 121 | 90 | 91 | 94 |
| | *** | 779 | 790 | 1432 | 278 | 286 | 456 | 164 | 168 | 241 | 116 | 119 | 153 | 91 | 92 | 108 |
| 0.1 | *** | 1419 | 1427 | 1604 | 439 | 448 | 495 | 236 | 243 | 263 | 157 | 162 | 172 | 117 | 120 | 126 |
| | *** | 1422 | 1444 | 2265 | 442 | 460 | 651 | 239 | 250 | 322 | 159 | 166 | 196 | 118 | 123 | 133 |
| 0.15 | *** | 1962 | 1977 | 2351 | 568 | 584 | 679 | 292 | 304 | 342 | 188 | 197 | 215 | 137 | 142 | 153 |
| | *** | 1967 | 2006 | 2994 | 574 | 607 | 821 | 297 | 317 | 391 | 192 | 204 | 232 | 139 | 147 | 154 |
| 0.2 | *** | 2382 | 2404 | 3033 | 666 | 689 | 841 | 334 | 352 | 411 | 212 | 223 | 252 | 151 | 159 | 175 |
| | *** | 2389 | 2448 | 3619 | 674 | 723 | 964 | 341 | 370 | 449 | 217 | 234 | 261 | 154 | 165 | 170 |
| 0.25 | *** | 2672 | 2704 | 3629 | 731 | 764 | 980 | 362 | 386 | 467 | 227 | 243 | 281 | 160 | 171 | 191 |
| | *** | 2683 | 2767 | 4140 | 743 | 811 | 1081 | 372 | 411 | 495 | 234 | 257 | 284 | 165 | 179 | 183 |
| 0.3 | *** | 2839 | 2882 | 4127 | 768 | 811 | 1092 | 379 | 409 | 512 | 236 | 256 | 303 | 166 | 178 | 203 |
| | *** | 2853 | 2967 | 4556 | 783 | 871 | 1172 | 391 | 440 | 530 | 244 | 272 | 300 | 171 | 188 | 191 |
| 0.35 | *** | 2892 | 2949 | 4519 | 780 | 834 | 1177 | 385 | 421 | 544 | 240 | 262 | 318 | 168 | 182 | 211 |
| | *** | 2911 | 3061 | 4869 | 799 | 907 | 1237 | 400 | 458 | 553 | 249 | 282 | 310 | 174 | 193 | 195 |
| 0.4 | *** | 2846 | 2920 | 4802 | 771 | 836 | 1234 | 383 | 424 | 564 | 239 | 264 | 325 | 167 | 182 | 214 |
| | *** | 2871 | 3064 | 5077 | 795 | 922 | 1276 | 400 | 466 | 565 | 249 | 286 | 313 | 173 | 194 | 195 |
| 0.45 | *** | 2717 | 2812 | 4973 | 745 | 822 | 1263 | 374 | 419 | 570 | 234 | 260 | 326 | 163 | 179 | 212 |
| | *** | 2749 | 2993 | 5181 | 773 | 919 | 1289 | 392 | 465 | 565 | 245 | 284 | 310 | 170 | 192 | 191 |
| 0.5 | *** | 2523 | 2643 | 5031 | 706 | 793 | 1264 | 359 | 407 | 564 | 225 | 252 | 319 | 156 | 172 | 205 |
| | *** | 2563 | 2864 | 5181 | 739 | 899 | 1276 | 379 | 455 | 553 | 236 | 276 | 300 | 163 | 185 | 183 |
| 0.55 | *** | 2281 | 2432 | 4975 | 659 | 754 | 1236 | 339 | 389 | 546 | 213 | 240 | 305 | 147 | 163 | 194 |
| | *** | 2332 | 2693 | 5077 | 695 | 864 | 1237 | 360 | 438 | 530 | 224 | 264 | 284 | 154 | 175 | 170 |
| 0.6 | *** | 2012 | 2197 | 4806 | 605 | 705 | 1180 | 315 | 365 | 515 | 197 | 224 | 284 | 135 | 150 | 178 |
| | *** | 2076 | 2493 | 4869 | 644 | 817 | 1172 | 336 | 412 | 495 | 209 | 246 | 261 | 142 | 162 | 154 |
| 0.65 | *** | 1735 | 1953 | 4524 | 548 | 648 | 1095 | 288 | 335 | 471 | 179 | 203 | 256 | 122 | 135 | 158 |
| | *** | 1813 | 2274 | 4556 | 587 | 757 | 1081 | 307 | 379 | 449 | 190 | 223 | 232 | 127 | 144 | 133 |
| 0.7 | *** | 1468 | 1710 | 4130 | 487 | 583 | 983 | 256 | 299 | 415 | 158 | 178 | 221 | 105 | 116 | 134 |
| | *** | 1558 | 2039 | 4140 | 525 | 685 | 964 | 274 | 338 | 391 | 167 | 195 | 196 | 110 | 123 | 108 |
| 0.75 | *** | 1222 | 1471 | 3626 | 422 | 509 | 843 | 220 | 256 | 347 | 132 | 148 | 179 | . | . | . |
| | *** | 1316 | 1791 | 3619 | 457 | 599 | 821 | 235 | 288 | 322 | 139 | 161 | 153 | . | . | . |
| 0.8 | *** | 996 | 1233 | 3011 | 351 | 425 | 676 | 178 | 205 | 266 | . | . | . | . | . | . |
| | *** | 1087 | 1523 | 2994 | 382 | 498 | 651 | 190 | 228 | 241 | . | . | . | . | . | . |
| 0.85 | *** | 782 | 986 | 2288 | 271 | 325 | 482 | . | . | . | . | . | . | . | . | . |
| | *** | 862 | 1226 | 2265 | 294 | 375 | 456 | . | . | . | . | . | . | . | . | . |
| 0.9 | *** | 560 | 709 | 1458 | . | . | . | . | . | . | . | . | . | . | . | . |
| | *** | 619 | 874 | 1432 | . | . | . | . | . | . | . | . | . | . | . | . |

TABLE 4: ALPHA= 0.01  POWER= 0.9    EXPECTED ACCRUAL THRU MINIMUM FOLLOW-UP= 160

| | | DEL=.05 | | | DEL=.10 | | | DEL=.15 | | | DEL=.20 | | | DEL=.25 | | |
|---|---|---|---|---|---|---|---|---|---|---|---|---|---|---|---|---|
| FACT= | | 1.0 .75 | .50 .25 | .00 BIN | 1.0 .75 | .50 .25 | .00 BIN | 1.0 .75 | .50 .25 | .00 BIN | 1.0 75 | .50 .25 | .00 BIN | 1.0 .75 | .50 .25 | .00 BIN |
| PCONT=*** | | | | | REQUIRED | NUMBER OF | PATIENTS | | | | | | | | | |
| 0.05 | *** | 778 | 783 | 832 | 277 | 281 | 296 | 163 | 166 | 172 | 116 | 118 | 121 | 90 | 92 | 94 |
| | *** | 780 | 790 | 1432 | 279 | 286 | 456 | 164 | 168 | 241 | 116 | 119 | 153 | 91 | 93 | 108 |
| 0.1 | *** | 1419 | 1429 | 1604 | 439 | 449 | 495 | 236 | 244 | 263 | 158 | 162 | 172 | 117 | 120 | 126 |
| | *** | 1422 | 1447 | 2265 | 443 | 462 | 651 | 239 | 250 | 322 | 160 | 166 | 196 | 119 | 123 | 133 |
| 0.15 | *** | 1963 | 1979 | 2351 | 570 | 586 | 679 | 293 | 306 | 342 | 189 | 198 | 216 | 137 | 143 | 153 |
| | *** | 1968 | 2010 | 2994 | 575 | 609 | 821 | 298 | 318 | 391 | 193 | 204 | 232 | 140 | 147 | 154 |
| 0.2 | *** | 2383 | 2407 | 3033 | 667 | 692 | 841 | 336 | 354 | 411 | 213 | 225 | 252 | 152 | 160 | 175 |
| | *** | 2391 | 2454 | 3619 | 676 | 727 | 964 | 343 | 372 | 449 | 218 | 235 | 261 | 155 | 166 | 170 |
| 0.25 | *** | 2674 | 2708 | 3629 | 734 | 768 | 980 | 365 | 389 | 467 | 229 | 244 | 281 | 162 | 172 | 191 |
| | *** | 2686 | 2775 | 4140 | 746 | 815 | 1081 | 374 | 414 | 495 | 235 | 258 | 284 | 166 | 180 | 183 |
| 0.3 | *** | 2842 | 2888 | 4127 | 771 | 816 | 1092 | 382 | 412 | 512 | 238 | 257 | 303 | 167 | 179 | 204 |
| | *** | 2857 | 2978 | 4556 | 787 | 877 | 1172 | 394 | 443 | 530 | 246 | 274 | 300 | 173 | 189 | 191 |
| 0.35 | *** | 2896 | 2957 | 4519 | 784 | 840 | 1177 | 388 | 425 | 544 | 242 | 264 | 318 | 169 | 183 | 211 |
| | *** | 2916 | 3076 | 4869 | 804 | 915 | 1237 | 403 | 462 | 553 | 252 | 284 | 310 | 175 | 194 | 195 |
| 0.4 | *** | 2851 | 2930 | 4802 | 776 | 844 | 1235 | 387 | 428 | 564 | 241 | 266 | 325 | 168 | 184 | 214 |
| | *** | 2878 | 3082 | 5077 | 801 | 931 | 1276 | 403 | 470 | 565 | 252 | 287 | 313 | 175 | 195 | 195 |
| 0.45 | *** | 2724 | 2825 | 4973 | 751 | 830 | 1263 | 378 | 424 | 570 | 236 | 263 | 326 | 164 | 180 | 212 |
| | *** | 2757 | 3015 | 5181 | 781 | 928 | 1289 | 397 | 469 | 565 | 247 | 286 | 310 | 171 | 193 | 191 |
| 0.5 | *** | 2531 | 2659 | 5031 | 713 | 803 | 1264 | 363 | 412 | 564 | 227 | 255 | 319 | 158 | 174 | 205 |
| | *** | 2574 | 2890 | 5181 | 747 | 909 | 1276 | 383 | 460 | 553 | 239 | 278 | 300 | 165 | 186 | 183 |
| 0.55 | *** | 2291 | 2451 | 4975 | 667 | 764 | 1236 | 344 | 394 | 546 | 215 | 243 | 305 | 149 | 164 | 194 |
| | *** | 2346 | 2723 | 5077 | 704 | 875 | 1237 | 364 | 442 | 530 | 227 | 266 | 284 | 155 | 176 | 170 |
| 0.6 | *** | 2025 | 2220 | 4806 | 614 | 715 | 1180 | 320 | 370 | 515 | 200 | 226 | 284 | 137 | 152 | 178 |
| | *** | 2093 | 2526 | 4869 | 654 | 828 | 1172 | 341 | 416 | 495 | 211 | 248 | 261 | 143 | 162 | 154 |
| 0.65 | *** | 1751 | 1979 | 4524 | 556 | 658 | 1095 | 292 | 339 | 471 | 182 | 205 | 256 | 123 | 136 | 158 |
| | *** | 1833 | 2308 | 4556 | 597 | 768 | 1081 | 312 | 383 | 449 | 192 | 225 | 232 | 129 | 145 | 133 |
| 0.7 | *** | 1487 | 1738 | 4130 | 495 | 592 | 983 | 260 | 303 | 415 | 160 | 180 | 221 | 106 | 116 | 134 |
| | *** | 1580 | 2074 | 4140 | 534 | 694 | 964 | 278 | 341 | 391 | 169 | 196 | 196 | 111 | 124 | 108 |
| 0.75 | *** | 1242 | 1498 | 3626 | 430 | 518 | 843 | 223 | 260 | 347 | 134 | 150 | 179 | . | . | . |
| | *** | 1339 | 1823 | 3619 | 466 | 608 | 821 | 239 | 291 | 322 | 141 | 162 | 153 | . | . | . |
| 0.8 | *** | 1015 | 1258 | 3011 | 358 | 432 | 676 | 181 | 208 | 266 | . | . | . | . | . | . |
| | *** | 1109 | 1552 | 2994 | 388 | 504 | 651 | 192 | 230 | 241 | . | . | . | . | . | . |
| 0.85 | *** | 799 | 1008 | 2288 | 276 | 330 | 482 | . | . | . | . | . | . | . | . | . |
| | *** | 881 | 1250 | 2265 | 299 | 380 | 456 | . | . | . | . | . | . | . | . | . |
| 0.9 | *** | 573 | 724 | 1458 | . | . | . | . | . | . | . | . | . | . | . | . |
| | *** | 633 | 890 | 1432 | . | . | . | . | . | . | . | . | . | . | . | . |

## TABLE 4: ALPHA= 0.01  POWER= 0.9    EXPECTED ACCRUAL THRU MINIMUM FOLLOW-UP= 170

| | | DEL=.05 | | | DEL=.10 | | | DEL=.15 | | | DEL=.20 | | | DEL=.25 | |
|---|---|---|---|---|---|---|---|---|---|---|---|---|---|---|---|---|
| FACT= | 1.0 .75 | .50 .25 | .00 BIN | 1.0 .75 | .50 .25 | .00 BIN | 1.0 .75 | .50 .25 | .00 BIN | 1.0 75 | .50 .25 | .00 BIN | 1.0 .75 | .50 .25 | .00 BIN |
| PCONT=*** | | | | REQUIRED | NUMBER | OF PATIENTS | | | | | | | | | |
| 0.05  *** | 779 | 783 | 832 | 277 | 282 | 296 | 163 | 166 | 172 | 116 | 118 | 121 | 90 | 92 | 94 |
|        *** | 780 | 791 | 1432 | 279 | 286 | 456 | 164 | 169 | 241 | 117 | 119 | 153 | 91 | 93 | 108 |
| 0.1   *** | 1420 | 1430 | 1604 | 440 | 450 | 495 | 237 | 244 | 263 | 158 | 163 | 172 | 117 | 121 | 126 |
|        *** | 1423 | 1449 | 2265 | 444 | 463 | 651 | 240 | 251 | 322 | 160 | 167 | 196 | 119 | 123 | 133 |
| 0.15  *** | 1964 | 1981 | 2351 | 571 | 588 | 679 | 294 | 307 | 342 | 190 | 198 | 215 | 138 | 143 | 153 |
|        *** | 1970 | 2014 | 2994 | 577 | 611 | 821 | 299 | 319 | 391 | 194 | 205 | 232 | 140 | 147 | 154 |
| 0.2   *** | 2385 | 2410 | 3033 | 669 | 695 | 841 | 337 | 355 | 411 | 214 | 225 | 252 | 152 | 160 | 175 |
|        *** | 2393 | 2460 | 3619 | 678 | 730 | 964 | 344 | 374 | 449 | 219 | 235 | 261 | 156 | 166 | 170 |
| 0.25  *** | 2677 | 2712 | 3629 | 736 | 771 | 980 | 366 | 391 | 467 | 230 | 246 | 281 | 162 | 172 | 191 |
|        *** | 2688 | 2783 | 4140 | 749 | 820 | 1081 | 376 | 416 | 495 | 237 | 259 | 284 | 167 | 180 | 183 |
| 0.3   *** | 2845 | 2893 | 4127 | 774 | 821 | 1092 | 384 | 415 | 512 | 240 | 259 | 303 | 168 | 180 | 203 |
|        *** | 2861 | 2989 | 4556 | 791 | 883 | 1172 | 396 | 446 | 530 | 248 | 275 | 300 | 174 | 190 | 191 |
| 0.35  *** | 2900 | 2964 | 4519 | 788 | 846 | 1177 | 391 | 428 | 544 | 244 | 266 | 318 | 171 | 184 | 211 |
|        *** | 2921 | 3090 | 4869 | 809 | 922 | 1237 | 406 | 465 | 553 | 254 | 285 | 310 | 177 | 195 | 195 |
| 0.4   *** | 2856 | 2940 | 4802 | 781 | 851 | 1235 | 390 | 432 | 564 | 244 | 268 | 325 | 170 | 185 | 214 |
|        *** | 2884 | 3100 | 5077 | 807 | 939 | 1276 | 407 | 473 | 565 | 254 | 289 | 313 | 176 | 196 | 195 |
| 0.45  *** | 2730 | 2837 | 4973 | 757 | 838 | 1263 | 382 | 428 | 570 | 239 | 265 | 326 | 166 | 181 | 212 |
|        *** | 2766 | 3037 | 5181 | 787 | 937 | 1289 | 401 | 473 | 565 | 250 | 287 | 310 | 173 | 194 | 191 |
| 0.5   *** | 2539 | 2674 | 5031 | 720 | 811 | 1264 | 368 | 416 | 564 | 230 | 257 | 319 | 159 | 175 | 205 |
|        *** | 2585 | 2916 | 5181 | 755 | 918 | 1276 | 388 | 463 | 553 | 242 | 280 | 300 | 166 | 187 | 183 |
| 0.55  *** | 2302 | 2470 | 4975 | 674 | 773 | 1236 | 348 | 398 | 546 | 218 | 245 | 305 | 150 | 165 | 194 |
|        *** | 2359 | 2753 | 5077 | 713 | 885 | 1237 | 369 | 446 | 530 | 229 | 267 | 284 | 157 | 177 | 170 |
| 0.6   *** | 2038 | 2242 | 4806 | 622 | 725 | 1180 | 324 | 374 | 515 | 202 | 228 | 284 | 138 | 153 | 178 |
|        *** | 2109 | 2558 | 4869 | 662 | 837 | 1172 | 345 | 420 | 495 | 214 | 249 | 261 | 145 | 163 | 154 |
| 0.65  *** | 1767 | 2004 | 4524 | 565 | 667 | 1095 | 296 | 344 | 471 | 184 | 207 | 256 | 124 | 137 | 158 |
|        *** | 1853 | 2341 | 4556 | 606 | 777 | 1081 | 316 | 386 | 449 | 194 | 226 | 232 | 130 | 146 | 133 |
| 0.7   *** | 1505 | 1764 | 4130 | 503 | 601 | 983 | 264 | 307 | 415 | 161 | 182 | 221 | 107 | 117 | 134 |
|        *** | 1601 | 2107 | 4140 | 543 | 703 | 964 | 282 | 344 | 391 | 170 | 197 | 196 | 112 | 124 | 108 |
| 0.75  *** | 1261 | 1524 | 3626 | 437 | 526 | 843 | 227 | 263 | 347 | 135 | 151 | 179 | . | . | . |
|        *** | 1361 | 1854 | 3619 | 473 | 615 | 821 | 242 | 293 | 322 | 142 | 163 | 153 | . | . | . |
| 0.8   *** | 1034 | 1282 | 3011 | 364 | 439 | 676 | 183 | 210 | 266 | . | . | . | . | . | . |
|        *** | 1130 | 1580 | 2994 | 395 | 510 | 651 | 195 | 232 | 241 | . | . | . | . | . | . |
| 0.85  *** | 816 | 1028 | 2288 | 281 | 335 | 482 | . | . | . | . | . | . | . | . | . |
|        *** | 899 | 1272 | 2265 | 304 | 384 | 456 | . | . | . | . | . | . | . | . | . |
| 0.9   *** | 585 | 738 | 1458 | . | . | . | . | . | . | . | . | . | . | . | . |
|        *** | 646 | 905 | 1432 | . | . | . | . | . | . | . | . | . | . | . | . |

TABLE 4: ALPHA= 0.01  POWER= 0.9    EXPECTED ACCRUAL THRU MINIMUM FOLLOW-UP= 180

| | | DEL=.05 | | | DEL=.10 | | | DEL=.15 | | | DEL=.20 | | | DEL=.25 | |
|---|---|---|---|---|---|---|---|---|---|---|---|---|---|---|---|
| FACT= | 1.0 .75 | .50 .25 | .00 BIN | 1.0 .75 | .50 .25 | .00 BIN | 1.0 .75 | .50 .25 | .00 BIN | 1.0 75 | .50 .25 | .00 BIN | 1.0 .75 | .50 .25 | .00 BIN |

PCONT=***    REQUIRED NUMBER OF PATIENTS

| PCONT | | DEL=.05 1.0/.75 | .50/.25 | .00/BIN | DEL=.10 1.0/.75 | .50/.25 | .00/BIN | DEL=.15 1.0/.75 | .50/.25 | .00/BIN | DEL=.20 1.0/.75 | .50/.25 | .00/BIN | DEL=.25 1.0/.75 | .50/.25 | .00/BIN |
|---|---|---|---|---|---|---|---|---|---|---|---|---|---|---|---|---|
| 0.05 | *** | 779 | 784 | 832 | 278 | 282 | 296 | 163 | 166 | 172 | 116 | 118 | 121 | 90 | 92 | 94 |
| | *** | 780 | 792 | 1432 | 279 | 287 | 456 | 165 | 169 | 241 | 117 | 119 | 153 | 91 | 93 | 108 |
| 0.1 | *** | 1420 | 1431 | 1604 | 441 | 451 | 495 | 238 | 245 | 263 | 158 | 163 | 172 | 118 | 121 | 126 |
| | *** | 1424 | 1451 | 2265 | 444 | 464 | 651 | 240 | 251 | 322 | 160 | 167 | 196 | 119 | 123 | 133 |
| 0.15 | *** | 1965 | 1983 | 2351 | 572 | 590 | 679 | 295 | 308 | 342 | 191 | 199 | 216 | 138 | 144 | 153 |
| | *** | 1971 | 2018 | 2994 | 578 | 613 | 821 | 300 | 320 | 391 | 194 | 205 | 232 | 141 | 147 | 154 |
| 0.2 | *** | 2386 | 2413 | 3033 | 671 | 697 | 841 | 338 | 357 | 411 | 215 | 226 | 252 | 153 | 161 | 175 |
| | *** | 2395 | 2466 | 3619 | 680 | 733 | 964 | 346 | 375 | 449 | 220 | 236 | 261 | 156 | 166 | 170 |
| 0.25 | *** | 2679 | 2717 | 3629 | 738 | 775 | 980 | 368 | 393 | 467 | 231 | 247 | 281 | 163 | 173 | 191 |
| | *** | 2691 | 2791 | 4140 | 751 | 824 | 1081 | 378 | 417 | 495 | 238 | 260 | 284 | 168 | 181 | 183 |
| 0.3 | *** | 2847 | 2899 | 4127 | 777 | 825 | 1092 | 386 | 417 | 512 | 242 | 260 | 303 | 169 | 181 | 204 |
| | *** | 2865 | 3000 | 4556 | 795 | 888 | 1172 | 399 | 448 | 530 | 249 | 276 | 300 | 175 | 190 | 191 |
| 0.35 | *** | 2904 | 2972 | 4519 | 792 | 852 | 1177 | 394 | 431 | 544 | 246 | 268 | 318 | 172 | 185 | 211 |
| | *** | 2926 | 3104 | 4869 | 814 | 928 | 1237 | 409 | 467 | 553 | 255 | 287 | 310 | 178 | 196 | 195 |
| 0.4 | *** | 2861 | 2949 | 4802 | 785 | 857 | 1235 | 393 | 436 | 564 | 246 | 270 | 325 | 171 | 186 | 214 |
| | *** | 2891 | 3118 | 5077 | 812 | 946 | 1276 | 411 | 477 | 565 | 256 | 291 | 313 | 177 | 197 | 195 |
| 0.45 | *** | 2736 | 2850 | 4973 | 762 | 846 | 1263 | 386 | 432 | 570 | 241 | 267 | 326 | 167 | 183 | 212 |
| | *** | 2774 | 3059 | 5181 | 794 | 945 | 1289 | 404 | 476 | 565 | 252 | 289 | 310 | 174 | 194 | 191 |
| 0.5 | *** | 2547 | 2690 | 5031 | 727 | 820 | 1264 | 371 | 420 | 564 | 232 | 259 | 319 | 161 | 176 | 205 |
| | *** | 2595 | 2941 | 5181 | 763 | 927 | 1276 | 392 | 467 | 553 | 244 | 282 | 300 | 168 | 188 | 183 |
| 0.55 | *** | 2312 | 2489 | 4975 | 682 | 782 | 1236 | 352 | 402 | 546 | 220 | 247 | 305 | 151 | 167 | 194 |
| | *** | 2373 | 2781 | 5077 | 721 | 894 | 1237 | 373 | 449 | 530 | 232 | 269 | 284 | 158 | 178 | 170 |
| 0.6 | *** | 2051 | 2264 | 4806 | 630 | 734 | 1180 | 328 | 378 | 515 | 205 | 230 | 284 | 140 | 154 | 178 |
| | *** | 2126 | 2589 | 4869 | 671 | 847 | 1172 | 349 | 423 | 495 | 216 | 251 | 261 | 146 | 164 | 154 |
| 0.65 | *** | 1783 | 2028 | 4524 | 573 | 676 | 1095 | 300 | 347 | 471 | 186 | 209 | 256 | 125 | 138 | 158 |
| | *** | 1872 | 2373 | 4556 | 614 | 786 | 1081 | 320 | 389 | 449 | 196 | 227 | 232 | 131 | 146 | 133 |
| 0.7 | *** | 1523 | 1789 | 4130 | 511 | 610 | 983 | 267 | 310 | 415 | 163 | 183 | 221 | 108 | 118 | 134 |
| | *** | 1622 | 2138 | 4140 | 551 | 711 | 964 | 285 | 347 | 391 | 172 | 198 | 196 | 112 | 125 | 108 |
| 0.75 | *** | 1280 | 1549 | 3626 | 444 | 533 | 843 | 230 | 265 | 347 | 137 | 152 | 179 | . | . | . |
| | *** | 1383 | 1884 | 3619 | 481 | 622 | 821 | 245 | 295 | 322 | 144 | 163 | 153 | . | . | . |
| 0.8 | *** | 1053 | 1305 | 3011 | 370 | 445 | 676 | 186 | 212 | 266 | . | . | . | . | . | . |
| | *** | 1151 | 1606 | 2994 | 401 | 516 | 651 | 197 | 233 | 241 | . | . | . | . | . | . |
| 0.85 | *** | 832 | 1047 | 2288 | 285 | 339 | 482 | . | . | . | . | . | . | . | . | . |
| | *** | 916 | 1293 | 2265 | 308 | 387 | 456 | . | . | . | . | . | . | . | . | . |
| 0.9 | *** | 597 | 752 | 1458 | . | . | . | . | . | . | . | . | . | . | . | . |
| | *** | 659 | 918 | 1432 | . | . | . | . | . | . | . | . | . | . | . | . |

## TABLE 4: ALPHA= 0.01 POWER= 0.9 EXPECTED ACCRUAL THRU MINIMUM FOLLOW-UP= 190

| | | DEL=.05 | | | DEL=.10 | | | DEL=.15 | | | DEL=.20 | | | DEL=.25 | | |
|---|---|---|---|---|---|---|---|---|---|---|---|---|---|---|---|---|
| FACT= | | 1.0 .75 | .50 .25 | .00 BIN | 1.0 .75 | .50 .25 | .00 BIN | 1.0 .75 | .50 .25 | .00 BIN | 1.0 75 | .50 .25 | .00 BIN | 1.0 .75 | .50 .25 | .00 BIN |
| PCONT=*** | | | | | REQUIRED NUMBER OF PATIENTS | | | | | | | | | | | |
| 0.05 | *** | 779 | 784 | 832 | 278 | 282 | 296 | 164 | 167 | 172 | 116 | 118 | 121 | 90 | 92 | 94 |
| | *** | 781 | 793 | 1432 | 280 | 287 | 456 | 165 | 169 | 241 | 117 | 119 | 153 | 91 | 93 | 108 |
| 0.1 | *** | 1421 | 1432 | 1604 | 441 | 452 | 495 | 238 | 245 | 263 | 159 | 163 | 172 | 118 | 121 | 126 |
| | *** | 1425 | 1453 | 2265 | 445 | 465 | 651 | 241 | 252 | 322 | 161 | 167 | 196 | 119 | 123 | 133 |
| 0.15 | *** | 1966 | 1985 | 2351 | 573 | 591 | 679 | 296 | 309 | 342 | 191 | 199 | 215 | 139 | 144 | 153 |
| | *** | 1972 | 2021 | 2994 | 580 | 615 | 821 | 301 | 321 | 391 | 195 | 206 | 232 | 141 | 148 | 154 |
| 0.2 | *** | 2388 | 2416 | 3033 | 672 | 700 | 841 | 340 | 358 | 411 | 216 | 227 | 252 | 154 | 161 | 174 |
| | *** | 2397 | 2472 | 3619 | 682 | 736 | 964 | 347 | 376 | 449 | 221 | 237 | 261 | 157 | 167 | 170 |
| 0.25 | *** | 2681 | 2721 | 3629 | 740 | 778 | 980 | 370 | 395 | 467 | 233 | 248 | 281 | 164 | 174 | 191 |
| | *** | 2694 | 2799 | 4140 | 754 | 828 | 1081 | 380 | 419 | 495 | 239 | 260 | 284 | 168 | 181 | 183 |
| 0.3 | *** | 2850 | 2905 | 4127 | 780 | 830 | 1092 | 389 | 420 | 512 | 243 | 262 | 303 | 170 | 182 | 203 |
| | *** | 2868 | 3011 | 4556 | 799 | 893 | 1172 | 401 | 450 | 530 | 251 | 277 | 300 | 176 | 191 | 191 |
| 0.35 | *** | 2907 | 2979 | 4519 | 796 | 857 | 1177 | 397 | 434 | 544 | 248 | 269 | 318 | 173 | 186 | 211 |
| | *** | 2931 | 3118 | 4869 | 819 | 934 | 1237 | 412 | 470 | 553 | 257 | 288 | 310 | 179 | 196 | 195 |
| 0.4 | *** | 2866 | 2959 | 4802 | 790 | 864 | 1234 | 397 | 439 | 564 | 248 | 272 | 325 | 172 | 187 | 214 |
| | *** | 2897 | 3136 | 5077 | 818 | 954 | 1276 | 414 | 479 | 565 | 258 | 292 | 313 | 179 | 198 | 195 |
| 0.45 | *** | 2743 | 2862 | 4973 | 768 | 853 | 1263 | 389 | 435 | 570 | 243 | 269 | 326 | 168 | 184 | 212 |
| | *** | 2783 | 3080 | 5181 | 801 | 953 | 1289 | 408 | 479 | 565 | 254 | 290 | 310 | 175 | 195 | 191 |
| 0.5 | *** | 2555 | 2705 | 5031 | 733 | 828 | 1264 | 375 | 424 | 564 | 234 | 261 | 319 | 162 | 177 | 205 |
| | *** | 2606 | 2966 | 5181 | 770 | 936 | 1276 | 396 | 470 | 553 | 246 | 283 | 300 | 169 | 189 | 183 |
| 0.55 | *** | 2322 | 2508 | 4975 | 689 | 790 | 1236 | 356 | 406 | 546 | 222 | 249 | 305 | 153 | 168 | 194 |
| | *** | 2386 | 2808 | 5077 | 729 | 903 | 1237 | 377 | 453 | 530 | 234 | 270 | 284 | 159 | 179 | 170 |
| 0.6 | *** | 2063 | 2286 | 4806 | 637 | 743 | 1180 | 332 | 382 | 515 | 207 | 232 | 284 | 141 | 155 | 178 |
| | *** | 2142 | 2618 | 4869 | 679 | 856 | 1172 | 353 | 426 | 495 | 218 | 252 | 261 | 147 | 165 | 154 |
| 0.65 | *** | 1798 | 2052 | 4524 | 580 | 685 | 1095 | 304 | 351 | 471 | 188 | 211 | 256 | 126 | 138 | 158 |
| | *** | 1890 | 2404 | 4556 | 622 | 794 | 1081 | 324 | 392 | 449 | 198 | 229 | 232 | 132 | 147 | 133 |
| 0.7 | *** | 1541 | 1813 | 4130 | 518 | 618 | 983 | 271 | 313 | 415 | 165 | 185 | 221 | 109 | 118 | 134 |
| | *** | 1643 | 2168 | 4140 | 559 | 719 | 964 | 289 | 349 | 391 | 174 | 199 | 196 | 113 | 125 | 108 |
| 0.75 | *** | 1298 | 1573 | 3626 | 451 | 540 | 843 | 233 | 268 | 347 | 138 | 153 | 179 | . | . | . |
| | *** | 1404 | 1912 | 3619 | 488 | 629 | 821 | 248 | 297 | 322 | 145 | 164 | 153 | . | . | . |
| 0.8 | *** | 1070 | 1327 | 3011 | 376 | 450 | 676 | 188 | 214 | 266 | . | . | . | . | . | . |
| | *** | 1170 | 1631 | 2994 | 407 | 521 | 651 | 199 | 234 | 241 | . | . | . | . | . | . |
| 0.85 | *** | 847 | 1065 | 2288 | 290 | 343 | 482 | . | . | . | . | . | . | . | . | . |
| | *** | 933 | 1313 | 2265 | 312 | 391 | 456 | . | . | . | . | . | . | . | . | . |
| 0.9 | *** | 609 | 764 | 1458 | . | . | . | . | . | . | . | . | . | . | . | . |
| | *** | 671 | 931 | 1432 | . | . | . | . | . | . | . | . | . | . | . | . |

TABLE 4: ALPHA= 0.01  POWER= 0.9    EXPECTED ACCRUAL THRU MINIMUM FOLLOW-UP= 200

| | DEL=.05 | | | DEL=.10 | | | DEL=.15 | | | DEL=.20 | | | DEL=.25 | | |
|---|---|---|---|---|---|---|---|---|---|---|---|---|---|---|---|
| FACT= | 1.0 .75 | .50 .25 | .00 BIN | 1.0 .75 | .50 .25 | .00 BIN | 1.0 .75 | .50 .25 | .00 BIN | 1.0 75 | .50 .25 | .00 BIN | 1.0 .75 | .50 .25 | .00 BIN |
| PCONT=*** | | | REQUIRED NUMBER OF PATIENTS | | | | | | | | | | | | |
| 0.05 *** | 779 | 785 | 832 | 278 | 283 | 296 | 164 | 167 | 172 | 116 | 118 | 121 | 91 | 92 | 94 |
| *** | 781 | 794 | 1432 | 280 | 287 | 456 | 165 | 169 | 241 | 117 | 119 | 153 | 91 | 93 | 108 |
| 0.1 *** | 1422 | 1433 | 1604 | 442 | 453 | 495 | 239 | 246 | 263 | 159 | 164 | 172 | 118 | 121 | 126 |
| *** | 1425 | 1455 | 2265 | 446 | 466 | 651 | 242 | 252 | 322 | 161 | 167 | 196 | 120 | 124 | 133 |
| 0.15 *** | 1967 | 1987 | 2351 | 574 | 593 | 679 | 297 | 310 | 342 | 192 | 200 | 216 | 139 | 144 | 153 |
| *** | 1974 | 2025 | 2994 | 581 | 617 | 821 | 302 | 321 | 391 | 195 | 206 | 232 | 141 | 148 | 154 |
| 0.2 *** | 2389 | 2419 | 3033 | 674 | 702 | 841 | 341 | 360 | 411 | 217 | 228 | 252 | 154 | 162 | 175 |
| *** | 2399 | 2477 | 3619 | 684 | 739 | 964 | 349 | 378 | 449 | 221 | 237 | 261 | 158 | 167 | 170 |
| 0.25 *** | 2683 | 2725 | 3629 | 743 | 782 | 980 | 372 | 397 | 467 | 234 | 249 | 281 | 165 | 175 | 191 |
| *** | 2697 | 2807 | 4140 | 757 | 832 | 1081 | 382 | 421 | 495 | 240 | 261 | 284 | 169 | 182 | 183 |
| 0.3 *** | 2853 | 2910 | 4127 | 783 | 834 | 1092 | 391 | 422 | 512 | 244 | 263 | 303 | 171 | 183 | 204 |
| *** | 2872 | 3022 | 4556 | 802 | 898 | 1172 | 404 | 452 | 530 | 252 | 278 | 300 | 176 | 191 | 191 |
| 0.35 *** | 2911 | 2987 | 4519 | 799 | 863 | 1177 | 400 | 437 | 544 | 249 | 271 | 318 | 174 | 187 | 211 |
| *** | 2936 | 3132 | 4869 | 823 | 940 | 1237 | 415 | 472 | 553 | 259 | 289 | 310 | 180 | 197 | 195 |
| 0.4 *** | 2871 | 2969 | 4802 | 795 | 870 | 1235 | 400 | 442 | 564 | 249 | 273 | 325 | 173 | 188 | 214 |
| *** | 2904 | 3153 | 5077 | 823 | 960 | 1276 | 417 | 482 | 565 | 260 | 293 | 313 | 180 | 198 | 195 |
| 0.45 *** | 2749 | 2874 | 4973 | 773 | 860 | 1263 | 392 | 439 | 570 | 245 | 271 | 326 | 170 | 185 | 212 |
| *** | 2791 | 3100 | 5181 | 807 | 961 | 1289 | 412 | 482 | 565 | 256 | 292 | 310 | 176 | 196 | 191 |
| 0.5 *** | 2563 | 2721 | 5031 | 739 | 836 | 1264 | 379 | 428 | 564 | 237 | 263 | 319 | 163 | 178 | 205 |
| *** | 2617 | 2990 | 5181 | 777 | 944 | 1276 | 399 | 473 | 553 | 248 | 284 | 300 | 170 | 189 | 183 |
| 0.55 *** | 2332 | 2526 | 4975 | 696 | 799 | 1236 | 360 | 410 | 546 | 224 | 251 | 305 | 154 | 169 | 194 |
| *** | 2399 | 2835 | 5077 | 736 | 911 | 1237 | 381 | 456 | 530 | 236 | 272 | 284 | 160 | 179 | 170 |
| 0.6 *** | 2076 | 2307 | 4806 | 644 | 751 | 1180 | 336 | 385 | 515 | 209 | 234 | 284 | 142 | 156 | 178 |
| *** | 2158 | 2647 | 4869 | 687 | 864 | 1172 | 357 | 430 | 495 | 220 | 253 | 261 | 148 | 165 | 154 |
| 0.65 *** | 1813 | 2074 | 4524 | 588 | 693 | 1095 | 307 | 354 | 471 | 190 | 212 | 256 | 127 | 139 | 158 |
| *** | 1909 | 2433 | 4556 | 630 | 802 | 1081 | 327 | 395 | 449 | 200 | 230 | 232 | 133 | 147 | 133 |
| 0.7 *** | 1558 | 1837 | 4130 | 525 | 625 | 983 | 274 | 316 | 415 | 167 | 186 | 221 | 110 | 119 | 134 |
| *** | 1663 | 2197 | 4140 | 566 | 726 | 964 | 292 | 352 | 391 | 175 | 200 | 196 | 114 | 125 | 108 |
| 0.75 *** | 1316 | 1596 | 3626 | 457 | 547 | 843 | 235 | 270 | 347 | 139 | 154 | 179 | . | . | . |
| *** | 1424 | 1940 | 3619 | 494 | 635 | 821 | 250 | 299 | 322 | 146 | 165 | 153 | . | . | . |
| 0.8 *** | 1087 | 1348 | 3011 | 382 | 456 | 676 | 190 | 216 | 266 | . | . | . | . | . | . |
| *** | 1189 | 1655 | 2994 | 412 | 526 | 651 | 201 | 236 | 241 | . | . | . | . | . | . |
| 0.85 *** | 862 | 1082 | 2288 | 294 | 347 | 482 | . | . | . | . | . | . | . | . | . |
| *** | 949 | 1332 | 2265 | 316 | 394 | 456 | . | . | . | . | . | . | . | . | . |
| 0.9 *** | 619 | 777 | 1458 | . | . | . | . | . | . | . | . | . | . | . | . |
| *** | 683 | 944 | 1432 | . | . | . | . | . | . | . | . | . | . | . | . |

## TABLE 4: ALPHA= 0.01 POWER= 0.9    EXPECTED ACCRUAL THRU MINIMUM FOLLOW-UP= 225

| PCONT=*** | | DEL=.05 | | | DEL=.10 | | | DEL=.15 | | | DEL=.20 | | | DEL=.25 | | |
|---|---|---|---|---|---|---|---|---|---|---|---|---|---|---|---|---|
| FACT= | | 1.0 .75 | .50 .25 | .00 BIN | 1.0 .75 | .50 .25 | .00 BIN | 1.0 .75 | .50 .25 | .00 BIN | 1.0 75 | .50 .25 | .00 BIN | 1.0 .75 | .50 .25 | .00 BIN |
| | | | | | REQUIRED NUMBER OF PATIENTS | | | | | | | | | | | |
| 0.05 | *** | 780 | 786 | 831 | 279 | 284 | 296 | 164 | 167 | 172 | 117 | 118 | 121 | 91 | 92 | 94 |
| | *** | 782 | 795 | 1432 | 281 | 288 | 456 | 165 | 169 | 241 | 117 | 120 | 153 | 91 | 93 | 108 |
| 0.1 | *** | 1423 | 1436 | 1604 | 444 | 455 | 495 | 240 | 247 | 263 | 160 | 164 | 172 | 119 | 122 | 126 |
| | *** | 1427 | 1460 | 2265 | 448 | 468 | 651 | 243 | 253 | 322 | 162 | 168 | 196 | 120 | 124 | 133 |
| 0.15 | *** | 1969 | 1992 | 2351 | 577 | 597 | 678 | 299 | 312 | 342 | 193 | 201 | 216 | 140 | 145 | 153 |
| | *** | 1977 | 2034 | 2994 | 584 | 621 | 821 | 304 | 323 | 391 | 197 | 207 | 232 | 142 | 149 | 154 |
| 0.2 | *** | 2393 | 2426 | 3033 | 678 | 708 | 841 | 344 | 363 | 411 | 219 | 230 | 252 | 156 | 163 | 174 |
| | *** | 2404 | 2491 | 3619 | 689 | 745 | 964 | 352 | 380 | 449 | 223 | 239 | 261 | 159 | 168 | 170 |
| 0.25 | *** | 2688 | 2735 | 3629 | 748 | 790 | 980 | 376 | 401 | 467 | 236 | 251 | 281 | 167 | 176 | 191 |
| | *** | 2704 | 2827 | 4140 | 764 | 841 | 1081 | 386 | 424 | 495 | 243 | 263 | 284 | 171 | 183 | 183 |
| 0.3 | *** | 2860 | 2925 | 4127 | 791 | 844 | 1092 | 396 | 428 | 512 | 248 | 266 | 303 | 174 | 185 | 203 |
| | *** | 2882 | 3048 | 4556 | 811 | 910 | 1172 | 409 | 457 | 530 | 255 | 281 | 300 | 178 | 192 | 191 |
| 0.35 | *** | 2921 | 3006 | 4519 | 809 | 875 | 1177 | 406 | 443 | 544 | 253 | 275 | 318 | 176 | 189 | 211 |
| | *** | 2949 | 3165 | 4869 | 834 | 954 | 1237 | 421 | 478 | 553 | 262 | 291 | 310 | 182 | 198 | 195 |
| 0.4 | *** | 2883 | 2993 | 4802 | 806 | 885 | 1235 | 407 | 449 | 564 | 254 | 277 | 325 | 176 | 190 | 214 |
| | *** | 2920 | 3194 | 5077 | 836 | 976 | 1276 | 424 | 488 | 565 | 264 | 296 | 313 | 182 | 200 | 195 |
| 0.45 | *** | 2765 | 2905 | 4973 | 787 | 877 | 1263 | 400 | 447 | 570 | 249 | 275 | 326 | 173 | 187 | 212 |
| | *** | 2812 | 3150 | 5181 | 822 | 978 | 1289 | 419 | 489 | 565 | 260 | 294 | 310 | 179 | 197 | 191 |
| 0.5 | *** | 2583 | 2758 | 5031 | 754 | 854 | 1264 | 387 | 436 | 564 | 241 | 267 | 319 | 166 | 181 | 205 |
| | *** | 2643 | 3047 | 5181 | 793 | 962 | 1276 | 408 | 480 | 553 | 252 | 287 | 300 | 173 | 191 | 183 |
| 0.55 | *** | 2358 | 2570 | 4975 | 712 | 818 | 1236 | 368 | 418 | 546 | 229 | 255 | 305 | 157 | 171 | 194 |
| | *** | 2432 | 2898 | 5077 | 754 | 930 | 1237 | 389 | 462 | 530 | 240 | 275 | 284 | 163 | 181 | 170 |
| 0.6 | *** | 2107 | 2357 | 4806 | 661 | 770 | 1180 | 344 | 393 | 515 | 213 | 237 | 284 | 145 | 158 | 178 |
| | *** | 2197 | 2714 | 4869 | 705 | 883 | 1172 | 365 | 436 | 495 | 224 | 256 | 261 | 150 | 166 | 154 |
| 0.65 | *** | 1850 | 2129 | 4524 | 605 | 712 | 1095 | 315 | 362 | 471 | 194 | 216 | 256 | 130 | 141 | 158 |
| | *** | 1953 | 2502 | 4556 | 648 | 820 | 1081 | 335 | 401 | 449 | 203 | 232 | 232 | 135 | 148 | 133 |
| 0.7 | *** | 1599 | 1893 | 4130 | 542 | 643 | 983 | 282 | 323 | 415 | 170 | 189 | 221 | 111 | 120 | 134 |
| | *** | 1710 | 2265 | 4140 | 583 | 743 | 964 | 299 | 357 | 391 | 178 | 202 | 196 | 116 | 126 | 108 |
| 0.75 | *** | 1359 | 1650 | 3626 | 472 | 563 | 843 | 242 | 276 | 347 | 142 | 156 | 179 | . | . | . |
| | *** | 1471 | 2003 | 3619 | 509 | 649 | 821 | 257 | 303 | 322 | 149 | 166 | 153 | . | . | . |
| 0.8 | *** | 1128 | 1397 | 3011 | 394 | 468 | 676 | 194 | 219 | 266 | . | . | . | . | . | . |
| | *** | 1233 | 1710 | 2994 | 425 | 536 | 651 | 205 | 238 | 241 | . | . | . | . | . | . |
| 0.85 | *** | 897 | 1123 | 2288 | 303 | 356 | 482 | . | . | . | . | . | . | . | . | . |
| | *** | 986 | 1376 | 2265 | 325 | 401 | 456 | . | . | . | . | . | . | . | . | . |
| 0.9 | *** | 645 | 805 | 1458 | . | . | . | . | . | . | . | . | . | . | . | . |
| | *** | 709 | 972 | 1432 | . | . | . | . | . | . | . | . | . | . | . | . |

TABLE 4: ALPHA= 0.01  POWER= 0.9    EXPECTED ACCRUAL THRU MINIMUM FOLLOW-UP= 250

| | | DEL=.05 | | | DEL=.10 | | | DEL=.15 | | | DEL=.20 | | | DEL=.25 | | |
|---|---|---|---|---|---|---|---|---|---|---|---|---|---|---|---|---|
| FACT= | | 1.0 .75 | .50 .25 | .00 BIN | 1.0 .75 | .50 .25 | .00 BIN | 1.0 .75 | .50 .25 | .00 BIN | 1.0 75 | .50 .25 | .00 BIN | 1.0 .75 | .50 .25 | .00 BIN |
| PCONT=*** | | | | | REQUIRED NUMBER OF PATIENTS | | | | | | | | | | | |
| 0.05 | *** | 781 | 787 | 832 | 280 | 284 | 296 | 165 | 168 | 172 | 117 | 119 | 121 | 91 | 92 | 94 |
| | *** | 783 | 797 | 1432 | 282 | 289 | 456 | 166 | 170 | 241 | 118 | 120 | 153 | 92 | 93 | 108 |
| 0.1 | *** | 1424 | 1439 | 1604 | 445 | 457 | 495 | 241 | 248 | 263 | 161 | 165 | 172 | 119 | 122 | 126 |
| | *** | 1429 | 1465 | 2265 | 450 | 470 | 651 | 244 | 254 | 322 | 163 | 168 | 196 | 121 | 124 | 133 |
| 0.15 | *** | 1972 | 1997 | 2351 | 579 | 600 | 679 | 301 | 314 | 342 | 195 | 202 | 216 | 141 | 146 | 153 |
| | *** | 1980 | 2043 | 2994 | 587 | 624 | 821 | 306 | 325 | 391 | 198 | 208 | 232 | 143 | 149 | 154 |
| 0.2 | *** | 2397 | 2434 | 3033 | 682 | 714 | 841 | 347 | 366 | 411 | 220 | 231 | 252 | 157 | 164 | 175 |
| | *** | 2409 | 2504 | 3619 | 694 | 751 | 964 | 355 | 382 | 449 | 225 | 240 | 261 | 160 | 168 | 170 |
| 0.25 | *** | 2693 | 2746 | 3629 | 754 | 797 | 980 | 380 | 405 | 467 | 239 | 253 | 281 | 168 | 177 | 191 |
| | *** | 2711 | 2846 | 4140 | 770 | 849 | 1081 | 390 | 428 | 495 | 245 | 264 | 284 | 172 | 183 | 183 |
| 0.3 | *** | 2867 | 2939 | 4127 | 798 | 854 | 1092 | 401 | 432 | 512 | 251 | 269 | 303 | 175 | 186 | 204 |
| | *** | 2891 | 3073 | 4556 | 819 | 919 | 1172 | 414 | 461 | 530 | 258 | 282 | 300 | 180 | 193 | 191 |
| 0.35 | *** | 2930 | 3024 | 4519 | 817 | 887 | 1177 | 411 | 449 | 544 | 257 | 277 | 318 | 179 | 191 | 211 |
| | *** | 2962 | 3198 | 4869 | 844 | 966 | 1237 | 427 | 482 | 553 | 266 | 293 | 310 | 184 | 199 | 195 |
| 0.4 | *** | 2896 | 3017 | 4802 | 817 | 898 | 1234 | 413 | 456 | 564 | 257 | 280 | 325 | 178 | 192 | 214 |
| | *** | 2937 | 3234 | 5077 | 848 | 990 | 1276 | 431 | 494 | 565 | 267 | 298 | 313 | 184 | 201 | 195 |
| 0.45 | *** | 2781 | 2935 | 4973 | 799 | 892 | 1264 | 407 | 454 | 570 | 254 | 278 | 326 | 175 | 189 | 212 |
| | *** | 2833 | 3197 | 5181 | 835 | 993 | 1289 | 427 | 494 | 565 | 264 | 297 | 310 | 181 | 199 | 191 |
| 0.5 | *** | 2603 | 2794 | 5031 | 768 | 870 | 1264 | 394 | 443 | 564 | 245 | 271 | 319 | 168 | 182 | 205 |
| | *** | 2669 | 3100 | 5181 | 809 | 979 | 1276 | 415 | 486 | 553 | 256 | 290 | 300 | 175 | 192 | 183 |
| 0.55 | *** | 2383 | 2613 | 4975 | 727 | 835 | 1236 | 376 | 426 | 546 | 233 | 258 | 305 | 159 | 172 | 194 |
| | *** | 2464 | 2957 | 5077 | 770 | 947 | 1237 | 397 | 468 | 530 | 244 | 277 | 284 | 165 | 182 | 170 |
| 0.6 | *** | 2138 | 2405 | 4806 | 677 | 787 | 1180 | 352 | 400 | 515 | 217 | 241 | 284 | 147 | 159 | 178 |
| | *** | 2235 | 2776 | 4869 | 722 | 899 | 1172 | 373 | 442 | 495 | 228 | 258 | 261 | 152 | 167 | 154 |
| 0.65 | *** | 1886 | 2180 | 4524 | 620 | 728 | 1095 | 323 | 368 | 471 | 197 | 219 | 256 | 132 | 142 | 158 |
| | *** | 1996 | 2565 | 4556 | 664 | 836 | 1081 | 342 | 406 | 449 | 207 | 234 | 232 | 136 | 149 | 133 |
| 0.7 | *** | 1638 | 1945 | 4130 | 557 | 658 | 983 | 288 | 328 | 415 | 173 | 191 | 221 | 113 | 122 | 134 |
| | *** | 1755 | 2326 | 4140 | 599 | 757 | 964 | 305 | 361 | 391 | 181 | 204 | 196 | 117 | 127 | 108 |
| 0.75 | *** | 1399 | 1701 | 3626 | 486 | 576 | 843 | 247 | 280 | 347 | 144 | 158 | 179 | . | . | . |
| | *** | 1516 | 2060 | 3619 | 523 | 661 | 821 | 262 | 306 | 322 | 151 | 167 | 153 | . | . | . |
| 0.8 | *** | 1165 | 1443 | 3011 | 406 | 479 | 676 | 199 | 223 | 266 | . | . | . | . | . | . |
| | *** | 1274 | 1760 | 2994 | 437 | 545 | 651 | 209 | 241 | 241 | . | . | . | . | . | . |
| 0.85 | *** | 929 | 1160 | 2288 | 311 | 363 | 482 | . | . | . | . | . | . | . | . | . |
| | *** | 1021 | 1415 | 2265 | 333 | 406 | 456 | . | . | . | . | . | . | . | . | . |
| 0.9 | *** | 668 | 830 | 1458 | . | . | . | . | . | . | . | . | . | . | . | . |
| | *** | 734 | 997 | 1432 | . | . | . | . | . | . | . | . | . | . | . | . |

## TABLE 4: ALPHA= 0.01  POWER= 0.9    EXPECTED ACCRUAL THRU MINIMUM FOLLOW-UP= 275

|  |  | DEL=.05 | | | DEL=.10 | | | DEL=.15 | | | DEL=.20 | | | DEL=.25 | | |
|---|---|---|---|---|---|---|---|---|---|---|---|---|---|---|---|---|
| FACT= | | 1.0 .75 | .50 .25 | .00 BIN | 1.0 .75 | .50 .25 | .00 BIN | 1.0 .75 | .50 .25 | .00 BIN | 1.0 75 | .50 .25 | .00 BIN | 1.0 .75 | .50 .25 | .00 BIN |
| PCONT=*** | | | | | REQUIRED NUMBER OF PATIENTS | | | | | | | | | | | |
| 0.05 | *** | 781 | 788 | 832 | 280 | 285 | 296 | 165 | 168 | 172 | 117 | 119 | 121 | 91 | 92 | 94 |
|  | *** | 784 | 799 | 1432 | 282 | 289 | 456 | 166 | 170 | 241 | 118 | 120 | 153 | 92 | 93 | 108 |
| 0.1 | *** | 1426 | 1442 | 1604 | 447 | 459 | 495 | 242 | 249 | 263 | 161 | 166 | 172 | 120 | 122 | 126 |
|  | *** | 1431 | 1470 | 2265 | 451 | 471 | 651 | 245 | 255 | 322 | 163 | 168 | 196 | 121 | 124 | 133 |
| 0.15 | *** | 1974 | 2001 | 2351 | 582 | 604 | 679 | 303 | 315 | 342 | 196 | 203 | 216 | 142 | 146 | 153 |
|  | *** | 1983 | 2051 | 2994 | 590 | 628 | 821 | 308 | 326 | 391 | 199 | 208 | 232 | 144 | 149 | 154 |
| 0.2 | *** | 2400 | 2441 | 3033 | 685 | 718 | 841 | 349 | 368 | 411 | 222 | 233 | 252 | 158 | 165 | 175 |
|  | *** | 2414 | 2517 | 3619 | 698 | 756 | 964 | 357 | 384 | 449 | 227 | 241 | 261 | 161 | 169 | 170 |
| 0.25 | *** | 2699 | 2756 | 3629 | 759 | 804 | 980 | 383 | 408 | 467 | 241 | 255 | 281 | 169 | 178 | 191 |
|  | *** | 2718 | 2864 | 4140 | 776 | 855 | 1081 | 394 | 430 | 495 | 247 | 266 | 284 | 173 | 184 | 183 |
| 0.3 | *** | 2875 | 2953 | 4127 | 804 | 863 | 1092 | 405 | 436 | 512 | 253 | 271 | 303 | 177 | 187 | 204 |
|  | *** | 2901 | 3097 | 4556 | 827 | 928 | 1172 | 418 | 464 | 530 | 261 | 284 | 300 | 182 | 194 | 191 |
| 0.35 | *** | 2939 | 3043 | 4519 | 826 | 897 | 1177 | 417 | 454 | 544 | 260 | 280 | 318 | 180 | 192 | 211 |
|  | *** | 2974 | 3228 | 4869 | 854 | 977 | 1237 | 432 | 486 | 553 | 268 | 295 | 310 | 186 | 200 | 195 |
| 0.4 | *** | 2908 | 3041 | 4802 | 827 | 911 | 1234 | 419 | 461 | 564 | 261 | 283 | 325 | 180 | 193 | 213 |
|  | *** | 2953 | 3271 | 5077 | 860 | 1002 | 1276 | 437 | 498 | 565 | 271 | 300 | 313 | 186 | 202 | 195 |
| 0.45 | *** | 2796 | 2964 | 4973 | 811 | 906 | 1264 | 414 | 460 | 570 | 257 | 281 | 326 | 177 | 190 | 212 |
|  | *** | 2854 | 3241 | 5181 | 848 | 1007 | 1289 | 433 | 499 | 565 | 268 | 299 | 310 | 183 | 199 | 191 |
| 0.5 | *** | 2623 | 2830 | 5030 | 781 | 885 | 1264 | 401 | 450 | 564 | 249 | 274 | 319 | 171 | 184 | 205 |
|  | *** | 2695 | 3150 | 5181 | 823 | 993 | 1276 | 422 | 491 | 553 | 260 | 292 | 300 | 177 | 193 | 183 |
| 0.55 | *** | 2408 | 2654 | 4975 | 741 | 850 | 1236 | 383 | 432 | 546 | 237 | 261 | 305 | 161 | 174 | 194 |
|  | *** | 2495 | 3011 | 5077 | 785 | 961 | 1237 | 404 | 473 | 530 | 248 | 279 | 284 | 167 | 183 | 170 |
| 0.6 | *** | 2168 | 2450 | 4806 | 692 | 803 | 1180 | 359 | 407 | 515 | 221 | 244 | 284 | 149 | 160 | 178 |
|  | *** | 2271 | 2833 | 4869 | 737 | 914 | 1172 | 379 | 446 | 495 | 231 | 260 | 261 | 154 | 168 | 154 |
| 0.65 | *** | 1920 | 2228 | 4524 | 635 | 744 | 1095 | 329 | 374 | 471 | 200 | 221 | 256 | 133 | 143 | 158 |
|  | *** | 2036 | 2623 | 4556 | 679 | 850 | 1081 | 348 | 410 | 449 | 210 | 236 | 232 | 138 | 150 | 133 |
| 0.7 | *** | 1675 | 1994 | 4130 | 570 | 672 | 983 | 294 | 333 | 415 | 176 | 193 | 221 | 114 | 122 | 134 |
|  | *** | 1797 | 2383 | 4140 | 612 | 769 | 964 | 311 | 365 | 391 | 184 | 205 | 196 | 118 | 127 | 108 |
| 0.75 | *** | 1436 | 1747 | 3626 | 498 | 588 | 843 | 252 | 285 | 347 | 147 | 160 | 179 | . | . | . |
|  | *** | 1557 | 2112 | 3619 | 536 | 671 | 821 | 266 | 309 | 322 | 153 | 168 | 153 | . | . | . |
| 0.8 | *** | 1200 | 1484 | 3011 | 416 | 489 | 676 | 202 | 226 | 266 | . | . | . | . | . | . |
|  | *** | 1312 | 1806 | 2994 | 447 | 553 | 651 | 213 | 243 | 241 | . | . | . | . | . | . |
| 0.85 | *** | 959 | 1195 | 2288 | 319 | 370 | 482 | . | . | . | . | . | . | . | . | . |
|  | *** | 1053 | 1451 | 2265 | 341 | 411 | 456 | . | . | . | . | . | . | . | . | . |
| 0.9 | *** | 689 | 853 | 1458 | . | . | . | . | . | . | . | . | . | . | . | . |
|  | *** | 756 | 1019 | 1432 | . | . | . | . | . | . | . | . | . | . | . | . |

TABLE 4: ALPHA= 0.01  POWER= 0.9    EXPECTED ACCRUAL THRU MINIMUM FOLLOW-UP= 300

| | | DEL=.05 | | | DEL=.10 | | | DEL=.15 | | | DEL=.20 | | | DEL=.25 | | |
|---|---|---|---|---|---|---|---|---|---|---|---|---|---|---|---|---|
| FACT= | | 1.0 .75 | .50 .25 | .00 BIN | 1.0 .75 | .50 .25 | .00 BIN | 1.0 .75 | .50 .25 | .00 BIN | 1.0 75 | .50 .25 | .00 BIN | 1.0 .75 | .50 .25 | .00 BIN |
| PCONT=*** | | | | | REQUIRED NUMBER OF PATIENTS | | | | | | | | | | | |
| 0.05 | *** | 782 | 790 | 832 | 281 | 286 | 295 | 166 | 168 | 172 | 117 | 119 | 121 | 91 | 92 | 94 |
| | *** | 785 | 800 | 1432 | 283 | 289 | 456 | 167 | 170 | 241 | 118 | 120 | 153 | 92 | 93 | 108 |
| 0.1 | *** | 1427 | 1444 | 1604 | 448 | 460 | 495 | 243 | 250 | 262 | 162 | 166 | 172 | 120 | 123 | 126 |
| | *** | 1433 | 1474 | 2265 | 453 | 473 | 651 | 246 | 255 | 322 | 164 | 169 | 196 | 121 | 124 | 133 |
| 0.15 | *** | 1977 | 2006 | 2351 | 584 | 607 | 679 | 304 | 317 | 342 | 197 | 204 | 215 | 142 | 147 | 153 |
| | *** | 1987 | 2059 | 2994 | 593 | 630 | 821 | 310 | 327 | 391 | 200 | 209 | 232 | 144 | 149 | 154 |
| 0.2 | *** | 2404 | 2448 | 3033 | 689 | 723 | 841 | 352 | 370 | 411 | 223 | 234 | 252 | 159 | 165 | 175 |
| | *** | 2419 | 2530 | 3619 | 702 | 760 | 964 | 360 | 386 | 449 | 228 | 241 | 261 | 162 | 169 | 170 |
| 0.25 | *** | 2704 | 2767 | 3629 | 764 | 811 | 980 | 386 | 411 | 467 | 243 | 257 | 281 | 171 | 179 | 191 |
| | *** | 2725 | 2882 | 4140 | 782 | 862 | 1081 | 397 | 433 | 495 | 249 | 267 | 284 | 175 | 184 | 183 |
| 0.3 | *** | 2882 | 2967 | 4127 | 811 | 871 | 1092 | 409 | 440 | 512 | 256 | 272 | 303 | 178 | 188 | 203 |
| | *** | 2910 | 3121 | 4556 | 834 | 936 | 1172 | 422 | 467 | 530 | 263 | 285 | 300 | 183 | 195 | 191 |
| 0.35 | *** | 2949 | 3061 | 4519 | 834 | 907 | 1177 | 421 | 458 | 544 | 262 | 282 | 318 | 182 | 193 | 211 |
| | *** | 2987 | 3258 | 4869 | 862 | 986 | 1237 | 437 | 490 | 553 | 271 | 297 | 310 | 187 | 201 | 195 |
| 0.4 | *** | 2920 | 3064 | 4802 | 836 | 922 | 1234 | 424 | 466 | 564 | 264 | 286 | 325 | 182 | 194 | 214 |
| | *** | 2969 | 3307 | 5077 | 870 | 1013 | 1276 | 442 | 502 | 565 | 273 | 302 | 313 | 188 | 203 | 195 |
| 0.45 | *** | 2812 | 2993 | 4973 | 822 | 919 | 1263 | 419 | 465 | 570 | 260 | 284 | 326 | 179 | 192 | 212 |
| | *** | 2874 | 3283 | 5181 | 860 | 1019 | 1289 | 439 | 504 | 565 | 271 | 301 | 310 | 185 | 200 | 191 |
| 0.5 | *** | 2643 | 2864 | 5031 | 793 | 899 | 1264 | 407 | 455 | 564 | 252 | 276 | 319 | 172 | 185 | 205 |
| | *** | 2721 | 3197 | 5181 | 836 | 1006 | 1276 | 428 | 496 | 553 | 263 | 294 | 300 | 178 | 194 | 183 |
| 0.55 | *** | 2432 | 2693 | 4975 | 754 | 864 | 1236 | 389 | 438 | 546 | 240 | 264 | 305 | 163 | 175 | 194 |
| | *** | 2526 | 3062 | 5077 | 799 | 975 | 1237 | 410 | 478 | 530 | 251 | 281 | 284 | 169 | 183 | 170 |
| 0.6 | *** | 2197 | 2493 | 4806 | 705 | 817 | 1180 | 365 | 412 | 515 | 224 | 246 | 284 | 150 | 162 | 178 |
| | *** | 2306 | 2887 | 4869 | 751 | 927 | 1172 | 385 | 451 | 495 | 234 | 262 | 261 | 155 | 169 | 154 |
| 0.65 | *** | 1953 | 2274 | 4524 | 648 | 757 | 1095 | 335 | 379 | 471 | 203 | 223 | 256 | 135 | 144 | 158 |
| | *** | 2074 | 2677 | 4556 | 693 | 862 | 1081 | 354 | 414 | 449 | 212 | 237 | 232 | 139 | 151 | 133 |
| 0.7 | *** | 1710 | 2039 | 4130 | 583 | 685 | 983 | 299 | 338 | 415 | 178 | 195 | 221 | 115 | 123 | 133 |
| | *** | 1837 | 2435 | 4140 | 625 | 780 | 964 | 316 | 368 | 391 | 186 | 206 | 196 | 119 | 128 | 108 |
| 0.75 | *** | 1471 | 1791 | 3626 | 509 | 599 | 843 | 256 | 288 | 347 | 148 | 161 | 179 | . | . | . |
| | *** | 1596 | 2160 | 3619 | 547 | 681 | 821 | 270 | 312 | 322 | 154 | 169 | 153 | . | . | . |
| 0.8 | *** | 1233 | 1523 | 3011 | 425 | 498 | 676 | 205 | 228 | 266 | . | . | . | . | . | . |
| | *** | 1348 | 1847 | 2994 | 456 | 560 | 651 | 216 | 244 | 241 | . | . | . | . | . | . |
| 0.85 | *** | 986 | 1226 | 2288 | 325 | 375 | 482 | . | . | . | . | . | . | . | . | . |
| | *** | 1082 | 1483 | 2265 | 347 | 416 | 456 | . | . | . | . | . | . | . | . | . |
| 0.9 | *** | 709 | 874 | 1458 | . | . | . | . | . | . | . | . | . | . | . | . |
| | *** | 777 | 1039 | 1432 | . | . | . | . | . | . | . | . | . | . | . | . |

## TABLE 4: ALPHA= 0.01  POWER= 0.9    EXPECTED ACCRUAL THRU MINIMUM FOLLOW-UP= 325

|  |  | DEL=.05 | | | DEL=.10 | | | DEL=.15 | | | DEL=.20 | | | DEL=.25 | | |
|---|---|---|---|---|---|---|---|---|---|---|---|---|---|---|---|---|
| FACT= | | 1.0 .75 | .50 .25 | .00 BIN | 1.0 .75 | .50 .25 | .00 BIN | 1.0 .75 | .50 .25 | .00 BIN | 1.0 75 | .50 .25 | .00 BIN | 1.0 .75 | .50 .25 | .00 BIN |
| PCONT=*** | | | | | REQUIRED NUMBER OF PATIENTS | | | | | | | | | | | |
| 0.05 | *** | 783 | 791 | 832 | 281 | 286 | 296 | 166 | 168 | 172 | 118 | 119 | 121 | 92 | 93 | 94 |
|  | *** | 785 | 802 | 1432 | 283 | 290 | 456 | 167 | 170 | 241 | 118 | 120 | 153 | 92 | 93 | 108 |
| 0.1 | *** | 1429 | 1447 | 1604 | 449 | 462 | 495 | 244 | 250 | 263 | 162 | 166 | 172 | 121 | 123 | 126 |
|  | *** | 1435 | 1478 | 2265 | 454 | 474 | 651 | 247 | 255 | 322 | 164 | 169 | 196 | 122 | 125 | 133 |
| 0.15 | *** | 1979 | 2011 | 2351 | 587 | 610 | 679 | 306 | 318 | 342 | 198 | 205 | 216 | 143 | 147 | 153 |
|  | *** | 1990 | 2067 | 2994 | 596 | 633 | 821 | 311 | 328 | 391 | 201 | 209 | 232 | 145 | 150 | 154 |
| 0.2 | *** | 2408 | 2456 | 3033 | 693 | 727 | 841 | 354 | 372 | 411 | 225 | 235 | 252 | 160 | 166 | 175 |
|  | *** | 2424 | 2542 | 3619 | 706 | 764 | 964 | 362 | 388 | 449 | 229 | 242 | 261 | 162 | 170 | 170 |
| 0.25 | *** | 2709 | 2777 | 3629 | 769 | 816 | 980 | 389 | 414 | 467 | 245 | 258 | 281 | 172 | 180 | 191 |
|  | *** | 2732 | 2899 | 4140 | 787 | 867 | 1081 | 400 | 435 | 495 | 251 | 268 | 284 | 175 | 185 | 183 |
| 0.3 | *** | 2889 | 2981 | 4127 | 817 | 879 | 1092 | 413 | 444 | 512 | 258 | 274 | 303 | 180 | 189 | 203 |
|  | *** | 2920 | 3143 | 4556 | 841 | 944 | 1172 | 426 | 470 | 530 | 265 | 286 | 300 | 184 | 196 | 191 |
| 0.35 | *** | 2959 | 3079 | 4519 | 842 | 916 | 1177 | 426 | 462 | 544 | 265 | 284 | 318 | 184 | 194 | 211 |
|  | *** | 2999 | 3286 | 4869 | 871 | 995 | 1237 | 441 | 493 | 553 | 273 | 298 | 310 | 188 | 202 | 195 |
| 0.4 | *** | 2932 | 3087 | 4802 | 845 | 933 | 1235 | 429 | 471 | 564 | 266 | 288 | 325 | 184 | 196 | 214 |
|  | *** | 2985 | 3342 | 5077 | 880 | 1023 | 1276 | 447 | 506 | 565 | 276 | 303 | 313 | 189 | 203 | 195 |
| 0.45 | *** | 2828 | 3021 | 4973 | 832 | 930 | 1263 | 425 | 470 | 570 | 263 | 286 | 326 | 181 | 193 | 212 |
|  | *** | 2895 | 3322 | 5181 | 872 | 1030 | 1289 | 444 | 508 | 565 | 273 | 302 | 310 | 186 | 201 | 191 |
| 0.5 | *** | 2663 | 2897 | 5031 | 805 | 911 | 1264 | 413 | 460 | 564 | 255 | 279 | 319 | 174 | 186 | 205 |
|  | *** | 2746 | 3242 | 5181 | 848 | 1018 | 1276 | 433 | 499 | 553 | 266 | 295 | 300 | 180 | 195 | 183 |
| 0.55 | *** | 2456 | 2731 | 4975 | 766 | 877 | 1236 | 395 | 443 | 546 | 243 | 266 | 305 | 164 | 177 | 194 |
|  | *** | 2556 | 3110 | 5077 | 811 | 987 | 1237 | 416 | 482 | 530 | 253 | 282 | 284 | 170 | 184 | 170 |
| 0.6 | *** | 2226 | 2534 | 4806 | 718 | 830 | 1180 | 371 | 417 | 515 | 227 | 248 | 284 | 152 | 163 | 178 |
|  | *** | 2340 | 2937 | 4869 | 764 | 938 | 1172 | 391 | 454 | 495 | 236 | 263 | 261 | 157 | 170 | 154 |
| 0.65 | *** | 1985 | 2317 | 4524 | 660 | 770 | 1095 | 340 | 384 | 471 | 206 | 225 | 256 | 136 | 145 | 158 |
|  | *** | 2111 | 2727 | 4556 | 706 | 873 | 1081 | 359 | 418 | 449 | 215 | 238 | 232 | 140 | 151 | 133 |
| 0.7 | *** | 1744 | 2082 | 4130 | 595 | 697 | 983 | 304 | 342 | 415 | 181 | 196 | 221 | 117 | 124 | 134 |
|  | *** | 1875 | 2484 | 4140 | 637 | 790 | 964 | 320 | 371 | 391 | 188 | 207 | 196 | 120 | 128 | 108 |
| 0.75 | *** | 1505 | 1831 | 3626 | 520 | 609 | 843 | 260 | 291 | 347 | 150 | 162 | 179 | . | . | . |
|  | *** | 1633 | 2205 | 3619 | 558 | 689 | 821 | 274 | 314 | 322 | 156 | 170 | 153 | . | . | . |
| 0.8 | *** | 1264 | 1559 | 3011 | 434 | 506 | 676 | 208 | 230 | 266 | . | . | . | . | . | . |
|  | *** | 1381 | 1886 | 2994 | 464 | 567 | 651 | 218 | 246 | 241 | . | . | . | . | . | . |
| 0.85 | *** | 1013 | 1255 | 2288 | 331 | 381 | 482 | . | . | . | . | . | . | . | . | . |
|  | *** | 1110 | 1512 | 2265 | 353 | 420 | 456 | . | . | . | . | . | . | . | . | . |
| 0.9 | *** | 728 | 894 | 1458 | . | . | . | . | . | . | . | . | . | . | . | . |
|  | *** | 796 | 1057 | 1432 | . | . | . | . | . | . | . | . | . | . | . | . |

## TABLE 4: ALPHA= 0.01  POWER= 0.9     EXPECTED ACCRUAL THRU MINIMUM FOLLOW-UP= 350

|  |  | DEL=.05 | | | DEL=.10 | | | DEL=.15 | | | DEL=.20 | | | DEL=.25 | | |
|---|---|---|---|---|---|---|---|---|---|---|---|---|---|---|---|---|
| FACT= | | 1.0 .75 | .50 .25 | .00 BIN | 1.0 .75 | .50 .25 | .00 BIN | 1.0 .75 | .50 .25 | .00 BIN | 1.0 75 | .50 .25 | .00 BIN | 1.0 .75 | .50 .25 | .00 BIN |
| PCONT=*** | | | | | REQUIRED NUMBER OF PATIENTS | | | | | | | | | | | |
| 0.05 | *** | 783 | 792 | 832 | 282 | 286 | 296 | 166 | 169 | 172 | 118 | 119 | 121 | 92 | 93 | 94 |
|  | *** | 786 | 803 | 1432 | 284 | 290 | 456 | 167 | 170 | 241 | 118 | 120 | 153 | 92 | 93 | 108 |
| 0.1 | *** | 1430 | 1450 | 1604 | 451 | 463 | 495 | 244 | 251 | 263 | 163 | 167 | 172 | 121 | 123 | 126 |
|  | *** | 1437 | 1482 | 2265 | 456 | 475 | 651 | 247 | 256 | 322 | 165 | 169 | 196 | 122 | 125 | 133 |
| 0.15 | *** | 1982 | 2016 | 2351 | 589 | 612 | 678 | 307 | 319 | 342 | 199 | 205 | 216 | 143 | 147 | 153 |
|  | *** | 1993 | 2074 | 2994 | 598 | 635 | 821 | 313 | 329 | 391 | 202 | 210 | 232 | 145 | 150 | 154 |
| 0.2 | *** | 2411 | 2463 | 3033 | 696 | 731 | 841 | 356 | 374 | 411 | 226 | 236 | 252 | 160 | 166 | 174 |
|  | *** | 2429 | 2554 | 3619 | 710 | 768 | 964 | 364 | 389 | 449 | 230 | 243 | 261 | 163 | 170 | 170 |
| 0.25 | *** | 2714 | 2787 | 3629 | 773 | 822 | 980 | 392 | 416 | 467 | 246 | 259 | 281 | 173 | 180 | 191 |
|  | *** | 2739 | 2915 | 4140 | 792 | 872 | 1081 | 402 | 436 | 495 | 252 | 269 | 284 | 176 | 185 | 183 |
| 0.3 | *** | 2896 | 2995 | 4127 | 823 | 886 | 1092 | 416 | 447 | 512 | 260 | 276 | 303 | 181 | 190 | 204 |
|  | *** | 2929 | 3165 | 4556 | 848 | 950 | 1172 | 429 | 472 | 530 | 267 | 287 | 300 | 185 | 196 | 191 |
| 0.35 | *** | 2968 | 3097 | 4519 | 849 | 925 | 1177 | 430 | 466 | 544 | 267 | 286 | 318 | 185 | 195 | 211 |
|  | *** | 3012 | 3314 | 4869 | 879 | 1003 | 1237 | 445 | 496 | 553 | 275 | 299 | 310 | 190 | 202 | 195 |
| 0.4 | *** | 2945 | 3109 | 4802 | 854 | 943 | 1235 | 434 | 475 | 564 | 269 | 290 | 325 | 185 | 197 | 214 |
|  | *** | 3001 | 3374 | 5077 | 890 | 1032 | 1276 | 451 | 509 | 565 | 278 | 305 | 313 | 190 | 204 | 195 |
| 0.45 | *** | 2843 | 3048 | 4973 | 842 | 941 | 1263 | 430 | 474 | 570 | 266 | 288 | 326 | 182 | 194 | 212 |
|  | *** | 2915 | 3360 | 5181 | 882 | 1040 | 1289 | 449 | 511 | 565 | 276 | 304 | 310 | 188 | 202 | 191 |
| 0.5 | *** | 2682 | 2929 | 5031 | 816 | 923 | 1264 | 418 | 465 | 565 | 258 | 281 | 319 | 176 | 188 | 205 |
|  | *** | 2770 | 3284 | 5181 | 859 | 1028 | 1276 | 439 | 503 | 553 | 268 | 297 | 300 | 181 | 195 | 183 |
| 0.55 | *** | 2480 | 2767 | 4975 | 778 | 890 | 1236 | 400 | 447 | 546 | 246 | 268 | 305 | 166 | 177 | 194 |
|  | *** | 2585 | 3156 | 5077 | 824 | 998 | 1237 | 421 | 485 | 530 | 256 | 284 | 284 | 171 | 185 | 170 |
| 0.6 | *** | 2253 | 2574 | 4806 | 729 | 842 | 1180 | 376 | 422 | 515 | 229 | 250 | 284 | 153 | 164 | 178 |
|  | *** | 2373 | 2984 | 4869 | 776 | 949 | 1172 | 396 | 458 | 495 | 239 | 265 | 261 | 158 | 170 | 154 |
| 0.65 | *** | 2016 | 2357 | 4524 | 672 | 782 | 1095 | 345 | 388 | 471 | 208 | 227 | 256 | 137 | 146 | 158 |
|  | *** | 2147 | 2774 | 4556 | 717 | 883 | 1081 | 364 | 421 | 449 | 217 | 239 | 232 | 141 | 152 | 133 |
| 0.7 | *** | 1776 | 2123 | 4130 | 606 | 707 | 983 | 308 | 345 | 415 | 183 | 198 | 221 | 118 | 124 | 134 |
|  | *** | 1911 | 2529 | 4140 | 648 | 799 | 964 | 325 | 373 | 391 | 190 | 208 | 196 | 121 | 129 | 108 |
| 0.75 | *** | 1537 | 1869 | 3626 | 530 | 619 | 843 | 264 | 294 | 347 | 152 | 163 | 179 | . | . | . |
|  | *** | 1668 | 2246 | 3619 | 567 | 696 | 821 | 277 | 316 | 322 | 157 | 170 | 153 | . | . | . |
| 0.8 | *** | 1294 | 1593 | 3011 | 442 | 513 | 676 | 211 | 232 | 266 | . | . | . | . | . | . |
|  | *** | 1413 | 1921 | 2994 | 472 | 572 | 651 | 221 | 247 | 241 | . | . | . | . | . | . |
| 0.85 | *** | 1037 | 1282 | 2288 | 337 | 385 | 482 | . | . | . | . | . | . | . | . | . |
|  | *** | 1136 | 1539 | 2265 | 358 | 423 | 456 | . | . | . | . | . | . | . | . | . |
| 0.9 | *** | 745 | 911 | 1458 | . | . | . | . | . | . | . | . | . | . | . | . |
|  | *** | 813 | 1073 | 1432 | . | . | . | . | . | . | . | . | . | . | . | . |

TABLE 4: ALPHA= 0.01  POWER= 0.9     EXPECTED ACCRUAL THRU MINIMUM FOLLOW-UP= 375

| | | DEL=.05 | | | DEL=.10 | | | DEL=.15 | | | DEL=.20 | | | DEL=.25 | | |
|---|---|---|---|---|---|---|---|---|---|---|---|---|---|---|---|---|---|
| FACT= | | 1.0 .75 | .50 .25 | .00 BIN | 1.0 .75 | .50 .25 | .00 BIN | 1.0 .75 | .50 .25 | .00 BIN | 1.0 75 | .50 .25 | .00 BIN | 1.0 .75 | .50 .25 | .00 BIN |
| PCONT=*** | | | | | REQUIRED NUMBER OF PATIENTS | | | | | | | | | | | |
| 0.05 | *** | 784 | 793 | 831 | 282 | 287 | 296 | 167 | 169 | 172 | 118 | 119 | 121 | 92 | 93 | 94 |
| | *** | 787 | 804 | 1432 | 284 | 290 | 456 | 167 | 170 | 241 | 118 | 120 | 153 | 92 | 93 | 108 |
| 0.1 | *** | 1432 | 1453 | 1604 | 452 | 465 | 495 | 245 | 252 | 263 | 163 | 167 | 172 | 121 | 123 | 126 |
| | *** | 1439 | 1486 | 2265 | 457 | 476 | 651 | 248 | 256 | 322 | 165 | 169 | 196 | 122 | 125 | 133 |
| 0.15 | *** | 1984 | 2020 | 2351 | 591 | 615 | 679 | 309 | 320 | 342 | 199 | 206 | 215 | 144 | 148 | 153 |
| | *** | 1997 | 2081 | 2994 | 600 | 637 | 821 | 314 | 329 | 391 | 202 | 210 | 232 | 146 | 150 | 154 |
| 0.2 | *** | 2415 | 2470 | 3033 | 699 | 735 | 841 | 358 | 376 | 410 | 227 | 237 | 252 | 161 | 167 | 175 |
| | *** | 2434 | 2565 | 3619 | 714 | 771 | 964 | 366 | 390 | 449 | 231 | 243 | 261 | 164 | 170 | 170 |
| 0.25 | *** | 2720 | 2797 | 3629 | 778 | 827 | 980 | 394 | 419 | 467 | 248 | 260 | 281 | 174 | 181 | 191 |
| | *** | 2746 | 2931 | 4140 | 797 | 877 | 1081 | 405 | 438 | 495 | 253 | 269 | 284 | 177 | 186 | 183 |
| 0.3 | *** | 2903 | 3008 | 4127 | 829 | 892 | 1092 | 419 | 450 | 512 | 261 | 277 | 303 | 182 | 191 | 204 |
| | *** | 2939 | 3185 | 4556 | 854 | 956 | 1172 | 432 | 474 | 530 | 268 | 288 | 300 | 186 | 197 | 191 |
| 0.35 | *** | 2977 | 3115 | 4519 | 856 | 933 | 1177 | 433 | 469 | 544 | 269 | 287 | 318 | 186 | 196 | 211 |
| | *** | 3024 | 3340 | 4869 | 887 | 1010 | 1237 | 449 | 498 | 553 | 277 | 300 | 310 | 191 | 203 | 195 |
| 0.4 | *** | 2957 | 3131 | 4802 | 862 | 952 | 1235 | 438 | 479 | 564 | 271 | 291 | 325 | 186 | 197 | 214 |
| | *** | 3017 | 3405 | 5077 | 898 | 1041 | 1276 | 455 | 512 | 565 | 280 | 306 | 313 | 192 | 205 | 195 |
| 0.45 | *** | 2859 | 3074 | 4973 | 851 | 951 | 1263 | 434 | 478 | 570 | 268 | 290 | 326 | 183 | 195 | 212 |
| | *** | 2935 | 3396 | 5181 | 892 | 1049 | 1289 | 453 | 514 | 565 | 278 | 305 | 310 | 189 | 202 | 191 |
| 0.5 | *** | 2702 | 2960 | 5030 | 826 | 934 | 1264 | 423 | 469 | 565 | 261 | 283 | 319 | 177 | 189 | 205 |
| | *** | 2794 | 3323 | 5181 | 870 | 1038 | 1276 | 443 | 506 | 553 | 271 | 298 | 300 | 182 | 196 | 183 |
| 0.55 | *** | 2503 | 2801 | 4975 | 788 | 901 | 1236 | 405 | 452 | 546 | 248 | 270 | 305 | 167 | 178 | 194 |
| | *** | 2613 | 3198 | 5077 | 835 | 1007 | 1237 | 425 | 488 | 530 | 258 | 285 | 284 | 172 | 185 | 170 |
| 0.6 | *** | 2280 | 2611 | 4806 | 740 | 853 | 1180 | 381 | 426 | 515 | 232 | 252 | 284 | 154 | 164 | 178 |
| | *** | 2405 | 3028 | 4869 | 787 | 959 | 1172 | 400 | 461 | 495 | 241 | 266 | 261 | 159 | 171 | 154 |
| 0.65 | *** | 2046 | 2396 | 4524 | 683 | 792 | 1095 | 350 | 392 | 471 | 210 | 228 | 256 | 138 | 147 | 158 |
| | *** | 2180 | 2818 | 4556 | 728 | 892 | 1081 | 368 | 423 | 449 | 219 | 240 | 232 | 142 | 152 | 133 |
| 0.7 | *** | 1807 | 2161 | 4130 | 616 | 717 | 983 | 312 | 349 | 415 | 184 | 199 | 221 | 118 | 125 | 133 |
| | *** | 1945 | 2571 | 4140 | 658 | 808 | 964 | 328 | 376 | 391 | 191 | 209 | 196 | 122 | 129 | 108 |
| 0.75 | *** | 1567 | 1905 | 3626 | 539 | 627 | 843 | 267 | 297 | 347 | 153 | 164 | 179 | . | . | . |
| | *** | 1701 | 2285 | 3619 | 576 | 703 | 821 | 280 | 317 | 322 | 158 | 171 | 153 | . | . | . |
| 0.8 | *** | 1322 | 1625 | 3011 | 449 | 520 | 676 | 213 | 234 | 266 | . | . | . | . | . | . |
| | *** | 1443 | 1954 | 2994 | 479 | 577 | 651 | 223 | 248 | 241 | . | . | . | . | . | . |
| 0.85 | *** | 1060 | 1308 | 2288 | 342 | 390 | 482 | . | . | . | . | . | . | . | . | . |
| | *** | 1160 | 1564 | 2265 | 363 | 426 | 456 | . | . | . | . | . | . | . | . | . |
| 0.9 | *** | 761 | 928 | 1458 | . | . | . | . | . | . | . | . | . | . | . | . |
| | *** | 830 | 1088 | 1432 | . | . | . | . | . | . | . | . | . | . | . | . |

TABLE 4: ALPHA= 0.01  POWER= 0.9    EXPECTED ACCRUAL THRU MINIMUM FOLLOW-UP= 400

| | | DEL=.05 | | | DEL=.10 | | | DEL=.15 | | | DEL=.20 | | | DEL=.25 | | |
|---|---|---|---|---|---|---|---|---|---|---|---|---|---|---|---|---|---|
| FACT= | | 1.0 .75 | .50 .25 | .00 BIN | 1.0 .75 | .50 .25 | .00 BIN | 1.0 .75 | .50 .25 | .00 BIN | 1.0 75 | .50 .25 | .00 BIN | 1.0 .75 | .50 .25 | .00 BIN |
| PCONT=*** | | | | | | | REQUIRED NUMBER OF PATIENTS | | | | | | | | | |
| 0.05 | *** | 785 | 794 | 832 | 283 | 287 | 296 | 167 | 169 | 172 | 118 | 119 | 121 | 92 | 93 | 94 |
| | *** | 788 | 805 | 1432 | 285 | 291 | 456 | 168 | 171 | 241 | 119 | 120 | 153 | 92 | 93 | 108 |
| 0.1 | *** | 1433 | 1455 | 1604 | 453 | 466 | 495 | 246 | 252 | 263 | 164 | 167 | 172 | 121 | 124 | 126 |
| | *** | 1441 | 1489 | 2265 | 458 | 477 | 651 | 249 | 257 | 322 | 165 | 170 | 196 | 122 | 125 | 133 |
| 0.15 | *** | 1987 | 2025 | 2351 | 593 | 617 | 679 | 310 | 321 | 342 | 200 | 206 | 216 | 144 | 148 | 153 |
| | *** | 2000 | 2088 | 2994 | 603 | 639 | 821 | 315 | 330 | 391 | 203 | 210 | 232 | 146 | 150 | 154 |
| 0.2 | *** | 2419 | 2477 | 3033 | 702 | 739 | 841 | 360 | 378 | 411 | 228 | 237 | 252 | 162 | 167 | 175 |
| | *** | 2439 | 2575 | 3619 | 717 | 774 | 964 | 367 | 391 | 449 | 232 | 244 | 261 | 164 | 171 | 170 |
| 0.25 | *** | 2725 | 2807 | 3629 | 782 | 832 | 980 | 397 | 421 | 467 | 249 | 261 | 281 | 175 | 182 | 191 |
| | *** | 2753 | 2946 | 4140 | 802 | 881 | 1081 | 407 | 440 | 495 | 255 | 270 | 284 | 178 | 186 | 183 |
| 0.3 | *** | 2910 | 3022 | 4127 | 834 | 898 | 1092 | 422 | 452 | 512 | 263 | 278 | 303 | 183 | 191 | 204 |
| | *** | 2948 | 3206 | 4556 | 860 | 962 | 1172 | 435 | 476 | 530 | 270 | 289 | 300 | 187 | 197 | 191 |
| 0.35 | *** | 2987 | 3132 | 4519 | 863 | 940 | 1177 | 437 | 472 | 544 | 271 | 289 | 318 | 187 | 197 | 211 |
| | *** | 3037 | 3364 | 4869 | 894 | 1017 | 1237 | 452 | 501 | 553 | 279 | 301 | 310 | 192 | 203 | 195 |
| 0.4 | *** | 2969 | 3153 | 4802 | 870 | 960 | 1235 | 442 | 482 | 564 | 273 | 293 | 325 | 188 | 198 | 214 |
| | *** | 3033 | 3435 | 5077 | 907 | 1048 | 1276 | 459 | 514 | 565 | 282 | 307 | 313 | 193 | 205 | 195 |
| 0.45 | *** | 2874 | 3100 | 4973 | 860 | 961 | 1263 | 439 | 482 | 570 | 271 | 292 | 326 | 185 | 196 | 212 |
| | *** | 2954 | 3430 | 5181 | 901 | 1058 | 1289 | 458 | 517 | 565 | 280 | 306 | 310 | 190 | 203 | 191 |
| 0.5 | *** | 2721 | 2990 | 5031 | 836 | 944 | 1264 | 428 | 473 | 564 | 263 | 284 | 319 | 178 | 189 | 205 |
| | *** | 2818 | 3361 | 5181 | 880 | 1047 | 1276 | 448 | 509 | 553 | 273 | 299 | 300 | 183 | 196 | 183 |
| 0.55 | *** | 2526 | 2835 | 4975 | 799 | 911 | 1236 | 410 | 456 | 546 | 251 | 272 | 305 | 169 | 179 | 194 |
| | *** | 2640 | 3239 | 5077 | 845 | 1017 | 1237 | 430 | 491 | 530 | 260 | 286 | 284 | 173 | 186 | 170 |
| 0.6 | *** | 2307 | 2647 | 4806 | 751 | 864 | 1180 | 385 | 430 | 515 | 234 | 253 | 284 | 156 | 165 | 178 |
| | *** | 2435 | 3070 | 4869 | 798 | 968 | 1172 | 405 | 463 | 495 | 243 | 267 | 261 | 160 | 171 | 154 |
| 0.65 | *** | 2074 | 2433 | 4524 | 693 | 802 | 1095 | 354 | 395 | 471 | 212 | 230 | 256 | 139 | 147 | 158 |
| | *** | 2213 | 2860 | 4556 | 739 | 901 | 1081 | 372 | 426 | 449 | 220 | 241 | 232 | 143 | 152 | 133 |
| 0.7 | *** | 1837 | 2197 | 4130 | 625 | 726 | 983 | 316 | 352 | 415 | 186 | 200 | 221 | 119 | 125 | 134 |
| | *** | 1978 | 2611 | 4140 | 668 | 815 | 964 | 332 | 378 | 391 | 193 | 210 | 196 | 122 | 129 | 108 |
| 0.75 | *** | 1596 | 1940 | 3626 | 547 | 635 | 843 | 270 | 299 | 347 | 154 | 165 | 179 | . | . | . |
| | *** | 1732 | 2321 | 3619 | 584 | 709 | 821 | 283 | 319 | 322 | 159 | 171 | 153 | . | . | . |
| 0.8 | *** | 1348 | 1655 | 3011 | 456 | 526 | 676 | 216 | 236 | 266 | . | . | . | . | . | . |
| | *** | 1471 | 1985 | 2994 | 486 | 582 | 651 | 225 | 249 | 241 | . | . | . | . | . | . |
| 0.85 | *** | 1082 | 1332 | 2288 | 347 | 394 | 482 | . | . | . | . | . | . | . | . | . |
| | *** | 1184 | 1588 | 2265 | 368 | 429 | 456 | . | . | . | . | . | . | . | . | . |
| 0.9 | *** | 777 | 944 | 1458 | . | . | . | . | . | . | . | . | . | . | . | . |
| | *** | 846 | 1102 | 1432 | . | . | . | . | . | . | . | . | . | . | . | . |

## TABLE 4: ALPHA= 0.01  POWER= 0.9  EXPECTED ACCRUAL THRU MINIMUM FOLLOW-UP= 425

| | | DEL=.05 | | | DEL=.10 | | | DEL=.15 | | | DEL=.20 | | | DEL=.25 | | |
|---|---|---|---|---|---|---|---|---|---|---|---|---|---|---|---|---|
| FACT= | | 1.0 .75 | .50 .25 | .00 BIN | 1.0 .75 | .50 .25 | .00 BIN | 1.0 .75 | .50 .25 | .00 BIN | 1.0 75 | .50 .25 | .00 BIN | 1.0 .75 | .50 .25 | .00 BIN |
| PCONT=*** | | | | | REQUIRED NUMBER OF PATIENTS | | | | | | | | | | | |
| 0.05 | *** | 785 | 795 | 832 | 283 | 288 | 295 | 167 | 169 | 172 | 118 | 120 | 121 | 92 | 93 | 94 |
| | *** | 789 | 806 | 1432 | 285 | 291 | 456 | 168 | 171 | 241 | 119 | 120 | 153 | 93 | 93 | 108 |
| 0.1 | *** | 1434 | 1458 | 1604 | 454 | 467 | 495 | 247 | 253 | 263 | 164 | 167 | 172 | 121 | 124 | 126 |
| | *** | 1443 | 1493 | 2265 | 459 | 478 | 651 | 249 | 257 | 322 | 166 | 170 | 196 | 122 | 125 | 133 |
| 0.15 | *** | 1989 | 2029 | 2351 | 595 | 619 | 679 | 311 | 322 | 342 | 201 | 207 | 215 | 145 | 148 | 153 |
| | *** | 2003 | 2095 | 2994 | 605 | 641 | 821 | 316 | 331 | 391 | 203 | 211 | 232 | 146 | 150 | 154 |
| 0.2 | *** | 2423 | 2484 | 3033 | 705 | 742 | 841 | 361 | 379 | 410 | 229 | 238 | 252 | 162 | 167 | 175 |
| | *** | 2444 | 2586 | 3619 | 720 | 777 | 964 | 369 | 392 | 449 | 233 | 244 | 261 | 165 | 171 | 170 |
| 0.25 | *** | 2730 | 2817 | 3629 | 786 | 836 | 980 | 399 | 423 | 467 | 250 | 262 | 281 | 175 | 182 | 191 |
| | *** | 2760 | 2960 | 4140 | 806 | 885 | 1081 | 409 | 441 | 495 | 256 | 271 | 284 | 178 | 186 | 183 |
| 0.3 | *** | 2917 | 3035 | 4127 | 839 | 904 | 1092 | 425 | 455 | 512 | 265 | 280 | 303 | 184 | 192 | 204 |
| | *** | 2958 | 3224 | 4556 | 866 | 967 | 1172 | 438 | 478 | 530 | 271 | 290 | 300 | 188 | 197 | 191 |
| 0.35 | *** | 2996 | 3149 | 4519 | 869 | 947 | 1177 | 440 | 475 | 544 | 273 | 290 | 318 | 188 | 198 | 211 |
| | *** | 3049 | 3388 | 4869 | 901 | 1023 | 1237 | 455 | 503 | 553 | 281 | 302 | 310 | 193 | 204 | 195 |
| 0.4 | *** | 2981 | 3174 | 4802 | 878 | 969 | 1234 | 446 | 485 | 563 | 275 | 295 | 325 | 189 | 199 | 214 |
| | *** | 3049 | 3463 | 5077 | 915 | 1055 | 1276 | 463 | 516 | 565 | 284 | 308 | 313 | 193 | 206 | 195 |
| 0.45 | *** | 2890 | 3125 | 4973 | 869 | 970 | 1263 | 443 | 486 | 570 | 273 | 293 | 326 | 186 | 197 | 212 |
| | *** | 2974 | 3462 | 5181 | 910 | 1065 | 1289 | 461 | 519 | 565 | 282 | 307 | 310 | 191 | 203 | 191 |
| 0.5 | *** | 2739 | 3019 | 5031 | 845 | 953 | 1264 | 432 | 477 | 564 | 265 | 286 | 319 | 179 | 190 | 205 |
| | *** | 2841 | 3397 | 5181 | 890 | 1055 | 1276 | 452 | 511 | 553 | 274 | 300 | 300 | 184 | 197 | 183 |
| 0.55 | *** | 2548 | 2867 | 4975 | 808 | 921 | 1236 | 414 | 459 | 546 | 253 | 273 | 305 | 170 | 180 | 194 |
| | *** | 2667 | 3277 | 5077 | 855 | 1025 | 1237 | 434 | 494 | 530 | 262 | 287 | 284 | 174 | 186 | 170 |
| 0.6 | *** | 2332 | 2681 | 4806 | 761 | 873 | 1180 | 390 | 433 | 515 | 236 | 255 | 284 | 156 | 166 | 178 |
| | *** | 2465 | 3109 | 4869 | 808 | 976 | 1172 | 409 | 466 | 495 | 244 | 268 | 261 | 161 | 171 | 154 |
| 0.65 | *** | 2102 | 2468 | 4524 | 703 | 811 | 1096 | 358 | 398 | 471 | 214 | 231 | 256 | 140 | 148 | 158 |
| | *** | 2244 | 2899 | 4556 | 748 | 908 | 1081 | 376 | 428 | 449 | 222 | 242 | 232 | 144 | 153 | 133 |
| 0.7 | *** | 1866 | 2232 | 4130 | 634 | 734 | 983 | 319 | 354 | 415 | 187 | 201 | 221 | 120 | 126 | 133 |
| | *** | 2009 | 2648 | 4140 | 677 | 822 | 964 | 335 | 379 | 391 | 194 | 210 | 196 | 122 | 129 | 108 |
| 0.75 | *** | 1624 | 1972 | 3626 | 555 | 642 | 843 | 273 | 301 | 347 | 155 | 165 | 179 | . | . | . |
| | *** | 1762 | 2355 | 3619 | 592 | 715 | 821 | 286 | 320 | 322 | 160 | 172 | 153 | . | . | . |
| 0.8 | *** | 1373 | 1684 | 3011 | 462 | 531 | 676 | 218 | 237 | 266 | . | . | . | . | . | . |
| | *** | 1498 | 2013 | 2994 | 492 | 586 | 651 | 226 | 250 | 241 | . | . | . | . | . | . |
| 0.85 | *** | 1104 | 1354 | 2288 | 351 | 397 | 482 | . | . | . | . | . | . | . | . | . |
| | *** | 1206 | 1609 | 2265 | 372 | 431 | 456 | . | . | . | . | . | . | . | . | . |
| 0.9 | *** | 791 | 958 | 1458 | . | . | . | . | . | . | . | . | . | . | . | . |
| | *** | 860 | 1115 | 1432 | . | . | . | . | . | . | . | . | . | . | . | . |

TABLE 4: ALPHA= 0.01  POWER= 0.9    EXPECTED ACCRUAL THRU MINIMUM FOLLOW-UP= 450

| | | DEL=.05 | | | DEL=.10 | | | DEL=.15 | | | DEL=.20 | | | DEL=.25 | | |
|---|---|---|---|---|---|---|---|---|---|---|---|---|---|---|---|---|---|
| FACT= | | 1.0 .75 | .50 .25 | .00 BIN | 1.0 .75 | .50 .25 | .00 BIN | 1.0 .75 | .50 .25 | .00 BIN | 1.0 75 | .50 .25 | .00 BIN | 1.0 .75 | .50 .25 | .00 BIN |
| PCONT=*** | | | | | REQUIRED | NUMBER OF | PATIENTS | | | | | | | | | |
| 0.05 | *** | 786 | 795 | 831 | 284 | 288 | 296 | 167 | 169 | 172 | 118 | 120 | 121 | 92 | 93 | 94 |
| | *** | 789 | 807 | 1432 | 285 | 291 | 456 | 168 | 171 | 241 | 119 | 120 | 153 | 93 | 93 | 108 |
| 0.1 | *** | 1436 | 1460 | 1604 | 455 | 468 | 495 | 247 | 253 | 262 | 164 | 168 | 172 | 122 | 124 | 126 |
| | *** | 1445 | 1496 | 2265 | 460 | 479 | 651 | 250 | 257 | 322 | 166 | 170 | 196 | 123 | 125 | 133 |
| 0.15 | *** | 1992 | 2034 | 2351 | 597 | 621 | 678 | 312 | 323 | 342 | 201 | 207 | 216 | 145 | 149 | 153 |
| | *** | 2006 | 2101 | 2994 | 607 | 642 | 821 | 317 | 331 | 391 | 204 | 211 | 232 | 147 | 150 | 154 |
| 0.2 | *** | 2426 | 2491 | 3033 | 708 | 745 | 841 | 363 | 380 | 411 | 230 | 239 | 252 | 163 | 168 | 174 |
| | *** | 2448 | 2595 | 3619 | 723 | 779 | 964 | 370 | 393 | 449 | 234 | 244 | 261 | 165 | 171 | 170 |
| 0.25 | *** | 2736 | 2827 | 3629 | 790 | 841 | 980 | 401 | 424 | 468 | 251 | 263 | 281 | 176 | 183 | 191 |
| | *** | 2767 | 2975 | 4140 | 811 | 889 | 1081 | 411 | 442 | 495 | 257 | 271 | 284 | 179 | 186 | 183 |
| 0.3 | *** | 2925 | 3048 | 4127 | 844 | 910 | 1092 | 428 | 457 | 512 | 266 | 280 | 303 | 185 | 192 | 203 |
| | *** | 2967 | 3243 | 4556 | 871 | 972 | 1172 | 440 | 479 | 530 | 273 | 290 | 300 | 188 | 198 | 191 |
| 0.35 | *** | 3006 | 3165 | 4519 | 875 | 954 | 1177 | 443 | 478 | 544 | 275 | 291 | 318 | 189 | 198 | 211 |
| | *** | 3061 | 3411 | 4869 | 907 | 1029 | 1237 | 458 | 504 | 553 | 282 | 303 | 310 | 193 | 204 | 195 |
| 0.4 | *** | 2993 | 3194 | 4802 | 885 | 976 | 1234 | 449 | 488 | 564 | 277 | 296 | 325 | 190 | 200 | 213 |
| | *** | 3064 | 3490 | 5077 | 922 | 1062 | 1276 | 466 | 518 | 565 | 285 | 309 | 313 | 194 | 206 | 195 |
| 0.45 | *** | 2905 | 3150 | 4973 | 877 | 978 | 1263 | 447 | 489 | 570 | 275 | 294 | 326 | 187 | 197 | 212 |
| | *** | 2993 | 3493 | 5181 | 919 | 1073 | 1289 | 465 | 522 | 565 | 284 | 308 | 310 | 192 | 204 | 191 |
| 0.5 | *** | 2758 | 3047 | 5031 | 854 | 962 | 1264 | 436 | 480 | 564 | 267 | 287 | 319 | 181 | 191 | 205 |
| | *** | 2864 | 3431 | 5181 | 899 | 1063 | 1276 | 455 | 514 | 553 | 276 | 301 | 300 | 185 | 197 | 183 |
| 0.55 | *** | 2570 | 2898 | 4975 | 818 | 930 | 1236 | 418 | 462 | 546 | 255 | 275 | 305 | 171 | 181 | 194 |
| | *** | 2693 | 3313 | 5077 | 864 | 1033 | 1237 | 438 | 496 | 530 | 264 | 288 | 284 | 175 | 186 | 170 |
| 0.6 | *** | 2357 | 2714 | 4806 | 770 | 883 | 1180 | 393 | 436 | 515 | 237 | 256 | 284 | 158 | 166 | 178 |
| | *** | 2493 | 3146 | 4869 | 817 | 984 | 1172 | 412 | 468 | 495 | 246 | 268 | 261 | 162 | 172 | 154 |
| 0.65 | *** | 2129 | 2502 | 4524 | 712 | 820 | 1095 | 362 | 401 | 471 | 216 | 232 | 256 | 141 | 148 | 158 |
| | *** | 2274 | 2936 | 4556 | 757 | 915 | 1081 | 379 | 430 | 449 | 223 | 243 | 232 | 144 | 153 | 133 |
| 0.7 | *** | 1893 | 2265 | 4130 | 643 | 743 | 983 | 323 | 357 | 415 | 189 | 202 | 221 | 120 | 126 | 134 |
| | *** | 2039 | 2683 | 4140 | 685 | 828 | 964 | 338 | 381 | 391 | 195 | 211 | 196 | 123 | 130 | 108 |
| 0.75 | *** | 1650 | 2003 | 3626 | 563 | 649 | 843 | 276 | 303 | 347 | 156 | 166 | 179 | . | . | . |
| | *** | 1791 | 2387 | 3619 | 599 | 720 | 821 | 288 | 322 | 322 | 161 | 172 | 153 | . | . | . |
| 0.8 | *** | 1397 | 1710 | 3011 | 468 | 536 | 676 | 219 | 238 | 266 | . | . | . | . | . | . |
| | *** | 1523 | 2040 | 2994 | 498 | 590 | 651 | 228 | 251 | 241 | . | . | . | . | . | . |
| 0.85 | *** | 1123 | 1376 | 2288 | 356 | 401 | 482 | . | . | . | . | . | . | . | . | . |
| | *** | 1226 | 1630 | 2265 | 375 | 434 | 456 | . | . | . | . | . | . | . | . | . |
| 0.9 | *** | 805 | 972 | 1458 | . | . | . | . | . | . | . | . | . | . | . | . |
| | *** | 874 | 1127 | 1432 | . | . | . | . | . | . | . | . | . | . | . | . |

TABLE 4: ALPHA= 0.01  POWER= 0.9      EXPECTED ACCRUAL THRU MINIMUM FOLLOW-UP= 475

| | | DEL=.05 | | | DEL=.10 | | | DEL=.15 | | | DEL=.20 | | | DEL=.25 | | |
|---|---|---|---|---|---|---|---|---|---|---|---|---|---|---|---|---|---|
| FACT= | | 1.0 .75 | .50 .25 | .00 BIN | 1.0 .75 | .50 .25 | .00 BIN | 1.0 .75 | .50 .25 | .00 BIN | 1.0 75 | .50 .25 | .00 BIN | 1.0 .75 | .50 .25 | .00 BIN |
| PCONT=*** | | | | | REQUIRED NUMBER OF PATIENTS | | | | | | | | | | | |
| 0.05 | *** | 786 | 796 | 832 | 284 | 288 | 296 | 167 | 169 | 172 | 118 | 120 | 121 | 92 | 93 | 94 |
| | *** | 790 | 808 | 1432 | 286 | 291 | 456 | 168 | 171 | 241 | 119 | 120 | 153 | 93 | 93 | 108 |
| 0.1 | *** | 1438 | 1463 | 1604 | 456 | 469 | 495 | 248 | 254 | 262 | 165 | 168 | 172 | 122 | 124 | 126 |
| | *** | 1446 | 1499 | 2265 | 461 | 479 | 651 | 250 | 257 | 322 | 166 | 170 | 196 | 123 | 125 | 133 |
| 0.15 | *** | 1994 | 2038 | 2351 | 599 | 623 | 679 | 313 | 324 | 342 | 202 | 207 | 216 | 145 | 149 | 153 |
| | *** | 2009 | 2107 | 2994 | 609 | 644 | 821 | 318 | 332 | 391 | 204 | 211 | 232 | 147 | 150 | 154 |
| 0.2 | *** | 2430 | 2498 | 3033 | 711 | 748 | 841 | 364 | 381 | 411 | 231 | 239 | 252 | 163 | 168 | 175 |
| | *** | 2453 | 2605 | 3619 | 726 | 782 | 964 | 372 | 394 | 449 | 235 | 245 | 261 | 166 | 171 | 170 |
| 0.25 | *** | 2740 | 2836 | 3629 | 794 | 845 | 980 | 403 | 426 | 467 | 252 | 264 | 281 | 176 | 183 | 191 |
| | *** | 2773 | 2988 | 4140 | 814 | 892 | 1081 | 413 | 443 | 495 | 257 | 271 | 284 | 179 | 187 | 183 |
| 0.3 | *** | 2932 | 3060 | 4127 | 849 | 915 | 1092 | 430 | 459 | 512 | 267 | 281 | 303 | 185 | 193 | 203 |
| | *** | 2976 | 3261 | 4556 | 876 | 976 | 1172 | 443 | 481 | 530 | 274 | 291 | 300 | 189 | 198 | 191 |
| 0.35 | *** | 3015 | 3182 | 4519 | 881 | 960 | 1177 | 446 | 480 | 544 | 276 | 292 | 318 | 190 | 199 | 211 |
| | *** | 3073 | 3433 | 4869 | 913 | 1034 | 1237 | 461 | 506 | 553 | 283 | 303 | 310 | 194 | 204 | 195 |
| 0.4 | *** | 3005 | 3214 | 4802 | 892 | 983 | 1234 | 452 | 491 | 564 | 279 | 297 | 325 | 191 | 200 | 213 |
| | *** | 3079 | 3516 | 5077 | 929 | 1068 | 1276 | 469 | 520 | 565 | 287 | 309 | 313 | 195 | 206 | 195 |
| 0.45 | *** | 2920 | 3173 | 4973 | 885 | 986 | 1264 | 450 | 492 | 570 | 276 | 296 | 326 | 188 | 198 | 212 |
| | *** | 3011 | 3523 | 5181 | 927 | 1079 | 1289 | 469 | 523 | 565 | 285 | 309 | 310 | 192 | 204 | 191 |
| 0.5 | *** | 2776 | 3074 | 5031 | 862 | 971 | 1264 | 440 | 483 | 564 | 269 | 289 | 319 | 181 | 191 | 205 |
| | *** | 2886 | 3463 | 5181 | 907 | 1070 | 1276 | 459 | 516 | 553 | 278 | 302 | 300 | 186 | 198 | 183 |
| 0.55 | *** | 2592 | 2928 | 4975 | 826 | 939 | 1236 | 422 | 466 | 546 | 257 | 276 | 305 | 172 | 181 | 194 |
| | *** | 2718 | 3348 | 5077 | 873 | 1040 | 1237 | 441 | 498 | 530 | 265 | 289 | 284 | 176 | 187 | 170 |
| 0.6 | *** | 2381 | 2746 | 4806 | 779 | 891 | 1180 | 397 | 439 | 514 | 239 | 257 | 284 | 158 | 167 | 178 |
| | *** | 2521 | 3182 | 5077 | 826 | 990 | 1172 | 416 | 470 | 495 | 248 | 269 | 261 | 162 | 172 | 154 |
| 0.65 | *** | 2155 | 2534 | 4524 | 720 | 828 | 1096 | 365 | 403 | 471 | 217 | 233 | 256 | 141 | 149 | 158 |
| | *** | 2303 | 2971 | 4556 | 766 | 922 | 1081 | 382 | 431 | 449 | 224 | 243 | 232 | 145 | 153 | 133 |
| 0.7 | *** | 1920 | 2296 | 4130 | 651 | 750 | 983 | 326 | 359 | 415 | 190 | 203 | 221 | 121 | 127 | 134 |
| | *** | 2068 | 2716 | 4140 | 693 | 834 | 964 | 340 | 383 | 391 | 196 | 211 | 196 | 124 | 130 | 108 |
| 0.75 | *** | 1676 | 2032 | 3626 | 569 | 655 | 843 | 278 | 305 | 347 | 157 | 167 | 179 | . | . | . |
| | *** | 1818 | 2417 | 3619 | 606 | 725 | 821 | 290 | 323 | 322 | 162 | 172 | 153 | . | . | . |
| 0.8 | *** | 1421 | 1736 | 3011 | 474 | 541 | 676 | 221 | 240 | 266 | . | . | . | . | . | . |
| | *** | 1548 | 2065 | 2994 | 503 | 593 | 651 | 229 | 251 | 241 | . | . | . | . | . | . |
| 0.85 | *** | 1142 | 1396 | 2288 | 359 | 403 | 482 | . | . | . | . | . | . | . | . | . |
| | *** | 1246 | 1649 | 2265 | 379 | 436 | 456 | . | . | . | . | . | . | . | . | . |
| 0.9 | *** | 818 | 984 | 1458 | . | . | . | . | . | . | . | . | . | . | . | . |
| | *** | 887 | 1138 | 1432 | . | . | . | . | . | . | . | . | . | . | . | . |

TABLE 4: ALPHA= 0.01  POWER= 0.9    EXPECTED ACCRUAL THRU MINIMUM FOLLOW-UP= 500

| | | DEL=.05 | | | DEL=.10 | | | DEL=.15 | | | DEL=.20 | | | DEL=.25 | | |
|---|---|---|---|---|---|---|---|---|---|---|---|---|---|---|---|---|---|
| FACT= | | 1.0 .75 | .50 .25 | .00 BIN | 1.0 .75 | .50 .25 | .00 BIN | 1.0 .75 | .50 .25 | .00 BIN | 1.0 75 | .50 .25 | .00 BIN | 1.0 .75 | .50 .25 | .00 BIN |
| PCONT=*** | | REQUIRED NUMBER OF PATIENTS | | | | | | | | | | | | | | |
| 0.05 | *** | 787 | 797 | 832 | 284 | 288 | 296 | 168 | 170 | 172 | 118 | 120 | 121 | 92 | 93 | 94 |
| | *** | 791 | 808 | 1432 | 286 | 292 | 456 | 168 | 171 | 241 | 119 | 120 | 153 | 93 | 93 | 108 |
| 0.1 | *** | 1439 | 1465 | 1604 | 457 | 470 | 495 | 248 | 254 | 263 | 165 | 168 | 172 | 122 | 124 | 126 |
| | *** | 1448 | 1502 | 2265 | 463 | 480 | 651 | 251 | 258 | 322 | 167 | 170 | 196 | 123 | 125 | 133 |
| 0.15 | *** | 1997 | 2043 | 2351 | 600 | 624 | 678 | 314 | 325 | 342 | 202 | 208 | 216 | 146 | 149 | 153 |
| | *** | 2013 | 2113 | 2994 | 610 | 645 | 821 | 319 | 332 | 391 | 205 | 211 | 232 | 147 | 151 | 154 |
| 0.2 | *** | 2434 | 2504 | 3033 | 713 | 751 | 841 | 366 | 383 | 411 | 231 | 240 | 252 | 164 | 168 | 175 |
| | *** | 2458 | 2614 | 3619 | 729 | 784 | 964 | 373 | 394 | 449 | 235 | 245 | 261 | 166 | 171 | 170 |
| 0.25 | *** | 2746 | 2846 | 3629 | 797 | 848 | 980 | 405 | 428 | 468 | 253 | 264 | 281 | 177 | 183 | 191 |
| | *** | 2780 | 3001 | 4140 | 818 | 895 | 1081 | 415 | 444 | 495 | 258 | 272 | 284 | 180 | 187 | 183 |
| 0.3 | *** | 2939 | 3073 | 4127 | 854 | 919 | 1092 | 432 | 461 | 512 | 268 | 282 | 303 | 186 | 193 | 203 |
| | *** | 2985 | 3278 | 4556 | 881 | 980 | 1172 | 445 | 482 | 530 | 275 | 292 | 300 | 189 | 198 | 191 |
| 0.35 | *** | 3024 | 3198 | 4519 | 887 | 966 | 1177 | 449 | 483 | 544 | 277 | 293 | 318 | 191 | 199 | 211 |
| | *** | 3085 | 3454 | 4869 | 919 | 1039 | 1237 | 463 | 508 | 553 | 285 | 304 | 310 | 195 | 205 | 195 |
| 0.4 | *** | 3017 | 3234 | 4802 | 898 | 990 | 1234 | 456 | 493 | 563 | 280 | 298 | 325 | 192 | 201 | 213 |
| | *** | 3094 | 3541 | 5077 | 936 | 1073 | 1276 | 472 | 522 | 565 | 288 | 310 | 313 | 196 | 207 | 195 |
| 0.45 | *** | 2935 | 3197 | 4973 | 892 | 993 | 1263 | 453 | 494 | 570 | 278 | 297 | 326 | 189 | 198 | 212 |
| | *** | 3030 | 3551 | 5181 | 934 | 1086 | 1289 | 472 | 525 | 565 | 287 | 310 | 310 | 193 | 204 | 191 |
| 0.5 | *** | 2794 | 3100 | 5031 | 870 | 978 | 1264 | 443 | 486 | 564 | 271 | 290 | 319 | 182 | 192 | 205 |
| | *** | 2908 | 3494 | 5181 | 915 | 1076 | 1276 | 462 | 518 | 553 | 279 | 303 | 300 | 187 | 198 | 183 |
| 0.55 | *** | 2613 | 2957 | 4975 | 835 | 947 | 1236 | 426 | 468 | 546 | 258 | 277 | 305 | 173 | 182 | 194 |
| | *** | 2743 | 3380 | 5077 | 882 | 1047 | 1237 | 444 | 500 | 530 | 267 | 289 | 284 | 177 | 187 | 170 |
| 0.6 | *** | 2405 | 2776 | 4806 | 787 | 899 | 1180 | 400 | 442 | 515 | 241 | 258 | 284 | 159 | 168 | 178 |
| | *** | 2548 | 3215 | 4869 | 834 | 997 | 1172 | 419 | 472 | 495 | 249 | 270 | 261 | 163 | 173 | 154 |
| 0.65 | *** | 2180 | 2565 | 4524 | 728 | 836 | 1095 | 368 | 406 | 471 | 218 | 234 | 256 | 142 | 149 | 158 |
| | *** | 2330 | 3004 | 4556 | 774 | 928 | 1081 | 385 | 433 | 449 | 226 | 244 | 232 | 145 | 153 | 133 |
| 0.7 | *** | 1945 | 2326 | 4130 | 658 | 757 | 983 | 328 | 361 | 415 | 191 | 204 | 221 | 122 | 127 | 133 |
| | *** | 2096 | 2748 | 4140 | 700 | 839 | 964 | 343 | 384 | 391 | 197 | 212 | 196 | 124 | 130 | 108 |
| 0.75 | *** | 1701 | 2060 | 3626 | 576 | 661 | 843 | 280 | 306 | 347 | 158 | 167 | 179 | . | . | . |
| | *** | 1844 | 2445 | 3619 | 613 | 729 | 821 | 292 | 324 | 322 | 162 | 173 | 153 | . | . | . |
| 0.8 | *** | 1443 | 1760 | 3011 | 479 | 545 | 676 | 223 | 241 | 266 | . | . | . | . | . | . |
| | *** | 1571 | 2089 | 2994 | 508 | 597 | 651 | 231 | 252 | 241 | . | . | . | . | . | . |
| 0.85 | *** | 1160 | 1415 | 2288 | 363 | 406 | 482 | . | . | . | . | . | . | . | . | . |
| | *** | 1265 | 1666 | 2265 | 382 | 438 | 456 | . | . | . | . | . | . | . | . | . |
| 0.9 | *** | 830 | 997 | 1458 | . | . | . | . | . | . | . | . | . | . | . | . |
| | *** | 900 | 1148 | 1432 | . | . | . | . | . | . | . | . | . | . | . | . |

## TABLE 4: ALPHA= 0.01  POWER= 0.9    EXPECTED ACCRUAL THRU MINIMUM FOLLOW-UP= 550

| | | DEL=.02 | | | DEL=.05 | | | DEL=.10 | | | DEL=.15 | | | DEL=.20 | | |
|---|---|---|---|---|---|---|---|---|---|---|---|---|---|---|---|---|---|
| FACT= | | 1.0 .75 | .50 .25 | .00 BIN | 1.0 .75 | .50 .25 | .00 BIN | 1.0 .75 | .50 .25 | .00 BIN | 1.0 75 | .50 .25 | .00 BIN | 1.0 .75 | .50 .25 | .00 BIN |
| PCONT=*** | | | | | REQUIRED NUMBER OF PATIENTS | | | | | | | | | | | |
| 0.05 | *** | 3702 | 3713 | 3921 | 788 | 799 | 831 | 285 | 289 | 296 | 168 | 170 | 172 | 119 | 120 | 121 |
| | *** | 3706 | 3736 | 7329 | 792 | 810 | 1432 | 287 | 292 | 456 | 169 | 171 | 241 | 119 | 121 | 153 |
| 0.1 | *** | 7701 | 7728 | 8615 | 1442 | 1470 | 1604 | 459 | 471 | 495 | 249 | 255 | 263 | 166 | 168 | 172 |
| | *** | 7710 | 7782 | 12731 | 1452 | 1507 | 2265 | 464 | 481 | 651 | 252 | 258 | 322 | 167 | 170 | 196 |
| 0.15 | *** | 11247 | 11295 | 13324 | 2001 | 2051 | 2351 | 604 | 628 | 679 | 316 | 326 | 342 | 203 | 208 | 215 |
| | *** | 11263 | 11390 | 17482 | 2019 | 2123 | 2994 | 614 | 648 | 821 | 320 | 333 | 391 | 206 | 212 | 232 |
| 0.2 | *** | 14068 | 14142 | 17703 | 2441 | 2517 | 3033 | 718 | 756 | 841 | 368 | 384 | 411 | 233 | 241 | 252 |
| | *** | 14093 | 14289 | 21583 | 2468 | 2631 | 3619 | 734 | 788 | 964 | 375 | 396 | 449 | 236 | 246 | 261 |
| 0.25 | *** | 16089 | 16195 | 21585 | 2756 | 2864 | 3629 | 804 | 855 | 980 | 408 | 430 | 467 | 255 | 266 | 281 |
| | *** | 16124 | 16406 | 25032 | 2794 | 3025 | 4140 | 825 | 901 | 1081 | 418 | 446 | 495 | 260 | 272 | 284 |
| 0.3 | *** | 17321 | 17466 | 24877 | 2953 | 3097 | 4127 | 863 | 928 | 1092 | 437 | 464 | 512 | 270 | 284 | 303 |
| | *** | 17369 | 17757 | 27831 | 3004 | 3309 | 4556 | 890 | 987 | 1172 | 448 | 484 | 530 | 277 | 292 | 300 |
| 0.35 | *** | 17820 | 18013 | 27524 | 3043 | 3228 | 4519 | 897 | 976 | 1177 | 454 | 486 | 544 | 280 | 295 | 318 |
| | *** | 17884 | 18400 | 29979 | 3109 | 3493 | 4869 | 930 | 1048 | 1237 | 468 | 510 | 553 | 287 | 305 | 310 |
| 0.4 | *** | 17665 | 17918 | 29494 | 3041 | 3271 | 4802 | 911 | 1002 | 1234 | 461 | 498 | 564 | 283 | 300 | 325 |
| | *** | 17749 | 18422 | 31475 | 3124 | 3588 | 5077 | 949 | 1084 | 1276 | 477 | 525 | 565 | 291 | 311 | 313 |
| 0.45 | *** | 16952 | 17278 | 30769 | 2964 | 3241 | 4973 | 906 | 1007 | 1264 | 459 | 499 | 570 | 281 | 299 | 326 |
| | *** | 17061 | 17926 | 32322 | 3066 | 3604 | 5181 | 948 | 1097 | 1289 | 477 | 529 | 565 | 289 | 311 | 310 |
| 0.5 | *** | 15785 | 16200 | 31340 | 2830 | 3150 | 5030 | 885 | 993 | 1264 | 450 | 491 | 564 | 274 | 292 | 319 |
| | *** | 15923 | 17023 | 32517 | 2950 | 3553 | 5181 | 930 | 1088 | 1276 | 468 | 521 | 553 | 282 | 304 | 300 |
| 0.55 | *** | 14272 | 14802 | 31203 | 2654 | 3011 | 4975 | 850 | 961 | 1236 | 432 | 473 | 546 | 261 | 279 | 305 |
| | *** | 14449 | 15831 | 32061 | 2790 | 3442 | 5077 | 897 | 1058 | 1237 | 450 | 503 | 530 | 269 | 291 | 284 |
| 0.6 | *** | 12530 | 13204 | 30357 | 2450 | 2833 | 4806 | 803 | 914 | 1180 | 407 | 446 | 514 | 244 | 260 | 284 |
| | *** | 12755 | 14457 | 30955 | 2599 | 3278 | 4869 | 850 | 1009 | 1172 | 424 | 475 | 495 | 251 | 271 | 261 |
| 0.65 | *** | 10679 | 11529 | 28807 | 2228 | 2623 | 4524 | 743 | 850 | 1095 | 374 | 410 | 471 | 221 | 236 | 256 |
| | *** | 10967 | 12996 | 29197 | 2384 | 3066 | 4556 | 789 | 939 | 1081 | 390 | 436 | 449 | 228 | 245 | 232 |
| 0.7 | *** | 8847 | 9885 | 26555 | 1994 | 2383 | 4130 | 672 | 769 | 983 | 333 | 365 | 415 | 193 | 205 | 221 |
| | *** | 9210 | 11507 | 26789 | 2148 | 2807 | 4140 | 714 | 849 | 964 | 347 | 386 | 391 | 199 | 212 | 196 |
| 0.75 | *** | 7155 | 8339 | 23608 | 1747 | 2112 | 3626 | 588 | 671 | 843 | 285 | 309 | 347 | 159 | 168 | 179 |
| | *** | 7586 | 10017 | 23730 | 1894 | 2498 | 3619 | 624 | 737 | 821 | 296 | 326 | 322 | 164 | 173 | 153 |
| 0.8 | *** | 5676 | 6901 | 19973 | 1484 | 1806 | 3011 | 489 | 553 | 676 | 225 | 243 | 266 | . | . | . |
| | *** | 6137 | 8513 | 20021 | 1614 | 2133 | 2994 | 517 | 602 | 651 | 233 | 253 | 241 | . | . | . |
| 0.85 | *** | 4392 | 5528 | 15656 | 1194 | 1451 | 2288 | 369 | 411 | 482 | . | . | . | . | . | . |
| | *** | 4828 | 6947 | 15660 | 1300 | 1699 | 2265 | 388 | 441 | 456 | . | . | . | . | . | . |
| 0.9 | *** | 3207 | 4120 | 10667 | 853 | 1019 | 1458 | . | . | . | . | . | . | . | . | . |
| | *** | 3563 | 5209 | 10648 | 923 | 1167 | 1432 | . | . | . | . | . | . | . | . | . |
| 0.95 | *** | 1914 | 2443 | 5011 | . | . | . | . | . | . | . | . | . | . | . | . |
| | *** | 2125 | 3022 | 4986 | . | . | . | . | . | . | . | . | . | . | . | . |

TABLE 4: ALPHA= 0.01  POWER= 0.9   EXPECTED ACCRUAL THRU MINIMUM FOLLOW-UP= 600

| | | DEL=.02 | | | DEL=.05 | | | DEL=.10 | | | DEL=.15 | | | DEL=.20 | | |
|---|---|---|---|---|---|---|---|---|---|---|---|---|---|---|---|---|
| FACT= | | 1.0 .75 | .50 .25 | .00 BIN | 1.0 .75 | .50 .25 | .00 BIN | 1.0 .75 | .50 .25 | .00 BIN | 1.0 75 | .50 .25 | .00 BIN | 1.0 .75 | .50 .25 | .00 BIN |
| PCONT=*** | | REQUIRED NUMBER OF PATIENTS | | | | | | | | | | | | | | |
| 0.05 | *** | 3703 | 3715 | 3921 | 790 | 800 | 832 | 286 | 289 | 295 | 168 | 170 | 172 | 119 | 120 | 121 |
| | *** | 3707 | 3740 | 7329 | 794 | 811 | 1432 | 287 | 292 | 456 | 169 | 171 | 241 | 119 | 121 | 153 |
| 0.1 | *** | 7703 | 7733 | 8615 | 1444 | 1474 | 1604 | 460 | 473 | 495 | 250 | 255 | 262 | 166 | 169 | 172 |
| | *** | 7713 | 7792 | 12731 | 1455 | 1511 | 2265 | 466 | 482 | 651 | 252 | 258 | 322 | 167 | 170 | 196 |
| 0.15 | *** | 11251 | 11303 | 13324 | 2006 | 2059 | 2351 | 607 | 630 | 679 | 317 | 327 | 342 | 204 | 209 | 215 |
| | *** | 11269 | 11408 | 17482 | 2025 | 2133 | 2994 | 617 | 649 | 821 | 321 | 334 | 391 | 206 | 212 | 232 |
| 0.2 | *** | 14075 | 14155 | 17703 | 2448 | 2530 | 3033 | 723 | 760 | 841 | 370 | 386 | 410 | 234 | 241 | 252 |
| | *** | 14101 | 14316 | 21583 | 2477 | 2647 | 3619 | 739 | 791 | 964 | 377 | 397 | 449 | 237 | 246 | 261 |
| 0.25 | *** | 16098 | 16214 | 21586 | 2767 | 2882 | 3629 | 811 | 862 | 980 | 411 | 433 | 467 | 257 | 267 | 281 |
| | *** | 16137 | 16445 | 25032 | 2807 | 3047 | 4140 | 832 | 905 | 1081 | 421 | 447 | 495 | 261 | 273 | 284 |
| 0.3 | *** | 17334 | 17492 | 24877 | 2967 | 3121 | 4127 | 871 | 936 | 1092 | 440 | 467 | 512 | 272 | 285 | 303 |
| | *** | 17387 | 17809 | 27831 | 3022 | 3339 | 4556 | 898 | 993 | 1172 | 452 | 486 | 530 | 278 | 293 | 300 |
| 0.35 | *** | 17837 | 18048 | 27524 | 3061 | 3258 | 4519 | 907 | 986 | 1177 | 458 | 490 | 544 | 282 | 297 | 318 |
| | *** | 17908 | 18470 | 29979 | 3132 | 3530 | 4869 | 940 | 1055 | 1237 | 472 | 513 | 553 | 289 | 306 | 310 |
| 0.4 | *** | 17688 | 17963 | 29494 | 3064 | 3307 | 4802 | 922 | 1013 | 1234 | 466 | 502 | 563 | 286 | 302 | 325 |
| | *** | 17780 | 18514 | 31475 | 3152 | 3631 | 5077 | 960 | 1093 | 1276 | 482 | 528 | 565 | 293 | 312 | 313 |
| 0.45 | *** | 16982 | 17337 | 30769 | 2993 | 3283 | 4973 | 919 | 1019 | 1263 | 465 | 503 | 570 | 284 | 301 | 326 |
| | *** | 17100 | 18043 | 32322 | 3100 | 3653 | 5181 | 961 | 1106 | 1289 | 482 | 532 | 565 | 292 | 312 | 310 |
| 0.5 | *** | 15823 | 16276 | 31340 | 2864 | 3197 | 5030 | 899 | 1006 | 1264 | 455 | 496 | 564 | 276 | 294 | 319 |
| | *** | 15974 | 17169 | 32517 | 2990 | 3606 | 5181 | 944 | 1098 | 1276 | 473 | 524 | 553 | 284 | 305 | 300 |
| 0.55 | *** | 14320 | 14898 | 31203 | 2693 | 3062 | 4975 | 864 | 975 | 1236 | 437 | 478 | 546 | 263 | 281 | 305 |
| | *** | 14513 | 16008 | 32061 | 2835 | 3498 | 5077 | 911 | 1069 | 1237 | 455 | 506 | 530 | 271 | 292 | 284 |
| 0.6 | *** | 12591 | 13324 | 30358 | 2493 | 2887 | 4806 | 817 | 926 | 1180 | 412 | 451 | 515 | 246 | 262 | 284 |
| | *** | 12837 | 14665 | 30955 | 2647 | 3335 | 4869 | 864 | 1019 | 1172 | 430 | 478 | 495 | 253 | 272 | 261 |
| 0.65 | *** | 10758 | 11676 | 28807 | 2273 | 2677 | 4524 | 757 | 862 | 1095 | 379 | 414 | 471 | 223 | 237 | 256 |
| | *** | 11071 | 13228 | 29197 | 2433 | 3122 | 4556 | 802 | 948 | 1081 | 395 | 439 | 449 | 230 | 245 | 232 |
| 0.7 | *** | 8947 | 10056 | 26555 | 2039 | 2435 | 4130 | 685 | 780 | 983 | 338 | 368 | 415 | 195 | 206 | 221 |
| | *** | 9338 | 11752 | 26789 | 2197 | 2860 | 4140 | 726 | 857 | 964 | 352 | 388 | 391 | 200 | 213 | 196 |
| 0.75 | *** | 7277 | 8522 | 23608 | 1790 | 2160 | 3626 | 599 | 680 | 843 | 288 | 311 | 347 | 161 | 169 | 179 |
| | *** | 7733 | 10261 | 23730 | 1939 | 2545 | 3619 | 635 | 744 | 821 | 299 | 327 | 322 | 164 | 174 | 153 |
| 0.8 | *** | 5808 | 7082 | 19973 | 1523 | 1847 | 3011 | 498 | 560 | 676 | 228 | 244 | 266 | . | . | . |
| | *** | 6289 | 8741 | 20021 | 1655 | 2173 | 2994 | 526 | 607 | 651 | 235 | 254 | 241 | . | . | . |
| 0.85 | *** | 4519 | 5691 | 15656 | 1226 | 1483 | 2288 | 375 | 416 | 482 | . | . | . | . | . | . |
| | *** | 4970 | 7143 | 15660 | 1332 | 1728 | 2265 | 394 | 444 | 456 | . | . | . | . | . | . |
| 0.9 | *** | 3311 | 4248 | 10666 | 874 | 1039 | 1457 | . | . | . | . | . | . | . | . | . |
| | *** | 3677 | 5356 | 10648 | 944 | 1183 | 1432 | . | . | . | . | . | . | . | . | . |
| 0.95 | *** | 1976 | 2513 | 5011 | . | . | . | . | . | . | . | . | . | . | . | . |
| | *** | 2191 | 3095 | 4986 | . | . | . | . | . | . | . | . | . | . | . | . |

# TABLE 4: ALPHA= 0.01  POWER= 0.9     EXPECTED ACCRUAL THRU MINIMUM FOLLOW-UP= 650

|       |        | DEL=.02 | | | DEL=.05 | | | DEL=.10 | | | DEL=.15 | | | DEL=.20 | | |
|-------|--------|------|------|------|------|------|------|------|------|------|------|------|------|------|------|------|
| FACT= |        | 1.0 .75 | .50 .25 | .00 BIN | 1.0 .75 | .50 .25 | .00 BIN | 1.0 .75 | .50 .25 | .00 BIN | 1.0 75 | .50 .25 | .00 BIN | 1.0 .75 | .50 .25 | .00 BIN |
| PCONT=*** | | REQUIRED NUMBER OF PATIENTS | | | | | | | | | | | | | | |
| 0.05 | *** | 3704 | 3717 | 3921 | 790 | 802 | 831 | 286 | 290 | 296 | 168 | 170 | 172 | 119 | 120 | 121 |
|      | *** | 3708 | 3744 | 7329 | 795 | 812 | 1432 | 288 | 292 | 456 | 169 | 171 | 241 | 120 | 120 | 153 |
| 0.1 | *** | 7706 | 7738 | 8615 | 1447 | 1478 | 1604 | 462 | 474 | 495 | 250 | 255 | 263 | 166 | 169 | 172 |
|     | *** | 7717 | 7802 | 12731 | 1459 | 1516 | 2265 | 467 | 483 | 651 | 253 | 259 | 322 | 168 | 171 | 196 |
| 0.15 | *** | 11256 | 11312 | 13324 | 2011 | 2067 | 2351 | 610 | 633 | 679 | 318 | 328 | 342 | 205 | 210 | 216 |
|      | *** | 11274 | 11425 | 17482 | 2031 | 2142 | 2994 | 619 | 652 | 821 | 322 | 334 | 391 | 207 | 212 | 232 |
| 0.2 | *** | 14081 | 14169 | 17703 | 2456 | 2542 | 3033 | 727 | 764 | 841 | 372 | 387 | 411 | 235 | 242 | 252 |
|     | *** | 14111 | 14343 | 21583 | 2486 | 2662 | 3619 | 743 | 794 | 964 | 379 | 398 | 449 | 238 | 246 | 261 |
| 0.25 | *** | 16108 | 16233 | 21586 | 2777 | 2899 | 3629 | 816 | 867 | 980 | 414 | 435 | 467 | 258 | 268 | 281 |
|      | *** | 16149 | 16483 | 25032 | 2820 | 3069 | 4140 | 838 | 910 | 1081 | 423 | 449 | 495 | 262 | 274 | 284 |
| 0.3 | *** | 17347 | 17519 | 24877 | 2981 | 3143 | 4127 | 879 | 944 | 1092 | 444 | 470 | 512 | 274 | 286 | 303 |
|     | *** | 17404 | 17862 | 27831 | 3039 | 3366 | 4556 | 906 | 999 | 1172 | 455 | 488 | 530 | 280 | 294 | 300 |
| 0.35 | *** | 17855 | 18083 | 27524 | 3079 | 3286 | 4519 | 916 | 995 | 1177 | 462 | 493 | 544 | 284 | 298 | 318 |
|      | *** | 17931 | 18540 | 29979 | 3154 | 3564 | 4869 | 950 | 1062 | 1237 | 476 | 515 | 553 | 291 | 307 | 310 |
| 0.4 | *** | 17711 | 18010 | 29494 | 3087 | 3342 | 4802 | 933 | 1023 | 1234 | 471 | 506 | 564 | 288 | 303 | 325 |
|     | *** | 17811 | 18605 | 31475 | 3180 | 3671 | 5077 | 971 | 1100 | 1276 | 487 | 530 | 565 | 295 | 314 | 313 |
| 0.45 | *** | 17012 | 17396 | 30769 | 3021 | 3322 | 4973 | 930 | 1030 | 1263 | 470 | 508 | 570 | 286 | 302 | 326 |
|      | *** | 17140 | 18158 | 32322 | 3134 | 3698 | 5181 | 973 | 1115 | 1289 | 487 | 534 | 565 | 294 | 313 | 310 |
| 0.5 | *** | 15860 | 16352 | 31340 | 2897 | 3242 | 5030 | 912 | 1017 | 1264 | 461 | 500 | 565 | 279 | 295 | 319 |
|     | *** | 16024 | 17313 | 32517 | 3028 | 3655 | 5181 | 957 | 1108 | 1276 | 478 | 527 | 553 | 286 | 306 | 300 |
| 0.55 | *** | 14368 | 14994 | 31203 | 2731 | 3110 | 4975 | 877 | 987 | 1236 | 443 | 482 | 546 | 266 | 282 | 305 |
|      | *** | 14577 | 16181 | 32061 | 2877 | 3550 | 5077 | 924 | 1078 | 1237 | 460 | 509 | 530 | 274 | 293 | 284 |
| 0.6 | *** | 12653 | 13444 | 30358 | 2534 | 2937 | 4806 | 830 | 938 | 1180 | 417 | 454 | 515 | 248 | 263 | 284 |
|     | *** | 12919 | 14866 | 30955 | 2692 | 3388 | 4869 | 877 | 1028 | 1172 | 434 | 480 | 495 | 255 | 273 | 261 |
| 0.65 | *** | 10837 | 11821 | 28807 | 2317 | 2727 | 4524 | 770 | 873 | 1095 | 384 | 418 | 471 | 225 | 238 | 256 |
|      | *** | 11175 | 13450 | 29197 | 2480 | 3174 | 4556 | 814 | 957 | 1081 | 399 | 441 | 449 | 231 | 246 | 232 |
| 0.7 | *** | 9047 | 10221 | 26555 | 2082 | 2484 | 4130 | 697 | 790 | 983 | 342 | 371 | 415 | 197 | 207 | 221 |
|     | *** | 9464 | 11985 | 26789 | 2243 | 2908 | 4140 | 737 | 864 | 964 | 355 | 390 | 391 | 201 | 214 | 196 |
| 0.75 | *** | 7395 | 8699 | 23608 | 1831 | 2205 | 3626 | 609 | 689 | 843 | 291 | 314 | 347 | 162 | 170 | 179 |
|      | *** | 7875 | 10491 | 23730 | 1982 | 2589 | 3619 | 644 | 750 | 821 | 302 | 328 | 322 | 166 | 174 | 153 |
| 0.8 | *** | 5935 | 7255 | 19973 | 1559 | 1886 | 3011 | 506 | 567 | 676 | 230 | 246 | 266 | . | . | . |
|     | *** | 6435 | 8956 | 20021 | 1693 | 2209 | 2994 | 533 | 612 | 651 | 237 | 255 | 241 | . | . | . |
| 0.85 | *** | 4639 | 5845 | 15656 | 1255 | 1512 | 2288 | 380 | 419 | 482 | . | . | . | . | . | . |
|      | *** | 5104 | 7327 | 15660 | 1362 | 1754 | 2265 | 398 | 446 | 456 | . | . | . | . | . | . |
| 0.9 | *** | 3410 | 4368 | 10666 | 894 | 1057 | 1458 | . | . | . | . | . | . | . | . | . |
|     | *** | 3785 | 5493 | 10648 | 963 | 1198 | 1432 | . | . | . | . | . | . | . | . | . |
| 0.95 | *** | 2034 | 2579 | 5011 | . | . | . | . | . | . | . | . | . | . | . | . |
|      | *** | 2253 | 3162 | 4986 | . | . | . | . | . | . | . | . | . | . | . | . |

TABLE 4: ALPHA= 0.01  POWER= 0.9    EXPECTED ACCRUAL THRU MINIMUM FOLLOW-UP= 700

| | | DEL=.02 | | | DEL=.05 | | | DEL=.10 | | | DEL=.15 | | | DEL=.20 | | |
|---|---|---|---|---|---|---|---|---|---|---|---|---|---|---|---|---|---|
| FACT= | | 1.0 .75 | .50 .25 | .00 BIN | 1.0 .75 | .50 .25 | .00 BIN | 1.0 .75 | .50 .25 | .00 BIN | 1.0 75 | .50 .25 | .00 BIN | 1.0 .75 | .50 .25 | .00 BIN |
| PCONT=*** | | | | | REQUIRED NUMBER OF PATIENTS | | | | | | | | | | | |
| 0.05 | *** | 3705 | 3719 | 3921 | 792 | 803 | 831 | 286 | 290 | 296 | 169 | 170 | 172 | 119 | 120 | 121 |
| | *** | 3710 | 3747 | 7329 | 796 | 814 | 1432 | 288 | 292 | 456 | 170 | 171 | 241 | 120 | 121 | 153 |
| 0.1 | *** | 7708 | 7743 | 8615 | 1450 | 1482 | 1604 | 464 | 475 | 495 | 251 | 256 | 263 | 166 | 169 | 172 |
| | *** | 7720 | 7812 | 12731 | 1462 | 1520 | 2265 | 468 | 484 | 651 | 254 | 259 | 322 | 168 | 170 | 196 |
| 0.15 | *** | 11260 | 11321 | 13323 | 2016 | 2074 | 2351 | 612 | 635 | 678 | 319 | 329 | 342 | 205 | 210 | 215 |
| | *** | 11280 | 11443 | 17482 | 2037 | 2150 | 2994 | 622 | 653 | 821 | 324 | 335 | 391 | 207 | 212 | 232 |
| 0.2 | *** | 14088 | 14182 | 17703 | 2463 | 2553 | 3033 | 731 | 768 | 841 | 374 | 389 | 411 | 236 | 243 | 252 |
| | *** | 14120 | 14370 | 21583 | 2495 | 2675 | 3619 | 747 | 797 | 964 | 381 | 398 | 449 | 239 | 247 | 261 |
| 0.25 | *** | 16118 | 16252 | 21586 | 2787 | 2915 | 3629 | 822 | 872 | 980 | 416 | 436 | 467 | 259 | 268 | 281 |
| | *** | 16162 | 16522 | 25032 | 2833 | 3088 | 4140 | 843 | 914 | 1081 | 425 | 450 | 495 | 264 | 274 | 284 |
| 0.3 | *** | 17360 | 17545 | 24877 | 2994 | 3165 | 4127 | 886 | 950 | 1092 | 447 | 472 | 512 | 276 | 287 | 303 |
| | *** | 17422 | 17915 | 27831 | 3056 | 3392 | 4556 | 913 | 1004 | 1172 | 458 | 489 | 530 | 281 | 294 | 300 |
| 0.35 | *** | 17872 | 18118 | 27524 | 3097 | 3313 | 4519 | 925 | 1003 | 1177 | 466 | 496 | 544 | 286 | 299 | 318 |
| | *** | 17954 | 18610 | 29979 | 3176 | 3595 | 4869 | 958 | 1068 | 1237 | 479 | 516 | 553 | 292 | 308 | 310 |
| 0.4 | *** | 17734 | 18055 | 29494 | 3109 | 3374 | 4802 | 943 | 1032 | 1234 | 475 | 509 | 564 | 290 | 305 | 325 |
| | *** | 17841 | 18695 | 31475 | 3208 | 3708 | 5077 | 981 | 1108 | 1276 | 490 | 532 | 565 | 297 | 314 | 313 |
| 0.45 | *** | 17041 | 17455 | 30769 | 3048 | 3360 | 4973 | 941 | 1040 | 1263 | 474 | 511 | 570 | 288 | 304 | 326 |
| | *** | 17179 | 18273 | 32322 | 3166 | 3740 | 5181 | 983 | 1123 | 1289 | 491 | 536 | 565 | 296 | 314 | 310 |
| 0.5 | *** | 15898 | 16427 | 31341 | 2929 | 3284 | 5031 | 923 | 1028 | 1264 | 465 | 503 | 565 | 281 | 297 | 319 |
| | *** | 16074 | 17455 | 32517 | 3065 | 3701 | 5181 | 968 | 1116 | 1276 | 482 | 529 | 553 | 288 | 307 | 300 |
| 0.55 | *** | 14417 | 15089 | 31203 | 2767 | 3155 | 4975 | 890 | 998 | 1236 | 447 | 485 | 546 | 268 | 284 | 305 |
| | *** | 14642 | 16350 | 32061 | 2918 | 3597 | 5077 | 936 | 1087 | 1237 | 464 | 511 | 530 | 275 | 293 | 284 |
| 0.6 | *** | 12714 | 13563 | 30357 | 2574 | 2984 | 4806 | 842 | 949 | 1180 | 422 | 458 | 515 | 250 | 264 | 284 |
| | *** | 13001 | 15061 | 30955 | 2735 | 3436 | 4869 | 888 | 1036 | 1172 | 438 | 482 | 495 | 257 | 274 | 261 |
| 0.65 | *** | 10915 | 11963 | 28807 | 2357 | 2774 | 4524 | 782 | 883 | 1095 | 388 | 421 | 471 | 227 | 240 | 256 |
| | *** | 11277 | 13663 | 29197 | 2523 | 3222 | 4556 | 825 | 964 | 1081 | 403 | 443 | 449 | 233 | 247 | 232 |
| 0.7 | *** | 9145 | 10382 | 26555 | 2123 | 2529 | 4130 | 707 | 799 | 983 | 345 | 373 | 415 | 198 | 208 | 221 |
| | *** | 9588 | 12206 | 26789 | 2286 | 2953 | 4140 | 747 | 871 | 964 | 358 | 392 | 391 | 203 | 214 | 196 |
| 0.75 | *** | 7511 | 8867 | 23608 | 1869 | 2246 | 3626 | 618 | 696 | 843 | 294 | 316 | 347 | 163 | 170 | 179 |
| | *** | 8013 | 10710 | 23730 | 2022 | 2628 | 3619 | 653 | 755 | 821 | 304 | 330 | 322 | 166 | 174 | 153 |
| 0.8 | *** | 6057 | 7419 | 19973 | 1593 | 1921 | 3011 | 513 | 572 | 676 | 232 | 247 | 266 | . | . | . |
| | *** | 6575 | 9158 | 20021 | 1727 | 2242 | 2994 | 539 | 615 | 651 | 239 | 256 | 241 | . | . | . |
| 0.85 | *** | 4755 | 5991 | 15656 | 1283 | 1539 | 2288 | 385 | 423 | 482 | . | . | . | . | . | . |
| | *** | 5232 | 7499 | 15660 | 1389 | 1778 | 2265 | 402 | 449 | 456 | . | . | . | . | . | . |
| 0.9 | *** | 3503 | 4481 | 10666 | 912 | 1073 | 1458 | . | . | . | . | . | . | . | . | . |
| | *** | 3887 | 5620 | 10648 | 980 | 1211 | 1432 | . | . | . | . | . | . | . | . | . |
| 0.95 | *** | 2089 | 2641 | 5011 | . | . | . | . | . | . | . | . | . | . | . | . |
| | *** | 2311 | 3225 | 4986 | . | . | . | . | . | . | . | . | . | . | . | . |

# TABLE 4: ALPHA= 0.01  POWER= 0.9     EXPECTED ACCRUAL THRU MINIMUM FOLLOW-UP= 750

| | | DEL=.02 | | | DEL=.05 | | | DEL=.10 | | | DEL=.15 | | | DEL=.20 | | |
|---|---|---|---|---|---|---|---|---|---|---|---|---|---|---|---|---|
| FACT= | | 1.0 .75 | .50 .25 | .00 BIN | 1.0 .75 | .50 .25 | .00 BIN | 1.0 .75 | .50 .25 | .00 BIN | 1.0 75 | .50 .25 | .00 BIN | 1.0 .75 | .50 .25 | .00 BIN |
| PCONT=*** | | | | | REQUIRED NUMBER OF PATIENTS | | | | | | | | | | | |
| 0.05 | *** | 3706 | 3722 | 3921 | 793 | 804 | 831 | 287 | 290 | 295 | 169 | 170 | 172 | 119 | 120 | 121 |
| | *** | 3711 | 3751 | 7329 | 797 | 814 | 1432 | 289 | 293 | 456 | 169 | 171 | 241 | 120 | 121 | 153 |
| 0.1 | *** | 7711 | 7748 | 8615 | 1452 | 1486 | 1604 | 465 | 476 | 495 | 251 | 256 | 263 | 167 | 169 | 172 |
| | *** | 7723 | 7822 | 12731 | 1465 | 1523 | 2265 | 470 | 484 | 651 | 254 | 259 | 322 | 168 | 171 | 196 |
| 0.15 | *** | 11265 | 11330 | 13324 | 2020 | 2081 | 2351 | 615 | 637 | 679 | 320 | 329 | 342 | 205 | 210 | 215 |
| | *** | 11286 | 11460 | 17482 | 2043 | 2158 | 2994 | 625 | 654 | 821 | 325 | 335 | 391 | 208 | 213 | 232 |
| 0.2 | *** | 14095 | 14195 | 17704 | 2470 | 2565 | 3033 | 735 | 771 | 841 | 376 | 390 | 410 | 236 | 243 | 252 |
| | *** | 14128 | 14396 | 21583 | 2504 | 2688 | 3619 | 751 | 799 | 964 | 382 | 399 | 449 | 240 | 247 | 261 |
| 0.25 | *** | 16127 | 16271 | 21586 | 2797 | 2931 | 3629 | 827 | 877 | 979 | 419 | 438 | 468 | 260 | 269 | 281 |
| | *** | 16175 | 16560 | 25032 | 2845 | 3106 | 4140 | 849 | 917 | 1081 | 428 | 451 | 495 | 265 | 274 | 284 |
| 0.3 | *** | 17374 | 17572 | 24877 | 3008 | 3185 | 4127 | 892 | 956 | 1092 | 450 | 474 | 512 | 277 | 288 | 303 |
| | *** | 17440 | 17967 | 27831 | 3073 | 3416 | 4556 | 919 | 1009 | 1172 | 460 | 490 | 530 | 282 | 295 | 300 |
| 0.35 | *** | 17890 | 18154 | 27524 | 3115 | 3340 | 4519 | 933 | 1010 | 1177 | 469 | 499 | 544 | 288 | 300 | 318 |
| | *** | 17978 | 18679 | 29979 | 3198 | 3625 | 4869 | 966 | 1074 | 1237 | 483 | 518 | 553 | 293 | 308 | 310 |
| 0.4 | *** | 17757 | 18101 | 29494 | 3131 | 3405 | 4802 | 952 | 1041 | 1234 | 479 | 512 | 564 | 291 | 306 | 325 |
| | *** | 17872 | 18785 | 31475 | 3234 | 3743 | 5077 | 990 | 1114 | 1276 | 493 | 534 | 565 | 298 | 315 | 313 |
| 0.45 | *** | 17071 | 17514 | 30769 | 3074 | 3396 | 4973 | 951 | 1049 | 1264 | 478 | 514 | 570 | 290 | 305 | 325 |
| | *** | 17219 | 18386 | 32322 | 3197 | 3779 | 5181 | 994 | 1130 | 1289 | 494 | 538 | 565 | 297 | 314 | 310 |
| 0.5 | *** | 15936 | 16503 | 31340 | 2960 | 3323 | 5030 | 934 | 1038 | 1264 | 469 | 506 | 565 | 282 | 298 | 319 |
| | *** | 16125 | 17594 | 32517 | 3100 | 3743 | 5181 | 979 | 1123 | 1276 | 486 | 531 | 553 | 290 | 308 | 300 |
| 0.55 | *** | 14465 | 15184 | 31203 | 2801 | 3198 | 4975 | 901 | 1008 | 1236 | 452 | 488 | 546 | 270 | 285 | 305 |
| | *** | 14706 | 16516 | 32061 | 2957 | 3642 | 5077 | 947 | 1094 | 1237 | 469 | 513 | 530 | 277 | 294 | 284 |
| 0.6 | *** | 12776 | 13680 | 30358 | 2611 | 3028 | 4806 | 853 | 959 | 1180 | 426 | 460 | 514 | 252 | 265 | 284 |
| | *** | 13082 | 15249 | 30955 | 2776 | 3482 | 4869 | 899 | 1043 | 1172 | 442 | 484 | 495 | 259 | 274 | 261 |
| 0.65 | *** | 10993 | 12102 | 28807 | 2396 | 2818 | 4524 | 792 | 892 | 1095 | 392 | 423 | 471 | 228 | 240 | 256 |
| | *** | 11379 | 13868 | 29197 | 2565 | 3265 | 4556 | 835 | 971 | 1081 | 406 | 444 | 449 | 234 | 248 | 232 |
| 0.7 | *** | 9243 | 10538 | 26555 | 2161 | 2571 | 4130 | 717 | 807 | 983 | 349 | 376 | 415 | 199 | 209 | 221 |
| | *** | 9708 | 12419 | 26789 | 2326 | 2994 | 4140 | 757 | 877 | 964 | 361 | 393 | 391 | 204 | 214 | 196 |
| 0.75 | *** | 7624 | 9030 | 23608 | 1905 | 2285 | 3625 | 627 | 703 | 843 | 296 | 318 | 347 | 164 | 171 | 179 |
| | *** | 8146 | 10917 | 23730 | 2060 | 2665 | 3619 | 661 | 760 | 821 | 306 | 331 | 322 | 167 | 175 | 153 |
| 0.8 | *** | 6175 | 7576 | 19973 | 1625 | 1954 | 3011 | 520 | 577 | 676 | 234 | 248 | 266 | . | . | . |
| | *** | 6709 | 9349 | 20021 | 1760 | 2271 | 2994 | 545 | 619 | 651 | 241 | 257 | 241 | . | . | . |
| 0.85 | *** | 4864 | 6130 | 15656 | 1308 | 1564 | 2288 | 390 | 426 | 482 | . | . | . | . | . | . |
| | *** | 5354 | 7662 | 15660 | 1415 | 1799 | 2265 | 406 | 450 | 456 | . | . | . | . | . | . |
| 0.9 | *** | 3592 | 4588 | 10667 | 928 | 1088 | 1458 | . | . | . | . | . | . | . | . | . |
| | *** | 3984 | 5740 | 10648 | 997 | 1222 | 1432 | . | . | . | . | . | . | . | . | . |
| 0.95 | *** | 2141 | 2698 | 5011 | . | . | . | . | . | . | . | . | . | . | . | . |
| | *** | 2366 | 3282 | 4986 | . | . | . | . | . | . | . | . | . | . | . | . |

TABLE 4: ALPHA= 0.01  POWER= 0.9     EXPECTED ACCRUAL THRU MINIMUM FOLLOW-UP= 800

| PCONT | FACT | DEL=.02 1.0/.75 | DEL=.02 .50/.25 | DEL=.02 .00/BIN | DEL=.05 1.0/.75 | DEL=.05 .50/.25 | DEL=.05 .00/BIN | DEL=.10 1.0/.75 | DEL=.10 .50/.25 | DEL=.10 .00/BIN | DEL=.15 1.0/.75 | DEL=.15 .50/.25 | DEL=.15 .00/BIN | DEL=.20 1.0/.75 | DEL=.20 .50/.25 | DEL=.20 .00/BIN |
|---|---|---|---|---|---|---|---|---|---|---|---|---|---|---|---|---|
| | | | | | REQUIRED NUMBER OF PATIENTS | | | | | | | | | | | |
| 0.05 | *** | 3707 | 3724 | 3921 | 794 | 805 | 832 | 287 | 291 | 296 | 169 | 171 | 172 | 119 | 120 | 121 |
| | *** | 3713 | 3755 | 7329 | 798 | 815 | 1432 | 289 | 293 | 456 | 170 | 171 | 241 | 120 | 121 | 153 |
| 0.1 | *** | 7713 | 7753 | 8615 | 1455 | 1489 | 1604 | 466 | 477 | 495 | 252 | 257 | 263 | 167 | 170 | 172 |
| | *** | 7726 | 7831 | 12731 | 1468 | 1527 | 2265 | 471 | 485 | 651 | 254 | 259 | 322 | 168 | 171 | 196 |
| 0.15 | *** | 11269 | 11338 | 13324 | 2025 | 2088 | 2351 | 617 | 639 | 679 | 321 | 330 | 342 | 206 | 210 | 216 |
| | *** | 11292 | 11477 | 17482 | 2048 | 2165 | 2994 | 627 | 656 | 821 | 325 | 336 | 391 | 208 | 213 | 232 |
| 0.2 | *** | 14102 | 14209 | 17703 | 2477 | 2575 | 3033 | 739 | 774 | 841 | 378 | 391 | 411 | 237 | 244 | 252 |
| | *** | 14137 | 14423 | 21583 | 2513 | 2700 | 3619 | 754 | 801 | 964 | 384 | 400 | 449 | 240 | 247 | 261 |
| 0.25 | *** | 16137 | 16291 | 21586 | 2807 | 2946 | 3629 | 832 | 881 | 980 | 421 | 440 | 467 | 261 | 270 | 281 |
| | *** | 16188 | 16598 | 25032 | 2858 | 3123 | 4140 | 853 | 920 | 1081 | 429 | 452 | 495 | 265 | 275 | 284 |
| 0.3 | *** | 17387 | 17598 | 24877 | 3022 | 3206 | 4127 | 898 | 962 | 1092 | 452 | 476 | 512 | 278 | 289 | 303 |
| | *** | 17457 | 18020 | 27831 | 3089 | 3438 | 4556 | 926 | 1013 | 1172 | 463 | 492 | 530 | 283 | 295 | 300 |
| 0.35 | *** | 17908 | 18189 | 27524 | 3132 | 3364 | 4519 | 940 | 1017 | 1177 | 472 | 501 | 544 | 289 | 301 | 318 |
| | *** | 18001 | 18749 | 29979 | 3218 | 3652 | 4869 | 973 | 1079 | 1237 | 485 | 520 | 553 | 295 | 309 | 310 |
| 0.4 | *** | 17780 | 18147 | 29494 | 3153 | 3435 | 4802 | 960 | 1048 | 1235 | 482 | 514 | 564 | 293 | 307 | 325 |
| | *** | 17903 | 18874 | 31475 | 3259 | 3775 | 5077 | 998 | 1120 | 1276 | 497 | 536 | 565 | 300 | 315 | 313 |
| 0.45 | *** | 17100 | 17573 | 30769 | 3100 | 3430 | 4973 | 961 | 1058 | 1263 | 482 | 517 | 570 | 292 | 306 | 326 |
| | *** | 17258 | 18499 | 32322 | 3226 | 3815 | 5181 | 1003 | 1136 | 1289 | 498 | 540 | 565 | 298 | 315 | 310 |
| 0.5 | *** | 15974 | 16578 | 31340 | 2990 | 3361 | 5031 | 944 | 1047 | 1264 | 473 | 509 | 564 | 284 | 299 | 319 |
| | *** | 16175 | 17731 | 32517 | 3134 | 3782 | 5181 | 988 | 1130 | 1276 | 489 | 533 | 553 | 291 | 308 | 300 |
| 0.55 | *** | 14513 | 15279 | 31203 | 2835 | 3239 | 4975 | 911 | 1017 | 1236 | 456 | 491 | 546 | 272 | 286 | 305 |
| | *** | 14770 | 16677 | 32061 | 2993 | 3683 | 5077 | 957 | 1101 | 1237 | 472 | 515 | 530 | 278 | 295 | 284 |
| 0.6 | *** | 12837 | 13796 | 30358 | 2647 | 3070 | 4806 | 864 | 968 | 1180 | 430 | 463 | 515 | 253 | 267 | 284 |
| | *** | 13163 | 15432 | 30955 | 2815 | 3523 | 4869 | 909 | 1050 | 1172 | 445 | 486 | 495 | 260 | 275 | 261 |
| 0.65 | *** | 11071 | 12238 | 28807 | 2433 | 2860 | 4524 | 802 | 901 | 1095 | 395 | 426 | 471 | 230 | 241 | 256 |
| | *** | 11479 | 14065 | 29197 | 2604 | 3306 | 4556 | 845 | 977 | 1081 | 409 | 446 | 449 | 235 | 248 | 232 |
| 0.7 | *** | 9338 | 10688 | 26555 | 2197 | 2611 | 4130 | 726 | 815 | 983 | 352 | 378 | 415 | 200 | 210 | 221 |
| | *** | 9827 | 12621 | 26789 | 2365 | 3032 | 4140 | 765 | 882 | 964 | 364 | 394 | 391 | 205 | 215 | 196 |
| 0.75 | *** | 7733 | 9186 | 23608 | 1940 | 2321 | 3626 | 635 | 709 | 821 | 299 | 319 | 347 | 165 | 171 | 179 |
| | *** | 8276 | 11115 | 23730 | 2095 | 2699 | 3619 | 668 | 764 | 821 | 308 | 332 | 322 | 168 | 175 | 153 |
| 0.8 | *** | 6289 | 7726 | 19973 | 1655 | 1985 | 3011 | 526 | 582 | 676 | 236 | 249 | 266 | . | . | . |
| | *** | 6838 | 9531 | 20021 | 1791 | 2299 | 2994 | 551 | 622 | 651 | 242 | 257 | 241 | . | . | . |
| 0.85 | *** | 4970 | 6262 | 15656 | 1332 | 1588 | 2288 | 394 | 429 | 482 | . | . | . | . | . | . |
| | *** | 5471 | 7816 | 15660 | 1439 | 1819 | 2265 | 410 | 452 | 456 | . | . | . | . | . | . |
| 0.9 | *** | 3677 | 4690 | 10667 | 944 | 1102 | 1458 | . | . | . | . | . | . | . | . | . |
| | *** | 4076 | 5852 | 10648 | 1012 | 1233 | 1432 | . | . | . | . | . | . | . | . | . |
| 0.95 | *** | 2191 | 2753 | 5011 | . | . | . | . | . | . | . | . | . | . | . | . |
| | *** | 2418 | 3336 | 4986 | . | . | . | . | . | . | . | . | . | . | . | . |

## TABLE 4: ALPHA= 0.01  POWER= 0.9    EXPECTED ACCRUAL THRU MINIMUM FOLLOW-UP= 850

| | | DEL=.02 | | | DEL=.05 | | | DEL=.10 | | | DEL=.15 | | | DEL=.20 | | |
|---|---|---|---|---|---|---|---|---|---|---|---|---|---|---|---|---|
| FACT= | | 1.0 .75 | .50 .25 | .00 BIN | 1.0 .75 | .50 .25 | .00 BIN | 1.0 .75 | .50 .25 | .00 BIN | 1.0 75 | .50 .25 | .00 BIN | 1.0 .75 | .50 .25 | .00 BIN |
| PCONT=*** | | | | | REQUIRED NUMBER OF PATIENTS | | | | | | | | | | | |
| 0.05 | *** | 3708 | 3726 | 3921 | 794 | 806 | 832 | 288 | 291 | 295 | 169 | 171 | 172 | 120 | 120 | 121 |
| | *** | 3714 | 3758 | 7329 | 799 | 816 | 1432 | 289 | 293 | 456 | 170 | 171 | 241 | 120 | 121 | 153 |
| 0.1 | *** | 7716 | 7757 | 8615 | 1458 | 1493 | 1604 | 467 | 478 | 495 | 253 | 257 | 263 | 168 | 170 | 172 |
| | *** | 7730 | 7841 | 12731 | 1471 | 1530 | 2265 | 472 | 485 | 651 | 255 | 259 | 322 | 169 | 171 | 196 |
| 0.15 | *** | 11273 | 11347 | 13323 | 2029 | 2095 | 2351 | 619 | 641 | 679 | 322 | 331 | 342 | 207 | 210 | 215 |
| | *** | 11298 | 11494 | 17482 | 2054 | 2171 | 2994 | 629 | 657 | 821 | 326 | 336 | 391 | 208 | 213 | 232 |
| 0.2 | *** | 14108 | 14222 | 17703 | 2484 | 2586 | 3033 | 742 | 777 | 841 | 379 | 392 | 410 | 238 | 244 | 252 |
| | *** | 14146 | 14450 | 21583 | 2521 | 2711 | 3619 | 757 | 803 | 964 | 385 | 400 | 449 | 241 | 248 | 261 |
| 0.25 | *** | 16147 | 16310 | 21585 | 2817 | 2960 | 3629 | 836 | 885 | 980 | 423 | 441 | 467 | 262 | 271 | 281 |
| | *** | 16201 | 16637 | 25032 | 2870 | 3139 | 4140 | 858 | 923 | 1081 | 431 | 453 | 495 | 266 | 275 | 284 |
| 0.3 | *** | 17400 | 17624 | 24877 | 3035 | 3224 | 4127 | 904 | 967 | 1092 | 454 | 478 | 512 | 280 | 290 | 303 |
| | *** | 17475 | 18072 | 27831 | 3105 | 3459 | 4556 | 931 | 1017 | 1172 | 465 | 493 | 530 | 284 | 295 | 300 |
| 0.35 | *** | 17925 | 18224 | 27524 | 3149 | 3388 | 4519 | 947 | 1023 | 1177 | 475 | 503 | 544 | 290 | 302 | 318 |
| | *** | 18025 | 18818 | 29979 | 3239 | 3678 | 4869 | 980 | 1083 | 1237 | 488 | 521 | 553 | 295 | 309 | 310 |
| 0.4 | *** | 17803 | 18193 | 29494 | 3174 | 3463 | 4802 | 969 | 1055 | 1234 | 485 | 516 | 563 | 294 | 308 | 325 |
| | *** | 17933 | 18963 | 31475 | 3284 | 3805 | 5077 | 1006 | 1125 | 1276 | 499 | 537 | 565 | 301 | 316 | 313 |
| 0.45 | *** | 17130 | 17632 | 30769 | 3126 | 3462 | 4973 | 970 | 1065 | 1263 | 486 | 519 | 570 | 293 | 307 | 326 |
| | *** | 17298 | 18609 | 32322 | 3255 | 3849 | 5181 | 1011 | 1142 | 1289 | 501 | 542 | 565 | 300 | 316 | 310 |
| 0.5 | *** | 16012 | 16653 | 31340 | 3019 | 3397 | 5031 | 953 | 1055 | 1264 | 477 | 511 | 564 | 286 | 300 | 319 |
| | *** | 16226 | 17866 | 32517 | 3166 | 3819 | 5181 | 997 | 1136 | 1276 | 493 | 535 | 553 | 292 | 309 | 300 |
| 0.55 | *** | 14561 | 15372 | 31203 | 2867 | 3277 | 4975 | 921 | 1025 | 1236 | 459 | 494 | 546 | 273 | 287 | 305 |
| | *** | 14834 | 16835 | 32061 | 3029 | 3722 | 5077 | 966 | 1107 | 1237 | 475 | 516 | 530 | 280 | 295 | 284 |
| 0.6 | *** | 12899 | 13910 | 30357 | 2681 | 3109 | 4806 | 873 | 976 | 1179 | 433 | 465 | 514 | 255 | 267 | 284 |
| | *** | 13244 | 15608 | 30955 | 2852 | 3562 | 4869 | 918 | 1056 | 1172 | 448 | 487 | 495 | 261 | 275 | 261 |
| 0.65 | *** | 11149 | 12371 | 28807 | 2468 | 2899 | 4524 | 811 | 908 | 1096 | 398 | 428 | 471 | 231 | 242 | 256 |
| | *** | 11578 | 14255 | 29197 | 2641 | 3344 | 4556 | 854 | 983 | 1081 | 412 | 447 | 449 | 236 | 248 | 232 |
| 0.7 | *** | 9433 | 10835 | 26555 | 2232 | 2648 | 4130 | 734 | 821 | 983 | 354 | 379 | 415 | 201 | 210 | 221 |
| | *** | 9943 | 12816 | 26789 | 2401 | 3067 | 4140 | 773 | 887 | 964 | 366 | 395 | 391 | 205 | 215 | 196 |
| 0.75 | *** | 7840 | 9336 | 23608 | 1972 | 2355 | 3625 | 642 | 715 | 843 | 301 | 321 | 346 | 165 | 172 | 179 |
| | *** | 8401 | 11305 | 23730 | 2129 | 2730 | 3619 | 674 | 768 | 821 | 310 | 332 | 322 | 169 | 175 | 153 |
| 0.8 | *** | 6399 | 7870 | 19973 | 1684 | 2013 | 3011 | 531 | 586 | 676 | 237 | 250 | 266 | . | . | . |
| | *** | 6962 | 9705 | 20021 | 1820 | 2324 | 2994 | 556 | 624 | 651 | 243 | 257 | 241 | . | . | . |
| 0.85 | *** | 5071 | 6388 | 15656 | 1354 | 1609 | 2288 | 397 | 431 | 481 | . | . | . | . | . | . |
| | *** | 5583 | 7962 | 15660 | 1462 | 1837 | 2265 | 413 | 454 | 456 | . | . | . | . | . | . |
| 0.9 | *** | 3758 | 4786 | 10667 | 958 | 1115 | 1458 | . | . | . | . | . | . | . | . | . |
| | *** | 4164 | 5959 | 10648 | 1025 | 1243 | 1432 | . | . | . | . | . | . | . | . | . |
| 0.95 | *** | 2238 | 2804 | 5012 | . | . | . | . | . | . | . | . | . | . | . | . |
| | *** | 2467 | 3386 | 4986 | . | . | . | . | . | . | . | . | . | . | . | . |

TABLE 4: ALPHA= 0.01  POWER= 0.9    EXPECTED ACCRUAL THRU MINIMUM FOLLOW-UP= 900

| | | DEL=.02 | | | DEL=.05 | | | DEL=.10 | | | DEL=.15 | | | DEL=.20 | |
|---|---|---|---|---|---|---|---|---|---|---|---|---|---|---|---|---|
| FACT= | 1.0 .75 | .50 .25 | .00 BIN | 1.0 .75 | .50 .25 | .00 BIN | 1.0 .75 | .50 .25 | .00 BIN | 1.0 75 | .50 .25 | .00 BIN | 1.0 .75 | .50 .25 | .00 BIN |
| PCONT=*** | | | | REQUIRED NUMBER OF PATIENTS | | | | | | | | | | | |
| 0.05 *** | 3709 | 3728 | 3921 | 795 | 807 | 831 | 288 | 291 | 296 | 170 | 171 | 172 | 119 | 120 | 121 |
| *** | 3716 | 3762 | 7329 | 800 | 816 | 1432 | 289 | 293 | 456 | 170 | 171 | 241 | 120 | 120 | 153 |
| 0.1 *** | 7718 | 7763 | 8615 | 1460 | 1496 | 1604 | 468 | 479 | 495 | 253 | 257 | 262 | 168 | 170 | 172 |
| *** | 7733 | 7850 | 12731 | 1474 | 1532 | 2265 | 473 | 486 | 651 | 255 | 260 | 322 | 169 | 171 | 196 |
| 0.15 *** | 11278 | 11356 | 13323 | 2034 | 2101 | 2351 | 621 | 642 | 678 | 323 | 332 | 342 | 207 | 211 | 216 |
| *** | 11304 | 11511 | 17482 | 2060 | 2178 | 2994 | 630 | 658 | 821 | 327 | 336 | 391 | 209 | 213 | 232 |
| 0.2 *** | 14115 | 14236 | 17703 | 2491 | 2595 | 3033 | 745 | 779 | 841 | 380 | 393 | 411 | 239 | 244 | 252 |
| *** | 14156 | 14476 | 21583 | 2530 | 2721 | 3619 | 760 | 805 | 964 | 386 | 401 | 449 | 242 | 248 | 261 |
| 0.25 *** | 16156 | 16329 | 21585 | 2827 | 2975 | 3629 | 840 | 889 | 980 | 424 | 442 | 468 | 263 | 271 | 281 |
| *** | 16214 | 16675 | 25032 | 2882 | 3154 | 4140 | 861 | 926 | 1081 | 433 | 453 | 495 | 267 | 276 | 284 |
| 0.3 *** | 17413 | 17651 | 24877 | 3048 | 3243 | 4127 | 910 | 972 | 1092 | 457 | 479 | 512 | 280 | 290 | 303 |
| *** | 17492 | 18124 | 27831 | 3121 | 3479 | 4556 | 936 | 1019 | 1172 | 467 | 494 | 530 | 285 | 296 | 300 |
| 0.35 *** | 17943 | 18260 | 27524 | 3165 | 3411 | 4519 | 954 | 1028 | 1178 | 478 | 504 | 544 | 291 | 303 | 318 |
| *** | 18048 | 18887 | 29979 | 3258 | 3702 | 4869 | 986 | 1088 | 1237 | 490 | 522 | 553 | 297 | 309 | 310 |
| 0.4 *** | 17826 | 18239 | 29494 | 3194 | 3491 | 4802 | 976 | 1062 | 1234 | 488 | 518 | 564 | 296 | 308 | 325 |
| *** | 17964 | 19051 | 31475 | 3307 | 3834 | 5077 | 1013 | 1130 | 1276 | 502 | 539 | 565 | 302 | 316 | 313 |
| 0.45 *** | 17159 | 17691 | 30770 | 3150 | 3493 | 4973 | 978 | 1073 | 1263 | 489 | 522 | 570 | 294 | 308 | 326 |
| *** | 17337 | 18719 | 32322 | 3282 | 3881 | 5181 | 1019 | 1147 | 1289 | 504 | 543 | 565 | 301 | 316 | 310 |
| 0.5 *** | 16049 | 16727 | 31340 | 3047 | 3431 | 5031 | 962 | 1063 | 1264 | 480 | 514 | 564 | 287 | 301 | 319 |
| *** | 16276 | 17997 | 32517 | 3197 | 3854 | 5181 | 1006 | 1142 | 1276 | 496 | 536 | 553 | 294 | 309 | 300 |
| 0.55 *** | 14609 | 15465 | 31203 | 2898 | 3313 | 4975 | 930 | 1033 | 1236 | 462 | 496 | 546 | 275 | 288 | 305 |
| *** | 14898 | 16989 | 32061 | 3062 | 3758 | 5077 | 975 | 1113 | 1237 | 478 | 518 | 530 | 281 | 296 | 284 |
| 0.6 *** | 12960 | 14023 | 30358 | 2714 | 3146 | 4806 | 883 | 983 | 1180 | 436 | 468 | 515 | 256 | 269 | 284 |
| *** | 13325 | 15780 | 30955 | 2887 | 3599 | 4869 | 927 | 1061 | 1172 | 451 | 488 | 495 | 262 | 276 | 261 |
| 0.65 *** | 11226 | 12502 | 28807 | 2502 | 2936 | 4524 | 820 | 915 | 1095 | 401 | 430 | 471 | 232 | 243 | 256 |
| *** | 11676 | 14438 | 29197 | 2677 | 3379 | 4556 | 862 | 987 | 1081 | 414 | 448 | 449 | 237 | 249 | 232 |
| 0.7 *** | 9526 | 10977 | 26555 | 2265 | 2683 | 4130 | 743 | 828 | 983 | 357 | 381 | 415 | 202 | 210 | 221 |
| *** | 10056 | 13002 | 26789 | 2435 | 3100 | 4140 | 780 | 891 | 964 | 368 | 396 | 391 | 206 | 216 | 196 |
| 0.75 *** | 7945 | 9482 | 23608 | 2003 | 2387 | 3626 | 649 | 720 | 843 | 303 | 322 | 347 | 166 | 172 | 179 |
| *** | 8523 | 11485 | 23730 | 2160 | 2759 | 3619 | 681 | 771 | 821 | 312 | 333 | 322 | 169 | 176 | 153 |
| 0.8 *** | 6506 | 8008 | 19973 | 1710 | 2040 | 3011 | 536 | 590 | 676 | 238 | 251 | 266 | . | . | . |
| *** | 7082 | 9870 | 20021 | 1847 | 2348 | 2994 | 560 | 627 | 651 | 244 | 258 | 241 | . | . | . |
| 0.85 *** | 5169 | 6509 | 15656 | 1376 | 1630 | 2288 | 401 | 434 | 482 | . | . | . | . | . | . |
| *** | 5691 | 8101 | 15660 | 1483 | 1854 | 2265 | 416 | 455 | 456 | . | . | . | . | . | . |
| 0.9 *** | 3836 | 4879 | 10666 | 972 | 1127 | 1458 | . | . | . | . | . | . | . | . | . |
| *** | 4248 | 6059 | 10648 | 1038 | 1252 | 1432 | . | . | . | . | . | . | . | . | . |
| 0.95 *** | 2282 | 2852 | 5012 | . | . | . | . | . | . | . | . | . | . | . | . |
| *** | 2513 | 3432 | 4986 | . | . | . | . | . | . | . | . | . | . | . | . |

## TABLE 4: ALPHA= 0.01 POWER= 0.9   EXPECTED ACCRUAL THRU MINIMUM FOLLOW-UP= 950

| | | DEL=.02 | | | DEL=.05 | | | DEL=.10 | | | DEL=.15 | | | DEL=.20 | | |
|---|---|---|---|---|---|---|---|---|---|---|---|---|---|---|---|---|---|
| FACT= | | 1.0 .75 | .50 .25 | .00 BIN | 1.0 .75 | .50 .25 | .00 BIN | 1.0 .75 | .50 .25 | .00 BIN | 1.0 75 | .50 .25 | .00 BIN | 1.0 .75 | .50 .25 | .00 BIN |
| PCONT=*** | | | | | | REQUIRED NUMBER OF PATIENTS | | | | | | | | | | |
| 0.05 | *** | 3710 | 3730 | 3921 | 796 | 808 | 831 | 288 | 291 | 296 | 169 | 171 | 172 | 120 | 120 | 121 |
| | *** | 3717 | 3765 | 7329 | 801 | 817 | 1432 | 290 | 293 | 456 | 170 | 172 | 241 | 120 | 121 | 153 |
| 0.1 | *** | 7721 | 7767 | 8615 | 1463 | 1499 | 1604 | 469 | 479 | 495 | 254 | 257 | 262 | 168 | 170 | 172 |
| | *** | 7736 | 7860 | 12731 | 1477 | 1535 | 2265 | 473 | 486 | 651 | 255 | 260 | 322 | 169 | 171 | 196 |
| 0.15 | *** | 11282 | 11364 | 13323 | 2039 | 2107 | 2351 | 622 | 644 | 679 | 324 | 331 | 342 | 207 | 211 | 216 |
| | *** | 11309 | 11528 | 17482 | 2065 | 2183 | 2994 | 632 | 659 | 821 | 327 | 336 | 391 | 209 | 213 | 232 |
| 0.2 | *** | 14122 | 14249 | 17703 | 2497 | 2605 | 3033 | 748 | 781 | 841 | 381 | 394 | 410 | 239 | 245 | 252 |
| | *** | 14164 | 14503 | 21583 | 2538 | 2731 | 3619 | 762 | 806 | 964 | 387 | 401 | 449 | 242 | 248 | 261 |
| 0.25 | *** | 16165 | 16348 | 21585 | 2837 | 2988 | 3629 | 844 | 892 | 980 | 426 | 443 | 467 | 264 | 272 | 281 |
| | *** | 16227 | 16712 | 25032 | 2893 | 3168 | 4140 | 865 | 928 | 1081 | 434 | 454 | 495 | 267 | 276 | 284 |
| 0.3 | *** | 17426 | 17677 | 24877 | 3060 | 3260 | 4127 | 914 | 976 | 1092 | 458 | 481 | 512 | 281 | 291 | 303 |
| | *** | 17510 | 18175 | 27831 | 3136 | 3497 | 4556 | 941 | 1022 | 1172 | 469 | 495 | 530 | 286 | 296 | 300 |
| 0.35 | *** | 17961 | 18294 | 27524 | 3181 | 3433 | 4519 | 960 | 1034 | 1177 | 480 | 506 | 544 | 292 | 304 | 318 |
| | *** | 18071 | 18954 | 29979 | 3277 | 3725 | 4869 | 992 | 1091 | 1237 | 492 | 523 | 553 | 298 | 310 | 310 |
| 0.4 | *** | 17849 | 18285 | 29494 | 3214 | 3516 | 4802 | 983 | 1068 | 1235 | 491 | 520 | 564 | 297 | 310 | 325 |
| | *** | 17994 | 19138 | 31475 | 3331 | 3860 | 5077 | 1020 | 1134 | 1276 | 504 | 539 | 565 | 303 | 317 | 313 |
| 0.45 | *** | 17189 | 17750 | 30769 | 3173 | 3523 | 4973 | 986 | 1079 | 1264 | 492 | 523 | 570 | 296 | 309 | 325 |
| | *** | 17376 | 18827 | 32322 | 3309 | 3911 | 5181 | 1027 | 1152 | 1289 | 506 | 544 | 565 | 302 | 317 | 310 |
| 0.5 | *** | 16087 | 16802 | 31340 | 3073 | 3464 | 5030 | 971 | 1070 | 1264 | 483 | 516 | 564 | 289 | 302 | 319 |
| | *** | 16327 | 18127 | 32517 | 3227 | 3886 | 5181 | 1014 | 1147 | 1276 | 498 | 538 | 553 | 295 | 310 | 300 |
| 0.55 | *** | 14657 | 15558 | 31203 | 2928 | 3348 | 4974 | 939 | 1040 | 1236 | 466 | 498 | 546 | 276 | 289 | 305 |
| | *** | 14962 | 17138 | 32061 | 3095 | 3792 | 5077 | 983 | 1117 | 1237 | 481 | 519 | 530 | 281 | 296 | 284 |
| 0.6 | *** | 13021 | 14134 | 30357 | 2746 | 3181 | 4806 | 891 | 990 | 1180 | 439 | 470 | 514 | 257 | 269 | 284 |
| | *** | 13404 | 15947 | 30955 | 2921 | 3633 | 5077 | 935 | 1066 | 1237 | 453 | 490 | 495 | 262 | 276 | 261 |
| 0.65 | *** | 11303 | 12630 | 28806 | 2534 | 2971 | 4524 | 828 | 922 | 1096 | 403 | 431 | 471 | 233 | 243 | 256 |
| | *** | 11773 | 14615 | 29197 | 2711 | 3412 | 4556 | 869 | 992 | 1081 | 416 | 449 | 449 | 238 | 249 | 232 |
| 0.7 | *** | 9618 | 11115 | 26555 | 2296 | 2717 | 4130 | 749 | 834 | 983 | 359 | 382 | 415 | 203 | 211 | 221 |
| | *** | 10167 | 13182 | 26789 | 2468 | 3131 | 4140 | 787 | 895 | 964 | 370 | 397 | 391 | 207 | 216 | 196 |
| 0.75 | *** | 8047 | 9622 | 23608 | 2032 | 2417 | 3625 | 655 | 725 | 843 | 305 | 323 | 347 | 166 | 172 | 179 |
| | *** | 8640 | 11658 | 23730 | 2191 | 2786 | 3619 | 686 | 774 | 821 | 313 | 334 | 322 | 169 | 176 | 153 |
| 0.8 | *** | 6609 | 8141 | 19973 | 1736 | 2065 | 3011 | 541 | 593 | 676 | 239 | 251 | 266 | . | . | . |
| | *** | 7198 | 10027 | 20021 | 1873 | 2370 | 2994 | 565 | 629 | 651 | 245 | 258 | 241 | . | . | . |
| 0.85 | *** | 5263 | 6625 | 15656 | 1396 | 1648 | 2288 | 403 | 436 | 482 | . | . | . | . | . | . |
| | *** | 5795 | 8234 | 15660 | 1502 | 1870 | 2265 | 418 | 456 | 456 | . | . | . | . | . | . |
| 0.9 | *** | 3911 | 4967 | 10666 | 984 | 1138 | 1458 | . | . | . | . | . | . | . | . | . |
| | *** | 4328 | 6154 | 10648 | 1051 | 1260 | 1432 | . | . | . | . | . | . | . | . | . |
| 0.95 | *** | 2325 | 2898 | 5011 | . | . | . | . | . | . | . | . | . | . | . | . |
| | *** | 2558 | 3477 | 4986 | . | . | . | . | . | . | . | . | . | . | . | . |

TABLE 4: ALPHA= 0.01  POWER= 0.9    EXPECTED ACCRUAL THRU MINIMUM FOLLOW-UP= 1000

| | | DEL=.02 | | | DEL=.05 | | | DEL=.10 | | | DEL=.15 | | | DEL=.20 | | |
|---|---|---|---|---|---|---|---|---|---|---|---|---|---|---|---|---|---|
| FACT= | | 1.0 .75 | .50 .25 | .00 BIN | 1.0 .75 | .50 .25 | .00 BIN | 1.0 .75 | .50 .25 | .00 BIN | 1.0 75 | .50 .25 | .00 BIN | 1.0 .75 | .50 .25 | .00 BIN |
| PCONT=*** | | | | | REQUIRED NUMBER OF PATIENTS | | | | | | | | | | | |
| 0.05 | *** | 3711 | 3732 | 3921 | 797 | 808 | 831 | 288 | 291 | 296 | 170 | 171 | 172 | 120 | 120 | 121 |
| | *** | 3718 | 3768 | 7329 | 802 | 818 | 1432 | 290 | 293 | 456 | 170 | 171 | 241 | 120 | 121 | 153 |
| 0.1 | *** | 7723 | 7773 | 8615 | 1465 | 1501 | 1604 | 470 | 480 | 495 | 254 | 258 | 263 | 168 | 170 | 172 |
| | *** | 7740 | 7869 | 12731 | 1480 | 1538 | 2265 | 475 | 487 | 651 | 256 | 260 | 322 | 169 | 171 | 196 |
| 0.15 | *** | 11286 | 11373 | 13323 | 2043 | 2113 | 2351 | 625 | 645 | 678 | 325 | 332 | 342 | 208 | 211 | 216 |
| | *** | 11315 | 11545 | 17482 | 2070 | 2189 | 2994 | 634 | 660 | 821 | 328 | 337 | 391 | 210 | 213 | 232 |
| 0.2 | *** | 14128 | 14263 | 17703 | 2505 | 2614 | 3033 | 751 | 784 | 841 | 383 | 395 | 411 | 240 | 245 | 252 |
| | *** | 14173 | 14529 | 21583 | 2546 | 2740 | 3619 | 765 | 808 | 964 | 388 | 402 | 449 | 242 | 248 | 261 |
| 0.25 | *** | 16175 | 16368 | 21586 | 2846 | 3001 | 3629 | 848 | 895 | 980 | 428 | 444 | 468 | 265 | 272 | 281 |
| | *** | 16240 | 16750 | 25032 | 2905 | 3181 | 4140 | 869 | 930 | 1081 | 435 | 455 | 495 | 268 | 276 | 284 |
| 0.3 | *** | 17440 | 17704 | 24877 | 3073 | 3278 | 4127 | 920 | 980 | 1092 | 461 | 482 | 512 | 282 | 291 | 303 |
| | *** | 17528 | 18227 | 27831 | 3151 | 3515 | 4556 | 946 | 1026 | 1172 | 470 | 495 | 530 | 286 | 297 | 300 |
| 0.35 | *** | 17978 | 18330 | 27524 | 3198 | 3454 | 4519 | 966 | 1039 | 1177 | 483 | 508 | 544 | 293 | 304 | 318 |
| | *** | 18095 | 19022 | 29979 | 3296 | 3747 | 4869 | 998 | 1095 | 1237 | 494 | 524 | 553 | 298 | 311 | 310 |
| 0.4 | *** | 17872 | 18331 | 29494 | 3234 | 3541 | 4802 | 990 | 1073 | 1235 | 493 | 522 | 563 | 298 | 310 | 325 |
| | *** | 18025 | 19224 | 31475 | 3353 | 3886 | 5077 | 1026 | 1138 | 1276 | 506 | 541 | 565 | 304 | 317 | 313 |
| 0.45 | *** | 17219 | 17809 | 30770 | 3196 | 3551 | 4973 | 993 | 1086 | 1263 | 495 | 525 | 570 | 297 | 310 | 326 |
| | *** | 17416 | 18933 | 32322 | 3335 | 3940 | 5181 | 1034 | 1156 | 1289 | 509 | 545 | 565 | 303 | 317 | 310 |
| 0.5 | *** | 16125 | 16876 | 31340 | 3100 | 3495 | 5031 | 978 | 1076 | 1264 | 486 | 518 | 565 | 290 | 303 | 319 |
| | *** | 16377 | 18254 | 32517 | 3256 | 3917 | 5181 | 1021 | 1151 | 1276 | 501 | 539 | 553 | 296 | 310 | 300 |
| 0.55 | *** | 14706 | 15650 | 31203 | 2956 | 3380 | 4975 | 947 | 1046 | 1236 | 468 | 500 | 546 | 277 | 290 | 305 |
| | *** | 15026 | 17285 | 32061 | 3126 | 3824 | 5077 | 991 | 1123 | 1237 | 483 | 521 | 530 | 283 | 296 | 284 |
| 0.6 | *** | 13082 | 14243 | 30358 | 2776 | 3215 | 4806 | 899 | 997 | 1180 | 441 | 472 | 515 | 258 | 270 | 284 |
| | *** | 13484 | 16108 | 30955 | 2953 | 3665 | 4869 | 942 | 1071 | 1172 | 456 | 491 | 495 | 264 | 276 | 261 |
| 0.65 | *** | 11378 | 12755 | 28807 | 2565 | 3004 | 4524 | 836 | 928 | 1095 | 406 | 433 | 471 | 234 | 244 | 256 |
| | *** | 11869 | 14786 | 29197 | 2743 | 3444 | 4556 | 876 | 996 | 1081 | 418 | 450 | 449 | 239 | 250 | 232 |
| 0.7 | *** | 9708 | 11250 | 26555 | 2326 | 2748 | 4130 | 756 | 839 | 983 | 361 | 384 | 415 | 204 | 211 | 221 |
| | *** | 10276 | 13355 | 26789 | 2499 | 3160 | 4140 | 793 | 899 | 964 | 372 | 398 | 391 | 208 | 216 | 196 |
| 0.75 | *** | 8146 | 9758 | 23608 | 2060 | 2445 | 3626 | 661 | 730 | 843 | 306 | 324 | 346 | 167 | 173 | 179 |
| | *** | 8756 | 11825 | 23730 | 2219 | 2811 | 3619 | 691 | 778 | 821 | 315 | 335 | 322 | 170 | 176 | 153 |
| 0.8 | *** | 6709 | 8270 | 19973 | 1760 | 2090 | 3011 | 545 | 596 | 676 | 241 | 252 | 266 | . | . | . |
| | *** | 7310 | 10178 | 20021 | 1898 | 2390 | 2994 | 569 | 631 | 651 | 246 | 259 | 241 | . | . | . |
| 0.85 | *** | 5355 | 6736 | 15656 | 1415 | 1666 | 2288 | 406 | 438 | 482 | . | . | . | . | . | . |
| | *** | 5895 | 8360 | 15660 | 1521 | 1884 | 2265 | 421 | 458 | 456 | . | . | . | . | . | . |
| 0.9 | *** | 3983 | 5051 | 10666 | 996 | 1148 | 1458 | . | . | . | . | . | . | . | . | . |
| | *** | 4406 | 6245 | 10648 | 1063 | 1268 | 1432 | . | . | . | . | . | . | . | . | . |
| 0.95 | *** | 2366 | 2941 | 5011 | . | . | . | . | . | . | . | . | . | . | . | . |
| | *** | 2600 | 3518 | 4986 | . | . | . | . | . | . | . | . | . | . | . | . |

## TABLE 4: ALPHA= 0.01  POWER= 0.9    EXPECTED ACCRUAL THRU MINIMUM FOLLOW-UP= 1100

| | | DEL=.02 | | | DEL=.05 | | | DEL=.10 | | | DEL=.15 | | | DEL=.20 | | |
|---|---|---|---|---|---|---|---|---|---|---|---|---|---|---|---|---|
| FACT= | | 1.0 .75 | .50 .25 | .00 BIN | 1.0 .75 | .50 .25 | .00 BIN | 1.0 .75 | .50 .25 | .00 BIN | 1.0 75 | .50 .25 | .00 BIN | 1.0 .75 | .50 .25 | .00 BIN |
| PCONT=*** | | | | | | REQUIRED | NUMBER | OF PATIENTS | | | | | | | | |
| 0.05 | *** | 3713 | 3736 | 3921 | 799 | 810 | 831 | 289 | 291 | 296 | 170 | 170 | 172 | 120 | 120 | 121 |
| | *** | 3721 | 3774 | 7329 | 804 | 819 | 1432 | 290 | 294 | 456 | 170 | 171 | 241 | 120 | 121 | 153 |
| 0.1 | *** | 7728 | 7782 | 8615 | 1470 | 1506 | 1604 | 471 | 481 | 495 | 254 | 258 | 263 | 169 | 170 | 172 |
| | *** | 7746 | 7887 | 12731 | 1484 | 1542 | 2265 | 476 | 488 | 651 | 257 | 260 | 322 | 169 | 171 | 196 |
| 0.15 | *** | 11295 | 11390 | 13324 | 2051 | 2123 | 2351 | 628 | 648 | 679 | 326 | 333 | 342 | 208 | 212 | 215 |
| | *** | 11327 | 11579 | 17482 | 2079 | 2199 | 2994 | 637 | 661 | 821 | 329 | 337 | 391 | 210 | 213 | 232 |
| 0.2 | *** | 14142 | 14289 | 17703 | 2517 | 2631 | 3033 | 756 | 788 | 841 | 384 | 395 | 411 | 241 | 246 | 252 |
| | *** | 14191 | 14581 | 21583 | 2561 | 2756 | 3619 | 770 | 811 | 964 | 389 | 402 | 449 | 243 | 248 | 261 |
| 0.25 | *** | 16195 | 16406 | 21586 | 2864 | 3025 | 3629 | 855 | 901 | 980 | 430 | 445 | 467 | 265 | 272 | 280 |
| | *** | 16265 | 16825 | 25032 | 2925 | 3205 | 4140 | 875 | 934 | 1081 | 437 | 456 | 495 | 269 | 276 | 284 |
| 0.3 | *** | 17466 | 17757 | 24877 | 3097 | 3309 | 4127 | 928 | 987 | 1092 | 464 | 484 | 512 | 284 | 292 | 302 |
| | *** | 17563 | 18329 | 27831 | 3178 | 3547 | 4556 | 954 | 1031 | 1172 | 473 | 496 | 530 | 288 | 297 | 300 |
| 0.35 | *** | 18013 | 18400 | 27524 | 3228 | 3493 | 4519 | 976 | 1048 | 1177 | 486 | 510 | 544 | 295 | 305 | 318 |
| | *** | 18142 | 19156 | 29979 | 3331 | 3786 | 4869 | 1008 | 1101 | 1237 | 497 | 525 | 553 | 300 | 311 | 310 |
| 0.4 | *** | 17918 | 18422 | 29494 | 3271 | 3587 | 4802 | 1002 | 1083 | 1234 | 498 | 525 | 564 | 300 | 312 | 325 |
| | *** | 18086 | 19393 | 31475 | 3395 | 3932 | 5077 | 1038 | 1145 | 1276 | 510 | 543 | 565 | 305 | 318 | 313 |
| 0.45 | *** | 17278 | 17926 | 30769 | 3241 | 3604 | 4973 | 1006 | 1097 | 1264 | 499 | 529 | 570 | 299 | 311 | 326 |
| | *** | 17494 | 19141 | 32322 | 3384 | 3992 | 5181 | 1046 | 1164 | 1289 | 513 | 547 | 565 | 305 | 318 | 310 |
| 0.5 | *** | 16200 | 17023 | 31340 | 3150 | 3552 | 5031 | 993 | 1088 | 1264 | 491 | 521 | 565 | 291 | 304 | 319 |
| | *** | 16477 | 18501 | 32517 | 3310 | 3973 | 5181 | 1035 | 1159 | 1276 | 505 | 540 | 553 | 298 | 311 | 300 |
| 0.55 | *** | 14802 | 15830 | 31203 | 3011 | 3442 | 4975 | 961 | 1058 | 1236 | 473 | 503 | 546 | 279 | 291 | 305 |
| | *** | 15152 | 17566 | 32061 | 3184 | 3882 | 5077 | 1005 | 1131 | 1237 | 488 | 522 | 530 | 285 | 297 | 284 |
| 0.6 | *** | 13204 | 14458 | 30357 | 2833 | 3278 | 4806 | 914 | 1009 | 1180 | 446 | 475 | 514 | 260 | 271 | 284 |
| | *** | 13641 | 16417 | 30955 | 3013 | 3724 | 4869 | 956 | 1079 | 1172 | 459 | 493 | 495 | 265 | 277 | 261 |
| 0.65 | *** | 11529 | 12996 | 28807 | 2623 | 3066 | 4524 | 850 | 939 | 1095 | 411 | 436 | 471 | 236 | 245 | 256 |
| | *** | 12056 | 15111 | 29197 | 2804 | 3501 | 4556 | 889 | 1004 | 1081 | 422 | 452 | 449 | 240 | 250 | 232 |
| 0.7 | *** | 9885 | 11507 | 26555 | 2383 | 2806 | 4130 | 769 | 848 | 983 | 364 | 386 | 415 | 205 | 213 | 221 |
| | *** | 10487 | 13682 | 26789 | 2557 | 3213 | 4140 | 804 | 906 | 964 | 375 | 400 | 391 | 208 | 217 | 196 |
| 0.75 | *** | 8339 | 10017 | 23608 | 2112 | 2498 | 3626 | 671 | 737 | 843 | 309 | 326 | 346 | 168 | 173 | 179 |
| | *** | 8976 | 12139 | 23730 | 2272 | 2857 | 3619 | 701 | 782 | 821 | 317 | 335 | 322 | 170 | 176 | 153 |
| 0.8 | *** | 6901 | 8513 | 19973 | 1805 | 2133 | 3011 | 554 | 602 | 676 | 243 | 253 | 266 | . | . | . |
| | *** | 7524 | 10462 | 20021 | 1943 | 2428 | 2994 | 576 | 635 | 651 | 247 | 259 | 241 | . | . | . |
| 0.85 | *** | 5527 | 6946 | 15657 | 1451 | 1699 | 2288 | 411 | 441 | 482 | . | . | . | . | . | . |
| | *** | 6084 | 8596 | 15660 | 1556 | 1910 | 2265 | 425 | 459 | 456 | . | . | . | . | . | . |
| 0.9 | *** | 4120 | 5209 | 10667 | 1019 | 1167 | 1457 | . | . | . | . | . | . | . | . | . |
| | *** | 4553 | 6413 | 10648 | 1083 | 1281 | 1432 | . | . | . | . | . | . | . | . | . |
| 0.95 | *** | 2443 | 3022 | 5011 | . | . | . | . | . | . | . | . | . | . | . | . |
| | *** | 2679 | 3593 | 4986 | . | . | . | . | . | . | . | . | . | . | . | . |

TABLE 4: ALPHA= 0.01  POWER= 0.9    EXPECTED ACCRUAL THRU MINIMUM FOLLOW-UP= 1200

| | DEL=.02 | | | DEL=.05 | | | DEL=.10 | | | DEL=.15 | | | DEL=.20 | | |
|---|---|---|---|---|---|---|---|---|---|---|---|---|---|---|---|
| FACT= | 1.0 .75 | .50 .25 | .00 BIN | 1.0 .75 | .50 .25 | .00 BIN | 1.0 .75 | .50 .25 | .00 BIN | 1.0 75 | .50 .25 | .00 BIN | 1.0 .75 | .50 .25 | .00 BIN |
| PCONT=*** | REQUIRED NUMBER OF PATIENTS | | | | | | | | | | | | | | |
| 0.05 *** | 3715 | 3739 | 3921 | 800 | 811 | 832 | 289 | 292 | 295 | 169 | 171 | 172 | 120 | 121 | 121 |
| *** | 3724 | 3780 | 7329 | 805 | 820 | 1432 | 291 | 294 | 456 | 170 | 172 | 241 | 120 | 121 | 153 |
| 0.1 *** | 7733 | 7792 | 8615 | 1474 | 1511 | 1603 | 472 | 482 | 495 | 255 | 258 | 262 | 169 | 170 | 172 |
| *** | 7753 | 7905 | 12731 | 1489 | 1546 | 2265 | 477 | 488 | 651 | 256 | 260 | 322 | 169 | 171 | 196 |
| 0.15 *** | 11303 | 11408 | 13324 | 2059 | 2133 | 2350 | 630 | 649 | 679 | 327 | 334 | 342 | 208 | 211 | 215 |
| *** | 11338 | 11611 | 17482 | 2088 | 2207 | 2994 | 639 | 662 | 821 | 330 | 337 | 391 | 210 | 214 | 232 |
| 0.2 *** | 14155 | 14316 | 17703 | 2530 | 2647 | 3033 | 760 | 791 | 841 | 386 | 397 | 410 | 241 | 246 | 252 |
| *** | 14209 | 14632 | 21583 | 2575 | 2771 | 3619 | 774 | 813 | 964 | 391 | 403 | 449 | 244 | 249 | 261 |
| 0.25 *** | 16213 | 16444 | 21586 | 2881 | 3047 | 3629 | 862 | 905 | 979 | 433 | 447 | 467 | 267 | 273 | 280 |
| *** | 16291 | 16899 | 25032 | 2946 | 3227 | 4140 | 881 | 937 | 1081 | 439 | 457 | 495 | 270 | 277 | 284 |
| 0.3 *** | 17492 | 17809 | 24877 | 3121 | 3339 | 4126 | 936 | 993 | 1092 | 467 | 486 | 512 | 285 | 293 | 303 |
| *** | 17598 | 18429 | 27831 | 3205 | 3575 | 4556 | 961 | 1035 | 1172 | 475 | 498 | 530 | 289 | 298 | 300 |
| 0.35 *** | 18048 | 18470 | 27523 | 3258 | 3529 | 4519 | 986 | 1055 | 1177 | 490 | 513 | 544 | 297 | 306 | 318 |
| *** | 18189 | 19287 | 29979 | 3364 | 3822 | 4869 | 1017 | 1106 | 1237 | 500 | 527 | 553 | 301 | 311 | 310 |
| 0.4 *** | 17963 | 18514 | 29494 | 3307 | 3631 | 4802 | 1013 | 1093 | 1234 | 502 | 528 | 563 | 301 | 312 | 325 |
| *** | 18147 | 19558 | 31475 | 3435 | 3973 | 5077 | 1048 | 1151 | 1276 | 514 | 544 | 565 | 307 | 319 | 313 |
| 0.45 *** | 17337 | 18043 | 30769 | 3283 | 3652 | 4972 | 1019 | 1106 | 1263 | 503 | 532 | 570 | 301 | 312 | 325 |
| *** | 17573 | 19342 | 32322 | 3430 | 4039 | 5181 | 1057 | 1171 | 1289 | 517 | 549 | 565 | 306 | 319 | 310 |
| 0.5 *** | 16276 | 17169 | 31340 | 3197 | 3606 | 5030 | 1006 | 1098 | 1264 | 496 | 524 | 564 | 294 | 305 | 319 |
| *** | 16578 | 18737 | 32517 | 3361 | 4024 | 5181 | 1047 | 1166 | 1276 | 508 | 542 | 553 | 299 | 311 | 300 |
| 0.55 *** | 14898 | 16008 | 31203 | 3062 | 3498 | 4975 | 975 | 1069 | 1236 | 478 | 506 | 546 | 280 | 292 | 305 |
| *** | 15278 | 17834 | 32061 | 3238 | 3935 | 5077 | 1016 | 1138 | 1237 | 491 | 524 | 530 | 286 | 298 | 284 |
| 0.6 *** | 13324 | 14665 | 30358 | 2887 | 3335 | 4806 | 926 | 1018 | 1180 | 451 | 478 | 514 | 262 | 271 | 284 |
| *** | 13795 | 16708 | 30955 | 3070 | 3777 | 4869 | 967 | 1086 | 1172 | 463 | 494 | 495 | 266 | 277 | 261 |
| 0.65 *** | 11676 | 13228 | 28807 | 2677 | 3122 | 4524 | 862 | 948 | 1095 | 414 | 439 | 471 | 237 | 245 | 256 |
| *** | 12238 | 15416 | 29197 | 2860 | 3552 | 4556 | 901 | 1010 | 1081 | 425 | 453 | 449 | 241 | 250 | 232 |
| 0.7 *** | 10056 | 11752 | 26554 | 2435 | 2860 | 4130 | 780 | 857 | 983 | 368 | 388 | 415 | 206 | 213 | 221 |
| *** | 10688 | 13987 | 26789 | 2611 | 3259 | 4140 | 814 | 910 | 964 | 377 | 400 | 391 | 209 | 217 | 196 |
| 0.75 *** | 8522 | 10261 | 23608 | 2160 | 2545 | 3625 | 680 | 744 | 843 | 311 | 327 | 346 | 169 | 174 | 179 |
| *** | 9186 | 12431 | 23730 | 2321 | 2898 | 3619 | 709 | 787 | 821 | 319 | 336 | 322 | 171 | 176 | 153 |
| 0.8 *** | 7082 | 8741 | 19972 | 1847 | 2173 | 3011 | 560 | 607 | 676 | 244 | 254 | 266 | . | . | . |
| *** | 7726 | 10726 | 20021 | 1984 | 2460 | 2994 | 582 | 637 | 651 | 249 | 260 | 241 | . | . | . |
| 0.85 *** | 5691 | 7143 | 15656 | 1483 | 1728 | 2288 | 415 | 444 | 481 | . | . | . | . | . | . |
| *** | 6262 | 8814 | 15660 | 1588 | 1933 | 2265 | 429 | 461 | 456 | . | . | . | . | . | . |
| 0.9 *** | 4248 | 5356 | 10666 | 1039 | 1183 | 1457 | . | . | . | . | . | . | . | . | . |
| *** | 4690 | 6567 | 10648 | 1102 | 1292 | 1432 | . | . | . | . | . | . | . | . | . |
| 0.95 *** | 2513 | 3095 | 5011 | . | . | . | . | . | . | . | . | . | . | . | . |
| *** | 2752 | 3661 | 4986 | . | . | . | . | . | . | . | . | . | . | . | . |

TABLE 4: ALPHA= 0.01  POWER= 0.9    EXPECTED ACCRUAL THRU MINIMUM FOLLOW-UP= 1300

| | | DEL=.02 | | | DEL=.05 | | | DEL=.10 | | | DEL=.15 | | | DEL=.20 | | |
|---|---|---|---|---|---|---|---|---|---|---|---|---|---|---|---|---|
| FACT= | | 1.0 .75 | .50 .25 | .00 BIN | 1.0 .75 | .50 .25 | .00 BIN | 1.0 .75 | .50 .25 | .00 BIN | 1.0 75 | .50 .25 | .00 BIN | 1.0 .75 | .50 .25 | .00 BIN |
| PCONT=*** | | | | | REQUIRED | NUMBER OF | PATIENTS | | | | | | | | | |
| 0.05 | *** | 3717 | 3744 | 3921 | 802 | 812 | 831 | 290 | 292 | 296 | 170 | 172 | 172 | 120 | 120 | 121 |
| | *** | 3726 | 3786 | 7329 | 806 | 821 | 1432 | 291 | 294 | 456 | 171 | 172 | 241 | 120 | 121 | 153 |
| 0.1 | *** | 7738 | 7803 | 8615 | 1478 | 1515 | 1604 | 474 | 483 | 495 | 255 | 258 | 263 | 169 | 171 | 172 |
| | *** | 7759 | 7922 | 12731 | 1493 | 1550 | 2265 | 478 | 488 | 651 | 257 | 261 | 322 | 170 | 172 | 196 |
| 0.15 | *** | 11313 | 11425 | 13323 | 2067 | 2142 | 2351 | 633 | 652 | 679 | 328 | 334 | 342 | 210 | 212 | 215 |
| | *** | 11350 | 11644 | 17482 | 2097 | 2215 | 2994 | 641 | 664 | 821 | 331 | 338 | 391 | 211 | 214 | 232 |
| 0.2 | *** | 14168 | 14343 | 17704 | 2542 | 2662 | 3033 | 764 | 794 | 841 | 388 | 397 | 410 | 242 | 246 | 252 |
| | *** | 14227 | 14683 | 21583 | 2589 | 2785 | 3619 | 778 | 815 | 964 | 393 | 404 | 449 | 245 | 249 | 261 |
| 0.25 | *** | 16233 | 16483 | 21586 | 2899 | 3069 | 3630 | 867 | 910 | 980 | 435 | 448 | 467 | 267 | 274 | 281 |
| | *** | 16317 | 16971 | 25032 | 2965 | 3247 | 4140 | 887 | 940 | 1081 | 441 | 458 | 495 | 271 | 277 | 284 |
| 0.3 | *** | 17519 | 17862 | 24877 | 3144 | 3366 | 4127 | 943 | 999 | 1092 | 470 | 487 | 512 | 286 | 294 | 303 |
| | *** | 17633 | 18528 | 27831 | 3230 | 3602 | 4556 | 968 | 1038 | 1172 | 478 | 499 | 530 | 290 | 298 | 300 |
| 0.35 | *** | 18083 | 18540 | 27524 | 3287 | 3564 | 4519 | 994 | 1062 | 1177 | 493 | 514 | 544 | 298 | 307 | 318 |
| | *** | 18236 | 19415 | 29979 | 3396 | 3854 | 4869 | 1025 | 1111 | 1237 | 503 | 528 | 553 | 302 | 312 | 310 |
| 0.4 | *** | 18010 | 18605 | 29494 | 3342 | 3671 | 4802 | 1023 | 1100 | 1234 | 505 | 530 | 564 | 303 | 314 | 325 |
| | *** | 18208 | 19719 | 31475 | 3473 | 4011 | 5077 | 1058 | 1156 | 1276 | 517 | 545 | 565 | 308 | 319 | 313 |
| 0.45 | *** | 17396 | 18159 | 30769 | 3322 | 3698 | 4972 | 1030 | 1116 | 1264 | 508 | 534 | 570 | 302 | 313 | 326 |
| | *** | 17652 | 19537 | 32322 | 3473 | 4081 | 5181 | 1068 | 1177 | 1289 | 520 | 551 | 565 | 307 | 319 | 310 |
| 0.5 | *** | 16352 | 17313 | 31341 | 3242 | 3655 | 5030 | 1017 | 1108 | 1264 | 500 | 526 | 565 | 295 | 306 | 318 |
| | *** | 16677 | 18965 | 32517 | 3409 | 4070 | 5181 | 1058 | 1173 | 1276 | 512 | 544 | 553 | 301 | 312 | 300 |
| 0.55 | *** | 14994 | 16181 | 31203 | 3110 | 3550 | 4975 | 986 | 1078 | 1236 | 482 | 509 | 546 | 282 | 292 | 305 |
| | *** | 15403 | 18089 | 32061 | 3289 | 3983 | 5077 | 1028 | 1144 | 1237 | 494 | 526 | 530 | 287 | 298 | 284 |
| 0.6 | *** | 13445 | 14865 | 30358 | 2937 | 3388 | 4806 | 939 | 1028 | 1180 | 454 | 480 | 514 | 263 | 273 | 284 |
| | *** | 13947 | 16985 | 30955 | 3122 | 3825 | 4869 | 978 | 1092 | 1172 | 466 | 496 | 495 | 268 | 278 | 261 |
| 0.65 | *** | 11821 | 13449 | 28806 | 2728 | 3174 | 4524 | 873 | 957 | 1095 | 418 | 440 | 471 | 238 | 246 | 256 |
| | *** | 12415 | 15703 | 29197 | 2911 | 3598 | 4556 | 911 | 1016 | 1081 | 428 | 455 | 449 | 242 | 251 | 232 |
| 0.7 | *** | 10221 | 11985 | 26555 | 2484 | 2908 | 4130 | 791 | 864 | 983 | 370 | 390 | 415 | 207 | 214 | 221 |
| | *** | 10883 | 14274 | 26789 | 2660 | 3302 | 4140 | 824 | 916 | 964 | 380 | 401 | 391 | 211 | 217 | 196 |
| 0.75 | *** | 8699 | 10491 | 23608 | 2205 | 2589 | 3625 | 689 | 750 | 843 | 314 | 328 | 347 | 170 | 174 | 179 |
| | *** | 9385 | 12704 | 23730 | 2366 | 2935 | 3619 | 717 | 791 | 821 | 321 | 337 | 322 | 172 | 176 | 153 |
| 0.8 | *** | 7255 | 8955 | 19973 | 1886 | 2208 | 3011 | 566 | 612 | 676 | 245 | 255 | 266 | . | . | . |
| | *** | 7916 | 10970 | 20021 | 2022 | 2489 | 2994 | 588 | 640 | 651 | 250 | 260 | 241 | . | . | . |
| 0.85 | *** | 5845 | 7327 | 15656 | 1512 | 1754 | 2288 | 419 | 446 | 482 | . | . | . | . | . | . |
| | *** | 6428 | 9015 | 15660 | 1616 | 1953 | 2265 | 432 | 462 | 456 | . | . | . | . | . | . |
| 0.9 | *** | 4368 | 5492 | 10666 | 1057 | 1198 | 1458 | . | . | . | . | . | . | . | . | . |
| | *** | 4817 | 6708 | 10648 | 1119 | 1303 | 1432 | . | . | . | . | . | . | . | . | . |
| 0.95 | *** | 2579 | 3162 | 5011 | . | . | . | . | . | . | . | . | . | . | . | . |
| | *** | 2820 | 3722 | 4986 | . | . | . | . | . | . | . | . | . | . | . | . |

TABLE 4: ALPHA= 0.01 POWER= 0.9     EXPECTED ACCRUAL THRU MINIMUM FOLLOW-UP= 1400

| | | DEL=.02 | | | DEL=.05 | | | DEL=.10 | | | DEL=.15 | | | DEL=.20 | | |
|---|---|---|---|---|---|---|---|---|---|---|---|---|---|---|---|---|
| FACT= | | 1.0 .75 | .50 .25 | .00 BIN | 1.0 .75 | .50 .25 | .00 BIN | 1.0 .75 | .50 .25 | .00 BIN | 1.0 75 | .50 .25 | .00 BIN | 1.0 .75 | .50 .25 | .00 BIN |
| PCONT=*** | | | | | REQUIRED NUMBER OF PATIENTS | | | | | | | | | | | |
| 0.05 | *** *** | 3720 3729 | 3748 3790 | 3921 7329 | 802 808 | 814 821 | 831 1432 | 290 291 | 292 294 | 296 456 | 171 171 | 171 171 | 172 241 | 120 121 | 121 121 | 121 153 |
| 0.1 | *** *** | 7743 7766 | 7812 7939 | 8615 12731 | 1482 1498 | 1520 1552 | 1604 2265 | 475 479 | 484 489 | 495 651 | 256 257 | 259 261 | 262 322 | 169 170 | 171 171 | 172 196 |
| 0.15 | *** *** | 11321 11362 | 11442 11675 | 13324 17482 | 2075 2105 | 2150 2222 | 2351 2994 | 635 643 | 653 664 | 678 821 | 329 332 | 335 339 | 342 391 | 210 211 | 213 213 | 215 232 |
| 0.2 | *** *** | 14182 14245 | 14370 14733 | 17703 21583 | 2553 2602 | 2675 2796 | 3033 3619 | 767 780 | 797 816 | 841 964 | 388 394 | 398 404 | 410 449 | 242 245 | 247 249 | 252 261 |
| 0.25 | *** *** | 16252 16342 | 16522 17043 | 21585 25032 | 2915 2984 | 3088 3265 | 3629 4140 | 872 891 | 913 942 | 980 1081 | 437 443 | 450 458 | 467 495 | 269 271 | 274 277 | 281 284 |
| 0.3 | *** *** | 17545 17669 | 17915 18624 | 24877 27831 | 3165 3255 | 3392 3625 | 4126 4556 | 950 975 | 1004 1042 | 1092 1172 | 472 480 | 489 500 | 512 530 | 287 290 | 294 298 | 303 300 |
| 0.35 | *** *** | 18119 18282 | 18609 19540 | 27524 29979 | 3314 3426 | 3595 3883 | 4519 4869 | 1003 1032 | 1068 1115 | 1177 1237 | 496 506 | 516 529 | 544 553 | 299 304 | 308 312 | 318 310 |
| 0.4 | *** *** | 18056 18270 | 18695 19876 | 29494 31475 | 3374 3508 | 3708 4046 | 4802 5077 | 1032 1066 | 1108 1161 | 1235 1276 | 508 520 | 532 547 | 563 565 | 304 309 | 314 319 | 325 313 |
| 0.45 | *** *** | 17455 17730 | 18273 19725 | 30769 32322 | 3360 3513 | 3740 4119 | 4973 5181 | 1040 1077 | 1123 1182 | 1263 1289 | 511 522 | 536 552 | 570 565 | 304 309 | 314 319 | 325 310 |
| 0.5 | *** *** | 16427 16777 | 17454 19183 | 31341 32517 | 3284 3453 | 3700 4111 | 5030 5181 | 1028 1067 | 1116 1178 | 1263 1276 | 503 515 | 529 545 | 564 553 | 297 302 | 307 312 | 318 300 |
| 0.55 | *** *** | 15089 15528 | 16350 18334 | 31203 32061 | 3155 3336 | 3597 4026 | 4974 5077 | 997 1038 | 1087 1150 | 1236 1237 | 485 497 | 511 527 | 546 530 | 283 289 | 293 299 | 305 284 |
| 0.6 | *** *** | 13562 14097 | 15060 17248 | 30357 30955 | 2984 3170 | 3436 3867 | 4805 4869 | 949 988 | 1036 1097 | 1179 1172 | 458 469 | 482 497 | 514 495 | 264 269 | 274 278 | 284 261 |
| 0.65 | *** *** | 11963 12587 | 13663 15975 | 28807 29197 | 2775 2959 | 3222 3639 | 4524 4556 | 883 920 | 964 1020 | 1095 1081 | 421 430 | 443 456 | 471 449 | 240 243 | 247 251 | 256 232 |
| 0.7 | *** *** | 10382 11070 | 12206 14543 | 26554 26789 | 2529 2705 | 2953 3340 | 4130 4140 | 799 832 | 871 920 | 983 964 | 374 382 | 392 402 | 415 391 | 208 211 | 214 217 | 221 196 |
| 0.75 | *** *** | 8867 9576 | 10710 12959 | 23608 23730 | 2246 2407 | 2628 2968 | 3626 3619 | 696 724 | 755 794 | 843 821 | 316 322 | 330 338 | 346 322 | 171 172 | 174 177 | 179 153 |
| 0.8 | *** *** | 7419 8097 | 9158 11198 | 19973 20021 | 1921 2057 | 2242 2516 | 3011 2994 | 572 592 | 615 643 | 676 651 | 247 251 | 255 261 | 266 241 | . . | . . | . . |
| 0.85 | *** *** | 5991 6587 | 7500 9202 | 15656 15660 | 1539 1642 | 1778 1970 | 2288 2265 | 423 435 | 449 464 | 482 456 | . . | . . | . . | . . | . . | . . |
| 0.9 | *** *** | 4481 4938 | 5620 6839 | 10666 10648 | 1073 1134 | 1211 1312 | 1458 1432 | . . | . . | . . | . . | . . | . . | . . | . . | . . |
| 0.95 | *** *** | 2641 2882 | 3225 3777 | 5011 4986 | . . | . . | . . | . . | . . | . . | . . | . . | . . | . . | . . | . . |

## TABLE 4: ALPHA= 0.01  POWER= 0.9    EXPECTED ACCRUAL THRU MINIMUM FOLLOW-UP= 1500

| | | DEL=.02 | | | DEL=.05 | | | DEL=.10 | | | DEL=.15 | | | DEL=.20 | | |
|---|---|---|---|---|---|---|---|---|---|---|---|---|---|---|---|---|
| FACT= | | 1.0 .75 | .50 .25 | .00 BIN | 1.0 .75 | .50 .25 | .00 BIN | 1.0 .75 | .50 .25 | .00 BIN | 1.0 75 | .50 .25 | .00 BIN | 1.0 .75 | .50 .25 | .00 BIN |
| PCONT=*** | | REQUIRED NUMBER OF PATIENTS | | | | | | | | | | | | | | |
| 0.05 | *** | 3722 3751 3922 | | | 804 815 832 | | | 290 292 295 | | | 170 172 172 | | | 120 121 121 | | |
| | *** | 3732 3795 7329 | | | 808 822 1432 | | | 292 294 456 | | | 170 172 241 | | | 120 121 153 | | |
| 0.1 | *** | 7747 7822 8615 | | | 1486 1523 1604 | | | 476 485 495 | | | 256 260 262 | | | 170 170 172 | | |
| | *** | 7773 7955 12731 | | | 1502 1555 2265 | | | 480 489 651 | | | 258 260 322 | | | 170 172 196 | | |
| 0.15 | *** | 11330 11460 13324 | | | 2081 2158 2351 | | | 637 654 679 | | | 329 335 342 | | | 210 213 215 | | |
| | *** | 11373 11707 17482 | | | 2112 2228 2994 | | | 645 665 821 | | | 332 338 391 | | | 211 214 232 | | |
| 0.2 | *** | 14195 14396 17704 | | | 2565 2688 3033 | | | 770 799 841 | | | 390 399 410 | | | 243 247 252 | | |
| | *** | 14262 14782 21583 | | | 2614 2808 3619 | | | 784 817 964 | | | 395 405 449 | | | 245 249 261 | | |
| 0.25 | *** | 16271 16560 21586 | | | 2930 3106 3629 | | | 877 917 980 | | | 438 451 468 | | | 269 275 281 | | |
| | *** | 16368 17113 25032 | | | 3001 3280 4140 | | | 895 945 1081 | | | 444 458 495 | | | 272 277 284 | | |
| 0.3 | *** | 17572 17967 24877 | | | 3185 3416 4127 | | | 956 1009 1092 | | | 474 490 512 | | | 288 295 303 | | |
| | *** | 17704 18719 27831 | | | 3277 3647 4556 | | | 980 1044 1172 | | | 482 500 530 | | | 292 299 300 | | |
| 0.35 | *** | 18154 18680 27524 | | | 3339 3624 4519 | | | 1010 1073 1177 | | | 499 518 544 | | | 300 308 318 | | |
| | *** | 18330 19662 29979 | | | 3454 3910 4869 | | | 1039 1118 1237 | | | 507 530 553 | | | 304 313 310 | | |
| 0.4 | *** | 18101 18785 29494 | | | 3405 3742 4802 | | | 1040 1114 1235 | | | 512 534 563 | | | 305 315 325 | | |
| | *** | 18331 20027 31475 | | | 3541 4077 5077 | | | 1073 1165 1276 | | | 522 547 565 | | | 310 320 313 | | |
| 0.45 | *** | 17514 18386 30770 | | | 3395 3779 4972 | | | 1049 1130 1264 | | | 514 538 570 | | | 305 314 325 | | |
| | *** | 17809 19907 32322 | | | 3551 4155 5181 | | | 1085 1187 1289 | | | 525 553 565 | | | 309 320 313 | | |
| 0.5 | *** | 16503 17594 31340 | | | 3323 3742 5030 | | | 1038 1123 1264 | | | 506 532 564 | | | 298 307 319 | | |
| | *** | 16876 19392 32517 | | | 3494 4148 5181 | | | 1076 1183 1276 | | | 517 547 553 | | | 303 313 300 | | |
| 0.55 | *** | 15184 16516 31203 | | | 3198 3642 4974 | | | 1008 1094 1235 | | | 488 513 545 | | | 285 294 305 | | |
| | *** | 15650 18566 32061 | | | 3380 4065 5077 | | | 1046 1155 1237 | | | 500 529 530 | | | 290 299 284 | | |
| 0.6 | *** | 13680 15249 30358 | | | 3028 3482 4805 | | | 959 1043 1179 | | | 460 484 515 | | | 265 274 284 | | |
| | *** | 14243 17497 30955 | | | 3215 3907 4869 | | | 997 1102 1172 | | | 472 499 495 | | | 270 278 261 | | |
| 0.65 | *** | 12102 13867 28807 | | | 2818 3265 4524 | | | 892 971 1095 | | | 423 444 470 | | | 240 247 256 | | |
| | *** | 12755 16232 29197 | | | 3004 3677 4556 | | | 928 1025 1081 | | | 433 457 449 | | | 244 251 232 | | |
| 0.7 | *** | 10537 12419 26555 | | | 2570 2993 4130 | | | 807 877 983 | | | 376 393 415 | | | 209 215 221 | | |
| | *** | 11250 14797 26789 | | | 2748 3375 4140 | | | 839 923 964 | | | 384 403 391 | | | 212 217 196 | | |
| 0.75 | *** | 9030 10917 23608 | | | 2285 2665 3625 | | | 703 760 843 | | | 318 331 347 | | | 170 174 179 | | |
| | *** | 9757 13199 23730 | | | 2445 2997 3619 | | | 729 797 821 | | | 323 338 322 | | | 172 177 153 | | |
| 0.8 | *** | 7576 9350 19972 | | | 1954 2272 3011 | | | 577 619 676 | | | 248 257 266 | | | . . . | | |
| | *** | 8270 11413 20021 | | | 2090 2539 2994 | | | 596 645 651 | | | 252 262 241 | | | . . . | | |
| 0.85 | *** | 6129 7662 15656 | | | 1565 1799 2288 | | | 427 450 482 | | | . . . | | | . . . | | |
| | *** | 6736 9378 15660 | | | 1666 1987 2265 | | | 438 465 456 | | | . . . | | | . . . | | |
| 0.9 | *** | 4588 5740 10667 | | | 1088 1222 1458 | | | . . . | | | . . . | | | . . . | | |
| | *** | 5051 6959 10648 | | | 1148 1320 1432 | | | . . . | | | . . . | | | . . . | | |
| 0.95 | *** | 2698 3282 5011 | | | . . . | | | . . . | | | . . . | | | . . . | | |
| | *** | 2941 3828 4986 | | | . . . | | | . . . | | | . . . | | | . . . | | |

TABLE 4: ALPHA= 0.01  POWER= 0.9   EXPECTED ACCRUAL THRU MINIMUM FOLLOW-UP= 1600

| | DEL=.02 | | | DEL=.05 | | | DEL=.10 | | | DEL=.15 | | | DEL=.20 | | |
|---|---|---|---|---|---|---|---|---|---|---|---|---|---|---|---|
| FACT= | 1.0 .75 | .50 .25 | .00 BIN | 1.0 .75 | .50 .25 | .00 BIN | 1.0 .75 | .50 .25 | .00 BIN | 1.0 75 | .50 .25 | .00 BIN | 1.0 .75 | .50 .25 | .00 BIN |

PCONT=***                    REQUIRED NUMBER OF PATIENTS

| PCONT | DEL=.02 1.0/.75 | .50/.25 | .00/BIN | DEL=.05 1.0/.75 | .50/.25 | .00/BIN | DEL=.10 1.0/.75 | .50/.25 | .00/BIN | DEL=.15 1.0/.75 | .50/.25 | .00/BIN | DEL=.20 1.0/.75 | .50/.25 | .00/BIN |
|---|---|---|---|---|---|---|---|---|---|---|---|---|---|---|---|
| 0.05 *** | 3724 | 3755 | 3921 | 805 | 815 | 832 | 291 | 293 | 296 | 171 | 171 | 172 | 120 | 121 | 121 |
| *** | 3735 | 3799 | 7329 | 810 | 822 | 1432 | 292 | 294 | 456 | 171 | 172 | 241 | 120 | 121 | 153 |
| 0.1 *** | 7753 | 7831 | 8615 | 1489 | 1527 | 1604 | 477 | 485 | 495 | 257 | 259 | 263 | 170 | 171 | 172 |
| *** | 7779 | 7970 | 12731 | 1505 | 1557 | 2265 | 481 | 490 | 651 | 258 | 261 | 322 | 170 | 172 | 196 |
| 0.15 *** | 11338 | 11477 | 13324 | 2088 | 2165 | 2351 | 639 | 656 | 679 | 330 | 336 | 342 | 210 | 213 | 216 |
| *** | 11385 | 11737 | 17482 | 2120 | 2234 | 2994 | 647 | 666 | 821 | 333 | 339 | 391 | 212 | 214 | 232 |
| 0.2 *** | 14209 | 14423 | 17703 | 2575 | 2700 | 3033 | 774 | 801 | 841 | 391 | 400 | 411 | 244 | 247 | 252 |
| *** | 14280 | 14830 | 21583 | 2626 | 2817 | 3619 | 787 | 819 | 964 | 395 | 405 | 449 | 246 | 250 | 261 |
| 0.25 *** | 16291 | 16598 | 21586 | 2946 | 3123 | 3629 | 881 | 920 | 980 | 440 | 452 | 467 | 270 | 275 | 281 |
| *** | 16394 | 17182 | 25032 | 3017 | 3295 | 4140 | 899 | 947 | 1081 | 445 | 459 | 495 | 272 | 278 | 284 |
| 0.3 *** | 17598 | 18020 | 24877 | 3206 | 3438 | 4127 | 962 | 1013 | 1092 | 476 | 492 | 512 | 289 | 295 | 303 |
| *** | 17739 | 18812 | 27831 | 3299 | 3667 | 4556 | 985 | 1047 | 1172 | 483 | 501 | 530 | 292 | 299 | 300 |
| 0.35 *** | 18189 | 18749 | 27524 | 3364 | 3652 | 4519 | 1017 | 1079 | 1177 | 501 | 520 | 544 | 301 | 309 | 318 |
| *** | 18376 | 19782 | 29979 | 3480 | 3935 | 4869 | 1045 | 1121 | 1237 | 510 | 531 | 553 | 305 | 313 | 310 |
| 0.4 *** | 18147 | 18874 | 29494 | 3435 | 3775 | 4802 | 1048 | 1120 | 1235 | 514 | 536 | 564 | 307 | 315 | 325 |
| *** | 18392 | 20175 | 31475 | 3573 | 4106 | 5077 | 1080 | 1169 | 1276 | 524 | 549 | 565 | 311 | 320 | 313 |
| 0.45 *** | 17573 | 18499 | 30769 | 3430 | 3815 | 4973 | 1058 | 1136 | 1263 | 517 | 540 | 570 | 306 | 315 | 326 |
| *** | 17887 | 20082 | 32322 | 3587 | 4187 | 5181 | 1093 | 1191 | 1289 | 528 | 554 | 565 | 311 | 320 | 310 |
| 0.5 *** | 16578 | 17731 | 31340 | 3361 | 3782 | 5031 | 1047 | 1130 | 1264 | 509 | 533 | 564 | 299 | 308 | 319 |
| *** | 16975 | 19594 | 32517 | 3534 | 4184 | 5181 | 1084 | 1187 | 1276 | 520 | 548 | 565 | 304 | 313 | 300 |
| 0.55 *** | 15279 | 16677 | 31203 | 3239 | 3683 | 4975 | 1017 | 1101 | 1236 | 491 | 515 | 546 | 286 | 295 | 305 |
| *** | 15771 | 18790 | 32061 | 3422 | 4101 | 5077 | 1055 | 1159 | 1237 | 502 | 529 | 530 | 290 | 300 | 284 |
| 0.6 *** | 13796 | 15432 | 30358 | 3070 | 3523 | 4806 | 968 | 1050 | 1180 | 463 | 486 | 515 | 267 | 275 | 284 |
| *** | 14387 | 17735 | 30955 | 3258 | 3943 | 4869 | 1005 | 1106 | 1172 | 474 | 499 | 495 | 271 | 279 | 261 |
| 0.65 *** | 12238 | 14065 | 28807 | 2860 | 3306 | 4524 | 901 | 977 | 1095 | 426 | 446 | 471 | 241 | 248 | 256 |
| *** | 12917 | 16476 | 29197 | 3046 | 3712 | 4556 | 935 | 1029 | 1081 | 435 | 458 | 449 | 245 | 252 | 232 |
| 0.7 *** | 10688 | 12621 | 26555 | 2611 | 3032 | 4130 | 815 | 882 | 983 | 378 | 394 | 415 | 210 | 215 | 221 |
| *** | 11423 | 15039 | 26789 | 2788 | 3406 | 4140 | 846 | 927 | 964 | 386 | 404 | 391 | 212 | 218 | 196 |
| 0.75 *** | 9186 | 11115 | 23608 | 2321 | 2699 | 3626 | 709 | 764 | 843 | 319 | 332 | 347 | 171 | 175 | 179 |
| *** | 9932 | 13426 | 23730 | 2481 | 3025 | 3619 | 735 | 800 | 821 | 325 | 339 | 322 | 173 | 177 | 153 |
| 0.8 *** | 7726 | 9531 | 19973 | 1985 | 2299 | 3011 | 582 | 622 | 676 | 249 | 257 | 266 | . | . | . |
| *** | 8434 | 11614 | 20021 | 2119 | 2560 | 2994 | 601 | 647 | 651 | 253 | 262 | 241 | . | . | . |
| 0.85 *** | 6262 | 7816 | 15656 | 1588 | 1819 | 2288 | 429 | 452 | 482 | . | . | . | . | . | . |
| *** | 6878 | 9541 | 15660 | 1689 | 2001 | 2265 | 440 | 466 | 456 | . | . | . | . | . | . |
| 0.9 *** | 4690 | 5852 | 10667 | 1102 | 1233 | 1458 | . | . | . | . | . | . | . | . | . |
| *** | 5158 | 7072 | 10648 | 1161 | 1327 | 1432 | . | . | . | . | . | . | . | . | . |
| 0.95 *** | 2753 | 3336 | 5011 | . | . | . | . | . | . | . | . | . | . | . | . |
| *** | 2996 | 3874 | 4986 | . | . | . | . | . | . | . | . | . | . | . | . |

TABLE 4: ALPHA= 0.01  POWER= 0.9    EXPECTED ACCRUAL THRU MINIMUM FOLLOW-UP= 1700

| | DEL=.02 | | | DEL=.05 | | | DEL=.10 | | | DEL=.15 | | | DEL=.20 | | |
|---|---|---|---|---|---|---|---|---|---|---|---|---|---|---|---|
| FACT= | 1.0 .75 | .50 .25 | .00 BIN | 1.0 .75 | .50 .25 | .00 BIN | 1.0 .75 | .50 .25 | .00 BIN | 1.0 75 | .50 .25 | .00 BIN | 1.0 .75 | .50 .25 | .00 BIN |

PCONT=***                REQUIRED NUMBER OF PATIENTS

| PCONT | DEL=.02 1.0/.75 | .50/.25 | .00/BIN | DEL=.05 1.0/.75 | .50/.25 | .00/BIN | DEL=.10 1.0/.75 | .50/.25 | .00/BIN | DEL=.15 1.0/75 | .50/.25 | .00/BIN | DEL=.20 1.0/.75 | .50/.25 | .00/BIN |
|---|---|---|---|---|---|---|---|---|---|---|---|---|---|---|---|
| 0.05 *** | 3726 | 3758 | 3922 | 806 | 816 | 832 | 291 | 293 | 295 | 171 | 171 | 172 | 120 | 121 | 121 |
| *** | 3738 | 3803 | 7329 | 811 | 822 | 1432 | 292 | 294 | 456 | 171 | 172 | 241 | 120 | 121 | 153 |
| 0.1 *** | 7757 | 7841 | 8614 | 1493 | 1530 | 1604 | 478 | 486 | 495 | 257 | 259 | 262 | 170 | 171 | 172 |
| *** | 7786 | 7985 | 12731 | 1508 | 1559 | 2265 | 481 | 490 | 651 | 258 | 261 | 322 | 170 | 171 | 196 |
| 0.15 *** | 11347 | 11494 | 13323 | 2095 | 2171 | 2351 | 641 | 656 | 679 | 330 | 335 | 342 | 210 | 212 | 216 |
| *** | 11396 | 11766 | 17482 | 2126 | 2239 | 2994 | 648 | 667 | 821 | 333 | 339 | 391 | 211 | 214 | 232 |
| 0.2 *** | 14222 | 14450 | 17703 | 2586 | 2710 | 3033 | 777 | 803 | 841 | 392 | 401 | 410 | 244 | 248 | 252 |
| *** | 14298 | 14877 | 21583 | 2637 | 2826 | 3619 | 789 | 820 | 964 | 396 | 405 | 449 | 245 | 250 | 261 |
| 0.25 *** | 16310 | 16636 | 21585 | 2960 | 3138 | 3629 | 885 | 923 | 979 | 441 | 452 | 467 | 271 | 275 | 280 |
| *** | 16419 | 17250 | 25032 | 3032 | 3308 | 4140 | 902 | 947 | 1081 | 446 | 460 | 495 | 273 | 278 | 284 |
| 0.3 *** | 17624 | 18072 | 24877 | 3225 | 3459 | 4126 | 967 | 1017 | 1092 | 478 | 493 | 512 | 290 | 295 | 303 |
| *** | 17775 | 18903 | 27831 | 3319 | 3684 | 4556 | 989 | 1049 | 1172 | 484 | 501 | 530 | 292 | 299 | 300 |
| 0.35 *** | 18224 | 18818 | 27524 | 3388 | 3678 | 4519 | 1023 | 1083 | 1177 | 503 | 520 | 544 | 301 | 309 | 318 |
| *** | 18423 | 19897 | 29979 | 3506 | 3958 | 4869 | 1051 | 1124 | 1237 | 511 | 531 | 553 | 306 | 313 | 310 |
| 0.4 *** | 18193 | 18963 | 29494 | 3463 | 3805 | 4802 | 1055 | 1125 | 1234 | 516 | 537 | 563 | 308 | 316 | 325 |
| *** | 18452 | 20317 | 31475 | 3603 | 4133 | 5077 | 1087 | 1172 | 1276 | 526 | 549 | 565 | 311 | 321 | 313 |
| 0.45 *** | 17632 | 18610 | 30769 | 3463 | 3849 | 4972 | 1066 | 1142 | 1263 | 520 | 542 | 571 | 307 | 316 | 326 |
| *** | 17964 | 20251 | 32322 | 3621 | 4217 | 5181 | 1100 | 1194 | 1289 | 530 | 554 | 565 | 311 | 321 | 310 |
| 0.5 *** | 16653 | 17866 | 31341 | 3397 | 3820 | 5031 | 1055 | 1136 | 1264 | 511 | 534 | 564 | 301 | 309 | 318 |
| *** | 17072 | 19787 | 32517 | 3571 | 4216 | 5181 | 1091 | 1191 | 1276 | 522 | 548 | 553 | 305 | 313 | 300 |
| 0.55 *** | 15372 | 16835 | 31203 | 3276 | 3722 | 4974 | 1025 | 1107 | 1236 | 494 | 516 | 546 | 287 | 295 | 305 |
| *** | 15890 | 19003 | 32061 | 3461 | 4134 | 5077 | 1062 | 1163 | 1237 | 505 | 530 | 530 | 291 | 299 | 284 |
| 0.6 *** | 13910 | 15608 | 30357 | 3109 | 3563 | 4806 | 976 | 1056 | 1179 | 465 | 488 | 514 | 267 | 275 | 284 |
| *** | 14528 | 17962 | 30955 | 3298 | 3976 | 4869 | 1013 | 1110 | 1172 | 476 | 500 | 495 | 271 | 279 | 261 |
| 0.65 *** | 12371 | 14254 | 28806 | 2898 | 3344 | 4524 | 908 | 983 | 1095 | 428 | 447 | 471 | 242 | 248 | 256 |
| *** | 13074 | 16708 | 29197 | 3085 | 3743 | 4556 | 942 | 1032 | 1081 | 437 | 458 | 449 | 245 | 252 | 232 |
| 0.7 *** | 10835 | 12816 | 26555 | 2647 | 3067 | 4130 | 821 | 887 | 983 | 379 | 395 | 415 | 210 | 216 | 221 |
| *** | 11591 | 15267 | 26789 | 2825 | 3435 | 4140 | 852 | 930 | 964 | 386 | 405 | 391 | 212 | 218 | 196 |
| 0.75 *** | 9336 | 11305 | 23608 | 2354 | 2730 | 3625 | 715 | 768 | 843 | 321 | 333 | 346 | 172 | 175 | 180 |
| *** | 10100 | 13640 | 23730 | 2514 | 3049 | 3619 | 739 | 802 | 821 | 326 | 339 | 322 | 173 | 177 | 153 |
| 0.8 *** | 7870 | 9705 | 19973 | 2013 | 2324 | 3011 | 586 | 624 | 675 | 250 | 257 | 267 | . | . | . |
| *** | 8590 | 11804 | 20021 | 2147 | 2579 | 2994 | 605 | 648 | 651 | 254 | 261 | 241 | . | . | . |
| 0.85 *** | 6387 | 7962 | 15656 | 1610 | 1837 | 2288 | 431 | 454 | 481 | . | . | . | . | . | . |
| *** | 7014 | 9695 | 15660 | 1710 | 2014 | 2265 | 442 | 466 | 456 | . | . | . | . | . | . |
| 0.9 *** | 4787 | 5958 | 10666 | 1115 | 1243 | 1457 | . | . | . | . | . | . | . | . | . |
| *** | 5259 | 7177 | 10648 | 1172 | 1333 | 1432 | . | . | . | . | . | . | . | . | . |
| 0.95 *** | 2804 | 3386 | 5012 | . | . | . | . | . | . | . | . | . | . | . | . |
| *** | 3047 | 3917 | 4986 | . | . | . | . | . | . | . | . | . | . | . | . |

TABLE 4: ALPHA= 0.01 POWER= 0.9    EXPECTED ACCRUAL THRU MINIMUM FOLLOW-UP= 1800

| | | DEL=.02 | | | DEL=.05 | | | DEL=.10 | | | DEL=.15 | | | DEL=.20 | | |
|---|---|---|---|---|---|---|---|---|---|---|---|---|---|---|---|---|---|
| FACT= | | 1.0 .75 | .50 .25 | .00 BIN | 1.0 .75 | .50 .25 | .00 BIN | 1.0 .75 | .50 .25 | .00 BIN | 1.0 75 | .50 .25 | .00 BIN | 1.0 .75 | .50 .25 | .00 BIN |
| PCONT=*** | | | | REQUIRED NUMBER OF PATIENTS | | | | | | | | | | | | |
| 0.05 | *** | 3728 | 3762 | 3921 | 807 | 816 | 831 | 291 | 294 | 296 | 171 | 171 | 172 | 120 | 120 | 121 |
| | *** | 3739 | 3807 | 7329 | 811 | 823 | 1432 | 292 | 294 | 456 | 171 | 172 | 241 | 120 | 121 | 153 |
| 0.1 | *** | 7762 | 7850 | 8615 | 1496 | 1532 | 1604 | 479 | 486 | 495 | 258 | 260 | 262 | 170 | 171 | 172 |
| | *** | 7793 | 7998 | 12731 | 1512 | 1561 | 2265 | 483 | 490 | 651 | 258 | 261 | 322 | 171 | 172 | 196 |
| 0.15 | *** | 11355 | 11511 | 13323 | 2101 | 2178 | 2351 | 642 | 658 | 678 | 332 | 336 | 342 | 211 | 213 | 216 |
| | *** | 11409 | 11794 | 17482 | 2133 | 2244 | 2994 | 649 | 667 | 821 | 334 | 339 | 391 | 211 | 215 | 232 |
| 0.2 | *** | 14235 | 14476 | 17703 | 2595 | 2721 | 3033 | 780 | 805 | 841 | 393 | 400 | 411 | 244 | 247 | 252 |
| | *** | 14316 | 14922 | 21583 | 2647 | 2835 | 3619 | 791 | 821 | 964 | 397 | 406 | 449 | 246 | 249 | 261 |
| 0.25 | *** | 16329 | 16674 | 21585 | 2974 | 3154 | 3629 | 888 | 926 | 980 | 442 | 453 | 468 | 271 | 276 | 281 |
| | *** | 16445 | 17315 | 25032 | 3048 | 3321 | 4140 | 906 | 949 | 1081 | 447 | 460 | 495 | 273 | 278 | 284 |
| 0.3 | *** | 17651 | 18123 | 24877 | 3243 | 3478 | 4126 | 972 | 1019 | 1092 | 479 | 494 | 512 | 290 | 296 | 303 |
| | *** | 17810 | 18991 | 27831 | 3339 | 3701 | 4556 | 993 | 1052 | 1172 | 486 | 503 | 530 | 294 | 299 | 300 |
| 0.35 | *** | 18260 | 18886 | 27524 | 3411 | 3702 | 4519 | 1028 | 1088 | 1178 | 504 | 522 | 544 | 303 | 309 | 318 |
| | *** | 18470 | 20011 | 29979 | 3530 | 3978 | 4869 | 1055 | 1127 | 1237 | 513 | 532 | 553 | 306 | 314 | 310 |
| 0.4 | *** | 18240 | 19050 | 29494 | 3491 | 3834 | 4803 | 1062 | 1129 | 1234 | 519 | 539 | 564 | 308 | 316 | 325 |
| | *** | 18514 | 20456 | 31475 | 3631 | 4157 | 5077 | 1092 | 1176 | 1276 | 528 | 550 | 565 | 312 | 321 | 313 |
| 0.45 | *** | 17691 | 18719 | 30770 | 3493 | 3881 | 4972 | 1073 | 1147 | 1263 | 522 | 543 | 570 | 308 | 316 | 326 |
| | *** | 18042 | 20415 | 32322 | 3653 | 4245 | 5181 | 1107 | 1198 | 1289 | 532 | 555 | 565 | 312 | 321 | 310 |
| 0.5 | *** | 16728 | 17997 | 31340 | 3431 | 3854 | 5031 | 1063 | 1142 | 1264 | 514 | 537 | 564 | 301 | 309 | 319 |
| | *** | 17169 | 19974 | 32517 | 3606 | 4245 | 5181 | 1098 | 1194 | 1276 | 524 | 549 | 553 | 305 | 314 | 300 |
| 0.55 | *** | 15465 | 16989 | 31203 | 3313 | 3757 | 4974 | 1032 | 1113 | 1236 | 496 | 519 | 546 | 288 | 296 | 305 |
| | *** | 16008 | 19208 | 32061 | 3498 | 4164 | 5077 | 1068 | 1167 | 1237 | 506 | 531 | 530 | 291 | 300 | 284 |
| 0.6 | *** | 14023 | 15780 | 30358 | 3147 | 3599 | 4806 | 983 | 1061 | 1180 | 468 | 488 | 515 | 269 | 276 | 285 |
| | *** | 14665 | 18179 | 30955 | 3336 | 4007 | 4869 | 1019 | 1113 | 1172 | 478 | 501 | 495 | 272 | 280 | 261 |
| 0.65 | *** | 12502 | 14438 | 28806 | 2936 | 3379 | 4524 | 915 | 987 | 1095 | 429 | 447 | 471 | 243 | 249 | 256 |
| | *** | 13227 | 16929 | 29197 | 3122 | 3772 | 4556 | 948 | 1035 | 1081 | 438 | 459 | 449 | 245 | 252 | 232 |
| 0.7 | *** | 10977 | 13002 | 26554 | 2683 | 3100 | 4130 | 828 | 891 | 983 | 381 | 396 | 415 | 210 | 216 | 222 |
| | *** | 11751 | 15483 | 26789 | 2859 | 3462 | 4140 | 857 | 933 | 964 | 388 | 405 | 391 | 213 | 218 | 196 |
| 0.75 | *** | 9481 | 11485 | 23608 | 2387 | 2758 | 3626 | 720 | 771 | 843 | 321 | 333 | 346 | 172 | 175 | 179 |
| | *** | 10261 | 13843 | 23730 | 2546 | 3072 | 3619 | 744 | 804 | 821 | 327 | 339 | 322 | 174 | 177 | 153 |
| 0.8 | *** | 8007 | 9870 | 19973 | 2040 | 2348 | 3012 | 589 | 627 | 676 | 251 | 258 | 267 | . | . | . |
| | *** | 8741 | 11983 | 20021 | 2173 | 2598 | 2994 | 607 | 649 | 651 | 254 | 262 | 241 | . | . | . |
| 0.85 | *** | 6509 | 8101 | 15657 | 1630 | 1854 | 2288 | 434 | 456 | 481 | . | . | . | . | . | . |
| | *** | 7143 | 9840 | 15660 | 1728 | 2026 | 2265 | 444 | 468 | 456 | . | . | . | . | . | . |
| 0.9 | *** | 4879 | 6059 | 10666 | 1127 | 1252 | 1458 | . | . | . | . | . | . | . | . | . |
| | *** | 5356 | 7275 | 10648 | 1183 | 1340 | 1432 | . | . | . | . | . | . | . | . | . |
| 0.95 | *** | 2852 | 3432 | 5012 | . | . | . | . | . | . | . | . | . | . | . | . |
| | *** | 3095 | 3957 | 4986 | . | . | . | . | . | . | . | . | . | . | . | . |

## TABLE 4: ALPHA= 0.01  POWER= 0.9    EXPECTED ACCRUAL THRU MINIMUM FOLLOW-UP= 1900

| | | DEL=.02 | | | DEL=.05 | | | DEL=.10 | | | DEL=.15 | | | DEL=.20 | | |
|---|---|---|---|---|---|---|---|---|---|---|---|---|---|---|---|---|---|
| FACT= | | 1.0 .75 | .50 .25 | .00 BIN | 1.0 .75 | .50 .25 | .00 BIN | 1.0 .75 | .50 .25 | .00 BIN | 1.0 75 | .50 .25 | .00 BIN | 1.0 .75 | .50 .25 | .00 BIN |
| PCONT=*** | | | | | REQUIRED NUMBER OF PATIENTS | | | | | | | | | | | |
| 0.05 | *** | 3730 | 3765 | 3921 | 807 | 817 | 831 | 291 | 293 | 296 | 171 | 172 | 172 | 120 | 121 | 121 |
| | *** | 3743 | 3811 | 7329 | 812 | 824 | 1432 | 292 | 294 | 456 | 171 | 172 | 241 | 121 | 121 | 153 |
| 0.1 | *** | 7767 | 7860 | 8615 | 1498 | 1535 | 1604 | 479 | 486 | 495 | 258 | 260 | 262 | 170 | 171 | 172 |
| | *** | 7799 | 8013 | 12731 | 1514 | 1564 | 2265 | 483 | 490 | 651 | 258 | 261 | 322 | 171 | 172 | 196 |
| 0.15 | *** | 11364 | 11528 | 13323 | 2106 | 2184 | 2351 | 643 | 659 | 679 | 331 | 336 | 342 | 211 | 213 | 216 |
| | *** | 11420 | 11821 | 17482 | 2139 | 2249 | 2994 | 650 | 668 | 821 | 334 | 339 | 391 | 212 | 215 | 232 |
| 0.2 | *** | 14249 | 14503 | 17703 | 2605 | 2731 | 3032 | 781 | 806 | 840 | 394 | 401 | 410 | 244 | 248 | 251 |
| | *** | 14334 | 14967 | 21583 | 2656 | 2842 | 3619 | 793 | 823 | 964 | 398 | 406 | 449 | 247 | 250 | 261 |
| 0.25 | *** | 16348 | 16712 | 21585 | 2987 | 3168 | 3629 | 892 | 928 | 980 | 443 | 453 | 467 | 272 | 275 | 281 |
| | *** | 16470 | 17379 | 25032 | 3061 | 3333 | 4140 | 908 | 951 | 1081 | 448 | 460 | 495 | 273 | 277 | 284 |
| 0.3 | *** | 17677 | 18175 | 24877 | 3260 | 3497 | 4126 | 976 | 1022 | 1092 | 481 | 495 | 512 | 291 | 296 | 303 |
| | *** | 17844 | 19077 | 27831 | 3357 | 3716 | 4556 | 997 | 1053 | 1172 | 486 | 503 | 530 | 293 | 299 | 300 |
| 0.35 | *** | 18294 | 18954 | 27523 | 3433 | 3725 | 4519 | 1034 | 1091 | 1177 | 505 | 524 | 543 | 304 | 310 | 318 |
| | *** | 18517 | 20121 | 29979 | 3553 | 3997 | 4869 | 1060 | 1129 | 1237 | 514 | 533 | 553 | 306 | 313 | 310 |
| 0.4 | *** | 18285 | 19137 | 29494 | 3516 | 3860 | 4802 | 1067 | 1134 | 1235 | 520 | 539 | 564 | 310 | 317 | 325 |
| | *** | 18574 | 20591 | 31475 | 3657 | 4180 | 5077 | 1098 | 1178 | 1276 | 529 | 551 | 565 | 313 | 320 | 313 |
| 0.45 | *** | 17750 | 18826 | 30769 | 3523 | 3911 | 4973 | 1079 | 1151 | 1263 | 524 | 543 | 570 | 308 | 317 | 325 |
| | *** | 18120 | 20573 | 32322 | 3683 | 4270 | 5181 | 1113 | 1200 | 1289 | 533 | 557 | 565 | 312 | 320 | 310 |
| 0.5 | *** | 16802 | 18127 | 31340 | 3464 | 3887 | 5030 | 1070 | 1147 | 1263 | 516 | 538 | 564 | 301 | 310 | 319 |
| | *** | 17265 | 20153 | 32517 | 3640 | 4272 | 5181 | 1104 | 1198 | 1276 | 526 | 550 | 553 | 306 | 315 | 300 |
| 0.55 | *** | 15558 | 17138 | 31202 | 3347 | 3792 | 4974 | 1040 | 1117 | 1236 | 498 | 519 | 546 | 288 | 296 | 305 |
| | *** | 16123 | 19405 | 32061 | 3533 | 4193 | 5077 | 1075 | 1170 | 1237 | 508 | 532 | 530 | 292 | 300 | 284 |
| 0.6 | *** | 14133 | 15947 | 30357 | 3181 | 3632 | 4806 | 990 | 1066 | 1180 | 470 | 490 | 514 | 269 | 277 | 284 |
| | *** | 14800 | 18386 | 30955 | 3371 | 4035 | 4869 | 1025 | 1116 | 1172 | 479 | 501 | 495 | 273 | 280 | 261 |
| 0.65 | *** | 12630 | 14614 | 28806 | 2971 | 3412 | 4524 | 921 | 992 | 1096 | 431 | 448 | 471 | 243 | 249 | 256 |
| | *** | 13377 | 17140 | 29197 | 3157 | 3800 | 4556 | 954 | 1037 | 1081 | 440 | 459 | 449 | 246 | 253 | 232 |
| 0.7 | *** | 11115 | 13182 | 26554 | 2717 | 3131 | 4130 | 833 | 895 | 983 | 382 | 398 | 415 | 211 | 216 | 220 |
| | *** | 11908 | 15690 | 26789 | 2892 | 3486 | 4140 | 862 | 934 | 964 | 389 | 406 | 391 | 213 | 218 | 196 |
| 0.75 | *** | 9622 | 11658 | 23609 | 2416 | 2785 | 3625 | 725 | 774 | 843 | 323 | 334 | 346 | 172 | 175 | 179 |
| | *** | 10415 | 14036 | 23730 | 2574 | 3093 | 3619 | 748 | 806 | 821 | 327 | 339 | 322 | 174 | 178 | 153 |
| 0.8 | *** | 8141 | 10027 | 19972 | 2065 | 2370 | 3011 | 593 | 629 | 676 | 251 | 258 | 266 | . | . | . |
| | *** | 8886 | 12154 | 20021 | 2196 | 2614 | 2994 | 610 | 650 | 651 | 255 | 262 | 241 | . | . | . |
| 0.85 | *** | 6625 | 8234 | 15656 | 1648 | 1870 | 2288 | 436 | 456 | 482 | . | . | . | . | . | . |
| | *** | 7267 | 9977 | 15660 | 1745 | 2037 | 2265 | 445 | 469 | 456 | . | . | . | . | . | . |
| 0.9 | *** | 4967 | 6155 | 10666 | 1137 | 1260 | 1458 | . | . | . | . | . | . | . | . | . |
| | *** | 5448 | 7367 | 10648 | 1193 | 1344 | 1432 | . | . | . | . | . | . | . | . | . |
| 0.95 | *** | 2897 | 3477 | 5011 | . | . | . | . | . | . | . | . | . | . | . | . |
| | *** | 3141 | 3993 | 4986 | . | . | . | . | . | . | . | . | . | . | . | . |

TABLE 4: ALPHA= 0.01  POWER= 0.9     EXPECTED ACCRUAL THRU MINIMUM FOLLOW-UP= 2000

| PCONT=*** | FACT= | DEL=.02 1.0 / .75 | .50 / .25 | .00 / BIN | DEL=.05 1.0 / .75 | .50 / .25 | .00 / BIN | DEL=.10 1.0 / .75 | .50 / .25 | .00 / BIN | DEL=.15 1.0 / 75 | .50 / .25 | .00 / BIN | DEL=.20 1.0 / .75 | .50 / .25 | .00 / BIN |
|---|---|---|---|---|---|---|---|---|---|---|---|---|---|---|---|---|
| | | REQUIRED NUMBER OF PATIENTS | | | | | | | | | | | | | | |
| 0.05 | *** | 3732 | 3769 | 3921 | 809 | 817 | 831 | 291 | 294 | 296 | 171 | 171 | 172 | 120 | 121 | 121 |
| | *** | 3745 | 3814 | 7329 | 812 | 824 | 1432 | 292 | 295 | 456 | 171 | 172 | 241 | 121 | 121 | 153 |
| 0.1 | *** | 7772 | 7869 | 8615 | 1501 | 1537 | 1604 | 480 | 487 | 495 | 257 | 260 | 262 | 170 | 171 | 172 |
| | *** | 7805 | 8026 | 12731 | 1517 | 1565 | 2265 | 484 | 491 | 651 | 259 | 261 | 322 | 171 | 171 | 196 |
| 0.15 | *** | 11374 | 11545 | 13324 | 2112 | 2189 | 2351 | 645 | 660 | 679 | 332 | 337 | 342 | 211 | 214 | 216 |
| | *** | 11431 | 11849 | 17482 | 2145 | 2252 | 2994 | 652 | 669 | 821 | 335 | 340 | 391 | 212 | 215 | 232 |
| 0.2 | *** | 14262 | 14529 | 17704 | 2614 | 2740 | 3034 | 784 | 809 | 841 | 395 | 402 | 411 | 245 | 249 | 252 |
| | *** | 14352 | 15010 | 21583 | 2666 | 2850 | 3619 | 795 | 824 | 964 | 397 | 406 | 449 | 246 | 250 | 261 |
| 0.25 | *** | 16367 | 16750 | 21586 | 3001 | 3181 | 3629 | 895 | 930 | 980 | 444 | 455 | 467 | 272 | 276 | 281 |
| | *** | 16496 | 17441 | 25032 | 3075 | 3344 | 4140 | 911 | 952 | 1081 | 449 | 461 | 495 | 274 | 279 | 284 |
| 0.3 | *** | 17704 | 18227 | 24877 | 3277 | 3515 | 4127 | 980 | 1026 | 1092 | 482 | 495 | 512 | 291 | 297 | 302 |
| | *** | 17880 | 19161 | 27831 | 3375 | 3731 | 4556 | 1001 | 1055 | 1172 | 489 | 504 | 530 | 294 | 300 | 300 |
| 0.35 | *** | 18330 | 19022 | 27524 | 3454 | 3747 | 4519 | 1039 | 1095 | 1177 | 507 | 524 | 544 | 304 | 311 | 317 |
| | *** | 18564 | 20227 | 29979 | 3575 | 4016 | 4869 | 1065 | 1131 | 1237 | 515 | 534 | 553 | 307 | 314 | 310 |
| 0.4 | *** | 18331 | 19224 | 29494 | 3541 | 3886 | 4802 | 1074 | 1137 | 1235 | 522 | 541 | 564 | 310 | 317 | 325 |
| | *** | 18635 | 20721 | 31475 | 3684 | 4201 | 5077 | 1102 | 1181 | 1276 | 531 | 551 | 565 | 314 | 321 | 313 |
| 0.45 | *** | 17809 | 18934 | 30770 | 3551 | 3940 | 4972 | 1086 | 1156 | 1264 | 525 | 545 | 570 | 310 | 317 | 326 |
| | *** | 18196 | 20727 | 32322 | 3712 | 4294 | 5181 | 1119 | 1204 | 1289 | 535 | 557 | 565 | 314 | 321 | 310 |
| 0.5 | *** | 16876 | 18254 | 31340 | 3495 | 3917 | 5031 | 1076 | 1151 | 1264 | 517 | 539 | 565 | 302 | 310 | 319 |
| | *** | 17360 | 20326 | 32517 | 3671 | 4299 | 5181 | 1110 | 1201 | 1276 | 527 | 551 | 553 | 306 | 315 | 300 |
| 0.55 | *** | 15650 | 17285 | 31204 | 3380 | 3824 | 4975 | 1046 | 1122 | 1236 | 500 | 521 | 546 | 290 | 296 | 305 |
| | *** | 16239 | 19594 | 32061 | 3566 | 4220 | 5077 | 1081 | 1172 | 1237 | 510 | 532 | 530 | 292 | 301 | 284 |
| 0.6 | *** | 14244 | 16107 | 30357 | 3215 | 3665 | 4806 | 997 | 1071 | 1180 | 472 | 491 | 515 | 270 | 276 | 284 |
| | *** | 14931 | 18585 | 30955 | 3405 | 4061 | 4869 | 1031 | 1119 | 1172 | 481 | 502 | 495 | 274 | 280 | 261 |
| 0.65 | *** | 12755 | 14786 | 28807 | 3004 | 3444 | 4524 | 929 | 996 | 1095 | 434 | 450 | 471 | 244 | 250 | 256 |
| | *** | 13521 | 17342 | 29197 | 3190 | 3825 | 4556 | 960 | 1041 | 1081 | 441 | 460 | 449 | 246 | 252 | 232 |
| 0.7 | *** | 11250 | 13355 | 26555 | 2749 | 3160 | 4130 | 839 | 899 | 984 | 384 | 399 | 415 | 211 | 216 | 221 |
| | *** | 12060 | 15887 | 26789 | 2924 | 3510 | 4140 | 867 | 937 | 964 | 391 | 406 | 391 | 214 | 219 | 196 |
| 0.75 | *** | 9757 | 11825 | 23609 | 2445 | 2811 | 3626 | 730 | 777 | 844 | 324 | 335 | 346 | 172 | 176 | 179 |
| | *** | 10565 | 14220 | 23730 | 2602 | 3112 | 3619 | 752 | 807 | 821 | 329 | 340 | 322 | 175 | 177 | 153 |
| 0.8 | *** | 8270 | 10179 | 19972 | 2090 | 2390 | 3011 | 596 | 631 | 676 | 252 | 259 | 266 | . | . | . |
| | *** | 9024 | 12315 | 20021 | 2220 | 2629 | 2994 | 612 | 652 | 651 | 255 | 262 | 241 | . | . | . |
| 0.85 | *** | 6736 | 8360 | 15656 | 1666 | 1884 | 2289 | 437 | 457 | 482 | . | . | . | . | . | . |
| | *** | 7386 | 10106 | 15660 | 1762 | 2047 | 2265 | 447 | 469 | 456 | . | . | . | . | . | . |
| 0.9 | *** | 5051 | 6245 | 10666 | 1149 | 1267 | 1457 | . | . | . | . | . | . | . | . | . |
| | *** | 5536 | 7454 | 10648 | 1202 | 1350 | 1432 | . | . | . | . | . | . | . | . | . |
| 0.95 | *** | 2941 | 3517 | 5011 | . | . | . | . | . | . | . | . | . | . | . | . |
| | *** | 3184 | 4027 | 4986 | . | . | . | . | . | . | . | . | . | . | . | . |

## TABLE 4: ALPHA= 0.01  POWER= 0.9    EXPECTED ACCRUAL THRU MINIMUM FOLLOW-UP= 2250

| | | DEL=.02 | | | DEL=.05 | | | DEL=.10 | | | DEL=.15 | | | DEL=.20 | | |
|---|---|---|---|---|---|---|---|---|---|---|---|---|---|---|---|---|---|
| FACT= | | 1.0 .75 | .50 .25 | .00 BIN | 1.0 .75 | .50 .25 | .00 BIN | 1.0 .75 | .50 .25 | .00 BIN | 1.0 75 | .50 .25 | .00 BIN | 1.0 .75 | .50 .25 | .00 BIN |
| PCONT=*** | | | | REQUIRED NUMBER OF PATIENTS | | | | | | | | | | | | |
| 0.05 | *** | 3737 | 3776 | 3922 | 809 | 820 | 831 | 292 | 294 | 295 | 171 | 171 | 173 | 120 | 120 | 120 |
| | *** | 3751 | 3822 | 7329 | 814 | 825 | 1432 | 292 | 295 | 456 | 171 | 171 | 241 | 120 | 120 | 153 |
| 0.1 | *** | 7784 | 7891 | 8614 | 1507 | 1542 | 1604 | 480 | 488 | 494 | 258 | 260 | 263 | 170 | 171 | 173 |
| | *** | 7821 | 8057 | 12731 | 1523 | 1569 | 2265 | 485 | 491 | 651 | 260 | 261 | 322 | 171 | 171 | 196 |
| 0.15 | *** | 11395 | 11587 | 13324 | 2126 | 2201 | 2351 | 648 | 662 | 679 | 333 | 337 | 342 | 212 | 213 | 215 |
| | *** | 11459 | 11912 | 17482 | 2158 | 2261 | 2994 | 654 | 669 | 821 | 336 | 340 | 391 | 212 | 215 | 232 |
| 0.2 | *** | 14295 | 14594 | 17703 | 2635 | 2760 | 3033 | 789 | 811 | 840 | 396 | 403 | 410 | 246 | 249 | 252 |
| | *** | 14397 | 15114 | 21583 | 2688 | 2865 | 3619 | 798 | 825 | 964 | 399 | 406 | 449 | 247 | 250 | 261 |
| 0.25 | *** | 16416 | 16844 | 21585 | 3030 | 3211 | 3629 | 902 | 935 | 980 | 447 | 455 | 468 | 272 | 277 | 281 |
| | *** | 16559 | 17592 | 25032 | 3106 | 3368 | 4140 | 916 | 955 | 1081 | 451 | 461 | 495 | 274 | 278 | 284 |
| 0.3 | *** | 17769 | 18354 | 24878 | 3317 | 3554 | 4127 | 988 | 1032 | 1092 | 485 | 497 | 511 | 292 | 298 | 303 |
| | *** | 17967 | 19362 | 27831 | 3416 | 3763 | 4556 | 1008 | 1059 | 1172 | 491 | 505 | 530 | 295 | 300 | 300 |
| 0.35 | *** | 18417 | 19189 | 27524 | 3503 | 3795 | 4519 | 1050 | 1102 | 1177 | 511 | 525 | 544 | 305 | 312 | 317 |
| | *** | 18679 | 20483 | 29979 | 3625 | 4055 | 4869 | 1074 | 1136 | 1237 | 519 | 534 | 553 | 308 | 314 | 310 |
| 0.4 | *** | 18446 | 19436 | 29494 | 3598 | 3943 | 4802 | 1085 | 1147 | 1234 | 525 | 542 | 564 | 312 | 317 | 326 |
| | *** | 18784 | 21030 | 31475 | 3743 | 4248 | 5077 | 1113 | 1186 | 1276 | 534 | 552 | 565 | 314 | 322 | 313 |
| 0.45 | *** | 17954 | 19192 | 30770 | 3616 | 4003 | 4972 | 1099 | 1166 | 1264 | 530 | 548 | 570 | 311 | 317 | 326 |
| | *** | 18387 | 21088 | 32322 | 3778 | 4347 | 5181 | 1130 | 1209 | 1289 | 538 | 558 | 565 | 314 | 322 | 310 |
| 0.5 | *** | 17060 | 18561 | 31341 | 3566 | 3987 | 5030 | 1091 | 1161 | 1264 | 522 | 541 | 565 | 305 | 311 | 319 |
| | *** | 17593 | 20733 | 32517 | 3743 | 4355 | 5181 | 1123 | 1208 | 1276 | 531 | 552 | 553 | 308 | 314 | 300 |
| 0.55 | *** | 15875 | 17634 | 31203 | 3456 | 3897 | 4975 | 1062 | 1133 | 1236 | 505 | 523 | 545 | 291 | 298 | 305 |
| | *** | 16516 | 20036 | 32061 | 3642 | 4279 | 5077 | 1094 | 1178 | 1237 | 513 | 534 | 530 | 294 | 300 | 284 |
| 0.6 | *** | 14509 | 16491 | 30358 | 3293 | 3737 | 4806 | 1011 | 1081 | 1180 | 475 | 493 | 514 | 271 | 277 | 284 |
| | *** | 15249 | 19049 | 30955 | 3481 | 4120 | 4869 | 1043 | 1124 | 1172 | 483 | 503 | 495 | 274 | 281 | 261 |
| 0.65 | *** | 13055 | 15189 | 28807 | 3081 | 3514 | 4524 | 942 | 1005 | 1095 | 437 | 452 | 471 | 244 | 250 | 255 |
| | *** | 13868 | 17811 | 29197 | 3265 | 3880 | 4556 | 972 | 1046 | 1081 | 444 | 461 | 449 | 247 | 253 | 232 |
| 0.7 | *** | 11570 | 13760 | 26555 | 2820 | 3225 | 4130 | 851 | 907 | 983 | 387 | 401 | 415 | 212 | 216 | 221 |
| | *** | 12418 | 16343 | 26789 | 2994 | 3560 | 4140 | 877 | 942 | 964 | 393 | 407 | 391 | 215 | 219 | 196 |
| 0.75 | *** | 10079 | 12214 | 23608 | 2510 | 2868 | 3625 | 739 | 784 | 843 | 326 | 336 | 347 | 173 | 176 | 179 |
| | *** | 10918 | 14644 | 23730 | 2665 | 3155 | 3619 | 761 | 811 | 821 | 330 | 342 | 322 | 174 | 178 | 153 |
| 0.8 | *** | 8571 | 10529 | 19973 | 2144 | 2435 | 3011 | 603 | 635 | 676 | 253 | 260 | 267 | . | . | . |
| | *** | 9350 | 12687 | 20021 | 2271 | 2662 | 2994 | 618 | 655 | 651 | 257 | 263 | 241 | . | . | . |
| 0.85 | *** | 6997 | 8652 | 15657 | 1707 | 1917 | 2288 | 441 | 460 | 482 | . | . | . | . | . | . |
| | *** | 7662 | 10402 | 15660 | 1799 | 2069 | 2265 | 449 | 471 | 456 | . | . | . | . | . | . |
| 0.9 | *** | 5248 | 6453 | 10666 | 1171 | 1284 | 1458 | . | . | . | . | . | . | . | . | . |
| | *** | 5740 | 7651 | 10648 | 1222 | 1360 | 1432 | . | . | . | . | . | . | . | . | . |
| 0.95 | *** | 3040 | 3611 | 5011 | . | . | . | . | . | . | . | . | . | . | . | . |
| | *** | 3282 | 4103 | 4986 | . | . | . | . | . | . | . | . | . | . | . | . |

TABLE 4: ALPHA= 0.01 POWER= 0.9    EXPECTED ACCRUAL THRU MINIMUM FOLLOW-UP= 2500

| | | DEL=.02 | | | DEL=.05 | | | DEL=.10 | | | DEL=.15 | | | DEL=.20 | | |
|---|---|---|---|---|---|---|---|---|---|---|---|---|---|---|---|---|
| FACT= | | 1.0 .75 | .50 .25 | .00 BIN | 1.0 .75 | .50 .25 | .00 BIN | 1.0 .75 | .50 .25 | .00 BIN | 1.0 75 | .50 .25 | .00 BIN | 1.0 .75 | .50 .25 | .00 BIN |
| PCONT=*** | | | | | | REQUIRED | NUMBER | OF PATIENTS | | | | | | | | |
| 0.05 | *** | 3742 | 3783 | 3921 | 812 | 820 | 831 | 292 | 293 | 295 | 171 | 171 | 171 | 120 | 121 | 121 |
| | *** | 3758 | 3827 | 7329 | 815 | 824 | 1432 | 293 | 295 | 456 | 171 | 171 | 241 | 120 | 121 | 153 |
| 0.1 | *** | 7796 | 7914 | 8615 | 1514 | 1548 | 1604 | 483 | 489 | 495 | 259 | 261 | 262 | 170 | 171 | 171 |
| | *** | 7837 | 8086 | 12731 | 1529 | 1571 | 2265 | 486 | 492 | 651 | 259 | 262 | 322 | 171 | 171 | 196 |
| 0.15 | *** | 11417 | 11627 | 13323 | 2137 | 2212 | 2351 | 649 | 662 | 677 | 334 | 337 | 342 | 212 | 214 | 215 |
| | *** | 11489 | 11971 | 17482 | 2170 | 2268 | 2994 | 656 | 670 | 821 | 336 | 340 | 391 | 212 | 215 | 232 |
| 0.2 | *** | 14329 | 14658 | 17702 | 2654 | 2777 | 3033 | 793 | 814 | 842 | 396 | 402 | 411 | 246 | 249 | 251 |
| | *** | 14440 | 15211 | 21583 | 2708 | 2879 | 3619 | 802 | 826 | 964 | 399 | 408 | 449 | 248 | 249 | 261 |
| 0.25 | *** | 16464 | 16936 | 21586 | 3059 | 3237 | 3629 | 908 | 939 | 979 | 448 | 458 | 467 | 273 | 276 | 281 |
| | *** | 16624 | 17733 | 25032 | 3134 | 3387 | 4140 | 921 | 958 | 1081 | 452 | 462 | 495 | 274 | 279 | 284 |
| 0.3 | *** | 17836 | 18479 | 24877 | 3352 | 3589 | 4126 | 996 | 1037 | 1092 | 487 | 498 | 512 | 293 | 298 | 302 |
| | *** | 18054 | 19549 | 27831 | 3452 | 3790 | 4556 | 1015 | 1062 | 1172 | 492 | 504 | 530 | 295 | 299 | 300 |
| 0.35 | *** | 18504 | 19351 | 27523 | 3546 | 3839 | 4518 | 1059 | 1109 | 1177 | 514 | 527 | 543 | 306 | 312 | 318 |
| | *** | 18795 | 20720 | 29979 | 3670 | 4089 | 4869 | 1083 | 1140 | 1237 | 520 | 536 | 553 | 309 | 315 | 310 |
| 0.4 | *** | 18559 | 19639 | 29493 | 3651 | 3993 | 4801 | 1096 | 1154 | 1234 | 529 | 545 | 564 | 312 | 318 | 324 |
| | *** | 18934 | 21318 | 31475 | 3795 | 4289 | 5077 | 1123 | 1190 | 1276 | 537 | 554 | 565 | 315 | 321 | 313 |
| 0.45 | *** | 18101 | 19440 | 30770 | 3676 | 4061 | 4973 | 1111 | 1174 | 1264 | 533 | 549 | 570 | 312 | 318 | 326 |
| | *** | 18573 | 21421 | 32322 | 3839 | 4392 | 5181 | 1140 | 1214 | 1289 | 540 | 559 | 565 | 315 | 321 | 310 |
| 0.5 | *** | 17242 | 18851 | 31340 | 3631 | 4046 | 5031 | 1102 | 1170 | 1264 | 526 | 543 | 564 | 306 | 312 | 318 |
| | *** | 17821 | 21108 | 32517 | 3808 | 4402 | 5181 | 1134 | 1212 | 1276 | 534 | 552 | 553 | 309 | 315 | 300 |
| 0.55 | *** | 16095 | 17964 | 31202 | 3524 | 3959 | 4974 | 1073 | 1142 | 1236 | 508 | 524 | 546 | 292 | 298 | 304 |
| | *** | 16783 | 20439 | 32061 | 3709 | 4327 | 5077 | 1104 | 1184 | 1237 | 515 | 536 | 530 | 295 | 301 | 284 |
| 0.6 | *** | 14767 | 16849 | 30358 | 3362 | 3801 | 4806 | 1023 | 1089 | 1179 | 479 | 495 | 515 | 271 | 277 | 284 |
| | *** | 15549 | 19470 | 30955 | 3549 | 4170 | 4869 | 1054 | 1129 | 1172 | 487 | 504 | 495 | 274 | 281 | 261 |
| 0.65 | *** | 13340 | 15562 | 28808 | 3148 | 3574 | 4524 | 952 | 1014 | 1095 | 440 | 454 | 471 | 246 | 251 | 256 |
| | *** | 14192 | 18236 | 29197 | 3331 | 3927 | 4556 | 981 | 1051 | 1081 | 446 | 462 | 449 | 248 | 252 | 232 |
| 0.7 | *** | 11870 | 14133 | 26554 | 2884 | 3281 | 4131 | 861 | 914 | 983 | 389 | 401 | 415 | 214 | 217 | 221 |
| | *** | 12751 | 16754 | 26789 | 3056 | 3602 | 4140 | 886 | 945 | 964 | 395 | 408 | 391 | 215 | 218 | 196 |
| 0.75 | *** | 10377 | 12570 | 23608 | 2567 | 2917 | 3626 | 746 | 789 | 843 | 327 | 337 | 346 | 174 | 176 | 179 |
| | *** | 11242 | 15024 | 23730 | 2720 | 3192 | 3619 | 767 | 814 | 821 | 333 | 342 | 322 | 174 | 177 | 153 |
| 0.8 | *** | 8849 | 10849 | 19973 | 2192 | 2474 | 3011 | 609 | 639 | 676 | 254 | 261 | 267 | . | . | . |
| | *** | 9648 | 13018 | 20021 | 2317 | 2690 | 2994 | 623 | 656 | 651 | 258 | 264 | 241 | . | . | . |
| 0.85 | *** | 7237 | 8917 | 15656 | 1742 | 1943 | 2289 | 445 | 462 | 483 | . | . | . | . | . | . |
| | *** | 7914 | 10664 | 15660 | 1831 | 2087 | 2265 | 452 | 471 | 456 | . | . | . | . | . | . |
| 0.9 | *** | 5426 | 6639 | 10667 | 1190 | 1298 | 1458 | . | . | . | . | . | . | . | . | . |
| | *** | 5923 | 7823 | 10648 | 1240 | 1368 | 1432 | . | . | . | . | . | . | . | . | . |
| 0.95 | *** | 3129 | 3692 | 5011 | . | . | . | . | . | . | . | . | . | . | . | . |
| | *** | 3370 | 4167 | 4986 | . | . | . | . | . | . | . | . | . | . | . | . |

## TABLE 4: ALPHA= 0.01  POWER= 0.9    EXPECTED ACCRUAL THRU MINIMUM FOLLOW-UP= 2750

| | | DEL=.02 | | | DEL=.05 | | | DEL=.10 | | | DEL=.15 | | | DEL=.20 | | |
|---|---|---|---|---|---|---|---|---|---|---|---|---|---|---|---|---|
| | FACT= | 1.0 .75 | .50 .25 | .00 BIN | 1.0 .75 | .50 .25 | .00 BIN | 1.0 .75 | .50 .25 | .00 BIN | 1.0 75 | .50 .25 | .00 BIN | 1.0 .75 | .50 .25 | .00 BIN |
| PCONT=*** | | REQUIRED NUMBER OF PATIENTS | | | | | | | | | | | | | | |
| 0.05 | *** | 3746 | 3789 | 3921 | 813 | 821 | 831 | 291 | 294 | 295 | 171 | 171 | 171 | 120 | 122 | 122 |
| | *** | 3762 | 3834 | 7329 | 816 | 826 | 1432 | 294 | 295 | 456 | 171 | 171 | 241 | 120 | 122 | 153 |
| 0.1 | *** | 7809 | 7935 | 8616 | 1519 | 1552 | 1603 | 484 | 489 | 494 | 259 | 260 | 263 | 170 | 171 | 171 |
| | *** | 7854 | 8110 | 12731 | 1532 | 1574 | 2265 | 486 | 491 | 651 | 259 | 260 | 322 | 171 | 171 | 196 |
| 0.15 | *** | 11438 | 11668 | 13323 | 2148 | 2220 | 2350 | 652 | 665 | 679 | 335 | 338 | 342 | 212 | 214 | 216 |
| | *** | 11517 | 12027 | 17482 | 2179 | 2275 | 2994 | 658 | 672 | 821 | 336 | 340 | 391 | 212 | 214 | 232 |
| 0.2 | *** | 14363 | 14721 | 17702 | 2672 | 2794 | 3033 | 795 | 816 | 841 | 398 | 404 | 410 | 247 | 249 | 252 |
| | *** | 14485 | 15302 | 21583 | 2724 | 2890 | 3619 | 806 | 828 | 964 | 401 | 407 | 449 | 249 | 250 | 261 |
| 0.25 | *** | 16512 | 17025 | 21585 | 3083 | 3260 | 3629 | 912 | 941 | 979 | 450 | 459 | 467 | 274 | 278 | 281 |
| | *** | 16687 | 17864 | 25032 | 3158 | 3404 | 4140 | 926 | 958 | 1081 | 453 | 462 | 495 | 276 | 280 | 284 |
| 0.3 | *** | 17902 | 18600 | 24876 | 3385 | 3619 | 4126 | 1003 | 1041 | 1092 | 489 | 500 | 511 | 294 | 298 | 302 |
| | *** | 18141 | 19726 | 27831 | 3485 | 3814 | 4556 | 1020 | 1065 | 1172 | 494 | 505 | 530 | 297 | 300 | 300 |
| 0.35 | *** | 18593 | 19509 | 27523 | 3588 | 3877 | 4520 | 1067 | 1113 | 1177 | 517 | 529 | 544 | 307 | 312 | 318 |
| | *** | 18909 | 20943 | 29979 | 3710 | 4117 | 4869 | 1089 | 1143 | 1237 | 522 | 535 | 553 | 311 | 315 | 310 |
| 0.4 | *** | 18672 | 19837 | 29493 | 3698 | 4037 | 4801 | 1106 | 1160 | 1233 | 532 | 546 | 563 | 314 | 319 | 326 |
| | *** | 19079 | 21585 | 31475 | 3842 | 4322 | 5077 | 1130 | 1194 | 1276 | 539 | 555 | 565 | 315 | 322 | 313 |
| 0.45 | *** | 18244 | 19678 | 30768 | 3729 | 4110 | 4972 | 1122 | 1180 | 1263 | 535 | 551 | 570 | 314 | 319 | 326 |
| | *** | 18754 | 21731 | 32322 | 3890 | 4430 | 5181 | 1149 | 1218 | 1289 | 542 | 560 | 565 | 315 | 322 | 310 |
| 0.5 | *** | 17419 | 19129 | 31341 | 3690 | 4100 | 5030 | 1113 | 1177 | 1264 | 529 | 544 | 565 | 307 | 312 | 319 |
| | *** | 18041 | 21451 | 32517 | 3865 | 4446 | 5181 | 1143 | 1216 | 1276 | 535 | 555 | 553 | 309 | 315 | 300 |
| 0.55 | *** | 16309 | 18273 | 31204 | 3587 | 4014 | 4975 | 1084 | 1147 | 1235 | 510 | 527 | 546 | 294 | 298 | 305 |
| | *** | 17039 | 20810 | 32061 | 3769 | 4372 | 5077 | 1115 | 1189 | 1237 | 518 | 535 | 530 | 295 | 302 | 284 |
| 0.6 | *** | 15013 | 17183 | 30358 | 3425 | 3856 | 4805 | 1034 | 1096 | 1180 | 483 | 496 | 515 | 273 | 278 | 283 |
| | *** | 15836 | 19856 | 30955 | 3611 | 4212 | 4869 | 1064 | 1134 | 1172 | 489 | 505 | 495 | 276 | 281 | 261 |
| 0.65 | *** | 13610 | 15908 | 29808 | 3210 | 3629 | 4523 | 962 | 1019 | 1096 | 441 | 455 | 470 | 247 | 250 | 256 |
| | *** | 14497 | 18622 | 29197 | 3391 | 3968 | 4556 | 989 | 1055 | 1081 | 448 | 463 | 449 | 249 | 254 | 232 |
| 0.7 | *** | 12153 | 14478 | 26554 | 2942 | 3330 | 4130 | 869 | 919 | 982 | 391 | 401 | 415 | 214 | 218 | 221 |
| | *** | 13062 | 17128 | 26789 | 3110 | 3640 | 4140 | 893 | 948 | 964 | 397 | 408 | 391 | 216 | 219 | 196 |
| 0.75 | *** | 10655 | 12897 | 23608 | 2619 | 2959 | 3626 | 754 | 793 | 844 | 329 | 338 | 346 | 175 | 177 | 178 |
| | *** | 11544 | 15370 | 23730 | 2769 | 3222 | 3619 | 773 | 816 | 821 | 333 | 342 | 322 | 175 | 178 | 153 |
| 0.8 | *** | 9109 | 11142 | 19973 | 2234 | 2509 | 3010 | 615 | 642 | 676 | 256 | 260 | 266 | . | . | . |
| | *** | 9923 | 13316 | 20021 | 2356 | 2714 | 2994 | 627 | 658 | 651 | 257 | 264 | 241 | . | . | . |
| 0.85 | *** | 7457 | 9157 | 15656 | 1772 | 1965 | 2289 | 448 | 463 | 483 | . | . | . | . | . | . |
| | *** | 8146 | 10898 | 15660 | 1859 | 2103 | 2265 | 455 | 472 | 456 | . | . | . | . | . | . |
| 0.9 | *** | 5589 | 6808 | 10666 | 1208 | 1309 | 1457 | . | . | . | . | . | . | . | . | . |
| | *** | 6090 | 7974 | 10648 | 1254 | 1376 | 1432 | . | . | . | . | . | . | . | . | . |
| 0.95 | *** | 3210 | 3763 | 5011 | . | . | . | . | . | . | . | . | . | . | . | . |
| | *** | 3447 | 4223 | 4986 | . | . | . | . | . | . | . | . | . | . | . | . |

**TABLE 4: ALPHA= 0.01  POWER= 0.9    EXPECTED ACCRUAL THRU MINIMUM FOLLOW-UP= 3000**

| | | DEL=.01 | | | DEL=.02 | | | DEL=.05 | | | DEL=.10 | | | DEL=.15 | | |
|---|---|---|---|---|---|---|---|---|---|---|---|---|---|---|---|---|
| FACT= | | 1.0 .75 | .50 .25 | .00 BIN | 1.0 .75 | .50 .25 | .00 BIN | 1.0 .75 | .50 .25 | .00 BIN | 1.0 75 | .50 .25 | .00 BIN | 1.0 .75 | .50 .25 | .00 BIN |
| PCONT=*** | | | | REQUIRED NUMBER OF PATIENTS | | | | | | | | | | | | |
| 0.01 | *** | 1990 | 1993 | 2008 | 730 | 733 | 737 | 242 | 242 | 242 | 122 | 122 | 122 | 85 | 85 | 85 |
| | *** | 1990 | 2000 | 7680 | 733 | 733 | 2539 | 242 | 242 | 691 | 122 | 122 | 281 | 85 | 85 | 167 |
| 0.02 | *** | 4390 | 4408 | 4480 | 1412 | 1420 | 1430 | 385 | 385 | 385 | 167 | 167 | 167 | 110 | 110 | 110 |
| | *** | 4397 | 4430 | 12679 | 1412 | 1423 | 3775 | 385 | 385 | 883 | 167 | 167 | 326 | 110 | 110 | 186 |
| 0.05 | *** | 13285 | 13340 | 13993 | 3752 | 3793 | 3920 | 815 | 823 | 830 | 290 | 295 | 295 | 170 | 170 | 170 |
| | *** | 13303 | 13445 | 27050 | 3767 | 3838 | 7329 | 815 | 827 | 1432 | 295 | 295 | 456 | 170 | 170 | 241 |
| 0.1 | *** | 29297 | 29435 | 32570 | 7820 | 7955 | 8615 | 1525 | 1555 | 1603 | 485 | 490 | 493 | 260 | 260 | 260 |
| | *** | 29342 | 29713 | 48918 | 7870 | 8135 | 12731 | 1535 | 1577 | 2265 | 485 | 493 | 651 | 260 | 260 | 322 |
| 0.15 | *** | 43735 | 43985 | 51455 | 11458 | 11705 | 13322 | 2158 | 2230 | 2350 | 655 | 665 | 677 | 335 | 340 | 343 |
| | *** | 43817 | 44480 | 68183 | 11545 | 12077 | 17482 | 2188 | 2278 | 2994 | 658 | 670 | 821 | 335 | 340 | 391 |
| 0.2 | *** | 55352 | 55742 | 69130 | 14395 | 14780 | 17702 | 2687 | 2807 | 3032 | 797 | 815 | 842 | 400 | 403 | 410 |
| | *** | 55483 | 56515 | 84845 | 14530 | 15385 | 21583 | 2740 | 2900 | 3619 | 808 | 827 | 964 | 403 | 407 | 449 |
| 0.25 | *** | 63797 | 64355 | 84868 | 16558 | 17113 | 21587 | 3107 | 3280 | 3628 | 917 | 943 | 980 | 452 | 460 | 467 |
| | *** | 63980 | 65473 | 98903 | 16750 | 17987 | 25032 | 3182 | 3418 | 4140 | 928 | 962 | 1081 | 455 | 463 | 495 |
| 0.3 | *** | 69080 | 69853 | 98278 | 17968 | 18718 | 24875 | 3415 | 3647 | 4127 | 1007 | 1045 | 1093 | 490 | 500 | 512 |
| | *** | 69340 | 71390 | 110358 | 18227 | 19892 | 27831 | 3515 | 3835 | 4556 | 1025 | 1067 | 1172 | 493 | 505 | 530 |
| 0.35 | *** | 71425 | 72452 | 109123 | 18680 | 19663 | 27523 | 3625 | 3910 | 4517 | 1075 | 1120 | 1175 | 520 | 530 | 542 |
| | *** | 71765 | 74500 | 119210 | 19022 | 21152 | 29979 | 3748 | 4142 | 4869 | 1093 | 1145 | 1237 | 523 | 538 | 553 |
| 0.4 | *** | 71135 | 72478 | 117275 | 18785 | 20027 | 29492 | 3740 | 4078 | 4802 | 1112 | 1165 | 1235 | 535 | 545 | 565 |
| | *** | 71582 | 75148 | 125458 | 19225 | 21835 | 31475 | 3887 | 4352 | 5077 | 1138 | 1198 | 1276 | 542 | 553 | 565 |
| 0.45 | *** | 68593 | 70325 | 122657 | 18385 | 19907 | 30770 | 3778 | 4153 | 4970 | 1130 | 1187 | 1262 | 538 | 553 | 568 |
| | *** | 69170 | 73735 | 129102 | 18932 | 22018 | 32322 | 3940 | 4465 | 5181 | 1157 | 1220 | 1289 | 545 | 560 | 565 |
| 0.5 | *** | 64213 | 66430 | 125222 | 17593 | 19393 | 31340 | 3740 | 4150 | 5030 | 1123 | 1183 | 1262 | 530 | 545 | 565 |
| | *** | 64952 | 70705 | 130144 | 18253 | 21770 | 32517 | 3917 | 4480 | 5181 | 1150 | 1220 | 1276 | 538 | 553 | 553 |
| 0.55 | *** | 58445 | 61258 | 124955 | 16517 | 18565 | 31202 | 3643 | 4063 | 4975 | 1093 | 1153 | 1235 | 512 | 527 | 545 |
| | *** | 59387 | 66493 | 128582 | 17285 | 21152 | 32061 | 3823 | 4408 | 5077 | 1123 | 1190 | 1237 | 520 | 535 | 530 |
| 0.6 | *** | 51755 | 55295 | 121855 | 15250 | 17495 | 30358 | 3482 | 3905 | 4805 | 1045 | 1100 | 1180 | 482 | 497 | 515 |
| | *** | 52952 | 61487 | 124416 | 16108 | 20210 | 30955 | 3665 | 4250 | 4869 | 1070 | 1138 | 1172 | 490 | 505 | 495 |
| 0.65 | *** | 44642 | 49000 | 115933 | 13865 | 16232 | 28805 | 3265 | 3677 | 4525 | 970 | 1025 | 1093 | 445 | 455 | 470 |
| | *** | 46153 | 56000 | 117648 | 14785 | 18977 | 29197 | 3445 | 4003 | 4556 | 995 | 1055 | 1081 | 448 | 463 | 449 |
| 0.7 | *** | 37610 | 42730 | 107203 | 12418 | 14795 | 26555 | 2995 | 3373 | 4130 | 875 | 925 | 985 | 392 | 403 | 415 |
| | *** | 39445 | 50230 | 108275 | 13355 | 17470 | 26789 | 3160 | 3670 | 4140 | 898 | 950 | 964 | 400 | 407 | 391 |
| 0.75 | *** | 31075 | 36677 | 95695 | 10918 | 13198 | 23608 | 2665 | 2998 | 3625 | 760 | 797 | 842 | 332 | 340 | 347 |
| | *** | 33152 | 44252 | 96300 | 11825 | 15685 | 23730 | 2810 | 3250 | 3619 | 778 | 820 | 821 | 335 | 343 | 322 |
| 0.8 | *** | 25220 | 30850 | 81425 | 9350 | 11413 | 19970 | 2270 | 2537 | 3010 | 617 | 643 | 677 | 257 | 260 | 265 |
| | *** | 27362 | 38012 | 81721 | 10180 | 13585 | 20021 | 2390 | 2732 | 2994 | 632 | 658 | 651 | 257 | 265 | 241 |
| 0.85 | *** | 19940 | 25078 | 64430 | 7663 | 9377 | 15655 | 1798 | 1985 | 2290 | 448 | 463 | 482 | . | . | . |
| | *** | 21928 | 31330 | 64538 | 8360 | 11110 | 15660 | 1885 | 2117 | 2265 | 455 | 475 | 456 | . | . | . |
| 0.9 | *** | 14867 | 18985 | 44740 | 5740 | 6958 | 10667 | 1220 | 1318 | 1457 | . | . | . | . | . | . |
| | *** | 16480 | 23770 | 44753 | 6245 | 8110 | 10648 | 1265 | 1382 | 1432 | . | . | . | . | . | . |
| 0.95 | *** | 9212 | 11653 | 22385 | 3283 | 3827 | 5012 | . | . | . | . | . | . | . | . | . |
| | *** | 10190 | 14260 | 22364 | 3515 | 4270 | 4986 | . | . | . | . | . | . | . | . | . |
| 0.98 | *** | 4453 | 5353 | 7705 | . | . | . | . | . | . | . | . | . | . | . | . |
| | *** | 4832 | 6148 | 7680 | . | . | . | . | . | . | . | . | . | . | . | . |

## TABLE 4: ALPHA= 0.01  POWER= 0.9     EXPECTED ACCRUAL THRU MINIMUM FOLLOW-UP= 3250

| | DEL=.01 | | | DEL=.02 | | | DEL=.05 | | | DEL=.10 | | | DEL=.15 | | |
|---|---|---|---|---|---|---|---|---|---|---|---|---|---|---|---|
| FACT= | 1.0 .75 | .50 .25 | .00 BIN | 1.0 .75 | .50 .25 | .00 BIN | 1.0 .75 | .50 .25 | .00 BIN | 1.0 75 | .50 .25 | .00 BIN | 1.0 .75 | .50 .25 | .00 BIN |

PCONT=***                    REQUIRED NUMBER OF PATIENTS

| PCONT | 1.0/.75 | .50/.25 | .00/BIN | 1.0/.75 | .50/.25 | .00/BIN | 1.0/.75 | .50/.25 | .00/BIN | 1.0/75 | .50/.25 | .00/BIN | 1.0/.75 | .50/.25 | .00/BIN |
|---|---|---|---|---|---|---|---|---|---|---|---|---|---|---|---|
| 0.01 | 1988 | 1993 | 2009 | 729 | 734 | 737 | 241 | 241 | 241 | 119 | 119 | 119 | 87 | 87 | 87 |
| | 1993 | 2001 | 7680 | 734 | 734 | 2539 | 241 | 241 | 691 | 119 | 119 | 281 | 87 | 87 | 167 |
| 0.02 | 4393 | 4409 | 4479 | 1411 | 1419 | 1433 | 384 | 384 | 384 | 168 | 168 | 168 | 111 | 111 | 111 |
| | 4398 | 4434 | 12679 | 1416 | 1424 | 3775 | 384 | 384 | 883 | 168 | 168 | 326 | 111 | 111 | 186 |
| 0.05 | 13290 | 13352 | 13994 | 3756 | 3800 | 3922 | 815 | 823 | 831 | 290 | 295 | 295 | 173 | 173 | 173 |
| | 13311 | 13461 | 27050 | 3773 | 3846 | 7329 | 818 | 826 | 1432 | 295 | 295 | 456 | 173 | 173 | 241 |
| 0.1 | 29309 | 29459 | 32571 | 7835 | 7973 | 8615 | 1525 | 1557 | 1603 | 485 | 490 | 493 | 257 | 263 | 263 |
| | 29358 | 29759 | 48918 | 7884 | 8155 | 12731 | 1541 | 1579 | 2265 | 485 | 493 | 651 | 257 | 263 | 322 |
| 0.15 | 43756 | 44027 | 51453 | 11483 | 11743 | 13322 | 2167 | 2237 | 2351 | 656 | 664 | 677 | 336 | 339 | 344 |
| | 43845 | 44563 | 68183 | 11573 | 12125 | 17482 | 2196 | 2286 | 2994 | 661 | 672 | 821 | 336 | 339 | 391 |
| 0.2 | 55386 | 55805 | 69130 | 14427 | 14842 | 17702 | 2703 | 2817 | 3033 | 802 | 818 | 839 | 401 | 404 | 409 |
| | 55524 | 56645 | 84845 | 14571 | 15464 | 21583 | 2752 | 2906 | 3619 | 810 | 831 | 964 | 401 | 409 | 449 |
| 0.25 | 63841 | 64450 | 84868 | 16610 | 17198 | 21586 | 3126 | 3296 | 3629 | 921 | 945 | 981 | 452 | 458 | 466 |
| | 64044 | 65656 | 98903 | 16813 | 18100 | 25032 | 3199 | 3431 | 4140 | 932 | 961 | 1081 | 458 | 461 | 495 |
| 0.3 | 69146 | 69983 | 98277 | 18032 | 18836 | 24876 | 3442 | 3670 | 4125 | 1013 | 1046 | 1091 | 490 | 501 | 509 |
| | 69426 | 71644 | 110358 | 18311 | 20047 | 27831 | 3540 | 3849 | 4556 | 1029 | 1067 | 1172 | 498 | 506 | 530 |
| 0.35 | 71511 | 72624 | 109124 | 18766 | 19811 | 27522 | 3659 | 3938 | 4520 | 1078 | 1124 | 1176 | 517 | 531 | 542 |
| | 71879 | 74837 | 119210 | 19132 | 21347 | 29979 | 3781 | 4166 | 4869 | 1099 | 1148 | 1237 | 526 | 539 | 553 |
| 0.4 | 71246 | 72700 | 117279 | 18896 | 20209 | 29491 | 3781 | 4114 | 4799 | 1119 | 1167 | 1232 | 534 | 547 | 563 |
| | 71733 | 75584 | 125458 | 19364 | 22070 | 31475 | 3922 | 4377 | 5077 | 1143 | 1200 | 1276 | 542 | 555 | 565 |
| 0.45 | 68735 | 70612 | 122658 | 18528 | 20123 | 30767 | 3824 | 4195 | 4970 | 1135 | 1192 | 1262 | 539 | 555 | 571 |
| | 69361 | 74284 | 129102 | 19107 | 22284 | 32322 | 3984 | 4496 | 5181 | 1164 | 1224 | 1289 | 547 | 563 | 565 |
| 0.5 | 64396 | 66793 | 125220 | 17764 | 19644 | 31341 | 3792 | 4190 | 5032 | 1132 | 1189 | 1265 | 534 | 547 | 563 |
| | 65198 | 71376 | 130144 | 18457 | 22065 | 32517 | 3962 | 4512 | 5181 | 1156 | 1221 | 1276 | 539 | 555 | 553 |
| 0.55 | 58681 | 61720 | 124957 | 16716 | 18844 | 31203 | 3691 | 4109 | 4975 | 1102 | 1159 | 1238 | 514 | 531 | 547 |
| | 59700 | 67286 | 128582 | 17520 | 21469 | 32061 | 3873 | 4442 | 5077 | 1127 | 1197 | 1237 | 523 | 539 | 530 |
| 0.6 | 52054 | 55865 | 121856 | 15476 | 17791 | 30358 | 3532 | 3951 | 4804 | 1051 | 1108 | 1181 | 485 | 498 | 514 |
| | 53351 | 62386 | 124416 | 16366 | 20537 | 30955 | 3716 | 4284 | 4869 | 1078 | 1140 | 1172 | 493 | 506 | 495 |
| 0.65 | 45023 | 49671 | 115933 | 14111 | 16537 | 28806 | 3318 | 3719 | 4523 | 978 | 1029 | 1094 | 444 | 458 | 469 |
| | 46643 | 56978 | 117648 | 15058 | 19302 | 29197 | 3491 | 4036 | 4556 | 1002 | 1059 | 1081 | 452 | 466 | 449 |
| 0.7 | 38079 | 43474 | 107204 | 12669 | 15094 | 26555 | 3041 | 3415 | 4130 | 883 | 929 | 981 | 396 | 404 | 417 |
| | 40026 | 51239 | 108275 | 13628 | 17783 | 26789 | 3204 | 3699 | 4140 | 904 | 953 | 964 | 401 | 409 | 391 |
| 0.75 | 31617 | 37454 | 95694 | 11161 | 13482 | 23609 | 2708 | 3033 | 3626 | 766 | 799 | 842 | 331 | 339 | 347 |
| | 33794 | 45237 | 96300 | 12087 | 15971 | 23730 | 2849 | 3272 | 3619 | 783 | 818 | 821 | 336 | 344 | 322 |
| 0.8 | 25786 | 31601 | 81426 | 9574 | 11662 | 19974 | 2305 | 2565 | 3012 | 623 | 647 | 677 | 257 | 263 | 266 |
| | 28004 | 38929 | 81721 | 10419 | 13834 | 20021 | 2419 | 2752 | 2994 | 631 | 661 | 651 | 257 | 263 | 241 |
| 0.85 | 20472 | 25746 | 64434 | 7854 | 9582 | 15654 | 1823 | 2004 | 2289 | 452 | 466 | 482 | . | . | . |
| | 22517 | 32113 | 64538 | 8558 | 11299 | 15660 | 1907 | 2126 | 2265 | 458 | 474 | 456 | . | . | . |
| 0.9 | 15302 | 19506 | 44742 | 5880 | 7099 | 10666 | 1238 | 1327 | 1457 | . | . | . | . | . | . |
| | 16954 | 24353 | 44753 | 6384 | 8233 | 10648 | 1278 | 1387 | 1432 | . | . | . | . | . | . |
| 0.95 | 9476 | 11954 | 22387 | 3350 | 3886 | 5011 | . | . | . | . | . | . | . | . | . |
| | 10476 | 14557 | 22364 | 3581 | 4312 | 4986 | . | . | . | . | . | . | . | . | . |
| 0.98 | 4561 | 5449 | 7705 | . | . | . | . | . | . | . | . | . | . | . | . |
| | 4937 | 6229 | 7680 | . | . | . | . | . | . | . | . | . | . | . | . |

TABLE 4: ALPHA= 0.01  POWER= 0.9    EXPECTED ACCRUAL THRU MINIMUM FOLLOW-UP= 3500

| | | DEL=.01 | | | DEL=.02 | | | DEL=.05 | | | DEL=.10 | | | DEL=.15 | | |
|---|---|---|---|---|---|---|---|---|---|---|---|---|---|---|---|---|---|
| FACT= | | 1.0 .75 | .50 .25 | .00 BIN | 1.0 .75 | .50 .25 | .00 BIN | 1.0 .75 | .50 .25 | .00 BIN | 1.0 75 | .50 .25 | .00 BIN | 1.0 .75 | .50 .25 | .00 BIN |
| PCONT=*** | | | | | | | REQUIRED NUMBER OF PATIENTS | | | | | | | | | |
| 0.01 | *** | 1989 | 1992 | 2006 | 732 | 732 | 738 | 242 | 242 | 242 | 120 | 120 | 120 | 85 | 85 | 85 |
| | *** | 1992 | 2001 | 7680 | 732 | 732 | 2539 | 242 | 242 | 691 | 120 | 120 | 281 | 85 | 85 | 167 |
| 0.02 | *** | 4395 | 4413 | 4483 | 1411 | 1420 | 1432 | 382 | 382 | 388 | 169 | 169 | 169 | 111 | 111 | 111 |
| | *** | 4398 | 4433 | 12679 | 1415 | 1423 | 3775 | 382 | 382 | 883 | 169 | 169 | 326 | 111 | 111 | 186 |
| 0.05 | *** | 13294 | 13358 | 13994 | 3760 | 3803 | 3923 | 816 | 825 | 828 | 291 | 295 | 295 | 172 | 172 | 172 |
| | *** | 13315 | 13478 | 27050 | 3777 | 3847 | 7329 | 820 | 825 | 1432 | 295 | 295 | 456 | 172 | 172 | 241 |
| 0.1 | *** | 29318 | 29481 | 32570 | 7846 | 7991 | 8616 | 1528 | 1560 | 1604 | 484 | 487 | 496 | 260 | 260 | 260 |
| | *** | 29376 | 29805 | 48918 | 7898 | 8175 | 12731 | 1543 | 1581 | 2265 | 487 | 493 | 651 | 260 | 260 | 322 |
| 0.15 | *** | 43779 | 44068 | 51453 | 11503 | 11780 | 13323 | 2173 | 2243 | 2351 | 659 | 668 | 676 | 335 | 338 | 344 |
| | *** | 43875 | 44645 | 68183 | 11600 | 12168 | 17482 | 2202 | 2290 | 2994 | 662 | 671 | 821 | 338 | 338 | 391 |
| 0.2 | *** | 55416 | 55871 | 69128 | 14461 | 14898 | 17704 | 2715 | 2829 | 3033 | 802 | 820 | 843 | 400 | 405 | 408 |
| | *** | 55568 | 56773 | 84845 | 14615 | 15543 | 21583 | 2768 | 2916 | 3619 | 811 | 828 | 964 | 400 | 408 | 449 |
| 0.25 | *** | 63890 | 64543 | 84869 | 16654 | 17284 | 21583 | 3147 | 3313 | 3628 | 925 | 948 | 977 | 452 | 458 | 466 |
| | *** | 64105 | 65841 | 98903 | 16873 | 18211 | 25032 | 3217 | 3441 | 4140 | 933 | 965 | 1081 | 458 | 461 | 495 |
| 0.3 | *** | 69210 | 70108 | 98277 | 18098 | 18946 | 24879 | 3468 | 3695 | 4127 | 1018 | 1053 | 1091 | 493 | 501 | 510 |
| | *** | 69513 | 71896 | 110358 | 18395 | 20192 | 27831 | 3567 | 3865 | 4556 | 1035 | 1070 | 1172 | 496 | 505 | 530 |
| 0.35 | *** | 71595 | 72794 | 109124 | 18850 | 19953 | 27525 | 3690 | 3966 | 4518 | 1082 | 1126 | 1175 | 522 | 531 | 545 |
| | *** | 71992 | 75174 | 119210 | 19244 | 21528 | 29979 | 3809 | 4185 | 4869 | 1105 | 1149 | 1237 | 528 | 536 | 553 |
| 0.4 | *** | 71359 | 72925 | 117279 | 19008 | 20385 | 29493 | 3818 | 4145 | 4801 | 1126 | 1175 | 1236 | 536 | 548 | 563 |
| | *** | 71878 | 76014 | 125458 | 19501 | 22289 | 31475 | 3961 | 4404 | 5077 | 1149 | 1201 | 1276 | 545 | 557 | 565 |
| 0.45 | *** | 68883 | 70898 | 122655 | 18666 | 20332 | 30768 | 3865 | 4229 | 4973 | 1143 | 1196 | 1263 | 540 | 554 | 571 |
| | *** | 69556 | 74824 | 129102 | 19273 | 22537 | 32322 | 4022 | 4521 | 5181 | 1170 | 1228 | 1289 | 548 | 563 | 565 |
| 0.5 | *** | 64581 | 67162 | 125224 | 17931 | 19883 | 31340 | 3835 | 4229 | 5028 | 1140 | 1193 | 1263 | 536 | 548 | 563 |
| | *** | 65444 | 72033 | 130144 | 18658 | 22345 | 32517 | 4005 | 4544 | 5181 | 1166 | 1228 | 1276 | 540 | 557 | 553 |
| 0.55 | *** | 58916 | 62180 | 124956 | 16911 | 19107 | 31205 | 3739 | 4150 | 4973 | 1108 | 1166 | 1236 | 519 | 531 | 545 |
| | *** | 60013 | 68055 | 128582 | 17748 | 21764 | 32061 | 3917 | 4474 | 5077 | 1135 | 1196 | 1237 | 522 | 536 | 530 |
| 0.6 | *** | 52354 | 56423 | 121855 | 15695 | 18071 | 30356 | 3581 | 3993 | 4806 | 1056 | 1108 | 1178 | 487 | 501 | 513 |
| | *** | 53745 | 63256 | 124416 | 16613 | 20840 | 30955 | 3760 | 4311 | 4869 | 1082 | 1143 | 1172 | 493 | 505 | 495 |
| 0.65 | *** | 45401 | 50324 | 115935 | 14347 | 16820 | 28808 | 3363 | 3756 | 4521 | 986 | 1035 | 1096 | 449 | 458 | 470 |
| | *** | 47130 | 57910 | 117648 | 15315 | 19606 | 29197 | 3532 | 4063 | 4556 | 1009 | 1061 | 1081 | 452 | 466 | 449 |
| 0.7 | *** | 38541 | 44199 | 107202 | 12909 | 15376 | 26553 | 3083 | 3450 | 4127 | 890 | 930 | 983 | 396 | 405 | 414 |
| | *** | 40597 | 52196 | 108275 | 13889 | 18075 | 26789 | 3243 | 3721 | 4140 | 907 | 956 | 964 | 400 | 408 | 391 |
| 0.75 | *** | 32145 | 38200 | 95693 | 11395 | 13743 | 23610 | 2745 | 3060 | 3625 | 767 | 802 | 843 | 330 | 338 | 347 |
| | *** | 34411 | 46171 | 96300 | 12335 | 16234 | 23730 | 2885 | 3293 | 3619 | 785 | 820 | 821 | 335 | 344 | 322 |
| 0.8 | *** | 26331 | 32316 | 81425 | 9788 | 11894 | 19973 | 2333 | 2587 | 3013 | 624 | 650 | 676 | 256 | 260 | 265 |
| | *** | 28624 | 39789 | 81721 | 10637 | 14058 | 20021 | 2447 | 2768 | 2994 | 636 | 662 | 651 | 260 | 265 | 241 |
| 0.85 | *** | 20980 | 26378 | 64432 | 8030 | 9768 | 15656 | 1843 | 2018 | 2286 | 452 | 466 | 484 | . | . | . |
| | *** | 23076 | 32845 | 64538 | 8744 | 11477 | 15660 | 1922 | 2138 | 2265 | 461 | 475 | 456 | . | . | . |
| 0.9 | *** | 15712 | 19996 | 44741 | 6008 | 7225 | 10663 | 1248 | 1336 | 1458 | . | . | . | . | . | . |
| | *** | 17401 | 24896 | 44753 | 6516 | 8341 | 10648 | 1289 | 1394 | 1432 | . | . | . | . | . | . |
| 0.95 | *** | 9727 | 12230 | 22385 | 3410 | 3935 | 5011 | . | . | . | . | . | . | . | . | . |
| | *** | 10739 | 14834 | 22364 | 3637 | 4351 | 4986 | . | . | . | . | . | . | . | . | . |
| 0.98 | *** | 4658 | 5541 | 7706 | . | . | . | . | . | . | . | . | . | . | . | . |
| | *** | 5034 | 6303 | 7680 | . | . | . | . | . | . | . | . | . | . | . | . |

TABLE 4: ALPHA= 0.01  POWER= 0.9     EXPECTED ACCRUAL THRU MINIMUM FOLLOW-UP= 3750

| | | DEL=.01 | | | DEL=.02 | | | DEL=.05 | | | DEL=.10 | | | DEL=.15 | | |
|---|---|---|---|---|---|---|---|---|---|---|---|---|---|---|---|---|---|
| FACT= | | 1.0 .75 | .50 .25 | .00 BIN | 1.0 .75 | .50 .25 | .00 BIN | 1.0 .75 | .50 .25 | .00 BIN | 1.0 75 | .50 .25 | .00 BIN | 1.0 .75 | .50 .25 | .00 BIN |
| PCONT=*** | | | | REQUIRED NUMBER OF PATIENTS | | | | | | | | | | | | |
| 0.01 | *** | 1990 | 1994 | 2009 | 734 | 734 | 734 | 241 | 241 | 241 | 119 | 119 | 119 | 87 | 87 | 87 |
| | *** | 1994 | 2000 | 7680 | 734 | 734 | 2539 | 241 | 241 | 691 | 119 | 119 | 281 | 87 | 87 | 167 |
| 0.02 | *** | 4394 | 4413 | 4478 | 1413 | 1418 | 1431 | 381 | 381 | 387 | 166 | 166 | 166 | 109 | 109 | 109 |
| | *** | 4403 | 4437 | 12679 | 1418 | 1422 | 3775 | 381 | 387 | 883 | 166 | 166 | 326 | 109 | 109 | 186 |
| 0.05 | *** | 13300 | 13366 | 13994 | 3762 | 3809 | 3922 | 818 | 822 | 831 | 293 | 293 | 293 | 172 | 172 | 172 |
| | *** | 13325 | 13488 | 27050 | 3781 | 3850 | 7329 | 818 | 828 | 1432 | 293 | 293 | 456 | 172 | 172 | 241 |
| 0.1 | *** | 29331 | 29506 | 32572 | 7859 | 8009 | 8613 | 1534 | 1563 | 1606 | 484 | 490 | 494 | 259 | 259 | 259 |
| | *** | 29388 | 29847 | 48918 | 7915 | 8191 | 12731 | 1550 | 1581 | 2265 | 490 | 494 | 651 | 259 | 259 | 322 |
| 0.15 | *** | 43797 | 44106 | 51453 | 11525 | 11815 | 13325 | 2181 | 2247 | 2350 | 659 | 668 | 678 | 334 | 340 | 340 |
| | *** | 43900 | 44725 | 68183 | 11628 | 12209 | 17482 | 2209 | 2290 | 2994 | 663 | 672 | 821 | 334 | 340 | 391 |
| 0.2 | *** | 55450 | 55934 | 69128 | 14497 | 14956 | 17703 | 2725 | 2838 | 3031 | 803 | 822 | 841 | 400 | 406 | 409 |
| | *** | 55609 | 56900 | 84845 | 14656 | 15612 | 21583 | 2778 | 2922 | 3619 | 813 | 831 | 964 | 400 | 406 | 449 |
| 0.25 | *** | 63934 | 64634 | 84869 | 16703 | 17365 | 21584 | 3162 | 3331 | 3631 | 925 | 950 | 978 | 453 | 462 | 466 |
| | *** | 64169 | 66025 | 98903 | 16934 | 18312 | 25032 | 3237 | 3453 | 4140 | 940 | 963 | 1081 | 456 | 462 | 495 |
| 0.3 | *** | 69275 | 70240 | 98275 | 18162 | 19056 | 24878 | 3494 | 3715 | 4128 | 1019 | 1053 | 1090 | 494 | 503 | 513 |
| | *** | 69597 | 72153 | 110358 | 18481 | 20328 | 27831 | 3588 | 3878 | 4556 | 1038 | 1072 | 1172 | 500 | 509 | 530 |
| 0.35 | *** | 71678 | 72963 | 109122 | 18934 | 20093 | 27522 | 3719 | 3991 | 4516 | 1090 | 1128 | 1178 | 522 | 531 | 541 |
| | *** | 72109 | 75509 | 119210 | 19353 | 21700 | 29979 | 3837 | 4203 | 4869 | 1109 | 1150 | 1237 | 528 | 537 | 553 |
| 0.4 | *** | 71472 | 73150 | 117278 | 19118 | 20556 | 29491 | 3856 | 4175 | 4803 | 1131 | 1178 | 1234 | 537 | 550 | 565 |
| | *** | 72031 | 76441 | 125458 | 19638 | 22493 | 31475 | 3991 | 4422 | 5077 | 1156 | 1203 | 1276 | 547 | 556 | 565 |
| 0.45 | *** | 69025 | 71187 | 122656 | 18800 | 20534 | 30772 | 3903 | 4263 | 4972 | 1150 | 1197 | 1263 | 541 | 556 | 569 |
| | *** | 69747 | 75359 | 129102 | 19441 | 22769 | 32322 | 4062 | 4544 | 5181 | 1175 | 1231 | 1289 | 550 | 565 | 565 |
| 0.5 | *** | 64769 | 67525 | 125225 | 18097 | 20106 | 31338 | 3878 | 4263 | 5031 | 1147 | 1197 | 1263 | 537 | 550 | 565 |
| | *** | 65693 | 72678 | 130144 | 18850 | 22600 | 32517 | 4047 | 4568 | 5181 | 1169 | 1225 | 1276 | 541 | 556 | 553 |
| 0.55 | *** | 59150 | 62631 | 124956 | 17103 | 19356 | 31203 | 3784 | 4188 | 4975 | 1118 | 1169 | 1234 | 518 | 531 | 547 |
| | *** | 60325 | 68800 | 128582 | 17965 | 22038 | 32061 | 3959 | 4497 | 5077 | 1141 | 1197 | 1237 | 522 | 537 | 530 |
| 0.6 | *** | 52653 | 56975 | 121853 | 15906 | 18334 | 30359 | 3625 | 4028 | 4806 | 1066 | 1113 | 1178 | 490 | 500 | 513 |
| | *** | 54138 | 64090 | 124416 | 16850 | 21125 | 30955 | 3800 | 4338 | 4869 | 1090 | 1147 | 1172 | 494 | 509 | 495 |
| 0.65 | *** | 45781 | 50959 | 115934 | 14572 | 17088 | 28806 | 3406 | 3794 | 4525 | 991 | 1038 | 1094 | 447 | 456 | 472 |
| | *** | 47609 | 58803 | 117648 | 15559 | 19887 | 29197 | 3575 | 4084 | 4556 | 1015 | 1066 | 1081 | 453 | 466 | 449 |
| 0.7 | *** | 38997 | 44890 | 107206 | 13137 | 15640 | 26553 | 3125 | 3481 | 4131 | 893 | 934 | 981 | 397 | 406 | 415 |
| | *** | 41150 | 53106 | 108275 | 14131 | 18344 | 26789 | 3278 | 3743 | 4140 | 912 | 959 | 964 | 400 | 409 | 391 |
| 0.75 | *** | 32656 | 38909 | 95693 | 11613 | 13990 | 23609 | 2778 | 3087 | 3625 | 775 | 803 | 841 | 334 | 340 | 344 |
| | *** | 35003 | 47059 | 96300 | 12569 | 16478 | 23730 | 2918 | 3312 | 3619 | 790 | 822 | 821 | 334 | 344 | 322 |
| 0.8 | *** | 26856 | 32997 | 81428 | 9987 | 12109 | 19972 | 2365 | 2609 | 3012 | 631 | 650 | 678 | 259 | 259 | 265 |
| | *** | 29215 | 40600 | 81721 | 10850 | 14266 | 20021 | 2472 | 2781 | 2994 | 640 | 663 | 651 | 259 | 265 | 241 |
| 0.85 | *** | 21462 | 26978 | 64431 | 8200 | 9944 | 15653 | 1863 | 2031 | 2290 | 456 | 466 | 481 | . | . | . |
| | *** | 23613 | 33531 | 64538 | 8918 | 11637 | 15660 | 1943 | 2144 | 2265 | 462 | 475 | 456 | . | . | . |
| 0.9 | *** | 16103 | 20463 | 44740 | 6128 | 7343 | 10666 | 1259 | 1343 | 1456 | . | . | . | . | . | . |
| | *** | 17825 | 25400 | 44753 | 6640 | 8444 | 10648 | 1297 | 1394 | 1432 | . | . | . | . | . | . |
| 0.95 | *** | 9968 | 12490 | 22384 | 3466 | 3981 | 5009 | . | . | . | . | . | . | . | . | . |
| | *** | 10984 | 15087 | 22364 | 3691 | 4384 | 4986 | . | . | . | . | . | . | . | . | . |
| 0.98 | *** | 4747 | 5622 | 7703 | . | . | . | . | . | . | . | . | . | . | . | . |
| | *** | 5122 | 6368 | 7680 | . | . | . | . | . | . | . | . | . | . | . | . |

TABLE 4: ALPHA= 0.01  POWER= 0.9     EXPECTED ACCRUAL THRU MINIMUM FOLLOW-UP= 4000

|  | DEL=.01 | | | DEL=.02 | | | DEL=.05 | | | DEL=.10 | | | DEL=.15 | | |
|---|---|---|---|---|---|---|---|---|---|---|---|---|---|---|---|
| FACT= | 1.0 .75 | .50 .25 | .00 BIN | 1.0 .75 | .50 .25 | .00 BIN | 1.0 .75 | .50 .25 | .00 BIN | 1.0 75 | .50 .25 | .00 BIN | 1.0 .75 | .50 .25 | .00 BIN |
| PCONT=*** | | | | REQUIRED NUMBER OF PATIENTS | | | | | | | | | | | |
| 0.01 *** | 1993 | 1997 | 2007 | 733 | 733 | 737 | 243 | 243 | 243 | 123 | 123 | 123 | 87 | 87 | 87 |
| *** | 1993 | 2003 | 7680 | 733 | 733 | 2539 | 243 | 243 | 691 | 123 | 123 | 281 | 87 | 87 | 167 |
| 0.02 *** | 4397 | 4417 | 4483 | 1413 | 1423 | 1433 | 383 | 383 | 387 | 167 | 167 | 167 | 113 | 113 | 113 |
| *** | 4403 | 4437 | 12679 | 1417 | 1427 | 3775 | 383 | 383 | 883 | 167 | 167 | 326 | 113 | 113 | 186 |
| 0.05 *** | 13303 | 13377 | 13993 | 3767 | 3813 | 3923 | 817 | 823 | 833 | 293 | 293 | 297 | 173 | 173 | 173 |
| *** | 13327 | 13503 | 27050 | 3787 | 3853 | 7329 | 823 | 827 | 1432 | 293 | 293 | 456 | 173 | 173 | 241 |
| 0.1 *** | 29343 | 29527 | 32573 | 7867 | 8027 | 8613 | 1537 | 1563 | 1603 | 487 | 493 | 493 | 257 | 263 | 263 |
| *** | 29407 | 29893 | 48918 | 7927 | 8207 | 12731 | 1547 | 1583 | 2265 | 487 | 493 | 651 | 263 | 263 | 322 |
| 0.15 *** | 43817 | 44153 | 51453 | 11543 | 11847 | 13323 | 2187 | 2253 | 2353 | 657 | 667 | 677 | 337 | 337 | 343 |
| *** | 43927 | 44807 | 68183 | 11653 | 12247 | 17482 | 2217 | 2297 | 2994 | 663 | 673 | 821 | 337 | 343 | 391 |
| 0.2 *** | 55483 | 55997 | 69127 | 14527 | 15007 | 17703 | 2737 | 2847 | 3033 | 807 | 823 | 843 | 403 | 407 | 413 |
| *** | 55653 | 57027 | 84845 | 14697 | 15677 | 21583 | 2787 | 2927 | 3619 | 813 | 833 | 964 | 403 | 407 | 449 |
| 0.25 *** | 63983 | 64727 | 84867 | 16747 | 17443 | 21587 | 3183 | 3343 | 3627 | 927 | 953 | 977 | 453 | 463 | 467 |
| *** | 64233 | 66207 | 98903 | 16997 | 18407 | 25032 | 3253 | 3463 | 4140 | 943 | 963 | 1081 | 457 | 463 | 495 |
| 0.3 *** | 69337 | 70367 | 98277 | 18227 | 19163 | 24877 | 3513 | 3733 | 4127 | 1027 | 1053 | 1093 | 493 | 503 | 513 |
| *** | 69683 | 72403 | 110358 | 18563 | 20457 | 27831 | 3607 | 3893 | 4556 | 1037 | 1073 | 1172 | 497 | 507 | 530 |
| 0.35 *** | 71767 | 73137 | 109123 | 19023 | 20227 | 27523 | 3747 | 4017 | 4517 | 1093 | 1133 | 1177 | 523 | 533 | 543 |
| *** | 72223 | 75837 | 119210 | 19457 | 21863 | 29979 | 3863 | 4217 | 4869 | 1113 | 1153 | 1237 | 527 | 537 | 553 |
| 0.4 *** | 71583 | 73373 | 117277 | 19223 | 20723 | 29493 | 3887 | 4203 | 4803 | 1137 | 1183 | 1233 | 543 | 553 | 563 |
| *** | 72177 | 76863 | 125458 | 19773 | 22683 | 31475 | 4023 | 4443 | 5077 | 1157 | 1207 | 1276 | 547 | 557 | 565 |
| 0.45 *** | 69167 | 71477 | 122657 | 18933 | 20727 | 30767 | 3937 | 4293 | 4973 | 1157 | 1203 | 1263 | 543 | 557 | 567 |
| *** | 69937 | 75883 | 129102 | 19597 | 22993 | 32322 | 4093 | 4563 | 5181 | 1177 | 1233 | 1289 | 553 | 563 | 565 |
| 0.5 *** | 64953 | 67887 | 125223 | 18253 | 20327 | 31337 | 3917 | 4297 | 5033 | 1153 | 1203 | 1263 | 537 | 553 | 563 |
| *** | 65937 | 73303 | 130144 | 19037 | 22843 | 32517 | 4083 | 4593 | 5181 | 1173 | 1227 | 1276 | 543 | 557 | 553 |
| 0.55 *** | 59387 | 63083 | 124957 | 17283 | 19593 | 31203 | 3823 | 4217 | 4973 | 1123 | 1173 | 1237 | 523 | 533 | 547 |
| *** | 60637 | 69527 | 128582 | 18173 | 22297 | 32061 | 3997 | 4523 | 5077 | 1147 | 1203 | 1237 | 527 | 537 | 530 |
| 0.6 *** | 52953 | 57513 | 121857 | 16107 | 18583 | 30357 | 3663 | 4063 | 4807 | 1073 | 1117 | 1177 | 493 | 503 | 513 |
| *** | 54527 | 64893 | 124416 | 17073 | 21387 | 30955 | 3837 | 4363 | 4869 | 1093 | 1147 | 1172 | 497 | 507 | 495 |
| 0.65 *** | 46153 | 51577 | 115933 | 14787 | 17343 | 28807 | 3443 | 3823 | 4523 | 997 | 1043 | 1093 | 447 | 457 | 473 |
| *** | 48077 | 59657 | 117648 | 15797 | 20153 | 29197 | 3613 | 4107 | 4556 | 1017 | 1067 | 1081 | 453 | 463 | 449 |
| 0.7 *** | 39443 | 45563 | 107203 | 13353 | 15887 | 26553 | 3157 | 3507 | 4127 | 897 | 937 | 983 | 397 | 407 | 413 |
| *** | 41687 | 53977 | 108275 | 14367 | 18593 | 26789 | 3313 | 3763 | 4140 | 917 | 957 | 964 | 403 | 407 | 391 |
| 0.75 *** | 33153 | 39593 | 95693 | 11823 | 14217 | 23607 | 2813 | 3113 | 3627 | 777 | 807 | 843 | 333 | 337 | 347 |
| *** | 35583 | 47903 | 96300 | 12787 | 16707 | 23730 | 2947 | 3327 | 3619 | 793 | 823 | 821 | 337 | 343 | 322 |
| 0.8 *** | 27363 | 33647 | 81427 | 10177 | 12313 | 19973 | 2387 | 2627 | 3013 | 633 | 653 | 677 | 257 | 263 | 267 |
| *** | 29783 | 41373 | 81721 | 11047 | 14463 | 20021 | 2497 | 2793 | 2994 | 643 | 663 | 651 | 263 | 263 | 241 |
| 0.85 *** | 21927 | 27547 | 64433 | 8357 | 10107 | 15657 | 1883 | 2047 | 2287 | 457 | 467 | 483 | . | . | . |
| *** | 24123 | 34183 | 64538 | 9077 | 11783 | 15660 | 1957 | 2153 | 2265 | 463 | 473 | 456 | . | . | . |
| 0.9 *** | 16483 | 20903 | 44743 | 6243 | 7453 | 10667 | 1267 | 1347 | 1457 | . | . | . | . | . | . |
| *** | 18227 | 25877 | 44753 | 6753 | 8533 | 10648 | 1307 | 1397 | 1432 | . | . | . | . | . | . |
| 0.95 *** | 10193 | 12733 | 22387 | 3517 | 4027 | 5013 | . | . | . | . | . | . | . | . | . |
| *** | 11223 | 15323 | 22364 | 3743 | 4417 | 4986 | . | . | . | . | . | . | . | . | . |
| 0.98 *** | 4833 | 5703 | 7707 | . | . | . | . | . | . | . | . | . | . | . | . |
| *** | 5203 | 6427 | 7680 | . | . | . | . | . | . | . | . | . | . | . | . |

## TABLE 4: ALPHA= 0.01  POWER= 0.9    EXPECTED ACCRUAL THRU MINIMUM FOLLOW-UP= 4250

| | | DEL=.01 | | | DEL=.02 | | | DEL=.05 | | | DEL=.10 | | | DEL=.15 | |
|---|---|---|---|---|---|---|---|---|---|---|---|---|---|---|---|---|
| **FACT=** | 1.0 .75 | .50 .25 | .00 BIN | 1.0 .75 | .50 .25 | .00 BIN | 1.0 .75 | .50 .25 | .00 BIN | 1.0 75 | .50 .25 | .00 BIN | 1.0 .75 | .50 .25 | .00 BIN | |
| **PCONT=*** | | | | REQUIRED NUMBER OF PATIENTS | | | | | | | | | | | | |
| 0.01 *** | 1990 | 1994 | 2005 | 730 | 736 | 736 | 241 | 241 | 241 | 120 | 120 | 120 | 88 | 88 | 88 |
| *** | 1994 | 2001 | 7680 | 730 | 736 | 2539 | 241 | 241 | 691 | 120 | 120 | 281 | 88 | 88 | 167 |
| 0.02 *** | 4395 | 4417 | 4480 | 1416 | 1420 | 1431 | 386 | 386 | 386 | 167 | 167 | 167 | 109 | 109 | 109 |
| *** | 4406 | 4438 | 12679 | 1416 | 1427 | 3775 | 386 | 386 | 883 | 167 | 167 | 326 | 109 | 109 | 186 |
| 0.05 *** | 13310 | 13384 | 13996 | 3768 | 3818 | 3924 | 815 | 825 | 832 | 294 | 294 | 294 | 173 | 173 | 173 |
| *** | 13338 | 13518 | 27050 | 3790 | 3860 | 7329 | 821 | 825 | 1432 | 294 | 294 | 456 | 173 | 173 | 241 |
| 0.1 *** | 29353 | 29551 | 32573 | 7880 | 8040 | 8613 | 1537 | 1565 | 1601 | 485 | 492 | 496 | 258 | 262 | 262 |
| *** | 29424 | 29934 | 48918 | 7940 | 8227 | 12731 | 1554 | 1586 | 2265 | 485 | 492 | 651 | 258 | 262 | 322 |
| 0.15 *** | 43842 | 44193 | 51453 | 11567 | 11882 | 13320 | 2196 | 2256 | 2351 | 662 | 666 | 677 | 337 | 337 | 343 |
| *** | 43959 | 44887 | 68183 | 11680 | 12286 | 17482 | 2224 | 2298 | 2994 | 666 | 673 | 821 | 337 | 343 | 391 |
| 0.2 *** | 55512 | 56065 | 69129 | 14559 | 15063 | 17704 | 2748 | 2855 | 3031 | 811 | 825 | 843 | 400 | 407 | 411 |
| *** | 55699 | 57155 | 84845 | 14740 | 15739 | 21583 | 2798 | 2936 | 3619 | 815 | 832 | 964 | 400 | 407 | 449 |
| 0.25 *** | 64029 | 64820 | 84869 | 16795 | 17517 | 21587 | 3195 | 3354 | 3630 | 932 | 953 | 981 | 453 | 460 | 464 |
| *** | 64295 | 66392 | 98903 | 17056 | 18501 | 25032 | 3265 | 3471 | 4140 | 942 | 963 | 1081 | 460 | 464 | 495 |
| 0.3 *** | 69406 | 70493 | 98278 | 18289 | 19260 | 24876 | 3535 | 3747 | 4126 | 1027 | 1055 | 1091 | 496 | 503 | 513 |
| *** | 69767 | 72650 | 110358 | 18639 | 20577 | 27831 | 3630 | 3907 | 4556 | 1044 | 1076 | 1172 | 503 | 507 | 530 |
| 0.35 *** | 71853 | 73309 | 109126 | 19107 | 20354 | 27522 | 3768 | 4034 | 4519 | 1098 | 1133 | 1176 | 524 | 534 | 545 |
| *** | 72338 | 76163 | 119210 | 19557 | 22012 | 29979 | 3885 | 4232 | 4869 | 1112 | 1155 | 1237 | 528 | 538 | 553 |
| 0.4 *** | 71694 | 73596 | 117275 | 19330 | 20881 | 29492 | 3913 | 4225 | 4799 | 1140 | 1183 | 1236 | 538 | 549 | 560 |
| *** | 72328 | 77279 | 125458 | 19897 | 22868 | 31475 | 4051 | 4459 | 5077 | 1161 | 1208 | 1276 | 545 | 556 | 565 |
| 0.45 *** | 69314 | 71764 | 122658 | 19064 | 20913 | 30767 | 3970 | 4321 | 4969 | 1161 | 1208 | 1261 | 545 | 556 | 570 |
| *** | 70132 | 76390 | 129102 | 19755 | 23198 | 32322 | 4126 | 4583 | 5181 | 1183 | 1236 | 1289 | 549 | 566 | 565 |
| 0.5 *** | 65138 | 68252 | 125223 | 18410 | 20535 | 31340 | 3949 | 4328 | 5029 | 1155 | 1204 | 1261 | 538 | 549 | 566 |
| *** | 66180 | 73915 | 130144 | 19217 | 23074 | 32517 | 4115 | 4608 | 5181 | 1176 | 1229 | 1276 | 545 | 556 | 553 |
| 0.55 *** | 59620 | 63530 | 124957 | 17460 | 19819 | 31202 | 3860 | 4247 | 4976 | 1129 | 1176 | 1236 | 524 | 534 | 545 |
| *** | 60948 | 70228 | 128582 | 18374 | 22539 | 32061 | 4030 | 4544 | 5077 | 1151 | 1204 | 1237 | 528 | 538 | 530 |
| 0.6 *** | 53249 | 58041 | 121855 | 16302 | 18820 | 30359 | 3701 | 4094 | 4806 | 1076 | 1123 | 1176 | 492 | 503 | 513 |
| *** | 54913 | 65670 | 124416 | 17290 | 21640 | 30955 | 3875 | 4381 | 4869 | 1098 | 1151 | 1172 | 496 | 507 | 495 |
| 0.65 *** | 46519 | 52183 | 115933 | 14988 | 17581 | 28808 | 3482 | 3853 | 4523 | 1002 | 1044 | 1098 | 449 | 460 | 471 |
| *** | 48542 | 60474 | 117648 | 16019 | 20397 | 29197 | 3648 | 4130 | 4556 | 1023 | 1066 | 1081 | 453 | 464 | 449 |
| 0.7 *** | 39883 | 46211 | 107203 | 13561 | 16121 | 26555 | 3195 | 3535 | 4130 | 900 | 938 | 981 | 400 | 407 | 418 |
| *** | 42216 | 54807 | 108275 | 14585 | 18824 | 26789 | 3343 | 3779 | 4140 | 921 | 959 | 964 | 400 | 411 | 391 |
| 0.75 *** | 33635 | 40251 | 95692 | 12024 | 14436 | 23605 | 2840 | 3138 | 3626 | 779 | 811 | 843 | 333 | 343 | 347 |
| *** | 36139 | 48702 | 96300 | 12998 | 16918 | 23730 | 2972 | 3343 | 3619 | 793 | 825 | 821 | 337 | 343 | 322 |
| 0.8 *** | 27851 | 34269 | 81427 | 10356 | 12509 | 19972 | 2415 | 2649 | 3010 | 634 | 651 | 677 | 258 | 262 | 269 |
| *** | 30327 | 42099 | 81721 | 11234 | 14638 | 20021 | 2521 | 2802 | 2994 | 641 | 662 | 651 | 262 | 262 | 241 |
| 0.85 *** | 22373 | 28096 | 64433 | 8507 | 10256 | 15654 | 1898 | 2058 | 2288 | 460 | 471 | 481 | . | . | . |
| *** | 24611 | 34793 | 64538 | 9230 | 11918 | 15660 | 1973 | 2160 | 2265 | 464 | 475 | 456 | . | . | . |
| 0.9 *** | 16837 | 21321 | 44738 | 6350 | 7558 | 10664 | 1278 | 1353 | 1459 | . | . | . | . | . | . |
| *** | 18612 | 26325 | 44753 | 6860 | 8620 | 10648 | 1314 | 1399 | 1432 | . | . | . | . | . | . |
| 0.95 *** | 10405 | 12959 | 22383 | 3567 | 4066 | 5012 | . | . | . | . | . | . | . | . | . |
| *** | 11446 | 15541 | 22364 | 3786 | 4444 | 4986 | . | . | . | . | . | . | . | . | . |
| 0.98 *** | 4912 | 5773 | 7706 | . | . | . | . | . | . | . | . | . | . | . | . |
| *** | 5277 | 6484 | 7680 | . | . | . | . | . | . | . | . | . | . | . | . |

TABLE 4: ALPHA= 0.01  POWER= 0.9    EXPECTED ACCRUAL THRU MINIMUM FOLLOW-UP= 4500

| | DEL=.01 | | | DEL=.02 | | | DEL=.05 | | | DEL=.10 | | | DEL=.15 | | |
|---|---|---|---|---|---|---|---|---|---|---|---|---|---|---|---|
| FACT= | 1.0 .75 | .50 .25 | .00 BIN | 1.0 .75 | .50 .25 | .00 BIN | 1.0 .75 | .50 .25 | .00 BIN | 1.0 75 | .50 .25 | .00 BIN | 1.0 .75 | .50 .25 | .00 BIN |
| PCONT=*** | | | | | | REQUIRED NUMBER OF PATIENTS | | | | | | | | | |
| 0.01 *** | 1995 | 1999 | 2006 | 735 | 735 | 735 | 240 | 240 | 244 | 120 | 120 | 120 | 86 | 86 | 86 |
| *** | 1995 | 1999 | 7680 | 735 | 735 | 2539 | 240 | 240 | 691 | 120 | 120 | 281 | 86 | 86 | 167 |
| 0.02 *** | 4402 | 4418 | 4481 | 1414 | 1421 | 1432 | 386 | 386 | 386 | 165 | 165 | 165 | 109 | 109 | 109 |
| *** | 4406 | 4440 | 12679 | 1421 | 1425 | 3775 | 386 | 386 | 883 | 165 | 165 | 326 | 109 | 109 | 186 |
| 0.05 *** | 13312 | 13395 | 13991 | 3776 | 3821 | 3923 | 818 | 825 | 829 | 296 | 296 | 296 | 172 | 172 | 172 |
| *** | 13339 | 13530 | 27050 | 3795 | 3862 | 7329 | 825 | 829 | 1432 | 296 | 296 | 456 | 172 | 172 | 241 |
| 0.1 *** | 29366 | 29573 | 32572 | 7890 | 8058 | 8614 | 1545 | 1567 | 1605 | 487 | 491 | 491 | 262 | 262 | 262 |
| *** | 29438 | 29973 | 48918 | 7957 | 8238 | 12731 | 1556 | 1583 | 2265 | 487 | 491 | 651 | 262 | 262 | 322 |
| 0.15 *** | 43860 | 44231 | 51454 | 11584 | 11910 | 13323 | 2201 | 2258 | 2348 | 660 | 667 | 678 | 334 | 341 | 341 |
| *** | 43984 | 44970 | 68183 | 11708 | 12315 | 17482 | 2231 | 2303 | 2994 | 667 | 671 | 821 | 341 | 341 | 391 |
| 0.2 *** | 55549 | 56130 | 69128 | 14595 | 15112 | 17704 | 2760 | 2865 | 3034 | 813 | 825 | 840 | 401 | 408 | 408 |
| *** | 55740 | 57277 | 84845 | 14779 | 15798 | 21583 | 2809 | 2940 | 3619 | 818 | 829 | 964 | 401 | 408 | 449 |
| 0.25 *** | 64076 | 64916 | 84866 | 16845 | 17591 | 21585 | 3210 | 3367 | 3630 | 937 | 953 | 982 | 453 | 458 | 469 |
| *** | 64353 | 66570 | 98903 | 17115 | 18588 | 25032 | 3281 | 3480 | 4140 | 941 | 964 | 1081 | 458 | 465 | 495 |
| 0.3 *** | 69465 | 70624 | 98276 | 18352 | 19365 | 24877 | 3551 | 3761 | 4125 | 1031 | 1061 | 1095 | 498 | 503 | 510 |
| *** | 69855 | 72896 | 110358 | 18716 | 20692 | 27831 | 3648 | 3911 | 4556 | 1043 | 1072 | 1172 | 498 | 510 | 530 |
| 0.35 *** | 71936 | 73477 | 109121 | 19189 | 20483 | 27525 | 3795 | 4053 | 4519 | 1099 | 1133 | 1178 | 525 | 532 | 543 |
| *** | 72453 | 76485 | 119210 | 19661 | 22159 | 29979 | 3911 | 4245 | 4869 | 1117 | 1155 | 1237 | 532 | 536 | 553 |
| 0.4 *** | 71805 | 73819 | 117278 | 19436 | 21030 | 29494 | 3941 | 4249 | 4800 | 1144 | 1185 | 1234 | 543 | 555 | 566 |
| *** | 72480 | 77689 | 125458 | 20028 | 23036 | 31475 | 4076 | 4474 | 5077 | 1166 | 1207 | 1276 | 548 | 559 | 565 |
| 0.45 *** | 69461 | 72048 | 122655 | 19189 | 21086 | 30772 | 4001 | 4346 | 4969 | 1166 | 1207 | 1263 | 548 | 559 | 570 |
| *** | 70327 | 76897 | 129102 | 19905 | 23396 | 32322 | 4155 | 4605 | 5181 | 1185 | 1234 | 1289 | 555 | 566 | 565 |
| 0.5 *** | 65321 | 68610 | 125220 | 18559 | 20730 | 31339 | 3986 | 4357 | 5032 | 1162 | 1207 | 1263 | 543 | 555 | 566 |
| *** | 66428 | 74512 | 130144 | 19391 | 23291 | 32517 | 4148 | 4631 | 5181 | 1185 | 1234 | 1276 | 548 | 559 | 553 |
| 0.55 *** | 59858 | 63971 | 124957 | 17632 | 20033 | 31204 | 3896 | 4278 | 4976 | 1133 | 1178 | 1234 | 521 | 532 | 543 |
| *** | 61260 | 70912 | 128582 | 18566 | 22766 | 32061 | 4065 | 4564 | 5077 | 1155 | 1207 | 1237 | 525 | 536 | 530 |
| 0.6 *** | 53546 | 58564 | 121856 | 16489 | 19050 | 30356 | 3738 | 4121 | 4807 | 1083 | 1121 | 1178 | 491 | 503 | 514 |
| *** | 55297 | 66416 | 124416 | 17497 | 21873 | 30955 | 3907 | 4402 | 4869 | 1099 | 1151 | 1172 | 498 | 510 | 495 |
| 0.65 *** | 46886 | 52770 | 115935 | 15191 | 17812 | 28808 | 3513 | 3878 | 4526 | 1005 | 1043 | 1095 | 453 | 458 | 469 |
| *** | 49001 | 61264 | 117648 | 16230 | 20629 | 29197 | 3675 | 4148 | 4556 | 1027 | 1072 | 1081 | 458 | 465 | 449 |
| 0.7 *** | 40312 | 46841 | 107205 | 13762 | 16343 | 26553 | 3225 | 3558 | 4132 | 908 | 941 | 982 | 401 | 408 | 413 |
| *** | 42731 | 55601 | 108275 | 14797 | 19043 | 26789 | 3371 | 3799 | 4140 | 926 | 960 | 964 | 401 | 408 | 391 |
| 0.75 *** | 34102 | 40886 | 95696 | 12214 | 14644 | 23606 | 2865 | 3153 | 3626 | 784 | 813 | 840 | 334 | 341 | 345 |
| *** | 36678 | 49470 | 96300 | 13200 | 17115 | 23730 | 2996 | 3356 | 3619 | 795 | 825 | 821 | 341 | 345 | 322 |
| 0.8 *** | 28320 | 34867 | 81424 | 10526 | 12686 | 19972 | 2433 | 2663 | 3011 | 633 | 656 | 678 | 262 | 262 | 266 |
| *** | 30851 | 42798 | 81721 | 11411 | 14808 | 20021 | 2539 | 2816 | 2994 | 645 | 667 | 651 | 262 | 262 | 241 |
| 0.85 *** | 22800 | 28616 | 64432 | 8655 | 10403 | 15656 | 1916 | 2066 | 2287 | 458 | 469 | 480 | . | . | . |
| *** | 25080 | 35378 | 64538 | 9379 | 12045 | 15660 | 1988 | 2168 | 2265 | 465 | 476 | 456 | . | . | . |
| 0.9 *** | 17182 | 21720 | 44738 | 6454 | 7653 | 10668 | 1286 | 1358 | 1459 | . | . | . | . | . | . |
| *** | 18982 | 26749 | 44753 | 6960 | 8693 | 10648 | 1320 | 1403 | 1432 | . | . | . | . | . | . |
| 0.95 *** | 10605 | 13177 | 22384 | 3608 | 4103 | 5010 | . | . | . | . | . | . | . | . | . |
| *** | 11651 | 15746 | 22364 | 3828 | 4470 | 4986 | . | . | . | . | . | . | . | . | . |
| 0.98 *** | 4987 | 5835 | 7703 | . | . | . | . | . | . | . | . | . | . | . | . |
| *** | 5351 | 6533 | 7680 | . | . | . | . | . | . | . | . | . | . | . | . |

## TABLE 4: ALPHA= 0.01  POWER= 0.9    EXPECTED ACCRUAL THRU MINIMUM FOLLOW-UP= 4750

|  |  | DEL=.01 | | | DEL=.02 | | | DEL=.05 | | | DEL=.10 | | | DEL=.15 | | |
|---|---|---|---|---|---|---|---|---|---|---|---|---|---|---|---|---|
| FACT= | | 1.0 .75 | .50 .25 | .00 BIN | 1.0 .75 | .50 .25 | .00 BIN | 1.0 .75 | .50 .25 | .00 BIN | 1.0 75 | .50 .25 | .00 BIN | 1.0 .75 | .50 .25 | .00 BIN |
| PCONT=*** | | REQUIRED NUMBER OF PATIENTS | | | | | | | | | | | | | | |
| 0.01 | *** | 1991 1998 | 2010 | | 732 732 | 732 | | 241 241 | 241 | | 122 122 | 122 | | 87 87 | 87 | |
|  | *** | 1991 2003 | 7680 | | 732 732 | 2539 | | 241 241 | 691 | | 122 122 | 281 | | 87 87 | 167 | |
| 0.02 | *** | 4402 4421 | 4480 | | 1417 1421 | 1433 | | 383 383 | 383 | | 170 170 | 170 | | 110 110 | 110 | |
|  | *** | 4409 4445 | 12679 | | 1417 1428 | 3775 | | 383 383 | 883 | | 170 170 | 326 | | 110 110 | 186 | |
| 0.05 | *** | 13315 13403 | 13992 | | 3780 3827 | 3922 | | 815 823 | 827 | | 293 293 | 293 | | 170 170 | 170 | |
|  | *** | 13344 13541 | 27050 | | 3796 3863 | 7329 | | 823 827 | 1432 | | 293 293 | 456 | | 170 170 | 241 | |
| 0.1 | *** | 29375 29600 | 32569 | | 7900 8071 | 8613 | | 1547 1571 | 1607 | | 490 490 | 495 | | 257 257 | 265 | |
|  | *** | 29453 30016 | 48918 | | 7964 8249 | 12731 | | 1559 1587 | 2265 | | 490 490 | 651 | | 257 265 | 322 | |
| 0.15 | *** | 43882 44273 | 51450 | | 11605 11942 | 13320 | | 2205 2264 | 2347 | | 661 668 | 680 | | 336 340 | 340 | |
|  | *** | 44012 45045 | 68183 | | 11729 12346 | 17482 | | 2236 2300 | 2994 | | 668 673 | 821 | | 336 340 | 391 | |
| 0.2 | *** | 55578 56196 | 69128 | | 14626 15160 | 17702 | | 2770 2870 | 3032 | | 811 823 | 839 | | 400 407 | 412 | |
|  | *** | 55785 57400 | 84845 | | 14823 15849 | 21583 | | 2818 2941 | 3619 | | 815 835 | 964 | | 407 407 | 449 | |
| 0.25 | *** | 64121 65007 | 84867 | | 16890 17662 | 21585 | | 3222 3376 | 3630 | | 934 953 | 977 | | 455 459 | 467 | |
|  | *** | 64418 66753 | 98903 | | 17167 18671 | 25032 | | 3293 3483 | 4140 | | 946 965 | 1081 | | 459 467 | 495 | |
| 0.3 | *** | 69532 70747 | 98274 | | 18414 19455 | 24874 | | 3570 3780 | 4124 | | 1037 1060 | 1089 | | 495 502 | 514 | |
|  | *** | 69940 73142 | 110358 | | 18794 20801 | 27831 | | 3661 3922 | 4556 | | 1048 1077 | 1172 | | 502 507 | 530 | |
| 0.35 | *** | 72025 73652 | 109123 | | 19269 20607 | 27522 | | 3815 4069 | 4520 | | 1108 1136 | 1179 | | 526 538 | 542 | |
|  | *** | 72564 76804 | 119210 | | 19763 22293 | 29979 | | 3927 4259 | 4869 | | 1120 1155 | 1237 | | 530 538 | 553 | |
| 0.4 | *** | 71918 74044 | 117274 | | 19538 21177 | 29494 | | 3970 4267 | 4801 | | 1148 1191 | 1231 | | 542 554 | 562 | |
|  | *** | 72631 78093 | 125458 | | 20148 23200 | 31475 | | 4100 4492 | 5077 | | 1167 1207 | 1276 | | 550 554 | 565 | |
| 0.45 | *** | 69603 72334 | 122653 | | 19317 21260 | 30772 | | 4034 4366 | 4972 | | 1172 1215 | 1262 | | 550 562 | 566 | |
|  | *** | 70517 77393 | 129102 | | 20053 23580 | 32322 | | 4183 4615 | 5181 | | 1191 1238 | 1289 | | 554 566 | 565 | |
| 0.5 | *** | 65506 68966 | 125225 | | 18707 20927 | 31342 | | 4017 4378 | 5031 | | 1167 1207 | 1262 | | 542 554 | 562 | |
|  | *** | 66674 75094 | 130144 | | 19562 23492 | 32517 | | 4176 4647 | 5181 | | 1184 1231 | 1276 | | 550 554 | 553 | |
| 0.55 | *** | 60091 64402 | 124957 | | 17804 20243 | 31204 | | 3927 4302 | 4972 | | 1136 1179 | 1238 | | 526 530 | 542 | |
|  | *** | 61563 71574 | 128582 | | 18754 22982 | 32061 | | 4093 4580 | 5077 | | 1160 1207 | 1237 | | 530 538 | 530 | |
| 0.6 | *** | 53845 59074 | 121857 | | 16676 19265 | 30356 | | 3768 4148 | 4805 | | 1084 1124 | 1179 | | 495 502 | 514 | |
|  | *** | 55673 67137 | 124416 | | 17697 22091 | 30955 | | 3939 4421 | 4869 | | 1108 1155 | 1172 | | 495 507 | 495 | |
| 0.65 | *** | 47247 53346 | 115932 | | 15382 18030 | 28805 | | 3547 3903 | 4520 | | 1005 1048 | 1096 | | 455 459 | 471 | |
|  | *** | 49451 62027 | 117648 | | 16438 20844 | 29197 | | 3708 4164 | 4556 | | 1029 1072 | 1081 | | 455 467 | 449 | |
| 0.7 | *** | 40735 47449 | 107204 | | 13949 16557 | 26556 | | 3257 3582 | 4129 | | 910 942 | 982 | | 400 407 | 412 | |
|  | *** | 43228 56362 | 108275 | | 15002 19253 | 26789 | | 3400 3815 | 4140 | | 922 965 | 964 | | 400 412 | 391 | |
| 0.75 | *** | 34560 41495 | 95692 | | 12394 14840 | 23611 | | 2894 3174 | 3625 | | 787 811 | 839 | | 336 340 | 348 | |
|  | *** | 37200 50199 | 96300 | | 13387 17298 | 23730 | | 3020 3369 | 3619 | | 799 827 | 821 | | 336 340 | 322 | |
| 0.8 | *** | 28777 35443 | 81423 | | 10695 12857 | 19970 | | 2454 2675 | 3012 | | 637 657 | 673 | | 257 265 | 265 | |
|  | *** | 31353 43459 | 81721 | | 11582 14966 | 20021 | | 2557 2822 | 2994 | | 645 661 | 651 | | 257 265 | 241 | |
| 0.85 | *** | 23212 29114 | 64430 | | 8784 10537 | 15655 | | 1927 2074 | 2288 | | 459 471 | 483 | | . . | . | |
|  | *** | 25527 35937 | 64538 | | 9515 12163 | 15660 | | 1998 2169 | 2265 | | 467 478 | 456 | | . . | . | |
| 0.9 | *** | 17507 22095 | 44741 | | 6547 7739 | 10667 | | 1290 1362 | 1457 | | . . | . | | . . | . | |
|  | *** | 19336 27150 | 44753 | | 7050 8767 | 10648 | | 1326 1409 | 1432 | | . . | . | | . . | . | |
| 0.95 | *** | 10802 13379 | 22388 | | 3654 4136 | 5007 | | . . | . | | . . | . | | . . | . | |
|  | *** | 11855 15940 | 22364 | | 3867 4492 | 4986 | | . . | . | | . . | . | | . . | . | |
| 0.98 | *** | 5055 5898 | 7703 | | . . | . | | . . | . | | . . | . | | . . | . | |
|  | *** | 5418 6575 | 7680 | | . . | . | | . . | . | | . . | . | | . . | . | |

TABLE 4: ALPHA= 0.01  POWER= 0.9    EXPECTED ACCRUAL THRU MINIMUM FOLLOW-UP= 5000

| | | DEL=.01 | | | DEL=.02 | | | DEL=.05 | | | DEL=.10 | | | DEL=.15 | | |
|---|---|---|---|---|---|---|---|---|---|---|---|---|---|---|---|---|
| FACT= | | 1.0 .75 | .50 .25 | .00 BIN | 1.0 .75 | .50 .25 | .00 BIN | 1.0 .75 | .50 .25 | .00 BIN | 1.0 75 | .50 .25 | .00 BIN | 1.0 .75 | .50 .25 | .00 BIN |
| PCONT=*** | | | | | | REQUIRED | NUMBER | OF | PATIENTS | | | | | | |
| 0.01 | *** | 1991 | 1996 | 2008 | 733 | 733 | 733 | 241 | 241 | 241 | 121 | 121 | 121 | 83 | 83 | 83 |
|  | *** | 1996 | 2004 | 7680 | 733 | 733 | 2539 | 241 | 241 | 691 | 121 | 121 | 281 | 83 | 83 | 167 |
| 0.02 | *** | 4404 | 4421 | 4479 | 1416 | 1421 | 1429 | 383 | 383 | 383 | 166 | 166 | 166 | 108 | 108 | 108 |
|  | *** | 4408 | 4446 | 12679 | 1421 | 1429 | 3775 | 383 | 383 | 883 | 166 | 166 | 326 | 108 | 108 | 186 |
| 0.05 | *** | 13321 | 13408 | 13991 | 3783 | 3829 | 3921 | 821 | 821 | 829 | 291 | 296 | 296 | 171 | 171 | 171 |
|  | *** | 13354 | 13554 | 27050 | 3804 | 3866 | 7329 | 821 | 829 | 1432 | 296 | 296 | 456 | 171 | 171 | 241 |
| 0.1 | *** | 29391 | 29621 | 32571 | 7916 | 8083 | 8616 | 1546 | 1571 | 1604 | 491 | 491 | 496 | 258 | 258 | 258 |
|  | *** | 29466 | 30054 | 48918 | 7979 | 8266 | 12731 | 1558 | 1583 | 2265 | 491 | 491 | 651 | 258 | 258 | 322 |
| 0.15 | *** | 43904 | 44316 | 51454 | 11629 | 11971 | 13321 | 2208 | 2266 | 2354 | 658 | 671 | 679 | 333 | 341 | 341 |
|  | *** | 44041 | 45121 | 68183 | 11754 | 12379 | 17482 | 2233 | 2304 | 2994 | 666 | 671 | 821 | 341 | 341 | 391 |
| 0.2 | *** | 55608 | 56258 | 69129 | 14658 | 15208 | 17704 | 2779 | 2879 | 3033 | 816 | 829 | 841 | 404 | 408 | 408 |
|  | *** | 55829 | 57521 | 84845 | 14858 | 15904 | 21583 | 2821 | 2946 | 3619 | 821 | 833 | 964 | 404 | 408 | 449 |
| 0.25 | *** | 64166 | 65104 | 84866 | 16933 | 17733 | 21583 | 3233 | 3383 | 3629 | 941 | 958 | 979 | 458 | 458 | 466 |
|  | *** | 64479 | 66929 | 98903 | 17229 | 18746 | 25032 | 3304 | 3491 | 4140 | 946 | 966 | 1081 | 458 | 466 | 495 |
| 0.3 | *** | 69596 | 70879 | 98279 | 18479 | 19546 | 24879 | 3591 | 3791 | 4129 | 1033 | 1058 | 1091 | 496 | 504 | 508 |
|  | *** | 70021 | 73379 | 110358 | 18871 | 20904 | 27831 | 3679 | 3933 | 4556 | 1046 | 1079 | 1172 | 504 | 508 | 530 |
| 0.35 | *** | 72108 | 73821 | 109121 | 19354 | 20721 | 27521 | 3841 | 4091 | 4516 | 1108 | 1141 | 1179 | 529 | 533 | 541 |
|  | *** | 72679 | 77121 | 119210 | 19858 | 22421 | 29979 | 3946 | 4271 | 4869 | 1121 | 1158 | 1237 | 529 | 541 | 553 |
| 0.4 | *** | 72029 | 74266 | 117279 | 19641 | 21316 | 29491 | 3991 | 4291 | 4804 | 1154 | 1191 | 1233 | 546 | 554 | 566 |
|  | *** | 72779 | 78491 | 125458 | 20271 | 23354 | 31475 | 4121 | 4504 | 5077 | 1171 | 1208 | 1276 | 546 | 558 | 565 |
| 0.45 | *** | 69746 | 72616 | 122658 | 19441 | 21421 | 30771 | 4058 | 4391 | 4971 | 1171 | 1216 | 1266 | 546 | 558 | 571 |
|  | *** | 70708 | 77871 | 129102 | 20196 | 23754 | 32322 | 4208 | 4633 | 5181 | 1191 | 1233 | 1289 | 554 | 566 | 565 |
| 0.5 | *** | 65691 | 69321 | 125221 | 18854 | 21108 | 31341 | 4046 | 4404 | 5029 | 1171 | 1208 | 1266 | 541 | 554 | 566 |
|  | *** | 66916 | 75658 | 130144 | 19721 | 23683 | 32517 | 4204 | 4666 | 5181 | 1191 | 1233 | 1276 | 546 | 558 | 553 |
| 0.55 | *** | 60321 | 64833 | 124954 | 17966 | 20441 | 31204 | 3958 | 4329 | 4971 | 1141 | 1183 | 1233 | 521 | 533 | 546 |
|  | *** | 61871 | 72216 | 128582 | 18933 | 23183 | 32061 | 4121 | 4596 | 5077 | 1158 | 1208 | 1237 | 529 | 541 | 530 |
| 0.6 | *** | 54133 | 59579 | 121854 | 16846 | 19471 | 30358 | 3804 | 4171 | 4804 | 1091 | 1129 | 1179 | 496 | 504 | 516 |
|  | *** | 56054 | 67841 | 124416 | 17883 | 22296 | 30955 | 3966 | 4433 | 4869 | 1108 | 1154 | 1172 | 496 | 508 | 495 |
| 0.65 | *** | 47608 | 53904 | 115933 | 15558 | 18233 | 28808 | 3571 | 3929 | 4521 | 1016 | 1054 | 1096 | 454 | 458 | 471 |
|  | *** | 49891 | 62754 | 117648 | 16633 | 21046 | 29197 | 3733 | 4179 | 4556 | 1029 | 1071 | 1081 | 458 | 466 | 449 |
| 0.7 | *** | 41146 | 48041 | 107204 | 14133 | 16754 | 26554 | 3279 | 3604 | 4129 | 916 | 946 | 983 | 404 | 408 | 416 |
|  | *** | 43721 | 57096 | 108275 | 15191 | 19446 | 26789 | 3429 | 3829 | 4140 | 929 | 966 | 964 | 404 | 408 | 391 |
| 0.75 | *** | 35004 | 42079 | 95696 | 12571 | 15021 | 23608 | 2916 | 3191 | 3629 | 791 | 816 | 841 | 333 | 341 | 346 |
|  | *** | 37708 | 50896 | 96300 | 13571 | 17479 | 23730 | 3041 | 3379 | 3619 | 804 | 829 | 821 | 341 | 341 | 322 |
| 0.8 | *** | 29216 | 35991 | 81429 | 10846 | 13016 | 19971 | 2471 | 2691 | 3008 | 641 | 654 | 679 | 258 | 266 | 266 |
|  | *** | 31846 | 44091 | 81721 | 11741 | 15108 | 20021 | 2571 | 2829 | 2994 | 646 | 666 | 651 | 258 | 266 | 241 |
| 0.85 | *** | 23608 | 29591 | 64433 | 8916 | 10666 | 15654 | 1941 | 2083 | 2291 | 458 | 471 | 483 | . | . | . |
|  | *** | 25958 | 36466 | 64538 | 9646 | 12271 | 15660 | 2008 | 2179 | 2265 | 466 | 479 | 456 | . | . | . |
| 0.9 | *** | 17829 | 22458 | 44741 | 6641 | 7821 | 10666 | 1296 | 1366 | 1458 | . | . | . | . | . | . |
|  | *** | 19671 | 27529 | 44753 | 7141 | 8833 | 10648 | 1329 | 1408 | 1432 | . | . | . | . | . | . |
| 0.95 | *** | 10983 | 13571 | 22383 | 3691 | 4166 | 5008 | . | . | . | . | . | . | . | . | . |
|  | *** | 12046 | 16121 | 22364 | 3904 | 4516 | 4986 | . | . | . | . | . | . | . | . | . |
| 0.98 | *** | 5121 | 5954 | 7704 | . | . | . | . | . | . | . | . | . | . | . | . |
|  | *** | 5483 | 6621 | 7680 | . | . | . | . | . | . | . | . | . | . | . | . |

## TABLE 4: ALPHA= 0.01  POWER= 0.9     EXPECTED ACCRUAL THRU MINIMUM FOLLOW-UP= 5500

| | | DEL=.01 | | | DEL=.02 | | | DEL=.05 | | | DEL=.10 | | | DEL=.15 | | |
|---|---|---|---|---|---|---|---|---|---|---|---|---|---|---|---|---|---|
| | FACT= | 1.0 .75 | .50 .25 | .00 BIN | 1.0 .75 | .50 .25 | .00 BIN | 1.0 .75 | .50 .25 | .00 BIN | 1.0 75 | .50 .25 | .00 BIN | 1.0 .75 | .50 .25 | .00 BIN |
| PCONT=*** | | | | | REQUIRED NUMBER OF PATIENTS | | | | | | | | | | | |
| 0.01 | *** | 1989 1998 | 733 733 | 243 243 | 119 119 | 86 86 | | | | | | | | | | |
| 0.01 | *** | 1989 | 1998 | 2003 | 733 | 733 | 733 | 243 | 243 | 243 | 119 | 119 | 119 | 86 | 86 | 86 |
| | *** | 1998 | 2003 | 7680 | 733 | 733 | 2539 | 243 | 243 | 691 | 119 | 119 | 281 | 86 | 86 | 167 |
| 0.02 | *** | 4404 | 4423 | 4478 | 1420 | 1420 | 1434 | 380 | 380 | 389 | 169 | 169 | 169 | 114 | 114 | 114 |
| | *** | 4418 | 4445 | 12679 | 1420 | 1425 | 3775 | 380 | 380 | 883 | 169 | 169 | 326 | 114 | 114 | 186 |
| 0.05 | *** | 13333 | 13429 | 13993 | 3790 | 3832 | 3923 | 820 | 829 | 829 | 293 | 293 | 293 | 169 | 169 | 169 |
| | *** | 13369 | 13575 | 27050 | 3804 | 3868 | 7329 | 820 | 829 | 1432 | 293 | 293 | 456 | 169 | 169 | 241 |
| 0.1 | *** | 29415 | 29668 | 32569 | 7938 | 8108 | 8617 | 1549 | 1571 | 1604 | 490 | 490 | 490 | 257 | 257 | 265 |
| | *** | 29498 | 30135 | 48918 | 8006 | 8287 | 12731 | 1563 | 1585 | 2265 | 490 | 490 | 651 | 257 | 265 | 322 |
| 0.15 | *** | 43940 | 44403 | 51456 | 11669 | 12027 | 13319 | 2218 | 2273 | 2347 | 664 | 669 | 678 | 339 | 339 | 339 |
| | *** | 44092 | 45274 | 68183 | 11801 | 12434 | 17482 | 2245 | 2305 | 2994 | 669 | 678 | 821 | 339 | 339 | 391 |
| 0.2 | *** | 55678 | 56384 | 69130 | 14722 | 15299 | 17700 | 2795 | 2891 | 3034 | 815 | 829 | 843 | 403 | 408 | 408 |
| | *** | 55911 | 57768 | 84845 | 14936 | 15995 | 21583 | 2836 | 2952 | 3619 | 820 | 834 | 964 | 403 | 408 | 449 |
| 0.25 | *** | 64263 | 65289 | 84869 | 17026 | 17865 | 21583 | 3263 | 3405 | 3625 | 939 | 958 | 980 | 458 | 463 | 463 |
| | *** | 64601 | 67274 | 98903 | 17334 | 18888 | 25032 | 3323 | 3502 | 4140 | 953 | 966 | 1081 | 458 | 463 | 495 |
| 0.3 | *** | 69722 | 71133 | 98275 | 18599 | 19727 | 24878 | 3620 | 3813 | 4129 | 1040 | 1063 | 1090 | 499 | 504 | 513 |
| | *** | 70198 | 73855 | 110358 | 19020 | 21096 | 27831 | 3708 | 3950 | 4556 | 1049 | 1076 | 1172 | 504 | 504 | 530 |
| 0.35 | *** | 72279 | 74163 | 109124 | 19507 | 20945 | 27523 | 3873 | 4115 | 4519 | 1109 | 1145 | 1178 | 526 | 532 | 545 |
| | *** | 72906 | 77738 | 119210 | 20043 | 22664 | 29979 | 3983 | 4285 | 4869 | 1123 | 1159 | 1237 | 532 | 540 | 553 |
| 0.4 | *** | 72252 | 74708 | 117278 | 19837 | 21583 | 29489 | 4038 | 4321 | 4803 | 1159 | 1192 | 1233 | 545 | 554 | 559 |
| | *** | 73077 | 79264 | 125458 | 20497 | 23640 | 31475 | 4162 | 4528 | 5077 | 1178 | 1214 | 1276 | 545 | 559 | 565 |
| 0.45 | *** | 70038 | 73181 | 122654 | 19680 | 21729 | 30768 | 4107 | 4431 | 4973 | 1178 | 1219 | 1260 | 554 | 559 | 568 |
| | *** | 71091 | 78810 | 129102 | 20469 | 24080 | 32322 | 4253 | 4657 | 5181 | 1200 | 1241 | 1289 | 554 | 568 | 565 |
| 0.5 | *** | 66059 | 70019 | 125225 | 19130 | 21454 | 31340 | 4101 | 4445 | 5028 | 1178 | 1214 | 1260 | 545 | 554 | 568 |
| | *** | 67406 | 76756 | 130144 | 20038 | 24039 | 32517 | 4253 | 4693 | 5181 | 1192 | 1241 | 1276 | 545 | 559 | 553 |
| 0.55 | *** | 60793 | 65674 | 124955 | 18269 | 20808 | 31203 | 4010 | 4368 | 4973 | 1145 | 1186 | 1233 | 526 | 532 | 545 |
| | *** | 62484 | 73443 | 128582 | 19273 | 23558 | 32061 | 4175 | 4624 | 5077 | 1164 | 1214 | 1237 | 532 | 540 | 530 |
| 0.6 | *** | 54720 | 60550 | 121856 | 17183 | 19859 | 30355 | 3854 | 4211 | 4803 | 1095 | 1131 | 1178 | 499 | 504 | 513 |
| | *** | 56791 | 69166 | 124416 | 18250 | 22683 | 30955 | 4019 | 4464 | 4869 | 1118 | 1159 | 1172 | 499 | 513 | 495 |
| 0.65 | *** | 48313 | 54976 | 115935 | 15904 | 18621 | 28810 | 3625 | 3969 | 4519 | 1021 | 1054 | 1095 | 458 | 463 | 471 |
| | *** | 50747 | 64139 | 117648 | 16999 | 21426 | 29197 | 3785 | 4203 | 4556 | 1035 | 1076 | 1081 | 458 | 463 | 449 |
| 0.7 | *** | 41955 | 49165 | 107204 | 14474 | 17128 | 26555 | 3331 | 3639 | 4129 | 917 | 944 | 980 | 403 | 408 | 416 |
| | *** | 44664 | 58474 | 108275 | 15555 | 19795 | 26789 | 3469 | 3854 | 4140 | 930 | 966 | 964 | 403 | 408 | 391 |
| 0.75 | *** | 35864 | 43198 | 95695 | 12893 | 15368 | 23604 | 2960 | 3221 | 3625 | 793 | 815 | 843 | 339 | 339 | 348 |
| | *** | 38674 | 52218 | 96300 | 13910 | 17796 | 23730 | 3075 | 3400 | 3619 | 801 | 829 | 821 | 339 | 348 | 322 |
| 0.8 | *** | 30053 | 37038 | 81423 | 11141 | 13314 | 19974 | 2506 | 2713 | 3007 | 642 | 655 | 678 | 257 | 265 | 265 |
| | *** | 32775 | 45283 | 81721 | 12040 | 15376 | 20021 | 2603 | 2842 | 2994 | 650 | 664 | 651 | 265 | 265 | 241 |
| 0.85 | *** | 24369 | 30493 | 64428 | 9153 | 10899 | 15657 | 1962 | 2099 | 2286 | 463 | 471 | 485 | . | . | . |
| | *** | 26780 | 37450 | 64538 | 9882 | 12475 | 15660 | 2030 | 2190 | 2265 | 463 | 477 | 456 | . | . | . |
| 0.9 | *** | 18420 | 23145 | 44738 | 6810 | 7970 | 10665 | 1310 | 1379 | 1453 | . | . | . | . | . | . |
| | *** | 20313 | 28233 | 44753 | 7305 | 8955 | 10648 | 1338 | 1412 | 1432 | . | . | . | . | . | . |
| 0.95 | *** | 11334 | 13933 | 22389 | 3763 | 4225 | 5009 | . | . | . | . | . | . | . | . | . |
| | *** | 12406 | 16449 | 22364 | 3969 | 4555 | 4986 | . | . | . | . | . | . | . | . | . |
| 0.98 | *** | 5243 | 6059 | 7704 | . | . | . | . | . | . | . | . | . | . | . | . |
| | *** | 5600 | 6700 | 7680 | . | . | . | . | . | . | . | . | . | . | . | . |

TABLE 4: ALPHA= 0.01  POWER= 0.9    EXPECTED ACCRUAL THRU MINIMUM FOLLOW-UP= 6000

| | | DEL=.01 | | | DEL=.02 | | | DEL=.05 | | | DEL=.10 | | | DEL=.15 | | |
|---|---|---|---|---|---|---|---|---|---|---|---|---|---|---|---|---|---|
| FACT= | | 1.0 | .50 | .00 | 1.0 | .50 | .00 | 1.0 | .50 | .00 | 1.0 | .50 | .00 | 1.0 | .50 | .00 |
| | | .75 | .25 | BIN | .75 | .25 | BIN | .75 | .25 | BIN | 75 | .25 | BIN | .75 | .25 | BIN |
| PCONT=*** | | | | | REQUIRED NUMBER OF PATIENTS | | | | | | | | | | | |
| 0.01 | *** | 1990 | 1999 | 2005 | 730 | 730 | 739 | 244 | 244 | 244 | 124 | 124 | 124 | 85 | 85 | 85 |
| | *** | 1999 | 1999 | 7680 | 730 | 730 | 2539 | 244 | 244 | 691 | 124 | 124 | 281 | 85 | 85 | 167 |
| 0.02 | *** | 4405 | 4429 | 4480 | 1420 | 1420 | 1429 | 385 | 385 | 385 | 169 | 169 | 169 | 109 | 109 | 109 |
| | *** | 4414 | 4450 | 12679 | 1420 | 1429 | 3775 | 385 | 385 | 883 | 169 | 169 | 326 | 109 | 109 | 186 |
| 0.05 | *** | 13339 | 13444 | 13990 | 3790 | 3835 | 3919 | 820 | 829 | 829 | 295 | 295 | 295 | 169 | 169 | 169 |
| | *** | 13375 | 13594 | 27050 | 3814 | 3874 | 7329 | 820 | 829 | 1432 | 295 | 295 | 456 | 169 | 169 | 241 |
| 0.1 | *** | 29434 | 29710 | 32569 | 7954 | 8134 | 8614 | 1555 | 1579 | 1600 | 490 | 490 | 490 | 259 | 259 | 259 |
| | *** | 29530 | 30205 | 48918 | 8029 | 8305 | 12731 | 1564 | 1585 | 2265 | 490 | 490 | 651 | 259 | 259 | 322 |
| 0.15 | *** | 43984 | 44479 | 51454 | 11704 | 12079 | 13324 | 2230 | 2275 | 2350 | 664 | 670 | 679 | 340 | 340 | 340 |
| | *** | 44149 | 45424 | 68183 | 11845 | 12484 | 17482 | 2254 | 2314 | 2994 | 670 | 670 | 821 | 340 | 340 | 391 |
| 0.2 | *** | 55744 | 56515 | 69130 | 14779 | 15385 | 17704 | 2809 | 2899 | 3034 | 814 | 829 | 844 | 400 | 409 | 409 |
| | *** | 55999 | 58000 | 84845 | 15010 | 16084 | 21583 | 2845 | 2959 | 3619 | 820 | 835 | 964 | 409 | 409 | 449 |
| 0.25 | *** | 64354 | 65470 | 84865 | 17110 | 17989 | 21589 | 3280 | 3415 | 3625 | 940 | 964 | 979 | 460 | 460 | 469 |
| | *** | 64729 | 67615 | 98903 | 17440 | 19015 | 25032 | 3340 | 3514 | 4140 | 949 | 970 | 1081 | 460 | 460 | 495 |
| 0.3 | *** | 69850 | 71389 | 98275 | 18715 | 19894 | 24874 | 3649 | 3835 | 4129 | 1045 | 1069 | 1090 | 499 | 505 | 514 |
| | *** | 70369 | 74320 | 110358 | 19159 | 21274 | 27831 | 3730 | 3964 | 4556 | 1054 | 1075 | 1172 | 505 | 505 | 530 |
| 0.35 | *** | 72454 | 74500 | 109120 | 19660 | 21154 | 27520 | 3910 | 4144 | 4519 | 1120 | 1144 | 1174 | 529 | 535 | 544 |
| | *** | 73135 | 78340 | 119210 | 20224 | 22879 | 29979 | 4015 | 4309 | 4869 | 1129 | 1159 | 1237 | 535 | 535 | 553 |
| 0.4 | *** | 72475 | 75145 | 117274 | 20029 | 21835 | 29494 | 4075 | 4354 | 4804 | 1165 | 1195 | 1234 | 544 | 550 | 565 |
| | *** | 73375 | 80014 | 125458 | 20719 | 23899 | 31475 | 4204 | 4540 | 5077 | 1180 | 1210 | 1276 | 550 | 559 | 565 |
| 0.45 | *** | 70324 | 73735 | 122659 | 19909 | 22015 | 30769 | 4150 | 4465 | 4969 | 1189 | 1219 | 1264 | 550 | 559 | 565 |
| | *** | 71479 | 79705 | 129102 | 20725 | 24370 | 32322 | 4294 | 4684 | 5181 | 1204 | 1240 | 1289 | 559 | 565 | 565 |
| 0.5 | *** | 66430 | 70705 | 125224 | 19390 | 21769 | 31339 | 4150 | 4480 | 5029 | 1180 | 1219 | 1264 | 544 | 550 | 565 |
| | *** | 67885 | 77794 | 130144 | 20329 | 24355 | 32517 | 4300 | 4714 | 5181 | 1204 | 1240 | 1276 | 550 | 559 | 553 |
| 0.55 | *** | 61255 | 66490 | 124954 | 18565 | 21154 | 31204 | 4060 | 4405 | 4975 | 1150 | 1189 | 1234 | 529 | 535 | 544 |
| | *** | 63085 | 74605 | 128582 | 19594 | 23899 | 32061 | 4219 | 4645 | 5077 | 1174 | 1210 | 1237 | 529 | 544 | 530 |
| 0.6 | *** | 55294 | 61489 | 121855 | 17494 | 20209 | 30355 | 3904 | 4249 | 4804 | 1099 | 1135 | 1180 | 499 | 505 | 514 |
| | *** | 57514 | 70420 | 124416 | 18580 | 23029 | 30955 | 4060 | 4489 | 4869 | 1120 | 1159 | 1172 | 499 | 505 | 495 |
| 0.65 | *** | 49000 | 55999 | 115930 | 16234 | 18979 | 28804 | 3679 | 4000 | 4525 | 1024 | 1054 | 1090 | 454 | 460 | 469 |
| | *** | 51580 | 65434 | 117648 | 17344 | 21760 | 29197 | 3820 | 4225 | 4556 | 1039 | 1075 | 1081 | 460 | 469 | 449 |
| 0.7 | *** | 42730 | 50230 | 107200 | 14794 | 17470 | 26554 | 3370 | 3670 | 4129 | 925 | 949 | 985 | 400 | 409 | 415 |
| | *** | 45565 | 59764 | 108275 | 15889 | 20119 | 26789 | 3505 | 3874 | 4140 | 934 | 964 | 964 | 409 | 409 | 391 |
| 0.75 | *** | 36679 | 44254 | 95695 | 13195 | 15685 | 23605 | 2995 | 3250 | 3625 | 799 | 820 | 844 | 340 | 340 | 349 |
| | *** | 39595 | 53434 | 96300 | 14215 | 18079 | 23730 | 3109 | 3415 | 3619 | 805 | 829 | 821 | 340 | 340 | 322 |
| 0.8 | *** | 30850 | 38014 | 81424 | 11410 | 13585 | 19969 | 2539 | 2734 | 3010 | 640 | 655 | 679 | 259 | 265 | 265 |
| | *** | 33649 | 46375 | 81721 | 12310 | 15610 | 20021 | 2629 | 2860 | 2994 | 649 | 664 | 651 | 259 | 265 | 241 |
| 0.85 | *** | 25075 | 31330 | 64429 | 9379 | 11110 | 15655 | 1984 | 2119 | 2290 | 460 | 475 | 484 | . | . | . |
| | *** | 27550 | 38350 | 64538 | 10105 | 12649 | 15660 | 2044 | 2194 | 2265 | 469 | 475 | 456 | . | . | . |
| 0.9 | *** | 18985 | 23770 | 44740 | 6955 | 8110 | 10669 | 1315 | 1384 | 1459 | . | . | . | . | . | . |
| | *** | 20905 | 28870 | 44753 | 7450 | 9055 | 10648 | 1345 | 1414 | 1432 | . | . | . | . | . | . |
| 0.95 | *** | 11650 | 14260 | 22384 | 3829 | 4270 | 5014 | . | . | . | . | . | . | . | . | . |
| | *** | 12730 | 16744 | 22364 | 4024 | 4585 | 4986 | . | . | . | . | . | . | . | . | . |
| 0.98 | *** | 5350 | 6145 | 7705 | . | . | . | . | . | . | . | . | . | . | . | . |
| | *** | 5704 | 6760 | 7680 | . | . | . | . | . | . | . | . | . | . | . | . |

## TABLE 4: ALPHA= 0.01  POWER= 0.9    EXPECTED ACCRUAL THRU MINIMUM FOLLOW-UP= 6500

| | | DEL=.01 | | | DEL=.02 | | | DEL=.05 | | | DEL=.10 | | | DEL=.15 | | |
|---|---|---|---|---|---|---|---|---|---|---|---|---|---|---|---|---|
| FACT= | | 1.0 .75 | .50 .25 | .00 BIN | 1.0 .75 | .50 .25 | .00 BIN | 1.0 .75 | .50 .25 | .00 BIN | 1.0 75 | .50 .25 | .00 BIN | 1.0 .75 | .50 .25 | .00 BIN |
| PCONT=*** | | | | REQUIRED | NUMBER OF | PATIENTS | | | | | | | | | | |
| 0.01 | *** | 1993 | 2003 | 2009 | 736 | 736 | 736 | 238 | 238 | 238 | 118 | 118 | 118 | 86 | 86 | 86 |
| | *** | 1993 | 2003 | 7680 | 736 | 736 | 2539 | 238 | 238 | 691 | 118 | 118 | 281 | 86 | 86 | 167 |
| 0.02 | *** | 4408 | 4431 | 4479 | 1418 | 1424 | 1435 | 384 | 384 | 384 | 167 | 167 | 167 | 108 | 108 | 108 |
| | *** | 4414 | 4447 | 12679 | 1418 | 1424 | 3775 | 384 | 384 | 883 | 167 | 167 | 326 | 108 | 108 | 186 |
| 0.05 | *** | 13352 | 13460 | 13996 | 3797 | 3846 | 3921 | 823 | 823 | 833 | 297 | 297 | 297 | 173 | 173 | 173 |
| | *** | 13384 | 13612 | 27050 | 3813 | 3878 | 7329 | 823 | 823 | 1432 | 297 | 297 | 456 | 173 | 173 | 241 |
| 0.1 | *** | 29456 | 29758 | 32570 | 7973 | 8152 | 8617 | 1554 | 1581 | 1603 | 492 | 492 | 492 | 265 | 265 | 265 |
| | *** | 29563 | 30278 | 48918 | 8048 | 8325 | 12731 | 1565 | 1587 | 2265 | 492 | 492 | 651 | 265 | 265 | 322 |
| 0.15 | *** | 44026 | 44562 | 51452 | 11743 | 12127 | 13319 | 2237 | 2286 | 2351 | 661 | 671 | 677 | 336 | 336 | 346 |
| | *** | 44205 | 45559 | 68183 | 11889 | 12523 | 17482 | 2253 | 2312 | 2994 | 671 | 677 | 821 | 336 | 336 | 391 |
| 0.2 | *** | 55807 | 56642 | 69132 | 14841 | 15464 | 17701 | 2816 | 2903 | 3033 | 817 | 833 | 839 | 401 | 411 | 411 |
| | *** | 56083 | 58228 | 84845 | 15074 | 16157 | 21583 | 2865 | 2962 | 3619 | 823 | 833 | 964 | 401 | 411 | 449 |
| 0.25 | *** | 64452 | 65655 | 84868 | 17197 | 18097 | 21585 | 3293 | 3433 | 3628 | 947 | 963 | 980 | 460 | 460 | 466 |
| | *** | 64848 | 67946 | 98903 | 17544 | 19131 | 25032 | 3358 | 3521 | 4140 | 953 | 969 | 1081 | 460 | 466 | 495 |
| 0.3 | *** | 69983 | 71641 | 98274 | 18838 | 20047 | 24873 | 3667 | 3846 | 4122 | 1045 | 1067 | 1093 | 498 | 508 | 508 |
| | *** | 70536 | 74771 | 110358 | 19293 | 21428 | 27831 | 3748 | 3970 | 4556 | 1061 | 1077 | 1172 | 498 | 508 | 530 |
| 0.35 | *** | 72626 | 74836 | 109123 | 19813 | 21347 | 27522 | 3937 | 4165 | 4522 | 1126 | 1148 | 1175 | 531 | 541 | 541 |
| | *** | 73363 | 78921 | 119210 | 20398 | 23080 | 29979 | 4041 | 4317 | 4869 | 1132 | 1158 | 1237 | 531 | 541 | 553 |
| 0.4 | *** | 72697 | 75583 | 117281 | 20209 | 22072 | 29488 | 4116 | 4376 | 4798 | 1164 | 1197 | 1229 | 547 | 557 | 563 |
| | *** | 73672 | 80735 | 125458 | 20924 | 24136 | 31475 | 4230 | 4561 | 5077 | 1181 | 1213 | 1276 | 547 | 557 | 565 |
| 0.45 | *** | 70611 | 74283 | 122660 | 20122 | 22283 | 30766 | 4197 | 4496 | 4967 | 1191 | 1223 | 1262 | 557 | 563 | 573 |
| | *** | 71862 | 80572 | 129102 | 20967 | 24640 | 32322 | 4327 | 4701 | 5181 | 1207 | 1240 | 1289 | 557 | 563 | 565 |
| 0.5 | *** | 66792 | 71375 | 125217 | 19641 | 22062 | 31341 | 4187 | 4512 | 5032 | 1191 | 1223 | 1262 | 547 | 557 | 563 |
| | *** | 68368 | 78785 | 130144 | 20599 | 24656 | 32517 | 4333 | 4733 | 5181 | 1207 | 1240 | 1276 | 547 | 557 | 553 |
| 0.55 | *** | 61722 | 67286 | 124957 | 18844 | 21471 | 31205 | 4106 | 4441 | 4977 | 1158 | 1197 | 1240 | 531 | 541 | 547 |
| | *** | 63672 | 75703 | 128582 | 19895 | 24207 | 32061 | 4262 | 4668 | 5077 | 1175 | 1213 | 1237 | 531 | 541 | 530 |
| 0.6 | *** | 55862 | 62388 | 121853 | 17788 | 20534 | 30360 | 3953 | 4284 | 4804 | 1110 | 1142 | 1181 | 498 | 508 | 514 |
| | *** | 58218 | 71592 | 124416 | 18893 | 23340 | 30955 | 4100 | 4506 | 4869 | 1126 | 1158 | 1172 | 498 | 508 | 495 |
| 0.65 | *** | 49671 | 56977 | 115932 | 16537 | 19299 | 28806 | 3716 | 4035 | 4522 | 1028 | 1061 | 1093 | 460 | 466 | 466 |
| | *** | 52378 | 66646 | 117648 | 17658 | 22072 | 29197 | 3862 | 4246 | 4556 | 1045 | 1077 | 1081 | 460 | 466 | 449 |
| 0.7 | *** | 43473 | 51241 | 107206 | 15091 | 17782 | 26557 | 3417 | 3699 | 4132 | 931 | 953 | 980 | 401 | 411 | 417 |
| | *** | 46421 | 60958 | 108275 | 16196 | 20404 | 26789 | 3547 | 3888 | 4140 | 937 | 969 | 964 | 411 | 411 | 391 |
| 0.75 | *** | 37451 | 45234 | 95691 | 13482 | 15968 | 23606 | 3033 | 3271 | 3628 | 801 | 817 | 839 | 336 | 346 | 346 |
| | *** | 40467 | 54572 | 96300 | 14506 | 18335 | 23730 | 3141 | 3433 | 3619 | 807 | 833 | 821 | 336 | 346 | 322 |
| 0.8 | *** | 31601 | 38929 | 81423 | 11662 | 13833 | 19976 | 2562 | 2751 | 3011 | 644 | 661 | 677 | 265 | 265 | 265 |
| | *** | 34471 | 47390 | 81721 | 12566 | 15822 | 20021 | 2653 | 2871 | 2994 | 655 | 671 | 651 | 265 | 265 | 241 |
| 0.85 | *** | 25745 | 32115 | 64436 | 9582 | 11298 | 15653 | 2003 | 2123 | 2286 | 466 | 476 | 482 | . | . | . |
| | *** | 28269 | 39183 | 64538 | 10307 | 12810 | 15660 | 2058 | 2198 | 2265 | 466 | 476 | 456 | . | . | . |
| 0.9 | *** | 19505 | 24353 | 44741 | 7096 | 8233 | 10665 | 1327 | 1386 | 1457 | . | . | . | . | . | . |
| | *** | 21455 | 29456 | 44753 | 7583 | 9153 | 10648 | 1353 | 1418 | 1432 | . | . | . | . | . | . |
| 0.95 | *** | 11954 | 14554 | 22387 | 3888 | 4311 | 5010 | . | . | . | . | . | . | . | . | . |
| | *** | 13037 | 17008 | 22364 | 4073 | 4609 | 4986 | . | . | . | . | . | . | . | . | . |
| 0.98 | *** | 5448 | 6228 | 7707 | . | . | . | . | . | . | . | . | . | . | . | . |
| | *** | 5796 | 6819 | 7680 | . | . | . | . | . | . | . | . | . | . | . | . |

## TABLE 4: ALPHA= 0.01  POWER= 0.9    EXPECTED ACCRUAL THRU MINIMUM FOLLOW-UP= 7000

| | | DEL=.01 | | | DEL=.02 | | | DEL=.05 | | | DEL=.10 | | | DEL=.15 | | |
|---|---|---|---|---|---|---|---|---|---|---|---|---|---|---|---|---|
| FACT= | | 1.0 .75 | .50 .25 | .00 BIN | 1.0 .75 | .50 .25 | .00 BIN | 1.0 .75 | .50 .25 | .00 BIN | 1.0 75 | .50 .25 | .00 BIN | 1.0 .75 | .50 .25 | .00 BIN |
| PCONT=*** | | | | | REQUIRED | NUMBER OF | PATIENTS | | | | | | | | | |
| 0.01 | *** | 1989 | 2000 | 2006 | 729 | 729 | 740 | 239 | 239 | 239 | 116 | 116 | 116 | 81 | 81 | 81 |
| | *** | 2000 | 2000 | 7680 | 729 | 729 | 2539 | 239 | 239 | 691 | 116 | 116 | 281 | 81 | 81 | 167 |
| 0.02 | *** | 4415 | 4432 | 4485 | 1422 | 1422 | 1429 | 379 | 379 | 390 | 169 | 169 | 169 | 110 | 110 | 110 |
| | *** | 4421 | 4450 | 12679 | 1422 | 1429 | 3775 | 379 | 379 | 883 | 169 | 169 | 326 | 110 | 110 | 186 |
| 0.05 | *** | 13357 | 13480 | 13994 | 3802 | 3844 | 3925 | 827 | 827 | 827 | 291 | 291 | 291 | 169 | 169 | 169 |
| | *** | 13399 | 13626 | 27050 | 3820 | 3879 | 7329 | 827 | 827 | 1432 | 291 | 291 | 456 | 169 | 169 | 241 |
| 0.1 | *** | 29481 | 29807 | 32572 | 7991 | 8177 | 8615 | 1562 | 1580 | 1604 | 484 | 495 | 495 | 256 | 256 | 256 |
| | *** | 29586 | 30350 | 48918 | 8061 | 8341 | 12731 | 1569 | 1586 | 2265 | 495 | 495 | 651 | 256 | 256 | 322 |
| 0.15 | *** | 44070 | 44647 | 51455 | 11782 | 12167 | 13322 | 2245 | 2286 | 2350 | 670 | 670 | 676 | 337 | 337 | 344 |
| | *** | 44262 | 45697 | 68183 | 11929 | 12559 | 17482 | 2262 | 2315 | 2994 | 670 | 676 | 821 | 337 | 337 | 391 |
| 0.2 | *** | 55871 | 56775 | 69130 | 14897 | 15545 | 17704 | 2829 | 2916 | 3032 | 816 | 827 | 845 | 407 | 407 | 407 |
| | *** | 56169 | 58455 | 84845 | 15149 | 16227 | 21583 | 2864 | 2969 | 3619 | 827 | 834 | 964 | 407 | 407 | 449 |
| 0.25 | *** | 64545 | 65840 | 84869 | 17284 | 18211 | 21582 | 3312 | 3441 | 3627 | 950 | 967 | 974 | 460 | 460 | 466 |
| | *** | 64971 | 68272 | 98903 | 17634 | 19237 | 25032 | 3371 | 3529 | 4140 | 956 | 967 | 1081 | 460 | 466 | 495 |
| 0.3 | *** | 70110 | 71895 | 98274 | 18946 | 20189 | 24879 | 3697 | 3861 | 4124 | 1055 | 1072 | 1090 | 501 | 501 | 512 |
| | *** | 70705 | 75202 | 110358 | 19430 | 21571 | 27831 | 3774 | 3984 | 4556 | 1061 | 1079 | 1172 | 501 | 512 | 530 |
| 0.35 | *** | 72794 | 75174 | 109124 | 19955 | 21530 | 27521 | 3966 | 4187 | 4520 | 1125 | 1149 | 1177 | 530 | 536 | 547 |
| | *** | 73592 | 79479 | 119210 | 20567 | 23262 | 29797 | 4065 | 4334 | 4869 | 1131 | 1160 | 1237 | 536 | 536 | 553 |
| 0.4 | *** | 72927 | 76014 | 117279 | 20381 | 22289 | 29492 | 4141 | 4404 | 4800 | 1177 | 1201 | 1236 | 547 | 554 | 565 |
| | *** | 73966 | 81421 | 125458 | 21127 | 24347 | 31475 | 4264 | 4579 | 5077 | 1184 | 1219 | 1276 | 554 | 554 | 565 |
| 0.45 | *** | 70897 | 74824 | 122651 | 20329 | 22534 | 30770 | 4229 | 4520 | 4975 | 1195 | 1230 | 1265 | 554 | 565 | 571 |
| | *** | 72234 | 81397 | 129102 | 21204 | 24890 | 32322 | 4362 | 4719 | 5181 | 1212 | 1247 | 1289 | 554 | 565 | 565 |
| 0.5 | *** | 67159 | 72035 | 125224 | 19885 | 22341 | 31336 | 4229 | 4544 | 5027 | 1195 | 1230 | 1265 | 547 | 554 | 565 |
| | *** | 68850 | 79724 | 130144 | 20865 | 24914 | 32517 | 4369 | 4754 | 5181 | 1212 | 1247 | 1276 | 554 | 554 | 553 |
| 0.55 | *** | 62182 | 68051 | 124955 | 19104 | 21764 | 31207 | 4152 | 4474 | 4975 | 1166 | 1195 | 1236 | 530 | 536 | 547 |
| | *** | 64254 | 76749 | 128582 | 20171 | 24487 | 32061 | 4292 | 4684 | 5077 | 1177 | 1212 | 1237 | 536 | 536 | 530 |
| 0.6 | *** | 56425 | 63256 | 121857 | 18071 | 20836 | 30356 | 3995 | 4310 | 4806 | 1107 | 1142 | 1177 | 501 | 501 | 512 |
| | *** | 58910 | 72706 | 124416 | 19191 | 23619 | 30955 | 4135 | 4526 | 4869 | 1125 | 1160 | 1172 | 501 | 512 | 495 |
| 0.65 | *** | 50324 | 57912 | 115931 | 16822 | 19605 | 28810 | 3756 | 4065 | 4520 | 1037 | 1061 | 1096 | 460 | 466 | 466 |
| | *** | 53152 | 67782 | 117648 | 17960 | 22352 | 29197 | 3896 | 4264 | 4556 | 1044 | 1079 | 1081 | 460 | 466 | 449 |
| 0.7 | *** | 44199 | 52196 | 107199 | 15376 | 18071 | 26552 | 3452 | 3721 | 4124 | 932 | 956 | 985 | 407 | 407 | 414 |
| | *** | 47244 | 62084 | 108275 | 16490 | 20672 | 26789 | 3575 | 3907 | 4140 | 939 | 967 | 964 | 407 | 414 | 391 |
| 0.75 | *** | 38196 | 46170 | 95695 | 13742 | 16234 | 23612 | 3056 | 3295 | 3627 | 799 | 816 | 845 | 337 | 344 | 344 |
| | *** | 41294 | 55626 | 96300 | 14775 | 18572 | 23730 | 3172 | 3441 | 3619 | 810 | 834 | 821 | 337 | 344 | 322 |
| 0.8 | *** | 32316 | 39789 | 81421 | 11894 | 14057 | 19972 | 2584 | 2770 | 3015 | 652 | 659 | 676 | 256 | 267 | 267 |
| | *** | 35250 | 48329 | 81721 | 12797 | 16017 | 20021 | 2671 | 2875 | 2994 | 652 | 670 | 651 | 267 | 267 | 241 |
| 0.85 | *** | 26377 | 32841 | 64429 | 9770 | 11474 | 15656 | 2017 | 2140 | 2286 | 466 | 477 | 484 | . | . | . |
| | *** | 28950 | 39957 | 64538 | 10494 | 12944 | 15660 | 2076 | 2210 | 2265 | 466 | 477 | 456 | . | . | . |
| 0.9 | *** | 19996 | 24896 | 44741 | 7221 | 8341 | 10662 | 1335 | 1394 | 1457 | . | . | . | . | . | . |
| | *** | 21974 | 30000 | 44753 | 7711 | 9227 | 10648 | 1359 | 1422 | 1432 | . | . | . | . | . | . |
| 0.95 | *** | 12226 | 14834 | 22387 | 3931 | 4351 | 5010 | . | . | . | . | . | . | . | . | . |
| | *** | 13311 | 17242 | 22364 | 4124 | 4631 | 4986 | . | . | . | . | . | . | . | . | . |
| 0.98 | *** | 5541 | 6305 | 7705 | . | . | . | . | . | . | . | . | . | . | . | . |
| | *** | 5874 | 6871 | 7680 | . | . | . | . | . | . | . | . | . | . | . | . |

## TABLE 4: ALPHA= 0.01  POWER= 0.9   EXPECTED ACCRUAL THRU MINIMUM FOLLOW-UP= 7500

| | | DEL=.01 | | | DEL=.02 | | | DEL=.05 | | | DEL=.10 | | | DEL=.15 | | |
|---|---|---|---|---|---|---|---|---|---|---|---|---|---|---|---|---|---|
| FACT= | | 1.0 .75 | .50 .25 | .00 BIN | 1.0 .75 | .50 .25 | .00 BIN | 1.0 .75 | .50 .25 | .00 BIN | 1.0 75 | .50 .25 | .00 BIN | 1.0 .75 | .50 .25 | .00 BIN |
| PCONT=*** | | | | REQUIRED NUMBER OF PATIENTS | | | | | | | | | | | | |
| 0.01 | *** | 1993 | 2000 | 2011 | 736 | 736 | 736 | 237 | 237 | 237 | 118 | 118 | 118 | 87 | 87 | 87 |
| | *** | 2000 | 2000 | 7680 | 736 | 736 | 2539 | 237 | 237 | 691 | 118 | 118 | 281 | 87 | 87 | 167 |
| 0.02 | *** | 4411 | 4437 | 4475 | 1418 | 1418 | 1430 | 380 | 387 | 387 | 162 | 162 | 162 | 106 | 106 | 106 |
| | *** | 4418 | 4456 | 12679 | 1418 | 1430 | 3775 | 380 | 387 | 883 | 162 | 162 | 326 | 106 | 106 | 186 |
| 0.05 | *** | 13362 | 13486 | 13993 | 3811 | 3849 | 3924 | 818 | 830 | 830 | 293 | 293 | 293 | 174 | 174 | 174 |
| | *** | 13411 | 13643 | 27050 | 3830 | 3886 | 7329 | 818 | 830 | 1432 | 293 | 293 | 456 | 174 | 174 | 241 |
| 0.1 | *** | 29506 | 29843 | 32574 | 8011 | 8187 | 8611 | 1561 | 1580 | 1606 | 493 | 493 | 493 | 256 | 256 | 256 |
| | *** | 29618 | 30406 | 48918 | 8086 | 8356 | 12731 | 1568 | 1587 | 2265 | 493 | 493 | 651 | 256 | 256 | 322 |
| 0.15 | *** | 44105 | 44724 | 51455 | 11818 | 12211 | 13325 | 2243 | 2293 | 2349 | 668 | 668 | 680 | 343 | 343 | 343 |
| | *** | 44318 | 45830 | 68183 | 11968 | 12593 | 17482 | 2262 | 2318 | 2994 | 668 | 680 | 821 | 343 | 343 | 391 |
| 0.2 | *** | 55936 | 56900 | 69125 | 14956 | 15612 | 17705 | 2836 | 2918 | 3031 | 818 | 830 | 837 | 406 | 406 | 406 |
| | *** | 56255 | 58662 | 84845 | 15211 | 16299 | 21583 | 2881 | 2975 | 3619 | 830 | 837 | 964 | 406 | 406 | 449 |
| 0.25 | *** | 64636 | 66024 | 84868 | 17368 | 18312 | 21586 | 3331 | 3455 | 3631 | 950 | 961 | 980 | 462 | 462 | 462 |
| | *** | 65105 | 68581 | 98903 | 17731 | 19336 | 25032 | 3387 | 3530 | 4140 | 961 | 968 | 1081 | 462 | 462 | 495 |
| 0.3 | *** | 70243 | 72155 | 98274 | 19055 | 20330 | 24875 | 3718 | 3875 | 4130 | 1055 | 1074 | 1093 | 500 | 511 | 511 |
| | *** | 70880 | 75624 | 110358 | 19550 | 21706 | 27831 | 3793 | 3987 | 4556 | 1062 | 1081 | 1172 | 500 | 511 | 530 |
| 0.35 | *** | 72961 | 75511 | 109118 | 20093 | 21699 | 27518 | 3987 | 4205 | 4512 | 1130 | 1149 | 1175 | 530 | 537 | 537 |
| | *** | 73824 | 80030 | 119210 | 20724 | 23431 | 29979 | 4093 | 4343 | 4869 | 1137 | 1168 | 1237 | 537 | 537 | 553 |
| 0.4 | *** | 73149 | 76437 | 117275 | 20555 | 22493 | 29487 | 4175 | 4418 | 4805 | 1175 | 1205 | 1231 | 549 | 556 | 568 |
| | *** | 74262 | 82093 | 125458 | 21312 | 24549 | 31475 | 4287 | 4587 | 5077 | 1186 | 1212 | 1276 | 556 | 556 | 565 |
| 0.45 | *** | 71187 | 75361 | 122656 | 20536 | 22768 | 30774 | 4261 | 4543 | 4974 | 1193 | 1231 | 1261 | 556 | 568 | 568 |
| | *** | 72612 | 82186 | 129102 | 21418 | 25111 | 32322 | 4393 | 4730 | 5181 | 1212 | 1243 | 1289 | 556 | 568 | 565 |
| 0.5 | *** | 67524 | 72680 | 125225 | 20105 | 22599 | 31336 | 4261 | 4568 | 5030 | 1193 | 1224 | 1261 | 549 | 556 | 568 |
| | *** | 69324 | 80630 | 130144 | 21106 | 25168 | 32517 | 4400 | 4768 | 5181 | 1212 | 1243 | 1276 | 549 | 556 | 553 |
| 0.55 | *** | 62630 | 68799 | 124955 | 19355 | 22036 | 31205 | 4186 | 4493 | 4974 | 1168 | 1193 | 1231 | 530 | 537 | 549 |
| | *** | 64831 | 77743 | 128582 | 20443 | 24743 | 32061 | 4325 | 4711 | 5077 | 1186 | 1212 | 1237 | 537 | 537 | 530 |
| 0.6 | *** | 56975 | 64093 | 121850 | 18331 | 21125 | 30361 | 4025 | 4336 | 4805 | 1111 | 1149 | 1175 | 500 | 511 | 511 |
| | *** | 59574 | 73756 | 124416 | 19468 | 23881 | 30955 | 4168 | 4543 | 4869 | 1130 | 1156 | 1172 | 500 | 511 | 495 |
| 0.65 | *** | 50956 | 58805 | 115936 | 17086 | 19887 | 28805 | 3793 | 4081 | 4524 | 1036 | 1062 | 1093 | 455 | 462 | 474 |
| | *** | 53900 | 68855 | 117648 | 18237 | 22606 | 29197 | 3924 | 4280 | 4556 | 1055 | 1081 | 1081 | 462 | 462 | 449 |
| 0.7 | *** | 44893 | 53105 | 107206 | 15643 | 18343 | 26555 | 3481 | 3743 | 4130 | 931 | 961 | 980 | 406 | 406 | 418 |
| | *** | 48043 | 63143 | 108275 | 16756 | 20911 | 26789 | 3605 | 3912 | 4140 | 943 | 968 | 964 | 406 | 406 | 391 |
| 0.75 | *** | 38911 | 47056 | 95693 | 13993 | 16475 | 23611 | 3087 | 3312 | 3624 | 800 | 818 | 837 | 343 | 343 | 343 |
| | *** | 42080 | 56618 | 96300 | 15024 | 18781 | 23730 | 3193 | 3455 | 3619 | 811 | 830 | 821 | 343 | 343 | 322 |
| 0.8 | *** | 32993 | 40599 | 81425 | 12106 | 14262 | 19974 | 2611 | 2780 | 3012 | 650 | 661 | 680 | 256 | 268 | 268 |
| | *** | 35993 | 49212 | 81721 | 13018 | 16193 | 20021 | 2686 | 2881 | 2994 | 650 | 668 | 651 | 268 | 268 | 241 |
| 0.85 | *** | 26975 | 33530 | 64430 | 9943 | 11637 | 15650 | 2030 | 2143 | 2293 | 462 | 474 | 481 | . | . | . |
| | *** | 29593 | 40674 | 64538 | 10662 | 13074 | 15660 | 2086 | 2206 | 2265 | 474 | 474 | 456 | . | . | . |
| 0.9 | *** | 20461 | 25400 | 44743 | 7343 | 8443 | 10662 | 1343 | 1393 | 1456 | . | . | . | . | . | . |
| | *** | 22456 | 30493 | 44753 | 7824 | 9305 | 10648 | 1362 | 1418 | 1432 | . | . | . | . | . | . |
| 0.95 | *** | 12493 | 15087 | 22381 | 3980 | 4381 | 5011 | . | . | . | . | . | . | . | . | . |
| | *** | 13568 | 17461 | 22364 | 4168 | 4655 | 4986 | . | . | . | . | . | . | . | . | . |
| 0.98 | *** | 5618 | 6368 | 7700 | . | . | . | . | . | . | . | . | . | . | . | . |
| | *** | 5956 | 6912 | 7680 | . | . | . | . | . | . | . | . | . | . | . | . |

TABLE 4: ALPHA= 0.01  POWER= 0.9   EXPECTED ACCRUAL THRU MINIMUM FOLLOW-UP= 8000

| | | DEL=.01 | | | DEL=.02 | | | DEL=.05 | | | DEL=.10 | | | DEL=.15 | |
|---|---|---|---|---|---|---|---|---|---|---|---|---|---|---|---|---|
| FACT= | 1.0 .75 | .50 .25 | .00 BIN | 1.0 .75 | .50 .25 | .00 BIN | 1.0 .75 | .50 .25 | .00 BIN | 1.0 75 | .50 .25 | .00 BIN | 1.0 .75 | .50 .25 | .00 BIN |
| PCONT=*** | | | REQUIRED NUMBER OF PATIENTS | | | | | | | | | | | | |
| 0.01 *** | 1993 | 2005 | 2005 | 733 | 733 | 733 | 245 | 245 | 245 | 125 | 125 | 125 | 85 | 85 | 85 |
| *** | 1993 | 2005 | 7680 | 733 | 733 | 2539 | 245 | 245 | 691 | 125 | 125 | 281 | 85 | 85 | 167 |
| 0.02 *** | 4413 | 4433 | 4485 | 1425 | 1425 | 1433 | 385 | 385 | 385 | 165 | 165 | 165 | 113 | 113 | 113 |
| *** | 4425 | 4453 | 12679 | 1425 | 1425 | 3775 | 385 | 385 | 883 | 165 | 165 | 326 | 113 | 113 | 186 |
| 0.05 *** | 13373 | 13505 | 13993 | 3813 | 3853 | 3925 | 825 | 825 | 833 | 293 | 293 | 293 | 173 | 173 | 173 |
| *** | 13425 | 13653 | 27050 | 3833 | 3885 | 7329 | 825 | 825 | 1432 | 293 | 293 | 456 | 173 | 173 | 241 |
| 0.1 *** | 29525 | 29893 | 32573 | 8025 | 8205 | 8613 | 1565 | 1585 | 1605 | 493 | 493 | 493 | 265 | 265 | 265 |
| *** | 29653 | 30473 | 48918 | 8105 | 8365 | 12731 | 1573 | 1593 | 2265 | 493 | 493 | 651 | 265 | 265 | 322 |
| 0.15 *** | 44153 | 44805 | 51453 | 11845 | 12245 | 13325 | 2253 | 2293 | 2353 | 665 | 673 | 673 | 333 | 345 | 345 |
| *** | 44373 | 45965 | 68183 | 12005 | 12633 | 17482 | 2273 | 2325 | 2994 | 673 | 673 | 821 | 333 | 345 | 391 |
| 0.2 *** | 55993 | 57025 | 69125 | 15005 | 15673 | 17705 | 2845 | 2925 | 3033 | 825 | 833 | 845 | 405 | 405 | 413 |
| *** | 56345 | 58873 | 84845 | 15273 | 16353 | 21583 | 2885 | 2973 | 3619 | 825 | 833 | 964 | 405 | 405 | 449 |
| 0.25 *** | 64725 | 66205 | 84865 | 17445 | 18405 | 21585 | 3345 | 3465 | 3625 | 953 | 965 | 973 | 465 | 465 | 465 |
| *** | 65225 | 68885 | 98903 | 17825 | 19425 | 25032 | 3393 | 3533 | 4140 | 953 | 973 | 1081 | 465 | 465 | 495 |
| 0.3 *** | 70365 | 72405 | 98273 | 19165 | 20453 | 24873 | 3733 | 3893 | 4125 | 1053 | 1073 | 1093 | 505 | 505 | 513 |
| *** | 71045 | 76033 | 110358 | 19665 | 21825 | 27831 | 3805 | 3993 | 4556 | 1065 | 1085 | 1172 | 505 | 505 | 530 |
| 0.35 *** | 73133 | 75833 | 109125 | 20225 | 21865 | 27525 | 4013 | 4213 | 4513 | 1133 | 1153 | 1173 | 533 | 533 | 545 |
| *** | 74045 | 80553 | 119210 | 20865 | 23585 | 29979 | 4105 | 4353 | 4869 | 1145 | 1165 | 1237 | 533 | 545 | 553 |
| 0.4 *** | 73373 | 76865 | 117273 | 20725 | 22685 | 29493 | 4205 | 4445 | 4805 | 1185 | 1205 | 1233 | 553 | 553 | 565 |
| *** | 74553 | 82733 | 125458 | 21493 | 24733 | 31475 | 4313 | 4605 | 5077 | 1193 | 1213 | 1276 | 553 | 553 | 565 |
| 0.45 *** | 71473 | 75885 | 122653 | 20725 | 22993 | 30765 | 4293 | 4565 | 4973 | 1205 | 1233 | 1265 | 553 | 565 | 565 |
| *** | 72993 | 82945 | 129102 | 21633 | 25313 | 32322 | 4413 | 4745 | 5181 | 1213 | 1245 | 1289 | 553 | 565 | 565 |
| 0.5 *** | 67885 | 73305 | 125225 | 20325 | 22845 | 31333 | 4293 | 4593 | 5033 | 1205 | 1225 | 1265 | 553 | 553 | 565 |
| *** | 69785 | 81493 | 130144 | 21333 | 25393 | 32517 | 4433 | 4785 | 5181 | 1213 | 1245 | 1276 | 553 | 565 | 553 |
| 0.55 *** | 63085 | 69525 | 124953 | 19593 | 22293 | 31205 | 4213 | 4525 | 4973 | 1173 | 1205 | 1233 | 533 | 533 | 545 |
| *** | 65393 | 78685 | 128582 | 20685 | 24985 | 32061 | 4353 | 4725 | 5077 | 1185 | 1213 | 1237 | 533 | 545 | 530 |
| 0.6 *** | 57513 | 64893 | 121853 | 18585 | 21385 | 30353 | 4065 | 4365 | 4805 | 1113 | 1145 | 1173 | 505 | 505 | 513 |
| *** | 60233 | 74753 | 124416 | 19733 | 24125 | 30955 | 4193 | 4553 | 4869 | 1133 | 1165 | 1172 | 505 | 513 | 495 |
| 0.65 *** | 51573 | 59653 | 115933 | 17345 | 20153 | 28805 | 3825 | 4105 | 4525 | 1045 | 1065 | 1093 | 453 | 465 | 473 |
| *** | 54625 | 69873 | 117648 | 18493 | 22833 | 29197 | 3953 | 4293 | 4556 | 1053 | 1073 | 1081 | 465 | 465 | 449 |
| 0.7 *** | 45565 | 53973 | 107205 | 15885 | 18593 | 26553 | 3505 | 3765 | 4125 | 933 | 953 | 985 | 405 | 405 | 413 |
| *** | 48793 | 64133 | 108275 | 17005 | 21125 | 26789 | 3625 | 3925 | 4140 | 945 | 973 | 964 | 405 | 413 | 391 |
| 0.75 *** | 39593 | 47905 | 95693 | 14213 | 16705 | 23605 | 3113 | 3325 | 3625 | 805 | 825 | 845 | 333 | 345 | 345 |
| *** | 42833 | 57553 | 96300 | 15253 | 18973 | 23730 | 3213 | 3465 | 3619 | 813 | 833 | 821 | 345 | 345 | 322 |
| 0.8 *** | 33645 | 41373 | 81425 | 12313 | 14465 | 19973 | 2625 | 2793 | 3013 | 653 | 665 | 673 | 265 | 265 | 265 |
| *** | 36693 | 50045 | 81721 | 13213 | 16353 | 20021 | 2705 | 2893 | 2994 | 653 | 665 | 651 | 265 | 265 | 241 |
| 0.85 *** | 27545 | 34185 | 64433 | 10105 | 11785 | 15653 | 2045 | 2153 | 2285 | 465 | 473 | 485 | . | . | . |
| *** | 30193 | 41345 | 64538 | 10825 | 13193 | 15660 | 2093 | 2213 | 2265 | 473 | 473 | 456 | . | . | . |
| 0.9 *** | 20905 | 25873 | 44745 | 7453 | 8533 | 10665 | 1345 | 1393 | 1453 | . | . | . | . | . | . |
| *** | 22925 | 30953 | 44753 | 7925 | 9373 | 10648 | 1373 | 1425 | 1432 | . | . | . | . | . | . |
| 0.95 *** | 12733 | 15325 | 22385 | 4025 | 4413 | 5013 | . | . | . | . | . | . | . | . | . |
| *** | 13813 | 17665 | 22364 | 4205 | 4673 | 4986 | . | . | . | . | . | . | . | . | . |
| 0.98 *** | 5705 | 6425 | 7705 | . | . | . | . | . | . | . | . | . | . | . | . |
| *** | 6025 | 6953 | 7680 | . | . | . | . | . | . | . | . | . | . | . | . |

# TABLE 4: ALPHA= 0.01  POWER= 0.9    EXPECTED ACCRUAL THRU MINIMUM FOLLOW-UP= 8500

| | | DEL=.01 | | | DEL=.02 | | | DEL=.05 | | | DEL=.10 | | | DEL=.15 | | |
|---|---|---|---|---|---|---|---|---|---|---|---|---|---|---|---|---|---|
| FACT= | | 1.0 .75 | .50 .25 | .00 BIN | 1.0 .75 | .50 .25 | .00 BIN | 1.0 .75 | .50 .25 | .00 BIN | 1.0 75 | .50 .25 | .00 BIN | 1.0 .75 | .50 .25 | .00 BIN |
| PCONT=*** | | | | | REQUIRED NUMBER OF PATIENTS | | | | | | | | | | | |
| 0.01 | *** | 1990 | 2003 | 2003 | 736 | 736 | 736 | 240 | 240 | 240 | 120 | 120 | 120 | 91 | 91 | 91 |
| | *** | 2003 | 2003 | 7680 | 736 | 736 | 2539 | 240 | 240 | 691 | 120 | 120 | 281 | 91 | 91 | 167 |
| 0.02 | *** | 4413 | 4434 | 4476 | 1416 | 1430 | 1430 | 388 | 388 | 388 | 163 | 163 | 163 | 112 | 112 | 112 |
| | *** | 4426 | 4455 | 12679 | 1416 | 1430 | 3775 | 388 | 388 | 883 | 163 | 163 | 326 | 112 | 112 | 186 |
| 0.05 | *** | 13380 | 13521 | 13996 | 3818 | 3860 | 3924 | 821 | 821 | 835 | 290 | 290 | 290 | 176 | 176 | 176 |
| | *** | 13436 | 13670 | 27050 | 3831 | 3881 | 7329 | 821 | 835 | 1432 | 290 | 290 | 456 | 176 | 176 | 241 |
| 0.1 | *** | 29551 | 29934 | 32569 | 8038 | 8230 | 8612 | 1565 | 1586 | 1600 | 495 | 495 | 495 | 261 | 261 | 261 |
| | *** | 29679 | 30529 | 48918 | 8123 | 8378 | 12731 | 1578 | 1586 | 2265 | 495 | 495 | 651 | 261 | 261 | 322 |
| 0.15 | *** | 44193 | 44886 | 51452 | 11885 | 12288 | 13316 | 2258 | 2301 | 2351 | 665 | 673 | 673 | 333 | 346 | 346 |
| | *** | 44426 | 46084 | 68183 | 12041 | 12658 | 17482 | 2280 | 2322 | 2994 | 673 | 673 | 821 | 333 | 346 | 391 |
| 0.2 | *** | 56063 | 57155 | 69132 | 15059 | 15739 | 17707 | 2853 | 2938 | 3031 | 821 | 835 | 843 | 410 | 410 | 410 |
| | *** | 56433 | 59081 | 84845 | 15327 | 16411 | 21583 | 2896 | 2981 | 3619 | 821 | 835 | 964 | 410 | 410 | 449 |
| 0.25 | *** | 64818 | 66391 | 84865 | 17516 | 18501 | 21583 | 3350 | 3470 | 3626 | 949 | 962 | 983 | 460 | 460 | 460 |
| | *** | 65350 | 69183 | 98903 | 17906 | 19513 | 25032 | 3406 | 3541 | 4140 | 962 | 970 | 1081 | 460 | 460 | 495 |
| 0.3 | *** | 70492 | 72646 | 98274 | 19258 | 20576 | 24876 | 3746 | 3903 | 4128 | 1055 | 1076 | 1090 | 503 | 503 | 516 |
| | *** | 71223 | 76429 | 110358 | 19776 | 21936 | 27831 | 3818 | 4001 | 4556 | 1068 | 1076 | 1172 | 503 | 503 | 530 |
| 0.35 | *** | 73305 | 76166 | 109125 | 20350 | 22008 | 27525 | 4030 | 4235 | 4519 | 1132 | 1153 | 1175 | 537 | 537 | 545 |
| | *** | 74275 | 81061 | 119210 | 21009 | 23721 | 29979 | 4128 | 4362 | 4869 | 1140 | 1161 | 1237 | 537 | 537 | 553 |
| 0.4 | *** | 73595 | 77279 | 117271 | 20881 | 22871 | 29488 | 4221 | 4455 | 4795 | 1183 | 1204 | 1238 | 545 | 558 | 558 |
| | *** | 74856 | 83356 | 125458 | 21668 | 24898 | 31475 | 4328 | 4617 | 5077 | 1196 | 1217 | 1276 | 558 | 558 | 565 |
| 0.45 | *** | 71767 | 76386 | 122661 | 20916 | 23198 | 30763 | 4320 | 4583 | 4965 | 1204 | 1238 | 1260 | 558 | 566 | 566 |
| | *** | 73361 | 83667 | 129102 | 21830 | 25514 | 32322 | 4447 | 4753 | 5181 | 1217 | 1246 | 1289 | 558 | 566 | 565 |
| 0.5 | *** | 68248 | 73913 | 125219 | 20533 | 23070 | 31336 | 4328 | 4604 | 5029 | 1204 | 1225 | 1260 | 545 | 558 | 566 |
| | *** | 70245 | 82315 | 130144 | 21561 | 25599 | 32517 | 4455 | 4795 | 5181 | 1217 | 1246 | 1276 | 558 | 558 | 553 |
| 0.55 | *** | 63530 | 70224 | 124956 | 19819 | 22539 | 31201 | 4243 | 4540 | 4978 | 1175 | 1204 | 1238 | 537 | 537 | 545 |
| | *** | 65945 | 79574 | 128582 | 20924 | 25208 | 32061 | 4383 | 4731 | 5077 | 1183 | 1217 | 1237 | 537 | 545 | 530 |
| 0.6 | *** | 58040 | 65668 | 121853 | 18820 | 21638 | 30359 | 4094 | 4383 | 4808 | 1119 | 1153 | 1175 | 503 | 503 | 516 |
| | *** | 60866 | 75698 | 124416 | 19981 | 24345 | 30955 | 4221 | 4575 | 4869 | 1132 | 1161 | 1172 | 503 | 516 | 495 |
| 0.65 | *** | 52183 | 60470 | 115933 | 17580 | 20393 | 28808 | 3852 | 4128 | 4519 | 1047 | 1068 | 1098 | 460 | 460 | 473 |
| | *** | 55320 | 70832 | 117648 | 18748 | 23062 | 29197 | 3980 | 4306 | 4556 | 1055 | 1076 | 1081 | 460 | 473 | 449 |
| 0.7 | *** | 46211 | 54810 | 107199 | 16121 | 18820 | 26555 | 3533 | 3775 | 4128 | 941 | 962 | 983 | 410 | 410 | 418 |
| | *** | 49526 | 65081 | 108275 | 17248 | 21328 | 26789 | 3648 | 3937 | 4140 | 949 | 970 | 964 | 410 | 410 | 391 |
| 0.75 | *** | 40253 | 48698 | 95695 | 14435 | 16921 | 23601 | 3138 | 3342 | 3626 | 813 | 821 | 843 | 346 | 346 | 346 |
| | *** | 43555 | 58443 | 96300 | 15476 | 19152 | 23730 | 3236 | 3470 | 3619 | 813 | 835 | 821 | 346 | 346 | 322 |
| 0.8 | *** | 34269 | 42102 | 81423 | 12509 | 14634 | 19968 | 2649 | 2798 | 3010 | 651 | 665 | 673 | 261 | 261 | 269 |
| | *** | 37371 | 50823 | 81721 | 13401 | 16496 | 20021 | 2726 | 2896 | 2994 | 651 | 673 | 651 | 261 | 261 | 241 |
| 0.85 | *** | 28098 | 34792 | 64436 | 10256 | 11914 | 15654 | 2054 | 2160 | 2288 | 473 | 473 | 481 | . | . | . |
| | *** | 30776 | 41975 | 64538 | 10971 | 13295 | 15660 | 2110 | 2216 | 2265 | 473 | 481 | 456 | . | . | . |
| 0.9 | *** | 21320 | 26321 | 44737 | 7558 | 8620 | 10660 | 1353 | 1395 | 1459 | . | . | . | . | . | . |
| | *** | 23360 | 31379 | 44753 | 8017 | 9428 | 10648 | 1374 | 1430 | 1432 | . | . | . | . | . | . |
| 0.95 | *** | 12955 | 15540 | 22382 | 4065 | 4447 | 5008 | . | . | . | . | . | . | . | . | . |
| | *** | 14039 | 17843 | 22364 | 4235 | 4689 | 4986 | . | . | . | . | . | . | . | . | . |
| 0.98 | *** | 5773 | 6487 | 7706 | . | . | . | . | . | . | . | . | . | . | . | . |
| | *** | 6091 | 6997 | 7680 | . | . | . | . | . | . | . | . | . | . | . | . |

TABLE 4: ALPHA= 0.01  POWER= 0.9    EXPECTED ACCRUAL THRU MINIMUM FOLLOW-UP= 9000

| | | DEL=.01 | | | DEL=.02 | | | DEL=.05 | | | DEL=.10 | | | DEL=.15 | |
|---|---|---|---|---|---|---|---|---|---|---|---|---|---|---|---|
| FACT= | 1.0 .75 | .50 .25 | .00 BIN | 1.0 .75 | .50 .25 | .00 BIN | 1.0 .75 | .50 .25 | .00 BIN | 1.0 75 | .50 .25 | .00 BIN | 1.0 .75 | .50 .25 | .00 BIN |
| PCONT=*** | | | | REQUIRED NUMBER OF PATIENTS | | | | | | | | | | | |
| 0.01 *** | 1995 1995 | 2009 | | 735 735 | 735 | | 240 240 | 240 | | 119 119 | 119 | | 82 82 | 82 | |
| *** | 1995 2009 | 7680 | | 735 735 | 2539 | | 240 240 | 691 | | 119 119 | 281 | | 82 82 | 167 | |
| 0.02 *** | 4416 4439 | 4484 | | 1424 1424 | 1432 | | 389 389 | 389 | | 164 164 | 164 | | 105 105 | 105 | |
| *** | 4425 4461 | 12679 | | 1424 1424 | 3775 | | 389 389 | 883 | | 164 164 | 326 | | 105 105 | 186 | |
| 0.05 *** | 13394 13529 | 13987 | | 3817 3862 | 3921 | | 825 825 | 825 | | 299 299 | 299 | | 172 172 | 172 | |
| *** | 13447 13686 | 27050 | | 3840 3885 | 7329 | | 825 825 | 1432 | | 299 299 | 456 | | 172 172 | 241 | |
| 0.1 *** | 29571 29976 | 32572 | | 8061 8241 | 8610 | | 1567 1581 | 1604 | | 487 487 | 487 | | 262 262 | 262 | |
| *** | 29715 30584 | 48918 | | 8137 8385 | 12731 | | 1581 1590 | 2265 | | 487 487 | 651 | | 262 262 | 322 | |
| 0.15 *** | 44227 44970 | 51450 | | 11909 12314 | 13326 | | 2256 2301 | 2346 | | 667 667 | 681 | | 344 344 | 344 | |
| *** | 44475 46199 | 68183 | | 12075 12682 | 17482 | | 2279 2324 | 2994 | | 667 681 | 821 | | 344 344 | 391 | |
| 0.2 *** | 56130 57277 | 69126 | | 15112 15801 | 17700 | | 2864 2940 | 3030 | | 825 825 | 839 | | 411 411 | 411 | |
| *** | 56512 59280 | 84845 | | 15382 16454 | 21583 | | 2895 2985 | 3619 | | 825 839 | 964 | | 411 411 | 449 | |
| 0.25 *** | 64919 66570 | 84862 | | 17587 18591 | 21584 | | 3367 3480 | 3629 | | 951 960 | 982 | | 456 465 | 465 | |
| *** | 65467 69472 | 98903 | | 17984 19581 | 25032 | | 3412 3547 | 4140 | | 960 974 | 1081 | | 465 465 | 495 | |
| 0.3 *** | 70620 72892 | 98272 | | 19365 20692 | 24877 | | 3764 3907 | 4124 | | 1064 1072 | 1095 | | 501 510 | 510 | |
| *** | 71385 76821 | 110358 | | 19896 22042 | 27831 | | 3831 4011 | 4556 | | 1064 1086 | 1172 | | 501 510 | 530 | |
| 0.35 *** | 73477 76484 | 109117 | | 20481 22155 | 27524 | | 4056 4245 | 4515 | | 1131 1154 | 1176 | | 532 532 | 546 | |
| *** | 74504 81546 | 119210 | | 21156 23856 | 29979 | | 4146 4371 | 4869 | | 1140 1162 | 1237 | | 532 546 | 553 | |
| 0.4 *** | 73815 77685 | 117276 | | 21030 23032 | 29490 | | 4245 4470 | 4799 | | 1185 1207 | 1230 | | 555 555 | 569 | |
| *** | 75142 83954 | 125458 | | 21831 25057 | 31475 | | 4349 4619 | 5077 | | 1199 1221 | 1276 | | 555 555 | 565 | |
| 0.45 *** | 72051 76897 | 122654 | | 21089 23392 | 30772 | | 4349 4605 | 4965 | | 1207 1230 | 1266 | | 555 569 | 569 | |
| *** | 73739 84367 | 129102 | | 22020 25687 | 32322 | | 4461 4762 | 5181 | | 1221 1244 | 1289 | | 555 569 | 565 | |
| 0.5 *** | 68609 74512 | 125219 | | 20729 23294 | 31335 | | 4357 4627 | 5032 | | 1207 1230 | 1266 | | 555 555 | 569 | |
| *** | 70701 83099 | 130144 | | 21772 25791 | 32517 | | 4484 4807 | 5181 | | 1221 1244 | 1276 | | 555 555 | 553 | |
| 0.55 *** | 63974 70912 | 124957 | | 20031 22762 | 31200 | | 4281 4560 | 4979 | | 1176 1207 | 1230 | | 532 532 | 546 | |
| *** | 66494 80444 | 128582 | | 21156 25409 | 32061 | | 4402 4740 | 5077 | | 1185 1221 | 1237 | | 532 546 | 530 | |
| 0.6 *** | 58560 66412 | 121852 | | 19050 21876 | 30359 | | 4124 4402 | 4807 | | 1117 1154 | 1176 | | 501 510 | 510 | |
| *** | 61485 76596 | 124416 | | 20211 24554 | 30955 | | 4245 4582 | 4869 | | 1140 1162 | 1172 | | 501 510 | 495 | |
| 0.65 *** | 52769 61260 | 115935 | | 17812 20625 | 28806 | | 3876 4146 | 4529 | | 1041 1072 | 1095 | | 456 465 | 465 | |
| *** | 55995 71745 | 117648 | | 18974 23257 | 29197 | | 3997 4312 | 4556 | | 1050 1086 | 1081 | | 465 465 | 449 | |
| 0.7 *** | 46837 55604 | 107205 | | 16341 19041 | 26556 | | 3561 3795 | 4132 | | 937 960 | 982 | | 411 411 | 411 | |
| *** | 50226 65976 | 108275 | | 17466 21516 | 26789 | | 3674 3952 | 4140 | | 951 974 | 964 | | 411 411 | 391 | |
| 0.75 *** | 40889 49470 | 95699 | | 14640 17115 | 23609 | | 3156 3359 | 3629 | | 816 825 | 839 | | 344 344 | 344 | |
| *** | 44250 59271 | 96300 | | 15689 19320 | 23730 | | 3246 3480 | 3619 | | 816 839 | 821 | | 344 344 | 322 | |
| 0.8 *** | 34867 42801 | 81420 | | 12682 14811 | 19972 | | 2661 2819 | 3007 | | 659 667 | 681 | | 262 262 | 262 | |
| *** | 38009 51554 | 81721 | | 13582 16634 | 20021 | | 2729 2909 | 2994 | | 659 667 | 651 | | 262 262 | 241 | |
| 0.85 *** | 28612 35376 | 64432 | | 10401 12044 | 15652 | | 2062 2166 | 2287 | | 465 479 | 479 | | . . | . | |
| *** | 31326 42562 | 64538 | | 11107 13394 | 15660 | | 2121 2220 | 2265 | | 479 479 | 456 | | . . | . | |
| 0.9 *** | 21719 26745 | 44736 | | 7656 8691 | 10671 | | 1356 1401 | 1455 | | . . | . | | . . | . | |
| *** | 23766 31785 | 44753 | | 8106 9487 | 10648 | | 1379 1432 | 1432 | | . . | . | | . . | . | |
| 0.95 *** | 13177 15742 | 22380 | | 4101 4470 | 5010 | | . . | . | | . . | . | | . . | . | |
| *** | 14257 18015 | 22364 | | 4267 4709 | 4986 | | . . | . | | . . | . | | . . | . | |
| 0.98 *** | 5834 6531 | 7701 | | . . | . | | . . | . | | . . | . | | . . | . | |
| *** | 6149 7026 | 7680 | | . . | . | | . . | . | | . . | . | | . . | . | |

TABLE 4: ALPHA= 0.01  POWER= 0.9    EXPECTED ACCRUAL THRU MINIMUM FOLLOW-UP= 9500

| | | DEL=.01 | | | DEL=.02 | | | DEL=.05 | | | DEL=.10 | | | DEL=.15 | | |
|---|---|---|---|---|---|---|---|---|---|---|---|---|---|---|---|---|---|
| FACT= | | 1.0 .75 | .50 .25 | .00 BIN | 1.0 .75 | .50 .25 | .00 BIN | 1.0 .75 | .50 .25 | .00 BIN | 1.0 75 | .50 .25 | .00 BIN | 1.0 .75 | .50 .25 | .00 BIN |
| PCONT=*** | | | | | | | REQUIRED NUMBER OF PATIENTS | | | | | | | | | |
| 0.01 | *** | 2001 | 2001 | 2010 | 728 | 728 | 728 | 244 | 244 | 244 | 125 | 125 | 125 | 87 | 87 | 87 |
| | *** | 2001 | 2001 | 7680 | 728 | 728 | 2539 | 244 | 244 | 691 | 125 | 125 | 281 | 87 | 87 | 167 |
| 0.02 | *** | 4424 | 4448 | 4480 | 1417 | 1431 | 1431 | 386 | 386 | 386 | 173 | 173 | 173 | 110 | 110 | 110 |
| | *** | 4433 | 4457 | 12679 | 1417 | 1431 | 3775 | 386 | 386 | 883 | 173 | 173 | 326 | 110 | 110 | 186 |
| 0.05 | *** | 13401 | 13544 | 13995 | 3830 | 3863 | 3925 | 823 | 823 | 823 | 291 | 291 | 291 | 173 | 173 | 173 |
| | *** | 13458 | 13695 | 27050 | 3839 | 3887 | 7329 | 823 | 823 | 1432 | 291 | 291 | 456 | 173 | 173 | 241 |
| 0.1 | *** | 29599 | 30012 | 32568 | 8067 | 8248 | 8613 | 1574 | 1583 | 1607 | 490 | 490 | 490 | 253 | 268 | 268 |
| | *** | 29741 | 30629 | 48918 | 8153 | 8399 | 12731 | 1574 | 1598 | 2265 | 490 | 490 | 651 | 268 | 268 | 322 |
| 0.15 | *** | 44276 | 45045 | 51449 | 11938 | 12342 | 13315 | 2263 | 2295 | 2343 | 671 | 671 | 680 | 339 | 339 | 339 |
| | *** | 44538 | 46319 | 68183 | 12104 | 12713 | 17482 | 2286 | 2319 | 2994 | 671 | 671 | 821 | 339 | 339 | 391 |
| 0.2 | *** | 56199 | 57395 | 69128 | 15159 | 15848 | 17700 | 2865 | 2937 | 3032 | 823 | 838 | 838 | 410 | 410 | 410 |
| | *** | 56603 | 59462 | 84845 | 15444 | 16498 | 21583 | 2904 | 2984 | 3619 | 823 | 838 | 964 | 410 | 410 | 449 |
| 0.25 | *** | 65010 | 66753 | 84865 | 17662 | 18674 | 21580 | 3379 | 3483 | 3625 | 956 | 965 | 980 | 458 | 467 | 467 |
| | *** | 65589 | 69745 | 98903 | 18065 | 19657 | 25032 | 3426 | 3554 | 4140 | 956 | 965 | 1081 | 458 | 467 | 495 |
| 0.3 | *** | 70743 | 73142 | 98269 | 19458 | 20797 | 24873 | 3783 | 3925 | 4124 | 1060 | 1075 | 1084 | 505 | 505 | 514 |
| | *** | 71565 | 77194 | 110358 | 19989 | 22141 | 27831 | 3839 | 4020 | 4556 | 1060 | 1084 | 1172 | 505 | 505 | 530 |
| 0.35 | *** | 73655 | 76799 | 109123 | 20607 | 22293 | 27518 | 4068 | 4258 | 4519 | 1132 | 1155 | 1179 | 538 | 538 | 538 |
| | *** | 74724 | 82024 | 119210 | 21286 | 23979 | 29979 | 4163 | 4376 | 4869 | 1146 | 1170 | 1237 | 538 | 538 | 553 |
| 0.4 | *** | 74044 | 78096 | 117269 | 21177 | 23195 | 29489 | 4267 | 4495 | 4804 | 1194 | 1203 | 1227 | 553 | 553 | 562 |
| | *** | 75436 | 84533 | 125458 | 21984 | 25205 | 31475 | 4376 | 4623 | 5077 | 1194 | 1218 | 1276 | 553 | 562 | 565 |
| 0.45 | *** | 72334 | 77393 | 122651 | 21263 | 23575 | 30772 | 4362 | 4614 | 4970 | 1218 | 1241 | 1265 | 562 | 562 | 562 |
| | *** | 74106 | 85040 | 129102 | 22198 | 25855 | 32322 | 4480 | 4780 | 5181 | 1227 | 1250 | 1289 | 562 | 562 | 565 |
| 0.5 | *** | 68962 | 75089 | 125225 | 20930 | 23495 | 31342 | 4376 | 4647 | 5027 | 1203 | 1227 | 1265 | 553 | 553 | 562 |
| | *** | 71147 | 83853 | 130144 | 21975 | 25974 | 32517 | 4504 | 4813 | 5181 | 1218 | 1250 | 1276 | 553 | 562 | 553 |
| 0.55 | *** | 64402 | 71574 | 124955 | 20241 | 22982 | 31199 | 4305 | 4575 | 4970 | 1179 | 1203 | 1241 | 529 | 538 | 538 |
| | *** | 67029 | 81255 | 128582 | 21367 | 25594 | 32061 | 4433 | 4756 | 5077 | 1194 | 1218 | 1237 | 538 | 538 | 530 |
| 0.6 | *** | 59073 | 67133 | 121853 | 19268 | 22094 | 30359 | 4148 | 4424 | 4804 | 1123 | 1155 | 1179 | 505 | 505 | 514 |
| | *** | 62089 | 77464 | 124416 | 20431 | 24754 | 30955 | 4267 | 4590 | 4869 | 1132 | 1170 | 1172 | 505 | 514 | 495 |
| 0.65 | *** | 53349 | 62027 | 115930 | 18033 | 20844 | 28800 | 3901 | 4163 | 4519 | 1051 | 1075 | 1099 | 458 | 467 | 467 |
| | *** | 56659 | 72619 | 117648 | 19196 | 23448 | 29197 | 4020 | 4329 | 4556 | 1060 | 1084 | 1081 | 467 | 467 | 449 |
| 0.7 | *** | 47444 | 56365 | 107199 | 16560 | 19253 | 26559 | 3578 | 3815 | 4124 | 942 | 965 | 980 | 410 | 410 | 410 |
| | *** | 50903 | 66815 | 108275 | 17676 | 21690 | 26789 | 3688 | 3958 | 4140 | 956 | 965 | 964 | 410 | 410 | 391 |
| 0.75 | *** | 41498 | 50199 | 95695 | 14835 | 17296 | 23614 | 3174 | 3364 | 3625 | 814 | 823 | 838 | 339 | 339 | 348 |
| | *** | 44918 | 60055 | 96300 | 15880 | 19467 | 23730 | 3260 | 3483 | 3619 | 823 | 838 | 821 | 339 | 348 | 322 |
| 0.8 | *** | 35441 | 43454 | 81421 | 12855 | 14969 | 19965 | 2675 | 2818 | 3008 | 657 | 657 | 671 | 268 | 268 | 268 |
| | *** | 38633 | 52242 | 81721 | 13758 | 16759 | 20021 | 2747 | 2913 | 2994 | 657 | 671 | 651 | 268 | 268 | 241 |
| 0.85 | *** | 29109 | 35940 | 64425 | 10537 | 12166 | 15658 | 2073 | 2168 | 2286 | 467 | 481 | 481 | . | . | . |
| | *** | 31855 | 43122 | 64538 | 11240 | 13482 | 15660 | 2120 | 2224 | 2265 | 467 | 481 | 456 | . | . | . |
| 0.9 | *** | 22094 | 27153 | 44737 | 7734 | 8770 | 10670 | 1360 | 1408 | 1455 | . | . | . | . | . | . |
| | *** | 24160 | 32164 | 44753 | 8185 | 9530 | 10648 | 1384 | 1431 | 1432 | . | . | . | . | . | . |
| 0.95 | *** | 13378 | 15943 | 22388 | 4139 | 4495 | 5003 | . | . | . | . | . | . | . | . | . |
| | *** | 14455 | 18175 | 22364 | 4305 | 4718 | 4986 | . | . | . | . | . | . | . | . | . |
| 0.98 | *** | 5896 | 6570 | 7701 | . | . | . | . | . | . | . | . | . | . | . | . |
| | *** | 6205 | 7060 | 7680 | . | . | . | . | . | . | . | . | . | . | . | . |

## TABLE 4: ALPHA= 0.01  POWER= 0.9    EXPECTED ACCRUAL THRU MINIMUM FOLLOW-UP= 10000

| | | DEL=.01 | | | DEL=.02 | | | DEL=.05 | | | DEL=.10 | | | DEL=.15 | | |
|---|---|---|---|---|---|---|---|---|---|---|---|---|---|---|---|---|
| FACT= | | 1.0 .75 | .50 .25 | .00 BIN | 1.0 .75 | .50 .25 | .00 BIN | 1.0 .75 | .50 .25 | .00 BIN | 1.0 75 | .50 .25 | .00 BIN | 1.0 .75 | .50 .25 | .00 BIN |
| PCONT=*** | | | | | REQUIRED NUMBER OF PATIENTS | | | | | | | | | | | |
| 0.01 | *** | 1991 | 2007 | 2007 | 732 | 732 | 732 | 241 | 241 | 241 | 116 | 116 | 116 | 82 | 82 | 82 |
| | *** | 1991 | 2007 | 7680 | 732 | 732 | 2539 | 241 | 241 | 691 | 116 | 116 | 281 | 82 | 82 | 167 |
| 0.02 | *** | 4416 | 4441 | 4482 | 1416 | 1432 | 1432 | 382 | 382 | 382 | 166 | 166 | 166 | 107 | 107 | 107 |
| | *** | 4432 | 4457 | 12679 | 1416 | 1432 | 3775 | 382 | 382 | 883 | 166 | 166 | 326 | 107 | 107 | 186 |
| 0.05 | *** | 13407 | 13557 | 13991 | 3832 | 3866 | 3916 | 816 | 832 | 832 | 291 | 291 | 291 | 166 | 166 | 166 |
| | *** | 13466 | 13707 | 27050 | 3841 | 3891 | 7329 | 832 | 832 | 1432 | 291 | 291 | 456 | 166 | 166 | 241 |
| 0.1 | *** | 29616 | 30057 | 32566 | 8082 | 8266 | 8616 | 1566 | 1582 | 1607 | 491 | 491 | 491 | 257 | 257 | 257 |
| | *** | 29766 | 30682 | 48918 | 8157 | 8407 | 12731 | 1582 | 1591 | 2265 | 491 | 491 | 651 | 257 | 257 | 322 |
| 0.15 | *** | 44316 | 45116 | 51457 | 11966 | 12382 | 13316 | 2266 | 2307 | 2357 | 666 | 666 | 682 | 341 | 341 | 341 |
| | *** | 44591 | 46432 | 68183 | 12141 | 12732 | 17482 | 2282 | 2332 | 2994 | 666 | 682 | 821 | 341 | 341 | 391 |
| 0.2 | *** | 56257 | 57516 | 69132 | 15207 | 15907 | 17707 | 2882 | 2941 | 3032 | 832 | 832 | 841 | 407 | 407 | 407 |
| | *** | 56682 | 59641 | 84845 | 15491 | 16541 | 21583 | 2907 | 2982 | 3619 | 832 | 832 | 964 | 407 | 407 | 449 |
| 0.25 | *** | 65107 | 66932 | 84866 | 17732 | 18741 | 21582 | 3382 | 3491 | 3632 | 957 | 966 | 982 | 457 | 466 | 466 |
| | *** | 65716 | 70016 | 98903 | 18141 | 19716 | 25032 | 3432 | 3557 | 4140 | 957 | 966 | 1081 | 466 | 466 | 495 |
| 0.3 | *** | 70882 | 73382 | 98282 | 19541 | 20907 | 24882 | 3791 | 3932 | 4132 | 1057 | 1082 | 1091 | 507 | 507 | 507 |
| | *** | 71732 | 77557 | 110358 | 20091 | 22232 | 27831 | 3857 | 4016 | 4556 | 1066 | 1082 | 1172 | 507 | 507 | 530 |
| 0.35 | *** | 73816 | 77116 | 109116 | 20716 | 22416 | 27516 | 4091 | 4266 | 4516 | 1141 | 1157 | 1182 | 532 | 541 | 541 |
| | *** | 74957 | 82482 | 119210 | 21407 | 24091 | 29979 | 4166 | 4382 | 4869 | 1141 | 1166 | 1237 | 532 | 541 | 553 |
| 0.4 | *** | 74266 | 78491 | 117282 | 21316 | 23357 | 29491 | 4291 | 4507 | 4807 | 1191 | 1207 | 1232 | 557 | 557 | 566 |
| | *** | 75732 | 85091 | 125458 | 22141 | 25341 | 31475 | 4382 | 4641 | 5077 | 1207 | 1216 | 1276 | 557 | 557 | 565 |
| 0.45 | *** | 72616 | 77866 | 122657 | 21416 | 23757 | 30766 | 4391 | 4632 | 4966 | 1216 | 1232 | 1266 | 557 | 566 | 566 |
| | *** | 74466 | 85682 | 129102 | 22366 | 26007 | 32322 | 4507 | 4782 | 5181 | 1232 | 1241 | 1289 | 557 | 566 | 565 |
| 0.5 | *** | 69316 | 75657 | 125216 | 21107 | 23682 | 31341 | 4407 | 4666 | 5032 | 1207 | 1232 | 1266 | 557 | 557 | 566 |
| | *** | 71591 | 84582 | 130144 | 22157 | 26141 | 32517 | 4516 | 4832 | 5181 | 1216 | 1241 | 1276 | 557 | 557 | 553 |
| 0.55 | *** | 64832 | 72216 | 124957 | 20441 | 23182 | 31207 | 4332 | 4591 | 4966 | 1182 | 1207 | 1232 | 532 | 541 | 541 |
| | *** | 67541 | 82041 | 128582 | 21566 | 25766 | 32061 | 4457 | 4766 | 5077 | 1191 | 1216 | 1237 | 532 | 541 | 530 |
| 0.6 | *** | 59582 | 67841 | 121857 | 19466 | 22291 | 30357 | 4166 | 4432 | 4807 | 1132 | 1157 | 1182 | 507 | 507 | 516 |
| | *** | 62682 | 78282 | 124416 | 20641 | 24932 | 30955 | 4291 | 4607 | 4869 | 1141 | 1166 | 1172 | 507 | 507 | 495 |
| 0.65 | *** | 53907 | 62757 | 115932 | 18232 | 21041 | 28807 | 3932 | 4182 | 4516 | 1057 | 1066 | 1091 | 457 | 466 | 466 |
| | *** | 57291 | 73441 | 117648 | 19407 | 23616 | 29197 | 4041 | 4332 | 4556 | 1057 | 1082 | 1081 | 466 | 466 | 449 |
| 0.7 | *** | 48041 | 57091 | 107207 | 16757 | 19441 | 26557 | 3607 | 3832 | 4132 | 941 | 966 | 982 | 407 | 407 | 416 |
| | *** | 51566 | 67632 | 108275 | 17882 | 21857 | 26789 | 3707 | 3966 | 4140 | 957 | 966 | 964 | 407 | 416 | 391 |
| 0.75 | *** | 42082 | 50891 | 95691 | 15016 | 17482 | 23607 | 3191 | 3382 | 3632 | 816 | 832 | 841 | 341 | 341 | 341 |
| | *** | 45557 | 60807 | 96300 | 16057 | 19607 | 23730 | 3282 | 3491 | 3619 | 816 | 832 | 821 | 341 | 341 | 322 |
| 0.8 | *** | 35991 | 44091 | 81432 | 13016 | 15107 | 19966 | 2691 | 2832 | 3007 | 657 | 666 | 682 | 266 | 266 | 266 |
| | *** | 39216 | 52907 | 81721 | 13907 | 16866 | 20021 | 2757 | 2916 | 2994 | 657 | 666 | 651 | 266 | 266 | 241 |
| 0.85 | *** | 29591 | 36466 | 64432 | 10666 | 12266 | 15657 | 2082 | 2182 | 2291 | 466 | 482 | 482 | . | . | . |
| | *** | 32357 | 43641 | 64538 | 11357 | 13566 | 15660 | 2132 | 2232 | 2265 | 466 | 482 | 456 | . | . | . |
| 0.9 | *** | 22457 | 27532 | 44741 | 7816 | 8832 | 10666 | 1366 | 1407 | 1457 | . | . | . | . | . | . |
| | *** | 24532 | 32516 | 44753 | 8266 | 9582 | 10648 | 1391 | 1432 | 1432 | . | . | . | . | . | . |
| 0.95 | *** | 13566 | 16116 | 22382 | 4166 | 4516 | 5007 | . | . | . | . | . | . | . | . | . |
| | *** | 14657 | 18316 | 22364 | 4332 | 4732 | 4986 | . | . | . | . | . | . | . | . | . |
| 0.98 | *** | 5957 | 6616 | 7707 | . | . | . | . | . | . | . | . | . | . | . | . |
| | *** | 6257 | 7082 | 7680 | . | . | . | . | . | . | . | . | . | . | . | . |

## TABLE 4: ALPHA= 0.01  POWER= 0.9  EXPECTED ACCRUAL THRU MINIMUM FOLLOW-UP= 11000

| | | DEL=.01 | | | DEL=.02 | | | DEL=.05 | | | DEL=.10 | | | DEL=.15 | | |
|---|---|---|---|---|---|---|---|---|---|---|---|---|---|---|---|---|
| FACT= | | 1.0 .75 | .50 .25 | .00 BIN | 1.0 .75 | .50 .25 | .00 BIN | 1.0 .75 | .50 .25 | .00 BIN | 1.0 75 | .50 .25 | .00 BIN | 1.0 .75 | .50 .25 | .00 BIN |
| PCONT=*** | | | | | | REQUIRED NUMBER OF PATIENTS | | | | | | | | | | |
| 0.01 | *** | 1998 1998 | 1998 | | 733 733 | 733 | | 238 238 | 238 | | 117 117 | 117 | | 90 90 | 90 | |
| | *** | 1998 1998 | 7680 | | 733 733 | 2539 | | 238 238 | 691 | | 117 117 | 281 | | 90 90 | 167 | |
| 0.02 | *** | 4418 4445 | 4473 | | 1420 1420 | 1437 | | 375 375 | 392 | | 172 172 | 172 | | 117 117 | 117 | |
| | *** | 4435 4462 | 12679 | | 1420 1420 | 3775 | | 375 375 | 883 | | 172 172 | 326 | | 117 117 | 186 | |
| 0.05 | *** | 13427 13575 | 13988 | | 3830 3868 | 3923 | | 832 832 | 832 | | 293 293 | 293 | | 172 172 | 172 | |
| | *** | 13482 13713 | 27050 | | 3857 3895 | 7329 | | 832 832 | 1432 | | 293 293 | 456 | | 172 172 | 241 | |
| 0.1 | *** | 29663 30130 | 32567 | | 8103 8285 | 8615 | | 1575 1585 | 1602 | | 485 485 | 485 | | 255 265 | 265 | |
| | *** | 29828 30780 | 48918 | | 8185 8422 | 12731 | | 1575 1602 | 2265 | | 485 485 | 651 | | 265 265 | 322 | |
| 0.15 | *** | 44403 45272 | 51460 | | 12025 12437 | 13317 | | 2273 2300 | 2345 | | 667 678 | 678 | | 337 337 | 337 | |
| | *** | 44695 46630 | 68183 | | 12200 12778 | 17482 | | 2290 2328 | 2994 | | 667 678 | 821 | | 337 337 | 391 | |
| 0.2 | *** | 56382 57768 | 69125 | | 15297 15995 | 17700 | | 2895 2950 | 3032 | | 832 832 | 843 | | 403 403 | 403 | |
| | *** | 56860 59995 | 84845 | | 15583 16628 | 21583 | | 2922 2988 | 3619 | | 832 832 | 964 | | 403 403 | 449 | |
| 0.25 | *** | 65292 67272 | 84872 | | 17865 18883 | 21578 | | 3400 3500 | 3620 | | 953 970 | 980 | | 458 458 | 458 | |
| | *** | 65963 70528 | 98903 | | 18278 19835 | 25032 | | 3445 3555 | 4140 | | 970 970 | 1081 | | 458 458 | 495 | |
| 0.3 | *** | 71133 73855 | 98275 | | 19725 21100 | 24878 | | 3813 3950 | 4132 | | 1063 1080 | 1090 | | 502 502 | 513 | |
| | *** | 72068 78245 | 110358 | | 20285 22392 | 27831 | | 3868 4033 | 4556 | | 1063 1080 | 1172 | | 502 513 | 530 | |
| 0.35 | *** | 74158 77733 | 109127 | | 20945 22667 | 27518 | | 4115 4280 | 4517 | | 1145 1162 | 1173 | | 530 540 | 540 | |
| | *** | 75395 83360 | 119210 | | 21650 24300 | 29979 | | 4198 4390 | 4869 | | 1145 1162 | 1237 | | 540 540 | 553 | |
| 0.4 | *** | 74708 79262 | 117278 | | 21578 23640 | 29487 | | 4325 4528 | 4803 | | 1190 1217 | 1228 | | 557 557 | 557 | |
| | *** | 76303 86137 | 125458 | | 22420 25593 | 31475 | | 4418 4655 | 5077 | | 1200 1217 | 1276 | | 557 557 | 565 | |
| 0.45 | *** | 73185 78805 | 122657 | | 21732 24080 | 30763 | | 4435 4655 | 4968 | | 1217 1245 | 1255 | | 557 568 | 568 | |
| | *** | 75175 86907 | 129102 | | 22695 26297 | 32322 | | 4528 4803 | 5181 | | 1228 1245 | 1289 | | 557 568 | 565 | |
| 0.5 | *** | 70022 76760 | 125225 | | 21457 24042 | 31340 | | 4445 4693 | 5023 | | 1217 1245 | 1255 | | 557 557 | 568 | |
| | *** | 72470 85945 | 130144 | | 22513 26445 | 32517 | | 4555 4847 | 5181 | | 1228 1245 | 1276 | | 557 557 | 553 | |
| 0.55 | *** | 65677 73443 | 124950 | | 20808 23558 | 31203 | | 4363 4627 | 4968 | | 1190 1217 | 1228 | | 530 540 | 540 | |
| | *** | 68548 83525 | 128582 | | 21952 26088 | 32061 | | 4490 4775 | 5077 | | 1200 1217 | 1237 | | 540 540 | 530 | |
| 0.6 | *** | 60545 69170 | 121860 | | 19862 22678 | 30350 | | 4215 4462 | 4803 | | 1135 1162 | 1173 | | 502 513 | 513 | |
| | *** | 63818 79823 | 124416 | | 21028 25252 | 30955 | | 4325 4610 | 4869 | | 1145 1162 | 1172 | | 502 513 | 495 | |
| 0.65 | *** | 54980 64137 | 115930 | | 18625 21430 | 28810 | | 3967 4198 | 4517 | | 1052 1080 | 1090 | | 458 458 | 475 | |
| | *** | 58510 75000 | 117648 | | 19790 23932 | 29197 | | 4077 4352 | 4556 | | 1063 1080 | 1081 | | 458 475 | 449 | |
| 0.7 | *** | 49160 58472 | 107202 | | 17123 19790 | 26555 | | 3637 3857 | 4132 | | 942 970 | 980 | | 403 403 | 420 | |
| | *** | 52807 69125 | 108275 | | 18250 22145 | 26789 | | 3730 3978 | 4140 | | 953 970 | 964 | | 403 420 | 391 | |
| 0.75 | *** | 43193 52213 | 95690 | | 15363 17800 | 23602 | | 3225 3400 | 3620 | | 815 832 | 843 | | 337 348 | 348 | |
| | *** | 46768 62195 | 96300 | | 16397 19862 | 23730 | | 3307 3500 | 3619 | | 815 832 | 821 | | 337 348 | 322 | |
| 0.8 | *** | 37033 45283 | 81418 | | 13317 15380 | 19972 | | 2713 2840 | 3005 | | 650 667 | 678 | | 265 265 | 265 | |
| | *** | 40333 54110 | 81721 | | 14197 17068 | 20021 | | 2768 2922 | 2994 | | 667 667 | 651 | | 265 265 | 241 | |
| 0.85 | *** | 30488 37445 | 64423 | | 10897 12475 | 15655 | | 2097 2190 | 2290 | | 475 475 | 485 | | . . | . | |
| | *** | 33310 44612 | 64538 | | 11585 13713 | 15660 | | 2135 2235 | 2265 | | 475 475 | 456 | | . . | . | |
| 0.9 | *** | 23145 28233 | 44733 | | 7965 8955 | 10660 | | 1382 1410 | 1448 | | . . | . | | . . | . | |
| | *** | 25235 33155 | 44753 | | 8405 9660 | 10648 | | 1393 1437 | 1432 | | . . | . | | . . | . | |
| 0.95 | *** | 13933 16452 | 22392 | | 4225 4555 | 5012 | | . . | . | | . . | . | | . . | . | |
| | *** | 15005 18580 | 22364 | | 4380 4765 | 4986 | | . . | . | | . . | . | | . . | . | |
| 0.98 | *** | 6057 6700 | 7707 | | . . | . | | . . | . | | . . | . | | . . | . | |
| | *** | 6343 7130 | 7680 | | . . | . | | . . | . | | . . | . | | . . | . | |

TABLE 4: ALPHA= 0.01  POWER= 0.9    EXPECTED ACCRUAL THRU MINIMUM FOLLOW-UP= 12000

| | | DEL=.01 | | | DEL=.02 | | | DEL=.05 | | | DEL=.10 | | | DEL=.15 | | |
|---|---|---|---|---|---|---|---|---|---|---|---|---|---|---|---|---|---|
| FACT= | | 1.0 .75 | .50 .25 | .00 BIN | 1.0 .75 | .50 .25 | .00 BIN | 1.0 .75 | .50 .25 | .00 BIN | 1.0 75 | .50 .25 | .00 BIN | 1.0 .75 | .50 .25 | .00 BIN |
| PCONT=*** | | | | | REQUIRED NUMBER OF PATIENTS | | | | | | | | | | | |
| 0.01 | *** | 1999 | 1999 | 1999 | 728 | 728 | 739 | 248 | 248 | 248 | 128 | 128 | 128 | 79 | 79 | 79 |
| | *** | 1999 | 1999 | 7680 | 728 | 739 | 2539 | 248 | 248 | 691 | 128 | 128 | 281 | 79 | 79 | 167 |
| 0.02 | *** | 4429 | 4448 | 4478 | 1418 | 1429 | 1429 | 379 | 379 | 379 | 169 | 169 | 169 | 109 | 109 | 109 |
| | *** | 4429 | 4459 | 12679 | 1429 | 1429 | 3775 | 379 | 379 | 883 | 169 | 169 | 326 | 109 | 109 | 186 |
| 0.05 | *** | 13448 | 13598 | 13988 | 3829 | 3878 | 3919 | 829 | 829 | 829 | 289 | 289 | 289 | 169 | 169 | 169 |
| | *** | 13508 | 13729 | 27050 | 3848 | 3889 | 7329 | 829 | 829 | 1432 | 289 | 289 | 456 | 169 | 169 | 241 |
| 0.1 | *** | 29708 | 30199 | 32569 | 8138 | 8299 | 8618 | 1579 | 1579 | 1598 | 488 | 488 | 488 | 259 | 259 | 259 |
| | *** | 29888 | 30859 | 48918 | 8209 | 8438 | 12731 | 1579 | 1598 | 2265 | 488 | 488 | 651 | 259 | 259 | 322 |
| 0.15 | *** | 44479 | 45428 | 51458 | 12079 | 12488 | 13328 | 2269 | 2318 | 2348 | 668 | 668 | 679 | 338 | 338 | 338 |
| | *** | 44809 | 46819 | 68183 | 12248 | 12818 | 17482 | 2299 | 2329 | 2994 | 668 | 679 | 821 | 338 | 338 | 391 |
| 0.2 | *** | 56509 | 57998 | 69128 | 15379 | 16088 | 17708 | 2899 | 2959 | 3038 | 829 | 829 | 848 | 409 | 409 | 409 |
| | *** | 57019 | 60319 | 84845 | 15679 | 16688 | 21583 | 2929 | 2989 | 3619 | 829 | 829 | 964 | 409 | 409 | 449 |
| 0.25 | *** | 65468 | 67609 | 84859 | 17989 | 19009 | 21589 | 3409 | 3518 | 3619 | 968 | 968 | 979 | 458 | 458 | 469 |
| | *** | 66199 | 70999 | 98903 | 18409 | 19939 | 25032 | 3458 | 3559 | 4140 | 968 | 968 | 1081 | 458 | 469 | 495 |
| 0.3 | *** | 71389 | 74318 | 98269 | 19898 | 21278 | 24878 | 3829 | 3968 | 4129 | 1069 | 1069 | 1088 | 499 | 499 | 518 |
| | *** | 72398 | 78878 | 110358 | 20449 | 22538 | 27831 | 3889 | 4039 | 4556 | 1069 | 1088 | 1172 | 499 | 499 | 530 |
| 0.35 | *** | 74498 | 78338 | 109118 | 21158 | 22879 | 27518 | 4148 | 4309 | 4519 | 1148 | 1159 | 1178 | 529 | 529 | 548 |
| | *** | 75829 | 84169 | 119210 | 21859 | 24488 | 29979 | 4219 | 4399 | 4869 | 1148 | 1159 | 1237 | 529 | 548 | 553 |
| 0.4 | *** | 75139 | 80018 | 117278 | 21829 | 23899 | 29498 | 4358 | 4538 | 4808 | 1189 | 1208 | 1238 | 548 | 559 | 559 |
| | *** | 76868 | 87128 | 125458 | 22688 | 25808 | 31475 | 4448 | 4658 | 5077 | 1208 | 1219 | 1276 | 559 | 559 | 565 |
| 0.45 | *** | 73729 | 79699 | 122659 | 22009 | 24368 | 30769 | 4459 | 4688 | 4969 | 1219 | 1238 | 1268 | 559 | 559 | 559 |
| | *** | 75878 | 88039 | 129102 | 22988 | 26539 | 32322 | 4568 | 4808 | 5181 | 1238 | 1249 | 1289 | 559 | 559 | 565 |
| 0.5 | *** | 70699 | 77798 | 125228 | 21769 | 24349 | 31339 | 4478 | 4718 | 5029 | 1219 | 1238 | 1268 | 548 | 559 | 559 |
| | *** | 73298 | 87218 | 130144 | 22838 | 26719 | 32517 | 4598 | 4849 | 5181 | 1219 | 1249 | 1276 | 559 | 559 | 553 |
| 0.55 | *** | 66488 | 74599 | 124958 | 21158 | 23899 | 31208 | 4399 | 4639 | 4969 | 1189 | 1208 | 1238 | 529 | 548 | 548 |
| | *** | 69529 | 84878 | 128582 | 22298 | 26378 | 32061 | 4519 | 4789 | 5077 | 1208 | 1219 | 1237 | 529 | 548 | 530 |
| 0.6 | *** | 61489 | 70418 | 121849 | 20209 | 23029 | 30349 | 4249 | 4489 | 4808 | 1129 | 1159 | 1178 | 499 | 499 | 518 |
| | *** | 64898 | 81229 | 124416 | 21379 | 25538 | 30955 | 4358 | 4628 | 4869 | 1148 | 1159 | 1172 | 499 | 518 | 495 |
| 0.65 | *** | 55999 | 65438 | 115928 | 18979 | 21758 | 28808 | 3998 | 4219 | 4519 | 1058 | 1069 | 1088 | 458 | 469 | 469 |
| | *** | 59659 | 76418 | 117648 | 20149 | 24218 | 29197 | 4099 | 4358 | 4556 | 1069 | 1088 | 1081 | 458 | 469 | 449 |
| 0.7 | *** | 50228 | 59768 | 107198 | 17468 | 20119 | 26558 | 3668 | 3878 | 4129 | 949 | 968 | 979 | 409 | 409 | 409 |
| | *** | 53978 | 70508 | 108275 | 18589 | 22399 | 26789 | 3758 | 3998 | 4140 | 949 | 968 | 964 | 409 | 409 | 391 |
| 0.75 | *** | 44258 | 53438 | 95689 | 15679 | 18079 | 23599 | 3248 | 3409 | 3619 | 818 | 829 | 848 | 338 | 338 | 349 |
| | *** | 47899 | 63469 | 96300 | 16699 | 20089 | 23730 | 3319 | 3518 | 3619 | 818 | 829 | 821 | 338 | 349 | 322 |
| 0.8 | *** | 38018 | 46369 | 81428 | 13579 | 15608 | 19969 | 2738 | 2858 | 3008 | 649 | 668 | 679 | 259 | 259 | 259 |
| | *** | 41378 | 55219 | 81721 | 14468 | 17258 | 20021 | 2798 | 2929 | 2994 | 668 | 668 | 651 | 259 | 259 | 241 |
| 0.85 | *** | 31328 | 38348 | 64429 | 11108 | 12649 | 15649 | 2119 | 2198 | 2288 | 469 | 469 | 488 | . | . | . |
| | *** | 34178 | 45488 | 64538 | 11779 | 13838 | 15660 | 2149 | 2239 | 2265 | 469 | 469 | 456 | . | . | . |
| 0.9 | *** | 23768 | 28868 | 44738 | 8108 | 9049 | 10669 | 1388 | 1418 | 1459 | . | . | . | . | . | . |
| | *** | 25879 | 33728 | 44753 | 8528 | 9728 | 10648 | 1399 | 1429 | 1432 | . | . | . | . | . | . |
| 0.95 | *** | 14258 | 16748 | 22388 | 4268 | 4579 | 5018 | . | . | . | . | . | . | . | . | . |
| | *** | 15319 | 18799 | 22364 | 4418 | 4778 | 4986 | . | . | . | . | . | . | . | . | . |
| 0.98 | *** | 6139 | 6758 | 7699 | . | . | . | . | . | . | . | . | . | . | . | . |
| | *** | 6428 | 7178 | 7680 | . | . | . | . | . | . | . | . | . | . | . | . |

## TABLE 4: ALPHA= 0.01 POWER= 0.9 EXPECTED ACCRUAL THRU MINIMUM FOLLOW-UP= 13000

| PCONT=*** | | DEL=.01 | | | DEL=.02 | | | DEL=.05 | | | DEL=.10 | | | DEL=.15 | | |
|---|---|---|---|---|---|---|---|---|---|---|---|---|---|---|---|---|
| FACT= | | 1.0 .75 | .50 .25 | .00 BIN | 1.0 .75 | .50 .25 | .00 BIN | 1.0 .75 | .50 .25 | .00 BIN | 1.0 75 | .50 .25 | .00 BIN | 1.0 .75 | .50 .25 | .00 BIN |

REQUIRED NUMBER OF PATIENTS

| PCONT | | 1.0 | .50 | .00 | 1.0 | .50 | .00 | 1.0 | .50 | .00 | 1.0 | .50 | .00 | 1.0 | .50 | .00 |
|---|---|---|---|---|---|---|---|---|---|---|---|---|---|---|---|---|
| 0.01 | *** | 2003 | 2003 | 2003 | 736 | 736 | 736 | 236 | 236 | 236 | 118 | 118 | 118 | 86 | 86 | 86 |
|  | *** | 2003 | 2003 | 7680 | 736 | 736 | 2539 | 236 | 236 | 691 | 118 | 118 | 281 | 86 | 86 | 167 |
| 0.02 | *** | 4429 | 4441 | 4473 | 1418 | 1418 | 1439 | 378 | 378 | 378 | 171 | 171 | 171 | 106 | 106 | 106 |
|  | *** | 4441 | 4461 | 12679 | 1418 | 1418 | 3775 | 378 | 378 | 883 | 171 | 171 | 326 | 106 | 106 | 186 |
| 0.05 | *** | 13464 | 13606 | 13996 | 3844 | 3876 | 3921 | 821 | 821 | 833 | 301 | 301 | 301 | 171 | 171 | 171 |
|  | *** | 13529 | 13756 | 27050 | 3856 | 3888 | 7329 | 821 | 833 | 1432 | 301 | 301 | 456 | 171 | 171 | 241 |
| 0.1 | *** | 29758 | 30278 | 32574 | 8146 | 8329 | 8621 | 1581 | 1581 | 1601 | 496 | 496 | 496 | 269 | 269 | 269 |
|  | *** | 29941 | 30949 | 48918 | 8231 | 8438 | 12731 | 1581 | 1601 | 2265 | 496 | 496 | 651 | 269 | 269 | 322 |
| 0.15 | *** | 44566 | 45553 | 51456 | 12131 | 12521 | 13313 | 2284 | 2316 | 2349 | 671 | 671 | 671 | 334 | 334 | 346 |
|  | *** | 44903 | 47004 | 68183 | 12294 | 12846 | 17482 | 2296 | 2328 | 2994 | 671 | 671 | 821 | 334 | 334 | 391 |
| 0.2 | *** | 56636 | 58228 | 69136 | 15458 | 16161 | 17701 | 2901 | 2966 | 3031 | 833 | 833 | 833 | 411 | 411 | 411 |
|  | *** | 57188 | 60621 | 84845 | 15751 | 16746 | 21583 | 2934 | 2999 | 3619 | 833 | 833 | 964 | 411 | 411 | 449 |
| 0.25 | *** | 65659 | 67946 | 84866 | 18091 | 19131 | 21589 | 3433 | 3519 | 3628 | 963 | 963 | 984 | 464 | 464 | 464 |
|  | *** | 66451 | 71444 | 98903 | 18534 | 20041 | 25032 | 3466 | 3563 | 4140 | 963 | 963 | 1081 | 464 | 464 | 495 |
| 0.3 | *** | 71639 | 74771 | 98268 | 20041 | 21426 | 24871 | 3844 | 3974 | 4116 | 1061 | 1081 | 1093 | 508 | 508 | 508 |
|  | *** | 72723 | 79483 | 110358 | 20614 | 22673 | 27831 | 3909 | 4039 | 4556 | 1081 | 1081 | 1172 | 508 | 508 | 530 |
| 0.35 | *** | 74836 | 78919 | 109123 | 21341 | 23084 | 27516 | 4169 | 4311 | 4526 | 1146 | 1158 | 1179 | 541 | 541 | 541 |
|  | *** | 76266 | 84931 | 119210 | 22056 | 24644 | 29979 | 4234 | 4408 | 4869 | 1158 | 1158 | 1237 | 541 | 541 | 553 |
| 0.4 | *** | 75583 | 80739 | 117281 | 22076 | 24136 | 29486 | 4376 | 4559 | 4798 | 1191 | 1211 | 1223 | 561 | 561 | 561 |
|  | *** | 77424 | 88031 | 125458 | 22921 | 26009 | 31475 | 4461 | 4668 | 5077 | 1211 | 1223 | 1276 | 561 | 561 | 565 |
| 0.45 | *** | 74283 | 80576 | 122664 | 22283 | 24644 | 30766 | 4494 | 4701 | 4961 | 1223 | 1244 | 1256 | 561 | 561 | 573 |
|  | *** | 76558 | 89103 | 129102 | 23258 | 26768 | 32322 | 4591 | 4819 | 5181 | 1223 | 1256 | 1289 | 561 | 561 | 565 |
| 0.5 | *** | 71379 | 78789 | 125211 | 22056 | 24656 | 31339 | 4506 | 4733 | 5026 | 1223 | 1244 | 1256 | 561 | 561 | 561 |
|  | *** | 74109 | 88388 | 130144 | 23149 | 26963 | 32517 | 4624 | 4863 | 5181 | 1223 | 1256 | 1276 | 561 | 561 | 553 |
| 0.55 | *** | 67284 | 75701 | 124951 | 21471 | 24201 | 31209 | 4441 | 4668 | 4981 | 1191 | 1211 | 1244 | 541 | 541 | 541 |
|  | *** | 70448 | 86146 | 128582 | 22608 | 26638 | 32061 | 4538 | 4819 | 5077 | 1211 | 1223 | 1237 | 541 | 541 | 530 |
| 0.6 | *** | 62388 | 71586 | 121851 | 20528 | 23344 | 30364 | 4278 | 4506 | 4798 | 1146 | 1158 | 1179 | 508 | 508 | 508 |
|  | *** | 65919 | 82538 | 124416 | 21719 | 25793 | 30955 | 4396 | 4636 | 4869 | 1146 | 1158 | 1172 | 508 | 508 | 495 |
| 0.65 | *** | 56981 | 66646 | 115936 | 19293 | 22076 | 28804 | 4039 | 4246 | 4526 | 1061 | 1081 | 1093 | 464 | 464 | 464 |
|  | *** | 60751 | 77728 | 117648 | 20484 | 24461 | 29197 | 4136 | 4376 | 4556 | 1061 | 1081 | 1081 | 464 | 464 | 449 |
| 0.7 | *** | 51241 | 60958 | 107206 | 17786 | 20398 | 26561 | 3693 | 3888 | 4136 | 951 | 963 | 984 | 411 | 411 | 411 |
|  | *** | 55076 | 71769 | 108275 | 18903 | 22629 | 26789 | 3791 | 4006 | 4140 | 963 | 963 | 964 | 411 | 411 | 391 |
| 0.75 | *** | 45228 | 54576 | 95689 | 15966 | 18339 | 23604 | 3271 | 3433 | 3628 | 821 | 833 | 833 | 346 | 346 | 346 |
|  | *** | 48954 | 64631 | 96300 | 16986 | 20289 | 23730 | 3336 | 3519 | 3619 | 821 | 833 | 821 | 346 | 346 | 322 |
| 0.8 | *** | 38923 | 47394 | 81421 | 13833 | 15816 | 19976 | 2751 | 2869 | 3011 | 659 | 671 | 671 | 269 | 269 | 269 |
|  | *** | 42336 | 56213 | 81721 | 14699 | 17408 | 20021 | 2804 | 2934 | 2994 | 659 | 671 | 651 | 269 | 269 | 241 |
| 0.85 | *** | 32119 | 39183 | 64436 | 11298 | 12814 | 15653 | 2121 | 2198 | 2284 | 476 | 476 | 476 | . | . | . |
|  | *** | 34991 | 46268 | 64538 | 11969 | 13951 | 15660 | 2166 | 2251 | 2265 | 476 | 476 | 456 | . | . | . |
| 0.9 | *** | 24351 | 29454 | 44741 | 8231 | 9153 | 10669 | 1386 | 1418 | 1451 | . | . | . | . | . | . |
|  | *** | 26464 | 34243 | 44753 | 8633 | 9791 | 10648 | 1406 | 1439 | 1432 | . | . | . | . | . | . |
| 0.95 | *** | 14548 | 17006 | 22381 | 4311 | 4603 | 5014 | . | . | . | . | . | . | . | . | . |
|  | *** | 15609 | 19001 | 22364 | 4461 | 4798 | 4986 | . | . | . | . | . | . | . | . | . |
| 0.98 | *** | 6228 | 6813 | 7711 | . | . | . | . | . | . | . | . | . | . | . | . |
|  | *** | 6488 | 7203 | 7680 | . | . | . | . | . | . | . | . | . | . | . | . |

TABLE 4: ALPHA= 0.01  POWER= 0.9     EXPECTED ACCRUAL THRU MINIMUM FOLLOW-UP= 14000

| | | DEL=.01 | | | DEL=.02 | | | DEL=.05 | | | DEL=.10 | | | DEL=.15 | | |
|---|---|---|---|---|---|---|---|---|---|---|---|---|---|---|---|---|
| FACT= | | 1.0 .75 | .50 .25 | .00 BIN | 1.0 .75 | .50 .25 | .00 BIN | 1.0 .75 | .50 .25 | .00 BIN | 1.0 75 | .50 .25 | .00 BIN | 1.0 .75 | .50 .25 | .00 BIN |
| PCONT=*** | | | | | | | REQUIRED | NUMBER | OF PATIENTS | | | | | | |
| 0.01 | *** | 2004 | 2004 | 2004 | 722 | 722 | 744 | 232 | 232 | 232 | 114 | 114 | 114 | 79 | 79 | 79 |
| | *** | 2004 | 2004 | 7680 | 722 | 744 | 2539 | 232 | 232 | 691 | 114 | 114 | 281 | 79 | 79 | 167 |
| 0.02 | *** | 4432 | 4454 | 4489 | 1422 | 1422 | 1422 | 372 | 372 | 394 | 162 | 162 | 162 | 114 | 114 | 114 |
| | *** | 4432 | 4467 | 12679 | 1422 | 1422 | 3775 | 372 | 394 | 883 | 162 | 162 | 326 | 114 | 114 | 186 |
| 0.05 | *** | 13484 | 13624 | 13987 | 3837 | 3872 | 3929 | 827 | 827 | 827 | 289 | 289 | 289 | 162 | 162 | 162 |
| | *** | 13532 | 13764 | 27050 | 3859 | 3894 | 7329 | 827 | 827 | 1432 | 289 | 289 | 456 | 162 | 162 | 241 |
| 0.1 | *** | 29807 | 30354 | 32572 | 8177 | 8339 | 8619 | 1584 | 1584 | 1597 | 499 | 499 | 499 | 254 | 254 | 254 |
| | *** | 30004 | 31019 | 48918 | 8247 | 8457 | 12731 | 1584 | 1597 | 2265 | 499 | 499 | 651 | 254 | 254 | 322 |
| 0.15 | *** | 44647 | 45697 | 51459 | 12167 | 12552 | 13322 | 2284 | 2319 | 2354 | 674 | 674 | 674 | 337 | 337 | 337 |
| | *** | 45019 | 47167 | 68183 | 12342 | 12867 | 17482 | 2297 | 2332 | 2994 | 674 | 674 | 821 | 337 | 337 | 391 |
| 0.2 | *** | 56779 | 58459 | 69134 | 15549 | 16227 | 17697 | 2914 | 2962 | 3032 | 827 | 827 | 849 | 407 | 407 | 407 |
| | *** | 57352 | 60909 | 84845 | 15829 | 16809 | 21583 | 2949 | 2997 | 3619 | 827 | 827 | 964 | 407 | 407 | 449 |
| 0.25 | *** | 65844 | 68272 | 84862 | 18209 | 19237 | 21582 | 3439 | 3522 | 3627 | 967 | 967 | 967 | 464 | 464 | 464 |
| | *** | 66684 | 71864 | 98903 | 18642 | 20112 | 25032 | 3487 | 3579 | 4140 | 967 | 967 | 1081 | 464 | 464 | 495 |
| 0.3 | *** | 71899 | 75202 | 98267 | 20182 | 21569 | 24872 | 3859 | 3977 | 4117 | 1072 | 1072 | 1094 | 499 | 512 | 512 |
| | *** | 73054 | 80054 | 110358 | 20764 | 22794 | 27831 | 3929 | 4047 | 4556 | 1072 | 1094 | 1172 | 512 | 512 | 530 |
| 0.35 | *** | 75167 | 79472 | 109117 | 21534 | 23262 | 27519 | 4187 | 4327 | 4524 | 1142 | 1164 | 1177 | 534 | 534 | 547 |
| | *** | 76694 | 85654 | 119210 | 22247 | 24789 | 29979 | 4257 | 4419 | 4869 | 1164 | 1164 | 1237 | 534 | 534 | 553 |
| 0.4 | *** | 76007 | 81419 | 117272 | 22282 | 24347 | 29492 | 4397 | 4572 | 4804 | 1199 | 1212 | 1234 | 547 | 547 | 569 |
| | *** | 77954 | 88909 | 125458 | 23144 | 26189 | 31475 | 4489 | 4677 | 5077 | 1212 | 1234 | 1276 | 547 | 569 | 565 |
| 0.45 | *** | 74817 | 81397 | 122649 | 22527 | 24894 | 30774 | 4524 | 4712 | 4979 | 1234 | 1247 | 1269 | 569 | 569 | 569 |
| | *** | 77219 | 90099 | 129102 | 23507 | 26959 | 32322 | 4607 | 4839 | 5181 | 1234 | 1247 | 1289 | 569 | 569 | 565 |
| 0.5 | *** | 72039 | 79717 | 125217 | 22339 | 24907 | 31334 | 4537 | 4747 | 5027 | 1234 | 1247 | 1269 | 547 | 547 | 569 |
| | *** | 74909 | 89482 | 130144 | 23424 | 27182 | 32517 | 4642 | 4874 | 5181 | 1234 | 1247 | 1276 | 547 | 569 | 553 |
| 0.55 | *** | 68049 | 76742 | 124959 | 21757 | 24487 | 31207 | 4467 | 4677 | 4979 | 1199 | 1212 | 1234 | 534 | 534 | 547 |
| | *** | 71352 | 87312 | 128582 | 22912 | 26854 | 32061 | 4572 | 4817 | 5077 | 1199 | 1234 | 1237 | 534 | 547 | 530 |
| 0.6 | *** | 63254 | 72704 | 121857 | 20834 | 23612 | 30354 | 4314 | 4524 | 4804 | 1142 | 1164 | 1177 | 499 | 512 | 512 |
| | *** | 66894 | 83764 | 124416 | 22024 | 26027 | 30955 | 4419 | 4664 | 4869 | 1142 | 1164 | 1172 | 512 | 512 | 495 |
| 0.65 | *** | 57912 | 67782 | 115929 | 19609 | 22352 | 28814 | 4069 | 4257 | 4524 | 1059 | 1072 | 1094 | 464 | 464 | 464 |
| | *** | 61762 | 78947 | 117648 | 20777 | 24684 | 29197 | 4152 | 4384 | 4556 | 1072 | 1094 | 1081 | 464 | 464 | 449 |
| 0.7 | *** | 52194 | 62077 | 107192 | 18069 | 20672 | 26552 | 3719 | 3907 | 4117 | 954 | 967 | 989 | 407 | 407 | 407 |
| | *** | 56114 | 72927 | 108275 | 19189 | 22829 | 26789 | 3802 | 4012 | 4140 | 954 | 967 | 964 | 407 | 407 | 391 |
| 0.75 | *** | 46174 | 55624 | 95699 | 16227 | 18572 | 23612 | 3299 | 3439 | 3627 | 814 | 827 | 849 | 337 | 337 | 337 |
| | *** | 49954 | 65704 | 96300 | 17242 | 20462 | 23730 | 3369 | 3522 | 3619 | 827 | 827 | 821 | 337 | 337 | 322 |
| 0.8 | *** | 39782 | 48322 | 81419 | 14057 | 16017 | 19972 | 2774 | 2879 | 3019 | 652 | 674 | 674 | 267 | 267 | 267 |
| | *** | 43234 | 57142 | 81721 | 14919 | 17557 | 20021 | 2822 | 2949 | 2994 | 652 | 674 | 651 | 267 | 267 | 241 |
| 0.85 | *** | 32839 | 39957 | 64422 | 11467 | 12937 | 15654 | 2144 | 2214 | 2284 | 477 | 477 | 477 | . | . | . |
| | *** | 35757 | 46992 | 64538 | 12119 | 14044 | 15660 | 2179 | 2249 | 2265 | 477 | 477 | 456 | . | . | . |
| 0.9 | *** | 24894 | 30004 | 44739 | 8339 | 9227 | 10662 | 1387 | 1422 | 1457 | . | . | . | . | . | . |
| | *** | 27007 | 34707 | 44753 | 8737 | 9844 | 10648 | 1409 | 1444 | 1432 | . | . | . | . | . | . |
| 0.95 | *** | 14827 | 17242 | 22387 | 4349 | 4629 | 5014 | . | . | . | . | . | . | . | . | . |
| | *** | 15877 | 19189 | 22364 | 4489 | 4804 | 4986 | . | . | . | . | . | . | . | . | . |
| 0.98 | *** | 6309 | 6869 | 7709 | . | . | . | . | . | . | . | . | . | . | . | . |
| | *** | 6567 | 7232 | 7680 | . | . | . | . | . | . | . | . | . | . | . | . |

TABLE 4: ALPHA= 0.01  POWER= 0.9    EXPECTED ACCRUAL THRU MINIMUM FOLLOW-UP= 15000

| | | DEL=.01 | | | DEL=.02 | | | DEL=.05 | | | DEL=.10 | | | DEL=.15 | | |
|---|---|---|---|---|---|---|---|---|---|---|---|---|---|---|---|---|---|
| FACT= | | 1.0 .75 | .50 .25 | .00 BIN | 1.0 .75 | .50 .25 | .00 BIN | 1.0 .75 | .50 .25 | .00 BIN | 1.0 75 | .50 .25 | .00 BIN | 1.0 .75 | .50 .25 | .00 BIN |
| PCONT=*** | | | | | REQUIRED NUMBER OF PATIENTS | | | | | | | | | | | |
| 0.01 | *** | 1997 | 1997 | 2011 | 736 | 736 | 736 | 235 | 235 | 235 | 122 | 122 | 122 | 85 | 85 | 85 |
| | *** | 1997 | 1997 | 7680 | 736 | 736 | 2539 | 235 | 235 | 691 | 122 | 122 | 281 | 85 | 85 | 167 |
| 0.02 | *** | 4435 | 4449 | 4472 | 1411 | 1435 | 1435 | 385 | 385 | 385 | 160 | 160 | 160 | 99 | 99 | 99 |
| | *** | 4449 | 4472 | 12679 | 1435 | 1435 | 3775 | 385 | 385 | 883 | 160 | 160 | 326 | 99 | 99 | 186 |
| 0.05 | *** | 13486 | 13636 | 13997 | 3849 | 3886 | 3924 | 835 | 835 | 835 | 286 | 286 | 286 | 174 | 174 | 174 |
| | *** | 13547 | 13772 | 27050 | 3872 | 3886 | 7329 | 835 | 835 | 1432 | 286 | 286 | 456 | 174 | 174 | 241 |
| 0.1 | *** | 29836 | 30399 | 32574 | 8185 | 8349 | 8611 | 1585 | 1585 | 1599 | 497 | 497 | 497 | 249 | 249 | 249 |
| | *** | 30047 | 31074 | 48918 | 8260 | 8461 | 12731 | 1585 | 1599 | 2265 | 497 | 497 | 651 | 249 | 249 | 322 |
| 0.15 | *** | 44724 | 45835 | 51460 | 12211 | 12586 | 13322 | 2297 | 2311 | 2349 | 661 | 685 | 685 | 347 | 347 | 347 |
| | *** | 45122 | 47311 | 68183 | 12385 | 12886 | 17482 | 2297 | 2335 | 2994 | 661 | 685 | 821 | 347 | 347 | 391 |
| 0.2 | *** | 56897 | 58660 | 69122 | 15610 | 16299 | 17710 | 2911 | 2972 | 3024 | 835 | 835 | 835 | 399 | 399 | 399 |
| | *** | 57511 | 61172 | 84845 | 15910 | 16847 | 21583 | 2949 | 3010 | 3619 | 835 | 835 | 964 | 399 | 399 | 449 |
| 0.25 | *** | 66024 | 68574 | 84872 | 18310 | 19336 | 21586 | 3460 | 3535 | 3624 | 961 | 961 | 985 | 460 | 460 | 460 |
| | *** | 66924 | 72272 | 98903 | 18736 | 20199 | 25032 | 3497 | 3572 | 4140 | 961 | 985 | 1081 | 460 | 460 | 495 |
| 0.3 | *** | 72160 | 75624 | 98274 | 20335 | 21699 | 24872 | 3872 | 3985 | 4135 | 1074 | 1074 | 1097 | 511 | 511 | 511 |
| | *** | 73374 | 80597 | 110358 | 20897 | 22885 | 27831 | 3924 | 4060 | 4556 | 1074 | 1074 | 1172 | 511 | 511 | 530 |
| 0.35 | *** | 75511 | 80035 | 109111 | 21699 | 23424 | 27511 | 4210 | 4336 | 4510 | 1149 | 1172 | 1172 | 535 | 535 | 535 |
| | *** | 77124 | 86311 | 119210 | 22411 | 24924 | 29979 | 4261 | 4435 | 4869 | 1149 | 1172 | 1237 | 535 | 535 | 553 |
| 0.4 | *** | 76435 | 82097 | 117272 | 22486 | 24549 | 29485 | 4411 | 4585 | 4810 | 1210 | 1210 | 1224 | 549 | 549 | 572 |
| | *** | 78497 | 89710 | 125458 | 23349 | 26335 | 31475 | 4510 | 4697 | 5077 | 1210 | 1224 | 1276 | 549 | 549 | 565 |
| 0.45 | *** | 75361 | 82186 | 122649 | 22772 | 25111 | 30774 | 4547 | 4735 | 4974 | 1224 | 1247 | 1261 | 572 | 572 | 572 |
| | *** | 77874 | 91022 | 129102 | 23747 | 27136 | 32322 | 4636 | 4847 | 5181 | 1224 | 1247 | 1289 | 572 | 572 | 565 |
| 0.5 | *** | 72685 | 80635 | 125222 | 22599 | 25172 | 31336 | 4561 | 4772 | 5035 | 1224 | 1247 | 1261 | 549 | 549 | 572 |
| | *** | 75661 | 90511 | 130144 | 23686 | 27385 | 32517 | 4660 | 4885 | 5181 | 1224 | 1247 | 1276 | 549 | 549 | 553 |
| 0.55 | *** | 68799 | 77747 | 124960 | 22036 | 24736 | 31210 | 4486 | 4711 | 4974 | 1186 | 1210 | 1224 | 535 | 535 | 549 |
| | *** | 72211 | 88411 | 128582 | 23185 | 27061 | 32061 | 4599 | 4824 | 5077 | 1210 | 1224 | 1237 | 535 | 535 | 530 |
| 0.6 | *** | 64097 | 73749 | 121847 | 21122 | 23874 | 30361 | 4336 | 4547 | 4810 | 1149 | 1149 | 1172 | 511 | 511 | 511 |
| | *** | 67847 | 84886 | 124416 | 22299 | 26222 | 30955 | 4435 | 4660 | 4869 | 1149 | 1172 | 1172 | 511 | 511 | 495 |
| 0.65 | *** | 58810 | 68860 | 115936 | 19885 | 22599 | 28810 | 4074 | 4285 | 4524 | 1060 | 1074 | 1097 | 460 | 460 | 474 |
| | *** | 62747 | 80072 | 117648 | 21047 | 24872 | 29197 | 4172 | 4397 | 4556 | 1074 | 1074 | 1081 | 460 | 474 | 449 |
| 0.7 | *** | 53110 | 63136 | 107199 | 18347 | 20911 | 26560 | 3736 | 3910 | 4135 | 961 | 961 | 985 | 399 | 399 | 422 |
| | *** | 57099 | 74011 | 108275 | 19449 | 23011 | 26789 | 3835 | 4022 | 4140 | 961 | 985 | 964 | 399 | 422 | 391 |
| 0.75 | *** | 47049 | 56611 | 95686 | 16472 | 18774 | 23611 | 3310 | 3460 | 3624 | 811 | 835 | 835 | 347 | 347 | 347 |
| | *** | 50897 | 66699 | 96300 | 17485 | 20611 | 23730 | 3385 | 3535 | 3619 | 835 | 835 | 821 | 347 | 347 | 322 |
| 0.8 | *** | 40599 | 49210 | 81422 | 14260 | 16186 | 19974 | 2785 | 2874 | 3010 | 661 | 661 | 685 | 272 | 272 | 272 |
| | *** | 44086 | 57999 | 81721 | 15099 | 17672 | 20021 | 2822 | 2949 | 2994 | 661 | 661 | 651 | 272 | 272 | 241 |
| 0.85 | *** | 33535 | 40674 | 64435 | 11635 | 13074 | 15647 | 2147 | 2199 | 2297 | 474 | 474 | 474 | . | . | . |
| | *** | 36460 | 47649 | 64538 | 12272 | 14124 | 15660 | 2185 | 2236 | 2265 | 474 | 474 | 456 | . | . | . |
| 0.9 | *** | 25397 | 30497 | 44747 | 8447 | 9310 | 10660 | 1397 | 1411 | 1449 | . | . | . | . | . | . |
| | *** | 27535 | 35147 | 44753 | 8836 | 9886 | 10648 | 1411 | 1435 | 1432 | . | . | . | . | . | . |
| 0.95 | *** | 15085 | 17461 | 22374 | 4374 | 4660 | 5011 | . | . | . | . | . | . | . | . | . |
| | *** | 16111 | 19360 | 22364 | 4510 | 4824 | 4986 | . | . | . | . | . | . | . | . | . |
| 0.98 | *** | 6361 | 6910 | 7697 | . | . | . | . | . | . | . | . | . | . | . | . |
| | *** | 6624 | 7261 | 7680 | . | . | . | . | . | . | . | . | . | . | . | . |

TABLE 4: ALPHA= 0.01  POWER= 0.9    EXPECTED ACCRUAL THRU MINIMUM FOLLOW-UP= 17000

| | | DEL=.01 | | | DEL=.02 | | | DEL=.05 | | | DEL=.10 | | | DEL=.15 | | |
|---|---|---|---|---|---|---|---|---|---|---|---|---|---|---|---|---|---|
| FACT= | | 1.0 .75 | .50 .25 | .00 BIN | 1.0 .75 | .50 .25 | .00 BIN | 1.0 .75 | .50 .25 | .00 BIN | 1.0 75 | .50 .25 | .00 BIN | 1.0 .75 | .50 .25 | .00 BIN |
| PCONT=*** | | | | REQUIRED NUMBER OF PATIENTS | | | | | | | | | | | | |
| 0.01 | *** | 2009 | 2009 | 2009 | 734 | 734 | 734 | 240 | 240 | 240 | 112 | 112 | 112 | 96 | 96 | 96 |
| | *** | 2009 | 2009 | 7680 | 734 | 734 | 2539 | 240 | 240 | 691 | 112 | 112 | 281 | 96 | 96 | 167 |
| 0.02 | *** | 4431 | 4447 | 4474 | 1430 | 1430 | 1430 | 394 | 394 | 394 | 155 | 155 | 155 | 112 | 112 | 112 |
| | *** | 4447 | 4474 | 12679 | 1430 | 1430 | 3775 | 394 | 394 | 883 | 155 | 155 | 326 | 112 | 112 | 186 |
| 0.05 | *** | 13526 | 13670 | 13994 | 3852 | 3879 | 3921 | 819 | 835 | 835 | 282 | 282 | 282 | 181 | 181 | 181 |
| | *** | 13585 | 13797 | 27050 | 3879 | 3895 | 7329 | 819 | 835 | 1432 | 282 | 282 | 456 | 181 | 181 | 241 |
| 0.1 | *** | 29931 | 30526 | 32566 | 8230 | 8384 | 8612 | 1584 | 1584 | 1600 | 495 | 495 | 495 | 266 | 266 | 266 |
| | *** | 30160 | 31206 | 48918 | 8299 | 8485 | 12731 | 1584 | 1600 | 2265 | 495 | 495 | 651 | 266 | 266 | 322 |
| 0.15 | *** | 44891 | 46081 | 51452 | 12294 | 12650 | 13314 | 2306 | 2322 | 2349 | 665 | 665 | 665 | 351 | 351 | 351 |
| | *** | 45316 | 47611 | 68183 | 12437 | 12931 | 17482 | 2306 | 2322 | 2994 | 665 | 665 | 821 | 351 | 351 | 391 |
| 0.2 | *** | 57147 | 59086 | 69132 | 15736 | 16416 | 17707 | 2944 | 2986 | 3029 | 835 | 835 | 835 | 410 | 410 | 410 |
| | *** | 57854 | 61652 | 84845 | 16034 | 16926 | 21583 | 2960 | 3002 | 3619 | 835 | 835 | 964 | 410 | 410 | 449 |
| 0.25 | *** | 66396 | 69175 | 84857 | 18499 | 19519 | 21575 | 3470 | 3539 | 3624 | 962 | 962 | 989 | 452 | 452 | 452 |
| | *** | 67390 | 72984 | 98903 | 18924 | 20326 | 25032 | 3496 | 3581 | 4140 | 962 | 962 | 1081 | 452 | 452 | 495 |
| 0.3 | *** | 72644 | 76426 | 98271 | 20581 | 21941 | 24874 | 3895 | 4006 | 4134 | 1074 | 1074 | 1090 | 495 | 495 | 521 |
| | *** | 74004 | 81569 | 110358 | 21150 | 23062 | 27831 | 3964 | 4065 | 4556 | 1074 | 1090 | 1172 | 495 | 521 | 530 |
| 0.35 | *** | 76171 | 81059 | 109125 | 22000 | 23726 | 27525 | 4235 | 4362 | 4516 | 1159 | 1159 | 1175 | 537 | 537 | 537 |
| | *** | 77930 | 87561 | 119210 | 22749 | 25145 | 29979 | 4304 | 4431 | 4869 | 1159 | 1175 | 1237 | 537 | 537 | 553 |
| 0.4 | *** | 77276 | 83354 | 117269 | 22876 | 24890 | 29480 | 4447 | 4617 | 4787 | 1201 | 1217 | 1244 | 564 | 564 | 564 |
| | *** | 79502 | 91190 | 125458 | 23726 | 26616 | 31475 | 4532 | 4702 | 5077 | 1217 | 1217 | 1276 | 564 | 564 | 565 |
| 0.45 | *** | 76384 | 83667 | 122666 | 23190 | 25511 | 30755 | 4575 | 4745 | 4957 | 1244 | 1244 | 1260 | 564 | 564 | 564 |
| | *** | 79104 | 92720 | 129102 | 24167 | 27466 | 32322 | 4660 | 4856 | 5181 | 1244 | 1260 | 1289 | 564 | 564 | 565 |
| 0.5 | *** | 73919 | 82307 | 125216 | 23062 | 25596 | 31334 | 4601 | 4787 | 5026 | 1217 | 1244 | 1260 | 564 | 564 | 564 |
| | *** | 77106 | 92380 | 130144 | 24151 | 27721 | 32517 | 4702 | 4899 | 5181 | 1244 | 1260 | 1276 | 564 | 564 | 553 |
| 0.55 | *** | 70221 | 79571 | 124961 | 22536 | 25214 | 31206 | 4532 | 4729 | 4984 | 1201 | 1217 | 1244 | 537 | 537 | 537 |
| | *** | 73834 | 90409 | 128582 | 23684 | 27424 | 32061 | 4644 | 4856 | 5077 | 1201 | 1217 | 1237 | 537 | 537 | 530 |
| 0.6 | *** | 65674 | 75704 | 121859 | 21644 | 24337 | 30356 | 4389 | 4575 | 4814 | 1159 | 1159 | 1175 | 495 | 521 | 521 |
| | *** | 69600 | 86940 | 124416 | 22791 | 26590 | 30955 | 4474 | 4686 | 4869 | 1159 | 1175 | 1172 | 495 | 521 | 495 |
| 0.65 | *** | 60462 | 70832 | 115925 | 20385 | 23062 | 28800 | 4134 | 4304 | 4516 | 1074 | 1074 | 1090 | 452 | 479 | 479 |
| | *** | 64585 | 82121 | 117648 | 21532 | 25214 | 29197 | 4219 | 4405 | 4556 | 1074 | 1090 | 1081 | 452 | 479 | 449 |
| 0.7 | *** | 54810 | 65079 | 107196 | 18812 | 21320 | 26547 | 3767 | 3937 | 4134 | 962 | 962 | 989 | 410 | 410 | 410 |
| | *** | 58916 | 75959 | 108275 | 19901 | 23317 | 26789 | 3852 | 4022 | 4140 | 962 | 962 | 964 | 410 | 410 | 391 |
| 0.75 | *** | 48690 | 58449 | 95695 | 16926 | 19152 | 23599 | 3342 | 3470 | 3624 | 819 | 835 | 835 | 351 | 351 | 351 |
| | *** | 52626 | 68479 | 96300 | 17904 | 20895 | 23730 | 3411 | 3539 | 3619 | 835 | 835 | 821 | 351 | 351 | 322 |
| 0.8 | *** | 42102 | 50815 | 81415 | 14631 | 16501 | 19960 | 2790 | 2901 | 3002 | 665 | 665 | 665 | 266 | 266 | 266 |
| | *** | 45656 | 59511 | 81721 | 15455 | 17904 | 20021 | 2859 | 2944 | 2994 | 665 | 665 | 651 | 266 | 266 | 241 |
| 0.85 | *** | 34792 | 41975 | 64441 | 11911 | 13287 | 15651 | 2152 | 2221 | 2280 | 479 | 479 | 479 | . | . | . |
| | *** | 37751 | 48817 | 64538 | 12522 | 14291 | 15660 | 2195 | 2264 | 2265 | 479 | 479 | 456 | . | . | . |
| 0.9 | *** | 26319 | 31376 | 44737 | 8612 | 9420 | 10652 | 1387 | 1430 | 1456 | . | . | . | . | . | . |
| | *** | 28444 | 35897 | 44753 | 8995 | 9972 | 10648 | 1414 | 1430 | 1432 | . | . | . | . | . | . |
| 0.95 | *** | 15540 | 17835 | 22382 | 4447 | 4686 | 5000 | . | . | . | . | . | . | . | . | . |
| | *** | 16544 | 19620 | 22364 | 4559 | 4830 | 4986 | . | . | . | . | . | . | . | . | . |
| 0.98 | *** | 6487 | 6997 | 7704 | . | . | . | . | . | . | . | . | . | . | . | . |
| | *** | 6726 | 7321 | 7680 | . | . | . | . | . | . | . | . | . | . | . | . |

TABLE 4: ALPHA= 0.01  POWER= 0.9    EXPECTED ACCRUAL THRU MINIMUM FOLLOW-UP= 20000

| | | DEL=.01 | | | DEL=.02 | | | DEL=.05 | | | DEL=.10 | | | DEL=.15 | | |
|---|---|---|---|---|---|---|---|---|---|---|---|---|---|---|---|---|---|
| FACT= | | 1.0 .75 | .50 .25 | .00 BIN | 1.0 .75 | .50 .25 | .00 BIN | 1.0 .75 | .50 .25 | .00 BIN | 1.0 75 | .50 .25 | .00 BIN | 1.0 .75 | .50 .25 | .00 BIN |
| PCONT=*** | | | | REQUIRED | NUMBER | OF PATIENTS | | | | | | | | | |
| 0.01 | *** | 2013 | 2013 | 2013 | 732 | 732 | 732 | 232 | 232 | 232 | 113 | 113 | 113 | 82 | 82 | 82 |
| | *** | 2013 | 2013 | 7680 | 732 | 732 | 2539 | 232 | 232 | 691 | 113 | 113 | 281 | 82 | 82 | 167 |
| 0.02 | *** | 4432 | 4463 | 4482 | 1432 | 1432 | 1432 | 382 | 382 | 382 | 163 | 163 | 163 | 113 | 113 | 113 |
| | *** | 4463 | 4463 | 12679 | 1432 | 1432 | 3775 | 382 | 382 | 883 | 163 | 163 | 326 | 113 | 113 | 186 |
| 0.05 | *** | 13563 | 13713 | 13982 | 3863 | 3882 | 3913 | 832 | 832 | 832 | 282 | 282 | 282 | 163 | 163 | 163 |
| | *** | 13613 | 13813 | 27050 | 3882 | 3913 | 7329 | 832 | 832 | 1432 | 282 | 282 | 456 | 163 | 163 | 241 |
| 0.1 | *** | 30063 | 30682 | 32563 | 8263 | 8413 | 8613 | 1582 | 1582 | 1613 | 482 | 482 | 482 | 263 | 263 | 263 |
| | *** | 30313 | 31332 | 48918 | 8332 | 8513 | 12731 | 1582 | 1582 | 2265 | 482 | 482 | 651 | 263 | 263 | 322 |
| 0.15 | *** | 45113 | 46432 | 51463 | 12382 | 12732 | 13313 | 2313 | 2332 | 2363 | 663 | 682 | 682 | 332 | 332 | 332 |
| | *** | 45613 | 47963 | 68183 | 12532 | 12982 | 17482 | 2313 | 2332 | 2994 | 663 | 682 | 821 | 332 | 332 | 391 |
| 0.2 | *** | 57513 | 59632 | 69132 | 15913 | 16532 | 17713 | 2932 | 2982 | 3032 | 832 | 832 | 832 | 413 | 413 | 413 |
| | *** | 58313 | 62282 | 84845 | 16182 | 17032 | 21583 | 2963 | 3013 | 3619 | 832 | 832 | 964 | 413 | 413 | 449 |
| 0.25 | *** | 66932 | 70013 | 84863 | 18732 | 19713 | 21582 | 3482 | 3563 | 3632 | 963 | 963 | 982 | 463 | 463 | 463 |
| | *** | 68063 | 73932 | 98903 | 19163 | 20482 | 25032 | 3513 | 3582 | 4140 | 963 | 982 | 1081 | 463 | 463 | 495 |
| 0.3 | *** | 73382 | 77563 | 98282 | 20913 | 22232 | 24882 | 3932 | 4013 | 4132 | 1082 | 1082 | 1082 | 513 | 513 | 513 |
| | *** | 74913 | 82832 | 110358 | 21482 | 23282 | 27831 | 3982 | 4063 | 4556 | 1082 | 1082 | 1172 | 513 | 513 | 530 |
| 0.35 | *** | 77113 | 82482 | 109113 | 22413 | 24082 | 27513 | 4263 | 4382 | 4513 | 1163 | 1163 | 1182 | 532 | 532 | 532 |
| | *** | 79113 | 89163 | 119210 | 23132 | 25432 | 29979 | 4313 | 4432 | 4869 | 1163 | 1163 | 1237 | 532 | 532 | 553 |
| 0.4 | *** | 78482 | 85082 | 117282 | 23363 | 25332 | 29482 | 4513 | 4632 | 4813 | 1213 | 1213 | 1232 | 563 | 563 | 563 |
| | *** | 80963 | 93113 | 125458 | 24213 | 26932 | 31475 | 4563 | 4713 | 5077 | 1213 | 1232 | 1276 | 563 | 563 | 565 |
| 0.45 | *** | 77863 | 85682 | 122663 | 23763 | 26013 | 30763 | 4632 | 4782 | 4963 | 1232 | 1232 | 1263 | 563 | 563 | 563 |
| | *** | 80832 | 94913 | 129102 | 24732 | 27832 | 32322 | 4713 | 4863 | 5181 | 1232 | 1263 | 1289 | 563 | 563 | 565 |
| 0.5 | *** | 75663 | 84582 | 125213 | 23682 | 26132 | 31332 | 4663 | 4832 | 5032 | 1232 | 1232 | 1263 | 563 | 563 | 563 |
| | *** | 79113 | 94813 | 130144 | 24732 | 28132 | 32517 | 4732 | 4913 | 5181 | 1232 | 1263 | 1276 | 563 | 563 | 553 |
| 0.55 | *** | 72213 | 82032 | 124963 | 23182 | 25763 | 31213 | 4582 | 4763 | 4963 | 1213 | 1213 | 1232 | 532 | 532 | 532 |
| | *** | 76063 | 92982 | 128582 | 24313 | 27863 | 32061 | 4682 | 4863 | 5077 | 1213 | 1232 | 1237 | 532 | 532 | 530 |
| 0.6 | *** | 67832 | 78282 | 121863 | 22282 | 24932 | 30363 | 4432 | 4613 | 4813 | 1163 | 1163 | 1182 | 513 | 513 | 513 |
| | *** | 71963 | 89582 | 124416 | 23432 | 27013 | 30955 | 4513 | 4682 | 4869 | 1163 | 1163 | 1172 | 513 | 513 | 495 |
| 0.65 | *** | 62763 | 73432 | 115932 | 21032 | 23613 | 28813 | 4182 | 4332 | 4513 | 1063 | 1082 | 1082 | 463 | 463 | 463 |
| | *** | 67032 | 84732 | 117648 | 22163 | 25632 | 29197 | 4263 | 4413 | 4556 | 1082 | 1082 | 1081 | 463 | 463 | 449 |
| 0.7 | *** | 57082 | 67632 | 107213 | 19432 | 21863 | 26563 | 3832 | 3963 | 4132 | 963 | 963 | 982 | 413 | 413 | 413 |
| | *** | 61332 | 78463 | 108275 | 20482 | 23713 | 26789 | 3882 | 4032 | 4140 | 963 | 982 | 964 | 413 | 413 | 391 |
| 0.75 | *** | 50882 | 60813 | 95682 | 17482 | 19613 | 23613 | 3382 | 3482 | 3632 | 832 | 832 | 832 | 332 | 332 | 332 |
| | *** | 54932 | 70732 | 96300 | 18413 | 21213 | 23730 | 3432 | 3563 | 3619 | 832 | 832 | 821 | 332 | 332 | 322 |
| 0.8 | *** | 44082 | 52913 | 81432 | 15113 | 16863 | 19963 | 2832 | 2913 | 3013 | 663 | 663 | 682 | 263 | 263 | 263 |
| | *** | 47713 | 61432 | 81721 | 15882 | 18163 | 20021 | 2863 | 2963 | 2994 | 663 | 663 | 651 | 263 | 263 | 241 |
| 0.85 | *** | 36463 | 43632 | 64432 | 12263 | 13563 | 15663 | 2182 | 2232 | 2282 | 482 | 482 | 482 | . | . | . |
| | *** | 39463 | 50282 | 64538 | 12863 | 14463 | 15660 | 2213 | 2263 | 2265 | 482 | 482 | 456 | . | . | . |
| 0.9 | *** | 27532 | 32513 | 44732 | 8832 | 9582 | 10663 | 1413 | 1432 | 1463 | . | . | . | . | . | . |
| | *** | 29632 | 36813 | 44753 | 9182 | 10063 | 10648 | 1413 | 1432 | 1432 | . | . | . | . | . | . |
| 0.95 | *** | 16113 | 18313 | 22382 | 4513 | 4732 | 5013 | . | . | . | . | . | . | . | . | . |
| | *** | 17082 | 19963 | 22364 | 4613 | 4863 | 4986 | . | . | . | . | . | . | . | . | . |
| 0.98 | *** | 6613 | 7082 | 7713 | . | . | . | . | . | . | . | . | . | . | . | . |
| | *** | 6832 | 7363 | 7680 | . | . | . | . | . | . | . | . | . | . | . | . |

TABLE 4: ALPHA= 0.01  POWER= 0.9    EXPECTED ACCRUAL THRU MINIMUM FOLLOW-UP= 25000

| | DEL=.01 | | | DEL=.02 | | | DEL=.05 | | | DEL=.10 | | | DEL=.15 | | |
|---|---|---|---|---|---|---|---|---|---|---|---|---|---|---|---|
| FACT= | 1.0 .75 | .50 .25 | .00 BIN | 1.0 .75 | .50 .25 | .00 BIN | 1.0 .75 | .50 .25 | .00 BIN | 1.0 75 | .50 .25 | .00 BIN | 1.0 .75 | .50 .25 | .00 BIN |

PCONT=***                    REQUIRED NUMBER OF PATIENTS

| PCONT | 1.0/.75 | .50/.25 | .00/BIN | 1.0/.75 | .50/.25 | .00/BIN | 1.0/.75 | .50/.25 | .00/BIN | 1.0/.75 | .50/.25 | .00/BIN | 1.0/.75 | .50/.25 | .00/BIN |
|---|---|---|---|---|---|---|---|---|---|---|---|---|---|---|---|
| 0.01 *** | 2016 | 2016 | 2016 | 727 | 727 | 727 | 227 | 227 | 227 | 102 | 102 | 102 | 79 | 79 | 79 |
| *** | 2016 | 2016 | 7680 | 727 | 727 | 2539 | 227 | 227 | 691 | 102 | 102 | 281 | 79 | 79 | 167 |
| 0.02 *** | 4454 | 4454 | 4477 | 1415 | 1415 | 1415 | 391 | 391 | 391 | 165 | 165 | 165 | 102 | 102 | 102 |
| *** | 4454 | 4477 | 12679 | 1415 | 1415 | 3775 | 391 | 391 | 883 | 165 | 165 | 326 | 102 | 102 | 186 |
| 0.05 *** | 13602 | 13727 | 13977 | 3852 | 3891 | 3915 | 829 | 829 | 829 | 290 | 290 | 290 | 165 | 165 | 165 |
| *** | 13665 | 13852 | 27050 | 3891 | 3915 | 7329 | 829 | 829 | 1432 | 290 | 290 | 456 | 165 | 165 | 241 |
| 0.1 *** | 30227 | 30891 | 32579 | 8329 | 8454 | 8602 | 1579 | 1602 | 1602 | 477 | 477 | 477 | 266 | 266 | 266 |
| *** | 30516 | 31516 | 48918 | 8391 | 8516 | 12731 | 1579 | 1602 | 2265 | 477 | 477 | 651 | 266 | 266 | 322 |
| 0.15 *** | 45477 | 46915 | 51454 | 12516 | 12829 | 13329 | 2329 | 2329 | 2352 | 665 | 665 | 665 | 329 | 329 | 329 |
| *** | 46040 | 48415 | 68183 | 12641 | 13040 | 17482 | 2329 | 2329 | 2994 | 665 | 665 | 821 | 329 | 329 | 391 |
| 0.2 *** | 58102 | 60477 | 69141 | 16102 | 16727 | 17704 | 2954 | 2977 | 3040 | 829 | 829 | 829 | 415 | 415 | 415 |
| *** | 59016 | 63141 | 84845 | 16391 | 17141 | 21583 | 2977 | 3016 | 3619 | 829 | 829 | 964 | 415 | 415 | 449 |
| 0.25 *** | 67790 | 71227 | 84852 | 19079 | 19977 | 21579 | 3516 | 3579 | 3641 | 977 | 977 | 977 | 454 | 454 | 454 |
| *** | 69079 | 75204 | 98903 | 19477 | 20665 | 25032 | 3540 | 3602 | 4140 | 977 | 977 | 1081 | 454 | 454 | 495 |
| 0.3 *** | 74540 | 79204 | 98266 | 21352 | 22602 | 24891 | 3954 | 4040 | 4141 | 1079 | 1079 | 1079 | 516 | 516 | 516 |
| *** | 76290 | 84579 | 110358 | 21891 | 23540 | 27831 | 4016 | 4079 | 4556 | 1079 | 1079 | 1172 | 516 | 516 | 530 |
| 0.35 *** | 78641 | 84540 | 109102 | 22977 | 24579 | 27516 | 4329 | 4415 | 4516 | 1165 | 1165 | 1165 | 540 | 540 | 540 |
| *** | 80891 | 91352 | 119210 | 23665 | 25766 | 29979 | 4352 | 4454 | 4869 | 1165 | 1165 | 1237 | 540 | 540 | 553 |
| 0.4 *** | 80391 | 87579 | 117266 | 24016 | 25915 | 29477 | 4540 | 4665 | 4790 | 1204 | 1227 | 1227 | 540 | 540 | 579 |
| *** | 83141 | 95727 | 125458 | 24852 | 27352 | 31475 | 4602 | 4727 | 5077 | 1227 | 1227 | 1276 | 540 | 540 | 565 |
| 0.45 *** | 80141 | 88579 | 122665 | 24516 | 26665 | 30766 | 4704 | 4829 | 4977 | 1227 | 1266 | 1266 | 579 | 579 | 579 |
| *** | 83415 | 97891 | 129102 | 25454 | 28290 | 32322 | 4766 | 4891 | 5181 | 1227 | 1266 | 1289 | 579 | 579 | 565 |
| 0.5 *** | 78290 | 87829 | 125227 | 24516 | 26852 | 31329 | 4727 | 4852 | 5016 | 1227 | 1266 | 1266 | 540 | 540 | 579 |
| *** | 82040 | 98079 | 130144 | 25540 | 28641 | 32517 | 4790 | 4954 | 5181 | 1227 | 1266 | 1276 | 540 | 579 | 553 |
| 0.55 *** | 75165 | 85516 | 124954 | 24040 | 26516 | 31204 | 4665 | 4790 | 4977 | 1204 | 1227 | 1227 | 540 | 540 | 540 |
| *** | 79290 | 96454 | 128582 | 25141 | 28391 | 32061 | 4727 | 4891 | 5077 | 1227 | 1227 | 1237 | 540 | 540 | 530 |
| 0.6 *** | 71016 | 81891 | 121852 | 23165 | 25665 | 30352 | 4477 | 4641 | 4790 | 1165 | 1165 | 1165 | 516 | 516 | 516 |
| *** | 75391 | 93141 | 124416 | 24266 | 27540 | 30955 | 4579 | 4727 | 4869 | 1165 | 1165 | 1172 | 516 | 516 | 495 |
| 0.65 *** | 66040 | 77079 | 115915 | 21915 | 24329 | 28790 | 4227 | 4352 | 4516 | 1079 | 1079 | 1102 | 454 | 454 | 477 |
| *** | 70516 | 88227 | 117648 | 22977 | 26141 | 29197 | 4290 | 4454 | 4556 | 1079 | 1079 | 1081 | 454 | 477 | 449 |
| 0.7 *** | 60352 | 71141 | 107204 | 20266 | 22516 | 26540 | 3891 | 3977 | 4141 | 954 | 977 | 977 | 415 | 415 | 415 |
| *** | 64766 | 81766 | 108275 | 21266 | 24165 | 26789 | 3915 | 4040 | 4140 | 977 | 977 | 964 | 415 | 415 | 391 |
| 0.75 *** | 54016 | 64079 | 95704 | 18204 | 20204 | 23602 | 3415 | 3516 | 3641 | 829 | 829 | 829 | 352 | 352 | 352 |
| *** | 58141 | 73704 | 96300 | 19102 | 21602 | 23730 | 3454 | 3579 | 3619 | 829 | 829 | 821 | 352 | 352 | 322 |
| 0.8 *** | 46891 | 55727 | 81415 | 15727 | 17329 | 19977 | 2852 | 2915 | 3016 | 665 | 665 | 665 | 266 | 266 | 266 |
| *** | 50579 | 63954 | 81721 | 16454 | 18454 | 20021 | 2891 | 2977 | 2994 | 665 | 665 | 651 | 266 | 266 | 241 |
| 0.85 *** | 38766 | 45891 | 64415 | 12727 | 13891 | 15641 | 2204 | 2227 | 2290 | 477 | 477 | 477 | . | . | . |
| *** | 41766 | 52204 | 64538 | 13266 | 14665 | 15660 | 2227 | 2266 | 2265 | 477 | 477 | 456 | . | . | . |
| 0.9 *** | 29165 | 33977 | 44727 | 9102 | 9766 | 10665 | 1415 | 1415 | 1454 | . | . | . | . | . | . |
| *** | 31227 | 37977 | 44753 | 9415 | 10165 | 10648 | 1415 | 1454 | 1432 | . | . | . | . | . | . |
| 0.95 *** | 16891 | 18915 | 22391 | 4602 | 4790 | 5016 | . | . | . | . | . | . | . | . | . |
| *** | 17790 | 20352 | 22364 | 4704 | 4891 | 4986 | . | . | . | . | . | . | . | . | . |
| 0.98 *** | 6790 | 7204 | 7704 | . | . | . | . | . | . | . | . | . | . | . | . |
| *** | 6977 | 7415 | 7680 | . | . | . | . | . | . | . | . | . | . | . | . |

TABLE 5: ALPHA= 0.025 POWER= 0.8    EXPECTED ACCRUAL THRU MINIMUM FOLLOW-UP= 30

| | | DEL=.10 | | | DEL=.15 | | | DEL=.20 | | | DEL=.25 | | | DEL=.30 | | |
|---|---|---|---|---|---|---|---|---|---|---|---|---|---|---|---|---|---|
| FACT= | | 1.0 .75 | .50 .25 | .00 BIN | 1.0 .75 | .50 .25 | .00 BIN | 1.0 .75 | .50 .25 | .00 BIN | 1.0 75 | .50 .25 | .00 BIN | 1.0 .75 | .50 .25 | .00 BIN |
| PCONT=*** | | | | | REQUIRED NUMBER OF PATIENTS | | | | | | | | | | | |
| 0.05 | *** | 165 | 166 | 178 | 96 | 97 | 104 | 68 | 69 | 73 | 53 | 54 | 57 | 44 | 45 | 47 |
| | *** | 165 | 168 | 275 | 97 | 99 | 145 | 68 | 70 | 93 | 53 | 55 | 65 | 44 | 45 | 48 |
| 0.1 | *** | 260 | 263 | 299 | 138 | 140 | 159 | 91 | 93 | 104 | 67 | 69 | 76 | 53 | 55 | 60 |
| | *** | 261 | 267 | 393 | 139 | 144 | 194 | 92 | 96 | 118 | 68 | 71 | 80 | 54 | 57 | 58 |
| 0.15 | *** | 336 | 339 | 409 | 169 | 173 | 206 | 107 | 111 | 130 | 77 | 80 | 92 | 60 | 63 | 71 |
| | *** | 337 | 346 | 495 | 171 | 179 | 236 | 109 | 116 | 140 | 78 | 84 | 93 | 61 | 65 | 66 |
| 0.2 | *** | 391 | 396 | 507 | 191 | 197 | 248 | 119 | 124 | 152 | 84 | 88 | 105 | 64 | 68 | 79 |
| | *** | 393 | 406 | 581 | 193 | 206 | 271 | 120 | 131 | 157 | 85 | 93 | 103 | 65 | 71 | 72 |
| 0.25 | *** | 427 | 434 | 591 | 205 | 212 | 282 | 125 | 132 | 170 | 87 | 93 | 116 | 66 | 71 | 85 |
| | *** | 429 | 448 | 652 | 207 | 224 | 299 | 128 | 141 | 171 | 90 | 100 | 110 | 68 | 75 | 76 |
| 0.3 | *** | 444 | 454 | 659 | 210 | 220 | 309 | 128 | 136 | 183 | 89 | 96 | 123 | 67 | 72 | 89 |
| | *** | 447 | 472 | 707 | 214 | 236 | 320 | 131 | 147 | 181 | 91 | 103 | 115 | 69 | 78 | 79 |
| 0.35 | *** | 445 | 458 | 710 | 209 | 222 | 328 | 127 | 137 | 192 | 88 | 96 | 127 | 66 | 72 | 92 |
| | *** | 450 | 482 | 746 | 214 | 241 | 334 | 131 | 150 | 187 | 91 | 105 | 118 | 69 | 79 | 80 |
| 0.4 | *** | 433 | 449 | 745 | 203 | 219 | 340 | 123 | 136 | 196 | 85 | 95 | 129 | 64 | 71 | 92 |
| | *** | 438 | 479 | 770 | 209 | 241 | 341 | 128 | 150 | 189 | 89 | 105 | 118 | 67 | 78 | 79 |
| 0.45 | *** | 409 | 430 | 762 | 193 | 211 | 344 | 118 | 132 | 197 | 82 | 92 | 128 | 61 | 69 | 90 |
| | *** | 416 | 466 | 778 | 200 | 237 | 341 | 123 | 148 | 187 | 86 | 102 | 115 | 64 | 76 | 76 |
| 0.5 | *** | 377 | 403 | 762 | 180 | 201 | 341 | 111 | 126 | 193 | 77 | 88 | 124 | 58 | 65 | 86 |
| | *** | 386 | 446 | 770 | 188 | 228 | 334 | 117 | 143 | 181 | 82 | 99 | 110 | 61 | 72 | 72 |
| 0.55 | *** | 340 | 371 | 745 | 165 | 188 | 329 | 103 | 118 | 184 | 72 | 82 | 117 | 54 | 61 | 81 |
| | *** | 351 | 419 | 746 | 174 | 217 | 320 | 109 | 135 | 171 | 76 | 93 | 103 | 57 | 68 | 66 |
| 0.6 | *** | 300 | 336 | 712 | 149 | 174 | 311 | 94 | 109 | 171 | 66 | 76 | 108 | 49 | 56 | 73 |
| | *** | 313 | 388 | 707 | 159 | 202 | 299 | 100 | 126 | 157 | 70 | 86 | 93 | 52 | 62 | 58 |
| 0.65 | *** | 260 | 300 | 661 | 133 | 157 | 284 | 84 | 99 | 155 | 59 | 68 | 96 | 43 | 49 | 64 |
| | *** | 275 | 354 | 652 | 142 | 185 | 271 | 90 | 114 | 140 | 63 | 77 | 80 | 46 | 55 | 48 |
| 0.7 | *** | 221 | 263 | 593 | 116 | 139 | 250 | 73 | 87 | 133 | 51 | 59 | 81 | . | . | . |
| | *** | 237 | 317 | 581 | 125 | 165 | 236 | 79 | 101 | 118 | 54 | 66 | 65 | . | . | . |
| 0.75 | *** | 185 | 226 | 509 | 99 | 120 | 209 | 62 | 73 | 108 | . | . | . | . | . | . |
| | *** | 201 | 276 | 495 | 107 | 142 | 194 | 66 | 84 | 93 | . | . | . | . | . | . |
| 0.8 | *** | 151 | 187 | 408 | 80 | 97 | 161 | . | . | . | . | . | . | . | . | . |
| | *** | 165 | 230 | 393 | 87 | 115 | 145 | . | . | . | . | . | . | . | . | . |
| 0.85 | *** | 116 | 145 | 291 | . | . | . | . | . | . | . | . | . | . | . | . |
| | *** | 127 | 177 | 275 | . | . | . | . | . | . | . | . | . | . | . | . |

TABLE 5: ALPHA= 0.025 POWER= 0.8    EXPECTED ACCRUAL THRU MINIMUM FOLLOW-UP= 40

| PCONT | | DEL=.10 | | | DEL=.15 | | | DEL=.20 | | | DEL=.25 | | | DEL=.30 | | |
|---|---|---|---|---|---|---|---|---|---|---|---|---|---|---|---|---|
| FACT= | | 1.0 .75 | .50 .25 | .00 BIN | 1.0 .75 | .50 .25 | .00 BIN | 1.0 .75 | .50 .25 | .00 BIN | 1.0 75 | .50 .25 | .00 BIN | 1.0 .75 | .50 .25 | .00 BIN |
| PCONT=*** | | | | | REQUIRED NUMBER OF PATIENTS | | | | | | | | | | | |
| 0.05 | *** | 165 | 167 | 178 | 97 | 98 | 104 | 68 | 70 | 73 | 53 | 54 | 57 | 44 | 45 | 47 |
| | *** | 166 | 169 | 275 | 97 | 100 | 145 | 69 | 71 | 93 | 54 | 55 | 65 | 44 | 46 | 48 |
| 0.1 | *** | 261 | 264 | 299 | 139 | 142 | 159 | 92 | 94 | 104 | 68 | 70 | 76 | 54 | 56 | 60 |
| | *** | 262 | 269 | 393 | 140 | 146 | 194 | 93 | 97 | 118 | 69 | 72 | 80 | 55 | 57 | 58 |
| 0.15 | *** | 337 | 342 | 409 | 171 | 175 | 207 | 109 | 113 | 130 | 78 | 82 | 92 | 61 | 64 | 71 |
| | *** | 339 | 350 | 495 | 172 | 182 | 236 | 110 | 118 | 140 | 80 | 85 | 93 | 62 | 66 | 66 |
| 0.2 | *** | 393 | 400 | 507 | 193 | 200 | 248 | 121 | 127 | 152 | 85 | 90 | 105 | 65 | 69 | 79 |
| | *** | 395 | 413 | 581 | 196 | 210 | 271 | 123 | 134 | 157 | 87 | 95 | 103 | 67 | 73 | 72 |
| 0.25 | *** | 429 | 439 | 591 | 207 | 217 | 282 | 128 | 136 | 170 | 90 | 96 | 116 | 68 | 73 | 85 |
| | *** | 432 | 457 | 652 | 210 | 230 | 299 | 131 | 145 | 171 | 92 | 102 | 110 | 70 | 77 | 76 |
| 0.3 | *** | 447 | 460 | 659 | 214 | 226 | 309 | 131 | 141 | 183 | 91 | 99 | 123 | 69 | 75 | 89 |
| | *** | 452 | 484 | 707 | 218 | 243 | 320 | 135 | 152 | 181 | 94 | 107 | 115 | 71 | 80 | 79 |
| 0.35 | *** | 450 | 466 | 710 | 214 | 229 | 328 | 131 | 143 | 192 | 91 | 100 | 127 | 69 | 75 | 92 |
| | *** | 455 | 496 | 746 | 219 | 250 | 334 | 135 | 156 | 187 | 95 | 109 | 118 | 71 | 81 | 80 |
| 0.4 | *** | 438 | 460 | 745 | 209 | 227 | 340 | 128 | 142 | 196 | 89 | 99 | 129 | 67 | 74 | 92 |
| | *** | 446 | 496 | 770 | 216 | 251 | 341 | 133 | 157 | 189 | 93 | 109 | 118 | 70 | 80 | 79 |
| 0.45 | *** | 416 | 443 | 762 | 200 | 221 | 344 | 123 | 138 | 197 | 86 | 96 | 128 | 64 | 72 | 90 |
| | *** | 425 | 486 | 778 | 208 | 248 | 341 | 129 | 154 | 187 | 90 | 106 | 115 | 68 | 78 | 76 |
| 0.5 | *** | 386 | 418 | 762 | 188 | 212 | 341 | 117 | 133 | 193 | 82 | 92 | 124 | 61 | 68 | 86 |
| | *** | 397 | 468 | 770 | 197 | 241 | 334 | 123 | 150 | 181 | 86 | 103 | 110 | 64 | 75 | 72 |
| 0.55 | *** | 351 | 389 | 746 | 174 | 200 | 329 | 109 | 125 | 184 | 76 | 87 | 117 | 57 | 64 | 81 |
| | *** | 364 | 444 | 746 | 184 | 230 | 320 | 116 | 142 | 171 | 81 | 97 | 103 | 60 | 70 | 66 |
| 0.6 | *** | 313 | 356 | 712 | 159 | 185 | 311 | 100 | 116 | 171 | 70 | 80 | 108 | 52 | 58 | 73 |
| | *** | 329 | 414 | 707 | 169 | 215 | 299 | 107 | 133 | 157 | 74 | 89 | 93 | 55 | 64 | 58 |
| 0.65 | *** | 275 | 321 | 661 | 142 | 169 | 284 | 90 | 105 | 155 | 63 | 72 | 96 | 46 | 52 | 64 |
| | *** | 292 | 380 | 652 | 153 | 197 | 271 | 96 | 120 | 140 | 66 | 80 | 80 | 48 | 56 | 48 |
| 0.7 | *** | 237 | 284 | 593 | 125 | 150 | 250 | 79 | 93 | 133 | 54 | 62 | 81 | . | . | . |
| | *** | 255 | 341 | 581 | 135 | 176 | 236 | 85 | 106 | 118 | 58 | 69 | 65 | . | . | . |
| 0.75 | *** | 201 | 246 | 509 | 107 | 129 | 209 | 67 | 78 | 108 | . | . | . | . | . | . |
| | *** | 219 | 298 | 495 | 116 | 151 | 194 | 71 | 88 | 93 | . | . | . | . | . | . |
| 0.8 | *** | 165 | 205 | 408 | 87 | 104 | 161 | . | . | . | . | . | . | . | . | . |
| | *** | 181 | 249 | 393 | 94 | 121 | 145 | . | . | . | . | . | . | . | . | . |
| 0.85 | *** | 127 | 158 | 291 | . | . | . | . | . | . | . | . | . | . | . | . |
| | *** | 140 | 191 | 275 | . | . | . | . | . | . | . | . | . | . | . | . |

## TABLE 5: ALPHA= 0.025 POWER= 0.8    EXPECTED ACCRUAL THRU MINIMUM FOLLOW-UP= 50

|  |  | DEL=.10 | | | DEL=.15 | | | DEL=.20 | | | DEL=.25 | | | DEL=.30 | | |
|---|---|---|---|---|---|---|---|---|---|---|---|---|---|---|---|---|
| FACT= | | 1.0 .75 | .50 .25 | .00 BIN | 1.0 .75 | .50 .25 | .00 BIN | 1.0 .75 | .50 .25 | .00 BIN | 1.0 75 | .50 .25 | .00 BIN | 1.0 .75 | .50 .25 | .00 BIN |
| PCONT=*** | | | | | REQUIRED NUMBER OF PATIENTS | | | | | | | | | | | |
| 0.05 | *** | 166 | 167 | 178 | 97 | 99 | 104 | 69 | 70 | 73 | 54 | 55 | 57 | 44 | 45 | 47 |
|  | *** | 166 | 170 | 275 | 98 | 100 | 145 | 69 | 71 | 93 | 54 | 55 | 65 | 45 | 46 | 48 |
| 0.1 | *** | 262 | 265 | 299 | 140 | 143 | 159 | 93 | 95 | 104 | 69 | 71 | 76 | 55 | 56 | 60 |
|  | *** | 263 | 271 | 393 | 141 | 147 | 194 | 94 | 98 | 118 | 70 | 73 | 80 | 55 | 58 | 58 |
| 0.15 | *** | 338 | 344 | 409 | 172 | 177 | 207 | 110 | 115 | 130 | 80 | 83 | 92 | 62 | 65 | 71 |
|  | *** | 340 | 354 | 495 | 174 | 185 | 236 | 112 | 120 | 140 | 81 | 86 | 93 | 63 | 67 | 66 |
| 0.2 | *** | 395 | 403 | 507 | 195 | 203 | 248 | 122 | 129 | 152 | 87 | 92 | 105 | 67 | 70 | 79 |
|  | *** | 398 | 418 | 581 | 198 | 214 | 271 | 125 | 136 | 157 | 89 | 97 | 103 | 68 | 74 | 72 |
| 0.25 | *** | 432 | 443 | 591 | 210 | 221 | 282 | 130 | 139 | 170 | 92 | 98 | 116 | 70 | 74 | 85 |
|  | *** | 436 | 464 | 652 | 214 | 235 | 299 | 133 | 148 | 171 | 94 | 104 | 110 | 72 | 78 | 76 |
| 0.3 | *** | 451 | 466 | 659 | 217 | 231 | 309 | 134 | 144 | 183 | 94 | 101 | 123 | 71 | 76 | 89 |
|  | *** | 456 | 494 | 707 | 222 | 250 | 320 | 138 | 156 | 181 | 97 | 109 | 115 | 73 | 81 | 79 |
| 0.35 | *** | 454 | 474 | 710 | 218 | 235 | 328 | 134 | 147 | 192 | 94 | 103 | 127 | 71 | 77 | 92 |
|  | *** | 461 | 509 | 746 | 225 | 257 | 334 | 139 | 160 | 187 | 98 | 111 | 118 | 73 | 82 | 80 |
| 0.4 | *** | 444 | 470 | 745 | 214 | 235 | 340 | 132 | 147 | 196 | 92 | 102 | 129 | 69 | 76 | 92 |
|  | *** | 453 | 511 | 770 | 222 | 260 | 341 | 138 | 161 | 189 | 96 | 111 | 118 | 72 | 82 | 79 |
| 0.45 | *** | 423 | 455 | 762 | 206 | 230 | 344 | 128 | 144 | 197 | 89 | 100 | 128 | 67 | 74 | 90 |
|  | *** | 434 | 504 | 778 | 215 | 257 | 341 | 134 | 159 | 187 | 94 | 109 | 115 | 70 | 80 | 76 |
| 0.5 | *** | 395 | 433 | 762 | 195 | 221 | 341 | 122 | 138 | 193 | 85 | 96 | 124 | 63 | 71 | 86 |
|  | *** | 408 | 487 | 770 | 205 | 250 | 334 | 128 | 155 | 181 | 90 | 105 | 110 | 67 | 77 | 72 |
| 0.55 | *** | 361 | 405 | 746 | 182 | 209 | 329 | 114 | 131 | 184 | 80 | 90 | 117 | 59 | 66 | 81 |
|  | *** | 377 | 464 | 746 | 192 | 239 | 320 | 121 | 147 | 171 | 84 | 100 | 103 | 62 | 72 | 66 |
| 0.6 | *** | 325 | 373 | 712 | 167 | 195 | 311 | 105 | 122 | 171 | 73 | 83 | 108 | 54 | 60 | 73 |
|  | *** | 343 | 435 | 707 | 178 | 225 | 299 | 112 | 137 | 157 | 77 | 92 | 93 | 57 | 65 | 58 |
| 0.65 | *** | 288 | 339 | 661 | 150 | 178 | 284 | 95 | 110 | 155 | 66 | 75 | 96 | 48 | 53 | 64 |
|  | *** | 307 | 400 | 652 | 161 | 206 | 271 | 101 | 125 | 140 | 70 | 82 | 80 | 50 | 58 | 48 |
| 0.7 | *** | 251 | 302 | 593 | 133 | 158 | 250 | 83 | 97 | 133 | 57 | 65 | 81 | . | . | . |
|  | *** | 271 | 361 | 581 | 143 | 184 | 236 | 89 | 109 | 118 | 60 | 71 | 65 | . | . | . |
| 0.75 | *** | 215 | 262 | 509 | 114 | 136 | 209 | 70 | 81 | 108 | . | . | . | . | . | . |
|  | *** | 233 | 315 | 495 | 123 | 158 | 194 | 75 | 91 | 93 | . | . | . | . | . | . |
| 0.8 | *** | 177 | 218 | 408 | 92 | 110 | 161 | . | . | . | . | . | . | . | . | . |
|  | *** | 194 | 263 | 393 | 100 | 126 | 145 | . | . | . | . | . | . | . | . | . |
| 0.85 | *** | 137 | 169 | 291 | . | . | . | . | . | . | . | . | . | . | . | . |
|  | *** | 150 | 201 | 275 | . | . | . | . | . | . | . | . | . | . | . | . |

TABLE 5: ALPHA= 0.025 POWER= 0.8    EXPECTED ACCRUAL THRU MINIMUM FOLLOW-UP= 60

| | | DEL=.10 | | | DEL=.15 | | | DEL=.20 | | | DEL=.25 | | | DEL=.30 | | |
|---|---|---|---|---|---|---|---|---|---|---|---|---|---|---|---|---|
| FACT= | | 1.0 .75 | .50 .25 | .00 BIN | 1.0 .75 | .50 .25 | .00 BIN | 1.0 .75 | .50 .25 | .00 BIN | 1.0 75 | .50 .25 | .00 BIN | 1.0 .75 | .50 .25 | .00 BIN |
| PCONT=*** | | REQUIRED NUMBER OF PATIENTS | | | | | | | | | | | | | | |
| 0.05 | *** | 166 | 168 | 178 | 97 | 99 | 104 | 69 | 70 | 73 | 54 | 55 | 57 | 44 | 45 | 47 |
| | *** | 167 | 171 | 275 | 98 | 101 | 145 | 70 | 71 | 93 | 54 | 56 | 65 | 45 | 46 | 48 |
| 0.1 | *** | 263 | 267 | 299 | 140 | 144 | 159 | 93 | 96 | 104 | 69 | 71 | 76 | 55 | 57 | 60 |
| | *** | 264 | 273 | 393 | 142 | 148 | 194 | 94 | 99 | 118 | 70 | 73 | 80 | 56 | 58 | 58 |
| 0.15 | *** | 340 | 346 | 409 | 173 | 179 | 206 | 111 | 116 | 130 | 80 | 84 | 92 | 63 | 65 | 71 |
| | *** | 342 | 358 | 495 | 175 | 187 | 236 | 113 | 121 | 140 | 82 | 87 | 93 | 64 | 67 | 66 |
| 0.2 | *** | 396 | 406 | 507 | 197 | 206 | 248 | 124 | 131 | 152 | 88 | 93 | 105 | 68 | 71 | 79 |
| | *** | 400 | 423 | 581 | 200 | 217 | 271 | 127 | 138 | 157 | 90 | 98 | 103 | 69 | 74 | 72 |
| 0.25 | *** | 434 | 448 | 591 | 212 | 224 | 282 | 132 | 141 | 170 | 93 | 100 | 116 | 71 | 75 | 85 |
| | *** | 439 | 471 | 652 | 217 | 239 | 299 | 136 | 150 | 171 | 96 | 105 | 110 | 73 | 79 | 76 |
| 0.3 | *** | 454 | 472 | 659 | 220 | 236 | 309 | 136 | 148 | 183 | 96 | 103 | 123 | 72 | 78 | 89 |
| | *** | 460 | 503 | 707 | 226 | 255 | 320 | 141 | 159 | 181 | 99 | 110 | 115 | 75 | 82 | 79 |
| 0.35 | *** | 458 | 482 | 710 | 222 | 241 | 328 | 137 | 151 | 192 | 96 | 105 | 127 | 72 | 79 | 92 |
| | *** | 466 | 520 | 746 | 229 | 263 | 334 | 143 | 164 | 187 | 100 | 113 | 118 | 75 | 84 | 80 |
| 0.4 | *** | 449 | 479 | 745 | 219 | 241 | 340 | 136 | 150 | 196 | 95 | 105 | 129 | 71 | 78 | 92 |
| | *** | 460 | 525 | 770 | 227 | 267 | 341 | 142 | 165 | 189 | 99 | 113 | 118 | 74 | 83 | 79 |
| 0.45 | *** | 430 | 466 | 762 | 211 | 237 | 344 | 132 | 148 | 197 | 92 | 102 | 128 | 69 | 76 | 90 |
| | *** | 443 | 519 | 778 | 221 | 265 | 341 | 138 | 163 | 187 | 96 | 112 | 115 | 72 | 81 | 76 |
| 0.5 | *** | 403 | 446 | 762 | 201 | 228 | 341 | 126 | 143 | 193 | 88 | 99 | 124 | 65 | 72 | 86 |
| | *** | 418 | 504 | 770 | 212 | 258 | 334 | 133 | 159 | 181 | 92 | 108 | 110 | 68 | 78 | 72 |
| 0.55 | *** | 371 | 419 | 745 | 188 | 217 | 329 | 118 | 135 | 184 | 82 | 93 | 117 | 61 | 68 | 81 |
| | *** | 389 | 481 | 746 | 200 | 247 | 320 | 125 | 151 | 171 | 87 | 102 | 103 | 64 | 73 | 66 |
| 0.6 | *** | 336 | 388 | 712 | 174 | 202 | 311 | 109 | 126 | 171 | 76 | 86 | 108 | 56 | 62 | 73 |
| | *** | 356 | 452 | 707 | 185 | 232 | 299 | 116 | 141 | 157 | 80 | 94 | 93 | 58 | 66 | 58 |
| 0.65 | *** | 300 | 354 | 661 | 157 | 185 | 284 | 99 | 114 | 155 | 68 | 77 | 96 | 49 | 55 | 64 |
| | *** | 321 | 418 | 652 | 169 | 214 | 271 | 105 | 128 | 140 | 72 | 84 | 80 | 52 | 58 | 48 |
| 0.7 | *** | 263 | 317 | 593 | 139 | 165 | 250 | 87 | 101 | 133 | 59 | 66 | 81 | . | . | . |
| | *** | 284 | 377 | 581 | 150 | 191 | 236 | 93 | 112 | 118 | 62 | 72 | 65 | . | . | . |
| 0.75 | *** | 226 | 276 | 509 | 120 | 142 | 209 | 73 | 84 | 108 | . | . | . | . | . | . |
| | *** | 246 | 330 | 495 | 129 | 163 | 194 | 78 | 93 | 93 | . | . | . | . | . | . |
| 0.8 | *** | 187 | 230 | 408 | 97 | 115 | 161 | . | . | . | . | . | . | . | . | . |
| | *** | 205 | 275 | 393 | 104 | 130 | 145 | . | . | . | . | . | . | . | . | . |
| 0.85 | *** | 145 | 177 | 291 | . | . | . | . | . | . | . | . | . | . | . | . |
| | *** | 158 | 209 | 275 | . | . | . | . | . | . | . | . | . | . | . | . |

TABLE 5: ALPHA= 0.025 POWER= 0.8     EXPECTED ACCRUAL THRU MINIMUM FOLLOW-UP= 70

|  |  | DEL=.10 | | | DEL=.15 | | | DEL=.20 | | | DEL=.25 | | | DEL=.30 | | |
|---|---|---|---|---|---|---|---|---|---|---|---|---|---|---|---|---|
| FACT= | | 1.0 .75 | .50 .25 | .00 BIN | 1.0 .75 | .50 .25 | .00 BIN | 1.0 .75 | .50 .25 | .00 BIN | 1.0 75 | .50 .25 | .00 BIN | 1.0 .75 | .50 .25 | .00 BIN |
| PCONT=*** | | REQUIRED NUMBER OF PATIENTS | | | | | | | | | | | | | | |
| 0.05 | *** | 166 | 169 | 178 | 98 | 99 | 104 | 69 | 71 | 73 | 54 | 55 | 57 | 45 | 45 | 47 |
|  | *** | 167 | 171 | 275 | 98 | 101 | 145 | 70 | 72 | 93 | 54 | 56 | 65 | 45 | 46 | 48 |
| 0.1 | *** | 263 | 268 | 299 | 141 | 145 | 159 | 94 | 97 | 104 | 70 | 72 | 76 | 55 | 57 | 60 |
|  | *** | 265 | 275 | 393 | 143 | 149 | 194 | 95 | 99 | 118 | 71 | 74 | 80 | 56 | 58 | 58 |
| 0.15 | *** | 341 | 348 | 409 | 174 | 181 | 206 | 112 | 117 | 130 | 81 | 85 | 92 | 63 | 66 | 71 |
|  | *** | 343 | 361 | 495 | 177 | 189 | 236 | 114 | 122 | 140 | 83 | 88 | 93 | 64 | 68 | 66 |
| 0.2 | *** | 398 | 410 | 507 | 198 | 208 | 248 | 125 | 132 | 152 | 89 | 94 | 105 | 68 | 72 | 79 |
|  | *** | 402 | 428 | 581 | 202 | 220 | 271 | 128 | 139 | 157 | 91 | 99 | 103 | 70 | 75 | 72 |
| 0.25 | *** | 436 | 452 | 591 | 214 | 227 | 282 | 134 | 143 | 170 | 95 | 101 | 116 | 72 | 76 | 85 |
|  | *** | 442 | 478 | 652 | 219 | 243 | 299 | 138 | 152 | 171 | 97 | 106 | 110 | 74 | 80 | 76 |
| 0.3 | *** | 457 | 478 | 659 | 223 | 240 | 309 | 139 | 150 | 183 | 97 | 105 | 123 | 74 | 79 | 89 |
|  | *** | 464 | 511 | 707 | 229 | 259 | 320 | 143 | 161 | 181 | 101 | 112 | 115 | 76 | 83 | 79 |
| 0.35 | *** | 462 | 489 | 710 | 226 | 246 | 328 | 140 | 153 | 192 | 98 | 107 | 127 | 74 | 80 | 92 |
|  | *** | 472 | 530 | 746 | 233 | 268 | 334 | 146 | 166 | 187 | 102 | 115 | 118 | 76 | 84 | 80 |
| 0.4 | *** | 454 | 488 | 745 | 223 | 247 | 340 | 139 | 154 | 196 | 97 | 107 | 129 | 73 | 79 | 92 |
|  | *** | 466 | 536 | 770 | 232 | 272 | 341 | 145 | 168 | 189 | 101 | 115 | 118 | 75 | 84 | 79 |
| 0.45 | *** | 436 | 477 | 762 | 217 | 243 | 344 | 135 | 151 | 197 | 94 | 105 | 128 | 70 | 77 | 90 |
|  | *** | 451 | 532 | 778 | 227 | 271 | 341 | 142 | 166 | 187 | 99 | 113 | 115 | 73 | 82 | 76 |
| 0.5 | *** | 411 | 457 | 762 | 207 | 235 | 341 | 130 | 146 | 193 | 90 | 101 | 124 | 67 | 74 | 86 |
|  | *** | 428 | 518 | 770 | 218 | 264 | 334 | 137 | 162 | 181 | 95 | 109 | 110 | 70 | 79 | 72 |
| 0.55 | *** | 380 | 432 | 745 | 194 | 224 | 329 | 122 | 139 | 184 | 85 | 95 | 117 | 63 | 69 | 81 |
|  | *** | 400 | 496 | 746 | 206 | 254 | 320 | 129 | 154 | 171 | 89 | 103 | 103 | 65 | 74 | 66 |
| 0.6 | *** | 346 | 402 | 712 | 180 | 209 | 311 | 113 | 130 | 171 | 78 | 88 | 108 | 57 | 63 | 73 |
|  | *** | 368 | 468 | 707 | 192 | 239 | 299 | 120 | 144 | 157 | 82 | 95 | 93 | 60 | 67 | 58 |
| 0.65 | *** | 311 | 368 | 661 | 163 | 192 | 284 | 102 | 118 | 155 | 70 | 79 | 96 | 51 | 56 | 64 |
|  | *** | 333 | 432 | 652 | 175 | 219 | 271 | 109 | 131 | 140 | 74 | 85 | 80 | 53 | 59 | 48 |
| 0.7 | *** | 274 | 330 | 593 | 145 | 171 | 250 | 90 | 103 | 133 | 61 | 68 | 81 | . | . | . |
|  | *** | 296 | 391 | 581 | 156 | 196 | 236 | 96 | 114 | 118 | 64 | 73 | 65 | . | . | . |
| 0.75 | *** | 237 | 287 | 509 | 125 | 147 | 209 | 76 | 86 | 108 | . | . | . | . | . | . |
|  | *** | 257 | 342 | 495 | 134 | 167 | 194 | 80 | 95 | 93 | . | . | . | . | . | . |
| 0.8 | *** | 197 | 240 | 408 | 101 | 118 | 161 | . | . | . | . | . | . | . | . | . |
|  | *** | 214 | 285 | 393 | 108 | 133 | 145 | . | . | . | . | . | . | . | . | . |
| 0.85 | *** | 152 | 184 | 291 | . | . | . | . | . | . | . | . | . | . | . | . |
|  | *** | 165 | 216 | 275 | . | . | . | . | . | . | . | . | . | . | . | . |

TABLE 5: ALPHA= 0.025 POWER= 0.8    EXPECTED ACCRUAL THRU MINIMUM FOLLOW-UP= 80

| | | DEL=.10 | | | DEL=.15 | | | DEL=.20 | | | DEL=.25 | | | DEL=.30 | |
|---|---|---|---|---|---|---|---|---|---|---|---|---|---|---|---|---|
| FACT= | 1.0 .75 | .50 .25 | .00 BIN | 1.0 .75 | .50 .25 | .00 BIN | 1.0 .75 | .50 .25 | .00 BIN | 1.0 75 | .50 .25 | .00 BIN | 1.0 .75 | .50 .25 | .00 BIN |
| PCONT=*** | | | | | REQUIRED NUMBER OF PATIENTS | | | | | | | | | | |
| 0.05 *** | 167 | 169 | 178 | 98 | 100 | 104 | 70 | 71 | 73 | 54 | 55 | 57 | 45 | 46 | 47 |
| *** | 168 | 172 | 275 | 99 | 101 | 145 | 70 | 72 | 93 | 55 | 56 | 65 | 45 | 46 | 48 |
| 0.1 *** | 264 | 269 | 299 | 142 | 146 | 159 | 94 | 97 | 104 | 70 | 72 | 76 | 56 | 57 | 60 |
| *** | 266 | 276 | 393 | 143 | 150 | 194 | 96 | 100 | 118 | 71 | 74 | 80 | 57 | 59 | 58 |
| 0.15 *** | 342 | 350 | 409 | 175 | 182 | 207 | 113 | 118 | 130 | 82 | 85 | 92 | 64 | 66 | 71 |
| *** | 345 | 364 | 495 | 178 | 190 | 236 | 115 | 122 | 140 | 83 | 88 | 93 | 65 | 68 | 66 |
| 0.2 *** | 400 | 413 | 507 | 200 | 210 | 248 | 127 | 134 | 152 | 90 | 95 | 105 | 69 | 73 | 79 |
| *** | 404 | 432 | 581 | 204 | 222 | 271 | 129 | 140 | 157 | 92 | 99 | 103 | 71 | 75 | 72 |
| 0.25 *** | 439 | 457 | 591 | 217 | 230 | 282 | 136 | 145 | 170 | 96 | 102 | 116 | 73 | 77 | 85 |
| *** | 445 | 484 | 652 | 222 | 246 | 299 | 139 | 154 | 171 | 99 | 107 | 110 | 75 | 80 | 76 |
| 0.3 *** | 460 | 484 | 659 | 226 | 243 | 309 | 141 | 152 | 183 | 99 | 107 | 123 | 75 | 80 | 89 |
| *** | 468 | 518 | 707 | 233 | 262 | 320 | 146 | 163 | 181 | 102 | 113 | 115 | 77 | 84 | 79 |
| 0.35 *** | 466 | 496 | 710 | 229 | 250 | 328 | 143 | 156 | 192 | 100 | 109 | 127 | 75 | 81 | 92 |
| *** | 477 | 539 | 746 | 237 | 273 | 334 | 148 | 168 | 187 | 104 | 116 | 118 | 78 | 85 | 80 |
| 0.4 *** | 460 | 496 | 745 | 227 | 251 | 340 | 142 | 157 | 196 | 99 | 109 | 129 | 74 | 80 | 92 |
| *** | 473 | 547 | 770 | 237 | 277 | 341 | 148 | 170 | 189 | 103 | 116 | 118 | 77 | 85 | 79 |
| 0.45 *** | 443 | 486 | 762 | 221 | 248 | 344 | 138 | 154 | 197 | 96 | 106 | 128 | 72 | 78 | 90 |
| *** | 459 | 543 | 778 | 232 | 276 | 341 | 145 | 169 | 187 | 101 | 115 | 115 | 75 | 83 | 76 |
| 0.5 *** | 418 | 468 | 762 | 212 | 241 | 341 | 133 | 150 | 193 | 92 | 103 | 124 | 68 | 75 | 86 |
| *** | 437 | 530 | 770 | 223 | 270 | 334 | 140 | 164 | 181 | 97 | 111 | 110 | 71 | 80 | 72 |
| 0.55 *** | 389 | 444 | 746 | 200 | 230 | 329 | 125 | 142 | 184 | 87 | 97 | 117 | 64 | 70 | 81 |
| *** | 410 | 509 | 746 | 212 | 259 | 320 | 133 | 157 | 171 | 91 | 105 | 103 | 67 | 75 | 66 |
| 0.6 *** | 356 | 414 | 712 | 185 | 215 | 311 | 116 | 133 | 171 | 80 | 89 | 108 | 58 | 64 | 73 |
| *** | 378 | 481 | 707 | 197 | 244 | 299 | 123 | 146 | 157 | 84 | 97 | 93 | 61 | 68 | 58 |
| 0.65 *** | 321 | 380 | 661 | 169 | 197 | 284 | 105 | 120 | 155 | 72 | 80 | 96 | 52 | 56 | 64 |
| *** | 344 | 445 | 652 | 180 | 224 | 271 | 112 | 133 | 140 | 76 | 86 | 80 | 54 | 60 | 48 |
| 0.7 *** | 284 | 341 | 593 | 150 | 176 | 250 | 93 | 106 | 133 | 62 | 69 | 81 | . | . | . |
| *** | 307 | 402 | 581 | 161 | 200 | 236 | 98 | 116 | 118 | 65 | 74 | 65 | . | . | . |
| 0.75 *** | 246 | 298 | 509 | 129 | 151 | 209 | 78 | 88 | 108 | . | . | . | . | . | . |
| *** | 267 | 352 | 495 | 138 | 171 | 194 | 82 | 96 | 93 | . | . | . | . | . | . |
| 0.8 *** | 205 | 249 | 408 | 104 | 121 | 161 | . | . | . | . | . | . | . | . | . |
| *** | 222 | 293 | 393 | 112 | 136 | 145 | . | . | . | . | . | . | . | . | . |
| 0.85 *** | 158 | 191 | 291 | . | . | . | . | . | . | . | . | . | . | . | . |
| *** | 172 | 222 | 275 | . | . | . | . | . | . | . | . | . | . | . | . |

## TABLE 5: ALPHA= 0.025 POWER= 0.8   EXPECTED ACCRUAL THRU MINIMUM FOLLOW-UP= 90

| | | DEL=.10 | | | DEL=.15 | | | DEL=.20 | | | DEL=.25 | | | DEL=.30 | | |
|---|---|---|---|---|---|---|---|---|---|---|---|---|---|---|---|---|---|
| FACT= | | 1.0 .75 | .50 .25 | .00 BIN | 1.0 .75 | .50 .25 | .00 BIN | 1.0 .75 | .50 .25 | .00 BIN | 1.0 75 | .50 .25 | .00 BIN | 1.0 .75 | .50 .25 | .00 BIN |
| PCONT=*** | | | | | | | REQUIRED NUMBER OF PATIENTS | | | | | | | | | |
| 0.05 | *** | 167 | 170 | 178 | 98 | 100 | 104 | 70 | 71 | 73 | 54 | 55 | 57 | 45 | 46 | 47 |
| | *** | 168 | 172 | 275 | 99 | 102 | 145 | 70 | 72 | 93 | 55 | 56 | 65 | 45 | 46 | 48 |
| 0.1 | *** | 265 | 270 | 299 | 142 | 147 | 159 | 95 | 98 | 104 | 71 | 73 | 76 | 56 | 58 | 60 |
| | *** | 267 | 278 | 393 | 144 | 151 | 194 | 96 | 100 | 118 | 72 | 74 | 80 | 57 | 59 | 58 |
| 0.15 | *** | 343 | 352 | 409 | 176 | 184 | 207 | 114 | 119 | 130 | 83 | 86 | 92 | 64 | 67 | 71 |
| | *** | 346 | 366 | 495 | 179 | 191 | 236 | 116 | 123 | 140 | 84 | 89 | 93 | 65 | 68 | 66 |
| 0.2 | *** | 401 | 416 | 507 | 202 | 212 | 248 | 128 | 135 | 152 | 91 | 96 | 105 | 70 | 73 | 79 |
| | *** | 406 | 436 | 581 | 206 | 224 | 271 | 131 | 141 | 157 | 93 | 100 | 103 | 71 | 76 | 72 |
| 0.25 | *** | 441 | 461 | 591 | 219 | 233 | 282 | 137 | 147 | 170 | 97 | 103 | 116 | 74 | 78 | 85 |
| | *** | 448 | 489 | 652 | 224 | 248 | 299 | 141 | 155 | 171 | 100 | 108 | 110 | 75 | 81 | 76 |
| 0.3 | *** | 463 | 489 | 659 | 229 | 247 | 309 | 143 | 154 | 183 | 100 | 108 | 123 | 76 | 81 | 89 |
| | *** | 472 | 525 | 707 | 236 | 266 | 320 | 147 | 164 | 181 | 103 | 114 | 115 | 78 | 84 | 79 |
| 0.35 | *** | 470 | 503 | 710 | 232 | 254 | 328 | 145 | 158 | 192 | 101 | 110 | 127 | 76 | 82 | 92 |
| | *** | 482 | 547 | 746 | 241 | 276 | 334 | 150 | 170 | 187 | 105 | 117 | 118 | 79 | 86 | 80 |
| 0.4 | *** | 465 | 504 | 745 | 231 | 256 | 340 | 144 | 159 | 196 | 101 | 110 | 129 | 75 | 81 | 92 |
| | *** | 479 | 556 | 770 | 241 | 281 | 341 | 150 | 172 | 189 | 105 | 117 | 118 | 78 | 86 | 79 |
| 0.45 | *** | 449 | 495 | 762 | 226 | 253 | 344 | 141 | 157 | 197 | 98 | 108 | 128 | 73 | 79 | 90 |
| | *** | 466 | 554 | 778 | 237 | 280 | 341 | 148 | 171 | 187 | 102 | 116 | 115 | 76 | 84 | 76 |
| 0.5 | *** | 426 | 478 | 762 | 216 | 246 | 341 | 136 | 152 | 192 | 94 | 104 | 124 | 70 | 76 | 86 |
| | *** | 446 | 542 | 770 | 228 | 275 | 334 | 143 | 167 | 181 | 99 | 112 | 110 | 72 | 80 | 72 |
| 0.55 | *** | 397 | 454 | 745 | 205 | 235 | 329 | 128 | 145 | 184 | 89 | 98 | 117 | 65 | 71 | 81 |
| | *** | 419 | 521 | 746 | 217 | 264 | 320 | 135 | 159 | 171 | 93 | 106 | 103 | 68 | 75 | 66 |
| 0.6 | *** | 365 | 425 | 712 | 190 | 220 | 310 | 119 | 135 | 171 | 82 | 91 | 108 | 59 | 65 | 73 |
| | *** | 388 | 492 | 707 | 202 | 249 | 299 | 126 | 148 | 157 | 86 | 98 | 93 | 62 | 68 | 58 |
| 0.65 | *** | 330 | 390 | 661 | 173 | 202 | 284 | 108 | 123 | 155 | 73 | 81 | 96 | 53 | 57 | 64 |
| | *** | 354 | 456 | 652 | 185 | 229 | 271 | 114 | 135 | 140 | 77 | 87 | 80 | 55 | 60 | 48 |
| 0.7 | *** | 293 | 351 | 593 | 154 | 180 | 250 | 95 | 108 | 133 | 63 | 70 | 81 | . | . | . |
| | *** | 317 | 413 | 581 | 165 | 204 | 236 | 101 | 118 | 118 | 66 | 74 | 65 | . | . | . |
| 0.75 | *** | 254 | 307 | 509 | 133 | 155 | 209 | 80 | 90 | 108 | . | . | . | . | . | . |
| | *** | 276 | 361 | 495 | 142 | 174 | 194 | 84 | 97 | 93 | . | . | . | . | . | . |
| 0.8 | *** | 212 | 256 | 408 | 107 | 124 | 161 | . | . | . | . | . | . | . | . | . |
| | *** | 230 | 300 | 393 | 115 | 138 | 145 | . | . | . | . | . | . | . | . | . |
| 0.85 | *** | 164 | 196 | 291 | . | . | . | . | . | . | . | . | . | . | . | . |
| | *** | 177 | 226 | 275 | . | . | . | . | . | . | . | . | . | . | . | . |

TABLE 5: ALPHA= 0.025 POWER= 0.8     EXPECTED ACCRUAL THRU MINIMUM FOLLOW-UP= 100

| | | DEL=.10 | | | DEL=.15 | | | DEL=.20 | | | DEL=.25 | | | DEL=.30 | | |
|---|---|---|---|---|---|---|---|---|---|---|---|---|---|---|---|---|
| FACT= | | 1.0 .75 | .50 .25 | .00 BIN | 1.0 .75 | .50 .25 | .00 BIN | 1.0 .75 | .50 .25 | .00 BIN | 1.0 75 | .50 .25 | .00 BIN | 1.0 .75 | .50 .25 | .00 BIN |
| PCONT=*** | | | | | REQUIRED | NUMBER OF | PATIENTS | | | | | | | | | |
| 0.05 | *** | 167 | 170 | 178 | 99 | 100 | 104 | 70 | 71 | 73 | 55 | 55 | 57 | 45 | 46 | 47 |
| | *** | 168 | 173 | 275 | 99 | 102 | 145 | 70 | 72 | 93 | 55 | 56 | 65 | 45 | 46 | 48 |
| 0.1 | *** | 265 | 271 | 299 | 143 | 147 | 159 | 95 | 98 | 104 | 71 | 73 | 76 | 56 | 58 | 60 |
| | *** | 268 | 279 | 393 | 145 | 151 | 194 | 97 | 101 | 118 | 72 | 74 | 80 | 57 | 59 | 58 |
| 0.15 | *** | 344 | 354 | 409 | 177 | 185 | 207 | 115 | 120 | 130 | 83 | 86 | 92 | 65 | 67 | 71 |
| | *** | 348 | 368 | 495 | 180 | 192 | 236 | 117 | 124 | 140 | 85 | 89 | 93 | 66 | 69 | 66 |
| 0.2 | *** | 403 | 418 | 507 | 203 | 214 | 248 | 129 | 136 | 152 | 92 | 97 | 105 | 70 | 74 | 79 |
| | *** | 409 | 440 | 581 | 207 | 225 | 271 | 132 | 142 | 157 | 94 | 100 | 103 | 72 | 76 | 72 |
| 0.25 | *** | 443 | 464 | 591 | 221 | 235 | 282 | 139 | 148 | 170 | 98 | 104 | 116 | 74 | 78 | 85 |
| | *** | 451 | 493 | 652 | 226 | 250 | 299 | 143 | 156 | 171 | 101 | 109 | 110 | 76 | 81 | 76 |
| 0.3 | *** | 466 | 494 | 659 | 231 | 250 | 309 | 144 | 156 | 183 | 101 | 109 | 123 | 76 | 81 | 89 |
| | *** | 476 | 531 | 707 | 238 | 268 | 320 | 149 | 166 | 181 | 105 | 114 | 115 | 79 | 85 | 79 |
| 0.35 | *** | 474 | 509 | 710 | 235 | 257 | 328 | 147 | 160 | 192 | 103 | 111 | 127 | 77 | 82 | 92 |
| | *** | 487 | 554 | 746 | 244 | 280 | 334 | 153 | 172 | 187 | 106 | 118 | 118 | 79 | 86 | 80 |
| 0.4 | *** | 470 | 511 | 745 | 235 | 260 | 340 | 147 | 161 | 196 | 102 | 111 | 129 | 76 | 82 | 92 |
| | *** | 485 | 564 | 770 | 245 | 285 | 341 | 153 | 174 | 189 | 106 | 118 | 118 | 79 | 86 | 79 |
| 0.45 | *** | 455 | 504 | 762 | 230 | 257 | 344 | 144 | 159 | 197 | 100 | 109 | 128 | 74 | 80 | 90 |
| | *** | 473 | 563 | 778 | 241 | 284 | 341 | 150 | 173 | 187 | 104 | 117 | 115 | 77 | 84 | 76 |
| 0.5 | *** | 433 | 487 | 762 | 221 | 250 | 341 | 138 | 155 | 193 | 96 | 105 | 124 | 71 | 77 | 86 |
| | *** | 454 | 552 | 770 | 233 | 279 | 334 | 145 | 169 | 181 | 100 | 113 | 110 | 73 | 81 | 72 |
| 0.55 | *** | 405 | 464 | 746 | 209 | 239 | 329 | 131 | 147 | 184 | 90 | 100 | 117 | 66 | 72 | 81 |
| | *** | 428 | 531 | 746 | 222 | 268 | 320 | 138 | 161 | 171 | 94 | 107 | 103 | 69 | 76 | 66 |
| 0.6 | *** | 373 | 435 | 712 | 195 | 225 | 311 | 122 | 137 | 171 | 83 | 92 | 108 | 60 | 65 | 73 |
| | *** | 397 | 503 | 707 | 207 | 253 | 299 | 128 | 150 | 157 | 87 | 98 | 93 | 63 | 69 | 58 |
| 0.65 | *** | 339 | 400 | 661 | 178 | 206 | 284 | 110 | 125 | 155 | 75 | 82 | 96 | 53 | 58 | 64 |
| | *** | 363 | 466 | 652 | 190 | 232 | 271 | 117 | 136 | 140 | 78 | 88 | 80 | 55 | 60 | 48 |
| 0.7 | *** | 302 | 361 | 593 | 158 | 184 | 250 | 97 | 109 | 133 | 65 | 71 | 81 | . | . | . |
| | *** | 325 | 422 | 581 | 169 | 207 | 236 | 103 | 119 | 118 | 67 | 75 | 65 | . | . | . |
| 0.75 | *** | 262 | 315 | 509 | 136 | 158 | 209 | 81 | 91 | 108 | . | . | . | . | . | . |
| | *** | 284 | 369 | 495 | 145 | 176 | 194 | 86 | 98 | 93 | . | . | . | . | . | . |
| 0.8 | *** | 218 | 263 | 408 | 110 | 126 | 161 | . | . | . | . | . | . | . | . | . |
| | *** | 237 | 306 | 393 | 117 | 139 | 145 | . | . | . | . | . | . | . | . | . |
| 0.85 | *** | 169 | 201 | 291 | . | . | . | . | . | . | . | . | . | . | . | . |
| | *** | 182 | 231 | 275 | . | . | . | . | . | . | . | . | . | . | . | . |

## TABLE 5: ALPHA= 0.025 POWER= 0.8    EXPECTED ACCRUAL THRU MINIMUM FOLLOW-UP= 110

| | | DEL=.05 | | | DEL=.10 | | | DEL=.15 | | | DEL=.20 | | | DEL=.25 | | |
|---|---|---|---|---|---|---|---|---|---|---|---|---|---|---|---|---|
| FACT= | | 1.0 .75 | .50 .25 | .00 BIN | 1.0 .75 | .50 .25 | .00 BIN | 1.0 .75 | .50 .25 | .00 BIN | 1.0 75 | .50 .25 | .00 BIN | 1.0 .75 | .50 .25 | .00 BIN |
| PCONT=*** | | | | | REQUIRED NUMBER OF PATIENTS | | | | | | | | | | | |
| 0.05 | *** | 470 | 473 | 502 | 168 | 170 | 178 | 99 | 100 | 104 | 70 | 71 | 73 | 55 | 56 | 57 |
| | *** | 471 | 478 | 864 | 169 | 173 | 275 | 100 | 102 | 145 | 71 | 72 | 93 | 55 | 56 | 65 |
| 0.1 | *** | 857 | 863 | 967 | 266 | 272 | 299 | 144 | 148 | 159 | 96 | 99 | 104 | 71 | 73 | 76 |
| | *** | 859 | 875 | 1366 | 268 | 280 | 393 | 145 | 152 | 194 | 97 | 101 | 118 | 72 | 75 | 80 |
| 0.15 | *** | 1185 | 1196 | 1418 | 345 | 356 | 409 | 178 | 186 | 207 | 115 | 120 | 130 | 84 | 87 | 92 |
| | *** | 1189 | 1217 | 1806 | 349 | 370 | 495 | 181 | 193 | 236 | 117 | 124 | 140 | 85 | 89 | 93 |
| 0.2 | *** | 1439 | 1456 | 1829 | 405 | 421 | 507 | 204 | 216 | 248 | 130 | 137 | 152 | 93 | 97 | 105 |
| | *** | 1445 | 1488 | 2182 | 411 | 443 | 581 | 209 | 226 | 271 | 133 | 143 | 157 | 95 | 101 | 103 |
| 0.25 | *** | 1616 | 1639 | 2188 | 446 | 468 | 591 | 223 | 237 | 282 | 140 | 149 | 170 | 99 | 105 | 116 |
| | *** | 1623 | 1684 | 2496 | 454 | 498 | 652 | 229 | 252 | 299 | 144 | 157 | 171 | 101 | 109 | 110 |
| 0.3 | *** | 1718 | 1749 | 2489 | 469 | 498 | 659 | 234 | 252 | 309 | 146 | 157 | 183 | 102 | 110 | 123 |
| | *** | 1728 | 1811 | 2748 | 480 | 537 | 707 | 241 | 271 | 320 | 151 | 167 | 181 | 106 | 115 | 115 |
| 0.35 | *** | 1752 | 1793 | 2725 | 478 | 515 | 710 | 238 | 261 | 328 | 149 | 162 | 192 | 104 | 112 | 127 |
| | *** | 1765 | 1874 | 2936 | 492 | 561 | 746 | 247 | 282 | 334 | 154 | 173 | 187 | 108 | 118 | 118 |
| 0.4 | *** | 1726 | 1780 | 2896 | 474 | 518 | 745 | 238 | 263 | 340 | 149 | 163 | 196 | 104 | 112 | 129 |
| | *** | 1744 | 1883 | 3062 | 491 | 572 | 770 | 248 | 288 | 341 | 155 | 176 | 189 | 107 | 119 | 118 |
| 0.45 | *** | 1651 | 1720 | 2999 | 461 | 511 | 762 | 233 | 261 | 344 | 146 | 161 | 197 | 101 | 111 | 128 |
| | *** | 1674 | 1848 | 3124 | 480 | 571 | 778 | 245 | 288 | 341 | 152 | 175 | 187 | 105 | 118 | 115 |
| 0.5 | *** | 1537 | 1624 | 3034 | 439 | 496 | 762 | 225 | 254 | 341 | 141 | 157 | 193 | 97 | 107 | 124 |
| | *** | 1567 | 1777 | 3124 | 461 | 561 | 770 | 237 | 282 | 334 | 148 | 170 | 181 | 101 | 114 | 110 |
| 0.55 | *** | 1396 | 1504 | 3000 | 412 | 473 | 746 | 213 | 243 | 329 | 133 | 149 | 184 | 92 | 101 | 117 |
| | *** | 1433 | 1681 | 3062 | 436 | 541 | 746 | 226 | 272 | 320 | 140 | 163 | 171 | 96 | 108 | 103 |
| 0.6 | *** | 1238 | 1369 | 2898 | 381 | 444 | 712 | 199 | 229 | 311 | 124 | 139 | 171 | 85 | 93 | 108 |
| | *** | 1284 | 1565 | 2936 | 406 | 512 | 707 | 211 | 256 | 299 | 131 | 152 | 157 | 88 | 99 | 93 |
| 0.65 | *** | 1077 | 1227 | 2728 | 347 | 409 | 661 | 182 | 210 | 284 | 113 | 127 | 155 | 76 | 83 | 96 |
| | *** | 1132 | 1436 | 2748 | 372 | 475 | 652 | 194 | 235 | 271 | 119 | 137 | 140 | 79 | 88 | 80 |
| 0.7 | *** | 921 | 1083 | 2491 | 309 | 369 | 593 | 162 | 188 | 250 | 99 | 111 | 133 | 65 | 71 | 81 |
| | *** | 982 | 1294 | 2496 | 333 | 430 | 581 | 173 | 210 | 236 | 104 | 120 | 118 | 68 | 75 | 65 |
| 0.75 | *** | 775 | 938 | 2186 | 269 | 323 | 509 | 139 | 161 | 209 | 83 | 92 | 108 | . | . | . |
| | *** | 837 | 1140 | 2182 | 291 | 376 | 495 | 148 | 178 | 194 | 87 | 99 | 93 | . | . | . |
| 0.8 | *** | 638 | 790 | 1816 | 224 | 269 | 408 | 112 | 128 | 161 | . | . | . | . | . | . |
| | *** | 697 | 972 | 1806 | 243 | 312 | 393 | 119 | 141 | 145 | . | . | . | . | . | . |
| 0.85 | *** | 504 | 634 | 1380 | 173 | 205 | 291 | . | . | . | . | . | . | . | . | . |
| | *** | 555 | 783 | 1366 | 187 | 234 | 275 | . | . | . | . | . | . | . | . | . |
| 0.9 | *** | 362 | 455 | 879 | . | . | . | . | . | . | . | . | . | . | . | . |
| | *** | 399 | 556 | 864 | . | . | . | . | . | . | . | . | . | . | . | . |

TABLE 5: ALPHA= 0.025 POWER= 0.8    EXPECTED ACCRUAL THRU MINIMUM FOLLOW-UP= 120

| PCONT | | DEL=.05 | | | DEL=.10 | | | DEL=.15 | | | DEL=.20 | | | DEL=.25 | | |
|---|---|---|---|---|---|---|---|---|---|---|---|---|---|---|---|---|
| FACT= | | 1.0 .75 | .50 .25 | .00 BIN | 1.0 .75 | .50 .25 | .00 BIN | 1.0 .75 | .50 .25 | .00 BIN | 1.0 75 | .50 .25 | .00 BIN | 1.0 .75 | .50 .25 | .00 BIN |
| PCONT=*** | | | | | REQUIRED NUMBER OF PATIENTS | | | | | | | | | | | |
| 0.05 | *** | 470 | 473 | 502 | 168 | 171 | 178 | 99 | 101 | 104 | 70 | 71 | 73 | 55 | 56 | 57 |
| | *** | 471 | 479 | 864 | 169 | 173 | 275 | 100 | 102 | 145 | 71 | 72 | 93 | 55 | 56 | 65 |
| 0.1 | *** | 857 | 864 | 967 | 267 | 273 | 299 | 144 | 148 | 159 | 96 | 99 | 104 | 71 | 73 | 76 |
| | *** | 860 | 878 | 1366 | 269 | 281 | 393 | 146 | 152 | 194 | 97 | 101 | 118 | 72 | 75 | 80 |
| 0.15 | *** | 1186 | 1198 | 1418 | 346 | 358 | 409 | 179 | 187 | 206 | 116 | 121 | 130 | 84 | 87 | 92 |
| | *** | 1190 | 1221 | 1806 | 350 | 372 | 495 | 182 | 194 | 236 | 118 | 124 | 140 | 85 | 89 | 93 |
| 0.2 | *** | 1441 | 1459 | 1829 | 406 | 423 | 507 | 206 | 217 | 248 | 131 | 138 | 152 | 93 | 98 | 105 |
| | *** | 1447 | 1493 | 2182 | 413 | 445 | 581 | 210 | 228 | 271 | 134 | 143 | 157 | 95 | 101 | 103 |
| 0.25 | *** | 1618 | 1643 | 2188 | 448 | 471 | 591 | 224 | 239 | 282 | 141 | 150 | 170 | 100 | 105 | 116 |
| | *** | 1626 | 1692 | 2496 | 457 | 502 | 652 | 230 | 254 | 299 | 145 | 158 | 171 | 102 | 110 | 110 |
| 0.3 | *** | 1720 | 1755 | 2489 | 472 | 503 | 659 | 236 | 255 | 309 | 148 | 159 | 183 | 103 | 110 | 123 |
| | *** | 1732 | 1821 | 2748 | 484 | 542 | 707 | 243 | 273 | 320 | 152 | 168 | 181 | 106 | 116 | 115 |
| 0.35 | *** | 1755 | 1801 | 2725 | 482 | 520 | 710 | 241 | 263 | 328 | 151 | 164 | 192 | 105 | 113 | 127 |
| | *** | 1770 | 1888 | 2936 | 496 | 567 | 746 | 250 | 285 | 334 | 156 | 174 | 187 | 109 | 119 | 118 |
| 0.4 | *** | 1731 | 1790 | 2896 | 479 | 525 | 745 | 241 | 267 | 340 | 150 | 165 | 196 | 105 | 113 | 129 |
| | *** | 1751 | 1900 | 3062 | 496 | 579 | 770 | 251 | 291 | 341 | 157 | 177 | 189 | 109 | 120 | 118 |
| 0.45 | *** | 1657 | 1733 | 2999 | 466 | 519 | 762 | 237 | 265 | 344 | 148 | 163 | 197 | 102 | 112 | 128 |
| | *** | 1683 | 1868 | 3124 | 486 | 579 | 778 | 248 | 291 | 341 | 154 | 176 | 187 | 106 | 118 | 115 |
| 0.5 | *** | 1545 | 1640 | 3034 | 446 | 504 | 762 | 228 | 258 | 340 | 143 | 159 | 193 | 99 | 108 | 124 |
| | *** | 1577 | 1801 | 3124 | 468 | 569 | 770 | 241 | 285 | 334 | 150 | 172 | 181 | 103 | 114 | 110 |
| 0.55 | *** | 1406 | 1522 | 3000 | 419 | 481 | 745 | 217 | 247 | 329 | 135 | 151 | 184 | 93 | 102 | 117 |
| | *** | 1446 | 1708 | 3062 | 444 | 549 | 746 | 229 | 275 | 320 | 142 | 164 | 171 | 97 | 108 | 103 |
| 0.6 | *** | 1251 | 1390 | 2898 | 388 | 452 | 712 | 202 | 232 | 310 | 126 | 141 | 171 | 86 | 94 | 108 |
| | *** | 1300 | 1504 | 2936 | 414 | 521 | 707 | 215 | 259 | 299 | 133 | 153 | 157 | 89 | 100 | 93 |
| 0.65 | *** | 1093 | 1250 | 2728 | 354 | 418 | 661 | 185 | 214 | 284 | 114 | 128 | 155 | 77 | 84 | 96 |
| | *** | 1150 | 1465 | 2748 | 380 | 483 | 652 | 197 | 238 | 271 | 120 | 139 | 140 | 80 | 89 | 80 |
| 0.7 | *** | 938 | 1107 | 2491 | 317 | 377 | 593 | 165 | 191 | 250 | 101 | 112 | 133 | 66 | 72 | 81 |
| | *** | 1002 | 1323 | 2496 | 341 | 438 | 581 | 176 | 212 | 236 | 106 | 121 | 118 | 69 | 76 | 65 |
| 0.75 | *** | 793 | 961 | 2186 | 276 | 330 | 509 | 142 | 163 | 209 | 84 | 93 | 108 | . | . | . |
| | *** | 857 | 1168 | 2182 | 298 | 383 | 495 | 151 | 180 | 194 | 88 | 99 | 93 | . | . | . |
| 0.8 | *** | 655 | 812 | 1816 | 230 | 275 | 408 | 115 | 130 | 161 | . | . | . | . | . | . |
| | *** | 716 | 997 | 1806 | 249 | 317 | 393 | 121 | 142 | 145 | . | . | . | . | . | . |
| 0.85 | *** | 519 | 652 | 1380 | 177 | 209 | 291 | . | . | . | . | . | . | . | . | . |
| | *** | 571 | 802 | 1366 | 191 | 237 | 275 | . | . | . | . | . | . | . | . | . |
| 0.9 | *** | 373 | 468 | 879 | . | . | . | . | . | . | . | . | . | . | . | . |
| | *** | 411 | 568 | 864 | . | . | . | . | . | . | . | . | . | . | . | . |

## TABLE 5: ALPHA= 0.025 POWER= 0.8    EXPECTED ACCRUAL THRU MINIMUM FOLLOW-UP= 130

| | | DEL=.05 | | | DEL=.10 | | | DEL=.15 | | | DEL=.20 | | | DEL=.25 | | |
|---|---|---|---|---|---|---|---|---|---|---|---|---|---|---|---|---|
| FACT= | | 1.0 .75 | .50 .25 | .00 BIN | 1.0 .75 | .50 .25 | .00 BIN | 1.0 .75 | .50 .25 | .00 BIN | 1.0 75 | .50 .25 | .00 BIN | 1.0 .75 | .50 .25 | .00 BIN |
| PCONT=*** | | | | | REQUIRED NUMBER OF PATIENTS | | | | | | | | | | | |
| 0.05 | *** | 470 | 474 | 502 | 168 | 171 | 178 | 99 | 101 | 104 | 70 | 72 | 73 | 55 | 56 | 57 |
| | *** | 472 | 479 | 864 | 169 | 174 | 275 | 100 | 102 | 145 | 71 | 72 | 93 | 55 | 56 | 65 |
| 0.1 | *** | 858 | 865 | 967 | 267 | 274 | 299 | 145 | 149 | 159 | 96 | 99 | 104 | 72 | 74 | 76 |
| | *** | 860 | 880 | 1366 | 270 | 282 | 393 | 146 | 153 | 194 | 98 | 101 | 118 | 73 | 75 | 80 |
| 0.15 | *** | 1187 | 1200 | 1418 | 347 | 359 | 409 | 180 | 188 | 206 | 116 | 121 | 130 | 84 | 87 | 92 |
| | *** | 1192 | 1225 | 1806 | 352 | 374 | 495 | 183 | 195 | 236 | 119 | 125 | 140 | 86 | 90 | 93 |
| 0.2 | *** | 1442 | 1461 | 1829 | 408 | 426 | 507 | 207 | 218 | 248 | 132 | 138 | 152 | 94 | 98 | 105 |
| | *** | 1449 | 1499 | 2182 | 415 | 448 | 581 | 212 | 229 | 271 | 135 | 144 | 157 | 96 | 101 | 103 |
| 0.25 | *** | 1620 | 1647 | 2188 | 450 | 475 | 591 | 226 | 241 | 282 | 142 | 151 | 170 | 100 | 106 | 116 |
| | *** | 1629 | 1700 | 2496 | 459 | 505 | 652 | 232 | 255 | 299 | 146 | 158 | 171 | 103 | 110 | 110 |
| 0.3 | *** | 1723 | 1760 | 2489 | 475 | 507 | 659 | 238 | 257 | 309 | 149 | 160 | 183 | 104 | 111 | 123 |
| | *** | 1736 | 1832 | 2748 | 487 | 546 | 707 | 246 | 275 | 320 | 154 | 169 | 181 | 107 | 116 | 115 |
| 0.35 | *** | 1759 | 1808 | 2725 | 486 | 525 | 710 | 243 | 266 | 328 | 152 | 165 | 192 | 106 | 114 | 127 |
| | *** | 1776 | 1901 | 2936 | 501 | 572 | 746 | 253 | 287 | 334 | 158 | 175 | 187 | 109 | 119 | 118 |
| 0.4 | *** | 1736 | 1800 | 2896 | 484 | 531 | 745 | 244 | 270 | 340 | 152 | 167 | 196 | 106 | 114 | 129 |
| | *** | 1757 | 1917 | 3062 | 502 | 585 | 770 | 254 | 293 | 341 | 158 | 178 | 189 | 109 | 120 | 118 |
| 0.45 | *** | 1664 | 1745 | 2999 | 472 | 525 | 762 | 240 | 268 | 344 | 150 | 165 | 197 | 104 | 112 | 128 |
| | *** | 1691 | 1888 | 3124 | 492 | 586 | 778 | 251 | 294 | 341 | 156 | 177 | 187 | 108 | 119 | 115 |
| 0.5 | *** | 1553 | 1655 | 3034 | 452 | 511 | 762 | 232 | 261 | 341 | 145 | 160 | 193 | 100 | 109 | 124 |
| | *** | 1588 | 1825 | 3124 | 475 | 577 | 770 | 244 | 288 | 334 | 151 | 173 | 181 | 104 | 115 | 110 |
| 0.55 | *** | 1416 | 1540 | 3000 | 426 | 489 | 746 | 220 | 251 | 329 | 137 | 153 | 184 | 94 | 103 | 117 |
| | *** | 1459 | 1734 | 3062 | 451 | 557 | 746 | 233 | 278 | 320 | 144 | 165 | 171 | 98 | 109 | 103 |
| 0.6 | *** | 1264 | 1410 | 2898 | 395 | 460 | 712 | 206 | 236 | 310 | 128 | 143 | 171 | 87 | 95 | 108 |
| | *** | 1316 | 1622 | 2936 | 421 | 528 | 707 | 218 | 262 | 299 | 134 | 154 | 157 | 90 | 100 | 93 |
| 0.65 | *** | 1107 | 1272 | 2728 | 361 | 425 | 661 | 189 | 217 | 284 | 116 | 129 | 155 | 78 | 85 | 96 |
| | *** | 1168 | 1493 | 2748 | 387 | 491 | 652 | 200 | 241 | 271 | 122 | 140 | 140 | 81 | 89 | 80 |
| 0.7 | *** | 955 | 1129 | 2491 | 323 | 384 | 593 | 168 | 193 | 250 | 102 | 113 | 133 | 67 | 73 | 81 |
| | *** | 1021 | 1351 | 2496 | 348 | 444 | 581 | 179 | 214 | 236 | 107 | 122 | 118 | 70 | 76 | 65 |
| 0.75 | *** | 810 | 983 | 2186 | 282 | 336 | 509 | 145 | 165 | 209 | 85 | 94 | 108 | . | . | . |
| | *** | 877 | 1194 | 2182 | 304 | 388 | 495 | 154 | 182 | 194 | 89 | 100 | 93 | . | . | . |
| 0.8 | *** | 671 | 832 | 1816 | 235 | 280 | 408 | 116 | 132 | 161 | . | . | . | . | . | . |
| | *** | 734 | 1019 | 1806 | 254 | 321 | 393 | 123 | 143 | 145 | . | . | . | . | . | . |
| 0.85 | *** | 533 | 669 | 1380 | 181 | 213 | 291 | . | . | . | . | . | . | . | . | . |
| | *** | 587 | 820 | 1366 | 194 | 240 | 275 | . | . | . | . | . | . | . | . | . |
| 0.9 | *** | 383 | 479 | 879 | . | . | . | . | . | . | . | . | . | . | . | . |
| | *** | 422 | 580 | 864 | . | . | . | . | . | . | . | . | . | . | . | . |

## TABLE 5: ALPHA= 0.025 POWER= 0.8　　EXPECTED ACCRUAL THRU MINIMUM FOLLOW-UP= 140

| | | DEL=.05 | | | DEL=.10 | | | DEL=.15 | | | DEL=.20 | | | DEL=.25 | | |
|---|---|---|---|---|---|---|---|---|---|---|---|---|---|---|---|---|---|
| FACT= | | 1.0 .75 | .50 .25 | .00 BIN | 1.0 .75 | .50 .25 | .00 BIN | 1.0 .75 | .50 .25 | .00 BIN | 1.0 75 | .50 .25 | .00 BIN | 1.0 .75 | .50 .25 | .00 BIN |
| PCONT=*** | | REQUIRED NUMBER OF PATIENTS | | | | | | | | | | | | | | |
| 0.05 | *** | 471 | 474 | 502 | 169 | 171 | 178 | 99 | 101 | 104 | 71 | 72 | 73 | 55 | 56 | 57 |
| | *** | 472 | 480 | 864 | 170 | 174 | 275 | 100 | 102 | 145 | 71 | 72 | 93 | 55 | 56 | 65 |
| 0.1 | *** | 858 | 867 | 967 | 268 | 275 | 299 | 145 | 149 | 159 | 97 | 99 | 104 | 72 | 74 | 76 |
| | *** | 861 | 882 | 1366 | 271 | 283 | 393 | 147 | 153 | 194 | 98 | 101 | 118 | 73 | 75 | 80 |
| 0.15 | *** | 1188 | 1202 | 1418 | 348 | 361 | 409 | 181 | 189 | 207 | 117 | 122 | 130 | 85 | 88 | 92 |
| | *** | 1193 | 1228 | 1806 | 353 | 375 | 495 | 184 | 195 | 236 | 119 | 125 | 140 | 86 | 90 | 93 |
| 0.2 | *** | 1444 | 1464 | 1829 | 410 | 428 | 507 | 208 | 220 | 248 | 132 | 139 | 152 | 94 | 99 | 105 |
| | *** | 1451 | 1504 | 2182 | 417 | 450 | 581 | 213 | 230 | 271 | 135 | 144 | 157 | 96 | 102 | 103 |
| 0.25 | *** | 1622 | 1651 | 2188 | 452 | 478 | 591 | 228 | 243 | 282 | 143 | 152 | 170 | 101 | 106 | 116 |
| | *** | 1632 | 1708 | 2496 | 462 | 509 | 652 | 234 | 257 | 299 | 147 | 159 | 171 | 103 | 110 | 110 |
| 0.3 | *** | 1726 | 1766 | 2489 | 478 | 511 | 659 | 240 | 259 | 309 | 150 | 161 | 183 | 105 | 112 | 123 |
| | *** | 1740 | 1842 | 2748 | 491 | 550 | 707 | 248 | 276 | 320 | 155 | 170 | 181 | 108 | 116 | 115 |
| 0.35 | *** | 1763 | 1816 | 2725 | 489 | 530 | 710 | 246 | 268 | 328 | 153 | 166 | 192 | 107 | 115 | 127 |
| | *** | 1781 | 1915 | 2936 | 505 | 578 | 746 | 255 | 289 | 334 | 159 | 176 | 187 | 110 | 120 | 118 |
| 0.4 | *** | 1741 | 1809 | 2896 | 488 | 536 | 745 | 247 | 272 | 340 | 154 | 168 | 196 | 107 | 115 | 129 |
| | *** | 1764 | 1933 | 3062 | 507 | 591 | 770 | 257 | 296 | 341 | 160 | 179 | 189 | 110 | 121 | 118 |
| 0.45 | *** | 1670 | 1757 | 2999 | 477 | 532 | 762 | 243 | 271 | 344 | 151 | 166 | 197 | 105 | 113 | 128 |
| | *** | 1699 | 1908 | 3124 | 498 | 593 | 778 | 254 | 296 | 341 | 158 | 178 | 187 | 109 | 119 | 115 |
| 0.5 | *** | 1561 | 1670 | 3033 | 457 | 518 | 762 | 235 | 264 | 341 | 146 | 162 | 193 | 101 | 109 | 124 |
| | *** | 1598 | 1847 | 3124 | 481 | 583 | 770 | 247 | 291 | 334 | 153 | 174 | 181 | 105 | 116 | 110 |
| 0.55 | *** | 1426 | 1558 | 3000 | 432 | 496 | 746 | 224 | 254 | 329 | 139 | 154 | 184 | 95 | 103 | 117 |
| | *** | 1472 | 1758 | 3062 | 458 | 564 | 746 | 236 | 280 | 320 | 146 | 166 | 171 | 99 | 109 | 103 |
| 0.6 | *** | 1276 | 1430 | 2898 | 402 | 468 | 712 | 209 | 239 | 311 | 130 | 144 | 171 | 88 | 95 | 108 |
| | *** | 1332 | 1648 | 2936 | 428 | 535 | 707 | 222 | 264 | 299 | 136 | 155 | 157 | 91 | 101 | 93 |
| 0.65 | *** | 1122 | 1293 | 2728 | 368 | 432 | 661 | 192 | 219 | 284 | 118 | 131 | 155 | 79 | 85 | 96 |
| | *** | 1185 | 1520 | 2748 | 394 | 498 | 652 | 204 | 243 | 271 | 123 | 140 | 140 | 82 | 90 | 80 |
| 0.7 | *** | 971 | 1151 | 2491 | 330 | 391 | 593 | 171 | 196 | 250 | 103 | 114 | 133 | 68 | 73 | 81 |
| | *** | 1039 | 1377 | 2496 | 355 | 450 | 581 | 182 | 216 | 236 | 108 | 122 | 118 | 70 | 76 | 65 |
| 0.75 | *** | 827 | 1004 | 2186 | 287 | 342 | 509 | 147 | 167 | 209 | 86 | 95 | 108 | . | . | . |
| | *** | 895 | 1218 | 2182 | 310 | 393 | 495 | 156 | 183 | 194 | 90 | 101 | 93 | . | . | . |
| 0.8 | *** | 687 | 851 | 1816 | 240 | 285 | 408 | 118 | 133 | 161 | . | . | . | . | . | . |
| | *** | 751 | 1040 | 1806 | 259 | 325 | 393 | 125 | 144 | 145 | . | . | . | . | . | . |
| 0.85 | *** | 547 | 684 | 1380 | 184 | 216 | 291 | . | . | . | . | . | . | . | . | . |
| | *** | 601 | 837 | 1366 | 198 | 243 | 275 | . | . | . | . | . | . | . | . | . |
| 0.9 | *** | 393 | 490 | 879 | . | . | . | . | . | . | . | . | . | . | . | . |
| | *** | 432 | 591 | 864 | . | . | . | . | . | . | . | . | . | . | . | . |

## TABLE 5: ALPHA= 0.025 POWER= 0.8    EXPECTED ACCRUAL THRU MINIMUM FOLLOW-UP= 150

|  |  | DEL=.05 | | | DEL=.10 | | | DEL=.15 | | | DEL=.20 | | | DEL=.25 | | |
|---|---|---|---|---|---|---|---|---|---|---|---|---|---|---|---|---|
| FACT= | | 1.0 .75 | .50 .25 | .00 BIN | 1.0 .75 | .50 .25 | .00 BIN | 1.0 .75 | .50 .25 | .00 BIN | 1.0 75 | .50 .25 | .00 BIN | 1.0 .75 | .50 .25 | .00 BIN |
| PCONT=*** | | | | | REQUIRED | NUMBER OF | PATIENTS | | | | | | | | | |
| 0.05 | *** | 471 | 475 | 502 | 169 | 172 | 178 | 100 | 101 | 104 | 71 | 72 | 73 | 55 | 56 | 57 |
|  | *** | 472 | 481 | 864 | 170 | 174 | 275 | 100 | 102 | 145 | 71 | 72 | 93 | 55 | 56 | 65 |
| 0.1 | *** | 859 | 868 | 967 | 269 | 276 | 299 | 145 | 150 | 158 | 97 | 100 | 104 | 72 | 74 | 76 |
|  | *** | 862 | 883 | 1366 | 271 | 283 | 393 | 147 | 153 | 194 | 98 | 102 | 118 | 73 | 75 | 80 |
| 0.15 | *** | 1189 | 1204 | 1418 | 349 | 362 | 409 | 182 | 189 | 206 | 118 | 122 | 130 | 85 | 88 | 92 |
|  | *** | 1194 | 1232 | 1806 | 354 | 377 | 495 | 185 | 196 | 236 | 119 | 125 | 140 | 86 | 90 | 93 |
| 0.2 | *** | 1445 | 1467 | 1829 | 411 | 430 | 507 | 209 | 221 | 248 | 133 | 140 | 152 | 95 | 99 | 105 |
|  | *** | 1453 | 1510 | 2182 | 418 | 453 | 581 | 214 | 231 | 271 | 136 | 145 | 157 | 97 | 102 | 103 |
| 0.25 | *** | 1624 | 1656 | 2188 | 454 | 481 | 591 | 229 | 244 | 282 | 144 | 153 | 170 | 102 | 107 | 116 |
|  | *** | 1635 | 1715 | 2496 | 464 | 512 | 652 | 235 | 258 | 299 | 148 | 160 | 171 | 104 | 111 | 110 |
| 0.3 | *** | 1729 | 1772 | 2489 | 481 | 515 | 659 | 242 | 261 | 309 | 151 | 162 | 183 | 106 | 112 | 123 |
|  | *** | 1743 | 1852 | 2748 | 494 | 554 | 707 | 250 | 278 | 320 | 156 | 170 | 181 | 109 | 117 | 115 |
| 0.35 | *** | 1767 | 1823 | 2725 | 493 | 535 | 710 | 248 | 271 | 328 | 155 | 167 | 192 | 108 | 115 | 127 |
|  | *** | 1786 | 1927 | 2936 | 509 | 582 | 746 | 257 | 291 | 334 | 160 | 177 | 187 | 111 | 120 | 118 |
| 0.4 | *** | 1746 | 1819 | 2896 | 492 | 542 | 745 | 249 | 275 | 340 | 155 | 169 | 196 | 108 | 116 | 129 |
|  | *** | 1770 | 1949 | 3062 | 511 | 597 | 770 | 260 | 298 | 341 | 161 | 180 | 189 | 111 | 121 | 118 |
| 0.45 | *** | 1676 | 1769 | 2999 | 482 | 538 | 762 | 245 | 273 | 344 | 153 | 168 | 197 | 106 | 114 | 128 |
|  | *** | 1708 | 1926 | 3124 | 504 | 599 | 778 | 257 | 298 | 341 | 159 | 179 | 187 | 109 | 120 | 115 |
| 0.5 | *** | 1569 | 1684 | 3034 | 463 | 524 | 762 | 238 | 267 | 341 | 148 | 163 | 193 | 102 | 110 | 124 |
|  | *** | 1609 | 1868 | 3124 | 487 | 590 | 770 | 250 | 293 | 334 | 155 | 175 | 181 | 105 | 116 | 110 |
| 0.55 | *** | 1436 | 1574 | 3000 | 438 | 503 | 745 | 227 | 257 | 329 | 141 | 156 | 184 | 96 | 104 | 117 |
|  | *** | 1485 | 1781 | 3062 | 464 | 571 | 746 | 239 | 282 | 320 | 147 | 167 | 171 | 100 | 110 | 103 |
| 0.6 | *** | 1288 | 1449 | 2898 | 408 | 474 | 712 | 212 | 241 | 310 | 131 | 145 | 171 | 89 | 96 | 108 |
|  | *** | 1347 | 1672 | 2936 | 435 | 542 | 707 | 225 | 266 | 299 | 137 | 156 | 157 | 92 | 101 | 93 |
| 0.65 | *** | 1136 | 1313 | 2728 | 374 | 439 | 661 | 195 | 222 | 284 | 119 | 132 | 155 | 79 | 86 | 95 |
|  | *** | 1202 | 1545 | 2748 | 400 | 504 | 652 | 206 | 245 | 271 | 125 | 141 | 140 | 82 | 90 | 80 |
| 0.7 | *** | 987 | 1172 | 2491 | 335 | 397 | 593 | 174 | 198 | 250 | 105 | 115 | 133 | 68 | 73 | 81 |
|  | *** | 1057 | 1401 | 2496 | 361 | 456 | 581 | 184 | 218 | 236 | 109 | 123 | 118 | 71 | 77 | 65 |
| 0.75 | *** | 842 | 1024 | 2186 | 293 | 347 | 509 | 149 | 169 | 209 | 87 | 95 | 108 | . | . | . |
|  | *** | 913 | 1241 | 2182 | 315 | 398 | 495 | 158 | 185 | 194 | 91 | 101 | 93 | . | . | . |
| 0.8 | *** | 702 | 869 | 1816 | 244 | 289 | 408 | 120 | 134 | 161 | . | . | . | . | . | . |
|  | *** | 767 | 1060 | 1806 | 263 | 329 | 393 | 126 | 145 | 145 | . | . | . | . | . | . |
| 0.85 | *** | 559 | 699 | 1380 | 188 | 219 | 291 | . | . | . | . | . | . | . | . | . |
|  | *** | 615 | 852 | 1366 | 201 | 245 | 275 | . | . | . | . | . | . | . | . | . |
| 0.9 | *** | 402 | 500 | 879 | . | . | . | . | . | . | . | . | . | . | . | . |
|  | *** | 442 | 600 | 864 | . | . | . | . | . | . | . | . | . | . | . | . |

TABLE 5: ALPHA= 0.025 POWER= 0.8    EXPECTED ACCRUAL THRU MINIMUM FOLLOW-UP= 160

| PCONT=*** | DEL=.05 1.0 / .75 | .50 / .25 | .00 / BIN | DEL=.10 1.0 / .75 | .50 / .25 | .00 / BIN | DEL=.15 1.0 / .75 | .50 / .25 | .00 / BIN | DEL=.20 1.0 / 75 | .50 / .25 | .00 / BIN | DEL=.25 1.0 / .75 | .50 / .25 | .00 / BIN |
|---|---|---|---|---|---|---|---|---|---|---|---|---|---|---|---|
| | | | | REQUIRED NUMBER OF PATIENTS | | | | | | | | | | | |
| 0.05 *** | 471 | 475 | 502 | 169 | 172 | 178 | 100 | 101 | 104 | 71 | 72 | 73 | 55 | 56 | 57 |
| *** | 473 | 482 | 864 | 170 | 174 | 275 | 100 | 103 | 145 | 71 | 72 | 93 | 56 | 56 | 65 |
| 0.1 *** | 860 | 869 | 967 | 269 | 276 | 299 | 146 | 150 | 159 | 97 | 100 | 104 | 72 | 74 | 76 |
| *** | 863 | 885 | 1366 | 272 | 284 | 393 | 148 | 154 | 194 | 98 | 102 | 118 | 73 | 75 | 80 |
| 0.15 *** | 1190 | 1206 | 1418 | 350 | 364 | 409 | 182 | 190 | 207 | 118 | 122 | 130 | 85 | 88 | 92 |
| *** | 1195 | 1235 | 1806 | 355 | 378 | 495 | 186 | 196 | 236 | 120 | 126 | 140 | 87 | 90 | 93 |
| 0.2 *** | 1447 | 1470 | 1829 | 413 | 432 | 507 | 210 | 222 | 248 | 134 | 140 | 152 | 95 | 99 | 105 |
| *** | 1455 | 1515 | 2182 | 420 | 455 | 581 | 215 | 232 | 271 | 137 | 145 | 157 | 97 | 102 | 103 |
| 0.25 *** | 1626 | 1660 | 2188 | 457 | 484 | 591 | 230 | 246 | 282 | 145 | 154 | 170 | 102 | 107 | 116 |
| *** | 1637 | 1723 | 2496 | 467 | 514 | 652 | 237 | 259 | 299 | 149 | 160 | 171 | 105 | 111 | 110 |
| 0.3 *** | 1732 | 1777 | 2489 | 484 | 518 | 659 | 243 | 262 | 309 | 152 | 163 | 183 | 107 | 113 | 123 |
| *** | 1747 | 1862 | 2748 | 497 | 558 | 707 | 251 | 279 | 320 | 157 | 171 | 181 | 109 | 117 | 115 |
| 0.35 *** | 1770 | 1831 | 2725 | 496 | 539 | 710 | 250 | 273 | 328 | 156 | 168 | 192 | 109 | 116 | 127 |
| *** | 1791 | 1940 | 2936 | 513 | 587 | 746 | 260 | 293 | 334 | 161 | 178 | 187 | 112 | 121 | 118 |
| 0.4 *** | 1751 | 1828 | 2896 | 496 | 547 | 745 | 251 | 277 | 340 | 157 | 170 | 196 | 109 | 116 | 129 |
| *** | 1777 | 1964 | 3062 | 516 | 602 | 770 | 262 | 300 | 341 | 163 | 181 | 189 | 112 | 122 | 118 |
| 0.45 *** | 1683 | 1781 | 2999 | 486 | 543 | 762 | 248 | 276 | 344 | 154 | 169 | 197 | 106 | 115 | 128 |
| *** | 1716 | 1944 | 3124 | 509 | 604 | 778 | 260 | 300 | 341 | 161 | 180 | 187 | 110 | 120 | 115 |
| 0.5 *** | 1577 | 1698 | 3034 | 468 | 530 | 762 | 241 | 270 | 341 | 150 | 164 | 193 | 103 | 111 | 124 |
| *** | 1619 | 1888 | 3124 | 493 | 596 | 770 | 253 | 295 | 334 | 156 | 176 | 181 | 106 | 116 | 110 |
| 0.55 *** | 1446 | 1591 | 3000 | 444 | 509 | 746 | 230 | 259 | 329 | 142 | 157 | 184 | 97 | 105 | 117 |
| *** | 1498 | 1803 | 3062 | 470 | 577 | 746 | 242 | 285 | 320 | 149 | 168 | 171 | 100 | 110 | 103 |
| 0.6 *** | 1300 | 1467 | 2898 | 414 | 481 | 712 | 215 | 244 | 311 | 133 | 146 | 171 | 89 | 97 | 108 |
| *** | 1361 | 1696 | 2936 | 441 | 548 | 707 | 227 | 268 | 299 | 139 | 157 | 157 | 93 | 101 | 93 |
| 0.65 *** | 1150 | 1333 | 2728 | 380 | 445 | 661 | 197 | 224 | 284 | 120 | 133 | 155 | 80 | 86 | 96 |
| *** | 1219 | 1569 | 2748 | 406 | 509 | 652 | 209 | 247 | 271 | 126 | 142 | 140 | 83 | 90 | 80 |
| 0.7 *** | 1002 | 1191 | 2491 | 341 | 402 | 593 | 176 | 200 | 250 | 106 | 116 | 133 | 69 | 74 | 81 |
| *** | 1074 | 1424 | 2496 | 366 | 461 | 581 | 186 | 219 | 236 | 110 | 124 | 118 | 71 | 77 | 65 |
| 0.75 *** | 858 | 1043 | 2186 | 298 | 352 | 509 | 151 | 171 | 209 | 88 | 96 | 108 | . | . | . |
| *** | 930 | 1262 | 2182 | 320 | 403 | 495 | 160 | 186 | 194 | 92 | 101 | 93 | . | . | . |
| 0.8 *** | 716 | 886 | 1816 | 249 | 293 | 408 | 121 | 136 | 161 | . | . | . | . | . | . |
| *** | 783 | 1079 | 1806 | 267 | 332 | 393 | 128 | 146 | 145 | . | . | . | . | . | . |
| 0.85 *** | 571 | 713 | 1380 | 191 | 222 | 291 | . | . | . | . | . | . | . | . | . |
| *** | 628 | 867 | 1366 | 204 | 247 | 275 | . | . | . | . | . | . | . | . | . |
| 0.9 *** | 411 | 509 | 879 | . | . | . | . | . | . | . | . | . | . | . | . |
| *** | 451 | 610 | 864 | . | . | . | . | . | . | . | . | . | . | . | . |

## TABLE 5: ALPHA= 0.025 POWER= 0.8    EXPECTED ACCRUAL THRU MINIMUM FOLLOW-UP= 170

| | | DEL=.05 | | | DEL=.10 | | | DEL=.15 | | | DEL=.20 | | | DEL=.25 | | |
|---|---|---|---|---|---|---|---|---|---|---|---|---|---|---|---|---|---|
| FACT= | | 1.0 .75 | .50 .25 | .00 BIN | 1.0 .75 | .50 .25 | .00 BIN | 1.0 .75 | .50 .25 | .00 BIN | 1.0 75 | .50 .25 | .00 BIN | 1.0 .75 | .50 .25 | .00 BIN |
| PCONT=*** | | | | | REQUIRED NUMBER OF PATIENTS | | | | | | | | | | | |
| 0.05 | *** | 471 | 476 | 502 | 169 | 172 | 178 | 100 | 101 | 104 | 71 | 72 | 73 | 55 | 56 | 57 |
| | *** | 473 | 482 | 864 | 170 | 175 | 275 | 101 | 103 | 145 | 71 | 72 | 93 | 56 | 56 | 65 |
| 0.1 | *** | 860 | 870 | 967 | 270 | 277 | 299 | 146 | 150 | 159 | 98 | 100 | 104 | 72 | 74 | 76 |
| | *** | 864 | 887 | 1366 | 273 | 285 | 393 | 148 | 154 | 194 | 99 | 102 | 118 | 73 | 75 | 80 |
| 0.15 | *** | 1191 | 1208 | 1418 | 351 | 365 | 409 | 183 | 191 | 206 | 118 | 123 | 130 | 86 | 88 | 92 |
| | *** | 1197 | 1238 | 1806 | 357 | 379 | 495 | 186 | 197 | 236 | 120 | 126 | 140 | 87 | 90 | 93 |
| 0.2 | *** | 1448 | 1473 | 1829 | 414 | 434 | 507 | 211 | 223 | 248 | 134 | 141 | 152 | 96 | 99 | 105 |
| | *** | 1457 | 1520 | 2182 | 422 | 457 | 581 | 216 | 232 | 271 | 137 | 145 | 157 | 97 | 102 | 103 |
| 0.25 | *** | 1628 | 1664 | 2188 | 459 | 486 | 591 | 232 | 247 | 282 | 146 | 154 | 170 | 103 | 108 | 116 |
| | *** | 1640 | 1730 | 2496 | 469 | 517 | 652 | 238 | 260 | 299 | 150 | 161 | 171 | 105 | 111 | 110 |
| 0.3 | *** | 1735 | 1783 | 2489 | 486 | 522 | 659 | 245 | 264 | 309 | 153 | 164 | 183 | 107 | 113 | 123 |
| | *** | 1751 | 1872 | 2748 | 500 | 561 | 707 | 253 | 280 | 320 | 158 | 172 | 181 | 110 | 117 | 115 |
| 0.35 | *** | 1774 | 1838 | 2725 | 500 | 543 | 710 | 252 | 275 | 328 | 157 | 169 | 192 | 109 | 116 | 127 |
| | *** | 1796 | 1952 | 2936 | 516 | 591 | 746 | 262 | 294 | 334 | 163 | 178 | 187 | 112 | 121 | 118 |
| 0.4 | *** | 1756 | 1838 | 2896 | 500 | 551 | 745 | 254 | 279 | 340 | 158 | 171 | 196 | 109 | 117 | 129 |
| | *** | 1783 | 1979 | 3062 | 520 | 606 | 770 | 264 | 301 | 341 | 164 | 181 | 189 | 113 | 122 | 118 |
| 0.45 | *** | 1689 | 1792 | 2999 | 491 | 549 | 762 | 251 | 278 | 344 | 156 | 170 | 197 | 107 | 115 | 128 |
| | *** | 1724 | 1962 | 3124 | 514 | 609 | 778 | 262 | 302 | 341 | 162 | 181 | 187 | 111 | 121 | 115 |
| 0.5 | *** | 1585 | 1712 | 3033 | 473 | 536 | 762 | 243 | 272 | 341 | 151 | 166 | 193 | 103 | 111 | 124 |
| | *** | 1630 | 1908 | 3124 | 498 | 601 | 770 | 256 | 297 | 334 | 157 | 177 | 181 | 107 | 117 | 110 |
| 0.55 | *** | 1456 | 1607 | 3000 | 449 | 515 | 745 | 232 | 262 | 329 | 144 | 158 | 184 | 98 | 105 | 117 |
| | *** | 1510 | 1825 | 3062 | 476 | 582 | 746 | 245 | 286 | 320 | 150 | 169 | 171 | 101 | 110 | 103 |
| 0.6 | *** | 1312 | 1485 | 2898 | 419 | 487 | 712 | 218 | 246 | 310 | 134 | 147 | 171 | 90 | 97 | 108 |
| | *** | 1376 | 1718 | 2936 | 447 | 553 | 707 | 230 | 270 | 299 | 140 | 157 | 157 | 93 | 102 | 93 |
| 0.65 | *** | 1164 | 1351 | 2728 | 385 | 451 | 661 | 200 | 227 | 284 | 122 | 134 | 155 | 81 | 87 | 96 |
| | *** | 1234 | 1591 | 2748 | 412 | 515 | 652 | 211 | 248 | 271 | 127 | 143 | 140 | 84 | 91 | 80 |
| 0.7 | *** | 1016 | 1210 | 2491 | 346 | 408 | 593 | 178 | 202 | 250 | 107 | 117 | 133 | 69 | 74 | 81 |
| | *** | 1091 | 1446 | 2496 | 372 | 466 | 581 | 189 | 221 | 236 | 111 | 124 | 118 | 72 | 77 | 65 |
| 0.75 | *** | 872 | 1061 | 2186 | 303 | 357 | 509 | 153 | 172 | 209 | 89 | 97 | 108 | . | . | . |
| | *** | 946 | 1282 | 2182 | 325 | 407 | 495 | 161 | 187 | 194 | 92 | 102 | 93 | . | . | . |
| 0.8 | *** | 730 | 902 | 1816 | 252 | 297 | 408 | 123 | 137 | 161 | . | . | . | . | . | . |
| | *** | 798 | 1096 | 1806 | 271 | 335 | 393 | 129 | 147 | 145 | . | . | . | . | . | . |
| 0.85 | *** | 583 | 726 | 1380 | 194 | 224 | 291 | . | . | . | . | . | . | . | . | . |
| | *** | 640 | 880 | 1366 | 207 | 249 | 275 | . | . | . | . | . | . | . | . | . |
| 0.9 | *** | 419 | 518 | 879 | . | . | . | . | . | . | . | . | . | . | . | . |
| | *** | 460 | 618 | 864 | . | . | . | . | . | . | . | . | . | . | . | . |

TABLE 5: ALPHA= 0.025 POWER= 0.8    EXPECTED ACCRUAL THRU MINIMUM FOLLOW-UP= 180

| | DEL=.05 | | | DEL=.10 | | | DEL=.15 | | | DEL=.20 | | | DEL=.25 | | |
|---|---|---|---|---|---|---|---|---|---|---|---|---|---|---|---|
| FACT= | 1.0 .75 | .50 .25 | .00 BIN | 1.0 .75 | .50 .25 | .00 BIN | 1.0 .75 | .50 .25 | .00 BIN | 1.0 75 | .50 .25 | .00 BIN | 1.0 .75 | .50 .25 | .00 BIN |
| PCONT=*** | | | | REQUIRED NUMBER OF PATIENTS | | | | | | | | | | | |
| 0.05 *** | 472 | 476 | 502 | 170 | 172 | 178 | 100 | 102 | 104 | 71 | 72 | 73 | 55 | 56 | 57 |
| *** | 473 | 483 | 864 | 171 | 175 | 275 | 101 | 103 | 145 | 71 | 73 | 93 | 56 | 56 | 65 |
| 0.1 *** | 861 | 871 | 967 | 270 | 278 | 299 | 147 | 151 | 159 | 98 | 100 | 104 | 73 | 74 | 76 |
| *** | 864 | 889 | 1366 | 273 | 285 | 393 | 148 | 154 | 194 | 99 | 102 | 118 | 73 | 75 | 80 |
| 0.15 *** | 1192 | 1210 | 1418 | 352 | 366 | 409 | 184 | 191 | 207 | 119 | 123 | 130 | 86 | 89 | 92 |
| *** | 1198 | 1242 | 1806 | 358 | 380 | 495 | 187 | 197 | 236 | 121 | 126 | 140 | 87 | 90 | 93 |
| 0.2 *** | 1450 | 1476 | 1829 | 416 | 436 | 507 | 212 | 224 | 248 | 135 | 141 | 152 | 96 | 100 | 105 |
| *** | 1459 | 1525 | 2182 | 423 | 458 | 581 | 217 | 233 | 271 | 138 | 146 | 157 | 98 | 102 | 103 |
| 0.25 *** | 1630 | 1668 | 2188 | 461 | 489 | 591 | 233 | 248 | 282 | 147 | 155 | 170 | 103 | 108 | 116 |
| *** | 1643 | 1737 | 2496 | 471 | 519 | 652 | 239 | 261 | 299 | 150 | 161 | 171 | 105 | 111 | 110 |
| 0.3 *** | 1738 | 1789 | 2489 | 489 | 525 | 659 | 247 | 266 | 309 | 154 | 164 | 183 | 108 | 114 | 123 |
| *** | 1755 | 1881 | 2748 | 503 | 564 | 707 | 255 | 282 | 320 | 159 | 172 | 181 | 110 | 118 | 115 |
| 0.35 *** | 1778 | 1845 | 2725 | 503 | 547 | 710 | 254 | 276 | 328 | 158 | 170 | 192 | 110 | 117 | 127 |
| *** | 1801 | 1964 | 2936 | 520 | 595 | 746 | 263 | 296 | 334 | 164 | 179 | 187 | 113 | 121 | 118 |
| 0.4 *** | 1761 | 1847 | 2896 | 504 | 556 | 745 | 256 | 281 | 340 | 159 | 172 | 196 | 110 | 117 | 129 |
| *** | 1790 | 1993 | 3062 | 525 | 611 | 770 | 267 | 303 | 341 | 165 | 182 | 189 | 113 | 122 | 118 |
| 0.45 *** | 1695 | 1804 | 2999 | 495 | 554 | 762 | 253 | 280 | 344 | 157 | 171 | 197 | 108 | 116 | 128 |
| *** | 1733 | 1978 | 3124 | 519 | 614 | 778 | 265 | 304 | 341 | 163 | 182 | 187 | 112 | 121 | 115 |
| 0.5 *** | 1593 | 1726 | 3034 | 478 | 542 | 762 | 246 | 275 | 341 | 152 | 167 | 192 | 104 | 112 | 124 |
| *** | 1640 | 1926 | 3124 | 504 | 606 | 770 | 258 | 299 | 334 | 159 | 177 | 181 | 108 | 117 | 110 |
| 0.55 *** | 1466 | 1623 | 3000 | 454 | 521 | 746 | 235 | 264 | 329 | 145 | 159 | 184 | 98 | 106 | 117 |
| *** | 1522 | 1845 | 3062 | 481 | 588 | 746 | 247 | 288 | 320 | 151 | 169 | 171 | 102 | 111 | 103 |
| 0.6 *** | 1324 | 1502 | 2898 | 425 | 492 | 712 | 220 | 249 | 310 | 135 | 148 | 171 | 91 | 98 | 108 |
| *** | 1390 | 1739 | 2936 | 452 | 559 | 707 | 232 | 272 | 299 | 141 | 158 | 157 | 94 | 102 | 93 |
| 0.65 *** | 1177 | 1370 | 2728 | 390 | 456 | 661 | 202 | 229 | 284 | 123 | 135 | 155 | 81 | 87 | 96 |
| *** | 1250 | 1613 | 2748 | 418 | 519 | 652 | 213 | 250 | 271 | 128 | 143 | 140 | 84 | 91 | 80 |
| 0.7 *** | 1030 | 1228 | 2491 | 351 | 413 | 593 | 180 | 204 | 250 | 108 | 118 | 134 | 70 | 74 | 81 |
| *** | 1107 | 1467 | 2496 | 377 | 470 | 581 | 191 | 222 | 236 | 112 | 125 | 118 | 72 | 77 | 65 |
| 0.75 *** | 886 | 1078 | 2186 | 307 | 361 | 509 | 155 | 174 | 209 | 90 | 97 | 108 | . | . | . |
| *** | 961 | 1301 | 2182 | 330 | 410 | 495 | 163 | 188 | 194 | 93 | 102 | 93 | . | . | . |
| 0.8 *** | 743 | 917 | 1816 | 256 | 300 | 408 | 124 | 138 | 161 | . | . | . | . | . | . |
| *** | 812 | 1113 | 1806 | 275 | 338 | 393 | 130 | 147 | 145 | . | . | . | . | . | . |
| 0.85 *** | 594 | 738 | 1380 | 196 | 226 | 291 | . | . | . | . | . | . | . | . | . |
| *** | 652 | 893 | 1366 | 209 | 251 | 275 | . | . | . | . | . | . | . | . | . |
| 0.9 *** | 427 | 527 | 879 | . | . | . | . | . | . | . | . | . | . | . | . |
| *** | 468 | 626 | 864 | . | . | . | . | . | . | . | . | . | . | . | . |

TABLE 5: ALPHA= 0.025 POWER= 0.8     EXPECTED ACCRUAL THRU MINIMUM FOLLOW-UP= 190

|  |  | DEL=.05 | | | DEL=.10 | | | DEL=.15 | | | DEL=.20 | | | DEL=.25 | | |
|---|---|---|---|---|---|---|---|---|---|---|---|---|---|---|---|---|
| FACT= |  | 1.0 .75 | .50 .25 | .00 BIN | 1.0 .75 | .50 .25 | .00 BIN | 1.0 .75 | .50 .25 | .00 BIN | 1.0 75 | .50 .25 | .00 BIN | 1.0 .75 | .50 .25 | .00 BIN |
| PCONT=*** | | | | | | REQUIRED NUMBER OF PATIENTS | | | | | | | | | | |
| 0.05 | *** | 472 | 477 | 502 | 170 | 173 | 178 | 100 | 102 | 104 | 71 | 72 | 73 | 55 | 56 | 57 |
|  | *** | 474 | 483 | 864 | 171 | 175 | 275 | 101 | 103 | 145 | 71 | 73 | 93 | 56 | 56 | 65 |
| 0.1 | *** | 861 | 872 | 967 | 271 | 278 | 299 | 147 | 151 | 158 | 98 | 100 | 104 | 73 | 74 | 76 |
|  | *** | 865 | 891 | 1366 | 274 | 286 | 393 | 149 | 154 | 194 | 99 | 102 | 118 | 73 | 75 | 80 |
| 0.15 | *** | 1193 | 1212 | 1418 | 353 | 367 | 409 | 184 | 192 | 206 | 119 | 123 | 130 | 86 | 89 | 92 |
|  | *** | 1199 | 1245 | 1806 | 359 | 381 | 495 | 187 | 198 | 236 | 121 | 126 | 140 | 87 | 90 | 93 |
| 0.2 | *** | 1451 | 1479 | 1829 | 417 | 438 | 507 | 213 | 224 | 248 | 135 | 142 | 152 | 96 | 100 | 105 |
|  | *** | 1461 | 1530 | 2182 | 425 | 460 | 581 | 218 | 234 | 271 | 138 | 146 | 157 | 98 | 102 | 103 |
| 0.25 | *** | 1633 | 1672 | 2188 | 462 | 491 | 591 | 234 | 249 | 282 | 147 | 155 | 170 | 104 | 108 | 116 |
|  | *** | 1646 | 1744 | 2496 | 474 | 522 | 652 | 241 | 262 | 299 | 151 | 161 | 171 | 106 | 112 | 110 |
| 0.3 | *** | 1740 | 1794 | 2489 | 491 | 528 | 659 | 248 | 267 | 309 | 155 | 165 | 183 | 108 | 114 | 123 |
|  | *** | 1759 | 1890 | 2748 | 506 | 567 | 707 | 256 | 283 | 320 | 160 | 173 | 181 | 111 | 118 | 115 |
| 0.35 | *** | 1782 | 1853 | 2725 | 506 | 551 | 710 | 256 | 278 | 328 | 159 | 171 | 192 | 111 | 117 | 127 |
|  | *** | 1806 | 1975 | 2936 | 523 | 598 | 746 | 265 | 297 | 334 | 165 | 180 | 187 | 114 | 122 | 118 |
| 0.4 | *** | 1765 | 1856 | 2896 | 508 | 560 | 744 | 258 | 283 | 340 | 160 | 173 | 196 | 111 | 118 | 129 |
|  | *** | 1796 | 2007 | 3062 | 529 | 615 | 770 | 269 | 304 | 341 | 166 | 183 | 189 | 114 | 123 | 118 |
| 0.45 | *** | 1702 | 1815 | 2999 | 500 | 558 | 762 | 255 | 282 | 344 | 158 | 172 | 197 | 109 | 116 | 128 |
|  | *** | 1741 | 1994 | 3124 | 523 | 619 | 778 | 267 | 305 | 341 | 164 | 182 | 187 | 112 | 121 | 115 |
| 0.5 | *** | 1601 | 1739 | 3034 | 483 | 547 | 762 | 248 | 277 | 341 | 154 | 168 | 193 | 105 | 112 | 124 |
|  | *** | 1650 | 1944 | 3124 | 509 | 611 | 770 | 260 | 301 | 334 | 160 | 178 | 181 | 108 | 117 | 110 |
| 0.55 | *** | 1475 | 1638 | 3000 | 459 | 526 | 745 | 237 | 266 | 329 | 146 | 160 | 184 | 99 | 106 | 117 |
|  | *** | 1534 | 1864 | 3062 | 486 | 592 | 746 | 249 | 290 | 320 | 152 | 170 | 171 | 102 | 111 | 103 |
| 0.6 | *** | 1335 | 1519 | 2898 | 430 | 498 | 712 | 222 | 251 | 310 | 136 | 149 | 171 | 91 | 98 | 108 |
|  | *** | 1403 | 1759 | 2936 | 458 | 563 | 707 | 235 | 273 | 299 | 142 | 159 | 157 | 94 | 102 | 93 |
| 0.65 | *** | 1190 | 1387 | 2728 | 396 | 462 | 661 | 204 | 230 | 284 | 124 | 135 | 155 | 82 | 88 | 96 |
|  | *** | 1265 | 1633 | 2748 | 423 | 524 | 652 | 216 | 251 | 271 | 129 | 144 | 140 | 84 | 91 | 80 |
| 0.7 | *** | 1044 | 1246 | 2491 | 356 | 418 | 593 | 182 | 205 | 250 | 109 | 118 | 133 | 70 | 75 | 81 |
|  | *** | 1122 | 1486 | 2496 | 382 | 474 | 581 | 192 | 223 | 236 | 113 | 125 | 118 | 72 | 78 | 65 |
| 0.75 | *** | 900 | 1095 | 2186 | 311 | 365 | 509 | 156 | 175 | 209 | 90 | 98 | 108 | . | . | . |
|  | *** | 976 | 1319 | 2182 | 334 | 414 | 495 | 165 | 189 | 194 | 94 | 102 | 93 | . | . | . |
| 0.8 | *** | 755 | 932 | 1816 | 260 | 303 | 408 | 125 | 139 | 161 | . | . | . | . | . | . |
|  | *** | 825 | 1128 | 1806 | 278 | 341 | 393 | 131 | 148 | 145 | . | . | . | . | . | . |
| 0.85 | *** | 605 | 750 | 1380 | 199 | 229 | 291 | . | . | . | . | . | . | . | . | . |
|  | *** | 663 | 905 | 1366 | 212 | 252 | 275 | . | . | . | . | . | . | . | . | . |
| 0.9 | *** | 435 | 535 | 879 | . | . | . | . | . | . | . | . | . | . | . | . |
|  | *** | 476 | 633 | 864 | . | . | . | . | . | . | . | . | . | . | . | . |

TABLE 5: ALPHA= 0.025 POWER= 0.8    EXPECTED ACCRUAL THRU MINIMUM FOLLOW-UP= 200

| | | DEL=.05 | | | DEL=.10 | | | DEL=.15 | | | DEL=.20 | | | DEL=.25 | | |
|---|---|---|---|---|---|---|---|---|---|---|---|---|---|---|---|---|---|
| FACT= | | 1.0 .75 | .50 .25 | .00 BIN | 1.0 .75 | .50 .25 | .00 BIN | 1.0 .75 | .50 .25 | .00 BIN | 1.0 75 | .50 .25 | .00 BIN | 1.0 .75 | .50 .25 | .00 BIN |
| PCONT=*** | | | | REQUIRED | NUMBER | OF PATIENTS | | | | | | | | | | |
| 0.05 | *** | 472 | 477 | 502 | 170 | 173 | 178 | 100 | 102 | 104 | 71 | 72 | 73 | 55 | 56 | 57 |
| | *** | 474 | 484 | 864 | 171 | 175 | 275 | 101 | 103 | 145 | 72 | 73 | 93 | 56 | 56 | 65 |
| 0.1 | *** | 862 | 873 | 967 | 271 | 279 | 299 | 147 | 151 | 159 | 98 | 101 | 104 | 73 | 74 | 76 |
| | *** | 866 | 892 | 1366 | 274 | 286 | 393 | 149 | 154 | 194 | 99 | 102 | 118 | 74 | 75 | 80 |
| 0.15 | *** | 1194 | 1214 | 1418 | 354 | 368 | 409 | 185 | 192 | 207 | 120 | 124 | 130 | 86 | 89 | 92 |
| | *** | 1201 | 1248 | 1806 | 360 | 382 | 495 | 188 | 198 | 236 | 121 | 126 | 140 | 88 | 90 | 93 |
| 0.2 | *** | 1453 | 1482 | 1829 | 418 | 440 | 507 | 214 | 225 | 248 | 136 | 142 | 152 | 97 | 100 | 105 |
| | *** | 1463 | 1535 | 2182 | 427 | 462 | 581 | 219 | 234 | 271 | 139 | 146 | 157 | 98 | 103 | 103 |
| 0.25 | *** | 1635 | 1676 | 2188 | 464 | 493 | 591 | 235 | 250 | 282 | 148 | 156 | 170 | 104 | 109 | 116 |
| | *** | 1649 | 1751 | 2496 | 476 | 524 | 652 | 242 | 263 | 299 | 152 | 162 | 171 | 106 | 112 | 110 |
| 0.3 | *** | 1743 | 1800 | 2489 | 494 | 531 | 659 | 250 | 268 | 309 | 156 | 166 | 183 | 109 | 114 | 123 |
| | *** | 1762 | 1899 | 2748 | 508 | 570 | 707 | 258 | 284 | 320 | 160 | 173 | 181 | 111 | 118 | 115 |
| 0.35 | *** | 1786 | 1860 | 2725 | 509 | 554 | 710 | 257 | 280 | 328 | 160 | 172 | 192 | 111 | 118 | 127 |
| | *** | 1811 | 1986 | 2936 | 527 | 601 | 746 | 267 | 298 | 334 | 165 | 180 | 187 | 114 | 122 | 118 |
| 0.4 | *** | 1770 | 1865 | 2896 | 511 | 564 | 745 | 260 | 285 | 340 | 161 | 174 | 196 | 111 | 118 | 129 |
| | *** | 1803 | 2020 | 3062 | 532 | 619 | 770 | 270 | 306 | 341 | 167 | 183 | 189 | 114 | 123 | 118 |
| 0.45 | *** | 1708 | 1826 | 2999 | 504 | 563 | 762 | 257 | 284 | 344 | 159 | 173 | 197 | 109 | 117 | 128 |
| | *** | 1749 | 2010 | 3124 | 527 | 623 | 778 | 269 | 307 | 341 | 165 | 183 | 187 | 113 | 122 | 115 |
| 0.5 | *** | 1609 | 1752 | 3034 | 487 | 552 | 762 | 250 | 279 | 341 | 155 | 169 | 193 | 105 | 113 | 124 |
| | *** | 1660 | 1962 | 3124 | 513 | 616 | 770 | 262 | 302 | 334 | 161 | 179 | 181 | 109 | 118 | 110 |
| 0.55 | *** | 1485 | 1653 | 3000 | 464 | 531 | 746 | 239 | 268 | 329 | 147 | 161 | 184 | 100 | 107 | 117 |
| | *** | 1546 | 1883 | 3062 | 491 | 597 | 746 | 252 | 291 | 320 | 153 | 171 | 171 | 103 | 111 | 103 |
| 0.6 | *** | 1347 | 1535 | 2898 | 435 | 503 | 712 | 225 | 253 | 311 | 137 | 150 | 171 | 92 | 98 | 108 |
| | *** | 1417 | 1779 | 2936 | 463 | 568 | 707 | 237 | 275 | 299 | 143 | 159 | 157 | 95 | 103 | 93 |
| 0.65 | *** | 1202 | 1404 | 2728 | 400 | 466 | 661 | 206 | 232 | 284 | 125 | 136 | 155 | 82 | 88 | 96 |
| | *** | 1279 | 1652 | 2748 | 428 | 528 | 652 | 218 | 252 | 271 | 130 | 144 | 140 | 85 | 91 | 80 |
| 0.7 | *** | 1057 | 1262 | 2491 | 361 | 422 | 593 | 184 | 207 | 250 | 109 | 119 | 133 | 71 | 75 | 81 |
| | *** | 1137 | 1505 | 2496 | 386 | 478 | 581 | 194 | 224 | 236 | 114 | 125 | 118 | 73 | 78 | 65 |
| 0.75 | *** | 913 | 1111 | 2186 | 315 | 369 | 509 | 158 | 176 | 209 | 91 | 98 | 108 | . | . | . |
| | *** | 991 | 1337 | 2182 | 338 | 417 | 495 | 166 | 190 | 194 | 94 | 103 | 93 | . | . | . |
| 0.8 | *** | 767 | 946 | 1816 | 263 | 306 | 408 | 126 | 139 | 161 | . | . | . | . | . | . |
| | *** | 838 | 1143 | 1806 | 282 | 343 | 393 | 132 | 149 | 145 | . | . | . | . | . | . |
| 0.85 | *** | 615 | 762 | 1380 | 201 | 231 | 291 | . | . | . | . | . | . | . | . | . |
| | *** | 674 | 917 | 1366 | 214 | 254 | 275 | . | . | . | . | . | . | . | . | . |
| 0.9 | *** | 442 | 542 | 879 | . | . | . | . | . | . | . | . | . | . | . | . |
| | *** | 483 | 640 | 864 | . | . | . | . | . | . | . | . | . | . | . | . |

# TABLE 5: ALPHA= 0.025 POWER= 0.8    EXPECTED ACCRUAL THRU MINIMUM FOLLOW-UP= 225

| FACT= | DEL=.05 | | | DEL=.10 | | | DEL=.15 | | | DEL=.20 | | | DEL=.25 | | |
|---|---|---|---|---|---|---|---|---|---|---|---|---|---|---|---|
| | 1.0 .75 | .50 .25 | .00 BIN | 1.0 .75 | .50 .25 | .00 BIN | 1.0 .75 | .50 .25 | .00 BIN | 1.0 75 | .50 .25 | .00 BIN | 1.0 .75 | .50 .25 | .00 BIN |

PCONT=***        REQUIRED NUMBER OF PATIENTS

| PCONT | DEL=.05 1.0/.75 | .50/.25 | .00/BIN | DEL=.10 1.0/.75 | .50/.25 | .00/BIN | DEL=.15 1.0/.75 | .50/.25 | .00/BIN | DEL=.20 1.0/75 | .50/.25 | .00/BIN | DEL=.25 1.0/.75 | .50/.25 | .00/BIN |
|---|---|---|---|---|---|---|---|---|---|---|---|---|---|---|---|
| 0.05 *** | 473 | 478 | 502 | 170 | 173 | 178 | 101 | 102 | 104 | 71 | 72 | 73 | 56 | 56 | 57 |
| *** | 475 | 485 | 864 | 172 | 175 | 275 | 101 | 103 | 145 | 72 | 73 | 93 | 56 | 56 | 65 |
| 0.1 *** | 863 | 876 | 967 | 273 | 280 | 299 | 148 | 152 | 158 | 99 | 101 | 104 | 73 | 75 | 76 |
| *** | 868 | 896 | 1366 | 276 | 287 | 393 | 150 | 155 | 194 | 100 | 102 | 118 | 74 | 75 | 80 |
| 0.15 *** | 1197 | 1218 | 1418 | 356 | 371 | 409 | 186 | 193 | 206 | 120 | 124 | 130 | 87 | 89 | 92 |
| *** | 1204 | 1255 | 1806 | 362 | 384 | 495 | 189 | 199 | 236 | 122 | 127 | 140 | 88 | 91 | 93 |
| 0.2 *** | 1456 | 1489 | 1829 | 422 | 443 | 507 | 216 | 227 | 248 | 137 | 143 | 152 | 97 | 101 | 105 |
| *** | 1467 | 1546 | 2182 | 430 | 465 | 581 | 221 | 235 | 271 | 140 | 147 | 157 | 99 | 103 | 103 |
| 0.25 *** | 1640 | 1686 | 2188 | 469 | 499 | 591 | 238 | 253 | 282 | 149 | 157 | 170 | 105 | 109 | 116 |
| *** | 1656 | 1767 | 2496 | 481 | 529 | 652 | 244 | 264 | 299 | 153 | 163 | 171 | 107 | 112 | 110 |
| 0.3 *** | 1751 | 1813 | 2489 | 500 | 538 | 659 | 253 | 271 | 309 | 158 | 167 | 183 | 110 | 115 | 123 |
| *** | 1772 | 1920 | 2748 | 515 | 577 | 707 | 261 | 286 | 320 | 162 | 174 | 181 | 112 | 119 | 115 |
| 0.35 *** | 1795 | 1877 | 2725 | 516 | 562 | 710 | 261 | 283 | 328 | 162 | 173 | 192 | 112 | 118 | 127 |
| *** | 1823 | 2013 | 2936 | 534 | 609 | 746 | 271 | 300 | 334 | 167 | 181 | 187 | 115 | 122 | 118 |
| 0.4 *** | 1783 | 1887 | 2896 | 520 | 574 | 745 | 264 | 289 | 340 | 164 | 176 | 196 | 113 | 119 | 129 |
| *** | 1819 | 2052 | 3062 | 542 | 627 | 770 | 275 | 309 | 341 | 169 | 185 | 189 | 116 | 124 | 118 |
| 0.45 *** | 1723 | 1853 | 2999 | 513 | 573 | 762 | 262 | 289 | 344 | 162 | 175 | 197 | 111 | 118 | 128 |
| *** | 1769 | 2046 | 3124 | 538 | 633 | 778 | 273 | 310 | 341 | 168 | 184 | 187 | 114 | 122 | 115 |
| 0.5 *** | 1628 | 1784 | 3034 | 498 | 563 | 762 | 255 | 283 | 341 | 157 | 171 | 192 | 107 | 114 | 124 |
| *** | 1684 | 2002 | 3124 | 524 | 626 | 770 | 267 | 305 | 334 | 163 | 180 | 181 | 110 | 118 | 110 |
| 0.55 *** | 1508 | 1688 | 3000 | 475 | 543 | 745 | 244 | 272 | 329 | 150 | 163 | 184 | 101 | 108 | 117 |
| *** | 1574 | 1927 | 3062 | 503 | 607 | 746 | 257 | 294 | 320 | 156 | 172 | 171 | 104 | 112 | 103 |
| 0.6 *** | 1374 | 1573 | 2898 | 446 | 514 | 712 | 230 | 257 | 311 | 140 | 152 | 171 | 93 | 99 | 108 |
| *** | 1449 | 1824 | 2936 | 474 | 578 | 707 | 241 | 278 | 299 | 145 | 160 | 157 | 96 | 103 | 93 |
| 0.65 *** | 1232 | 1443 | 2728 | 411 | 477 | 661 | 211 | 236 | 284 | 127 | 138 | 155 | 84 | 89 | 95 |
| *** | 1313 | 1698 | 2748 | 439 | 538 | 652 | 222 | 255 | 271 | 132 | 145 | 140 | 86 | 92 | 80 |
| 0.7 *** | 1089 | 1301 | 2491 | 371 | 432 | 593 | 188 | 210 | 250 | 111 | 120 | 133 | 72 | 75 | 81 |
| *** | 1172 | 1549 | 2496 | 397 | 487 | 581 | 198 | 227 | 236 | 115 | 126 | 118 | 73 | 78 | 65 |
| 0.75 *** | 944 | 1148 | 2186 | 325 | 378 | 509 | 161 | 179 | 209 | 92 | 99 | 108 | . | . | . |
| *** | 1024 | 1376 | 2182 | 347 | 424 | 495 | 169 | 192 | 194 | 95 | 103 | 93 | . | . | . |
| 0.8 *** | 796 | 979 | 1816 | 271 | 313 | 408 | 129 | 141 | 161 | . | . | . | . | . | . |
| *** | 869 | 1177 | 1806 | 289 | 348 | 393 | 134 | 150 | 145 | . | . | . | . | . | . |
| 0.85 *** | 639 | 788 | 1380 | 206 | 235 | 291 | . | . | . | . | . | . | . | . | . |
| *** | 699 | 942 | 1366 | 219 | 257 | 275 | . | . | . | . | . | . | . | . | . |
| 0.9 *** | 459 | 559 | 879 | . | . | . | . | . | . | . | . | . | . | . | . |
| *** | 500 | 656 | 864 | . | . | . | . | . | . | . | . | . | . | . | . |

TABLE 5: ALPHA= 0.025 POWER= 0.8    EXPECTED ACCRUAL THRU MINIMUM FOLLOW-UP= 250

| | DEL=.05 | | | DEL=.10 | | | DEL=.15 | | | DEL=.20 | | | DEL=.25 | | |
|---|---|---|---|---|---|---|---|---|---|---|---|---|---|---|---|
| FACT= | 1.0 .75 | .50 .25 | .00 BIN | 1.0 .75 | .50 .25 | .00 BIN | 1.0 .75 | .50 .25 | .00 BIN | 1.0 75 | .50 .25 | .00 BIN | 1.0 .75 | .50 .25 | .00 BIN |
| PCONT=*** | | | | | | | REQUIRED NUMBER OF PATIENTS | | | | | | | | |
| 0.05 *** | 474 | 479 | 502 | 171 | 174 | 178 | 101 | 102 | 104 | 72 | 72 | 73 | 56 | 56 | 57 |
| *** | 476 | 486 | 864 | 172 | 176 | 275 | 101 | 103 | 145 | 72 | 73 | 93 | 56 | 57 | 65 |
| 0.1 *** | 865 | 879 | 967 | 274 | 282 | 299 | 149 | 152 | 159 | 99 | 101 | 104 | 74 | 75 | 76 |
| *** | 870 | 899 | 1366 | 277 | 288 | 393 | 150 | 155 | 194 | 100 | 102 | 118 | 74 | 76 | 80 |
| 0.15 *** | 1199 | 1223 | 1418 | 359 | 373 | 409 | 187 | 194 | 207 | 121 | 125 | 130 | 87 | 89 | 92 |
| *** | 1207 | 1262 | 1806 | 364 | 386 | 495 | 190 | 199 | 236 | 123 | 127 | 140 | 88 | 91 | 93 |
| 0.2 *** | 1460 | 1496 | 1829 | 425 | 447 | 507 | 218 | 228 | 248 | 138 | 144 | 152 | 98 | 101 | 105 |
| *** | 1472 | 1557 | 2182 | 434 | 468 | 581 | 222 | 236 | 271 | 141 | 147 | 157 | 99 | 103 | 103 |
| 0.25 *** | 1645 | 1696 | 2189 | 473 | 503 | 591 | 240 | 255 | 282 | 151 | 158 | 170 | 106 | 110 | 116 |
| *** | 1662 | 1782 | 2496 | 485 | 533 | 652 | 247 | 266 | 299 | 154 | 163 | 171 | 108 | 112 | 110 |
| 0.3 *** | 1758 | 1827 | 2489 | 505 | 544 | 659 | 256 | 274 | 309 | 159 | 168 | 183 | 111 | 116 | 123 |
| *** | 1781 | 1940 | 2748 | 521 | 582 | 707 | 264 | 288 | 320 | 163 | 175 | 181 | 113 | 119 | 115 |
| 0.35 *** | 1804 | 1895 | 2725 | 523 | 570 | 710 | 265 | 286 | 328 | 164 | 175 | 192 | 113 | 119 | 127 |
| *** | 1836 | 2037 | 2936 | 542 | 616 | 746 | 274 | 303 | 334 | 169 | 182 | 187 | 116 | 123 | 118 |
| 0.4 *** | 1795 | 1909 | 2896 | 528 | 582 | 745 | 268 | 292 | 340 | 166 | 177 | 196 | 114 | 120 | 129 |
| *** | 1834 | 2081 | 3062 | 550 | 635 | 770 | 279 | 311 | 341 | 171 | 186 | 189 | 117 | 124 | 118 |
| 0.45 *** | 1739 | 1878 | 2999 | 522 | 583 | 762 | 266 | 292 | 344 | 164 | 177 | 197 | 112 | 119 | 128 |
| *** | 1788 | 2080 | 3124 | 547 | 641 | 778 | 278 | 313 | 341 | 170 | 185 | 187 | 115 | 123 | 115 |
| 0.5 *** | 1647 | 1813 | 3034 | 507 | 573 | 762 | 260 | 287 | 341 | 159 | 172 | 193 | 108 | 115 | 124 |
| *** | 1708 | 2040 | 3124 | 534 | 634 | 770 | 272 | 308 | 334 | 165 | 181 | 181 | 111 | 119 | 110 |
| 0.55 *** | 1531 | 1721 | 3000 | 485 | 553 | 746 | 249 | 276 | 329 | 152 | 164 | 184 | 102 | 109 | 117 |
| *** | 1602 | 1967 | 3062 | 513 | 616 | 746 | 261 | 297 | 320 | 158 | 173 | 171 | 105 | 112 | 103 |
| 0.6 *** | 1400 | 1608 | 2898 | 456 | 524 | 712 | 234 | 260 | 311 | 142 | 154 | 172 | 94 | 100 | 108 |
| *** | 1479 | 1865 | 2936 | 485 | 587 | 707 | 246 | 280 | 299 | 147 | 161 | 157 | 97 | 104 | 93 |
| 0.65 *** | 1261 | 1480 | 2728 | 422 | 487 | 661 | 215 | 239 | 284 | 129 | 139 | 155 | 84 | 89 | 96 |
| *** | 1345 | 1739 | 2748 | 449 | 546 | 652 | 226 | 258 | 271 | 134 | 146 | 140 | 87 | 92 | 80 |
| 0.7 *** | 1118 | 1337 | 2491 | 380 | 441 | 593 | 192 | 213 | 250 | 113 | 121 | 134 | 72 | 76 | 81 |
| *** | 1204 | 1588 | 2496 | 406 | 494 | 581 | 201 | 229 | 236 | 117 | 127 | 118 | 74 | 78 | 65 |
| 0.75 *** | 972 | 1181 | 2186 | 333 | 386 | 509 | 164 | 181 | 209 | 94 | 100 | 108 | . | . | . |
| *** | 1055 | 1412 | 2182 | 355 | 430 | 495 | 172 | 193 | 194 | 97 | 104 | 93 | . | . | . |
| 0.8 *** | 822 | 1008 | 1816 | 277 | 319 | 408 | 131 | 143 | 161 | . | . | . | . | . | . |
| *** | 897 | 1207 | 1806 | 295 | 353 | 393 | 136 | 151 | 145 | . | . | . | . | . | . |
| 0.85 *** | 660 | 811 | 1380 | 211 | 239 | 291 | . | . | . | . | . | . | . | . | . |
| *** | 722 | 965 | 1366 | 223 | 260 | 275 | . | . | . | . | . | . | . | . | . |
| 0.9 *** | 474 | 574 | 879 | . | . | . | . | . | . | . | . | . | . | . | . |
| *** | 515 | 669 | 864 | . | . | . | . | . | . | . | . | . | . | . | . |

## TABLE 5: ALPHA= 0.025 POWER= 0.8     EXPECTED ACCRUAL THRU MINIMUM FOLLOW-UP= 275

| | DEL=.05 | | | DEL=.10 | | | DEL=.15 | | | DEL=.20 | | | DEL=.25 | | |
|---|---|---|---|---|---|---|---|---|---|---|---|---|---|---|---|
| FACT= | 1.0 .75 | .50 .25 | .00 BIN | 1.0 .75 | .50 .25 | .00 BIN | 1.0 .75 | .50 .25 | .00 BIN | 1.0 75 | .50 .25 | .00 BIN | 1.0 .75 | .50 .25 | .00 BIN |

PCONT=***     REQUIRED NUMBER OF PATIENTS

| PCONT | 1.0/.75 | .50/.25 | .00/BIN | 1.0/.75 | .50/.25 | .00/BIN | 1.0/.75 | .50/.25 | .00/BIN | 1.0/75 | .50/.25 | .00/BIN | 1.0/.75 | .50/.25 | .00/BIN |
|---|---|---|---|---|---|---|---|---|---|---|---|---|---|---|---|
| 0.05 *** | 474 | 480 | 502 | 171 | 174 | 178 | 101 | 102 | 104 | 72 | 72 | 73 | 56 | 56 | 57 |
| *** | 476 | 487 | 864 | 172 | 176 | 275 | 102 | 103 | 145 | 72 | 73 | 93 | 56 | 56 | 65 |
| 0.1 *** | 866 | 881 | 967 | 275 | 282 | 299 | 149 | 153 | 158 | 99 | 101 | 104 | 74 | 75 | 76 |
| *** | 871 | 903 | 1366 | 278 | 289 | 393 | 151 | 155 | 194 | 100 | 103 | 118 | 74 | 76 | 80 |
| 0.15 *** | 1201 | 1227 | 1418 | 360 | 375 | 409 | 188 | 195 | 206 | 122 | 125 | 130 | 88 | 90 | 92 |
| *** | 1210 | 1268 | 1806 | 366 | 388 | 495 | 191 | 200 | 236 | 123 | 127 | 140 | 89 | 91 | 93 |
| 0.2 *** | 1464 | 1503 | 1829 | 428 | 450 | 507 | 219 | 230 | 248 | 139 | 144 | 152 | 98 | 101 | 105 |
| *** | 1477 | 1567 | 2182 | 437 | 470 | 581 | 224 | 237 | 271 | 141 | 148 | 157 | 100 | 103 | 103 |
| 0.25 *** | 1650 | 1706 | 2189 | 477 | 508 | 591 | 242 | 256 | 282 | 152 | 159 | 169 | 106 | 110 | 116 |
| *** | 1669 | 1796 | 2496 | 490 | 537 | 652 | 249 | 267 | 299 | 155 | 164 | 171 | 108 | 113 | 110 |
| 0.3 *** | 1765 | 1840 | 2489 | 510 | 549 | 659 | 258 | 276 | 309 | 161 | 169 | 183 | 112 | 116 | 123 |
| *** | 1790 | 1958 | 2748 | 526 | 587 | 707 | 266 | 289 | 320 | 165 | 175 | 181 | 114 | 119 | 115 |
| 0.35 *** | 1814 | 1911 | 2725 | 529 | 576 | 710 | 268 | 289 | 328 | 166 | 176 | 192 | 114 | 120 | 127 |
| *** | 1848 | 2060 | 2936 | 548 | 621 | 746 | 277 | 305 | 334 | 171 | 183 | 187 | 117 | 123 | 118 |
| 0.4 *** | 1807 | 1929 | 2896 | 535 | 590 | 745 | 272 | 295 | 340 | 168 | 179 | 196 | 115 | 121 | 129 |
| *** | 1850 | 2109 | 3062 | 557 | 641 | 770 | 282 | 313 | 341 | 173 | 186 | 189 | 118 | 124 | 118 |
| 0.45 *** | 1754 | 1903 | 2999 | 530 | 591 | 762 | 270 | 295 | 344 | 166 | 178 | 197 | 113 | 119 | 128 |
| *** | 1807 | 2111 | 3124 | 555 | 648 | 778 | 281 | 315 | 341 | 171 | 186 | 187 | 116 | 123 | 115 |
| 0.5 *** | 1666 | 1841 | 3033 | 516 | 582 | 762 | 264 | 290 | 341 | 161 | 174 | 193 | 109 | 115 | 124 |
| *** | 1730 | 2074 | 3124 | 543 | 642 | 770 | 275 | 310 | 334 | 167 | 182 | 181 | 112 | 119 | 110 |
| 0.55 *** | 1553 | 1752 | 3000 | 495 | 562 | 745 | 253 | 279 | 329 | 154 | 166 | 184 | 103 | 109 | 117 |
| *** | 1628 | 2003 | 3062 | 523 | 624 | 746 | 265 | 300 | 320 | 159 | 174 | 171 | 106 | 113 | 103 |
| 0.6 *** | 1425 | 1641 | 2898 | 466 | 534 | 712 | 238 | 264 | 310 | 144 | 155 | 171 | 95 | 101 | 108 |
| *** | 1508 | 1903 | 2936 | 494 | 594 | 707 | 249 | 283 | 299 | 149 | 162 | 157 | 98 | 104 | 93 |
| 0.65 *** | 1288 | 1513 | 2728 | 431 | 496 | 661 | 219 | 242 | 284 | 131 | 140 | 155 | 85 | 90 | 96 |
| *** | 1375 | 1776 | 2748 | 458 | 553 | 652 | 229 | 260 | 271 | 135 | 147 | 140 | 87 | 92 | 80 |
| 0.7 *** | 1146 | 1370 | 2491 | 389 | 449 | 593 | 195 | 216 | 250 | 114 | 122 | 133 | 73 | 76 | 81 |
| *** | 1234 | 1623 | 2496 | 414 | 500 | 581 | 204 | 230 | 236 | 118 | 127 | 118 | 74 | 78 | 65 |
| 0.75 *** | 999 | 1212 | 2186 | 340 | 392 | 509 | 167 | 183 | 209 | 95 | 100 | 108 | . | . | . |
| *** | 1084 | 1444 | 2182 | 363 | 435 | 495 | 174 | 194 | 194 | 97 | 104 | 93 | . | . | . |
| 0.8 *** | 846 | 1035 | 1816 | 283 | 324 | 408 | 133 | 144 | 161 | . | . | . | . | . | . |
| *** | 922 | 1234 | 1806 | 301 | 356 | 393 | 138 | 151 | 145 | . | . | . | . | . | . |
| 0.85 *** | 680 | 833 | 1380 | 215 | 242 | 291 | . | . | . | . | . | . | . | . | . |
| *** | 742 | 986 | 1366 | 227 | 262 | 275 | . | . | . | . | . | . | . | . | . |
| 0.9 *** | 487 | 588 | 879 | . | . | . | . | . | . | . | . | . | . | . | . |
| *** | 529 | 681 | 864 | . | . | . | . | . | . | . | . | . | . | . | . |

## TABLE 5: ALPHA= 0.025 POWER= 0.8   EXPECTED ACCRUAL THRU MINIMUM FOLLOW-UP= 300

| | | DEL=.05 | | | DEL=.10 | | | DEL=.15 | | | DEL=.20 | | | DEL=.25 | | |
|---|---|---|---|---|---|---|---|---|---|---|---|---|---|---|---|---|---|
| FACT= | | 1.0 .75 | .50 .25 | .00 BIN | 1.0 .75 | .50 .25 | .00 BIN | 1.0 .75 | .50 .25 | .00 BIN | 1.0 75 | .50 .25 | .00 BIN | 1.0 .75 | .50 .25 | .00 BIN |
| PCONT=*** | | REQUIRED NUMBER OF PATIENTS | | | | | | | | | | | | | | |
| 0.05 | *** | 475 | 481 | 502 | 172 | 174 | 178 | 101 | 102 | 104 | 72 | 72 | 73 | 56 | 56 | 57 |
| | *** | 477 | 488 | 864 | 173 | 176 | 275 | 102 | 103 | 145 | 72 | 73 | 93 | 56 | 56 | 65 |
| 0.1 | *** | 868 | 883 | 967 | 276 | 283 | 299 | 150 | 153 | 158 | 100 | 102 | 104 | 74 | 75 | 76 |
| | *** | 873 | 905 | 1366 | 279 | 289 | 393 | 151 | 156 | 194 | 100 | 103 | 118 | 74 | 76 | 80 |
| 0.15 | *** | 1204 | 1232 | 1418 | 362 | 377 | 409 | 189 | 196 | 206 | 122 | 125 | 130 | 88 | 90 | 92 |
| | *** | 1213 | 1274 | 1806 | 368 | 389 | 495 | 192 | 200 | 236 | 124 | 127 | 140 | 89 | 91 | 93 |
| 0.2 | *** | 1467 | 1510 | 1829 | 430 | 453 | 507 | 221 | 231 | 248 | 140 | 145 | 152 | 99 | 102 | 105 |
| | *** | 1482 | 1576 | 2182 | 439 | 473 | 581 | 225 | 238 | 271 | 142 | 148 | 157 | 100 | 103 | 103 |
| 0.25 | *** | 1656 | 1715 | 2188 | 481 | 511 | 591 | 244 | 258 | 282 | 153 | 160 | 169 | 107 | 111 | 115 |
| | *** | 1676 | 1809 | 2496 | 493 | 540 | 652 | 250 | 268 | 299 | 156 | 164 | 171 | 109 | 113 | 110 |
| 0.3 | *** | 1772 | 1852 | 2488 | 515 | 554 | 659 | 261 | 278 | 309 | 162 | 170 | 183 | 112 | 117 | 123 |
| | *** | 1800 | 1975 | 2748 | 531 | 591 | 707 | 268 | 291 | 320 | 166 | 176 | 181 | 114 | 120 | 115 |
| 0.35 | *** | 1823 | 1927 | 2725 | 535 | 582 | 710 | 271 | 291 | 328 | 167 | 177 | 192 | 115 | 120 | 127 |
| | *** | 1860 | 2081 | 2936 | 554 | 626 | 746 | 280 | 306 | 334 | 172 | 184 | 187 | 118 | 124 | 118 |
| 0.4 | *** | 1819 | 1949 | 2896 | 541 | 597 | 745 | 275 | 298 | 340 | 169 | 180 | 196 | 116 | 121 | 129 |
| | *** | 1865 | 2134 | 3062 | 564 | 647 | 770 | 285 | 315 | 341 | 174 | 187 | 189 | 118 | 125 | 118 |
| 0.45 | *** | 1769 | 1926 | 2999 | 538 | 599 | 762 | 273 | 298 | 344 | 168 | 179 | 197 | 114 | 120 | 128 |
| | *** | 1826 | 2140 | 3124 | 563 | 654 | 778 | 284 | 317 | 341 | 173 | 187 | 187 | 117 | 124 | 115 |
| 0.5 | *** | 1684 | 1868 | 3034 | 524 | 590 | 762 | 267 | 293 | 340 | 163 | 175 | 193 | 110 | 116 | 124 |
| | *** | 1752 | 2105 | 3124 | 552 | 649 | 770 | 279 | 312 | 334 | 169 | 183 | 181 | 113 | 120 | 110 |
| 0.55 | *** | 1574 | 1781 | 3000 | 503 | 571 | 745 | 256 | 282 | 329 | 156 | 167 | 184 | 104 | 110 | 117 |
| | *** | 1653 | 2037 | 3062 | 531 | 631 | 746 | 268 | 301 | 320 | 161 | 175 | 171 | 107 | 113 | 103 |
| 0.6 | *** | 1449 | 1672 | 2898 | 474 | 542 | 712 | 241 | 266 | 310 | 145 | 156 | 171 | 96 | 101 | 108 |
| | *** | 1535 | 1937 | 2936 | 503 | 601 | 707 | 253 | 285 | 299 | 150 | 163 | 157 | 98 | 104 | 93 |
| 0.65 | *** | 1313 | 1545 | 2728 | 439 | 504 | 661 | 222 | 245 | 284 | 132 | 141 | 154 | 86 | 90 | 95 |
| | *** | 1404 | 1810 | 2748 | 466 | 559 | 652 | 232 | 261 | 271 | 136 | 147 | 140 | 88 | 93 | 80 |
| 0.7 | *** | 1171 | 1401 | 2491 | 397 | 456 | 593 | 198 | 218 | 250 | 115 | 123 | 133 | 73 | 77 | 81 |
| | *** | 1262 | 1655 | 2496 | 422 | 506 | 581 | 207 | 232 | 236 | 119 | 128 | 118 | 75 | 79 | 65 |
| 0.75 | *** | 1024 | 1241 | 2186 | 347 | 398 | 509 | 169 | 185 | 209 | 95 | 101 | 108 | . | . | . |
| | *** | 1111 | 1473 | 2182 | 369 | 440 | 495 | 176 | 195 | 194 | 98 | 104 | 93 | . | . | . |
| 0.8 | *** | 869 | 1060 | 1816 | 289 | 329 | 408 | 134 | 145 | 161 | . | . | . | . | . | . |
| | *** | 946 | 1259 | 1806 | 306 | 360 | 393 | 139 | 152 | 145 | . | . | . | . | . | . |
| 0.85 | *** | 699 | 852 | 1380 | 219 | 245 | 291 | . | . | . | . | . | . | . | . | . |
| | *** | 762 | 1004 | 1366 | 230 | 264 | 275 | . | . | . | . | . | . | . | . | . |
| 0.9 | *** | 500 | 600 | 879 | . | . | . | . | . | . | . | . | . | . | . | . |
| | *** | 542 | 692 | 864 | . | . | . | . | . | . | . | . | . | . | . | . |

# TABLE 5: ALPHA= 0.025 POWER= 0.8    EXPECTED ACCRUAL THRU MINIMUM FOLLOW-UP= 325

| | | DEL=.05 | | | DEL=.10 | | | DEL=.15 | | | DEL=.20 | | | DEL=.25 | | |
|---|---|---|---|---|---|---|---|---|---|---|---|---|---|---|---|---|
| FACT= | | 1.0 .75 | .50 .25 | .00 BIN | 1.0 .75 | .50 .25 | .00 BIN | 1.0 .75 | .50 .25 | .00 BIN | 1.0 75 | .50 .25 | .00 BIN | 1.0 .75 | .50 .25 | .00 BIN |
| PCONT=*** | | | | REQUIRED | NUMBER | OF PATIENTS | | | | | | | | | | |
| 0.05 | *** | 476 | 482 | 502 | 172 | 174 | 178 | 101 | 103 | 104 | 72 | 73 | 73 | 56 | 56 | 57 |
| | *** | 478 | 489 | 864 | 173 | 176 | 275 | 102 | 103 | 145 | 72 | 73 | 93 | 56 | 56 | 65 |
| 0.1 | *** | 869 | 886 | 967 | 277 | 284 | 299 | 150 | 154 | 159 | 100 | 102 | 104 | 74 | 75 | 76 |
| | *** | 875 | 908 | 1366 | 280 | 290 | 393 | 152 | 156 | 194 | 101 | 103 | 118 | 75 | 76 | 80 |
| 0.15 | *** | 1206 | 1236 | 1418 | 364 | 378 | 409 | 190 | 197 | 207 | 122 | 126 | 130 | 88 | 90 | 92 |
| | *** | 1217 | 1279 | 1806 | 370 | 390 | 495 | 193 | 201 | 236 | 124 | 128 | 140 | 89 | 91 | 93 |
| 0.2 | *** | 1471 | 1516 | 1829 | 433 | 455 | 507 | 222 | 232 | 248 | 140 | 145 | 152 | 99 | 102 | 105 |
| | *** | 1487 | 1585 | 2182 | 442 | 475 | 581 | 226 | 239 | 271 | 143 | 148 | 157 | 101 | 104 | 103 |
| 0.25 | *** | 1661 | 1725 | 2188 | 484 | 515 | 591 | 246 | 259 | 282 | 154 | 160 | 170 | 107 | 111 | 116 |
| | *** | 1683 | 1821 | 2496 | 497 | 543 | 652 | 252 | 269 | 299 | 157 | 164 | 171 | 109 | 113 | 110 |
| 0.3 | *** | 1779 | 1865 | 2489 | 519 | 559 | 659 | 263 | 280 | 309 | 163 | 171 | 183 | 113 | 117 | 123 |
| | *** | 1809 | 1992 | 2748 | 536 | 595 | 707 | 270 | 292 | 320 | 167 | 176 | 181 | 115 | 120 | 115 |
| 0.35 | *** | 1832 | 1943 | 2725 | 540 | 588 | 710 | 273 | 293 | 328 | 169 | 178 | 192 | 116 | 121 | 127 |
| | *** | 1872 | 2101 | 2936 | 560 | 631 | 746 | 282 | 307 | 334 | 173 | 184 | 187 | 118 | 124 | 118 |
| 0.4 | *** | 1831 | 1968 | 2896 | 548 | 603 | 745 | 278 | 300 | 340 | 171 | 181 | 196 | 116 | 122 | 129 |
| | *** | 1880 | 2158 | 3062 | 571 | 652 | 770 | 287 | 316 | 341 | 175 | 188 | 189 | 119 | 125 | 118 |
| 0.45 | *** | 1784 | 1949 | 2999 | 545 | 606 | 762 | 277 | 301 | 344 | 169 | 180 | 197 | 115 | 120 | 128 |
| | *** | 1844 | 2166 | 3124 | 570 | 660 | 778 | 287 | 318 | 341 | 174 | 187 | 187 | 117 | 124 | 115 |
| 0.5 | *** | 1702 | 1893 | 3033 | 532 | 597 | 762 | 271 | 296 | 341 | 165 | 176 | 193 | 111 | 117 | 124 |
| | *** | 1773 | 2135 | 3124 | 559 | 655 | 770 | 282 | 314 | 334 | 170 | 183 | 181 | 114 | 120 | 110 |
| 0.55 | *** | 1595 | 1809 | 3000 | 511 | 578 | 745 | 260 | 285 | 329 | 157 | 168 | 184 | 105 | 110 | 117 |
| | *** | 1676 | 2068 | 3062 | 539 | 637 | 746 | 271 | 303 | 320 | 162 | 175 | 171 | 107 | 113 | 103 |
| 0.6 | *** | 1472 | 1701 | 2898 | 482 | 549 | 712 | 245 | 269 | 311 | 147 | 157 | 171 | 97 | 102 | 108 |
| | *** | 1561 | 1969 | 2936 | 511 | 607 | 707 | 255 | 286 | 299 | 151 | 164 | 157 | 99 | 104 | 93 |
| 0.65 | *** | 1338 | 1574 | 2728 | 447 | 511 | 661 | 225 | 247 | 284 | 133 | 142 | 155 | 86 | 91 | 95 |
| | *** | 1430 | 1841 | 2748 | 474 | 565 | 652 | 235 | 263 | 271 | 137 | 148 | 140 | 88 | 93 | 80 |
| 0.7 | *** | 1196 | 1430 | 2491 | 404 | 463 | 593 | 201 | 220 | 250 | 116 | 124 | 133 | 74 | 77 | 81 |
| | *** | 1289 | 1685 | 2496 | 429 | 511 | 581 | 209 | 233 | 236 | 120 | 128 | 118 | 75 | 79 | 65 |
| 0.75 | *** | 1048 | 1267 | 2186 | 353 | 404 | 509 | 171 | 186 | 209 | 96 | 102 | 108 | . | . | . |
| | *** | 1136 | 1500 | 2182 | 375 | 444 | 495 | 178 | 196 | 194 | 99 | 105 | 93 | . | . | . |
| 0.8 | *** | 890 | 1083 | 1816 | 294 | 333 | 408 | 136 | 146 | 161 | . | . | . | . | . | . |
| | *** | 968 | 1281 | 1806 | 311 | 363 | 393 | 141 | 153 | 145 | . | . | . | . | . | . |
| 0.85 | *** | 716 | 870 | 1380 | 222 | 248 | 291 | . | . | . | . | . | . | . | . | . |
| | *** | 779 | 1020 | 1366 | 234 | 266 | 275 | . | . | . | . | . | . | . | . | . |
| 0.9 | *** | 512 | 612 | 879 | . | . | . | . | . | . | . | . | . | . | . | . |
| | *** | 554 | 701 | 864 | . | . | . | . | . | . | . | . | . | . | . | . |

TABLE 5: ALPHA= 0.025 POWER= 0.8    EXPECTED ACCRUAL THRU MINIMUM FOLLOW-UP= 350

| PCONT | FACT= | DEL=.05 1.0/.75 | .50/.25 | .00/BIN | DEL=.10 1.0/.75 | .50/.25 | .00/BIN | DEL=.15 1.0/.75 | .50/.25 | .00/BIN | DEL=.20 1.0/75 | .50/.25 | .00/BIN | DEL=.25 1.0/.75 | .50/.25 | .00/BIN |
|---|---|---|---|---|---|---|---|---|---|---|---|---|---|---|---|---|
| | | | | | | | REQUIRED NUMBER OF PATIENTS | | | | | | | | |
| 0.05 | *** | 476 | 482 | 502 | 172 | 175 | 178 | 101 | 103 | 104 | 72 | 73 | 73 | 56 | 56 | 57 |
| | *** | 479 | 489 | 864 | 173 | 176 | 275 | 102 | 103 | 145 | 72 | 73 | 93 | 56 | 57 | 65 |
| 0.1 | *** | 871 | 888 | 967 | 278 | 285 | 299 | 151 | 154 | 159 | 100 | 102 | 104 | 74 | 75 | 76 |
| | *** | 877 | 911 | 1366 | 281 | 291 | 393 | 152 | 156 | 194 | 101 | 103 | 118 | 75 | 76 | 80 |
| 0.15 | *** | 1209 | 1240 | 1418 | 365 | 380 | 409 | 191 | 197 | 206 | 123 | 126 | 130 | 89 | 90 | 92 |
| | *** | 1220 | 1284 | 1806 | 371 | 391 | 495 | 194 | 201 | 236 | 124 | 128 | 140 | 89 | 91 | 93 |
| 0.2 | *** | 1475 | 1523 | 1829 | 435 | 458 | 507 | 223 | 232 | 248 | 141 | 146 | 152 | 100 | 102 | 105 |
| | *** | 1492 | 1593 | 2182 | 444 | 476 | 581 | 227 | 239 | 271 | 143 | 148 | 157 | 101 | 104 | 103 |
| 0.25 | *** | 1666 | 1734 | 2189 | 488 | 518 | 591 | 248 | 260 | 282 | 155 | 161 | 170 | 108 | 111 | 116 |
| | *** | 1690 | 1833 | 2496 | 500 | 545 | 652 | 253 | 270 | 299 | 157 | 165 | 171 | 110 | 113 | 110 |
| 0.3 | *** | 1786 | 1876 | 2489 | 523 | 563 | 659 | 265 | 281 | 309 | 164 | 172 | 183 | 113 | 118 | 123 |
| | *** | 1818 | 2007 | 2748 | 540 | 598 | 707 | 272 | 293 | 320 | 168 | 177 | 181 | 115 | 120 | 115 |
| 0.35 | *** | 1842 | 1958 | 2725 | 545 | 593 | 710 | 276 | 295 | 328 | 170 | 179 | 192 | 117 | 121 | 127 |
| | *** | 1883 | 2120 | 2936 | 565 | 635 | 746 | 284 | 309 | 334 | 174 | 185 | 187 | 119 | 124 | 118 |
| 0.4 | *** | 1842 | 1986 | 2896 | 554 | 608 | 745 | 280 | 302 | 340 | 172 | 182 | 196 | 117 | 122 | 129 |
| | *** | 1895 | 2180 | 3062 | 577 | 657 | 770 | 290 | 318 | 341 | 176 | 188 | 189 | 120 | 125 | 118 |
| 0.45 | *** | 1798 | 1970 | 2999 | 551 | 612 | 762 | 279 | 303 | 344 | 171 | 181 | 197 | 115 | 121 | 128 |
| | *** | 1861 | 2192 | 3124 | 577 | 665 | 778 | 290 | 320 | 341 | 176 | 188 | 187 | 118 | 124 | 115 |
| 0.5 | *** | 1719 | 1917 | 3034 | 539 | 604 | 762 | 273 | 298 | 341 | 166 | 177 | 192 | 112 | 117 | 124 |
| | *** | 1793 | 2162 | 3124 | 566 | 660 | 770 | 284 | 316 | 334 | 171 | 184 | 181 | 114 | 120 | 110 |
| 0.55 | *** | 1615 | 1835 | 3000 | 518 | 585 | 745 | 263 | 287 | 329 | 159 | 169 | 184 | 106 | 111 | 117 |
| | *** | 1699 | 2096 | 3062 | 546 | 642 | 746 | 274 | 305 | 320 | 163 | 176 | 171 | 108 | 114 | 103 |
| 0.6 | *** | 1494 | 1729 | 2898 | 489 | 556 | 712 | 248 | 271 | 311 | 148 | 158 | 171 | 97 | 102 | 108 |
| | *** | 1585 | 1998 | 2936 | 518 | 612 | 707 | 258 | 288 | 299 | 152 | 164 | 157 | 99 | 105 | 93 |
| 0.65 | *** | 1361 | 1602 | 2728 | 454 | 517 | 661 | 228 | 249 | 284 | 134 | 143 | 155 | 87 | 91 | 96 |
| | *** | 1456 | 1870 | 2748 | 481 | 570 | 652 | 237 | 264 | 271 | 138 | 148 | 140 | 89 | 93 | 80 |
| 0.7 | *** | 1219 | 1457 | 2491 | 410 | 468 | 593 | 203 | 221 | 250 | 117 | 124 | 133 | 74 | 77 | 81 |
| | *** | 1314 | 1712 | 2496 | 435 | 515 | 581 | 211 | 234 | 236 | 120 | 129 | 118 | 76 | 79 | 65 |
| 0.75 | *** | 1070 | 1292 | 2186 | 359 | 408 | 509 | 173 | 188 | 209 | 97 | 102 | 108 | . | . | . |
| | *** | 1159 | 1524 | 2182 | 381 | 447 | 495 | 180 | 197 | 194 | 99 | 105 | 93 | . | . | . |
| 0.8 | *** | 910 | 1104 | 1816 | 298 | 337 | 408 | 137 | 147 | 161 | . | . | . | . | . | . |
| | *** | 989 | 1301 | 1806 | 315 | 365 | 393 | 142 | 153 | 145 | . | . | . | . | . | . |
| 0.85 | *** | 732 | 887 | 1380 | 225 | 250 | 291 | . | . | . | . | . | . | . | . | . |
| | *** | 796 | 1035 | 1366 | 236 | 267 | 275 | . | . | . | . | . | . | . | . | . |
| 0.9 | *** | 523 | 622 | 879 | . | . | . | . | . | . | . | . | . | . | . | . |
| | *** | 564 | 710 | 864 | . | . | . | . | . | . | . | . | . | . | . | . |

TABLE 5: ALPHA= 0.025 POWER= 0.8     EXPECTED ACCRUAL THRU MINIMUM FOLLOW-UP= 375

| | | DEL=.05 | | | DEL=.10 | | | DEL=.15 | | | DEL=.20 | | | DEL=.25 | |
|---|---|---|---|---|---|---|---|---|---|---|---|---|---|---|---|---|
| FACT= | 1.0 .75 | .50 .25 | .00 BIN | 1.0 .75 | .50 .25 | .00 BIN | 1.0 .75 | .50 .25 | .00 BIN | 1.0 75 | .50 .25 | .00 BIN | 1.0 .75 | .50 .25 | .00 BIN |
| PCONT=*** | | | | REQUIRED NUMBER OF PATIENTS | | | | | | | | | | | |
| 0.05 *** | 477 | 483 | 502 | 172 | 175 | 178 | 102 | 103 | 104 | 72 | 73 | 73 | 56 | 56 | 57 |
| *** | 479 | 490 | 864 | 174 | 176 | 275 | 102 | 103 | 145 | 72 | 73 | 93 | 56 | 57 | 65 |
| 0.1 *** | 872 | 890 | 967 | 278 | 286 | 299 | 151 | 154 | 159 | 100 | 102 | 104 | 74 | 75 | 76 |
| *** | 879 | 913 | 1366 | 281 | 291 | 393 | 152 | 156 | 194 | 101 | 103 | 118 | 75 | 76 | 80 |
| 0.15 *** | 1211 | 1244 | 1418 | 367 | 381 | 409 | 192 | 197 | 206 | 123 | 126 | 130 | 89 | 90 | 92 |
| *** | 1223 | 1289 | 1806 | 373 | 392 | 495 | 194 | 201 | 236 | 125 | 128 | 140 | 89 | 91 | 93 |
| 0.2 *** | 1478 | 1529 | 1829 | 437 | 460 | 507 | 224 | 233 | 248 | 141 | 146 | 152 | 100 | 102 | 105 |
| *** | 1496 | 1600 | 2182 | 447 | 478 | 581 | 228 | 240 | 271 | 144 | 149 | 157 | 101 | 104 | 103 |
| 0.25 *** | 1671 | 1742 | 2188 | 490 | 521 | 591 | 249 | 261 | 282 | 155 | 161 | 170 | 108 | 111 | 116 |
| *** | 1696 | 1843 | 2496 | 503 | 547 | 652 | 255 | 270 | 299 | 158 | 165 | 171 | 110 | 113 | 110 |
| 0.3 *** | 1793 | 1888 | 2488 | 527 | 567 | 659 | 267 | 283 | 309 | 165 | 172 | 183 | 114 | 118 | 123 |
| *** | 1827 | 2021 | 2748 | 544 | 601 | 707 | 274 | 294 | 320 | 168 | 177 | 181 | 116 | 120 | 115 |
| 0.35 *** | 1851 | 1972 | 2725 | 550 | 597 | 710 | 278 | 296 | 328 | 171 | 179 | 192 | 117 | 122 | 127 |
| *** | 1895 | 2138 | 2936 | 570 | 638 | 746 | 286 | 310 | 334 | 175 | 185 | 187 | 119 | 124 | 118 |
| 0.4 *** | 1854 | 2004 | 2896 | 559 | 614 | 745 | 283 | 304 | 340 | 173 | 183 | 196 | 118 | 123 | 129 |
| *** | 1909 | 2200 | 3062 | 582 | 661 | 770 | 292 | 319 | 341 | 178 | 189 | 189 | 120 | 125 | 118 |
| 0.45 *** | 1812 | 1990 | 2999 | 557 | 618 | 762 | 282 | 305 | 344 | 172 | 182 | 197 | 116 | 121 | 128 |
| *** | 1878 | 2215 | 3124 | 583 | 670 | 778 | 292 | 321 | 341 | 177 | 189 | 187 | 118 | 124 | 115 |
| 0.5 *** | 1736 | 1940 | 3033 | 545 | 610 | 762 | 276 | 300 | 340 | 167 | 178 | 193 | 112 | 117 | 124 |
| *** | 1813 | 2188 | 3124 | 573 | 665 | 770 | 287 | 317 | 334 | 172 | 184 | 181 | 115 | 120 | 110 |
| 0.55 *** | 1634 | 1860 | 3000 | 525 | 591 | 745 | 265 | 289 | 329 | 160 | 170 | 184 | 106 | 111 | 117 |
| *** | 1721 | 2123 | 3062 | 553 | 647 | 746 | 276 | 306 | 320 | 164 | 176 | 171 | 108 | 114 | 103 |
| 0.6 *** | 1515 | 1754 | 2898 | 496 | 562 | 711 | 250 | 273 | 310 | 149 | 159 | 171 | 98 | 102 | 108 |
| *** | 1608 | 2026 | 2936 | 524 | 617 | 707 | 260 | 289 | 299 | 153 | 164 | 157 | 100 | 105 | 93 |
| 0.65 *** | 1383 | 1628 | 2728 | 460 | 523 | 661 | 230 | 251 | 284 | 135 | 144 | 155 | 88 | 91 | 95 |
| *** | 1480 | 1897 | 2748 | 487 | 574 | 652 | 239 | 265 | 271 | 139 | 148 | 140 | 89 | 93 | 80 |
| 0.7 *** | 1241 | 1482 | 2491 | 416 | 473 | 593 | 205 | 223 | 250 | 118 | 125 | 133 | 75 | 77 | 81 |
| *** | 1337 | 1738 | 2496 | 441 | 519 | 581 | 213 | 235 | 236 | 121 | 129 | 118 | 76 | 79 | 65 |
| 0.75 *** | 1091 | 1315 | 2186 | 364 | 413 | 509 | 175 | 189 | 209 | 97 | 102 | 108 | . | . | . |
| *** | 1181 | 1547 | 2182 | 385 | 450 | 495 | 181 | 198 | 194 | 100 | 105 | 93 | . | . | . |
| 0.8 *** | 928 | 1124 | 1816 | 302 | 340 | 408 | 138 | 148 | 161 | . | . | . | . | . | . |
| *** | 1008 | 1320 | 1806 | 319 | 368 | 393 | 143 | 154 | 145 | . | . | . | . | . | . |
| 0.85 *** | 747 | 902 | 1380 | 228 | 252 | 291 | . | . | . | . | . | . | . | . | . |
| *** | 811 | 1049 | 1366 | 239 | 268 | 275 | . | . | . | . | . | . | . | . | . |
| 0.9 *** | 533 | 631 | 879 | . | . | . | . | . | . | . | . | . | . | . | . |
| *** | 574 | 718 | 864 | . | . | . | . | . | . | . | . | . | . | . | . |

TABLE 5: ALPHA= 0.025 POWER= 0.8    EXPECTED ACCRUAL THRU MINIMUM FOLLOW-UP= 400

| | | DEL=.05 | | | DEL=.10 | | | DEL=.15 | | | DEL=.20 | | | DEL=.25 | | |
|---|---|---|---|---|---|---|---|---|---|---|---|---|---|---|---|---|---|
| FACT= | | 1.0 .75 | .50 .25 | .00 BIN | 1.0 .75 | .50 .25 | .00 BIN | 1.0 .75 | .50 .25 | .00 BIN | 1.0 75 | .50 .25 | .00 BIN | 1.0 .75 | .50 .25 | .00 BIN |
| PCONT=*** | | | | | REQUIRED NUMBER OF PATIENTS | | | | | | | | | | | |
| 0.05 | *** | 477 | 484 | 502 | 173 | 175 | 178 | 102 | 103 | 104 | 72 | 73 | 73 | 56 | 56 | 57 |
| | *** | 480 | 490 | 864 | 174 | 177 | 275 | 102 | 103 | 145 | 72 | 73 | 93 | 56 | 57 | 65 |
| 0.1 | *** | 873 | 892 | 967 | 279 | 286 | 299 | 151 | 154 | 159 | 101 | 102 | 104 | 74 | 75 | 76 |
| | *** | 880 | 915 | 1366 | 282 | 292 | 393 | 153 | 156 | 194 | 101 | 103 | 118 | 75 | 76 | 80 |
| 0.15 | *** | 1214 | 1248 | 1418 | 368 | 382 | 409 | 192 | 198 | 207 | 124 | 126 | 130 | 89 | 90 | 92 |
| | *** | 1226 | 1293 | 1806 | 374 | 393 | 495 | 195 | 202 | 236 | 125 | 128 | 140 | 90 | 91 | 93 |
| 0.2 | *** | 1482 | 1535 | 1829 | 440 | 462 | 507 | 225 | 234 | 248 | 142 | 146 | 152 | 100 | 103 | 105 |
| | *** | 1501 | 1607 | 2182 | 449 | 479 | 581 | 229 | 240 | 271 | 144 | 149 | 157 | 101 | 104 | 103 |
| 0.25 | *** | 1676 | 1751 | 2188 | 493 | 524 | 591 | 250 | 263 | 282 | 156 | 162 | 170 | 109 | 112 | 116 |
| | *** | 1703 | 1854 | 2496 | 506 | 550 | 652 | 256 | 271 | 299 | 159 | 165 | 171 | 110 | 114 | 110 |
| 0.3 | *** | 1800 | 1899 | 2489 | 531 | 570 | 659 | 268 | 284 | 309 | 166 | 173 | 183 | 114 | 118 | 123 |
| | *** | 1835 | 2034 | 2748 | 548 | 603 | 707 | 275 | 295 | 320 | 169 | 177 | 181 | 116 | 120 | 115 |
| 0.35 | *** | 1860 | 1986 | 2725 | 554 | 601 | 710 | 280 | 298 | 328 | 172 | 180 | 192 | 118 | 122 | 127 |
| | *** | 1906 | 2154 | 2936 | 574 | 642 | 746 | 288 | 311 | 334 | 176 | 185 | 187 | 120 | 124 | 118 |
| 0.4 | *** | 1865 | 2020 | 2896 | 564 | 619 | 745 | 285 | 306 | 340 | 174 | 183 | 196 | 118 | 123 | 129 |
| | *** | 1922 | 2220 | 3062 | 587 | 665 | 770 | 294 | 320 | 341 | 178 | 189 | 189 | 121 | 126 | 118 |
| 0.45 | *** | 1826 | 2010 | 2999 | 563 | 623 | 762 | 284 | 307 | 344 | 173 | 183 | 197 | 117 | 122 | 128 |
| | *** | 1895 | 2237 | 3124 | 588 | 674 | 778 | 294 | 323 | 341 | 178 | 189 | 187 | 119 | 125 | 115 |
| 0.5 | *** | 1752 | 1962 | 3034 | 552 | 616 | 762 | 279 | 302 | 341 | 169 | 179 | 193 | 113 | 118 | 124 |
| | *** | 1832 | 2212 | 3124 | 579 | 669 | 770 | 289 | 318 | 334 | 173 | 185 | 181 | 115 | 121 | 110 |
| 0.55 | *** | 1653 | 1883 | 3000 | 531 | 597 | 746 | 268 | 291 | 329 | 161 | 171 | 184 | 107 | 111 | 117 |
| | *** | 1742 | 2148 | 3062 | 559 | 652 | 746 | 278 | 307 | 320 | 165 | 177 | 171 | 109 | 114 | 103 |
| 0.6 | *** | 1535 | 1779 | 2898 | 503 | 568 | 712 | 253 | 275 | 311 | 150 | 159 | 171 | 98 | 103 | 108 |
| | *** | 1631 | 2051 | 2936 | 531 | 621 | 707 | 263 | 290 | 299 | 154 | 165 | 157 | 100 | 105 | 93 |
| 0.65 | *** | 1404 | 1652 | 2728 | 466 | 528 | 661 | 232 | 252 | 284 | 136 | 144 | 155 | 88 | 91 | 96 |
| | *** | 1503 | 1922 | 2748 | 493 | 578 | 652 | 241 | 266 | 271 | 140 | 149 | 140 | 90 | 93 | 80 |
| 0.7 | *** | 1262 | 1505 | 2491 | 422 | 478 | 593 | 207 | 224 | 250 | 119 | 125 | 133 | 75 | 78 | 81 |
| | *** | 1360 | 1761 | 2496 | 446 | 523 | 581 | 215 | 236 | 236 | 122 | 129 | 118 | 76 | 79 | 65 |
| 0.75 | *** | 1111 | 1337 | 2186 | 369 | 417 | 509 | 176 | 190 | 209 | 98 | 103 | 108 | . | . | . |
| | *** | 1202 | 1568 | 2182 | 390 | 453 | 495 | 183 | 199 | 194 | 100 | 105 | 93 | . | . | . |
| 0.8 | *** | 946 | 1143 | 1816 | 306 | 343 | 408 | 139 | 149 | 161 | . | . | . | . | . | . |
| | *** | 1027 | 1337 | 1806 | 323 | 370 | 393 | 144 | 154 | 145 | . | . | . | . | . | . |
| 0.85 | *** | 762 | 917 | 1380 | 231 | 254 | 291 | . | . | . | . | . | . | . | . | . |
| | *** | 826 | 1062 | 1366 | 241 | 270 | 275 | . | . | . | . | . | . | . | . | . |
| 0.9 | *** | 542 | 640 | 879 | . | . | . | . | . | . | . | . | . | . | . | . |
| | *** | 584 | 725 | 864 | . | . | . | . | . | . | . | . | . | . | . | . |

TABLE 5: ALPHA= 0.025 POWER= 0.8    EXPECTED ACCRUAL THRU MINIMUM FOLLOW-UP= 425

| | | DEL=.05 | | | DEL=.10 | | | DEL=.15 | | | DEL=.20 | | | DEL=.25 | | |
|---|---|---|---|---|---|---|---|---|---|---|---|---|---|---|---|---|---|
| FACT= | | 1.0 .75 | .50 .25 | .00 BIN | 1.0 .75 | .50 .25 | .00 BIN | 1.0 .75 | .50 .25 | .00 BIN | 1.0 75 | .50 .25 | .00 BIN | 1.0 .75 | .50 .25 | .00 BIN | |
| PCONT=*** | | | | | REQUIRED | NUMBER | OF | PATIENTS | | | | | | | | | |
| 0.05 | *** | 478 | 484 | 502 | 173 | 175 | 178 | 102 | 103 | 104 | 72 | 73 | 73 | 56 | 56 | 57 | |
| | *** | 480 | 491 | 864 | 174 | 177 | 275 | 102 | 103 | 145 | 72 | 73 | 93 | 56 | 57 | 65 | |
| 0.1 | *** | 875 | 894 | 967 | 280 | 287 | 299 | 152 | 155 | 159 | 101 | 102 | 104 | 74 | 75 | 76 | |
| | *** | 882 | 917 | 1366 | 283 | 292 | 393 | 153 | 156 | 194 | 102 | 103 | 118 | 75 | 76 | 80 | |
| 0.15 | *** | 1216 | 1251 | 1418 | 370 | 383 | 409 | 193 | 198 | 206 | 124 | 127 | 130 | 89 | 91 | 93 | |
| | *** | 1229 | 1297 | 1806 | 375 | 394 | 495 | 195 | 202 | 236 | 125 | 128 | 140 | 90 | 91 | 93 | |
| 0.2 | *** | 1486 | 1541 | 1829 | 442 | 463 | 507 | 226 | 235 | 248 | 142 | 147 | 152 | 101 | 103 | 105 | |
| | *** | 1505 | 1614 | 2182 | 451 | 481 | 581 | 230 | 240 | 271 | 144 | 149 | 157 | 102 | 104 | 103 | |
| 0.25 | *** | 1681 | 1759 | 2189 | 496 | 527 | 591 | 251 | 263 | 282 | 156 | 162 | 170 | 109 | 112 | 116 | |
| | *** | 1709 | 1863 | 2496 | 509 | 552 | 652 | 257 | 272 | 299 | 159 | 166 | 171 | 110 | 114 | 110 | |
| 0.3 | *** | 1807 | 1910 | 2488 | 535 | 574 | 659 | 270 | 285 | 309 | 167 | 173 | 183 | 115 | 118 | 123 | |
| | *** | 1844 | 2047 | 2748 | 551 | 606 | 707 | 277 | 295 | 320 | 170 | 178 | 181 | 116 | 120 | 115 | |
| 0.35 | *** | 1869 | 2000 | 2725 | 558 | 605 | 710 | 281 | 299 | 328 | 173 | 181 | 192 | 118 | 122 | 127 | |
| | *** | 1917 | 2170 | 2936 | 578 | 645 | 746 | 289 | 312 | 334 | 176 | 186 | 187 | 120 | 125 | 118 | |
| 0.4 | *** | 1876 | 2037 | 2896 | 569 | 623 | 745 | 287 | 307 | 340 | 175 | 184 | 196 | 119 | 123 | 129 | |
| | *** | 1936 | 2238 | 3062 | 592 | 668 | 770 | 296 | 321 | 341 | 179 | 190 | 189 | 121 | 126 | 118 | |
| 0.45 | *** | 1839 | 2028 | 2999 | 568 | 628 | 762 | 286 | 308 | 344 | 174 | 183 | 197 | 117 | 122 | 128 | |
| | *** | 1911 | 2258 | 3124 | 594 | 678 | 778 | 297 | 324 | 341 | 178 | 189 | 187 | 119 | 125 | 115 | |
| 0.5 | *** | 1768 | 1982 | 3034 | 557 | 621 | 762 | 281 | 304 | 341 | 170 | 179 | 192 | 113 | 118 | 124 | |
| | *** | 1850 | 2234 | 3124 | 584 | 673 | 770 | 291 | 319 | 334 | 174 | 185 | 181 | 116 | 121 | 110 | |
| 0.55 | *** | 1671 | 1905 | 3000 | 537 | 602 | 745 | 270 | 293 | 329 | 162 | 171 | 184 | 107 | 112 | 117 | |
| | *** | 1762 | 2172 | 3062 | 565 | 656 | 746 | 281 | 308 | 320 | 166 | 177 | 171 | 109 | 114 | 103 | |
| 0.6 | *** | 1554 | 1802 | 2898 | 509 | 573 | 712 | 255 | 276 | 311 | 151 | 160 | 171 | 99 | 103 | 108 | |
| | *** | 1652 | 2075 | 2936 | 536 | 625 | 707 | 265 | 291 | 299 | 155 | 165 | 157 | 101 | 105 | 93 | |
| 0.65 | *** | 1424 | 1676 | 2728 | 472 | 533 | 661 | 234 | 254 | 284 | 137 | 145 | 155 | 88 | 91 | 95 | |
| | *** | 1524 | 1945 | 2748 | 499 | 582 | 652 | 243 | 267 | 271 | 141 | 149 | 140 | 90 | 93 | 80 | |
| 0.7 | *** | 1282 | 1527 | 2491 | 427 | 483 | 593 | 209 | 226 | 250 | 120 | 126 | 133 | 75 | 78 | 81 | |
| | *** | 1381 | 1783 | 2496 | 451 | 526 | 581 | 216 | 237 | 236 | 122 | 129 | 118 | 77 | 79 | 65 | |
| 0.75 | *** | 1130 | 1357 | 2186 | 374 | 421 | 509 | 178 | 191 | 209 | 99 | 103 | 108 | . | . | . | |
| | *** | 1222 | 1587 | 2182 | 394 | 456 | 495 | 184 | 199 | 194 | 101 | 105 | 93 | . | . | . | |
| 0.8 | *** | 963 | 1160 | 1816 | 310 | 346 | 408 | 140 | 149 | 161 | . | . | . | . | . | . | |
| | *** | 1044 | 1353 | 1806 | 326 | 371 | 393 | 145 | 154 | 145 | . | . | . | . | . | . | |
| 0.85 | *** | 775 | 930 | 1380 | 233 | 255 | 291 | . | . | . | . | . | . | . | . | . | |
| | *** | 839 | 1073 | 1366 | 243 | 271 | 275 | . | . | . | . | . | . | . | . | . | |
| 0.9 | *** | 551 | 648 | 879 | . | . | . | . | . | . | . | . | . | . | . | . | |
| | *** | 592 | 731 | 864 | . | . | . | . | . | . | . | . | . | . | . | . | |

TABLE 5: ALPHA= 0.025 POWER= 0.8     EXPECTED ACCRUAL THRU MINIMUM FOLLOW-UP= 450

|  |  | DEL=.05 | | | DEL=.10 | | | DEL=.15 | | | DEL=.20 | | | DEL=.25 | | |
|---|---|---|---|---|---|---|---|---|---|---|---|---|---|---|---|---|
| FACT= | | 1.0 .75 | .50 .25 | .00 BIN | 1.0 .75 | .50 .25 | .00 BIN | 1.0 .75 | .50 .25 | .00 BIN | 1.0 75 | .50 .25 | .00 BIN | 1.0 .75 | .50 .25 | .00 BIN |
| PCONT=*** | | REQUIRED NUMBER OF PATIENTS | | | | | | | | | | | | | | |
| 0.05 | *** | 478 | 485 | 501 | 173 | 175 | 178 | 102 | 103 | 104 | 72 | 73 | 73 | 56 | 56 | 57 |
|  | *** | 481 | 491 | 864 | 174 | 177 | 275 | 102 | 104 | 145 | 72 | 73 | 93 | 56 | 57 | 65 |
| 0.1 | *** | 876 | 896 | 967 | 280 | 287 | 299 | 152 | 155 | 158 | 101 | 102 | 104 | 75 | 75 | 76 |
|  | *** | 883 | 919 | 1366 | 283 | 292 | 393 | 153 | 156 | 194 | 102 | 103 | 118 | 75 | 76 | 80 |
| 0.15 | *** | 1218 | 1255 | 1418 | 371 | 384 | 409 | 193 | 199 | 207 | 124 | 127 | 130 | 89 | 91 | 92 |
|  | *** | 1232 | 1301 | 1806 | 377 | 395 | 495 | 196 | 202 | 236 | 126 | 128 | 140 | 90 | 91 | 93 |
| 0.2 | *** | 1489 | 1546 | 1829 | 443 | 465 | 507 | 227 | 235 | 248 | 143 | 147 | 152 | 101 | 103 | 105 |
|  | *** | 1510 | 1620 | 2182 | 453 | 482 | 581 | 231 | 241 | 271 | 145 | 149 | 157 | 102 | 104 | 103 |
| 0.25 | *** | 1686 | 1767 | 2188 | 499 | 529 | 591 | 253 | 264 | 282 | 157 | 163 | 170 | 109 | 112 | 116 |
|  | *** | 1715 | 1872 | 2496 | 512 | 553 | 652 | 258 | 272 | 299 | 159 | 166 | 171 | 111 | 114 | 110 |
| 0.3 | *** | 1813 | 1920 | 2489 | 538 | 577 | 659 | 271 | 286 | 309 | 167 | 174 | 183 | 115 | 119 | 123 |
|  | *** | 1852 | 2059 | 2748 | 554 | 608 | 707 | 278 | 296 | 320 | 170 | 178 | 181 | 117 | 121 | 115 |
| 0.35 | *** | 1877 | 2013 | 2725 | 562 | 609 | 710 | 283 | 300 | 328 | 173 | 181 | 192 | 118 | 122 | 127 |
|  | *** | 1927 | 2184 | 2936 | 582 | 648 | 746 | 291 | 312 | 334 | 177 | 186 | 187 | 120 | 125 | 118 |
| 0.4 | *** | 1887 | 2052 | 2896 | 574 | 627 | 744 | 289 | 309 | 340 | 176 | 185 | 196 | 119 | 123 | 129 |
|  | *** | 1949 | 2255 | 3062 | 597 | 672 | 770 | 298 | 322 | 341 | 180 | 190 | 189 | 121 | 126 | 118 |
| 0.45 | *** | 1853 | 2046 | 2999 | 573 | 633 | 762 | 289 | 310 | 344 | 175 | 184 | 197 | 118 | 122 | 128 |
|  | *** | 1926 | 2277 | 3124 | 599 | 681 | 778 | 298 | 325 | 341 | 179 | 190 | 187 | 120 | 125 | 115 |
| 0.5 | *** | 1783 | 2002 | 3034 | 563 | 626 | 762 | 283 | 305 | 341 | 171 | 180 | 192 | 114 | 118 | 124 |
|  | *** | 1868 | 2255 | 3124 | 590 | 677 | 770 | 293 | 320 | 334 | 175 | 186 | 181 | 116 | 121 | 110 |
| 0.55 | *** | 1688 | 1927 | 3000 | 543 | 607 | 745 | 272 | 294 | 329 | 163 | 172 | 184 | 108 | 112 | 117 |
|  | *** | 1781 | 2194 | 3062 | 571 | 660 | 746 | 282 | 309 | 320 | 167 | 177 | 171 | 110 | 114 | 103 |
| 0.6 | *** | 1573 | 1824 | 2898 | 514 | 578 | 712 | 257 | 278 | 311 | 152 | 160 | 171 | 99 | 103 | 108 |
|  | *** | 1672 | 2098 | 2936 | 542 | 629 | 707 | 266 | 292 | 299 | 156 | 165 | 157 | 101 | 105 | 93 |
| 0.65 | *** | 1443 | 1698 | 2728 | 477 | 538 | 661 | 236 | 255 | 284 | 138 | 145 | 154 | 89 | 92 | 95 |
|  | *** | 1545 | 1967 | 2748 | 504 | 585 | 652 | 245 | 268 | 271 | 141 | 149 | 140 | 90 | 93 | 80 |
| 0.7 | *** | 1301 | 1549 | 2491 | 432 | 487 | 593 | 210 | 227 | 250 | 120 | 126 | 133 | 75 | 78 | 81 |
|  | *** | 1401 | 1804 | 2496 | 456 | 529 | 581 | 218 | 237 | 236 | 123 | 129 | 118 | 77 | 79 | 65 |
| 0.75 | *** | 1148 | 1376 | 2187 | 378 | 424 | 509 | 179 | 192 | 209 | 99 | 103 | 108 | . | . | . |
|  | *** | 1241 | 1605 | 2182 | 398 | 458 | 495 | 185 | 199 | 194 | 101 | 105 | 93 | . | . | . |
| 0.8 | *** | 979 | 1177 | 1816 | 313 | 348 | 408 | 141 | 150 | 161 | . | . | . | . | . | . |
|  | *** | 1060 | 1369 | 1806 | 329 | 373 | 393 | 145 | 155 | 145 | . | . | . | . | . | . |
| 0.85 | *** | 788 | 942 | 1380 | 235 | 257 | 291 | . | . | . | . | . | . | . | . | . |
|  | *** | 852 | 1084 | 1366 | 245 | 272 | 275 | . | . | . | . | . | . | . | . | . |
| 0.9 | *** | 559 | 656 | 879 | . | . | . | . | . | . | . | . | . | . | . | . |
|  | *** | 600 | 737 | 864 | . | . | . | . | . | . | . | . | . | . | . | . |

# TABLE 5: ALPHA= 0.025 POWER= 0.8   EXPECTED ACCRUAL THRU MINIMUM FOLLOW-UP= 475

| | | DEL=.05 | | | DEL=.10 | | | DEL=.15 | | | DEL=.20 | | | DEL=.25 | | |
|---|---|---|---|---|---|---|---|---|---|---|---|---|---|---|---|---|
| FACT= | | 1.0 .75 | .50 .25 | .00 BIN | 1.0 .75 | .50 .25 | .00 BIN | 1.0 .75 | .50 .25 | .00 BIN | 1.0 75 | .50 .25 | .00 BIN | 1.0 .75 | .50 .25 | .00 BIN |
| PCONT=*** | | | | | | | REQUIRED NUMBER OF PATIENTS | | | | | | | | |
| 0.05 | *** | 479 | 485 | 502 | 173 | 175 | 178 | 102 | 103 | 104 | 72 | 73 | 73 | 56 | 56 | 57 |
| | *** | 481 | 492 | 864 | 174 | 177 | 275 | 102 | 104 | 145 | 72 | 73 | 93 | 56 | 57 | 65 |
| 0.1 | *** | 877 | 898 | 967 | 281 | 288 | 299 | 152 | 155 | 159 | 101 | 102 | 104 | 74 | 75 | 76 |
| | *** | 885 | 920 | 1366 | 284 | 292 | 393 | 153 | 156 | 194 | 102 | 103 | 118 | 75 | 76 | 80 |
| 0.15 | *** | 1220 | 1258 | 1418 | 372 | 385 | 409 | 194 | 199 | 206 | 124 | 127 | 130 | 89 | 91 | 92 |
| | *** | 1234 | 1305 | 1806 | 378 | 395 | 495 | 196 | 203 | 236 | 126 | 129 | 140 | 90 | 91 | 93 |
| 0.2 | *** | 1493 | 1552 | 1829 | 445 | 466 | 507 | 227 | 236 | 248 | 143 | 147 | 152 | 101 | 103 | 105 |
| | *** | 1514 | 1626 | 2182 | 454 | 483 | 581 | 231 | 241 | 271 | 145 | 149 | 157 | 102 | 104 | 103 |
| 0.25 | *** | 1691 | 1774 | 2189 | 501 | 531 | 591 | 254 | 265 | 282 | 158 | 163 | 169 | 110 | 112 | 115 |
| | *** | 1722 | 1881 | 2496 | 514 | 555 | 652 | 259 | 273 | 299 | 160 | 166 | 171 | 111 | 114 | 110 |
| 0.3 | *** | 1820 | 1930 | 2488 | 541 | 579 | 659 | 273 | 287 | 309 | 168 | 174 | 183 | 115 | 119 | 123 |
| | *** | 1860 | 2070 | 2748 | 557 | 610 | 707 | 279 | 297 | 320 | 171 | 178 | 181 | 117 | 121 | 115 |
| 0.35 | *** | 1886 | 2025 | 2725 | 566 | 612 | 710 | 285 | 302 | 328 | 174 | 182 | 192 | 119 | 123 | 127 |
| | *** | 1938 | 2198 | 2936 | 586 | 650 | 746 | 292 | 313 | 334 | 178 | 186 | 187 | 121 | 125 | 118 |
| 0.4 | *** | 1898 | 2067 | 2896 | 578 | 631 | 745 | 290 | 310 | 340 | 177 | 185 | 196 | 120 | 124 | 129 |
| | *** | 1962 | 2272 | 3062 | 601 | 675 | 770 | 299 | 323 | 341 | 181 | 190 | 189 | 122 | 126 | 118 |
| 0.45 | *** | 1866 | 2063 | 2999 | 578 | 637 | 762 | 290 | 311 | 344 | 176 | 185 | 197 | 118 | 122 | 128 |
| | *** | 1941 | 2295 | 3124 | 603 | 685 | 778 | 300 | 325 | 341 | 180 | 190 | 187 | 120 | 125 | 115 |
| 0.5 | *** | 1799 | 2021 | 3034 | 568 | 630 | 762 | 285 | 307 | 340 | 171 | 181 | 192 | 114 | 118 | 124 |
| | *** | 1885 | 2275 | 3124 | 595 | 680 | 770 | 295 | 321 | 334 | 175 | 186 | 181 | 116 | 121 | 110 |
| 0.55 | *** | 1705 | 1947 | 3000 | 548 | 612 | 745 | 274 | 296 | 329 | 164 | 172 | 184 | 108 | 112 | 117 |
| | *** | 1800 | 2215 | 3062 | 576 | 663 | 746 | 284 | 311 | 320 | 168 | 178 | 171 | 110 | 115 | 103 |
| 0.6 | *** | 1591 | 1845 | 2898 | 520 | 583 | 712 | 259 | 279 | 311 | 153 | 161 | 171 | 100 | 103 | 108 |
| | *** | 1692 | 2119 | 2936 | 547 | 632 | 707 | 268 | 293 | 299 | 156 | 166 | 157 | 101 | 105 | 93 |
| 0.65 | *** | 1462 | 1719 | 2728 | 482 | 542 | 661 | 238 | 257 | 284 | 138 | 146 | 154 | 89 | 92 | 96 |
| | *** | 1565 | 1988 | 2748 | 509 | 588 | 652 | 246 | 269 | 271 | 142 | 150 | 140 | 90 | 93 | 80 |
| 0.7 | *** | 1320 | 1569 | 2491 | 437 | 490 | 593 | 212 | 228 | 250 | 121 | 127 | 133 | 76 | 78 | 81 |
| | *** | 1421 | 1823 | 2496 | 460 | 531 | 581 | 219 | 238 | 236 | 124 | 130 | 118 | 77 | 79 | 65 |
| 0.75 | *** | 1165 | 1394 | 2186 | 382 | 427 | 509 | 180 | 192 | 209 | 99 | 103 | 108 | . | . | . |
| | *** | 1258 | 1622 | 2182 | 402 | 460 | 495 | 186 | 200 | 194 | 101 | 106 | 93 | . | . | . |
| 0.8 | *** | 994 | 1192 | 1816 | 316 | 350 | 408 | 142 | 150 | 161 | . | . | . | . | . | . |
| | *** | 1076 | 1383 | 1806 | 332 | 375 | 393 | 146 | 155 | 145 | . | . | . | . | . | . |
| 0.85 | *** | 800 | 954 | 1380 | 237 | 258 | 291 | . | . | . | . | . | . | . | . | . |
| | *** | 865 | 1094 | 1366 | 247 | 273 | 275 | . | . | . | . | . | . | . | . | . |
| 0.9 | *** | 567 | 663 | 879 | . | . | . | . | . | . | . | . | . | . | . | . |
| | *** | 608 | 742 | 864 | . | . | . | . | . | . | . | . | . | . | . | . |

TABLE 5: ALPHA= 0.025 POWER= 0.8    EXPECTED ACCRUAL THRU MINIMUM FOLLOW-UP= 500

| PCONT=*** | | DEL=.05 | | | DEL=.10 | | | DEL=.15 | | | DEL=.20 | | | DEL=.25 | | |
|---|---|---|---|---|---|---|---|---|---|---|---|---|---|---|---|---|
| FACT= | | 1.0 .75 | .50 .25 | .00 BIN | 1.0 .75 | .50 .25 | .00 BIN | 1.0 .75 | .50 .25 | .00 BIN | 1.0 75 | .50 .25 | .00 BIN | 1.0 .75 | .50 .25 | .00 BIN |
| PCONT=*** | | | | | | REQUIRED NUMBER OF PATIENTS | | | | | | | | | | |
| 0.05 | *** | 479 | 486 | 502 | 173 | 176 | 178 | 102 | 103 | 104 | 72 | 73 | 73 | 56 | 57 | 57 |
| | *** | 482 | 492 | 864 | 174 | 177 | 275 | 103 | 103 | 145 | 73 | 73 | 93 | 56 | 57 | 65 |
| 0.1 | *** | 878 | 899 | 967 | 282 | 288 | 299 | 153 | 155 | 158 | 101 | 103 | 104 | 75 | 76 | 76 |
| | *** | 887 | 922 | 1366 | 284 | 293 | 393 | 154 | 157 | 194 | 102 | 103 | 118 | 75 | 76 | 80 |
| 0.15 | *** | 1223 | 1262 | 1418 | 373 | 386 | 409 | 194 | 199 | 207 | 125 | 127 | 130 | 89 | 91 | 93 |
| | *** | 1237 | 1308 | 1806 | 379 | 396 | 495 | 197 | 203 | 236 | 126 | 128 | 140 | 90 | 92 | 93 |
| 0.2 | *** | 1496 | 1557 | 1829 | 447 | 468 | 508 | 228 | 236 | 248 | 143 | 147 | 152 | 101 | 103 | 105 |
| | *** | 1518 | 1632 | 2182 | 456 | 484 | 581 | 232 | 242 | 271 | 145 | 149 | 157 | 102 | 104 | 103 |
| 0.25 | *** | 1696 | 1782 | 2188 | 503 | 533 | 591 | 255 | 266 | 282 | 158 | 163 | 170 | 110 | 113 | 116 |
| | *** | 1728 | 1889 | 2496 | 516 | 556 | 652 | 260 | 273 | 299 | 160 | 166 | 171 | 111 | 114 | 110 |
| 0.3 | *** | 1827 | 1940 | 2488 | 544 | 582 | 659 | 274 | 288 | 309 | 168 | 175 | 183 | 116 | 119 | 123 |
| | *** | 1868 | 2081 | 2748 | 560 | 612 | 707 | 280 | 297 | 320 | 171 | 178 | 181 | 117 | 121 | 115 |
| 0.35 | *** | 1895 | 2037 | 2725 | 570 | 616 | 710 | 286 | 303 | 328 | 175 | 182 | 192 | 119 | 123 | 127 |
| | *** | 1948 | 2212 | 2936 | 589 | 652 | 746 | 294 | 314 | 334 | 178 | 187 | 187 | 121 | 125 | 118 |
| 0.4 | *** | 1909 | 2081 | 2896 | 582 | 635 | 745 | 292 | 311 | 340 | 178 | 186 | 196 | 120 | 124 | 129 |
| | *** | 1974 | 2287 | 3062 | 605 | 677 | 770 | 301 | 324 | 341 | 181 | 191 | 189 | 122 | 126 | 118 |
| 0.45 | *** | 1878 | 2080 | 2999 | 583 | 641 | 762 | 292 | 313 | 344 | 177 | 185 | 197 | 118 | 123 | 128 |
| | *** | 1956 | 2313 | 3124 | 608 | 688 | 778 | 302 | 326 | 341 | 181 | 190 | 187 | 121 | 125 | 115 |
| 0.5 | *** | 1813 | 2040 | 3033 | 573 | 634 | 762 | 287 | 308 | 341 | 172 | 181 | 193 | 115 | 119 | 124 |
| | *** | 1901 | 2294 | 3124 | 599 | 684 | 770 | 297 | 322 | 334 | 176 | 186 | 181 | 117 | 121 | 110 |
| 0.55 | *** | 1721 | 1967 | 3000 | 553 | 616 | 746 | 276 | 297 | 329 | 164 | 173 | 184 | 108 | 113 | 117 |
| | *** | 1818 | 2235 | 3062 | 580 | 666 | 746 | 286 | 311 | 320 | 168 | 178 | 171 | 110 | 115 | 103 |
| 0.6 | *** | 1608 | 1865 | 2898 | 524 | 587 | 712 | 260 | 280 | 311 | 153 | 161 | 172 | 100 | 103 | 108 |
| | *** | 1711 | 2138 | 2936 | 552 | 635 | 707 | 270 | 294 | 299 | 157 | 166 | 157 | 102 | 106 | 93 |
| 0.65 | *** | 1480 | 1738 | 2728 | 487 | 546 | 661 | 239 | 258 | 284 | 139 | 146 | 155 | 89 | 92 | 96 |
| | *** | 1584 | 2007 | 2748 | 513 | 591 | 652 | 248 | 269 | 271 | 142 | 150 | 140 | 91 | 94 | 80 |
| 0.7 | *** | 1338 | 1588 | 2491 | 441 | 494 | 593 | 213 | 228 | 250 | 121 | 127 | 133 | 76 | 78 | 81 |
| | *** | 1439 | 1841 | 2496 | 464 | 534 | 581 | 220 | 238 | 236 | 124 | 130 | 118 | 77 | 79 | 65 |
| 0.75 | *** | 1181 | 1412 | 2186 | 386 | 430 | 509 | 181 | 193 | 209 | 100 | 104 | 108 | . | . | . |
| | *** | 1276 | 1638 | 2182 | 405 | 463 | 495 | 187 | 200 | 194 | 102 | 106 | 93 | . | . | . |
| 0.8 | *** | 1008 | 1207 | 1816 | 319 | 353 | 408 | 143 | 151 | 161 | . | . | . | . | . | . |
| | *** | 1090 | 1396 | 1806 | 334 | 376 | 393 | 147 | 155 | 145 | . | . | . | . | . | . |
| 0.85 | *** | 811 | 965 | 1380 | 239 | 260 | 291 | . | . | . | . | . | . | . | . | . |
| | *** | 876 | 1104 | 1366 | 248 | 273 | 275 | . | . | . | . | . | . | . | . | . |
| 0.9 | *** | 574 | 669 | 879 | . | . | . | . | . | . | . | . | . | . | . | . |
| | *** | 615 | 747 | 864 | . | . | . | . | . | . | . | . | . | . | . | . |

## TABLE 5: ALPHA= 0.025 POWER= 0.8    EXPECTED ACCRUAL THRU MINIMUM FOLLOW-UP= 550

| | | DEL=.02 | | | DEL=.05 | | | DEL=.10 | | | DEL=.15 | | | DEL=.20 | | |
|---|---|---|---|---|---|---|---|---|---|---|---|---|---|---|---|---|---|
| FACT= | | 1.0 .75 | .50 .25 | .00 BIN | 1.0 .75 | .50 .25 | .00 BIN | 1.0 .75 | .50 .25 | .00 BIN | 1.0 75 | .50 .25 | .00 BIN | 1.0 .75 | .50 .25 | .00 BIN |
| PCONT=*** | | | | | REQUIRED NUMBER OF PATIENTS | | | | | | | | | | | |
| 0.05 | *** | 2237 | 2248 | 2365 | 480 | 487 | 501 | 174 | 176 | 178 | 102 | 103 | 104 | 72 | 73 | 73 |
| | *** | 2241 | 2269 | 4419 | 483 | 492 | 864 | 175 | 177 | 275 | 103 | 103 | 145 | 72 | 73 | 93 |
| 0.1 | *** | 4654 | 4681 | 5195 | 881 | 903 | 967 | 283 | 289 | 299 | 153 | 155 | 158 | 101 | 103 | 104 |
| | *** | 4664 | 4735 | 7677 | 890 | 925 | 1366 | 285 | 293 | 393 | 154 | 157 | 194 | 102 | 103 | 118 |
| 0.15 | *** | 6801 | 6849 | 8034 | 1227 | 1268 | 1418 | 375 | 388 | 409 | 195 | 200 | 206 | 125 | 127 | 130 |
| | *** | 6817 | 6944 | 10542 | 1243 | 1314 | 1806 | 380 | 397 | 495 | 197 | 203 | 236 | 126 | 129 | 140 |
| 0.2 | *** | 8512 | 8586 | 10675 | 1503 | 1567 | 1829 | 450 | 470 | 507 | 230 | 237 | 248 | 144 | 148 | 152 |
| | *** | 8537 | 8733 | 13014 | 1527 | 1642 | 2182 | 459 | 486 | 581 | 233 | 242 | 271 | 146 | 150 | 157 |
| 0.25 | *** | 9743 | 9849 | 13016 | 1706 | 1796 | 2189 | 508 | 536 | 591 | 256 | 267 | 282 | 159 | 164 | 169 |
| | *** | 9779 | 10060 | 15094 | 1739 | 1904 | 2496 | 520 | 558 | 652 | 261 | 274 | 299 | 161 | 166 | 171 |
| 0.3 | *** | 10502 | 10647 | 15001 | 1840 | 1958 | 2489 | 549 | 587 | 659 | 276 | 289 | 309 | 169 | 175 | 183 |
| | *** | 10550 | 10936 | 16781 | 1884 | 2101 | 2748 | 565 | 616 | 707 | 282 | 298 | 320 | 172 | 179 | 181 |
| 0.35 | *** | 10822 | 11015 | 16596 | 1911 | 2060 | 2725 | 576 | 621 | 710 | 289 | 305 | 328 | 176 | 183 | 192 |
| | *** | 10886 | 11398 | 18076 | 1968 | 2236 | 2936 | 596 | 657 | 746 | 296 | 315 | 334 | 179 | 187 | 187 |
| 0.4 | *** | 10752 | 11005 | 17784 | 1929 | 2109 | 2896 | 590 | 641 | 745 | 295 | 313 | 340 | 179 | 186 | 196 |
| | *** | 10836 | 11500 | 18979 | 1998 | 2316 | 3062 | 612 | 682 | 770 | 303 | 325 | 341 | 182 | 191 | 189 |
| 0.45 | *** | 10351 | 10676 | 18553 | 1903 | 2111 | 2999 | 591 | 648 | 762 | 295 | 315 | 344 | 178 | 186 | 197 |
| | *** | 10460 | 11303 | 19489 | 1983 | 2345 | 3124 | 616 | 693 | 778 | 304 | 328 | 341 | 182 | 191 | 187 |
| 0.5 | *** | 9683 | 10097 | 18898 | 1841 | 2074 | 3033 | 582 | 642 | 762 | 290 | 310 | 341 | 173 | 182 | 192 |
| | *** | 9822 | 10871 | 19607 | 1933 | 2329 | 3124 | 608 | 689 | 770 | 299 | 324 | 334 | 177 | 187 | 181 |
| 0.55 | *** | 8816 | 9339 | 18815 | 1752 | 2003 | 3000 | 562 | 624 | 745 | 279 | 300 | 329 | 166 | 174 | 184 |
| | *** | 8993 | 10266 | 19332 | 1851 | 2271 | 3062 | 589 | 672 | 746 | 289 | 313 | 320 | 170 | 179 | 171 |
| 0.6 | *** | 7824 | 8472 | 18305 | 1641 | 1903 | 2898 | 533 | 594 | 712 | 264 | 283 | 310 | 155 | 162 | 171 |
| | *** | 8046 | 9540 | 18665 | 1746 | 2175 | 2936 | 560 | 641 | 707 | 272 | 295 | 299 | 158 | 166 | 157 |
| 0.65 | *** | 6780 | 7557 | 17370 | 1513 | 1776 | 2728 | 496 | 553 | 661 | 242 | 259 | 284 | 140 | 147 | 155 |
| | *** | 7055 | 8732 | 17606 | 1619 | 2043 | 2748 | 521 | 596 | 652 | 250 | 270 | 271 | 143 | 150 | 140 |
| 0.7 | *** | 5758 | 6639 | 16012 | 1370 | 1623 | 2491 | 449 | 500 | 593 | 215 | 230 | 250 | 122 | 127 | 133 |
| | *** | 6080 | 7867 | 16153 | 1473 | 1874 | 2496 | 472 | 538 | 581 | 222 | 239 | 236 | 125 | 130 | 118 |
| 0.75 | *** | 4806 | 5738 | 14235 | 1212 | 1444 | 2186 | 392 | 435 | 509 | 183 | 194 | 209 | 100 | 104 | 108 |
| | *** | 5156 | 6951 | 14309 | 1307 | 1668 | 2182 | 411 | 466 | 495 | 188 | 201 | 194 | 102 | 106 | 93 |
| 0.8 | *** | 3938 | 4848 | 12043 | 1035 | 1234 | 1816 | 324 | 356 | 408 | 144 | 151 | 161 | . | . | . |
| | *** | 4288 | 5975 | 12072 | 1118 | 1419 | 1806 | 339 | 378 | 393 | 147 | 156 | 145 | . | . | . |
| 0.85 | *** | 3131 | 3942 | 9441 | 833 | 985 | 1380 | 242 | 262 | 291 | . | . | . | . | . | . |
| | *** | 3447 | 4905 | 9443 | 897 | 1121 | 1366 | 251 | 275 | 275 | . | . | . | . | . | . |
| 0.9 | *** | 2325 | 2955 | 6432 | 588 | 681 | 879 | . | . | . | . | . | . | . | . | . |
| | *** | 2574 | 3668 | 6421 | 628 | 756 | 864 | . | . | . | . | . | . | . | . | . |
| 0.95 | *** | 1383 | 1727 | 3022 | . | . | . | . | . | . | . | . | . | . | . | . |
| | *** | 1522 | 2076 | 3007 | . | . | . | . | . | . | . | . | . | . | . | . |

TABLE 5: ALPHA= 0.025 POWER= 0.8    EXPECTED ACCRUAL THRU MINIMUM FOLLOW-UP= 600

| | | DEL=.02 | | | DEL=.05 | | | DEL=.10 | | | DEL=.15 | | | DEL=.20 | | |
|---|---|---|---|---|---|---|---|---|---|---|---|---|---|---|---|---|
| FACT= | | 1.0 .75 | .50 .25 | .00 BIN | 1.0 .75 | .50 .25 | .00 BIN | 1.0 .75 | .50 .25 | .00 BIN | 1.0 75 | .50 .25 | .00 BIN | 1.0 .75 | .50 .25 | .00 BIN |
| PCONT=*** | | | | | REQUIRED | NUMBER OF | PATIENTS | | | | | | | | | |
| 0.05 | *** | 2238 | 2250 | 2365 | 481 | 488 | 502 | 174 | 176 | 178 | 102 | 103 | 104 | 72 | 73 | 73 |
| | *** | 2242 | 2272 | 4419 | 484 | 493 | 864 | 175 | 177 | 275 | 103 | 104 | 145 | 73 | 73 | 93 |
| 0.1 | *** | 4657 | 4687 | 5195 | 883 | 905 | 967 | 283 | 289 | 299 | 153 | 155 | 158 | 101 | 103 | 104 |
| | *** | 4667 | 4744 | 7677 | 892 | 927 | 1366 | 286 | 293 | 393 | 154 | 157 | 194 | 102 | 103 | 118 |
| 0.15 | *** | 6805 | 6857 | 8034 | 1232 | 1274 | 1418 | 377 | 389 | 409 | 196 | 200 | 206 | 125 | 127 | 130 |
| | *** | 6823 | 6961 | 10542 | 1248 | 1320 | 1806 | 382 | 398 | 495 | 198 | 203 | 236 | 126 | 129 | 140 |
| 0.2 | *** | 8519 | 8599 | 10675 | 1510 | 1576 | 1829 | 452 | 473 | 507 | 230 | 238 | 248 | 145 | 148 | 152 |
| | *** | 8546 | 8759 | 13014 | 1535 | 1652 | 2182 | 461 | 487 | 581 | 234 | 242 | 271 | 146 | 150 | 157 |
| 0.25 | *** | 9753 | 9868 | 13016 | 1715 | 1809 | 2188 | 511 | 540 | 591 | 258 | 268 | 282 | 160 | 164 | 169 |
| | *** | 9791 | 10098 | 15094 | 1751 | 1918 | 2496 | 524 | 561 | 652 | 262 | 274 | 299 | 162 | 167 | 171 |
| 0.3 | *** | 10515 | 10673 | 15000 | 1852 | 1975 | 2488 | 554 | 591 | 659 | 278 | 290 | 309 | 170 | 176 | 183 |
| | *** | 10568 | 10987 | 16781 | 1899 | 2118 | 2748 | 570 | 618 | 707 | 284 | 299 | 320 | 173 | 179 | 181 |
| 0.35 | *** | 10839 | 11050 | 16596 | 1927 | 2081 | 2725 | 582 | 626 | 710 | 291 | 306 | 328 | 177 | 184 | 192 |
| | *** | 10910 | 11466 | 18076 | 1986 | 2258 | 2936 | 601 | 660 | 746 | 298 | 316 | 334 | 180 | 187 | 187 |
| 0.4 | *** | 10775 | 11050 | 17784 | 1949 | 2134 | 2896 | 596 | 647 | 745 | 298 | 315 | 340 | 180 | 187 | 196 |
| | *** | 10867 | 11587 | 18979 | 2020 | 2342 | 3062 | 619 | 686 | 770 | 305 | 326 | 341 | 183 | 191 | 189 |
| 0.45 | *** | 10381 | 10735 | 18553 | 1926 | 2140 | 2999 | 599 | 654 | 762 | 298 | 317 | 344 | 179 | 187 | 197 |
| | *** | 10499 | 11410 | 19489 | 2009 | 2374 | 3124 | 623 | 697 | 778 | 307 | 329 | 341 | 183 | 191 | 187 |
| 0.5 | *** | 9721 | 10172 | 18898 | 1868 | 2105 | 3034 | 590 | 649 | 762 | 293 | 312 | 340 | 175 | 182 | 193 |
| | *** | 9872 | 10999 | 19607 | 1962 | 2360 | 3124 | 616 | 694 | 770 | 302 | 325 | 334 | 178 | 187 | 181 |
| 0.55 | *** | 8864 | 9431 | 18815 | 1781 | 2036 | 3000 | 571 | 631 | 745 | 282 | 301 | 329 | 167 | 175 | 184 |
| | *** | 9056 | 10414 | 19332 | 1883 | 2304 | 3062 | 597 | 677 | 746 | 291 | 314 | 320 | 170 | 179 | 171 |
| 0.6 | *** | 7885 | 8582 | 18305 | 1672 | 1937 | 2898 | 542 | 601 | 712 | 266 | 284 | 310 | 156 | 163 | 171 |
| | *** | 8126 | 9703 | 18665 | 1779 | 2208 | 2936 | 568 | 646 | 707 | 275 | 296 | 299 | 159 | 167 | 157 |
| 0.65 | *** | 6857 | 7683 | 17370 | 1545 | 1810 | 2728 | 503 | 559 | 661 | 245 | 261 | 284 | 141 | 147 | 154 |
| | *** | 7151 | 8905 | 17606 | 1652 | 2075 | 2748 | 528 | 601 | 652 | 252 | 272 | 271 | 144 | 151 | 140 |
| 0.7 | *** | 5849 | 6775 | 16012 | 1401 | 1655 | 2491 | 456 | 506 | 593 | 218 | 232 | 250 | 123 | 128 | 133 |
| | *** | 6190 | 8042 | 16153 | 1505 | 1904 | 2496 | 478 | 542 | 581 | 224 | 240 | 236 | 125 | 130 | 118 |
| 0.75 | *** | 4906 | 5876 | 14235 | 1241 | 1473 | 2186 | 398 | 440 | 509 | 185 | 195 | 209 | 101 | 104 | 108 |
| | *** | 5273 | 7121 | 14309 | 1336 | 1694 | 2182 | 417 | 469 | 495 | 190 | 202 | 194 | 103 | 106 | 93 |
| 0.8 | *** | 4040 | 4979 | 12043 | 1060 | 1259 | 1816 | 329 | 360 | 408 | 145 | 152 | 161 | . | . | . |
| | *** | 4402 | 6129 | 12072 | 1143 | 1440 | 1806 | 343 | 380 | 393 | 148 | 156 | 145 | . | . | . |
| 0.85 | *** | 3223 | 4055 | 9440 | 852 | 1004 | 1380 | 245 | 264 | 290 | . | . | . | . | . | . |
| | *** | 3548 | 5033 | 9443 | 916 | 1135 | 1366 | 254 | 276 | 275 | . | . | . | . | . | . |
| 0.9 | *** | 2398 | 3041 | 6432 | 600 | 692 | 879 | . | . | . | . | . | . | . | . | . |
| | *** | 2653 | 3760 | 6421 | 640 | 764 | 864 | . | . | . | . | . | . | . | . | . |
| 0.95 | *** | 1424 | 1771 | 3022 | . | . | . | . | . | . | . | . | . | . | . | . |
| | *** | 1565 | 2119 | 3007 | . | . | . | . | . | . | . | . | . | . | . | . |

## TABLE 5: ALPHA= 0.025 POWER= 0.8    EXPECTED ACCRUAL THRU MINIMUM FOLLOW-UP= 650

|  |  | DEL=.02 | | | DEL=.05 | | | DEL=.10 | | | DEL=.15 | | | DEL=.20 | | |
|---|---|---|---|---|---|---|---|---|---|---|---|---|---|---|---|---|
| FACT= | | 1.0 .75 | .50 .25 | .00 BIN | 1.0 .75 | .50 .25 | .00 BIN | 1.0 .75 | .50 .25 | .00 BIN | 1.0 75 | .50 .25 | .00 BIN | 1.0 .75 | .50 .25 | .00 BIN |
| PCONT=*** | | REQUIRED NUMBER OF PATIENTS | | | | | | | | | | | | | | |
| 0.05 | *** | 2239 | 2252 | 2365 | 482 | 489 | 502 | 175 | 176 | 178 | 103 | 103 | 104 | 73 | 73 | 73 |
|  | *** | 2244 | 2275 | 4419 | 484 | 494 | 864 | 175 | 177 | 275 | 103 | 103 | 145 | 73 | 73 | 93 |
| 0.1 | *** | 4660 | 4692 | 5195 | 886 | 908 | 967 | 284 | 290 | 299 | 153 | 156 | 159 | 102 | 103 | 104 |
|  | *** | 4670 | 4753 | 7677 | 895 | 929 | 1366 | 287 | 294 | 393 | 155 | 157 | 194 | 102 | 103 | 118 |
| 0.15 | *** | 6809 | 6866 | 8034 | 1236 | 1279 | 1418 | 378 | 390 | 409 | 197 | 201 | 207 | 126 | 128 | 130 |
|  | *** | 6828 | 6978 | 10542 | 1253 | 1325 | 1806 | 384 | 399 | 495 | 198 | 203 | 236 | 127 | 129 | 140 |
| 0.2 | *** | 8525 | 8613 | 10675 | 1516 | 1585 | 1829 | 455 | 475 | 507 | 232 | 239 | 248 | 145 | 148 | 152 |
|  | *** | 8555 | 8785 | 13014 | 1542 | 1660 | 2182 | 464 | 489 | 581 | 235 | 243 | 271 | 146 | 150 | 157 |
| 0.25 | *** | 9762 | 9888 | 13016 | 1725 | 1821 | 2188 | 515 | 543 | 591 | 259 | 269 | 282 | 160 | 164 | 170 |
|  | *** | 9804 | 10135 | 15094 | 1761 | 1930 | 2496 | 527 | 563 | 652 | 263 | 275 | 299 | 162 | 167 | 171 |
| 0.3 | *** | 10528 | 10700 | 15000 | 1865 | 1992 | 2489 | 559 | 595 | 659 | 280 | 292 | 309 | 171 | 176 | 183 |
|  | *** | 10585 | 11039 | 16781 | 1913 | 2135 | 2748 | 575 | 621 | 707 | 285 | 300 | 320 | 174 | 179 | 181 |
| 0.35 | *** | 10857 | 11086 | 16596 | 1943 | 2101 | 2725 | 588 | 631 | 710 | 293 | 307 | 328 | 178 | 184 | 192 |
|  | *** | 10933 | 11533 | 18076 | 2004 | 2278 | 2936 | 606 | 663 | 746 | 300 | 317 | 334 | 181 | 188 | 187 |
| 0.4 | *** | 10798 | 11096 | 17784 | 1968 | 2157 | 2896 | 603 | 652 | 744 | 300 | 316 | 340 | 181 | 188 | 197 |
|  | *** | 10897 | 11671 | 18979 | 2042 | 2365 | 3062 | 625 | 690 | 770 | 307 | 327 | 341 | 184 | 192 | 189 |
| 0.45 | *** | 10410 | 10793 | 18553 | 1949 | 2166 | 2999 | 606 | 660 | 762 | 301 | 318 | 344 | 180 | 188 | 197 |
|  | *** | 10538 | 11515 | 19489 | 2034 | 2400 | 3124 | 630 | 701 | 778 | 309 | 330 | 341 | 184 | 192 | 187 |
| 0.5 | *** | 9759 | 10246 | 18898 | 1893 | 2135 | 3033 | 597 | 655 | 762 | 296 | 314 | 341 | 176 | 184 | 192 |
|  | *** | 9922 | 11123 | 19607 | 1989 | 2389 | 3124 | 622 | 698 | 770 | 304 | 326 | 334 | 179 | 188 | 181 |
| 0.55 | *** | 8913 | 9522 | 18815 | 1809 | 2068 | 3000 | 578 | 637 | 745 | 285 | 303 | 329 | 168 | 175 | 184 |
|  | *** | 9120 | 10555 | 19332 | 1913 | 2334 | 3062 | 604 | 681 | 746 | 294 | 315 | 320 | 172 | 179 | 171 |
| 0.6 | *** | 7946 | 8690 | 18305 | 1701 | 1969 | 2898 | 549 | 607 | 712 | 269 | 286 | 311 | 157 | 164 | 171 |
|  | *** | 8205 | 9859 | 18665 | 1810 | 2238 | 2936 | 575 | 650 | 707 | 277 | 297 | 299 | 160 | 167 | 157 |
| 0.65 | *** | 6932 | 7805 | 17370 | 1575 | 1841 | 2728 | 510 | 565 | 661 | 247 | 263 | 284 | 142 | 148 | 155 |
|  | *** | 7245 | 9069 | 17606 | 1683 | 2104 | 2748 | 535 | 604 | 652 | 254 | 272 | 271 | 145 | 151 | 140 |
| 0.7 | *** | 5937 | 6905 | 16012 | 1430 | 1685 | 2491 | 463 | 511 | 593 | 220 | 233 | 250 | 124 | 128 | 133 |
|  | *** | 6295 | 8208 | 16153 | 1535 | 1931 | 2496 | 484 | 545 | 581 | 226 | 241 | 236 | 126 | 131 | 118 |
| 0.75 | *** | 5003 | 6007 | 14235 | 1267 | 1500 | 2186 | 404 | 444 | 509 | 186 | 197 | 209 | 101 | 105 | 108 |
|  | *** | 5384 | 7279 | 14309 | 1364 | 1717 | 2182 | 422 | 471 | 495 | 191 | 202 | 194 | 103 | 106 | 93 |
| 0.8 | *** | 4136 | 5102 | 12043 | 1083 | 1281 | 1816 | 333 | 363 | 408 | 146 | 153 | 161 | . | . | . |
|  | *** | 4509 | 6272 | 12072 | 1166 | 1459 | 1806 | 346 | 383 | 393 | 149 | 157 | 145 | . | . | . |
| 0.85 | *** | 3311 | 4162 | 9441 | 870 | 1020 | 1380 | 248 | 266 | 291 | . | . | . | . | . | . |
|  | *** | 3644 | 5153 | 9443 | 934 | 1149 | 1366 | 256 | 277 | 275 | . | . | . | . | . | . |
| 0.9 | *** | 2467 | 3121 | 6432 | 612 | 701 | 879 | . | . | . | . | . | . | . | . | . |
|  | *** | 2727 | 3846 | 6421 | 651 | 771 | 864 | . | . | . | . | . | . | . | . | . |
| 0.95 | *** | 1463 | 1812 | 3022 | . | . | . | . | . | . | . | . | . | . | . | . |
|  | *** | 1606 | 2157 | 3007 | . | . | . | . | . | . | . | . | . | . | . | . |

TABLE 5: ALPHA= 0.025 POWER= 0.8    EXPECTED ACCRUAL THRU MINIMUM FOLLOW-UP= 700

| | | DEL=.02 | | | DEL=.05 | | | DEL=.10 | | | DEL=.15 | | | DEL=.20 | | |
|---|---|---|---|---|---|---|---|---|---|---|---|---|---|---|---|---|---|
| FACT= | | 1.0 .75 | .50 .25 | .00 BIN | 1.0 .75 | .50 .25 | .00 BIN | 1.0 .75 | .50 .25 | .00 BIN | 1.0 75 | .50 .25 | .00 BIN | 1.0 .75 | .50 .25 | .00 BIN |
| PCONT=*** | | | | | REQUIRED NUMBER OF PATIENTS | | | | | | | | | | | |
| 0.05 | *** | 2240 | 2254 | 2364 | 482 | 489 | 502 | 175 | 176 | 178 | 103 | 103 | 104 | 72 | 73 | 73 |
| | *** | 2245 | 2278 | 4419 | 485 | 494 | 864 | 175 | 177 | 275 | 103 | 103 | 145 | 73 | 73 | 93 |
| 0.1 | *** | 4662 | 4696 | 5195 | 888 | 911 | 967 | 285 | 291 | 299 | 154 | 156 | 159 | 102 | 103 | 104 |
| | *** | 4673 | 4762 | 7677 | 897 | 931 | 1366 | 288 | 294 | 393 | 155 | 157 | 194 | 102 | 103 | 118 |
| 0.15 | *** | 6814 | 6875 | 8034 | 1240 | 1284 | 1418 | 380 | 391 | 409 | 197 | 201 | 206 | 126 | 128 | 130 |
| | *** | 6834 | 6994 | 10542 | 1257 | 1329 | 1806 | 385 | 399 | 495 | 199 | 204 | 236 | 127 | 129 | 140 |
| 0.2 | *** | 8532 | 8626 | 10675 | 1523 | 1593 | 1829 | 457 | 476 | 507 | 233 | 239 | 248 | 145 | 149 | 152 |
| | *** | 8563 | 8811 | 13014 | 1550 | 1668 | 2182 | 466 | 490 | 581 | 236 | 243 | 271 | 147 | 150 | 157 |
| 0.25 | *** | 9772 | 9907 | 13016 | 1734 | 1832 | 2189 | 518 | 545 | 591 | 261 | 270 | 282 | 161 | 165 | 170 |
| | *** | 9817 | 10173 | 15094 | 1772 | 1941 | 2496 | 530 | 565 | 652 | 265 | 275 | 299 | 163 | 167 | 171 |
| 0.3 | *** | 10541 | 10726 | 15000 | 1876 | 2007 | 2489 | 563 | 598 | 659 | 281 | 293 | 309 | 172 | 177 | 183 |
| | *** | 10603 | 11089 | 16781 | 1927 | 2150 | 2748 | 578 | 623 | 707 | 286 | 300 | 320 | 174 | 180 | 181 |
| 0.35 | *** | 10874 | 11121 | 16596 | 1958 | 2120 | 2725 | 593 | 635 | 710 | 295 | 309 | 328 | 179 | 184 | 192 |
| | *** | 10957 | 11599 | 18076 | 2021 | 2297 | 2936 | 611 | 666 | 746 | 301 | 317 | 334 | 181 | 188 | 187 |
| 0.4 | *** | 10821 | 11142 | 17784 | 1986 | 2179 | 2896 | 608 | 657 | 744 | 302 | 318 | 340 | 182 | 188 | 196 |
| | *** | 10928 | 11755 | 18979 | 2062 | 2387 | 3062 | 630 | 693 | 770 | 309 | 328 | 341 | 185 | 192 | 189 |
| 0.45 | *** | 10440 | 10852 | 18553 | 1970 | 2192 | 2999 | 612 | 665 | 762 | 303 | 320 | 344 | 181 | 188 | 197 |
| | *** | 10578 | 11616 | 19489 | 2058 | 2425 | 3124 | 635 | 705 | 778 | 311 | 331 | 341 | 184 | 192 | 187 |
| 0.5 | *** | 9797 | 10319 | 18898 | 1917 | 2162 | 3033 | 604 | 660 | 762 | 298 | 316 | 341 | 177 | 184 | 192 |
| | *** | 9973 | 11243 | 19607 | 2015 | 2415 | 3124 | 628 | 702 | 770 | 306 | 327 | 334 | 180 | 188 | 181 |
| 0.55 | *** | 8961 | 9611 | 18815 | 1835 | 2096 | 3000 | 585 | 642 | 745 | 287 | 305 | 329 | 169 | 176 | 184 |
| | *** | 9183 | 10691 | 19332 | 1941 | 2361 | 3062 | 611 | 684 | 746 | 296 | 316 | 320 | 172 | 180 | 171 |
| 0.6 | *** | 8006 | 8794 | 18305 | 1729 | 1998 | 2898 | 556 | 612 | 712 | 271 | 288 | 310 | 158 | 164 | 171 |
| | *** | 8282 | 10008 | 18665 | 1838 | 2266 | 2936 | 581 | 653 | 707 | 279 | 298 | 299 | 161 | 167 | 157 |
| 0.65 | *** | 7006 | 7922 | 17370 | 1602 | 1870 | 2728 | 517 | 570 | 661 | 249 | 264 | 284 | 143 | 148 | 155 |
| | *** | 7337 | 9225 | 17606 | 1712 | 2130 | 2748 | 541 | 608 | 652 | 256 | 273 | 271 | 145 | 151 | 140 |
| 0.7 | *** | 6024 | 7030 | 16012 | 1457 | 1712 | 2490 | 468 | 515 | 593 | 221 | 234 | 250 | 124 | 128 | 133 |
| | *** | 6398 | 8364 | 16153 | 1562 | 1955 | 2496 | 489 | 548 | 581 | 227 | 242 | 236 | 126 | 131 | 118 |
| 0.75 | *** | 5096 | 6130 | 14235 | 1292 | 1524 | 2186 | 408 | 447 | 509 | 187 | 197 | 209 | 102 | 105 | 108 |
| | *** | 5490 | 7429 | 14309 | 1388 | 1738 | 2182 | 426 | 474 | 495 | 192 | 203 | 194 | 103 | 107 | 93 |
| 0.8 | *** | 4229 | 5218 | 12043 | 1104 | 1301 | 1816 | 337 | 365 | 408 | 147 | 153 | 161 | . | . | . |
| | *** | 4612 | 6407 | 12072 | 1187 | 1476 | 1806 | 350 | 384 | 393 | 150 | 157 | 145 | . | . | . |
| 0.85 | *** | 3394 | 4262 | 9441 | 887 | 1035 | 1380 | 250 | 267 | 291 | . | . | . | . | . | . |
| | *** | 3735 | 5265 | 9443 | 950 | 1160 | 1366 | 258 | 278 | 275 | . | . | . | . | . | . |
| 0.9 | *** | 2532 | 3196 | 6432 | 622 | 710 | 879 | . | . | . | . | . | . | . | . | . |
| | *** | 2796 | 3925 | 6421 | 660 | 777 | 864 | . | . | . | . | . | . | . | . | . |
| 0.95 | *** | 1500 | 1850 | 3022 | . | . | . | . | . | . | . | . | . | . | . | . |
| | *** | 1643 | 2192 | 3007 | . | . | . | . | . | . | . | . | . | . | . | . |

## TABLE 5: ALPHA= 0.025 POWER= 0.8 EXPECTED ACCRUAL THRU MINIMUM FOLLOW-UP= 750

|  |  | DEL=.02 | | | DEL=.05 | | | DEL=.10 | | | DEL=.15 | | | DEL=.20 | | |
|---|---|---|---|---|---|---|---|---|---|---|---|---|---|---|---|---|
| FACT= | | 1.0 .75 | .50 .25 | .00 BIN | 1.0 .75 | .50 .25 | .00 BIN | 1.0 .75 | .50 .25 | .00 BIN | 1.0 75 | .50 .25 | .00 BIN | 1.0 .75 | .50 .25 | .00 BIN |
| PCONT=*** | | | | | REQUIRED | NUMBER OF | PATIENTS | | | | | | | | | |
| 0.05 | *** | 2241 | 2256 | 2365 | 483 | 490 | 502 | 175 | 176 | 178 | 103 | 103 | 104 | 72 | 73 | 73 |
| | *** | 2246 | 2281 | 4419 | 486 | 495 | 864 | 175 | 177 | 275 | 103 | 104 | 145 | 73 | 73 | 93 |
| 0.1 | *** | 4664 | 4701 | 5195 | 890 | 913 | 967 | 286 | 291 | 299 | 154 | 156 | 159 | 102 | 103 | 104 |
| | *** | 4676 | 4771 | 7677 | 899 | 933 | 1366 | 288 | 295 | 393 | 155 | 157 | 194 | 102 | 103 | 118 |
| 0.15 | *** | 6818 | 6883 | 8034 | 1244 | 1289 | 1418 | 381 | 392 | 409 | 198 | 201 | 206 | 126 | 128 | 130 |
| | *** | 6840 | 7010 | 10542 | 1262 | 1333 | 1806 | 386 | 400 | 495 | 199 | 204 | 236 | 127 | 129 | 140 |
| 0.2 | *** | 8539 | 8640 | 10675 | 1529 | 1600 | 1829 | 460 | 478 | 507 | 233 | 240 | 248 | 146 | 149 | 152 |
| | *** | 8573 | 8837 | 13014 | 1557 | 1675 | 2182 | 468 | 491 | 581 | 236 | 244 | 271 | 147 | 150 | 157 |
| 0.25 | *** | 9782 | 9926 | 13015 | 1742 | 1843 | 2188 | 521 | 547 | 591 | 261 | 270 | 282 | 161 | 165 | 169 |
| | *** | 9830 | 10209 | 15094 | 1781 | 1951 | 2496 | 533 | 566 | 652 | 265 | 276 | 299 | 163 | 167 | 171 |
| 0.3 | *** | 10555 | 10753 | 15000 | 1888 | 2021 | 2488 | 567 | 601 | 659 | 282 | 294 | 309 | 172 | 177 | 183 |
| | *** | 10621 | 11139 | 16781 | 1940 | 2163 | 2748 | 582 | 625 | 707 | 288 | 301 | 320 | 175 | 180 | 181 |
| 0.35 | *** | 10892 | 11155 | 16596 | 1972 | 2138 | 2725 | 597 | 638 | 710 | 296 | 310 | 328 | 179 | 185 | 192 |
| | *** | 10980 | 11664 | 18076 | 2037 | 2314 | 2936 | 616 | 668 | 746 | 303 | 319 | 334 | 182 | 188 | 187 |
| 0.4 | *** | 10844 | 11187 | 17784 | 2004 | 2200 | 2896 | 614 | 661 | 745 | 304 | 319 | 340 | 183 | 189 | 196 |
| | *** | 10959 | 11836 | 18979 | 2081 | 2407 | 3062 | 635 | 696 | 770 | 311 | 329 | 341 | 185 | 192 | 189 |
| 0.45 | *** | 10470 | 10910 | 18553 | 1990 | 2215 | 2999 | 618 | 670 | 762 | 305 | 321 | 344 | 182 | 189 | 197 |
| | *** | 10617 | 11715 | 19489 | 2080 | 2447 | 3124 | 641 | 708 | 778 | 312 | 332 | 341 | 185 | 192 | 187 |
| 0.5 | *** | 9834 | 10391 | 18897 | 1940 | 2188 | 3034 | 610 | 665 | 762 | 300 | 317 | 340 | 178 | 184 | 192 |
| | *** | 10023 | 11359 | 19607 | 2040 | 2439 | 3124 | 634 | 705 | 770 | 308 | 328 | 334 | 181 | 188 | 181 |
| 0.55 | *** | 9009 | 9699 | 18815 | 1860 | 2123 | 3000 | 591 | 647 | 745 | 289 | 306 | 329 | 170 | 176 | 184 |
| | *** | 9246 | 10822 | 19332 | 1967 | 2386 | 3062 | 616 | 688 | 746 | 297 | 317 | 320 | 173 | 180 | 171 |
| 0.6 | *** | 8066 | 8896 | 18305 | 1754 | 2026 | 2898 | 562 | 617 | 711 | 273 | 289 | 310 | 159 | 164 | 171 |
| | *** | 8359 | 10150 | 18665 | 1865 | 2290 | 2936 | 587 | 656 | 707 | 280 | 299 | 299 | 161 | 168 | 157 |
| 0.65 | *** | 7079 | 8035 | 17370 | 1628 | 1897 | 2728 | 523 | 574 | 661 | 251 | 265 | 284 | 144 | 148 | 154 |
| | *** | 7427 | 9373 | 17606 | 1738 | 2154 | 2748 | 546 | 611 | 652 | 258 | 274 | 271 | 146 | 151 | 140 |
| 0.7 | *** | 6108 | 7149 | 16012 | 1481 | 1737 | 2491 | 473 | 519 | 593 | 223 | 235 | 250 | 125 | 129 | 133 |
| | *** | 6497 | 8511 | 16153 | 1588 | 1977 | 2496 | 494 | 550 | 581 | 229 | 242 | 236 | 127 | 131 | 118 |
| 0.75 | *** | 5186 | 6249 | 14235 | 1315 | 1547 | 2186 | 413 | 450 | 509 | 189 | 198 | 209 | 102 | 105 | 108 |
| | *** | 5592 | 7569 | 14309 | 1412 | 1758 | 2182 | 430 | 476 | 495 | 193 | 203 | 194 | 104 | 107 | 93 |
| 0.8 | *** | 4317 | 5329 | 12043 | 1124 | 1320 | 1816 | 340 | 368 | 408 | 148 | 154 | 160 | . | . | . |
| | *** | 4710 | 6534 | 12072 | 1207 | 1491 | 1806 | 353 | 385 | 393 | 151 | 157 | 145 | . | . | . |
| 0.85 | *** | 3473 | 4357 | 9440 | 902 | 1049 | 1380 | 252 | 268 | 291 | . | . | . | . | . | . |
| | *** | 3820 | 5369 | 9443 | 965 | 1171 | 1366 | 259 | 279 | 275 | . | . | . | . | . | . |
| 0.9 | *** | 2594 | 3267 | 6432 | 631 | 717 | 879 | . | . | . | . | . | . | . | . | . |
| | *** | 2862 | 3998 | 6421 | 669 | 783 | 864 | . | . | . | . | . | . | . | . | . |
| 0.95 | *** | 1534 | 1885 | 3022 | . | . | . | . | . | . | . | . | . | . | . | . |
| | *** | 1678 | 2224 | 3007 | . | . | . | . | . | . | . | . | . | . | . | . |

TABLE 5: ALPHA= 0.025 POWER= 0.8     EXPECTED ACCRUAL THRU MINIMUM FOLLOW-UP= 800

| | | DEL=.02 | | | DEL=.05 | | | DEL=.10 | | | DEL=.15 | | | DEL=.20 | | |
|---|---|---|---|---|---|---|---|---|---|---|---|---|---|---|---|---|
| FACT= | | 1.0 .75 | .50 .25 | .00 BIN | 1.0 .75 | .50 .25 | .00 BIN | 1.0 .75 | .50 .25 | .00 BIN | 1.0 75 | .50 .25 | .00 BIN | 1.0 .75 | .50 .25 | .00 BIN |
| PCONT=*** | | | | REQUIRED NUMBER OF PATIENTS | | | | | | | | | | | | |
| 0.05 | *** | 2242 | 2258 | 2365 | 484 | 490 | 502 | 175 | 177 | 178 | 103 | 103 | 104 | 73 | 73 | 73 |
| | *** | 2248 | 2283 | 4419 | 487 | 495 | 864 | 176 | 177 | 275 | 103 | 104 | 145 | 73 | 73 | 93 |
| 0.1 | *** | 4667 | 4706 | 5195 | 892 | 915 | 967 | 286 | 292 | 299 | 154 | 156 | 159 | 102 | 103 | 104 |
| | *** | 4680 | 4780 | 7677 | 901 | 935 | 1366 | 289 | 295 | 393 | 155 | 157 | 194 | 103 | 104 | 118 |
| 0.15 | *** | 6823 | 6892 | 8034 | 1248 | 1293 | 1418 | 382 | 393 | 409 | 198 | 202 | 207 | 126 | 128 | 130 |
| | *** | 6846 | 7026 | 10542 | 1266 | 1337 | 1806 | 387 | 400 | 495 | 200 | 204 | 236 | 127 | 129 | 140 |
| 0.2 | *** | 8546 | 8653 | 10675 | 1535 | 1607 | 1829 | 462 | 479 | 507 | 234 | 240 | 248 | 146 | 149 | 152 |
| | *** | 8582 | 8862 | 13014 | 1563 | 1681 | 2182 | 470 | 492 | 581 | 237 | 244 | 271 | 148 | 150 | 157 |
| 0.25 | *** | 9791 | 9945 | 13016 | 1751 | 1854 | 2188 | 524 | 550 | 591 | 263 | 271 | 282 | 162 | 165 | 170 |
| | *** | 9843 | 10245 | 15094 | 1791 | 1961 | 2496 | 535 | 567 | 652 | 267 | 276 | 299 | 163 | 167 | 171 |
| 0.3 | *** | 10568 | 10779 | 15000 | 1899 | 2034 | 2489 | 570 | 603 | 659 | 284 | 295 | 309 | 173 | 177 | 183 |
| | *** | 10638 | 11188 | 16781 | 1952 | 2176 | 2748 | 585 | 627 | 707 | 289 | 301 | 320 | 175 | 180 | 181 |
| 0.35 | *** | 10910 | 11191 | 16596 | 1986 | 2154 | 2725 | 601 | 642 | 710 | 298 | 311 | 328 | 180 | 185 | 192 |
| | *** | 11003 | 11727 | 18076 | 2053 | 2329 | 2936 | 619 | 671 | 746 | 304 | 319 | 334 | 183 | 188 | 187 |
| 0.4 | *** | 10867 | 11233 | 17784 | 2020 | 2220 | 2896 | 619 | 665 | 745 | 306 | 320 | 340 | 183 | 189 | 196 |
| | *** | 10989 | 11916 | 18979 | 2100 | 2425 | 3062 | 639 | 698 | 770 | 312 | 329 | 341 | 186 | 193 | 189 |
| 0.45 | *** | 10499 | 10968 | 18553 | 2010 | 2237 | 2999 | 623 | 674 | 762 | 307 | 323 | 344 | 183 | 189 | 197 |
| | *** | 10657 | 11811 | 19489 | 2101 | 2467 | 3124 | 646 | 711 | 778 | 314 | 332 | 341 | 186 | 193 | 187 |
| 0.5 | *** | 9872 | 10462 | 18898 | 1962 | 2212 | 3034 | 616 | 669 | 762 | 302 | 318 | 341 | 179 | 185 | 193 |
| | *** | 10073 | 11471 | 19607 | 2063 | 2461 | 3124 | 640 | 708 | 770 | 310 | 329 | 334 | 182 | 189 | 181 |
| 0.55 | *** | 9056 | 9785 | 18815 | 1883 | 2148 | 3000 | 597 | 652 | 746 | 291 | 307 | 329 | 171 | 177 | 184 |
| | *** | 9308 | 10948 | 19332 | 1991 | 2409 | 3062 | 621 | 691 | 746 | 299 | 318 | 320 | 174 | 180 | 171 |
| 0.6 | *** | 8126 | 8996 | 18305 | 1779 | 2051 | 2898 | 568 | 621 | 712 | 275 | 290 | 311 | 159 | 165 | 171 |
| | *** | 8435 | 10285 | 18665 | 1891 | 2313 | 2936 | 592 | 659 | 707 | 282 | 300 | 299 | 162 | 168 | 157 |
| 0.65 | *** | 7151 | 8145 | 17370 | 1652 | 1922 | 2728 | 528 | 578 | 661 | 252 | 266 | 284 | 144 | 149 | 155 |
| | *** | 7514 | 9514 | 17606 | 1764 | 2176 | 2748 | 551 | 613 | 652 | 259 | 275 | 271 | 146 | 152 | 140 |
| 0.7 | *** | 6190 | 7263 | 16012 | 1505 | 1761 | 2491 | 478 | 523 | 593 | 224 | 236 | 250 | 125 | 129 | 133 |
| | *** | 6593 | 8652 | 16153 | 1612 | 1998 | 2496 | 498 | 553 | 581 | 230 | 243 | 236 | 127 | 131 | 118 |
| 0.75 | *** | 5273 | 6362 | 14235 | 1337 | 1568 | 2186 | 417 | 453 | 509 | 190 | 199 | 209 | 103 | 105 | 108 |
| | *** | 5691 | 7702 | 14309 | 1434 | 1775 | 2182 | 434 | 478 | 495 | 194 | 204 | 194 | 104 | 107 | 93 |
| 0.8 | *** | 4402 | 5433 | 12043 | 1143 | 1337 | 1816 | 343 | 370 | 408 | 149 | 154 | 161 | . | . | . |
| | *** | 4803 | 6653 | 12072 | 1225 | 1506 | 1806 | 355 | 387 | 393 | 151 | 157 | 145 | . | . | . |
| 0.85 | *** | 3549 | 4447 | 9441 | 917 | 1062 | 1380 | 254 | 270 | 291 | . | . | . | . | . | . |
| | *** | 3903 | 5467 | 9443 | 979 | 1181 | 1366 | 261 | 279 | 275 | . | . | . | . | . | . |
| 0.9 | *** | 2653 | 3333 | 6432 | 640 | 725 | 879 | . | . | . | . | . | . | . | . | . |
| | *** | 2925 | 4067 | 6421 | 677 | 787 | 864 | . | . | . | . | . | . | . | . | . |
| 0.95 | *** | 1566 | 1918 | 3022 | . | . | . | . | . | . | . | . | . | . | . | . |
| | *** | 1711 | 2254 | 3007 | . | . | . | . | . | . | . | . | . | . | . | . |

## TABLE 5: ALPHA= 0.025 POWER= 0.8    EXPECTED ACCRUAL THRU MINIMUM FOLLOW-UP= 850

| | | DEL=.02 | | | DEL=.05 | | | DEL=.10 | | | DEL=.15 | | | DEL=.20 | | |
|---|---|---|---|---|---|---|---|---|---|---|---|---|---|---|---|---|
| FACT= | | 1.0 .75 | .50 .25 | .00 BIN | 1.0 .75 | .50 .25 | .00 BIN | 1.0 .75 | .50 .25 | .00 BIN | 1.0 75 | .50 .25 | .00 BIN | 1.0 .75 | .50 .25 | .00 BIN |
| PCONT=*** | | | | REQUIRED NUMBER OF PATIENTS | | | | | | | | | | | | |
| 0.05 | *** | 2243 | 2260 | 2365 | 484 | 491 | 502 | 175 | 176 | 178 | 103 | 103 | 104 | 72 | 73 | 73 |
| | *** | 2249 | 2286 | 4419 | 487 | 495 | 864 | 176 | 178 | 275 | 103 | 104 | 145 | 73 | 73 | 93 |
| 0.1 | *** | 4669 | 4711 | 5195 | 894 | 917 | 967 | 287 | 292 | 299 | 155 | 156 | 158 | 102 | 103 | 104 |
| | *** | 4683 | 4788 | 7677 | 903 | 936 | 1366 | 289 | 295 | 393 | 155 | 157 | 194 | 103 | 103 | 118 |
| 0.15 | *** | 6827 | 6901 | 8034 | 1251 | 1297 | 1417 | 383 | 394 | 409 | 198 | 202 | 206 | 127 | 128 | 130 |
| | *** | 6852 | 7042 | 10542 | 1270 | 1341 | 1806 | 388 | 401 | 495 | 200 | 204 | 236 | 128 | 129 | 140 |
| 0.2 | *** | 8552 | 8667 | 10675 | 1541 | 1614 | 1829 | 463 | 481 | 508 | 235 | 240 | 248 | 147 | 149 | 152 |
| | *** | 8590 | 8887 | 13014 | 1570 | 1687 | 2182 | 471 | 493 | 581 | 238 | 244 | 271 | 148 | 151 | 157 |
| 0.25 | *** | 9801 | 9965 | 13016 | 1759 | 1863 | 2188 | 527 | 552 | 591 | 263 | 272 | 282 | 162 | 165 | 170 |
| | *** | 9855 | 10281 | 15094 | 1800 | 1970 | 2496 | 538 | 569 | 652 | 267 | 276 | 299 | 164 | 168 | 171 |
| 0.3 | *** | 10581 | 10805 | 15000 | 1909 | 2047 | 2488 | 573 | 606 | 658 | 285 | 295 | 309 | 173 | 178 | 183 |
| | *** | 10656 | 11236 | 16781 | 1964 | 2187 | 2748 | 588 | 629 | 707 | 290 | 301 | 320 | 175 | 180 | 181 |
| 0.35 | *** | 10928 | 11225 | 16596 | 2000 | 2170 | 2725 | 605 | 645 | 710 | 299 | 311 | 328 | 181 | 186 | 192 |
| | *** | 11027 | 11790 | 18076 | 2067 | 2344 | 2936 | 623 | 672 | 746 | 305 | 320 | 334 | 183 | 189 | 187 |
| 0.4 | *** | 10890 | 11278 | 17784 | 2037 | 2238 | 2895 | 623 | 668 | 745 | 307 | 321 | 340 | 184 | 190 | 196 |
| | *** | 11020 | 11994 | 18979 | 2117 | 2442 | 3062 | 644 | 700 | 770 | 314 | 329 | 341 | 187 | 193 | 189 |
| 0.45 | *** | 10528 | 11025 | 18553 | 2028 | 2258 | 2998 | 628 | 678 | 762 | 308 | 324 | 344 | 184 | 189 | 197 |
| | *** | 10696 | 11904 | 19489 | 2121 | 2486 | 3124 | 650 | 713 | 778 | 316 | 333 | 341 | 186 | 193 | 187 |
| 0.5 | *** | 9910 | 10533 | 18898 | 1982 | 2234 | 3034 | 621 | 673 | 763 | 304 | 320 | 341 | 179 | 185 | 192 |
| | *** | 10122 | 11579 | 19607 | 2085 | 2481 | 3124 | 644 | 711 | 770 | 311 | 329 | 334 | 182 | 189 | 181 |
| 0.55 | *** | 9104 | 9869 | 18815 | 1905 | 2172 | 3000 | 602 | 656 | 746 | 293 | 308 | 329 | 171 | 177 | 184 |
| | *** | 9370 | 11069 | 19332 | 2015 | 2430 | 3062 | 627 | 694 | 746 | 300 | 318 | 320 | 174 | 180 | 171 |
| 0.6 | *** | 8185 | 9093 | 18305 | 1802 | 2075 | 2898 | 573 | 626 | 712 | 276 | 291 | 310 | 159 | 165 | 171 |
| | *** | 8509 | 10415 | 18665 | 1914 | 2334 | 2936 | 597 | 662 | 707 | 283 | 300 | 299 | 162 | 168 | 157 |
| 0.65 | *** | 7222 | 8250 | 17370 | 1676 | 1945 | 2728 | 533 | 582 | 661 | 254 | 267 | 284 | 145 | 149 | 155 |
| | *** | 7600 | 9648 | 17606 | 1787 | 2197 | 2748 | 555 | 616 | 652 | 260 | 275 | 271 | 147 | 152 | 140 |
| 0.7 | *** | 6270 | 7373 | 16012 | 1528 | 1783 | 2491 | 482 | 526 | 593 | 225 | 237 | 250 | 125 | 129 | 134 |
| | *** | 6685 | 8785 | 16153 | 1634 | 2016 | 2496 | 502 | 555 | 581 | 231 | 243 | 236 | 127 | 131 | 118 |
| 0.75 | *** | 5357 | 6470 | 14235 | 1357 | 1587 | 2186 | 420 | 456 | 509 | 191 | 199 | 209 | 103 | 105 | 108 |
| | *** | 5785 | 7829 | 14309 | 1454 | 1791 | 2182 | 437 | 479 | 495 | 195 | 204 | 194 | 104 | 107 | 93 |
| 0.8 | *** | 4483 | 5534 | 12043 | 1160 | 1353 | 1816 | 345 | 372 | 408 | 149 | 154 | 161 | . | . | . |
| | *** | 4893 | 6766 | 12072 | 1243 | 1518 | 1806 | 358 | 388 | 393 | 152 | 157 | 145 | . | . | . |
| 0.85 | *** | 3621 | 4532 | 9440 | 930 | 1073 | 1380 | 255 | 271 | 291 | . | . | . | . | . | . |
| | *** | 3981 | 5560 | 9443 | 992 | 1189 | 1366 | 263 | 280 | 275 | . | . | . | . | . | . |
| 0.9 | *** | 2708 | 3397 | 6432 | 648 | 731 | 879 | . | . | . | . | . | . | . | . | . |
| | *** | 2984 | 4131 | 6421 | 685 | 792 | 864 | . | . | . | . | . | . | . | . | . |
| 0.95 | *** | 1596 | 1948 | 3022 | . | . | . | . | . | . | . | . | . | . | . | . |
| | *** | 1742 | 2281 | 3007 | . | . | . | . | . | . | . | . | . | . | . | . |

TABLE 5: ALPHA= 0.025 POWER= 0.8     EXPECTED ACCRUAL THRU MINIMUM FOLLOW-UP= 900

| | | DEL=.02 | | | DEL=.05 | | | DEL=.10 | | | DEL=.15 | | | DEL=.20 | | |
|---|---|---|---|---|---|---|---|---|---|---|---|---|---|---|---|---|---|
| FACT= | | 1.0 .75 | .50 .25 | .00 BIN | 1.0 .75 | .50 .25 | .00 BIN | 1.0 .75 | .50 .25 | .00 BIN | 1.0 75 | .50 .25 | .00 BIN | 1.0 .75 | .50 .25 | .00 BIN |
| PCONT=*** | | REQUIRED NUMBER OF PATIENTS | | | | | | | | | | | | | | |
| 0.05 | *** | 2244 | 2262 | 2364 | 485 | 491 | 501 | 175 | 177 | 179 | 103 | 104 | 104 | 73 | 73 | 73 |
| | *** | 2250 | 2288 | 4419 | 488 | 496 | 864 | 176 | 177 | 275 | 103 | 104 | 145 | 73 | 73 | 93 |
| 0.1 | *** | 4672 | 4716 | 5195 | 896 | 919 | 967 | 287 | 292 | 299 | 155 | 156 | 158 | 102 | 103 | 104 |
| | *** | 4686 | 4796 | 7677 | 905 | 938 | 1366 | 289 | 295 | 393 | 155 | 158 | 194 | 102 | 104 | 118 |
| 0.15 | *** | 6831 | 6909 | 8034 | 1255 | 1301 | 1418 | 384 | 395 | 409 | 199 | 202 | 207 | 127 | 128 | 130 |
| | *** | 6858 | 7057 | 10542 | 1274 | 1343 | 1806 | 389 | 401 | 495 | 200 | 204 | 236 | 127 | 129 | 140 |
| 0.2 | *** | 8559 | 8679 | 10675 | 1546 | 1620 | 1829 | 465 | 482 | 507 | 235 | 241 | 248 | 147 | 149 | 152 |
| | *** | 8599 | 8911 | 13014 | 1576 | 1693 | 2182 | 473 | 494 | 581 | 238 | 244 | 271 | 148 | 150 | 157 |
| 0.25 | *** | 9811 | 9984 | 13016 | 1767 | 1872 | 2188 | 529 | 553 | 591 | 264 | 272 | 282 | 163 | 165 | 170 |
| | *** | 9869 | 10316 | 15094 | 1809 | 1977 | 2496 | 540 | 569 | 652 | 268 | 277 | 299 | 164 | 168 | 171 |
| 0.3 | *** | 10594 | 10832 | 15000 | 1920 | 2059 | 2489 | 577 | 608 | 659 | 286 | 296 | 309 | 174 | 178 | 183 |
| | *** | 10674 | 11283 | 16781 | 1976 | 2198 | 2748 | 591 | 630 | 707 | 290 | 302 | 320 | 176 | 180 | 181 |
| 0.35 | *** | 10945 | 11260 | 16596 | 2013 | 2184 | 2725 | 609 | 648 | 710 | 300 | 312 | 328 | 181 | 186 | 192 |
| | *** | 11051 | 11851 | 18076 | 2081 | 2357 | 2936 | 626 | 674 | 746 | 306 | 320 | 334 | 183 | 189 | 187 |
| 0.4 | *** | 10913 | 11323 | 17784 | 2052 | 2255 | 2896 | 627 | 672 | 744 | 308 | 322 | 340 | 185 | 190 | 197 |
| | *** | 11051 | 12069 | 18979 | 2134 | 2457 | 3062 | 647 | 703 | 770 | 315 | 330 | 341 | 187 | 193 | 189 |
| 0.45 | *** | 10558 | 11081 | 18553 | 2046 | 2277 | 2999 | 632 | 681 | 762 | 310 | 325 | 344 | 184 | 190 | 197 |
| | *** | 10735 | 11996 | 19489 | 2140 | 2504 | 3124 | 654 | 716 | 778 | 317 | 334 | 341 | 187 | 193 | 187 |
| 0.5 | *** | 9947 | 10603 | 18897 | 2002 | 2255 | 3034 | 626 | 677 | 762 | 305 | 320 | 341 | 180 | 186 | 192 |
| | *** | 10172 | 11684 | 19607 | 2106 | 2501 | 3124 | 649 | 713 | 770 | 312 | 330 | 334 | 182 | 189 | 181 |
| 0.55 | *** | 9152 | 9951 | 18815 | 1927 | 2194 | 3000 | 607 | 659 | 746 | 294 | 309 | 329 | 172 | 177 | 184 |
| | *** | 9431 | 11186 | 19332 | 2036 | 2449 | 3062 | 631 | 696 | 746 | 302 | 318 | 320 | 174 | 181 | 171 |
| 0.6 | *** | 8244 | 9187 | 18305 | 1824 | 2098 | 2898 | 578 | 629 | 712 | 278 | 292 | 311 | 161 | 165 | 171 |
| | *** | 8582 | 10540 | 18665 | 1937 | 2354 | 2936 | 601 | 665 | 707 | 285 | 300 | 299 | 163 | 168 | 157 |
| 0.65 | *** | 7291 | 8353 | 17370 | 1698 | 1967 | 2728 | 538 | 585 | 660 | 255 | 268 | 284 | 145 | 149 | 154 |
| | *** | 7683 | 9776 | 17606 | 1810 | 2216 | 2748 | 559 | 618 | 652 | 261 | 275 | 271 | 147 | 152 | 140 |
| 0.7 | *** | 6347 | 7479 | 16012 | 1549 | 1803 | 2491 | 487 | 529 | 593 | 227 | 237 | 251 | 126 | 129 | 134 |
| | *** | 6776 | 8912 | 16153 | 1656 | 2034 | 2496 | 506 | 557 | 581 | 231 | 243 | 236 | 128 | 131 | 118 |
| 0.75 | *** | 5438 | 6574 | 14235 | 1376 | 1605 | 2187 | 424 | 458 | 509 | 191 | 199 | 209 | 103 | 105 | 108 |
| | *** | 5876 | 7948 | 14309 | 1473 | 1806 | 2182 | 440 | 480 | 495 | 195 | 204 | 194 | 104 | 107 | 93 |
| 0.8 | *** | 4562 | 5629 | 12043 | 1177 | 1369 | 1816 | 348 | 373 | 408 | 150 | 155 | 161 | . | . | . |
| | *** | 4979 | 6872 | 12072 | 1259 | 1530 | 1806 | 360 | 389 | 393 | 152 | 158 | 145 | . | . | . |
| 0.85 | *** | 3690 | 4613 | 9441 | 942 | 1084 | 1380 | 257 | 272 | 290 | . | . | . | . | . | . |
| | *** | 4055 | 5647 | 9443 | 1004 | 1197 | 1366 | 264 | 280 | 275 | . | . | . | . | . | . |
| 0.9 | *** | 2762 | 3456 | 6432 | 656 | 737 | 879 | . | . | . | . | . | . | . | . | . |
| | *** | 3041 | 4191 | 6421 | 692 | 795 | 864 | . | . | . | . | . | . | . | . | . |
| 0.95 | *** | 1625 | 1977 | 3022 | . | . | . | . | . | . | . | . | . | . | . | . |
| | *** | 1771 | 2306 | 3007 | . | . | . | . | . | . | . | . | . | . | . | . |

## TABLE 5: ALPHA= 0.025 POWER= 0.8     EXPECTED ACCRUAL THRU MINIMUM FOLLOW-UP= 950

| | | DEL=.02 | | | DEL=.05 | | | DEL=.10 | | | DEL=.15 | | | DEL=.20 | | |
|---|---|---|---|---|---|---|---|---|---|---|---|---|---|---|---|---|---|
| FACT= | | 1.0 .75 | .50 .25 | .00 BIN | 1.0 .75 | .50 .25 | .00 BIN | 1.0 .75 | .50 .25 | .00 BIN | 1.0 75 | .50 .25 | .00 BIN | 1.0 .75 | .50 .25 | .00 BIN |
| PCONT=*** | | REQUIRED NUMBER OF PATIENTS | | | | | | | | | | | | | | |
| 0.05 | *** | 2245 2252 | 2263 2290 | 2364 4419 | 485 488 | 492 496 | 502 864 | 175 176 | 177 178 | 178 275 | 103 103 | 103 103 | 104 145 | 72 72 | 73 73 | 73 93 |
| 0.1 | *** | 4674 4689 | 4721 4803 | 5195 7677 | 898 907 | 920 939 | 967 1366 | 287 290 | 292 295 | 299 393 | 155 156 | 156 158 | 159 194 | 102 103 | 103 103 | 104 118 |
| 0.15 | *** | 6835 6863 | 6918 7072 | 8034 10542 | 1258 1277 | 1305 1347 | 1417 1806 | 386 390 | 395 401 | 409 495 | 199 201 | 203 204 | 206 236 | 127 128 | 128 129 | 130 140 |
| 0.2 | *** | 8565 8608 | 8693 8935 | 10674 13014 | 1552 1582 | 1626 1698 | 1829 2182 | 466 474 | 483 494 | 507 581 | 236 238 | 241 244 | 248 271 | 147 148 | 149 150 | 152 157 |
| 0.25 | *** | 9820 9881 | 10003 10350 | 13016 15094 | 1774 1817 | 1881 1985 | 2189 2496 | 531 542 | 555 571 | 591 652 | 265 268 | 273 277 | 282 299 | 163 164 | 166 167 | 169 171 |
| 0.3 | *** | 10608 10691 | 10858 11330 | 15001 16781 | 1930 1986 | 2070 2208 | 2489 2748 | 579 593 | 610 631 | 659 707 | 287 292 | 296 302 | 309 320 | 174 176 | 178 181 | 183 181 |
| 0.35 | *** | 10963 11073 | 11295 11911 | 16596 18076 | 2025 2095 | 2198 2369 | 2725 2936 | 612 629 | 650 676 | 710 746 | 302 307 | 313 320 | 329 334 | 182 184 | 186 189 | 192 187 |
| 0.4 | *** | 10936 11081 | 11368 12143 | 17784 18979 | 2067 2149 | 2272 2472 | 2896 3062 | 631 651 | 675 704 | 745 770 | 310 316 | 323 331 | 340 341 | 185 188 | 190 193 | 196 189 |
| 0.45 | *** | 10588 10774 | 11138 12084 | 18553 19489 | 2063 2158 | 2295 2520 | 2998 3124 | 637 658 | 685 717 | 762 778 | 311 318 | 325 334 | 344 341 | 185 187 | 190 193 | 197 187 |
| 0.5 | *** | 9985 10221 | 10672 11786 | 18897 19607 | 2021 2125 | 2275 2518 | 3034 3124 | 630 653 | 680 716 | 762 770 | 306 314 | 321 330 | 340 334 | 181 183 | 186 189 | 192 181 |
| 0.55 | *** | 9199 9492 | 10033 11297 | 18815 19332 | 1947 2058 | 2215 2468 | 3000 3062 | 612 635 | 663 698 | 745 746 | 296 303 | 311 319 | 329 320 | 172 175 | 178 181 | 184 171 |
| 0.6 | *** | 8301 8654 | 9279 10660 | 18305 18665 | 1845 1958 | 2119 2373 | 2898 2936 | 583 605 | 633 666 | 711 707 | 279 286 | 293 301 | 311 299 | 161 163 | 166 168 | 171 157 |
| 0.65 | *** | 7360 7765 | 8452 9900 | 17370 17606 | 1718 1831 | 1988 2233 | 2728 2748 | 542 563 | 589 620 | 660 652 | 257 262 | 268 276 | 284 271 | 146 147 | 150 152 | 154 140 |
| 0.7 | *** | 6423 6863 | 7581 9033 | 16012 16153 | 1569 1675 | 1823 2050 | 2491 2496 | 490 509 | 532 558 | 593 581 | 228 232 | 238 243 | 250 236 | 127 128 | 129 131 | 133 118 |
| 0.75 | *** | 5516 5964 | 6674 8063 | 14235 14309 | 1394 1491 | 1622 1820 | 2186 2182 | 427 443 | 460 482 | 508 495 | 192 196 | 200 204 | 209 194 | 103 105 | 106 107 | 108 93 |
| 0.8 | *** | 4637 5062 | 5721 6974 | 12043 12072 | 1192 1274 | 1382 1541 | 1816 1806 | 350 362 | 375 390 | 408 393 | 150 153 | 155 158 | 160 145 | . . | . . | . . |
| 0.85 | *** | 3757 4127 | 4691 5730 | 9441 9443 | 954 1015 | 1094 1205 | 1380 1366 | 258 265 | 273 281 | 291 275 | . . | . . | . . | . . | . . | . . |
| 0.9 | *** | 2813 3095 | 3513 4248 | 6432 6421 | 663 698 | 742 799 | 879 864 | . . | . . | . . | . . | . . | . . | . . | . . | . . |
| 0.95 | *** | 1652 1799 | 2004 2329 | 3022 3007 | . . | . . | . . | . . | . . | . . | . . | . . | . . | . . | . . | . . |

TABLE 5: ALPHA= 0.025 POWER= 0.8    EXPECTED ACCRUAL THRU MINIMUM FOLLOW-UP= 1000

| | DEL=.02 | | | DEL=.05 | | | DEL=.10 | | | DEL=.15 | | | DEL=.20 | | |
|---|---|---|---|---|---|---|---|---|---|---|---|---|---|---|---|
| FACT= | 1.0 .75 | .50 .25 | .00 BIN | 1.0 .75 | .50 .25 | .00 BIN | 1.0 .75 | .50 .25 | .00 BIN | 1.0 75 | .50 .25 | .00 BIN | 1.0 .75 | .50 .25 | .00 BIN |

PCONT=***    REQUIRED NUMBER OF PATIENTS

| PCONT | DEL=.02 1.0/.75 | .50/.25 | .00/BIN | DEL=.05 1.0/.75 | .50/.25 | .00/BIN | DEL=.10 1.0/.75 | .50/.25 | .00/BIN | DEL=.15 1.0/.75 | .50/.25 | .00/BIN | DEL=.20 1.0/.75 | .50/.25 | .00/BIN |
|---|---|---|---|---|---|---|---|---|---|---|---|---|---|---|---|
| 0.05 | 2246 | 2266 | 2365 | 486 | 492 | 501 | 176 | 177 | 178 | 103 | 103 | 104 | 73 | 73 | 73 |
| | 2253 | 2293 | 4419 | 489 | 496 | 864 | 176 | 178 | 275 | 103 | 104 | 145 | 73 | 73 | 93 |
| 0.1 | 4676 | 4726 | 5195 | 900 | 922 | 967 | 288 | 293 | 299 | 155 | 156 | 158 | 103 | 103 | 104 |
| | 4693 | 4811 | 7677 | 909 | 940 | 1366 | 290 | 296 | 393 | 156 | 158 | 194 | 103 | 104 | 118 |
| 0.15 | 6840 | 6926 | 8034 | 1261 | 1308 | 1418 | 386 | 396 | 410 | 200 | 203 | 206 | 127 | 128 | 130 |
| | 6869 | 7088 | 10542 | 1281 | 1349 | 1806 | 391 | 402 | 495 | 201 | 205 | 236 | 128 | 130 | 140 |
| 0.2 | 8573 | 8706 | 10675 | 1557 | 1632 | 1829 | 468 | 484 | 508 | 236 | 241 | 248 | 147 | 150 | 152 |
| | 8617 | 8959 | 13014 | 1587 | 1702 | 2182 | 475 | 495 | 581 | 239 | 245 | 271 | 148 | 151 | 157 |
| 0.25 | 9830 | 10022 | 13016 | 1781 | 1889 | 2188 | 533 | 556 | 591 | 266 | 273 | 282 | 163 | 166 | 170 |
| | 9894 | 10385 | 15094 | 1825 | 1992 | 2496 | 543 | 571 | 652 | 269 | 277 | 299 | 165 | 168 | 171 |
| 0.3 | 10621 | 10884 | 15000 | 1940 | 2081 | 2488 | 582 | 612 | 659 | 288 | 297 | 309 | 175 | 178 | 183 |
| | 10709 | 11376 | 16781 | 1996 | 2218 | 2748 | 596 | 633 | 707 | 292 | 303 | 320 | 176 | 181 | 181 |
| 0.35 | 10980 | 11330 | 16596 | 2037 | 2211 | 2725 | 616 | 652 | 710 | 303 | 314 | 328 | 182 | 186 | 192 |
| | 11097 | 11970 | 18076 | 2108 | 2381 | 2936 | 632 | 678 | 746 | 308 | 321 | 334 | 185 | 189 | 187 |
| 0.4 | 10959 | 11412 | 17785 | 2081 | 2287 | 2896 | 635 | 677 | 745 | 311 | 324 | 340 | 186 | 191 | 196 |
| | 11111 | 12216 | 18979 | 2165 | 2486 | 3062 | 654 | 706 | 770 | 317 | 331 | 341 | 188 | 193 | 189 |
| 0.45 | 10617 | 11194 | 18553 | 2080 | 2313 | 2999 | 641 | 688 | 762 | 313 | 326 | 344 | 185 | 190 | 196 |
| | 10813 | 12170 | 19489 | 2175 | 2536 | 3124 | 662 | 720 | 778 | 319 | 335 | 341 | 188 | 193 | 187 |
| 0.5 | 10023 | 10739 | 18898 | 2040 | 2294 | 3033 | 635 | 684 | 762 | 308 | 322 | 341 | 181 | 186 | 193 |
| | 10270 | 11883 | 19607 | 2144 | 2535 | 3124 | 656 | 718 | 770 | 315 | 331 | 334 | 183 | 190 | 181 |
| 0.55 | 9246 | 10112 | 18815 | 1966 | 2235 | 3000 | 616 | 666 | 746 | 297 | 311 | 330 | 173 | 178 | 184 |
| | 9551 | 11406 | 19332 | 2078 | 2485 | 3062 | 639 | 700 | 746 | 304 | 320 | 320 | 175 | 181 | 171 |
| 0.6 | 8359 | 9368 | 18305 | 1865 | 2138 | 2898 | 586 | 635 | 711 | 280 | 294 | 311 | 161 | 166 | 171 |
| | 8725 | 10775 | 18665 | 1979 | 2390 | 2936 | 609 | 668 | 707 | 286 | 301 | 299 | 163 | 169 | 157 |
| 0.65 | 7427 | 8548 | 17370 | 1738 | 2007 | 2728 | 546 | 591 | 661 | 258 | 270 | 284 | 146 | 150 | 155 |
| | 7845 | 10018 | 17606 | 1851 | 2250 | 2748 | 566 | 621 | 652 | 263 | 276 | 271 | 148 | 152 | 140 |
| 0.7 | 6497 | 7680 | 16012 | 1588 | 1841 | 2491 | 494 | 534 | 593 | 228 | 238 | 250 | 126 | 130 | 133 |
| | 6948 | 9150 | 16153 | 1695 | 2065 | 2496 | 512 | 560 | 581 | 233 | 244 | 236 | 128 | 131 | 118 |
| 0.75 | 5593 | 6770 | 14235 | 1412 | 1638 | 2186 | 430 | 463 | 509 | 193 | 200 | 210 | 104 | 106 | 108 |
| | 6048 | 8172 | 14309 | 1508 | 1833 | 2182 | 445 | 483 | 495 | 196 | 205 | 194 | 105 | 107 | 93 |
| 0.8 | 4710 | 5809 | 12043 | 1207 | 1396 | 1816 | 353 | 376 | 408 | 151 | 155 | 161 | . | . | . |
| | 5141 | 7071 | 12072 | 1288 | 1551 | 1806 | 363 | 391 | 393 | 153 | 158 | 145 | . | . | . |
| 0.85 | 3821 | 4765 | 9441 | 965 | 1104 | 1380 | 260 | 273 | 291 | . | . | . | . | . | . |
| | 4196 | 5808 | 9443 | 1026 | 1211 | 1366 | 266 | 281 | 275 | . | . | . | . | . | . |
| 0.9 | 2863 | 3567 | 6432 | 670 | 747 | 879 | . | . | . | . | . | . | . | . | . |
| | 3146 | 4302 | 6421 | 704 | 803 | 864 | . | . | . | . | . | . | . | . | . |
| 0.95 | 1678 | 2030 | 3022 | . | . | . | . | . | . | . | . | . | . | . | . |
| | 1825 | 2351 | 3007 | . | . | . | . | . | . | . | . | . | . | . | . |

## TABLE 5: ALPHA= 0.025 POWER= 0.8    EXPECTED ACCRUAL THRU MINIMUM FOLLOW-UP= 1100

| | DEL=.02 | | | DEL=.05 | | | DEL=.10 | | | DEL=.15 | | | DEL=.20 | | |
|---|---|---|---|---|---|---|---|---|---|---|---|---|---|---|---|
| FACT= | 1.0 .75 | .50 .25 | .00 BIN | 1.0 .75 | .50 .25 | .00 BIN | 1.0 .75 | .50 .25 | .00 BIN | 1.0 75 | .50 .25 | .00 BIN | 1.0 .75 | .50 .25 | .00 BIN |
| PCONT=*** | REQUIRED NUMBER OF PATIENTS | | | | | | | | | | | | | | |
| 0.05 *** | 2248 | 2269 | 2364 | 487 | 492 | 501 | 176 | 177 | 178 | 103 | 103 | 104 | 73 | 73 | 73 |
| *** | 2256 | 2296 | 4419 | 489 | 496 | 864 | 176 | 177 | 275 | 103 | 104 | 145 | 73 | 73 | 93 |
| 0.1 *** | 4681 | 4735 | 5195 | 903 | 925 | 967 | 289 | 293 | 298 | 155 | 157 | 158 | 103 | 103 | 104 |
| *** | 4700 | 4826 | 7677 | 912 | 942 | 1366 | 291 | 296 | 393 | 156 | 158 | 194 | 103 | 104 | 118 |
| 0.15 *** | 6849 | 6944 | 8034 | 1268 | 1314 | 1418 | 388 | 397 | 409 | 200 | 203 | 206 | 127 | 129 | 130 |
| *** | 6880 | 7116 | 10542 | 1287 | 1354 | 1806 | 392 | 402 | 495 | 202 | 204 | 236 | 128 | 129 | 140 |
| 0.2 *** | 8585 | 8733 | 10675 | 1567 | 1643 | 1829 | 470 | 485 | 507 | 237 | 242 | 247 | 148 | 150 | 152 |
| *** | 8635 | 9004 | 13014 | 1598 | 1710 | 2182 | 477 | 496 | 581 | 239 | 245 | 271 | 148 | 151 | 157 |
| 0.25 *** | 9849 | 10060 | 13016 | 1796 | 1904 | 2188 | 536 | 558 | 591 | 267 | 274 | 282 | 164 | 166 | 169 |
| *** | 9920 | 10450 | 15094 | 1840 | 2005 | 2496 | 547 | 573 | 652 | 270 | 278 | 299 | 165 | 168 | 171 |
| 0.3 *** | 10647 | 10936 | 15001 | 1958 | 2100 | 2489 | 587 | 615 | 659 | 290 | 298 | 309 | 175 | 179 | 183 |
| *** | 10744 | 11464 | 16781 | 2017 | 2234 | 2748 | 599 | 635 | 707 | 294 | 303 | 320 | 177 | 181 | 181 |
| 0.35 *** | 11015 | 11398 | 16596 | 2060 | 2236 | 2725 | 621 | 657 | 710 | 305 | 315 | 328 | 183 | 187 | 192 |
| *** | 11144 | 12082 | 18076 | 2132 | 2402 | 2936 | 637 | 680 | 746 | 309 | 321 | 334 | 185 | 189 | 187 |
| 0.4 *** | 11005 | 11500 | 17784 | 2109 | 2315 | 2896 | 642 | 682 | 745 | 313 | 324 | 340 | 186 | 191 | 196 |
| *** | 11172 | 12354 | 18979 | 2193 | 2510 | 3062 | 660 | 709 | 770 | 318 | 332 | 341 | 188 | 193 | 189 |
| 0.45 *** | 10676 | 11303 | 18553 | 2111 | 2345 | 2999 | 648 | 692 | 762 | 315 | 328 | 344 | 186 | 191 | 197 |
| *** | 10891 | 12334 | 19489 | 2208 | 2563 | 3124 | 668 | 723 | 778 | 321 | 335 | 341 | 188 | 194 | 187 |
| 0.5 *** | 10097 | 10872 | 18897 | 2073 | 2329 | 3033 | 642 | 689 | 763 | 310 | 324 | 340 | 181 | 187 | 192 |
| *** | 10367 | 12071 | 19607 | 2179 | 2564 | 3124 | 664 | 721 | 770 | 316 | 331 | 334 | 184 | 190 | 181 |
| 0.55 *** | 9339 | 10266 | 18815 | 2003 | 2271 | 3000 | 624 | 672 | 745 | 300 | 313 | 329 | 174 | 179 | 184 |
| *** | 9670 | 11611 | 19332 | 2115 | 2516 | 3062 | 646 | 704 | 746 | 306 | 320 | 320 | 176 | 181 | 171 |
| 0.6 *** | 8472 | 9540 | 18305 | 1902 | 2175 | 2898 | 594 | 641 | 712 | 283 | 295 | 310 | 162 | 166 | 171 |
| *** | 8863 | 10993 | 18665 | 2017 | 2420 | 2936 | 615 | 672 | 707 | 288 | 302 | 299 | 164 | 169 | 157 |
| 0.65 *** | 7557 | 8732 | 17370 | 1776 | 2043 | 2728 | 553 | 596 | 661 | 259 | 270 | 284 | 147 | 150 | 155 |
| *** | 7998 | 10240 | 17606 | 1888 | 2279 | 2748 | 573 | 625 | 652 | 265 | 277 | 271 | 148 | 152 | 140 |
| 0.7 *** | 6639 | 7867 | 16012 | 1623 | 1874 | 2491 | 500 | 538 | 593 | 230 | 239 | 250 | 127 | 130 | 133 |
| *** | 7110 | 9367 | 16153 | 1729 | 2091 | 2496 | 518 | 562 | 581 | 235 | 245 | 236 | 129 | 132 | 118 |
| 0.75 *** | 5738 | 6951 | 14235 | 1444 | 1668 | 2186 | 435 | 466 | 509 | 194 | 201 | 209 | 104 | 106 | 108 |
| *** | 6210 | 8376 | 14309 | 1539 | 1856 | 2182 | 450 | 485 | 495 | 197 | 205 | 194 | 105 | 107 | 93 |
| 0.8 *** | 4848 | 5974 | 12043 | 1234 | 1419 | 1816 | 356 | 378 | 408 | 151 | 155 | 161 | . | . | . |
| *** | 5292 | 7251 | 12072 | 1314 | 1569 | 1806 | 367 | 392 | 393 | 153 | 158 | 145 | . | . | . |
| 0.85 *** | 3942 | 4905 | 9441 | 985 | 1121 | 1380 | 262 | 275 | 291 | . | . | . | . | . | . |
| *** | 4326 | 5954 | 9443 | 1045 | 1224 | 1366 | 268 | 282 | 275 | . | . | . | . | . | . |
| 0.9 *** | 2955 | 3668 | 6432 | 681 | 756 | 879 | . | . | . | . | . | . | . | . | . |
| *** | 3244 | 4401 | 6421 | 715 | 808 | 864 | . | . | . | . | . | . | . | . | . |
| 0.95 *** | 1726 | 2076 | 3022 | . | . | . | . | . | . | . | . | . | . | . | . |
| *** | 1874 | 2391 | 3007 | . | . | . | . | . | . | . | . | . | . | . | . |

TABLE 5: ALPHA= 0.025 POWER= 0.8    EXPECTED ACCRUAL THRU MINIMUM FOLLOW-UP= 1200

| | | DEL=.02 | | | DEL=.05 | | | DEL=.10 | | | DEL=.15 | | | DEL=.20 | | |
|---|---|---|---|---|---|---|---|---|---|---|---|---|---|---|---|---|
| FACT= | | 1.0 .75 | .50 .25 | .00 BIN | 1.0 .75 | .50 .25 | .00 BIN | 1.0 .75 | .50 .25 | .00 BIN | 1.0 75 | .50 .25 | .00 BIN | 1.0 .75 | .50 .25 | .00 BIN |
| PCONT=*** | | | | | REQUIRED NUMBER OF PATIENTS | | | | | | | | | | | |
| 0.05 | *** | 2250 | 2272 | 2365 | 487 | 493 | 502 | 176 | 177 | 178 | 103 | 103 | 104 | 73 | 73 | 73 |
| | *** | 2258 | 2299 | 4419 | 490 | 497 | 864 | 176 | 178 | 275 | 103 | 103 | 145 | 73 | 73 | 93 |
| 0.1 | *** | 4687 | 4744 | 5194 | 905 | 927 | 967 | 289 | 293 | 298 | 155 | 157 | 158 | 103 | 103 | 104 |
| | *** | 4706 | 4839 | 7677 | 915 | 943 | 1366 | 292 | 296 | 393 | 156 | 157 | 194 | 103 | 103 | 118 |
| 0.15 | *** | 6857 | 6961 | 8034 | 1273 | 1320 | 1417 | 389 | 397 | 409 | 200 | 203 | 206 | 127 | 129 | 130 |
| | *** | 6892 | 7143 | 10542 | 1293 | 1358 | 1806 | 393 | 403 | 495 | 202 | 205 | 236 | 128 | 129 | 140 |
| 0.2 | *** | 8599 | 8759 | 10675 | 1576 | 1651 | 1829 | 472 | 487 | 507 | 238 | 242 | 247 | 148 | 150 | 152 |
| | *** | 8653 | 9048 | 13014 | 1607 | 1718 | 2182 | 479 | 496 | 581 | 240 | 245 | 271 | 148 | 151 | 157 |
| 0.25 | *** | 9868 | 10098 | 13015 | 1809 | 1918 | 2188 | 540 | 561 | 591 | 268 | 274 | 282 | 164 | 166 | 169 |
| | *** | 9945 | 10513 | 15094 | 1853 | 2015 | 2496 | 550 | 574 | 652 | 271 | 277 | 299 | 165 | 168 | 171 |
| 0.3 | *** | 10673 | 10987 | 15000 | 1975 | 2118 | 2488 | 591 | 618 | 658 | 290 | 298 | 309 | 175 | 179 | 183 |
| | *** | 10779 | 11548 | 16781 | 2034 | 2249 | 2748 | 603 | 636 | 707 | 295 | 304 | 320 | 177 | 181 | 181 |
| 0.35 | *** | 11050 | 11466 | 16596 | 2081 | 2258 | 2725 | 626 | 660 | 710 | 306 | 316 | 328 | 184 | 187 | 192 |
| | *** | 11191 | 12190 | 18076 | 2154 | 2420 | 2936 | 641 | 682 | 746 | 310 | 322 | 334 | 185 | 190 | 187 |
| 0.4 | *** | 11050 | 11587 | 17784 | 2134 | 2341 | 2896 | 647 | 686 | 745 | 315 | 326 | 340 | 187 | 191 | 196 |
| | *** | 11233 | 12487 | 18979 | 2220 | 2532 | 3062 | 664 | 712 | 770 | 320 | 332 | 341 | 189 | 193 | 189 |
| 0.45 | *** | 10735 | 11410 | 18553 | 2140 | 2374 | 2998 | 654 | 697 | 762 | 316 | 329 | 344 | 187 | 191 | 196 |
| | *** | 10968 | 12489 | 19489 | 2236 | 2587 | 3124 | 674 | 726 | 778 | 322 | 336 | 341 | 189 | 193 | 187 |
| 0.5 | *** | 10171 | 10999 | 18898 | 2105 | 2360 | 3034 | 649 | 694 | 762 | 312 | 325 | 340 | 182 | 187 | 193 |
| | *** | 10462 | 12247 | 19607 | 2212 | 2590 | 3124 | 669 | 724 | 770 | 318 | 332 | 334 | 184 | 190 | 181 |
| 0.55 | *** | 9431 | 10414 | 18814 | 2036 | 2304 | 3000 | 631 | 676 | 745 | 301 | 313 | 329 | 175 | 179 | 184 |
| | *** | 9784 | 11803 | 19332 | 2148 | 2543 | 3062 | 652 | 707 | 746 | 307 | 321 | 320 | 177 | 181 | 171 |
| 0.6 | *** | 8582 | 9703 | 18305 | 1937 | 2208 | 2898 | 601 | 646 | 712 | 284 | 296 | 310 | 163 | 166 | 171 |
| | *** | 8995 | 11194 | 18665 | 2051 | 2447 | 2936 | 621 | 675 | 707 | 290 | 303 | 299 | 165 | 169 | 157 |
| 0.65 | *** | 7683 | 8905 | 17370 | 1810 | 2074 | 2728 | 559 | 601 | 661 | 261 | 271 | 284 | 147 | 151 | 154 |
| | *** | 8145 | 10445 | 17606 | 1921 | 2305 | 2748 | 578 | 628 | 652 | 266 | 277 | 271 | 148 | 152 | 140 |
| 0.7 | *** | 6775 | 8042 | 16012 | 1655 | 1903 | 2491 | 505 | 541 | 593 | 232 | 240 | 250 | 127 | 130 | 133 |
| | *** | 7263 | 9568 | 16153 | 1761 | 2115 | 2496 | 523 | 565 | 581 | 235 | 245 | 236 | 129 | 132 | 118 |
| 0.75 | *** | 5875 | 7120 | 14235 | 1473 | 1693 | 2186 | 439 | 469 | 508 | 195 | 202 | 209 | 104 | 106 | 108 |
| | *** | 6362 | 8564 | 14309 | 1567 | 1876 | 2182 | 453 | 487 | 495 | 199 | 205 | 194 | 105 | 107 | 93 |
| 0.8 | *** | 4978 | 6129 | 12043 | 1258 | 1440 | 1816 | 360 | 380 | 408 | 152 | 156 | 160 | . | . | . |
| | *** | 5433 | 7417 | 12072 | 1337 | 1585 | 1806 | 370 | 393 | 393 | 154 | 158 | 145 | . | . | . |
| 0.85 | *** | 4055 | 5033 | 9440 | 1003 | 1135 | 1380 | 264 | 276 | 290 | . | . | . | . | . | . |
| | *** | 4447 | 6086 | 9443 | 1062 | 1234 | 1366 | 269 | 283 | 275 | . | . | . | . | . | . |
| 0.9 | *** | 3040 | 3760 | 6432 | 691 | 764 | 879 | . | . | . | . | . | . | . | . | . |
| | *** | 3333 | 4489 | 6421 | 724 | 814 | 864 | . | . | . | . | . | . | . | . | . |
| 0.95 | *** | 1771 | 2119 | 3022 | . | . | . | . | . | . | . | . | . | . | . | . |
| | *** | 1918 | 2426 | 3007 | . | . | . | . | . | . | . | . | . | . | . | . |

TABLE 5: ALPHA= 0.025 POWER= 0.8    EXPECTED ACCRUAL THRU MINIMUM FOLLOW-UP= 1300

|  |  | DEL=.02 | | | DEL=.05 | | | DEL=.10 | | | DEL=.15 | | | DEL=.20 | | |
|---|---|---|---|---|---|---|---|---|---|---|---|---|---|---|---|---|
| FACT= |  | 1.0 .75 | .50 .25 | .00 BIN | 1.0 .75 | .50 .25 | .00 BIN | 1.0 .75 | .50 .25 | .00 BIN | 1.0 75 | .50 .25 | .00 BIN | 1.0 .75 | .50 .25 | .00 BIN |
| PCONT=*** |  | | | | | | | REQUIRED NUMBER OF PATIENTS | | | | | | | | |
| 0.05 | *** | 2252 | 2275 | 2364 | 488 | 494 | 501 | 176 | 177 | 178 | 103 | 103 | 104 | 73 | 73 | 73 |
|  | *** | 2260 | 2303 | 4419 | 491 | 497 | 864 | 176 | 178 | 275 | 103 | 104 | 145 | 73 | 73 | 93 |
| 0.1 | *** | 4691 | 4753 | 5195 | 908 | 929 | 967 | 290 | 294 | 299 | 156 | 157 | 159 | 102 | 103 | 104 |
|  | *** | 4712 | 4852 | 7677 | 917 | 945 | 1366 | 292 | 297 | 393 | 156 | 158 | 194 | 103 | 104 | 118 |
| 0.15 | *** | 6867 | 6978 | 8034 | 1279 | 1324 | 1418 | 390 | 399 | 409 | 201 | 203 | 206 | 128 | 129 | 130 |
|  | *** | 6904 | 7169 | 10542 | 1298 | 1362 | 1806 | 394 | 404 | 495 | 202 | 205 | 236 | 128 | 129 | 140 |
| 0.2 | *** | 8612 | 8786 | 10675 | 1584 | 1660 | 1829 | 474 | 488 | 507 | 239 | 243 | 248 | 148 | 150 | 152 |
|  | *** | 8671 | 9090 | 13014 | 1616 | 1725 | 2182 | 481 | 497 | 581 | 240 | 245 | 271 | 149 | 151 | 157 |
| 0.25 | *** | 9887 | 10135 | 13016 | 1821 | 1930 | 2188 | 543 | 563 | 591 | 269 | 275 | 282 | 164 | 167 | 170 |
|  | *** | 9971 | 10574 | 15094 | 1866 | 2026 | 2496 | 552 | 575 | 652 | 271 | 278 | 299 | 166 | 168 | 171 |
| 0.3 | *** | 10700 | 11039 | 15000 | 1992 | 2135 | 2489 | 595 | 621 | 659 | 292 | 300 | 309 | 176 | 180 | 183 |
|  | *** | 10814 | 11630 | 16781 | 2051 | 2262 | 2748 | 607 | 638 | 707 | 296 | 304 | 320 | 178 | 181 | 181 |
| 0.35 | *** | 11086 | 11533 | 16596 | 2101 | 2278 | 2725 | 630 | 663 | 710 | 307 | 317 | 328 | 185 | 188 | 192 |
|  | *** | 11237 | 12294 | 18076 | 2175 | 2437 | 2936 | 646 | 684 | 746 | 312 | 323 | 334 | 186 | 189 | 187 |
| 0.4 | *** | 11096 | 11672 | 17784 | 2157 | 2365 | 2896 | 653 | 690 | 744 | 316 | 327 | 340 | 188 | 192 | 197 |
|  | *** | 11293 | 12613 | 18979 | 2244 | 2551 | 3062 | 669 | 714 | 770 | 322 | 333 | 341 | 189 | 194 | 189 |
| 0.45 | *** | 10793 | 11515 | 18554 | 2166 | 2400 | 2999 | 660 | 701 | 762 | 318 | 330 | 344 | 188 | 192 | 197 |
|  | *** | 11043 | 12636 | 19489 | 2265 | 2610 | 3124 | 679 | 728 | 778 | 324 | 336 | 341 | 189 | 194 | 187 |
| 0.5 | *** | 10246 | 11123 | 18898 | 2135 | 2389 | 3033 | 655 | 698 | 762 | 315 | 326 | 341 | 184 | 188 | 193 |
|  | *** | 10556 | 12413 | 19607 | 2241 | 2614 | 3124 | 674 | 726 | 770 | 319 | 333 | 334 | 185 | 190 | 181 |
| 0.55 | *** | 9522 | 10555 | 18815 | 2068 | 2333 | 3000 | 637 | 681 | 745 | 303 | 315 | 329 | 175 | 180 | 185 |
|  | *** | 9896 | 11984 | 19332 | 2179 | 2567 | 3062 | 657 | 709 | 746 | 309 | 322 | 320 | 177 | 182 | 171 |
| 0.6 | *** | 8690 | 9859 | 18305 | 1969 | 2239 | 2898 | 607 | 650 | 712 | 286 | 297 | 310 | 163 | 167 | 172 |
|  | *** | 9124 | 11384 | 18665 | 2083 | 2472 | 2936 | 627 | 678 | 707 | 292 | 303 | 299 | 165 | 169 | 157 |
| 0.65 | *** | 7805 | 9069 | 17370 | 1841 | 2104 | 2728 | 565 | 604 | 661 | 263 | 272 | 284 | 148 | 151 | 154 |
|  | *** | 8285 | 10637 | 17606 | 1953 | 2328 | 2748 | 583 | 630 | 652 | 267 | 278 | 271 | 149 | 153 | 140 |
| 0.7 | *** | 6906 | 8208 | 16012 | 1685 | 1930 | 2490 | 511 | 545 | 593 | 233 | 240 | 250 | 128 | 131 | 133 |
|  | *** | 7409 | 9755 | 16153 | 1790 | 2136 | 2496 | 526 | 567 | 581 | 237 | 245 | 236 | 129 | 132 | 118 |
| 0.75 | *** | 6007 | 7279 | 14235 | 1500 | 1717 | 2187 | 444 | 471 | 509 | 197 | 202 | 209 | 105 | 107 | 108 |
|  | *** | 6506 | 8738 | 14309 | 1593 | 1894 | 2182 | 457 | 488 | 495 | 199 | 206 | 194 | 106 | 107 | 93 |
| 0.8 | *** | 5102 | 6272 | 12043 | 1280 | 1459 | 1816 | 362 | 383 | 408 | 153 | 157 | 161 | . | . | . |
|  | *** | 5566 | 7569 | 12072 | 1358 | 1598 | 1806 | 372 | 394 | 393 | 154 | 159 | 145 | . | . | . |
| 0.85 | *** | 4162 | 5153 | 9441 | 1020 | 1149 | 1380 | 266 | 277 | 291 | . | . | . | . | . | . |
|  | *** | 4560 | 6207 | 9443 | 1077 | 1243 | 1366 | 271 | 284 | 275 | . | . | . | . | . | . |
| 0.9 | *** | 3121 | 3846 | 6432 | 701 | 771 | 879 | . | . | . | . | . | . | . | . | . |
|  | *** | 3417 | 4570 | 6421 | 733 | 818 | 864 | . | . | . | . | . | . | . | . | . |
| 0.95 | *** | 1812 | 2157 | 3022 | . | . | . | . | . | . | . | . | . | . | . | . |
|  | *** | 1958 | 2458 | 3007 | . | . | . | . | . | . | . | . | . | . | . | . |

TABLE 5: ALPHA= 0.025 POWER= 0.8     EXPECTED ACCRUAL THRU MINIMUM FOLLOW-UP= 1400

| | | DEL=.02 | | | DEL=.05 | | | DEL=.10 | | | DEL=.15 | | | DEL=.20 | | |
|---|---|---|---|---|---|---|---|---|---|---|---|---|---|---|---|---|---|
| FACT= | | 1.0 .75 | .50 .25 | .00 BIN | 1.0 .75 | .50 .25 | .00 BIN | 1.0 .75 | .50 .25 | .00 BIN | 1.0 75 | .50 .25 | .00 BIN | 1.0 .75 | .50 .25 | .00 BIN |
| PCONT=*** | | | | REQUIRED NUMBER OF PATIENTS | | | | | | | | | | | | |
| 0.05 | *** | 2254 | 2278 | 2364 | 489 | 494 | 501 | 176 | 178 | 178 | 103 | 103 | 104 | 73 | 73 | 73 |
| | *** | 2263 | 2306 | 4419 | 492 | 498 | 864 | 177 | 178 | 275 | 103 | 104 | 145 | 73 | 73 | 93 |
| 0.1 | *** | 4696 | 4763 | 5195 | 911 | 931 | 967 | 290 | 294 | 298 | 156 | 157 | 158 | 103 | 103 | 104 |
| | *** | 4719 | 4863 | 7677 | 920 | 947 | 1366 | 292 | 297 | 393 | 157 | 157 | 194 | 103 | 103 | 118 |
| 0.15 | *** | 6875 | 6994 | 8034 | 1284 | 1329 | 1417 | 391 | 399 | 409 | 201 | 204 | 206 | 128 | 129 | 130 |
| | *** | 6915 | 7193 | 10542 | 1304 | 1365 | 1806 | 395 | 404 | 495 | 202 | 205 | 236 | 129 | 129 | 140 |
| 0.2 | *** | 8626 | 8811 | 10675 | 1592 | 1668 | 1829 | 476 | 490 | 507 | 239 | 243 | 248 | 149 | 150 | 152 |
| | *** | 8689 | 9131 | 13014 | 1624 | 1731 | 2182 | 483 | 498 | 581 | 241 | 245 | 271 | 150 | 151 | 157 |
| 0.25 | *** | 9907 | 10173 | 13016 | 1832 | 1941 | 2188 | 545 | 564 | 591 | 269 | 276 | 282 | 164 | 167 | 170 |
| | *** | 9997 | 10632 | 15094 | 1878 | 2034 | 2496 | 554 | 577 | 652 | 272 | 278 | 299 | 166 | 168 | 171 |
| 0.3 | *** | 10727 | 11089 | 15000 | 2006 | 2150 | 2488 | 598 | 623 | 659 | 293 | 300 | 309 | 177 | 179 | 183 |
| | *** | 10849 | 11708 | 16781 | 2067 | 2274 | 2748 | 610 | 640 | 707 | 297 | 304 | 320 | 178 | 181 | 181 |
| 0.35 | *** | 11120 | 11599 | 16596 | 2120 | 2297 | 2725 | 634 | 666 | 710 | 309 | 318 | 328 | 185 | 188 | 192 |
| | *** | 11283 | 12393 | 18076 | 2194 | 2452 | 2936 | 649 | 686 | 746 | 313 | 323 | 334 | 186 | 190 | 187 |
| 0.4 | *** | 11142 | 11755 | 17784 | 2180 | 2387 | 2895 | 657 | 693 | 745 | 318 | 328 | 340 | 188 | 192 | 196 |
| | *** | 11353 | 12732 | 18979 | 2266 | 2569 | 3062 | 674 | 716 | 770 | 323 | 333 | 341 | 190 | 194 | 189 |
| 0.45 | *** | 10852 | 11616 | 18553 | 2192 | 2425 | 2999 | 665 | 704 | 762 | 320 | 331 | 344 | 188 | 192 | 197 |
| | *** | 11119 | 12775 | 19489 | 2289 | 2629 | 3124 | 683 | 731 | 778 | 325 | 337 | 341 | 190 | 194 | 187 |
| 0.5 | *** | 10319 | 11243 | 18897 | 2162 | 2415 | 3034 | 660 | 702 | 762 | 316 | 327 | 340 | 184 | 188 | 192 |
| | *** | 10649 | 12568 | 19607 | 2269 | 2635 | 3124 | 679 | 729 | 770 | 321 | 333 | 334 | 185 | 190 | 181 |
| 0.55 | *** | 9611 | 10692 | 18815 | 2096 | 2361 | 2999 | 642 | 684 | 745 | 304 | 316 | 329 | 176 | 179 | 184 |
| | *** | 10006 | 12153 | 19332 | 2208 | 2589 | 3062 | 661 | 712 | 746 | 310 | 322 | 320 | 178 | 182 | 171 |
| 0.6 | *** | 8795 | 10007 | 18305 | 1998 | 2265 | 2898 | 612 | 654 | 711 | 288 | 298 | 311 | 164 | 167 | 171 |
| | *** | 9248 | 11561 | 18665 | 2111 | 2494 | 2936 | 631 | 680 | 707 | 292 | 304 | 299 | 165 | 170 | 157 |
| 0.65 | *** | 7922 | 9225 | 17370 | 1870 | 2130 | 2728 | 570 | 608 | 661 | 264 | 273 | 284 | 148 | 151 | 155 |
| | *** | 8419 | 10816 | 17606 | 1981 | 2348 | 2748 | 587 | 632 | 652 | 269 | 278 | 271 | 150 | 153 | 140 |
| 0.7 | *** | 7030 | 8364 | 16012 | 1712 | 1955 | 2490 | 515 | 548 | 593 | 234 | 241 | 250 | 129 | 131 | 133 |
| | *** | 7548 | 9929 | 16153 | 1816 | 2154 | 2496 | 530 | 569 | 581 | 238 | 246 | 236 | 129 | 132 | 118 |
| 0.75 | *** | 6130 | 7429 | 14235 | 1524 | 1739 | 2187 | 447 | 473 | 508 | 197 | 203 | 209 | 105 | 107 | 108 |
| | *** | 6641 | 8899 | 14309 | 1617 | 1909 | 2182 | 459 | 490 | 495 | 199 | 206 | 194 | 106 | 108 | 93 |
| 0.8 | *** | 5218 | 6407 | 12043 | 1301 | 1476 | 1816 | 365 | 384 | 408 | 153 | 157 | 161 | . | . | . |
| | *** | 5691 | 7710 | 12072 | 1378 | 1611 | 1806 | 374 | 395 | 393 | 155 | 158 | 145 | . | . | . |
| 0.85 | *** | 4262 | 5265 | 9440 | 1035 | 1160 | 1380 | 267 | 278 | 290 | . | . | . | . | . | . |
| | *** | 4665 | 6319 | 9443 | 1091 | 1251 | 1366 | 272 | 284 | 275 | . | . | . | . | . | . |
| 0.9 | *** | 3196 | 3924 | 6432 | 710 | 777 | 879 | . | . | . | . | . | . | . | . | . |
| | *** | 3494 | 4644 | 6421 | 740 | 822 | 864 | . | . | . | . | . | . | . | . | . |
| 0.95 | *** | 1850 | 2192 | 3022 | . | . | . | . | . | . | . | . | . | . | . | . |
| | *** | 1995 | 2486 | 3007 | . | . | . | . | . | . | . | . | . | . | . | . |

TABLE 5: ALPHA= 0.025 POWER= 0.8    EXPECTED ACCRUAL THRU MINIMUM FOLLOW-UP= 1500

| | | DEL=.02 | | | DEL=.05 | | | DEL=.10 | | | DEL=.15 | | | DEL=.20 | | |
|---|---|---|---|---|---|---|---|---|---|---|---|---|---|---|---|---|---|
| FACT= | | 1.0 .75 | .50 .25 | .00 BIN | 1.0 .75 | .50 .25 | .00 BIN | 1.0 .75 | .50 .25 | .00 BIN | 1.0 75 | .50 .25 | .00 BIN | 1.0 .75 | .50 .25 | .00 BIN |
| PCONT=*** | | | | REQUIRED NUMBER OF PATIENTS | | | | | | | | | | | | |
| 0.05 | *** | 2257 | 2281 | 2364 | 489 | 495 | 502 | 176 | 177 | 178 | 103 | 104 | 104 | 73 | 73 | 73 |
| | *** | 2266 | 2308 | 4419 | 492 | 498 | 864 | 177 | 178 | 275 | 103 | 104 | 145 | 73 | 73 | 93 |
| 0.1 | *** | 4702 | 4771 | 5195 | 913 | 933 | 967 | 290 | 294 | 299 | 157 | 157 | 158 | 103 | 103 | 104 |
| | *** | 4726 | 4875 | 7677 | 922 | 948 | 1366 | 292 | 296 | 393 | 157 | 157 | 194 | 103 | 104 | 118 |
| 0.15 | *** | 6883 | 7010 | 8034 | 1289 | 1333 | 1417 | 392 | 400 | 410 | 202 | 203 | 206 | 128 | 129 | 130 |
| | *** | 6926 | 7217 | 10542 | 1308 | 1368 | 1806 | 395 | 404 | 495 | 202 | 205 | 236 | 128 | 129 | 140 |
| 0.2 | *** | 8640 | 8837 | 10674 | 1600 | 1674 | 1829 | 478 | 491 | 507 | 240 | 244 | 247 | 149 | 150 | 152 |
| | *** | 8707 | 9170 | 13014 | 1632 | 1735 | 2182 | 484 | 499 | 581 | 242 | 245 | 271 | 149 | 151 | 157 |
| 0.25 | *** | 9926 | 10209 | 13015 | 1843 | 1951 | 2188 | 547 | 566 | 590 | 270 | 275 | 282 | 165 | 167 | 170 |
| | *** | 10022 | 10688 | 15094 | 1889 | 2042 | 2496 | 556 | 577 | 652 | 273 | 278 | 299 | 166 | 169 | 171 |
| 0.3 | *** | 10753 | 11138 | 15000 | 2021 | 2163 | 2488 | 601 | 625 | 659 | 293 | 301 | 308 | 177 | 180 | 183 |
| | *** | 10884 | 11782 | 16781 | 2081 | 2285 | 2748 | 612 | 640 | 707 | 297 | 305 | 320 | 178 | 181 | 181 |
| 0.35 | *** | 11155 | 11663 | 16597 | 2137 | 2314 | 2725 | 638 | 668 | 710 | 310 | 319 | 328 | 185 | 188 | 192 |
| | *** | 11330 | 12487 | 18076 | 2212 | 2465 | 2936 | 652 | 687 | 746 | 314 | 323 | 334 | 187 | 190 | 187 |
| 0.4 | *** | 11187 | 11836 | 17784 | 2200 | 2407 | 2896 | 661 | 695 | 744 | 319 | 329 | 340 | 188 | 192 | 196 |
| | *** | 11412 | 12847 | 18979 | 2287 | 2585 | 3062 | 677 | 718 | 770 | 323 | 334 | 341 | 190 | 194 | 189 |
| 0.45 | *** | 10910 | 11715 | 18553 | 2215 | 2447 | 2999 | 669 | 708 | 762 | 322 | 332 | 344 | 188 | 192 | 197 |
| | *** | 11194 | 12907 | 19489 | 2313 | 2647 | 3124 | 687 | 732 | 778 | 326 | 337 | 341 | 190 | 194 | 187 |
| 0.5 | *** | 10391 | 11359 | 18897 | 2188 | 2438 | 3034 | 665 | 705 | 762 | 317 | 328 | 340 | 185 | 188 | 192 |
| | *** | 10739 | 12716 | 19607 | 2294 | 2654 | 3124 | 683 | 731 | 770 | 322 | 334 | 334 | 187 | 190 | 181 |
| 0.55 | *** | 9698 | 10822 | 18815 | 2123 | 2386 | 3000 | 647 | 688 | 745 | 307 | 317 | 329 | 176 | 180 | 184 |
| | *** | 10112 | 12313 | 19332 | 2235 | 2609 | 3062 | 667 | 714 | 746 | 311 | 322 | 320 | 178 | 182 | 171 |
| 0.6 | *** | 8896 | 10149 | 18305 | 2026 | 2290 | 2898 | 617 | 656 | 712 | 289 | 299 | 310 | 164 | 168 | 172 |
| | *** | 9367 | 11728 | 18665 | 2138 | 2512 | 2936 | 635 | 682 | 707 | 293 | 305 | 299 | 166 | 170 | 157 |
| 0.65 | *** | 8035 | 9373 | 17370 | 1897 | 2154 | 2728 | 575 | 611 | 661 | 265 | 274 | 284 | 148 | 151 | 155 |
| | *** | 8548 | 10984 | 17606 | 2007 | 2367 | 2748 | 592 | 634 | 652 | 269 | 278 | 271 | 150 | 153 | 140 |
| 0.7 | *** | 7148 | 8512 | 16012 | 1737 | 1977 | 2491 | 519 | 550 | 593 | 235 | 242 | 250 | 128 | 131 | 133 |
| | *** | 7680 | 10091 | 16153 | 1841 | 2171 | 2496 | 533 | 570 | 581 | 238 | 245 | 236 | 130 | 132 | 118 |
| 0.75 | *** | 6249 | 7569 | 14235 | 1547 | 1758 | 2186 | 450 | 476 | 509 | 198 | 203 | 209 | 105 | 107 | 108 |
| | *** | 6770 | 9050 | 14309 | 1639 | 1924 | 2182 | 462 | 491 | 495 | 200 | 206 | 194 | 106 | 108 | 93 |
| 0.8 | *** | 5329 | 6533 | 12043 | 1320 | 1492 | 1816 | 367 | 385 | 408 | 154 | 157 | 160 | . | . | . |
| | *** | 5809 | 7840 | 12072 | 1396 | 1621 | 1806 | 376 | 395 | 393 | 155 | 158 | 145 | . | . | . |
| 0.85 | *** | 4357 | 5369 | 9440 | 1049 | 1171 | 1380 | 268 | 278 | 290 | . | . | . | . | . | . |
| | *** | 4765 | 6423 | 9443 | 1103 | 1258 | 1366 | 274 | 284 | 275 | . | . | . | . | . | . |
| 0.9 | *** | 3267 | 3998 | 6432 | 717 | 783 | 879 | . | . | . | . | . | . | . | . | . |
| | *** | 3567 | 4712 | 6421 | 747 | 825 | 864 | . | . | . | . | . | . | . | . | . |
| 0.95 | *** | 1884 | 2224 | 3022 | . | . | . | . | . | . | . | . | . | . | . | . |
| | *** | 2030 | 2510 | 3007 | . | . | . | . | . | . | . | . | . | . | . | . |

## TABLE 5: ALPHA= 0.025 POWER= 0.8    EXPECTED ACCRUAL THRU MINIMUM FOLLOW-UP= 1600

| | | DEL=.02 | | | DEL=.05 | | | DEL=.10 | | | DEL=.15 | | | DEL=.20 | | |
|---|---|---|---|---|---|---|---|---|---|---|---|---|---|---|---|---|---|
| FACT= | | 1.0 .75 | .50 .25 | .00 BIN | 1.0 .75 | .50 .25 | .00 BIN | 1.0 .75 | .50 .25 | .00 BIN | 1.0 75 | .50 .25 | .00 BIN | 1.0 .75 | .50 .25 | .00 BIN |
| PCONT=*** | | | | REQUIRED | NUMBER | OF PATIENTS | | | | | | | | | | |
| 0.05 | *** | 2258 | 2283 | 2365 | 490 | 495 | 502 | 177 | 177 | 178 | 103 | 104 | 104 | 73 | 73 | 73 |
| | *** | 2268 | 2311 | 4419 | 493 | 498 | 864 | 177 | 178 | 275 | 104 | 104 | 145 | 73 | 73 | 93 |
| 0.1 | *** | 4706 | 4780 | 5195 | 915 | 935 | 967 | 292 | 295 | 299 | 156 | 157 | 159 | 103 | 104 | 104 |
| | *** | 4732 | 4885 | 7677 | 924 | 949 | 1366 | 293 | 297 | 393 | 157 | 158 | 194 | 103 | 104 | 118 |
| 0.15 | *** | 6892 | 7026 | 8034 | 1293 | 1337 | 1418 | 393 | 400 | 409 | 202 | 204 | 207 | 128 | 129 | 130 |
| | *** | 6938 | 7240 | 10542 | 1312 | 1371 | 1806 | 397 | 405 | 495 | 203 | 205 | 236 | 129 | 130 | 140 |
| 0.2 | *** | 8653 | 8862 | 10675 | 1607 | 1681 | 1829 | 479 | 492 | 507 | 240 | 244 | 248 | 149 | 150 | 152 |
| | *** | 8724 | 9206 | 13014 | 1639 | 1740 | 2182 | 485 | 499 | 581 | 242 | 246 | 271 | 150 | 151 | 157 |
| 0.25 | *** | 9945 | 10245 | 13016 | 1854 | 1961 | 2188 | 550 | 567 | 591 | 271 | 276 | 282 | 165 | 167 | 170 |
| | *** | 10048 | 10741 | 15094 | 1899 | 2049 | 2496 | 558 | 578 | 652 | 273 | 279 | 299 | 166 | 168 | 171 |
| 0.3 | *** | 10779 | 11188 | 15000 | 2034 | 2176 | 2489 | 603 | 627 | 659 | 295 | 301 | 309 | 177 | 180 | 183 |
| | *** | 10919 | 11854 | 16781 | 2094 | 2294 | 2748 | 614 | 642 | 707 | 298 | 305 | 320 | 179 | 181 | 181 |
| 0.35 | *** | 11191 | 11727 | 16596 | 2154 | 2329 | 2725 | 642 | 671 | 710 | 311 | 319 | 328 | 185 | 188 | 192 |
| | *** | 11376 | 12578 | 18076 | 2228 | 2477 | 2936 | 655 | 689 | 746 | 315 | 323 | 334 | 187 | 190 | 187 |
| 0.4 | *** | 11233 | 11916 | 17784 | 2220 | 2425 | 2896 | 665 | 698 | 745 | 320 | 329 | 340 | 189 | 193 | 196 |
| | *** | 11471 | 12955 | 18979 | 2307 | 2599 | 3062 | 680 | 719 | 770 | 325 | 334 | 341 | 191 | 194 | 189 |
| 0.45 | *** | 10968 | 11811 | 18553 | 2237 | 2467 | 2999 | 674 | 711 | 762 | 323 | 332 | 344 | 189 | 193 | 197 |
| | *** | 11267 | 13033 | 19489 | 2335 | 2663 | 3124 | 691 | 734 | 778 | 327 | 338 | 341 | 191 | 195 | 187 |
| 0.5 | *** | 10462 | 11471 | 18898 | 2212 | 2461 | 3034 | 669 | 708 | 762 | 318 | 329 | 341 | 185 | 189 | 193 |
| | *** | 10828 | 12857 | 19607 | 2318 | 2671 | 3124 | 687 | 733 | 770 | 323 | 334 | 334 | 187 | 190 | 181 |
| 0.55 | *** | 9785 | 10948 | 18815 | 2148 | 2409 | 3000 | 652 | 691 | 746 | 307 | 318 | 329 | 177 | 180 | 184 |
| | *** | 10215 | 12464 | 19332 | 2260 | 2627 | 3062 | 670 | 716 | 746 | 312 | 323 | 320 | 178 | 182 | 171 |
| 0.6 | *** | 8996 | 10285 | 18305 | 2051 | 2313 | 2898 | 621 | 659 | 712 | 290 | 300 | 311 | 165 | 168 | 171 |
| | *** | 9483 | 11885 | 18665 | 2164 | 2531 | 2936 | 639 | 683 | 707 | 295 | 305 | 299 | 166 | 170 | 157 |
| 0.65 | *** | 8145 | 9514 | 17370 | 1922 | 2176 | 2728 | 578 | 613 | 661 | 266 | 275 | 284 | 149 | 152 | 155 |
| | *** | 8672 | 11142 | 17606 | 2031 | 2384 | 2748 | 595 | 635 | 652 | 270 | 279 | 271 | 150 | 153 | 140 |
| 0.7 | *** | 7263 | 8652 | 16012 | 1761 | 1998 | 2491 | 523 | 553 | 593 | 236 | 243 | 250 | 129 | 131 | 133 |
| | *** | 7806 | 10244 | 16153 | 1864 | 2186 | 2496 | 537 | 571 | 581 | 239 | 246 | 236 | 130 | 132 | 118 |
| 0.75 | *** | 6362 | 7702 | 14235 | 1568 | 1775 | 2186 | 453 | 478 | 509 | 199 | 204 | 209 | 105 | 107 | 108 |
| | *** | 6892 | 9190 | 14309 | 1658 | 1937 | 2182 | 465 | 492 | 495 | 201 | 206 | 194 | 106 | 107 | 93 |
| 0.8 | *** | 5433 | 6653 | 12043 | 1337 | 1506 | 1816 | 370 | 387 | 408 | 154 | 157 | 161 | . | . | . |
| | *** | 5921 | 7962 | 12072 | 1412 | 1631 | 1806 | 378 | 397 | 393 | 156 | 159 | 145 | . | . | . |
| 0.85 | *** | 4447 | 5467 | 9441 | 1062 | 1181 | 1380 | 270 | 279 | 291 | . | . | . | . | . | . |
| | *** | 4859 | 6519 | 9443 | 1115 | 1265 | 1366 | 274 | 285 | 275 | . | . | . | . | . | . |
| 0.9 | *** | 3333 | 4067 | 6432 | 725 | 787 | 879 | . | . | . | . | . | . | . | . | . |
| | *** | 3635 | 4775 | 6421 | 753 | 828 | 864 | . | . | . | . | . | . | . | . | . |
| 0.95 | *** | 1918 | 2254 | 3022 | . | . | . | . | . | . | . | . | . | . | . | . |
| | *** | 2061 | 2534 | 3007 | . | . | . | . | . | . | . | . | . | . | . | . |

## TABLE 5: ALPHA= 0.025 POWER= 0.8     EXPECTED ACCRUAL THRU MINIMUM FOLLOW-UP= 1700

| | | DEL=.02 | | | DEL=.05 | | | DEL=.10 | | | DEL=.15 | | | DEL=.20 | | |
|---|---|---|---|---|---|---|---|---|---|---|---|---|---|---|---|---|
| FACT= | | 1.0 / .75 | .50 / .25 | .00 / BIN | 1.0 / .75 | .50 / .25 | .00 / BIN | 1.0 / .75 | .50 / .25 | .00 / BIN | 1.0 / 75 | .50 / .25 | .00 / BIN | 1.0 / .75 | .50 / .25 | .00 / BIN |

PCONT=***           REQUIRED NUMBER OF PATIENTS

| PCONT | | DEL=.02 1.0 | .50 | .00 | DEL=.05 1.0 | .50 | .00 | DEL=.10 1.0 | .50 | .00 | DEL=.15 1.0 | .50 | .00 | DEL=.20 1.0 | .50 | .00 |
|---|---|---|---|---|---|---|---|---|---|---|---|---|---|---|---|---|
| | | .75 | .25 | BIN | .75 | .25 | BIN | .75 | .25 | BIN | .75 | .25 | BIN | .75 | .25 | BIN |
| 0.05 | *** | 2260 | 2285 | 2365 | 491 | 495 | 501 | 176 | 177 | 178 | 103 | 104 | 104 | 73 | 73 | 73 |
| | *** | 2269 | 2313 | 4419 | 493 | 498 | 864 | 177 | 178 | 275 | 104 | 104 | 145 | 73 | 73 | 93 |
| 0.1 | *** | 4711 | 4787 | 5195 | 917 | 936 | 967 | 292 | 295 | 299 | 156 | 157 | 158 | 103 | 103 | 104 |
| | *** | 4738 | 4895 | 7677 | 925 | 950 | 1366 | 293 | 296 | 393 | 157 | 158 | 194 | 103 | 104 | 118 |
| 0.15 | *** | 6901 | 7042 | 8034 | 1297 | 1341 | 1417 | 394 | 401 | 409 | 202 | 204 | 206 | 129 | 129 | 131 |
| | *** | 6950 | 7261 | 10542 | 1316 | 1372 | 1806 | 397 | 405 | 495 | 203 | 205 | 236 | 129 | 129 | 140 |
| 0.2 | *** | 8667 | 8886 | 10675 | 1614 | 1687 | 1829 | 481 | 493 | 508 | 240 | 244 | 248 | 148 | 151 | 152 |
| | *** | 8742 | 9241 | 13014 | 1646 | 1744 | 2182 | 486 | 499 | 581 | 242 | 245 | 271 | 150 | 151 | 157 |
| 0.25 | *** | 9965 | 10280 | 13015 | 1863 | 1970 | 2188 | 551 | 568 | 590 | 272 | 276 | 282 | 165 | 168 | 170 |
| | *** | 10072 | 10793 | 15094 | 1908 | 2056 | 2496 | 560 | 579 | 652 | 274 | 279 | 299 | 167 | 169 | 171 |
| 0.3 | *** | 10805 | 11236 | 15000 | 2047 | 2188 | 2488 | 605 | 629 | 658 | 295 | 301 | 309 | 177 | 180 | 182 |
| | *** | 10953 | 11922 | 16781 | 2107 | 2303 | 2748 | 616 | 643 | 707 | 299 | 305 | 320 | 178 | 182 | 181 |
| 0.35 | *** | 11225 | 11789 | 16596 | 2169 | 2344 | 2725 | 645 | 673 | 709 | 311 | 320 | 328 | 186 | 189 | 192 |
| | *** | 11421 | 12664 | 18076 | 2244 | 2488 | 2936 | 658 | 690 | 746 | 316 | 324 | 334 | 187 | 190 | 187 |
| 0.4 | *** | 11278 | 11993 | 17784 | 2237 | 2441 | 2895 | 668 | 700 | 745 | 321 | 329 | 340 | 190 | 193 | 197 |
| | *** | 11529 | 13059 | 18979 | 2324 | 2611 | 3062 | 683 | 720 | 770 | 325 | 335 | 341 | 191 | 194 | 189 |
| 0.45 | *** | 11024 | 11904 | 18553 | 2258 | 2486 | 2998 | 678 | 713 | 762 | 324 | 333 | 344 | 189 | 193 | 197 |
| | *** | 11339 | 13153 | 19489 | 2356 | 2677 | 3124 | 695 | 735 | 778 | 328 | 338 | 341 | 191 | 194 | 187 |
| 0.5 | *** | 10533 | 11579 | 18897 | 2234 | 2481 | 3033 | 673 | 711 | 763 | 320 | 329 | 341 | 185 | 189 | 192 |
| | *** | 10915 | 12990 | 19607 | 2339 | 2687 | 3124 | 690 | 734 | 770 | 324 | 335 | 334 | 187 | 190 | 181 |
| 0.55 | *** | 9868 | 11069 | 18814 | 2171 | 2430 | 2999 | 656 | 694 | 746 | 308 | 318 | 329 | 177 | 180 | 184 |
| | *** | 10316 | 12607 | 19332 | 2282 | 2642 | 3062 | 673 | 717 | 746 | 313 | 324 | 320 | 178 | 182 | 171 |
| 0.6 | *** | 9093 | 10414 | 18304 | 2075 | 2334 | 2898 | 626 | 662 | 712 | 291 | 299 | 310 | 165 | 168 | 171 |
| | *** | 9595 | 12034 | 18665 | 2186 | 2547 | 2936 | 643 | 684 | 707 | 295 | 305 | 299 | 167 | 170 | 157 |
| 0.65 | *** | 8250 | 9649 | 17369 | 1945 | 2197 | 2728 | 582 | 616 | 661 | 267 | 275 | 284 | 148 | 152 | 155 |
| | *** | 8791 | 11290 | 17606 | 2054 | 2399 | 2748 | 598 | 636 | 652 | 271 | 279 | 271 | 151 | 153 | 140 |
| 0.7 | *** | 7373 | 8784 | 16012 | 1783 | 2016 | 2490 | 526 | 554 | 593 | 237 | 243 | 250 | 129 | 131 | 134 |
| | *** | 7926 | 10387 | 16153 | 1885 | 2200 | 2496 | 539 | 573 | 581 | 240 | 246 | 236 | 131 | 133 | 118 |
| 0.75 | *** | 6470 | 7828 | 14235 | 1587 | 1791 | 2186 | 456 | 479 | 509 | 199 | 204 | 209 | 105 | 107 | 108 |
| | *** | 7009 | 9322 | 14309 | 1676 | 1948 | 2182 | 467 | 493 | 495 | 202 | 206 | 194 | 106 | 107 | 93 |
| 0.8 | *** | 5533 | 6766 | 12043 | 1353 | 1518 | 1816 | 372 | 388 | 408 | 154 | 157 | 160 | . | . | . |
| | *** | 6028 | 8076 | 12072 | 1427 | 1640 | 1806 | 379 | 397 | 393 | 156 | 159 | 145 | . | . | . |
| 0.85 | *** | 4532 | 5560 | 9440 | 1073 | 1189 | 1380 | 271 | 280 | 291 | . | . | . | . | . | . |
| | *** | 4949 | 6608 | 9443 | 1126 | 1270 | 1366 | 275 | 284 | 275 | . | . | . | . | . | . |
| 0.9 | *** | 3397 | 4131 | 6432 | 731 | 792 | 879 | . | . | . | . | . | . | . | . | . |
| | *** | 3699 | 4832 | 6421 | 758 | 831 | 864 | . | . | . | . | . | . | . | . | . |
| 0.95 | *** | 1948 | 2281 | 3021 | . | . | . | . | . | . | . | . | . | . | . | . |
| | *** | 2091 | 2555 | 3007 | . | . | . | . | . | . | . | . | . | . | . | . |

TABLE 5: ALPHA= 0.025 POWER= 0.8     EXPECTED ACCRUAL THRU MINIMUM FOLLOW-UP= 1800

| | | DEL=.02 | | | DEL=.05 | | | DEL=.10 | | | DEL=.15 | | | DEL=.20 | | |
|---|---|---|---|---|---|---|---|---|---|---|---|---|---|---|---|---|
| FACT= | | 1.0 .75 | .50 .25 | .00 BIN | 1.0 .75 | .50 .25 | .00 BIN | 1.0 .75 | .50 .25 | .00 BIN | 1.0 75 | .50 .25 | .00 BIN | 1.0 .75 | .50 .25 | .00 BIN |
| PCONT=*** | | | | | REQUIRED NUMBER OF PATIENTS | | | | | | | | | | | |
| 0.05 | *** | 2262 | 2288 | 2364 | 492 | 496 | 501 | 177 | 177 | 179 | 103 | 103 | 105 | 73 | 73 | 73 |
| | *** | 2272 | 2315 | 4419 | 494 | 498 | 864 | 177 | 177 | 275 | 103 | 103 | 145 | 73 | 73 | 93 |
| 0.1 | *** | 4716 | 4796 | 5195 | 919 | 938 | 967 | 292 | 294 | 299 | 156 | 157 | 159 | 103 | 103 | 105 |
| | *** | 4744 | 4904 | 7677 | 927 | 951 | 1366 | 294 | 297 | 393 | 157 | 159 | 194 | 103 | 103 | 118 |
| 0.15 | *** | 6909 | 7057 | 8034 | 1302 | 1343 | 1417 | 395 | 402 | 409 | 202 | 204 | 207 | 128 | 129 | 130 |
| | *** | 6960 | 7281 | 10542 | 1320 | 1374 | 1806 | 398 | 405 | 495 | 204 | 206 | 236 | 129 | 129 | 140 |
| 0.2 | *** | 8679 | 8911 | 10675 | 1620 | 1693 | 1829 | 481 | 494 | 507 | 240 | 244 | 247 | 150 | 150 | 152 |
| | *** | 8759 | 9276 | 13014 | 1651 | 1748 | 2182 | 487 | 499 | 581 | 243 | 246 | 271 | 150 | 152 | 157 |
| 0.25 | *** | 9984 | 10316 | 13016 | 1872 | 1977 | 2188 | 553 | 569 | 591 | 272 | 276 | 282 | 165 | 168 | 170 |
| | *** | 10098 | 10842 | 15094 | 1918 | 2061 | 2496 | 561 | 579 | 652 | 274 | 279 | 299 | 166 | 168 | 171 |
| 0.3 | *** | 10831 | 11283 | 15000 | 2058 | 2198 | 2488 | 609 | 630 | 659 | 296 | 301 | 309 | 177 | 180 | 183 |
| | *** | 10988 | 11988 | 16781 | 2118 | 2310 | 2748 | 618 | 643 | 707 | 299 | 305 | 320 | 179 | 181 | 181 |
| 0.35 | *** | 11260 | 11850 | 16596 | 2184 | 2357 | 2724 | 648 | 674 | 710 | 312 | 319 | 328 | 186 | 189 | 192 |
| | *** | 11466 | 12746 | 18076 | 2258 | 2499 | 2936 | 660 | 690 | 746 | 316 | 324 | 334 | 188 | 190 | 187 |
| 0.4 | *** | 11323 | 12069 | 17784 | 2256 | 2457 | 2895 | 672 | 703 | 744 | 321 | 330 | 339 | 190 | 193 | 197 |
| | *** | 11586 | 13158 | 18979 | 2342 | 2623 | 3062 | 686 | 722 | 770 | 326 | 335 | 341 | 191 | 195 | 189 |
| 0.45 | *** | 11081 | 11996 | 18553 | 2277 | 2504 | 2999 | 681 | 715 | 762 | 325 | 334 | 344 | 190 | 193 | 197 |
| | *** | 11409 | 13267 | 19489 | 2373 | 2691 | 3124 | 697 | 737 | 778 | 330 | 339 | 341 | 191 | 195 | 187 |
| 0.5 | *** | 10603 | 11684 | 18897 | 2256 | 2501 | 3034 | 677 | 713 | 762 | 321 | 330 | 341 | 186 | 189 | 192 |
| | *** | 10999 | 13116 | 19607 | 2360 | 2701 | 3124 | 694 | 735 | 770 | 325 | 335 | 334 | 188 | 191 | 181 |
| 0.55 | *** | 9951 | 11186 | 18814 | 2193 | 2449 | 3000 | 659 | 696 | 746 | 309 | 318 | 330 | 177 | 181 | 184 |
| | *** | 10414 | 12743 | 19332 | 2304 | 2657 | 3062 | 677 | 719 | 746 | 314 | 324 | 320 | 179 | 182 | 171 |
| 0.6 | *** | 9186 | 10540 | 18305 | 2098 | 2355 | 2898 | 629 | 665 | 712 | 292 | 300 | 310 | 165 | 168 | 171 |
| | *** | 9703 | 12174 | 18665 | 2208 | 2562 | 2936 | 645 | 686 | 707 | 296 | 306 | 299 | 166 | 170 | 157 |
| 0.65 | *** | 8353 | 9776 | 17370 | 1968 | 2216 | 2728 | 585 | 618 | 660 | 267 | 276 | 285 | 150 | 152 | 154 |
| | *** | 8905 | 11431 | 17606 | 2074 | 2413 | 2748 | 600 | 638 | 652 | 272 | 280 | 271 | 150 | 153 | 140 |
| 0.7 | *** | 7479 | 8912 | 16012 | 1803 | 2034 | 2490 | 528 | 557 | 593 | 237 | 243 | 251 | 129 | 132 | 134 |
| | *** | 8043 | 10522 | 16153 | 1903 | 2213 | 2496 | 542 | 573 | 581 | 240 | 246 | 236 | 130 | 132 | 118 |
| 0.75 | *** | 6574 | 7948 | 14235 | 1605 | 1806 | 2187 | 458 | 480 | 508 | 199 | 204 | 209 | 105 | 107 | 108 |
| | *** | 7121 | 9447 | 14309 | 1694 | 1959 | 2182 | 469 | 494 | 495 | 201 | 207 | 194 | 105 | 108 | 93 |
| 0.8 | *** | 5629 | 6873 | 12043 | 1369 | 1530 | 1815 | 373 | 389 | 408 | 155 | 157 | 161 | . | . | . |
| | *** | 6129 | 8183 | 12072 | 1440 | 1648 | 1806 | 380 | 398 | 393 | 156 | 159 | 145 | . | . | . |
| 0.85 | *** | 4614 | 5647 | 9441 | 1084 | 1197 | 1380 | 272 | 280 | 290 | . | . | . | . | . | . |
| | *** | 5033 | 6691 | 9443 | 1135 | 1275 | 1366 | 276 | 285 | 275 | . | . | . | . | . | . |
| 0.9 | *** | 3456 | 4191 | 6432 | 737 | 795 | 879 | . | . | . | . | . | . | . | . | . |
| | *** | 3761 | 4886 | 6421 | 764 | 834 | 864 | . | . | . | . | . | . | . | . | . |
| 0.95 | *** | 1977 | 2306 | 3021 | . | . | . | . | . | . | . | . | . | . | . | . |
| | *** | 2118 | 2574 | 3007 | . | . | . | . | . | . | . | . | . | . | . | . |

# TABLE 5: ALPHA= 0.025 POWER= 0.8    EXPECTED ACCRUAL THRU MINIMUM FOLLOW-UP= 1900

| PCONT | FACT | DEL=.02 1.0/.75 | DEL=.02 .50/.25 | DEL=.02 .00/BIN | DEL=.05 1.0/.75 | DEL=.05 .50/.25 | DEL=.05 .00/BIN | DEL=.10 1.0/.75 | DEL=.10 .50/.25 | DEL=.10 .00/BIN | DEL=.15 1.0/75 | DEL=.15 .50/.25 | DEL=.15 .00/BIN | DEL=.20 1.0/.75 | DEL=.20 .50/.25 | DEL=.20 .00/BIN |
|---|---|---|---|---|---|---|---|---|---|---|---|---|---|---|---|---|
| | | | | | | | REQUIRED NUMBER OF PATIENTS | | | | | | | | |
| 0.05 | *** | 2263 | 2291 | 2364 | 491 | 496 | 502 | 177 | 178 | 178 | 103 | 103 | 104 | 73 | 73 | 73 |
| | *** | 2274 | 2317 | 4419 | 494 | 498 | 864 | 177 | 178 | 275 | 103 | 104 | 145 | 73 | 73 | 93 |
| 0.1 | *** | 4721 | 4803 | 5195 | 920 | 939 | 968 | 292 | 296 | 299 | 156 | 158 | 159 | 103 | 103 | 104 |
| | *** | 4751 | 4913 | 7677 | 928 | 951 | 1366 | 294 | 296 | 393 | 156 | 158 | 194 | 103 | 104 | 118 |
| 0.15 | *** | 6918 | 7072 | 8034 | 1305 | 1346 | 1417 | 395 | 401 | 410 | 203 | 204 | 206 | 128 | 129 | 130 |
| | *** | 6972 | 7300 | 10542 | 1322 | 1377 | 1806 | 399 | 405 | 495 | 203 | 205 | 236 | 129 | 129 | 140 |
| 0.2 | *** | 8694 | 8934 | 10674 | 1626 | 1698 | 1828 | 483 | 494 | 507 | 241 | 244 | 248 | 149 | 151 | 152 |
| | *** | 8777 | 9307 | 13014 | 1657 | 1751 | 2182 | 488 | 500 | 581 | 242 | 246 | 271 | 149 | 152 | 157 |
| 0.25 | *** | 10003 | 10350 | 13016 | 1881 | 1985 | 2188 | 554 | 571 | 591 | 273 | 277 | 282 | 166 | 167 | 170 |
| | *** | 10123 | 10888 | 15094 | 1926 | 2066 | 2496 | 562 | 581 | 652 | 274 | 279 | 299 | 167 | 168 | 171 |
| 0.3 | *** | 10858 | 11330 | 15000 | 2070 | 2208 | 2489 | 610 | 631 | 659 | 296 | 303 | 308 | 178 | 180 | 182 |
| | *** | 11022 | 12050 | 16781 | 2129 | 2319 | 2748 | 619 | 643 | 707 | 299 | 305 | 320 | 179 | 182 | 181 |
| 0.35 | *** | 11295 | 11910 | 16596 | 2198 | 2369 | 2725 | 649 | 676 | 710 | 313 | 320 | 329 | 186 | 189 | 192 |
| | *** | 11510 | 12825 | 18076 | 2272 | 2507 | 2936 | 662 | 692 | 746 | 317 | 324 | 334 | 187 | 190 | 187 |
| 0.4 | *** | 11368 | 12143 | 17784 | 2272 | 2472 | 2896 | 674 | 704 | 744 | 323 | 331 | 339 | 190 | 193 | 196 |
| | *** | 11643 | 13252 | 18979 | 2357 | 2635 | 3062 | 688 | 723 | 770 | 326 | 334 | 341 | 192 | 194 | 189 |
| 0.45 | *** | 11137 | 12084 | 18553 | 2295 | 2519 | 2998 | 685 | 717 | 762 | 325 | 334 | 344 | 190 | 193 | 197 |
| | *** | 11480 | 13376 | 19489 | 2391 | 2702 | 3124 | 700 | 738 | 778 | 330 | 339 | 341 | 191 | 194 | 187 |
| 0.5 | *** | 10672 | 11786 | 18897 | 2275 | 2517 | 3034 | 680 | 716 | 762 | 322 | 330 | 341 | 186 | 189 | 192 |
| | *** | 11083 | 13237 | 19607 | 2379 | 2714 | 3124 | 697 | 737 | 770 | 325 | 334 | 334 | 187 | 191 | 181 |
| 0.55 | *** | 10033 | 11297 | 18814 | 2215 | 2467 | 2999 | 662 | 698 | 745 | 311 | 319 | 329 | 178 | 180 | 184 |
| | *** | 10509 | 12871 | 19332 | 2324 | 2671 | 3062 | 679 | 719 | 746 | 315 | 324 | 320 | 179 | 182 | 171 |
| 0.6 | *** | 9279 | 10660 | 18305 | 2118 | 2372 | 2897 | 633 | 666 | 711 | 293 | 301 | 311 | 166 | 168 | 171 |
| | *** | 9807 | 12307 | 18665 | 2229 | 2574 | 2936 | 648 | 687 | 707 | 296 | 305 | 299 | 167 | 170 | 157 |
| 0.65 | *** | 8452 | 9900 | 17369 | 1987 | 2234 | 2728 | 589 | 619 | 660 | 268 | 275 | 284 | 149 | 152 | 154 |
| | *** | 9015 | 11563 | 17606 | 2094 | 2426 | 2748 | 603 | 638 | 652 | 272 | 280 | 271 | 151 | 153 | 140 |
| 0.7 | *** | 7581 | 9033 | 16012 | 1823 | 2049 | 2491 | 532 | 558 | 592 | 237 | 243 | 250 | 129 | 132 | 133 |
| | *** | 8153 | 10651 | 16153 | 1922 | 2224 | 2496 | 543 | 574 | 581 | 241 | 247 | 236 | 130 | 133 | 118 |
| 0.75 | *** | 6673 | 8063 | 14235 | 1622 | 1820 | 2186 | 460 | 482 | 508 | 201 | 204 | 209 | 106 | 106 | 108 |
| | *** | 7227 | 9563 | 14309 | 1710 | 1968 | 2182 | 470 | 495 | 495 | 201 | 206 | 194 | 106 | 108 | 93 |
| 0.8 | *** | 5721 | 6974 | 12043 | 1382 | 1541 | 1816 | 375 | 389 | 408 | 155 | 158 | 160 | . | . | . |
| | *** | 6226 | 8284 | 12072 | 1453 | 1655 | 1806 | 382 | 399 | 393 | 156 | 159 | 145 | . | . | . |
| 0.85 | *** | 4690 | 5730 | 9440 | 1094 | 1205 | 1379 | 273 | 281 | 291 | . | . | . | . | . | . |
| | *** | 5114 | 6770 | 9443 | 1144 | 1280 | 1366 | 277 | 286 | 275 | . | . | . | . | . | . |
| 0.9 | *** | 3512 | 4248 | 6431 | 742 | 799 | 878 | . | . | . | . | . | . | . | . | . |
| | *** | 3818 | 4936 | 6421 | 768 | 836 | 864 | . | . | . | . | . | . | . | . | . |
| 0.95 | *** | 2004 | 2329 | 3022 | . | . | . | . | . | . | . | . | . | . | . | . |
| | *** | 2144 | 2592 | 3007 | . | . | . | . | . | . | . | . | . | . | . | . |

TABLE 5: ALPHA= 0.025 POWER= 0.8     EXPECTED ACCRUAL THRU MINIMUM FOLLOW-UP= 2000

| | | DEL=.02 | | | DEL=.05 | | | DEL=.10 | | | DEL=.15 | | | DEL=.20 | |
|---|---|---|---|---|---|---|---|---|---|---|---|---|---|---|---|---|
| FACT= | 1.0<br>.75 | .50<br>.25 | .00<br>BIN | 1.0<br>.75 | .50<br>.25 | .00<br>BIN | 1.0<br>.75 | .50<br>.25 | .00<br>BIN | 1.0<br>75 | .50<br>.25 | .00<br>BIN | 1.0<br>.75 | .50<br>.25 | .00<br>BIN |
| PCONT=*** | | | | | REQUIRED NUMBER OF PATIENTS | | | | | | | | | | | |
| 0.05 *** | 2266 | 2292 | 2365 | 492 | 496 | 501 | 177 | 177 | 179 | 104 | 104 | 104 | 72 | 74 | 74 |
| *** | 2276 | 2319 | 4419 | 494 | 499 | 864 | 177 | 179 | 275 | 104 | 104 | 145 | 74 | 74 | 93 |
| 0.1 *** | 4726 | 4811 | 5195 | 922 | 940 | 967 | 292 | 296 | 299 | 156 | 157 | 159 | 104 | 104 | 104 |
| *** | 4756 | 4921 | 7677 | 930 | 952 | 1366 | 294 | 297 | 393 | 157 | 159 | 194 | 104 | 104 | 118 |
| 0.15 *** | 6926 | 7087 | 8034 | 1309 | 1349 | 1417 | 396 | 402 | 410 | 202 | 205 | 206 | 129 | 130 | 130 |
| *** | 6984 | 7319 | 10542 | 1326 | 1379 | 1806 | 399 | 406 | 495 | 204 | 205 | 236 | 129 | 130 | 140 |
| 0.2 *** | 8706 | 8959 | 10675 | 1632 | 1702 | 1829 | 484 | 495 | 507 | 241 | 245 | 247 | 150 | 151 | 152 |
| *** | 8794 | 9339 | 13014 | 1662 | 1755 | 2182 | 489 | 501 | 581 | 242 | 246 | 271 | 150 | 151 | 157 |
| 0.25 *** | 10022 | 10385 | 13016 | 1889 | 1992 | 2189 | 556 | 571 | 591 | 272 | 277 | 282 | 166 | 167 | 170 |
| *** | 10147 | 10934 | 15094 | 1934 | 2071 | 2496 | 564 | 581 | 652 | 275 | 280 | 299 | 167 | 169 | 171 |
| 0.3 *** | 10884 | 11376 | 15000 | 2081 | 2217 | 2489 | 612 | 632 | 659 | 297 | 302 | 309 | 179 | 181 | 182 |
| *** | 11056 | 12111 | 16781 | 2140 | 2325 | 2748 | 622 | 645 | 707 | 300 | 306 | 320 | 180 | 181 | 181 |
| 0.35 *** | 11330 | 11970 | 16596 | 2211 | 2381 | 2725 | 652 | 677 | 710 | 314 | 321 | 329 | 186 | 189 | 192 |
| *** | 11555 | 12901 | 18076 | 2285 | 2516 | 2936 | 664 | 692 | 746 | 317 | 325 | 334 | 187 | 190 | 187 |
| 0.4 *** | 11412 | 12216 | 17785 | 2287 | 2486 | 2896 | 677 | 706 | 745 | 324 | 331 | 340 | 191 | 194 | 196 |
| *** | 11700 | 13342 | 18979 | 2372 | 2645 | 3062 | 691 | 724 | 770 | 327 | 336 | 341 | 192 | 195 | 189 |
| 0.45 *** | 11194 | 12170 | 18554 | 2312 | 2536 | 2999 | 687 | 720 | 762 | 326 | 335 | 344 | 190 | 194 | 196 |
| *** | 11549 | 13480 | 19489 | 2409 | 2715 | 3124 | 702 | 739 | 778 | 330 | 339 | 341 | 192 | 195 | 187 |
| 0.5 *** | 10739 | 11884 | 18897 | 2294 | 2535 | 3034 | 684 | 717 | 762 | 322 | 331 | 341 | 186 | 190 | 192 |
| *** | 11164 | 13352 | 19607 | 2397 | 2726 | 3124 | 700 | 739 | 770 | 326 | 335 | 334 | 187 | 191 | 181 |
| 0.55 *** | 10112 | 11406 | 18815 | 2235 | 2485 | 3000 | 666 | 700 | 746 | 311 | 320 | 330 | 179 | 181 | 184 |
| *** | 10601 | 12995 | 19332 | 2344 | 2684 | 3062 | 682 | 721 | 746 | 315 | 325 | 320 | 180 | 182 | 171 |
| 0.6 *** | 9367 | 10775 | 18305 | 2139 | 2390 | 2897 | 635 | 669 | 711 | 294 | 301 | 311 | 166 | 169 | 171 |
| *** | 9910 | 12435 | 18665 | 2247 | 2587 | 2936 | 651 | 689 | 707 | 297 | 306 | 299 | 167 | 170 | 157 |
| 0.65 *** | 8549 | 10017 | 17370 | 2007 | 2250 | 2729 | 591 | 621 | 661 | 270 | 276 | 284 | 150 | 152 | 155 |
| *** | 9122 | 11691 | 17606 | 2112 | 2437 | 2748 | 606 | 640 | 652 | 272 | 280 | 271 | 151 | 154 | 140 |
| 0.7 *** | 7680 | 9150 | 16012 | 1841 | 2065 | 2491 | 534 | 560 | 594 | 239 | 244 | 250 | 130 | 131 | 134 |
| *** | 8261 | 10771 | 16153 | 1939 | 2235 | 2496 | 546 | 575 | 581 | 241 | 247 | 236 | 131 | 132 | 118 |
| 0.75 *** | 6770 | 8172 | 14235 | 1639 | 1832 | 2186 | 462 | 484 | 509 | 200 | 205 | 210 | 106 | 107 | 109 |
| *** | 7330 | 9674 | 14309 | 1725 | 1977 | 2182 | 472 | 495 | 495 | 202 | 207 | 194 | 106 | 107 | 93 |
| 0.8 *** | 5809 | 7071 | 12044 | 1396 | 1551 | 1816 | 376 | 391 | 407 | 155 | 159 | 161 | . | . | . |
| *** | 6319 | 8379 | 12072 | 1465 | 1662 | 1806 | 384 | 399 | 393 | 156 | 160 | 145 | . | . | . |
| 0.85 *** | 4765 | 5809 | 9441 | 1104 | 1211 | 1380 | 274 | 281 | 291 | . | . | . | . | . | . |
| *** | 5191 | 6844 | 9443 | 1152 | 1285 | 1366 | 277 | 286 | 275 | . | . | . | . | . | . |
| 0.9 *** | 3567 | 4302 | 6432 | 747 | 802 | 879 | . | . | . | . | . | . | . | . | . |
| *** | 3872 | 4982 | 6421 | 774 | 837 | 864 | . | . | . | . | . | . | . | . | . |
| 0.95 *** | 2030 | 2351 | 3022 | . | . | . | . | . | . | . | . | . | . | . | . |
| *** | 2169 | 2609 | 3007 | . | . | . | . | . | . | . | . | . | . | . | . |

## TABLE 5: ALPHA= 0.025 POWER= 0.8    EXPECTED ACCRUAL THRU MINIMUM FOLLOW-UP= 2250

| PCONT= *** | | DEL=.02 | | | DEL=.05 | | | DEL=.10 | | | DEL=.15 | | | DEL=.20 | | |
|---|---|---|---|---|---|---|---|---|---|---|---|---|---|---|---|---|
| FACT= | | 1.0 .75 | .50 .25 | .00 BIN | 1.0 .75 | .50 .25 | .00 BIN | 1.0 .75 | .50 .25 | .00 BIN | 1.0 75 | .50 .25 | .00 BIN | 1.0 .75 | .50 .25 | .00 BIN |
| | | | | | REQUIRED NUMBER OF PATIENTS | | | | | | | | | | | |
| 0.05 | *** | 2269 | 2297 | 2365 | 493 | 496 | 502 | 177 | 178 | 178 | 104 | 104 | 104 | 73 | 73 | 73 |
| | *** | 2280 | 2323 | 4419 | 494 | 499 | 864 | 177 | 178 | 275 | 104 | 104 | 145 | 73 | 73 | 93 |
| 0.1 | *** | 4737 | 4829 | 5194 | 925 | 942 | 967 | 294 | 297 | 299 | 157 | 157 | 159 | 104 | 104 | 104 |
| | *** | 4771 | 4940 | 7677 | 933 | 953 | 1366 | 295 | 298 | 393 | 157 | 159 | 194 | 104 | 104 | 118 |
| 0.15 | *** | 6948 | 7122 | 8034 | 1316 | 1355 | 1417 | 398 | 403 | 409 | 204 | 205 | 207 | 129 | 129 | 131 |
| | *** | 7010 | 7362 | 10542 | 1333 | 1382 | 1806 | 401 | 406 | 495 | 204 | 205 | 236 | 129 | 129 | 140 |
| 0.2 | *** | 8740 | 9015 | 10675 | 1645 | 1712 | 1829 | 486 | 496 | 507 | 241 | 244 | 247 | 150 | 150 | 151 |
| | *** | 8836 | 9410 | 13014 | 1675 | 1762 | 2182 | 491 | 502 | 581 | 243 | 246 | 271 | 150 | 151 | 157 |
| 0.25 | *** | 10070 | 10467 | 13016 | 1908 | 2008 | 2188 | 559 | 573 | 590 | 274 | 278 | 282 | 167 | 168 | 170 |
| | *** | 10209 | 11039 | 15094 | 1951 | 2082 | 2496 | 567 | 582 | 652 | 275 | 280 | 299 | 167 | 168 | 171 |
| 0.3 | *** | 10949 | 11486 | 15000 | 2105 | 2238 | 2489 | 615 | 635 | 659 | 298 | 303 | 309 | 178 | 181 | 182 |
| | *** | 11139 | 12251 | 16781 | 2162 | 2339 | 2748 | 626 | 646 | 707 | 300 | 306 | 320 | 179 | 181 | 181 |
| 0.35 | *** | 11415 | 12110 | 16596 | 2241 | 2407 | 2725 | 658 | 680 | 710 | 314 | 322 | 329 | 187 | 190 | 192 |
| | *** | 11663 | 13077 | 18076 | 2313 | 2534 | 2936 | 668 | 694 | 746 | 319 | 325 | 334 | 188 | 191 | 187 |
| 0.4 | *** | 11522 | 12389 | 17785 | 2323 | 2516 | 2895 | 683 | 710 | 745 | 325 | 331 | 340 | 191 | 194 | 196 |
| | *** | 11836 | 13553 | 18979 | 2407 | 2666 | 3062 | 696 | 727 | 770 | 329 | 336 | 341 | 192 | 195 | 189 |
| 0.45 | *** | 11330 | 12373 | 18554 | 2352 | 2569 | 2999 | 694 | 724 | 762 | 327 | 336 | 344 | 191 | 194 | 196 |
| | *** | 11715 | 13721 | 19489 | 2446 | 2739 | 3124 | 708 | 741 | 778 | 331 | 340 | 341 | 192 | 195 | 187 |
| 0.5 | *** | 10904 | 12116 | 18897 | 2337 | 2570 | 3033 | 690 | 721 | 762 | 325 | 331 | 340 | 187 | 190 | 192 |
| | *** | 11359 | 13618 | 19607 | 2438 | 2753 | 3124 | 705 | 741 | 770 | 327 | 336 | 334 | 188 | 191 | 181 |
| 0.55 | *** | 10303 | 11660 | 18815 | 2279 | 2522 | 2999 | 673 | 704 | 745 | 313 | 320 | 329 | 178 | 181 | 184 |
| | *** | 10822 | 13277 | 19332 | 2386 | 2711 | 3062 | 687 | 724 | 746 | 316 | 325 | 320 | 179 | 182 | 171 |
| 0.6 | *** | 9582 | 11044 | 18305 | 2184 | 2427 | 2898 | 642 | 673 | 711 | 295 | 302 | 311 | 167 | 168 | 171 |
| | *** | 10150 | 12726 | 18665 | 2291 | 2614 | 2936 | 657 | 690 | 707 | 299 | 306 | 299 | 167 | 170 | 157 |
| 0.65 | *** | 8776 | 10292 | 17369 | 2052 | 2286 | 2728 | 597 | 626 | 660 | 271 | 277 | 284 | 150 | 153 | 154 |
| | *** | 9372 | 11981 | 17606 | 2154 | 2463 | 2748 | 612 | 642 | 652 | 274 | 281 | 271 | 151 | 153 | 140 |
| 0.7 | *** | 7911 | 9419 | 16013 | 1881 | 2098 | 2490 | 539 | 564 | 593 | 240 | 244 | 250 | 131 | 132 | 133 |
| | *** | 8512 | 11049 | 16153 | 1977 | 2258 | 2496 | 551 | 578 | 581 | 241 | 247 | 236 | 131 | 132 | 118 |
| 0.75 | *** | 6994 | 8425 | 14235 | 1675 | 1861 | 2187 | 466 | 486 | 509 | 201 | 205 | 209 | 106 | 106 | 108 |
| | *** | 7570 | 9927 | 14309 | 1757 | 1996 | 2182 | 477 | 496 | 495 | 204 | 207 | 194 | 106 | 108 | 93 |
| 0.8 | *** | 6014 | 7294 | 12043 | 1424 | 1573 | 1815 | 379 | 392 | 407 | 156 | 159 | 160 | . | . | . |
| | *** | 6533 | 8594 | 12072 | 1492 | 1676 | 1806 | 385 | 399 | 393 | 157 | 160 | 145 | . | . | . |
| 0.85 | *** | 4938 | 5987 | 9440 | 1124 | 1226 | 1379 | 275 | 282 | 291 | . | . | . | . | . | . |
| | *** | 5369 | 7010 | 9443 | 1171 | 1293 | 1366 | 278 | 286 | 275 | . | . | . | . | . | . |
| 0.9 | *** | 3691 | 4424 | 6432 | 758 | 809 | 879 | . | . | . | . | . | . | . | . | . |
| | *** | 3998 | 5086 | 6421 | 783 | 842 | 864 | . | . | . | . | . | . | . | . | . |
| 0.95 | *** | 2088 | 2400 | 3022 | . | . | . | . | . | . | . | . | . | . | . | . |
| | *** | 2224 | 2643 | 3007 | . | . | . | . | . | . | . | . | . | . | . | . |

TABLE 5: ALPHA= 0.025 POWER= 0.8    EXPECTED ACCRUAL THRU MINIMUM FOLLOW-UP= 2500

| | DEL=.02 | | | DEL=.05 | | | DEL=.10 | | | DEL=.15 | | | DEL=.20 | | |
|---|---|---|---|---|---|---|---|---|---|---|---|---|---|---|---|
| FACT= | 1.0 .75 | .50 .25 | .00 BIN | 1.0 .75 | .50 .25 | .00 BIN | 1.0 .75 | .50 .25 | .00 BIN | 1.0 75 | .50 .25 | .00 BIN | 1.0 .75 | .50 .25 | .00 BIN |
| PCONT=*** | | | | | | REQUIRED | NUMBER OF | PATIENTS | | | | | | |
| 0.05 *** | 2273 | 2301 | 2365 | 493 | 496 | 501 | 177 | 177 | 177 | 104 | 104 | 104 | 73 | 73 | 73 |
| *** | 2286 | 2326 | 4419 | 495 | 499 | 864 | 177 | 177 | 275 | 104 | 104 | 145 | 73 | 73 | 93 |
| 0.1 *** | 4749 | 4845 | 5195 | 927 | 945 | 967 | 293 | 296 | 298 | 158 | 158 | 159 | 102 | 104 | 104 |
| *** | 4786 | 4956 | 7677 | 936 | 954 | 1366 | 295 | 298 | 393 | 158 | 158 | 194 | 102 | 104 | 118 |
| 0.15 *** | 6968 | 7156 | 8034 | 1321 | 1361 | 1418 | 398 | 402 | 409 | 202 | 204 | 206 | 129 | 129 | 129 |
| *** | 7037 | 7398 | 10542 | 1339 | 1386 | 1806 | 401 | 406 | 495 | 204 | 206 | 236 | 129 | 129 | 140 |
| 0.2 *** | 8773 | 9070 | 10674 | 1656 | 1721 | 1829 | 489 | 496 | 508 | 242 | 245 | 248 | 149 | 151 | 151 |
| *** | 8877 | 9474 | 13014 | 1686 | 1768 | 2182 | 492 | 501 | 581 | 243 | 246 | 271 | 149 | 151 | 157 |
| 0.25 *** | 10117 | 10543 | 13015 | 1923 | 2020 | 2189 | 562 | 574 | 590 | 274 | 277 | 283 | 167 | 168 | 170 |
| *** | 10268 | 11134 | 15094 | 1967 | 2092 | 2496 | 568 | 583 | 652 | 276 | 279 | 299 | 167 | 168 | 171 |
| 0.3 *** | 11014 | 11590 | 14999 | 2126 | 2256 | 2489 | 620 | 637 | 659 | 299 | 304 | 309 | 179 | 181 | 183 |
| *** | 11220 | 12379 | 16781 | 2184 | 2352 | 2748 | 627 | 646 | 707 | 301 | 306 | 320 | 179 | 183 | 181 |
| 0.35 *** | 11499 | 12243 | 16596 | 2268 | 2429 | 2724 | 662 | 683 | 711 | 317 | 321 | 327 | 187 | 190 | 192 |
| *** | 11768 | 13237 | 18076 | 2339 | 2549 | 2936 | 671 | 696 | 746 | 318 | 324 | 334 | 189 | 190 | 187 |
| 0.4 *** | 11629 | 12551 | 17784 | 2354 | 2542 | 2895 | 689 | 714 | 745 | 326 | 333 | 340 | 192 | 193 | 196 |
| *** | 11968 | 13743 | 18979 | 2436 | 2686 | 3062 | 699 | 727 | 770 | 329 | 336 | 341 | 193 | 195 | 189 |
| 0.45 *** | 11462 | 12564 | 18552 | 2387 | 2599 | 2998 | 699 | 727 | 762 | 329 | 336 | 343 | 192 | 193 | 196 |
| *** | 11873 | 13937 | 19489 | 2481 | 2759 | 3124 | 712 | 743 | 778 | 333 | 340 | 341 | 193 | 195 | 187 |
| 0.5 *** | 11062 | 12331 | 18898 | 2374 | 2602 | 3034 | 696 | 724 | 762 | 324 | 333 | 340 | 187 | 190 | 192 |
| *** | 11543 | 13858 | 19607 | 2474 | 2776 | 3124 | 711 | 743 | 770 | 329 | 337 | 334 | 189 | 192 | 181 |
| 0.55 *** | 10486 | 11895 | 18815 | 2320 | 2556 | 2999 | 679 | 709 | 745 | 314 | 321 | 329 | 179 | 181 | 184 |
| *** | 11029 | 13531 | 19332 | 2423 | 2734 | 3062 | 693 | 726 | 746 | 318 | 324 | 320 | 181 | 183 | 171 |
| 0.6 *** | 9783 | 11290 | 18304 | 2223 | 2461 | 2898 | 648 | 676 | 712 | 296 | 302 | 311 | 167 | 168 | 171 |
| *** | 10371 | 12987 | 18665 | 2327 | 2637 | 2936 | 661 | 693 | 707 | 299 | 308 | 299 | 168 | 170 | 157 |
| 0.65 *** | 8989 | 10543 | 17370 | 2090 | 2317 | 2727 | 602 | 629 | 661 | 271 | 277 | 284 | 151 | 152 | 154 |
| *** | 9604 | 12239 | 17606 | 2190 | 2484 | 2748 | 615 | 643 | 652 | 274 | 281 | 271 | 151 | 152 | 140 |
| 0.7 *** | 8126 | 9664 | 16012 | 1918 | 2126 | 2490 | 543 | 565 | 593 | 240 | 245 | 249 | 131 | 133 | 134 |
| *** | 8742 | 11295 | 16153 | 2011 | 2276 | 2496 | 554 | 579 | 581 | 243 | 248 | 236 | 131 | 133 | 118 |
| 0.75 *** | 7201 | 8652 | 14236 | 1706 | 1886 | 2186 | 470 | 487 | 509 | 202 | 206 | 209 | 106 | 108 | 108 |
| *** | 7787 | 10149 | 14309 | 1786 | 2012 | 2182 | 479 | 498 | 495 | 204 | 208 | 194 | 108 | 108 | 93 |
| 0.8 *** | 6201 | 7493 | 12043 | 1449 | 1592 | 1815 | 381 | 393 | 408 | 156 | 159 | 161 | . | . | . |
| *** | 6729 | 8784 | 12072 | 1514 | 1689 | 1806 | 387 | 401 | 393 | 158 | 159 | 145 | . | . | . |
| 0.85 *** | 5095 | 6148 | 9440 | 1142 | 1239 | 1379 | 276 | 283 | 290 | . | . | . | . | . | . |
| *** | 5529 | 7154 | 9443 | 1187 | 1301 | 1366 | 279 | 287 | 275 | . | . | . | . | . | . |
| 0.9 *** | 3804 | 4531 | 6433 | 767 | 815 | 879 | . | . | . | . | . | . | . | . | . |
| *** | 4111 | 5176 | 6421 | 790 | 845 | 864 | . | . | . | . | . | . | . | . | . |
| 0.95 *** | 2139 | 2442 | 3021 | . | . | . | . | . | . | . | . | . | . | . | . |
| *** | 2271 | 2673 | 3007 | . | . | . | . | . | . | . | . | . | . | . | . |

## TABLE 5: ALPHA= 0.025 POWER= 0.8    EXPECTED ACCRUAL THRU MINIMUM FOLLOW-UP= 2750

|  |  | DEL=.02 | | | DEL=.05 | | | DEL=.10 | | | DEL=.15 | | | DEL=.20 | | |
|---|---|---|---|---|---|---|---|---|---|---|---|---|---|---|---|---|
| FACT= | | 1.0 .75 | .50 .25 | .00 BIN | 1.0 .75 | .50 .25 | .00 BIN | 1.0 .75 | .50 .25 | .00 BIN | 1.0 75 | .50 .25 | .00 BIN | 1.0 .75 | .50 .25 | .00 BIN |
| PCONT=*** | | REQUIRED NUMBER OF PATIENTS | | | | | | | | | | | | | | |
| 0.05 | *** | 2277 | 2304 | 2364 | 494 | 498 | 501 | 177 | 178 | 178 | 104 | 104 | 104 | 74 | 74 | 74 |
|  | *** | 2289 | 2329 | 4419 | 496 | 500 | 864 | 178 | 178 | 275 | 104 | 104 | 145 | 74 | 74 | 93 |
| 0.1 | *** | 4760 | 4860 | 5195 | 931 | 947 | 967 | 294 | 297 | 298 | 157 | 157 | 157 | 102 | 104 | 104 |
|  | *** | 4798 | 4970 | 7677 | 938 | 955 | 1366 | 295 | 297 | 393 | 157 | 157 | 194 | 102 | 104 | 118 |
| 0.15 | *** | 6990 | 7187 | 8035 | 1328 | 1364 | 1418 | 398 | 404 | 408 | 204 | 205 | 205 | 129 | 130 | 130 |
|  | *** | 7062 | 7431 | 10542 | 1345 | 1388 | 1806 | 401 | 407 | 495 | 204 | 205 | 236 | 129 | 130 | 140 |
| 0.2 | *** | 8805 | 9121 | 10675 | 1666 | 1728 | 1828 | 489 | 498 | 507 | 243 | 245 | 247 | 150 | 150 | 153 |
|  | *** | 8920 | 9534 | 13014 | 1694 | 1773 | 2182 | 493 | 503 | 581 | 243 | 247 | 271 | 150 | 150 | 157 |
| 0.25 | *** | 10163 | 10618 | 13016 | 1938 | 2033 | 2189 | 563 | 577 | 590 | 274 | 278 | 281 | 166 | 168 | 170 |
|  | *** | 10328 | 11219 | 15094 | 1979 | 2098 | 2496 | 570 | 584 | 652 | 276 | 280 | 299 | 168 | 168 | 171 |
| 0.3 | *** | 11077 | 11689 | 15000 | 2146 | 2271 | 2488 | 621 | 639 | 658 | 300 | 304 | 309 | 180 | 181 | 184 |
|  | *** | 11298 | 12495 | 16781 | 2201 | 2363 | 2748 | 630 | 648 | 707 | 302 | 307 | 320 | 180 | 181 | 181 |
| 0.35 | *** | 11582 | 12369 | 16595 | 2292 | 2449 | 2725 | 665 | 685 | 709 | 318 | 322 | 328 | 188 | 190 | 192 |
|  | *** | 11871 | 13381 | 18076 | 2361 | 2562 | 2936 | 675 | 697 | 746 | 319 | 326 | 334 | 188 | 190 | 187 |
| 0.4 | *** | 11734 | 12703 | 17784 | 2381 | 2564 | 2896 | 692 | 716 | 744 | 328 | 333 | 340 | 192 | 194 | 195 |
|  | *** | 12094 | 13916 | 18979 | 2463 | 2701 | 3062 | 703 | 730 | 770 | 331 | 336 | 341 | 194 | 195 | 189 |
| 0.45 | *** | 11590 | 12741 | 18554 | 2419 | 2624 | 2999 | 704 | 730 | 762 | 331 | 336 | 343 | 192 | 194 | 197 |
|  | *** | 12026 | 14134 | 19489 | 2509 | 2777 | 3124 | 716 | 745 | 778 | 333 | 340 | 341 | 194 | 195 | 187 |
| 0.5 | *** | 11212 | 12531 | 18897 | 2409 | 2629 | 3033 | 700 | 728 | 762 | 326 | 333 | 340 | 188 | 190 | 192 |
|  | *** | 11718 | 14072 | 19607 | 2505 | 2794 | 3124 | 714 | 744 | 770 | 329 | 336 | 334 | 188 | 192 | 181 |
| 0.55 | *** | 10658 | 12112 | 18815 | 2354 | 2584 | 3000 | 683 | 711 | 745 | 315 | 322 | 329 | 180 | 181 | 184 |
|  | *** | 11223 | 13760 | 19332 | 2456 | 2755 | 3062 | 697 | 727 | 746 | 319 | 326 | 320 | 180 | 184 | 171 |
| 0.6 | *** | 9971 | 11518 | 18304 | 2260 | 2488 | 2897 | 652 | 679 | 711 | 298 | 304 | 311 | 168 | 170 | 171 |
|  | *** | 10580 | 13222 | 18665 | 2361 | 2656 | 2936 | 665 | 694 | 707 | 300 | 307 | 299 | 168 | 170 | 157 |
| 0.65 | *** | 9186 | 10772 | 17369 | 2124 | 2344 | 2727 | 606 | 632 | 661 | 273 | 278 | 285 | 150 | 153 | 154 |
|  | *** | 9819 | 12470 | 17606 | 2222 | 2504 | 2748 | 618 | 645 | 652 | 276 | 281 | 271 | 153 | 154 | 140 |
| 0.7 | *** | 8325 | 9885 | 16011 | 1948 | 2150 | 2490 | 548 | 569 | 593 | 242 | 245 | 250 | 130 | 132 | 133 |
|  | *** | 8953 | 11515 | 16153 | 2040 | 2292 | 2496 | 558 | 580 | 581 | 243 | 249 | 236 | 132 | 132 | 118 |
| 0.75 | *** | 7392 | 8860 | 14236 | 1734 | 1906 | 2185 | 474 | 489 | 508 | 202 | 205 | 209 | 106 | 108 | 108 |
|  | *** | 7987 | 10348 | 14309 | 1811 | 2026 | 2182 | 480 | 498 | 495 | 204 | 208 | 194 | 106 | 108 | 93 |
| 0.8 | *** | 6374 | 7675 | 12043 | 1473 | 1608 | 1816 | 383 | 395 | 407 | 156 | 159 | 161 | . | . | . |
|  | *** | 6907 | 8953 | 12072 | 1534 | 1697 | 1806 | 390 | 401 | 393 | 157 | 159 | 145 | . | . | . |
| 0.85 | *** | 5238 | 6292 | 9441 | 1158 | 1249 | 1380 | 278 | 283 | 290 | . | . | . | . | . | . |
|  | *** | 5675 | 7282 | 9443 | 1199 | 1308 | 1366 | 281 | 287 | 275 | . | . | . | . | . | . |
| 0.9 | *** | 3906 | 4626 | 6431 | 775 | 821 | 879 | . | . | . | . | . | . | . | . | . |
|  | *** | 4210 | 5254 | 6421 | 797 | 848 | 864 | . | . | . | . | . | . | . | . | . |
| 0.95 | *** | 2184 | 2480 | 3021 | . | . | . | . | . | . | . | . | . | . | . | . |
|  | *** | 2315 | 2700 | 3007 | . | . | . | . | . | . | . | . | . | . | . | . |

TABLE 5: ALPHA= 0.025 POWER= 0.8    EXPECTED ACCRUAL THRU MINIMUM FOLLOW-UP= 3000

| | | DEL=.01 | | | DEL=.02 | | | DEL=.05 | | | DEL=.10 | | | DEL=.15 | | |
|---|---|---|---|---|---|---|---|---|---|---|---|---|---|---|---|---|---|
| FACT= | | 1.0 .75 | .50 .25 | .00 BIN | 1.0 .75 | .50 .25 | .00 BIN | 1.0 .75 | .50 .25 | .00 BIN | 1.0 75 | .50 .25 | .00 BIN | 1.0 .75 | .50 .25 | .00 BIN |
| PCONT=*** | | | | | | REQUIRED NUMBER OF PATIENTS | | | | | | | | | | |
| 0.01 | *** | 1202 | 1205 | 1210 | 440 | 440 | 445 | 145 | 145 | 145 | 73 | 73 | 73 | 50 | 50 | 50 |
| | *** | 1202 | 1205 | 4631 | 440 | 445 | 1531 | 145 | 145 | 417 | 73 | 73 | 170 | 50 | 50 | 101 |
| 0.02 | *** | 2653 | 2668 | 2702 | 853 | 857 | 865 | 230 | 230 | 230 | 100 | 100 | 103 | 65 | 65 | 65 |
| | *** | 2660 | 2680 | 7645 | 857 | 860 | 2277 | 230 | 230 | 532 | 100 | 103 | 197 | 65 | 65 | 113 |
| 0.05 | *** | 8035 | 8087 | 8440 | 2282 | 2308 | 2365 | 493 | 497 | 500 | 178 | 178 | 178 | 103 | 103 | 103 |
| | *** | 8050 | 8170 | 16310 | 2293 | 2330 | 4419 | 497 | 500 | 864 | 178 | 178 | 275 | 103 | 103 | 145 |
| 0.1 | *** | 17720 | 17860 | 19640 | 4772 | 4873 | 5195 | 932 | 947 | 965 | 295 | 295 | 298 | 155 | 155 | 160 |
| | *** | 17765 | 18122 | 29497 | 4810 | 4982 | 7677 | 940 | 958 | 1366 | 295 | 298 | 393 | 155 | 160 | 194 |
| 0.15 | *** | 26470 | 26720 | 31025 | 7010 | 7217 | 8035 | 1333 | 1367 | 1415 | 400 | 403 | 410 | 205 | 205 | 205 |
| | *** | 26552 | 27205 | 41113 | 7085 | 7460 | 10542 | 1348 | 1390 | 1806 | 403 | 407 | 495 | 205 | 205 | 236 |
| 0.2 | *** | 33530 | 33917 | 41683 | 8837 | 9170 | 10675 | 1675 | 1735 | 1828 | 490 | 497 | 508 | 242 | 245 | 245 |
| | *** | 33658 | 34678 | 51159 | 8957 | 9587 | 13014 | 1700 | 1775 | 2182 | 493 | 500 | 581 | 245 | 245 | 271 |
| 0.25 | *** | 38690 | 39250 | 51175 | 10210 | 10690 | 13015 | 1952 | 2042 | 2188 | 565 | 575 | 590 | 275 | 280 | 283 |
| | *** | 38875 | 40345 | 59636 | 10385 | 11297 | 15094 | 1993 | 2105 | 2496 | 572 | 583 | 652 | 275 | 280 | 299 |
| 0.3 | *** | 41960 | 42730 | 59260 | 11140 | 11780 | 14998 | 2162 | 2285 | 2488 | 625 | 640 | 658 | 302 | 305 | 310 |
| | *** | 42215 | 44233 | 66543 | 11375 | 12598 | 16781 | 2218 | 2372 | 2748 | 632 | 647 | 707 | 302 | 305 | 320 |
| 0.35 | *** | 43475 | 44503 | 65800 | 11665 | 12485 | 16595 | 2312 | 2465 | 2725 | 670 | 688 | 710 | 317 | 325 | 328 |
| | *** | 43817 | 46483 | 71881 | 11968 | 13513 | 18076 | 2380 | 2575 | 2936 | 677 | 700 | 746 | 320 | 325 | 334 |
| 0.4 | *** | 43427 | 44765 | 70715 | 11837 | 12845 | 17785 | 2405 | 2585 | 2897 | 695 | 718 | 745 | 328 | 332 | 340 |
| | *** | 43873 | 47305 | 75648 | 12215 | 14072 | 18979 | 2485 | 2713 | 3062 | 707 | 730 | 770 | 332 | 335 | 341 |
| 0.45 | *** | 42047 | 43768 | 73960 | 11713 | 12905 | 18553 | 2447 | 2645 | 2998 | 707 | 733 | 763 | 332 | 335 | 343 |
| | *** | 42625 | 46925 | 77846 | 12170 | 14315 | 19489 | 2537 | 2792 | 3124 | 718 | 745 | 778 | 335 | 340 | 341 |
| 0.5 | *** | 39598 | 41777 | 75505 | 11357 | 12715 | 18898 | 2440 | 2653 | 3032 | 703 | 730 | 763 | 328 | 332 | 340 |
| | *** | 40333 | 45587 | 78474 | 11882 | 14270 | 19607 | 2533 | 2810 | 3124 | 718 | 745 | 770 | 332 | 335 | 334 |
| 0.55 | *** | 36362 | 39065 | 75343 | 10820 | 12313 | 18815 | 2387 | 2608 | 2998 | 688 | 715 | 745 | 317 | 320 | 328 |
| | *** | 37288 | 43505 | 77532 | 11405 | 13967 | 19332 | 2485 | 2770 | 3062 | 700 | 730 | 746 | 320 | 325 | 320 |
| 0.6 | *** | 32627 | 35893 | 73475 | 10150 | 11728 | 18305 | 2290 | 2510 | 2897 | 655 | 680 | 710 | 298 | 305 | 310 |
| | *** | 33775 | 40862 | 75020 | 10775 | 13435 | 18665 | 2390 | 2672 | 2936 | 670 | 695 | 707 | 302 | 305 | 299 |
| 0.65 | *** | 28685 | 32470 | 69905 | 9373 | 10982 | 17368 | 2155 | 2368 | 2728 | 610 | 632 | 662 | 272 | 280 | 283 |
| | *** | 30058 | 37798 | 70939 | 10018 | 12680 | 17606 | 2248 | 2518 | 2748 | 620 | 647 | 652 | 275 | 280 | 271 |
| 0.7 | *** | 24790 | 28930 | 64640 | 8510 | 10090 | 16010 | 1978 | 2170 | 2492 | 550 | 568 | 595 | 242 | 245 | 250 |
| | *** | 26335 | 34385 | 65287 | 9148 | 11713 | 16153 | 2065 | 2308 | 2496 | 560 | 580 | 581 | 242 | 250 | 236 |
| 0.75 | *** | 21080 | 25340 | 57700 | 7570 | 9050 | 14233 | 1757 | 1922 | 2185 | 475 | 490 | 508 | 205 | 205 | 208 |
| | *** | 22705 | 30650 | 58067 | 8173 | 10528 | 14309 | 1832 | 2038 | 2182 | 482 | 500 | 495 | 205 | 208 | 194 |
| 0.8 | *** | 17590 | 21670 | 49097 | 6535 | 7840 | 12043 | 1490 | 1622 | 1817 | 385 | 395 | 407 | 155 | 160 | 160 |
| | *** | 19172 | 26552 | 49276 | 7070 | 9103 | 12072 | 1550 | 1708 | 1806 | 392 | 400 | 393 | 160 | 160 | 145 |
| 0.85 | *** | 14215 | 17815 | 38852 | 5368 | 6422 | 9440 | 1172 | 1258 | 1378 | 280 | 283 | 290 | . | . | . |
| | *** | 15628 | 21955 | 38915 | 5807 | 7393 | 9443 | 1210 | 1315 | 1366 | 280 | 287 | 275 | . | . | . |
| 0.9 | *** | 10730 | 13520 | 26980 | 4000 | 4712 | 6433 | 782 | 823 | 880 | . | . | . | . | . | . |
| | *** | 11845 | 16577 | 26985 | 4303 | 5323 | 6421 | 800 | 850 | 864 | . | . | . | . | . | . |
| 0.95 | *** | 6613 | 8173 | 13498 | 2222 | 2510 | 3020 | . | . | . | . | . | . | . | . | . |
| | *** | 7250 | 9710 | 13485 | 2350 | 2720 | 3007 | . | . | . | . | . | . | . | . | . |
| 0.98 | *** | 3085 | 3587 | 4648 | . | . | . | . | . | . | . | . | . | . | . | . |
| | *** | 3302 | 3988 | 4631 | . | . | . | . | . | . | . | . | . | . | . | . |

## TABLE 5: ALPHA= 0.025 POWER= 0.8    EXPECTED ACCRUAL THRU MINIMUM FOLLOW-UP= 3250

| PCONT | FACT= | DEL=.01 1.0 .75 | .50 .25 | .00 BIN | DEL=.02 1.0 .75 | .50 .25 | .00 BIN | DEL=.05 1.0 .75 | .50 .25 | .00 BIN | DEL=.10 1.0 75 | .50 .25 | .00 BIN | DEL=.15 1.0 .75 | .50 .25 | .00 BIN |
|---|---|---|---|---|---|---|---|---|---|---|---|---|---|---|---|---|

PCONT=***                                   REQUIRED NUMBER OF PATIENTS

| PCONT | FACT | 1.0/.75 | .50/.25 | .00/BIN | 1.0/.75 | .50/.25 | .00/BIN | 1.0/.75 | .50/.25 | .00/BIN | 1.0/75 | .50/.25 | .00/BIN | 1.0/.75 | .50/.25 | .00/BIN |
|---|---|---|---|---|---|---|---|---|---|---|---|---|---|---|---|---|
| 0.01 | *** | 1200 | 1205 | 1208 | 441 | 441 | 444 | 144 | 144 | 144 | 76 | 76 | 76 | 51 | 51 | 51 |
|  | *** | 1205 | 1208 | 4631 | 441 | 444 | 1531 | 144 | 144 | 417 | 76 | 76 | 170 | 51 | 51 | 101 |
| 0.02 | *** | 2654 | 2668 | 2700 | 856 | 859 | 864 | 230 | 233 | 233 | 100 | 100 | 100 | 68 | 68 | 68 |
|  | *** | 2662 | 2684 | 7645 | 856 | 859 | 2277 | 230 | 233 | 532 | 100 | 100 | 197 | 68 | 68 | 113 |
| 0.05 | *** | 8038 | 8095 | 8436 | 2286 | 2310 | 2362 | 493 | 498 | 501 | 176 | 176 | 176 | 103 | 103 | 103 |
|  | *** | 8057 | 8179 | 16310 | 2294 | 2334 | 4419 | 498 | 498 | 864 | 176 | 176 | 275 | 103 | 103 | 145 |
| 0.1 | *** | 17731 | 17881 | 19641 | 4780 | 4886 | 5194 | 937 | 948 | 964 | 295 | 295 | 298 | 157 | 157 | 157 |
|  | *** | 17783 | 18162 | 29497 | 4824 | 4994 | 7677 | 940 | 956 | 1366 | 295 | 298 | 393 | 157 | 157 | 194 |
| 0.15 | *** | 26490 | 26761 | 31027 | 7031 | 7245 | 8033 | 1338 | 1371 | 1416 | 401 | 404 | 409 | 206 | 206 | 206 |
|  | *** | 26579 | 27278 | 41113 | 7112 | 7489 | 10542 | 1351 | 1392 | 1806 | 401 | 409 | 495 | 206 | 206 | 236 |
| 0.2 | *** | 33562 | 33981 | 41684 | 8867 | 9216 | 10674 | 1684 | 1741 | 1831 | 490 | 498 | 506 | 241 | 246 | 246 |
|  | *** | 33705 | 34797 | 51159 | 8997 | 9634 | 13014 | 1709 | 1782 | 2182 | 493 | 501 | 581 | 246 | 246 | 271 |
| 0.25 | *** | 38734 | 39344 | 51174 | 10256 | 10755 | 13014 | 1964 | 2050 | 2188 | 566 | 579 | 591 | 274 | 279 | 282 |
|  | *** | 38938 | 40522 | 59636 | 10438 | 11369 | 15094 | 2001 | 2110 | 2496 | 571 | 582 | 652 | 279 | 279 | 299 |
| 0.3 | *** | 42025 | 42857 | 59258 | 11199 | 11873 | 15001 | 2180 | 2297 | 2489 | 628 | 639 | 661 | 303 | 303 | 306 |
|  | *** | 42304 | 44471 | 66543 | 11451 | 12697 | 16781 | 2232 | 2378 | 2748 | 636 | 647 | 707 | 303 | 306 | 320 |
| 0.35 | *** | 43561 | 44674 | 65799 | 11743 | 12599 | 16597 | 2334 | 2481 | 2724 | 672 | 688 | 709 | 319 | 322 | 328 |
|  | *** | 43929 | 46794 | 71881 | 12063 | 13636 | 18076 | 2399 | 2581 | 2936 | 680 | 696 | 746 | 319 | 328 | 334 |
| 0.4 | *** | 43536 | 44986 | 70714 | 11933 | 12981 | 17783 | 2427 | 2603 | 2895 | 696 | 721 | 745 | 328 | 336 | 339 |
|  | *** | 44024 | 47691 | 75648 | 12331 | 14216 | 18979 | 2505 | 2724 | 3062 | 709 | 729 | 770 | 331 | 336 | 341 |
| 0.45 | *** | 42191 | 44051 | 73959 | 11836 | 13062 | 18552 | 2473 | 2668 | 3001 | 712 | 734 | 761 | 331 | 339 | 344 |
|  | *** | 42816 | 47399 | 77846 | 12307 | 14476 | 19489 | 2557 | 2806 | 3124 | 721 | 745 | 778 | 336 | 339 | 341 |
| 0.5 | *** | 39783 | 42126 | 75503 | 11499 | 12892 | 18896 | 2464 | 2676 | 3033 | 709 | 734 | 761 | 328 | 336 | 339 |
|  | *** | 40579 | 46139 | 78474 | 12039 | 14449 | 19607 | 2557 | 2825 | 3124 | 721 | 745 | 770 | 331 | 336 | 334 |
| 0.55 | *** | 36592 | 39490 | 75346 | 10979 | 12499 | 18815 | 2416 | 2630 | 3001 | 693 | 718 | 745 | 319 | 322 | 328 |
|  | *** | 37592 | 44124 | 77532 | 11576 | 14159 | 19332 | 2508 | 2784 | 3062 | 704 | 729 | 746 | 319 | 328 | 320 |
| 0.6 | *** | 32917 | 36381 | 73477 | 10316 | 11922 | 18303 | 2318 | 2532 | 2898 | 661 | 685 | 712 | 298 | 303 | 311 |
|  | *** | 34147 | 41532 | 75020 | 10958 | 13628 | 18665 | 2416 | 2687 | 2936 | 672 | 696 | 707 | 303 | 306 | 299 |
| 0.65 | *** | 29041 | 33009 | 69905 | 9549 | 11177 | 17369 | 2180 | 2386 | 2727 | 615 | 636 | 661 | 274 | 279 | 282 |
|  | *** | 30488 | 38494 | 70939 | 10202 | 12873 | 17606 | 2272 | 2532 | 2748 | 623 | 647 | 652 | 279 | 282 | 271 |
| 0.7 | *** | 25193 | 29499 | 64640 | 8683 | 10281 | 16012 | 2001 | 2188 | 2489 | 555 | 571 | 591 | 241 | 246 | 249 |
|  | *** | 26807 | 35081 | 65287 | 9333 | 11892 | 16153 | 2086 | 2318 | 2496 | 563 | 582 | 581 | 246 | 249 | 236 |
| 0.75 | *** | 21512 | 25905 | 57701 | 7732 | 9224 | 14232 | 1777 | 1939 | 2188 | 477 | 493 | 509 | 206 | 206 | 209 |
|  | *** | 23194 | 31316 | 58067 | 8342 | 10690 | 14309 | 1850 | 2045 | 2182 | 485 | 501 | 495 | 206 | 209 | 194 |
| 0.8 | *** | 18016 | 22200 | 49097 | 6681 | 7989 | 12044 | 1509 | 1631 | 1814 | 387 | 396 | 409 | 157 | 160 | 160 |
|  | *** | 19641 | 27151 | 49276 | 7221 | 9236 | 12072 | 1566 | 1712 | 1806 | 393 | 401 | 393 | 157 | 160 | 145 |
| 0.85 | *** | 14595 | 18271 | 38851 | 5490 | 6543 | 9439 | 1184 | 1265 | 1379 | 279 | 287 | 290 | . | . | . |
|  | *** | 16044 | 22455 | 38915 | 5929 | 7497 | 9443 | 1221 | 1319 | 1366 | 282 | 287 | 275 | . | . | . |
| 0.9 | *** | 11031 | 13867 | 26978 | 4081 | 4788 | 6432 | 786 | 826 | 880 | . | . | . | . | . | . |
|  | *** | 12166 | 16935 | 26985 | 4385 | 5384 | 6421 | 807 | 851 | 864 | . | . | . | . | . | . |
| 0.95 | *** | 6790 | 8355 | 13498 | 2261 | 2538 | 3020 | . | . | . | . | . | . | . | . | . |
|  | *** | 7432 | 9877 | 13485 | 2383 | 2741 | 3007 | . | . | . | . | . | . | . | . | . |
| 0.98 | *** | 3147 | 3637 | 4645 | . | . | . | . | . | . | . | . | . | . | . | . |
|  | *** | 3361 | 4027 | 4631 | . | . | . | . | . | . | . | . | . | . | . | . |

## TABLE 5: ALPHA= 0.025 POWER= 0.8    EXPECTED ACCRUAL THRU MINIMUM FOLLOW-UP= 3500

| | | DEL=.01 | | | DEL=.02 | | | DEL=.05 | | | DEL=.10 | | | DEL=.15 | |
|---|---|---|---|---|---|---|---|---|---|---|---|---|---|---|---|
| FACT= | 1.0 .75 | .50 .25 | .00 BIN | 1.0 .75 | .50 .25 | .00 BIN | 1.0 .75 | .50 .25 | .00 BIN | 1.0 75 | .50 .25 | .00 BIN | 1.0 .75 | .50 .25 | .00 BIN |
| PCONT=*** | | | | REQUIRED NUMBER OF PATIENTS | | | | | | | | | | | |
| 0.01 *** | 1201 | 1205 | 1210 | 440 | 443 | 443 | 146 | 146 | 146 | 73 | 73 | 73 | 50 | 50 | 50 |
| *** | 1205 | 1205 | 4631 | 443 | 443 | 1531 | 146 | 146 | 417 | 73 | 73 | 170 | 50 | 50 | 101 |
| 0.02 *** | 2657 | 2671 | 2701 | 855 | 860 | 863 | 230 | 230 | 233 | 102 | 102 | 102 | 67 | 67 | 67 |
| *** | 2663 | 2683 | 7645 | 855 | 860 | 2277 | 230 | 233 | 532 | 102 | 102 | 197 | 67 | 67 | 113 |
| 0.05 *** | 8044 | 8105 | 8438 | 2286 | 2313 | 2365 | 496 | 496 | 501 | 178 | 178 | 178 | 102 | 102 | 102 |
| *** | 8065 | 8193 | 16310 | 2298 | 2333 | 4419 | 496 | 501 | 864 | 178 | 178 | 275 | 102 | 102 | 145 |
| 0.1 *** | 17742 | 17905 | 19641 | 4792 | 4897 | 5195 | 939 | 951 | 965 | 295 | 295 | 300 | 155 | 155 | 160 |
| *** | 17800 | 18197 | 29497 | 4833 | 5002 | 7677 | 942 | 956 | 1366 | 295 | 295 | 393 | 155 | 160 | 194 |
| 0.15 *** | 26510 | 26804 | 31025 | 7050 | 7268 | 8035 | 1341 | 1371 | 1415 | 400 | 405 | 408 | 204 | 204 | 207 |
| *** | 26606 | 27355 | 41113 | 7134 | 7513 | 10542 | 1359 | 1394 | 1806 | 405 | 405 | 495 | 204 | 204 | 236 |
| 0.2 *** | 33594 | 34049 | 41682 | 8896 | 9260 | 10672 | 1691 | 1747 | 1826 | 493 | 501 | 505 | 242 | 248 | 248 |
| *** | 33746 | 34918 | 51159 | 9033 | 9680 | 13014 | 1718 | 1782 | 2182 | 496 | 501 | 581 | 242 | 248 | 271 |
| 0.25 *** | 38783 | 39433 | 51173 | 10296 | 10818 | 13014 | 1975 | 2059 | 2190 | 566 | 580 | 589 | 277 | 277 | 283 |
| *** | 39001 | 40690 | 59636 | 10494 | 11439 | 15094 | 2010 | 2115 | 2496 | 575 | 583 | 652 | 277 | 283 | 299 |
| 0.3 *** | 42090 | 42986 | 59258 | 11258 | 11955 | 15000 | 2193 | 2307 | 2488 | 627 | 641 | 659 | 300 | 303 | 309 |
| *** | 42388 | 44701 | 66543 | 11521 | 12786 | 16781 | 2243 | 2386 | 2748 | 636 | 650 | 707 | 303 | 309 | 320 |
| 0.35 *** | 43648 | 44841 | 65797 | 11818 | 12702 | 16596 | 2351 | 2491 | 2724 | 671 | 688 | 711 | 318 | 321 | 326 |
| *** | 44045 | 47095 | 71881 | 12156 | 13749 | 18076 | 2412 | 2593 | 2936 | 680 | 697 | 746 | 321 | 326 | 334 |
| 0.4 *** | 43651 | 45208 | 70715 | 12028 | 13110 | 17783 | 2447 | 2619 | 2893 | 703 | 720 | 746 | 330 | 335 | 338 |
| *** | 44173 | 48070 | 75648 | 12445 | 14353 | 18979 | 2526 | 2736 | 3062 | 711 | 732 | 770 | 330 | 338 | 341 |
| 0.45 *** | 42335 | 44330 | 73958 | 11950 | 13210 | 18553 | 2496 | 2683 | 2998 | 715 | 738 | 764 | 335 | 338 | 344 |
| *** | 43009 | 47851 | 77846 | 12436 | 14627 | 19489 | 2578 | 2815 | 3124 | 723 | 746 | 778 | 335 | 338 | 341 |
| 0.5 *** | 39967 | 42475 | 75506 | 11631 | 13052 | 18897 | 2491 | 2692 | 3033 | 711 | 732 | 764 | 330 | 335 | 338 |
| *** | 40821 | 46666 | 78474 | 12186 | 14615 | 19607 | 2584 | 2838 | 3124 | 723 | 746 | 770 | 330 | 338 | 334 |
| 0.55 *** | 36826 | 39903 | 75343 | 11127 | 12676 | 18815 | 2438 | 2648 | 2998 | 694 | 720 | 746 | 318 | 321 | 330 |
| *** | 37893 | 44715 | 77532 | 11740 | 14335 | 19332 | 2535 | 2797 | 3062 | 706 | 732 | 746 | 321 | 326 | 320 |
| 0.6 *** | 33209 | 36858 | 73476 | 10476 | 12104 | 18302 | 2342 | 2552 | 2899 | 662 | 685 | 711 | 300 | 303 | 309 |
| *** | 34507 | 42172 | 75020 | 11127 | 13805 | 18665 | 2438 | 2701 | 2936 | 671 | 697 | 707 | 303 | 309 | 299 |
| 0.65 *** | 29385 | 33527 | 69906 | 9715 | 11360 | 17371 | 2208 | 2403 | 2727 | 615 | 636 | 659 | 274 | 277 | 283 |
| *** | 30908 | 39153 | 70939 | 10380 | 13043 | 17606 | 2295 | 2543 | 2748 | 627 | 650 | 652 | 277 | 283 | 271 |
| 0.7 *** | 25582 | 30041 | 64642 | 8849 | 10453 | 16010 | 2024 | 2208 | 2491 | 554 | 571 | 592 | 242 | 248 | 251 |
| *** | 27262 | 35738 | 65287 | 9505 | 12060 | 16153 | 2106 | 2330 | 2496 | 563 | 583 | 581 | 242 | 248 | 236 |
| 0.75 *** | 21925 | 26440 | 57700 | 7890 | 9386 | 14233 | 1800 | 1954 | 2185 | 478 | 493 | 510 | 204 | 207 | 207 |
| *** | 23663 | 31940 | 58067 | 8502 | 10835 | 14309 | 1870 | 2053 | 2182 | 487 | 501 | 495 | 204 | 207 | 194 |
| 0.8 *** | 18416 | 22695 | 49099 | 6819 | 8131 | 12043 | 1525 | 1642 | 1814 | 388 | 396 | 408 | 155 | 160 | 160 |
| *** | 20087 | 27714 | 49276 | 7361 | 9360 | 12072 | 1578 | 1721 | 1806 | 391 | 400 | 393 | 160 | 160 | 145 |
| 0.85 *** | 14956 | 18696 | 38853 | 5603 | 6653 | 9438 | 1193 | 1271 | 1380 | 277 | 286 | 291 | . | . | . |
| *** | 16435 | 22919 | 38915 | 6043 | 7589 | 9443 | 1231 | 1324 | 1366 | 283 | 286 | 275 | . | . | . |
| 0.9 *** | 11316 | 14186 | 26979 | 4162 | 4859 | 6434 | 793 | 834 | 878 | . | . | . | . | . | . |
| *** | 12466 | 17261 | 26985 | 4460 | 5436 | 6421 | 811 | 855 | 864 | . | . | . | . | . | . |
| 0.95 *** | 6953 | 8525 | 13498 | 2295 | 2566 | 3021 | . | . | . | . | . | . | . | . | . |
| *** | 7601 | 10030 | 13485 | 2412 | 2759 | 3007 | . | . | . | . | . | . | . | . | . |
| 0.98 *** | 3200 | 3686 | 4649 | . | . | . | . | . | . | . | . | . | . | . | . |
| *** | 3415 | 4063 | 4631 | . | . | . | . | . | . | . | . | . | . | . | . |

## TABLE 5: ALPHA= 0.025 POWER= 0.8     EXPECTED ACCRUAL THRU MINIMUM FOLLOW-UP= 3750

PCONT=***                              REQUIRED NUMBER OF PATIENTS

|  |  | DEL=.01 | | | DEL=.02 | | | DEL=.05 | | | DEL=.10 | | | DEL=.15 | | |
|---|---|---|---|---|---|---|---|---|---|---|---|---|---|---|---|---|
| FACT= | | 1.0 .75 | .50 .25 | .00 BIN | 1.0 .75 | .50 .25 | .00 BIN | 1.0 .75 | .50 .25 | .00 BIN | 1.0 75 | .50 .25 | .00 BIN | 1.0 .75 | .50 .25 | .00 BIN |
| 0.01 | *** | 1203 | 1206 | 1212 | 443 | 443 | 443 | 147 | 147 | 147 | 72 | 72 | 72 | 53 | 53 | 53 |
|  | *** | 1203 | 1206 | 4631 | 443 | 443 | 1531 | 147 | 147 | 417 | 72 | 72 | 170 | 53 | 53 | 101 |
| 0.02 | *** | 2659 | 2669 | 2703 | 856 | 859 | 865 | 231 | 231 | 231 | 100 | 100 | 100 | 68 | 68 | 68 |
|  | *** | 2665 | 2684 | 7645 | 856 | 859 | 2277 | 231 | 231 | 532 | 100 | 100 | 197 | 68 | 68 | 113 |
| 0.05 | *** | 8047 | 8112 | 8440 | 2290 | 2318 | 2365 | 494 | 500 | 500 | 175 | 175 | 175 | 106 | 106 | 106 |
|  | *** | 8069 | 8200 | 16310 | 2300 | 2337 | 4419 | 494 | 500 | 864 | 175 | 175 | 275 | 106 | 106 | 145 |
| 0.1 | *** | 17753 | 17928 | 19638 | 4803 | 4909 | 5197 | 940 | 950 | 968 | 293 | 297 | 297 | 156 | 156 | 156 |
|  | *** | 17815 | 18231 | 29497 | 4844 | 5013 | 7677 | 944 | 959 | 1366 | 297 | 297 | 393 | 156 | 156 | 194 |
| 0.15 | *** | 26534 | 26843 | 31025 | 7066 | 7297 | 8031 | 1347 | 1375 | 1418 | 400 | 406 | 409 | 203 | 203 | 203 |
|  | *** | 26637 | 27425 | 41113 | 7156 | 7540 | 10542 | 1362 | 1394 | 1806 | 400 | 406 | 495 | 203 | 203 | 236 |
| 0.2 | *** | 33625 | 34113 | 41684 | 8928 | 9297 | 10675 | 1694 | 1750 | 1831 | 494 | 500 | 509 | 247 | 247 | 247 |
|  | *** | 33790 | 35031 | 51159 | 9068 | 9719 | 13014 | 1722 | 1784 | 2182 | 494 | 503 | 581 | 247 | 247 | 271 |
| 0.25 | *** | 38828 | 39528 | 51172 | 10343 | 10878 | 13015 | 1981 | 2065 | 2187 | 569 | 578 | 588 | 275 | 278 | 284 |
|  | *** | 39063 | 40859 | 59636 | 10544 | 11497 | 15094 | 2018 | 2122 | 2496 | 575 | 584 | 652 | 278 | 278 | 299 |
| 0.3 | *** | 42153 | 43113 | 59256 | 11318 | 12034 | 14997 | 2206 | 2318 | 2487 | 631 | 644 | 659 | 303 | 306 | 306 |
|  | *** | 42475 | 44931 | 66543 | 11590 | 12869 | 16781 | 2256 | 2393 | 2748 | 634 | 650 | 707 | 303 | 306 | 320 |
| 0.35 | *** | 43731 | 45012 | 65800 | 11894 | 12803 | 16597 | 2365 | 2506 | 2725 | 678 | 691 | 709 | 322 | 325 | 325 |
|  | *** | 44159 | 47393 | 71881 | 12241 | 13850 | 18076 | 2431 | 2600 | 2936 | 681 | 700 | 746 | 322 | 325 | 334 |
| 0.4 | *** | 43759 | 45428 | 70713 | 12125 | 13231 | 17781 | 2468 | 2631 | 2894 | 706 | 725 | 743 | 331 | 334 | 340 |
|  | *** | 44322 | 48438 | 75648 | 12550 | 14472 | 18979 | 2543 | 2744 | 3062 | 715 | 734 | 770 | 331 | 334 | 341 |
| 0.45 | *** | 42481 | 44609 | 73956 | 12063 | 13347 | 18550 | 2515 | 2697 | 2997 | 715 | 738 | 762 | 334 | 340 | 344 |
|  | *** | 43197 | 48293 | 77846 | 12565 | 14768 | 19489 | 2600 | 2828 | 3124 | 728 | 747 | 778 | 334 | 340 | 341 |
| 0.5 | *** | 40150 | 42813 | 75503 | 11759 | 13206 | 18897 | 2515 | 2712 | 3034 | 715 | 738 | 762 | 331 | 334 | 340 |
|  | *** | 41065 | 47172 | 78474 | 12331 | 14768 | 19607 | 2603 | 2847 | 3124 | 725 | 747 | 770 | 331 | 334 | 334 |
| 0.55 | *** | 37056 | 40306 | 75344 | 11272 | 12841 | 18813 | 2463 | 2669 | 2997 | 697 | 719 | 743 | 316 | 325 | 331 |
|  | *** | 38197 | 45278 | 77532 | 11894 | 14491 | 19332 | 2556 | 2809 | 3062 | 709 | 734 | 746 | 322 | 325 | 320 |
| 0.6 | *** | 33494 | 37315 | 73475 | 10628 | 12275 | 18303 | 2369 | 2572 | 2900 | 663 | 687 | 709 | 303 | 306 | 312 |
|  | *** | 34868 | 42775 | 75020 | 11290 | 13972 | 18665 | 2459 | 2712 | 2936 | 678 | 697 | 707 | 303 | 306 | 299 |
| 0.65 | *** | 29725 | 34028 | 69906 | 9869 | 11528 | 17369 | 2228 | 2422 | 2725 | 622 | 640 | 659 | 275 | 278 | 284 |
|  | *** | 31315 | 39781 | 70939 | 10544 | 13206 | 17606 | 2318 | 2553 | 2748 | 631 | 650 | 652 | 278 | 284 | 271 |
| 0.7 | *** | 25966 | 30556 | 64643 | 9003 | 10619 | 16009 | 2047 | 2219 | 2491 | 556 | 575 | 593 | 241 | 247 | 250 |
|  | *** | 27706 | 36359 | 65287 | 9663 | 12209 | 16153 | 2125 | 2337 | 2496 | 565 | 584 | 581 | 247 | 247 | 236 |
| 0.75 | *** | 22325 | 26947 | 57700 | 8031 | 9531 | 14234 | 1816 | 1966 | 2187 | 481 | 494 | 509 | 203 | 209 | 209 |
|  | *** | 24106 | 32528 | 58067 | 8650 | 10972 | 14309 | 1887 | 2065 | 2182 | 484 | 500 | 495 | 203 | 209 | 194 |
| 0.8 | *** | 18803 | 23168 | 49100 | 6950 | 8256 | 12044 | 1540 | 1653 | 1816 | 391 | 397 | 406 | 156 | 156 | 162 |
|  | *** | 20509 | 28234 | 49276 | 7493 | 9472 | 12072 | 1591 | 1728 | 1806 | 391 | 400 | 393 | 156 | 162 | 145 |
| 0.85 | *** | 15303 | 19100 | 38853 | 5706 | 6753 | 9438 | 1203 | 1278 | 1381 | 278 | 284 | 288 | . | . | . |
|  | *** | 16806 | 23350 | 38915 | 6147 | 7672 | 9443 | 1240 | 1325 | 1366 | 284 | 288 | 275 | . | . | . |
| 0.9 | *** | 11584 | 14491 | 26978 | 4234 | 4925 | 6434 | 800 | 837 | 878 | . | . | . | . | . | . |
|  | *** | 12753 | 17566 | 26985 | 4531 | 5487 | 6421 | 813 | 856 | 864 | . | . | . | . | . | . |
| 0.95 | *** | 7109 | 8678 | 13497 | 2322 | 2584 | 3022 | . | . | . | . | . | . | . | . | . |
|  | *** | 7759 | 10165 | 13485 | 2440 | 2772 | 3007 | . | . | . | . | . | . | . | . | . |
| 0.98 | *** | 3256 | 3728 | 4647 | . | . | . | . | . | . | . | . | . | . | . | . |
|  | *** | 3462 | 4094 | 4631 | . | . | . | . | . | . | . | . | . | . | . | . |

TABLE 5: ALPHA= 0.025 POWER= 0.8     EXPECTED ACCRUAL THRU MINIMUM FOLLOW-UP= 4000

| | | DEL=.01 | | | DEL=.02 | | | DEL=.05 | | | DEL=.10 | | | DEL=.15 | | |
|---|---|---|---|---|---|---|---|---|---|---|---|---|---|---|---|---|---|
| FACT= | | 1.0 .75 | .50 .25 | .00 BIN | 1.0 .75 | .50 .25 | .00 BIN | 1.0 .75 | .50 .25 | .00 BIN | 1.0 75 | .50 .25 | .00 BIN | 1.0 .75 | .50 .25 | .00 BIN |
| PCONT=*** | | | | | REQUIRED NUMBER OF PATIENTS | | | | | | | | | | | |
| 0.01 | *** | 1203 | 1207 | 1213 | 443 | 443 | 443 | 147 | 147 | 147 | 73 | 73 | 73 | 53 | 53 | 53 |
| | *** | 1203 | 1207 | 4631 | 443 | 443 | 1531 | 147 | 147 | 417 | 73 | 73 | 170 | 53 | 53 | 101 |
| 0.02 | *** | 2657 | 2673 | 2703 | 857 | 857 | 863 | 233 | 233 | 233 | 103 | 103 | 103 | 67 | 67 | 67 |
| | *** | 2667 | 2683 | 7645 | 857 | 863 | 2277 | 233 | 233 | 532 | 103 | 103 | 197 | 67 | 67 | 113 |
| 0.05 | *** | 8053 | 8117 | 8437 | 2293 | 2317 | 2363 | 497 | 497 | 503 | 177 | 177 | 177 | 103 | 103 | 103 |
| | *** | 8077 | 8207 | 16310 | 2303 | 2337 | 4419 | 497 | 497 | 864 | 177 | 177 | 275 | 103 | 103 | 145 |
| 0.1 | *** | 17767 | 17953 | 19637 | 4813 | 4923 | 5193 | 937 | 953 | 967 | 297 | 297 | 297 | 157 | 157 | 157 |
| | *** | 17827 | 18267 | 29497 | 4857 | 5023 | 7677 | 947 | 957 | 1366 | 297 | 297 | 393 | 157 | 157 | 194 |
| 0.15 | *** | 26553 | 26883 | 31027 | 7087 | 7317 | 8033 | 1347 | 1377 | 1417 | 403 | 407 | 407 | 203 | 203 | 207 |
| | *** | 26663 | 27497 | 41113 | 7177 | 7557 | 10542 | 1363 | 1397 | 1806 | 403 | 407 | 495 | 203 | 207 | 236 |
| 0.2 | *** | 33657 | 34177 | 41683 | 8957 | 9337 | 10673 | 1703 | 1753 | 1827 | 493 | 503 | 507 | 243 | 247 | 247 |
| | *** | 33833 | 35147 | 51159 | 9103 | 9757 | 13014 | 1727 | 1787 | 2182 | 497 | 503 | 581 | 243 | 247 | 271 |
| 0.25 | *** | 38877 | 39617 | 51173 | 10383 | 10933 | 13017 | 1993 | 2073 | 2187 | 573 | 583 | 593 | 277 | 277 | 283 |
| | *** | 39123 | 41023 | 59636 | 10593 | 11553 | 15094 | 2027 | 2123 | 2496 | 577 | 587 | 652 | 277 | 283 | 299 |
| 0.3 | *** | 42217 | 43243 | 59257 | 11377 | 12113 | 14997 | 2217 | 2323 | 2487 | 633 | 643 | 657 | 303 | 307 | 307 |
| | *** | 42557 | 45153 | 66543 | 11657 | 12943 | 16781 | 2267 | 2397 | 2748 | 637 | 653 | 707 | 303 | 307 | 320 |
| 0.35 | *** | 43817 | 45183 | 65797 | 11967 | 12903 | 16597 | 2383 | 2517 | 2723 | 677 | 693 | 707 | 323 | 323 | 327 |
| | *** | 44273 | 47677 | 71881 | 12327 | 13947 | 18076 | 2443 | 2607 | 2936 | 683 | 703 | 746 | 323 | 327 | 334 |
| 0.4 | *** | 43873 | 45643 | 70717 | 12217 | 13343 | 17783 | 2487 | 2643 | 2897 | 707 | 723 | 743 | 333 | 337 | 337 |
| | *** | 44467 | 48793 | 75648 | 12653 | 14587 | 18979 | 2557 | 2753 | 3062 | 713 | 733 | 770 | 333 | 337 | 341 |
| 0.45 | *** | 42623 | 44877 | 73957 | 12167 | 13477 | 18553 | 2537 | 2713 | 2997 | 717 | 737 | 763 | 333 | 337 | 343 |
| | *** | 43387 | 48717 | 77846 | 12683 | 14897 | 19489 | 2617 | 2837 | 3124 | 727 | 747 | 778 | 337 | 343 | 341 |
| 0.5 | *** | 40333 | 43147 | 75507 | 11883 | 13353 | 18897 | 2533 | 2727 | 3033 | 717 | 737 | 763 | 333 | 333 | 343 |
| | *** | 41303 | 47663 | 78474 | 12463 | 14907 | 19607 | 2623 | 2857 | 3124 | 727 | 747 | 770 | 333 | 337 | 334 |
| 0.55 | *** | 37287 | 40697 | 75343 | 11407 | 12993 | 18813 | 2483 | 2683 | 2997 | 697 | 723 | 747 | 317 | 323 | 327 |
| | *** | 38487 | 45817 | 77532 | 12043 | 14643 | 19332 | 2573 | 2817 | 3062 | 707 | 733 | 746 | 323 | 327 | 320 |
| 0.6 | *** | 33777 | 37757 | 73477 | 10773 | 12433 | 18303 | 2387 | 2587 | 2897 | 667 | 687 | 713 | 303 | 307 | 313 |
| | *** | 35217 | 43353 | 75020 | 11443 | 14123 | 18665 | 2477 | 2723 | 2936 | 677 | 697 | 707 | 303 | 307 | 299 |
| 0.65 | *** | 30057 | 34507 | 69903 | 10017 | 11693 | 17367 | 2247 | 2437 | 2727 | 623 | 637 | 663 | 277 | 277 | 283 |
| | *** | 31713 | 40373 | 70939 | 10697 | 13353 | 17606 | 2333 | 2563 | 2748 | 627 | 647 | 652 | 277 | 283 | 271 |
| 0.7 | *** | 26333 | 31053 | 64643 | 9147 | 10773 | 16013 | 2063 | 2233 | 2493 | 557 | 573 | 593 | 243 | 247 | 247 |
| | *** | 28127 | 36943 | 65287 | 9813 | 12347 | 16153 | 2143 | 2347 | 2496 | 567 | 583 | 581 | 247 | 247 | 236 |
| 0.75 | *** | 22707 | 27433 | 57703 | 8173 | 9673 | 14233 | 1833 | 1977 | 2187 | 483 | 493 | 507 | 203 | 207 | 207 |
| | *** | 24533 | 33083 | 58067 | 8793 | 11097 | 14309 | 1897 | 2067 | 2182 | 487 | 503 | 495 | 207 | 207 | 194 |
| 0.8 | *** | 19173 | 23613 | 49097 | 7073 | 8377 | 12043 | 1553 | 1663 | 1817 | 393 | 397 | 407 | 157 | 157 | 163 |
| | *** | 20913 | 28733 | 49276 | 7617 | 9577 | 12072 | 1603 | 1733 | 1806 | 393 | 403 | 393 | 157 | 157 | 145 |
| 0.85 | *** | 15627 | 19483 | 38853 | 5807 | 6843 | 9443 | 1213 | 1283 | 1377 | 283 | 287 | 293 | . | . | . |
| | *** | 17157 | 23757 | 38915 | 6247 | 7747 | 9443 | 1247 | 1327 | 1366 | 283 | 287 | 275 | . | . | . |
| 0.9 | *** | 11843 | 14773 | 26977 | 4303 | 4983 | 6433 | 803 | 837 | 877 | . | . | . | . | . | . |
| | *** | 13023 | 17853 | 26985 | 4597 | 5533 | 6421 | 817 | 857 | 864 | . | . | . | . | . | . |
| 0.95 | *** | 7253 | 8823 | 13497 | 2353 | 2607 | 3023 | . | . | . | . | . | . | . | . | . |
| | *** | 7903 | 10293 | 13485 | 2467 | 2783 | 3007 | . | . | . | . | . | . | . | . | . |
| 0.98 | *** | 3303 | 3767 | 4647 | . | . | . | . | . | . | . | . | . | . | . | . |
| | *** | 3507 | 4123 | 4631 | . | . | . | . | . | . | . | . | . | . | . | . |

TABLE 5: ALPHA= 0.025 POWER= 0.8    EXPECTED ACCRUAL THRU MINIMUM FOLLOW-UP= 4250

| | DEL=.01 | | | DEL=.02 | | | DEL=.05 | | | DEL=.10 | | | DEL=.15 | | |
|---|---|---|---|---|---|---|---|---|---|---|---|---|---|---|---|
| FACT= | 1.0 | .50 | .00 | 1.0 | .50 | .00 | 1.0 | .50 | .00 | 1.0 | .50 | .00 | 1.0 | .50 | .00 |
| | .75 | .25 | BIN | .75 | .25 | BIN | .75 | .25 | BIN | 75 | .25 | BIN | .75 | .25 | BIN |

PCONT=***                    REQUIRED NUMBER OF PATIENTS

| PCONT | 1.0/.75 | .50/.25 | .00/BIN | 1.0/.75 | .50/.25 | .00/BIN | 1.0/.75 | .50/.25 | .00/BIN | 1.0/75 | .50/.25 | .00/BIN | 1.0/.75 | .50/.25 | .00/BIN |
|---|---|---|---|---|---|---|---|---|---|---|---|---|---|---|---|
| 0.01 *** | 1204 | 1204 | 1208 | 443 | 443 | 443 | 145 | 145 | 145 | 71 | 71 | 71 | 50 | 50 | 50 |
| *** | 1204 | 1208 | 4631 | 443 | 443 | 1531 | 145 | 145 | 417 | 71 | 71 | 170 | 50 | 50 | 101 |
| 0.02 *** | 2659 | 2674 | 2702 | 857 | 857 | 864 | 230 | 230 | 230 | 103 | 103 | 103 | 67 | 67 | 67 |
| *** | 2663 | 2685 | 7645 | 857 | 864 | 2277 | 230 | 230 | 532 | 103 | 103 | 197 | 67 | 67 | 113 |
| 0.05 *** | 8057 | 8125 | 8439 | 2292 | 2319 | 2366 | 496 | 496 | 503 | 177 | 177 | 177 | 103 | 103 | 103 |
| *** | 8082 | 8216 | 16310 | 2309 | 2341 | 4419 | 496 | 503 | 864 | 177 | 177 | 275 | 103 | 103 | 145 |
| 0.1 *** | 17779 | 17974 | 19638 | 4820 | 4933 | 5192 | 942 | 953 | 963 | 294 | 294 | 301 | 156 | 156 | 156 |
| *** | 17843 | 18303 | 29497 | 4863 | 5029 | 7677 | 949 | 959 | 1366 | 294 | 294 | 393 | 156 | 156 | 194 |
| 0.15 *** | 26576 | 26927 | 31028 | 7105 | 7338 | 8036 | 1353 | 1378 | 1416 | 400 | 407 | 407 | 205 | 205 | 205 |
| *** | 26693 | 27564 | 41113 | 7196 | 7579 | 10542 | 1363 | 1399 | 1806 | 400 | 407 | 495 | 205 | 205 | 236 |
| 0.2 *** | 33695 | 34241 | 41685 | 8985 | 9374 | 10675 | 1707 | 1756 | 1831 | 496 | 503 | 507 | 241 | 248 | 248 |
| *** | 33876 | 35257 | 51159 | 9134 | 9789 | 13014 | 1728 | 1788 | 2182 | 496 | 503 | 581 | 248 | 248 | 271 |
| 0.25 *** | 38923 | 39713 | 51173 | 10426 | 10989 | 13012 | 2001 | 2075 | 2185 | 570 | 581 | 592 | 279 | 279 | 279 |
| *** | 39188 | 41186 | 59636 | 10643 | 11606 | 15094 | 2037 | 2128 | 2496 | 577 | 588 | 652 | 279 | 279 | 299 |
| 0.3 *** | 42280 | 43368 | 59259 | 11429 | 12183 | 14999 | 2228 | 2334 | 2489 | 634 | 645 | 655 | 301 | 305 | 311 |
| *** | 42645 | 45372 | 66543 | 11723 | 13019 | 16781 | 2277 | 2404 | 2748 | 641 | 651 | 707 | 305 | 305 | 320 |
| 0.35 *** | 43906 | 45351 | 65797 | 12041 | 12991 | 16593 | 2394 | 2525 | 2723 | 677 | 694 | 708 | 322 | 322 | 326 |
| *** | 44388 | 47958 | 71881 | 12407 | 14039 | 18076 | 2451 | 2610 | 2936 | 687 | 698 | 746 | 322 | 326 | 334 |
| 0.4 *** | 43984 | 45861 | 70717 | 12300 | 13448 | 17783 | 2500 | 2653 | 2893 | 708 | 726 | 747 | 333 | 337 | 337 |
| *** | 44618 | 49137 | 75648 | 12753 | 14698 | 18979 | 2568 | 2759 | 3062 | 715 | 736 | 770 | 333 | 337 | 341 |
| 0.45 *** | 42769 | 45149 | 73957 | 12275 | 13603 | 18554 | 2553 | 2727 | 2999 | 719 | 740 | 762 | 333 | 337 | 343 |
| *** | 43580 | 49127 | 77846 | 12796 | 15020 | 19489 | 2632 | 2844 | 3124 | 730 | 751 | 778 | 337 | 343 | 341 |
| 0.5 *** | 40516 | 43474 | 75504 | 12003 | 13486 | 18898 | 2553 | 2738 | 3031 | 719 | 740 | 762 | 333 | 337 | 343 |
| *** | 41540 | 48128 | 78474 | 12594 | 15042 | 19607 | 2638 | 2865 | 3124 | 730 | 751 | 770 | 333 | 337 | 334 |
| 0.55 *** | 37520 | 41079 | 75345 | 11535 | 13140 | 18813 | 2504 | 2695 | 2999 | 704 | 719 | 747 | 322 | 326 | 326 |
| *** | 38778 | 46339 | 77532 | 12179 | 14783 | 19332 | 2589 | 2829 | 3062 | 708 | 730 | 746 | 322 | 326 | 320 |
| 0.6 *** | 34056 | 38189 | 73475 | 10915 | 12583 | 18303 | 2408 | 2600 | 2897 | 673 | 687 | 708 | 301 | 305 | 311 |
| *** | 35558 | 43899 | 75020 | 11588 | 14262 | 18665 | 2493 | 2727 | 2936 | 677 | 698 | 707 | 305 | 305 | 299 |
| 0.65 *** | 30380 | 34970 | 69905 | 10161 | 11839 | 17368 | 2266 | 2451 | 2727 | 623 | 641 | 662 | 279 | 279 | 283 |
| *** | 32095 | 40935 | 70939 | 10845 | 13490 | 17606 | 2351 | 2574 | 2748 | 630 | 651 | 652 | 279 | 283 | 271 |
| 0.7 *** | 26693 | 31528 | 64639 | 9289 | 10915 | 16008 | 2079 | 2245 | 2489 | 560 | 577 | 592 | 241 | 248 | 252 |
| *** | 28535 | 37499 | 65287 | 9959 | 12477 | 16153 | 2160 | 2355 | 2496 | 566 | 581 | 581 | 248 | 248 | 236 |
| 0.75 *** | 23074 | 27894 | 57701 | 8301 | 9803 | 14234 | 1845 | 1983 | 2185 | 485 | 496 | 507 | 205 | 205 | 209 |
| *** | 24944 | 33603 | 58067 | 8922 | 11213 | 14309 | 1909 | 2075 | 2182 | 492 | 503 | 495 | 205 | 209 | 194 |
| 0.8 *** | 19525 | 24041 | 49101 | 7186 | 8493 | 12041 | 1565 | 1671 | 1813 | 390 | 400 | 407 | 156 | 156 | 163 |
| *** | 21300 | 29194 | 49276 | 7732 | 9672 | 12072 | 1612 | 1735 | 1806 | 396 | 400 | 393 | 156 | 163 | 145 |
| 0.85 *** | 15941 | 19844 | 38852 | 5900 | 6931 | 9438 | 1218 | 1289 | 1378 | 279 | 283 | 290 | . | . | . |
| *** | 17492 | 24137 | 38915 | 6336 | 7817 | 9443 | 1250 | 1331 | 1366 | 283 | 290 | 275 | . | . | . |
| 0.9 *** | 12088 | 15042 | 26980 | 4363 | 5033 | 6431 | 804 | 836 | 878 | . | . | . | . | . | . |
| *** | 13278 | 18119 | 26985 | 4657 | 5571 | 6421 | 821 | 857 | 864 | . | . | . | . | . | . |
| 0.95 *** | 7388 | 8960 | 13497 | 2377 | 2628 | 3021 | . | . | . | . | . | . | . | . | . |
| *** | 8040 | 10409 | 13485 | 2489 | 2798 | 3007 | . | . | . | . | . | . | . | . | . |
| 0.98 *** | 3343 | 3807 | 4646 | . | . | . | . | . | . | . | . | . | . | . | . |
| *** | 3545 | 4147 | 4631 | . | . | . | . | . | . | . | . | . | . | . | . |

TABLE 5: ALPHA= 0.025 POWER= 0.8     EXPECTED ACCRUAL THRU MINIMUM FOLLOW-UP= 4500

| | | DEL=.01 | | | DEL=.02 | | | DEL=.05 | | | DEL=.10 | | | DEL=.15 | | |
|---|---|---|---|---|---|---|---|---|---|---|---|---|---|---|---|---|---|
| FACT= | | 1.0<br>.75 | .50<br>.25 | .00<br>BIN | 1.0<br>.75 | .50<br>.25 | .00<br>BIN | 1.0<br>.75 | .50<br>.25 | .00<br>BIN | 1.0<br>75 | .50<br>.25 | .00<br>BIN | 1.0<br>.75 | .50<br>.25 | .00<br>BIN |
| PCONT=*** | | | | | | REQUIRED NUMBER OF PATIENTS | | | | | | | | | | |
| 0.01 | *** | 1200 | 1207 | 1211 | 442 | 442 | 442 | 143 | 143 | 143 | 75 | 75 | 75 | 53 | 53 | 53 |
| | *** | 1207 | 1207 | 4631 | 442 | 442 | 1531 | 143 | 143 | 417 | 75 | 75 | 170 | 53 | 53 | 101 |
| 0.02 | *** | 2663 | 2674 | 2703 | 858 | 858 | 863 | 233 | 233 | 233 | 98 | 105 | 105 | 64 | 64 | 64 |
| | *** | 2670 | 2685 | 7645 | 858 | 863 | 2277 | 233 | 233 | 532 | 98 | 105 | 197 | 64 | 64 | 113 |
| 0.05 | *** | 8058 | 8130 | 8441 | 2298 | 2321 | 2366 | 498 | 498 | 503 | 176 | 176 | 176 | 105 | 105 | 105 |
| | *** | 8085 | 8227 | 16310 | 2310 | 2343 | 4419 | 498 | 498 | 864 | 176 | 176 | 275 | 105 | 105 | 145 |
| 0.1 | *** | 17790 | 17996 | 19639 | 4830 | 4942 | 5194 | 941 | 953 | 964 | 296 | 296 | 300 | 154 | 161 | 161 |
| | *** | 17861 | 18334 | 29497 | 4875 | 5036 | 7677 | 948 | 960 | 1366 | 296 | 296 | 393 | 154 | 161 | 194 |
| 0.15 | *** | 26591 | 26963 | 31024 | 7125 | 7361 | 8036 | 1353 | 1380 | 1414 | 401 | 408 | 408 | 206 | 206 | 206 |
| | *** | 26722 | 27633 | 41113 | 7215 | 7597 | 10542 | 1369 | 1398 | 1806 | 401 | 408 | 495 | 206 | 206 | 236 |
| 0.2 | *** | 33724 | 34305 | 41685 | 9015 | 9408 | 10673 | 1713 | 1763 | 1830 | 498 | 503 | 510 | 244 | 244 | 244 |
| | *** | 33915 | 35366 | 51159 | 9172 | 9825 | 13014 | 1736 | 1792 | 2182 | 498 | 503 | 581 | 244 | 244 | 271 |
| 0.25 | *** | 38966 | 39806 | 51173 | 10466 | 11040 | 13013 | 2006 | 2085 | 2186 | 570 | 581 | 588 | 278 | 278 | 285 |
| | *** | 39248 | 41340 | 59636 | 10691 | 11651 | 15094 | 2040 | 2130 | 2496 | 577 | 588 | 652 | 278 | 278 | 299 |
| 0.3 | *** | 42348 | 43496 | 59257 | 11483 | 12248 | 15000 | 2235 | 2336 | 2490 | 633 | 645 | 660 | 300 | 307 | 307 |
| | *** | 42731 | 45581 | 66543 | 11782 | 13080 | 16781 | 2287 | 2404 | 2748 | 638 | 649 | 707 | 307 | 307 | 320 |
| 0.35 | *** | 43991 | 45514 | 65798 | 12108 | 13076 | 16597 | 2404 | 2535 | 2726 | 678 | 694 | 712 | 323 | 323 | 330 |
| | *** | 44501 | 48232 | 71881 | 12484 | 14122 | 18076 | 2467 | 2618 | 2936 | 690 | 701 | 746 | 323 | 323 | 334 |
| 0.4 | *** | 44096 | 46072 | 70714 | 12390 | 13553 | 17783 | 2516 | 2663 | 2895 | 712 | 728 | 746 | 330 | 334 | 341 |
| | *** | 44767 | 49474 | 75648 | 12844 | 14790 | 18979 | 2584 | 2764 | 3062 | 716 | 735 | 770 | 334 | 334 | 341 |
| 0.45 | *** | 42911 | 45413 | 73961 | 12371 | 13721 | 18555 | 2568 | 2737 | 3000 | 723 | 739 | 761 | 334 | 341 | 345 |
| | *** | 43770 | 49519 | 77846 | 12907 | 15135 | 19489 | 2647 | 2854 | 3124 | 735 | 750 | 778 | 334 | 341 | 341 |
| 0.5 | *** | 40699 | 43793 | 75506 | 12113 | 13616 | 18896 | 2568 | 2753 | 3034 | 723 | 739 | 761 | 330 | 334 | 341 |
| | *** | 41779 | 48581 | 78474 | 12716 | 15161 | 19607 | 2651 | 2876 | 3124 | 728 | 750 | 770 | 334 | 341 | 334 |
| 0.55 | *** | 37747 | 41453 | 75345 | 11658 | 13278 | 18813 | 2523 | 2708 | 3000 | 705 | 723 | 746 | 318 | 323 | 330 |
| | *** | 39068 | 46830 | 77532 | 12311 | 14910 | 19332 | 2606 | 2838 | 3062 | 712 | 735 | 746 | 323 | 330 | 320 |
| 0.6 | *** | 34327 | 38606 | 73477 | 11044 | 12727 | 18307 | 2426 | 2613 | 2899 | 671 | 690 | 712 | 300 | 307 | 311 |
| | *** | 35895 | 44430 | 75020 | 11726 | 14392 | 18665 | 2512 | 2737 | 2936 | 683 | 701 | 707 | 307 | 307 | 299 |
| 0.65 | *** | 30698 | 35418 | 69904 | 10290 | 11978 | 17366 | 2287 | 2460 | 2726 | 626 | 645 | 660 | 278 | 278 | 285 |
| | *** | 32471 | 41471 | 70939 | 10983 | 13620 | 17606 | 2366 | 2580 | 2748 | 633 | 649 | 652 | 278 | 285 | 271 |
| 0.7 | *** | 27037 | 31980 | 64639 | 9420 | 11051 | 16012 | 2096 | 2258 | 2490 | 566 | 577 | 593 | 244 | 244 | 251 |
| | *** | 28931 | 38028 | 65287 | 10088 | 12596 | 16153 | 2168 | 2359 | 2496 | 570 | 581 | 581 | 244 | 251 | 236 |
| 0.75 | *** | 23430 | 28335 | 57698 | 8423 | 9926 | 14235 | 1860 | 1995 | 2186 | 487 | 498 | 510 | 206 | 206 | 210 |
| | *** | 25338 | 34102 | 58067 | 9048 | 11314 | 14309 | 1920 | 2085 | 2182 | 491 | 503 | 495 | 206 | 206 | 194 |
| 0.8 | *** | 19864 | 24443 | 49098 | 7293 | 8591 | 12041 | 1571 | 1673 | 1815 | 390 | 397 | 408 | 161 | 161 | 161 |
| | *** | 21671 | 29636 | 49276 | 7838 | 9757 | 12072 | 1623 | 1740 | 1806 | 397 | 401 | 393 | 161 | 161 | 145 |
| 0.85 | *** | 16241 | 20190 | 38850 | 5988 | 7012 | 9442 | 1223 | 1290 | 1380 | 285 | 285 | 289 | . | . | . |
| | *** | 17816 | 24495 | 38915 | 6420 | 7878 | 9443 | 1256 | 1335 | 1366 | 285 | 289 | 275 | . | . | . |
| 0.9 | *** | 12315 | 15296 | 26981 | 4425 | 5088 | 6431 | 806 | 840 | 881 | . | . | . | . | . | . |
| | *** | 13519 | 18368 | 26985 | 4710 | 5606 | 6421 | 825 | 858 | 864 | . | . | . | . | . | . |
| 0.95 | *** | 7518 | 9086 | 13496 | 2400 | 2640 | 3023 | . | . | . | . | . | . | . | . | . |
| | *** | 8175 | 10522 | 13485 | 2512 | 2809 | 3007 | . | . | . | . | . | . | . | . | . |
| 0.98 | *** | 3390 | 3840 | 4650 | . | . | . | . | . | . | . | . | . | . | . | . |
| | *** | 3585 | 4170 | 4631 | . | . | . | . | . | . | . | . | . | . | . | . |

# TABLE 5: ALPHA= 0.025 POWER= 0.8   EXPECTED ACCRUAL THRU MINIMUM FOLLOW-UP= 4750

| | | DEL=.01 | | | DEL=.02 | | | DEL=.05 | | | DEL=.10 | | | DEL=.15 | | |
|---|---|---|---|---|---|---|---|---|---|---|---|---|---|---|---|---|
| | FACT= | 1.0 .75 | .50 .25 | .00 BIN | 1.0 .75 | .50 .25 | .00 BIN | 1.0 .75 | .50 .25 | .00 BIN | 1.0 75 | .50 .25 | .00 BIN | 1.0 .75 | .50 .25 | .00 BIN |
| PCONT=*** | | | | | REQUIRED NUMBER OF PATIENTS | | | | | | | | | | | |
| 0.01 | *** | 1203 1203 | 1207 1207 | 1207 4631 | 443 443 | 443 443 | 443 1531 | 146 146 | 146 146 | 146 417 | 75 75 | 75 75 | 75 170 | 51 51 | 51 51 | 51 101 |
| 0.02 | *** | 2663 2668 | 2675 2687 | 2699 7645 | 858 858 | 858 863 | 863 2277 | 234 234 | 234 234 | 234 532 | 103 103 | 103 103 | 103 197 | 67 67 | 67 67 | 67 113 |
| 0.05 | *** | 8067 8090 | 8138 8233 | 8439 16310 | 2300 2312 | 2324 2343 | 2367 4419 | 495 495 | 495 502 | 502 864 | 174 174 | 174 174 | 174 275 | 103 103 | 103 103 | 103 145 |
| 0.1 | *** | 17804 17875 | 18018 18362 | 19637 29497 | 4837 4884 | 4948 5043 | 5193 7677 | 942 946 | 953 958 | 965 1366 | 293 293 | 293 300 | 300 393 | 158 158 | 158 158 | 158 194 |
| 0.15 | *** | 26615 26746 | 27007 27696 | 31025 41113 | 7140 7235 | 7378 7615 | 8035 10542 | 1357 1369 | 1385 1397 | 1417 1806 | 400 407 | 407 407 | 407 495 | 205 205 | 205 205 | 205 236 |
| 0.2 | *** | 33757 33959 | 34370 35474 | 41685 51159 | 9040 9199 | 9444 9852 | 10672 13014 | 1718 1737 | 1765 1797 | 1825 2182 | 495 495 | 502 502 | 507 581 | 245 245 | 245 245 | 245 271 |
| 0.25 | *** | 39017 39310 | 39896 41495 | 51173 59636 | 10505 10731 | 11087 11700 | 13018 15094 | 2015 2046 | 2086 2134 | 2188 2496 | 573 578 | 578 585 | 590 652 | 277 277 | 281 281 | 281 299 |
| 0.3 | *** | 42409 42817 | 43620 45786 | 59260 66543 | 11539 11843 | 12318 13142 | 15002 16781 | 2248 2295 | 2347 2407 | 2490 2748 | 637 637 | 645 649 | 657 707 | 305 305 | 305 305 | 305 320 |
| 0.35 | *** | 44076 44618 | 45679 48494 | 65795 71881 | 12175 12560 | 13161 14199 | 16597 18076 | 2419 2473 | 2545 2620 | 2723 2936 | 680 685 | 692 704 | 709 746 | 324 324 | 324 324 | 329 334 |
| 0.4 | *** | 44207 44915 | 46285 49795 | 70712 75648 | 12472 12935 | 13648 14887 | 17785 18979 | 2525 2597 | 2675 2775 | 2894 3062 | 709 720 | 728 732 | 744 770 | 329 336 | 336 336 | 340 341 |
| 0.45 | *** | 43055 43957 | 45675 49902 | 73961 77846 | 12472 13011 | 13830 15239 | 18552 19489 | 2585 2656 | 2751 2858 | 2996 3124 | 728 732 | 740 752 | 763 778 | 336 336 | 340 340 | 340 341 |
| 0.5 | *** | 40882 42010 | 44107 49012 | 75505 78474 | 12223 12833 | 13743 15279 | 18897 19607 | 2585 2668 | 2763 2882 | 3032 3124 | 720 732 | 740 752 | 763 770 | 329 336 | 336 336 | 340 334 |
| 0.55 | *** | 37972 39350 | 41815 47306 | 75343 77532 | 11776 12437 | 13410 15030 | 18813 19332 | 2537 2620 | 2723 2846 | 3000 3062 | 704 716 | 720 732 | 744 746 | 324 324 | 324 329 | 329 320 |
| 0.6 | *** | 34600 36222 | 39013 44931 | 73474 75020 | 11170 11859 | 12857 14515 | 18303 18665 | 2442 2525 | 2628 2747 | 2894 2936 | 673 680 | 692 704 | 709 707 | 300 305 | 305 305 | 312 299 |
| 0.65 | *** | 31009 32830 | 35847 41986 | 69904 70939 | 10418 11118 | 12116 13735 | 17369 17606 | 2300 2378 | 2473 2585 | 2727 2748 | 625 633 | 645 649 | 661 652 | 277 277 | 281 281 | 281 271 |
| 0.7 | *** | 27375 29311 | 32422 38530 | 64644 65287 | 9544 10220 | 11178 12710 | 16011 16153 | 2110 2181 | 2264 2367 | 2490 2496 | 566 573 | 578 585 | 590 581 | 245 245 | 245 245 | 253 236 |
| 0.75 | *** | 23777 25717 | 28757 34572 | 57704 58067 | 8542 9164 | 10042 11415 | 14234 14309 | 1872 1932 | 2003 2086 | 2188 2182 | 483 490 | 495 502 | 507 495 | 205 205 | 205 205 | 210 194 |
| 0.8 | *** | 20195 22024 | 24834 30052 | 49099 49276 | 7394 7940 | 8689 9836 | 12045 12072 | 1583 1630 | 1682 1742 | 1813 1806 | 395 395 | 400 400 | 407 393 | 158 158 | 158 158 | 158 145 |
| 0.85 | *** | 16526 18125 | 20516 24834 | 38851 38915 | 6072 6504 | 7085 7936 | 9437 9443 | 1231 1262 | 1298 1333 | 1381 1366 | 281 281 | 288 288 | 288 275 | . . | . . | . . |
| 0.9 | *** | 12543 13755 | 15536 18600 | 26976 26985 | 4480 4765 | 5133 5644 | 6432 6421 | 811 827 | 839 858 | 875 864 | . . | . . | . . | . . | . . | . . |
| 0.95 | *** | 7639 8297 | 9207 10624 | 13498 13485 | 2419 2533 | 2656 2818 | 3020 3007 | . . | . . | . . | . . | . . | . . | . . | . . | . . |
| 0.98 | *** | 3428 3625 | 3867 4188 | 4647 4631 | . . | . . | . . | . . | . . | . . | . . | . . | . . | . . | . . | . . |

TABLE 5: ALPHA= 0.025 POWER= 0.8     EXPECTED ACCRUAL THRU MINIMUM FOLLOW-UP= 5000

| | | DEL=.01 | | | DEL=.02 | | | DEL=.05 | | | DEL=.10 | | | DEL=.15 | | |
|---|---|---|---|---|---|---|---|---|---|---|---|---|---|---|---|---|---|
| FACT= | | 1.0 .75 | .50 .25 | .00 BIN | 1.0 .75 | .50 .25 | .00 BIN | 1.0 .75 | .50 .25 | .00 BIN | 1.0 75 | .50 .25 | .00 BIN | 1.0 .75 | .50 .25 | .00 BIN |
| PCONT=*** | | | | | | | REQUIRED NUMBER OF PATIENTS | | | | | | | | |
| 0.01 | *** | 1204 | 1208 | 1208 | 441 | 441 | 441 | 146 | 146 | 146 | 71 | 71 | 71 | 54 | 54 | 54 |
| | *** | 1204 | 1208 | 4631 | 441 | 441 | 1531 | 146 | 146 | 417 | 71 | 71 | 170 | 54 | 54 | 101 |
| 0.02 | *** | 2666 | 2679 | 2704 | 858 | 858 | 866 | 233 | 233 | 233 | 104 | 104 | 104 | 66 | 66 | 66 |
| | *** | 2671 | 2683 | 7645 | 858 | 858 | 2277 | 233 | 233 | 532 | 104 | 104 | 197 | 66 | 66 | 113 |
| 0.05 | *** | 8071 | 8146 | 8441 | 2304 | 2329 | 2366 | 496 | 496 | 504 | 179 | 179 | 179 | 104 | 104 | 104 |
| | *** | 8096 | 8241 | 16310 | 2308 | 2341 | 4419 | 496 | 496 | 864 | 179 | 179 | 275 | 104 | 104 | 145 |
| 0.1 | *** | 17816 | 18041 | 19641 | 4846 | 4954 | 5196 | 946 | 954 | 966 | 296 | 296 | 296 | 158 | 158 | 158 |
| | *** | 17891 | 18396 | 29497 | 4891 | 5046 | 7677 | 946 | 958 | 1366 | 296 | 296 | 393 | 158 | 158 | 194 |
| 0.15 | *** | 26633 | 27046 | 31029 | 7154 | 7396 | 8033 | 1358 | 1383 | 1416 | 404 | 404 | 408 | 204 | 204 | 204 |
| | *** | 26771 | 27758 | 41113 | 7254 | 7629 | 10542 | 1371 | 1404 | 1806 | 404 | 408 | 495 | 204 | 204 | 236 |
| 0.2 | *** | 33791 | 34429 | 41683 | 9071 | 9471 | 10671 | 1721 | 1766 | 1829 | 496 | 504 | 508 | 246 | 246 | 246 |
| | *** | 34004 | 35571 | 51159 | 9229 | 9879 | 13014 | 1741 | 1796 | 2182 | 496 | 504 | 581 | 246 | 246 | 271 |
| 0.25 | *** | 39058 | 39983 | 51171 | 10541 | 11133 | 13016 | 2021 | 2091 | 2191 | 571 | 583 | 591 | 279 | 279 | 283 |
| | *** | 39371 | 41641 | 59636 | 10779 | 11741 | 15094 | 2054 | 2133 | 2496 | 579 | 583 | 652 | 279 | 279 | 299 |
| 0.3 | *** | 42471 | 43741 | 59258 | 11591 | 12379 | 14996 | 2254 | 2354 | 2491 | 633 | 646 | 658 | 304 | 304 | 308 |
| | *** | 42904 | 45991 | 66543 | 11896 | 13204 | 16781 | 2296 | 2416 | 2748 | 641 | 654 | 707 | 304 | 308 | 320 |
| 0.35 | *** | 44158 | 45841 | 65796 | 12241 | 13233 | 16596 | 2429 | 2546 | 2721 | 683 | 696 | 708 | 321 | 321 | 329 |
| | *** | 44729 | 48754 | 71881 | 12633 | 14271 | 18076 | 2483 | 2629 | 2936 | 691 | 704 | 746 | 321 | 329 | 334 |
| 0.4 | *** | 44321 | 46496 | 70716 | 12554 | 13741 | 17783 | 2541 | 2683 | 2896 | 716 | 729 | 746 | 333 | 333 | 341 |
| | *** | 45058 | 50108 | 75648 | 13021 | 14971 | 18979 | 2608 | 2779 | 3062 | 721 | 733 | 770 | 333 | 341 | 341 |
| 0.45 | *** | 43196 | 45933 | 73958 | 12566 | 13933 | 18554 | 2596 | 2758 | 2996 | 729 | 741 | 758 | 333 | 341 | 341 |
| | *** | 44146 | 50271 | 77846 | 13116 | 15333 | 19489 | 2671 | 2866 | 3124 | 733 | 754 | 778 | 341 | 341 | 341 |
| 0.5 | *** | 41066 | 44416 | 75504 | 12329 | 13858 | 18896 | 2604 | 2779 | 3033 | 721 | 741 | 758 | 333 | 333 | 341 |
| | *** | 42241 | 49429 | 78474 | 12946 | 15383 | 19607 | 2683 | 2891 | 3124 | 733 | 754 | 770 | 333 | 341 | 334 |
| 0.55 | *** | 38196 | 42171 | 75346 | 11896 | 13529 | 18816 | 2554 | 2733 | 2996 | 708 | 729 | 746 | 321 | 321 | 329 |
| | *** | 39629 | 47766 | 77532 | 12558 | 15141 | 19332 | 2633 | 2854 | 3062 | 716 | 733 | 746 | 321 | 329 | 320 |
| 0.6 | *** | 34866 | 39404 | 73479 | 11291 | 12983 | 18304 | 2458 | 2633 | 2896 | 679 | 691 | 708 | 304 | 308 | 308 |
| | *** | 36541 | 45408 | 75020 | 11983 | 14629 | 18665 | 2541 | 2754 | 2936 | 683 | 704 | 707 | 304 | 308 | 299 |
| 0.65 | *** | 31316 | 36266 | 69904 | 10541 | 12241 | 17371 | 2316 | 2483 | 2729 | 629 | 641 | 658 | 279 | 279 | 283 |
| | *** | 33183 | 42471 | 70939 | 11241 | 13846 | 17606 | 2391 | 2591 | 2748 | 633 | 654 | 652 | 279 | 283 | 271 |
| 0.7 | *** | 27704 | 32841 | 64641 | 9666 | 11296 | 16008 | 2129 | 2279 | 2491 | 566 | 579 | 591 | 246 | 246 | 246 |
| | *** | 29683 | 39008 | 65287 | 10341 | 12808 | 16153 | 2196 | 2371 | 2496 | 571 | 583 | 581 | 246 | 246 | 236 |
| 0.75 | *** | 24108 | 29166 | 57704 | 8654 | 10146 | 14233 | 1883 | 2008 | 2183 | 483 | 496 | 508 | 204 | 208 | 208 |
| | *** | 26083 | 35021 | 58067 | 9279 | 11504 | 14309 | 1946 | 2091 | 2182 | 491 | 504 | 495 | 204 | 208 | 194 |
| 0.8 | *** | 20508 | 25204 | 49096 | 7491 | 8783 | 12041 | 1591 | 1691 | 1816 | 391 | 404 | 408 | 158 | 158 | 158 |
| | *** | 22366 | 30454 | 49276 | 8041 | 9908 | 12072 | 1633 | 1746 | 1806 | 396 | 404 | 393 | 158 | 158 | 145 |
| 0.85 | *** | 16804 | 20829 | 38854 | 6146 | 7154 | 9441 | 1241 | 1304 | 1379 | 283 | 283 | 291 | . | . | . |
| | *** | 18416 | 25154 | 38915 | 6579 | 7991 | 9443 | 1266 | 1341 | 1366 | 283 | 291 | 275 | . | . | . |
| 0.9 | *** | 12754 | 15766 | 26979 | 4529 | 5179 | 6433 | 816 | 846 | 879 | . | . | . | . | . | . |
| | *** | 13979 | 18816 | 26985 | 4816 | 5671 | 6421 | 829 | 858 | 864 | . | . | . | . | . | . |
| 0.95 | *** | 7758 | 9316 | 13496 | 2441 | 2671 | 3021 | . | . | . | . | . | . | . | . | . |
| | *** | 8416 | 10716 | 13485 | 2546 | 2829 | 3007 | . | . | . | . | . | . | . | . | . |
| 0.98 | *** | 3458 | 3896 | 4646 | . | . | . | . | . | . | . | . | . | . | . | . |
| | *** | 3654 | 4208 | 4631 | . | . | . | . | . | . | . | . | . | . | . | . |

## TABLE 5: ALPHA= 0.025 POWER= 0.8     EXPECTED ACCRUAL THRU MINIMUM FOLLOW-UP= 5500

| | | DEL=.01 | | | DEL=.02 | | | DEL=.05 | | | DEL=.10 | | | DEL=.15 | |
|---|---|---|---|---|---|---|---|---|---|---|---|---|---|---|---|---|
| FACT= | 1.0 .75 | .50 .25 | .00 BIN | 1.0 .75 | .50 .25 | .00 BIN | 1.0 .75 | .50 .25 | .00 BIN | 1.0 75 | .50 .25 | .00 BIN | 1.0 .75 | .50 .25 | .00 BIN | |

PCONT=***                    REQUIRED NUMBER OF PATIENTS

| PCONT | | 1.0/.75 | .50/.25 | .00/BIN | 1.0/.75 | .50/.25 | .00/BIN | 1.0/.75 | .50/.25 | .00/BIN | 1.0/75 | .50/.25 | .00/BIN | 1.0/.75 | .50/.25 | .00/BIN |
|---|---|---|---|---|---|---|---|---|---|---|---|---|---|---|---|---|
| 0.01 | *** | 1205 | 1205 | 1214 | 444 | 444 | 444 | 147 | 147 | 147 | 73 | 73 | 73 | 50 | 50 | 50 |
| | *** | 1205 | 1205 | 4631 | 444 | 444 | 1531 | 147 | 147 | 417 | 73 | 73 | 170 | 50 | 50 | 101 |
| 0.02 | *** | 2663 | 2677 | 2699 | 856 | 862 | 862 | 229 | 229 | 229 | 100 | 100 | 100 | 64 | 64 | 64 |
| | *** | 2671 | 2690 | 7645 | 856 | 862 | 2277 | 229 | 229 | 532 | 100 | 100 | 197 | 64 | 64 | 113 |
| 0.05 | *** | 8080 | 8158 | 8438 | 2305 | 2328 | 2360 | 499 | 499 | 499 | 174 | 174 | 174 | 105 | 105 | 105 |
| | *** | 8108 | 8254 | 16310 | 2314 | 2341 | 4419 | 499 | 499 | 864 | 174 | 174 | 275 | 105 | 105 | 145 |
| 0.1 | *** | 17838 | 18077 | 19639 | 4858 | 4968 | 5193 | 944 | 953 | 966 | 298 | 298 | 298 | 155 | 155 | 155 |
| | *** | 17920 | 18448 | 29497 | 4904 | 5064 | 7677 | 953 | 958 | 1366 | 298 | 298 | 393 | 155 | 155 | 194 |
| 0.15 | *** | 26679 | 27124 | 31024 | 7187 | 7429 | 8034 | 1365 | 1384 | 1420 | 403 | 408 | 408 | 202 | 202 | 202 |
| | *** | 26830 | 27875 | 41113 | 7283 | 7654 | 10542 | 1379 | 1398 | 1806 | 403 | 408 | 495 | 202 | 202 | 236 |
| 0.2 | *** | 33856 | 34558 | 41680 | 9120 | 9533 | 10674 | 1728 | 1769 | 1824 | 499 | 504 | 504 | 243 | 243 | 243 |
| | *** | 34090 | 35768 | 51159 | 9285 | 9931 | 13014 | 1750 | 1797 | 2182 | 499 | 504 | 581 | 243 | 243 | 271 |
| 0.25 | *** | 39155 | 40168 | 51173 | 10619 | 11215 | 13017 | 2030 | 2099 | 2190 | 573 | 581 | 587 | 279 | 279 | 279 |
| | *** | 39494 | 41928 | 59636 | 10858 | 11820 | 15094 | 2066 | 2140 | 2496 | 581 | 587 | 652 | 279 | 279 | 299 |
| 0.3 | *** | 42601 | 43990 | 59258 | 11691 | 12494 | 14997 | 2273 | 2360 | 2484 | 636 | 650 | 655 | 306 | 306 | 306 |
| | *** | 43069 | 46374 | 66543 | 12008 | 13305 | 16781 | 2314 | 2415 | 2748 | 642 | 650 | 707 | 306 | 306 | 320 |
| 0.35 | *** | 44334 | 46168 | 65798 | 12370 | 13383 | 16592 | 2451 | 2561 | 2726 | 683 | 697 | 710 | 320 | 325 | 325 |
| | *** | 44953 | 49243 | 71881 | 12769 | 14405 | 18076 | 2498 | 2635 | 2936 | 691 | 705 | 746 | 325 | 325 | 334 |
| 0.4 | *** | 44545 | 46905 | 70712 | 12700 | 13919 | 17783 | 2561 | 2699 | 2897 | 719 | 733 | 746 | 334 | 334 | 339 |
| | *** | 45357 | 50705 | 75648 | 13190 | 15129 | 18979 | 2630 | 2787 | 3062 | 719 | 738 | 770 | 334 | 339 | 341 |
| 0.45 | *** | 43487 | 46438 | 73957 | 12742 | 14130 | 18553 | 2622 | 2773 | 3001 | 733 | 746 | 760 | 334 | 339 | 339 |
| | *** | 44513 | 50975 | 77846 | 13305 | 15514 | 19489 | 2690 | 2878 | 3124 | 738 | 752 | 778 | 339 | 339 | 341 |
| 0.5 | *** | 41424 | 45013 | 75505 | 12530 | 14070 | 18896 | 2630 | 2795 | 3034 | 724 | 746 | 760 | 334 | 334 | 339 |
| | *** | 42698 | 50219 | 78474 | 13154 | 15583 | 19607 | 2704 | 2897 | 3124 | 738 | 752 | 770 | 334 | 339 | 334 |
| 0.55 | *** | 38633 | 42854 | 75345 | 12109 | 13759 | 18814 | 2580 | 2754 | 3001 | 710 | 724 | 746 | 320 | 325 | 325 |
| | *** | 40173 | 48624 | 77532 | 12783 | 15349 | 19332 | 2663 | 2864 | 3062 | 719 | 738 | 746 | 325 | 325 | 320 |
| 0.6 | *** | 35388 | 40154 | 73475 | 11518 | 13223 | 18305 | 2484 | 2658 | 2897 | 678 | 691 | 710 | 306 | 306 | 312 |
| | *** | 37162 | 46314 | 75020 | 12219 | 14832 | 18665 | 2567 | 2768 | 2936 | 683 | 705 | 707 | 306 | 306 | 299 |
| 0.65 | *** | 31904 | 37052 | 69900 | 10770 | 12467 | 17370 | 2341 | 2506 | 2726 | 628 | 642 | 664 | 279 | 279 | 284 |
| | *** | 33862 | 43390 | 70939 | 11477 | 14048 | 17606 | 2415 | 2603 | 2748 | 636 | 650 | 652 | 279 | 284 | 271 |
| 0.7 | *** | 28334 | 33642 | 64643 | 9882 | 11513 | 16009 | 2149 | 2292 | 2493 | 568 | 581 | 595 | 243 | 251 | 251 |
| | *** | 30391 | 39906 | 65287 | 10564 | 12998 | 16153 | 2218 | 2383 | 2496 | 573 | 587 | 581 | 243 | 251 | 236 |
| 0.75 | *** | 24740 | 29938 | 57699 | 8859 | 10349 | 14235 | 1907 | 2025 | 2182 | 490 | 499 | 504 | 202 | 210 | 210 |
| | *** | 26780 | 35855 | 58067 | 9483 | 11669 | 14309 | 1962 | 2099 | 2182 | 490 | 504 | 495 | 202 | 210 | 194 |
| 0.8 | *** | 21110 | 25900 | 49097 | 7676 | 8955 | 12040 | 1604 | 1695 | 1819 | 394 | 403 | 408 | 160 | 160 | 160 |
| | *** | 23013 | 31189 | 49276 | 8218 | 10047 | 12072 | 1654 | 1750 | 1806 | 394 | 403 | 393 | 160 | 160 | 145 |
| 0.85 | *** | 17329 | 21418 | 38853 | 6293 | 7283 | 9442 | 1247 | 1310 | 1379 | 284 | 284 | 293 | . | . | . |
| | *** | 18970 | 25749 | 38915 | 6719 | 8089 | 9443 | 1274 | 1343 | 1366 | 284 | 284 | 275 | . | . | . |
| 0.9 | *** | 13154 | 16188 | 26981 | 4624 | 5256 | 6430 | 820 | 848 | 875 | . | . | . | . | . | . |
| | *** | 14392 | 19218 | 26985 | 4904 | 5729 | 6421 | 834 | 862 | 864 | . | . | . | . | . | . |
| 0.95 | *** | 7970 | 9524 | 13498 | 2479 | 2699 | 3020 | . | . | . | . | . | . | . | . | . |
| | *** | 8630 | 10885 | 13485 | 2580 | 2842 | 3007 | . | . | . | . | . | . | . | . | . |
| 0.98 | *** | 3529 | 3942 | 4643 | . | . | . | . | . | . | . | . | . | . | . | . |
| | *** | 3716 | 4239 | 4631 | . | . | . | . | . | . | . | . | . | . | . | . |

TABLE 5: ALPHA= 0.025 POWER= 0.8    EXPECTED ACCRUAL THRU MINIMUM FOLLOW-UP= 6000

| | | DEL=.01 | | | DEL=.02 | | | DEL=.05 | | | DEL=.10 | | | DEL=.15 | | |
|---|---|---|---|---|---|---|---|---|---|---|---|---|---|---|---|---|
| FACT= | | 1.0 .75 | .50 .25 | .00 BIN | 1.0 .75 | .50 .25 | .00 BIN | 1.0 .75 | .50 .25 | .00 BIN | 1.0 75 | .50 .25 | .00 BIN | 1.0 .75 | .50 .25 | .00 BIN |
| PCONT=*** | | REQUIRED NUMBER OF PATIENTS | | | | | | | | | | | | | | |
| 0.01 | *** | 1204 1204 | 1210 | | 439 445 | 445 | | 145 145 | 145 | | 70 70 | 70 | | 49 49 | 49 | |
| | *** | 1204 1210 | 4631 | | 445 445 | 1531 | | 145 145 | 417 | | 70 70 | 170 | | 49 49 | 101 | |
| 0.02 | *** | 2665 2680 | 2704 | | 859 859 | 865 | | 229 229 | 229 | | 100 100 | 100 | | 64 64 | 64 | |
| | *** | 2674 2689 | 7645 | | 859 859 | 2277 | | 229 229 | 532 | | 100 100 | 197 | | 64 64 | 113 | |
| 0.05 | *** | 8089 8170 | 8440 | | 2305 2329 | 2365 | | 499 499 | 499 | | 175 175 | 175 | | 100 100 | 100 | |
| | *** | 8119 8260 | 16310 | | 2320 2344 | 4419 | | 499 499 | 864 | | 175 175 | 275 | | 100 100 | 145 | |
| 0.1 | *** | 17860 18124 | 19639 | | 4870 4984 | 5194 | | 949 955 | 964 | | 295 295 | 295 | | 154 160 | 160 | |
| | *** | 17950 18499 | 29497 | | 4924 5065 | 7677 | | 949 964 | 1366 | | 295 295 | 393 | | 160 160 | 194 | |
| 0.15 | *** | 26719 27205 | 31024 | | 7219 7459 | 8035 | | 1369 1390 | 1414 | | 400 409 | 409 | | 205 205 | 205 | |
| | *** | 26884 27985 | 41113 | | 7315 7675 | 10542 | | 1375 1405 | 1806 | | 409 409 | 495 | | 205 205 | 236 | |
| 0.2 | *** | 33919 34675 | 41680 | | 9169 9589 | 10675 | | 1735 1774 | 1825 | | 499 499 | 505 | | 244 244 | 244 | |
| | *** | 34174 35959 | 51159 | | 9340 9979 | 13014 | | 1750 1804 | 2182 | | 499 505 | 581 | | 244 244 | 271 | |
| 0.25 | *** | 39250 40345 | 51175 | | 10690 11299 | 13015 | | 2044 2104 | 2185 | | 574 580 | 589 | | 280 280 | 280 | |
| | *** | 39619 42199 | 59636 | | 10930 11890 | 15094 | | 2074 2140 | 2496 | | 580 589 | 652 | | 280 280 | 299 | |
| 0.3 | *** | 42730 44230 | 59260 | | 11779 12595 | 14995 | | 2284 2374 | 2485 | | 640 649 | 655 | | 304 304 | 310 | |
| | *** | 43240 46744 | 66543 | | 12109 13399 | 16781 | | 2320 2425 | 2748 | | 640 655 | 707 | | 304 304 | 320 | |
| 0.35 | *** | 44500 46480 | 65800 | | 12484 13510 | 16594 | | 2464 2575 | 2725 | | 685 700 | 709 | | 325 325 | 325 | |
| | *** | 45184 49705 | 71881 | | 12904 14524 | 18076 | | 2515 2644 | 2936 | | 694 700 | 746 | | 325 325 | 334 | |
| 0.4 | *** | 44764 47305 | 70714 | | 12844 14074 | 17785 | | 2584 2710 | 2899 | | 715 730 | 745 | | 334 334 | 340 | |
| | *** | 45640 51274 | 75648 | | 13339 15274 | 18979 | | 2644 2794 | 3062 | | 724 739 | 770 | | 334 340 | 341 | |
| 0.45 | *** | 43765 46924 | 73960 | | 12904 14314 | 18550 | | 2644 2794 | 2995 | | 730 745 | 760 | | 334 340 | 340 | |
| | *** | 44875 51625 | 77846 | | 13480 15679 | 19489 | | 2710 2884 | 3124 | | 739 754 | 778 | | 340 340 | 341 | |
| 0.5 | *** | 41779 45589 | 75505 | | 12715 14269 | 18895 | | 2650 2809 | 3034 | | 730 745 | 760 | | 334 334 | 340 | |
| | *** | 43144 50959 | 78474 | | 13354 15754 | 19607 | | 2725 2914 | 3124 | | 739 754 | 770 | | 334 340 | 334 | |
| 0.55 | *** | 39064 43504 | 75340 | | 12310 13969 | 18814 | | 2605 2770 | 2995 | | 715 730 | 745 | | 319 325 | 325 | |
| | *** | 40699 49420 | 77532 | | 12994 15529 | 19332 | | 2680 2875 | 3062 | | 724 739 | 746 | | 325 325 | 320 | |
| 0.6 | *** | 35890 40864 | 73474 | | 11725 13435 | 18304 | | 2509 2674 | 2899 | | 679 694 | 709 | | 304 304 | 310 | |
| | *** | 37759 47155 | 75020 | | 12430 15019 | 18665 | | 2584 2770 | 2936 | | 685 700 | 707 | | 304 310 | 299 | |
| 0.65 | *** | 32470 37795 | 69904 | | 10984 12679 | 17365 | | 2365 2515 | 2725 | | 634 649 | 664 | | 280 280 | 280 | |
| | *** | 34510 44239 | 70939 | | 11689 14230 | 17606 | | 2434 2614 | 2748 | | 640 655 | 652 | | 280 280 | 271 | |
| 0.7 | *** | 28930 34384 | 64639 | | 10090 11710 | 16009 | | 2170 2305 | 2494 | | 565 580 | 595 | | 244 250 | 250 | |
| | *** | 31054 40729 | 65287 | | 10774 13165 | 16153 | | 2230 2389 | 2496 | | 574 589 | 581 | | 244 250 | 236 | |
| 0.75 | *** | 25339 30649 | 57700 | | 9049 10525 | 14230 | | 1924 2035 | 2185 | | 490 499 | 505 | | 205 205 | 205 | |
| | *** | 27430 36625 | 58067 | | 9670 11815 | 14309 | | 1975 2104 | 2182 | | 490 505 | 495 | | 205 205 | 194 | |
| 0.8 | *** | 21670 26554 | 49099 | | 7840 9100 | 12040 | | 1624 1705 | 1819 | | 394 400 | 409 | | 160 160 | 160 | |
| | *** | 23614 31855 | 49276 | | 8380 10165 | 12072 | | 1660 1759 | 1806 | | 400 400 | 393 | | 160 160 | 145 | |
| 0.85 | *** | 17815 21955 | 38854 | | 6424 7390 | 9439 | | 1255 1315 | 1375 | | 280 289 | 289 | | . | . | |
| | *** | 19480 26284 | 38915 | | 6844 8170 | 9443 | | 1285 1345 | 1366 | | 289 289 | 275 | | . | . | |
| 0.9 | *** | 13519 16579 | 26980 | | 4714 5320 | 6430 | | 820 850 | 880 | | . | . | | . | . | |
| | *** | 14770 19585 | 26985 | | 4984 5770 | 6421 | | 835 865 | 864 | | . | . | | . | . | |
| 0.95 | *** | 8170 9709 | 13495 | | 2509 2719 | 3019 | | . | . | | . | . | | . | . | |
| | *** | 8824 11035 | 13485 | | 2605 2854 | 3007 | | . | . | | . | . | | . | . | |
| 0.98 | *** | 3589 3985 | 4645 | | . | . | | . | . | | . | . | | . | . | |
| | *** | 3769 4270 | 4631 | | . | . | | . | . | | . | . | | . | . | |

## TABLE 5: ALPHA= 0.025 POWER= 0.8    EXPECTED ACCRUAL THRU MINIMUM FOLLOW-UP= 6500

| | FACT= | DEL=.01 1.0 / .75 | .50 / .25 | .00 / BIN | DEL=.02 1.0 / .75 | .50 / .25 | .00 / BIN | DEL=.05 1.0 / .75 | .50 / .25 | .00 / BIN | DEL=.10 1.0 / 75 | .50 / .25 | .00 / BIN | DEL=.15 1.0 / .75 | .50 / .25 | .00 / BIN |
|---|---|---|---|---|---|---|---|---|---|---|---|---|---|---|---|---|
| PCONT=*** | | | | | REQUIRED NUMBER OF PATIENTS | | | | | | | | | | | |
| 0.01 | *** | 1207 | 1207 | 1207 | 443 | 443 | 443 | 141 | 141 | 141 | 76 | 76 | 76 | 53 | 53 | 53 |
|  | *** | 1207 | 1207 | 4631 | 443 | 443 | 1531 | 141 | 141 | 417 | 76 | 76 | 170 | 53 | 53 | 101 |
| 0.02 | *** | 2670 | 2686 | 2702 | 856 | 856 | 866 | 232 | 232 | 232 | 102 | 102 | 102 | 70 | 70 | 70 |
|  | *** | 2676 | 2692 | 7645 | 856 | 866 | 2277 | 232 | 232 | 532 | 102 | 102 | 197 | 70 | 70 | 113 |
| 0.05 | *** | 8097 | 8178 | 8438 | 2312 | 2334 | 2361 | 498 | 498 | 498 | 173 | 173 | 173 | 102 | 102 | 102 |
|  | *** | 8130 | 8276 | 16310 | 2318 | 2345 | 4419 | 498 | 498 | 864 | 173 | 173 | 275 | 102 | 102 | 145 |
| 0.1 | *** | 17880 | 18162 | 19641 | 4886 | 4993 | 5194 | 947 | 953 | 963 | 297 | 297 | 297 | 157 | 157 | 157 |
|  | *** | 17977 | 18546 | 29497 | 4934 | 5075 | 7677 | 953 | 963 | 1366 | 297 | 297 | 393 | 157 | 157 | 194 |
| 0.15 | *** | 26758 | 27278 | 31026 | 7242 | 7486 | 8032 | 1370 | 1392 | 1418 | 401 | 411 | 411 | 206 | 206 | 206 |
|  | *** | 26937 | 28091 | 41113 | 7350 | 7697 | 10542 | 1376 | 1402 | 1806 | 401 | 411 | 495 | 206 | 206 | 236 |
| 0.2 | *** | 33983 | 34796 | 41686 | 9218 | 9631 | 10671 | 1743 | 1782 | 1831 | 498 | 498 | 508 | 248 | 248 | 248 |
|  | *** | 34260 | 36134 | 51159 | 9387 | 10015 | 13014 | 1760 | 1798 | 2182 | 498 | 508 | 581 | 248 | 248 | 271 |
| 0.25 | *** | 39346 | 40522 | 51176 | 10752 | 11369 | 13011 | 2052 | 2107 | 2188 | 579 | 579 | 590 | 281 | 281 | 281 |
|  | *** | 39742 | 42456 | 59636 | 11006 | 11948 | 15094 | 2074 | 2150 | 2496 | 579 | 590 | 652 | 281 | 281 | 299 |
| 0.3 | *** | 42856 | 44471 | 59258 | 11873 | 12696 | 15003 | 2296 | 2377 | 2491 | 638 | 644 | 661 | 303 | 303 | 303 |
|  | *** | 43408 | 47087 | 66543 | 12208 | 13482 | 16781 | 2334 | 2426 | 2748 | 644 | 655 | 707 | 303 | 303 | 320 |
| 0.35 | *** | 44676 | 46794 | 65801 | 12598 | 13638 | 16596 | 2481 | 2578 | 2724 | 687 | 693 | 709 | 319 | 330 | 330 |
|  | *** | 45407 | 50142 | 71881 | 13021 | 14630 | 18076 | 2529 | 2643 | 2936 | 693 | 703 | 746 | 319 | 330 | 334 |
| 0.4 | *** | 44985 | 47688 | 70714 | 12978 | 14213 | 17782 | 2605 | 2724 | 2897 | 720 | 726 | 742 | 336 | 336 | 336 |
|  | *** | 45933 | 51799 | 75648 | 13482 | 15399 | 18979 | 2659 | 2800 | 3062 | 726 | 736 | 770 | 336 | 336 | 341 |
| 0.45 | *** | 44048 | 47396 | 73958 | 13059 | 14473 | 18552 | 2670 | 2806 | 3001 | 736 | 742 | 758 | 336 | 336 | 346 |
|  | *** | 45234 | 52248 | 77846 | 13644 | 15816 | 19489 | 2735 | 2897 | 3124 | 742 | 752 | 778 | 336 | 346 | 341 |
| 0.5 | *** | 42125 | 46138 | 75502 | 12891 | 14451 | 18893 | 2676 | 2822 | 3033 | 736 | 742 | 758 | 336 | 336 | 336 |
|  | *** | 43577 | 51647 | 78474 | 13531 | 15913 | 19607 | 2741 | 2919 | 3124 | 742 | 752 | 770 | 336 | 336 | 334 |
| 0.55 | *** | 39492 | 44123 | 75346 | 12501 | 14158 | 18812 | 2627 | 2783 | 3001 | 720 | 726 | 742 | 319 | 330 | 330 |
|  | *** | 41204 | 50168 | 77532 | 13183 | 15692 | 19332 | 2702 | 2881 | 3062 | 720 | 736 | 746 | 319 | 330 | 320 |
| 0.6 | *** | 36378 | 41529 | 73477 | 11922 | 13628 | 18302 | 2529 | 2686 | 2897 | 687 | 693 | 709 | 303 | 303 | 313 |
|  | *** | 38328 | 47932 | 75020 | 12631 | 15182 | 18665 | 2605 | 2783 | 2936 | 687 | 703 | 707 | 303 | 303 | 299 |
| 0.65 | *** | 33008 | 38491 | 69902 | 11174 | 12875 | 17366 | 2383 | 2529 | 2724 | 638 | 644 | 661 | 281 | 281 | 281 |
|  | *** | 35121 | 45023 | 70939 | 11889 | 14392 | 17606 | 2458 | 2621 | 2748 | 638 | 655 | 652 | 281 | 281 | 271 |
| 0.7 | *** | 29498 | 35078 | 64637 | 10281 | 11889 | 16011 | 2188 | 2318 | 2491 | 573 | 579 | 590 | 248 | 248 | 248 |
|  | *** | 31682 | 41491 | 65287 | 10957 | 13313 | 16153 | 2247 | 2399 | 2496 | 573 | 590 | 581 | 248 | 248 | 236 |
| 0.75 | *** | 25907 | 31318 | 57698 | 9224 | 10687 | 14229 | 1938 | 2042 | 2188 | 492 | 498 | 508 | 206 | 206 | 206 |
|  | *** | 28042 | 37331 | 58067 | 9842 | 11948 | 14309 | 1987 | 2107 | 2182 | 498 | 508 | 495 | 206 | 206 | 194 |
| 0.8 | *** | 22202 | 27148 | 49096 | 7989 | 9235 | 12046 | 1630 | 1711 | 1814 | 395 | 401 | 411 | 157 | 157 | 157 |
|  | *** | 24174 | 32472 | 49276 | 8526 | 10275 | 12072 | 1668 | 1760 | 1806 | 401 | 401 | 393 | 157 | 157 | 145 |
| 0.85 | *** | 18270 | 22452 | 38848 | 6543 | 7496 | 9436 | 1262 | 1321 | 1376 | 287 | 287 | 287 | . | . | . |
|  | *** | 19960 | 26774 | 38915 | 6960 | 8249 | 9443 | 1288 | 1343 | 1366 | 287 | 287 | 275 | . | . | . |
| 0.9 | *** | 13866 | 16937 | 26980 | 4788 | 5383 | 6429 | 823 | 850 | 882 | . | . | . | . | . | . |
|  | *** | 15123 | 19911 | 26985 | 5048 | 5812 | 6421 | 839 | 866 | 864 | . | . | . | . | . | . |
| 0.95 | *** | 8357 | 9874 | 13498 | 2540 | 2741 | 3017 | . | . | . | . | . | . | . | . | . |
|  | *** | 9007 | 11168 | 13485 | 2627 | 2865 | 3007 | . | . | . | . | . | . | . | . | . |
| 0.98 | *** | 3634 | 4024 | 4642 | . | . | . | . | . | . | . | . | . | . | . | . |
|  | *** | 3813 | 4295 | 4631 | . | . | . | . | . | . | . | . | . | . | . | . |

TABLE 5: ALPHA= 0.025 POWER= 0.8    EXPECTED ACCRUAL THRU MINIMUM FOLLOW-UP= 7000

| | | DEL=.01 | | | DEL=.02 | | | DEL=.05 | | | DEL=.10 | | | DEL=.15 | | |
|---|---|---|---|---|---|---|---|---|---|---|---|---|---|---|---|---|---|
| FACT= | | 1.0 .75 | .50 .25 | .00 BIN | 1.0 .75 | .50 .25 | .00 BIN | 1.0 .75 | .50 .25 | .00 BIN | 1.0 75 | .50 .25 | .00 BIN | 1.0 .75 | .50 .25 | .00 BIN |
| PCONT=*** | | | | | REQUIRED NUMBER OF PATIENTS | | | | | | | | | | | |
| 0.01 | *** | 1201 | 1201 | 1212 | 442 | 442 | 442 | 145 | 145 | 145 | 75 | 75 | 75 | 46 | 46 | 46 |
| | *** | 1201 | 1212 | 4631 | 442 | 442 | 1531 | 145 | 145 | 417 | 75 | 75 | 170 | 46 | 46 | 101 |
| 0.02 | *** | 2671 | 2682 | 2700 | 862 | 862 | 862 | 232 | 232 | 232 | 99 | 99 | 99 | 64 | 64 | 64 |
| | *** | 2671 | 2689 | 7645 | 862 | 862 | 2277 | 232 | 232 | 532 | 99 | 99 | 197 | 64 | 64 | 113 |
| 0.05 | *** | 8107 | 8195 | 8440 | 2315 | 2332 | 2367 | 495 | 501 | 501 | 180 | 180 | 180 | 99 | 99 | 99 |
| | *** | 8142 | 8282 | 16310 | 2321 | 2350 | 4419 | 495 | 501 | 864 | 180 | 180 | 275 | 99 | 99 | 145 |
| 0.1 | *** | 17907 | 18194 | 19640 | 4894 | 4999 | 5191 | 950 | 956 | 967 | 291 | 291 | 302 | 151 | 162 | 162 |
| | *** | 18012 | 18590 | 29497 | 4946 | 5086 | 7677 | 950 | 956 | 1366 | 291 | 302 | 393 | 162 | 162 | 194 |
| 0.15 | *** | 26804 | 27357 | 31021 | 7267 | 7512 | 8037 | 1370 | 1394 | 1411 | 407 | 407 | 407 | 204 | 204 | 204 |
| | *** | 26990 | 28186 | 41113 | 7372 | 7722 | 10542 | 1387 | 1405 | 1806 | 407 | 407 | 495 | 204 | 204 | 236 |
| 0.2 | *** | 34049 | 34917 | 41679 | 9262 | 9682 | 10669 | 1744 | 1779 | 1825 | 501 | 501 | 501 | 250 | 250 | 250 |
| | *** | 34346 | 36300 | 51159 | 9426 | 10050 | 13014 | 1761 | 1807 | 2182 | 501 | 501 | 581 | 250 | 250 | 271 |
| 0.25 | *** | 39432 | 40692 | 51175 | 10820 | 11439 | 13014 | 2059 | 2111 | 2192 | 582 | 582 | 589 | 274 | 285 | 285 |
| | *** | 39870 | 42705 | 59636 | 11071 | 11999 | 15094 | 2087 | 2146 | 2496 | 582 | 589 | 652 | 274 | 285 | 299 |
| 0.3 | *** | 42985 | 44700 | 59260 | 11957 | 12786 | 15002 | 2304 | 2385 | 2490 | 641 | 652 | 659 | 302 | 309 | 309 |
| | *** | 43580 | 47419 | 66543 | 12296 | 13556 | 16781 | 2339 | 2437 | 2748 | 641 | 652 | 707 | 302 | 309 | 320 |
| 0.35 | *** | 44840 | 47097 | 65794 | 12699 | 13749 | 16595 | 2490 | 2595 | 2724 | 687 | 694 | 711 | 320 | 326 | 326 |
| | *** | 45627 | 50562 | 71881 | 13130 | 14722 | 18076 | 2542 | 2654 | 2936 | 694 | 705 | 746 | 326 | 326 | 334 |
| 0.4 | *** | 45207 | 48066 | 70711 | 13112 | 14355 | 17785 | 2619 | 2735 | 2892 | 722 | 729 | 746 | 337 | 337 | 337 |
| | *** | 46211 | 52301 | 75648 | 13620 | 15510 | 18979 | 2671 | 2811 | 3062 | 729 | 740 | 770 | 337 | 337 | 341 |
| 0.45 | *** | 44332 | 47850 | 73960 | 13206 | 14624 | 18555 | 2682 | 2811 | 2997 | 740 | 746 | 764 | 337 | 337 | 344 |
| | *** | 45592 | 52826 | 77846 | 13795 | 15947 | 19489 | 2741 | 2899 | 3124 | 740 | 757 | 778 | 337 | 344 | 341 |
| 0.5 | *** | 42477 | 46666 | 75506 | 13049 | 14617 | 18894 | 2689 | 2840 | 3032 | 729 | 746 | 764 | 337 | 337 | 337 |
| | *** | 44000 | 52295 | 78474 | 13696 | 16052 | 19607 | 2759 | 2927 | 3124 | 740 | 757 | 770 | 337 | 337 | 334 |
| 0.55 | *** | 39905 | 44717 | 75342 | 12675 | 14337 | 18817 | 2647 | 2794 | 2997 | 722 | 729 | 746 | 320 | 326 | 326 |
| | *** | 41696 | 50866 | 77532 | 13364 | 15842 | 19332 | 2717 | 2892 | 3062 | 722 | 740 | 746 | 326 | 326 | 320 |
| 0.6 | *** | 36860 | 42169 | 73476 | 12104 | 13801 | 18299 | 2549 | 2700 | 2899 | 687 | 694 | 711 | 302 | 309 | 309 |
| | *** | 38879 | 48655 | 75020 | 12815 | 15335 | 18665 | 2619 | 2787 | 2936 | 687 | 705 | 707 | 302 | 309 | 299 |
| 0.65 | *** | 33524 | 39152 | 69906 | 11362 | 13042 | 17371 | 2402 | 2542 | 2724 | 635 | 652 | 659 | 274 | 285 | 285 |
| | *** | 35705 | 45750 | 70939 | 12069 | 14536 | 17606 | 2472 | 2630 | 2748 | 641 | 652 | 652 | 285 | 285 | 271 |
| 0.7 | *** | 30041 | 35740 | 64639 | 10452 | 12062 | 16006 | 2210 | 2332 | 2490 | 571 | 582 | 589 | 250 | 250 | 250 |
| | *** | 32275 | 42197 | 65287 | 11135 | 13445 | 16153 | 2262 | 2402 | 2496 | 571 | 589 | 581 | 250 | 250 | 236 |
| 0.75 | *** | 26436 | 31942 | 57702 | 9385 | 10837 | 14232 | 1954 | 2052 | 2181 | 495 | 501 | 512 | 204 | 204 | 204 |
| | *** | 28624 | 37980 | 58067 | 10004 | 12062 | 14309 | 2000 | 2111 | 2182 | 495 | 501 | 495 | 204 | 204 | 194 |
| 0.8 | *** | 22691 | 27714 | 49099 | 8131 | 9356 | 12045 | 1639 | 1720 | 1814 | 396 | 396 | 407 | 162 | 162 | 162 |
| | *** | 24704 | 33045 | 49276 | 8656 | 10365 | 12072 | 1685 | 1761 | 1806 | 396 | 407 | 393 | 162 | 162 | 145 |
| 0.85 | *** | 18695 | 22919 | 38855 | 6655 | 7589 | 9437 | 1271 | 1324 | 1376 | 285 | 285 | 291 | . | . | . |
| | *** | 20410 | 27224 | 38915 | 7057 | 8317 | 9443 | 1300 | 1352 | 1366 | 285 | 291 | 275 | . | . | . |
| 0.9 | *** | 14186 | 17260 | 26979 | 4859 | 5436 | 6434 | 834 | 851 | 880 | . | . | . | . | . | . |
| | *** | 15457 | 20206 | 26985 | 5115 | 5850 | 6421 | 845 | 862 | 864 | . | . | . | . | . | . |
| 0.95 | *** | 8527 | 10032 | 13497 | 2566 | 2759 | 3021 | . | . | . | . | . | . | . | . | . |
| | *** | 9164 | 11292 | 13485 | 2654 | 2875 | 3007 | . | . | . | . | . | . | . | . | . |
| 0.98 | *** | 3686 | 4065 | 4649 | . | . | . | . | . | . | . | . | . | . | . | . |
| | *** | 3855 | 4316 | 4631 | . | . | . | . | . | . | . | . | . | . | . | . |

## TABLE 5: ALPHA= 0.025 POWER= 0.8    EXPECTED ACCRUAL THRU MINIMUM FOLLOW-UP= 7500

|  |  | DEL=.01 | | | DEL=.02 | | | DEL=.05 | | | DEL=.10 | | | DEL=.15 | | |
|---|---|---|---|---|---|---|---|---|---|---|---|---|---|---|---|---|---|
| | FACT= | 1.0 .75 | .50 .25 | .00 BIN | 1.0 .75 | .50 .25 | .00 BIN | 1.0 .75 | .50 .25 | .00 BIN | 1.0 75 | .50 .25 | .00 BIN | 1.0 .75 | .50 .25 | .00 BIN |
| PCONT=*** | | | | | REQUIRED NUMBER OF PATIENTS | | | | | | | | | | | |
| 0.01 | *** | 1205 1205 | 1212 | 443 443 | 443 | 143 143 | 143 | 68 68 | 68 | 50 50 | 50 | | | | |
| | *** | 1205 1205 | 4631 | 443 443 | 1531 | 143 143 | 417 | 68 68 | 170 | 50 50 | 101 | | | | |
| 0.02 | *** | 2668 2686 | 2705 | 856 856 | 868 | 230 230 | 230 | 99 99 | 99 | 68 68 | 68 | | | | |
| | *** | 2675 2693 | 7645 | 856 856 | 2277 | 230 230 | 532 | 99 99 | 197 | 68 68 | 113 | | | | |
| 0.05 | *** | 8112 8199 | 8443 | 2318 2337 | 2368 | 500 500 | 500 | 174 174 | 174 | 106 106 | 106 | | | | |
| | *** | 8143 8293 | 16310 | 2330 2349 | 4419 | 500 500 | 864 | 174 174 | 275 | 106 106 | 145 | | | | |
| 0.1 | *** | 17930 18230 | 19636 | 4906 5011 | 5199 | 950 961 | 968 | 293 293 | 293 | 155 155 | 155 | | | | |
| | *** | 18043 18631 | 29497 | 4955 5086 | 7677 | 950 961 | 1366 | 293 293 | 393 | 155 155 | 194 | | | | |
| 0.15 | *** | 26843 27425 | 31025 | 7299 7543 | 8030 | 1374 1393 | 1418 | 406 406 | 406 | 200 200 | 200 | | | | |
| | *** | 27043 28280 | 41113 | 7400 7737 | 10542 | 1381 1400 | 1806 | 406 406 | 495 | 200 200 | 236 | | | | |
| 0.2 | *** | 34111 35030 | 41686 | 9293 9718 | 10674 | 1749 1786 | 1831 | 500 500 | 511 | 249 249 | 249 | | | | |
| | *** | 34430 36455 | 51159 | 9474 10081 | 13014 | 1768 1805 | 2182 | 500 500 | 581 | 249 249 | 271 | | | | |
| 0.25 | *** | 39530 40861 | 51174 | 10880 11499 | 13018 | 2068 2124 | 2187 | 575 586 | 586 | 275 275 | 286 | | | | |
| | *** | 39987 42931 | 59636 | 11131 12050 | 15094 | 2093 2150 | 2496 | 586 586 | 652 | 275 275 | 299 | | | | |
| 0.3 | *** | 43111 44930 | 59255 | 12031 12868 | 14993 | 2318 2393 | 2487 | 643 650 | 661 | 305 305 | 305 | | | | |
| | *** | 43737 47724 | 66543 | 12380 13625 | 16781 | 2349 2431 | 2748 | 643 650 | 707 | 305 305 | 320 | | | | |
| 0.35 | *** | 45012 47393 | 65799 | 12800 13850 | 16599 | 2506 2600 | 2724 | 687 699 | 706 | 324 324 | 324 | | | | |
| | *** | 45837 50956 | 71881 | 13231 14806 | 18076 | 2543 2656 | 2936 | 699 706 | 746 | 324 324 | 334 | | | | |
| 0.4 | *** | 45425 48436 | 70711 | 13231 14468 | 17780 | 2630 2743 | 2893 | 725 736 | 743 | 331 331 | 343 | | | | |
| | *** | 46493 52775 | 75648 | 13737 15612 | 18979 | 2686 2818 | 3062 | 725 736 | 770 | 331 343 | 341 | | | | |
| 0.45 | *** | 44611 48293 | 73955 | 13343 14768 | 18549 | 2693 2825 | 2993 | 736 743 | 762 | 343 343 | 343 | | | | |
| | *** | 45931 53375 | 77846 | 13936 16062 | 19489 | 2761 2900 | 3124 | 743 755 | 778 | 343 343 | 341 | | | | |
| 0.5 | *** | 42811 47168 | 75500 | 13205 14768 | 18893 | 2712 2843 | 3031 | 736 743 | 762 | 331 331 | 343 | | | | |
| | *** | 44412 52906 | 78474 | 13861 16175 | 19607 | 2780 2930 | 3124 | 743 755 | 770 | 331 343 | 334 | | | | |
| 0.55 | *** | 40306 45275 | 75343 | 12837 14487 | 18811 | 2668 2806 | 2993 | 718 736 | 743 | 324 324 | 331 | | | | |
| | *** | 42174 51518 | 77532 | 13531 15980 | 19332 | 2731 2893 | 3062 | 725 736 | 746 | 324 324 | 320 | | | | |
| 0.6 | *** | 37318 42774 | 73475 | 12275 13974 | 18305 | 2574 2712 | 2900 | 687 699 | 706 | 305 305 | 312 | | | | |
| | *** | 39406 49336 | 75020 | 12987 15474 | 18665 | 2637 2799 | 2936 | 687 706 | 707 | 305 305 | 299 | | | | |
| 0.65 | *** | 34025 39781 | 69905 | 11525 13205 | 17368 | 2424 2555 | 2724 | 643 650 | 661 | 275 286 | 286 | | | | |
| | *** | 36268 46430 | 70939 | 12237 14668 | 17606 | 2480 2637 | 2748 | 643 650 | 652 | 275 286 | 271 | | | | |
| 0.7 | *** | 30556 36361 | 64643 | 10618 12211 | 16006 | 2218 2337 | 2487 | 575 586 | 593 | 249 249 | 249 | | | | |
| | *** | 32843 42849 | 65287 | 11293 13568 | 16153 | 2274 2405 | 2496 | 575 586 | 581 | 249 249 | 236 | | | | |
| 0.75 | *** | 26949 32525 | 57699 | 9530 10974 | 14236 | 1962 2068 | 2187 | 493 500 | 511 | 211 211 | 211 | | | | |
| | *** | 29168 38581 | 58067 | 10149 12162 | 14309 | 2011 2124 | 2182 | 500 500 | 495 | 211 211 | 194 | | | | |
| 0.8 | *** | 23168 28231 | 49100 | 8255 9474 | 12043 | 1655 1730 | 1812 | 399 399 | 406 | 155 162 | 162 | | | | |
| | *** | 25205 33568 | 49276 | 8780 10449 | 12072 | 1693 1768 | 1806 | 399 406 | 393 | 155 162 | 145 | | | | |
| 0.85 | *** | 19100 23349 | 38855 | 6755 7674 | 9436 | 1280 1325 | 1381 | 286 286 | 286 | . . | . | | | | |
| | *** | 20825 27643 | 38915 | 7156 8375 | 9443 | 1299 1355 | 1366 | 286 286 | 275 | . . | . | | | | |
| 0.9 | *** | 14487 17562 | 26975 | 4925 5487 | 6436 | 837 856 | 875 | . . | . | . . | . | | | | |
| | *** | 15762 20480 | 26985 | 5180 5881 | 6421 | 849 868 | 864 | . . | . | . . | . | | | | |
| 0.95 | *** | 8675 10168 | 13493 | 2581 2768 | 3024 | . . | . | . . | . | . . | . | | | | |
| | *** | 9312 11393 | 13485 | 2675 2881 | 3007 | . . | . | . . | . | . . | . | | | | |
| 0.98 | *** | 3725 4093 | 4643 | . . | . | . . | . | . . | . | . . | . | | | | |
| | *** | 3893 4336 | 4631 | . . | . | . . | . | . . | . | . . | . | | | | |

TABLE 5: ALPHA= 0.025 POWER= 0.8    EXPECTED ACCRUAL THRU MINIMUM FOLLOW-UP= 8000

| | | DEL=.01 | | | DEL=.02 | | | DEL=.05 | | | DEL=.10 | | | DEL=.15 | | |
|---|---|---|---|---|---|---|---|---|---|---|---|---|---|---|---|---|
| FACT= | | 1.0 .75 | .50 .25 | .00 BIN | 1.0 .75 | .50 .25 | .00 BIN | 1.0 .75 | .50 .25 | .00 BIN | 1.0 75 | .50 .25 | .00 BIN | 1.0 .75 | .50 .25 | .00 BIN |
| PCONT=*** | | | | | REQUIRED NUMBER OF PATIENTS | | | | | | | | | | | |
| 0.01 | *** | 1205 | 1205 | 1213 | 445 | 445 | 445 | 145 | 145 | 145 | 73 | 73 | 73 | 53 | 53 | 53 |
| | *** | 1205 | 1205 | 4631 | 445 | 445 | 1531 | 145 | 145 | 417 | 73 | 73 | 170 | 53 | 53 | 101 |
| 0.02 | *** | 2673 | 2685 | 2705 | 853 | 865 | 865 | 233 | 233 | 233 | 105 | 105 | 105 | 65 | 65 | 65 |
| | *** | 2673 | 2693 | 7645 | 853 | 865 | 2277 | 233 | 233 | 532 | 105 | 105 | 197 | 65 | 65 | 113 |
| 0.05 | *** | 8113 | 8205 | 8433 | 2313 | 2333 | 2365 | 493 | 493 | 505 | 173 | 173 | 173 | 105 | 105 | 105 |
| | *** | 8153 | 8293 | 16310 | 2325 | 2345 | 4419 | 493 | 505 | 864 | 173 | 173 | 275 | 105 | 105 | 145 |
| 0.1 | *** | 17953 | 18265 | 19633 | 4925 | 5025 | 5193 | 953 | 953 | 965 | 293 | 293 | 293 | 153 | 153 | 153 |
| | *** | 18065 | 18665 | 29497 | 4965 | 5093 | 7677 | 953 | 965 | 1366 | 293 | 293 | 393 | 153 | 153 | 194 |
| 0.15 | *** | 26885 | 27493 | 31025 | 7313 | 7553 | 8033 | 1373 | 1393 | 1413 | 405 | 405 | 405 | 205 | 205 | 205 |
| | *** | 27093 | 28365 | 41113 | 7425 | 7753 | 10542 | 1385 | 1405 | 1806 | 405 | 405 | 495 | 205 | 205 | 236 |
| 0.2 | *** | 34173 | 35145 | 41685 | 9333 | 9753 | 10673 | 1753 | 1785 | 1825 | 505 | 505 | 505 | 245 | 245 | 245 |
| | *** | 34513 | 36605 | 51159 | 9513 | 10105 | 13014 | 1773 | 1805 | 2182 | 505 | 505 | 581 | 245 | 245 | 271 |
| 0.25 | *** | 39613 | 41025 | 51173 | 10933 | 11553 | 13013 | 2073 | 2125 | 2185 | 585 | 585 | 593 | 273 | 285 | 285 |
| | *** | 40105 | 43153 | 59636 | 11193 | 12093 | 15094 | 2093 | 2153 | 2496 | 585 | 585 | 652 | 273 | 285 | 299 |
| 0.3 | *** | 43245 | 45153 | 59253 | 12113 | 12945 | 14993 | 2325 | 2393 | 2485 | 645 | 653 | 653 | 305 | 305 | 305 |
| | *** | 43905 | 48025 | 66543 | 12453 | 13685 | 16781 | 2353 | 2433 | 2748 | 645 | 653 | 707 | 305 | 305 | 320 |
| 0.35 | *** | 45185 | 47673 | 65793 | 12905 | 13945 | 16593 | 2513 | 2605 | 2725 | 693 | 705 | 705 | 325 | 325 | 325 |
| | *** | 46053 | 51325 | 71881 | 13333 | 14885 | 18076 | 2553 | 2665 | 2936 | 693 | 705 | 746 | 325 | 325 | 334 |
| 0.4 | *** | 45645 | 48793 | 70713 | 13345 | 14585 | 17785 | 2645 | 2753 | 2893 | 725 | 733 | 745 | 333 | 333 | 333 |
| | *** | 46765 | 53225 | 75648 | 13853 | 15705 | 18979 | 2693 | 2813 | 3062 | 725 | 733 | 770 | 333 | 333 | 341 |
| 0.45 | *** | 44873 | 48713 | 73953 | 13473 | 14893 | 18553 | 2713 | 2833 | 2993 | 733 | 745 | 765 | 333 | 345 | 345 |
| | *** | 46273 | 53893 | 77846 | 14073 | 16173 | 19489 | 2773 | 2913 | 3124 | 745 | 753 | 778 | 333 | 345 | 341 |
| 0.5 | *** | 43145 | 47665 | 75505 | 13353 | 14905 | 18893 | 2725 | 2853 | 3033 | 733 | 745 | 765 | 333 | 333 | 345 |
| | *** | 44813 | 53473 | 78474 | 14005 | 16293 | 19607 | 2785 | 2933 | 3124 | 745 | 753 | 770 | 333 | 333 | 334 |
| 0.55 | *** | 40693 | 45813 | 75345 | 12993 | 14645 | 18813 | 2685 | 2813 | 2993 | 725 | 733 | 745 | 325 | 325 | 325 |
| | *** | 42633 | 52133 | 77532 | 13685 | 16093 | 19332 | 2745 | 2905 | 3062 | 725 | 733 | 746 | 325 | 325 | 320 |
| 0.6 | *** | 37753 | 43353 | 73473 | 12433 | 14125 | 18305 | 2585 | 2725 | 2893 | 685 | 693 | 713 | 305 | 305 | 313 |
| | *** | 39905 | 49973 | 75020 | 13145 | 15593 | 18665 | 2653 | 2805 | 2936 | 693 | 705 | 707 | 305 | 305 | 299 |
| 0.65 | *** | 34505 | 40373 | 69905 | 11693 | 13353 | 17365 | 2433 | 2565 | 2725 | 633 | 645 | 665 | 273 | 285 | 285 |
| | *** | 36793 | 47073 | 70939 | 12393 | 14785 | 17606 | 2493 | 2633 | 2748 | 645 | 653 | 652 | 285 | 285 | 271 |
| 0.7 | *** | 31053 | 36945 | 64645 | 10773 | 12345 | 16013 | 2233 | 2345 | 2493 | 573 | 585 | 593 | 245 | 245 | 245 |
| | *** | 33373 | 43465 | 65287 | 11445 | 13673 | 16153 | 2285 | 2413 | 2496 | 573 | 585 | 581 | 245 | 245 | 236 |
| 0.75 | *** | 27433 | 33085 | 57705 | 9673 | 11093 | 14233 | 1973 | 2065 | 2185 | 493 | 505 | 505 | 205 | 205 | 205 |
| | *** | 29685 | 39145 | 58067 | 10285 | 12265 | 14309 | 2025 | 2125 | 2182 | 493 | 505 | 495 | 205 | 205 | 194 |
| 0.8 | *** | 23613 | 28733 | 49093 | 8373 | 9573 | 12045 | 1665 | 1733 | 1813 | 393 | 405 | 405 | 153 | 153 | 165 |
| | *** | 25673 | 34053 | 49276 | 8893 | 10525 | 12072 | 1693 | 1773 | 1806 | 405 | 405 | 393 | 153 | 153 | 145 |
| 0.85 | *** | 19485 | 23753 | 38853 | 6845 | 7745 | 9445 | 1285 | 1325 | 1373 | 285 | 285 | 293 | . | . | . |
| | *** | 21225 | 28025 | 38915 | 7245 | 8425 | 9443 | 1305 | 1353 | 1366 | 285 | 285 | 275 | . | . | . |
| 0.9 | *** | 14773 | 17853 | 26973 | 4985 | 5533 | 6433 | 833 | 853 | 873 | . | . | . | . | . | . |
| | *** | 16053 | 20725 | 26985 | 5225 | 5913 | 6421 | 845 | 865 | 864 | . | . | . | . | . | . |
| 0.95 | *** | 8825 | 10293 | 13493 | 2605 | 2785 | 3025 | . | . | . | . | . | . | . | . | . |
| | *** | 9453 | 11493 | 13485 | 2693 | 2893 | 3007 | . | . | . | . | . | . | . | . | . |
| 0.98 | *** | 3765 | 4125 | 4645 | . | . | . | . | . | . | . | . | . | . | . | . |
| | *** | 3933 | 4353 | 4631 | . | . | . | . | . | . | . | . | . | . | . | . |

## TABLE 5: ALPHA= 0.025 POWER= 0.8     EXPECTED ACCRUAL THRU MINIMUM FOLLOW-UP= 8500

|  | | DEL=.01 | | | DEL=.02 | | | DEL=.05 | | | DEL=.10 | | | DEL=.15 | | |
|---|---|---|---|---|---|---|---|---|---|---|---|---|---|---|---|---|
| FACT= | | 1.0 .75 | .50 .25 | .00 BIN | 1.0 .75 | .50 .25 | .00 BIN | 1.0 .75 | .50 .25 | .00 BIN | 1.0 75 | .50 .25 | .00 BIN | 1.0 .75 | .50 .25 | .00 BIN |
| PCONT=*** | | | | | REQUIRED NUMBER OF PATIENTS | | | | | | | | | | | |
| 0.01 | *** | 1204 | 1204 | 1204 | 439 | 439 | 439 | 141 | 141 | 141 | 70 | 70 | 70 | 48 | 48 | 48 |
| | *** | 1204 | 1204 | 4631 | 439 | 439 | 1531 | 141 | 141 | 417 | 70 | 70 | 170 | 48 | 48 | 101 |
| 0.02 | *** | 2670 | 2683 | 2705 | 856 | 864 | 864 | 226 | 226 | 226 | 99 | 99 | 99 | 70 | 70 | 70 |
| | *** | 2683 | 2691 | 7645 | 856 | 864 | 2277 | 226 | 226 | 532 | 99 | 99 | 197 | 70 | 70 | 113 |
| 0.05 | *** | 8123 | 8216 | 8442 | 2322 | 2343 | 2365 | 495 | 503 | 503 | 176 | 176 | 176 | 99 | 99 | 99 |
| | *** | 8166 | 8301 | 16310 | 2330 | 2351 | 4419 | 495 | 503 | 864 | 176 | 176 | 275 | 99 | 99 | 145 |
| 0.1 | *** | 17970 | 18302 | 19641 | 4936 | 5029 | 5191 | 949 | 962 | 962 | 290 | 290 | 303 | 155 | 155 | 155 |
| | *** | 18090 | 18706 | 29497 | 4978 | 5106 | 7677 | 949 | 962 | 1366 | 290 | 303 | 393 | 155 | 155 | 194 |
| 0.15 | *** | 26930 | 27567 | 31031 | 7337 | 7579 | 8038 | 1374 | 1395 | 1416 | 410 | 410 | 410 | 205 | 205 | 205 |
| | *** | 27150 | 28446 | 41113 | 7443 | 7762 | 10542 | 1387 | 1408 | 1806 | 410 | 410 | 495 | 205 | 205 | 236 |
| 0.2 | *** | 34240 | 35260 | 41685 | 9377 | 9789 | 10673 | 1756 | 1791 | 1833 | 503 | 503 | 503 | 248 | 248 | 248 |
| | *** | 34601 | 36747 | 51159 | 9547 | 10129 | 13014 | 1770 | 1812 | 2182 | 503 | 503 | 581 | 248 | 248 | 271 |
| 0.25 | *** | 39709 | 41188 | 51176 | 10992 | 11608 | 13011 | 2075 | 2131 | 2181 | 580 | 588 | 588 | 282 | 282 | 282 |
| | *** | 40232 | 43364 | 59636 | 11247 | 12140 | 15094 | 2096 | 2152 | 2496 | 580 | 588 | 652 | 282 | 282 | 299 |
| 0.3 | *** | 43364 | 45375 | 59259 | 12182 | 13019 | 14995 | 2330 | 2407 | 2492 | 643 | 651 | 651 | 303 | 303 | 311 |
| | *** | 44065 | 48307 | 66543 | 12530 | 13741 | 16781 | 2365 | 2436 | 2748 | 651 | 651 | 707 | 303 | 303 | 320 |
| 0.35 | *** | 45353 | 47954 | 65796 | 12990 | 14039 | 16589 | 2521 | 2606 | 2726 | 694 | 694 | 707 | 325 | 325 | 325 |
| | *** | 46275 | 51686 | 71881 | 13423 | 14966 | 18076 | 2564 | 2662 | 2936 | 694 | 707 | 746 | 325 | 325 | 334 |
| 0.4 | *** | 45863 | 49136 | 70713 | 13444 | 14698 | 17779 | 2649 | 2755 | 2896 | 728 | 736 | 750 | 333 | 333 | 333 |
| | *** | 47040 | 53649 | 75648 | 13967 | 15795 | 18979 | 2705 | 2819 | 3062 | 728 | 736 | 770 | 333 | 333 | 341 |
| 0.45 | *** | 45149 | 49123 | 73956 | 13606 | 15016 | 18557 | 2726 | 2840 | 3002 | 736 | 750 | 758 | 333 | 346 | 346 |
| | *** | 46607 | 54385 | 77846 | 14201 | 16270 | 19489 | 2776 | 2917 | 3124 | 750 | 758 | 778 | 346 | 346 | 341 |
| 0.5 | *** | 43470 | 48124 | 75507 | 13486 | 15038 | 18897 | 2734 | 2861 | 3031 | 736 | 750 | 758 | 333 | 333 | 346 |
| | *** | 45205 | 54023 | 78474 | 14137 | 16398 | 19607 | 2798 | 2946 | 3124 | 750 | 758 | 770 | 333 | 333 | 334 |
| 0.55 | *** | 41082 | 46339 | 75345 | 13138 | 14783 | 18812 | 2691 | 2832 | 3002 | 715 | 728 | 750 | 325 | 325 | 325 |
| | *** | 43080 | 52714 | 77532 | 13826 | 16206 | 19332 | 2755 | 2904 | 3062 | 728 | 736 | 746 | 325 | 325 | 320 |
| 0.6 | *** | 38192 | 43895 | 73475 | 12586 | 14265 | 18302 | 2598 | 2726 | 2896 | 686 | 694 | 707 | 303 | 303 | 311 |
| | *** | 40389 | 50568 | 75020 | 13295 | 15710 | 18665 | 2662 | 2811 | 2936 | 694 | 707 | 707 | 303 | 311 | 299 |
| 0.65 | *** | 34970 | 40933 | 69905 | 11842 | 13486 | 17367 | 2450 | 2577 | 2726 | 643 | 651 | 665 | 282 | 282 | 282 |
| | *** | 37308 | 47670 | 70939 | 12543 | 14889 | 17606 | 2513 | 2641 | 2748 | 643 | 651 | 652 | 282 | 282 | 271 |
| 0.7 | *** | 31528 | 37499 | 64635 | 10915 | 12480 | 16007 | 2245 | 2351 | 2492 | 580 | 580 | 588 | 248 | 248 | 248 |
| | *** | 33886 | 44044 | 65287 | 11587 | 13776 | 16153 | 2301 | 2415 | 2496 | 580 | 588 | 581 | 248 | 248 | 236 |
| 0.75 | *** | 27894 | 33602 | 57700 | 9802 | 11213 | 14230 | 1982 | 2075 | 2181 | 495 | 503 | 503 | 205 | 205 | 205 |
| | *** | 30181 | 39680 | 58067 | 10405 | 12352 | 14309 | 2025 | 2131 | 2182 | 495 | 503 | 495 | 205 | 205 | 194 |
| 0.8 | *** | 24040 | 29190 | 49101 | 8493 | 9675 | 12041 | 1671 | 1735 | 1812 | 396 | 396 | 410 | 155 | 163 | 163 |
| | *** | 26122 | 34503 | 49276 | 9003 | 10588 | 12072 | 1706 | 1770 | 1806 | 396 | 410 | 393 | 155 | 163 | 145 |
| 0.85 | *** | 19840 | 24133 | 38851 | 6933 | 7813 | 9441 | 1289 | 1331 | 1374 | 282 | 290 | 290 | . | . | . |
| | *** | 21596 | 28375 | 38915 | 7316 | 8471 | 9443 | 1310 | 1353 | 1366 | 282 | 290 | 275 | . | . | . |
| 0.9 | *** | 15038 | 18119 | 26980 | 5029 | 5573 | 6431 | 835 | 856 | 877 | . | . | . | . | . | . |
| | *** | 16326 | 20958 | 26985 | 5276 | 5943 | 6421 | 843 | 864 | 864 | . | . | . | . | . | . |
| 0.95 | *** | 8960 | 10405 | 13500 | 2628 | 2798 | 3023 | . | . | . | . | . | . | . | . | . |
| | *** | 9590 | 11574 | 13485 | 2705 | 2896 | 3007 | . | . | . | . | . | . | . | . | . |
| 0.98 | *** | 3810 | 4150 | 4646 | . | . | . | . | . | . | . | . | . | . | . | . |
| | *** | 3958 | 4370 | 4631 | . | . | . | . | . | . | . | . | . | . | . | . |

TABLE 5: ALPHA= 0.025 POWER= 0.8     EXPECTED ACCRUAL THRU MINIMUM FOLLOW-UP= 9000

| | DEL=.01 | | | DEL=.02 | | | DEL=.05 | | | DEL=.10 | | | DEL=.15 | | |
|---|---|---|---|---|---|---|---|---|---|---|---|---|---|---|---|
| FACT= | 1.0 .75 | .50 .25 | .00 BIN | 1.0 .75 | .50 .25 | .00 BIN | 1.0 .75 | .50 .25 | .00 BIN | 1.0 75 | .50 .25 | .00 BIN | 1.0 .75 | .50 .25 | .00 BIN |
| PCONT=*** | | | | | REQUIRED NUMBER OF PATIENTS | | | | | | | | | | |
| 0.01 *** | 1207 | 1207 | 1207 | 442 | 442 | 442 | 141 | 141 | 141 | 74 | 74 | 74 | 51 | 51 | 51 |
| *** | 1207 | 1207 | 4631 | 442 | 442 | 1531 | 141 | 141 | 417 | 74 | 74 | 170 | 51 | 51 | 101 |
| 0.02 *** | 2670 | 2684 | 2706 | 861 | 861 | 861 | 231 | 231 | 231 | 105 | 105 | 105 | 60 | 60 | 60 |
| *** | 2684 | 2692 | 7645 | 861 | 861 | 2277 | 231 | 231 | 532 | 105 | 105 | 197 | 60 | 60 | 113 |
| 0.05 *** | 8129 | 8227 | 8444 | 2324 | 2346 | 2369 | 501 | 501 | 501 | 172 | 172 | 172 | 105 | 105 | 105 |
| *** | 8174 | 8309 | 16310 | 2332 | 2355 | 4419 | 501 | 501 | 864 | 172 | 172 | 275 | 105 | 105 | 145 |
| 0.1 *** | 17992 | 18330 | 19635 | 4942 | 5032 | 5190 | 951 | 960 | 960 | 299 | 299 | 299 | 164 | 164 | 164 |
| *** | 18119 | 18735 | 29497 | 4979 | 5100 | 7677 | 960 | 960 | 1366 | 299 | 299 | 393 | 164 | 164 | 194 |
| 0.15 *** | 26961 | 27636 | 31020 | 7364 | 7597 | 8039 | 1379 | 1401 | 1410 | 411 | 411 | 411 | 209 | 209 | 209 |
| *** | 27209 | 28522 | 41113 | 7462 | 7777 | 10542 | 1387 | 1410 | 1806 | 411 | 411 | 495 | 209 | 209 | 236 |
| 0.2 *** | 34305 | 35362 | 41685 | 9411 | 9825 | 10671 | 1761 | 1792 | 1829 | 501 | 501 | 510 | 240 | 240 | 240 |
| *** | 34679 | 36884 | 51159 | 9591 | 10162 | 13014 | 1770 | 1806 | 2182 | 501 | 501 | 581 | 240 | 240 | 271 |
| 0.25 *** | 39809 | 41339 | 51171 | 11040 | 11647 | 13011 | 2085 | 2130 | 2189 | 577 | 591 | 591 | 276 | 276 | 285 |
| *** | 40349 | 43552 | 59636 | 11301 | 12179 | 15094 | 2107 | 2152 | 2496 | 577 | 591 | 652 | 276 | 276 | 299 |
| 0.3 *** | 43499 | 45577 | 59257 | 12246 | 13079 | 15000 | 2332 | 2400 | 2490 | 645 | 645 | 659 | 307 | 307 | 307 |
| *** | 44227 | 48570 | 66543 | 12592 | 13799 | 16781 | 2369 | 2445 | 2748 | 645 | 659 | 707 | 307 | 307 | 320 |
| 0.35 *** | 45510 | 48232 | 65796 | 13079 | 14122 | 16597 | 2535 | 2616 | 2729 | 690 | 704 | 712 | 321 | 321 | 330 |
| *** | 46477 | 52026 | 71881 | 13515 | 15022 | 18076 | 2571 | 2670 | 2936 | 704 | 704 | 746 | 321 | 330 | 334 |
| 0.4 *** | 46072 | 49470 | 70710 | 13551 | 14789 | 17781 | 2661 | 2760 | 2895 | 726 | 735 | 749 | 330 | 330 | 344 |
| *** | 47301 | 54060 | 75648 | 14069 | 15877 | 18979 | 2715 | 2827 | 3062 | 726 | 735 | 770 | 330 | 344 | 341 |
| 0.45 *** | 45411 | 49515 | 73964 | 13717 | 15135 | 18555 | 2737 | 2850 | 2999 | 735 | 749 | 757 | 344 | 344 | 344 |
| *** | 46927 | 54839 | 77846 | 14316 | 16364 | 19489 | 2796 | 2917 | 3124 | 749 | 757 | 778 | 344 | 344 | 341 |
| 0.5 *** | 43791 | 48584 | 75502 | 13619 | 15157 | 18892 | 2751 | 2872 | 3030 | 735 | 749 | 757 | 330 | 344 | 344 |
| *** | 45591 | 54532 | 78474 | 14271 | 16499 | 19607 | 2805 | 2954 | 3124 | 749 | 757 | 770 | 330 | 344 | 334 |
| 0.55 *** | 41451 | 46829 | 75345 | 13281 | 14910 | 18816 | 2706 | 2841 | 2999 | 726 | 735 | 749 | 321 | 330 | 330 |
| *** | 43507 | 53264 | 77532 | 13965 | 16305 | 19332 | 2774 | 2909 | 3062 | 726 | 735 | 746 | 321 | 330 | 320 |
| 0.6 *** | 38602 | 44430 | 73477 | 12727 | 14392 | 18307 | 2616 | 2737 | 2895 | 690 | 704 | 712 | 307 | 307 | 307 |
| *** | 40866 | 51135 | 75020 | 13439 | 15810 | 18665 | 2670 | 2819 | 2936 | 690 | 704 | 707 | 307 | 307 | 299 |
| 0.65 *** | 35421 | 41474 | 69900 | 11976 | 13619 | 17362 | 2459 | 2580 | 2729 | 645 | 645 | 659 | 276 | 285 | 285 |
| *** | 37792 | 48232 | 70939 | 12682 | 14991 | 17606 | 2512 | 2647 | 2748 | 645 | 659 | 652 | 276 | 285 | 271 |
| 0.7 *** | 31979 | 38031 | 64635 | 11054 | 12592 | 16012 | 2256 | 2355 | 2490 | 577 | 577 | 591 | 240 | 254 | 254 |
| *** | 34386 | 44579 | 65287 | 11715 | 13866 | 16153 | 2310 | 2422 | 2496 | 577 | 591 | 581 | 254 | 254 | 236 |
| 0.75 *** | 28334 | 34102 | 57696 | 9929 | 11310 | 14235 | 1995 | 2085 | 2189 | 501 | 501 | 510 | 209 | 209 | 209 |
| *** | 30651 | 40169 | 58067 | 10522 | 12426 | 14309 | 2040 | 2130 | 2182 | 501 | 501 | 495 | 209 | 209 | 194 |
| 0.8 *** | 24441 | 29639 | 49101 | 8587 | 9757 | 12044 | 1671 | 1739 | 1815 | 397 | 397 | 411 | 164 | 164 | 164 |
| *** | 26556 | 34935 | 49276 | 9105 | 10657 | 12072 | 1702 | 1770 | 1806 | 397 | 411 | 393 | 164 | 164 | 145 |
| 0.85 *** | 20189 | 24495 | 38850 | 7012 | 7881 | 9442 | 1289 | 1334 | 1379 | 285 | 285 | 285 | . | . | . |
| *** | 21952 | 28702 | 38915 | 7395 | 8520 | 9443 | 1311 | 1356 | 1366 | 285 | 285 | 275 | . | . | . |
| 0.9 *** | 15292 | 18366 | 26984 | 5091 | 5609 | 6427 | 839 | 861 | 884 | . | . | . | . | . | . |
| *** | 16575 | 21179 | 26985 | 5325 | 5969 | 6421 | 847 | 870 | 864 | . | . | . | . | . | . |
| 0.95 *** | 9082 | 10522 | 13492 | 2639 | 2805 | 3021 | . | . | . | . | . | . | . | . | . |
| *** | 9712 | 11661 | 13485 | 2715 | 2909 | 3007 | . | . | . | . | . | . | . | . | . |
| 0.98 *** | 3840 | 4169 | 4650 | . | . | . | . | . | . | . | . | . | . | . | . |
| *** | 3989 | 4380 | 4631 | . | . | . | . | . | . | . | . | . | . | . | . |

## TABLE 5: ALPHA= 0.025 POWER= 0.8    EXPECTED ACCRUAL THRU MINIMUM FOLLOW-UP= 9500

|  | | DEL=.01 | | | DEL=.02 | | | DEL=.05 | | | DEL=.10 | | | DEL=.15 | |
|---|---|---|---|---|---|---|---|---|---|---|---|---|---|---|---|---|
| FACT= | | 1.0 .75 | .50 .25 | .00 BIN | 1.0 .75 | .50 .25 | .00 BIN | 1.0 .75 | .50 .25 | .00 BIN | 1.0 75 | .50 .25 | .00 BIN | 1.0 .75 | .50 .25 | .00 BIN |
| PCONT=*** | | | | | REQUIRED | NUMBER OF | PATIENTS | | | | | | | | | |
| 0.01 | *** | 1203 | 1203 | 1203 | 443 | 443 | 443 | 149 | 149 | 149 | 78 | 78 | 78 | 54 | 54 | 54 |
|  | *** | 1203 | 1203 | 4631 | 443 | 443 | 1531 | 149 | 149 | 417 | 78 | 78 | 170 | 54 | 54 | 101 |
| 0.02 | *** | 2675 | 2690 | 2699 | 861 | 861 | 861 | 229 | 229 | 229 | 101 | 101 | 101 | 63 | 63 | 63 |
|  | *** | 2675 | 2690 | 7645 | 861 | 861 | 2277 | 229 | 229 | 532 | 101 | 101 | 197 | 63 | 63 | 113 |
| 0.05 | *** | 8138 | 8233 | 8438 | 2319 | 2343 | 2367 | 490 | 505 | 505 | 173 | 173 | 173 | 101 | 101 | 101 |
|  | *** | 8176 | 8319 | 16310 | 2334 | 2358 | 4419 | 505 | 505 | 864 | 173 | 173 | 275 | 101 | 101 | 145 |
| 0.1 | *** | 18018 | 18365 | 19633 | 4946 | 5041 | 5193 | 956 | 956 | 965 | 291 | 300 | 300 | 158 | 158 | 158 |
|  | *** | 18151 | 18769 | 29497 | 4994 | 5113 | 7677 | 956 | 965 | 1366 | 300 | 300 | 393 | 158 | 158 | 194 |
| 0.15 | *** | 27010 | 27699 | 31024 | 7378 | 7615 | 8034 | 1384 | 1393 | 1417 | 410 | 410 | 410 | 205 | 205 | 205 |
|  | *** | 27257 | 28601 | 41113 | 7473 | 7782 | 10542 | 1393 | 1408 | 1806 | 410 | 410 | 495 | 205 | 205 | 236 |
| 0.2 | *** | 34373 | 35474 | 41688 | 9444 | 9848 | 10670 | 1764 | 1797 | 1820 | 505 | 505 | 505 | 244 | 244 | 244 |
|  | *** | 34762 | 37009 | 51159 | 9610 | 10180 | 13014 | 1773 | 1811 | 2182 | 505 | 505 | 581 | 244 | 244 | 271 |
| 0.25 | *** | 39892 | 41498 | 51173 | 11083 | 11700 | 13021 | 2082 | 2129 | 2191 | 576 | 585 | 585 | 277 | 277 | 277 |
|  | *** | 40462 | 43739 | 59636 | 11344 | 12214 | 15094 | 2105 | 2153 | 2496 | 585 | 585 | 652 | 277 | 277 | 299 |
| 0.3 | *** | 43620 | 45782 | 59263 | 12318 | 13140 | 15002 | 2343 | 2405 | 2485 | 648 | 648 | 657 | 300 | 300 | 300 |
|  | *** | 44395 | 48822 | 66543 | 12665 | 13838 | 16781 | 2381 | 2453 | 2748 | 648 | 657 | 707 | 300 | 300 | 320 |
| 0.35 | *** | 45678 | 48489 | 65794 | 13164 | 14194 | 16593 | 2548 | 2619 | 2723 | 695 | 704 | 704 | 324 | 324 | 324 |
|  | *** | 46684 | 52337 | 71881 | 13591 | 15088 | 18076 | 2580 | 2666 | 2936 | 695 | 704 | 746 | 324 | 324 | 334 |
| 0.4 | *** | 46280 | 49795 | 70710 | 13648 | 14883 | 17780 | 2675 | 2770 | 2889 | 728 | 728 | 743 | 339 | 339 | 339 |
|  | *** | 47563 | 54441 | 75648 | 14170 | 15943 | 18979 | 2723 | 2833 | 3062 | 728 | 743 | 770 | 339 | 339 | 341 |
| 0.45 | *** | 45678 | 49905 | 73964 | 13829 | 15239 | 18555 | 2747 | 2856 | 2999 | 743 | 752 | 766 | 339 | 339 | 339 |
|  | *** | 47245 | 55282 | 77846 | 14423 | 16441 | 19489 | 2794 | 2928 | 3124 | 743 | 752 | 778 | 339 | 339 | 341 |
| 0.5 | *** | 44110 | 49012 | 75508 | 13743 | 15278 | 18897 | 2761 | 2880 | 3032 | 743 | 752 | 766 | 339 | 339 | 339 |
|  | *** | 45963 | 55020 | 78474 | 14384 | 16593 | 19607 | 2818 | 2951 | 3124 | 743 | 752 | 770 | 339 | 339 | 334 |
| 0.55 | *** | 41815 | 47302 | 75341 | 13410 | 15025 | 18816 | 2723 | 2842 | 2999 | 719 | 728 | 743 | 324 | 324 | 324 |
|  | *** | 43920 | 53785 | 77532 | 14099 | 16403 | 19332 | 2785 | 2913 | 3062 | 728 | 743 | 746 | 324 | 324 | 320 |
| 0.6 | *** | 39013 | 44927 | 73474 | 12855 | 14518 | 18303 | 2628 | 2747 | 2889 | 695 | 704 | 704 | 300 | 300 | 315 |
|  | *** | 41317 | 51672 | 75020 | 13568 | 15904 | 18665 | 2675 | 2818 | 2936 | 695 | 704 | 707 | 300 | 315 | 299 |
| 0.65 | *** | 35845 | 41982 | 69903 | 12119 | 13734 | 17368 | 2476 | 2580 | 2723 | 648 | 648 | 657 | 277 | 277 | 277 |
|  | *** | 38268 | 48765 | 70939 | 12808 | 15088 | 17606 | 2524 | 2652 | 2748 | 648 | 657 | 652 | 277 | 277 | 271 |
| 0.7 | *** | 32425 | 38529 | 64639 | 11178 | 12713 | 16014 | 2263 | 2367 | 2485 | 576 | 585 | 585 | 244 | 244 | 253 |
|  | *** | 34857 | 45093 | 65287 | 11834 | 13948 | 16153 | 2310 | 2429 | 2496 | 576 | 585 | 581 | 244 | 244 | 236 |
| 0.75 | *** | 28753 | 34572 | 57704 | 10038 | 11415 | 14233 | 2001 | 2082 | 2191 | 490 | 505 | 505 | 205 | 205 | 205 |
|  | *** | 31095 | 40643 | 58067 | 10632 | 12499 | 14309 | 2049 | 2129 | 2182 | 505 | 505 | 495 | 205 | 205 | 194 |
| 0.8 | *** | 24834 | 30050 | 49098 | 8684 | 9839 | 12048 | 1678 | 1740 | 1811 | 395 | 395 | 410 | 158 | 158 | 158 |
|  | *** | 26948 | 35332 | 49276 | 9198 | 10718 | 12072 | 1716 | 1773 | 1806 | 395 | 410 | 393 | 158 | 158 | 145 |
| 0.85 | *** | 20512 | 24834 | 38847 | 7084 | 7939 | 9435 | 1298 | 1336 | 1384 | 291 | 291 | 291 | . | . | . |
|  | *** | 22293 | 29014 | 38915 | 7464 | 8556 | 9443 | 1313 | 1360 | 1366 | 291 | 291 | 275 | . | . | . |
| 0.9 | *** | 15539 | 18603 | 26972 | 5136 | 5644 | 6428 | 838 | 861 | 870 | . | . | . | . | . | . |
|  | *** | 16821 | 21367 | 26985 | 5359 | 5977 | 6421 | 847 | 870 | 864 | . | . | . | . | . | . |
| 0.95 | *** | 9207 | 10623 | 13496 | 2652 | 2818 | 3023 | . | . | . | . | . | . | . | . | . |
|  | *** | 9824 | 11739 | 13485 | 2738 | 2913 | 3007 | . | . | . | . | . | . | . | . | . |
| 0.98 | *** | 3863 | 4186 | 4647 | . | . | . | . | . | . | . | . | . | . | . | . |
|  | *** | 4020 | 4400 | 4631 | . | . | . | . | . | . | . | . | . | . | . | . |

TABLE 5: ALPHA= 0.025 POWER= 0.8    EXPECTED ACCRUAL THRU MINIMUM FOLLOW-UP= 10000

| | | DEL=.01 | | | DEL=.02 | | | DEL=.05 | | | DEL=.10 | | | DEL=.15 | | |
|---|---|---|---|---|---|---|---|---|---|---|---|---|---|---|---|---|
| FACT= | | 1.0 .75 | .50 .25 | .00 BIN | 1.0 .75 | .50 .25 | .00 BIN | 1.0 .75 | .50 .25 | .00 BIN | 1.0 75 | .50 .25 | .00 BIN | 1.0 .75 | .50 .25 | .00 BIN |
| PCONT=*** | | | | | | | REQUIRED NUMBER OF PATIENTS | | | | | | | | | |
| 0.01 | *** | 1207 1207 | 1207 | 441 441 | 441 | 141 141 | 141 | 66 66 | 66 | 57 57 | 57 | | | | |
| | *** | 1207 1207 | 4631 | 441 441 | 1531 | 141 141 | 417 | 66 66 | 170 | 57 57 | 101 | | | | |
| 0.02 | *** | 2682 2682 | 2707 | 857 857 | 866 | 232 232 | 232 | 107 107 | 107 | 66 66 | 66 | | | | |
| | *** | 2682 2691 | 7645 | 857 857 | 2277 | 232 232 | 532 | 107 107 | 197 | 66 66 | 113 | | | | |
| 0.05 | *** | 8141 8241 | 8441 | 2332 2341 | 2366 | 491 491 | 507 | 182 182 | 182 | 107 107 | 107 | | | | |
| | *** | 8182 8316 | 16310 | 2332 2357 | 4419 | 491 507 | 864 | 182 182 | 275 | 107 107 | 145 | | | | |
| 0.1 | *** | 18041 18391 | 19641 | 4957 5041 | 5191 | 957 957 | 966 | 291 291 | 291 | 157 157 | 157 | | | | |
| | *** | 18166 18791 | 29497 | 4991 5116 | 7677 | 957 966 | 1366 | 291 291 | 393 | 157 157 | 194 | | | | |
| 0.15 | *** | 27041 27757 | 31032 | 7391 7632 | 8032 | 1382 1407 | 1416 | 407 407 | 407 | 207 207 | 207 | | | | |
| | *** | 27307 28666 | 41113 | 7491 7791 | 10542 | 1391 1407 | 1806 | 407 407 | 495 | 207 207 | 236 | | | | |
| 0.2 | *** | 34432 35566 | 41682 | 9466 9882 | 10666 | 1766 1791 | 1832 | 507 507 | 507 | 241 241 | 241 | | | | |
| | *** | 34841 37132 | 51159 | 9641 10207 | 13014 | 1782 1807 | 2182 | 507 507 | 581 | 241 241 | 271 | | | | |
| 0.25 | *** | 39982 41641 | 51166 | 11132 11741 | 13016 | 2091 2132 | 2191 | 582 582 | 591 | 282 282 | 282 | | | | |
| | *** | 40582 43932 | 59636 | 11391 12241 | 15094 | 2107 2157 | 2496 | 582 591 | 652 | 282 282 | 299 | | | | |
| 0.3 | *** | 43741 45991 | 59257 | 12382 13207 | 14991 | 2357 2416 | 2491 | 641 657 | 657 | 307 307 | 307 | | | | |
| | *** | 44541 49066 | 66543 | 12732 13891 | 16781 | 2382 2441 | 2748 | 641 657 | 707 | 307 307 | 320 | | | | |
| 0.35 | *** | 45841 48757 | 65791 | 13232 14266 | 16591 | 2541 2632 | 2716 | 691 707 | 707 | 316 332 | 332 | | | | |
| | *** | 46891 52641 | 71881 | 13666 15141 | 18076 | 2582 2666 | 2936 | 691 707 | 746 | 332 332 | 334 | | | | |
| 0.4 | *** | 46491 50107 | 70716 | 13741 14966 | 17782 | 2682 2782 | 2891 | 732 732 | 741 | 332 341 | 341 | | | | |
| | *** | 47816 54807 | 75648 | 14266 16016 | 18979 | 2732 2832 | 3062 | 732 741 | 770 | 332 341 | 341 | | | | |
| 0.45 | *** | 45932 50266 | 73957 | 13932 15332 | 18557 | 2757 2866 | 2991 | 741 757 | 757 | 341 341 | 341 | | | | |
| | *** | 47557 55707 | 77846 | 14532 16516 | 19489 | 2807 2932 | 3124 | 741 757 | 778 | 341 341 | 341 | | | | |
| 0.5 | *** | 44416 49432 | 75507 | 13857 15382 | 18891 | 2782 2891 | 3032 | 741 757 | 757 | 332 341 | 341 | | | | |
| | *** | 46316 55482 | 78474 | 14507 16682 | 19607 | 2832 2957 | 3124 | 741 757 | 770 | 332 341 | 334 | | | | |
| 0.55 | *** | 42166 47766 | 75341 | 13532 15141 | 18816 | 2732 2857 | 2991 | 732 732 | 741 | 316 332 | 332 | | | | |
| | *** | 44332 54266 | 77532 | 14216 16491 | 19332 | 2791 2916 | 3062 | 732 741 | 746 | 332 332 | 320 | | | | |
| 0.6 | *** | 39407 45407 | 73482 | 12982 14632 | 18307 | 2632 2757 | 2891 | 691 707 | 707 | 307 307 | 307 | | | | |
| | *** | 41757 52182 | 75020 | 13691 15991 | 18665 | 2691 2816 | 2936 | 691 707 | 707 | 307 307 | 299 | | | | |
| 0.65 | *** | 36266 42466 | 69907 | 12241 13841 | 17366 | 2482 2591 | 2732 | 641 657 | 657 | 282 282 | 282 | | | | |
| | *** | 38716 49266 | 70939 | 12932 15166 | 17606 | 2532 2657 | 2748 | 641 657 | 652 | 282 282 | 271 | | | | |
| 0.7 | *** | 32841 39007 | 64641 | 11291 12807 | 16007 | 2282 2366 | 2491 | 582 582 | 591 | 241 241 | 241 | | | | |
| | *** | 35307 45566 | 65287 | 11957 14032 | 16153 | 2316 2432 | 2496 | 582 591 | 581 | 241 241 | 236 | | | | |
| 0.75 | *** | 29166 35016 | 57707 | 10141 11507 | 14232 | 2007 2091 | 2182 | 491 507 | 507 | 207 207 | 207 | | | | |
| | *** | 31532 41082 | 58067 | 10741 12566 | 14309 | 2041 2132 | 2182 | 491 507 | 495 | 207 207 | 194 | | | | |
| 0.8 | *** | 25207 30457 | 49091 | 8782 9907 | 12041 | 1691 1741 | 1816 | 407 407 | 407 | 157 157 | 157 | | | | |
| | *** | 27341 35707 | 49276 | 9282 10766 | 12072 | 1716 1782 | 1806 | 407 407 | 393 | 157 157 | 145 | | | | |
| 0.85 | *** | 20832 25157 | 38857 | 7157 7991 | 9441 | 1307 1341 | 1382 | 282 291 | 291 | . . | . | | | | |
| | *** | 22616 29307 | 38915 | 7532 8591 | 9443 | 1316 1357 | 1366 | 282 291 | 275 | . . | . | | | | |
| 0.9 | *** | 15766 18816 | 26982 | 5182 5666 | 6432 | 841 857 | 882 | . . | . | . . | . | | | | |
| | *** | 17041 21557 | 26985 | 5407 6007 | 6421 | 857 866 | 864 | . . | . | . . | . | | | | |
| 0.95 | *** | 9316 10716 | 13491 | 2666 2832 | 3016 | . . | . | . . | . | . . | . | | | | |
| | *** | 9932 11807 | 13485 | 2741 2916 | 3007 | . . | . | . . | . | . . | . | | | | |
| 0.98 | *** | 3891 4207 | 4641 | . . | . | . . | . | . . | . | . . | . | | | | |
| | *** | 4041 4407 | 4631 | . . | . | . . | . | . . | . | . . | . | | | | |

## TABLE 5: ALPHA= 0.025 POWER= 0.8   EXPECTED ACCRUAL THRU MINIMUM FOLLOW-UP= 11000

| | | DEL=.01 | | | DEL=.02 | | | DEL=.05 | | | DEL=.10 | | | DEL=.15 | | |
|---|---|---|---|---|---|---|---|---|---|---|---|---|---|---|---|---|---|
| FACT= | | 1.0 .75 | .50 .25 | .00 BIN | 1.0 .75 | .50 .25 | .00 BIN | 1.0 .75 | .50 .25 | .00 BIN | 1.0 75 | .50 .25 | .00 BIN | 1.0 .75 | .50 .25 | .00 BIN |
| PCONT=*** | | | | | REQUIRED NUMBER OF PATIENTS | | | | | | | | | | | |
| 0.01 | *** | 1200 | 1200 | 1217 | 447 | 447 | 447 | 145 | 145 | 145 | 73 | 73 | 73 | 45 | 45 | 45 |
| | *** | 1200 | 1200 | 4631 | 447 | 447 | 1531 | 145 | 145 | 417 | 73 | 73 | 170 | 45 | 45 | 101 |
| 0.02 | *** | 2675 | 2685 | 2702 | 860 | 860 | 860 | 227 | 227 | 227 | 100 | 100 | 100 | 62 | 62 | 62 |
| | *** | 2685 | 2685 | 7645 | 860 | 860 | 2277 | 227 | 227 | 532 | 100 | 100 | 197 | 62 | 62 | 113 |
| 0.05 | *** | 8158 | 8257 | 8433 | 2328 | 2345 | 2355 | 502 | 502 | 502 | 172 | 172 | 172 | 100 | 100 | 100 |
| | *** | 8202 | 8323 | 16310 | 2328 | 2355 | 4419 | 502 | 502 | 864 | 172 | 172 | 275 | 100 | 100 | 145 |
| 0.1 | *** | 18075 | 18443 | 19642 | 4968 | 5067 | 5188 | 953 | 953 | 970 | 293 | 293 | 293 | 155 | 155 | 155 |
| | *** | 18223 | 18845 | 29497 | 5012 | 5122 | 7677 | 953 | 970 | 1366 | 293 | 293 | 393 | 155 | 155 | 194 |
| 0.15 | *** | 27122 | 27875 | 31027 | 7432 | 7652 | 8037 | 1382 | 1393 | 1420 | 403 | 403 | 403 | 200 | 200 | 200 |
| | *** | 27397 | 28800 | 41113 | 7525 | 7817 | 10542 | 1393 | 1410 | 1806 | 403 | 403 | 495 | 200 | 200 | 236 |
| 0.2 | *** | 34558 | 35768 | 41680 | 9533 | 9935 | 10677 | 1767 | 1795 | 1822 | 502 | 502 | 502 | 238 | 238 | 238 |
| | *** | 34998 | 37352 | 51159 | 9698 | 10237 | 13014 | 1778 | 1805 | 2182 | 502 | 502 | 581 | 238 | 238 | 271 |
| 0.25 | *** | 40168 | 41928 | 51168 | 11210 | 11815 | 13015 | 2097 | 2135 | 2190 | 585 | 585 | 585 | 282 | 282 | 282 |
| | *** | 40800 | 44255 | 59636 | 11475 | 12300 | 15094 | 2125 | 2163 | 2496 | 585 | 585 | 652 | 282 | 282 | 299 |
| 0.3 | *** | 43990 | 46372 | 59253 | 12492 | 13300 | 14995 | 2355 | 2410 | 2482 | 650 | 650 | 650 | 310 | 310 | 310 |
| | *** | 44860 | 49518 | 66543 | 12833 | 13960 | 16781 | 2383 | 2455 | 2748 | 650 | 650 | 707 | 310 | 310 | 320 |
| 0.35 | *** | 46163 | 49243 | 65798 | 13383 | 14400 | 16590 | 2565 | 2630 | 2730 | 695 | 705 | 705 | 320 | 320 | 320 |
| | *** | 47290 | 53220 | 71881 | 13812 | 15242 | 18076 | 2592 | 2675 | 2936 | 695 | 705 | 746 | 320 | 320 | 334 |
| 0.4 | *** | 46905 | 50700 | 70710 | 13922 | 15132 | 17783 | 2702 | 2785 | 2895 | 733 | 733 | 750 | 337 | 337 | 337 |
| | *** | 48308 | 55485 | 75648 | 14428 | 16133 | 18979 | 2740 | 2840 | 3062 | 733 | 733 | 770 | 337 | 337 | 341 |
| 0.45 | *** | 46438 | 50975 | 73955 | 14125 | 15517 | 18553 | 2768 | 2878 | 3005 | 750 | 750 | 760 | 337 | 337 | 337 |
| | *** | 48143 | 56475 | 77846 | 14720 | 16655 | 19489 | 2823 | 2933 | 3124 | 750 | 760 | 778 | 337 | 337 | 341 |
| 0.5 | *** | 45008 | 50222 | 75505 | 14070 | 15583 | 18900 | 2795 | 2895 | 3032 | 750 | 750 | 760 | 337 | 337 | 337 |
| | *** | 47005 | 56338 | 78474 | 14720 | 16820 | 19607 | 2840 | 2960 | 3124 | 750 | 760 | 770 | 337 | 337 | 334 |
| 0.55 | *** | 42852 | 48627 | 75340 | 13757 | 15352 | 18817 | 2757 | 2867 | 3005 | 722 | 733 | 750 | 320 | 320 | 320 |
| | *** | 45090 | 55183 | 77532 | 14445 | 16655 | 19332 | 2812 | 2922 | 3062 | 733 | 733 | 746 | 320 | 320 | 320 |
| 0.6 | *** | 40157 | 46317 | 73470 | 13218 | 14830 | 18305 | 2658 | 2768 | 2895 | 695 | 705 | 705 | 310 | 310 | 310 |
| | *** | 42577 | 53120 | 75020 | 13922 | 16150 | 18665 | 2702 | 2823 | 2936 | 695 | 705 | 707 | 310 | 310 | 299 |
| 0.65 | *** | 37050 | 43385 | 69895 | 12465 | 14043 | 17370 | 2510 | 2603 | 2730 | 640 | 650 | 667 | 282 | 282 | 282 |
| | *** | 39580 | 50195 | 70939 | 13152 | 15325 | 17606 | 2548 | 2658 | 2748 | 650 | 650 | 652 | 282 | 282 | 271 |
| 0.7 | *** | 33640 | 39910 | 64643 | 11513 | 12998 | 16012 | 2290 | 2383 | 2493 | 585 | 585 | 595 | 255 | 255 | 255 |
| | *** | 36153 | 46455 | 65287 | 12162 | 14170 | 16153 | 2328 | 2427 | 2496 | 585 | 585 | 581 | 255 | 255 | 236 |
| 0.75 | *** | 29938 | 35850 | 57702 | 10347 | 11667 | 14235 | 2025 | 2097 | 2180 | 502 | 502 | 502 | 210 | 210 | 210 |
| | *** | 32330 | 41873 | 58067 | 10925 | 12685 | 14309 | 2053 | 2135 | 2182 | 502 | 502 | 495 | 210 | 210 | 194 |
| 0.8 | *** | 25895 | 31192 | 49095 | 8955 | 10045 | 12035 | 1695 | 1750 | 1822 | 403 | 403 | 403 | 155 | 155 | 155 |
| | *** | 28068 | 36390 | 49276 | 9440 | 10853 | 12072 | 1723 | 1778 | 1806 | 403 | 403 | 393 | 155 | 155 | 145 |
| 0.85 | *** | 21413 | 25747 | 38848 | 7278 | 8092 | 9440 | 1310 | 1338 | 1382 | 282 | 282 | 293 | . | . | . |
| | *** | 23217 | 29828 | 38915 | 7635 | 8653 | 9443 | 1327 | 1355 | 1366 | 282 | 293 | 275 | . | . | . |
| 0.9 | *** | 16188 | 19213 | 26985 | 5260 | 5727 | 6425 | 843 | 860 | 870 | . | . | . | . | . | . |
| | *** | 17470 | 21880 | 26985 | 5463 | 6040 | 6421 | 860 | 870 | 864 | . | . | . | . | . | . |
| 0.95 | *** | 9522 | 10880 | 13493 | 2702 | 2840 | 3015 | . | . | . | . | . | . | . | . | . |
| | *** | 10127 | 11925 | 13485 | 2768 | 2922 | 3007 | . | . | . | . | . | . | . | . | . |
| 0.98 | *** | 3940 | 4242 | 4638 | . | . | . | . | . | . | . | . | . | . | . | . |
| | *** | 4077 | 4418 | 4631 | . | . | . | . | . | . | . | . | . | . | . | . |

TABLE 5: ALPHA= 0.025 POWER= 0.8     EXPECTED ACCRUAL THRU MINIMUM FOLLOW-UP= 12000

| | | DEL=.01 | | | DEL=.02 | | | DEL=.05 | | | DEL=.10 | | | DEL=.15 | | |
|---|---|---|---|---|---|---|---|---|---|---|---|---|---|---|---|---|---|
| FACT= | | 1.0 .75 | .50 .25 | .00 BIN | 1.0 .75 | .50 .25 | .00 BIN | 1.0 .75 | .50 .25 | .00 BIN | 1.0 75 | .50 .25 | .00 BIN | 1.0 .75 | .50 .25 | .00 BIN |
| PCONT=*** | | | | | | REQUIRED NUMBER OF PATIENTS | | | | | | | | | | |
| 0.01 | *** | 1208 | 1208 | 1208 | 439 | 439 | 439 | 139 | 139 | 139 | 68 | 68 | 68 | 49 | 49 | 49 |
| | *** | 1208 | 1208 | 4631 | 439 | 439 | 1531 | 139 | 139 | 417 | 68 | 68 | 170 | 49 | 49 | 101 |
| 0.02 | *** | 2678 | 2689 | 2708 | 859 | 859 | 859 | 229 | 229 | 229 | 98 | 98 | 98 | 68 | 68 | 68 |
| | *** | 2678 | 2689 | 7645 | 859 | 859 | 2277 | 229 | 229 | 532 | 98 | 98 | 197 | 68 | 68 | 113 |
| 0.05 | *** | 8168 | 8258 | 8438 | 2329 | 2348 | 2359 | 499 | 499 | 499 | 169 | 169 | 169 | 98 | 98 | 98 |
| | *** | 8209 | 8329 | 16310 | 2329 | 2348 | 4419 | 499 | 499 | 864 | 169 | 169 | 275 | 98 | 98 | 145 |
| 0.1 | *** | 18128 | 18499 | 19639 | 4988 | 5059 | 5198 | 949 | 968 | 968 | 289 | 289 | 289 | 158 | 158 | 158 |
| | *** | 18259 | 18889 | 29497 | 5018 | 5119 | 7677 | 949 | 968 | 1366 | 289 | 289 | 393 | 158 | 158 | 194 |
| 0.15 | *** | 27199 | 27979 | 31028 | 7459 | 7669 | 8029 | 1388 | 1399 | 1418 | 409 | 409 | 409 | 199 | 199 | 199 |
| | *** | 27499 | 28909 | 41113 | 7549 | 7838 | 10542 | 1399 | 1399 | 1806 | 409 | 409 | 495 | 199 | 199 | 236 |
| 0.2 | *** | 34669 | 35959 | 41678 | 9589 | 9979 | 10669 | 1778 | 1808 | 1819 | 499 | 499 | 499 | 248 | 248 | 248 |
| | *** | 35149 | 37549 | 51159 | 9758 | 10268 | 13014 | 1789 | 1808 | 2182 | 499 | 499 | 581 | 248 | 248 | 271 |
| 0.25 | *** | 40339 | 42199 | 51169 | 11299 | 11888 | 13009 | 2108 | 2138 | 2179 | 578 | 589 | 589 | 278 | 278 | 278 |
| | *** | 41018 | 44558 | 59636 | 11558 | 12338 | 15094 | 2119 | 2168 | 2496 | 589 | 589 | 652 | 278 | 278 | 299 |
| 0.3 | *** | 44228 | 46748 | 59258 | 12589 | 13399 | 14989 | 2378 | 2419 | 2479 | 649 | 649 | 649 | 308 | 308 | 308 |
| | *** | 45158 | 49928 | 66543 | 12938 | 14029 | 16781 | 2389 | 2449 | 2748 | 649 | 649 | 707 | 308 | 308 | 320 |
| 0.35 | *** | 46478 | 49699 | 65798 | 13508 | 14528 | 16598 | 2569 | 2648 | 2719 | 698 | 698 | 709 | 319 | 319 | 319 |
| | *** | 47678 | 53738 | 71881 | 13939 | 15338 | 18076 | 2599 | 2678 | 2936 | 698 | 709 | 746 | 319 | 319 | 334 |
| 0.4 | *** | 47299 | 51278 | 70718 | 14078 | 15278 | 17779 | 2708 | 2798 | 2899 | 728 | 739 | 739 | 338 | 338 | 338 |
| | *** | 48788 | 56108 | 75648 | 14588 | 16238 | 18979 | 2749 | 2839 | 3062 | 728 | 739 | 770 | 338 | 338 | 341 |
| 0.45 | *** | 46928 | 51619 | 73958 | 14318 | 15679 | 18548 | 2798 | 2888 | 2989 | 739 | 758 | 758 | 338 | 338 | 338 |
| | *** | 48709 | 57188 | 77846 | 14899 | 16778 | 19489 | 2839 | 2929 | 3124 | 739 | 758 | 778 | 338 | 338 | 341 |
| 0.5 | *** | 45589 | 50959 | 75499 | 14269 | 15758 | 18889 | 2809 | 2918 | 3038 | 739 | 758 | 758 | 338 | 338 | 338 |
| | *** | 47659 | 57128 | 78474 | 14899 | 16958 | 19607 | 2858 | 2959 | 3124 | 739 | 758 | 770 | 338 | 338 | 334 |
| 0.55 | *** | 43508 | 49418 | 75338 | 13969 | 15529 | 18818 | 2768 | 2869 | 2989 | 728 | 739 | 739 | 319 | 319 | 319 |
| | *** | 45818 | 56018 | 77532 | 14648 | 16789 | 19332 | 2809 | 2929 | 3062 | 728 | 739 | 746 | 319 | 319 | 320 |
| 0.6 | *** | 40868 | 47149 | 73478 | 13429 | 15019 | 18308 | 2678 | 2768 | 2899 | 698 | 698 | 709 | 308 | 308 | 308 |
| | *** | 43358 | 53959 | 75020 | 14119 | 16279 | 18665 | 2719 | 2828 | 2936 | 698 | 709 | 707 | 308 | 308 | 299 |
| 0.65 | *** | 37789 | 44239 | 69908 | 12679 | 14228 | 17359 | 2509 | 2618 | 2719 | 649 | 649 | 668 | 278 | 278 | 278 |
| | *** | 40369 | 51038 | 70939 | 13358 | 15458 | 17606 | 2558 | 2659 | 2748 | 649 | 649 | 652 | 278 | 278 | 271 |
| 0.7 | *** | 34388 | 40729 | 64639 | 11708 | 13159 | 16009 | 2299 | 2389 | 2498 | 578 | 589 | 589 | 248 | 248 | 248 |
| | *** | 36938 | 47258 | 65287 | 12349 | 14288 | 16153 | 2348 | 2438 | 2496 | 578 | 589 | 581 | 248 | 248 | 236 |
| 0.75 | *** | 30649 | 36619 | 57698 | 10519 | 11809 | 14228 | 2029 | 2108 | 2179 | 499 | 499 | 499 | 199 | 199 | 199 |
| | *** | 33079 | 42608 | 58067 | 11089 | 12788 | 14309 | 2059 | 2138 | 2182 | 499 | 499 | 495 | 199 | 199 | 194 |
| 0.8 | *** | 26558 | 31849 | 49099 | 9098 | 10159 | 12038 | 1699 | 1759 | 1819 | 398 | 398 | 409 | 158 | 158 | 158 |
| | *** | 28729 | 37009 | 49276 | 9578 | 10939 | 12072 | 1729 | 1789 | 1806 | 398 | 409 | 393 | 158 | 158 | 145 |
| 0.85 | *** | 21949 | 26288 | 38858 | 7388 | 8168 | 9439 | 1309 | 1339 | 1369 | 289 | 289 | 289 | . | . | . |
| | *** | 23749 | 30308 | 38915 | 7748 | 8708 | 9443 | 1328 | 1358 | 1366 | 289 | 289 | 275 | . | . | . |
| 0.9 | *** | 16579 | 19579 | 26978 | 5318 | 5768 | 6428 | 848 | 859 | 878 | . | . | . | . | . | . |
| | *** | 17858 | 22178 | 26985 | 5528 | 6068 | 6421 | 859 | 878 | 864 | . | . | . | . | . | . |
| 0.95 | *** | 9709 | 11029 | 13489 | 2719 | 2858 | 3019 | . | . | . | . | . | . | . | . | . |
| | *** | 10298 | 12038 | 13485 | 2779 | 2929 | 3007 | . | . | . | . | . | . | . | . | . |
| 0.98 | *** | 3979 | 4268 | 4639 | . | . | . | . | . | . | . | . | . | . | . | . |
| | *** | 4118 | 4448 | 4631 | . | . | . | . | . | . | . | . | . | . | . | . |

## TABLE 5: ALPHA= 0.025 POWER= 0.8    EXPECTED ACCRUAL THRU MINIMUM FOLLOW-UP= 13000

| | | DEL=.01 | | | DEL=.02 | | | DEL=.05 | | | DEL=.10 | | | DEL=.15 | | |
|---|---|---|---|---|---|---|---|---|---|---|---|---|---|---|---|---|---|
| FACT= | | 1.0 .75 | .50 .25 | .00 BIN | 1.0 .75 | .50 .25 | .00 BIN | 1.0 .75 | .50 .25 | .00 BIN | 1.0 75 | .50 .25 | .00 BIN | 1.0 .75 | .50 .25 | .00 BIN |
| PCONT=*** | | | | | | | REQUIRED NUMBER OF PATIENTS | | | | | | | | |
| 0.01 | *** | 1211 | 1211 | 1211 | 443 | 443 | 443 | 139 | 139 | 139 | 74 | 74 | 74 | 53 | 53 | 53 |
| | *** | 1211 | 1211 | 4631 | 443 | 443 | 1531 | 139 | 139 | 417 | 74 | 74 | 170 | 53 | 53 | 101 |
| 0.02 | *** | 2686 | 2686 | 2706 | 854 | 866 | 866 | 236 | 236 | 236 | 106 | 106 | 106 | 74 | 74 | 74 |
| | *** | 2686 | 2686 | 7645 | 854 | 866 | 2277 | 236 | 236 | 532 | 106 | 106 | 197 | 74 | 74 | 113 |
| 0.05 | *** | 8178 | 8276 | 8438 | 2328 | 2349 | 2361 | 496 | 496 | 496 | 171 | 171 | 171 | 106 | 106 | 106 |
| | *** | 8211 | 8341 | 16310 | 2328 | 2349 | 4419 | 496 | 496 | 864 | 171 | 171 | 275 | 106 | 106 | 145 |
| 0.1 | *** | 18156 | 18546 | 19639 | 4993 | 5079 | 5188 | 951 | 963 | 963 | 301 | 301 | 301 | 151 | 151 | 151 |
| | *** | 18306 | 18936 | 29497 | 5026 | 5123 | 7677 | 963 | 963 | 1366 | 301 | 301 | 393 | 151 | 151 | 194 |
| 0.15 | *** | 27276 | 28089 | 31026 | 7484 | 7691 | 8036 | 1386 | 1406 | 1418 | 411 | 411 | 411 | 204 | 204 | 204 |
| | *** | 27581 | 29011 | 41113 | 7581 | 7841 | 10542 | 1406 | 1406 | 1806 | 411 | 411 | 495 | 204 | 204 | 236 |
| 0.2 | *** | 34796 | 36128 | 41686 | 9629 | 10019 | 10669 | 1776 | 1796 | 1829 | 496 | 508 | 508 | 248 | 248 | 248 |
| | *** | 35283 | 37741 | 51159 | 9803 | 10291 | 13014 | 1796 | 1808 | 2182 | 496 | 508 | 581 | 248 | 248 | 271 |
| 0.25 | *** | 40516 | 42454 | 51176 | 11363 | 11948 | 13009 | 2101 | 2154 | 2186 | 573 | 594 | 594 | 281 | 281 | 281 |
| | *** | 41231 | 44838 | 59636 | 11623 | 12391 | 15094 | 2121 | 2166 | 2496 | 594 | 594 | 652 | 281 | 281 | 299 |
| 0.3 | *** | 44469 | 47081 | 59256 | 12696 | 13476 | 15003 | 2381 | 2426 | 2491 | 638 | 659 | 659 | 301 | 301 | 301 |
| | *** | 45444 | 50298 | 66543 | 13041 | 14093 | 16781 | 2393 | 2458 | 2748 | 659 | 659 | 707 | 301 | 301 | 320 |
| 0.35 | *** | 46788 | 50136 | 65801 | 13638 | 14634 | 16596 | 2576 | 2641 | 2718 | 691 | 703 | 703 | 334 | 334 | 334 |
| | *** | 48044 | 54219 | 71881 | 14061 | 15414 | 18076 | 2609 | 2686 | 2936 | 703 | 703 | 746 | 334 | 334 | 334 |
| 0.4 | *** | 47686 | 51793 | 70708 | 14211 | 15393 | 17786 | 2718 | 2804 | 2901 | 724 | 736 | 736 | 334 | 334 | 334 |
| | *** | 49246 | 56668 | 75648 | 14731 | 16336 | 18979 | 2771 | 2848 | 3062 | 736 | 736 | 770 | 334 | 334 | 341 |
| 0.45 | *** | 47394 | 52248 | 73958 | 14471 | 15816 | 18546 | 2804 | 2901 | 2999 | 736 | 756 | 756 | 334 | 346 | 346 |
| | *** | 49258 | 57838 | 77846 | 15056 | 16888 | 19489 | 2848 | 2946 | 3124 | 756 | 756 | 778 | 346 | 346 | 341 |
| 0.5 | *** | 46138 | 51651 | 75506 | 14451 | 15913 | 18891 | 2816 | 2913 | 3031 | 736 | 756 | 756 | 334 | 334 | 334 |
| | *** | 48283 | 57838 | 78474 | 15089 | 17071 | 19607 | 2869 | 2966 | 3124 | 756 | 756 | 770 | 334 | 334 | 334 |
| 0.55 | *** | 44123 | 50168 | 75344 | 14158 | 15686 | 18806 | 2783 | 2881 | 2999 | 724 | 736 | 736 | 334 | 334 | 334 |
| | *** | 46496 | 56766 | 77532 | 14829 | 16909 | 19332 | 2836 | 2934 | 3062 | 736 | 736 | 746 | 334 | 334 | 320 |
| 0.6 | *** | 41523 | 47926 | 73471 | 13626 | 15186 | 18306 | 2686 | 2783 | 2901 | 691 | 703 | 703 | 301 | 301 | 313 |
| | *** | 44079 | 54739 | 75020 | 14309 | 16401 | 18665 | 2739 | 2836 | 2936 | 703 | 703 | 707 | 301 | 313 | 299 |
| 0.65 | *** | 38489 | 45021 | 69896 | 12879 | 14386 | 17364 | 2523 | 2621 | 2718 | 638 | 659 | 659 | 281 | 281 | 281 |
| | *** | 41121 | 51814 | 70939 | 13529 | 15556 | 17606 | 2576 | 2674 | 2748 | 659 | 659 | 652 | 281 | 281 | 271 |
| 0.7 | *** | 35076 | 41491 | 64631 | 11883 | 13313 | 16011 | 2316 | 2393 | 2491 | 573 | 594 | 594 | 248 | 248 | 248 |
| | *** | 37676 | 47991 | 65287 | 12521 | 14386 | 16153 | 2361 | 2446 | 2496 | 573 | 594 | 581 | 248 | 248 | 236 |
| 0.75 | *** | 31318 | 37331 | 57696 | 10681 | 11948 | 14223 | 2036 | 2101 | 2186 | 496 | 508 | 508 | 204 | 204 | 204 |
| | *** | 33776 | 43266 | 58067 | 11254 | 12879 | 14309 | 2068 | 2154 | 2182 | 496 | 508 | 495 | 204 | 204 | 194 |
| 0.8 | *** | 27146 | 32476 | 49096 | 9239 | 10279 | 12046 | 1711 | 1764 | 1808 | 399 | 399 | 411 | 151 | 151 | 151 |
| | *** | 29336 | 37558 | 49276 | 9694 | 11006 | 12072 | 1731 | 1796 | 1806 | 399 | 399 | 393 | 151 | 151 | 145 |
| 0.85 | *** | 22446 | 26768 | 38846 | 7496 | 8243 | 9434 | 1321 | 1341 | 1374 | 281 | 281 | 281 | . | . | . |
| | *** | 24254 | 30721 | 38915 | 7841 | 8763 | 9443 | 1321 | 1353 | 1366 | 281 | 281 | 275 | . | . | . |
| 0.9 | *** | 16941 | 19911 | 26984 | 5383 | 5806 | 6423 | 854 | 866 | 886 | . | . | . | . | . | . |
| | *** | 18209 | 22434 | 26985 | 5578 | 6086 | 6421 | 854 | 866 | 864 | . | . | . | . | . | . |
| 0.95 | *** | 9868 | 11168 | 13496 | 2739 | 2869 | 3011 | . | . | . | . | . | . | . | . | . |
| | *** | 10453 | 12111 | 13485 | 2804 | 2934 | 3007 | . | . | . | . | . | . | . | . | . |
| 0.98 | *** | 4018 | 4299 | 4636 | . | . | . | . | . | . | . | . | . | . | . | . |
| | *** | 4148 | 4461 | 4631 | . | . | . | . | . | . | . | . | . | . | . | . |

TABLE 5: ALPHA= 0.025 POWER= 0.8    EXPECTED ACCRUAL THRU MINIMUM FOLLOW-UP= 14000

| | | DEL=.01 | | | DEL=.02 | | | DEL=.05 | | | DEL=.10 | | | DEL=.15 | | |
|---|---|---|---|---|---|---|---|---|---|---|---|---|---|---|---|---|---|
| FACT= | | 1.0 .75 | .50 .25 | .00 BIN | 1.0 .75 | .50 .25 | .00 BIN | 1.0 .75 | .50 .25 | .00 BIN | 1.0 75 | .50 .25 | .00 BIN | 1.0 .75 | .50 .25 | .00 BIN |
| PCONT=*** | | | | | | REQUIRED NUMBER OF PATIENTS | | | | | | | | | | |
| 0.01 | *** | 1199 | 1212 | 1212 | 442 | 442 | 442 | 149 | 149 | 149 | 79 | 79 | 79 | 44 | 44 | 44 |
| | *** | 1212 | 1212 | 4631 | 442 | 442 | 1531 | 149 | 149 | 417 | 79 | 79 | 170 | 44 | 44 | 101 |
| 0.02 | *** | 2682 | 2682 | 2704 | 862 | 862 | 862 | 232 | 232 | 232 | 92 | 92 | 92 | 57 | 57 | 57 |
| | *** | 2682 | 2704 | 7645 | 862 | 862 | 2277 | 232 | 232 | 532 | 92 | 92 | 197 | 57 | 57 | 113 |
| 0.05 | *** | 8199 | 8282 | 8444 | 2332 | 2354 | 2367 | 499 | 499 | 499 | 184 | 184 | 184 | 92 | 92 | 92 |
| | *** | 8234 | 8339 | 16310 | 2332 | 2354 | 4419 | 499 | 499 | 864 | 184 | 184 | 275 | 92 | 92 | 145 |
| 0.1 | *** | 18187 | 18594 | 19644 | 4992 | 5084 | 5189 | 954 | 954 | 967 | 289 | 302 | 302 | 162 | 162 | 162 |
| | *** | 18349 | 18979 | 29497 | 5049 | 5132 | 7677 | 954 | 967 | 1366 | 302 | 302 | 393 | 162 | 162 | 194 |
| 0.15 | *** | 27357 | 28184 | 31019 | 7512 | 7722 | 8037 | 1387 | 1409 | 1409 | 407 | 407 | 407 | 197 | 197 | 197 |
| | *** | 27672 | 29107 | 41113 | 7604 | 7849 | 10542 | 1387 | 1409 | 1806 | 407 | 407 | 495 | 197 | 197 | 236 |
| 0.2 | *** | 34917 | 36304 | 41672 | 9682 | 10054 | 10662 | 1772 | 1807 | 1829 | 499 | 499 | 499 | 254 | 254 | 254 |
| | *** | 35429 | 37914 | 51159 | 9844 | 10312 | 13014 | 1794 | 1807 | 2182 | 499 | 499 | 581 | 254 | 254 | 271 |
| 0.25 | *** | 40692 | 42709 | 51179 | 11432 | 11992 | 13007 | 2109 | 2144 | 2192 | 582 | 582 | 582 | 289 | 289 | 289 |
| | *** | 41449 | 45102 | 59636 | 11677 | 12412 | 15094 | 2122 | 2157 | 2496 | 582 | 582 | 652 | 289 | 289 | 299 |
| 0.3 | *** | 44704 | 47412 | 59264 | 12784 | 13554 | 15002 | 2389 | 2437 | 2494 | 652 | 652 | 652 | 302 | 302 | 302 |
| | *** | 45719 | 50654 | 66543 | 13112 | 14149 | 16781 | 2402 | 2459 | 2748 | 652 | 652 | 707 | 302 | 302 | 320 |
| 0.35 | *** | 47097 | 50562 | 65787 | 13742 | 14722 | 16599 | 2599 | 2647 | 2717 | 687 | 709 | 709 | 324 | 324 | 324 |
| | *** | 48414 | 54644 | 71881 | 14162 | 15479 | 18076 | 2612 | 2682 | 2936 | 709 | 709 | 746 | 324 | 324 | 334 |
| 0.4 | *** | 48064 | 52299 | 70709 | 14359 | 15514 | 17789 | 2739 | 2809 | 2892 | 722 | 744 | 744 | 337 | 337 | 337 |
| | *** | 49687 | 57199 | 75648 | 14849 | 16424 | 18979 | 2774 | 2844 | 3062 | 722 | 744 | 770 | 337 | 337 | 341 |
| 0.45 | *** | 47854 | 52824 | 73964 | 14617 | 15947 | 18559 | 2809 | 2892 | 2997 | 744 | 757 | 757 | 337 | 337 | 337 |
| | *** | 49779 | 58437 | 77846 | 15199 | 16984 | 19489 | 2857 | 2949 | 3124 | 744 | 757 | 778 | 337 | 337 | 341 |
| 0.5 | *** | 46664 | 52299 | 75504 | 14617 | 16052 | 18887 | 2844 | 2927 | 3032 | 744 | 757 | 757 | 337 | 337 | 337 |
| | *** | 48869 | 58494 | 78474 | 15234 | 17172 | 19607 | 2879 | 2984 | 3124 | 744 | 757 | 770 | 337 | 337 | 334 |
| 0.55 | *** | 44717 | 50864 | 75342 | 14337 | 15842 | 18817 | 2787 | 2892 | 2997 | 722 | 744 | 744 | 324 | 324 | 324 |
| | *** | 47154 | 57457 | 77532 | 14989 | 17019 | 19332 | 2844 | 2949 | 3062 | 722 | 744 | 746 | 324 | 324 | 320 |
| 0.6 | *** | 42162 | 48659 | 73474 | 13799 | 15339 | 18292 | 2704 | 2787 | 2892 | 687 | 709 | 709 | 302 | 302 | 302 |
| | *** | 44752 | 55449 | 75020 | 14477 | 16507 | 18665 | 2739 | 2844 | 2936 | 709 | 709 | 707 | 302 | 302 | 299 |
| 0.65 | *** | 39152 | 45754 | 69904 | 13042 | 14534 | 17369 | 2542 | 2634 | 2717 | 652 | 652 | 652 | 289 | 289 | 289 |
| | *** | 41812 | 52509 | 70939 | 13694 | 15667 | 17606 | 2577 | 2669 | 2748 | 652 | 652 | 652 | 289 | 289 | 271 |
| 0.7 | *** | 35744 | 42197 | 64632 | 12062 | 13449 | 16004 | 2332 | 2402 | 2494 | 582 | 582 | 582 | 254 | 254 | 254 |
| | *** | 38369 | 48637 | 65287 | 12679 | 14477 | 16153 | 2367 | 2437 | 2496 | 582 | 582 | 581 | 254 | 254 | 236 |
| 0.75 | *** | 31942 | 37984 | 57702 | 10837 | 12062 | 14232 | 2052 | 2109 | 2179 | 499 | 499 | 512 | 197 | 197 | 197 |
| | *** | 34414 | 43864 | 58067 | 11384 | 12959 | 14309 | 2087 | 2144 | 2182 | 499 | 499 | 495 | 197 | 197 | 194 |
| 0.8 | *** | 27707 | 33049 | 49092 | 9354 | 10369 | 12049 | 1724 | 1759 | 1807 | 394 | 407 | 407 | 162 | 162 | 162 |
| | *** | 29912 | 38067 | 49276 | 9809 | 11069 | 12072 | 1737 | 1794 | 1806 | 407 | 407 | 393 | 162 | 162 | 145 |
| 0.85 | *** | 22912 | 27217 | 38859 | 7582 | 8317 | 9437 | 1317 | 1352 | 1374 | 289 | 289 | 289 | . | . | . |
| | *** | 24719 | 31102 | 38915 | 7919 | 8807 | 9443 | 1339 | 1352 | 1366 | 289 | 289 | 275 | . | . | . |
| 0.9 | *** | 17264 | 20204 | 26972 | 5434 | 5854 | 6427 | 849 | 862 | 884 | . | . | . | . | . | . |
| | *** | 18524 | 22667 | 26985 | 5622 | 6112 | 6421 | 862 | 862 | 864 | . | . | . | . | . | . |
| 0.95 | *** | 10032 | 11292 | 13497 | 2752 | 2879 | 3019 | . | . | . | . | . | . | . | . | . |
| | *** | 10592 | 12202 | 13485 | 2809 | 2949 | 3007 | . | . | . | . | . | . | . | . | . |
| 0.98 | *** | 4069 | 4314 | 4642 | . | . | . | . | . | . | . | . | . | . | . | . |
| | *** | 4174 | 4467 | 4631 | . | . | . | . | . | . | . | . | . | . | . | . |

## TABLE 5: ALPHA= 0.025 POWER= 0.8    EXPECTED ACCRUAL THRU MINIMUM FOLLOW-UP= 15000

| | | DEL=.01 | | | DEL=.02 | | | DEL=.05 | | | DEL=.10 | | | DEL=.15 | | |
|---|---|---|---|---|---|---|---|---|---|---|---|---|---|---|---|---|
| FACT= | | 1.0 .75 | .50 .25 | .00 BIN | 1.0 .75 | .50 .25 | .00 BIN | 1.0 .75 | .50 .25 | .00 BIN | 1.0 75 | .50 .25 | .00 BIN | 1.0 .75 | .50 .25 | .00 BIN |
| PCONT=*** | | | | | | REQUIRED | NUMBER | OF PATIENTS | | | | | | | | |
| 0.01 | *** | 1210 | 1210 | 1210 | 436 | 436 | 436 | 136 | 136 | 136 | 61 | 61 | 61 | 47 | 47 | 47 |
| | *** | 1210 | 1210 | 4631 | 436 | 436 | 1531 | 136 | 136 | 417 | 61 | 61 | 170 | 47 | 47 | 101 |
| 0.02 | *** | 2686 | 2686 | 2710 | 849 | 849 | 872 | 235 | 235 | 235 | 99 | 99 | 99 | 61 | 61 | 61 |
| | *** | 2686 | 2686 | 7645 | 849 | 849 | 2277 | 235 | 235 | 532 | 99 | 99 | 197 | 61 | 61 | 113 |
| 0.05 | *** | 8199 | 8297 | 8447 | 2335 | 2349 | 2372 | 497 | 497 | 497 | 174 | 174 | 174 | 99 | 99 | 99 |
| | *** | 8236 | 8349 | 16310 | 2335 | 2349 | 4419 | 497 | 497 | 864 | 174 | 174 | 275 | 99 | 99 | 145 |
| 0.1 | *** | 18235 | 18624 | 19636 | 5011 | 5086 | 5199 | 961 | 961 | 961 | 286 | 286 | 286 | 160 | 160 | 160 |
| | *** | 18399 | 18999 | 29497 | 5049 | 5147 | 7677 | 961 | 961 | 1366 | 286 | 286 | 393 | 160 | 160 | 194 |
| 0.15 | *** | 27422 | 28285 | 31022 | 7547 | 7735 | 8035 | 1397 | 1397 | 1411 | 399 | 399 | 399 | 197 | 197 | 197 |
| | *** | 27760 | 29185 | 41113 | 7622 | 7861 | 10542 | 1397 | 1411 | 1806 | 399 | 399 | 495 | 197 | 197 | 236 |
| 0.2 | *** | 35035 | 36460 | 41686 | 9722 | 10074 | 10674 | 1786 | 1810 | 1824 | 497 | 497 | 511 | 249 | 249 | 249 |
| | *** | 35574 | 38049 | 51159 | 9872 | 10336 | 13014 | 1786 | 1810 | 2182 | 497 | 497 | 581 | 249 | 249 | 271 |
| 0.25 | *** | 40861 | 42924 | 51174 | 11499 | 12047 | 13022 | 2124 | 2147 | 2185 | 586 | 586 | 586 | 272 | 272 | 286 |
| | *** | 41635 | 45324 | 59636 | 11747 | 12460 | 15094 | 2124 | 2161 | 2496 | 586 | 586 | 652 | 272 | 272 | 299 |
| 0.3 | *** | 44935 | 47724 | 59260 | 12872 | 13622 | 14986 | 2386 | 2424 | 2485 | 647 | 647 | 661 | 310 | 310 | 310 |
| | *** | 45985 | 50972 | 66543 | 13210 | 14185 | 16781 | 2410 | 2461 | 2748 | 647 | 647 | 707 | 310 | 310 | 320 |
| 0.35 | *** | 47386 | 50949 | 65799 | 13847 | 14799 | 16599 | 2597 | 2649 | 2724 | 699 | 699 | 699 | 324 | 324 | 324 |
| | *** | 48760 | 55060 | 71881 | 14274 | 15535 | 18076 | 2635 | 2686 | 2936 | 699 | 699 | 746 | 324 | 324 | 334 |
| 0.4 | *** | 48436 | 52772 | 70711 | 14461 | 15610 | 17785 | 2747 | 2822 | 2897 | 736 | 736 | 736 | 324 | 347 | 347 |
| | *** | 50110 | 57685 | 75648 | 14972 | 16486 | 18979 | 2785 | 2860 | 3062 | 736 | 736 | 770 | 347 | 347 | 341 |
| 0.45 | *** | 48286 | 53372 | 73960 | 14761 | 16060 | 18549 | 2822 | 2897 | 2986 | 736 | 760 | 760 | 347 | 347 | 347 |
| | *** | 50274 | 58997 | 77846 | 15324 | 17049 | 19489 | 2860 | 2949 | 3124 | 760 | 760 | 778 | 347 | 347 | 341 |
| 0.5 | *** | 47161 | 52899 | 75497 | 14761 | 16172 | 18886 | 2836 | 2935 | 3024 | 736 | 760 | 760 | 324 | 347 | 347 |
| | *** | 49435 | 59086 | 78474 | 15385 | 17260 | 19607 | 2897 | 2972 | 3124 | 760 | 760 | 770 | 347 | 347 | 334 |
| 0.55 | *** | 45272 | 51511 | 75347 | 14485 | 15985 | 18811 | 2799 | 2897 | 2986 | 736 | 736 | 736 | 324 | 324 | 324 |
| | *** | 47761 | 58111 | 77532 | 15136 | 17110 | 19332 | 2860 | 2949 | 3062 | 736 | 736 | 746 | 324 | 324 | 320 |
| 0.6 | *** | 42774 | 49336 | 73472 | 13974 | 15474 | 18310 | 2710 | 2799 | 2897 | 699 | 699 | 699 | 310 | 310 | 310 |
| | *** | 45399 | 56110 | 75020 | 14635 | 16599 | 18665 | 2747 | 2836 | 2936 | 699 | 699 | 707 | 310 | 310 | 299 |
| 0.65 | *** | 39774 | 46435 | 69910 | 13210 | 14672 | 17372 | 2560 | 2635 | 2724 | 647 | 647 | 661 | 286 | 286 | 286 |
| | *** | 42474 | 53147 | 70939 | 13847 | 15760 | 17606 | 2597 | 2672 | 2748 | 647 | 661 | 652 | 286 | 286 | 271 |
| 0.7 | *** | 36361 | 42849 | 64636 | 12211 | 13561 | 15999 | 2335 | 2410 | 2485 | 586 | 586 | 586 | 249 | 249 | 249 |
| | *** | 39010 | 49261 | 65287 | 12811 | 14574 | 16153 | 2372 | 2447 | 2496 | 586 | 586 | 581 | 249 | 249 | 236 |
| 0.75 | *** | 32522 | 38574 | 57699 | 10974 | 12160 | 14236 | 2072 | 2124 | 2185 | 497 | 497 | 511 | 211 | 211 | 211 |
| | *** | 35011 | 44410 | 58067 | 11499 | 13022 | 14309 | 2086 | 2147 | 2182 | 497 | 511 | 495 | 211 | 211 | 194 |
| 0.8 | *** | 28224 | 33572 | 49097 | 9474 | 10449 | 12047 | 1735 | 1772 | 1810 | 399 | 399 | 399 | 160 | 160 | 160 |
| | *** | 30460 | 38522 | 49276 | 9910 | 11124 | 12072 | 1749 | 1786 | 1806 | 399 | 399 | 393 | 160 | 160 | 145 |
| 0.85 | *** | 23349 | 27647 | 38860 | 7674 | 8372 | 9436 | 1322 | 1360 | 1374 | 286 | 286 | 286 | . | . | . |
| | *** | 25149 | 31449 | 38915 | 7997 | 8836 | 9443 | 1336 | 1360 | 1366 | 286 | 286 | 275 | . | . | . |
| 0.9 | *** | 17560 | 20485 | 26972 | 5485 | 5874 | 6436 | 849 | 872 | 872 | . | . | . | . | . | . |
| | *** | 18811 | 22885 | 26985 | 5672 | 6136 | 6421 | 849 | 872 | 864 | . | . | . | . | . | . |
| 0.95 | *** | 10172 | 11386 | 13486 | 2761 | 2874 | 3024 | . | . | . | . | . | . | . | . | . |
| | *** | 10711 | 12272 | 13485 | 2822 | 2949 | 3007 | . | . | . | . | . | . | . | . | . |
| 0.98 | *** | 4097 | 4336 | 4636 | . | . | . | . | . | . | . | . | . | . | . | . |
| | *** | 4210 | 4472 | 4631 | . | . | . | . | . | . | . | . | . | . | . | . |

TABLE 5: ALPHA= 0.025 POWER= 0.8    EXPECTED ACCRUAL THRU MINIMUM FOLLOW-UP= 17000

| | | DEL=.01 | | | DEL=.02 | | | DEL=.05 | | | DEL=.10 | | | DEL=.15 | | |
|---|---|---|---|---|---|---|---|---|---|---|---|---|---|---|---|---|
| FACT= | | 1.0 .75 | .50 .25 | .00 BIN | 1.0 .75 | .50 .25 | .00 BIN | 1.0 .75 | .50 .25 | .00 BIN | 1.0 75 | .50 .25 | .00 BIN | 1.0 .75 | .50 .25 | .00 BIN |
| PCONT=*** | | | | | REQUIRED NUMBER OF PATIENTS | | | | | | | | | | | |
| 0.01 | *** | 1201 | 1201 | 1201 | 436 | 436 | 436 | 139 | 139 | 139 | 70 | 70 | 70 | 54 | 54 | 54 |
| | *** | 1201 | 1201 | 4631 | 436 | 436 | 1531 | 139 | 139 | 417 | 70 | 70 | 170 | 54 | 54 | 101 |
| 0.02 | *** | 2689 | 2689 | 2705 | 861 | 861 | 861 | 224 | 224 | 224 | 96 | 96 | 96 | 70 | 70 | 70 |
| | *** | 2689 | 2689 | 7645 | 861 | 861 | 2277 | 224 | 224 | 532 | 96 | 96 | 197 | 70 | 70 | 113 |
| 0.05 | *** | 8214 | 8299 | 8442 | 2349 | 2349 | 2365 | 495 | 495 | 495 | 181 | 181 | 181 | 96 | 96 | 96 |
| | *** | 8256 | 8357 | 16310 | 2349 | 2349 | 4419 | 495 | 495 | 864 | 181 | 181 | 275 | 96 | 96 | 145 |
| 0.1 | *** | 18302 | 18711 | 19646 | 5026 | 5111 | 5196 | 962 | 962 | 962 | 282 | 309 | 309 | 155 | 155 | 155 |
| | *** | 18472 | 19067 | 29497 | 5069 | 5154 | 7677 | 962 | 962 | 1366 | 309 | 309 | 393 | 155 | 155 | 194 |
| 0.15 | *** | 27567 | 28444 | 31036 | 7576 | 7762 | 8044 | 1387 | 1414 | 1414 | 410 | 410 | 410 | 197 | 197 | 197 |
| | *** | 27907 | 29336 | 41113 | 7661 | 7890 | 10542 | 1387 | 1414 | 1806 | 410 | 410 | 495 | 197 | 197 | 236 |
| 0.2 | *** | 35260 | 36747 | 41677 | 9786 | 10126 | 10679 | 1796 | 1812 | 1839 | 495 | 495 | 495 | 240 | 240 | 240 |
| | *** | 35839 | 38346 | 51159 | 9956 | 10381 | 13014 | 1796 | 1812 | 2182 | 495 | 495 | 581 | 240 | 240 | 271 |
| 0.25 | *** | 41194 | 43361 | 51181 | 11614 | 12140 | 13016 | 2136 | 2152 | 2179 | 580 | 580 | 580 | 282 | 282 | 282 |
| | *** | 42017 | 45757 | 59636 | 11842 | 12506 | 15094 | 2136 | 2179 | 2496 | 580 | 580 | 652 | 282 | 282 | 299 |
| 0.3 | *** | 45375 | 48307 | 59256 | 13016 | 13739 | 14987 | 2407 | 2434 | 2492 | 649 | 649 | 649 | 309 | 309 | 309 |
| | *** | 46506 | 51564 | 66543 | 13330 | 14265 | 16781 | 2407 | 2450 | 2748 | 649 | 649 | 707 | 309 | 309 | 320 |
| 0.35 | *** | 47951 | 51691 | 65801 | 14036 | 14971 | 16586 | 2604 | 2662 | 2731 | 691 | 707 | 707 | 325 | 325 | 325 |
| | *** | 49396 | 55787 | 71881 | 14435 | 15625 | 18076 | 2646 | 2689 | 2936 | 707 | 707 | 746 | 325 | 325 | 334 |
| 0.4 | *** | 49141 | 53646 | 70705 | 14690 | 15795 | 17776 | 2747 | 2816 | 2901 | 734 | 734 | 750 | 325 | 325 | 325 |
| | *** | 50900 | 58550 | 75648 | 15184 | 16602 | 18979 | 2790 | 2859 | 3062 | 734 | 734 | 770 | 325 | 325 | 341 |
| 0.45 | *** | 49115 | 54385 | 73961 | 15014 | 16262 | 18557 | 2832 | 2917 | 3002 | 750 | 750 | 750 | 351 | 351 | 351 |
| | *** | 51197 | 59979 | 77846 | 15566 | 17197 | 19489 | 2875 | 2960 | 3124 | 750 | 750 | 778 | 351 | 351 | 341 |
| 0.5 | *** | 48121 | 54029 | 75507 | 15030 | 16390 | 18897 | 2859 | 2944 | 3029 | 750 | 750 | 750 | 325 | 325 | 351 |
| | *** | 50475 | 60191 | 78474 | 15651 | 17410 | 19607 | 2901 | 2986 | 3124 | 750 | 750 | 770 | 325 | 325 | 334 |
| 0.55 | *** | 46336 | 52711 | 75337 | 14775 | 16204 | 18812 | 2832 | 2901 | 3002 | 734 | 734 | 750 | 325 | 325 | 325 |
| | *** | 48902 | 59256 | 77532 | 15412 | 17266 | 19332 | 2859 | 2944 | 3062 | 734 | 734 | 746 | 325 | 325 | 320 |
| 0.6 | *** | 43887 | 50560 | 73467 | 14265 | 15710 | 18302 | 2731 | 2816 | 2901 | 691 | 707 | 707 | 309 | 309 | 309 |
| | *** | 46607 | 57275 | 75020 | 14902 | 16772 | 18665 | 2774 | 2859 | 2936 | 707 | 707 | 707 | 309 | 309 | 299 |
| 0.65 | *** | 40939 | 47670 | 69897 | 13484 | 14886 | 17367 | 2577 | 2646 | 2731 | 649 | 649 | 665 | 282 | 282 | 282 |
| | *** | 43675 | 54300 | 70939 | 14121 | 15906 | 17606 | 2604 | 2689 | 2748 | 649 | 649 | 652 | 282 | 282 | 271 |
| 0.7 | *** | 37496 | 44041 | 64627 | 12480 | 13781 | 16007 | 2349 | 2407 | 2492 | 580 | 580 | 580 | 240 | 240 | 240 |
| | *** | 40190 | 50331 | 65287 | 13059 | 14716 | 16153 | 2391 | 2450 | 2496 | 580 | 580 | 581 | 240 | 240 | 236 |
| 0.75 | *** | 33602 | 39680 | 57700 | 11205 | 12352 | 14222 | 2067 | 2136 | 2179 | 495 | 495 | 495 | 197 | 197 | 197 |
| | *** | 36110 | 45375 | 58067 | 11715 | 13144 | 14309 | 2094 | 2152 | 2182 | 495 | 495 | 495 | 197 | 197 | 194 |
| 0.8 | *** | 29182 | 34495 | 49099 | 9675 | 10594 | 12039 | 1727 | 1770 | 1812 | 394 | 410 | 410 | 155 | 155 | 155 |
| | *** | 31419 | 39324 | 49276 | 10084 | 11231 | 12072 | 1754 | 1796 | 1806 | 410 | 410 | 393 | 155 | 155 | 145 |
| 0.85 | *** | 24125 | 28375 | 38856 | 7805 | 8469 | 9446 | 1329 | 1345 | 1371 | 282 | 282 | 282 | . | . | . |
| | *** | 25936 | 32056 | 38915 | 8129 | 8910 | 9443 | 1345 | 1371 | 1366 | 282 | 282 | 275 | . | . | . |
| 0.9 | *** | 18116 | 20964 | 26972 | 5579 | 5935 | 6429 | 861 | 861 | 877 | . | . | . | . | . | . |
| | *** | 19349 | 23232 | 26985 | 5749 | 6174 | 6421 | 861 | 877 | 864 | . | . | . | . | . | . |
| 0.95 | *** | 10397 | 11571 | 13500 | 2790 | 2901 | 3029 | . | . | . | . | . | . | . | . | . |
| | *** | 10934 | 12395 | 13485 | 2832 | 2960 | 3007 | . | . | . | . | . | . | . | . | . |
| 0.98 | *** | 4150 | 4362 | 4644 | . | . | . | . | . | . | . | . | . | . | . | . |
| | *** | 4261 | 4490 | 4631 | . | . | . | . | . | . | . | . | . | . | . | . |

## TABLE 5: ALPHA= 0.025 POWER= 0.8    EXPECTED ACCRUAL THRU MINIMUM FOLLOW-UP= 20000

|  | FACT= | DEL=.01 | | | DEL=.02 | | | DEL=.05 | | | DEL=.10 | | | DEL=.15 | | |
|---|---|---|---|---|---|---|---|---|---|---|---|---|---|---|---|---|
|  |  | 1.0 .75 | .50 .25 | .00 BIN | 1.0 .75 | .50 .25 | .00 BIN | 1.0 .75 | .50 .25 | .00 BIN | 1.0 75 | .50 .25 | .00 BIN | 1.0 .75 | .50 .25 | .00 BIN |
| PCONT=*** |  | REQUIRED NUMBER OF PATIENTS | | | | | | | | | | | | | | |
| 0.01 | *** | 1213 | 1213 | 1213 | 432 | 432 | 432 | 132 | 132 | 132 | 63 | 63 | 63 | 63 | 63 | 63 |
|  | *** | 1213 | 1213 | 4631 | 432 | 432 | 1531 | 132 | 132 | 417 | 63 | 63 | 170 | 63 | 63 | 101 |
| 0.02 | *** | 2682 | 2682 | 2713 | 863 | 863 | 863 | 232 | 232 | 232 | 113 | 113 | 113 | 63 | 63 | 63 |
|  | *** | 2682 | 2682 | 7645 | 863 | 863 | 2277 | 232 | 232 | 532 | 113 | 113 | 197 | 63 | 63 | 113 |
| 0.05 | *** | 8232 | 8313 | 8432 | 2332 | 2363 | 2363 | 482 | 513 | 513 | 182 | 182 | 182 | 113 | 113 | 113 |
|  | *** | 8263 | 8363 | 16310 | 2332 | 2363 | 4419 | 513 | 513 | 864 | 182 | 182 | 275 | 113 | 113 | 145 |
| 0.1 | *** | 18382 | 18782 | 19632 | 5032 | 5113 | 5182 | 963 | 963 | 963 | 282 | 282 | 282 | 163 | 163 | 163 |
|  | *** | 18563 | 19132 | 29497 | 5082 | 5163 | 7677 | 963 | 963 | 1366 | 282 | 282 | 393 | 163 | 163 | 194 |
| 0.15 | *** | 27763 | 28663 | 31032 | 7632 | 7782 | 8032 | 1413 | 1413 | 1413 | 413 | 413 | 413 | 213 | 213 | 213 |
|  | *** | 28132 | 29532 | 41113 | 7713 | 7913 | 10542 | 1413 | 1413 | 1806 | 413 | 413 | 495 | 213 | 213 | 236 |
| 0.2 | *** | 35563 | 37132 | 41682 | 9882 | 10213 | 10663 | 1782 | 1813 | 1832 | 513 | 513 | 513 | 232 | 232 | 232 |
|  | *** | 36182 | 38682 | 51159 | 10032 | 10413 | 13014 | 1813 | 1813 | 2182 | 513 | 513 | 581 | 232 | 232 | 271 |
| 0.25 | *** | 41632 | 43932 | 51163 | 11732 | 12232 | 13013 | 2132 | 2163 | 2182 | 582 | 582 | 582 | 282 | 282 | 282 |
|  | *** | 42532 | 46282 | 59636 | 11963 | 12582 | 15094 | 2132 | 2163 | 2496 | 582 | 582 | 652 | 282 | 282 | 299 |
| 0.3 | *** | 45982 | 49063 | 59263 | 13213 | 13882 | 14982 | 2413 | 2432 | 2482 | 663 | 663 | 663 | 313 | 313 | 313 |
|  | *** | 47182 | 52282 | 66543 | 13513 | 14363 | 16781 | 2432 | 2463 | 2748 | 663 | 663 | 707 | 313 | 313 | 320 |
| 0.35 | *** | 48763 | 52632 | 65782 | 14263 | 15132 | 16582 | 2632 | 2663 | 2713 | 713 | 713 | 713 | 332 | 332 | 332 |
|  | *** | 50282 | 56713 | 71881 | 14663 | 15763 | 18076 | 2663 | 2682 | 2936 | 713 | 713 | 746 | 332 | 332 | 334 |
| 0.4 | *** | 50113 | 54813 | 70713 | 14963 | 16013 | 17782 | 2782 | 2832 | 2882 | 732 | 732 | 732 | 332 | 332 | 332 |
|  | *** | 51982 | 59663 | 75648 | 15432 | 16763 | 18979 | 2813 | 2863 | 3062 | 732 | 732 | 770 | 332 | 332 | 341 |
| 0.45 | *** | 50263 | 55713 | 73963 | 15332 | 16513 | 18563 | 2863 | 2932 | 2982 | 763 | 763 | 763 | 332 | 332 | 332 |
|  | *** | 52432 | 61232 | 77846 | 15863 | 17363 | 19489 | 2882 | 2963 | 3124 | 763 | 763 | 778 | 332 | 332 | 341 |
| 0.5 | *** | 49432 | 55482 | 75513 | 15382 | 16682 | 18882 | 2882 | 2963 | 3032 | 763 | 763 | 763 | 332 | 332 | 332 |
|  | *** | 51863 | 61563 | 78474 | 15963 | 17613 | 19607 | 2913 | 2982 | 3124 | 763 | 763 | 770 | 332 | 332 | 334 |
| 0.55 | *** | 47763 | 54263 | 75332 | 15132 | 16482 | 18813 | 2863 | 2913 | 2982 | 732 | 732 | 732 | 332 | 332 | 332 |
|  | *** | 50413 | 60682 | 77532 | 15732 | 17463 | 19332 | 2882 | 2963 | 3062 | 732 | 732 | 746 | 332 | 332 | 320 |
| 0.6 | *** | 45413 | 52182 | 73482 | 14632 | 15982 | 18313 | 2763 | 2813 | 2882 | 713 | 713 | 713 | 313 | 313 | 313 |
|  | *** | 48182 | 58732 | 75020 | 15232 | 16963 | 18665 | 2782 | 2863 | 2936 | 713 | 713 | 707 | 313 | 313 | 299 |
| 0.65 | *** | 42463 | 49263 | 69913 | 13832 | 15163 | 17363 | 2582 | 2663 | 2732 | 663 | 663 | 663 | 282 | 282 | 282 |
|  | *** | 45263 | 55732 | 70939 | 14432 | 16082 | 17606 | 2613 | 2682 | 2748 | 663 | 663 | 652 | 282 | 282 | 271 |
| 0.7 | *** | 39013 | 45563 | 64632 | 12813 | 14032 | 16013 | 2363 | 2432 | 2482 | 582 | 582 | 582 | 232 | 232 | 232 |
|  | *** | 41732 | 51682 | 65287 | 13363 | 14882 | 16153 | 2382 | 2463 | 2496 | 582 | 582 | 581 | 232 | 232 | 236 |
| 0.75 | *** | 35013 | 41082 | 57713 | 11513 | 12563 | 14232 | 2082 | 2132 | 2182 | 513 | 513 | 513 | 213 | 213 | 213 |
|  | *** | 37563 | 46582 | 58067 | 11982 | 13282 | 14309 | 2113 | 2163 | 2182 | 513 | 513 | 495 | 213 | 213 | 194 |
| 0.8 | *** | 30463 | 35713 | 49082 | 9913 | 10763 | 12032 | 1732 | 1782 | 1813 | 413 | 413 | 413 | 163 | 163 | 163 |
|  | *** | 32663 | 40313 | 49276 | 10313 | 11332 | 12072 | 1763 | 1782 | 1806 | 413 | 413 | 393 | 163 | 163 | 145 |
| 0.85 | *** | 25163 | 29313 | 38863 | 7982 | 8582 | 9432 | 1332 | 1363 | 1382 | 282 | 282 | 282 | . | . | . |
|  | *** | 26932 | 32782 | 38915 | 8263 | 8982 | 9443 | 1332 | 1363 | 1366 | 282 | 282 | 275 | . | . | . |
| 0.9 | *** | 18813 | 21563 | 26982 | 5663 | 6013 | 6432 | 863 | 863 | 882 | . | . | . | . | . | . |
|  | *** | 20013 | 23682 | 26985 | 5832 | 6213 | 6421 | 863 | 863 | 864 | . | . | . | . | . | . |
| 0.95 | *** | 10713 | 11813 | 13482 | 2832 | 2913 | 3013 | . | . | . | . | . | . | . | . | . |
|  | *** | 11213 | 12532 | 13485 | 2863 | 2963 | 3007 | . | . | . | . | . | . | . | . | . |
| 0.98 | *** | 4213 | 4413 | 4632 | . | . | . | . | . | . | . | . | . | . | . | . |
|  | *** | 4313 | 4513 | 4631 | . | . | . | . | . | . | . | . | . | . | . | . |

TABLE 5: ALPHA= 0.025 POWER= 0.8    EXPECTED ACCRUAL THRU MINIMUM FOLLOW-UP= 25000

| PCONT | | DEL=.01 | | | DEL=.02 | | | DEL=.05 | | | DEL=.10 | | | DEL=.15 | | |
|---|---|---|---|---|---|---|---|---|---|---|---|---|---|---|---|---|
| FACT= | | 1.0 .75 | .50 .25 | .00 BIN | 1.0 .75 | .50 .25 | .00 BIN | 1.0 .75 | .50 .25 | .00 BIN | 1.0 75 | .50 .25 | .00 BIN | 1.0 .75 | .50 .25 | .00 BIN |
| PCONT=*** | | | | REQUIRED NUMBER OF PATIENTS | | | | | | | | | | | | |
| 0.01 | *** | 1204 1204 | 1204 | 454 454 | 454 | 141 141 | 141 | 79 | 79 | 79 | 40 | 40 | 40 |
|  | *** | 1204 1204 | 4631 | 454 454 | 1531 | 141 141 | 417 | 79 | 79 | 170 | 40 | 40 | 101 |
| 0.02 | *** | 2704 2704 | 2704 | 852 852 | 852 | 227 227 | 227 | 102 | 102 | 102 | 79 | 79 | 79 |
|  | *** | 2704 2704 | 7645 | 852 852 | 2277 | 227 227 | 532 | 102 | 102 | 197 | 79 | 79 | 113 |
| 0.05 | *** | 8266 8329 | 8454 | 2352 2352 | 2352 | 516 516 | 516 | 165 | 165 | 165 | 102 | 102 | 102 |
|  | *** | 8290 8391 | 16310 | 2352 2352 | 4419 | 516 516 | 864 | 165 | 165 | 275 | 102 | 102 | 145 |
| 0.1 | *** | 18516 18915 | 19641 | 5079 5141 | 5204 | 954 954 | 954 | 290 | 290 | 290 | 165 | 165 | 165 |
|  | *** | 18704 19204 | 29497 | 5102 5165 | 7677 | 954 954 | 1366 | 290 | 290 | 393 | 165 | 165 | 194 |
| 0.15 | *** | 28040 28954 | 31016 | 7704 7829 | 8040 | 1391 1415 | 1415 | 415 | 415 | 415 | 204 | 204 | 204 |
|  | *** | 28415 29766 | 41113 | 7766 7915 | 10542 | 1415 1415 | 1806 | 415 | 415 | 495 | 204 | 204 | 236 |
| 0.2 | *** | 36040 37641 | 41665 | 9977 10266 | 10665 | 1790 1829 | 1829 | 516 | 516 | 516 | 227 | 227 | 227 |
|  | *** | 36704 39102 | 51159 | 10141 10454 | 13014 | 1790 1829 | 2182 | 516 | 516 | 581 | 227 | 227 | 271 |
| 0.25 | *** | 42329 44704 | 51165 | 11915 12352 | 13016 | 2141 2165 | 2204 | 579 | 579 | 579 | 266 | 266 | 290 |
|  | *** | 43290 46954 | 59636 | 12102 12665 | 15094 | 2141 2165 | 2496 | 579 | 579 | 652 | 266 | 290 | 299 |
| 0.3 | *** | 46915 50102 | 59266 | 13454 14079 | 14977 | 2415 2454 | 2477 | 641 | 641 | 665 | 290 | 290 | 290 |
|  | *** | 48204 53204 | 66543 | 13727 14477 | 16781 | 2454 2477 | 2748 | 641 | 665 | 707 | 290 | 290 | 320 |
| 0.35 | *** | 49915 53977 | 65790 | 14579 15352 | 16602 | 2641 2665 | 2727 | 704 | 704 | 704 | 329 | 329 | 329 |
|  | *** | 51579 57891 | 71881 | 14915 15915 | 18076 | 2665 2704 | 2936 | 704 | 704 | 746 | 329 | 329 | 334 |
| 0.4 | *** | 51540 56391 | 70704 | 15329 16290 | 17790 | 2790 2852 | 2891 | 727 | 727 | 727 | 329 | 329 | 329 |
|  | *** | 53516 61079 | 75648 | 15766 16954 | 18979 | 2829 2852 | 3062 | 727 | 727 | 770 | 329 | 329 | 341 |
| 0.45 | *** | 51954 57516 | 73954 | 15727 16829 | 18540 | 2891 2954 | 2977 | 766 | 766 | 766 | 329 | 329 | 329 |
|  | *** | 54227 62852 | 77846 | 16227 17579 | 19489 | 2915 2977 | 3124 | 766 | 766 | 778 | 329 | 329 | 341 |
| 0.5 | *** | 51290 57477 | 75516 | 15829 17016 | 18891 | 2915 2977 | 3040 | 766 | 766 | 766 | 329 | 329 | 329 |
|  | *** | 53852 63329 | 78474 | 16352 17829 | 19607 | 2954 3016 | 3124 | 766 | 766 | 770 | 329 | 329 | 334 |
| 0.55 | *** | 49790 56391 | 75352 | 15602 16852 | 18829 | 2891 2915 | 2977 | 727 | 727 | 727 | 329 | 329 | 329 |
|  | *** | 52516 62579 | 77532 | 16165 17704 | 19332 | 2915 2954 | 3062 | 727 | 727 | 746 | 329 | 329 | 320 |
| 0.6 | *** | 47540 54352 | 73477 | 15102 16352 | 18290 | 2766 2829 | 2891 | 704 | 704 | 704 | 290 | 290 | 290 |
|  | *** | 50391 60641 | 75020 | 15665 17204 | 18665 | 2790 2852 | 2936 | 704 | 704 | 707 | 290 | 290 | 299 |
| 0.65 | *** | 44641 51415 | 69891 | 14329 15516 | 17352 | 2602 2665 | 2727 | 641 | 665 | 665 | 290 | 290 | 290 |
|  | *** | 47477 57602 | 70939 | 14852 16329 | 17606 | 2641 2704 | 2748 | 641 | 665 | 652 | 290 | 290 | 271 |
| 0.7 | *** | 41102 47641 | 64641 | 13227 14329 | 16016 | 2391 2454 | 2477 | 579 | 579 | 579 | 227 | 227 | 227 |
|  | *** | 43852 53415 | 65287 | 13727 15079 | 16153 | 2415 2454 | 2496 | 579 | 579 | 581 | 227 | 227 | 236 |
| 0.75 | *** | 36977 42954 | 57704 | 11891 12829 | 14227 | 2102 2141 | 2165 | 516 | 516 | 516 | 204 | 204 | 204 |
|  | *** | 39516 48102 | 58067 | 12329 13454 | 14309 | 2141 2165 | 2182 | 516 | 516 | 495 | 204 | 204 | 194 |
| 0.8 | *** | 32165 37290 | 49102 | 10227 10977 | 12040 | 1766 1790 | 1829 | 391 | 391 | 415 | 165 | 165 | 165 |
|  | *** | 34352 41579 | 49276 | 10579 11454 | 12072 | 1766 1790 | 1806 | 391 | 415 | 393 | 165 | 165 | 145 |
| 0.85 | *** | 26540 30516 | 38852 | 8204 8727 | 9454 | 1352 1352 | 1391 | 290 | 290 | 290 | . | . | . |
|  | *** | 28266 33704 | 38915 | 8454 9040 | 9443 | 1352 1352 | 1366 | 290 | 290 | 275 | . | . | . |
| 0.9 | *** | 19766 22329 | 26977 | 5790 6079 | 6415 | 852 852 | 891 | . | . | . | . | . | . |
|  | *** | 20891 24204 | 26985 | 5915 6227 | 6421 | 852 891 | 864 | . | . | . | . | . | . |
| 0.95 | *** | 11102 12079 | 13477 | 2852 2915 | 3016 | . | . | . | . | . | . | . | . | . |
|  | *** | 11540 12704 | 13485 | 2891 2977 | 3007 | . | . | . | . | . | . | . | . | . |
| 0.98 | *** | 4290 4454 | 4641 | . | . | . | . | . | . | . | . | . | . | . | . |
|  | *** | 4352 4540 | 4631 | . | . | . | . | . | . | . | . | . | . | . | . |

## TABLE 6: ALPHA= 0.025 POWER= 0.9     EXPECTED ACCRUAL THRU MINIMUM FOLLOW-UP= 30

| | | DEL=.10 | | | DEL=.15 | | | DEL=.20 | | | DEL=.25 | | | DEL=.30 | | |
|---|---|---|---|---|---|---|---|---|---|---|---|---|---|---|---|---|---|
| FACT= | | 1.0 .75 | .50 .25 | .00 BIN | 1.0 .75 | .50 .25 | .00 BIN | 1.0 .75 | .50 .25 | .00 BIN | 1.0 75 | .50 .25 | .00 BIN | 1.0 .75 | .50 .25 | .00 BIN |
| PCONT=*** | | | | | REQUIRED NUMBER OF PATIENTS | | | | | | | | | | | |
| 0.05 | *** | 220 | 222 | 239 | 128 | 129 | 139 | 90 | 92 | 98 | 70 | 71 | 76 | 58 | 59 | 62 |
| | *** | 221 | 224 | 368 | 129 | 131 | 194 | 91 | 93 | 124 | 71 | 73 | 87 | 58 | 60 | 65 |
| 0.1 | *** | 348 | 350 | 400 | 184 | 186 | 212 | 121 | 123 | 139 | 89 | 91 | 102 | 71 | 73 | 80 |
| | *** | 348 | 354 | 526 | 185 | 190 | 260 | 122 | 127 | 158 | 90 | 94 | 107 | 71 | 75 | 78 |
| 0.15 | *** | 449 | 452 | 548 | 225 | 229 | 276 | 142 | 146 | 174 | 102 | 106 | 124 | 79 | 82 | 94 |
| | *** | 450 | 459 | 662 | 226 | 236 | 316 | 144 | 152 | 187 | 103 | 110 | 124 | 80 | 86 | 88 |
| 0.2 | *** | 522 | 527 | 679 | 254 | 260 | 332 | 157 | 162 | 203 | 110 | 115 | 141 | 84 | 88 | 106 |
| | *** | 524 | 537 | 778 | 256 | 270 | 362 | 159 | 171 | 211 | 112 | 122 | 138 | 85 | 93 | 96 |
| 0.25 | *** | 569 | 576 | 791 | 271 | 279 | 377 | 165 | 172 | 227 | 114 | 121 | 155 | 86 | 92 | 114 |
| | *** | 571 | 590 | 873 | 274 | 293 | 400 | 167 | 183 | 229 | 117 | 130 | 148 | 88 | 98 | 102 |
| 0.3 | *** | 591 | 601 | 882 | 278 | 288 | 413 | 167 | 177 | 245 | 115 | 124 | 164 | 86 | 93 | 120 |
| | *** | 594 | 620 | 946 | 281 | 306 | 428 | 171 | 191 | 242 | 118 | 134 | 154 | 89 | 101 | 106 |
| 0.35 | *** | 592 | 604 | 950 | 276 | 289 | 439 | 165 | 177 | 257 | 114 | 124 | 170 | 85 | 93 | 123 |
| | *** | 596 | 629 | 999 | 280 | 311 | 446 | 169 | 194 | 250 | 117 | 136 | 158 | 88 | 102 | 107 |
| 0.4 | *** | 574 | 590 | 997 | 266 | 283 | 455 | 159 | 174 | 263 | 110 | 121 | 173 | 82 | 91 | 123 |
| | *** | 579 | 622 | 1030 | 272 | 309 | 456 | 165 | 193 | 253 | 114 | 135 | 158 | 86 | 100 | 106 |
| 0.45 | *** | 541 | 561 | 1020 | 251 | 271 | 461 | 151 | 168 | 263 | 104 | 117 | 171 | 78 | 88 | 121 |
| | *** | 548 | 601 | 1041 | 258 | 302 | 456 | 157 | 189 | 250 | 109 | 131 | 154 | 82 | 97 | 102 |
| 0.5 | *** | 496 | 522 | 1020 | 232 | 256 | 456 | 141 | 159 | 258 | 98 | 111 | 166 | 73 | 83 | 116 |
| | *** | 505 | 569 | 1030 | 241 | 289 | 446 | 148 | 181 | 242 | 103 | 126 | 148 | 77 | 93 | 96 |
| 0.55 | *** | 443 | 476 | 998 | 211 | 238 | 441 | 130 | 149 | 246 | 90 | 104 | 157 | 68 | 77 | 108 |
| | *** | 454 | 531 | 999 | 221 | 273 | 428 | 137 | 171 | 229 | 96 | 119 | 138 | 72 | 87 | 88 |
| 0.6 | *** | 387 | 426 | 952 | 188 | 218 | 416 | 117 | 137 | 229 | 82 | 96 | 144 | 61 | 71 | 98 |
| | *** | 401 | 488 | 946 | 199 | 254 | 400 | 125 | 159 | 211 | 87 | 109 | 124 | 65 | 79 | 78 |
| 0.65 | *** | 331 | 376 | 884 | 166 | 196 | 380 | 104 | 124 | 207 | 73 | 86 | 128 | 54 | 63 | 86 |
| | *** | 347 | 441 | 873 | 177 | 232 | 362 | 112 | 144 | 187 | 78 | 98 | 107 | 58 | 70 | 65 |
| 0.7 | *** | 278 | 327 | 794 | 143 | 173 | 335 | 91 | 109 | 179 | 63 | 74 | 108 | . | . | . |
| | *** | 296 | 392 | 778 | 155 | 206 | 316 | 98 | 127 | 158 | 68 | 85 | 87 | . | . | . |
| 0.75 | *** | 229 | 278 | 681 | 121 | 148 | 280 | 76 | 91 | 145 | . | . | . | . | . | . |
| | *** | 248 | 340 | 662 | 132 | 177 | 260 | 82 | 107 | 124 | . | . | . | . | . | . |
| 0.8 | *** | 184 | 229 | 546 | 98 | 120 | 215 | . | . | . | . | . | . | . | . | . |
| | *** | 202 | 283 | 526 | 107 | 143 | 194 | . | . | . | . | . | . | . | . | . |
| 0.85 | *** | 140 | 177 | 389 | . | . | . | . | . | . | . | . | . | . | . | . |
| | *** | 155 | 219 | 368 | . | . | . | . | . | . | . | . | . | . | . | . |

TABLE 6: ALPHA= 0.025 POWER= 0.9    EXPECTED ACCRUAL THRU MINIMUM FOLLOW-UP= 40

| | | DEL=.10 | | | DEL=.15 | | | DEL=.20 | | | DEL=.25 | | | DEL=.30 | | |
|---|---|---|---|---|---|---|---|---|---|---|---|---|---|---|---|---|
| FACT= | | 1.0 .75 | .50 .25 | .00 BIN | 1.0 .75 | .50 .25 | .00 BIN | 1.0 .75 | .50 .25 | .00 BIN | 1.0 75 | .50 .25 | .00 BIN | 1.0 .75 | .50 .25 | .00 BIN |
| PCONT=*** | | | | | REQUIRED NUMBER OF PATIENTS | | | | | | | | | | | |
| 0.05 | *** | 221 | 222 | 239 | 129 | 130 | 139 | 91 | 92 | 98 | 71 | 72 | 76 | 58 | 59 | 62 |
| | *** | 221 | 225 | 368 | 129 | 132 | 194 | 91 | 94 | 124 | 71 | 73 | 87 | 59 | 60 | 65 |
| 0.1 | *** | 349 | 351 | 400 | 185 | 188 | 212 | 122 | 125 | 139 | 90 | 93 | 102 | 71 | 74 | 80 |
| | *** | 349 | 357 | 526 | 186 | 193 | 260 | 123 | 128 | 158 | 91 | 96 | 107 | 72 | 76 | 78 |
| 0.15 | *** | 450 | 454 | 548 | 226 | 232 | 276 | 144 | 149 | 174 | 103 | 107 | 124 | 80 | 84 | 94 |
| | *** | 451 | 463 | 662 | 228 | 240 | 316 | 145 | 155 | 187 | 105 | 112 | 124 | 81 | 87 | 88 |
| 0.2 | *** | 524 | 530 | 679 | 256 | 263 | 332 | 159 | 166 | 203 | 112 | 118 | 141 | 86 | 90 | 106 |
| | *** | 526 | 544 | 778 | 258 | 275 | 362 | 161 | 175 | 211 | 114 | 125 | 138 | 87 | 95 | 96 |
| 0.25 | *** | 571 | 581 | 791 | 274 | 284 | 377 | 167 | 177 | 227 | 117 | 124 | 155 | 88 | 95 | 114 |
| | *** | 574 | 599 | 873 | 277 | 300 | 400 | 171 | 189 | 229 | 120 | 133 | 148 | 91 | 101 | 102 |
| 0.3 | *** | 595 | 607 | 882 | 281 | 294 | 413 | 171 | 182 | 245 | 118 | 128 | 164 | 89 | 97 | 120 |
| | *** | 599 | 632 | 946 | 286 | 315 | 428 | 175 | 197 | 242 | 122 | 138 | 154 | 92 | 104 | 106 |
| 0.35 | *** | 596 | 613 | 950 | 280 | 297 | 439 | 169 | 184 | 257 | 117 | 128 | 170 | 88 | 97 | 123 |
| | *** | 602 | 645 | 999 | 286 | 322 | 446 | 175 | 201 | 250 | 122 | 140 | 158 | 92 | 105 | 107 |
| 0.4 | *** | 579 | 601 | 997 | 272 | 293 | 455 | 165 | 181 | 263 | 114 | 127 | 173 | 86 | 95 | 123 |
| | *** | 587 | 641 | 1030 | 279 | 322 | 456 | 171 | 201 | 253 | 119 | 140 | 158 | 89 | 104 | 106 |
| 0.45 | *** | 548 | 575 | 1020 | 258 | 283 | 461 | 157 | 176 | 263 | 109 | 123 | 171 | 82 | 92 | 121 |
| | *** | 557 | 624 | 1041 | 267 | 316 | 456 | 165 | 198 | 250 | 115 | 137 | 154 | 86 | 101 | 102 |
| 0.5 | *** | 505 | 539 | 1020 | 241 | 269 | 456 | 148 | 168 | 258 | 103 | 117 | 166 | 77 | 87 | 116 |
| | *** | 516 | 596 | 1030 | 251 | 305 | 446 | 156 | 191 | 242 | 109 | 132 | 148 | 81 | 97 | 96 |
| 0.55 | *** | 454 | 496 | 998 | 221 | 252 | 441 | 137 | 158 | 246 | 96 | 110 | 157 | 72 | 82 | 108 |
| | *** | 469 | 561 | 999 | 232 | 290 | 428 | 145 | 181 | 229 | 102 | 124 | 138 | 76 | 90 | 88 |
| 0.6 | *** | 401 | 449 | 952 | 199 | 232 | 416 | 125 | 146 | 229 | 87 | 101 | 144 | 65 | 74 | 98 |
| | *** | 418 | 519 | 946 | 212 | 271 | 400 | 133 | 168 | 211 | 93 | 115 | 124 | 69 | 83 | 78 |
| 0.65 | *** | 347 | 401 | 884 | 177 | 210 | 380 | 112 | 132 | 207 | 78 | 91 | 128 | 58 | 66 | 86 |
| | *** | 367 | 473 | 873 | 190 | 248 | 362 | 120 | 153 | 187 | 83 | 103 | 107 | 61 | 73 | 65 |
| 0.7 | *** | 296 | 352 | 794 | 155 | 186 | 335 | 98 | 116 | 179 | 68 | 79 | 108 | . | . | . |
| | *** | 317 | 423 | 778 | 167 | 221 | 316 | 105 | 134 | 158 | 72 | 89 | 87 | . | . | . |
| 0.75 | *** | 248 | 302 | 681 | 132 | 160 | 280 | 82 | 98 | 145 | . | . | . | . | . | . |
| | *** | 269 | 368 | 662 | 143 | 190 | 260 | 89 | 112 | 124 | . | . | . | . | . | . |
| 0.8 | *** | 202 | 251 | 546 | 107 | 130 | 215 | . | . | . | . | . | . | . | . | . |
| | *** | 221 | 307 | 526 | 116 | 153 | 194 | . | . | . | . | . | . | . | . | . |
| 0.85 | *** | 155 | 194 | 389 | . | . | . | . | . | . | . | . | . | . | . | . |
| | *** | 170 | 237 | 368 | . | . | . | . | . | . | . | . | . | . | . | . |

| TABLE 6: ALPHA= 0.025 POWER= 0.9 | EXPECTED ACCRUAL THRU MINIMUM FOLLOW-UP= 50 |
|---|---|

|  | DEL=.10 | | | DEL=.15 | | | DEL=.20 | | | DEL=.25 | | | DEL=.30 | | |
|---|---|---|---|---|---|---|---|---|---|---|---|---|---|---|---|
| FACT= | 1.0 / .75 | .50 / .25 | .00 / BIN | 1.0 / .75 | .50 / .25 | .00 / BIN | 1.0 / .75 | .50 / .25 | .00 / BIN | 1.0 / 75 | .50 / .25 | .00 / BIN | 1.0 / .75 | .50 / .25 | .00 / BIN |

PCONT=***      REQUIRED NUMBER OF PATIENTS

| PCONT | DEL.10 (1.0/.75) | DEL.10 (.50/.25) | DEL.10 (.00/BIN) | DEL.15 (1.0/.75) | DEL.15 (.50/.25) | DEL.15 (.00/BIN) | DEL.20 (1.0/.75) | DEL.20 (.50/.25) | DEL.20 (.00/BIN) | DEL.25 (1.0/75) | DEL.25 (.50/.25) | DEL.25 (.00/BIN) | DEL.30 (1.0/.75) | DEL.30 (.50/.25) | DEL.30 (.00/BIN) |
|---|---|---|---|---|---|---|---|---|---|---|---|---|---|---|---|
| 0.05 *** | 221 | 223 | 239 | 129 | 131 | 139 | 91 | 93 | 98 | 71 | 72 | 76 | 59 | 60 | 62 |
| *** | 222 | 226 | 368 | 130 | 133 | 194 | 92 | 94 | 124 | 72 | 74 | 87 | 59 | 61 | 65 |
| 0.1 *** | 349 | 353 | 400 | 185 | 189 | 212 | 122 | 126 | 139 | 91 | 94 | 102 | 72 | 74 | 80 |
| *** | 350 | 359 | 526 | 187 | 195 | 260 | 124 | 130 | 158 | 92 | 96 | 107 | 73 | 76 | 78 |
| 0.15 *** | 451 | 457 | 548 | 228 | 234 | 276 | 145 | 151 | 174 | 104 | 109 | 124 | 81 | 85 | 94 |
| *** | 453 | 468 | 662 | 230 | 243 | 316 | 147 | 157 | 187 | 106 | 114 | 124 | 83 | 88 | 88 |
| 0.2 *** | 525 | 534 | 679 | 258 | 267 | 332 | 161 | 168 | 203 | 114 | 120 | 141 | 87 | 92 | 106 |
| *** | 528 | 550 | 778 | 261 | 280 | 362 | 163 | 178 | 211 | 116 | 127 | 138 | 89 | 97 | 96 |
| 0.25 *** | 574 | 585 | 791 | 276 | 288 | 377 | 170 | 180 | 227 | 119 | 127 | 155 | 90 | 97 | 114 |
| *** | 578 | 608 |  | 280 | 306 | 400 | 174 | 193 | 229 | 122 | 136 | 148 | 93 | 103 | 102 |
| 0.3 *** | 598 | 614 | 882 | 285 | 300 | 413 | 174 | 187 | 245 | 121 | 131 | 164 | 91 | 99 | 120 |
| *** | 603 | 643 | 946 | 290 | 323 | 428 | 179 | 202 | 242 | 125 | 142 | 154 | 95 | 106 | 106 |
| 0.35 *** | 600 | 621 | 950 | 285 | 304 | 439 | 173 | 189 | 257 | 121 | 132 | 170 | 91 | 99 | 123 |
| *** | 607 | 659 | 999 | 292 | 332 | 446 | 179 | 207 | 250 | 125 | 144 | 158 | 94 | 107 | 107 |
| 0.4 *** | 585 | 611 | 997 | 277 | 301 | 455 | 170 | 188 | 263 | 118 | 131 | 173 | 89 | 98 | 123 |
| *** | 594 | 658 | 1030 | 286 | 333 | 456 | 177 | 208 | 253 | 123 | 144 | 158 | 92 | 107 | 106 |
| 0.45 *** | 554 | 588 | 1020 | 265 | 293 | 461 | 163 | 183 | 263 | 114 | 128 | 171 | 85 | 95 | 121 |
| *** | 566 | 644 | 1041 | 275 | 328 | 456 | 171 | 205 | 250 | 119 | 141 | 154 | 89 | 104 | 102 |
| 0.5 *** | 513 | 555 | 1020 | 249 | 280 | 456 | 154 | 175 | 258 | 108 | 122 | 166 | 80 | 90 | 116 |
| *** | 528 | 619 | 1030 | 260 | 318 | 446 | 163 | 198 | 242 | 114 | 136 | 148 | 85 | 99 | 96 |
| 0.55 *** | 465 | 514 | 998 | 230 | 263 | 441 | 143 | 165 | 246 | 100 | 115 | 157 | 75 | 85 | 108 |
| *** | 483 | 586 | 999 | 243 | 303 | 428 | 152 | 188 | 229 | 106 | 128 | 138 | 79 | 93 | 88 |
| 0.6 *** | 414 | 470 | 952 | 209 | 244 | 416 | 132 | 153 | 229 | 92 | 106 | 144 | 68 | 77 | 98 |
| *** | 434 | 546 | 946 | 223 | 284 | 400 | 140 | 175 | 211 | 98 | 118 | 124 | 72 | 85 | 78 |
| 0.65 *** | 362 | 422 | 884 | 187 | 222 | 380 | 118 | 139 | 207 | 82 | 95 | 128 | 60 | 68 | 86 |
| *** | 385 | 500 | 873 | 201 | 260 | 362 | 127 | 159 | 187 | 88 | 106 | 107 | 64 | 75 | 65 |
| 0.7 *** | 312 | 374 | 794 | 164 | 197 | 335 | 104 | 122 | 179 | 71 | 82 | 108 | . | . | . |
| *** | 336 | 448 | 778 | 178 | 232 | 316 | 111 | 140 | 158 | 76 | 91 | 87 | . | . | . |
| 0.75 *** | 264 | 323 | 681 | 140 | 169 | 280 | 87 | 103 | 145 | . | . | . | . | . | . |
| *** | 287 | 391 | 662 | 152 | 199 | 260 | 94 | 117 | 124 | . | . | . | . | . | . |
| 0.8 *** | 216 | 268 | 546 | 114 | 137 | 215 | . | . | . | . | . | . | . | . | . |
| *** | 237 | 327 | 526 | 123 | 160 | 194 | . | . | . | . | . | . | . | . | . |
| 0.85 *** | 167 | 207 | 389 | . | . | . | . | . | . | . | . | . | . | . | . |
| *** | 183 | 251 | 368 | . | . | . | . | . | . | . | . | . | . | . | . |

TABLE 6: ALPHA= 0.025 POWER= 0.9    EXPECTED ACCRUAL THRU MINIMUM FOLLOW-UP= 60

| | | DEL=.10 | | | DEL=.15 | | | DEL=.20 | | | DEL=.25 | | | DEL=.30 | | |
|---|---|---|---|---|---|---|---|---|---|---|---|---|---|---|---|---|---|
| FACT= | | 1.0 .75 | .50 .25 | .00 BIN | 1.0 .75 | .50 .25 | .00 BIN | 1.0 .75 | .50 .25 | .00 BIN | 1.0 75 | .50 .25 | .00 BIN | 1.0 .75 | .50 .25 | .00 BIN |
| PCONT=*** | | | | | REQUIRED NUMBER OF PATIENTS | | | | | | | | | | | |
| 0.05 | *** | 221 | 224 | 239 | 129 | 131 | 139 | 92 | 93 | 98 | 71 | 73 | 76 | 59 | 60 | 62 |
| | *** | 222 | 227 | 368 | 130 | 134 | 194 | 92 | 95 | 124 | 72 | 74 | 87 | 59 | 61 | 65 |
| 0.1 | *** | 350 | 354 | 400 | 186 | 190 | 212 | 123 | 127 | 139 | 91 | 94 | 102 | 73 | 75 | 80 |
| | *** | 351 | 362 | 526 | 188 | 196 | 260 | 125 | 131 | 158 | 93 | 97 | 107 | 74 | 77 | 78 |
| 0.15 | *** | 452 | 459 | 548 | 229 | 236 | 276 | 146 | 152 | 174 | 106 | 110 | 124 | 82 | 86 | 94 |
| | *** | 454 | 472 | 662 | 232 | 246 | 316 | 149 | 159 | 187 | 107 | 115 | 124 | 84 | 89 | 88 |
| 0.2 | *** | 527 | 537 | 679 | 260 | 270 | 332 | 162 | 171 | 203 | 115 | 122 | 141 | 88 | 93 | 106 |
| | *** | 530 | 556 | 778 | 263 | 284 | 362 | 166 | 180 | 211 | 118 | 128 | 138 | 90 | 98 | 96 |
| 0.25 | *** | 576 | 590 | 791 | 279 | 293 | 377 | 172 | 183 | 227 | 121 | 130 | 155 | 92 | 98 | 114 |
| | *** | 581 | 616 | 873 | 284 | 312 | 400 | 176 | 196 | 229 | 124 | 138 | 148 | 95 | 104 | 102 |
| 0.3 | *** | 601 | 620 | 882 | 288 | 306 | 413 | 177 | 191 | 245 | 124 | 134 | 164 | 93 | 101 | 120 |
| | *** | 607 | 654 | 946 | 294 | 330 | 428 | 182 | 206 | 242 | 128 | 144 | 154 | 97 | 108 | 106 |
| 0.35 | *** | 604 | 629 | 950 | 289 | 311 | 439 | 177 | 194 | 257 | 124 | 136 | 170 | 93 | 102 | 123 |
| | *** | 613 | 672 | 999 | 297 | 340 | 446 | 184 | 212 | 250 | 128 | 147 | 158 | 97 | 109 | 107 |
| 0.4 | *** | 590 | 622 | 997 | 283 | 309 | 455 | 174 | 193 | 263 | 121 | 135 | 173 | 91 | 100 | 123 |
| | *** | 601 | 674 | 1030 | 293 | 342 | 456 | 181 | 213 | 253 | 127 | 147 | 158 | 95 | 108 | 106 |
| 0.45 | *** | 561 | 601 | 1020 | 271 | 302 | 461 | 168 | 188 | 263 | 117 | 131 | 171 | 88 | 97 | 121 |
| | *** | 575 | 662 | 1041 | 283 | 338 | 456 | 176 | 210 | 250 | 123 | 144 | 154 | 92 | 106 | 102 |
| 0.5 | *** | 522 | 569 | 1020 | 256 | 289 | 456 | 159 | 181 | 258 | 111 | 126 | 166 | 83 | 93 | 116 |
| | *** | 539 | 639 | 1030 | 269 | 329 | 446 | 168 | 204 | 242 | 117 | 139 | 148 | 87 | 101 | 96 |
| 0.55 | *** | 476 | 531 | 998 | 238 | 273 | 441 | 149 | 171 | 246 | 104 | 119 | 157 | 77 | 87 | 108 |
| | *** | 496 | 607 | 999 | 252 | 314 | 428 | 158 | 194 | 229 | 110 | 131 | 138 | 82 | 95 | 88 |
| 0.6 | *** | 426 | 488 | 952 | 218 | 254 | 416 | 137 | 159 | 229 | 96 | 109 | 144 | 71 | 79 | 98 |
| | *** | 449 | 568 | 946 | 232 | 294 | 400 | 146 | 181 | 211 | 101 | 121 | 124 | 74 | 86 | 78 |
| 0.65 | *** | 376 | 441 | 884 | 196 | 232 | 380 | 124 | 144 | 207 | 86 | 98 | 128 | 63 | 70 | 86 |
| | *** | 401 | 522 | 873 | 210 | 270 | 362 | 132 | 164 | 187 | 91 | 109 | 107 | 66 | 76 | 65 |
| 0.7 | *** | 327 | 392 | 794 | 173 | 206 | 335 | 109 | 127 | 179 | 74 | 85 | 108 | . | . | . |
| | *** | 352 | 470 | 778 | 186 | 241 | 316 | 116 | 144 | 158 | 79 | 93 | 87 | . | . | . |
| 0.75 | *** | 278 | 340 | 681 | 148 | 177 | 280 | 91 | 107 | 145 | . | . | . | . | . | . |
| | *** | 302 | 410 | 662 | 160 | 207 | 260 | 98 | 120 | 124 | . | . | . | . | . | . |
| 0.8 | *** | 229 | 283 | 546 | 120 | 143 | 215 | . | . | . | . | . | . | . | . | . |
| | *** | 251 | 343 | 526 | 130 | 166 | 194 | . | . | . | . | . | . | . | . | . |
| 0.85 | *** | 177 | 219 | 389 | . | . | . | . | . | . | . | . | . | . | . | . |
| | *** | 194 | 262 | 368 | . | . | . | . | . | . | . | . | . | . | . | . |

## TABLE 6: ALPHA= 0.025  POWER= 0.9    EXPECTED ACCRUAL THRU MINIMUM FOLLOW-UP= 70

| | | DEL=.10 | | | DEL=.15 | | | DEL=.20 | | | DEL=.25 | | | DEL=.30 | | |
|---|---|---|---|---|---|---|---|---|---|---|---|---|---|---|---|---|---|
| FACT= | | 1.0 .75 | .50 .25 | .00 BIN | 1.0 .75 | .50 .25 | .00 BIN | 1.0 .75 | .50 .25 | .00 BIN | 1.0 75 | .50 .25 | .00 BIN | 1.0 .75 | .50 .25 | .00 BIN |
| PCONT=*** | | | | | REQUIRED NUMBER OF PATIENTS | | | | | | | | | | | |
| 0.05 | *** | 222 | 224 | 239 | 130 | 132 | 139 | 92 | 94 | 98 | 72 | 73 | 76 | 59 | 60 | 62 |
| | *** | 223 | 228 | 368 | 131 | 134 | 194 | 93 | 95 | 124 | 72 | 74 | 87 | 60 | 61 | 65 |
| 0.1 | *** | 351 | 355 | 400 | 187 | 192 | 212 | 124 | 128 | 139 | 92 | 95 | 102 | 73 | 75 | 80 |
| | *** | 352 | 364 | 526 | 189 | 197 | 260 | 125 | 132 | 158 | 93 | 98 | 107 | 74 | 77 | 78 |
| 0.15 | *** | 453 | 461 | 548 | 230 | 238 | 276 | 147 | 154 | 174 | 107 | 111 | 124 | 83 | 86 | 94 |
| | *** | 456 | 475 | 662 | 233 | 248 | 316 | 150 | 160 | 187 | 109 | 116 | 124 | 84 | 90 | 88 |
| 0.2 | *** | 529 | 541 | 679 | 261 | 273 | 332 | 164 | 173 | 203 | 117 | 123 | 141 | 89 | 94 | 106 |
| | *** | 533 | 562 | 778 | 265 | 287 | 362 | 167 | 182 | 211 | 119 | 130 | 138 | 92 | 99 | 96 |
| 0.25 | *** | 578 | 595 | 791 | 281 | 296 | 377 | 174 | 186 | 227 | 123 | 131 | 155 | 93 | 100 | 114 |
| | *** | 584 | 624 | 873 | 287 | 316 | 400 | 179 | 199 | 229 | 126 | 139 | 148 | 96 | 105 | 102 |
| 0.3 | *** | 604 | 626 | 882 | 291 | 311 | 413 | 180 | 194 | 245 | 126 | 136 | 164 | 95 | 103 | 120 |
| | *** | 612 | 664 | 946 | 298 | 336 | 428 | 185 | 209 | 242 | 130 | 146 | 154 | 98 | 109 | 106 |
| 0.35 | *** | 609 | 637 | 950 | 293 | 317 | 439 | 181 | 198 | 257 | 126 | 138 | 170 | 95 | 103 | 123 |
| | *** | 618 | 685 | 999 | 302 | 346 | 446 | 187 | 215 | 250 | 131 | 149 | 158 | 99 | 111 | 107 |
| 0.4 | *** | 596 | 632 | 997 | 288 | 316 | 455 | 178 | 197 | 263 | 124 | 137 | 172 | 93 | 102 | 123 |
| | *** | 608 | 689 | 1030 | 298 | 350 | 456 | 186 | 217 | 253 | 130 | 149 | 158 | 97 | 110 | 106 |
| 0.45 | *** | 568 | 612 | 1020 | 277 | 309 | 460 | 172 | 193 | 263 | 120 | 134 | 171 | 90 | 99 | 121 |
| | *** | 584 | 679 | 1041 | 290 | 347 | 456 | 181 | 215 | 250 | 126 | 147 | 154 | 94 | 107 | 102 |
| 0.5 | *** | 531 | 583 | 1020 | 263 | 298 | 456 | 164 | 186 | 258 | 115 | 129 | 166 | 85 | 95 | 116 |
| | *** | 549 | 657 | 1030 | 276 | 337 | 446 | 173 | 208 | 242 | 121 | 142 | 148 | 89 | 103 | 96 |
| 0.55 | *** | 486 | 546 | 998 | 245 | 282 | 441 | 154 | 177 | 246 | 107 | 122 | 157 | 80 | 89 | 108 |
| | *** | 508 | 627 | 999 | 260 | 323 | 428 | 163 | 198 | 229 | 113 | 134 | 138 | 84 | 96 | 88 |
| 0.6 | *** | 438 | 504 | 952 | 225 | 263 | 416 | 142 | 164 | 229 | 99 | 112 | 144 | 73 | 81 | 98 |
| | *** | 463 | 588 | 946 | 240 | 303 | 400 | 151 | 185 | 211 | 104 | 124 | 124 | 76 | 88 | 78 |
| 0.65 | *** | 389 | 458 | 884 | 203 | 240 | 380 | 128 | 149 | 207 | 88 | 101 | 128 | 64 | 72 | 86 |
| | *** | 416 | 541 | 873 | 218 | 278 | 362 | 137 | 168 | 187 | 94 | 111 | 107 | 68 | 77 | 65 |
| 0.7 | *** | 340 | 408 | 794 | 180 | 214 | 335 | 113 | 131 | 179 | 77 | 87 | 108 | . | . | . |
| | *** | 367 | 488 | 778 | 194 | 249 | 316 | 120 | 147 | 158 | 81 | 95 | 87 | . | . | . |
| 0.75 | *** | 291 | 355 | 681 | 154 | 184 | 280 | 95 | 110 | 145 | . | . | . | . | . | . |
| | *** | 316 | 427 | 662 | 166 | 213 | 260 | 101 | 122 | 124 | . | . | . | . | . | . |
| 0.8 | *** | 240 | 296 | 546 | 125 | 149 | 215 | . | . | . | . | . | . | . | . | . |
| | *** | 263 | 356 | 526 | 135 | 170 | 194 | . | . | . | . | . | . | . | . | . |
| 0.85 | *** | 186 | 228 | 389 | . | . | . | . | . | . | . | . | . | . | . | . |
| | *** | 203 | 272 | 368 | . | . | . | . | . | . | . | . | . | . | . | . |

## TABLE 6: ALPHA= 0.025 POWER= 0.9　　EXPECTED ACCRUAL THRU MINIMUM FOLLOW-UP= 80

| | | DEL=.10 | | | DEL=.15 | | | DEL=.20 | | | DEL=.25 | | | DEL=.30 | | |
|---|---|---|---|---|---|---|---|---|---|---|---|---|---|---|---|---|
| FACT= | | 1.0 .75 | .50 .25 | .00 BIN | 1.0 .75 | .50 .25 | .00 BIN | 1.0 .75 | .50 .25 | .00 BIN | 1.0 75 | .50 .25 | .00 BIN | 1.0 .75 | .50 .25 | .00 BIN |
| PCONT=*** | | REQUIRED NUMBER OF PATIENTS | | | | | | | | | | | | | | |
| 0.05 | *** | 222 | 225 | 239 | 130 | 132 | 139 | 92 | 94 | 98 | 72 | 73 | 76 | 59 | 60 | 62 |
| | *** | 223 | 228 | 368 | 131 | 135 | 194 | 93 | 95 | 124 | 72 | 74 | 87 | 60 | 61 | 65 |
| 0.1 | *** | 351 | 357 | 400 | 188 | 193 | 212 | 125 | 128 | 139 | 93 | 96 | 102 | 74 | 76 | 80 |
| | *** | 353 | 366 | 526 | 190 | 198 | 260 | 126 | 132 | 158 | 94 | 98 | 107 | 75 | 78 | 78 |
| 0.15 | *** | 454 | 463 | 548 | 232 | 240 | 276 | 149 | 155 | 174 | 107 | 112 | 124 | 84 | 87 | 94 |
| | *** | 457 | 479 | 662 | 235 | 250 | 316 | 151 | 161 | 187 | 109 | 116 | 124 | 85 | 90 | 88 |
| 0.2 | *** | 530 | 544 | 679 | 263 | 275 | 332 | 166 | 175 | 203 | 118 | 125 | 141 | 90 | 95 | 106 |
| | *** | 535 | 567 | 778 | 268 | 290 | 362 | 169 | 184 | 211 | 121 | 131 | 138 | 92 | 99 | 96 |
| 0.25 | *** | 581 | 599 | 791 | 284 | 300 | 377 | 177 | 189 | 227 | 124 | 133 | 155 | 95 | 101 | 114 |
| | *** | 587 | 631 | 873 | 290 | 320 | 400 | 181 | 201 | 229 | 128 | 141 | 148 | 97 | 106 | 102 |
| 0.3 | *** | 607 | 632 | 882 | 294 | 315 | 413 | 182 | 197 | 245 | 128 | 138 | 164 | 97 | 104 | 120 |
| | *** | 616 | 673 | 946 | 302 | 341 | 428 | 188 | 212 | 242 | 132 | 148 | 154 | 100 | 110 | 106 |
| 0.35 | *** | 613 | 645 | 950 | 297 | 322 | 439 | 184 | 201 | 257 | 128 | 140 | 170 | 97 | 105 | 123 |
| | *** | 624 | 696 | 999 | 307 | 352 | 446 | 191 | 219 | 250 | 133 | 151 | 158 | 100 | 112 | 107 |
| 0.4 | *** | 601 | 641 | 997 | 293 | 322 | 455 | 181 | 201 | 263 | 127 | 140 | 173 | 95 | 104 | 123 |
| | *** | 615 | 702 | 1030 | 304 | 357 | 456 | 189 | 221 | 253 | 132 | 152 | 158 | 99 | 111 | 106 |
| 0.45 | *** | 575 | 624 | 1020 | 283 | 316 | 461 | 176 | 198 | 263 | 123 | 137 | 171 | 92 | 101 | 121 |
| | *** | 592 | 694 | 1041 | 296 | 354 | 456 | 185 | 218 | 250 | 129 | 149 | 154 | 96 | 109 | 102 |
| 0.5 | *** | 539 | 596 | 1020 | 269 | 305 | 456 | 168 | 191 | 258 | 117 | 132 | 166 | 87 | 97 | 116 |
| | *** | 560 | 674 | 1030 | 283 | 345 | 446 | 177 | 212 | 242 | 123 | 144 | 148 | 91 | 104 | 96 |
| 0.55 | *** | 496 | 561 | 998 | 252 | 290 | 441 | 158 | 181 | 246 | 110 | 124 | 157 | 82 | 90 | 108 |
| | *** | 520 | 644 | 999 | 267 | 331 | 428 | 168 | 202 | 229 | 116 | 136 | 138 | 85 | 97 | 88 |
| 0.6 | *** | 449 | 519 | 952 | 232 | 271 | 416 | 146 | 168 | 229 | 101 | 115 | 144 | 74 | 83 | 98 |
| | *** | 476 | 605 | 946 | 248 | 311 | 400 | 155 | 189 | 211 | 107 | 126 | 124 | 78 | 89 | 78 |
| 0.65 | *** | 401 | 473 | 884 | 210 | 248 | 380 | 132 | 153 | 207 | 91 | 103 | 128 | 66 | 73 | 86 |
| | *** | 429 | 558 | 873 | 225 | 285 | 362 | 141 | 171 | 187 | 96 | 112 | 107 | 69 | 78 | 65 |
| 0.7 | *** | 352 | 423 | 794 | 186 | 221 | 335 | 116 | 134 | 179 | 79 | 89 | 108 | . | . | . |
| | *** | 380 | 504 | 778 | 200 | 255 | 316 | 124 | 150 | 158 | 83 | 96 | 87 | . | . | . |
| 0.75 | *** | 302 | 368 | 681 | 160 | 190 | 280 | 98 | 112 | 145 | . | . | . | . | . | . |
| | *** | 329 | 441 | 662 | 172 | 218 | 260 | 104 | 124 | 124 | . | . | . | . | . | . |
| 0.8 | *** | 251 | 307 | 546 | 130 | 153 | 215 | . | . | . | . | . | . | . | . | . |
| | *** | 273 | 367 | 526 | 139 | 174 | 194 | . | . | . | . | . | . | . | . | . |
| 0.85 | *** | 194 | 237 | 389 | . | . | . | . | . | . | . | . | . | . | . | . |
| | *** | 211 | 280 | 368 | . | . | . | . | . | . | . | . | . | . | . | . |

## TABLE 6: ALPHA= 0.025 POWER= 0.9    EXPECTED ACCRUAL THRU MINIMUM FOLLOW-UP= 90

| PCONT=*** | | DEL=.10 | | | DEL=.15 | | | DEL=.20 | | | DEL=.25 | | | DEL=.30 | | |
|---|---|---|---|---|---|---|---|---|---|---|---|---|---|---|---|---|
| FACT= | | 1.0 .75 | .50 .25 | .00 BIN | 1.0 .75 | .50 .25 | .00 BIN | 1.0 .75 | .50 .25 | .00 BIN | 1.0 75 | .50 .25 | .00 BIN | 1.0 .75 | .50 .25 | .00 BIN |
| | | REQUIRED NUMBER OF PATIENTS | | | | | | | | | | | | | | |
| 0.05 | *** | 223 | 225 | 239 | 130 | 133 | 139 | 92 | 94 | 98 | 72 | 73 | 76 | 60 | 61 | 62 |
| | *** | 224 | 229 | 368 | 131 | 135 | 194 | 93 | 96 | 124 | 73 | 74 | 87 | 60 | 61 | 65 |
| 0.1 | *** | 352 | 358 | 400 | 188 | 194 | 212 | 125 | 129 | 139 | 93 | 96 | 102 | 74 | 76 | 80 |
| | *** | 354 | 367 | 526 | 190 | 199 | 260 | 127 | 133 | 158 | 94 | 98 | 107 | 75 | 78 | 78 |
| 0.15 | *** | 455 | 465 | 548 | 233 | 241 | 276 | 150 | 156 | 174 | 108 | 113 | 124 | 84 | 88 | 94 |
| | *** | 459 | 482 | 662 | 236 | 252 | 316 | 152 | 162 | 187 | 110 | 117 | 124 | 86 | 90 | 88 |
| 0.2 | *** | 532 | 547 | 679 | 265 | 278 | 332 | 167 | 176 | 203 | 119 | 126 | 141 | 91 | 96 | 106 |
| | *** | 537 | 571 | 778 | 270 | 293 | 362 | 171 | 186 | 211 | 122 | 131 | 138 | 93 | 100 | 96 |
| 0.25 | *** | 583 | 604 | 791 | 286 | 303 | 377 | 178 | 191 | 227 | 126 | 135 | 155 | 96 | 102 | 114 |
| | *** | 590 | 637 | 873 | 292 | 324 | 400 | 183 | 203 | 229 | 130 | 142 | 148 | 98 | 107 | 102 |
| 0.3 | *** | 610 | 638 | 882 | 297 | 319 | 413 | 185 | 200 | 245 | 130 | 140 | 164 | 98 | 105 | 120 |
| | *** | 620 | 681 | 946 | 306 | 345 | 428 | 191 | 215 | 242 | 134 | 149 | 154 | 101 | 111 | 106 |
| 0.35 | *** | 617 | 652 | 950 | 301 | 327 | 439 | 186 | 204 | 257 | 130 | 142 | 170 | 98 | 106 | 123 |
| | *** | 629 | 706 | 999 | 311 | 357 | 446 | 194 | 221 | 250 | 136 | 153 | 158 | 102 | 113 | 107 |
| 0.4 | *** | 606 | 650 | 997 | 297 | 328 | 455 | 185 | 205 | 263 | 129 | 142 | 173 | 97 | 105 | 123 |
| | *** | 622 | 713 | 1030 | 309 | 362 | 456 | 193 | 224 | 253 | 135 | 153 | 158 | 100 | 112 | 106 |
| 0.45 | *** | 582 | 634 | 1020 | 288 | 323 | 461 | 180 | 201 | 258 | 125 | 139 | 171 | 93 | 103 | 120 |
| | *** | 601 | 707 | 1041 | 302 | 360 | 456 | 189 | 222 | 250 | 131 | 151 | 154 | 97 | 110 | 102 |
| 0.5 | *** | 547 | 608 | 1020 | 275 | 312 | 456 | 172 | 195 | 258 | 120 | 134 | 166 | 89 | 98 | 116 |
| | *** | 569 | 688 | 1030 | 289 | 352 | 446 | 181 | 215 | 242 | 126 | 146 | 148 | 93 | 105 | 96 |
| 0.55 | *** | 505 | 574 | 998 | 258 | 297 | 441 | 162 | 185 | 246 | 113 | 126 | 157 | 83 | 92 | 108 |
| | *** | 531 | 659 | 999 | 273 | 337 | 428 | 171 | 205 | 229 | 119 | 138 | 138 | 87 | 98 | 88 |
| 0.6 | *** | 460 | 533 | 952 | 238 | 278 | 416 | 150 | 172 | 229 | 104 | 117 | 144 | 76 | 84 | 98 |
| | *** | 488 | 620 | 946 | 254 | 317 | 400 | 159 | 192 | 211 | 109 | 127 | 124 | 79 | 90 | 78 |
| 0.65 | *** | 412 | 487 | 884 | 216 | 254 | 380 | 136 | 156 | 207 | 93 | 105 | 128 | 67 | 74 | 85 |
| | *** | 441 | 573 | 873 | 232 | 292 | 362 | 144 | 174 | 187 | 98 | 114 | 107 | 70 | 79 | 65 |
| 0.7 | *** | 363 | 436 | 794 | 192 | 227 | 335 | 119 | 137 | 179 | 80 | 90 | 108 | . | . | . |
| | *** | 392 | 518 | 778 | 206 | 260 | 316 | 127 | 152 | 158 | 85 | 97 | 87 | . | . | . |
| 0.75 | *** | 313 | 380 | 681 | 165 | 195 | 280 | 100 | 115 | 145 | . | . | . | . | . | . |
| | *** | 340 | 453 | 662 | 177 | 222 | 260 | 107 | 126 | 124 | . | . | . | . | . | . |
| 0.8 | *** | 260 | 317 | 546 | 134 | 157 | 215 | . | . | . | . | . | . | . | . | . |
| | *** | 283 | 377 | 526 | 143 | 177 | 194 | . | . | . | . | . | . | . | . | . |
| 0.85 | *** | 201 | 244 | 389 | . | . | . | . | . | . | . | . | . | . | . | . |
| | *** | 219 | 287 | 368 | . | . | . | . | . | . | . | . | . | . | . | . |

## TABLE 6: ALPHA= 0.025 POWER= 0.9     EXPECTED ACCRUAL THRU MINIMUM FOLLOW-UP= 100

|  |  | DEL=.10 | | | DEL=.15 | | | DEL=.20 | | | DEL=.25 | | | DEL=.30 | | |
|---|---|---|---|---|---|---|---|---|---|---|---|---|---|---|---|---|
| FACT= | | 1.0 .75 | .50 .25 | .00 BIN | 1.0 .75 | .50 .25 | .00 BIN | 1.0 .75 | .50 .25 | .00 BIN | 1.0 75 | .50 .25 | .00 BIN | 1.0 .75 | .50 .25 | .00 BIN |
| PCONT=*** | | | | | REQUIRED NUMBER OF PATIENTS | | | | | | | | | | | |
| 0.05 | *** | 223 | 226 | 239 | 131 | 133 | 139 | 93 | 94 | 98 | 72 | 74 | 76 | 60 | 61 | 62 |
|  | *** | 224 | 230 | 368 | 132 | 135 | 194 | 93 | 96 | 124 | 73 | 75 | 87 | 60 | 61 | 65 |
| 0.1 | *** | 353 | 359 | 400 | 189 | 195 | 212 | 126 | 130 | 139 | 94 | 96 | 102 | 74 | 76 | 80 |
|  | *** | 355 | 369 | 526 | 191 | 200 | 260 | 127 | 133 | 158 | 95 | 99 | 107 | 75 | 78 | 78 |
| 0.15 | *** | 457 | 468 | 548 | 234 | 243 | 276 | 151 | 157 | 174 | 109 | 114 | 124 | 85 | 88 | 94 |
|  | *** | 460 | 485 | 662 | 237 | 253 | 316 | 153 | 163 | 187 | 111 | 118 | 124 | 86 | 91 | 88 |
| 0.2 | *** | 534 | 550 | 679 | 267 | 280 | 332 | 168 | 178 | 203 | 120 | 127 | 141 | 92 | 97 | 106 |
|  | *** | 539 | 576 | 778 | 272 | 295 | 362 | 172 | 187 | 211 | 123 | 132 | 138 | 94 | 100 | 96 |
| 0.25 | *** | 585 | 608 | 791 | 288 | 306 | 377 | 180 | 193 | 227 | 127 | 136 | 155 | 97 | 103 | 114 |
|  | *** | 593 | 643 | 873 | 295 | 327 | 400 | 185 | 204 | 229 | 131 | 143 | 148 | 99 | 107 | 102 |
| 0.3 | *** | 614 | 643 | 882 | 300 | 323 | 413 | 187 | 202 | 245 | 131 | 142 | 164 | 99 | 106 | 120 |
|  | *** | 624 | 689 | 946 | 309 | 349 | 428 | 193 | 217 | 242 | 136 | 150 | 154 | 102 | 112 | 106 |
| 0.35 | *** | 621 | 659 | 950 | 304 | 332 | 439 | 189 | 207 | 257 | 132 | 144 | 170 | 99 | 107 | 123 |
|  | *** | 635 | 715 | 999 | 315 | 362 | 446 | 196 | 224 | 250 | 137 | 154 | 158 | 103 | 113 | 107 |
| 0.4 | *** | 611 | 658 | 997 | 301 | 333 | 455 | 188 | 208 | 263 | 131 | 144 | 173 | 98 | 107 | 123 |
|  | *** | 628 | 724 | 1030 | 314 | 367 | 456 | 196 | 226 | 253 | 137 | 155 | 158 | 102 | 113 | 106 |
| 0.45 | *** | 588 | 644 | 1020 | 293 | 328 | 461 | 183 | 205 | 263 | 128 | 141 | 171 | 95 | 104 | 121 |
|  | *** | 609 | 719 | 1041 | 307 | 366 | 456 | 192 | 224 | 250 | 133 | 152 | 154 | 99 | 111 | 102 |
| 0.5 | *** | 555 | 619 | 1020 | 280 | 318 | 456 | 175 | 198 | 258 | 122 | 136 | 166 | 90 | 99 | 116 |
|  | *** | 579 | 701 | 1030 | 295 | 357 | 446 | 185 | 218 | 242 | 128 | 147 | 148 | 94 | 106 | 96 |
| 0.55 | *** | 514 | 586 | 998 | 263 | 303 | 441 | 165 | 188 | 246 | 115 | 128 | 157 | 85 | 93 | 108 |
|  | *** | 541 | 673 | 999 | 279 | 343 | 428 | 175 | 208 | 229 | 121 | 139 | 138 | 88 | 99 | 88 |
| 0.6 | *** | 470 | 546 | 952 | 244 | 284 | 416 | 153 | 175 | 229 | 106 | 118 | 144 | 77 | 85 | 98 |
|  | *** | 499 | 634 | 946 | 260 | 323 | 400 | 163 | 194 | 211 | 111 | 128 | 124 | 81 | 90 | 78 |
| 0.65 | *** | 422 | 500 | 884 | 222 | 260 | 380 | 139 | 159 | 207 | 95 | 106 | 128 | 68 | 75 | 86 |
|  | *** | 453 | 587 | 873 | 238 | 297 | 362 | 148 | 176 | 187 | 100 | 115 | 107 | 71 | 79 | 65 |
| 0.7 | *** | 374 | 448 | 794 | 197 | 232 | 335 | 122 | 140 | 179 | 82 | 91 | 108 | . | . | . |
|  | *** | 403 | 530 | 778 | 212 | 265 | 316 | 130 | 154 | 158 | 86 | 98 | 87 | . | . | . |
| 0.75 | *** | 323 | 391 | 681 | 169 | 199 | 280 | 103 | 117 | 145 | . | . | . | . | . | . |
|  | *** | 350 | 464 | 662 | 182 | 226 | 260 | 109 | 128 | 124 | . | . | . | . | . | . |
| 0.8 | *** | 268 | 327 | 546 | 137 | 160 | 215 | . | . | . | . | . | . | . | . | . |
|  | *** | 292 | 386 | 526 | 147 | 180 | 194 | . | . | . | . | . | . | . | . | . |
| 0.85 | *** | 207 | 251 | 389 | . | . | . | . | . | . | . | . | . | . | . | . |
|  | *** | 225 | 293 | 368 | . | . | . | . | . | . | . | . | . | . | . | . |

TABLE 6: ALPHA= 0.025 POWER= 0.9     EXPECTED ACCRUAL THRU MINIMUM FOLLOW-UP= 110

| | | DEL=.05 | | | DEL=.10 | | | DEL=.15 | | | DEL=.20 | | | DEL=.25 | |
|---|---|---|---|---|---|---|---|---|---|---|---|---|---|---|---|
| FACT= | 1.0 .75 | .50 .25 | .00 BIN | 1.0 .75 | .50 .25 | .00 BIN | 1.0 .75 | .50 .25 | .00 BIN | 1.0 75 | .50 .25 | .00 BIN | 1.0 .75 | .50 .25 | .00 BIN |
| PCONT=*** | | | | | | REQUIRED NUMBER OF PATIENTS | | | | | | | | | |
| 0.05 *** | 628 | 631 | 671 | 223 | 226 | 239 | 131 | 133 | 139 | 93 | 95 | 98 | 72 | 74 | 76 |
| *** | 629 | 636 | 1156 | 224 | 230 | 368 | 132 | 136 | 194 | 94 | 96 | 124 | 73 | 75 | 87 |
| 0.1 *** | 1145 | 1151 | 1295 | 353 | 360 | 400 | 190 | 195 | 212 | 126 | 130 | 139 | 94 | 97 | 102 |
| *** | 1147 | 1164 | 1829 | 356 | 370 | 526 | 192 | 201 | 260 | 128 | 134 | 158 | 95 | 99 | 107 |
| 0.15 *** | 1583 | 1594 | 1898 | 458 | 470 | 548 | 235 | 244 | 276 | 151 | 158 | 174 | 110 | 114 | 124 |
| *** | 1586 | 1615 | 2417 | 462 | 487 | 662 | 239 | 255 | 316 | 154 | 164 | 187 | 112 | 118 | 124 |
| 0.2 *** | 1921 | 1937 | 2448 | 536 | 553 | 679 | 268 | 282 | 332 | 170 | 179 | 203 | 121 | 127 | 141 |
| *** | 1927 | 1970 | 2922 | 542 | 580 | 778 | 273 | 297 | 362 | 174 | 188 | 211 | 124 | 133 | 138 |
| 0.25 *** | 2155 | 2178 | 2930 | 588 | 612 | 791 | 290 | 309 | 377 | 182 | 194 | 227 | 128 | 137 | 155 |
| *** | 2163 | 2224 | 3342 | 596 | 649 | 873 | 298 | 329 | 400 | 187 | 206 | 229 | 132 | 144 | 148 |
| 0.3 *** | 2289 | 2320 | 3331 | 617 | 649 | 882 | 303 | 327 | 413 | 189 | 204 | 245 | 133 | 143 | 164 |
| *** | 2299 | 2383 | 3678 | 628 | 696 | 946 | 312 | 352 | 428 | 195 | 218 | 242 | 137 | 151 | 154 |
| 0.35 *** | 2331 | 2372 | 3648 | 625 | 666 | 950 | 308 | 336 | 439 | 192 | 209 | 257 | 134 | 146 | 170 |
| *** | 2344 | 2455 | 3930 | 640 | 724 | 999 | 319 | 366 | 446 | 199 | 226 | 250 | 139 | 155 | 158 |
| 0.4 *** | 2292 | 2346 | 3876 | 617 | 667 | 997 | 305 | 338 | 455 | 190 | 210 | 263 | 133 | 146 | 173 |
| *** | 2310 | 2453 | 4098 | 635 | 734 | 1030 | 318 | 372 | 456 | 199 | 229 | 253 | 138 | 156 | 158 |
| 0.45 *** | 2187 | 2256 | 4014 | 594 | 654 | 1020 | 297 | 333 | 461 | 186 | 207 | 263 | 129 | 143 | 171 |
| *** | 2210 | 2390 | 4182 | 616 | 730 | 1041 | 312 | 371 | 456 | 195 | 227 | 250 | 135 | 154 | 154 |
| 0.5 *** | 2027 | 2116 | 4061 | 562 | 630 | 1020 | 285 | 324 | 456 | 178 | 201 | 258 | 124 | 138 | 166 |
| *** | 2057 | 2281 | 4182 | 588 | 713 | 1030 | 300 | 363 | 446 | 188 | 221 | 242 | 130 | 148 | 148 |
| 0.55 *** | 1830 | 1941 | 4016 | 523 | 597 | 998 | 269 | 309 | 441 | 169 | 191 | 246 | 117 | 130 | 157 |
| *** | 1868 | 2139 | 4098 | 551 | 685 | 999 | 285 | 348 | 428 | 178 | 211 | 229 | 122 | 140 | 138 |
| 0.6 *** | 1610 | 1748 | 3879 | 479 | 557 | 952 | 249 | 289 | 416 | 156 | 178 | 229 | 108 | 120 | 144 |
| *** | 1657 | 1974 | 3930 | 509 | 647 | 946 | 266 | 328 | 400 | 166 | 197 | 211 | 113 | 130 | 124 |
| 0.65 *** | 1383 | 1547 | 3652 | 432 | 511 | 884 | 227 | 265 | 380 | 142 | 162 | 207 | 97 | 108 | 128 |
| *** | 1441 | 1795 | 3678 | 463 | 599 | 873 | 243 | 302 | 362 | 150 | 178 | 187 | 101 | 116 | 107 |
| 0.7 *** | 1164 | 1349 | 3334 | 383 | 460 | 794 | 202 | 237 | 335 | 125 | 142 | 179 | 83 | 92 | 108 |
| *** | 1232 | 1606 | 3342 | 414 | 542 | 778 | 217 | 269 | 316 | 132 | 156 | 158 | 87 | 99 | 87 |
| 0.75 *** | 963 | 1156 | 2927 | 331 | 401 | 681 | 174 | 203 | 280 | 105 | 118 | 145 | . | . | . |
| *** | 1036 | 1407 | 2922 | 360 | 474 | 662 | 186 | 229 | 260 | 111 | 129 | 124 | . | . | . |
| 0.8 *** | 781 | 966 | 2431 | 276 | 335 | 546 | 141 | 163 | 215 | . | . | . | . | . | . |
| *** | 852 | 1195 | 2417 | 300 | 394 | 526 | 150 | 182 | 194 | . | . | . | . | . | . |
| 0.85 *** | 611 | 772 | 1847 | 213 | 257 | 389 | . | . | . | . | . | . | . | . | . |
| *** | 674 | 962 | 1829 | 231 | 298 | 368 | . | . | . | . | . | . | . | . | . |
| 0.9 *** | 437 | 555 | 1177 | . | . | . | . | . | . | . | . | . | . | . | . |
| *** | 484 | 687 | 1156 | . | . | . | . | . | . | . | . | . | . | . | . |

TABLE 6: ALPHA= 0.025 POWER= 0.9     EXPECTED ACCRUAL THRU MINIMUM FOLLOW-UP= 120

| | | DEL=.05 | | | DEL=.10 | | | DEL=.15 | | | DEL=.20 | | | DEL=.25 | | |
|---|---|---|---|---|---|---|---|---|---|---|---|---|---|---|---|---|---|
| FACT= | | 1.0 .75 | .50 .25 | .00 BIN | 1.0 .75 | .50 .25 | .00 BIN | 1.0 .75 | .50 .25 | .00 BIN | 1.0 75 | .50 .25 | .00 BIN | 1.0 .75 | .50 .25 | .00 BIN |
| PCONT=*** | | | | | REQUIRED NUMBER OF PATIENTS | | | | | | | | | | | |
| 0.05 | *** | 628 | 631 | 671 | 223 | 227 | 239 | 131 | 134 | 139 | 93 | 95 | 98 | 73 | 74 | 76 |
| | *** | 629 | 637 | 1156 | 225 | 231 | 368 | 132 | 136 | 194 | 94 | 96 | 124 | 73 | 75 | 87 |
| 0.1 | *** | 1145 | 1152 | 1295 | 354 | 362 | 400 | 190 | 196 | 212 | 127 | 131 | 139 | 94 | 97 | 102 |
| | *** | 1147 | 1166 | 1829 | 357 | 372 | 526 | 193 | 202 | 260 | 128 | 134 | 158 | 96 | 99 | 107 |
| 0.15 | *** | 1584 | 1596 | 1898 | 459 | 472 | 548 | 236 | 246 | 276 | 152 | 159 | 174 | 110 | 115 | 124 |
| | *** | 1588 | 1619 | 2417 | 463 | 490 | 662 | 240 | 256 | 316 | 155 | 165 | 187 | 112 | 118 | 124 |
| 0.2 | *** | 1923 | 1940 | 2448 | 537 | 556 | 679 | 270 | 284 | 332 | 171 | 180 | 203 | 122 | 128 | 141 |
| | *** | 1928 | 1976 | 2922 | 544 | 583 | 778 | 275 | 299 | 362 | 175 | 189 | 211 | 125 | 133 | 138 |
| 0.25 | *** | 2157 | 2182 | 2930 | 590 | 616 | 791 | 292 | 312 | 377 | 183 | 196 | 227 | 130 | 138 | 155 |
| | *** | 2165 | 2232 | 3342 | 599 | 654 | 873 | 300 | 332 | 400 | 189 | 207 | 229 | 133 | 144 | 148 |
| 0.3 | *** | 2291 | 2326 | 3331 | 620 | 654 | 882 | 306 | 330 | 413 | 191 | 206 | 245 | 134 | 144 | 164 |
| | *** | 2303 | 2394 | 3678 | 632 | 702 | 946 | 315 | 355 | 428 | 197 | 220 | 242 | 138 | 152 | 154 |
| 0.35 | *** | 2334 | 2380 | 3648 | 629 | 672 | 950 | 311 | 340 | 439 | 194 | 212 | 257 | 136 | 147 | 170 |
| | *** | 2349 | 2469 | 3930 | 645 | 732 | 999 | 322 | 370 | 446 | 201 | 228 | 250 | 140 | 156 | 158 |
| 0.4 | *** | 2297 | 2356 | 3876 | 622 | 674 | 997 | 309 | 342 | 455 | 193 | 213 | 263 | 135 | 147 | 172 |
| | *** | 2317 | 2471 | 4098 | 641 | 744 | 1030 | 322 | 376 | 456 | 201 | 230 | 253 | 140 | 157 | 158 |
| 0.45 | *** | 2193 | 2269 | 4014 | 601 | 662 | 1020 | 302 | 338 | 460 | 188 | 210 | 263 | 131 | 144 | 171 |
| | *** | 2218 | 2413 | 4182 | 624 | 741 | 1041 | 316 | 375 | 456 | 198 | 229 | 250 | 137 | 155 | 154 |
| 0.5 | *** | 2036 | 2132 | 4061 | 569 | 639 | 1020 | 289 | 329 | 456 | 181 | 204 | 258 | 126 | 139 | 166 |
| | *** | 2068 | 2309 | 4182 | 596 | 724 | 1030 | 305 | 367 | 446 | 191 | 223 | 242 | 132 | 150 | 148 |
| 0.55 | *** | 1840 | 1961 | 4016 | 531 | 607 | 998 | 273 | 314 | 441 | 171 | 194 | 246 | 118 | 131 | 157 |
| | *** | 1881 | 2171 | 4098 | 561 | 697 | 999 | 290 | 353 | 428 | 181 | 213 | 229 | 124 | 141 | 138 |
| 0.6 | *** | 1623 | 1771 | 3879 | 488 | 568 | 952 | 254 | 294 | 415 | 159 | 181 | 229 | 109 | 121 | 144 |
| | *** | 1674 | 2009 | 3930 | 519 | 658 | 946 | 271 | 332 | 400 | 168 | 198 | 211 | 115 | 130 | 124 |
| 0.65 | *** | 1399 | 1574 | 3652 | 441 | 522 | 884 | 232 | 270 | 380 | 144 | 164 | 207 | 98 | 109 | 128 |
| | *** | 1461 | 1832 | 3678 | 473 | 610 | 873 | 248 | 306 | 362 | 153 | 180 | 187 | 103 | 116 | 107 |
| 0.7 | *** | 1183 | 1378 | 3334 | 392 | 470 | 794 | 206 | 241 | 335 | 127 | 144 | 178 | 85 | 93 | 108 |
| | *** | 1255 | 1642 | 3342 | 423 | 552 | 778 | 221 | 272 | 316 | 134 | 157 | 158 | 88 | 99 | 87 |
| 0.75 | *** | 984 | 1185 | 2927 | 340 | 410 | 681 | 177 | 207 | 280 | 106 | 120 | 145 | . | . | . |
| | *** | 1060 | 1442 | 2922 | 368 | 483 | 662 | 190 | 232 | 260 | 112 | 130 | 124 | . | . | . |
| 0.8 | *** | 802 | 993 | 2431 | 283 | 343 | 546 | 143 | 166 | 215 | . | . | . | . | . | . |
| | *** | 875 | 1226 | 2417 | 307 | 401 | 526 | 153 | 184 | 194 | . | . | . | . | . | . |
| 0.85 | *** | 629 | 794 | 1847 | 219 | 262 | 389 | . | . | . | . | . | . | . | . | . |
| | *** | 694 | 987 | 1829 | 237 | 303 | 368 | . | . | . | . | . | . | . | . | . |
| 0.9 | *** | 451 | 571 | 1177 | . | . | . | . | . | . | . | . | . | . | . | . |
| | *** | 499 | 704 | 1156 | . | . | . | . | . | . | . | . | . | . | . | . |

## TABLE 6: ALPHA= 0.025 POWER= 0.9 — EXPECTED ACCRUAL THRU MINIMUM FOLLOW-UP= 130

| | | DEL=.05 | | | DEL=.10 | | | DEL=.15 | | | DEL=.20 | | | DEL=.25 | | |
|---|---|---|---|---|---|---|---|---|---|---|---|---|---|---|---|---|
| FACT= | | 1.0 .75 | .50 .25 | .00 BIN | 1.0 .75 | .50 .25 | .00 BIN | 1.0 .75 | .50 .25 | .00 BIN | 1.0 75 | .50 .25 | .00 BIN | 1.0 .75 | .50 .25 | .00 BIN |
| PCONT=*** | | | | | REQUIRED NUMBER OF PATIENTS | | | | | | | | | | | |
| 0.05 | *** | 628 | 632 | 671 | 224 | 227 | 239 | 132 | 134 | 139 | 93 | 95 | 98 | 73 | 74 | 76 |
| | *** | 630 | 638 | 1156 | 225 | 231 | 368 | 133 | 136 | 194 | 94 | 96 | 124 | 73 | 75 | 87 |
| 0.1 | *** | 1146 | 1153 | 1295 | 355 | 363 | 400 | 191 | 197 | 212 | 127 | 131 | 139 | 95 | 97 | 102 |
| | *** | 1148 | 1168 | 1829 | 358 | 373 | 526 | 193 | 202 | 260 | 129 | 134 | 158 | 96 | 99 | 107 |
| 0.15 | *** | 1585 | 1598 | 1898 | 460 | 473 | 548 | 237 | 247 | 276 | 153 | 160 | 174 | 111 | 115 | 124 |
| | *** | 1589 | 1623 | 2417 | 465 | 492 | 662 | 241 | 257 | 316 | 156 | 165 | 187 | 113 | 119 | 124 |
| 0.2 | *** | 1924 | 1943 | 2448 | 539 | 559 | 679 | 271 | 286 | 332 | 172 | 181 | 203 | 123 | 129 | 141 |
| | *** | 1930 | 1982 | 2922 | 546 | 587 | 778 | 277 | 301 | 362 | 176 | 190 | 211 | 125 | 134 | 138 |
| 0.25 | *** | 2159 | 2186 | 2930 | 593 | 620 | 791 | 295 | 314 | 377 | 185 | 197 | 227 | 131 | 139 | 155 |
| | *** | 2168 | 2241 | 3342 | 602 | 659 | 873 | 302 | 334 | 400 | 190 | 208 | 229 | 134 | 145 | 148 |
| 0.3 | *** | 2294 | 2331 | 3331 | 623 | 659 | 882 | 308 | 333 | 413 | 193 | 208 | 245 | 135 | 145 | 164 |
| | *** | 2307 | 2405 | 3678 | 636 | 709 | 946 | 318 | 358 | 428 | 199 | 221 | 242 | 139 | 153 | 154 |
| 0.35 | *** | 2338 | 2387 | 3648 | 633 | 679 | 950 | 314 | 343 | 439 | 196 | 214 | 257 | 137 | 148 | 170 |
| | *** | 2355 | 2484 | 3930 | 650 | 739 | 999 | 326 | 373 | 446 | 203 | 229 | 250 | 142 | 157 | 158 |
| 0.4 | *** | 2302 | 2366 | 3876 | 627 | 682 | 997 | 313 | 346 | 455 | 195 | 215 | 263 | 136 | 148 | 173 |
| | *** | 2323 | 2490 | 4098 | 647 | 752 | 1030 | 326 | 380 | 455 | 204 | 232 | 253 | 141 | 158 | 158 |
| 0.45 | *** | 2199 | 2281 | 4014 | 607 | 671 | 1020 | 306 | 343 | 460 | 191 | 212 | 263 | 133 | 146 | 171 |
| | *** | 2227 | 2436 | 4182 | 631 | 750 | 1041 | 321 | 379 | 456 | 200 | 231 | 250 | 139 | 156 | 154 |
| 0.5 | *** | 2044 | 2148 | 4061 | 576 | 649 | 1020 | 294 | 333 | 456 | 184 | 206 | 258 | 128 | 141 | 166 |
| | *** | 2079 | 2335 | 4182 | 604 | 735 | 1030 | 310 | 371 | 446 | 193 | 225 | 242 | 133 | 151 | 148 |
| 0.55 | *** | 1851 | 1980 | 4016 | 539 | 617 | 998 | 278 | 318 | 441 | 174 | 196 | 246 | 120 | 133 | 157 |
| | *** | 1895 | 2201 | 4098 | 569 | 707 | 999 | 295 | 357 | 428 | 184 | 215 | 229 | 126 | 142 | 138 |
| 0.6 | *** | 1636 | 1794 | 3879 | 496 | 578 | 952 | 259 | 299 | 416 | 162 | 183 | 229 | 111 | 123 | 144 |
| | *** | 1691 | 2042 | 3930 | 529 | 669 | 946 | 275 | 336 | 400 | 171 | 200 | 211 | 116 | 131 | 124 |
| 0.65 | *** | 1415 | 1600 | 3652 | 450 | 532 | 884 | 236 | 274 | 380 | 147 | 166 | 207 | 99 | 110 | 128 |
| | *** | 1481 | 1866 | 3678 | 483 | 620 | 873 | 252 | 309 | 362 | 155 | 182 | 187 | 104 | 117 | 107 |
| 0.7 | *** | 1202 | 1405 | 3334 | 401 | 479 | 794 | 210 | 245 | 335 | 129 | 146 | 179 | 86 | 94 | 108 |
| | *** | 1277 | 1677 | 3342 | 432 | 561 | 778 | 225 | 276 | 316 | 136 | 159 | 158 | 89 | 100 | 87 |
| 0.75 | *** | 1004 | 1212 | 2927 | 348 | 419 | 681 | 181 | 210 | 280 | 108 | 121 | 145 | . | . | . |
| | *** | 1083 | 1475 | 2922 | 376 | 491 | 662 | 193 | 235 | 260 | 114 | 131 | 124 | . | . | . |
| 0.8 | *** | 821 | 1018 | 2431 | 290 | 349 | 546 | 146 | 168 | 215 | . | . | . | . | . | . |
| | *** | 897 | 1256 | 2417 | 314 | 408 | 526 | 156 | 186 | 194 | . | . | . | . | . | . |
| 0.85 | *** | 647 | 815 | 1847 | 224 | 267 | 389 | . | . | . | . | . | . | . | . | . |
| | *** | 713 | 1011 | 1829 | 242 | 307 | 368 | . | . | . | . | . | . | . | . | . |
| 0.9 | *** | 464 | 586 | 1177 | . | . | . | . | . | . | . | . | . | . | . | . |
| | *** | 512 | 720 | 1156 | . | . | . | . | . | . | . | . | . | . | . | . |

## TABLE 6: ALPHA= 0.025 POWER= 0.9    EXPECTED ACCRUAL THRU MINIMUM FOLLOW-UP= 140

| | DEL=.05 | | | DEL=.10 | | | DEL=.15 | | | DEL=.20 | | | DEL=.25 | | |
|---|---|---|---|---|---|---|---|---|---|---|---|---|---|---|---|
| FACT= | 1.0 .75 | .50 .25 | .00 BIN | 1.0 .75 | .50 .25 | .00 BIN | 1.0 .75 | .50 .25 | .00 BIN | 1.0 75 | .50 .25 | .00 BIN | 1.0 .75 | .50 .25 | .00 BIN |
| PCONT=*** | REQUIRED NUMBER OF PATIENTS | | | | | | | | | | | | | | |
| 0.05 *** | 629 | 632 | 671 | 224 | 228 | 239 | 132 | 134 | 139 | 94 | 95 | 98 | 73 | 74 | 76 |
| *** | 630 | 639 | 1156 | 225 | 231 | 368 | 133 | 136 | 194 | 94 | 96 | 124 | 74 | 75 | 87 |
| 0.1 *** | 1146 | 1154 | 1295 | 355 | 364 | 400 | 192 | 197 | 212 | 128 | 132 | 139 | 95 | 98 | 102 |
| *** | 1149 | 1170 | 1829 | 358 | 374 | 526 | 194 | 203 | 260 | 129 | 135 | 158 | 96 | 99 | 107 |
| 0.15 *** | 1586 | 1600 | 1898 | 461 | 475 | 548 | 238 | 248 | 276 | 154 | 160 | 174 | 111 | 116 | 124 |
| *** | 1590 | 1627 | 2417 | 466 | 494 | 662 | 242 | 258 | 316 | 156 | 166 | 187 | 113 | 119 | 124 |
| 0.2 *** | 1926 | 1946 | 2448 | 541 | 561 | 679 | 273 | 287 | 332 | 173 | 182 | 203 | 123 | 130 | 141 |
| *** | 1932 | 1987 | 2922 | 548 | 590 | 778 | 278 | 302 | 362 | 177 | 190 | 211 | 126 | 134 | 138 |
| 0.25 *** | 2161 | 2191 | 2930 | 595 | 624 | 791 | 296 | 316 | 377 | 186 | 199 | 227 | 132 | 139 | 155 |
| *** | 2171 | 2249 | 3342 | 605 | 663 | 873 | 304 | 336 | 400 | 191 | 209 | 229 | 135 | 146 | 148 |
| 0.3 *** | 2297 | 2337 | 3331 | 626 | 664 | 882 | 311 | 336 | 413 | 194 | 209 | 245 | 136 | 146 | 164 |
| *** | 2310 | 2416 | 3678 | 640 | 714 | 946 | 321 | 361 | 428 | 201 | 223 | 242 | 141 | 153 | 154 |
| 0.35 *** | 2342 | 2395 | 3648 | 637 | 685 | 950 | 317 | 346 | 439 | 198 | 216 | 257 | 138 | 149 | 170 |
| *** | 2360 | 2498 | 3930 | 655 | 746 | 999 | 329 | 376 | 446 | 205 | 231 | 250 | 143 | 158 | 158 |
| 0.4 *** | 2307 | 2376 | 3876 | 632 | 689 | 997 | 316 | 350 | 455 | 197 | 217 | 263 | 137 | 149 | 172 |
| *** | 2330 | 2508 | 4098 | 653 | 760 | 1030 | 330 | 383 | 456 | 206 | 234 | 253 | 143 | 159 | 158 |
| 0.45 *** | 2206 | 2294 | 4014 | 613 | 679 | 1020 | 309 | 347 | 461 | 193 | 215 | 263 | 134 | 147 | 171 |
| *** | 2235 | 2458 | 4182 | 638 | 759 | 1041 | 325 | 383 | 456 | 202 | 232 | 250 | 140 | 157 | 154 |
| 0.5 *** | 2052 | 2163 | 4061 | 583 | 657 | 1020 | 298 | 337 | 456 | 186 | 208 | 258 | 129 | 142 | 166 |
| *** | 2089 | 2361 | 4182 | 612 | 744 | 1030 | 314 | 375 | 446 | 196 | 227 | 242 | 135 | 151 | 148 |
| 0.55 *** | 1861 | 1999 | 4016 | 546 | 627 | 998 | 282 | 323 | 441 | 177 | 198 | 246 | 122 | 134 | 157 |
| *** | 1908 | 2230 | 4098 | 578 | 717 | 999 | 299 | 361 | 428 | 186 | 216 | 229 | 127 | 143 | 138 |
| 0.6 *** | 1649 | 1816 | 3879 | 504 | 588 | 952 | 263 | 303 | 416 | 164 | 185 | 229 | 112 | 124 | 144 |
| *** | 1707 | 2074 | 3930 | 537 | 679 | 946 | 280 | 340 | 400 | 173 | 202 | 211 | 117 | 132 | 124 |
| 0.65 *** | 1431 | 1624 | 3652 | 458 | 541 | 884 | 240 | 278 | 380 | 149 | 168 | 207 | 101 | 111 | 128 |
| *** | 1501 | 1899 | 3678 | 491 | 630 | 873 | 256 | 313 | 362 | 157 | 183 | 187 | 105 | 118 | 107 |
| 0.7 *** | 1220 | 1431 | 3334 | 408 | 488 | 794 | 214 | 249 | 335 | 131 | 147 | 179 | 87 | 95 | 108 |
| *** | 1299 | 1709 | 3342 | 440 | 570 | 778 | 229 | 279 | 316 | 138 | 160 | 158 | 90 | 100 | 87 |
| 0.75 *** | 1023 | 1237 | 2927 | 355 | 427 | 681 | 184 | 213 | 280 | 110 | 122 | 145 | . | . | . |
| *** | 1105 | 1505 | 2922 | 384 | 499 | 662 | 196 | 237 | 260 | 115 | 132 | 124 | . | . | . |
| 0.8 *** | 840 | 1042 | 2431 | 296 | 356 | 546 | 149 | 170 | 215 | . | . | . | . | . | . |
| *** | 918 | 1283 | 2417 | 321 | 413 | 526 | 158 | 187 | 194 | . | . | . | . | . | . |
| 0.85 *** | 663 | 835 | 1847 | 228 | 272 | 389 | . | . | . | . | . | . | . | . | . |
| *** | 731 | 1033 | 1829 | 246 | 311 | 368 | . | . | . | . | . | . | . | . | . |
| 0.9 *** | 476 | 600 | 1177 | . | . | . | . | . | . | . | . | . | . | . | . |
| *** | 525 | 734 | 1156 | . | . | . | . | . | . | . | . | . | . | . | . |

TABLE 6: ALPHA= 0.025 POWER= 0.9    EXPECTED ACCRUAL THRU MINIMUM FOLLOW-UP= 150

| | | DEL=.05 | | | DEL=.10 | | | DEL=.15 | | | DEL=.20 | | | DEL=.25 | | |
|---|---|---|---|---|---|---|---|---|---|---|---|---|---|---|---|---|---|
| FACT= | | 1.0 .75 | .50 .25 | .00 BIN | 1.0 .75 | .50 .25 | .00 BIN | 1.0 .75 | .50 .25 | .00 BIN | 1.0 75 | .50 .25 | .00 BIN | 1.0 .75 | .50 .25 | .00 BIN |
| PCONT=*** | | | | | REQUIRED NUMBER OF PATIENTS | | | | | | | | | | | |
| 0.05 | *** | 629 | 633 | 671 | 224 | 228 | 239 | 132 | 134 | 139 | 94 | 95 | 98 | 73 | 74 | 76 |
| | *** | 630 | 640 | 1156 | 226 | 232 | 368 | 133 | 136 | 194 | 94 | 96 | 124 | 74 | 75 | 87 |
| 0.1 | *** | 1147 | 1156 | 1295 | 356 | 365 | 400 | 192 | 198 | 212 | 128 | 132 | 139 | 95 | 98 | 102 |
| | *** | 1150 | 1172 | 1829 | 359 | 375 | 526 | 194 | 203 | 260 | 130 | 135 | 158 | 96 | 100 | 107 |
| 0.15 | *** | 1587 | 1601 | 1898 | 462 | 477 | 548 | 239 | 249 | 276 | 154 | 161 | 174 | 112 | 116 | 124 |
| | *** | 1592 | 1630 | 2417 | 467 | 496 | 662 | 243 | 259 | 316 | 157 | 166 | 187 | 114 | 119 | 124 |
| 0.2 | *** | 1927 | 1949 | 2448 | 542 | 564 | 679 | 274 | 289 | 332 | 174 | 183 | 203 | 124 | 130 | 141 |
| | *** | 1934 | 1993 | 2922 | 550 | 593 | 778 | 280 | 303 | 362 | 178 | 191 | 211 | 127 | 135 | 138 |
| 0.25 | *** | 2163 | 2195 | 2930 | 597 | 627 | 791 | 298 | 318 | 377 | 187 | 200 | 227 | 132 | 140 | 155 |
| | *** | 2174 | 2257 | 3342 | 608 | 667 | 873 | 306 | 338 | 400 | 193 | 210 | 229 | 136 | 146 | 148 |
| 0.3 | *** | 2300 | 2343 | 3331 | 629 | 668 | 882 | 313 | 338 | 413 | 196 | 211 | 245 | 137 | 147 | 164 |
| | *** | 2314 | 2427 | 3678 | 643 | 720 | 946 | 323 | 363 | 428 | 202 | 224 | 242 | 142 | 154 | 154 |
| 0.35 | *** | 2346 | 2402 | 3648 | 641 | 690 | 950 | 320 | 349 | 439 | 200 | 217 | 257 | 139 | 150 | 170 |
| | *** | 2365 | 2512 | 3930 | 659 | 752 | 999 | 332 | 379 | 446 | 207 | 232 | 250 | 144 | 158 | 158 |
| 0.4 | *** | 2312 | 2386 | 3876 | 636 | 695 | 997 | 319 | 353 | 455 | 199 | 219 | 263 | 139 | 151 | 172 |
| | *** | 2336 | 2525 | 4098 | 658 | 767 | 1030 | 333 | 386 | 456 | 208 | 235 | 253 | 144 | 159 | 158 |
| 0.45 | *** | 2212 | 2306 | 4014 | 618 | 686 | 1020 | 313 | 350 | 460 | 196 | 217 | 263 | 136 | 148 | 171 |
| | *** | 2243 | 2479 | 4182 | 644 | 767 | 1041 | 328 | 386 | 456 | 205 | 234 | 250 | 141 | 157 | 154 |
| 0.5 | *** | 2060 | 2179 | 4061 | 590 | 666 | 1020 | 302 | 341 | 456 | 189 | 210 | 258 | 130 | 143 | 166 |
| | *** | 2100 | 2386 | 4182 | 619 | 753 | 1030 | 318 | 379 | 446 | 198 | 228 | 242 | 136 | 152 | 148 |
| 0.55 | *** | 1871 | 2018 | 4016 | 554 | 635 | 998 | 286 | 327 | 441 | 179 | 200 | 246 | 123 | 135 | 157 |
| | *** | 1922 | 2258 | 4098 | 586 | 726 | 999 | 303 | 364 | 428 | 188 | 218 | 229 | 128 | 144 | 138 |
| 0.6 | *** | 1661 | 1838 | 3879 | 512 | 596 | 952 | 267 | 307 | 416 | 166 | 187 | 229 | 113 | 125 | 144 |
| | *** | 1724 | 2104 | 3930 | 545 | 688 | 946 | 284 | 343 | 400 | 175 | 203 | 211 | 118 | 133 | 124 |
| 0.65 | *** | 1446 | 1648 | 3652 | 466 | 550 | 884 | 244 | 282 | 380 | 151 | 170 | 207 | 102 | 112 | 128 |
| | *** | 1520 | 1930 | 3678 | 500 | 638 | 873 | 260 | 316 | 362 | 159 | 184 | 187 | 106 | 118 | 107 |
| 0.7 | *** | 1238 | 1456 | 3334 | 416 | 496 | 794 | 218 | 252 | 335 | 133 | 149 | 179 | 88 | 96 | 108 |
| | *** | 1319 | 1740 | 3342 | 448 | 578 | 778 | 232 | 281 | 316 | 140 | 161 | 158 | 91 | 101 | 87 |
| 0.75 | *** | 1042 | 1262 | 2927 | 362 | 434 | 681 | 187 | 215 | 280 | 111 | 123 | 145 | . | . | . |
| | *** | 1126 | 1534 | 2922 | 391 | 505 | 662 | 199 | 239 | 260 | 117 | 132 | 124 | . | . | . |
| 0.8 | *** | 858 | 1064 | 2431 | 302 | 362 | 546 | 151 | 172 | 215 | . | . | . | . | . | . |
| | *** | 938 | 1309 | 2417 | 327 | 419 | 526 | 160 | 189 | 194 | . | . | . | . | . | . |
| 0.85 | *** | 679 | 854 | 1847 | 233 | 276 | 389 | . | . | . | . | . | . | . | . | . |
| | *** | 748 | 1053 | 1829 | 251 | 314 | 368 | . | . | . | . | . | . | . | . | . |
| 0.9 | *** | 488 | 613 | 1177 | . | . | . | . | . | . | . | . | . | . | . | . |
| | *** | 538 | 748 | 1156 | . | . | . | . | . | . | . | . | . | . | . | . |

TABLE 6: ALPHA= 0.025 POWER= 0.9    EXPECTED ACCRUAL THRU MINIMUM FOLLOW-UP= 160

| | | DEL=.05 | | | DEL=.10 | | | DEL=.15 | | | DEL=.20 | | | DEL=.25 | | |
|---|---|---|---|---|---|---|---|---|---|---|---|---|---|---|---|---|---|
| FACT= | | 1.0 .75 | .50 .25 | .00 BIN | 1.0 .75 | .50 .25 | .00 BIN | 1.0 .75 | .50 .25 | .00 BIN | 1.0 75 | .50 .25 | .00 BIN | 1.0 .75 | .50 .25 | .00 BIN |
| PCONT=*** | | | | | REQUIRED | NUMBER OF | PATIENTS | | | | | | | | | |
| 0.05 | *** | 629 | 633 | 671 | 225 | 228 | 239 | 132 | 135 | 139 | 94 | 95 | 98 | 73 | 74 | 76 |
| | *** | 631 | 641 | 1156 | 226 | 232 | 368 | 133 | 137 | 194 | 95 | 97 | 124 | 74 | 75 | 87 |
| 0.1 | *** | 1148 | 1157 | 1295 | 357 | 366 | 400 | 193 | 198 | 212 | 128 | 132 | 139 | 96 | 98 | 102 |
| | *** | 1151 | 1175 | 1829 | 360 | 376 | 526 | 195 | 204 | 260 | 130 | 135 | 158 | 97 | 100 | 107 |
| 0.15 | *** | 1588 | 1603 | 1898 | 463 | 479 | 548 | 240 | 250 | 276 | 155 | 161 | 174 | 112 | 116 | 124 |
| | *** | 1593 | 1634 | 2417 | 469 | 498 | 662 | 244 | 259 | 316 | 158 | 167 | 187 | 114 | 120 | 124 |
| 0.2 | *** | 1929 | 1952 | 2448 | 544 | 567 | 679 | 275 | 290 | 332 | 175 | 184 | 203 | 125 | 131 | 141 |
| | *** | 1936 | 1999 | 2922 | 552 | 596 | 778 | 281 | 305 | 362 | 179 | 192 | 211 | 127 | 135 | 138 |
| 0.25 | *** | 2165 | 2199 | 2930 | 599 | 631 | 791 | 300 | 320 | 377 | 189 | 201 | 227 | 133 | 141 | 155 |
| | *** | 2177 | 2265 | 3342 | 611 | 671 | 873 | 308 | 340 | 400 | 194 | 211 | 229 | 137 | 147 | 148 |
| 0.3 | *** | 2303 | 2349 | 3331 | 632 | 673 | 882 | 315 | 341 | 413 | 197 | 212 | 245 | 138 | 148 | 164 |
| | *** | 2318 | 2438 | 3678 | 647 | 725 | 946 | 326 | 365 | 428 | 204 | 225 | 242 | 142 | 155 | 154 |
| 0.35 | *** | 2349 | 2410 | 3648 | 645 | 696 | 950 | 322 | 352 | 439 | 201 | 219 | 257 | 140 | 151 | 170 |
| | *** | 2370 | 2526 | 3930 | 664 | 758 | 999 | 335 | 381 | 446 | 209 | 233 | 250 | 145 | 159 | 158 |
| 0.4 | *** | 2317 | 2395 | 3876 | 641 | 702 | 997 | 322 | 357 | 455 | 201 | 221 | 263 | 140 | 152 | 173 |
| | *** | 2343 | 2543 | 4098 | 664 | 774 | 1030 | 336 | 389 | 456 | 209 | 237 | 253 | 145 | 160 | 158 |
| 0.45 | *** | 2218 | 2318 | 4014 | 624 | 694 | 1020 | 316 | 354 | 461 | 198 | 218 | 263 | 137 | 149 | 171 |
| | *** | 2252 | 2500 | 4182 | 651 | 775 | 1041 | 332 | 389 | 456 | 206 | 235 | 250 | 142 | 158 | 154 |
| 0.5 | *** | 2068 | 2194 | 4061 | 596 | 674 | 1020 | 305 | 345 | 456 | 191 | 212 | 258 | 132 | 144 | 166 |
| | *** | 2111 | 2410 | 4182 | 626 | 761 | 1030 | 322 | 382 | 446 | 200 | 229 | 242 | 137 | 153 | 148 |
| 0.55 | *** | 1881 | 2036 | 4016 | 561 | 644 | 998 | 290 | 331 | 441 | 181 | 202 | 246 | 124 | 136 | 157 |
| | *** | 1935 | 2285 | 4098 | 593 | 735 | 999 | 307 | 367 | 428 | 190 | 219 | 229 | 129 | 145 | 138 |
| 0.6 | *** | 1674 | 1859 | 3879 | 519 | 605 | 952 | 271 | 311 | 416 | 168 | 189 | 229 | 115 | 126 | 144 |
| | *** | 1740 | 2133 | 3930 | 553 | 696 | 946 | 287 | 346 | 400 | 177 | 204 | 211 | 119 | 133 | 124 |
| 0.65 | *** | 1461 | 1671 | 3652 | 473 | 558 | 884 | 248 | 285 | 380 | 153 | 171 | 207 | 103 | 112 | 128 |
| | *** | 1538 | 1960 | 3678 | 508 | 647 | 873 | 264 | 319 | 362 | 161 | 185 | 187 | 107 | 119 | 107 |
| 0.7 | *** | 1255 | 1480 | 3334 | 423 | 504 | 794 | 221 | 255 | 335 | 134 | 150 | 179 | 89 | 96 | 108 |
| | *** | 1339 | 1770 | 3342 | 456 | 585 | 778 | 235 | 284 | 316 | 141 | 162 | 158 | 92 | 101 | 87 |
| 0.75 | *** | 1060 | 1285 | 2927 | 368 | 441 | 681 | 190 | 218 | 280 | 112 | 124 | 145 | . | . | . |
| | *** | 1147 | 1562 | 2922 | 398 | 512 | 662 | 202 | 241 | 260 | 118 | 133 | 124 | . | . | . |
| 0.8 | *** | 875 | 1085 | 2431 | 307 | 367 | 546 | 153 | 174 | 215 | . | . | . | . | . | . |
| | *** | 957 | 1333 | 2417 | 332 | 424 | 526 | 162 | 190 | 194 | . | . | . | . | . | . |
| 0.85 | *** | 694 | 871 | 1847 | 237 | 280 | 389 | . | . | . | . | . | . | . | . | . |
| | *** | 764 | 1073 | 1829 | 255 | 317 | 368 | . | . | . | . | . | . | . | . | . |
| 0.9 | *** | 499 | 625 | 1177 | . | . | . | . | . | . | . | . | . | . | . | . |
| | *** | 549 | 760 | 1156 | . | . | . | . | . | . | . | . | . | . | . | . |

TABLE 6: ALPHA= 0.025 POWER= 0.9     EXPECTED ACCRUAL THRU MINIMUM FOLLOW-UP= 170

|  | | DEL=.05 | | | DEL=.10 | | | DEL=.15 | | | DEL=.20 | | | DEL=.25 | | |
|---|---|---|---|---|---|---|---|---|---|---|---|---|---|---|---|---|
| FACT= | | 1.0 .75 | .50 .25 | .00 BIN | 1.0 .75 | .50 .25 | .00 BIN | 1.0 .75 | .50 .25 | .00 BIN | 1.0 75 | .50 .25 | .00 BIN | 1.0 .75 | .50 .25 | .00 BIN |
| PCONT=*** | | | | | | | REQUIRED NUMBER OF PATIENTS | | | | | | | | |
| 0.05 | *** | 629 | 634 | 671 | 225 | 229 | 239 | 133 | 135 | 139 | 94 | 96 | 98 | 73 | 74 | 76 |
| | *** | 631 | 641 | 1156 | 226 | 232 | 368 | 134 | 137 | 194 | 95 | 97 | 124 | 74 | 75 | 87 |
| 0.1 | *** | 1148 | 1158 | 1295 | 357 | 366 | 400 | 193 | 199 | 212 | 129 | 133 | 139 | 96 | 98 | 102 |
| | *** | 1151 | 1177 | 1829 | 361 | 377 | 526 | 195 | 204 | 260 | 130 | 135 | 158 | 97 | 100 | 107 |
| 0.15 | *** | 1589 | 1605 | 1898 | 464 | 480 | 548 | 241 | 251 | 276 | 156 | 162 | 174 | 113 | 117 | 124 |
| | *** | 1594 | 1638 | 2417 | 470 | 500 | 662 | 245 | 260 | 316 | 158 | 167 | 187 | 115 | 120 | 124 |
| 0.2 | *** | 1930 | 1955 | 2448 | 545 | 569 | 679 | 276 | 292 | 331 | 176 | 185 | 203 | 125 | 131 | 141 |
| | *** | 1938 | 2004 | 2922 | 554 | 599 | 778 | 283 | 306 | 362 | 180 | 192 | 211 | 128 | 135 | 138 |
| 0.25 | *** | 2167 | 2203 | 2930 | 602 | 634 | 791 | 302 | 322 | 377 | 190 | 202 | 227 | 134 | 141 | 155 |
| | *** | 2179 | 2273 | 3342 | 613 | 675 | 873 | 310 | 341 | 400 | 195 | 212 | 229 | 137 | 147 | 148 |
| 0.3 | *** | 2306 | 2354 | 3331 | 635 | 677 | 882 | 317 | 343 | 413 | 199 | 213 | 245 | 139 | 148 | 164 |
| | *** | 2322 | 2448 | 3678 | 651 | 729 | 946 | 328 | 367 | 428 | 205 | 226 | 242 | 143 | 155 | 154 |
| 0.35 | *** | 2353 | 2418 | 3648 | 649 | 701 | 950 | 325 | 355 | 439 | 203 | 220 | 257 | 141 | 152 | 170 |
| | *** | 2375 | 2540 | 3930 | 668 | 764 | 999 | 337 | 383 | 446 | 210 | 234 | 250 | 146 | 160 | 158 |
| 0.4 | *** | 2322 | 2405 | 3876 | 645 | 708 | 997 | 325 | 359 | 455 | 203 | 222 | 263 | 141 | 152 | 173 |
| | *** | 2350 | 2559 | 4098 | 669 | 781 | 1030 | 339 | 392 | 456 | 211 | 238 | 253 | 146 | 161 | 158 |
| 0.45 | *** | 2224 | 2331 | 4014 | 629 | 700 | 1020 | 320 | 357 | 460 | 199 | 220 | 263 | 138 | 150 | 171 |
| | *** | 2260 | 2520 | 4182 | 657 | 782 | 1041 | 335 | 392 | 456 | 208 | 237 | 250 | 143 | 159 | 154 |
| 0.5 | *** | 2076 | 2209 | 4061 | 602 | 681 | 1020 | 309 | 348 | 456 | 193 | 214 | 258 | 133 | 145 | 166 |
| | *** | 2121 | 2433 | 4182 | 633 | 769 | 1030 | 325 | 385 | 446 | 202 | 231 | 242 | 138 | 154 | 148 |
| 0.55 | *** | 1891 | 2054 | 4016 | 567 | 651 | 998 | 293 | 334 | 441 | 183 | 204 | 246 | 125 | 137 | 157 |
| | *** | 1948 | 2311 | 4098 | 601 | 742 | 999 | 310 | 370 | 428 | 192 | 220 | 229 | 130 | 145 | 138 |
| 0.6 | *** | 1687 | 1879 | 3879 | 526 | 613 | 952 | 274 | 314 | 416 | 170 | 190 | 229 | 116 | 126 | 144 |
| | *** | 1756 | 2160 | 3930 | 561 | 704 | 946 | 291 | 349 | 400 | 179 | 206 | 211 | 120 | 134 | 124 |
| 0.65 | *** | 1476 | 1694 | 3652 | 480 | 566 | 884 | 251 | 289 | 380 | 155 | 173 | 207 | 104 | 113 | 128 |
| | *** | 1556 | 1988 | 3678 | 515 | 654 | 873 | 267 | 321 | 362 | 163 | 186 | 187 | 108 | 119 | 107 |
| 0.7 | *** | 1272 | 1503 | 3334 | 430 | 511 | 794 | 224 | 258 | 335 | 136 | 151 | 178 | 89 | 97 | 108 |
| | *** | 1359 | 1797 | 3342 | 463 | 592 | 778 | 238 | 286 | 316 | 143 | 162 | 158 | 93 | 102 | 87 |
| 0.75 | *** | 1077 | 1308 | 2927 | 375 | 447 | 681 | 192 | 220 | 280 | 114 | 125 | 145 | . | . | . |
| | *** | 1166 | 1588 | 2922 | 404 | 517 | 662 | 204 | 243 | 260 | 119 | 134 | 124 | . | . | . |
| 0.8 | *** | 892 | 1106 | 2431 | 313 | 373 | 546 | 155 | 176 | 215 | . | . | . | . | . | . |
| | *** | 976 | 1356 | 2417 | 338 | 428 | 526 | 164 | 191 | 194 | . | . | . | . | . | . |
| 0.85 | *** | 708 | 888 | 1847 | 241 | 283 | 389 | . | . | . | . | . | . | . | . | . |
| | *** | 779 | 1091 | 1829 | 259 | 320 | 368 | . | . | . | . | . | . | . | . | . |
| 0.9 | *** | 509 | 637 | 1177 | . | . | . | . | . | . | . | . | . | . | . | . |
| | *** | 560 | 772 | 1156 | . | . | . | . | . | . | . | . | . | . | . | . |

TABLE 6: ALPHA= 0.025 POWER= 0.9    EXPECTED ACCRUAL THRU MINIMUM FOLLOW-UP= 180

| | | DEL=.05 | | | DEL=.10 | | | DEL=.15 | | | DEL=.20 | | | DEL=.25 | | |
|---|---|---|---|---|---|---|---|---|---|---|---|---|---|---|---|---|---|
| FACT= | | 1.0 .75 | .50 .25 | .00 BIN | 1.0 .75 | .50 .25 | .00 BIN | 1.0 .75 | .50 .25 | .00 BIN | 1.0 75 | .50 .25 | .00 BIN | 1.0 .75 | .50 .25 | .00 BIN |
| PCONT=*** | | | | REQUIRED | NUMBER | OF PATIENTS | | | | | | | | | | |
| 0.05 | *** | 630 | 634 | 671 | 225 | 229 | 239 | 133 | 135 | 139 | 94 | 96 | 98 | 73 | 74 | 76 |
| | *** | 631 | 642 | 1156 | 227 | 233 | 368 | 134 | 137 | 194 | 95 | 97 | 124 | 74 | 75 | 87 |
| 0.1 | *** | 1149 | 1159 | 1295 | 358 | 367 | 400 | 194 | 199 | 212 | 129 | 133 | 139 | 96 | 98 | 102 |
| | *** | 1152 | 1179 | 1829 | 362 | 378 | 526 | 196 | 204 | 260 | 131 | 135 | 158 | 97 | 100 | 107 |
| 0.15 | *** | 1590 | 1607 | 1898 | 465 | 482 | 548 | 242 | 252 | 276 | 156 | 162 | 174 | 113 | 117 | 123 |
| | *** | 1596 | 1641 | 2417 | 471 | 501 | 662 | 246 | 261 | 316 | 159 | 167 | 187 | 115 | 120 | 124 |
| 0.2 | *** | 1932 | 1958 | 2448 | 547 | 571 | 679 | 278 | 293 | 332 | 176 | 186 | 203 | 126 | 132 | 141 |
| | *** | 1940 | 2010 | 2922 | 556 | 601 | 778 | 284 | 307 | 362 | 180 | 193 | 211 | 128 | 136 | 138 |
| 0.25 | *** | 2170 | 2207 | 2930 | 604 | 637 | 791 | 303 | 324 | 377 | 191 | 203 | 227 | 135 | 142 | 155 |
| | *** | 2182 | 2281 | 3342 | 616 | 678 | 873 | 312 | 343 | 400 | 196 | 212 | 229 | 138 | 147 | 148 |
| 0.3 | *** | 2309 | 2360 | 3331 | 638 | 681 | 882 | 319 | 345 | 413 | 200 | 215 | 245 | 140 | 149 | 164 |
| | *** | 2326 | 2459 | 3678 | 654 | 734 | 946 | 330 | 369 | 428 | 206 | 226 | 242 | 144 | 155 | 154 |
| 0.35 | *** | 2357 | 2425 | 3648 | 652 | 706 | 950 | 327 | 357 | 439 | 204 | 221 | 257 | 142 | 153 | 170 |
| | *** | 2380 | 2553 | 3930 | 672 | 769 | 999 | 340 | 386 | 446 | 212 | 235 | 250 | 147 | 160 | 158 |
| 0.4 | *** | 2327 | 2415 | 3876 | 650 | 713 | 997 | 328 | 362 | 455 | 205 | 224 | 263 | 142 | 153 | 173 |
| | *** | 2356 | 2576 | 4098 | 674 | 787 | 1030 | 342 | 394 | 456 | 213 | 239 | 253 | 147 | 161 | 158 |
| 0.45 | *** | 2231 | 2343 | 4014 | 634 | 707 | 1020 | 323 | 360 | 461 | 201 | 222 | 263 | 139 | 151 | 171 |
| | *** | 2269 | 2539 | 4182 | 663 | 789 | 1041 | 338 | 394 | 456 | 210 | 238 | 250 | 144 | 159 | 154 |
| 0.5 | *** | 2084 | 2224 | 4061 | 608 | 688 | 1020 | 312 | 352 | 456 | 195 | 215 | 258 | 134 | 146 | 166 |
| | *** | 2132 | 2456 | 4182 | 639 | 776 | 1030 | 329 | 387 | 446 | 204 | 232 | 242 | 139 | 154 | 148 |
| 0.55 | *** | 1901 | 2072 | 4016 | 574 | 659 | 998 | 297 | 337 | 441 | 185 | 205 | 246 | 126 | 138 | 157 |
| | *** | 1961 | 2335 | 4098 | 607 | 750 | 999 | 314 | 373 | 428 | 194 | 222 | 229 | 132 | 146 | 138 |
| 0.6 | *** | 1699 | 1899 | 3879 | 533 | 620 | 952 | 278 | 317 | 416 | 172 | 192 | 229 | 117 | 127 | 144 |
| | *** | 1771 | 2187 | 3930 | 568 | 711 | 946 | 294 | 352 | 400 | 181 | 207 | 211 | 121 | 134 | 124 |
| 0.65 | *** | 1491 | 1715 | 3652 | 487 | 573 | 884 | 254 | 292 | 380 | 156 | 174 | 207 | 105 | 114 | 128 |
| | *** | 1574 | 2015 | 3678 | 522 | 661 | 873 | 270 | 323 | 362 | 164 | 187 | 187 | 109 | 120 | 107 |
| 0.7 | *** | 1288 | 1525 | 3334 | 436 | 518 | 794 | 227 | 260 | 335 | 137 | 152 | 179 | 90 | 97 | 108 |
| | *** | 1378 | 1824 | 3342 | 470 | 598 | 778 | 241 | 288 | 316 | 144 | 163 | 158 | 93 | 102 | 87 |
| 0.75 | *** | 1094 | 1329 | 2927 | 380 | 453 | 681 | 195 | 222 | 280 | 115 | 126 | 145 | . | . | . |
| | *** | 1185 | 1613 | 2922 | 410 | 523 | 662 | 207 | 244 | 260 | 120 | 134 | 124 | . | . | . |
| 0.8 | *** | 908 | 1125 | 2431 | 317 | 377 | 546 | 157 | 177 | 215 | . | . | . | . | . | . |
| | *** | 993 | 1377 | 2417 | 343 | 432 | 526 | 166 | 192 | 194 | . | . | . | . | . | . |
| 0.85 | *** | 722 | 904 | 1847 | 244 | 287 | 389 | . | . | . | . | . | . | . | . | . |
| | *** | 794 | 1108 | 1829 | 262 | 323 | 368 | . | . | . | . | . | . | . | . | . |
| 0.9 | *** | 519 | 648 | 1177 | . | . | . | . | . | . | . | . | . | . | . | . |
| | *** | 571 | 783 | 1156 | . | . | . | . | . | . | . | . | . | . | . | . |

TABLE 6: ALPHA= 0.025 POWER= 0.9    EXPECTED ACCRUAL THRU MINIMUM FOLLOW-UP= 190

| | | DEL=.05 | | | DEL=.10 | | | DEL=.15 | | | DEL=.20 | | | DEL=.25 | | |
|---|---|---|---|---|---|---|---|---|---|---|---|---|---|---|---|---|---|
| FACT= | | 1.0 .75 | .50 .25 | .00 BIN | 1.0 .75 | .50 .25 | .00 BIN | 1.0 .75 | .50 .25 | .00 BIN | 1.0 75 | .50 .25 | .00 BIN | 1.0 .75 | .50 .25 | .00 BIN |
| PCONT=*** | | | | REQUIRED NUMBER OF PATIENTS | | | | | | | | | | | | |
| 0.05 | *** | 630 | 635 | 671 | 226 | 229 | 239 | 133 | 135 | 139 | 94 | 96 | 98 | 73 | 75 | 76 |
| | *** | 632 | 643 | 1156 | 227 | 233 | 368 | 134 | 137 | 194 | 95 | 97 | 124 | 74 | 75 | 87 |
| 0.1 | *** | 1149 | 1160 | 1295 | 359 | 368 | 400 | 194 | 200 | 212 | 130 | 133 | 139 | 96 | 98 | 102 |
| | *** | 1153 | 1181 | 1829 | 362 | 378 | 526 | 196 | 205 | 260 | 131 | 136 | 158 | 97 | 100 | 107 |
| 0.15 | *** | 1591 | 1609 | 1898 | 467 | 483 | 548 | 242 | 253 | 276 | 157 | 163 | 174 | 113 | 117 | 124 |
| | *** | 1597 | 1645 | 2417 | 473 | 502 | 662 | 246 | 261 | 316 | 159 | 168 | 187 | 115 | 120 | 124 |
| 0.2 | *** | 1933 | 1961 | 2448 | 549 | 573 | 679 | 279 | 294 | 331 | 177 | 186 | 203 | 126 | 132 | 141 |
| | *** | 1942 | 2015 | 2922 | 558 | 603 | 778 | 285 | 308 | 362 | 181 | 193 | 211 | 129 | 136 | 138 |
| 0.25 | *** | 2172 | 2212 | 2929 | 606 | 640 | 791 | 305 | 325 | 377 | 192 | 204 | 227 | 135 | 142 | 155 |
| | *** | 2185 | 2288 | 3342 | 619 | 681 | 873 | 313 | 344 | 400 | 197 | 213 | 229 | 138 | 148 | 148 |
| 0.3 | *** | 2311 | 2366 | 3331 | 641 | 685 | 882 | 321 | 347 | 413 | 201 | 216 | 245 | 141 | 150 | 164 |
| | *** | 2329 | 2469 | 3678 | 657 | 738 | 946 | 332 | 370 | 428 | 207 | 227 | 242 | 145 | 156 | 154 |
| 0.35 | *** | 2361 | 2432 | 3648 | 656 | 710 | 950 | 329 | 360 | 439 | 206 | 223 | 257 | 143 | 153 | 170 |
| | *** | 2385 | 2566 | 3930 | 677 | 774 | 999 | 342 | 387 | 446 | 213 | 236 | 250 | 148 | 160 | 158 |
| 0.4 | *** | 2332 | 2424 | 3876 | 654 | 719 | 997 | 331 | 365 | 455 | 206 | 225 | 263 | 143 | 154 | 173 |
| | *** | 2363 | 2592 | 4098 | 679 | 793 | 1030 | 345 | 396 | 456 | 214 | 240 | 253 | 148 | 162 | 158 |
| 0.45 | *** | 2237 | 2355 | 4014 | 639 | 713 | 1020 | 325 | 363 | 460 | 203 | 223 | 263 | 140 | 152 | 171 |
| | *** | 2277 | 2559 | 4182 | 668 | 795 | 1041 | 341 | 397 | 456 | 212 | 239 | 250 | 145 | 160 | 154 |
| 0.5 | *** | 2092 | 2239 | 4061 | 614 | 695 | 1020 | 315 | 355 | 456 | 196 | 217 | 258 | 135 | 146 | 166 |
| | *** | 2142 | 2478 | 4182 | 646 | 782 | 1030 | 332 | 390 | 446 | 205 | 233 | 242 | 140 | 155 | 148 |
| 0.55 | *** | 1912 | 2089 | 4016 | 580 | 666 | 998 | 300 | 340 | 441 | 187 | 207 | 246 | 127 | 139 | 157 |
| | *** | 1974 | 2359 | 4098 | 614 | 757 | 999 | 317 | 375 | 428 | 195 | 222 | 229 | 132 | 146 | 138 |
| 0.6 | *** | 1712 | 1919 | 3879 | 539 | 628 | 952 | 281 | 320 | 416 | 174 | 193 | 229 | 117 | 128 | 144 |
| | *** | 1786 | 2212 | 3930 | 575 | 718 | 946 | 297 | 354 | 400 | 182 | 208 | 211 | 122 | 135 | 124 |
| 0.65 | *** | 1506 | 1736 | 3652 | 493 | 580 | 884 | 257 | 294 | 380 | 158 | 175 | 207 | 105 | 114 | 128 |
| | *** | 1591 | 2041 | 3678 | 529 | 667 | 873 | 273 | 325 | 362 | 165 | 188 | 187 | 109 | 120 | 107 |
| 0.7 | *** | 1304 | 1546 | 3334 | 443 | 524 | 794 | 230 | 263 | 335 | 139 | 153 | 179 | 91 | 98 | 108 |
| | *** | 1396 | 1849 | 3342 | 476 | 604 | 778 | 244 | 290 | 316 | 145 | 164 | 158 | 94 | 102 | 87 |
| 0.75 | *** | 1110 | 1350 | 2927 | 386 | 459 | 681 | 197 | 224 | 280 | 116 | 127 | 145 | . | . | . |
| | *** | 1203 | 1636 | 2922 | 416 | 528 | 662 | 209 | 246 | 260 | 121 | 135 | 124 | . | . | . |
| 0.8 | *** | 923 | 1144 | 2431 | 322 | 382 | 546 | 158 | 178 | 215 | . | . | . | . | . | . |
| | *** | 1010 | 1398 | 2417 | 347 | 436 | 526 | 167 | 193 | 194 | . | . | . | . | . | . |
| 0.85 | *** | 735 | 920 | 1847 | 248 | 290 | 389 | . | . | . | . | . | . | . | . | . |
| | *** | 808 | 1124 | 1829 | 266 | 325 | 368 | . | . | . | . | . | . | . | . | . |
| 0.9 | *** | 529 | 658 | 1177 | . | . | . | . | . | . | . | . | . | . | . | . |
| | *** | 581 | 793 | 1156 | . | . | . | . | . | . | . | . | . | . | . | . |

TABLE 6: ALPHA= 0.025 POWER= 0.9    EXPECTED ACCRUAL THRU MINIMUM FOLLOW-UP= 200

| | | DEL=.05 | | | DEL=.10 | | | DEL=.15 | | | DEL=.20 | | | DEL=.25 | | |
|---|---|---|---|---|---|---|---|---|---|---|---|---|---|---|---|---|---|
| FACT= | | 1.0 .75 | .50 .25 | .00 BIN | 1.0 .75 | .50 .25 | .00 BIN | 1.0 .75 | .50 .25 | .00 BIN | 1.0 75 | .50 .25 | .00 BIN | 1.0 .75 | .50 .25 | .00 BIN |
| PCONT=*** | | | | | REQUIRED NUMBER OF PATIENTS | | | | | | | | | | | |
| 0.05 | *** | 630 | 635 | 671 | 226 | 230 | 239 | 133 | 135 | 139 | 94 | 96 | 98 | 74 | 75 | 76 |
| | *** | 632 | 644 | 1156 | 227 | 233 | 368 | 134 | 137 | 194 | 95 | 97 | 124 | 74 | 75 | 87 |
| 0.1 | *** | 1150 | 1161 | 1295 | 359 | 369 | 400 | 195 | 200 | 212 | 130 | 133 | 139 | 96 | 99 | 102 |
| | *** | 1154 | 1182 | 1829 | 363 | 379 | 526 | 197 | 205 | 260 | 131 | 136 | 158 | 97 | 100 | 107 |
| 0.15 | *** | 1592 | 1611 | 1898 | 468 | 485 | 548 | 243 | 253 | 276 | 157 | 163 | 174 | 114 | 118 | 124 |
| | *** | 1598 | 1648 | 2417 | 474 | 504 | 662 | 247 | 262 | 316 | 160 | 168 | 187 | 115 | 120 | 124 |
| 0.2 | *** | 1934 | 1964 | 2448 | 550 | 576 | 679 | 280 | 295 | 332 | 178 | 187 | 203 | 127 | 132 | 141 |
| | *** | 1944 | 2021 | 2922 | 560 | 606 | 778 | 286 | 309 | 362 | 182 | 194 | 211 | 129 | 136 | 138 |
| 0.25 | *** | 2174 | 2216 | 2930 | 608 | 643 | 791 | 306 | 327 | 377 | 193 | 204 | 227 | 136 | 143 | 155 |
| | *** | 2188 | 2296 | 3342 | 621 | 684 | 873 | 315 | 345 | 400 | 198 | 214 | 229 | 139 | 148 | 148 |
| 0.3 | *** | 2314 | 2371 | 3331 | 643 | 689 | 882 | 323 | 349 | 413 | 202 | 217 | 245 | 142 | 150 | 164 |
| | *** | 2333 | 2479 | 3678 | 661 | 742 | 946 | 334 | 372 | 428 | 208 | 228 | 242 | 145 | 156 | 154 |
| 0.35 | *** | 2365 | 2440 | 3648 | 659 | 715 | 950 | 332 | 362 | 439 | 207 | 224 | 257 | 144 | 154 | 170 |
| | *** | 2390 | 2579 | 3930 | 681 | 779 | 999 | 344 | 389 | 446 | 214 | 237 | 250 | 149 | 161 | 158 |
| 0.4 | *** | 2337 | 2434 | 3876 | 658 | 724 | 997 | 333 | 367 | 455 | 208 | 226 | 263 | 144 | 155 | 173 |
| | *** | 2369 | 2608 | 4098 | 684 | 798 | 1030 | 347 | 398 | 456 | 216 | 241 | 253 | 149 | 162 | 158 |
| 0.45 | *** | 2243 | 2367 | 4014 | 644 | 719 | 1020 | 328 | 366 | 461 | 205 | 224 | 263 | 141 | 152 | 171 |
| | *** | 2285 | 2577 | 4182 | 674 | 801 | 1041 | 344 | 399 | 456 | 213 | 240 | 250 | 146 | 160 | 154 |
| 0.5 | *** | 2100 | 2253 | 4061 | 619 | 701 | 1020 | 318 | 357 | 456 | 198 | 218 | 258 | 136 | 147 | 166 |
| | *** | 2153 | 2499 | 4182 | 652 | 789 | 1030 | 335 | 392 | 446 | 207 | 234 | 242 | 141 | 155 | 148 |
| 0.55 | *** | 1922 | 2106 | 4016 | 586 | 673 | 998 | 303 | 343 | 441 | 188 | 208 | 246 | 128 | 139 | 157 |
| | *** | 1987 | 2383 | 4098 | 621 | 763 | 999 | 320 | 378 | 428 | 197 | 223 | 229 | 133 | 147 | 138 |
| 0.6 | *** | 1724 | 1938 | 3879 | 546 | 634 | 952 | 284 | 323 | 416 | 175 | 194 | 229 | 118 | 128 | 144 |
| | *** | 1801 | 2237 | 3930 | 581 | 725 | 946 | 300 | 356 | 400 | 184 | 208 | 211 | 123 | 135 | 124 |
| 0.65 | *** | 1520 | 1756 | 3652 | 500 | 587 | 884 | 260 | 297 | 380 | 159 | 176 | 207 | 106 | 115 | 128 |
| | *** | 1608 | 2066 | 3678 | 535 | 674 | 873 | 276 | 327 | 362 | 167 | 189 | 187 | 110 | 120 | 107 |
| 0.7 | *** | 1319 | 1567 | 3334 | 448 | 530 | 794 | 232 | 265 | 335 | 140 | 154 | 179 | 91 | 98 | 108 |
| | *** | 1414 | 1874 | 3342 | 482 | 610 | 778 | 246 | 291 | 316 | 146 | 164 | 158 | 94 | 102 | 87 |
| 0.75 | *** | 1126 | 1369 | 2927 | 391 | 464 | 681 | 199 | 226 | 280 | 117 | 128 | 145 | . | . | . |
| | *** | 1221 | 1659 | 2922 | 422 | 533 | 662 | 211 | 247 | 260 | 122 | 135 | 124 | . | . | . |
| 0.8 | *** | 938 | 1161 | 2431 | 327 | 386 | 546 | 160 | 180 | 215 | . | . | . | . | . | . |
| | *** | 1026 | 1418 | 2417 | 352 | 440 | 526 | 169 | 194 | 194 | . | . | . | . | . | . |
| 0.85 | *** | 748 | 934 | 1847 | 251 | 293 | 389 | . | . | . | . | . | . | . | . | . |
| | *** | 822 | 1140 | 1829 | 269 | 328 | 368 | . | . | . | . | . | . | . | . | . |
| 0.9 | *** | 538 | 668 | 1177 | . | . | . | . | . | . | . | . | . | . | . | . |
| | *** | 591 | 803 | 1156 | . | . | . | . | . | . | . | . | . | . | . | . |

## TABLE 6: ALPHA= 0.025 POWER= 0.9    EXPECTED ACCRUAL THRU MINIMUM FOLLOW-UP= 225

| PCONT=*** | FACT= | DEL=.05 1.0/.75 | .50/.25 | .00/BIN | DEL=.10 1.0/.75 | .50/.25 | .00/BIN | DEL=.15 1.0/.75 | .50/.25 | .00/BIN | DEL=.20 1.0/75 | .50/.25 | .00/BIN | DEL=.25 1.0/.75 | .50/.25 | .00/BIN |
|---|---|---|---|---|---|---|---|---|---|---|---|---|---|---|---|---|
| | | | | | REQUIRED NUMBER OF PATIENTS | | | | | | | | | | | |
| 0.05 | *** | 631 | 637 | 671 | 226 | 230 | 239 | 133 | 136 | 139 | 95 | 96 | 98 | 74 | 75 | 76 |
| | *** | 633 | 645 | 1156 | 228 | 233 | 368 | 134 | 137 | 194 | 95 | 97 | 124 | 74 | 75 | 87 |
| 0.1 | *** | 1151 | 1164 | 1295 | 361 | 371 | 400 | 195 | 201 | 212 | 130 | 134 | 139 | 97 | 99 | 102 |
| | *** | 1156 | 1187 | 1829 | 365 | 381 | 526 | 198 | 206 | 260 | 132 | 136 | 158 | 98 | 100 | 107 |
| 0.15 | *** | 1594 | 1616 | 1898 | 470 | 488 | 548 | 245 | 255 | 276 | 158 | 164 | 174 | 114 | 118 | 124 |
| | *** | 1602 | 1657 | 2417 | 477 | 507 | 662 | 249 | 263 | 316 | 161 | 168 | 187 | 116 | 120 | 124 |
| 0.2 | *** | 1938 | 1971 | 2448 | 554 | 581 | 679 | 282 | 298 | 332 | 179 | 188 | 203 | 128 | 133 | 141 |
| | *** | 1949 | 2034 | 2922 | 564 | 611 | 778 | 289 | 311 | 362 | 183 | 194 | 211 | 130 | 137 | 138 |
| 0.25 | *** | 2179 | 2226 | 2930 | 613 | 650 | 791 | 310 | 330 | 377 | 195 | 206 | 227 | 137 | 144 | 155 |
| | *** | 2195 | 2314 | 3342 | 627 | 691 | 873 | 318 | 348 | 400 | 200 | 215 | 229 | 140 | 149 | 148 |
| 0.3 | *** | 2321 | 2385 | 3331 | 650 | 698 | 882 | 327 | 353 | 413 | 205 | 219 | 245 | 143 | 151 | 164 |
| | *** | 2343 | 2503 | 3678 | 668 | 750 | 946 | 338 | 375 | 428 | 211 | 229 | 242 | 147 | 157 | 154 |
| 0.35 | *** | 2374 | 2458 | 3648 | 668 | 726 | 950 | 337 | 367 | 439 | 210 | 226 | 257 | 146 | 155 | 170 |
| | *** | 2402 | 2610 | 3930 | 690 | 790 | 999 | 349 | 393 | 446 | 217 | 239 | 250 | 150 | 162 | 158 |
| 0.4 | *** | 2349 | 2457 | 3876 | 669 | 737 | 997 | 339 | 373 | 455 | 211 | 229 | 263 | 146 | 156 | 173 |
| | *** | 2386 | 2645 | 4182 | 695 | 810 | 1030 | 353 | 403 | 446 | 219 | 243 | 253 | 151 | 163 | 158 |
| 0.45 | *** | 2259 | 2396 | 4014 | 656 | 733 | 1020 | 335 | 372 | 461 | 208 | 227 | 263 | 143 | 154 | 171 |
| | *** | 2306 | 2621 | 4182 | 686 | 815 | 1041 | 350 | 404 | 456 | 217 | 242 | 250 | 148 | 161 | 154 |
| 0.5 | *** | 2120 | 2288 | 4061 | 632 | 716 | 1020 | 325 | 364 | 456 | 202 | 221 | 258 | 138 | 149 | 166 |
| | *** | 2179 | 2549 | 4182 | 666 | 803 | 1030 | 341 | 397 | 446 | 210 | 236 | 242 | 143 | 156 | 148 |
| 0.55 | *** | 1946 | 2147 | 4016 | 600 | 688 | 998 | 310 | 349 | 441 | 192 | 211 | 246 | 130 | 141 | 157 |
| | *** | 2018 | 2437 | 4098 | 635 | 778 | 999 | 327 | 383 | 428 | 200 | 226 | 229 | 135 | 148 | 138 |
| 0.6 | *** | 1754 | 1983 | 3879 | 560 | 650 | 952 | 291 | 329 | 416 | 179 | 197 | 229 | 120 | 130 | 144 |
| | *** | 1838 | 2294 | 3930 | 597 | 739 | 946 | 307 | 361 | 400 | 187 | 210 | 211 | 125 | 136 | 124 |
| 0.65 | *** | 1554 | 1805 | 3652 | 514 | 602 | 884 | 267 | 303 | 380 | 162 | 179 | 207 | 108 | 116 | 128 |
| | *** | 1648 | 2124 | 3678 | 550 | 687 | 873 | 282 | 332 | 362 | 170 | 191 | 187 | 111 | 121 | 107 |
| 0.7 | *** | 1356 | 1615 | 3334 | 462 | 545 | 794 | 238 | 270 | 335 | 142 | 156 | 179 | 93 | 99 | 108 |
| | *** | 1456 | 1930 | 3342 | 496 | 622 | 778 | 252 | 295 | 316 | 149 | 166 | 158 | 96 | 103 | 87 |
| 0.75 | *** | 1164 | 1416 | 2927 | 404 | 476 | 681 | 204 | 230 | 280 | 119 | 129 | 145 | . | . | . |
| | *** | 1262 | 1711 | 2922 | 434 | 543 | 662 | 216 | 250 | 260 | 123 | 136 | 124 | . | . | . |
| 0.8 | *** | 973 | 1203 | 2431 | 337 | 396 | 546 | 164 | 183 | 215 | . | . | . | . | . | . |
| | *** | 1064 | 1463 | 2417 | 362 | 448 | 526 | 172 | 196 | 194 | . | . | . | . | . | . |
| 0.85 | *** | 777 | 968 | 1847 | 258 | 299 | 389 | . | . | . | . | . | . | . | . | . |
| | *** | 854 | 1175 | 1829 | 276 | 333 | 368 | . | . | . | . | . | . | . | . | . |
| 0.9 | *** | 559 | 691 | 1177 | . | . | . | . | . | . | . | . | . | . | . | . |
| | *** | 613 | 825 | 1156 | . | . | . | . | . | . | . | . | . | . | . | . |

TABLE 6: ALPHA= 0.025 POWER= 0.9    EXPECTED ACCRUAL THRU MINIMUM FOLLOW-UP= 250

| PCONT= *** | | DEL=.05 | | | DEL=.10 | | | DEL=.15 | | | DEL=.20 | | | DEL=.25 | | |
|---|---|---|---|---|---|---|---|---|---|---|---|---|---|---|---|---|
| FACT= | | 1.0 .75 | .50 .25 | .00 BIN | 1.0 .75 | .50 .25 | .00 BIN | 1.0 .75 | .50 .25 | .00 BIN | 1.0 75 | .50 .25 | .00 BIN | 1.0 .75 | .50 .25 | .00 BIN |

REQUIRED NUMBER OF PATIENTS

| PCONT | | DEL=.05 1.0/.75 | .50/.25 | .00/BIN | DEL=.10 1.0/.75 | .50/.25 | .00/BIN | DEL=.15 1.0/.75 | .50/.25 | .00/BIN | DEL=.20 1.0/75 | .50/.25 | .00/BIN | DEL=.25 1.0/.75 | .50/.25 | .00/BIN |
|---|---|---|---|---|---|---|---|---|---|---|---|---|---|---|---|---|
| 0.05 | *** | 632 | 638 | 671 | 227 | 231 | 239 | 134 | 136 | 139 | 95 | 96 | 98 | 74 | 75 | 76 |
|  | *** | 634 | 647 | 1156 | 229 | 234 | 368 | 135 | 137 | 194 | 95 | 97 | 124 | 74 | 75 | 87 |
| 0.1 | *** | 1153 | 1167 | 1295 | 362 | 372 | 400 | 196 | 202 | 212 | 131 | 134 | 139 | 97 | 99 | 102 |
|  | *** | 1158 | 1191 | 1829 | 366 | 382 | 526 | 199 | 206 | 260 | 132 | 136 | 158 | 98 | 101 | 107 |
| 0.15 | *** | 1597 | 1621 | 1898 | 472 | 491 | 548 | 246 | 256 | 276 | 159 | 165 | 174 | 115 | 119 | 124 |
|  | *** | 1605 | 1665 | 2417 | 480 | 510 | 662 | 251 | 264 | 316 | 162 | 169 | 187 | 117 | 121 | 124 |
| 0.2 | *** | 1942 | 1979 | 2449 | 557 | 585 | 679 | 285 | 300 | 332 | 181 | 189 | 203 | 129 | 134 | 141 |
|  | *** | 1954 | 2046 | 2922 | 568 | 615 | 778 | 291 | 312 | 362 | 185 | 195 | 211 | 131 | 137 | 138 |
| 0.25 | *** | 2184 | 2237 | 2930 | 618 | 656 | 791 | 313 | 333 | 377 | 197 | 208 | 227 | 138 | 145 | 155 |
|  | *** | 2202 | 2332 | 3342 | 633 | 697 | 873 | 321 | 350 | 400 | 202 | 216 | 229 | 141 | 149 | 148 |
| 0.3 | *** | 2329 | 2399 | 3331 | 657 | 706 | 882 | 331 | 357 | 413 | 207 | 221 | 245 | 144 | 152 | 164 |
|  | *** | 2352 | 2526 | 3678 | 676 | 758 | 946 | 342 | 378 | 428 | 213 | 231 | 242 | 148 | 158 | 154 |
| 0.35 | *** | 2384 | 2477 | 3648 | 676 | 735 | 950 | 342 | 371 | 439 | 213 | 228 | 257 | 148 | 157 | 170 |
|  | *** | 2415 | 2639 | 3930 | 699 | 799 | 999 | 354 | 397 | 446 | 220 | 240 | 250 | 152 | 163 | 158 |
| 0.4 | *** | 2361 | 2481 | 3876 | 678 | 748 | 997 | 344 | 378 | 455 | 214 | 231 | 263 | 148 | 157 | 172 |
|  | *** | 2402 | 2681 | 4098 | 706 | 821 | 1030 | 359 | 407 | 456 | 222 | 244 | 253 | 152 | 164 | 158 |
| 0.45 | *** | 2275 | 2425 | 4014 | 667 | 745 | 1020 | 340 | 377 | 461 | 211 | 230 | 263 | 145 | 155 | 171 |
|  | *** | 2327 | 2663 | 4182 | 698 | 826 | 1041 | 356 | 408 | 456 | 219 | 244 | 250 | 150 | 162 | 154 |
| 0.5 | *** | 2140 | 2322 | 4061 | 644 | 730 | 1020 | 331 | 369 | 456 | 205 | 224 | 258 | 140 | 150 | 166 |
|  | *** | 2204 | 2595 | 4182 | 679 | 816 | 1030 | 347 | 401 | 446 | 213 | 238 | 242 | 144 | 157 | 148 |
| 0.55 | *** | 1971 | 2186 | 4016 | 612 | 702 | 998 | 316 | 355 | 441 | 195 | 214 | 246 | 132 | 142 | 157 |
|  | *** | 2049 | 2487 | 4098 | 649 | 791 | 999 | 333 | 387 | 428 | 203 | 227 | 229 | 137 | 148 | 138 |
| 0.6 | *** | 1783 | 2026 | 3879 | 573 | 664 | 952 | 297 | 334 | 416 | 182 | 199 | 229 | 122 | 131 | 144 |
|  | *** | 1873 | 2347 | 3930 | 610 | 752 | 946 | 313 | 365 | 400 | 190 | 212 | 211 | 126 | 137 | 124 |
| 0.65 | *** | 1587 | 1849 | 3652 | 527 | 615 | 884 | 272 | 308 | 380 | 165 | 181 | 207 | 109 | 117 | 128 |
|  | *** | 1686 | 2177 | 3678 | 564 | 699 | 873 | 288 | 336 | 362 | 172 | 192 | 187 | 113 | 122 | 107 |
| 0.7 | *** | 1392 | 1660 | 3334 | 474 | 557 | 794 | 243 | 274 | 335 | 145 | 158 | 179 | 94 | 100 | 108 |
|  | *** | 1495 | 1981 | 3342 | 509 | 633 | 778 | 257 | 298 | 316 | 151 | 167 | 158 | 97 | 104 | 87 |
| 0.75 | *** | 1199 | 1458 | 2927 | 415 | 487 | 681 | 208 | 234 | 280 | 120 | 130 | 145 | . | . | . |
|  | *** | 1300 | 1758 | 2922 | 445 | 552 | 662 | 219 | 252 | 260 | 125 | 137 | 124 | . | . | . |
| 0.8 | *** | 1006 | 1241 | 2431 | 346 | 404 | 546 | 167 | 185 | 215 | . | . | . | . | . | . |
|  | *** | 1099 | 1504 | 2417 | 371 | 455 | 526 | 175 | 198 | 194 | . | . | . | . | . | . |
| 0.85 | *** | 805 | 999 | 1847 | 265 | 305 | 389 | . | . | . | . | . | . | . | . | . |
|  | *** | 883 | 1207 | 1829 | 282 | 337 | 368 | . | . | . | . | . | . | . | . | . |
| 0.9 | *** | 579 | 712 | 1177 | . | . | . | . | . | . | . | . | . | . | . | . |
|  | *** | 633 | 844 | 1156 | . | . | . | . | . | . | . | . | . | . | . | . |

## TABLE 6: ALPHA= 0.025 POWER= 0.9    EXPECTED ACCRUAL THRU MINIMUM FOLLOW-UP= 275

| | | DEL=.05 | | | DEL=.10 | | | DEL=.15 | | | DEL=.20 | | | DEL=.25 | | |
|---|---|---|---|---|---|---|---|---|---|---|---|---|---|---|---|---|
| FACT= | | 1.0 .75 | .50 .25 | .00 BIN | 1.0 .75 | .50 .25 | .00 BIN | 1.0 .75 | .50 .25 | .00 BIN | 1.0 75 | .50 .25 | .00 BIN | 1.0 .75 | .50 .25 | .00 BIN |
| PCONT=*** | | | | | REQUIRED NUMBER OF PATIENTS | | | | | | | | | | | |
| 0.05 | *** | 632 | 639 | 671 | 227 | 231 | 239 | 134 | 136 | 139 | 95 | 96 | 98 | 74 | 75 | 76 |
| | *** | 635 | 648 | 1156 | 229 | 234 | 368 | 135 | 138 | 194 | 96 | 97 | 124 | 74 | 75 | 87 |
| 0.1 | *** | 1154 | 1170 | 1295 | 363 | 374 | 400 | 197 | 203 | 212 | 132 | 135 | 139 | 98 | 99 | 102 |
| | *** | 1159 | 1195 | 1829 | 367 | 383 | 526 | 200 | 207 | 260 | 133 | 136 | 158 | 98 | 101 | 107 |
| 0.15 | *** | 1599 | 1626 | 1898 | 475 | 494 | 548 | 248 | 257 | 276 | 160 | 166 | 174 | 116 | 119 | 123 |
| | *** | 1608 | 1672 | 2417 | 482 | 512 | 662 | 252 | 265 | 316 | 162 | 169 | 187 | 117 | 121 | 124 |
| 0.2 | *** | 1946 | 1986 | 2448 | 561 | 589 | 679 | 287 | 302 | 332 | 182 | 190 | 203 | 129 | 134 | 141 |
| | *** | 1959 | 2058 | 2922 | 572 | 619 | 778 | 293 | 314 | 362 | 186 | 196 | 211 | 132 | 137 | 138 |
| 0.25 | *** | 2190 | 2247 | 2929 | 623 | 662 | 791 | 316 | 336 | 377 | 198 | 209 | 227 | 139 | 145 | 155 |
| | *** | 2209 | 2348 | 3342 | 638 | 703 | 873 | 324 | 352 | 400 | 203 | 217 | 229 | 142 | 150 | 148 |
| 0.3 | *** | 2336 | 2413 | 3331 | 663 | 713 | 882 | 335 | 360 | 413 | 209 | 222 | 245 | 146 | 153 | 164 |
| | *** | 2362 | 2548 | 3678 | 682 | 765 | 946 | 345 | 380 | 428 | 215 | 232 | 242 | 149 | 158 | 154 |
| 0.35 | *** | 2393 | 2495 | 3648 | 683 | 744 | 950 | 346 | 375 | 439 | 215 | 230 | 257 | 149 | 157 | 170 |
| | *** | 2427 | 2667 | 3930 | 707 | 807 | 999 | 358 | 399 | 446 | 222 | 241 | 250 | 153 | 163 | 158 |
| 0.4 | *** | 2373 | 2503 | 3876 | 687 | 758 | 997 | 349 | 382 | 455 | 217 | 233 | 263 | 149 | 158 | 172 |
| | *** | 2418 | 2714 | 4098 | 715 | 831 | 1030 | 363 | 410 | 456 | 224 | 246 | 253 | 153 | 165 | 158 |
| 0.45 | *** | 2290 | 2452 | 4014 | 677 | 757 | 1020 | 346 | 382 | 461 | 214 | 232 | 263 | 147 | 156 | 171 |
| | *** | 2347 | 2701 | 4182 | 709 | 837 | 1041 | 361 | 411 | 456 | 222 | 245 | 250 | 151 | 163 | 154 |
| 0.5 | *** | 2159 | 2355 | 4061 | 655 | 742 | 1020 | 336 | 374 | 456 | 208 | 226 | 257 | 142 | 151 | 166 |
| | *** | 2229 | 2638 | 4182 | 690 | 827 | 1030 | 353 | 405 | 446 | 216 | 239 | 242 | 146 | 158 | 148 |
| 0.55 | *** | 1995 | 2223 | 4016 | 624 | 715 | 998 | 322 | 360 | 441 | 198 | 216 | 246 | 134 | 143 | 157 |
| | *** | 2078 | 2534 | 4098 | 661 | 802 | 999 | 338 | 391 | 428 | 206 | 229 | 229 | 138 | 149 | 138 |
| 0.6 | *** | 1811 | 2066 | 3879 | 585 | 676 | 952 | 302 | 339 | 415 | 184 | 201 | 229 | 123 | 132 | 144 |
| | *** | 1906 | 2395 | 3930 | 623 | 763 | 946 | 318 | 369 | 400 | 192 | 213 | 211 | 127 | 137 | 124 |
| 0.65 | *** | 1618 | 1891 | 3652 | 539 | 628 | 884 | 277 | 312 | 380 | 167 | 183 | 207 | 110 | 118 | 128 |
| | *** | 1722 | 2226 | 3678 | 576 | 710 | 873 | 292 | 339 | 362 | 174 | 193 | 187 | 114 | 122 | 107 |
| 0.7 | *** | 1424 | 1701 | 3334 | 486 | 568 | 794 | 248 | 278 | 335 | 147 | 159 | 178 | 95 | 100 | 108 |
| | *** | 1532 | 2028 | 3342 | 520 | 643 | 778 | 261 | 301 | 316 | 153 | 168 | 158 | 97 | 104 | 87 |
| 0.75 | *** | 1231 | 1498 | 2927 | 425 | 497 | 681 | 212 | 237 | 280 | 122 | 131 | 145 | . | . | . |
| | *** | 1336 | 1801 | 2922 | 455 | 560 | 662 | 223 | 254 | 260 | 126 | 137 | 124 | . | . | . |
| 0.8 | *** | 1036 | 1276 | 2431 | 354 | 412 | 546 | 170 | 187 | 215 | . | . | . | . | . | . |
| | *** | 1131 | 1540 | 2417 | 379 | 461 | 526 | 177 | 199 | 194 | . | . | . | . | . | . |
| 0.85 | *** | 830 | 1027 | 1847 | 271 | 310 | 389 | . | . | . | . | . | . | . | . | . |
| | *** | 909 | 1235 | 1829 | 288 | 341 | 368 | . | . | . | . | . | . | . | . | . |
| 0.9 | *** | 596 | 731 | 1177 | . | . | . | . | . | . | . | . | . | . | . | . |
| | *** | 651 | 862 | 1156 | . | . | . | . | . | . | . | . | . | . | . | . |

TABLE 6: ALPHA= 0.025 POWER= 0.9    EXPECTED ACCRUAL THRU MINIMUM FOLLOW-UP= 300

| | | DEL=.05 | | | DEL=.10 | | | DEL=.15 | | | DEL=.20 | | | DEL=.25 | | |
|---|---|---|---|---|---|---|---|---|---|---|---|---|---|---|---|---|---|
| FACT= | | 1.0 .75 | .50 .25 | .00 BIN | 1.0 .75 | .50 .25 | .00 BIN | 1.0 .75 | .50 .25 | .00 BIN | 1.0 75 | .50 .25 | .00 BIN | 1.0 .75 | .50 .25 | .00 BIN |
| PCONT=*** | | | | REQUIRED NUMBER OF PATIENTS | | | | | | | | | | | | |
| 0.05 | *** | 633 | 640 | 671 | 228 | 232 | 239 | 134 | 136 | 139 | 95 | 96 | 98 | 74 | 75 | 76 |
| | *** | 635 | 649 | 1156 | 229 | 235 | 368 | 135 | 138 | 194 | 96 | 97 | 124 | 75 | 75 | 87 |
| 0.1 | *** | 1156 | 1172 | 1295 | 365 | 375 | 400 | 198 | 203 | 212 | 132 | 135 | 139 | 98 | 100 | 102 |
| | *** | 1161 | 1199 | 1829 | 369 | 384 | 526 | 200 | 207 | 260 | 133 | 137 | 158 | 99 | 101 | 107 |
| 0.15 | *** | 1601 | 1630 | 1898 | 477 | 496 | 548 | 249 | 259 | 276 | 161 | 166 | 174 | 116 | 119 | 124 |
| | *** | 1611 | 1680 | 2417 | 484 | 514 | 662 | 253 | 266 | 316 | 163 | 170 | 187 | 118 | 121 | 124 |
| 0.2 | *** | 1949 | 1993 | 2448 | 564 | 593 | 679 | 289 | 303 | 331 | 183 | 191 | 203 | 130 | 135 | 141 |
| | *** | 1964 | 2069 | 2922 | 576 | 622 | 778 | 295 | 315 | 362 | 187 | 196 | 211 | 132 | 137 | 138 |
| 0.25 | *** | 2195 | 2257 | 2929 | 627 | 667 | 791 | 318 | 338 | 377 | 200 | 210 | 227 | 140 | 146 | 154 |
| | *** | 2216 | 2364 | 3342 | 643 | 707 | 873 | 327 | 353 | 400 | 204 | 217 | 229 | 143 | 150 | 148 |
| 0.3 | *** | 2343 | 2427 | 3331 | 668 | 720 | 882 | 338 | 363 | 413 | 211 | 224 | 245 | 147 | 154 | 164 |
| | *** | 2371 | 2569 | 3678 | 689 | 771 | 946 | 349 | 382 | 428 | 217 | 232 | 242 | 150 | 159 | 154 |
| 0.35 | *** | 2402 | 2512 | 3648 | 690 | 752 | 950 | 349 | 379 | 439 | 217 | 232 | 256 | 150 | 158 | 170 |
| | *** | 2440 | 2693 | 3930 | 715 | 815 | 999 | 362 | 402 | 446 | 224 | 242 | 250 | 154 | 164 | 158 |
| 0.4 | *** | 2386 | 2525 | 3876 | 695 | 767 | 997 | 353 | 386 | 455 | 219 | 235 | 263 | 151 | 159 | 172 |
| | *** | 2434 | 2746 | 4098 | 724 | 839 | 1030 | 367 | 413 | 456 | 226 | 247 | 253 | 155 | 165 | 158 |
| 0.45 | *** | 2306 | 2479 | 4014 | 686 | 767 | 1020 | 350 | 386 | 460 | 217 | 234 | 263 | 148 | 157 | 171 |
| | *** | 2367 | 2737 | 4182 | 719 | 846 | 1041 | 366 | 415 | 456 | 224 | 246 | 250 | 152 | 163 | 154 |
| 0.5 | *** | 2179 | 2386 | 4061 | 666 | 753 | 1020 | 341 | 379 | 456 | 210 | 228 | 258 | 143 | 152 | 166 |
| | *** | 2253 | 2679 | 4182 | 701 | 837 | 1030 | 357 | 408 | 446 | 218 | 241 | 242 | 147 | 158 | 148 |
| 0.55 | *** | 2018 | 2258 | 4016 | 635 | 726 | 998 | 327 | 364 | 441 | 200 | 218 | 246 | 135 | 144 | 157 |
| | *** | 2106 | 2577 | 4098 | 673 | 812 | 999 | 343 | 394 | 428 | 208 | 230 | 229 | 139 | 150 | 138 |
| 0.6 | *** | 1838 | 2104 | 3879 | 596 | 688 | 952 | 307 | 343 | 415 | 187 | 203 | 229 | 125 | 133 | 144 |
| | *** | 1938 | 2440 | 3930 | 634 | 773 | 946 | 323 | 372 | 400 | 194 | 214 | 211 | 128 | 138 | 124 |
| 0.65 | *** | 1648 | 1930 | 3652 | 550 | 638 | 884 | 282 | 316 | 380 | 170 | 184 | 207 | 112 | 118 | 128 |
| | *** | 1756 | 2270 | 3678 | 587 | 719 | 873 | 297 | 341 | 362 | 176 | 194 | 187 | 115 | 123 | 107 |
| 0.7 | *** | 1456 | 1740 | 3334 | 496 | 578 | 794 | 252 | 281 | 335 | 149 | 161 | 178 | 96 | 101 | 108 |
| | *** | 1567 | 2071 | 3342 | 530 | 651 | 778 | 265 | 303 | 316 | 154 | 169 | 158 | 98 | 104 | 87 |
| 0.75 | *** | 1262 | 1534 | 2927 | 434 | 505 | 681 | 215 | 239 | 280 | 123 | 132 | 145 | . | . | . |
| | *** | 1369 | 1840 | 2922 | 464 | 567 | 662 | 226 | 256 | 260 | 127 | 138 | 124 | . | . | . |
| 0.8 | *** | 1064 | 1309 | 2431 | 362 | 419 | 546 | 172 | 189 | 215 | . | . | . | . | . | . |
| | *** | 1161 | 1574 | 2417 | 386 | 466 | 526 | 180 | 200 | 194 | . | . | . | . | . | . |
| 0.85 | *** | 854 | 1053 | 1847 | 276 | 314 | 389 | . | . | . | . | . | . | . | . | . |
| | *** | 934 | 1260 | 1829 | 293 | 344 | 368 | . | . | . | . | . | . | . | . | . |
| 0.9 | *** | 613 | 748 | 1177 | . | . | . | . | . | . | . | . | . | . | . | . |
| | *** | 668 | 877 | 1156 | . | . | . | . | . | . | . | . | . | . | . | . |

TABLE 6: ALPHA= 0.025 POWER= 0.9     EXPECTED ACCRUAL THRU MINIMUM FOLLOW-UP= 325

| | | DEL=.05 | | | DEL=.10 | | | DEL=.15 | | | DEL=.20 | | | DEL=.25 | | |
|---|---|---|---|---|---|---|---|---|---|---|---|---|---|---|---|---|---|
| FACT= | | 1.0 .75 | .50 .25 | .00 BIN | 1.0 .75 | .50 .25 | .00 BIN | 1.0 .75 | .50 .25 | .00 BIN | 1.0 75 | .50 .25 | .00 BIN | 1.0 .75 | .50 .25 | .00 BIN |
| PCONT=*** | | | | | REQUIRED NUMBER OF PATIENTS | | | | | | | | | | | |
| 0.05 | *** | 634 | 641 | 671 | 229 | 232 | 239 | 135 | 136 | 139 | 95 | 96 | 98 | 74 | 75 | 76 |
| | *** | 636 | 650 | 1156 | 230 | 235 | 368 | 135 | 138 | 194 | 96 | 97 | 124 | 75 | 75 | 87 |
| 0.1 | *** | 1157 | 1175 | 1295 | 366 | 376 | 400 | 199 | 204 | 212 | 132 | 135 | 139 | 98 | 100 | 102 |
| | *** | 1163 | 1202 | 1829 | 370 | 385 | 526 | 201 | 207 | 260 | 134 | 137 | 158 | 99 | 101 | 107 |
| 0.15 | *** | 1604 | 1635 | 1898 | 479 | 498 | 548 | 250 | 260 | 276 | 161 | 167 | 174 | 117 | 120 | 123 |
| | *** | 1615 | 1686 | 2417 | 487 | 516 | 662 | 254 | 267 | 316 | 164 | 170 | 187 | 118 | 121 | 124 |
| 0.2 | *** | 1953 | 2000 | 2448 | 567 | 597 | 679 | 291 | 305 | 331 | 184 | 192 | 203 | 131 | 135 | 141 |
| | *** | 1969 | 2080 | 2922 | 579 | 625 | 778 | 297 | 316 | 362 | 188 | 197 | 211 | 133 | 138 | 138 |
| 0.25 | *** | 2200 | 2267 | 2930 | 632 | 672 | 791 | 321 | 340 | 377 | 201 | 211 | 227 | 141 | 147 | 155 |
| | *** | 2223 | 2379 | 3342 | 648 | 712 | 873 | 329 | 355 | 400 | 206 | 218 | 229 | 144 | 150 | 148 |
| 0.3 | *** | 2350 | 2440 | 3331 | 674 | 726 | 882 | 341 | 365 | 413 | 213 | 225 | 245 | 148 | 155 | 164 |
| | *** | 2381 | 2589 | 3678 | 695 | 777 | 946 | 352 | 385 | 428 | 218 | 233 | 242 | 151 | 159 | 154 |
| 0.35 | *** | 2412 | 2530 | 3648 | 697 | 760 | 950 | 353 | 382 | 439 | 219 | 233 | 257 | 151 | 159 | 170 |
| | *** | 2452 | 2718 | 3930 | 722 | 821 | 999 | 365 | 404 | 446 | 225 | 243 | 250 | 155 | 164 | 158 |
| 0.4 | *** | 2398 | 2547 | 3876 | 703 | 776 | 996 | 357 | 390 | 455 | 221 | 237 | 263 | 152 | 160 | 172 |
| | *** | 2450 | 2775 | 4098 | 733 | 847 | 1030 | 371 | 415 | 456 | 228 | 248 | 253 | 156 | 166 | 158 |
| 0.45 | *** | 2322 | 2505 | 4014 | 695 | 777 | 1020 | 355 | 390 | 460 | 219 | 236 | 263 | 149 | 158 | 171 |
| | *** | 2387 | 2772 | 4182 | 728 | 855 | 1041 | 370 | 417 | 456 | 226 | 247 | 250 | 153 | 164 | 154 |
| 0.5 | *** | 2198 | 2416 | 4061 | 676 | 763 | 1020 | 346 | 382 | 456 | 213 | 230 | 258 | 144 | 153 | 166 |
| | *** | 2277 | 2716 | 4182 | 711 | 846 | 1030 | 362 | 411 | 446 | 220 | 242 | 242 | 148 | 159 | 148 |
| 0.55 | *** | 2041 | 2291 | 4016 | 646 | 736 | 998 | 331 | 368 | 441 | 203 | 220 | 246 | 136 | 145 | 157 |
| | *** | 2134 | 2618 | 4098 | 683 | 821 | 999 | 348 | 397 | 428 | 210 | 231 | 229 | 140 | 150 | 138 |
| 0.6 | *** | 1864 | 2140 | 3879 | 607 | 698 | 952 | 312 | 347 | 416 | 189 | 205 | 229 | 126 | 133 | 144 |
| | *** | 1968 | 2481 | 3930 | 645 | 782 | 946 | 327 | 374 | 400 | 196 | 216 | 211 | 129 | 138 | 124 |
| 0.65 | *** | 1677 | 1967 | 3652 | 560 | 648 | 884 | 286 | 319 | 380 | 172 | 186 | 207 | 112 | 119 | 128 |
| | *** | 1789 | 2312 | 3678 | 597 | 728 | 873 | 301 | 344 | 362 | 178 | 195 | 187 | 116 | 123 | 107 |
| 0.7 | *** | 1485 | 1777 | 3334 | 506 | 587 | 794 | 255 | 284 | 335 | 150 | 162 | 179 | 96 | 101 | 108 |
| | *** | 1599 | 2111 | 3342 | 540 | 658 | 778 | 268 | 305 | 316 | 156 | 169 | 158 | 99 | 104 | 87 |
| 0.75 | *** | 1291 | 1568 | 2927 | 442 | 513 | 681 | 219 | 242 | 280 | 125 | 133 | 145 | . | . | . |
| | *** | 1401 | 1877 | 2922 | 472 | 573 | 662 | 229 | 258 | 260 | 129 | 138 | 124 | . | . | . |
| 0.8 | *** | 1090 | 1339 | 2431 | 369 | 425 | 546 | 174 | 190 | 215 | . | . | . | . | . | . |
| | *** | 1190 | 1604 | 2417 | 393 | 470 | 526 | 182 | 201 | 194 | . | . | . | . | . | . |
| 0.85 | *** | 876 | 1077 | 1847 | 281 | 318 | 389 | . | . | . | . | . | . | . | . | . |
| | *** | 957 | 1284 | 1829 | 297 | 346 | 368 | . | . | . | . | . | . | . | . | . |
| 0.9 | *** | 628 | 763 | 1177 | . | . | . | . | . | . | . | . | . | . | . | . |
| | *** | 684 | 891 | 1156 | . | . | . | . | . | . | . | . | . | . | . | . |

TABLE 6: ALPHA= 0.025 POWER= 0.9    EXPECTED ACCRUAL THRU MINIMUM FOLLOW-UP= 350

| | DEL=.05 | | | DEL=.10 | | | DEL=.15 | | | DEL=.20 | | | DEL=.25 | | |
|---|---|---|---|---|---|---|---|---|---|---|---|---|---|---|---|
| FACT= | 1.0 .75 | .50 .25 | .00 BIN | 1.0 .75 | .50 .25 | .00 BIN | 1.0 .75 | .50 .25 | .00 BIN | 1.0 75 | .50 .25 | .00 BIN | 1.0 .75 | .50 .25 | .00 BIN |
| PCONT=*** | | | REQUIRED NUMBER OF PATIENTS | | | | | | | | | | | | |
| 0.05 *** | 634 | 642 | 671 | 229 | 232 | 239 | 135 | 137 | 139 | 96 | 97 | 98 | 74 | 75 | 76 |
| *** | 637 | 651 | 1156 | 230 | 235 | 368 | 136 | 138 | 194 | 96 | 97 | 124 | 75 | 75 | 87 |
| 0.1 *** | 1158 | 1177 | 1295 | 367 | 377 | 400 | 199 | 204 | 212 | 133 | 135 | 139 | 98 | 100 | 102 |
| *** | 1165 | 1206 | 1829 | 371 | 386 | 526 | 201 | 208 | 260 | 134 | 137 | 158 | 99 | 101 | 107 |
| 0.15 *** | 1606 | 1640 | 1898 | 481 | 500 | 548 | 251 | 260 | 276 | 162 | 167 | 174 | 117 | 120 | 124 |
| *** | 1618 | 1693 | 2417 | 489 | 518 | 662 | 255 | 267 | 316 | 164 | 170 | 187 | 118 | 122 | 124 |
| 0.2 *** | 1957 | 2007 | 2448 | 570 | 600 | 679 | 292 | 306 | 332 | 185 | 192 | 203 | 131 | 135 | 141 |
| *** | 1974 | 2090 | 2922 | 582 | 628 | 778 | 298 | 317 | 362 | 188 | 197 | 211 | 133 | 138 | 138 |
| 0.25 *** | 2205 | 2277 | 2930 | 636 | 677 | 791 | 323 | 342 | 377 | 202 | 212 | 227 | 142 | 147 | 155 |
| *** | 2230 | 2394 | 3342 | 652 | 716 | 873 | 331 | 356 | 400 | 207 | 218 | 229 | 144 | 150 | 148 |
| 0.3 *** | 2357 | 2453 | 3331 | 679 | 731 | 882 | 344 | 368 | 413 | 214 | 226 | 245 | 149 | 155 | 164 |
| *** | 2390 | 2608 | 3678 | 700 | 782 | 946 | 354 | 386 | 428 | 219 | 234 | 242 | 152 | 159 | 154 |
| 0.35 *** | 2421 | 2546 | 3648 | 703 | 767 | 950 | 356 | 384 | 439 | 221 | 235 | 257 | 152 | 160 | 170 |
| *** | 2465 | 2741 | 3930 | 729 | 827 | 999 | 369 | 406 | 446 | 227 | 244 | 250 | 156 | 165 | 158 |
| 0.4 *** | 2410 | 2568 | 3876 | 711 | 784 | 997 | 361 | 393 | 455 | 223 | 238 | 263 | 153 | 161 | 173 |
| *** | 2465 | 2803 | 4098 | 741 | 854 | 1030 | 375 | 418 | 456 | 230 | 249 | 253 | 157 | 166 | 158 |
| 0.45 *** | 2337 | 2530 | 4014 | 704 | 785 | 1020 | 359 | 393 | 460 | 221 | 237 | 263 | 150 | 159 | 171 |
| *** | 2406 | 2804 | 4182 | 737 | 862 | 1041 | 374 | 420 | 456 | 228 | 248 | 250 | 154 | 164 | 154 |
| 0.5 *** | 2217 | 2445 | 4061 | 685 | 772 | 1020 | 350 | 386 | 456 | 215 | 231 | 258 | 145 | 154 | 166 |
| *** | 2300 | 2752 | 4182 | 721 | 854 | 1030 | 366 | 414 | 446 | 222 | 243 | 242 | 149 | 159 | 148 |
| 0.55 *** | 2063 | 2323 | 4016 | 655 | 746 | 998 | 336 | 372 | 441 | 205 | 221 | 246 | 137 | 145 | 157 |
| *** | 2160 | 2655 | 4098 | 693 | 830 | 999 | 351 | 399 | 428 | 212 | 232 | 229 | 141 | 151 | 138 |
| 0.6 *** | 1889 | 2173 | 3879 | 617 | 708 | 952 | 316 | 350 | 416 | 191 | 206 | 229 | 127 | 134 | 144 |
| *** | 1998 | 2520 | 3930 | 655 | 790 | 946 | 331 | 377 | 400 | 198 | 216 | 211 | 130 | 139 | 124 |
| 0.65 *** | 1704 | 2002 | 3652 | 570 | 657 | 884 | 290 | 322 | 380 | 173 | 187 | 207 | 113 | 120 | 128 |
| *** | 1820 | 2351 | 3678 | 607 | 735 | 873 | 304 | 346 | 362 | 180 | 196 | 187 | 116 | 123 | 107 |
| 0.7 *** | 1514 | 1811 | 3334 | 514 | 595 | 794 | 259 | 287 | 335 | 152 | 163 | 178 | 97 | 102 | 108 |
| *** | 1630 | 2148 | 3342 | 549 | 665 | 778 | 271 | 307 | 316 | 157 | 170 | 158 | 99 | 105 | 87 |
| 0.75 *** | 1318 | 1601 | 2927 | 450 | 520 | 681 | 221 | 244 | 280 | 126 | 134 | 145 | . | . | . |
| *** | 1430 | 1910 | 2922 | 480 | 579 | 662 | 231 | 259 | 260 | 129 | 139 | 124 | . | . | . |
| 0.8 *** | 1115 | 1367 | 2431 | 375 | 430 | 546 | 176 | 192 | 215 | . | . | . | . | . | . |
| *** | 1216 | 1633 | 2417 | 399 | 474 | 526 | 183 | 202 | 194 | . | . | . | . | . | . |
| 0.85 *** | 896 | 1099 | 1847 | 285 | 322 | 389 | . | . | . | . | . | . | . | . | . |
| *** | 979 | 1305 | 1829 | 301 | 349 | 368 | . | . | . | . | . | . | . | . | . |
| 0.9 *** | 643 | 777 | 1177 | . | . | . | . | . | . | . | . | . | . | . | . |
| *** | 699 | 903 | 1156 | . | . | . | . | . | . | . | . | . | . | . | . |

TABLE 6: ALPHA= 0.025 POWER= 0.9    EXPECTED ACCRUAL THRU MINIMUM FOLLOW-UP= 375

| | | DEL=.05 | | | DEL=.10 | | | DEL=.15 | | | DEL=.20 | | | DEL=.25 | | |
|---|---|---|---|---|---|---|---|---|---|---|---|---|---|---|---|---|---|
| FACT= | | 1.0 .75 | .50 .25 | .00 BIN | 1.0 .75 | .50 .25 | .00 BIN | 1.0 .75 | .50 .25 | .00 BIN | 1.0 75 | .50 .25 | .00 BIN | 1.0 .75 | .50 .25 | .00 BIN |
| PCONT=*** | | | | | REQUIRED NUMBER OF PATIENTS | | | | | | | | | | | |
| 0.05 | *** | 635 | 643 | 671 | 229 | 233 | 239 | 135 | 137 | 139 | 96 | 97 | 98 | 74 | 75 | 76 |
| | *** | 638 | 652 | 1156 | 231 | 235 | 368 | 136 | 138 | 194 | 96 | 97 | 124 | 75 | 75 | 87 |
| 0.1 | *** | 1160 | 1180 | 1295 | 368 | 378 | 400 | 200 | 205 | 212 | 133 | 136 | 139 | 99 | 100 | 102 |
| | *** | 1167 | 1209 | 1829 | 372 | 387 | 526 | 202 | 208 | 260 | 134 | 137 | 158 | 99 | 101 | 107 |
| 0.15 | *** | 1609 | 1644 | 1898 | 483 | 502 | 548 | 252 | 261 | 276 | 163 | 167 | 174 | 117 | 120 | 124 |
| | *** | 1621 | 1699 | 2417 | 491 | 519 | 662 | 256 | 268 | 316 | 165 | 170 | 187 | 118 | 122 | 124 |
| 0.2 | *** | 1960 | 2014 | 2448 | 573 | 603 | 679 | 294 | 307 | 332 | 186 | 193 | 203 | 132 | 136 | 141 |
| | *** | 1979 | 2100 | 2922 | 585 | 630 | 778 | 300 | 317 | 362 | 189 | 198 | 211 | 133 | 138 | 138 |
| 0.25 | *** | 2210 | 2286 | 2930 | 640 | 680 | 791 | 325 | 343 | 377 | 203 | 213 | 227 | 142 | 148 | 155 |
| | *** | 2237 | 2407 | 3342 | 656 | 719 | 873 | 333 | 358 | 400 | 208 | 219 | 229 | 145 | 151 | 148 |
| 0.3 | *** | 2364 | 2466 | 3331 | 684 | 737 | 882 | 346 | 370 | 413 | 215 | 227 | 245 | 149 | 156 | 164 |
| | *** | 2399 | 2626 | 3678 | 706 | 786 | 946 | 357 | 388 | 428 | 221 | 235 | 242 | 152 | 160 | 154 |
| 0.35 | *** | 2431 | 2563 | 3648 | 709 | 773 | 950 | 359 | 387 | 439 | 222 | 236 | 257 | 153 | 160 | 170 |
| | *** | 2477 | 2764 | 3930 | 735 | 833 | 999 | 371 | 408 | 446 | 228 | 245 | 250 | 156 | 165 | 158 |
| 0.4 | *** | 2422 | 2588 | 3876 | 718 | 791 | 997 | 364 | 395 | 455 | 225 | 239 | 263 | 154 | 162 | 172 |
| | *** | 2480 | 2830 | 4098 | 748 | 860 | 1030 | 378 | 419 | 456 | 231 | 250 | 253 | 157 | 167 | 158 |
| 0.45 | *** | 2352 | 2554 | 4014 | 712 | 793 | 1020 | 362 | 396 | 460 | 223 | 238 | 263 | 152 | 160 | 171 |
| | *** | 2425 | 2834 | 4182 | 745 | 869 | 1041 | 377 | 422 | 456 | 230 | 249 | 250 | 155 | 165 | 154 |
| 0.5 | *** | 2235 | 2472 | 4061 | 693 | 781 | 1020 | 354 | 389 | 456 | 216 | 233 | 257 | 146 | 154 | 166 |
| | *** | 2322 | 2785 | 4182 | 730 | 861 | 1030 | 369 | 416 | 446 | 224 | 243 | 242 | 150 | 160 | 148 |
| 0.55 | *** | 2085 | 2353 | 4016 | 664 | 755 | 998 | 340 | 375 | 441 | 207 | 222 | 246 | 138 | 146 | 157 |
| | *** | 2186 | 2691 | 4098 | 702 | 837 | 999 | 355 | 401 | 428 | 214 | 233 | 229 | 142 | 151 | 138 |
| 0.6 | *** | 1914 | 2206 | 3879 | 626 | 717 | 952 | 319 | 354 | 415 | 193 | 207 | 229 | 128 | 135 | 144 |
| | *** | 2026 | 2557 | 3930 | 664 | 797 | 946 | 334 | 379 | 400 | 199 | 217 | 211 | 131 | 139 | 124 |
| 0.65 | *** | 1731 | 2035 | 3652 | 579 | 666 | 884 | 294 | 325 | 380 | 175 | 188 | 207 | 114 | 120 | 128 |
| | *** | 1849 | 2387 | 3678 | 615 | 742 | 873 | 308 | 348 | 362 | 181 | 196 | 187 | 117 | 124 | 107 |
| 0.7 | *** | 1541 | 1843 | 3334 | 523 | 603 | 794 | 262 | 289 | 335 | 153 | 164 | 178 | 98 | 102 | 108 |
| | *** | 1660 | 2182 | 3342 | 557 | 671 | 778 | 274 | 309 | 316 | 158 | 170 | 158 | 100 | 105 | 87 |
| 0.75 | *** | 1345 | 1631 | 2927 | 457 | 527 | 681 | 224 | 245 | 280 | 127 | 134 | 145 | . | . | . |
| | *** | 1458 | 1941 | 2922 | 487 | 584 | 662 | 234 | 260 | 260 | 130 | 139 | 124 | . | . | . |
| 0.8 | *** | 1139 | 1393 | 2431 | 381 | 435 | 546 | 178 | 193 | 215 | . | . | . | . | . | . |
| | *** | 1241 | 1659 | 2417 | 404 | 478 | 526 | 185 | 203 | 194 | . | . | . | . | . | . |
| 0.85 | *** | 916 | 1120 | 1847 | 289 | 325 | 389 | . | . | . | . | . | . | . | . | . |
| | *** | 999 | 1325 | 1829 | 305 | 351 | 368 | . | . | . | . | . | . | . | . | . |
| 0.9 | *** | 656 | 791 | 1177 | . | . | . | . | . | . | . | . | . | . | . | . |
| | *** | 712 | 915 | 1156 | . | . | . | . | . | . | . | . | . | . | . | . |

TABLE 6: ALPHA= 0.025 POWER= 0.9     EXPECTED ACCRUAL THRU MINIMUM FOLLOW-UP= 400

| | | DEL=.05 | | | DEL=.10 | | | DEL=.15 | | | DEL=.20 | | | DEL=.25 | | |
|---|---|---|---|---|---|---|---|---|---|---|---|---|---|---|---|---|
| FACT= | | 1.0 .75 | .50 .25 | .00 BIN | 1.0 .75 | .50 .25 | .00 BIN | 1.0 .75 | .50 .25 | .00 BIN | 1.0 75 | .50 .25 | .00 BIN | 1.0 .75 | .50 .25 | .00 BIN |
| PCONT=*** | | | | | REQUIRED | NUMBER OF | PATIENTS | | | | | | | | | |
| 0.05 | *** | 635 | 644 | 671 | 230 | 233 | 239 | 135 | 137 | 139 | 96 | 97 | 98 | 75 | 75 | 76 |
| | *** | 638 | 653 | 1156 | 231 | 235 | 368 | 136 | 138 | 194 | 96 | 97 | 124 | 75 | 76 | 87 |
| 0.1 | *** | 1161 | 1182 | 1295 | 369 | 379 | 400 | 200 | 205 | 212 | 133 | 136 | 139 | 99 | 100 | 102 |
| | *** | 1169 | 1212 | 1829 | 373 | 387 | 526 | 202 | 208 | 260 | 134 | 137 | 158 | 99 | 101 | 107 |
| 0.15 | *** | 1611 | 1648 | 1898 | 485 | 504 | 548 | 253 | 262 | 276 | 163 | 168 | 174 | 118 | 120 | 124 |
| | *** | 1624 | 1705 | 2417 | 493 | 521 | 662 | 257 | 268 | 316 | 165 | 171 | 187 | 119 | 122 | 124 |
| 0.2 | *** | 1964 | 2021 | 2448 | 576 | 606 | 679 | 295 | 309 | 332 | 187 | 194 | 203 | 132 | 136 | 141 |
| | *** | 1984 | 2109 | 2922 | 588 | 633 | 778 | 301 | 318 | 362 | 190 | 198 | 211 | 134 | 138 | 138 |
| 0.25 | *** | 2216 | 2296 | 2930 | 643 | 684 | 791 | 327 | 345 | 377 | 204 | 214 | 227 | 143 | 148 | 155 |
| | *** | 2243 | 2421 | 3342 | 660 | 722 | 873 | 335 | 359 | 400 | 209 | 219 | 229 | 145 | 151 | 148 |
| 0.3 | *** | 2371 | 2479 | 3331 | 689 | 742 | 882 | 349 | 372 | 413 | 217 | 228 | 245 | 150 | 156 | 164 |
| | *** | 2409 | 2643 | 3678 | 711 | 790 | 946 | 359 | 389 | 428 | 222 | 235 | 242 | 153 | 160 | 154 |
| 0.35 | *** | 2440 | 2579 | 3648 | 715 | 779 | 950 | 362 | 389 | 439 | 224 | 237 | 257 | 154 | 161 | 170 |
| | *** | 2489 | 2785 | 3930 | 741 | 838 | 999 | 374 | 410 | 446 | 230 | 246 | 250 | 157 | 165 | 158 |
| 0.4 | *** | 2434 | 2608 | 3876 | 724 | 798 | 997 | 367 | 398 | 455 | 226 | 241 | 263 | 155 | 162 | 173 |
| | *** | 2496 | 2855 | 4098 | 755 | 866 | 1030 | 381 | 421 | 456 | 233 | 250 | 253 | 158 | 167 | 158 |
| 0.45 | *** | 2367 | 2577 | 4014 | 719 | 801 | 1020 | 366 | 399 | 461 | 224 | 240 | 263 | 152 | 160 | 171 |
| | *** | 2443 | 2863 | 4182 | 753 | 876 | 1041 | 380 | 424 | 456 | 231 | 250 | 250 | 156 | 165 | 154 |
| 0.5 | *** | 2253 | 2499 | 4061 | 701 | 789 | 1020 | 357 | 392 | 456 | 218 | 234 | 258 | 147 | 155 | 166 |
| | *** | 2344 | 2817 | 4182 | 738 | 868 | 1030 | 373 | 418 | 446 | 225 | 244 | 242 | 151 | 160 | 148 |
| 0.55 | *** | 2106 | 2383 | 4016 | 673 | 763 | 998 | 343 | 378 | 441 | 208 | 223 | 246 | 139 | 147 | 157 |
| | *** | 2211 | 2724 | 4098 | 711 | 844 | 999 | 358 | 403 | 428 | 215 | 234 | 229 | 143 | 151 | 138 |
| 0.6 | *** | 1938 | 2237 | 3879 | 634 | 725 | 952 | 323 | 356 | 416 | 194 | 208 | 229 | 128 | 135 | 144 |
| | *** | 2053 | 2591 | 3930 | 672 | 804 | 946 | 338 | 381 | 400 | 201 | 218 | 211 | 132 | 139 | 124 |
| 0.65 | *** | 1756 | 2066 | 3652 | 587 | 674 | 884 | 297 | 327 | 380 | 176 | 189 | 207 | 115 | 120 | 128 |
| | *** | 1877 | 2420 | 3678 | 624 | 748 | 873 | 311 | 350 | 362 | 182 | 197 | 187 | 117 | 124 | 107 |
| 0.7 | *** | 1567 | 1874 | 3334 | 530 | 610 | 794 | 265 | 291 | 335 | 154 | 164 | 179 | 98 | 102 | 108 |
| | *** | 1688 | 2214 | 3342 | 564 | 677 | 778 | 277 | 310 | 316 | 159 | 171 | 158 | 100 | 105 | 87 |
| 0.75 | *** | 1369 | 1659 | 2927 | 464 | 533 | 681 | 226 | 247 | 280 | 128 | 135 | 145 | . | . | . |
| | *** | 1485 | 1970 | 2922 | 494 | 588 | 662 | 236 | 261 | 260 | 131 | 140 | 124 | . | . | . |
| 0.8 | *** | 1161 | 1418 | 2431 | 386 | 440 | 546 | 180 | 194 | 215 | . | . | . | . | . | . |
| | *** | 1265 | 1683 | 2417 | 410 | 481 | 526 | 186 | 204 | 194 | . | . | . | . | . | . |
| 0.85 | *** | 934 | 1140 | 1847 | 293 | 328 | 389 | . | . | . | . | . | . | . | . | . |
| | *** | 1018 | 1343 | 1829 | 308 | 353 | 368 | . | . | . | . | . | . | . | . | . |
| 0.9 | *** | 668 | 803 | 1177 | . | . | . | . | . | . | . | . | . | . | . | . |
| | *** | 725 | 925 | 1156 | . | . | . | . | . | . | . | . | . | . | . | . |

TABLE 6: ALPHA= 0.025 POWER= 0.9     EXPECTED ACCRUAL THRU MINIMUM FOLLOW-UP= 425

|  | | DEL=.05 | | | DEL=.10 | | | DEL=.15 | | | DEL=.20 | | | DEL=.25 | | |
|---|---|---|---|---|---|---|---|---|---|---|---|---|---|---|---|---|
| FACT= | | 1.0 .75 | .50 .25 | .00 BIN | 1.0 .75 | .50 .25 | .00 BIN | 1.0 .75 | .50 .25 | .00 BIN | 1.0 75 | .50 .25 | .00 BIN | 1.0 .75 | .50 .25 | .00 BIN |
| PCONT=*** | | | | | REQUIRED NUMBER OF PATIENTS | | | | | | | | | | | |
| 0.05 | *** | 636 | 644 | 671 | 230 | 233 | 239 | 136 | 137 | 139 | 96 | 97 | 98 | 75 | 75 | 76 |
|  | *** | 639 | 654 | 1156 | 231 | 236 | 368 | 136 | 138 | 194 | 96 | 97 | 124 | 75 | 76 | 87 |
| 0.1 | *** | 1163 | 1185 | 1295 | 370 | 380 | 400 | 201 | 205 | 212 | 133 | 136 | 139 | 99 | 100 | 102 |
|  | *** | 1171 | 1215 | 1829 | 374 | 388 | 526 | 203 | 208 | 260 | 135 | 137 | 158 | 99 | 101 | 107 |
| 0.15 | *** | 1614 | 1652 | 1898 | 486 | 506 | 548 | 254 | 263 | 276 | 164 | 168 | 174 | 118 | 120 | 124 |
|  | *** | 1627 | 1710 | 2417 | 494 | 522 | 662 | 258 | 269 | 316 | 166 | 171 | 187 | 119 | 122 | 124 |
| 0.2 | *** | 1968 | 2027 | 2448 | 578 | 608 | 679 | 297 | 309 | 332 | 187 | 194 | 203 | 133 | 136 | 141 |
|  | *** | 1988 | 2118 | 2922 | 591 | 635 | 778 | 302 | 319 | 362 | 190 | 198 | 211 | 134 | 138 | 138 |
| 0.25 | *** | 2221 | 2305 | 2930 | 647 | 688 | 791 | 328 | 346 | 377 | 205 | 214 | 227 | 144 | 148 | 155 |
|  | *** | 2250 | 2433 | 3342 | 664 | 725 | 873 | 336 | 359 | 400 | 209 | 220 | 229 | 146 | 151 | 148 |
| 0.3 | *** | 2379 | 2491 | 3331 | 693 | 746 | 882 | 351 | 374 | 413 | 218 | 229 | 245 | 151 | 156 | 164 |
|  | *** | 2418 | 2660 | 3678 | 715 | 794 | 946 | 361 | 390 | 428 | 223 | 236 | 242 | 154 | 160 | 154 |
| 0.35 | *** | 2449 | 2594 | 3648 | 720 | 784 | 951 | 365 | 391 | 439 | 225 | 238 | 257 | 155 | 161 | 170 |
|  | *** | 2501 | 2805 | 3930 | 747 | 842 | 999 | 376 | 411 | 446 | 231 | 246 | 250 | 158 | 166 | 158 |
| 0.4 | *** | 2446 | 2627 | 3876 | 731 | 804 | 997 | 370 | 400 | 455 | 228 | 242 | 263 | 155 | 163 | 172 |
|  | *** | 2511 | 2879 | 4098 | 761 | 871 | 1030 | 384 | 423 | 456 | 234 | 251 | 253 | 159 | 167 | 158 |
| 0.45 | *** | 2382 | 2600 | 4014 | 726 | 808 | 1020 | 369 | 401 | 460 | 226 | 241 | 263 | 153 | 161 | 171 |
|  | *** | 2461 | 2890 | 4182 | 760 | 881 | 1041 | 383 | 426 | 456 | 233 | 251 | 250 | 157 | 166 | 154 |
| 0.5 | *** | 2271 | 2524 | 4061 | 709 | 796 | 1020 | 361 | 394 | 456 | 220 | 235 | 257 | 148 | 155 | 166 |
|  | *** | 2365 | 2846 | 4182 | 745 | 874 | 1030 | 376 | 420 | 446 | 227 | 245 | 242 | 152 | 160 | 148 |
| 0.55 | *** | 2127 | 2410 | 4016 | 681 | 771 | 998 | 346 | 380 | 441 | 210 | 224 | 246 | 140 | 147 | 156 |
|  | *** | 2235 | 2756 | 4098 | 719 | 850 | 999 | 361 | 405 | 428 | 217 | 234 | 229 | 143 | 152 | 138 |
| 0.6 | *** | 1961 | 2266 | 3879 | 642 | 732 | 952 | 326 | 359 | 416 | 196 | 209 | 229 | 129 | 136 | 144 |
|  | *** | 2079 | 2623 | 3930 | 680 | 810 | 946 | 341 | 382 | 400 | 202 | 218 | 211 | 132 | 139 | 124 |
| 0.65 | *** | 1781 | 2096 | 3652 | 595 | 681 | 884 | 300 | 330 | 380 | 178 | 190 | 207 | 115 | 121 | 128 |
|  | *** | 1904 | 2452 | 3678 | 631 | 754 | 873 | 313 | 351 | 362 | 183 | 197 | 187 | 118 | 124 | 107 |
| 0.7 | *** | 1591 | 1903 | 3334 | 538 | 616 | 794 | 267 | 293 | 335 | 155 | 165 | 179 | 99 | 103 | 108 |
|  | *** | 1715 | 2244 | 3342 | 571 | 682 | 778 | 279 | 311 | 316 | 160 | 171 | 158 | 101 | 105 | 87 |
| 0.75 | *** | 1393 | 1686 | 2927 | 470 | 538 | 681 | 228 | 249 | 280 | 128 | 136 | 145 | . | . | . |
|  | *** | 1510 | 1997 | 2922 | 500 | 592 | 662 | 238 | 262 | 260 | 132 | 140 | 124 | . | . | . |
| 0.8 | *** | 1183 | 1441 | 2431 | 391 | 444 | 546 | 181 | 195 | 215 | . | . | . | . | . | . |
|  | *** | 1287 | 1706 | 2417 | 414 | 484 | 526 | 188 | 204 | 194 | . | . | . | . | . | . |
| 0.85 | *** | 952 | 1158 | 1847 | 296 | 330 | 389 | . | . | . | . | . | . | . | . | . |
|  | *** | 1036 | 1360 | 1829 | 311 | 355 | 368 | . | . | . | . | . | . | . | . | . |
| 0.9 | *** | 680 | 814 | 1177 | . | . | . | . | . | . | . | . | . | . | . | . |
|  | *** | 736 | 935 | 1156 | . | . | . | . | . | . | . | . | . | . | . | . |

TABLE 6: ALPHA= 0.025 POWER= 0.9    EXPECTED ACCRUAL THRU MINIMUM FOLLOW-UP= 450

| | | DEL=.05 | | | DEL=.10 | | | DEL=.15 | | | DEL=.20 | | | DEL=.25 | | |
|---|---|---|---|---|---|---|---|---|---|---|---|---|---|---|---|---|
| FACT= | | 1.0 .75 | .50 .25 | .00 BIN | 1.0 .75 | .50 .25 | .00 BIN | 1.0 .75 | .50 .25 | .00 BIN | 1.0 75 | .50 .25 | .00 BIN | 1.0 .75 | .50 .25 | .00 BIN |
| PCONT=*** | | | | | REQUIRED NUMBER OF PATIENTS | | | | | | | | | | | |
| 0.05 | *** | 636 | 645 | 671 | 230 | 234 | 239 | 136 | 137 | 139 | 96 | 97 | 98 | 75 | 75 | 76 |
| | *** | 640 | 654 | 1156 | 231 | 236 | 368 | 136 | 138 | 194 | 96 | 97 | 124 | 75 | 75 | 87 |
| 0.1 | *** | 1164 | 1187 | 1295 | 371 | 381 | 400 | 201 | 206 | 212 | 134 | 136 | 139 | 99 | 100 | 102 |
| | *** | 1172 | 1217 | 1829 | 375 | 388 | 526 | 203 | 208 | 260 | 135 | 138 | 158 | 100 | 101 | 107 |
| 0.15 | *** | 1616 | 1657 | 1898 | 488 | 507 | 548 | 255 | 263 | 276 | 164 | 168 | 174 | 118 | 120 | 123 |
| | *** | 1630 | 1715 | 2417 | 496 | 523 | 662 | 259 | 269 | 316 | 166 | 171 | 187 | 119 | 122 | 124 |
| 0.2 | *** | 1971 | 2034 | 2448 | 581 | 611 | 679 | 298 | 311 | 332 | 188 | 194 | 203 | 133 | 136 | 141 |
| | *** | 1993 | 2126 | 2922 | 593 | 636 | 778 | 303 | 320 | 362 | 191 | 199 | 211 | 135 | 139 | 138 |
| 0.25 | *** | 2226 | 2314 | 2930 | 650 | 691 | 791 | 330 | 348 | 378 | 206 | 215 | 227 | 144 | 149 | 154 |
| | *** | 2257 | 2445 | 3342 | 667 | 728 | 873 | 338 | 360 | 400 | 210 | 220 | 229 | 146 | 151 | 148 |
| 0.3 | *** | 2385 | 2503 | 3331 | 698 | 750 | 882 | 353 | 375 | 414 | 219 | 229 | 245 | 151 | 157 | 164 |
| | *** | 2427 | 2675 | 3678 | 720 | 798 | 946 | 363 | 391 | 428 | 224 | 236 | 242 | 154 | 160 | 154 |
| 0.35 | *** | 2458 | 2610 | 3648 | 726 | 789 | 950 | 367 | 393 | 439 | 226 | 239 | 257 | 155 | 162 | 170 |
| | *** | 2512 | 2824 | 3930 | 752 | 847 | 999 | 379 | 412 | 446 | 232 | 247 | 250 | 158 | 166 | 158 |
| 0.4 | *** | 2457 | 2645 | 3876 | 737 | 810 | 996 | 373 | 402 | 455 | 229 | 243 | 263 | 156 | 163 | 172 |
| | *** | 2525 | 2901 | 4098 | 768 | 876 | 1030 | 386 | 424 | 456 | 235 | 252 | 253 | 159 | 167 | 158 |
| 0.45 | *** | 2396 | 2621 | 4014 | 733 | 815 | 1020 | 372 | 404 | 460 | 227 | 242 | 263 | 154 | 161 | 171 |
| | *** | 2479 | 2916 | 4182 | 767 | 887 | 1041 | 386 | 427 | 456 | 234 | 251 | 250 | 157 | 166 | 154 |
| 0.5 | *** | 2288 | 2549 | 4061 | 716 | 803 | 1020 | 364 | 397 | 456 | 221 | 236 | 258 | 149 | 156 | 166 |
| | *** | 2386 | 2874 | 4182 | 753 | 880 | 1030 | 379 | 421 | 446 | 228 | 246 | 242 | 152 | 160 | 148 |
| 0.55 | *** | 2147 | 2437 | 4016 | 688 | 778 | 998 | 349 | 383 | 441 | 211 | 226 | 246 | 141 | 148 | 157 |
| | *** | 2258 | 2785 | 4098 | 726 | 856 | 999 | 364 | 407 | 428 | 218 | 235 | 229 | 144 | 152 | 138 |
| 0.6 | *** | 1983 | 2294 | 3879 | 650 | 739 | 952 | 329 | 361 | 415 | 197 | 210 | 229 | 130 | 136 | 144 |
| | *** | 2104 | 2653 | 3930 | 688 | 816 | 946 | 343 | 384 | 400 | 203 | 219 | 211 | 133 | 140 | 124 |
| 0.65 | *** | 1805 | 2124 | 3652 | 602 | 687 | 884 | 303 | 332 | 380 | 179 | 190 | 207 | 116 | 121 | 128 |
| | *** | 1930 | 2482 | 3678 | 639 | 759 | 873 | 316 | 352 | 362 | 184 | 198 | 187 | 118 | 124 | 107 |
| 0.7 | *** | 1615 | 1930 | 3334 | 545 | 622 | 794 | 270 | 295 | 335 | 156 | 166 | 179 | 99 | 103 | 108 |
| | *** | 1740 | 2272 | 3342 | 578 | 686 | 778 | 281 | 312 | 316 | 161 | 172 | 158 | 101 | 105 | 87 |
| 0.75 | *** | 1416 | 1711 | 2927 | 477 | 543 | 681 | 230 | 250 | 280 | 129 | 136 | 145 | . | . | . |
| | *** | 1534 | 2022 | 2922 | 505 | 596 | 662 | 239 | 263 | 260 | 132 | 140 | 124 | . | . | . |
| 0.8 | *** | 1203 | 1463 | 2431 | 396 | 448 | 546 | 183 | 196 | 215 | . | . | . | . | . | . |
| | *** | 1308 | 1727 | 2417 | 419 | 487 | 526 | 189 | 204 | 194 | . | . | . | . | . | . |
| 0.85 | *** | 968 | 1175 | 1847 | 299 | 333 | 389 | . | . | . | . | . | . | . | . | . |
| | *** | 1053 | 1375 | 1829 | 314 | 356 | 368 | . | . | . | . | . | . | . | . | . |
| 0.9 | *** | 691 | 825 | 1177 | . | . | . | . | . | . | . | . | . | . | . | . |
| | *** | 748 | 944 | 1156 | . | . | . | . | . | . | . | . | . | . | . | . |

# TABLE 6: ALPHA= 0.025 POWER= 0.9    EXPECTED ACCRUAL THRU MINIMUM FOLLOW-UP= 475

| PCONT=*** | | DEL=.05 | | | DEL=.10 | | | DEL=.15 | | | DEL=.20 | | | DEL=.25 | | |
|---|---|---|---|---|---|---|---|---|---|---|---|---|---|---|---|---|
| FACT= | | 1.0 .75 | .50 .25 | .00 BIN | 1.0 .75 | .50 .25 | .00 BIN | 1.0 .75 | .50 .25 | .00 BIN | 1.0 75 | .50 .25 | .00 BIN | 1.0 .75 | .50 .25 | .00 BIN |
| | | | | | REQUIRED NUMBER OF PATIENTS | | | | | | | | | | | |
| 0.05 | *** | 637 | 646 | 671 | 230 | 234 | 239 | 136 | 137 | 139 | 96 | 97 | 98 | 75 | 75 | 76 |
| | *** | 641 | 655 | 1156 | 232 | 236 | 368 | 137 | 138 | 194 | 96 | 97 | 124 | 75 | 75 | 87 |
| 0.1 | *** | 1166 | 1189 | 1295 | 371 | 381 | 400 | 202 | 206 | 212 | 134 | 136 | 139 | 99 | 100 | 102 |
| | *** | 1174 | 1219 | 1829 | 376 | 389 | 526 | 204 | 209 | 260 | 135 | 137 | 158 | 100 | 101 | 107 |
| 0.15 | *** | 1619 | 1661 | 1898 | 489 | 509 | 548 | 256 | 264 | 276 | 165 | 169 | 174 | 118 | 121 | 124 |
| | *** | 1633 | 1720 | 2417 | 498 | 524 | 662 | 259 | 269 | 316 | 167 | 171 | 187 | 119 | 122 | 124 |
| 0.2 | *** | 1975 | 2040 | 2448 | 583 | 613 | 679 | 299 | 311 | 332 | 188 | 195 | 203 | 133 | 137 | 141 |
| | *** | 1998 | 2134 | 2922 | 596 | 638 | 778 | 304 | 320 | 362 | 191 | 199 | 211 | 135 | 139 | 138 |
| 0.25 | *** | 2231 | 2323 | 2930 | 653 | 694 | 791 | 332 | 349 | 377 | 207 | 215 | 227 | 144 | 149 | 155 |
| | *** | 2264 | 2456 | 3342 | 670 | 730 | 873 | 339 | 361 | 400 | 211 | 221 | 229 | 146 | 151 | 148 |
| 0.3 | *** | 2392 | 2515 | 3331 | 701 | 754 | 882 | 355 | 376 | 413 | 220 | 230 | 245 | 152 | 157 | 165 |
| | *** | 2436 | 2690 | 3678 | 724 | 801 | 946 | 365 | 392 | 428 | 224 | 237 | 242 | 154 | 161 | 154 |
| 0.35 | *** | 2468 | 2625 | 3648 | 731 | 794 | 950 | 369 | 395 | 439 | 227 | 239 | 257 | 156 | 162 | 170 |
| | *** | 2524 | 2843 | 3930 | 757 | 851 | 999 | 381 | 414 | 446 | 233 | 247 | 250 | 159 | 166 | 158 |
| 0.4 | *** | 2469 | 2663 | 3876 | 742 | 816 | 997 | 376 | 405 | 455 | 230 | 243 | 263 | 157 | 164 | 172 |
| | *** | 2540 | 2923 | 4098 | 773 | 881 | 1030 | 388 | 426 | 456 | 236 | 252 | 253 | 160 | 168 | 158 |
| 0.45 | *** | 2410 | 2642 | 4014 | 739 | 821 | 1020 | 374 | 406 | 460 | 229 | 243 | 263 | 155 | 162 | 171 |
| | *** | 2496 | 2940 | 4182 | 773 | 891 | 1041 | 389 | 429 | 456 | 235 | 252 | 250 | 158 | 166 | 154 |
| 0.5 | *** | 2306 | 2572 | 4061 | 723 | 810 | 1020 | 367 | 399 | 456 | 223 | 237 | 257 | 149 | 156 | 166 |
| | *** | 2406 | 2901 | 4182 | 760 | 885 | 1030 | 381 | 423 | 446 | 229 | 246 | 242 | 153 | 161 | 148 |
| 0.55 | *** | 2167 | 2463 | 4016 | 695 | 785 | 998 | 352 | 385 | 441 | 213 | 226 | 246 | 141 | 148 | 156 |
| | *** | 2280 | 2813 | 4098 | 733 | 861 | 999 | 367 | 408 | 428 | 219 | 235 | 229 | 145 | 152 | 138 |
| 0.6 | *** | 2005 | 2321 | 3879 | 657 | 746 | 952 | 332 | 363 | 416 | 198 | 211 | 229 | 130 | 136 | 144 |
| | *** | 2128 | 2682 | 3930 | 695 | 821 | 946 | 346 | 385 | 400 | 204 | 219 | 211 | 133 | 140 | 124 |
| 0.65 | *** | 1827 | 2151 | 3652 | 609 | 694 | 884 | 305 | 334 | 380 | 180 | 191 | 207 | 116 | 121 | 128 |
| | *** | 1955 | 2510 | 3678 | 645 | 764 | 873 | 318 | 354 | 362 | 185 | 198 | 187 | 119 | 124 | 107 |
| 0.7 | *** | 1638 | 1956 | 3334 | 551 | 628 | 794 | 272 | 297 | 335 | 157 | 166 | 178 | 99 | 103 | 108 |
| | *** | 1765 | 2299 | 3342 | 584 | 691 | 778 | 283 | 313 | 316 | 162 | 172 | 158 | 101 | 105 | 87 |
| 0.75 | *** | 1438 | 1735 | 2927 | 482 | 548 | 681 | 232 | 251 | 280 | 130 | 136 | 145 | . | . | . |
| | *** | 1557 | 2046 | 2922 | 511 | 599 | 662 | 241 | 264 | 260 | 133 | 140 | 124 | . | . | . |
| 0.8 | *** | 1223 | 1484 | 2431 | 400 | 451 | 546 | 184 | 197 | 215 | . | . | . | . | . | . |
| | *** | 1329 | 1747 | 2417 | 423 | 490 | 526 | 190 | 205 | 194 | . | . | . | . | . | . |
| 0.85 | *** | 984 | 1191 | 1847 | 302 | 335 | 389 | . | . | . | . | . | . | . | . | . |
| | *** | 1069 | 1390 | 1829 | 317 | 358 | 368 | . | . | . | . | . | . | . | . | . |
| 0.9 | *** | 702 | 835 | 1177 | . | . | . | . | . | . | . | . | . | . | . | . |
| | *** | 758 | 952 | 1156 | . | . | . | . | . | . | . | . | . | . | . | . |

TABLE 6: ALPHA= 0.025 POWER= 0.9    EXPECTED ACCRUAL THRU MINIMUM FOLLOW-UP= 500

| | | DEL=.05 | | | DEL=.10 | | | DEL=.15 | | | DEL=.20 | | | DEL=.25 | | |
|---|---|---|---|---|---|---|---|---|---|---|---|---|---|---|---|---|
| FACT= | | 1.0 .75 | .50 .25 | .00 BIN | 1.0 .75 | .50 .25 | .00 BIN | 1.0 .75 | .50 .25 | .00 BIN | 1.0 75 | .50 .25 | .00 BIN | 1.0 .75 | .50 .25 | .00 BIN |
| PCONT=*** | | REQUIRED NUMBER OF PATIENTS | | | | | | | | | | | | | | |
| 0.05 | *** | 638 | 647 | 671 | 231 | 234 | 239 | 136 | 137 | 139 | 96 | 97 | 98 | 75 | 75 | 76 |
| | *** | 641 | 655 | 1156 | 232 | 236 | 368 | 137 | 138 | 194 | 97 | 98 | 124 | 75 | 76 | 87 |
| 0.1 | *** | 1167 | 1191 | 1295 | 372 | 382 | 400 | 202 | 206 | 212 | 134 | 136 | 139 | 99 | 101 | 102 |
| | *** | 1176 | 1222 | 1829 | 377 | 389 | 526 | 204 | 209 | 260 | 135 | 138 | 158 | 100 | 101 | 107 |
| 0.15 | *** | 1621 | 1665 | 1898 | 491 | 510 | 548 | 256 | 264 | 276 | 165 | 169 | 174 | 118 | 121 | 123 |
| | *** | 1637 | 1725 | 2417 | 499 | 525 | 662 | 260 | 270 | 316 | 167 | 171 | 187 | 120 | 122 | 124 |
| 0.2 | *** | 1979 | 2046 | 2448 | 585 | 615 | 679 | 300 | 312 | 332 | 189 | 195 | 203 | 133 | 137 | 141 |
| | *** | 2003 | 2142 | 2922 | 598 | 640 | 778 | 305 | 321 | 362 | 192 | 199 | 211 | 135 | 139 | 138 |
| 0.25 | *** | 2237 | 2332 | 2930 | 656 | 698 | 791 | 333 | 350 | 378 | 208 | 216 | 227 | 145 | 149 | 155 |
| | *** | 2270 | 2467 | 3342 | 673 | 733 | 873 | 341 | 362 | 400 | 212 | 221 | 229 | 147 | 152 | 148 |
| 0.3 | *** | 2399 | 2526 | 3331 | 706 | 758 | 882 | 357 | 378 | 413 | 221 | 231 | 245 | 152 | 158 | 164 |
| | *** | 2445 | 2704 | 3678 | 728 | 804 | 946 | 366 | 393 | 428 | 225 | 237 | 242 | 155 | 161 | 154 |
| 0.35 | *** | 2477 | 2639 | 3648 | 735 | 799 | 950 | 371 | 397 | 439 | 228 | 240 | 257 | 157 | 163 | 170 |
| | *** | 2535 | 2860 | 3930 | 762 | 854 | 999 | 383 | 415 | 446 | 234 | 248 | 250 | 159 | 166 | 158 |
| 0.4 | *** | 2481 | 2681 | 3876 | 748 | 821 | 997 | 378 | 407 | 455 | 231 | 244 | 263 | 158 | 164 | 173 |
| | *** | 2554 | 2944 | 4098 | 779 | 885 | 1030 | 391 | 427 | 456 | 237 | 253 | 253 | 161 | 168 | 158 |
| 0.45 | *** | 2425 | 2663 | 4014 | 745 | 826 | 1020 | 377 | 408 | 461 | 230 | 243 | 263 | 155 | 162 | 171 |
| | *** | 2513 | 2963 | 4182 | 779 | 896 | 1041 | 391 | 430 | 456 | 236 | 252 | 250 | 158 | 166 | 154 |
| 0.5 | *** | 2322 | 2595 | 4061 | 730 | 816 | 1020 | 369 | 401 | 456 | 224 | 238 | 258 | 150 | 157 | 166 |
| | *** | 2426 | 2927 | 4182 | 766 | 890 | 1030 | 384 | 424 | 446 | 230 | 247 | 242 | 153 | 161 | 148 |
| 0.55 | *** | 2186 | 2488 | 4016 | 702 | 791 | 998 | 355 | 387 | 441 | 214 | 227 | 246 | 142 | 148 | 157 |
| | *** | 2302 | 2840 | 4098 | 740 | 866 | 999 | 369 | 410 | 428 | 220 | 236 | 229 | 145 | 152 | 138 |
| 0.6 | *** | 2026 | 2347 | 3879 | 664 | 752 | 953 | 334 | 365 | 416 | 199 | 212 | 229 | 131 | 137 | 144 |
| | *** | 2151 | 2709 | 3930 | 702 | 826 | 946 | 348 | 387 | 400 | 205 | 220 | 211 | 134 | 140 | 124 |
| 0.65 | *** | 1849 | 2177 | 3652 | 615 | 699 | 884 | 308 | 336 | 380 | 181 | 192 | 207 | 117 | 122 | 128 |
| | *** | 1979 | 2537 | 3678 | 652 | 768 | 873 | 320 | 355 | 362 | 186 | 199 | 187 | 119 | 125 | 107 |
| 0.7 | *** | 1660 | 1981 | 3334 | 557 | 633 | 794 | 274 | 298 | 335 | 158 | 167 | 178 | 100 | 103 | 108 |
| | *** | 1788 | 2324 | 3342 | 590 | 694 | 778 | 285 | 314 | 316 | 162 | 172 | 158 | 102 | 106 | 87 |
| 0.75 | *** | 1458 | 1758 | 2927 | 487 | 552 | 681 | 234 | 253 | 280 | 130 | 137 | 145 | . | . | . |
| | *** | 1579 | 2069 | 2922 | 516 | 603 | 662 | 242 | 265 | 260 | 133 | 141 | 124 | . | . | . |
| 0.8 | *** | 1241 | 1503 | 2431 | 404 | 455 | 546 | 185 | 198 | 215 | . | . | . | . | . | . |
| | *** | 1348 | 1766 | 2417 | 427 | 492 | 526 | 191 | 206 | 194 | . | . | . | . | . | . |
| 0.85 | *** | 999 | 1207 | 1847 | 305 | 337 | 389 | . | . | . | . | . | . | . | . | . |
| | *** | 1085 | 1403 | 1829 | 319 | 359 | 368 | . | . | . | . | . | . | . | . | . |
| 0.9 | *** | 712 | 844 | 1177 | . | . | . | . | . | . | . | . | . | . | . | . |
| | *** | 768 | 960 | 1156 | . | . | . | . | . | . | . | . | . | . | . | . |

TABLE 6: ALPHA= 0.025 POWER= 0.9    EXPECTED ACCRUAL THRU MINIMUM FOLLOW-UP= 550

|  | | DEL=.02 | | | DEL=.05 | | | DEL=.10 | | | DEL=.15 | | | DEL=.20 | | |
|---|---|---|---|---|---|---|---|---|---|---|---|---|---|---|---|---|
| FACT= | | 1.0 .75 | .50 .25 | .00 BIN | 1.0 .75 | .50 .25 | .00 BIN | 1.0 .75 | .50 .25 | .00 BIN | 1.0 75 | .50 .25 | .00 BIN | 1.0 .75 | .50 .25 | .00 BIN |
| PCONT=*** | | | | | | | REQUIRED NUMBER OF PATIENTS | | | | | | | | | |
| 0.05 | *** | 2991 | 3002 | 3165 | 639 | 648 | 671 | 231 | 234 | 239 | 136 | 137 | 139 | 96 | 97 | 98 |
|  | *** | 2994 | 3024 | 5916 | 642 | 657 | 1156 | 233 | 236 | 368 | 137 | 138 | 194 | 96 | 98 | 124 |
| 0.1 | *** | 6221 | 6249 | 6954 | 1170 | 1195 | 1295 | 374 | 383 | 400 | 203 | 206 | 212 | 135 | 136 | 139 |
|  | *** | 6231 | 6303 | 10277 | 1179 | 1226 | 1829 | 378 | 390 | 526 | 204 | 209 | 260 | 135 | 138 | 158 |
| 0.15 | *** | 9088 | 9136 | 10755 | 1626 | 1672 | 1898 | 494 | 512 | 548 | 257 | 265 | 276 | 166 | 169 | 174 |
|  | *** | 9104 | 9231 | 14112 | 1643 | 1733 | 2417 | 501 | 527 | 662 | 261 | 270 | 316 | 167 | 171 | 187 |
| 0.2 | *** | 11370 | 11444 | 14290 | 1986 | 2058 | 2448 | 589 | 619 | 679 | 302 | 313 | 332 | 190 | 196 | 203 |
|  | *** | 11395 | 11591 | 17422 | 2012 | 2156 | 2922 | 602 | 642 | 778 | 307 | 321 | 362 | 193 | 199 | 211 |
| 0.25 | *** | 13007 | 13113 | 17424 | 2247 | 2348 | 2929 | 662 | 703 | 791 | 335 | 352 | 377 | 209 | 217 | 227 |
|  | *** | 13043 | 13325 | 20206 | 2283 | 2487 | 3342 | 679 | 737 | 873 | 343 | 363 | 400 | 212 | 221 | 229 |
| 0.3 | *** | 14009 | 14155 | 20081 | 2413 | 2549 | 3331 | 713 | 765 | 882 | 360 | 380 | 413 | 222 | 232 | 245 |
|  | *** | 14058 | 14445 | 22465 | 2462 | 2731 | 3678 | 735 | 809 | 946 | 369 | 395 | 428 | 226 | 237 | 242 |
| 0.35 | *** | 14422 | 14615 | 22217 | 2494 | 2667 | 3648 | 744 | 807 | 950 | 375 | 399 | 439 | 230 | 241 | 257 |
|  | *** | 14486 | 15001 | 24199 | 2557 | 2893 | 3930 | 771 | 861 | 999 | 386 | 417 | 446 | 235 | 248 | 250 |
| 0.4 | *** | 14308 | 14561 | 23808 | 2503 | 2714 | 3876 | 758 | 831 | 996 | 382 | 410 | 455 | 233 | 246 | 263 |
|  | *** | 14392 | 15064 | 25407 | 2581 | 2982 | 4098 | 789 | 892 | 1030 | 395 | 429 | 456 | 239 | 253 | 253 |
| 0.45 | *** | 13747 | 14072 | 24838 | 2452 | 2701 | 4014 | 756 | 837 | 1020 | 382 | 411 | 461 | 232 | 245 | 263 |
|  | *** | 13855 | 14716 | 26090 | 2546 | 3007 | 4182 | 791 | 904 | 1041 | 395 | 432 | 456 | 238 | 253 | 250 |
| 0.5 | *** | 12822 | 13238 | 25298 | 2355 | 2638 | 4061 | 742 | 827 | 1020 | 374 | 405 | 456 | 226 | 239 | 257 |
|  | *** | 12961 | 14047 | 26248 | 2463 | 2974 | 4182 | 778 | 899 | 1030 | 388 | 426 | 446 | 232 | 247 | 242 |
| 0.55 | *** | 11623 | 12152 | 25187 | 2223 | 2534 | 4016 | 715 | 802 | 998 | 360 | 391 | 441 | 216 | 228 | 246 |
|  | *** | 11800 | 13148 | 25880 | 2344 | 2890 | 4098 | 752 | 875 | 999 | 374 | 412 | 428 | 222 | 237 | 229 |
| 0.6 | *** | 10245 | 10912 | 24505 | 2066 | 2395 | 3880 | 676 | 763 | 952 | 339 | 368 | 415 | 201 | 213 | 229 |
|  | *** | 10470 | 12099 | 24987 | 2195 | 2760 | 3930 | 714 | 834 | 946 | 353 | 389 | 400 | 207 | 221 | 211 |
| 0.65 | *** | 8787 | 9614 | 23253 | 1891 | 2226 | 3652 | 628 | 710 | 884 | 312 | 338 | 380 | 182 | 193 | 206 |
|  | *** | 9072 | 10966 | 23569 | 2024 | 2586 | 3678 | 663 | 776 | 873 | 324 | 357 | 362 | 188 | 199 | 187 |
| 0.7 | *** | 7353 | 8333 | 21436 | 1702 | 2028 | 3334 | 568 | 643 | 794 | 278 | 301 | 335 | 159 | 168 | 178 |
|  | *** | 7702 | 9787 | 21625 | 1832 | 2370 | 3342 | 600 | 701 | 778 | 288 | 316 | 316 | 163 | 173 | 158 |
| 0.75 | *** | 6029 | 7108 | 19057 | 1498 | 1801 | 2927 | 497 | 560 | 681 | 236 | 254 | 280 | 131 | 137 | 145 |
|  | *** | 6427 | 8580 | 19156 | 1621 | 2110 | 2922 | 525 | 608 | 662 | 245 | 266 | 260 | 134 | 141 | 124 |
| 0.8 | *** | 4853 | 5940 | 16122 | 1276 | 1540 | 2431 | 412 | 461 | 546 | 187 | 199 | 215 | . | . | . |
|  | *** | 5266 | 7332 | 16161 | 1384 | 1800 | 2417 | 433 | 496 | 526 | 192 | 206 | 194 | . | . | . |
| 0.85 | *** | 3804 | 4793 | 12638 | 1027 | 1235 | 1847 | 310 | 341 | 389 | . | . | . | . | . | . |
|  | *** | 4186 | 6003 | 12641 | 1113 | 1428 | 1829 | 324 | 362 | 368 | . | . | . | . | . | . |
| 0.9 | *** | 2800 | 3584 | 8610 | 731 | 862 | 1177 | . | . | . | . | . | . | . | . | . |
|  | *** | 3107 | 4499 | 8596 | 786 | 973 | 1156 | . | . | . | . | . | . | . | . | . |
| 0.95 | *** | 1671 | 2114 | 4045 | . | . | . | . | . | . | . | . | . | . | . | . |
|  | *** | 1848 | 2585 | 4025 | . | . | . | . | . | . | . | . | . | . | . | . |

TABLE 6: ALPHA= 0.025 POWER= 0.9     EXPECTED ACCRUAL THRU MINIMUM FOLLOW-UP= 600

| | DEL=.02 | | | DEL=.05 | | | DEL=.10 | | | DEL=.15 | | | DEL=.20 | | |
|---|---|---|---|---|---|---|---|---|---|---|---|---|---|---|---|
| FACT= | 1.0 .75 | .50 .25 | .00 BIN | 1.0 .75 | .50 .25 | .00 BIN | 1.0 .75 | .50 .25 | .00 BIN | 1.0 75 | .50 .25 | .00 BIN | 1.0 .75 | .50 .25 | .00 BIN |
| PCONT=*** | | | REQUIRED NUMBER OF PATIENTS | | | | | | | | | | | | |
| 0.05 *** | 2992 3004 | 3004 3028 | 3165 5916 | 640 643 | 649 657 | 671 1156 | 232 233 | 235 236 | 239 368 | 136 137 | 137 138 | 139 194 | 96 97 | 97 97 | 98 124 |
| 0.1 *** | 6224 6234 | 6254 6313 | 6954 10277 | 1172 1182 | 1199 1229 | 1295 1829 | 375 379 | 384 391 | 400 526 | 203 205 | 207 209 | 212 260 | 135 136 | 137 138 | 139 158 |
| 0.15 *** | 9092 9110 | 9145 9249 | 10755 14112 | 1630 1648 | 1679 1741 | 1898 2417 | 496 504 | 514 528 | 548 662 | 259 262 | 266 271 | 276 316 | 166 168 | 170 172 | 174 187 |
| 0.2 *** | 11377 11404 | 11457 11618 | 14290 17422 | 1993 2021 | 2069 2168 | 2448 2922 | 593 605 | 622 645 | 679 778 | 303 308 | 315 322 | 331 362 | 191 193 | 196 200 | 203 211 |
| 0.25 *** | 13017 13055 | 13133 13363 | 17424 20206 | 2257 2296 | 2364 2506 | 2929 3342 | 667 684 | 707 740 | 791 873 | 338 345 | 353 364 | 377 400 | 210 214 | 217 221 | 227 229 |
| 0.3 *** | 14023 14075 | 14181 14498 | 20081 22465 | 2427 2479 | 2569 2755 | 3331 3678 | 719 742 | 771 814 | 881 946 | 363 371 | 382 396 | 413 428 | 224 228 | 232 238 | 245 242 |
| 0.35 *** | 14439 14509 | 14650 15071 | 22217 24199 | 2512 2579 | 2693 2923 | 3648 3930 | 752 779 | 815 866 | 950 999 | 379 389 | 402 418 | 439 446 | 232 237 | 242 249 | 256 250 |
| 0.4 *** | 14331 14423 | 14607 15154 | 23808 25407 | 2525 2608 | 2746 3017 | 3876 4098 | 767 798 | 839 899 | 997 1030 | 386 398 | 413 431 | 455 456 | 235 241 | 247 254 | 263 253 |
| 0.45 *** | 13777 13895 | 14131 14830 | 24838 26090 | 2479 2577 | 2737 3046 | 4014 4182 | 767 801 | 846 911 | 1020 1041 | 386 399 | 415 434 | 460 456 | 234 239 | 246 254 | 263 250 |
| 0.5 *** | 12860 13011 | 13313 14187 | 25298 26248 | 2386 2498 | 2678 3017 | 4061 4182 | 753 789 | 837 906 | 1020 1030 | 379 392 | 408 429 | 455 446 | 228 234 | 241 248 | 257 242 |
| 0.55 *** | 11671 11864 | 12247 13314 | 25187 25880 | 2258 2383 | 2577 2935 | 4016 4098 | 726 763 | 812 883 | 998 999 | 364 377 | 394 414 | 440 428 | 218 223 | 230 237 | 246 229 |
| 0.6 *** | 10306 10551 | 11030 12289 | 24505 24987 | 2104 2236 | 2440 2806 | 3879 3930 | 688 725 | 773 841 | 952 946 | 343 356 | 371 391 | 415 400 | 203 208 | 214 221 | 229 211 |
| 0.65 *** | 8866 9174 | 9754 11173 | 23253 23569 | 1930 2066 | 2270 2631 | 3652 3678 | 638 674 | 719 783 | 884 873 | 316 327 | 341 358 | 380 362 | 184 189 | 194 200 | 206 187 |
| 0.7 *** | 7450 7824 | 8489 10002 | 21436 21625 | 1740 1874 | 2071 2413 | 3334 3342 | 578 610 | 651 707 | 794 778 | 281 291 | 303 317 | 335 316 | 161 164 | 169 173 | 178 158 |
| 0.75 *** | 6142 6562 | 7271 8791 | 19057 19156 | 1534 1659 | 1840 2147 | 2927 2922 | 505 532 | 567 613 | 681 662 | 239 247 | 256 267 | 280 260 | 132 135 | 138 141 | 145 124 |
| 0.8 *** | 4972 5401 | 6098 7527 | 16122 16161 | 1309 1417 | 1574 1830 | 2431 2417 | 419 440 | 466 499 | 546 526 | 189 194 | 200 207 | 215 194 | . . | . . | . . |
| 0.85 *** | 3915 4309 | 4933 6168 | 12638 12641 | 1053 1139 | 1260 1450 | 1847 1829 | 314 328 | 344 364 | 389 368 | . . | . . | . . | . . | . . | . . |
| 0.9 *** | 2890 3205 | 3692 4621 | 8610 8596 | 748 803 | 877 986 | 1177 1156 | . . | . . | . . | . . | . . | . . | . . | . . | . . |
| 0.95 *** | 1723 1904 | 2172 2644 | 4045 4025 | . . | . . | . . | . . | . . | . . | . . | . . | . . | . . | . . | . . |

## TABLE 6: ALPHA= 0.025 POWER= 0.9 EXPECTED ACCRUAL THRU MINIMUM FOLLOW-UP= 650

| | | DEL=.02 | | | DEL=.05 | | | DEL=.10 | | | DEL=.15 | | | DEL=.20 | | |
|---|---|---|---|---|---|---|---|---|---|---|---|---|---|---|---|---|
| FACT= | | 1.0 .75 | .50 .25 | .00 BIN | 1.0 .75 | .50 .25 | .00 BIN | 1.0 .75 | .50 .25 | .00 BIN | 1.0 75 | .50 .25 | .00 BIN | 1.0 .75 | .50 .25 | .00 BIN |
| PCONT=*** | | | | | REQUIRED | NUMBER | OF PATIENTS | | | | | | | | | |
| 0.05 | *** | 2993 | 3006 | 3165 | 641 | 650 | 671 | 232 | 235 | 239 | 136 | 138 | 139 | 97 | 97 | 98 |
| | *** | 2997 | 3031 | 5916 | 645 | 658 | 1156 | 233 | 237 | 368 | 137 | 138 | 194 | 97 | 97 | 124 |
| 0.1 | *** | 6226 | 6259 | 6954 | 1175 | 1202 | 1295 | 376 | 385 | 400 | 204 | 207 | 212 | 135 | 137 | 139 |
| | *** | 6237 | 6322 | 10277 | 1185 | 1233 | 1829 | 380 | 392 | 526 | 205 | 210 | 260 | 136 | 138 | 158 |
| 0.15 | *** | 9097 | 9154 | 10755 | 1635 | 1686 | 1898 | 498 | 516 | 548 | 259 | 267 | 276 | 166 | 170 | 174 |
| | *** | 9116 | 9266 | 14112 | 1654 | 1748 | 2417 | 506 | 529 | 662 | 263 | 271 | 316 | 168 | 172 | 187 |
| 0.2 | *** | 11384 | 11471 | 14290 | 2000 | 2080 | 2448 | 597 | 625 | 679 | 305 | 316 | 331 | 192 | 197 | 203 |
| | *** | 11413 | 11645 | 17422 | 2030 | 2180 | 2922 | 609 | 647 | 778 | 310 | 323 | 362 | 194 | 200 | 211 |
| 0.25 | *** | 13027 | 13152 | 17424 | 2267 | 2379 | 2930 | 672 | 712 | 791 | 340 | 355 | 377 | 211 | 218 | 227 |
| | *** | 13068 | 13402 | 20206 | 2308 | 2523 | 3342 | 689 | 743 | 873 | 347 | 365 | 400 | 214 | 222 | 229 |
| 0.3 | *** | 14036 | 14208 | 20081 | 2440 | 2589 | 3331 | 726 | 777 | 881 | 366 | 385 | 413 | 225 | 233 | 244 |
| | *** | 14093 | 14550 | 22465 | 2495 | 2777 | 3678 | 748 | 818 | 946 | 374 | 397 | 428 | 229 | 239 | 242 |
| 0.35 | *** | 14457 | 14685 | 22218 | 2530 | 2718 | 3648 | 760 | 821 | 951 | 382 | 405 | 439 | 233 | 243 | 257 |
| | *** | 14533 | 15140 | 24199 | 2600 | 2950 | 3930 | 786 | 871 | 999 | 392 | 419 | 446 | 238 | 249 | 250 |
| 0.4 | *** | 14354 | 14653 | 23808 | 2547 | 2775 | 3876 | 776 | 847 | 996 | 389 | 415 | 455 | 237 | 248 | 263 |
| | *** | 14454 | 15243 | 25407 | 2633 | 3050 | 4098 | 806 | 904 | 1030 | 401 | 432 | 456 | 242 | 255 | 253 |
| 0.45 | *** | 13806 | 14191 | 24838 | 2505 | 2772 | 4014 | 777 | 855 | 1020 | 390 | 418 | 461 | 236 | 247 | 263 |
| | *** | 13934 | 14942 | 26090 | 2607 | 3083 | 4182 | 810 | 918 | 1041 | 402 | 436 | 456 | 241 | 255 | 250 |
| 0.5 | *** | 12898 | 13388 | 25298 | 2416 | 2716 | 4061 | 763 | 846 | 1020 | 383 | 411 | 456 | 230 | 242 | 257 |
| | *** | 13061 | 14324 | 26248 | 2532 | 3057 | 4182 | 799 | 913 | 1030 | 396 | 431 | 446 | 236 | 249 | 242 |
| 0.55 | *** | 11719 | 12341 | 25188 | 2291 | 2618 | 4016 | 736 | 821 | 998 | 368 | 397 | 441 | 220 | 231 | 246 |
| | *** | 11928 | 13476 | 25880 | 2420 | 2976 | 4098 | 773 | 889 | 999 | 381 | 416 | 428 | 225 | 238 | 229 |
| 0.6 | *** | 10368 | 11146 | 24505 | 2140 | 2481 | 3880 | 698 | 782 | 952 | 347 | 374 | 415 | 205 | 216 | 229 |
| | *** | 10633 | 12472 | 24987 | 2275 | 2848 | 3930 | 735 | 848 | 946 | 359 | 392 | 400 | 210 | 222 | 211 |
| 0.65 | *** | 8943 | 9890 | 23253 | 1967 | 2312 | 3652 | 648 | 728 | 884 | 319 | 344 | 380 | 185 | 195 | 207 |
| | *** | 9275 | 11370 | 23569 | 2105 | 2672 | 3678 | 683 | 789 | 873 | 331 | 360 | 362 | 190 | 201 | 187 |
| 0.7 | *** | 7546 | 8640 | 21436 | 1777 | 2111 | 3334 | 587 | 658 | 794 | 284 | 305 | 335 | 162 | 169 | 179 |
| | *** | 7942 | 10205 | 21625 | 1912 | 2451 | 3342 | 619 | 712 | 778 | 294 | 318 | 316 | 165 | 174 | 158 |
| 0.75 | *** | 6252 | 7428 | 19057 | 1568 | 1877 | 2927 | 513 | 573 | 681 | 242 | 258 | 280 | 133 | 138 | 145 |
| | *** | 6691 | 8989 | 19156 | 1694 | 2181 | 2922 | 540 | 617 | 662 | 249 | 268 | 260 | 136 | 141 | 124 |
| 0.8 | *** | 5086 | 6249 | 16122 | 1338 | 1605 | 2431 | 425 | 470 | 546 | 190 | 201 | 215 | . | . | . |
| | *** | 5531 | 7709 | 16161 | 1448 | 1858 | 2417 | 445 | 502 | 526 | 195 | 207 | 194 | . | . | . |
| 0.85 | *** | 4020 | 5065 | 12638 | 1077 | 1284 | 1847 | 318 | 346 | 389 | . | . | . | . | . | . |
| | *** | 4426 | 6322 | 12641 | 1164 | 1470 | 1829 | 331 | 365 | 368 | . | . | . | . | . | . |
| 0.9 | *** | 2975 | 3794 | 8610 | 763 | 891 | 1177 | . | . | . | . | . | . | . | . | . |
| | *** | 3298 | 4734 | 8596 | 818 | 996 | 1156 | . | . | . | . | . | . | . | . | . |
| 0.95 | *** | 1773 | 2226 | 4045 | . | . | . | . | . | . | . | . | . | . | . | . |
| | *** | 1956 | 2697 | 4025 | . | . | . | . | . | . | . | . | . | . | . | . |

TABLE 6: ALPHA= 0.025 POWER= 0.9    EXPECTED ACCRUAL THRU MINIMUM FOLLOW-UP= 700

| | | DEL=.02 | | | DEL=.05 | | | DEL=.10 | | | DEL=.15 | | | DEL=.20 | |
|---|---|---|---|---|---|---|---|---|---|---|---|---|---|---|---|---|
| FACT= | 1.0 .75 | .50 .25 | .00 BIN | 1.0 .75 | .50 .25 | .00 BIN | 1.0 .75 | .50 .25 | .00 BIN | 1.0 75 | .50 .25 | .00 BIN | 1.0 .75 | .50 .25 | .00 BIN |
| PCONT=*** | | | | | REQUIRED NUMBER OF PATIENTS | | | | | | | | | | |
| 0.05 *** | 2994 | 3008 | 3166 | 642 | 651 | 671 | 233 | 235 | 239 | 137 | 138 | 139 | 96 | 97 | 98 |
| *** | 2998 | 3035 | 5916 | 646 | 659 | 1156 | 233 | 236 | 368 | 137 | 138 | 194 | 97 | 97 | 124 |
| 0.1 *** | 6229 | 6263 | 6954 | 1178 | 1206 | 1295 | 377 | 386 | 400 | 204 | 208 | 212 | 135 | 137 | 139 |
| *** | 6240 | 6332 | 10277 | 1188 | 1236 | 1829 | 381 | 392 | 526 | 206 | 210 | 260 | 136 | 138 | 158 |
| 0.15 *** | 9101 | 9162 | 10755 | 1640 | 1693 | 1898 | 500 | 518 | 548 | 261 | 267 | 276 | 167 | 170 | 174 |
| *** | 9122 | 9283 | 14112 | 1660 | 1755 | 2417 | 508 | 530 | 662 | 264 | 271 | 316 | 169 | 172 | 187 |
| 0.2 *** | 11390 | 11484 | 14290 | 2007 | 2090 | 2448 | 600 | 628 | 679 | 306 | 317 | 331 | 192 | 197 | 203 |
| *** | 11422 | 11671 | 17422 | 2038 | 2191 | 2922 | 612 | 649 | 778 | 311 | 324 | 362 | 195 | 200 | 211 |
| 0.25 *** | 13036 | 13171 | 17424 | 2277 | 2394 | 2930 | 677 | 716 | 791 | 342 | 356 | 377 | 212 | 219 | 227 |
| *** | 13081 | 13440 | 20206 | 2320 | 2538 | 3342 | 693 | 746 | 873 | 348 | 366 | 400 | 215 | 222 | 229 |
| 0.3 *** | 14049 | 14234 | 20081 | 2453 | 2608 | 3331 | 731 | 782 | 882 | 368 | 386 | 413 | 226 | 234 | 245 |
| *** | 14111 | 14602 | 22465 | 2511 | 2798 | 3678 | 753 | 821 | 946 | 376 | 398 | 428 | 230 | 239 | 242 |
| 0.35 *** | 14474 | 14720 | 22218 | 2546 | 2741 | 3648 | 767 | 828 | 950 | 384 | 406 | 439 | 235 | 244 | 257 |
| *** | 14556 | 15209 | 24199 | 2620 | 2976 | 3930 | 793 | 876 | 999 | 394 | 421 | 446 | 239 | 250 | 250 |
| 0.4 *** | 14377 | 14698 | 23808 | 2567 | 2803 | 3876 | 784 | 854 | 996 | 393 | 418 | 455 | 238 | 249 | 263 |
| *** | 14485 | 15332 | 25407 | 2657 | 3080 | 4098 | 814 | 909 | 1030 | 404 | 434 | 456 | 243 | 255 | 253 |
| 0.45 *** | 13836 | 14250 | 24838 | 2530 | 2804 | 4014 | 785 | 862 | 1020 | 393 | 420 | 460 | 237 | 248 | 263 |
| *** | 13974 | 15052 | 26090 | 2635 | 3117 | 4182 | 818 | 923 | 1041 | 405 | 438 | 456 | 242 | 255 | 250 |
| 0.5 *** | 12935 | 13463 | 25298 | 2445 | 2752 | 4061 | 772 | 854 | 1020 | 386 | 414 | 456 | 231 | 243 | 257 |
| *** | 13112 | 14458 | 26248 | 2564 | 3093 | 4182 | 807 | 919 | 1030 | 398 | 432 | 446 | 236 | 250 | 242 |
| 0.55 *** | 11768 | 12435 | 25188 | 2323 | 2655 | 4016 | 746 | 830 | 998 | 372 | 399 | 441 | 221 | 232 | 246 |
| *** | 11992 | 13632 | 25880 | 2454 | 3015 | 4098 | 782 | 895 | 999 | 384 | 418 | 428 | 226 | 239 | 229 |
| 0.6 *** | 10429 | 11260 | 24505 | 2173 | 2520 | 3880 | 708 | 790 | 952 | 350 | 376 | 415 | 206 | 216 | 229 |
| *** | 10713 | 12647 | 24987 | 2312 | 2886 | 3930 | 744 | 854 | 946 | 362 | 394 | 400 | 211 | 222 | 211 |
| 0.65 *** | 9021 | 10023 | 23253 | 2002 | 2350 | 3652 | 657 | 735 | 884 | 322 | 346 | 380 | 187 | 196 | 207 |
| *** | 9374 | 11558 | 23569 | 2142 | 2709 | 3678 | 691 | 795 | 873 | 333 | 361 | 362 | 191 | 201 | 187 |
| 0.7 *** | 7640 | 8786 | 21436 | 1811 | 2147 | 3334 | 595 | 665 | 794 | 287 | 307 | 335 | 163 | 170 | 178 |
| *** | 8057 | 10397 | 21625 | 1948 | 2485 | 3342 | 626 | 717 | 778 | 296 | 320 | 316 | 166 | 174 | 158 |
| 0.75 *** | 6358 | 7577 | 19057 | 1601 | 1910 | 2927 | 520 | 579 | 681 | 243 | 259 | 280 | 134 | 139 | 145 |
| *** | 6815 | 9176 | 19156 | 1727 | 2212 | 2922 | 546 | 621 | 662 | 251 | 269 | 260 | 136 | 142 | 124 |
| 0.8 *** | 5196 | 6392 | 16122 | 1367 | 1633 | 2431 | 430 | 474 | 546 | 192 | 202 | 215 | . | . | . |
| *** | 5654 | 7880 | 16161 | 1477 | 1883 | 2417 | 450 | 505 | 526 | 197 | 208 | 194 | . | . | . |
| 0.85 *** | 4121 | 5190 | 12638 | 1099 | 1305 | 1847 | 322 | 349 | 389 | . | . | . | . | . | . |
| *** | 4537 | 6466 | 12641 | 1186 | 1488 | 1829 | 334 | 367 | 368 | . | . | . | . | . | . |
| 0.9 *** | 3056 | 3890 | 8610 | 777 | 903 | 1177 | . | . | . | . | . | . | . | . | . |
| *** | 3385 | 4838 | 8596 | 831 | 1006 | 1156 | . | . | . | . | . | . | . | . | . |
| 0.95 *** | 1819 | 2277 | 4045 | . | . | . | . | . | . | . | . | . | . | . | . |
| *** | 2004 | 2746 | 4025 | . | . | . | . | . | . | . | . | . | . | . | . |

## TABLE 6: ALPHA= 0.025 POWER= 0.9     EXPECTED ACCRUAL THRU MINIMUM FOLLOW-UP= 750

| | | DEL=.02 | | | DEL=.05 | | | DEL=.10 | | | DEL=.15 | | | DEL=.20 | | |
|---|---|---|---|---|---|---|---|---|---|---|---|---|---|---|---|---|
| FACT= | | 1.0 .75 | .50 .25 | .00 BIN | 1.0 .75 | .50 .25 | .00 BIN | 1.0 .75 | .50 .25 | .00 BIN | 1.0 75 | .50 .25 | .00 BIN | 1.0 .75 | .50 .25 | .00 BIN |
| PCONT=*** | | | | | REQUIRED NUMBER OF PATIENTS | | | | | | | | | | | |
| 0.05 | *** | 2995 | 3010 | 3165 | 643 | 652 | 671 | 233 | 235 | 239 | 137 | 138 | 139 | 97 | 97 | 98 |
| | *** | 3000 | 3038 | 5916 | 647 | 660 | 1156 | 234 | 237 | 368 | 137 | 139 | 194 | 97 | 98 | 124 |
| 0.1 | *** | 6231 | 6268 | 6954 | 1180 | 1209 | 1295 | 378 | 387 | 400 | 205 | 208 | 212 | 136 | 137 | 139 |
| | *** | 6244 | 6341 | 10277 | 1191 | 1238 | 1829 | 382 | 393 | 526 | 206 | 210 | 260 | 136 | 138 | 158 |
| 0.15 | *** | 9106 | 9171 | 10755 | 1644 | 1699 | 1898 | 502 | 519 | 548 | 261 | 268 | 276 | 168 | 170 | 174 |
| | *** | 9127 | 9300 | 14112 | 1665 | 1761 | 2417 | 510 | 531 | 662 | 264 | 272 | 316 | 169 | 172 | 187 |
| 0.2 | *** | 11397 | 11498 | 14290 | 2014 | 2100 | 2449 | 603 | 630 | 679 | 307 | 318 | 332 | 193 | 198 | 203 |
| | *** | 11431 | 11698 | 17422 | 2046 | 2201 | 2922 | 615 | 650 | 778 | 312 | 324 | 362 | 195 | 200 | 211 |
| 0.25 | *** | 13046 | 13190 | 17424 | 2286 | 2407 | 2929 | 680 | 719 | 791 | 343 | 357 | 378 | 213 | 219 | 227 |
| | *** | 13094 | 13478 | 20206 | 2332 | 2553 | 3342 | 697 | 748 | 873 | 350 | 366 | 400 | 216 | 223 | 229 |
| 0.3 | *** | 14062 | 14260 | 20081 | 2466 | 2626 | 3331 | 737 | 786 | 881 | 370 | 387 | 413 | 227 | 235 | 244 |
| | *** | 14128 | 14654 | 22465 | 2526 | 2817 | 3678 | 758 | 825 | 946 | 378 | 399 | 428 | 230 | 239 | 242 |
| 0.35 | *** | 14492 | 14755 | 22218 | 2563 | 2764 | 3648 | 773 | 833 | 950 | 387 | 408 | 439 | 235 | 245 | 257 |
| | *** | 14580 | 15278 | 24199 | 2639 | 3000 | 3930 | 799 | 880 | 999 | 397 | 422 | 446 | 240 | 250 | 250 |
| 0.4 | *** | 14400 | 14744 | 23808 | 2588 | 2830 | 3876 | 791 | 860 | 997 | 395 | 419 | 455 | 239 | 250 | 263 |
| | *** | 14515 | 15419 | 25407 | 2680 | 3108 | 4098 | 821 | 914 | 1030 | 407 | 435 | 456 | 244 | 256 | 253 |
| 0.45 | *** | 13865 | 14308 | 24837 | 2554 | 2834 | 4014 | 793 | 869 | 1020 | 396 | 422 | 460 | 238 | 249 | 263 |
| | *** | 14013 | 15161 | 26090 | 2663 | 3147 | 4182 | 826 | 928 | 1041 | 408 | 439 | 456 | 244 | 256 | 250 |
| 0.5 | *** | 12973 | 13538 | 25298 | 2472 | 2785 | 4061 | 781 | 861 | 1020 | 389 | 416 | 456 | 233 | 244 | 258 |
| | *** | 13162 | 14589 | 26248 | 2595 | 3126 | 4182 | 816 | 924 | 1030 | 401 | 433 | 446 | 238 | 250 | 242 |
| 0.55 | *** | 11815 | 12528 | 25188 | 2353 | 2691 | 4016 | 755 | 837 | 998 | 375 | 401 | 441 | 222 | 233 | 246 |
| | *** | 12056 | 13784 | 25880 | 2487 | 3049 | 4098 | 791 | 901 | 999 | 387 | 419 | 428 | 227 | 239 | 229 |
| 0.6 | *** | 10490 | 11372 | 24505 | 2206 | 2557 | 3879 | 716 | 797 | 952 | 354 | 379 | 415 | 207 | 217 | 229 |
| | *** | 10793 | 12817 | 24987 | 2346 | 2921 | 3930 | 752 | 859 | 946 | 365 | 395 | 400 | 212 | 223 | 211 |
| 0.65 | *** | 9098 | 10152 | 23253 | 2035 | 2387 | 3652 | 666 | 742 | 884 | 325 | 348 | 380 | 188 | 196 | 206 |
| | *** | 9471 | 11738 | 23569 | 2177 | 2744 | 3678 | 700 | 799 | 873 | 335 | 363 | 362 | 192 | 201 | 187 |
| 0.7 | *** | 7733 | 8926 | 21436 | 1843 | 2182 | 3334 | 603 | 671 | 794 | 289 | 309 | 335 | 164 | 170 | 178 |
| | *** | 8170 | 10581 | 21625 | 1981 | 2517 | 3342 | 633 | 722 | 778 | 298 | 320 | 316 | 167 | 174 | 158 |
| 0.75 | *** | 6461 | 7720 | 19057 | 1630 | 1941 | 2927 | 527 | 584 | 681 | 245 | 260 | 280 | 134 | 139 | 145 |
| | *** | 6935 | 9353 | 19156 | 1759 | 2240 | 2922 | 552 | 625 | 662 | 252 | 269 | 260 | 137 | 142 | 124 |
| 0.8 | *** | 5300 | 6527 | 16122 | 1393 | 1659 | 2431 | 435 | 478 | 546 | 193 | 203 | 215 | . | . | . |
| | *** | 5772 | 8042 | 16161 | 1504 | 1906 | 2417 | 454 | 507 | 526 | 198 | 208 | 194 | . | . | . |
| 0.85 | *** | 4218 | 5309 | 12638 | 1120 | 1324 | 1847 | 325 | 351 | 389 | . | . | . | . | . | . |
| | *** | 4643 | 6602 | 12641 | 1206 | 1504 | 1829 | 337 | 368 | 368 | . | . | . | . | . | . |
| 0.9 | *** | 3132 | 3980 | 8610 | 790 | 915 | 1177 | . | . | . | . | . | . | . | . | . |
| | *** | 3468 | 4936 | 8596 | 844 | 1015 | 1156 | . | . | . | . | . | . | . | . | . |
| 0.95 | *** | 1863 | 2324 | 4045 | . | . | . | . | . | . | . | . | . | . | . | . |
| | *** | 2050 | 2792 | 4025 | . | . | . | . | . | . | . | . | . | . | . | . |

TABLE 6: ALPHA= 0.025 POWER= 0.9    EXPECTED ACCRUAL THRU MINIMUM FOLLOW-UP= 800

| | | DEL=.02 | | | DEL=.05 | | | DEL=.10 | | | DEL=.15 | | | DEL=.20 | | |
|---|---|---|---|---|---|---|---|---|---|---|---|---|---|---|---|---|---|
| FACT= | | 1.0 .75 | .50 .25 | .00 BIN | 1.0 .75 | .50 .25 | .00 BIN | 1.0 .75 | .50 .25 | .00 BIN | 1.0 75 | .50 .25 | .00 BIN | 1.0 .75 | .50 .25 | .00 BIN |
| PCONT=*** | | REQUIRED NUMBER OF PATIENTS | | | | | | | | | | | | | | | |
| 0.05 | *** | 2996 | 3012 | 3165 | 644 | 653 | 671 | 233 | 235 | 239 | 137 | 138 | 139 | 97 | 97 | 98 |
| | *** | 3001 | 3041 | 5916 | 647 | 660 | 1156 | 234 | 237 | 368 | 137 | 139 | 194 | 97 | 98 | 124 |
| 0.1 | *** | 6234 | 6274 | 6954 | 1182 | 1212 | 1295 | 379 | 387 | 400 | 205 | 208 | 212 | 136 | 137 | 139 |
| | *** | 6247 | 6351 | 10277 | 1194 | 1241 | 1829 | 383 | 393 | 526 | 206 | 210 | 260 | 137 | 138 | 158 |
| 0.15 | *** | 9110 | 9179 | 10755 | 1648 | 1705 | 1898 | 504 | 521 | 548 | 262 | 268 | 276 | 168 | 171 | 174 |
| | *** | 9133 | 9317 | 14112 | 1670 | 1766 | 2417 | 511 | 532 | 662 | 265 | 272 | 316 | 169 | 172 | 187 |
| 0.2 | *** | 11404 | 11511 | 14290 | 2021 | 2109 | 2448 | 606 | 633 | 679 | 309 | 318 | 332 | 194 | 198 | 203 |
| | *** | 11440 | 11724 | 17422 | 2054 | 2210 | 2922 | 618 | 652 | 778 | 313 | 324 | 362 | 196 | 201 | 211 |
| 0.25 | *** | 13056 | 13210 | 17424 | 2296 | 2421 | 2930 | 684 | 722 | 791 | 345 | 359 | 377 | 214 | 219 | 227 |
| | *** | 13107 | 13516 | 20206 | 2343 | 2566 | 3342 | 701 | 751 | 873 | 351 | 367 | 400 | 216 | 223 | 229 |
| 0.3 | *** | 14076 | 14287 | 20081 | 2479 | 2643 | 3331 | 742 | 790 | 882 | 372 | 389 | 413 | 228 | 235 | 245 |
| | *** | 14146 | 14706 | 22465 | 2541 | 2835 | 3678 | 763 | 828 | 946 | 380 | 400 | 428 | 231 | 240 | 242 |
| 0.35 | *** | 14509 | 14791 | 22218 | 2579 | 2785 | 3648 | 779 | 838 | 950 | 389 | 410 | 439 | 237 | 246 | 257 |
| | *** | 14603 | 15345 | 24199 | 2658 | 3022 | 3930 | 805 | 883 | 999 | 399 | 423 | 446 | 241 | 251 | 250 |
| 0.4 | *** | 14423 | 14790 | 23808 | 2608 | 2855 | 3876 | 798 | 866 | 997 | 398 | 421 | 455 | 241 | 250 | 263 |
| | *** | 14546 | 15506 | 25407 | 2703 | 3133 | 4098 | 828 | 918 | 1030 | 409 | 436 | 456 | 245 | 256 | 253 |
| 0.45 | *** | 13895 | 14367 | 24838 | 2577 | 2863 | 4014 | 801 | 876 | 1020 | 399 | 424 | 461 | 240 | 250 | 263 |
| | *** | 14053 | 15268 | 26090 | 2689 | 3176 | 4182 | 833 | 933 | 1041 | 410 | 440 | 456 | 245 | 256 | 250 |
| 0.5 | *** | 13011 | 13612 | 25298 | 2499 | 2817 | 4061 | 789 | 868 | 1020 | 392 | 418 | 456 | 234 | 244 | 258 |
| | *** | 13213 | 14717 | 26248 | 2624 | 3158 | 4182 | 823 | 929 | 1030 | 404 | 435 | 446 | 239 | 251 | 242 |
| 0.55 | *** | 11864 | 12620 | 25188 | 2383 | 2724 | 4016 | 763 | 844 | 998 | 378 | 403 | 441 | 223 | 234 | 246 |
| | *** | 12120 | 13932 | 25880 | 2519 | 3082 | 4098 | 799 | 905 | 999 | 390 | 420 | 428 | 228 | 240 | 229 |
| 0.6 | *** | 10551 | 11482 | 24505 | 2237 | 2591 | 3879 | 725 | 804 | 952 | 356 | 381 | 416 | 208 | 218 | 229 |
| | *** | 10873 | 12980 | 24987 | 2379 | 2954 | 3930 | 760 | 864 | 946 | 368 | 396 | 400 | 213 | 223 | 211 |
| 0.65 | *** | 9174 | 10278 | 23253 | 2066 | 2420 | 3652 | 674 | 748 | 884 | 327 | 350 | 380 | 189 | 197 | 207 |
| | *** | 9567 | 11911 | 23569 | 2210 | 2776 | 3678 | 707 | 804 | 873 | 338 | 363 | 362 | 193 | 202 | 187 |
| 0.7 | *** | 7824 | 9062 | 21436 | 1874 | 2214 | 3334 | 610 | 677 | 794 | 291 | 310 | 335 | 164 | 171 | 179 |
| | *** | 8279 | 10756 | 21625 | 2013 | 2547 | 3342 | 640 | 725 | 778 | 300 | 321 | 316 | 168 | 175 | 158 |
| 0.75 | *** | 6562 | 7857 | 19057 | 1659 | 1970 | 2927 | 533 | 588 | 681 | 247 | 261 | 280 | 135 | 140 | 145 |
| | *** | 7051 | 9522 | 19156 | 1787 | 2266 | 2922 | 558 | 627 | 662 | 254 | 270 | 260 | 137 | 142 | 124 |
| 0.8 | *** | 5401 | 6657 | 16122 | 1418 | 1683 | 2431 | 440 | 481 | 546 | 194 | 204 | 215 | . | . | . |
| | *** | 5885 | 8195 | 16161 | 1528 | 1927 | 2417 | 459 | 509 | 526 | 199 | 209 | 194 | . | . | . |
| 0.85 | *** | 4309 | 5422 | 12638 | 1140 | 1343 | 1847 | 328 | 353 | 389 | . | . | . | . | . | . |
| | *** | 4744 | 6730 | 12641 | 1226 | 1519 | 1829 | 339 | 369 | 368 | . | . | . | . | . | . |
| 0.9 | *** | 3205 | 4065 | 8610 | 803 | 925 | 1177 | . | . | . | . | . | . | . | . | . |
| | *** | 3546 | 5028 | 8596 | 856 | 1022 | 1156 | . | . | . | . | . | . | . | . | . |
| 0.95 | *** | 1904 | 2368 | 4045 | . | . | . | . | . | . | . | . | . | . | . | . |
| | *** | 2093 | 2834 | 4025 | . | . | . | . | . | . | . | . | . | . | . | . |

## TABLE 6: ALPHA= 0.025 POWER= 0.9    EXPECTED ACCRUAL THRU MINIMUM FOLLOW-UP= 850

|  |  | DEL=.02 | | | DEL=.05 | | | DEL=.10 | | | DEL=.15 | | | DEL=.20 | | |
|---|---|---|---|---|---|---|---|---|---|---|---|---|---|---|---|---|
| FACT= | | 1.0 .75 | .50 .25 | .00 BIN | 1.0 .75 | .50 .25 | .00 BIN | 1.0 .75 | .50 .25 | .00 BIN | 1.0 75 | .50 .25 | .00 BIN | 1.0 .75 | .50 .25 | .00 BIN |
| PCONT=*** | | | | | REQUIRED NUMBER OF PATIENTS | | | | | | | | | | | |
| 0.05 | *** | 2997 | 3014 | 3165 | 644 | 654 | 671 | 233 | 236 | 239 | 137 | 138 | 139 | 97 | 97 | 98 |
|  | *** | 3003 | 3044 | 5916 | 648 | 661 | 1156 | 235 | 237 | 368 | 137 | 138 | 194 | 97 | 97 | 124 |
| 0.1 | *** | 6237 | 6278 | 6954 | 1185 | 1215 | 1295 | 380 | 388 | 400 | 205 | 208 | 212 | 136 | 137 | 139 |
|  | *** | 6250 | 6360 | 10277 | 1196 | 1243 | 1829 | 384 | 393 | 526 | 207 | 210 | 260 | 137 | 138 | 158 |
| 0.15 | *** | 9114 | 9188 | 10755 | 1652 | 1710 | 1898 | 505 | 522 | 548 | 263 | 269 | 276 | 168 | 171 | 174 |
|  | *** | 9139 | 9334 | 14112 | 1675 | 1771 | 2417 | 513 | 533 | 662 | 265 | 272 | 316 | 169 | 172 | 187 |
| 0.2 | *** | 11410 | 11525 | 14290 | 2027 | 2118 | 2448 | 608 | 634 | 679 | 309 | 319 | 332 | 194 | 198 | 203 |
|  | *** | 11449 | 11750 | 17422 | 2062 | 2219 | 2922 | 620 | 654 | 778 | 314 | 325 | 362 | 196 | 201 | 211 |
| 0.25 | *** | 13065 | 13229 | 17424 | 2305 | 2433 | 2929 | 688 | 725 | 791 | 346 | 359 | 377 | 214 | 220 | 227 |
|  | *** | 13120 | 13553 | 20206 | 2354 | 2578 | 3342 | 705 | 752 | 873 | 352 | 368 | 400 | 217 | 223 | 229 |
| 0.3 | *** | 14089 | 14313 | 20081 | 2491 | 2660 | 3331 | 746 | 794 | 882 | 374 | 390 | 413 | 229 | 236 | 244 |
|  | *** | 14164 | 14757 | 22465 | 2555 | 2851 | 3678 | 767 | 830 | 946 | 381 | 401 | 428 | 232 | 240 | 242 |
| 0.35 | *** | 14527 | 14826 | 22218 | 2594 | 2805 | 3648 | 784 | 842 | 951 | 391 | 411 | 440 | 238 | 246 | 257 |
|  | *** | 14626 | 15412 | 24199 | 2675 | 3042 | 3930 | 810 | 886 | 999 | 400 | 424 | 446 | 242 | 251 | 250 |
| 0.4 | *** | 14446 | 14836 | 23808 | 2627 | 2879 | 3876 | 804 | 871 | 997 | 400 | 423 | 455 | 242 | 251 | 263 |
|  | *** | 14576 | 15591 | 25407 | 2725 | 3157 | 4098 | 834 | 922 | 1030 | 411 | 437 | 456 | 246 | 256 | 253 |
| 0.45 | *** | 13924 | 14426 | 24838 | 2600 | 2890 | 4014 | 808 | 882 | 1020 | 401 | 426 | 460 | 241 | 250 | 263 |
|  | *** | 14092 | 15373 | 26090 | 2713 | 3203 | 4182 | 840 | 937 | 1041 | 412 | 441 | 456 | 246 | 256 | 260 |
| 0.5 | *** | 13049 | 13686 | 25298 | 2524 | 2846 | 4061 | 797 | 874 | 1020 | 394 | 420 | 456 | 235 | 245 | 257 |
|  | *** | 13263 | 14841 | 26248 | 2652 | 3187 | 4182 | 831 | 933 | 1030 | 406 | 436 | 446 | 240 | 251 | 242 |
| 0.55 | *** | 11912 | 12710 | 25188 | 2411 | 2756 | 4016 | 771 | 850 | 998 | 380 | 405 | 441 | 224 | 234 | 246 |
|  | *** | 12183 | 14074 | 25880 | 2549 | 3112 | 4098 | 805 | 910 | 999 | 392 | 421 | 428 | 229 | 240 | 229 |
| 0.6 | *** | 10612 | 11590 | 24505 | 2266 | 2623 | 3879 | 732 | 810 | 952 | 359 | 382 | 416 | 209 | 219 | 229 |
|  | *** | 10952 | 13136 | 24987 | 2411 | 2985 | 3930 | 767 | 868 | 946 | 369 | 397 | 400 | 214 | 223 | 211 |
| 0.65 | *** | 9249 | 10400 | 23253 | 2096 | 2452 | 3652 | 681 | 754 | 884 | 329 | 351 | 380 | 190 | 197 | 207 |
|  | *** | 9661 | 12076 | 23569 | 2241 | 2805 | 3678 | 713 | 808 | 873 | 340 | 364 | 362 | 193 | 202 | 187 |
| 0.7 | *** | 7913 | 9192 | 21436 | 1903 | 2244 | 3334 | 616 | 682 | 794 | 293 | 311 | 335 | 165 | 171 | 179 |
|  | *** | 8385 | 10923 | 21625 | 2043 | 2574 | 3342 | 646 | 729 | 778 | 301 | 322 | 316 | 168 | 174 | 158 |
| 0.75 | *** | 6659 | 7989 | 19057 | 1686 | 1997 | 2927 | 538 | 593 | 681 | 249 | 262 | 280 | 136 | 140 | 145 |
|  | *** | 7163 | 9682 | 19156 | 1814 | 2290 | 2922 | 562 | 630 | 662 | 255 | 271 | 260 | 138 | 142 | 124 |
| 0.8 | *** | 5499 | 6781 | 16122 | 1441 | 1706 | 2431 | 444 | 484 | 546 | 195 | 204 | 215 | . | . | . |
|  | *** | 5994 | 8340 | 16161 | 1552 | 1946 | 2417 | 462 | 511 | 526 | 199 | 209 | 194 | . | . | . |
| 0.85 | *** | 4397 | 5529 | 12638 | 1158 | 1360 | 1847 | 330 | 355 | 389 | . | . | . | . | . | . |
|  | *** | 4840 | 6851 | 12641 | 1243 | 1532 | 1829 | 342 | 371 | 368 | . | . | . | . | . | . |
| 0.9 | *** | 3275 | 4147 | 8610 | 814 | 935 | 1177 | . | . | . | . | . | . | . | . | . |
|  | *** | 3621 | 5115 | 8596 | 867 | 1029 | 1156 | . | . | . | . | . | . | . | . | . |
| 0.95 | *** | 1943 | 2409 | 4045 | . | . | . | . | . | . | . | . | . | . | . | . |
|  | *** | 2134 | 2873 | 4025 | . | . | . | . | . | . | . | . | . | . | . | . |

## TABLE 6: ALPHA= 0.025 POWER= 0.9   EXPECTED ACCRUAL THRU MINIMUM FOLLOW-UP= 900

|        |       | DEL=.02 | | | DEL=.05 | | | DEL=.10 | | | DEL=.15 | | | DEL=.20 | | |
|--------|-------|------|------|------|------|------|------|------|------|------|------|------|------|------|------|------|
| FACT=  |       | 1.0 .75 | .50 .25 | .00 BIN | 1.0 .75 | .50 .25 | .00 BIN | 1.0 .75 | .50 .25 | .00 BIN | 1.0 75 | .50 .25 | .00 BIN | 1.0 .75 | .50 .25 | .00 BIN |
| PCONT=*** | | REQUIRED NUMBER OF PATIENTS | | | | | | | | | | | | | | |
| 0.05 | *** | 2998 | 3016 | 3165 | 645 | 654 | 671 | 234 | 236 | 239 | 137 | 138 | 139 | 97 | 98 | 98 |
|      | *** | 3004 | 3047 | 5916 | 649 | 661 | 1156 | 235 | 237 | 368 | 137 | 138 | 194 | 97 | 98 | 124 |
| 0.1  | *** | 6239 | 6283 | 6954 | 1187 | 1217 | 1295 | 381 | 388 | 399 | 206 | 208 | 212 | 136 | 137 | 139 |
|      | *** | 6254 | 6369 | 10277 | 1199 | 1245 | 1829 | 384 | 393 | 526 | 207 | 210 | 260 | 137 | 138 | 158 |
| 0.15 | *** | 9118 | 9197 | 10755 | 1657 | 1715 | 1898 | 507 | 523 | 548 | 263 | 269 | 276 | 168 | 171 | 174 |
|      | *** | 9145 | 9351 | 14112 | 1680 | 1776 | 2417 | 514 | 534 | 662 | 266 | 272 | 316 | 170 | 172 | 187 |
| 0.2  | *** | 11417 | 11538 | 14291 | 2034 | 2126 | 2448 | 611 | 636 | 679 | 311 | 320 | 332 | 194 | 199 | 203 |
|      | *** | 11457 | 11777 | 17422 | 2069 | 2227 | 2922 | 622 | 655 | 778 | 315 | 325 | 362 | 197 | 201 | 211 |
| 0.25 | *** | 13075 | 13248 | 17424 | 2314 | 2445 | 2930 | 692 | 728 | 791 | 348 | 360 | 378 | 215 | 220 | 227 |
|      | *** | 13133 | 13591 | 20206 | 2364 | 2591 | 3342 | 707 | 755 | 873 | 353 | 368 | 400 | 217 | 224 | 229 |
| 0.3  | *** | 14102 | 14340 | 20081 | 2503 | 2675 | 3331 | 750 | 798 | 882 | 375 | 391 | 414 | 229 | 236 | 245 |
|      | *** | 14181 | 14807 | 22465 | 2569 | 2867 | 3678 | 771 | 833 | 946 | 383 | 401 | 428 | 233 | 240 | 242 |
| 0.35 | *** | 14545 | 14861 | 22218 | 2610 | 2825 | 3648 | 789 | 847 | 950 | 393 | 413 | 440 | 239 | 246 | 257 |
|      | *** | 14650 | 15479 | 24199 | 2693 | 3061 | 3930 | 815 | 890 | 999 | 402 | 424 | 446 | 243 | 251 | 250 |
| 0.4  | *** | 14469 | 14882 | 23808 | 2645 | 2901 | 3876 | 810 | 876 | 996 | 402 | 424 | 455 | 243 | 252 | 263 |
|      | *** | 14607 | 15675 | 25407 | 2746 | 3179 | 4098 | 839 | 925 | 1030 | 413 | 438 | 456 | 247 | 257 | 253 |
| 0.45 | *** | 13954 | 14484 | 24837 | 2621 | 2916 | 4014 | 815 | 887 | 1020 | 404 | 427 | 460 | 242 | 251 | 263 |
|      | *** | 14131 | 15476 | 26090 | 2737 | 3228 | 4182 | 846 | 941 | 1041 | 415 | 442 | 456 | 246 | 257 | 250 |
| 0.5  | *** | 13087 | 13760 | 25299 | 2549 | 2874 | 4061 | 803 | 880 | 1020 | 397 | 422 | 456 | 236 | 245 | 258 |
|      | *** | 13313 | 14963 | 26248 | 2679 | 3214 | 4182 | 837 | 937 | 1030 | 408 | 437 | 446 | 240 | 251 | 242 |
| 0.55 | *** | 11960 | 12800 | 25188 | 2437 | 2785 | 4016 | 778 | 856 | 998 | 383 | 407 | 441 | 226 | 235 | 246 |
|      | *** | 12246 | 14213 | 25880 | 2577 | 3141 | 4098 | 812 | 914 | 999 | 394 | 422 | 428 | 230 | 240 | 229 |
| 0.6  | *** | 10673 | 11696 | 24505 | 2294 | 2654 | 3879 | 739 | 816 | 953 | 361 | 384 | 415 | 210 | 219 | 229 |
|      | *** | 11030 | 13288 | 24987 | 2440 | 3013 | 3930 | 773 | 872 | 946 | 371 | 398 | 400 | 215 | 224 | 211 |
| 0.65 | *** | 9324 | 10519 | 23253 | 2124 | 2482 | 3652 | 687 | 759 | 884 | 332 | 352 | 380 | 190 | 198 | 207 |
|      | *** | 9755 | 12236 | 23569 | 2270 | 2832 | 3678 | 720 | 811 | 873 | 342 | 365 | 362 | 194 | 202 | 187 |
| 0.7  | *** | 8000 | 9319 | 21435 | 1930 | 2272 | 3334 | 622 | 686 | 794 | 295 | 312 | 335 | 165 | 172 | 179 |
|      | *** | 8489 | 11082 | 21625 | 2071 | 2600 | 3342 | 651 | 731 | 778 | 303 | 323 | 316 | 168 | 175 | 158 |
| 0.75 | *** | 6753 | 8116 | 19056 | 1711 | 2022 | 2927 | 543 | 596 | 681 | 250 | 263 | 280 | 136 | 140 | 145 |
|      | *** | 7272 | 9835 | 19156 | 1841 | 2312 | 2922 | 567 | 632 | 662 | 256 | 271 | 260 | 138 | 143 | 124 |
| 0.8  | *** | 5593 | 6900 | 16122 | 1463 | 1727 | 2431 | 448 | 487 | 546 | 196 | 204 | 215 | . | . | . |
|      | *** | 6099 | 8479 | 16161 | 1574 | 1964 | 2417 | 466 | 513 | 526 | 200 | 209 | 194 | . | . | . |
| 0.85 | *** | 4482 | 5632 | 12638 | 1175 | 1375 | 1847 | 333 | 356 | 389 | . | . | . | . | . | . |
|      | *** | 4933 | 6966 | 12641 | 1260 | 1545 | 1829 | 344 | 371 | 368 | . | . | . | . | . | . |
| 0.9  | *** | 3342 | 4223 | 8610 | 825 | 944 | 1177 | . | . | . | . | . | . | . | . | . |
|      | *** | 3692 | 5196 | 8596 | 877 | 1036 | 1156 | . | . | . | . | . | . | . | . | . |
| 0.95 | *** | 1981 | 2448 | 4045 | . | . | . | . | . | . | . | . | . | . | . | . |
|      | *** | 2172 | 2909 | 4025 | . | . | . | . | . | . | . | . | . | . | . | . |

## TABLE 6: ALPHA= 0.025 POWER= 0.9    EXPECTED ACCRUAL THRU MINIMUM FOLLOW-UP= 950

| | | DEL=.02 | | | DEL=.05 | | | DEL=.10 | | | DEL=.15 | | | DEL=.20 | |
|---|---|---|---|---|---|---|---|---|---|---|---|---|---|---|---|---|
| FACT= | 1.0 .75 | .50 .25 | .00 BIN | 1.0 .75 | .50 .25 | .00 BIN | 1.0 .75 | .50 .25 | .00 BIN | 1.0 75 | .50 .25 | .00 BIN | 1.0 .75 | .50 .25 | .00 BIN |

PCONT=***   REQUIRED NUMBER OF PATIENTS

| PCONT | 1.0 (.02) | .50 (.02) | .00/BIN (.02) | 1.0 (.05) | .50 (.05) | .00/BIN (.05) | 1.0 (.10) | .50 (.10) | .00/BIN (.10) | 1.0 (.15) | .50 (.15) | .00/BIN (.15) | 1.0 (.20) | .50 (.20) | .00/BIN (.20) |
|---|---|---|---|---|---|---|---|---|---|---|---|---|---|---|---|
| 0.05 *** | 2998 | 3018 | 3165 | 646 | 654 | 671 | 234 | 236 | 239 | 137 | 138 | 139 | 97 | 97 | 98 |
| *** | 3006 | 3050 | 5916 | 650 | 661 | 1156 | 235 | 237 | 368 | 138 | 139 | 194 | 97 | 97 | 124 |
| 0.1 *** | 6241 | 6289 | 6954 | 1189 | 1219 | 1294 | 381 | 389 | 400 | 205 | 209 | 212 | 136 | 137 | 139 |
| *** | 6257 | 6378 | 10277 | 1201 | 1247 | 1829 | 385 | 394 | 526 | 207 | 210 | 260 | 137 | 139 | 158 |
| 0.15 *** | 9123 | 9206 | 10755 | 1661 | 1720 | 1898 | 508 | 524 | 547 | 264 | 269 | 276 | 169 | 171 | 174 |
| *** | 9150 | 9367 | 14112 | 1684 | 1780 | 2417 | 515 | 534 | 662 | 266 | 273 | 316 | 170 | 172 | 187 |
| 0.2 *** | 11424 | 11552 | 14290 | 2040 | 2134 | 2448 | 613 | 638 | 679 | 311 | 320 | 331 | 195 | 198 | 203 |
| *** | 11466 | 11802 | 17422 | 2077 | 2234 | 2922 | 624 | 656 | 778 | 315 | 325 | 362 | 197 | 201 | 211 |
| 0.25 *** | 13085 | 13268 | 17424 | 2323 | 2456 | 2930 | 694 | 730 | 791 | 349 | 361 | 377 | 215 | 220 | 227 |
| *** | 13146 | 13627 | 20206 | 2375 | 2601 | 3342 | 710 | 756 | 873 | 355 | 368 | 400 | 217 | 223 | 229 |
| 0.3 *** | 14115 | 14366 | 20081 | 2515 | 2690 | 3331 | 754 | 801 | 882 | 376 | 392 | 413 | 230 | 236 | 245 |
| *** | 14199 | 14858 | 22465 | 2583 | 2881 | 3678 | 775 | 834 | 946 | 384 | 401 | 428 | 233 | 241 | 242 |
| 0.35 *** | 14562 | 14896 | 22218 | 2624 | 2843 | 3648 | 794 | 850 | 950 | 395 | 413 | 439 | 239 | 247 | 257 |
| *** | 14674 | 15544 | 24199 | 2709 | 3079 | 3930 | 819 | 892 | 999 | 403 | 425 | 446 | 243 | 251 | 250 |
| 0.4 *** | 14492 | 14928 | 23808 | 2663 | 2923 | 3876 | 816 | 881 | 996 | 405 | 426 | 455 | 243 | 252 | 262 |
| *** | 14637 | 15757 | 25407 | 2765 | 3200 | 4098 | 844 | 928 | 1030 | 414 | 439 | 456 | 248 | 257 | 253 |
| 0.45 *** | 13984 | 14543 | 24837 | 2642 | 2940 | 4014 | 821 | 891 | 1020 | 406 | 429 | 460 | 242 | 252 | 263 |
| *** | 14170 | 15576 | 26090 | 2761 | 3251 | 4182 | 852 | 944 | 1041 | 416 | 443 | 456 | 247 | 257 | 250 |
| 0.5 *** | 13124 | 13832 | 25299 | 2572 | 2901 | 4061 | 809 | 885 | 1020 | 399 | 423 | 456 | 237 | 246 | 257 |
| *** | 13363 | 15081 | 26248 | 2704 | 3239 | 4182 | 843 | 941 | 1030 | 410 | 438 | 446 | 241 | 251 | 242 |
| 0.55 *** | 12008 | 12889 | 25188 | 2463 | 2813 | 4016 | 785 | 861 | 998 | 385 | 408 | 441 | 226 | 235 | 247 |
| *** | 12310 | 14347 | 25880 | 2604 | 3167 | 4098 | 818 | 918 | 999 | 395 | 423 | 428 | 230 | 241 | 229 |
| 0.6 *** | 10733 | 11800 | 24505 | 2320 | 2682 | 3879 | 746 | 821 | 952 | 363 | 386 | 416 | 211 | 219 | 229 |
| *** | 11107 | 13434 | 24987 | 2468 | 3040 | 3930 | 779 | 875 | 946 | 374 | 399 | 400 | 215 | 224 | 211 |
| 0.65 *** | 9398 | 10635 | 23253 | 2151 | 2510 | 3652 | 694 | 764 | 884 | 334 | 353 | 380 | 191 | 198 | 207 |
| *** | 9846 | 12389 | 23569 | 2299 | 2858 | 3678 | 725 | 814 | 873 | 343 | 366 | 362 | 194 | 202 | 187 |
| 0.7 *** | 8086 | 9442 | 21436 | 1957 | 2299 | 3334 | 628 | 691 | 793 | 296 | 313 | 335 | 166 | 172 | 178 |
| *** | 8590 | 11236 | 21625 | 2098 | 2623 | 3342 | 656 | 734 | 778 | 304 | 323 | 316 | 169 | 175 | 158 |
| 0.75 *** | 6846 | 8238 | 19057 | 1735 | 2046 | 2927 | 547 | 599 | 680 | 251 | 264 | 280 | 136 | 140 | 145 |
| *** | 7376 | 9982 | 19156 | 1865 | 2332 | 2922 | 571 | 635 | 662 | 257 | 272 | 260 | 139 | 143 | 124 |
| 0.8 *** | 5684 | 7015 | 16122 | 1484 | 1747 | 2431 | 451 | 489 | 546 | 197 | 205 | 215 | . | . | . |
| *** | 6200 | 8610 | 16161 | 1594 | 1980 | 2417 | 469 | 514 | 526 | 201 | 210 | 194 | . | . | . |
| 0.85 *** | 4564 | 5730 | 12638 | 1191 | 1389 | 1847 | 335 | 357 | 389 | . | . | . | . | . | . |
| *** | 5022 | 7075 | 12641 | 1276 | 1556 | 1829 | 346 | 372 | 368 | . | . | . | . | . | . |
| 0.9 *** | 3406 | 4297 | 8610 | 835 | 952 | 1177 | . | . | . | . | . | . | . | . | . |
| *** | 3761 | 5273 | 8596 | 887 | 1041 | 1156 | . | . | . | . | . | . | . | . | . |
| 0.95 *** | 2016 | 2485 | 4045 | . | . | . | . | . | . | . | . | . | . | . | . |
| *** | 2209 | 2943 | 4025 | . | . | . | . | . | . | . | . | . | . | . | . |

TABLE 6: ALPHA= 0.025 POWER= 0.9      EXPECTED ACCRUAL THRU MINIMUM FOLLOW-UP= 1000

| | | DEL=.02 | | | DEL=.05 | | | DEL=.10 | | | DEL=.15 | | | DEL=.20 | | |
|---|---|---|---|---|---|---|---|---|---|---|---|---|---|---|---|---|---|
| FACT= | | 1.0 | .50 | .00 | 1.0 | .50 | .00 | 1.0 | .50 | .00 | 1.0 | .50 | .00 | 1.0 | .50 | .00 |
| | | .75 | .25 | BIN | .75 | .25 | BIN | .75 | .25 | BIN | 75 | .25 | BIN | .75 | .25 | BIN |
| PCONT=*** | | REQUIRED NUMBER OF PATIENTS | | | | | | | | | | | | | | |
| 0.05 | *** | 3000 | 3020 | 3165 | 646 | 655 | 671 | 234 | 236 | 239 | 137 | 138 | 139 | 97 | 98 | 98 |
| | *** | 3007 | 3053 | 5916 | 650 | 662 | 1156 | 235 | 237 | 368 | 138 | 139 | 194 | 97 | 98 | 124 |
| 0.1 | *** | 6244 | 6293 | 6955 | 1191 | 1221 | 1295 | 382 | 390 | 400 | 206 | 209 | 212 | 136 | 138 | 139 |
| | *** | 6260 | 6386 | 10277 | 1204 | 1249 | 1829 | 386 | 394 | 526 | 208 | 210 | 260 | 137 | 138 | 158 |
| 0.15 | *** | 9127 | 9214 | 10755 | 1665 | 1725 | 1898 | 510 | 525 | 548 | 265 | 270 | 276 | 169 | 171 | 174 |
| | *** | 9156 | 9383 | 14112 | 1688 | 1785 | 2417 | 516 | 535 | 662 | 267 | 273 | 316 | 170 | 173 | 187 |
| 0.2 | *** | 11431 | 11565 | 14290 | 2046 | 2141 | 2448 | 615 | 640 | 679 | 312 | 321 | 331 | 195 | 199 | 203 |
| | *** | 11475 | 11828 | 17422 | 2083 | 2241 | 2922 | 626 | 657 | 778 | 316 | 326 | 362 | 197 | 201 | 211 |
| 0.25 | *** | 13094 | 13286 | 17424 | 2331 | 2467 | 2930 | 698 | 733 | 791 | 350 | 361 | 378 | 216 | 221 | 227 |
| | *** | 13158 | 13664 | 20206 | 2385 | 2611 | 3342 | 713 | 758 | 873 | 355 | 369 | 400 | 218 | 224 | 229 |
| 0.3 | *** | 14128 | 14393 | 20081 | 2526 | 2704 | 3331 | 758 | 804 | 881 | 378 | 393 | 413 | 231 | 237 | 245 |
| | *** | 14216 | 14908 | 22465 | 2596 | 2895 | 3678 | 778 | 836 | 946 | 385 | 402 | 428 | 234 | 241 | 242 |
| 0.35 | *** | 14580 | 14931 | 22218 | 2639 | 2860 | 3648 | 799 | 854 | 950 | 396 | 415 | 440 | 240 | 248 | 256 |
| | *** | 14697 | 15609 | 24199 | 2726 | 3096 | 3930 | 823 | 895 | 999 | 405 | 426 | 446 | 244 | 252 | 250 |
| 0.4 | *** | 14515 | 14973 | 23808 | 2681 | 2944 | 3876 | 821 | 885 | 996 | 406 | 427 | 455 | 245 | 253 | 263 |
| | *** | 14668 | 15839 | 25407 | 2785 | 3220 | 4098 | 850 | 931 | 1030 | 416 | 440 | 456 | 248 | 258 | 253 |
| 0.45 | *** | 14013 | 14601 | 24838 | 2663 | 2963 | 4014 | 826 | 896 | 1020 | 408 | 430 | 461 | 243 | 252 | 263 |
| | *** | 14210 | 15675 | 26090 | 2783 | 3274 | 4182 | 857 | 948 | 1041 | 418 | 444 | 456 | 248 | 258 | 250 |
| 0.5 | *** | 13162 | 13905 | 25298 | 2595 | 2926 | 4061 | 816 | 890 | 1020 | 401 | 424 | 456 | 238 | 246 | 258 |
| | *** | 13413 | 15197 | 26248 | 2728 | 3263 | 4182 | 849 | 944 | 1030 | 412 | 438 | 446 | 242 | 252 | 242 |
| 0.55 | *** | 12056 | 12976 | 25188 | 2488 | 2840 | 4016 | 791 | 866 | 998 | 387 | 410 | 441 | 227 | 236 | 246 |
| | *** | 12373 | 14478 | 25880 | 2630 | 3192 | 4098 | 825 | 921 | 999 | 398 | 424 | 428 | 231 | 241 | 229 |
| 0.6 | *** | 10793 | 11901 | 24505 | 2346 | 2710 | 3880 | 752 | 826 | 953 | 365 | 386 | 416 | 212 | 220 | 230 |
| | *** | 11184 | 13576 | 24987 | 2495 | 3065 | 3930 | 785 | 878 | 946 | 375 | 400 | 400 | 216 | 225 | 211 |
| 0.65 | *** | 9471 | 10748 | 23253 | 2177 | 2537 | 3652 | 700 | 768 | 885 | 336 | 355 | 380 | 192 | 199 | 206 |
| | *** | 9935 | 12536 | 23569 | 2325 | 2882 | 3678 | 730 | 817 | 873 | 345 | 366 | 362 | 195 | 203 | 187 |
| 0.7 | *** | 8170 | 9561 | 21436 | 1981 | 2324 | 3334 | 633 | 695 | 794 | 298 | 315 | 335 | 167 | 172 | 178 |
| | *** | 8690 | 11383 | 21625 | 2123 | 2645 | 3342 | 661 | 737 | 778 | 306 | 324 | 316 | 170 | 175 | 158 |
| 0.75 | *** | 6935 | 8356 | 19057 | 1758 | 2069 | 2927 | 552 | 603 | 681 | 253 | 265 | 280 | 136 | 141 | 145 |
| | *** | 7478 | 10121 | 19156 | 1888 | 2351 | 2922 | 575 | 636 | 662 | 258 | 272 | 260 | 138 | 143 | 124 |
| 0.8 | *** | 5772 | 7125 | 16122 | 1503 | 1766 | 2431 | 455 | 491 | 546 | 198 | 206 | 215 | . | . | . |
| | *** | 6297 | 8736 | 16161 | 1614 | 1995 | 2417 | 471 | 516 | 526 | 201 | 210 | 194 | . | . | . |
| 0.85 | *** | 4643 | 5825 | 12638 | 1206 | 1403 | 1847 | 337 | 359 | 389 | . | . | . | . | . | . |
| | *** | 5108 | 7180 | 12641 | 1291 | 1566 | 1829 | 348 | 373 | 368 | . | . | . | . | . | . |
| 0.9 | *** | 3468 | 4368 | 8610 | 845 | 960 | 1177 | . | . | . | . | . | . | . | . | . |
| | *** | 3826 | 5346 | 8596 | 895 | 1047 | 1156 | . | . | . | . | . | . | . | . | . |
| 0.95 | *** | 2050 | 2520 | 4045 | . | . | . | . | . | . | . | . | . | . | . | . |
| | *** | 2243 | 2975 | 4025 | . | . | . | . | . | . | . | . | . | . | . | . |

## TABLE 6: ALPHA= 0.025 POWER= 0.9    EXPECTED ACCRUAL THRU MINIMUM FOLLOW-UP= 1100

| | | DEL=.02 | | | DEL=.05 | | | DEL=.10 | | | DEL=.15 | | | DEL=.20 | | |
|---|---|---|---|---|---|---|---|---|---|---|---|---|---|---|---|---|---|
| FACT= | | 1.0 .75 | .50 .25 | .00 BIN | 1.0 .75 | .50 .25 | .00 BIN | 1.0 .75 | .50 .25 | .00 BIN | 1.0 75 | .50 .25 | .00 BIN | 1.0 .75 | .50 .25 | .00 BIN |
| PCONT=*** | | | | | REQUIRED | NUMBER | OF PATIENTS | | | | | | | | | |
| 0.05 | *** | 3002 | 3024 | 3165 | 648 | 657 | 671 | 235 | 236 | 239 | 137 | 138 | 139 | 97 | 98 | 98 |
| | *** | 3009 | 3058 | 5916 | 652 | 663 | 1156 | 235 | 237 | 368 | 137 | 139 | 194 | 97 | 98 | 124 |
| 0.1 | *** | 6249 | 6303 | 6954 | 1195 | 1226 | 1295 | 383 | 390 | 400 | 206 | 209 | 212 | 136 | 137 | 139 |
| | *** | 6267 | 6403 | 10277 | 1208 | 1252 | 1829 | 386 | 395 | 526 | 208 | 210 | 260 | 137 | 138 | 158 |
| 0.15 | *** | 9135 | 9231 | 10755 | 1672 | 1733 | 1897 | 512 | 527 | 548 | 265 | 270 | 276 | 169 | 171 | 174 |
| | *** | 9168 | 9415 | 14112 | 1697 | 1792 | 2417 | 518 | 536 | 662 | 268 | 273 | 316 | 170 | 173 | 187 |
| 0.2 | *** | 11444 | 11591 | 14290 | 2058 | 2155 | 2448 | 619 | 642 | 679 | 313 | 321 | 331 | 196 | 199 | 203 |
| | *** | 11493 | 11878 | 17422 | 2096 | 2254 | 2922 | 629 | 659 | 778 | 317 | 326 | 362 | 197 | 201 | 211 |
| 0.25 | *** | 13113 | 13325 | 17424 | 2348 | 2487 | 2930 | 703 | 736 | 791 | 352 | 363 | 378 | 217 | 221 | 227 |
| | *** | 13184 | 13736 | 20206 | 2403 | 2630 | 3342 | 718 | 760 | 873 | 357 | 369 | 400 | 219 | 224 | 229 |
| 0.3 | *** | 14155 | 14445 | 20081 | 2549 | 2731 | 3331 | 765 | 809 | 881 | 380 | 395 | 413 | 232 | 237 | 245 |
| | *** | 14252 | 15005 | 22465 | 2620 | 2919 | 3678 | 785 | 840 | 946 | 387 | 403 | 428 | 235 | 241 | 242 |
| 0.35 | *** | 14615 | 15001 | 22217 | 2667 | 2893 | 3648 | 807 | 861 | 950 | 400 | 417 | 439 | 241 | 248 | 257 |
| | *** | 14744 | 15735 | 24199 | 2756 | 3126 | 3930 | 831 | 899 | 999 | 408 | 427 | 446 | 245 | 252 | 250 |
| 0.4 | *** | 14561 | 15064 | 23808 | 2714 | 2982 | 3876 | 830 | 892 | 996 | 410 | 429 | 455 | 246 | 253 | 263 |
| | *** | 14729 | 15997 | 25407 | 2821 | 3256 | 4098 | 858 | 936 | 1030 | 419 | 441 | 456 | 250 | 258 | 253 |
| 0.45 | *** | 14073 | 14716 | 24837 | 2701 | 3007 | 4014 | 837 | 904 | 1020 | 411 | 433 | 461 | 245 | 253 | 263 |
| | *** | 14289 | 15866 | 26090 | 2824 | 3314 | 4182 | 867 | 953 | 1041 | 422 | 445 | 456 | 249 | 258 | 250 |
| 0.5 | *** | 13238 | 14047 | 25298 | 2638 | 2974 | 4060 | 827 | 899 | 1020 | 405 | 426 | 456 | 239 | 247 | 257 |
| | *** | 13513 | 15419 | 26248 | 2774 | 3306 | 4182 | 859 | 950 | 1030 | 415 | 440 | 446 | 243 | 252 | 242 |
| 0.55 | *** | 12152 | 13148 | 25187 | 2534 | 2890 | 4016 | 802 | 874 | 998 | 390 | 412 | 441 | 228 | 236 | 246 |
| | *** | 12497 | 14727 | 25880 | 2679 | 3237 | 4098 | 835 | 927 | 999 | 401 | 425 | 428 | 232 | 241 | 229 |
| 0.6 | *** | 10912 | 12099 | 24505 | 2395 | 2760 | 3880 | 763 | 834 | 952 | 368 | 389 | 415 | 213 | 221 | 229 |
| | *** | 11335 | 13845 | 24987 | 2545 | 3110 | 3930 | 795 | 884 | 946 | 378 | 401 | 400 | 217 | 225 | 211 |
| 0.65 | *** | 9614 | 10966 | 23253 | 2226 | 2586 | 3652 | 710 | 776 | 884 | 338 | 357 | 380 | 193 | 199 | 206 |
| | *** | 10109 | 12815 | 23569 | 2375 | 2925 | 3678 | 740 | 822 | 873 | 347 | 368 | 362 | 196 | 203 | 187 |
| 0.7 | *** | 8332 | 9787 | 21436 | 2028 | 2370 | 3334 | 643 | 701 | 793 | 301 | 316 | 335 | 168 | 173 | 178 |
| | *** | 8880 | 11660 | 21625 | 2171 | 2685 | 3342 | 669 | 741 | 778 | 308 | 324 | 316 | 170 | 175 | 158 |
| 0.75 | *** | 7107 | 8580 | 19057 | 1801 | 2110 | 2927 | 560 | 609 | 681 | 254 | 266 | 280 | 137 | 141 | 144 |
| | *** | 7673 | 10385 | 19156 | 1930 | 2386 | 2922 | 582 | 640 | 662 | 260 | 272 | 260 | 139 | 142 | 124 |
| 0.8 | *** | 5940 | 7332 | 16122 | 1540 | 1800 | 2431 | 461 | 496 | 546 | 199 | 206 | 215 | . | . | . |
| | *** | 6483 | 8973 | 16161 | 1650 | 2023 | 2417 | 477 | 518 | 526 | 202 | 210 | 194 | . | . | . |
| 0.85 | *** | 4793 | 6003 | 12638 | 1235 | 1428 | 1847 | 340 | 362 | 389 | . | . | . | . | . | . |
| | *** | 5270 | 7374 | 12641 | 1318 | 1585 | 1829 | 351 | 374 | 368 | . | . | . | . | . | . |
| 0.9 | *** | 3584 | 4499 | 8610 | 862 | 973 | 1176 | . | . | . | . | . | . | . | . | . |
| | *** | 3950 | 5482 | 8596 | 911 | 1056 | 1156 | . | . | . | . | . | . | . | . | . |
| 0.95 | *** | 2113 | 2585 | 4045 | . | . | . | . | . | . | . | . | . | . | . | . |
| | *** | 2309 | 3033 | 4025 | . | . | . | . | . | . | . | . | . | . | . | . |

## TABLE 6: ALPHA= 0.025 POWER= 0.9     EXPECTED ACCRUAL THRU MINIMUM FOLLOW-UP= 1200

| | | DEL=.02 | | | DEL=.05 | | | DEL=.10 | | | DEL=.15 | | | DEL=.20 | | |
|---|---|---|---|---|---|---|---|---|---|---|---|---|---|---|---|---|---|
| FACT= | | 1.0 / .75 | .50 / .25 | .00 / BIN | 1.0 / .75 | .50 / .25 | .00 / BIN | 1.0 / .75 | .50 / .25 | .00 / BIN | 1.0 / 75 | .50 / .25 | .00 / BIN | 1.0 / .75 | .50 / .25 | .00 / BIN |
| PCONT=*** | | | | | REQUIRED | NUMBER OF | PATIENTS | | | | | | | | | |
| 0.05 | *** | 3004 | 3028 | 3165 | 649 | 657 | 671 | 235 | 236 | 238 | 137 | 138 | 139 | 97 | 97 | 97 |
| | *** | 3012 | 3062 | 5916 | 652 | 663 | 1156 | 235 | 238 | 368 | 138 | 139 | 194 | 97 | 97 | 124 |
| 0.1 | *** | 6253 | 6313 | 6954 | 1199 | 1229 | 1294 | 384 | 391 | 400 | 207 | 209 | 212 | 136 | 138 | 139 |
| | *** | 6274 | 6419 | 10277 | 1211 | 1255 | 1829 | 387 | 395 | 526 | 208 | 211 | 260 | 137 | 138 | 158 |
| 0.15 | *** | 9145 | 9249 | 10755 | 1679 | 1741 | 1897 | 514 | 528 | 547 | 265 | 271 | 276 | 169 | 172 | 174 |
| | *** | 9179 | 9446 | 14112 | 1705 | 1798 | 2417 | 520 | 537 | 662 | 268 | 273 | 316 | 170 | 172 | 187 |
| 0.2 | *** | 11457 | 11618 | 14290 | 2069 | 2168 | 2448 | 622 | 645 | 679 | 315 | 322 | 331 | 196 | 199 | 203 |
| | *** | 11511 | 11927 | 17422 | 2109 | 2265 | 2922 | 632 | 660 | 778 | 318 | 326 | 362 | 198 | 201 | 211 |
| 0.25 | *** | 13132 | 13363 | 17424 | 2364 | 2506 | 2929 | 707 | 740 | 790 | 353 | 364 | 377 | 217 | 221 | 226 |
| | *** | 13210 | 13807 | 20206 | 2420 | 2647 | 3342 | 722 | 762 | 873 | 358 | 370 | 400 | 219 | 224 | 229 |
| 0.3 | *** | 14181 | 14497 | 20081 | 2569 | 2755 | 3331 | 771 | 814 | 881 | 382 | 396 | 413 | 232 | 238 | 244 |
| | *** | 14287 | 15100 | 22465 | 2643 | 2941 | 3678 | 790 | 843 | 946 | 388 | 404 | 428 | 235 | 241 | 242 |
| 0.35 | *** | 14650 | 15070 | 22217 | 2693 | 2923 | 3648 | 814 | 866 | 950 | 402 | 418 | 439 | 242 | 249 | 256 |
| | *** | 14791 | 15859 | 24199 | 2785 | 3154 | 3930 | 838 | 902 | 999 | 409 | 427 | 446 | 245 | 253 | 250 |
| 0.4 | *** | 14607 | 15154 | 23808 | 2746 | 3017 | 3876 | 839 | 898 | 997 | 412 | 430 | 455 | 247 | 254 | 262 |
| | *** | 14790 | 16150 | 25407 | 2854 | 3288 | 4098 | 865 | 940 | 1030 | 421 | 442 | 456 | 250 | 258 | 253 |
| 0.45 | *** | 14131 | 14830 | 24838 | 2737 | 3046 | 4014 | 846 | 911 | 1020 | 415 | 434 | 460 | 246 | 253 | 263 |
| | *** | 14367 | 16049 | 26090 | 2863 | 3350 | 4182 | 875 | 958 | 1041 | 424 | 446 | 456 | 250 | 258 | 250 |
| 0.5 | *** | 13313 | 14187 | 25298 | 2678 | 3016 | 4060 | 837 | 906 | 1020 | 408 | 429 | 455 | 241 | 248 | 257 |
| | *** | 13612 | 15631 | 26248 | 2816 | 3345 | 4182 | 868 | 955 | 1030 | 418 | 441 | 446 | 244 | 253 | 242 |
| 0.55 | *** | 12247 | 13314 | 25187 | 2577 | 2935 | 4015 | 812 | 883 | 997 | 394 | 414 | 440 | 229 | 237 | 246 |
| | *** | 12619 | 14962 | 25880 | 2724 | 3277 | 4098 | 844 | 931 | 999 | 403 | 426 | 428 | 233 | 241 | 229 |
| 0.6 | *** | 11030 | 12289 | 24505 | 2440 | 2806 | 3879 | 773 | 841 | 952 | 371 | 391 | 415 | 214 | 221 | 229 |
| | *** | 11482 | 14098 | 24987 | 2590 | 3150 | 3930 | 804 | 889 | 946 | 380 | 402 | 400 | 217 | 225 | 211 |
| 0.65 | *** | 9754 | 11173 | 23253 | 2270 | 2631 | 3652 | 719 | 783 | 884 | 341 | 358 | 380 | 194 | 199 | 206 |
| | *** | 10277 | 13075 | 23569 | 2420 | 2964 | 3678 | 748 | 826 | 873 | 349 | 368 | 362 | 196 | 203 | 187 |
| 0.7 | *** | 8489 | 10002 | 21436 | 2071 | 2413 | 3334 | 651 | 707 | 793 | 303 | 317 | 335 | 169 | 173 | 178 |
| | *** | 9061 | 11918 | 21625 | 2214 | 2720 | 3342 | 676 | 745 | 778 | 310 | 325 | 316 | 171 | 175 | 158 |
| 0.75 | *** | 7271 | 8791 | 19057 | 1840 | 2147 | 2926 | 567 | 613 | 681 | 256 | 267 | 280 | 138 | 141 | 145 |
| | *** | 7857 | 10629 | 19156 | 1969 | 2416 | 2922 | 588 | 643 | 662 | 261 | 273 | 260 | 139 | 142 | 124 |
| 0.8 | *** | 6098 | 7527 | 16122 | 1573 | 1830 | 2431 | 466 | 499 | 546 | 200 | 207 | 215 | . | . | . |
| | *** | 6657 | 9190 | 16161 | 1683 | 2047 | 2417 | 481 | 520 | 526 | 203 | 211 | 194 | . | . | . |
| 0.85 | *** | 4933 | 6168 | 12638 | 1260 | 1450 | 1847 | 343 | 364 | 388 | . | . | . | . | . | . |
| | *** | 5422 | 7551 | 12641 | 1342 | 1602 | 1829 | 353 | 375 | 368 | . | . | . | . | . | . |
| 0.9 | *** | 3692 | 4621 | 8610 | 877 | 985 | 1177 | . | . | . | . | . | . | . | . | . |
| | *** | 4065 | 5605 | 8596 | 925 | 1064 | 1156 | . | . | . | . | . | . | . | . | . |
| 0.95 | *** | 2172 | 2644 | 4045 | . | . | . | . | . | . | . | . | . | . | . | . |
| | *** | 2368 | 3085 | 4025 | . | . | . | . | . | . | . | . | . | . | . | . |

## TABLE 6: ALPHA= 0.025 POWER= 0.9    EXPECTED ACCRUAL THRU MINIMUM FOLLOW-UP= 1300

| | | DEL=.02 | | | DEL=.05 | | | DEL=.10 | | | DEL=.15 | | | DEL=.20 | |
|---|---|---|---|---|---|---|---|---|---|---|---|---|---|---|---|---|
| FACT= | 1.0 .75 | .50 .25 | .00 BIN | 1.0 .75 | .50 .25 | .00 BIN | 1.0 .75 | .50 .25 | .00 BIN | 1.0 75 | .50 .25 | .00 BIN | 1.0 .75 | .50 .25 | .00 BIN |

PCONT=*** REQUIRED NUMBER OF PATIENTS

| PCONT | | DEL=.02 1.0/.75 | .50/.25 | .00/BIN | DEL=.05 1.0/.75 | .50/.25 | .00/BIN | DEL=.10 1.0/.75 | .50/.25 | .00/BIN | DEL=.15 1.0/.75 | .50/.25 | .00/BIN | DEL=.20 1.0/.75 | .50/.25 | .00/BIN |
|---|---|---|---|---|---|---|---|---|---|---|---|---|---|---|---|---|
| 0.05 | *** | 3006 | 3032 | 3165 | 650 | 658 | 671 | 235 | 237 | 239 | 137 | 138 | 139 | 97 | 97 | 97 |
| | *** | 3015 | 3067 | 5916 | 653 | 664 | 1156 | 236 | 237 | 368 | 138 | 139 | 194 | 97 | 97 | 124 |
| 0.1 | *** | 6259 | 6322 | 6954 | 1202 | 1233 | 1294 | 385 | 392 | 400 | 207 | 210 | 212 | 136 | 138 | 139 |
| | *** | 6280 | 6435 | 10277 | 1215 | 1258 | 1829 | 388 | 396 | 526 | 208 | 211 | 260 | 137 | 138 | 158 |
| 0.15 | *** | 9154 | 9266 | 10755 | 1686 | 1748 | 1898 | 516 | 529 | 548 | 266 | 271 | 276 | 170 | 172 | 174 |
| | *** | 9191 | 9476 | 14112 | 1712 | 1804 | 2417 | 523 | 538 | 662 | 269 | 274 | 316 | 171 | 173 | 187 |
| 0.2 | *** | 11471 | 11645 | 14290 | 2080 | 2180 | 2448 | 625 | 647 | 679 | 316 | 323 | 331 | 197 | 200 | 203 |
| | *** | 11529 | 11975 | 17422 | 2121 | 2275 | 2922 | 635 | 661 | 778 | 319 | 327 | 362 | 198 | 201 | 211 |
| 0.25 | *** | 13152 | 13401 | 17424 | 2379 | 2523 | 2930 | 712 | 744 | 791 | 355 | 365 | 377 | 218 | 222 | 227 |
| | *** | 13236 | 13875 | 20206 | 2437 | 2661 | 3342 | 726 | 765 | 873 | 360 | 370 | 400 | 220 | 224 | 229 |
| 0.3 | *** | 14207 | 14550 | 20081 | 2590 | 2777 | 3331 | 777 | 817 | 882 | 384 | 397 | 414 | 233 | 239 | 245 |
| | *** | 14322 | 15193 | 22465 | 2665 | 2962 | 3678 | 796 | 846 | 946 | 390 | 405 | 428 | 236 | 241 | 242 |
| 0.35 | *** | 14685 | 15140 | 22218 | 2718 | 2950 | 3648 | 822 | 871 | 951 | 405 | 419 | 440 | 243 | 250 | 257 |
| | *** | 14838 | 15978 | 24199 | 2811 | 3178 | 3930 | 844 | 905 | 999 | 411 | 429 | 446 | 246 | 253 | 250 |
| 0.4 | *** | 14653 | 15243 | 23808 | 2775 | 3050 | 3877 | 847 | 904 | 996 | 415 | 432 | 455 | 248 | 254 | 263 |
| | *** | 14851 | 16297 | 25407 | 2887 | 3317 | 4098 | 873 | 944 | 1030 | 423 | 443 | 456 | 251 | 258 | 253 |
| 0.45 | *** | 14190 | 14942 | 24837 | 2772 | 3083 | 4014 | 855 | 918 | 1020 | 418 | 436 | 461 | 247 | 254 | 263 |
| | *** | 14446 | 16225 | 26090 | 2898 | 3383 | 4182 | 883 | 962 | 1041 | 426 | 448 | 456 | 251 | 258 | 250 |
| 0.5 | *** | 13388 | 14324 | 25298 | 2716 | 3057 | 4061 | 846 | 913 | 1020 | 411 | 431 | 456 | 241 | 249 | 258 |
| | *** | 13710 | 15833 | 26248 | 2856 | 3380 | 4182 | 876 | 959 | 1030 | 420 | 442 | 446 | 245 | 253 | 242 |
| 0.55 | *** | 12341 | 13476 | 25187 | 2618 | 2976 | 4015 | 822 | 889 | 998 | 396 | 416 | 440 | 231 | 238 | 246 |
| | *** | 12741 | 15186 | 25880 | 2766 | 3313 | 4098 | 852 | 936 | 999 | 406 | 427 | 428 | 234 | 242 | 229 |
| 0.6 | *** | 11146 | 12472 | 24505 | 2481 | 2848 | 3880 | 782 | 848 | 952 | 375 | 393 | 415 | 215 | 222 | 229 |
| | *** | 11625 | 14336 | 24987 | 2633 | 3186 | 3930 | 812 | 893 | 946 | 383 | 403 | 400 | 219 | 225 | 211 |
| 0.65 | *** | 9891 | 11370 | 23253 | 2312 | 2672 | 3652 | 728 | 789 | 884 | 344 | 360 | 380 | 195 | 201 | 206 |
| | *** | 10440 | 13320 | 23569 | 2462 | 2999 | 3678 | 756 | 830 | 873 | 352 | 370 | 362 | 198 | 203 | 187 |
| 0.7 | *** | 8640 | 10205 | 21435 | 2111 | 2450 | 3334 | 658 | 713 | 794 | 305 | 318 | 335 | 169 | 174 | 179 |
| | *** | 9235 | 12159 | 21625 | 2254 | 2752 | 3342 | 683 | 748 | 778 | 311 | 327 | 316 | 172 | 176 | 158 |
| 0.75 | *** | 7428 | 8989 | 19056 | 1877 | 2181 | 2927 | 573 | 617 | 681 | 258 | 268 | 279 | 138 | 141 | 145 |
| | *** | 8032 | 10856 | 19156 | 2005 | 2444 | 2922 | 593 | 646 | 662 | 263 | 274 | 260 | 140 | 143 | 124 |
| 0.8 | *** | 6249 | 7709 | 16123 | 1605 | 1858 | 2431 | 471 | 502 | 546 | 201 | 207 | 215 | . | . | . |
| | *** | 6821 | 9392 | 16161 | 1713 | 2069 | 2417 | 485 | 523 | 526 | 204 | 211 | 194 | . | . | . |
| 0.85 | *** | 5065 | 6322 | 12638 | 1284 | 1470 | 1847 | 346 | 365 | 389 | . | . | . | . | . | . |
| | *** | 5564 | 7715 | 12641 | 1365 | 1617 | 1829 | 355 | 376 | 368 | . | . | . | . | . | . |
| 0.9 | *** | 3794 | 4734 | 8610 | 890 | 996 | 1176 | . | . | . | . | . | . | . | . | . |
| | *** | 4172 | 5718 | 8596 | 938 | 1072 | 1156 | . | . | . | . | . | . | . | . | . |
| 0.95 | *** | 2226 | 2697 | 4046 | . | . | . | . | . | . | . | . | . | . | . | . |
| | *** | 2423 | 3131 | 4025 | . | . | . | . | . | . | . | . | . | . | . | . |

TABLE 6: ALPHA= 0.025 POWER= 0.9    EXPECTED ACCRUAL THRU MINIMUM FOLLOW-UP= 1400

| | | DEL=.02 | | | DEL=.05 | | | DEL=.10 | | | DEL=.15 | | | DEL=.20 | | |
|---|---|---|---|---|---|---|---|---|---|---|---|---|---|---|---|---|---|
| FACT= | | 1.0 .75 | .50 .25 | .00 BIN | 1.0 .75 | .50 .25 | .00 BIN | 1.0 .75 | .50 .25 | .00 BIN | 1.0 75 | .50 .25 | .00 BIN | 1.0 .75 | .50 .25 | .00 BIN |
| PCONT=*** | | | | | | REQUIRED | NUMBER | OF PATIENTS | | | | | | | | |
| 0.05 | *** | 3008 | 3034 | 3166 | 651 | 659 | 671 | 235 | 236 | 239 | 137 | 138 | 139 | 97 | 97 | 98 |
| | *** | 3018 | 3071 | 5916 | 654 | 664 | 1156 | 235 | 238 | 368 | 138 | 139 | 194 | 97 | 98 | 124 |
| 0.1 | *** | 6263 | 6331 | 6954 | 1206 | 1235 | 1295 | 386 | 392 | 400 | 207 | 210 | 212 | 137 | 138 | 139 |
| | *** | 6287 | 6450 | 10277 | 1219 | 1260 | 1829 | 388 | 395 | 526 | 208 | 211 | 260 | 137 | 138 | 158 |
| 0.15 | *** | 9162 | 9283 | 10755 | 1693 | 1754 | 1898 | 518 | 530 | 548 | 267 | 271 | 276 | 170 | 172 | 174 |
| | *** | 9202 | 9505 | 14112 | 1718 | 1809 | 2417 | 523 | 538 | 662 | 269 | 274 | 316 | 171 | 173 | 187 |
| 0.2 | *** | 11484 | 11672 | 14290 | 2090 | 2191 | 2448 | 627 | 649 | 679 | 317 | 324 | 332 | 197 | 200 | 203 |
| | *** | 11546 | 12022 | 17422 | 2131 | 2284 | 2922 | 638 | 662 | 778 | 320 | 327 | 362 | 199 | 201 | 211 |
| 0.25 | *** | 13171 | 13440 | 17424 | 2394 | 2538 | 2929 | 716 | 746 | 791 | 356 | 366 | 377 | 219 | 222 | 227 |
| | *** | 13261 | 13942 | 20206 | 2453 | 2675 | 3342 | 730 | 766 | 873 | 360 | 371 | 400 | 220 | 225 | 229 |
| 0.3 | *** | 14234 | 14602 | 20081 | 2608 | 2798 | 3331 | 781 | 822 | 882 | 386 | 398 | 413 | 234 | 239 | 245 |
| | *** | 14357 | 15283 | 22465 | 2685 | 2979 | 3678 | 800 | 848 | 946 | 392 | 405 | 428 | 236 | 241 | 242 |
| 0.35 | *** | 14720 | 15209 | 22218 | 2741 | 2976 | 3648 | 828 | 876 | 950 | 406 | 421 | 439 | 244 | 250 | 256 |
| | *** | 14885 | 16094 | 24199 | 2837 | 3201 | 3930 | 850 | 908 | 999 | 413 | 430 | 446 | 247 | 253 | 250 |
| 0.4 | *** | 14698 | 15332 | 23808 | 2803 | 3080 | 3876 | 854 | 909 | 997 | 417 | 434 | 455 | 248 | 255 | 262 |
| | *** | 14913 | 16439 | 25407 | 2916 | 3343 | 4098 | 879 | 948 | 1030 | 425 | 444 | 456 | 252 | 259 | 253 |
| 0.45 | *** | 14249 | 15053 | 24838 | 2803 | 3117 | 4014 | 862 | 923 | 1020 | 420 | 437 | 460 | 248 | 255 | 263 |
| | *** | 14523 | 16393 | 26090 | 2932 | 3412 | 4182 | 890 | 965 | 1041 | 428 | 448 | 456 | 251 | 259 | 250 |
| 0.5 | *** | 13463 | 14458 | 25298 | 2752 | 3093 | 4061 | 854 | 919 | 1020 | 414 | 432 | 456 | 242 | 249 | 257 |
| | *** | 13808 | 16025 | 26248 | 2893 | 3412 | 4182 | 883 | 962 | 1030 | 423 | 443 | 446 | 246 | 254 | 242 |
| 0.55 | *** | 12435 | 13632 | 25188 | 2656 | 3014 | 4015 | 829 | 895 | 997 | 399 | 417 | 441 | 232 | 239 | 246 |
| | *** | 12860 | 15397 | 25880 | 2804 | 3346 | 4098 | 859 | 940 | 999 | 408 | 428 | 428 | 235 | 242 | 229 |
| 0.6 | *** | 11259 | 12647 | 24505 | 2520 | 2886 | 3880 | 790 | 854 | 952 | 376 | 394 | 416 | 216 | 222 | 229 |
| | *** | 11765 | 14560 | 24987 | 2673 | 3218 | 3930 | 819 | 897 | 946 | 385 | 404 | 400 | 220 | 226 | 211 |
| 0.65 | *** | 10023 | 11558 | 23253 | 2350 | 2709 | 3652 | 735 | 794 | 885 | 346 | 361 | 381 | 196 | 200 | 206 |
| | *** | 10597 | 13549 | 23569 | 2501 | 3030 | 3678 | 762 | 834 | 873 | 353 | 370 | 362 | 198 | 204 | 187 |
| 0.7 | *** | 8786 | 10398 | 21436 | 2147 | 2485 | 3334 | 665 | 717 | 794 | 307 | 319 | 335 | 170 | 174 | 178 |
| | *** | 9401 | 12385 | 21625 | 2290 | 2781 | 3342 | 689 | 752 | 778 | 313 | 327 | 316 | 171 | 176 | 158 |
| 0.75 | *** | 7577 | 9176 | 19057 | 1910 | 2212 | 2927 | 578 | 621 | 681 | 259 | 269 | 280 | 139 | 142 | 144 |
| | *** | 8198 | 11068 | 19156 | 2039 | 2468 | 2922 | 598 | 648 | 662 | 263 | 274 | 260 | 140 | 143 | 124 |
| 0.8 | *** | 6392 | 7880 | 16122 | 1633 | 1883 | 2431 | 474 | 505 | 546 | 202 | 208 | 215 | . | . | . |
| | *** | 6977 | 9579 | 16161 | 1740 | 2088 | 2417 | 488 | 523 | 526 | 205 | 212 | 194 | . | . | . |
| 0.85 | *** | 5190 | 6466 | 12638 | 1305 | 1488 | 1847 | 349 | 367 | 388 | . | . | . | . | . | . |
| | *** | 5698 | 7867 | 12641 | 1385 | 1629 | 1829 | 357 | 377 | 368 | . | . | . | . | . | . |
| 0.9 | *** | 3889 | 4838 | 8610 | 903 | 1006 | 1177 | . | . | . | . | . | . | . | . | . |
| | *** | 4273 | 5821 | 8596 | 949 | 1078 | 1156 | . | . | . | . | . | . | . | . | . |
| 0.95 | *** | 2277 | 2747 | 4045 | . | . | . | . | . | . | . | . | . | . | . | . |
| | *** | 2474 | 3173 | 4025 | . | . | . | . | . | . | . | . | . | . | . | . |

## TABLE 6: ALPHA= 0.025 POWER= 0.9    EXPECTED ACCRUAL THRU MINIMUM FOLLOW-UP= 1500

| | | DEL=.02 | | | DEL=.05 | | | DEL=.10 | | | DEL=.15 | | | DEL=.20 | | |
|---|---|---|---|---|---|---|---|---|---|---|---|---|---|---|---|---|---|
| FACT= | | 1.0 .75 | .50 .25 | .00 BIN | 1.0 .75 | .50 .25 | .00 BIN | 1.0 .75 | .50 .25 | .00 BIN | 1.0 75 | .50 .25 | .00 BIN | 1.0 .75 | .50 .25 | .00 BIN |
| PCONT=*** | | | | | REQUIRED NUMBER OF PATIENTS | | | | | | | | | | | |
| 0.05 | *** | 3010 | 3038 | 3165 | 652 | 660 | 671 | 235 | 237 | 239 | 138 | 139 | 139 | 97 | 97 | 97 |
| | *** | 3020 | 3075 | 5916 | 655 | 665 | 1156 | 236 | 238 | 368 | 138 | 139 | 194 | 97 | 97 | 124 |
| 0.1 | *** | 6268 | 6341 | 6954 | 1208 | 1238 | 1295 | 387 | 393 | 399 | 208 | 210 | 212 | 137 | 138 | 139 |
| | *** | 6293 | 6464 | 10277 | 1222 | 1262 | 1829 | 389 | 395 | 526 | 209 | 211 | 260 | 138 | 139 | 158 |
| 0.15 | *** | 9170 | 9300 | 10755 | 1699 | 1760 | 1897 | 519 | 532 | 547 | 268 | 272 | 277 | 170 | 172 | 174 |
| | *** | 9214 | 9533 | 14112 | 1725 | 1814 | 2417 | 525 | 539 | 662 | 270 | 274 | 316 | 172 | 173 | 187 |
| 0.2 | *** | 11497 | 11698 | 14290 | 2100 | 2201 | 2449 | 630 | 650 | 679 | 318 | 324 | 332 | 198 | 200 | 203 |
| | *** | 11565 | 12067 | 17422 | 2141 | 2292 | 2922 | 639 | 664 | 778 | 320 | 327 | 362 | 199 | 202 | 211 |
| 0.25 | *** | 13190 | 13477 | 17424 | 2407 | 2553 | 2930 | 719 | 748 | 791 | 357 | 367 | 378 | 219 | 223 | 227 |
| | *** | 13286 | 14007 | 20206 | 2467 | 2687 | 3342 | 732 | 768 | 873 | 362 | 371 | 400 | 220 | 225 | 229 |
| 0.3 | *** | 14260 | 14654 | 20081 | 2626 | 2817 | 3331 | 787 | 825 | 881 | 387 | 399 | 413 | 234 | 239 | 245 |
| | *** | 14392 | 15370 | 22465 | 2704 | 2995 | 3678 | 803 | 850 | 946 | 393 | 406 | 428 | 237 | 242 | 242 |
| 0.35 | *** | 14755 | 15277 | 22218 | 2764 | 3000 | 3648 | 832 | 879 | 950 | 408 | 422 | 440 | 245 | 250 | 257 |
| | *** | 14932 | 16205 | 24199 | 2860 | 3220 | 3930 | 854 | 910 | 999 | 414 | 430 | 446 | 247 | 253 | 250 |
| 0.4 | *** | 14744 | 15419 | 23808 | 2829 | 3108 | 3877 | 860 | 914 | 997 | 419 | 435 | 455 | 249 | 256 | 262 |
| | *** | 14973 | 16576 | 25407 | 2944 | 3367 | 4098 | 885 | 950 | 1030 | 427 | 444 | 456 | 252 | 259 | 253 |
| 0.45 | *** | 14308 | 15161 | 24837 | 2834 | 3147 | 4014 | 869 | 928 | 1020 | 422 | 439 | 460 | 249 | 256 | 263 |
| | *** | 14600 | 16554 | 26090 | 2963 | 3439 | 4182 | 896 | 968 | 1041 | 430 | 449 | 456 | 252 | 259 | 250 |
| 0.5 | *** | 13537 | 14589 | 25298 | 2785 | 3127 | 4061 | 862 | 923 | 1020 | 416 | 433 | 455 | 244 | 250 | 258 |
| | *** | 13905 | 16208 | 26248 | 2927 | 3440 | 4182 | 890 | 965 | 1030 | 424 | 443 | 446 | 247 | 254 | 242 |
| 0.55 | *** | 12528 | 13784 | 25188 | 2690 | 3050 | 4016 | 837 | 901 | 997 | 401 | 419 | 440 | 232 | 239 | 247 |
| | *** | 12977 | 15598 | 25880 | 2840 | 3376 | 4098 | 866 | 943 | 999 | 410 | 429 | 428 | 236 | 243 | 229 |
| 0.6 | *** | 11372 | 12817 | 24505 | 2557 | 2921 | 3879 | 797 | 859 | 952 | 379 | 395 | 415 | 217 | 223 | 230 |
| | *** | 11902 | 14772 | 24987 | 2709 | 3247 | 3930 | 826 | 900 | 946 | 386 | 405 | 400 | 220 | 226 | 211 |
| 0.65 | *** | 10152 | 11738 | 23253 | 2387 | 2744 | 3652 | 742 | 800 | 884 | 348 | 363 | 380 | 196 | 202 | 206 |
| | *** | 10748 | 13766 | 23569 | 2537 | 3058 | 3678 | 769 | 837 | 873 | 354 | 371 | 362 | 199 | 203 | 187 |
| 0.7 | *** | 8926 | 10580 | 21436 | 2182 | 2517 | 3334 | 671 | 722 | 794 | 308 | 320 | 335 | 170 | 174 | 178 |
| | *** | 9560 | 12597 | 21625 | 2324 | 2807 | 3342 | 695 | 754 | 778 | 314 | 327 | 316 | 172 | 176 | 158 |
| 0.75 | *** | 7720 | 9353 | 19057 | 1940 | 2240 | 2927 | 584 | 624 | 680 | 260 | 269 | 280 | 139 | 142 | 144 |
| | *** | 8356 | 11266 | 19156 | 2069 | 2490 | 2922 | 603 | 650 | 662 | 264 | 275 | 260 | 140 | 143 | 124 |
| 0.8 | *** | 6527 | 8042 | 16122 | 1659 | 1906 | 2431 | 478 | 507 | 545 | 202 | 208 | 215 | . | . | . |
| | *** | 7124 | 9754 | 16161 | 1765 | 2105 | 2417 | 491 | 525 | 526 | 205 | 212 | 194 | . | . | . |
| 0.85 | *** | 5309 | 6602 | 12638 | 1325 | 1504 | 1847 | 352 | 368 | 389 | . | . | . | . | . | . |
| | *** | 5825 | 8008 | 12641 | 1403 | 1640 | 1829 | 359 | 378 | 368 | . | . | . | . | . | . |
| 0.9 | *** | 3980 | 4936 | 8610 | 915 | 1014 | 1177 | . | . | . | . | . | . | . | . | . |
| | *** | 4368 | 5917 | 8596 | 960 | 1084 | 1156 | . | . | . | . | . | . | . | . | . |
| 0.95 | *** | 2324 | 2792 | 4045 | . | . | . | . | . | . | . | . | . | . | . | . |
| | *** | 2520 | 3211 | 4025 | . | . | . | . | . | . | . | . | . | . | . | . |

TABLE 6: ALPHA= 0.025 POWER= 0.9   EXPECTED ACCRUAL THRU MINIMUM FOLLOW-UP= 1600

| | | DEL=.02 | | | DEL=.05 | | | DEL=.10 | | | DEL=.15 | | | DEL=.20 | | |
|---|---|---|---|---|---|---|---|---|---|---|---|---|---|---|---|---|---|
| FACT= | | 1.0 .75 | .50 .25 | .00 BIN | 1.0 .75 | .50 .25 | .00 BIN | 1.0 .75 | .50 .25 | .00 BIN | 1.0 75 | .50 .25 | .00 BIN | 1.0 .75 | .50 .25 | .00 BIN |
| PCONT=*** | | | | | REQUIRED NUMBER OF PATIENTS | | | | | | | | | | | |
| 0.05 | *** | 3012 | 3041 | 3165 | 653 | 660 | 671 | 235 | 237 | 239 | 138 | 139 | 139 | 97 | 98 | 98 |
| | *** | 3023 | 3078 | 5916 | 656 | 665 | 1156 | 236 | 238 | 368 | 138 | 139 | 194 | 97 | 98 | 124 |
| 0.1 | *** | 6274 | 6351 | 6954 | 1212 | 1241 | 1295 | 387 | 393 | 400 | 208 | 210 | 212 | 137 | 138 | 139 |
| | *** | 6300 | 6477 | 10277 | 1224 | 1263 | 1829 | 390 | 396 | 526 | 209 | 211 | 260 | 138 | 139 | 158 |
| 0.15 | *** | 9179 | 9317 | 10755 | 1705 | 1766 | 1898 | 521 | 532 | 548 | 268 | 272 | 276 | 171 | 172 | 174 |
| | *** | 9226 | 9561 | 14112 | 1731 | 1818 | 2417 | 526 | 540 | 662 | 270 | 274 | 316 | 171 | 173 | 187 |
| 0.2 | *** | 11511 | 11724 | 14290 | 2109 | 2210 | 2448 | 633 | 652 | 679 | 318 | 324 | 332 | 198 | 201 | 203 |
| | *** | 11583 | 12110 | 17422 | 2151 | 2299 | 2922 | 642 | 664 | 778 | 321 | 328 | 362 | 199 | 202 | 211 |
| 0.25 | *** | 13210 | 13516 | 17424 | 2421 | 2566 | 2930 | 722 | 751 | 791 | 359 | 367 | 377 | 219 | 223 | 227 |
| | *** | 13312 | 14070 | 20206 | 2481 | 2698 | 3342 | 735 | 769 | 873 | 363 | 372 | 400 | 221 | 225 | 229 |
| 0.3 | *** | 14287 | 14706 | 20081 | 2643 | 2835 | 3331 | 790 | 828 | 882 | 389 | 400 | 413 | 235 | 240 | 245 |
| | *** | 14428 | 15455 | 22465 | 2722 | 3010 | 3678 | 807 | 852 | 946 | 394 | 406 | 428 | 237 | 242 | 242 |
| 0.35 | *** | 14791 | 15345 | 22218 | 2785 | 3022 | 3648 | 838 | 883 | 950 | 410 | 423 | 439 | 246 | 251 | 257 |
| | *** | 14978 | 16313 | 24199 | 2882 | 3239 | 3930 | 859 | 913 | 999 | 416 | 431 | 446 | 248 | 254 | 250 |
| 0.4 | *** | 14790 | 15506 | 23808 | 2855 | 3133 | 3876 | 866 | 918 | 997 | 421 | 436 | 455 | 250 | 256 | 263 |
| | *** | 15034 | 16708 | 25407 | 2970 | 3388 | 4098 | 890 | 953 | 1030 | 428 | 445 | 456 | 253 | 259 | 253 |
| 0.45 | *** | 14367 | 15268 | 24838 | 2863 | 3176 | 4014 | 876 | 933 | 1020 | 424 | 440 | 461 | 250 | 256 | 263 |
| | *** | 14678 | 16709 | 26090 | 2993 | 3463 | 4182 | 902 | 971 | 1041 | 432 | 450 | 456 | 253 | 259 | 250 |
| 0.5 | *** | 13612 | 14717 | 25298 | 2817 | 3158 | 4061 | 868 | 929 | 1020 | 418 | 435 | 456 | 244 | 251 | 258 |
| | *** | 14000 | 16383 | 26248 | 2959 | 3466 | 4182 | 896 | 969 | 1030 | 426 | 445 | 446 | 247 | 254 | 242 |
| 0.55 | *** | 12620 | 13932 | 25188 | 2724 | 3082 | 4016 | 844 | 905 | 998 | 403 | 420 | 441 | 234 | 240 | 246 |
| | *** | 13091 | 15789 | 25880 | 2874 | 3403 | 4098 | 872 | 946 | 999 | 411 | 430 | 428 | 236 | 243 | 229 |
| 0.6 | *** | 11482 | 12980 | 24505 | 2591 | 2954 | 3879 | 804 | 864 | 952 | 381 | 396 | 416 | 218 | 223 | 229 |
| | *** | 12034 | 14974 | 24987 | 2744 | 3275 | 3930 | 831 | 903 | 946 | 388 | 405 | 400 | 220 | 226 | 211 |
| 0.65 | *** | 10278 | 11911 | 23253 | 2420 | 2776 | 3652 | 748 | 804 | 884 | 350 | 363 | 380 | 197 | 202 | 207 |
| | *** | 10894 | 13971 | 23569 | 2571 | 3084 | 3678 | 774 | 840 | 873 | 356 | 371 | 362 | 199 | 204 | 187 |
| 0.7 | *** | 9062 | 10756 | 21436 | 2214 | 2547 | 3334 | 677 | 725 | 794 | 310 | 321 | 335 | 171 | 175 | 179 |
| | *** | 9714 | 12797 | 21625 | 2356 | 2830 | 3342 | 699 | 756 | 778 | 315 | 328 | 316 | 173 | 176 | 158 |
| 0.75 | *** | 7857 | 9522 | 19057 | 1970 | 2266 | 2927 | 588 | 627 | 681 | 261 | 270 | 280 | 140 | 142 | 145 |
| | *** | 8507 | 11453 | 19156 | 2097 | 2510 | 2922 | 606 | 652 | 662 | 266 | 275 | 260 | 141 | 143 | 124 |
| 0.8 | *** | 6657 | 8195 | 16122 | 1683 | 1927 | 2431 | 481 | 509 | 546 | 204 | 209 | 215 | . | . | . |
| | *** | 7265 | 9918 | 16161 | 1789 | 2120 | 2417 | 495 | 526 | 526 | 206 | 212 | 194 | . | . | . |
| 0.85 | *** | 5422 | 6730 | 12638 | 1343 | 1519 | 1847 | 353 | 369 | 389 | . | . | . | . | . | . |
| | *** | 5945 | 8140 | 12641 | 1420 | 1651 | 1829 | 361 | 379 | 368 | . | . | . | . | . | . |
| 0.9 | *** | 4065 | 5028 | 8610 | 925 | 1022 | 1177 | . | . | . | . | . | . | . | . | . |
| | *** | 4457 | 6005 | 8596 | 969 | 1089 | 1156 | . | . | . | . | . | . | . | . | . |
| 0.95 | *** | 2368 | 2834 | 4045 | . | . | . | . | . | . | . | . | . | . | . | . |
| | *** | 2564 | 3246 | 4025 | . | . | . | . | . | . | . | . | . | . | . | . |

## TABLE 6: ALPHA= 0.025 POWER= 0.9    EXPECTED ACCRUAL THRU MINIMUM FOLLOW-UP= 1700

| | | DEL=.02 | | | DEL=.05 | | | DEL=.10 | | | DEL=.15 | | | DEL=.20 | | |
|---|---|---|---|---|---|---|---|---|---|---|---|---|---|---|---|---|---|
| | FACT= | 1.0 .75 | .50 .25 | .00 BIN | 1.0 .75 | .50 .25 | .00 BIN | 1.0 .75 | .50 .25 | .00 BIN | 1.0 75 | .50 .25 | .00 BIN | 1.0 .75 | .50 .25 | .00 BIN |
| PCONT=*** | | REQUIRED NUMBER OF PATIENTS | | | | | | | | | | | | | | | |
| 0.05 | *** | 3014 | 3044 | 3165 | 653 | 661 | 671 | 236 | 237 | 239 | 138 | 138 | 139 | 97 | 97 | 97 |
| | *** | 3025 | 3081 | 5916 | 656 | 665 | 1156 | 236 | 238 | 368 | 138 | 139 | 194 | 97 | 97 | 124 |
| 0.1 | *** | 6278 | 6360 | 6954 | 1214 | 1243 | 1295 | 388 | 393 | 399 | 208 | 210 | 212 | 137 | 138 | 139 |
| | *** | 6306 | 6489 | 10277 | 1227 | 1264 | 1829 | 391 | 396 | 526 | 209 | 211 | 260 | 138 | 139 | 158 |
| 0.15 | *** | 9188 | 9334 | 10754 | 1710 | 1771 | 1897 | 522 | 533 | 548 | 269 | 272 | 276 | 171 | 172 | 174 |
| | *** | 9237 | 9587 | 14112 | 1736 | 1821 | 2417 | 527 | 539 | 662 | 270 | 274 | 316 | 172 | 173 | 187 |
| 0.2 | *** | 11525 | 11750 | 14290 | 2118 | 2220 | 2448 | 634 | 653 | 679 | 318 | 325 | 331 | 199 | 201 | 203 |
| | *** | 11600 | 12153 | 17422 | 2160 | 2305 | 2922 | 644 | 665 | 778 | 322 | 328 | 362 | 199 | 202 | 211 |
| 0.25 | *** | 13229 | 13553 | 17424 | 2433 | 2579 | 2929 | 726 | 752 | 790 | 359 | 367 | 377 | 220 | 223 | 227 |
| | *** | 13338 | 14131 | 20206 | 2494 | 2707 | 3342 | 738 | 770 | 873 | 363 | 372 | 400 | 221 | 225 | 229 |
| 0.3 | *** | 14313 | 14757 | 20081 | 2659 | 2851 | 3331 | 794 | 830 | 882 | 390 | 401 | 413 | 236 | 240 | 244 |
| | *** | 14462 | 15537 | 22465 | 2739 | 3024 | 3678 | 811 | 853 | 946 | 395 | 407 | 428 | 238 | 242 | 242 |
| 0.35 | *** | 14826 | 15412 | 22218 | 2805 | 3042 | 3648 | 843 | 886 | 951 | 411 | 424 | 440 | 246 | 250 | 257 |
| | *** | 15025 | 16417 | 24199 | 2904 | 3255 | 3930 | 862 | 915 | 999 | 418 | 431 | 446 | 248 | 254 | 250 |
| 0.4 | *** | 14836 | 15591 | 23808 | 2879 | 3157 | 3876 | 871 | 922 | 996 | 423 | 437 | 454 | 250 | 256 | 262 |
| | *** | 15094 | 16835 | 25407 | 2994 | 3408 | 4098 | 894 | 955 | 1030 | 429 | 445 | 456 | 254 | 259 | 253 |
| 0.45 | *** | 14426 | 15373 | 24838 | 2890 | 3203 | 4014 | 882 | 937 | 1020 | 426 | 441 | 460 | 250 | 256 | 263 |
| | *** | 14754 | 16857 | 26090 | 3021 | 3485 | 4182 | 907 | 974 | 1041 | 433 | 450 | 456 | 254 | 259 | 250 |
| 0.5 | *** | 13686 | 14841 | 25298 | 2846 | 3186 | 4061 | 874 | 933 | 1020 | 420 | 435 | 456 | 245 | 250 | 257 |
| | *** | 14094 | 16551 | 26248 | 2989 | 3490 | 4182 | 901 | 972 | 1030 | 427 | 445 | 446 | 248 | 254 | 242 |
| 0.55 | *** | 12711 | 14074 | 25187 | 2756 | 3112 | 4016 | 850 | 909 | 998 | 405 | 420 | 441 | 233 | 240 | 246 |
| | *** | 13204 | 15971 | 25880 | 2906 | 3427 | 4098 | 877 | 949 | 999 | 413 | 430 | 428 | 237 | 243 | 229 |
| 0.6 | *** | 11589 | 13136 | 24505 | 2623 | 2985 | 3879 | 809 | 868 | 952 | 382 | 397 | 415 | 219 | 223 | 229 |
| | *** | 12163 | 15165 | 24987 | 2775 | 3299 | 3930 | 837 | 905 | 946 | 390 | 406 | 400 | 221 | 226 | 211 |
| 0.65 | *** | 10399 | 12076 | 23253 | 2452 | 2805 | 3652 | 754 | 807 | 884 | 350 | 364 | 380 | 197 | 202 | 207 |
| | *** | 11036 | 14164 | 23569 | 2602 | 3108 | 3678 | 779 | 843 | 873 | 357 | 372 | 362 | 199 | 204 | 187 |
| 0.7 | *** | 9192 | 10922 | 21436 | 2244 | 2574 | 3334 | 682 | 729 | 794 | 311 | 322 | 335 | 171 | 174 | 178 |
| | *** | 9861 | 12986 | 21625 | 2385 | 2851 | 3342 | 703 | 758 | 778 | 316 | 328 | 316 | 173 | 176 | 158 |
| 0.75 | *** | 7989 | 9683 | 19057 | 1997 | 2290 | 2927 | 593 | 630 | 681 | 262 | 271 | 280 | 140 | 142 | 144 |
| | *** | 8652 | 11629 | 19156 | 2123 | 2528 | 2922 | 610 | 653 | 662 | 267 | 275 | 260 | 141 | 143 | 124 |
| 0.8 | *** | 6781 | 8340 | 16122 | 1706 | 1946 | 2431 | 484 | 511 | 546 | 204 | 209 | 214 | . | . | . |
| | *** | 7399 | 10072 | 16161 | 1810 | 2135 | 2417 | 497 | 527 | 526 | 207 | 212 | 194 | . | . | . |
| 0.85 | *** | 5529 | 6851 | 12638 | 1360 | 1532 | 1848 | 355 | 371 | 389 | . | . | . | . | . | . |
| | *** | 6059 | 8263 | 12641 | 1436 | 1661 | 1829 | 362 | 379 | 368 | . | . | . | . | . | . |
| 0.9 | *** | 4147 | 5115 | 8610 | 935 | 1030 | 1177 | . | . | . | . | . | . | . | . | . |
| | *** | 4541 | 6087 | 8596 | 977 | 1093 | 1156 | . | . | . | . | . | . | . | . | . |
| 0.95 | *** | 2409 | 2873 | 4045 | . | . | . | . | . | . | . | . | . | . | . | . |
| | *** | 2605 | 3278 | 4025 | . | . | . | . | . | . | . | . | . | . | . | . |

TABLE 6: ALPHA= 0.025 POWER= 0.9    EXPECTED ACCRUAL THRU MINIMUM FOLLOW-UP= 1800

|  | | DEL=.02 | | | DEL=.05 | | | DEL=.10 | | | DEL=.15 | | | DEL=.20 | |
|---|---|---|---|---|---|---|---|---|---|---|---|---|---|---|---|
| FACT= | 1.0 .75 | .50 .25 | .00 BIN | 1.0 .75 | .50 .25 | .00 BIN | 1.0 .75 | .50 .25 | .00 BIN | 1.0 75 | .50 .25 | .00 BIN | 1.0 .75 | .50 .25 | .00 BIN |

PCONT=***                    REQUIRED NUMBER OF PATIENTS

| PCONT | | DEL=.02 | | | DEL=.05 | | | DEL=.10 | | | DEL=.15 | | | DEL=.20 | | |
|---|---|---|---|---|---|---|---|---|---|---|---|---|---|---|---|---|
| 0.05 | *** | 3016 | 3048 | 3165 | 654 | 661 | 672 | 236 | 237 | 238 | 138 | 138 | 139 | 98 | 98 | 98 |
|  | *** | 3027 | 3084 | 5916 | 657 | 666 | 1156 | 236 | 238 | 368 | 138 | 139 | 194 | 98 | 98 | 124 |
| 0.1 | *** | 6283 | 6369 | 6954 | 1217 | 1245 | 1295 | 388 | 393 | 399 | 208 | 210 | 213 | 137 | 138 | 139 |
|  | *** | 6312 | 6502 | 10277 | 1230 | 1266 | 1829 | 391 | 397 | 526 | 209 | 211 | 260 | 138 | 138 | 158 |
| 0.15 | *** | 9197 | 9351 | 10755 | 1716 | 1776 | 1898 | 523 | 534 | 548 | 269 | 272 | 276 | 171 | 172 | 174 |
|  | *** | 9249 | 9612 | 14112 | 1741 | 1824 | 2417 | 528 | 540 | 662 | 271 | 274 | 316 | 172 | 173 | 187 |
| 0.2 | *** | 11538 | 11776 | 14291 | 2126 | 2227 | 2448 | 636 | 654 | 679 | 319 | 325 | 332 | 199 | 201 | 204 |
|  | *** | 11618 | 12194 | 17422 | 2169 | 2312 | 2922 | 645 | 666 | 778 | 323 | 328 | 362 | 200 | 202 | 211 |
| 0.25 | *** | 13248 | 13591 | 17424 | 2445 | 2591 | 2929 | 728 | 755 | 791 | 360 | 368 | 378 | 220 | 224 | 227 |
|  | *** | 13364 | 14190 | 20206 | 2505 | 2717 | 3342 | 740 | 771 | 873 | 364 | 372 | 400 | 222 | 225 | 229 |
| 0.3 | *** | 14340 | 14807 | 20081 | 2675 | 2866 | 3331 | 798 | 832 | 882 | 391 | 402 | 414 | 236 | 240 | 245 |
|  | *** | 14498 | 15616 | 22465 | 2755 | 3036 | 3678 | 813 | 855 | 946 | 396 | 407 | 428 | 238 | 242 | 242 |
| 0.35 | *** | 14861 | 15479 | 22218 | 2825 | 3061 | 3648 | 847 | 890 | 951 | 413 | 424 | 440 | 246 | 251 | 256 |
|  | *** | 15070 | 16518 | 24199 | 2922 | 3271 | 3930 | 866 | 917 | 999 | 418 | 432 | 446 | 249 | 254 | 250 |
| 0.4 | *** | 14881 | 15675 | 23808 | 2901 | 3179 | 3876 | 876 | 924 | 996 | 424 | 438 | 456 | 252 | 256 | 263 |
|  | *** | 15153 | 16957 | 25407 | 3017 | 3426 | 4098 | 899 | 957 | 1030 | 431 | 447 | 456 | 254 | 260 | 253 |
| 0.45 | *** | 14484 | 15475 | 24837 | 2916 | 3228 | 4014 | 886 | 940 | 1020 | 427 | 442 | 460 | 251 | 256 | 263 |
|  | *** | 14829 | 17000 | 26090 | 3046 | 3505 | 4182 | 911 | 976 | 1041 | 434 | 451 | 456 | 254 | 260 | 250 |
| 0.5 | *** | 13760 | 14964 | 25299 | 2874 | 3214 | 4061 | 879 | 937 | 1020 | 422 | 436 | 456 | 245 | 251 | 258 |
|  | *** | 14187 | 16710 | 26248 | 3017 | 3512 | 4182 | 906 | 974 | 1030 | 429 | 445 | 446 | 249 | 254 | 242 |
| 0.55 | *** | 12800 | 14213 | 25188 | 2785 | 3141 | 4016 | 856 | 913 | 998 | 407 | 422 | 441 | 235 | 240 | 246 |
|  | *** | 13314 | 16146 | 25880 | 2935 | 3450 | 4098 | 883 | 951 | 999 | 414 | 431 | 428 | 237 | 243 | 229 |
| 0.6 | *** | 11695 | 13288 | 24504 | 2654 | 3012 | 3879 | 816 | 872 | 953 | 384 | 398 | 415 | 219 | 224 | 229 |
|  | *** | 12289 | 15347 | 24987 | 2805 | 3322 | 3930 | 841 | 908 | 946 | 390 | 406 | 400 | 222 | 226 | 211 |
| 0.65 | *** | 10518 | 12235 | 23253 | 2481 | 2832 | 3651 | 759 | 811 | 884 | 352 | 366 | 380 | 198 | 202 | 207 |
|  | *** | 11172 | 14348 | 23569 | 2631 | 3129 | 3678 | 783 | 843 | 873 | 359 | 372 | 362 | 200 | 204 | 187 |
| 0.7 | *** | 9319 | 11082 | 21435 | 2272 | 2600 | 3334 | 686 | 731 | 794 | 312 | 323 | 335 | 172 | 175 | 179 |
|  | *** | 10002 | 13164 | 21625 | 2413 | 2871 | 3342 | 708 | 759 | 778 | 317 | 328 | 316 | 173 | 177 | 158 |
| 0.75 | *** | 8115 | 9834 | 19056 | 2022 | 2312 | 2927 | 596 | 632 | 681 | 263 | 271 | 280 | 141 | 143 | 145 |
|  | *** | 8790 | 11796 | 19156 | 2148 | 2544 | 2922 | 613 | 654 | 662 | 267 | 276 | 260 | 141 | 144 | 124 |
| 0.8 | *** | 6900 | 8479 | 16122 | 1727 | 1964 | 2431 | 487 | 513 | 546 | 204 | 209 | 215 | . | . | . |
|  | *** | 7527 | 10218 | 16161 | 1830 | 2148 | 2417 | 499 | 528 | 526 | 207 | 213 | 194 | . | . | . |
| 0.85 | *** | 5631 | 6966 | 12638 | 1374 | 1545 | 1847 | 357 | 371 | 389 | . | . | . | . | . | . |
|  | *** | 6168 | 8379 | 12641 | 1450 | 1669 | 1829 | 363 | 380 | 368 | . | . | . | . | . | . |
| 0.9 | *** | 4223 | 5196 | 8610 | 944 | 1036 | 1176 | . | . | . | . | . | . | . | . | . |
|  | *** | 4621 | 6164 | 8596 | 985 | 1097 | 1156 | . | . | . | . | . | . | . | . | . |
| 0.95 | *** | 2448 | 2909 | 4045 | . | . | . | . | . | . | . | . | . | . | . | . |
|  | *** | 2643 | 3307 | 4025 | . | . | . | . | . | . | . | . | . | . | . | . |

TABLE 6: ALPHA= 0.025 POWER= 0.9    EXPECTED ACCRUAL THRU MINIMUM FOLLOW-UP= 1900

| | | DEL=.02 | | | DEL=.05 | | | DEL=.10 | | | DEL=.15 | | | DEL=.20 | | |
|---|---|---|---|---|---|---|---|---|---|---|---|---|---|---|---|---|---|
| FACT= | | 1.0 .75 | .50 .25 | .00 BIN | 1.0 .75 | .50 .25 | .00 BIN | 1.0 .75 | .50 .25 | .00 BIN | 1.0 75 | .50 .25 | .00 BIN | 1.0 .75 | .50 .25 | .00 BIN |
| PCONT=*** | | REQUIRED NUMBER OF PATIENTS | | | | | | | | | | | | | | |
| 0.05 | *** | 3018 | 3051 | 3165 | 654 | 661 | 671 | 236 | 237 | 239 | 137 | 139 | 139 | 97 | 97 | 98 |
| | *** | 3030 | 3087 | 5916 | 657 | 666 | 1156 | 236 | 237 | 368 | 139 | 139 | 194 | 97 | 97 | 124 |
| 0.1 | *** | 6289 | 6378 | 6954 | 1219 | 1246 | 1294 | 389 | 394 | 400 | 209 | 210 | 212 | 137 | 139 | 139 |
| | *** | 6319 | 6513 | 10277 | 1231 | 1267 | 1829 | 391 | 396 | 526 | 209 | 211 | 260 | 137 | 139 | 158 |
| 0.15 | *** | 9205 | 9367 | 10755 | 1721 | 1780 | 1897 | 524 | 534 | 547 | 269 | 273 | 277 | 171 | 172 | 174 |
| | *** | 9260 | 9636 | 14112 | 1745 | 1827 | 2417 | 529 | 540 | 662 | 270 | 274 | 316 | 172 | 173 | 187 |
| 0.2 | *** | 11552 | 11802 | 14290 | 2134 | 2234 | 2448 | 638 | 655 | 679 | 320 | 325 | 331 | 198 | 201 | 203 |
| | *** | 11636 | 12233 | 17422 | 2177 | 2318 | 2922 | 646 | 666 | 778 | 323 | 329 | 362 | 199 | 201 | 211 |
| 0.25 | *** | 13268 | 13627 | 17424 | 2455 | 2602 | 2929 | 730 | 756 | 790 | 361 | 368 | 377 | 220 | 223 | 227 |
| | *** | 13389 | 14247 | 20206 | 2517 | 2725 | 3342 | 742 | 771 | 873 | 364 | 372 | 400 | 222 | 225 | 229 |
| 0.3 | *** | 14366 | 14858 | 20082 | 2690 | 2880 | 3331 | 801 | 835 | 882 | 391 | 401 | 413 | 236 | 241 | 244 |
| | *** | 14532 | 15694 | 22465 | 2770 | 3047 | 3678 | 817 | 856 | 946 | 396 | 407 | 428 | 239 | 242 | 242 |
| 0.35 | *** | 14896 | 15544 | 22218 | 2842 | 3079 | 3648 | 850 | 892 | 950 | 413 | 425 | 439 | 247 | 251 | 256 |
| | *** | 15116 | 16615 | 24199 | 2941 | 3286 | 3930 | 869 | 918 | 999 | 419 | 432 | 446 | 249 | 254 | 250 |
| 0.4 | *** | 14928 | 15757 | 23808 | 2923 | 3200 | 3876 | 881 | 928 | 996 | 426 | 439 | 455 | 251 | 258 | 262 |
| | *** | 15213 | 17075 | 25407 | 3040 | 3443 | 4098 | 902 | 959 | 1030 | 432 | 446 | 456 | 254 | 260 | 253 |
| 0.45 | *** | 14543 | 15576 | 24837 | 2940 | 3251 | 4013 | 892 | 944 | 1020 | 429 | 443 | 460 | 251 | 258 | 263 |
| | *** | 14904 | 17137 | 26090 | 3070 | 3524 | 4182 | 915 | 978 | 1041 | 436 | 451 | 456 | 254 | 260 | 254 |
| 0.5 | *** | 13832 | 15081 | 25298 | 2901 | 3239 | 4061 | 885 | 940 | 1010 | 422 | 438 | 456 | 246 | 251 | 258 |
| | *** | 14278 | 16864 | 26248 | 3043 | 3533 | 4182 | 911 | 976 | 1030 | 429 | 446 | 446 | 249 | 254 | 242 |
| 0.55 | *** | 12889 | 14347 | 25188 | 2813 | 3167 | 4016 | 861 | 918 | 997 | 408 | 422 | 440 | 235 | 241 | 247 |
| | *** | 13422 | 16311 | 25880 | 2963 | 3471 | 4098 | 887 | 953 | 999 | 415 | 431 | 428 | 237 | 243 | 229 |
| 0.6 | *** | 11800 | 13434 | 24505 | 2682 | 3040 | 3879 | 820 | 875 | 952 | 386 | 399 | 415 | 220 | 224 | 229 |
| | *** | 12411 | 15522 | 24987 | 2834 | 3343 | 3930 | 847 | 909 | 946 | 391 | 407 | 400 | 222 | 227 | 211 |
| 0.65 | *** | 10635 | 12389 | 23253 | 2510 | 2858 | 3651 | 763 | 814 | 885 | 353 | 365 | 380 | 198 | 201 | 204 |
| | *** | 11305 | 14524 | 23569 | 2659 | 3149 | 3678 | 787 | 847 | 873 | 360 | 372 | 362 | 201 | 204 | 187 |
| 0.7 | *** | 9442 | 11236 | 21435 | 2299 | 2623 | 3334 | 691 | 733 | 793 | 313 | 323 | 334 | 172 | 175 | 178 |
| | *** | 10138 | 13334 | 21625 | 2438 | 2889 | 3342 | 711 | 761 | 778 | 318 | 329 | 316 | 173 | 177 | 158 |
| 0.75 | *** | 8238 | 9982 | 19057 | 2046 | 2332 | 2927 | 600 | 635 | 680 | 263 | 272 | 280 | 140 | 142 | 144 |
| | *** | 8924 | 11953 | 19156 | 2170 | 2560 | 2922 | 616 | 655 | 662 | 267 | 275 | 260 | 141 | 144 | 124 |
| 0.8 | *** | 7014 | 8610 | 16123 | 1747 | 1980 | 2431 | 489 | 514 | 546 | 205 | 210 | 215 | . | . | . |
| | *** | 7649 | 10355 | 16161 | 1849 | 2158 | 2417 | 501 | 529 | 526 | 208 | 212 | 194 | . | . | . |
| 0.85 | *** | 5730 | 7075 | 12638 | 1389 | 1557 | 1847 | 357 | 372 | 389 | . | . | . | . | . | . |
| | *** | 6272 | 8488 | 12641 | 1464 | 1676 | 1829 | 364 | 380 | 368 | . | . | . | . | . | . |
| 0.9 | *** | 4297 | 5274 | 8610 | 952 | 1041 | 1177 | . | . | . | . | . | . | . | . | . |
| | *** | 4696 | 6235 | 8596 | 992 | 1101 | 1156 | . | . | . | . | . | . | . | . | . |
| 0.95 | *** | 2485 | 2942 | 4046 | . | . | . | . | . | . | . | . | . | . | . | . |
| | *** | 2680 | 3334 | 4025 | . | . | . | . | . | . | . | . | . | . | . | . |

TABLE 6: ALPHA= 0.025 POWER= 0.9    EXPECTED ACCRUAL THRU MINIMUM FOLLOW-UP= 2000

| | DEL=.02 | | | DEL=.05 | | | DEL=.10 | | | DEL=.15 | | | DEL=.20 | | |
|---|---|---|---|---|---|---|---|---|---|---|---|---|---|---|---|
| FACT= | 1.0 .75 | .50 .25 | .00 BIN | 1.0 .75 | .50 .25 | .00 BIN | 1.0 .75 | .50 .25 | .00 BIN | 1.0 75 | .50 .25 | .00 BIN | 1.0 .75 | .50 .25 | .00 BIN |

PCONT=***                     REQUIRED NUMBER OF PATIENTS

| PCONT | | DEL=.02 1.0/.75 | .50/.25 | .00/BIN | DEL=.05 1.0/.75 | .50/.25 | .00/BIN | DEL=.10 1.0/.75 | .50/.25 | .00/BIN | DEL=.15 1.0/.75 | .50/.25 | .00/BIN | DEL=.20 1.0/.75 | .50/.25 | .00/BIN |
|---|---|---|---|---|---|---|---|---|---|---|---|---|---|---|---|---|
| 0.05 | *** | 3020 | 3052 | 3165 | 655 | 662 | 671 | 236 | 237 | 239 | 139 | 139 | 139 | 97 | 97 | 97 |
| | *** | 3032 | 3090 | 5916 | 659 | 666 | 1156 | 236 | 237 | 368 | 139 | 139 | 194 | 97 | 97 | 124 |
| 0.1 | *** | 6294 | 6386 | 6955 | 1221 | 1249 | 1295 | 390 | 394 | 400 | 209 | 210 | 212 | 137 | 139 | 139 |
| | *** | 6326 | 6525 | 10277 | 1234 | 1269 | 1829 | 392 | 397 | 526 | 210 | 211 | 260 | 139 | 139 | 158 |
| 0.15 | *** | 9214 | 9384 | 10755 | 1725 | 1785 | 1897 | 525 | 535 | 547 | 270 | 272 | 276 | 171 | 172 | 174 |
| | *** | 9272 | 9660 | 14112 | 1751 | 1831 | 2417 | 530 | 541 | 662 | 271 | 275 | 316 | 172 | 174 | 187 |
| 0.2 | *** | 11565 | 11827 | 14290 | 2141 | 2241 | 2449 | 640 | 657 | 679 | 321 | 326 | 331 | 199 | 201 | 204 |
| | *** | 11654 | 12272 | 17422 | 2184 | 2322 | 2922 | 647 | 667 | 778 | 324 | 329 | 362 | 200 | 202 | 211 |
| 0.25 | *** | 13286 | 13664 | 17424 | 2467 | 2611 | 2930 | 732 | 757 | 791 | 361 | 369 | 377 | 221 | 224 | 227 |
| | *** | 13415 | 14304 | 20206 | 2527 | 2732 | 3342 | 744 | 772 | 873 | 365 | 374 | 400 | 222 | 225 | 229 |
| 0.3 | *** | 14392 | 14907 | 20081 | 2704 | 2895 | 3331 | 804 | 836 | 881 | 394 | 402 | 414 | 237 | 241 | 245 |
| | *** | 14567 | 15767 | 22465 | 2785 | 3057 | 3678 | 819 | 857 | 946 | 397 | 407 | 428 | 239 | 242 | 242 |
| 0.35 | *** | 14931 | 15609 | 22217 | 2860 | 3096 | 3649 | 854 | 895 | 950 | 415 | 426 | 440 | 247 | 252 | 256 |
| | *** | 15164 | 16710 | 24199 | 2960 | 3299 | 3930 | 872 | 920 | 999 | 420 | 432 | 446 | 250 | 254 | 250 |
| 0.4 | *** | 14974 | 15839 | 23809 | 2944 | 3220 | 3876 | 885 | 931 | 996 | 427 | 440 | 455 | 252 | 257 | 262 |
| | *** | 15272 | 17189 | 25407 | 3060 | 3459 | 4098 | 906 | 961 | 1030 | 434 | 447 | 456 | 255 | 260 | 253 |
| 0.45 | *** | 14601 | 15675 | 24837 | 2964 | 3274 | 4014 | 896 | 947 | 1020 | 430 | 444 | 461 | 252 | 257 | 264 |
| | *** | 14979 | 17269 | 26090 | 3095 | 3541 | 4182 | 920 | 980 | 1041 | 436 | 452 | 456 | 255 | 260 | 250 |
| 0.5 | *** | 13905 | 15197 | 25299 | 2926 | 3262 | 4061 | 890 | 944 | 1020 | 424 | 439 | 456 | 246 | 252 | 257 |
| | *** | 14370 | 17012 | 26248 | 3069 | 3551 | 4182 | 915 | 979 | 1030 | 431 | 446 | 446 | 249 | 255 | 242 |
| 0.55 | *** | 12976 | 14477 | 25187 | 2840 | 3192 | 4016 | 866 | 921 | 997 | 410 | 424 | 441 | 236 | 241 | 246 |
| | *** | 13529 | 16471 | 25880 | 2990 | 3491 | 4098 | 891 | 956 | 999 | 416 | 432 | 428 | 239 | 244 | 229 |
| 0.6 | *** | 11901 | 13576 | 24505 | 2710 | 3065 | 3880 | 826 | 879 | 952 | 386 | 400 | 416 | 220 | 225 | 230 |
| | *** | 12531 | 15687 | 24987 | 2861 | 3362 | 3930 | 850 | 912 | 946 | 392 | 407 | 400 | 222 | 227 | 211 |
| 0.65 | *** | 10749 | 12536 | 23254 | 2537 | 2882 | 3652 | 769 | 817 | 885 | 355 | 366 | 380 | 199 | 202 | 206 |
| | *** | 11434 | 14691 | 23569 | 2685 | 3167 | 3678 | 791 | 847 | 873 | 360 | 374 | 362 | 201 | 205 | 187 |
| 0.7 | *** | 9561 | 11382 | 21436 | 2324 | 2645 | 3334 | 695 | 737 | 794 | 315 | 324 | 335 | 172 | 175 | 179 |
| | *** | 10270 | 13496 | 21625 | 2462 | 2905 | 3342 | 715 | 762 | 778 | 319 | 330 | 316 | 174 | 177 | 158 |
| 0.75 | *** | 8356 | 10121 | 19057 | 2069 | 2351 | 2927 | 602 | 636 | 681 | 265 | 272 | 280 | 141 | 142 | 145 |
| | *** | 9052 | 12102 | 19156 | 2191 | 2574 | 2922 | 619 | 657 | 662 | 269 | 276 | 260 | 141 | 144 | 124 |
| 0.8 | *** | 7125 | 8736 | 16122 | 1766 | 1995 | 2431 | 491 | 516 | 546 | 206 | 210 | 215 | . | . | . |
| | *** | 7767 | 10485 | 16161 | 1866 | 2170 | 2417 | 504 | 530 | 526 | 207 | 212 | 194 | . | . | . |
| 0.85 | *** | 5825 | 7180 | 12639 | 1404 | 1566 | 1847 | 359 | 372 | 389 | . | . | . | . | . | . |
| | *** | 6371 | 8590 | 12641 | 1476 | 1684 | 1829 | 366 | 381 | 368 | . | . | . | . | . | . |
| 0.9 | *** | 4367 | 5346 | 8610 | 960 | 1047 | 1177 | . | . | . | . | . | . | . | . | . |
| | *** | 4770 | 6302 | 8596 | 1000 | 1104 | 1156 | . | . | . | . | . | . | . | . | . |
| 0.95 | *** | 2520 | 2975 | 4045 | . | . | . | . | . | . | . | . | . | . | . | . |
| | *** | 2714 | 3360 | 4025 | . | . | . | . | . | . | . | . | . | . | . | . |

## TABLE 6: ALPHA= 0.025 POWER= 0.9    EXPECTED ACCRUAL THRU MINIMUM FOLLOW-UP= 2250

| | | DEL=.02 | | | DEL=.05 | | | DEL=.10 | | | DEL=.15 | | | DEL=.20 | |
|---|---|---|---|---|---|---|---|---|---|---|---|---|---|---|---|
| FACT= | 1.0 .75 | .50 .25 | .00 BIN | 1.0 .75 | .50 .25 | .00 BIN | 1.0 .75 | .50 .25 | .00 BIN | 1.0 75 | .50 .25 | .00 BIN | 1.0 .75 | .50 .25 | .00 BIN |
| PCONT=*** | | | | REQUIRED NUMBER OF PATIENTS | | | | | | | | | | | |
| 0.05 *** | 3025 | 3059 | 3165 | 657 | 663 | 672 | 236 | 237 | 239 | 139 | 139 | 139 | 97 | 98 | 98 |
| *** | 3039 | 3096 | 5916 | 659 | 666 | 1156 | 237 | 237 | 368 | 139 | 139 | 194 | 98 | 98 | 124 |
| 0.1 *** | 6305 | 6408 | 6954 | 1226 | 1253 | 1295 | 390 | 395 | 399 | 209 | 210 | 212 | 137 | 139 | 139 |
| *** | 6342 | 6550 | 10277 | 1239 | 1271 | 1829 | 392 | 398 | 526 | 209 | 210 | 260 | 137 | 139 | 158 |
| 0.15 *** | 9236 | 9423 | 10754 | 1735 | 1794 | 1898 | 527 | 537 | 548 | 269 | 272 | 277 | 171 | 173 | 174 |
| *** | 9300 | 9714 | 14112 | 1760 | 1838 | 2417 | 531 | 541 | 662 | 271 | 274 | 316 | 173 | 173 | 187 |
| 0.2 *** | 11598 | 11891 | 14290 | 2158 | 2257 | 2448 | 644 | 659 | 679 | 322 | 326 | 331 | 199 | 201 | 204 |
| *** | 11698 | 12362 | 17422 | 2201 | 2334 | 2922 | 651 | 668 | 778 | 325 | 329 | 362 | 201 | 202 | 211 |
| 0.25 *** | 13335 | 13754 | 17425 | 2491 | 2634 | 2929 | 738 | 761 | 792 | 362 | 370 | 378 | 222 | 223 | 226 |
| *** | 13477 | 14435 | 20206 | 2552 | 2750 | 3342 | 748 | 775 | 873 | 367 | 374 | 400 | 223 | 224 | 229 |
| 0.3 *** | 14459 | 15029 | 20081 | 2736 | 2924 | 3331 | 809 | 840 | 882 | 395 | 403 | 413 | 237 | 241 | 244 |
| *** | 14654 | 15944 | 22465 | 2817 | 3081 | 3678 | 825 | 859 | 946 | 399 | 407 | 428 | 239 | 243 | 242 |
| 0.35 *** | 15018 | 15766 | 22217 | 2901 | 3133 | 3647 | 862 | 899 | 950 | 417 | 427 | 440 | 249 | 253 | 257 |
| *** | 15277 | 16931 | 24199 | 2999 | 3328 | 3930 | 880 | 922 | 999 | 421 | 433 | 446 | 250 | 254 | 250 |
| 0.4 *** | 15086 | 16035 | 23807 | 2991 | 3264 | 3877 | 894 | 938 | 997 | 430 | 441 | 455 | 253 | 258 | 263 |
| *** | 15419 | 17456 | 25407 | 3107 | 3493 | 4098 | 914 | 964 | 1030 | 435 | 448 | 456 | 255 | 260 | 253 |
| 0.45 *** | 14744 | 15913 | 24837 | 3017 | 3324 | 4015 | 907 | 955 | 1019 | 433 | 446 | 461 | 253 | 258 | 263 |
| *** | 15161 | 17578 | 26090 | 3147 | 3580 | 4182 | 928 | 984 | 1041 | 438 | 452 | 456 | 255 | 260 | 250 |
| 0.5 *** | 14082 | 15474 | 25298 | 2985 | 3317 | 4061 | 899 | 950 | 1020 | 427 | 440 | 455 | 247 | 253 | 257 |
| *** | 14590 | 17355 | 26248 | 3126 | 3593 | 4182 | 924 | 983 | 1030 | 433 | 447 | 446 | 250 | 254 | 242 |
| 0.55 *** | 13190 | 14787 | 25187 | 2902 | 3248 | 4016 | 877 | 928 | 998 | 413 | 426 | 441 | 237 | 241 | 246 |
| *** | 13784 | 16841 | 25880 | 3050 | 3534 | 4098 | 901 | 960 | 999 | 419 | 433 | 428 | 239 | 244 | 229 |
| 0.6 *** | 12147 | 13909 | 24505 | 2772 | 3120 | 3880 | 837 | 885 | 952 | 389 | 402 | 416 | 221 | 224 | 229 |
| *** | 12816 | 16072 | 24987 | 2922 | 3405 | 3930 | 859 | 916 | 946 | 395 | 407 | 400 | 223 | 227 | 211 |
| 0.65 *** | 11018 | 12882 | 23253 | 2598 | 2936 | 3652 | 779 | 824 | 884 | 357 | 368 | 381 | 199 | 202 | 207 |
| *** | 11738 | 15077 | 23569 | 2743 | 3207 | 3678 | 800 | 852 | 873 | 362 | 374 | 362 | 201 | 205 | 187 |
| 0.7 *** | 9842 | 11727 | 21435 | 2382 | 2694 | 3334 | 703 | 742 | 794 | 316 | 325 | 334 | 173 | 176 | 178 |
| *** | 10580 | 13870 | 21625 | 2517 | 2941 | 3342 | 721 | 766 | 778 | 320 | 330 | 316 | 174 | 177 | 158 |
| 0.75 *** | 8634 | 10448 | 19057 | 2120 | 2395 | 2926 | 610 | 641 | 680 | 266 | 272 | 280 | 140 | 143 | 145 |
| *** | 9353 | 12447 | 19156 | 2240 | 2606 | 2922 | 624 | 659 | 662 | 269 | 277 | 260 | 142 | 143 | 124 |
| 0.8 *** | 7382 | 9028 | 16122 | 1808 | 2029 | 2431 | 496 | 519 | 545 | 207 | 210 | 215 | . | . | . |
| *** | 8042 | 10783 | 16161 | 1905 | 2193 | 2417 | 507 | 531 | 526 | 208 | 212 | 194 | . | . | . |
| 0.85 *** | 6045 | 7419 | 12638 | 1434 | 1590 | 1847 | 362 | 374 | 389 | . | . | . | . | . | . |
| *** | 6602 | 8824 | 12641 | 1504 | 1698 | 1829 | 368 | 381 | 368 | . | . | . | . | . | . |
| 0.9 *** | 4530 | 5514 | 8610 | 977 | 1059 | 1177 | . | . | . | . | . | . | . | . | . |
| *** | 4935 | 6454 | 8596 | 1015 | 1110 | 1156 | . | . | . | . | . | . | . | . | . |
| 0.95 *** | 2600 | 3047 | 4046 | . | . | . | . | . | . | . | . | . | . | . | . |
| *** | 2791 | 3416 | 4025 | . | . | . | . | . | . | . | . | . | . | . | . |

TABLE 6: ALPHA= 0.025 POWER= 0.9     EXPECTED ACCRUAL THRU MINIMUM FOLLOW-UP= 2500

| | DEL=.02 | | | DEL=.05 | | | DEL=.10 | | | DEL=.15 | | | DEL=.20 | | |
|---|---|---|---|---|---|---|---|---|---|---|---|---|---|---|---|
| FACT= | 1.0 .75 | .50 .25 | .00 BIN | 1.0 .75 | .50 .25 | .00 BIN | 1.0 .75 | .50 .25 | .00 BIN | 1.0 75 | .50 .25 | .00 BIN | 1.0 .75 | .50 .25 | .00 BIN |
| PCONT=*** | REQUIRED NUMBER OF PATIENTS | | | | | | | | | | | | | | |
| 0.05 *** | 3029 | 3065 | 3165 | 658 | 664 | 671 | 237 | 237 | 239 | 139 | 139 | 139 | 98 | 98 | 98 |
| *** | 3043 | 3101 | 5916 | 661 | 667 | 1156 | 237 | 239 | 368 | 139 | 139 | 194 | 98 | 98 | 124 |
| 0.1 *** | 6317 | 6427 | 6954 | 1231 | 1256 | 1295 | 392 | 395 | 399 | 209 | 211 | 212 | 137 | 139 | 139 |
| *** | 6358 | 6573 | 10277 | 1242 | 1273 | 1829 | 393 | 398 | 526 | 211 | 211 | 260 | 139 | 139 | 158 |
| 0.15 *** | 9258 | 9462 | 10754 | 1745 | 1801 | 1898 | 529 | 537 | 548 | 271 | 273 | 276 | 171 | 173 | 174 |
| *** | 9327 | 9765 | 14112 | 1770 | 1842 | 2417 | 533 | 542 | 662 | 271 | 274 | 316 | 171 | 173 | 187 |
| 0.2 *** | 11631 | 11951 | 14290 | 2174 | 2270 | 2448 | 646 | 661 | 679 | 323 | 326 | 331 | 199 | 201 | 202 |
| *** | 11742 | 12446 | 17422 | 2217 | 2343 | 2922 | 652 | 670 | 778 | 324 | 329 | 362 | 201 | 202 | 211 |
| 0.25 *** | 13383 | 13842 | 17424 | 2514 | 2654 | 2929 | 742 | 764 | 790 | 364 | 370 | 377 | 221 | 224 | 226 |
| *** | 13540 | 14556 | 20206 | 2574 | 2764 | 3342 | 751 | 776 | 873 | 367 | 373 | 400 | 223 | 226 | 229 |
| 0.3 *** | 14524 | 15146 | 20081 | 2767 | 2951 | 3331 | 815 | 845 | 881 | 396 | 404 | 414 | 239 | 242 | 245 |
| *** | 14740 | 16106 | 22465 | 2846 | 3101 | 3678 | 829 | 862 | 946 | 399 | 409 | 428 | 240 | 243 | 242 |
| 0.35 *** | 15106 | 15918 | 22218 | 2937 | 3167 | 3648 | 868 | 904 | 949 | 418 | 427 | 439 | 249 | 252 | 256 |
| *** | 15390 | 17136 | 24199 | 3036 | 3352 | 3930 | 886 | 924 | 999 | 423 | 434 | 446 | 251 | 254 | 250 |
| 0.4 *** | 15198 | 16224 | 23808 | 3034 | 3302 | 3876 | 901 | 942 | 996 | 433 | 442 | 454 | 254 | 259 | 262 |
| *** | 15562 | 17699 | 25407 | 3149 | 3521 | 4098 | 920 | 967 | 1030 | 437 | 448 | 456 | 256 | 261 | 253 |
| 0.45 *** | 14886 | 16139 | 24837 | 3065 | 3367 | 4014 | 915 | 959 | 1020 | 436 | 446 | 461 | 254 | 259 | 264 |
| *** | 15339 | 17859 | 26090 | 3195 | 3614 | 4182 | 936 | 987 | 1041 | 440 | 452 | 456 | 256 | 261 | 250 |
| 0.5 *** | 14256 | 15734 | 25298 | 3037 | 3364 | 4061 | 909 | 958 | 1020 | 429 | 442 | 456 | 248 | 252 | 258 |
| *** | 14799 | 17668 | 26248 | 3177 | 3627 | 4182 | 931 | 986 | 1030 | 436 | 448 | 446 | 251 | 256 | 242 |
| 0.55 *** | 13395 | 15076 | 25187 | 2956 | 3296 | 4015 | 886 | 934 | 998 | 415 | 426 | 440 | 237 | 242 | 246 |
| *** | 14027 | 17176 | 25880 | 3102 | 3570 | 4098 | 909 | 964 | 999 | 421 | 434 | 428 | 240 | 243 | 229 |
| 0.6 *** | 12381 | 14218 | 24504 | 2827 | 3168 | 3879 | 845 | 892 | 952 | 392 | 402 | 415 | 221 | 224 | 229 |
| *** | 13084 | 16418 | 24987 | 2974 | 3440 | 3930 | 867 | 920 | 946 | 396 | 409 | 400 | 223 | 227 | 211 |
| 0.65 *** | 11271 | 13199 | 23252 | 2652 | 2983 | 3651 | 786 | 829 | 884 | 359 | 368 | 381 | 199 | 202 | 206 |
| *** | 12021 | 15424 | 23569 | 2795 | 3242 | 3678 | 806 | 854 | 873 | 364 | 374 | 362 | 201 | 204 | 187 |
| 0.7 *** | 10104 | 12040 | 21436 | 2433 | 2737 | 3334 | 711 | 746 | 793 | 318 | 326 | 336 | 173 | 176 | 177 |
| *** | 10868 | 14202 | 21625 | 2565 | 2973 | 3342 | 727 | 768 | 778 | 321 | 331 | 316 | 174 | 177 | 158 |
| 0.75 *** | 8892 | 10745 | 19058 | 2165 | 2431 | 2926 | 615 | 645 | 681 | 267 | 273 | 279 | 142 | 143 | 145 |
| *** | 9629 | 12752 | 19156 | 2283 | 2631 | 2922 | 629 | 662 | 662 | 270 | 276 | 260 | 142 | 143 | 124 |
| 0.8 *** | 7620 | 9293 | 16121 | 1845 | 2058 | 2431 | 501 | 521 | 545 | 208 | 211 | 215 | . | . | . |
| *** | 8292 | 11046 | 16161 | 1940 | 2212 | 2417 | 511 | 533 | 526 | 209 | 214 | 194 | . | . | . |
| 0.85 *** | 6246 | 7636 | 12639 | 1461 | 1609 | 1846 | 364 | 376 | 389 | . | . | . | . | . | . |
| *** | 6812 | 9029 | 12641 | 1527 | 1712 | 1829 | 370 | 383 | 368 | . | . | . | . | . | . |
| 0.9 *** | 4677 | 5662 | 8611 | 992 | 1068 | 1176 | . | . | . | . | . | . | . | . | . |
| *** | 5087 | 6586 | 8596 | 1026 | 1117 | 1156 | . | . | . | . | . | . | . | . | . |
| 0.95 *** | 2671 | 3109 | 4045 | . | . | . | . | . | . | . | . | . | . | . | . |
| *** | 2861 | 3462 | 4025 | . | . | . | . | . | . | . | . | . | . | . | . |

## TABLE 6: ALPHA= 0.025 POWER= 0.9    EXPECTED ACCRUAL THRU MINIMUM FOLLOW-UP= 2750

|  |  | DEL=.02 | | | DEL=.05 | | | DEL=.10 | | | DEL=.15 | | | DEL=.20 | | |
|---|---|---|---|---|---|---|---|---|---|---|---|---|---|---|---|---|
| FACT= | | 1.0 .75 | .50 .25 | .00 BIN | 1.0 .75 | .50 .25 | .00 BIN | 1.0 .75 | .50 .25 | .00 BIN | 1.0 75 | .50 .25 | .00 BIN | 1.0 .75 | .50 .25 | .00 BIN |
| PCONT=*** | | | | | REQUIRED NUMBER OF PATIENTS | | | | | | | | | | | |
| 0.05 | *** | 3033 | 3069 | 3165 | 658 | 665 | 672 | 236 | 236 | 239 | 139 | 139 | 139 | 98 | 98 | 98 |
|  | *** | 3048 | 3105 | 5916 | 661 | 668 | 1156 | 236 | 239 | 368 | 139 | 139 | 194 | 98 | 98 | 124 |
| 0.1 | *** | 6330 | 6447 | 6953 | 1235 | 1259 | 1295 | 391 | 395 | 400 | 209 | 211 | 212 | 139 | 139 | 139 |
|  | *** | 6371 | 6594 | 10277 | 1246 | 1275 | 1829 | 393 | 398 | 526 | 211 | 211 | 260 | 139 | 139 | 158 |
| 0.15 | *** | 9279 | 9499 | 10755 | 1752 | 1807 | 1897 | 531 | 538 | 548 | 271 | 273 | 276 | 171 | 173 | 173 |
|  | *** | 9356 | 9810 | 14112 | 1776 | 1847 | 2417 | 534 | 542 | 662 | 273 | 274 | 316 | 173 | 173 | 187 |
| 0.2 | *** | 11665 | 12010 | 14291 | 2189 | 2282 | 2449 | 649 | 663 | 679 | 322 | 328 | 331 | 201 | 202 | 204 |
|  | *** | 11785 | 12522 | 17422 | 2229 | 2350 | 2922 | 654 | 670 | 778 | 324 | 329 | 362 | 201 | 202 | 211 |
| 0.25 | *** | 13430 | 13927 | 17424 | 2535 | 2670 | 2930 | 745 | 766 | 790 | 366 | 370 | 377 | 223 | 225 | 226 |
|  | *** | 13604 | 14669 | 20206 | 2593 | 2777 | 3342 | 754 | 778 | 873 | 367 | 374 | 400 | 223 | 226 | 229 |
| 0.3 | *** | 14590 | 15260 | 20081 | 2793 | 2975 | 3330 | 821 | 847 | 881 | 398 | 405 | 414 | 239 | 242 | 245 |
|  | *** | 14824 | 16255 | 22465 | 2872 | 3117 | 3678 | 833 | 864 | 946 | 401 | 408 | 428 | 240 | 243 | 242 |
| 0.35 | *** | 15192 | 16065 | 22218 | 2969 | 3195 | 3649 | 874 | 907 | 950 | 421 | 429 | 439 | 250 | 252 | 257 |
|  | *** | 15501 | 17324 | 24199 | 3068 | 3374 | 3930 | 890 | 927 | 999 | 424 | 434 | 446 | 250 | 254 | 250 |
| 0.4 | *** | 15310 | 16405 | 23807 | 3072 | 3337 | 3877 | 909 | 947 | 996 | 434 | 443 | 455 | 256 | 259 | 263 |
|  | *** | 15702 | 17926 | 25407 | 3186 | 3547 | 4098 | 926 | 969 | 1030 | 438 | 450 | 456 | 257 | 260 | 253 |
| 0.45 | *** | 15025 | 16351 | 24837 | 3109 | 3404 | 4014 | 923 | 964 | 1020 | 438 | 448 | 460 | 256 | 259 | 263 |
|  | *** | 15509 | 18118 | 26090 | 3236 | 3642 | 4182 | 941 | 989 | 1041 | 443 | 453 | 456 | 257 | 260 | 250 |
| 0.5 | *** | 14425 | 15977 | 25298 | 3085 | 3404 | 4061 | 917 | 962 | 1020 | 431 | 443 | 455 | 249 | 254 | 257 |
|  | *** | 15003 | 17955 | 26248 | 3222 | 3659 | 4182 | 938 | 989 | 1030 | 438 | 448 | 446 | 250 | 256 | 242 |
| 0.55 | *** | 13593 | 15344 | 25188 | 3006 | 3337 | 4016 | 893 | 938 | 998 | 417 | 428 | 441 | 239 | 242 | 247 |
|  | *** | 14258 | 17481 | 25880 | 3150 | 3602 | 4098 | 916 | 965 | 999 | 422 | 434 | 428 | 240 | 243 | 229 |
| 0.6 | *** | 12605 | 14505 | 24505 | 2876 | 3210 | 3879 | 852 | 896 | 951 | 393 | 404 | 415 | 223 | 226 | 230 |
|  | *** | 13337 | 16735 | 24987 | 3021 | 3471 | 3930 | 872 | 923 | 946 | 398 | 408 | 400 | 225 | 228 | 211 |
| 0.65 | *** | 11511 | 13494 | 23253 | 2700 | 3023 | 3652 | 793 | 833 | 885 | 360 | 370 | 379 | 201 | 204 | 205 |
|  | *** | 12287 | 15738 | 23569 | 2841 | 3270 | 3678 | 813 | 857 | 873 | 366 | 374 | 362 | 202 | 205 | 187 |
| 0.7 | *** | 10350 | 12330 | 21435 | 2476 | 2773 | 3334 | 716 | 751 | 793 | 319 | 326 | 335 | 173 | 177 | 178 |
|  | *** | 11133 | 14504 | 21625 | 2607 | 2999 | 3342 | 731 | 771 | 778 | 322 | 331 | 316 | 175 | 177 | 158 |
| 0.75 | *** | 9129 | 11016 | 19057 | 2205 | 2463 | 2927 | 620 | 648 | 680 | 267 | 274 | 280 | 142 | 144 | 144 |
|  | *** | 9884 | 13027 | 19156 | 2318 | 2653 | 2922 | 634 | 663 | 662 | 271 | 276 | 260 | 142 | 144 | 124 |
| 0.8 | *** | 7839 | 9534 | 16121 | 1876 | 2082 | 2432 | 505 | 524 | 546 | 208 | 211 | 214 | . | . | . |
|  | *** | 8523 | 11283 | 16161 | 1969 | 2229 | 2417 | 514 | 534 | 526 | 209 | 212 | 194 | . | . | . |
| 0.85 | *** | 6431 | 7830 | 12638 | 1483 | 1625 | 1847 | 366 | 377 | 390 | . | . | . | . | . | . |
|  | *** | 7004 | 9212 | 12641 | 1548 | 1721 | 1829 | 370 | 383 | 368 | . | . | . | . | . | . |
| 0.9 | *** | 4812 | 5795 | 8610 | 1003 | 1077 | 1177 | . | . | . | . | . | . | . | . | . |
|  | *** | 5223 | 6702 | 8596 | 1037 | 1122 | 1156 | . | . | . | . | . | . | . | . | . |
| 0.95 | *** | 2734 | 3164 | 4045 | . | . | . | . | . | . | . | . | . | . | . | . |
|  | *** | 2921 | 3502 | 4025 | . | . | . | . | . | . | . | . | . | . | . | . |

## TABLE 6: ALPHA= 0.025 POWER= 0.9 EXPECTED ACCRUAL THRU MINIMUM FOLLOW-UP= 3000

| | | DEL=.01 | | | DEL=.02 | | | DEL=.05 | | | DEL=.10 | | | DEL=.15 | | |
|---|---|---|---|---|---|---|---|---|---|---|---|---|---|---|---|---|
| FACT= | | 1.0 .75 | .50 .25 | .00 BIN | 1.0 .75 | .50 .25 | .00 BIN | 1.0 .75 | .50 .25 | .00 BIN | 1.0 75 | .50 .25 | .00 BIN | 1.0 .75 | .50 .25 | .00 BIN |
| PCONT=*** | | | | REQUIRED NUMBER OF PATIENTS | | | | | | | | | | | | |
| 0.01 | *** | 1607 | 1610 | 1622 | 590 | 590 | 595 | 193 | 197 | 197 | 100 | 100 | 100 | 70 | 70 | 70 |
| | *** | 1607 | 1615 | 6200 | 590 | 595 | 2049 | 193 | 197 | 558 | 100 | 100 | 227 | 70 | 70 | 135 |
| 0.02 | *** | 3550 | 3565 | 3617 | 1142 | 1145 | 1157 | 310 | 310 | 310 | 137 | 137 | 137 | 88 | 88 | 88 |
| | *** | 3553 | 3580 | 10235 | 1142 | 1150 | 3048 | 310 | 310 | 712 | 137 | 137 | 264 | 88 | 88 | 151 |
| 0.05 | *** | 10735 | 10790 | 11297 | 3040 | 3073 | 3163 | 658 | 665 | 670 | 238 | 238 | 238 | 137 | 137 | 137 |
| | *** | 10753 | 10888 | 21835 | 3050 | 3107 | 5916 | 662 | 665 | 1156 | 238 | 238 | 368 | 137 | 137 | 194 |
| 0.1 | *** | 23675 | 23815 | 26293 | 6340 | 6463 | 6955 | 1240 | 1262 | 1295 | 392 | 395 | 400 | 208 | 212 | 212 |
| | *** | 23720 | 24088 | 39487 | 6385 | 6613 | 10277 | 1247 | 1277 | 1829 | 392 | 395 | 526 | 208 | 212 | 260 |
| 0.15 | *** | 35353 | 35600 | 41533 | 9298 | 9535 | 10753 | 1760 | 1813 | 1895 | 530 | 538 | 545 | 272 | 272 | 275 |
| | *** | 35435 | 36095 | 55038 | 9385 | 9853 | 14112 | 1783 | 1850 | 2417 | 535 | 542 | 662 | 272 | 275 | 316 |
| 0.2 | *** | 44758 | 45145 | 55802 | 11698 | 12065 | 14290 | 2200 | 2293 | 2447 | 650 | 662 | 677 | 325 | 328 | 332 |
| | *** | 44885 | 45917 | 68488 | 11825 | 12595 | 17422 | 2240 | 2357 | 2922 | 658 | 670 | 778 | 325 | 328 | 362 |
| 0.25 | *** | 51605 | 52165 | 68507 | 13475 | 14008 | 17425 | 2552 | 2687 | 2930 | 748 | 767 | 790 | 365 | 370 | 377 |
| | *** | 51790 | 53278 | 79836 | 13663 | 14773 | 20206 | 2612 | 2788 | 3342 | 755 | 778 | 873 | 370 | 373 | 400 |
| 0.3 | *** | 55910 | 56683 | 79330 | 14653 | 15370 | 20080 | 2818 | 2995 | 3332 | 823 | 850 | 880 | 400 | 407 | 415 |
| | *** | 56170 | 58213 | 89082 | 14908 | 16393 | 22465 | 2893 | 3130 | 3678 | 835 | 865 | 946 | 403 | 410 | 428 |
| 0.35 | *** | 57853 | 58880 | 88085 | 15275 | 16205 | 22217 | 2998 | 3220 | 3647 | 880 | 910 | 950 | 422 | 430 | 440 |
| | *** | 58195 | 60913 | 96227 | 15610 | 17500 | 24199 | 3095 | 3392 | 3930 | 895 | 928 | 999 | 425 | 433 | 446 |
| 0.4 | *** | 57680 | 59023 | 94667 | 15418 | 16577 | 23807 | 3107 | 3365 | 3875 | 913 | 950 | 995 | 433 | 445 | 455 |
| | *** | 58127 | 61660 | 101271 | 15838 | 18133 | 25407 | 3220 | 3568 | 4098 | 932 | 973 | 1030 | 440 | 448 | 456 |
| 0.45 | *** | 55700 | 57433 | 99010 | 15160 | 16555 | 24838 | 3148 | 3437 | 4015 | 928 | 970 | 1018 | 437 | 448 | 460 |
| | *** | 56278 | 60770 | 104213 | 15673 | 18358 | 26090 | 3272 | 3665 | 4182 | 947 | 992 | 1041 | 445 | 455 | 456 |
| 0.5 | *** | 52262 | 54470 | 101080 | 14590 | 16210 | 25300 | 3125 | 3440 | 4060 | 925 | 965 | 1018 | 433 | 445 | 455 |
| | *** | 53000 | 58595 | 105054 | 15197 | 18220 | 26248 | 3260 | 3685 | 4182 | 943 | 992 | 1030 | 437 | 448 | 446 |
| 0.55 | *** | 47720 | 50507 | 100865 | 13783 | 15598 | 25187 | 3050 | 3377 | 4015 | 902 | 943 | 995 | 418 | 430 | 440 |
| | *** | 48662 | 55457 | 103793 | 14477 | 17762 | 25880 | 3193 | 3628 | 4098 | 920 | 970 | 999 | 422 | 433 | 428 |
| 0.6 | *** | 42470 | 45928 | 98365 | 12815 | 14773 | 24505 | 2920 | 3245 | 3880 | 857 | 898 | 950 | 395 | 403 | 415 |
| | *** | 43655 | 51643 | 100430 | 13577 | 17023 | 24987 | 3065 | 3497 | 3930 | 880 | 925 | 946 | 400 | 410 | 400 |
| 0.65 | *** | 36913 | 41068 | 93583 | 11740 | 13765 | 23252 | 2743 | 3058 | 3650 | 800 | 838 | 883 | 362 | 370 | 380 |
| | *** | 38380 | 47372 | 94967 | 12535 | 16025 | 23569 | 2882 | 3295 | 3678 | 815 | 857 | 873 | 365 | 373 | 362 |
| 0.7 | *** | 31430 | 36163 | 86537 | 10580 | 12598 | 21437 | 2518 | 2807 | 3332 | 722 | 752 | 793 | 320 | 328 | 335 |
| | *** | 33155 | 42770 | 87401 | 11383 | 14777 | 21625 | 2645 | 3020 | 3342 | 737 | 770 | 778 | 325 | 332 | 316 |
| 0.75 | *** | 26305 | 31333 | 77245 | 9355 | 11267 | 19055 | 2240 | 2488 | 2927 | 625 | 650 | 680 | 268 | 275 | 280 |
| | *** | 28195 | 37892 | 77734 | 10120 | 13277 | 19156 | 2350 | 2672 | 2922 | 635 | 665 | 662 | 272 | 275 | 260 |
| 0.8 | *** | 21625 | 26563 | 65728 | 8042 | 9752 | 16123 | 1907 | 2105 | 2432 | 508 | 523 | 545 | 208 | 212 | 215 |
| | *** | 23518 | 32687 | 65966 | 8735 | 11495 | 16161 | 1993 | 2245 | 2417 | 515 | 535 | 526 | 208 | 212 | 194 |
| 0.85 | *** | 17275 | 21715 | 52010 | 6602 | 8008 | 12640 | 1502 | 1640 | 1847 | 370 | 377 | 388 | . | . | . |
| | *** | 19003 | 26995 | 52096 | 7180 | 9377 | 12641 | 1565 | 1730 | 1829 | 373 | 385 | 368 | . | . | . |
| 0.9 | *** | 12958 | 16468 | 36115 | 4937 | 5915 | 8608 | 1015 | 1082 | 1175 | . | . | . | . | . | . |
| | *** | 14345 | 20450 | 36125 | 5345 | 6805 | 8596 | 1048 | 1127 | 1156 | . | . | . | . | . | . |
| 0.95 | *** | 8020 | 10052 | 18070 | 2792 | 3212 | 4045 | . | . | . | . | . | . | . | . | . |
| | *** | 8840 | 12152 | 18052 | 2975 | 3538 | 4025 | . | . | . | . | . | . | . | . | . |
| 0.98 | *** | 3823 | 4532 | 6220 | . | . | . | . | . | . | . | . | . | . | . | . |
| | *** | 4123 | 5135 | 6200 | . | . | . | . | . | . | . | . | . | . | . | . |

TABLE 6: ALPHA= 0.025 POWER= 0.9     EXPECTED ACCRUAL THRU MINIMUM FOLLOW-UP= 3250

| | FACT= | DEL=.01 | | | DEL=.02 | | | DEL=.05 | | | DEL=.10 | | | DEL=.15 | | |
|---|---|---|---|---|---|---|---|---|---|---|---|---|---|---|---|---|
| | | 1.0 .75 | .50 .25 | .00 BIN | 1.0 .75 | .50 .25 | .00 BIN | 1.0 .75 | .50 .25 | .00 BIN | 1.0 75 | .50 .25 | .00 BIN | 1.0 .75 | .50 .25 | .00 BIN |
| PCONT=*** | | | | | | | REQUIRED NUMBER OF PATIENTS | | | | | | | | |
| 0.01 | *** | 1606 | 1611 | 1619 | 591 | 591 | 596 | 192 | 198 | 198 | 100 | 100 | 100 | 71 | 71 | 71 |
| | *** | 1606 | 1614 | 6200 | 591 | 591 | 2049 | 192 | 198 | 558 | 100 | 100 | 227 | 71 | 71 | 135 |
| 0.02 | *** | 3548 | 3564 | 3618 | 1140 | 1148 | 1156 | 311 | 311 | 311 | 136 | 136 | 136 | 87 | 87 | 87 |
| | *** | 3556 | 3581 | 10235 | 1143 | 1151 | 3048 | 311 | 311 | 712 | 136 | 136 | 264 | 87 | 87 | 151 |
| 0.05 | *** | 10739 | 10801 | 11296 | 3041 | 3077 | 3166 | 661 | 664 | 672 | 238 | 238 | 238 | 136 | 141 | 141 |
| | *** | 10760 | 10901 | 21835 | 3058 | 3109 | 5916 | 664 | 669 | 1156 | 238 | 238 | 368 | 141 | 141 | 194 |
| 0.1 | *** | 23687 | 23836 | 26290 | 6351 | 6481 | 6952 | 1241 | 1262 | 1294 | 393 | 396 | 401 | 209 | 209 | 214 |
| | *** | 23739 | 24134 | 39487 | 6400 | 6627 | 10277 | 1254 | 1278 | 1829 | 396 | 396 | 526 | 209 | 209 | 260 |
| 0.15 | *** | 35374 | 35642 | 41532 | 9322 | 9566 | 10755 | 1766 | 1817 | 1899 | 531 | 539 | 547 | 271 | 274 | 274 |
| | *** | 35463 | 36175 | 55038 | 9411 | 9891 | 14112 | 1790 | 1855 | 2417 | 534 | 542 | 662 | 274 | 274 | 316 |
| 0.2 | *** | 44788 | 45210 | 55800 | 11730 | 12120 | 14289 | 2213 | 2302 | 2448 | 653 | 664 | 680 | 322 | 328 | 331 |
| | *** | 44929 | 46042 | 68488 | 11868 | 12656 | 17422 | 2253 | 2362 | 2922 | 656 | 672 | 778 | 328 | 331 | 362 |
| 0.25 | *** | 51653 | 52257 | 68507 | 13526 | 14086 | 17423 | 2570 | 2700 | 2931 | 750 | 769 | 791 | 368 | 371 | 376 |
| | *** | 51851 | 53460 | 79836 | 13726 | 14866 | 20206 | 2627 | 2798 | 3342 | 758 | 777 | 873 | 368 | 376 | 400 |
| 0.3 | *** | 55976 | 56813 | 79330 | 14717 | 15476 | 20079 | 2838 | 3012 | 3329 | 826 | 851 | 880 | 401 | 404 | 412 |
| | *** | 56255 | 58465 | 89082 | 14988 | 16524 | 22465 | 2914 | 3142 | 3678 | 839 | 867 | 946 | 404 | 409 | 428 |
| 0.35 | *** | 57937 | 59050 | 88086 | 15362 | 16337 | 22216 | 3025 | 3244 | 3646 | 883 | 913 | 948 | 425 | 428 | 441 |
| | *** | 58311 | 61244 | 96227 | 15716 | 17661 | 24199 | 3123 | 3407 | 3930 | 896 | 932 | 999 | 425 | 433 | 446 |
| 0.4 | *** | 57791 | 59245 | 94667 | 15524 | 16740 | 23809 | 3139 | 3394 | 3878 | 921 | 953 | 997 | 436 | 444 | 452 |
| | *** | 58278 | 62081 | 101271 | 15971 | 18327 | 25407 | 3247 | 3589 | 4098 | 937 | 972 | 1030 | 441 | 449 | 456 |
| 0.45 | *** | 55846 | 57723 | 99009 | 15294 | 16748 | 24836 | 3182 | 3467 | 4011 | 932 | 972 | 1018 | 441 | 449 | 461 |
| | *** | 56471 | 61298 | 104213 | 15833 | 18576 | 26090 | 3309 | 3686 | 4182 | 953 | 994 | 1041 | 444 | 452 | 456 |
| 0.5 | *** | 52444 | 54833 | 101081 | 14749 | 16426 | 25299 | 3163 | 3472 | 4060 | 929 | 969 | 1021 | 433 | 444 | 458 |
| | *** | 53246 | 59221 | 105054 | 15383 | 18463 | 26248 | 3301 | 3708 | 4182 | 948 | 994 | 1030 | 441 | 449 | 446 |
| 0.55 | *** | 47956 | 50957 | 100866 | 13969 | 15833 | 25185 | 3090 | 3410 | 4016 | 907 | 945 | 997 | 420 | 428 | 441 |
| | *** | 48972 | 56182 | 103793 | 14684 | 18019 | 25880 | 3228 | 3651 | 4098 | 924 | 969 | 999 | 425 | 433 | 428 |
| 0.6 | *** | 42767 | 46469 | 98364 | 13019 | 15021 | 24502 | 2960 | 3280 | 3878 | 864 | 904 | 953 | 396 | 404 | 417 |
| | *** | 44048 | 52449 | 100430 | 13802 | 17287 | 24987 | 3101 | 3521 | 3930 | 883 | 924 | 946 | 401 | 409 | 400 |
| 0.65 | *** | 37288 | 41687 | 93581 | 11954 | 14018 | 23251 | 2781 | 3090 | 3651 | 802 | 839 | 883 | 363 | 371 | 379 |
| | *** | 38851 | 48227 | 94967 | 12770 | 16288 | 23569 | 2919 | 3318 | 3678 | 823 | 859 | 873 | 368 | 376 | 362 |
| 0.7 | *** | 31877 | 36833 | 86537 | 10796 | 12843 | 21436 | 2554 | 2833 | 3334 | 726 | 758 | 794 | 322 | 328 | 336 |
| | *** | 33697 | 43642 | 87401 | 11616 | 15029 | 21625 | 2679 | 3041 | 3342 | 742 | 774 | 778 | 322 | 331 | 316 |
| 0.75 | *** | 26802 | 32018 | 77247 | 9561 | 11499 | 19056 | 2272 | 2513 | 2928 | 628 | 653 | 680 | 271 | 274 | 279 |
| | *** | 28768 | 38734 | 77734 | 10341 | 13506 | 19156 | 2378 | 2687 | 2922 | 639 | 664 | 662 | 271 | 279 | 260 |
| 0.8 | *** | 22127 | 27216 | 65729 | 8233 | 9956 | 16123 | 1931 | 2123 | 2432 | 509 | 526 | 547 | 209 | 214 | 214 |
| | *** | 24085 | 33456 | 65966 | 8935 | 11689 | 16161 | 2018 | 2256 | 2417 | 517 | 534 | 526 | 209 | 214 | 194 |
| 0.85 | *** | 17739 | 22284 | 52011 | 6763 | 8171 | 12637 | 1522 | 1652 | 1847 | 368 | 379 | 387 | . | . | . |
| | *** | 19514 | 27644 | 52096 | 7342 | 9525 | 12641 | 1582 | 1741 | 1829 | 371 | 384 | 368 | . | . | . |
| 0.9 | *** | 13336 | 16911 | 36113 | 5051 | 6026 | 8610 | 1021 | 1091 | 1176 | . | . | . | . | . | . |
| | *** | 14749 | 20927 | 36125 | 5457 | 6896 | 8596 | 1054 | 1132 | 1156 | . | . | . | . | . | . |
| 0.95 | *** | 8244 | 10297 | 18067 | 2841 | 3253 | 4044 | . | . | . | . | . | . | . | . | . |
| | *** | 9078 | 12388 | 18052 | 3025 | 3569 | 4025 | . | . | . | . | . | . | . | . | . |
| 0.98 | *** | 3906 | 4609 | 6221 | . | . | . | . | . | . | . | . | . | . | . | . |
| | *** | 4206 | 5194 | 6200 | . | . | . | . | . | . | . | . | . | . | . | . |

TABLE 6: ALPHA= 0.025 POWER= 0.9   EXPECTED ACCRUAL THRU MINIMUM FOLLOW-UP= 3500

| | | DEL=.01 | | | DEL=.02 | | | DEL=.05 | | | DEL=.10 | | | DEL=.15 | |
|---|---|---|---|---|---|---|---|---|---|---|---|---|---|---|---|---|
| FACT= | 1.0 .75 | .50 .25 | .00 BIN | 1.0 .75 | .50 .25 | .00 BIN | 1.0 .75 | .50 .25 | .00 BIN | 1.0 75 | .50 .25 | .00 BIN | 1.0 .75 | .50 .25 | .00 BIN |
| PCONT=*** | | | | | REQUIRED NUMBER OF PATIENTS | | | | | | | | | | |
| 0.01 *** | 1607 | 1613 | 1621 | 592 | 592 | 592 | 195 | 195 | 195 | 99 | 99 | 99 | 67 | 67 | 67 |
| *** | 1607 | 1616 | 6200 | 592 | 592 | 2049 | 195 | 195 | 558 | 99 | 99 | 227 | 67 | 67 | 135 |
| 0.02 *** | 3550 | 3567 | 3616 | 1140 | 1149 | 1158 | 309 | 309 | 312 | 134 | 134 | 137 | 90 | 90 | 90 |
| *** | 3558 | 3585 | 10235 | 1143 | 1152 | 3048 | 309 | 309 | 712 | 134 | 134 | 264 | 90 | 90 | 151 |
| 0.05 *** | 10742 | 10809 | 11293 | 3048 | 3083 | 3165 | 659 | 668 | 671 | 239 | 239 | 239 | 137 | 137 | 137 |
| *** | 10765 | 10914 | 21835 | 3060 | 3112 | 5916 | 662 | 668 | 1156 | 239 | 239 | 368 | 137 | 137 | 194 |
| 0.1 *** | 23698 | 23864 | 26291 | 6364 | 6495 | 6953 | 1245 | 1266 | 1292 | 391 | 396 | 400 | 207 | 213 | 213 |
| *** | 23753 | 24173 | 39487 | 6411 | 6644 | 10277 | 1254 | 1280 | 1829 | 396 | 396 | 526 | 213 | 213 | 260 |
| 0.15 *** | 35391 | 35685 | 41533 | 9342 | 9601 | 10756 | 1773 | 1823 | 1896 | 531 | 540 | 548 | 274 | 274 | 277 |
| *** | 35487 | 36257 | 55038 | 9435 | 9925 | 14112 | 1796 | 1858 | 2417 | 536 | 545 | 662 | 274 | 274 | 316 |
| 0.2 *** | 44820 | 45275 | 55801 | 11763 | 12174 | 14291 | 2225 | 2307 | 2447 | 653 | 668 | 680 | 326 | 326 | 330 |
| *** | 44972 | 46168 | 68488 | 11911 | 12720 | 17422 | 2260 | 2368 | 2922 | 659 | 671 | 778 | 326 | 330 | 362 |
| 0.25 *** | 51698 | 52348 | 68506 | 13574 | 14160 | 17424 | 2584 | 2710 | 2928 | 755 | 773 | 790 | 365 | 373 | 379 |
| *** | 51916 | 53640 | 79836 | 13784 | 14960 | 20206 | 2640 | 2803 | 3342 | 758 | 781 | 873 | 370 | 373 | 400 |
| 0.3 *** | 56041 | 56939 | 79330 | 14781 | 15578 | 20078 | 2858 | 3030 | 3331 | 828 | 855 | 881 | 400 | 405 | 414 |
| *** | 56338 | 58710 | 89082 | 15070 | 16645 | 22465 | 2934 | 3156 | 3678 | 843 | 869 | 946 | 405 | 408 | 428 |
| 0.35 *** | 58024 | 59223 | 88089 | 15446 | 16470 | 22219 | 3051 | 3261 | 3646 | 886 | 916 | 951 | 423 | 431 | 440 |
| *** | 58421 | 61571 | 96227 | 15817 | 17812 | 24199 | 3144 | 3418 | 3930 | 898 | 930 | 999 | 426 | 435 | 446 |
| 0.4 *** | 57905 | 59471 | 94669 | 15633 | 16893 | 23806 | 3170 | 3418 | 3873 | 921 | 956 | 995 | 435 | 443 | 452 |
| *** | 58426 | 62495 | 101271 | 16097 | 18509 | 25407 | 3278 | 3602 | 4098 | 939 | 974 | 1030 | 440 | 449 | 456 |
| 0.45 *** | 55988 | 58006 | 99009 | 15423 | 16928 | 24838 | 3214 | 3494 | 4013 | 939 | 974 | 1021 | 440 | 449 | 461 |
| *** | 56662 | 61807 | 104213 | 15989 | 18783 | 26090 | 3340 | 3704 | 4182 | 956 | 995 | 1041 | 443 | 452 | 456 |
| 0.5 *** | 52628 | 55192 | 101083 | 14904 | 16631 | 25299 | 3200 | 3503 | 4063 | 933 | 974 | 1021 | 435 | 443 | 458 |
| *** | 53491 | 59830 | 105054 | 15560 | 18684 | 26248 | 3331 | 3725 | 4182 | 951 | 995 | 1030 | 440 | 449 | 446 |
| 0.55 *** | 48192 | 51403 | 100864 | 14143 | 16059 | 25188 | 3126 | 3436 | 4013 | 913 | 951 | 995 | 423 | 431 | 440 |
| *** | 49283 | 56881 | 103793 | 14886 | 18258 | 25880 | 3266 | 3672 | 4098 | 930 | 974 | 999 | 426 | 435 | 428 |
| 0.6 *** | 43065 | 46999 | 98365 | 13210 | 15257 | 24506 | 2998 | 3310 | 3879 | 869 | 907 | 951 | 396 | 405 | 414 |
| *** | 44435 | 53220 | 100430 | 14015 | 17532 | 24987 | 3135 | 3541 | 3930 | 886 | 930 | 946 | 400 | 408 | 400 |
| 0.65 *** | 37654 | 42286 | 93584 | 12156 | 14256 | 23251 | 2820 | 3118 | 3651 | 808 | 843 | 886 | 365 | 370 | 379 |
| *** | 39311 | 49038 | 94967 | 12991 | 16531 | 23569 | 2951 | 3336 | 3678 | 825 | 863 | 873 | 370 | 373 | 362 |
| 0.7 *** | 32316 | 37479 | 86535 | 11001 | 13075 | 21435 | 2587 | 2858 | 3331 | 729 | 758 | 793 | 321 | 326 | 335 |
| *** | 34218 | 44465 | 87401 | 11833 | 15257 | 21625 | 2710 | 3056 | 3342 | 741 | 776 | 778 | 326 | 330 | 316 |
| 0.75 *** | 27280 | 32666 | 77248 | 9759 | 11713 | 19055 | 2298 | 2535 | 2925 | 633 | 653 | 680 | 268 | 274 | 277 |
| *** | 29324 | 39530 | 77734 | 10550 | 13714 | 19156 | 2409 | 2701 | 2922 | 641 | 668 | 662 | 274 | 277 | 260 |
| 0.8 *** | 22613 | 27831 | 65727 | 8411 | 10147 | 16120 | 1954 | 2141 | 2430 | 510 | 528 | 545 | 207 | 213 | 216 |
| *** | 24625 | 34180 | 65966 | 9120 | 11868 | 16161 | 2041 | 2263 | 2417 | 519 | 536 | 526 | 213 | 213 | 194 |
| 0.85 *** | 18180 | 22826 | 52013 | 6910 | 8318 | 12638 | 1537 | 1665 | 1849 | 370 | 379 | 388 | . | . | . |
| *** | 19996 | 28251 | 52096 | 7493 | 9657 | 12641 | 1595 | 1747 | 1829 | 373 | 382 | 368 | . | . | . |
| 0.9 *** | 13688 | 17322 | 36114 | 5156 | 6128 | 8607 | 1030 | 1096 | 1175 | . | . | . | . | . | . |
| *** | 15131 | 21370 | 36125 | 5562 | 6980 | 8596 | 1061 | 1131 | 1156 | . | . | . | . | . | . |
| 0.95 *** | 8455 | 10523 | 18071 | 2890 | 3293 | 4045 | . | . | . | . | . | . | . | . | . |
| *** | 9298 | 12603 | 18052 | 3068 | 3593 | 4025 | . | . | . | . | . | . | . | . | . |
| 0.98 *** | 3984 | 4675 | 6218 | . | . | . | . | . | . | . | . | . | . | . | . |
| *** | 4281 | 5247 | 6200 | . | . | . | . | . | . | . | . | . | . | . | . |

669

TABLE 6: ALPHA= 0.025 POWER= 0.9    EXPECTED ACCRUAL THRU MINIMUM FOLLOW-UP= 3750

| | | DEL=.01 | | | DEL=.02 | | | DEL=.05 | | | DEL=.10 | | | DEL=.15 | | |
|---|---|---|---|---|---|---|---|---|---|---|---|---|---|---|---|---|
| FACT= | | 1.0 .75 | .50 .25 | .00 BIN | 1.0 .75 | .50 .25 | .00 BIN | 1.0 .75 | .50 .25 | .00 BIN | 1.0 75 | .50 .25 | .00 BIN | 1.0 .75 | .50 .25 | .00 BIN |
| PCONT=*** | | | | REQUIRED NUMBER OF PATIENTS | | | | | | | | | | | | |
| 0.01 | *** | 1606 | 1609 | 1619 | 593 | 593 | 593 | 194 | 194 | 194 | 97 | 97 | 97 | 68 | 68 | 68 |
| | *** | 1609 | 1615 | 6200 | 593 | 593 | 2049 | 194 | 194 | 558 | 97 | 97 | 227 | 68 | 68 | 135 |
| 0.02 | *** | 3550 | 3569 | 3616 | 1141 | 1147 | 1156 | 312 | 312 | 312 | 134 | 134 | 134 | 87 | 87 | 87 |
| | *** | 3559 | 3588 | 10235 | 1147 | 1150 | 3048 | 312 | 312 | 712 | 134 | 134 | 264 | 87 | 87 | 151 |
| 0.05 | *** | 10747 | 10816 | 11294 | 3050 | 3087 | 3166 | 663 | 663 | 672 | 237 | 237 | 237 | 138 | 138 | 138 |
| | *** | 10769 | 10925 | 21835 | 3063 | 3119 | 5916 | 663 | 668 | 1156 | 237 | 237 | 368 | 138 | 138 | 194 |
| 0.1 | *** | 23712 | 23884 | 26290 | 6378 | 6509 | 6953 | 1244 | 1268 | 1297 | 391 | 397 | 400 | 209 | 209 | 213 |
| | *** | 23768 | 24213 | 39487 | 6428 | 6659 | 10277 | 1253 | 1278 | 1829 | 397 | 397 | 526 | 209 | 213 | 260 |
| 0.15 | *** | 35412 | 35725 | 41534 | 9363 | 9631 | 10756 | 1778 | 1825 | 1897 | 531 | 541 | 547 | 275 | 275 | 275 |
| | *** | 35519 | 36334 | 55038 | 9462 | 9959 | 14112 | 1803 | 1859 | 2417 | 537 | 541 | 662 | 275 | 275 | 316 |
| 0.2 | *** | 44853 | 45340 | 55803 | 11797 | 12222 | 14290 | 2234 | 2318 | 2450 | 653 | 668 | 678 | 325 | 325 | 331 |
| | *** | 45016 | 46291 | 68488 | 11950 | 12775 | 17422 | 2272 | 2375 | 2922 | 659 | 672 | 778 | 325 | 331 | 362 |
| 0.25 | *** | 51743 | 52441 | 68506 | 13619 | 14234 | 17425 | 2600 | 2722 | 2928 | 756 | 772 | 790 | 368 | 372 | 378 |
| | *** | 51978 | 53819 | 79836 | 13840 | 15040 | 20206 | 2656 | 2809 | 3342 | 762 | 781 | 873 | 368 | 372 | 400 |
| 0.3 | *** | 56106 | 57068 | 79328 | 14843 | 15672 | 20078 | 2875 | 3044 | 3331 | 831 | 856 | 878 | 400 | 406 | 415 |
| | *** | 56425 | 58956 | 89082 | 15147 | 16756 | 22465 | 2950 | 3166 | 3678 | 847 | 869 | 946 | 406 | 409 | 428 |
| 0.35 | *** | 58109 | 59393 | 88084 | 15528 | 16591 | 22216 | 3072 | 3284 | 3650 | 893 | 916 | 950 | 425 | 434 | 438 |
| | *** | 58534 | 61891 | 96227 | 15916 | 17950 | 24199 | 3166 | 3434 | 3930 | 903 | 931 | 999 | 428 | 434 | 446 |
| 0.4 | *** | 58015 | 59693 | 94666 | 15738 | 17047 | 23806 | 3194 | 3438 | 3875 | 925 | 959 | 997 | 438 | 447 | 453 |
| | *** | 58578 | 62903 | 101271 | 16225 | 18672 | 25407 | 3303 | 3622 | 4098 | 940 | 978 | 1030 | 443 | 453 | 456 |
| 0.45 | *** | 56134 | 58291 | 99012 | 15550 | 17103 | 24837 | 3247 | 3518 | 4015 | 944 | 978 | 1019 | 443 | 453 | 462 |
| | *** | 56856 | 62303 | 104213 | 16137 | 18972 | 26090 | 3368 | 3725 | 4182 | 959 | 997 | 1041 | 447 | 456 | 456 |
| 0.5 | *** | 52816 | 55550 | 101078 | 15053 | 16825 | 25297 | 3231 | 3528 | 4062 | 940 | 978 | 1019 | 438 | 447 | 456 |
| | *** | 53734 | 60419 | 105054 | 15734 | 18893 | 26248 | 3363 | 3747 | 4182 | 959 | 997 | 1030 | 443 | 453 | 446 |
| 0.55 | *** | 48425 | 51841 | 100863 | 14313 | 16272 | 25188 | 3162 | 3466 | 4015 | 916 | 953 | 997 | 425 | 428 | 438 |
| | *** | 49591 | 57550 | 103793 | 15078 | 18481 | 25880 | 3297 | 3691 | 4098 | 934 | 972 | 999 | 425 | 434 | 428 |
| 0.6 | *** | 43362 | 47515 | 98365 | 13400 | 15481 | 24503 | 3031 | 3334 | 3878 | 875 | 906 | 953 | 397 | 406 | 415 |
| | *** | 44815 | 53956 | 100430 | 14219 | 17759 | 24987 | 3166 | 3559 | 3930 | 893 | 931 | 946 | 400 | 409 | 400 |
| 0.65 | *** | 38018 | 42869 | 93584 | 12350 | 14481 | 23253 | 2853 | 3143 | 3650 | 813 | 847 | 884 | 363 | 372 | 381 |
| | *** | 39766 | 49812 | 94967 | 13197 | 16756 | 23569 | 2984 | 3353 | 3678 | 828 | 865 | 873 | 368 | 378 | 362 |
| 0.7 | *** | 32740 | 38097 | 86538 | 11197 | 13291 | 21434 | 2618 | 2884 | 3334 | 734 | 762 | 794 | 322 | 331 | 334 |
| | *** | 34728 | 45241 | 87401 | 12040 | 15472 | 21625 | 2734 | 3072 | 3342 | 747 | 775 | 778 | 325 | 331 | 316 |
| 0.75 | *** | 27743 | 33288 | 77243 | 9944 | 11913 | 19056 | 2328 | 2556 | 2928 | 634 | 653 | 681 | 269 | 275 | 278 |
| | *** | 29853 | 40278 | 77734 | 10747 | 13906 | 19156 | 2431 | 2716 | 2922 | 644 | 668 | 662 | 275 | 278 | 260 |
| 0.8 | *** | 23075 | 28418 | 65731 | 8575 | 10319 | 16122 | 1975 | 2153 | 2431 | 513 | 528 | 547 | 209 | 213 | 213 |
| | *** | 25141 | 34859 | 65966 | 9293 | 12025 | 16161 | 2056 | 2275 | 2417 | 522 | 537 | 526 | 209 | 213 | 194 |
| 0.85 | *** | 18603 | 23331 | 52009 | 7047 | 8459 | 12640 | 1553 | 1675 | 1844 | 372 | 378 | 387 | . | . | . |
| | *** | 20459 | 28822 | 52096 | 7634 | 9781 | 12641 | 1609 | 1750 | 1829 | 378 | 381 | 368 | . | . | . |
| 0.9 | *** | 14022 | 17712 | 36115 | 5253 | 6218 | 8609 | 1038 | 1100 | 1175 | . | . | . | . | . | . |
| | *** | 15490 | 21781 | 36125 | 5659 | 7053 | 8596 | 1066 | 1137 | 1156 | . | . | . | . | . | . |
| 0.95 | *** | 8656 | 10731 | 18068 | 2931 | 3325 | 4043 | . | . | . | . | . | . | . | . | . |
| | *** | 9503 | 12803 | 18052 | 3109 | 3622 | 4025 | . | . | . | . | . | . | . | . | . |
| 0.98 | *** | 4056 | 4741 | 6218 | . | . | . | . | . | . | . | . | . | . | . | . |
| | *** | 4353 | 5294 | 6200 | . | . | . | . | . | . | . | . | . | . | . | . |

TABLE 6: ALPHA= 0.025 POWER= 0.9    EXPECTED ACCRUAL THRU MINIMUM FOLLOW-UP= 4000

| | | DEL=.01 | | | DEL=.02 | | | DEL=.05 | | | DEL=.10 | | | DEL=.15 | | |
|---|---|---|---|---|---|---|---|---|---|---|---|---|---|---|---|---|
| FACT= | | 1.0 .75 | .50 .25 | .00 BIN | 1.0 .75 | .50 .25 | .00 BIN | 1.0 .75 | .50 .25 | .00 BIN | 1.0 75 | .50 .25 | .00 BIN | 1.0 .75 | .50 .25 | .00 BIN |
| PCONT=*** | | | | | | REQUIRED NUMBER OF PATIENTS | | | | | | | | | |
| 0.01 | *** | 1607 | 1613 | 1623 | 593 | 593 | 593 | 193 | 197 | 197 | 97 | 97 | 97 | 67 | 67 | 67 |
| | *** | 1607 | 1617 | 6200 | 593 | 593 | 2049 | 197 | 197 | 558 | 97 | 97 | 227 | 67 | 67 | 135 |
| 0.02 | *** | 3553 | 3573 | 3617 | 1143 | 1147 | 1157 | 307 | 313 | 313 | 137 | 137 | 137 | 87 | 87 | 87 |
| | *** | 3563 | 3587 | 10235 | 1147 | 1153 | 3048 | 307 | 313 | 712 | 137 | 137 | 264 | 87 | 87 | 151 |
| 0.05 | *** | 10753 | 10827 | 11297 | 3053 | 3087 | 3163 | 663 | 667 | 673 | 237 | 237 | 237 | 137 | 137 | 137 |
| | *** | 10777 | 10937 | 21835 | 3067 | 3117 | 5916 | 663 | 667 | 1156 | 237 | 237 | 368 | 137 | 137 | 194 |
| 0.1 | *** | 23723 | 23907 | 26293 | 6387 | 6523 | 6953 | 1247 | 1267 | 1293 | 393 | 397 | 397 | 207 | 213 | 213 |
| | *** | 23783 | 24257 | 39487 | 6437 | 6673 | 10277 | 1257 | 1283 | 1829 | 397 | 397 | 526 | 213 | 213 | 260 |
| 0.15 | *** | 35433 | 35767 | 41533 | 9383 | 9657 | 10753 | 1783 | 1833 | 1897 | 533 | 543 | 547 | 273 | 273 | 277 |
| | *** | 35547 | 36413 | 55038 | 9487 | 9987 | 14112 | 1807 | 1863 | 2417 | 537 | 543 | 662 | 273 | 273 | 316 |
| 0.2 | *** | 44887 | 45403 | 55803 | 11827 | 12273 | 14287 | 2243 | 2323 | 2447 | 657 | 667 | 677 | 327 | 327 | 333 |
| | *** | 45057 | 46417 | 68488 | 11993 | 12827 | 17422 | 2277 | 2377 | 2922 | 663 | 673 | 778 | 327 | 327 | 362 |
| 0.25 | *** | 51793 | 52537 | 68507 | 13663 | 14303 | 17423 | 2613 | 2733 | 2927 | 757 | 773 | 793 | 367 | 373 | 377 |
| | *** | 52037 | 53997 | 79836 | 13897 | 15117 | 20206 | 2667 | 2817 | 3342 | 763 | 783 | 873 | 373 | 373 | 400 |
| 0.3 | *** | 56167 | 57197 | 79327 | 14907 | 15767 | 20083 | 2893 | 3057 | 3333 | 837 | 857 | 883 | 403 | 407 | 413 |
| | *** | 56513 | 59197 | 89082 | 15223 | 16863 | 22465 | 2967 | 3173 | 3678 | 847 | 867 | 946 | 403 | 407 | 428 |
| 0.35 | *** | 58193 | 59563 | 88087 | 15607 | 16707 | 22217 | 3097 | 3297 | 3647 | 893 | 917 | 947 | 427 | 433 | 437 |
| | *** | 58653 | 62207 | 96227 | 16017 | 18083 | 24199 | 3187 | 3443 | 3930 | 907 | 933 | 999 | 427 | 437 | 446 |
| 0.4 | *** | 58127 | 59917 | 94667 | 15837 | 17187 | 23807 | 3217 | 3457 | 3877 | 933 | 963 | 997 | 437 | 447 | 453 |
| | *** | 58723 | 63303 | 101271 | 16343 | 18833 | 25407 | 3327 | 3633 | 4098 | 943 | 977 | 1030 | 443 | 453 | 456 |
| 0.45 | *** | 56277 | 58577 | 99007 | 15673 | 17267 | 24837 | 3273 | 3543 | 4013 | 947 | 977 | 1017 | 443 | 453 | 463 |
| | *** | 57047 | 62793 | 104213 | 16283 | 19153 | 26090 | 3393 | 3737 | 4182 | 963 | 997 | 1041 | 447 | 457 | 456 |
| 0.5 | *** | 52997 | 55907 | 101083 | 15197 | 17013 | 25297 | 3263 | 3553 | 4063 | 943 | 977 | 1017 | 437 | 447 | 457 |
| | *** | 53983 | 60993 | 105054 | 15897 | 19093 | 26248 | 3393 | 3763 | 4182 | 957 | 997 | 1030 | 443 | 453 | 446 |
| 0.55 | *** | 48663 | 52273 | 100867 | 14477 | 16473 | 25187 | 3193 | 3493 | 4017 | 923 | 957 | 997 | 423 | 433 | 443 |
| | *** | 49897 | 58203 | 103793 | 15257 | 18687 | 25880 | 3323 | 3707 | 4098 | 937 | 977 | 999 | 427 | 437 | 428 |
| 0.6 | *** | 43657 | 48017 | 98363 | 13577 | 15687 | 24503 | 3063 | 3363 | 3877 | 877 | 913 | 953 | 397 | 407 | 417 |
| | *** | 45193 | 54663 | 100430 | 14413 | 17973 | 24987 | 3197 | 3577 | 3930 | 893 | 933 | 946 | 403 | 413 | 400 |
| 0.65 | *** | 38377 | 43433 | 93583 | 12537 | 14693 | 23253 | 2883 | 3167 | 3653 | 817 | 847 | 883 | 367 | 373 | 377 |
| | *** | 40207 | 50553 | 94967 | 13397 | 16963 | 23569 | 3007 | 3373 | 3342 | 833 | 863 | 873 | 367 | 377 | 362 |
| 0.7 | *** | 33157 | 38693 | 86537 | 11383 | 13497 | 21437 | 2643 | 2903 | 3333 | 737 | 763 | 793 | 323 | 327 | 333 |
| | *** | 35223 | 45983 | 87401 | 12237 | 15667 | 21625 | 2763 | 3087 | 3342 | 747 | 777 | 778 | 327 | 333 | 316 |
| 0.75 | *** | 28193 | 33883 | 77247 | 10123 | 12103 | 19057 | 2353 | 2573 | 2927 | 637 | 657 | 683 | 273 | 277 | 277 |
| | *** | 30363 | 40987 | 77734 | 10927 | 14083 | 19156 | 2453 | 2727 | 2922 | 647 | 667 | 662 | 273 | 277 | 260 |
| 0.8 | *** | 23517 | 28977 | 65727 | 8737 | 10483 | 16123 | 1993 | 2167 | 2433 | 517 | 527 | 547 | 207 | 213 | 213 |
| | *** | 25637 | 35503 | 65966 | 9457 | 12177 | 16161 | 2073 | 2283 | 2417 | 523 | 537 | 526 | 213 | 213 | 194 |
| 0.85 | *** | 19003 | 23817 | 52013 | 7177 | 8587 | 12637 | 1567 | 1683 | 1847 | 373 | 383 | 387 | . | . | . |
| | *** | 20893 | 29357 | 52096 | 7767 | 9893 | 12641 | 1623 | 1757 | 1829 | 377 | 383 | 368 | . | . | . |
| 0.9 | *** | 14343 | 18077 | 36117 | 5347 | 6303 | 8607 | 1047 | 1103 | 1177 | . | . | . | . | . | . |
| | *** | 15833 | 22167 | 36125 | 5753 | 7123 | 8596 | 1073 | 1137 | 1156 | . | . | . | . | . | . |
| 0.95 | *** | 8843 | 10927 | 18067 | 2973 | 3357 | 4043 | . | . | . | . | . | . | . | . | . |
| | *** | 9697 | 12987 | 18052 | 3147 | 3643 | 4025 | . | . | . | . | . | . | . | . | . |
| 0.98 | *** | 4123 | 4797 | 6223 | . | . | . | . | . | . | . | . | . | . | . | . |
| | *** | 4417 | 5337 | 6200 | . | . | . | . | . | . | . | . | . | . | . | . |

TABLE 6: ALPHA= 0.025 POWER= 0.9     EXPECTED ACCRUAL THRU MINIMUM FOLLOW-UP= 4250

| | | DEL=.01 | | | DEL=.02 | | | DEL=.05 | | | DEL=.10 | | | DEL=.15 | | |
|---|---|---|---|---|---|---|---|---|---|---|---|---|---|---|---|---|
| FACT= | | 1.0 .75 | .50 .25 | .00 BIN | 1.0 .75 | .50 .25 | .00 BIN | 1.0 .75 | .50 .25 | .00 BIN | 1.0 75 | .50 .25 | .00 BIN | 1.0 .75 | .50 .25 | .00 BIN |
| PCONT=*** | | | | | REQUIRED | NUMBER | OF PATIENTS | | | | | | | | | |
| 0.01 | *** | 1608 | 1612 | 1618 | 592 | 592 | 592 | 194 | 194 | 194 | 99 | 99 | 99 | 71 | 71 | 71 |
| | *** | 1612 | 1618 | 6200 | 592 | 592 | 2049 | 194 | 194 | 558 | 99 | 99 | 227 | 71 | 71 | 135 |
| 0.02 | *** | 3556 | 3573 | 3616 | 1144 | 1151 | 1155 | 311 | 311 | 311 | 135 | 135 | 135 | 88 | 88 | 88 |
| | *** | 3563 | 3588 | 10235 | 1144 | 1151 | 3048 | 311 | 311 | 712 | 135 | 135 | 264 | 88 | 88 | 151 |
| 0.05 | *** | 10756 | 10834 | 11298 | 3057 | 3095 | 3163 | 662 | 666 | 673 | 237 | 237 | 237 | 141 | 141 | 141 |
| | *** | 10781 | 10947 | 21835 | 3074 | 3120 | 5916 | 662 | 666 | 1156 | 237 | 237 | 368 | 141 | 141 | 194 |
| 0.1 | *** | 23733 | 23931 | 26293 | 6399 | 6538 | 6952 | 1250 | 1268 | 1293 | 396 | 396 | 400 | 209 | 209 | 209 |
| | *** | 23797 | 24296 | 39487 | 6453 | 6680 | 10277 | 1261 | 1282 | 1829 | 396 | 396 | 526 | 209 | 209 | 260 |
| 0.15 | *** | 35452 | 35809 | 41536 | 9400 | 9687 | 10756 | 1788 | 1835 | 1898 | 534 | 538 | 549 | 273 | 273 | 273 |
| | *** | 35576 | 36489 | 55038 | 9513 | 10016 | 14112 | 1809 | 1863 | 2417 | 538 | 545 | 662 | 273 | 273 | 316 |
| 0.2 | *** | 44919 | 45468 | 55799 | 11861 | 12318 | 14287 | 2249 | 2330 | 2447 | 655 | 666 | 677 | 326 | 326 | 333 |
| | *** | 45100 | 46534 | 68488 | 12031 | 12881 | 17422 | 2288 | 2383 | 2922 | 662 | 673 | 778 | 326 | 333 | 362 |
| 0.25 | *** | 51836 | 52629 | 68507 | 13709 | 14368 | 17422 | 2621 | 2744 | 2929 | 758 | 772 | 789 | 368 | 375 | 375 |
| | *** | 52102 | 54173 | 79836 | 13954 | 15190 | 20206 | 2674 | 2823 | 3342 | 768 | 783 | 873 | 368 | 375 | 400 |
| 0.3 | *** | 56235 | 57325 | 79329 | 14967 | 15856 | 20078 | 2908 | 3067 | 3329 | 836 | 857 | 878 | 400 | 407 | 411 |
| | *** | 56596 | 59439 | 89082 | 15297 | 16961 | 22465 | 2982 | 3180 | 3678 | 847 | 868 | 946 | 407 | 411 | 428 |
| 0.35 | *** | 58281 | 59737 | 88084 | 15690 | 16823 | 22220 | 3116 | 3312 | 3648 | 896 | 921 | 949 | 428 | 432 | 439 |
| | *** | 58763 | 62521 | 96227 | 16111 | 18208 | 24199 | 3205 | 3456 | 3930 | 906 | 932 | 999 | 428 | 432 | 446 |
| 0.4 | *** | 58239 | 60134 | 94665 | 15941 | 17326 | 23807 | 3244 | 3478 | 3875 | 932 | 963 | 995 | 439 | 449 | 453 |
| | *** | 58876 | 63693 | 101271 | 16461 | 18979 | 25407 | 3343 | 3641 | 4098 | 949 | 981 | 1030 | 443 | 449 | 456 |
| 0.45 | *** | 56426 | 58859 | 99011 | 15796 | 17428 | 24838 | 3301 | 3563 | 4013 | 949 | 981 | 1017 | 443 | 453 | 460 |
| | *** | 57240 | 63264 | 104213 | 16419 | 19319 | 26090 | 3414 | 3754 | 4182 | 963 | 1002 | 1041 | 449 | 453 | 456 |
| 0.5 | *** | 53185 | 56256 | 101079 | 15335 | 17188 | 25295 | 3290 | 3573 | 4062 | 949 | 981 | 1017 | 439 | 449 | 453 |
| | *** | 54227 | 61547 | 105054 | 16058 | 19270 | 26248 | 3418 | 3775 | 4182 | 963 | 1002 | 1030 | 443 | 449 | 446 |
| 0.55 | *** | 48893 | 52697 | 100866 | 14634 | 16663 | 25188 | 3223 | 3513 | 4013 | 921 | 959 | 995 | 422 | 432 | 439 |
| | *** | 50206 | 58827 | 103793 | 15431 | 18877 | 25880 | 3350 | 3722 | 4098 | 938 | 974 | 999 | 428 | 439 | 428 |
| 0.6 | *** | 43948 | 48510 | 98363 | 13745 | 15881 | 24504 | 3095 | 3386 | 3881 | 878 | 910 | 953 | 400 | 407 | 418 |
| | *** | 45563 | 55338 | 100430 | 14595 | 18165 | 24987 | 3223 | 3594 | 3930 | 896 | 932 | 946 | 400 | 411 | 400 |
| 0.65 | *** | 38731 | 43973 | 93582 | 12711 | 14889 | 23251 | 2908 | 3191 | 3652 | 821 | 847 | 885 | 368 | 375 | 379 |
| | *** | 40644 | 51258 | 94967 | 13586 | 17156 | 23569 | 3035 | 3386 | 3678 | 836 | 864 | 873 | 368 | 375 | 362 |
| 0.7 | *** | 33561 | 39267 | 86537 | 11557 | 13688 | 21434 | 2670 | 2925 | 3333 | 740 | 762 | 793 | 322 | 326 | 333 |
| | *** | 35697 | 46689 | 87401 | 12417 | 15849 | 21625 | 2787 | 3099 | 3342 | 751 | 779 | 778 | 326 | 333 | 316 |
| 0.75 | *** | 28627 | 34453 | 77247 | 10288 | 12279 | 19058 | 2373 | 2589 | 2925 | 641 | 655 | 683 | 273 | 273 | 279 |
| | *** | 30858 | 41664 | 77734 | 11100 | 14245 | 19156 | 2472 | 2738 | 2922 | 645 | 666 | 662 | 273 | 279 | 260 |
| 0.8 | *** | 23945 | 29509 | 65729 | 8886 | 10639 | 16121 | 2011 | 2181 | 2430 | 517 | 528 | 545 | 209 | 209 | 216 |
| | *** | 26109 | 36111 | 65966 | 9608 | 12311 | 16161 | 2090 | 2292 | 2417 | 524 | 538 | 526 | 209 | 216 | 194 |
| 0.85 | *** | 19387 | 24281 | 52013 | 7303 | 8709 | 12636 | 1580 | 1693 | 1845 | 375 | 379 | 390 | . | . | . |
| | *** | 21310 | 29863 | 52096 | 7891 | 9995 | 12641 | 1633 | 1760 | 1829 | 375 | 386 | 368 | . | . | . |
| 0.9 | *** | 14648 | 18427 | 36118 | 5433 | 6382 | 8609 | 1055 | 1108 | 1176 | . | . | . | . | . | . |
| | *** | 16157 | 22528 | 36125 | 5836 | 7186 | 8596 | 1080 | 1140 | 1156 | . | . | . | . | . | . |
| 0.95 | *** | 9017 | 11117 | 18070 | 3010 | 3386 | 4045 | . | . | . | . | . | . | . | . | . |
| | *** | 9878 | 13157 | 18052 | 3180 | 3662 | 4025 | . | . | . | . | . | . | . | . | . |
| 0.98 | *** | 4189 | 4852 | 6219 | . | . | . | . | . | . | . | . | . | . | . | . |
| | *** | 4476 | 5379 | 6200 | . | . | . | . | . | . | . | . | . | . | . | . |

TABLE 6: ALPHA= 0.025 POWER= 0.9    EXPECTED ACCRUAL THRU MINIMUM FOLLOW-UP= 4500

| | | DEL=.01 | | | DEL=.02 | | | DEL=.05 | | | DEL=.10 | | | DEL=.15 | | |
|---|---|---|---|---|---|---|---|---|---|---|---|---|---|---|---|---|---|
| FACT= | | 1.0 .75 | .50 .25 | .00 BIN | 1.0 .75 | .50 .25 | .00 BIN | 1.0 .75 | .50 .25 | .00 BIN | 1.0 75 | .50 .25 | .00 BIN | 1.0 .75 | .50 .25 | .00 BIN |
| PCONT=*** | | | | | REQUIRED | NUMBER OF | PATIENTS | | | | | | | | | |
| 0.01 | *** | 1612 | 1612 | 1623 | 593 | 593 | 593 | 195 | 195 | 195 | 98 | 98 | 98 | 71 | 71 | 71 |
| | *** | 1612 | 1616 | 6200 | 593 | 593 | 2049 | 195 | 195 | 558 | 98 | 98 | 227 | 71 | 71 | 135 |
| 0.02 | *** | 3558 | 3574 | 3615 | 1144 | 1151 | 1155 | 311 | 311 | 311 | 138 | 138 | 138 | 86 | 86 | 86 |
| | *** | 3563 | 3592 | 10235 | 1144 | 1151 | 3048 | 311 | 311 | 712 | 138 | 138 | 264 | 86 | 86 | 151 |
| 0.05 | *** | 10763 | 10841 | 11298 | 3056 | 3097 | 3165 | 660 | 667 | 671 | 240 | 240 | 240 | 138 | 138 | 138 |
| | *** | 10792 | 10961 | 21835 | 3075 | 3124 | 5916 | 667 | 667 | 1156 | 240 | 240 | 368 | 138 | 138 | 194 |
| 0.1 | *** | 23745 | 23955 | 26295 | 6409 | 6551 | 6956 | 1252 | 1268 | 1297 | 397 | 397 | 397 | 210 | 210 | 210 |
| | *** | 23813 | 24330 | 39487 | 6465 | 6690 | 10277 | 1263 | 1279 | 1829 | 397 | 397 | 526 | 210 | 210 | 260 |
| 0.15 | *** | 35475 | 35850 | 41531 | 9424 | 9712 | 10751 | 1792 | 1837 | 1898 | 536 | 543 | 548 | 273 | 273 | 278 |
| | *** | 35603 | 36566 | 55038 | 9532 | 10043 | 14112 | 1815 | 1864 | 2417 | 536 | 543 | 662 | 273 | 273 | 316 |
| 0.2 | *** | 44951 | 45532 | 55803 | 11888 | 12360 | 14291 | 2258 | 2332 | 2449 | 660 | 667 | 678 | 323 | 330 | 330 |
| | *** | 45143 | 46657 | 68488 | 12068 | 12923 | 17422 | 2291 | 2381 | 2922 | 660 | 671 | 778 | 330 | 330 | 362 |
| 0.25 | *** | 51881 | 52721 | 68505 | 13755 | 14437 | 17423 | 2636 | 2748 | 2928 | 761 | 773 | 791 | 368 | 375 | 379 |
| | *** | 52163 | 54345 | 79836 | 14010 | 15263 | 20206 | 2685 | 2827 | 3342 | 768 | 784 | 873 | 368 | 375 | 400 |
| 0.3 | *** | 56298 | 57450 | 79331 | 15026 | 15945 | 20078 | 2921 | 3079 | 3333 | 840 | 858 | 881 | 401 | 408 | 413 |
| | *** | 56681 | 59673 | 89082 | 15371 | 17051 | 22465 | 2996 | 3187 | 3678 | 851 | 870 | 946 | 408 | 408 | 428 |
| 0.35 | *** | 58368 | 59903 | 88084 | 15765 | 16928 | 22215 | 3131 | 3326 | 3648 | 896 | 919 | 948 | 424 | 431 | 442 |
| | *** | 58879 | 62828 | 96227 | 16203 | 18323 | 24199 | 3221 | 3461 | 3930 | 908 | 937 | 999 | 431 | 435 | 446 |
| 0.4 | *** | 58350 | 60360 | 94665 | 16035 | 17456 | 23808 | 3266 | 3491 | 3878 | 937 | 964 | 998 | 442 | 446 | 453 |
| | *** | 59021 | 64076 | 101271 | 16575 | 19117 | 25407 | 3367 | 3653 | 4098 | 948 | 982 | 1030 | 442 | 453 | 456 |
| 0.45 | *** | 56568 | 59138 | 99008 | 15911 | 17576 | 24836 | 3322 | 3581 | 4013 | 953 | 982 | 1020 | 446 | 453 | 458 |
| | *** | 57345 | 63728 | 104213 | 16552 | 19477 | 26090 | 3439 | 3761 | 4182 | 971 | 998 | 1041 | 446 | 458 | 456 |
| 0.5 | *** | 53366 | 56602 | 101078 | 15472 | 17355 | 25298 | 3315 | 3592 | 4058 | 948 | 982 | 1020 | 442 | 446 | 453 |
| | *** | 54469 | 62085 | 105054 | 16208 | 19443 | 26248 | 3439 | 3788 | 4182 | 964 | 998 | 1030 | 442 | 453 | 446 |
| 0.55 | *** | 49125 | 53115 | 100864 | 14786 | 16838 | 25185 | 3248 | 3536 | 4013 | 926 | 960 | 998 | 424 | 431 | 442 |
| | *** | 50509 | 59430 | 103793 | 15596 | 19061 | 25880 | 3378 | 3738 | 4098 | 941 | 975 | 999 | 431 | 435 | 428 |
| 0.6 | *** | 44238 | 48990 | 98362 | 13908 | 16073 | 24506 | 3120 | 3405 | 3878 | 885 | 915 | 953 | 401 | 408 | 413 |
| | *** | 45930 | 55988 | 100430 | 14775 | 18352 | 24987 | 3248 | 3603 | 3930 | 896 | 930 | 946 | 401 | 413 | 400 |
| 0.65 | *** | 39086 | 44501 | 93581 | 12885 | 15078 | 23250 | 2933 | 3210 | 3653 | 825 | 851 | 885 | 368 | 375 | 379 |
| | *** | 41066 | 51933 | 94967 | 13766 | 17340 | 23569 | 3056 | 3394 | 3678 | 836 | 870 | 873 | 368 | 375 | 362 |
| 0.7 | *** | 33960 | 39817 | 86538 | 11726 | 13868 | 21435 | 2692 | 2940 | 3333 | 739 | 768 | 795 | 323 | 330 | 334 |
| | *** | 36161 | 47366 | 87401 | 12596 | 16023 | 21625 | 2805 | 3108 | 3342 | 750 | 780 | 778 | 330 | 334 | 316 |
| 0.75 | *** | 29051 | 35002 | 77246 | 10448 | 12446 | 19054 | 2393 | 2606 | 2928 | 638 | 660 | 678 | 273 | 278 | 278 |
| | *** | 31335 | 42303 | 77734 | 11265 | 14403 | 19156 | 2490 | 2748 | 2922 | 649 | 667 | 662 | 273 | 278 | 260 |
| 0.8 | *** | 24360 | 30018 | 65730 | 9026 | 10781 | 16125 | 2028 | 2190 | 2433 | 521 | 532 | 543 | 210 | 210 | 217 |
| | *** | 26565 | 36690 | 65966 | 9750 | 12439 | 16161 | 2107 | 2298 | 2417 | 525 | 536 | 526 | 210 | 210 | 194 |
| 0.85 | *** | 19758 | 24720 | 52012 | 7417 | 8823 | 12637 | 1590 | 1695 | 1848 | 375 | 379 | 390 | . | . | . |
| | *** | 21716 | 30345 | 52096 | 8006 | 10088 | 12641 | 1639 | 1770 | 1829 | 379 | 386 | 368 | . | . | . |
| 0.9 | *** | 14943 | 18757 | 36116 | 5516 | 6454 | 8610 | 1061 | 1110 | 1178 | . | . | . | . | . | . |
| | *** | 16466 | 22868 | 36125 | 5914 | 7241 | 8596 | 1083 | 1140 | 1156 | . | . | . | . | . | . |
| 0.95 | *** | 9188 | 11287 | 18071 | 3045 | 3416 | 4046 | . | . | . | . | . | . | . | . | . |
| | *** | 10054 | 13312 | 18052 | 3210 | 3675 | 4025 | . | . | . | . | . | . | . | . | . |
| 0.98 | *** | 4245 | 4901 | 6218 | . | . | . | . | . | . | . | . | . | . | . | . |
| | *** | 4530 | 5415 | 6200 | . | . | . | . | . | . | . | . | . | . | . | . |

# TABLE 6: ALPHA= 0.025 POWER= 0.9    EXPECTED ACCRUAL THRU MINIMUM FOLLOW-UP= 4750

|  |  | DEL=.01 | | | DEL=.02 | | | DEL=.05 | | | DEL=.10 | | | DEL=.15 | | |
|---|---|---|---|---|---|---|---|---|---|---|---|---|---|---|---|---|
| FACT= | | 1.0 .75 | .50 .25 | .00 BIN | 1.0 .75 | .50 .25 | .00 BIN | 1.0 .75 | .50 .25 | .00 BIN | 1.0 75 | .50 .25 | .00 BIN | 1.0 .75 | .50 .25 | .00 BIN |
| PCONT=*** | | | | | | REQUIRED | NUMBER | OF PATIENTS | | | | | | | | |
| 0.01 | *** | 1611 | 1611 | 1618 | 590 | 590 | 590 | 193 | 193 | 193 | 98 | 98 | 98 | 67 | 67 | 67 |
|  | *** | 1611 | 1618 | 6200 | 590 | 590 | 2049 | 193 | 193 | 558 | 98 | 98 | 227 | 67 | 67 | 135 |
| 0.02 | *** | 3559 | 3578 | 3618 | 1143 | 1148 | 1155 | 312 | 312 | 312 | 134 | 134 | 134 | 87 | 87 | 87 |
|  | *** | 3566 | 3590 | 10235 | 1148 | 1148 | 3048 | 312 | 312 | 712 | 134 | 134 | 264 | 87 | 87 | 151 |
| 0.05 | *** | 10767 | 10850 | 11297 | 3060 | 3095 | 3167 | 661 | 668 | 668 | 234 | 241 | 241 | 139 | 139 | 139 |
|  | *** | 10798 | 10969 | 21835 | 3079 | 3127 | 5916 | 661 | 668 | 1156 | 234 | 241 | 368 | 139 | 139 | 194 |
| 0.1 | *** | 23758 | 23979 | 26295 | 6416 | 6563 | 6955 | 1255 | 1274 | 1290 | 395 | 395 | 400 | 210 | 210 | 210 |
|  | *** | 23829 | 24371 | 39487 | 6475 | 6701 | 10277 | 1262 | 1279 | 1829 | 395 | 400 | 526 | 210 | 210 | 260 |
| 0.15 | *** | 35498 | 35890 | 41535 | 9444 | 9741 | 10755 | 1797 | 1837 | 1896 | 538 | 542 | 550 | 269 | 277 | 277 |
|  | *** | 35628 | 36638 | 55038 | 9555 | 10066 | 14112 | 1813 | 1868 | 2417 | 538 | 542 | 662 | 277 | 277 | 316 |
| 0.2 | *** | 44986 | 45596 | 55804 | 11919 | 12405 | 14289 | 2264 | 2335 | 2450 | 661 | 668 | 680 | 324 | 329 | 329 |
|  | *** | 45188 | 46772 |  | 12104 | 12964 | 17422 | 2295 | 2390 | 2922 | 661 | 673 | 778 | 329 | 329 | 362 |
| 0.25 | *** | 51933 | 52816 | 68503 | 13795 | 14495 | 17424 | 2644 | 2758 | 2929 | 763 | 775 | 792 | 372 | 372 | 376 |
|  | *** | 52222 | 54514 | 79836 | 14056 | 15327 | 20206 | 2692 | 2834 | 3342 | 768 | 780 | 873 | 372 | 376 | 400 |
| 0.3 | *** | 56362 | 57578 | 79328 | 15089 | 16027 | 20084 | 2937 | 3091 | 3328 | 839 | 858 | 882 | 400 | 407 | 412 |
|  | *** | 56766 | 59905 | 89082 | 15441 | 17139 | 22465 | 3008 | 3198 | 3678 | 851 | 870 | 946 | 407 | 412 | 428 |
| 0.35 | *** | 58452 | 60072 | 88085 | 15845 | 17037 | 22214 | 3150 | 3340 | 3649 | 899 | 922 | 946 | 424 | 431 | 435 |
|  | *** | 58991 | 63124 | 96227 | 16296 | 18433 | 24199 | 3233 | 3471 | 3930 | 910 | 934 | 999 | 431 | 435 | 446 |
| 0.4 | *** | 58464 | 60578 | 94664 | 16130 | 17578 | 23805 | 3285 | 3507 | 3875 | 942 | 965 | 994 | 443 | 447 | 455 |
|  | *** | 59169 | 64449 | 101271 | 16688 | 19245 | 25407 | 3380 | 3665 | 4098 | 953 | 982 | 1030 | 443 | 447 | 456 |
| 0.45 | *** | 56711 | 59419 | 99010 | 16027 | 17721 | 24839 | 3345 | 3594 | 4010 | 958 | 982 | 1017 | 447 | 455 | 459 |
|  | *** | 57625 | 64176 | 104213 | 16680 | 19621 | 26090 | 3459 | 3772 | 4182 | 970 | 1001 | 1041 | 447 | 455 | 456 |
| 0.5 | *** | 53552 | 56949 | 101083 | 15607 | 17519 | 25297 | 3340 | 3613 | 4057 | 953 | 982 | 1017 | 443 | 447 | 455 |
|  | *** | 54712 | 62608 | 105054 | 16355 | 19602 | 26248 | 3459 | 3803 | 4182 | 970 | 1001 | 1030 | 443 | 455 | 446 |
| 0.55 | *** | 49360 | 53524 | 100862 | 14935 | 17013 | 25190 | 3274 | 3554 | 4017 | 930 | 958 | 994 | 424 | 431 | 443 |
|  | *** | 50809 | 60012 | 103793 | 15754 | 19229 | 25880 | 3400 | 3749 | 4099 | 946 | 977 | 999 | 431 | 435 | 428 |
| 0.6 | *** | 44527 | 49463 | 98364 | 14068 | 16248 | 24506 | 3143 | 3423 | 3879 | 887 | 918 | 953 | 400 | 407 | 412 |
|  | *** | 46292 | 56616 | 100430 | 14942 | 18521 | 24987 | 3269 | 3618 | 3930 | 899 | 934 | 946 | 407 | 412 | 400 |
| 0.65 | *** | 39428 | 45014 | 93583 | 13042 | 15255 | 23255 | 2960 | 3226 | 3649 | 827 | 851 | 882 | 364 | 372 | 376 |
|  | *** | 41483 | 52579 | 94967 | 13937 | 17507 | 23569 | 3079 | 3412 | 3678 | 839 | 870 | 873 | 372 | 376 | 362 |
| 0.7 | *** | 34350 | 40355 | 86537 | 11883 | 14040 | 21438 | 2715 | 2960 | 3333 | 744 | 768 | 792 | 324 | 329 | 336 |
|  | *** | 36614 | 48007 | 87401 | 12762 | 16182 | 21625 | 2822 | 3119 | 3342 | 756 | 780 | 778 | 329 | 329 | 316 |
| 0.75 | *** | 29458 | 35526 | 77243 | 10600 | 12603 | 19055 | 2414 | 2616 | 2925 | 645 | 661 | 680 | 269 | 277 | 281 |
|  | *** | 31793 | 42912 | 77734 | 11420 | 14543 | 19156 | 2509 | 2751 | 2922 | 649 | 668 | 662 | 277 | 277 | 260 |
| 0.8 | *** | 24755 | 30510 | 65732 | 9164 | 10917 | 16122 | 2046 | 2205 | 2430 | 519 | 530 | 542 | 210 | 210 | 217 |
|  | *** | 27000 | 37236 | 65966 | 9888 | 12560 | 16161 | 2117 | 2307 | 2417 | 526 | 538 | 526 | 210 | 210 | 194 |
| 0.85 | *** | 20112 | 25135 | 52009 | 7532 | 8926 | 12638 | 1599 | 1706 | 1849 | 376 | 383 | 388 | . | . | . |
|  | *** | 22095 | 30795 | 52096 | 8119 | 10180 | 12641 | 1647 | 1773 | 1829 | 376 | 383 | 368 | . | . | . |
| 0.9 | *** | 15220 | 19075 | 36115 | 5589 | 6523 | 8613 | 1065 | 1112 | 1179 | . | . | . | . | . | . |
|  | *** | 16764 | 23188 | 36125 | 5988 | 7295 | 8596 | 1089 | 1143 | 1156 | . | . | . | . | . | . |
| 0.95 | *** | 9349 | 11451 | 18070 | 3079 | 3440 | 4045 | . | . | . | . | . | . | . | . | . |
|  | *** | 10216 | 13462 | 18052 | 3238 | 3697 | 4025 | . | . | . | . | . | . | . | . | . |
| 0.98 | *** | 4302 | 4948 | 6219 | . | . | . | . | . | . | . | . | . | . | . | . |
|  | *** | 4580 | 5447 | 6200 | . | . | . | . | . | . | . | . | . | . | . | . |

TABLE 6: ALPHA= 0.025 POWER= 0.9     EXPECTED ACCRUAL THRU MINIMUM FOLLOW-UP= 5000

| | | DEL=.01 | | | DEL=.02 | | | DEL=.05 | | | DEL=.10 | | | DEL=.15 | | |
|---|---|---|---|---|---|---|---|---|---|---|---|---|---|---|---|---|---|
| FACT= | | 1.0 .75 | .50 .25 | .00 BIN | 1.0 .75 | .50 .25 | .00 BIN | 1.0 .75 | .50 .25 | .00 BIN | 1.0 75 | .50 .25 | .00 BIN | 1.0 .75 | .50 .25 | .00 BIN |
| PCONT=*** | | | | REQUIRED | NUMBER | OF PATIENTS | | | | | | | | | |
| 0.01 | *** | 1608 | 1616 | 1621 | 591 | 591 | 591 | 196 | 196 | 196 | 96 | 96 | 96 | 71 | 71 | 71 |
| | *** | 1608 | 1616 | 6200 | 591 | 591 | 2049 | 196 | 196 | 558 | 96 | 96 | 227 | 71 | 71 | 135 |
| 0.02 | *** | 3558 | 3579 | 3616 | 1146 | 1146 | 1154 | 308 | 308 | 308 | 133 | 133 | 133 | 91 | 91 | 91 |
| | *** | 3566 | 3591 | 10235 | 1146 | 1154 | 3048 | 308 | 308 | 712 | 133 | 133 | 264 | 91 | 91 | 151 |
| 0.05 | *** | 10771 | 10858 | 11296 | 3066 | 3104 | 3166 | 666 | 666 | 671 | 233 | 241 | 241 | 141 | 141 | 141 |
| | *** | 10804 | 10979 | 21835 | 3079 | 3129 | 5916 | 666 | 666 | 1156 | 233 | 241 | 368 | 141 | 141 | 194 |
| 0.1 | *** | 23771 | 23996 | 26291 | 6429 | 6571 | 6954 | 1254 | 1271 | 1296 | 396 | 396 | 396 | 208 | 208 | 208 |
| | *** | 23846 | 24408 | 39487 | 6483 | 6708 | 10277 | 1266 | 1283 | 1829 | 396 | 396 | 526 | 208 | 208 | 260 |
| 0.15 | *** | 35516 | 35933 | 41533 | 9458 | 9766 | 10754 | 1804 | 1841 | 1896 | 533 | 541 | 546 | 271 | 271 | 279 |
| | *** | 35654 | 36708 | 55038 | 9579 | 10091 | 14112 | 1821 | 1866 | 2417 | 541 | 546 | 662 | 271 | 279 | 316 |
| 0.2 | *** | 45016 | 45658 | 55804 | 11954 | 12446 | 14291 | 2271 | 2341 | 2446 | 658 | 671 | 679 | 329 | 329 | 329 |
| | *** | 45229 | 46891 | 68488 | 12141 | 13008 | 17422 | 2304 | 2391 | 2922 | 666 | 671 | 778 | 329 | 329 | 362 |
| 0.25 | *** | 51979 | 52908 | 68508 | 13841 | 14554 | 17421 | 2654 | 2766 | 2929 | 766 | 779 | 791 | 371 | 371 | 379 |
| | *** | 52291 | 54683 | 79836 | 14108 | 15383 | 20206 | 2704 | 2833 | 3342 | 771 | 783 | 873 | 371 | 379 | 400 |
| 0.3 | *** | 56429 | 57708 | 79329 | 15146 | 16104 | 20079 | 2954 | 3104 | 3329 | 846 | 858 | 879 | 404 | 408 | 416 |
| | *** | 56854 | 60133 | 89082 | 15508 | 17221 | 22465 | 3016 | 3204 | 3678 | 854 | 871 | 946 | 404 | 408 | 428 |
| 0.35 | *** | 58533 | 60246 | 88083 | 15916 | 17133 | 22216 | 3166 | 3354 | 3646 | 904 | 921 | 946 | 429 | 433 | 441 |
| | *** | 59108 | 63421 | 96227 | 16383 | 18533 | 24199 | 3246 | 3479 | 3930 | 916 | 933 | 999 | 429 | 433 | 446 |
| 0.4 | *** | 58579 | 60796 | 94666 | 16221 | 17696 | 23808 | 3304 | 3521 | 3879 | 941 | 966 | 996 | 441 | 446 | 454 |
| | *** | 59321 | 64816 | 101271 | 16791 | 19366 | 25407 | 3404 | 3671 | 4098 | 954 | 979 | 1030 | 446 | 454 | 456 |
| 0.45 | *** | 56858 | 59691 | 99008 | 16141 | 17858 | 24833 | 3366 | 3616 | 4016 | 958 | 983 | 1021 | 446 | 454 | 458 |
| | *** | 57816 | 64616 | 104213 | 16808 | 19758 | 26090 | 3479 | 3783 | 4182 | 971 | 1004 | 1041 | 446 | 458 | 456 |
| 0.5 | *** | 53733 | 57283 | 101079 | 15733 | 17666 | 25296 | 3366 | 3629 | 4058 | 958 | 983 | 1021 | 441 | 446 | 454 |
| | *** | 54954 | 63108 | 105054 | 16496 | 19758 | 26248 | 3483 | 3816 | 4182 | 971 | 1004 | 1030 | 446 | 454 | 446 |
| 0.55 | *** | 49591 | 53921 | 100866 | 15079 | 17179 | 25183 | 3296 | 3571 | 4016 | 933 | 966 | 996 | 429 | 433 | 441 |
| | *** | 51108 | 60571 | 103793 | 15908 | 19391 | 25880 | 3421 | 3758 | 4098 | 946 | 979 | 999 | 429 | 433 | 428 |
| 0.6 | *** | 44816 | 49916 | 98366 | 14216 | 16416 | 24504 | 3166 | 3441 | 3879 | 891 | 921 | 954 | 404 | 408 | 416 |
| | *** | 46646 | 57216 | 100430 | 15104 | 18691 | 24987 | 3291 | 3629 | 3930 | 904 | 933 | 946 | 404 | 408 | 400 |
| 0.65 | *** | 39766 | 45516 | 93583 | 13196 | 15421 | 23254 | 2983 | 3241 | 3654 | 829 | 854 | 883 | 366 | 371 | 379 |
| | *** | 41891 | 53204 | 94967 | 14104 | 17666 | 23569 | 3096 | 3421 | 3678 | 841 | 866 | 873 | 371 | 379 | 362 |
| 0.7 | *** | 34729 | 40866 | 86533 | 12041 | 14204 | 21433 | 2733 | 2971 | 3333 | 746 | 766 | 791 | 329 | 329 | 333 |
| | *** | 37054 | 48621 | 87401 | 12921 | 16333 | 21625 | 2841 | 3129 | 3342 | 758 | 779 | 778 | 329 | 333 | 316 |
| 0.75 | *** | 29854 | 36033 | 77246 | 10746 | 12754 | 19058 | 2429 | 2629 | 2929 | 646 | 658 | 679 | 271 | 279 | 279 |
| | *** | 32233 | 43496 | 77734 | 11571 | 14679 | 19156 | 2521 | 2758 | 2922 | 654 | 671 | 662 | 271 | 279 | 260 |
| 0.8 | *** | 25141 | 30979 | 65729 | 9291 | 11046 | 16121 | 2058 | 2208 | 2429 | 521 | 533 | 546 | 208 | 216 | 216 |
| | *** | 27421 | 37758 | 65966 | 10021 | 12671 | 16161 | 2129 | 2308 | 2417 | 529 | 541 | 526 | 208 | 216 | 194 |
| 0.85 | *** | 20458 | 25541 | 52008 | 7633 | 9029 | 12641 | 1608 | 1708 | 1846 | 379 | 383 | 391 | . | . | . |
| | *** | 22466 | 31229 | 52096 | 8221 | 10258 | 12641 | 1658 | 1771 | 1829 | 379 | 383 | 368 | . | . | . |
| 0.9 | *** | 15491 | 19371 | 36116 | 5658 | 6583 | 8608 | 1066 | 1116 | 1179 | . | . | . | . | . | . |
| | *** | 17046 | 23496 | 36125 | 6058 | 7341 | 8596 | 1091 | 1146 | 1156 | . | . | . | . | . | . |
| 0.95 | *** | 9504 | 11608 | 18071 | 3108 | 3458 | 4046 | . | . | . | . | . | . | . | . | . |
| | *** | 10371 | 13604 | 18052 | 3266 | 3708 | 4025 | . | . | . | . | . | . | . | . | . |
| 0.98 | *** | 4354 | 4991 | 6221 | . | . | . | . | . | . | . | . | . | . | . | . |
| | *** | 4633 | 5479 | 6200 | . | . | . | . | . | . | . | . | . | . | . | . |

# TABLE 6: ALPHA= 0.025 POWER= 0.9    EXPECTED ACCRUAL THRU MINIMUM FOLLOW-UP= 5500

| | | DEL=.01 | | | DEL=.02 | | | DEL=.05 | | | DEL=.10 | | | DEL=.15 | | |
|---|---|---|---|---|---|---|---|---|---|---|---|---|---|---|---|---|
| FACT= | | 1.0 .75 | .50 .25 | .00 BIN | 1.0 .75 | .50 .25 | .00 BIN | 1.0 .75 | .50 .25 | .00 BIN | 1.0 75 | .50 .25 | .00 BIN | 1.0 .75 | .50 .25 | .00 BIN |
| PCONT=*** | | | | | REQUIRED NUMBER OF PATIENTS | | | | | | | | | | | |
| 0.01 | *** | 1613 | 1613 | 1618 | 595 | 595 | 595 | 196 | 196 | 196 | 100 | 100 | 100 | 73 | 73 | 73 |
| | *** | 1613 | 1618 | 6200 | 595 | 595 | 2049 | 196 | 196 | 558 | 100 | 100 | 227 | 73 | 73 | 135 |
| 0.02 | *** | 3557 | 3579 | 3620 | 1145 | 1150 | 1159 | 312 | 312 | 312 | 133 | 133 | 133 | 86 | 86 | 86 |
| | *** | 3570 | 3593 | 10235 | 1145 | 1150 | 3048 | 312 | 312 | 712 | 133 | 133 | 264 | 86 | 86 | 151 |
| 0.05 | *** | 10784 | 10872 | 11293 | 3070 | 3103 | 3166 | 664 | 669 | 669 | 238 | 238 | 238 | 141 | 141 | 141 |
| | *** | 10811 | 10995 | 21835 | 3084 | 3130 | 5916 | 664 | 669 | 1156 | 238 | 238 | 368 | 141 | 141 | 194 |
| 0.1 | *** | 23791 | 24044 | 26294 | 6444 | 6595 | 6953 | 1260 | 1274 | 1296 | 394 | 394 | 403 | 210 | 210 | 210 |
| | *** | 23879 | 24479 | 39487 | 6508 | 6728 | 10277 | 1269 | 1283 | 1829 | 394 | 394 | 526 | 210 | 210 | 260 |
| 0.15 | *** | 35561 | 36015 | 41534 | 9497 | 9808 | 10756 | 1805 | 1846 | 1893 | 540 | 540 | 545 | 270 | 270 | 279 |
| | *** | 35713 | 36845 | 55038 | 9620 | 10129 | 14112 | 1824 | 1865 | 2417 | 540 | 545 | 662 | 270 | 279 | 316 |
| 0.2 | *** | 45082 | 45791 | 55801 | 12008 | 12522 | 14290 | 2278 | 2347 | 2451 | 664 | 669 | 678 | 325 | 325 | 334 |
| | *** | 45315 | 47117 | 68488 | 12205 | 13080 | 17422 | 2314 | 2396 | 2922 | 664 | 678 | 778 | 325 | 325 | 362 |
| 0.25 | *** | 52067 | 53093 | 68506 | 13924 | 14667 | 17425 | 2671 | 2773 | 2933 | 765 | 779 | 788 | 367 | 375 | 375 |
| | *** | 52410 | 55009 | 79836 | 14208 | 15500 | 20206 | 2718 | 2842 | 3342 | 774 | 779 | 873 | 375 | 375 | 400 |
| 0.3 | *** | 56558 | 57960 | 79328 | 15258 | 16256 | 20079 | 2974 | 3117 | 3331 | 848 | 862 | 884 | 403 | 408 | 416 |
| | *** | 57025 | 60578 | 89082 | 15643 | 17370 | 22465 | 3043 | 3213 | 3678 | 856 | 870 | 946 | 408 | 408 | 428 |
| 0.35 | *** | 58708 | 60578 | 88086 | 16064 | 17320 | 22215 | 3194 | 3373 | 3648 | 903 | 925 | 953 | 430 | 435 | 435 |
| | *** | 59335 | 63988 | 96227 | 16550 | 18723 | 24199 | 3276 | 3496 | 3930 | 917 | 939 | 999 | 430 | 435 | 446 |
| 0.4 | *** | 58799 | 61233 | 94664 | 16408 | 17925 | 23805 | 3337 | 3543 | 3873 | 944 | 966 | 994 | 444 | 449 | 458 |
| | *** | 59615 | 65523 | 101271 | 16999 | 19589 | 25407 | 3433 | 3689 | 4098 | 958 | 980 | 1030 | 444 | 449 | 456 |
| 0.45 | *** | 57149 | 60234 | 99009 | 16353 | 18118 | 24836 | 3405 | 3639 | 4010 | 966 | 985 | 1021 | 449 | 449 | 458 |
| | *** | 58199 | 65454 | 104213 | 17045 | 20015 | 26090 | 3510 | 3804 | 4182 | 980 | 1008 | 1041 | 449 | 458 | 456 |
| 0.5 | *** | 54102 | 57952 | 101080 | 15973 | 17953 | 25295 | 3405 | 3661 | 4060 | 958 | 985 | 1021 | 444 | 449 | 458 |
| | *** | 55430 | 64079 | 105054 | 16765 | 20038 | 26248 | 3515 | 3832 | 4182 | 972 | 999 | 1030 | 444 | 449 | 446 |
| 0.55 | *** | 50054 | 54707 | 100865 | 15340 | 17480 | 25185 | 3337 | 3598 | 4019 | 939 | 966 | 999 | 430 | 435 | 444 |
| | *** | 51695 | 61645 | 103793 | 16201 | 19685 | 25880 | 3455 | 3777 | 4098 | 953 | 980 | 999 | 430 | 435 | 428 |
| 0.6 | *** | 45379 | 50802 | 98363 | 14502 | 16738 | 24506 | 3208 | 3469 | 3881 | 898 | 925 | 953 | 403 | 408 | 416 |
| | *** | 47345 | 58359 | 100430 | 15404 | 18984 | 24987 | 3331 | 3648 | 3930 | 911 | 939 | 946 | 408 | 408 | 400 |
| 0.65 | *** | 40429 | 46470 | 93586 | 13493 | 15739 | 23255 | 3020 | 3268 | 3653 | 834 | 856 | 884 | 367 | 375 | 380 |
| | *** | 42675 | 54377 | 94967 | 14405 | 17961 | 23569 | 3139 | 3433 | 3678 | 843 | 870 | 873 | 375 | 375 | 362 |
| 0.7 | *** | 35465 | 41850 | 86538 | 12329 | 14502 | 21432 | 2773 | 3001 | 3331 | 752 | 774 | 793 | 325 | 334 | 334 |
| | *** | 37890 | 49784 | 87401 | 13223 | 16605 | 21625 | 2878 | 3144 | 3342 | 760 | 779 | 778 | 325 | 334 | 316 |
| 0.75 | *** | 30611 | 36997 | 77243 | 11018 | 13025 | 19053 | 2465 | 2649 | 2924 | 650 | 664 | 678 | 270 | 279 | 279 |
| | *** | 33086 | 44595 | 77734 | 11848 | 14923 | 19156 | 2548 | 2773 | 2922 | 655 | 669 | 662 | 270 | 279 | 260 |
| 0.8 | *** | 25873 | 31863 | 65729 | 9533 | 11284 | 16119 | 2080 | 2231 | 2429 | 526 | 532 | 545 | 210 | 210 | 215 |
| | *** | 28224 | 38738 | 65966 | 10261 | 12874 | 16161 | 2149 | 2319 | 2417 | 526 | 540 | 526 | 210 | 215 | 194 |
| 0.85 | *** | 21110 | 26294 | 52012 | 7828 | 9208 | 12640 | 1626 | 1723 | 1846 | 375 | 380 | 389 | . | . | . |
| | *** | 23164 | 32028 | 52096 | 8419 | 10413 | 12641 | 1673 | 1778 | 1829 | 380 | 389 | 368 | . | . | . |
| 0.9 | *** | 15995 | 19933 | 36117 | 5793 | 6700 | 8611 | 1076 | 1123 | 1178 | . | . | . | . | . | . |
| | *** | 17582 | 24058 | 36125 | 6191 | 7429 | 8596 | 1095 | 1145 | 1156 | . | . | . | . | . | . |
| 0.95 | *** | 9785 | 11889 | 18071 | 3166 | 3502 | 4046 | . | . | . | . | . | . | . | . | . |
| | *** | 10665 | 13850 | 18052 | 3318 | 3735 | 4025 | . | . | . | . | . | . | . | . | . |
| 0.98 | *** | 4445 | 5064 | 6219 | . | . | . | . | . | . | . | . | . | . | . | . |
| | *** | 4720 | 5531 | 6200 | . | . | . | . | . | . | . | . | . | . | . | . |

TABLE 6: ALPHA= 0.025 POWER= 0.9    EXPECTED ACCRUAL THRU MINIMUM FOLLOW-UP= 6000

| | FACT= | DEL=.01 1.0 .75 | .50 .25 | .00 BIN | DEL=.02 1.0 .75 | .50 .25 | .00 BIN | DEL=.05 1.0 .75 | .50 .25 | .00 BIN | DEL=.10 1.0 75 | .50 .25 | .00 BIN | DEL=.15 1.0 .75 | .50 .25 | .00 BIN |
|---|---|---|---|---|---|---|---|---|---|---|---|---|---|---|---|---|
| PCONT=*** | | | | REQUIRED NUMBER OF PATIENTS | | | | | | | | | | | |
| 0.01 | *** | 1609 | 1615 | 1624 | 589 | 595 | 595 | 199 | 199 | 199 | 100 | 100 | 100 | 70 | 70 | 70 |
| | *** | 1609 | 1615 | 6200 | 589 | 595 | 2049 | 199 | 199 | 558 | 100 | 100 | 227 | 70 | 70 | 135 |
| 0.02 | *** | 3565 | 3580 | 3619 | 1144 | 1150 | 1159 | 310 | 310 | 310 | 139 | 139 | 139 | 85 | 85 | 85 |
| | *** | 3574 | 3595 | 10235 | 1150 | 1150 | 3048 | 310 | 310 | 712 | 139 | 139 | 264 | 85 | 85 | 151 |
| 0.05 | *** | 10789 | 10885 | 11299 | 3070 | 3109 | 3160 | 664 | 664 | 670 | 235 | 235 | 235 | 139 | 139 | 139 |
| | *** | 10825 | 11014 | 21835 | 3085 | 3130 | 5916 | 664 | 670 | 1156 | 235 | 235 | 368 | 139 | 139 | 194 |
| 0.1 | *** | 23815 | 24085 | 26290 | 6460 | 6610 | 6955 | 1264 | 1279 | 1294 | 394 | 394 | 400 | 214 | 214 | 214 |
| | *** | 23905 | 24544 | 39487 | 6520 | 6745 | 10277 | 1270 | 1285 | 1829 | 394 | 400 | 526 | 214 | 214 | 260 |
| 0.15 | *** | 35599 | 36094 | 41530 | 9535 | 9850 | 10750 | 1810 | 1849 | 1894 | 535 | 544 | 544 | 274 | 274 | 274 |
| | *** | 35764 | 36985 | 55038 | 9655 | 10165 | 14112 | 1834 | 1870 | 2417 | 544 | 544 | 662 | 274 | 274 | 316 |
| 0.2 | *** | 45145 | 45919 | 55804 | 12064 | 12595 | 14290 | 2290 | 2359 | 2449 | 664 | 670 | 679 | 325 | 325 | 334 |
| | *** | 45400 | 47335 | 68488 | 12274 | 13144 | 17422 | 2320 | 2395 | 2922 | 664 | 670 | 778 | 325 | 334 | 362 |
| 0.25 | *** | 52165 | 53275 | 68509 | 14005 | 14770 | 17425 | 2689 | 2785 | 2929 | 769 | 775 | 790 | 370 | 370 | 379 |
| | *** | 52534 | 55330 | 79836 | 14305 | 15595 | 20206 | 2734 | 2854 | 3342 | 769 | 784 | 873 | 370 | 379 | 400 |
| 0.3 | *** | 56680 | 58210 | 79330 | 15370 | 16390 | 20080 | 2995 | 3130 | 3334 | 850 | 865 | 880 | 409 | 409 | 415 |
| | *** | 57199 | 61000 | 89082 | 15769 | 17509 | 22465 | 3055 | 3220 | 3678 | 859 | 874 | 946 | 409 | 409 | 428 |
| 0.35 | *** | 58879 | 60910 | 88084 | 16204 | 17500 | 22219 | 3220 | 3394 | 3649 | 910 | 925 | 949 | 430 | 430 | 439 |
| | *** | 59560 | 64540 | 96227 | 16705 | 18895 | 24199 | 3295 | 3505 | 3930 | 919 | 940 | 999 | 430 | 439 | 446 |
| 0.4 | *** | 59020 | 61660 | 94669 | 16579 | 18130 | 23809 | 3364 | 3565 | 3874 | 949 | 970 | 994 | 445 | 445 | 454 |
| | *** | 59914 | 66199 | 101271 | 17185 | 19795 | 25407 | 3460 | 3700 | 4098 | 964 | 985 | 1030 | 445 | 454 | 456 |
| 0.45 | *** | 57430 | 60769 | 99010 | 16555 | 18355 | 24835 | 3439 | 3664 | 4015 | 970 | 994 | 1015 | 445 | 454 | 460 |
| | *** | 58579 | 66259 | 104213 | 17269 | 20245 | 26090 | 3544 | 3820 | 4182 | 979 | 1009 | 1041 | 454 | 454 | 456 |
| 0.5 | *** | 54469 | 58594 | 101080 | 16210 | 18220 | 25300 | 3439 | 3685 | 4060 | 964 | 994 | 1015 | 445 | 445 | 454 |
| | *** | 55909 | 64990 | 105054 | 17014 | 20284 | 26248 | 3550 | 3850 | 4182 | 979 | 1000 | 1030 | 445 | 454 | 446 |
| 0.55 | *** | 50509 | 55459 | 100864 | 15595 | 17764 | 25189 | 3379 | 3625 | 4015 | 940 | 970 | 994 | 430 | 430 | 439 |
| | *** | 52270 | 62644 | 103793 | 16474 | 19945 | 25880 | 3490 | 3799 | 4098 | 955 | 979 | 999 | 430 | 439 | 428 |
| 0.6 | *** | 45925 | 51640 | 98365 | 14770 | 17020 | 24505 | 3244 | 3499 | 3880 | 895 | 925 | 949 | 400 | 409 | 415 |
| | *** | 48019 | 59425 | 100430 | 15685 | 19255 | 24987 | 3364 | 3664 | 3930 | 910 | 940 | 946 | 409 | 409 | 400 |
| 0.65 | *** | 41065 | 47374 | 93580 | 13765 | 16024 | 23254 | 3055 | 3295 | 3649 | 835 | 859 | 880 | 370 | 370 | 379 |
| | *** | 43429 | 55465 | 94967 | 14689 | 18220 | 23569 | 3169 | 3454 | 3678 | 844 | 874 | 873 | 370 | 379 | 362 |
| 0.7 | *** | 36160 | 42769 | 86539 | 12595 | 14779 | 21439 | 2809 | 3019 | 3334 | 754 | 769 | 790 | 325 | 334 | 334 |
| | *** | 38689 | 50854 | 87401 | 13495 | 16849 | 21625 | 2905 | 3160 | 3342 | 760 | 784 | 778 | 325 | 334 | 316 |
| 0.75 | *** | 31330 | 37894 | 77245 | 11269 | 13279 | 19054 | 2485 | 2674 | 2929 | 649 | 664 | 679 | 274 | 274 | 280 |
| | *** | 33880 | 45604 | 77734 | 12100 | 15139 | 19156 | 2575 | 2785 | 2922 | 655 | 670 | 662 | 274 | 280 | 260 |
| 0.8 | *** | 26560 | 32689 | 65725 | 9754 | 11494 | 16120 | 2104 | 2245 | 2434 | 520 | 535 | 544 | 214 | 214 | 214 |
| | *** | 28975 | 39634 | 65966 | 10480 | 13054 | 16161 | 2170 | 2329 | 2417 | 529 | 535 | 526 | 214 | 214 | 194 |
| 0.85 | *** | 21715 | 26995 | 52009 | 8005 | 9379 | 12640 | 1639 | 1729 | 1849 | 379 | 385 | 385 | . | . | . |
| | *** | 23815 | 32755 | 52096 | 8590 | 10540 | 12641 | 1684 | 1789 | 1829 | 379 | 385 | 368 | . | . | . |
| 0.9 | *** | 16465 | 20449 | 36115 | 5914 | 6805 | 8605 | 1084 | 1129 | 1174 | . | . | . | . | . | . |
| | *** | 18079 | 24565 | 36125 | 6304 | 7504 | 8596 | 1105 | 1150 | 1156 | . | . | . | . | . | . |
| 0.95 | *** | 10054 | 12154 | 18070 | 3214 | 3535 | 4045 | . | . | . | . | . | . | . | . | . |
| | *** | 10930 | 14074 | 18052 | 3355 | 3760 | 4025 | . | . | . | . | . | . | . | . | . |
| 0.98 | *** | 4534 | 5134 | 6220 | . | . | . | . | . | . | . | . | . | . | . | . |
| | *** | 4795 | 5575 | 6200 | . | . | . | . | . | . | . | . | . | . | . | . |

## TABLE 6: ALPHA= 0.025 POWER= 0.9    EXPECTED ACCRUAL THRU MINIMUM FOLLOW-UP= 6500

| | | DEL=.01 | | | DEL=.02 | | | DEL=.05 | | | DEL=.10 | | | DEL=.15 | | |
|---|---|---|---|---|---|---|---|---|---|---|---|---|---|---|---|---|
| FACT= | | 1.0 .75 | .50 .25 | .00 BIN | 1.0 .75 | .50 .25 | .00 BIN | 1.0 .75 | .50 .25 | .00 BIN | 1.0 75 | .50 .25 | .00 BIN | 1.0 .75 | .50 .25 | .00 BIN |
| PCONT=*** | | | | REQUIRED NUMBER OF PATIENTS | | | | | | | | | | | | |
| 0.01 | *** | 1613 | 1613 | 1619 | 590 | 590 | 596 | 200 | 200 | 200 | 102 | 102 | 102 | 70 | 70 | 70 |
| | *** | 1613 | 1619 | 6200 | 590 | 596 | 2049 | 200 | 200 | 558 | 102 | 102 | 227 | 70 | 70 | 135 |
| 0.02 | *** | 3563 | 3580 | 3618 | 1148 | 1148 | 1158 | 313 | 313 | 313 | 135 | 135 | 135 | 86 | 86 | 86 |
| | *** | 3569 | 3596 | 10235 | 1148 | 1148 | 3048 | 313 | 313 | 712 | 135 | 135 | 264 | 86 | 86 | 151 |
| 0.05 | *** | 10801 | 10898 | 11298 | 3076 | 3108 | 3163 | 661 | 671 | 671 | 238 | 238 | 238 | 141 | 141 | 141 |
| | *** | 10833 | 11022 | 21835 | 3092 | 3131 | 5916 | 661 | 671 | 1156 | 238 | 238 | 368 | 141 | 141 | 194 |
| 0.1 | *** | 23833 | 24136 | 26287 | 6478 | 6624 | 6949 | 1262 | 1278 | 1294 | 395 | 395 | 401 | 206 | 206 | 216 |
| | *** | 23941 | 24597 | 39487 | 6543 | 6754 | 10277 | 1272 | 1288 | 1829 | 395 | 401 | 526 | 206 | 216 | 260 |
| 0.15 | *** | 35641 | 36177 | 41529 | 9566 | 9891 | 10752 | 1814 | 1857 | 1896 | 541 | 541 | 547 | 271 | 271 | 271 |
| | *** | 35820 | 37109 | 55038 | 9696 | 10199 | 14112 | 1831 | 1873 | 2417 | 541 | 547 | 662 | 271 | 271 | 316 |
| 0.2 | *** | 45212 | 46041 | 55797 | 12117 | 12653 | 14288 | 2302 | 2361 | 2448 | 661 | 671 | 677 | 330 | 330 | 330 |
| | *** | 45488 | 47542 | 68488 | 12328 | 13206 | 17422 | 2328 | 2399 | 2922 | 671 | 677 | 778 | 330 | 330 | 362 |
| 0.25 | *** | 52254 | 53457 | 68504 | 14083 | 14863 | 17425 | 2702 | 2800 | 2930 | 768 | 774 | 791 | 368 | 378 | 378 |
| | *** | 52661 | 55634 | 79836 | 14392 | 15686 | 20206 | 2741 | 2854 | 3342 | 774 | 785 | 873 | 368 | 378 | 400 |
| 0.3 | *** | 56815 | 58462 | 79327 | 15475 | 16521 | 20079 | 3011 | 3141 | 3326 | 850 | 866 | 882 | 401 | 411 | 411 |
| | *** | 57367 | 61413 | 89082 | 15887 | 17626 | 22465 | 3076 | 3228 | 3678 | 856 | 872 | 946 | 411 | 411 | 428 |
| 0.35 | *** | 59047 | 61241 | 88086 | 16336 | 17658 | 22218 | 3244 | 3407 | 3645 | 915 | 931 | 947 | 427 | 433 | 443 |
| | *** | 59788 | 65070 | 96227 | 16856 | 19050 | 24199 | 3320 | 3515 | 3930 | 921 | 937 | 999 | 433 | 433 | 446 |
| 0.4 | *** | 59242 | 62080 | 94667 | 16742 | 18324 | 23811 | 3391 | 3586 | 3878 | 953 | 969 | 996 | 443 | 449 | 449 |
| | *** | 60211 | 66841 | 101271 | 17366 | 19976 | 25407 | 3482 | 3716 | 4098 | 963 | 986 | 1030 | 449 | 449 | 456 |
| 0.45 | *** | 57725 | 61300 | 99006 | 16748 | 18578 | 24835 | 3466 | 3683 | 4008 | 969 | 996 | 1018 | 449 | 449 | 460 |
| | *** | 58949 | 67009 | 104213 | 17479 | 20453 | 26090 | 3569 | 3829 | 4098 | 980 | 1002 | 1041 | 449 | 460 | 456 |
| 0.5 | *** | 54832 | 59220 | 101080 | 16423 | 18465 | 25296 | 3472 | 3710 | 4057 | 969 | 996 | 1018 | 443 | 449 | 460 |
| | *** | 56376 | 65850 | 105054 | 17246 | 20512 | 26248 | 3580 | 3862 | 4182 | 980 | 1002 | 1030 | 449 | 449 | 446 |
| 0.55 | *** | 50954 | 56181 | 100868 | 15832 | 18016 | 25182 | 3407 | 3651 | 4018 | 947 | 969 | 996 | 427 | 433 | 443 |
| | *** | 52833 | 63591 | 103793 | 16716 | 20187 | 25880 | 3521 | 3813 | 4098 | 953 | 986 | 999 | 433 | 433 | 428 |
| 0.6 | *** | 46469 | 52449 | 98366 | 15020 | 17284 | 24499 | 3277 | 3521 | 3878 | 904 | 921 | 953 | 401 | 411 | 417 |
| | *** | 48673 | 60422 | 100430 | 15946 | 19494 | 24987 | 3391 | 3677 | 3930 | 915 | 937 | 946 | 411 | 411 | 400 |
| 0.65 | *** | 41686 | 48224 | 93578 | 14018 | 16287 | 23248 | 3092 | 3320 | 3651 | 839 | 856 | 882 | 368 | 378 | 378 |
| | *** | 44156 | 56490 | 94967 | 14955 | 18454 | 23569 | 3196 | 3466 | 3678 | 850 | 872 | 873 | 368 | 378 | 362 |
| 0.7 | *** | 36833 | 43642 | 86536 | 12842 | 15026 | 21438 | 2832 | 3043 | 3336 | 758 | 774 | 791 | 330 | 330 | 336 |
| | *** | 39449 | 51858 | 87401 | 13752 | 17073 | 21625 | 2930 | 3173 | 3342 | 768 | 785 | 778 | 330 | 330 | 316 |
| 0.75 | *** | 32017 | 38734 | 77247 | 11499 | 13508 | 19056 | 2513 | 2686 | 2930 | 655 | 661 | 677 | 271 | 281 | 281 |
| | *** | 34639 | 46534 | 77734 | 12338 | 15334 | 19156 | 2594 | 2800 | 2922 | 661 | 671 | 662 | 271 | 281 | 260 |
| 0.8 | *** | 27213 | 33453 | 65726 | 9956 | 11688 | 16125 | 2123 | 2253 | 2432 | 525 | 531 | 547 | 216 | 216 | 216 |
| | *** | 29683 | 40457 | 65966 | 10687 | 13216 | 16161 | 2182 | 2334 | 2417 | 531 | 541 | 526 | 216 | 216 | 194 |
| 0.85 | *** | 22283 | 27646 | 52011 | 8168 | 9527 | 12637 | 1652 | 1743 | 1847 | 378 | 384 | 384 | . | . | . |
| | *** | 24428 | 33431 | 52096 | 8747 | 10654 | 12641 | 1695 | 1792 | 1829 | 378 | 384 | 368 | . | . | . |
| 0.9 | *** | 16911 | 20924 | 36112 | 6023 | 6895 | 8607 | 1093 | 1132 | 1175 | . | . | . | . | . | . |
| | *** | 18536 | 25019 | 36125 | 6407 | 7567 | 8596 | 1110 | 1148 | 1156 | . | . | . | . | . | . |
| 0.95 | *** | 10297 | 12387 | 18064 | 3255 | 3569 | 4041 | . | . | . | . | . | . | . | . | . |
| | *** | 11174 | 14272 | 18052 | 3401 | 3775 | 4025 | . | . | . | . | . | . | . | . | . |
| 0.98 | *** | 4609 | 5194 | 6218 | . | . | . | . | . | . | . | . | . | . | . | . |
| | *** | 4869 | 5617 | 6200 | . | . | . | . | . | . | . | . | . | . | . | . |

TABLE 6: ALPHA= 0.025 POWER= 0.9    EXPECTED ACCRUAL THRU MINIMUM FOLLOW-UP= 7000

|  | | DEL=.01 | | | DEL=.02 | | | DEL=.05 | | | DEL=.10 | | | DEL=.15 | |
|---|---|---|---|---|---|---|---|---|---|---|---|---|---|---|---|---|
| FACT= | | 1.0 .75 | .50 .25 | .00 BIN | 1.0 .75 | .50 .25 | .00 BIN | 1.0 .75 | .50 .25 | .00 BIN | 1.0 75 | .50 .25 | .00 BIN | 1.0 .75 | .50 .25 | .00 BIN |
| PCONT=*** | | | | REQUIRED | NUMBER | OF PATIENTS | | | | | | | | | | |
| 0.01 | *** | 1615 1615 | 1615 1615 | 1621 6200 | 589 589 | 589 589 | 589 2049 | 197 197 | 197 197 | 197 558 | 99 99 | 99 99 | 99 227 | 64 64 | 64 64 | 64 135 |
| 0.02 | *** | 3564 3575 | 3581 3599 | 3616 10235 | 1149 1149 | 1149 1149 | 1160 3048 | 309 309 | 309 309 | 309 712 | 134 134 | 134 134 | 134 264 | 92 92 | 92 92 | 92 151 |
| 0.05 | *** | 10809 10844 | 10914 11036 | 11292 21835 | 3085 3091 | 3109 3137 | 3161 5916 | 670 670 | 670 670 | 670 1156 | 239 239 | 239 239 | 239 368 | 134 134 | 134 134 | 134 194 |
| 0.1 | *** | 23864 23969 | 24172 24662 | 26290 39487 | 6497 6556 | 6644 6766 | 6952 10277 | 1265 1271 | 1282 1282 | 1289 1829 | 396 396 | 396 396 | 396 526 | 215 215 | 215 215 | 215 260 |
| 0.15 | *** | 35687 35880 | 36254 37234 | 41532 55038 | 9601 9735 | 9927 10225 | 10756 14112 | 1825 1842 | 1860 1877 | 1895 2417 | 536 536 | 547 547 | 547 662 | 274 274 | 274 274 | 274 316 |
| 0.2 | *** | 45277 45575 | 46170 47745 | 55801 68488 | 12174 12395 | 12716 13259 | 14291 17422 | 2304 2339 | 2367 2402 | 2444 2922 | 670 670 | 670 676 | 676 778 | 326 326 | 326 326 | 326 362 |
| 0.25 | *** | 52347 52785 | 53642 55924 | 68506 79836 | 14162 14477 | 14956 15772 | 17424 20206 | 2706 2752 | 2805 2857 | 2927 3342 | 775 775 | 781 781 | 792 873 | 372 372 | 372 372 | 379 400 |
| 0.3 | *** | 56939 57534 | 58706 61804 | 79332 89082 | 15580 16000 | 16647 17739 | 20077 22465 | 3032 3085 | 3155 3231 | 3330 3678 | 851 862 | 869 869 | 880 946 | 407 407 | 407 407 | 414 428 |
| 0.35 | *** | 59225 60019 | 61570 65566 | 88089 96227 | 16472 16997 | 17809 19185 | 22219 24199 | 3260 3336 | 3417 3522 | 3645 3930 | 915 921 | 932 939 | 950 999 | 431 431 | 431 431 | 442 446 |
| 0.4 | *** | 59470 60502 | 62497 67456 | 94669 101271 | 16892 17540 | 18509 20147 | 23805 25407 | 3417 3505 | 3599 3721 | 3872 4098 | 956 967 | 974 985 | 991 1030 | 442 449 | 449 449 | 449 456 |
| 0.45 | *** | 58006 59319 | 61804 67736 | 99009 104213 | 16927 17669 | 18782 20644 | 24837 26090 | 3494 3592 | 3704 3844 | 4012 4182 | 974 985 | 991 1009 | 1020 1041 | 449 449 | 449 460 | 460 456 |
| 0.5 | *** | 55189 56834 | 59826 66669 | 101085 105054 | 16630 17459 | 18684 20714 | 25299 26248 | 3505 3599 | 3721 3872 | 4065 4182 | 974 985 | 991 1009 | 1020 1030 | 442 449 | 449 449 | 460 446 |
| 0.55 | *** | 51402 53386 | 56880 64481 | 100864 103793 | 16059 16951 | 18257 20399 | 25187 25880 | 3435 3546 | 3669 3826 | 4012 4098 | 950 956 | 974 985 | 991 999 | 431 431 | 431 442 | 442 428 |
| 0.6 | *** | 46999 49302 | 53222 61360 | 98361 100430 | 15254 16192 | 17529 19716 | 24505 24987 | 3312 3417 | 3540 3697 | 3879 3930 | 904 915 | 932 939 | 950 946 | 407 407 | 407 414 | 414 400 |
| 0.65 | *** | 42285 44846 | 49040 57440 | 93584 94967 | 14256 15195 | 16531 18666 | 23251 23569 | 3120 3214 | 3336 3476 | 3651 3678 | 845 851 | 862 869 | 886 873 | 372 372 | 372 379 | 379 362 |
| 0.7 | *** | 37479 40174 | 44461 52785 | 86531 87401 | 13077 13987 | 15254 17266 | 21431 21625 | 2857 2951 | 3056 3179 | 3330 3342 | 757 764 | 775 781 | 792 778 | 326 326 | 326 337 | 337 316 |
| 0.75 | *** | 32666 35355 | 39526 47412 | 77250 77734 | 11712 12552 | 13714 15510 | 19051 19156 | 2531 2612 | 2700 2805 | 2927 2922 | 652 659 | 670 670 | 676 662 | 274 274 | 274 274 | 274 260 |
| 0.8 | *** | 27830 30350 | 34182 41224 | 65724 65966 | 10144 10872 | 11870 13357 | 16122 16161 | 2140 2199 | 2262 2339 | 2426 2417 | 530 530 | 536 536 | 547 526 | 215 215 | 215 215 | 215 194 |
| 0.85 | *** | 22825 25001 | 28250 34049 | 52015 52096 | 8317 8895 | 9654 10756 | 12640 12641 | 1667 1702 | 1744 1790 | 1849 1829 | 379 379 | 379 390 | 390 368 | . . | . . | . . |
| 0.9 | *** | 17319 18964 | 21372 25450 | 36114 36125 | 6130 6497 | 6976 7624 | 8604 8596 | 1096 1114 | 1131 1149 | 1177 1156 | . . | . . | . . | . . | . . | . . |
| 0.95 | *** | 10522 11397 | 12605 14449 | 18071 18052 | 3295 3435 | 3592 3791 | 4047 4025 | . . | . . | . . | . . | . . | . . | . . | . . | . . |
| 0.98 | *** | 4677 4929 | 5244 5657 | 6217 6200 | . . | . . | . . | . . | . . | . . | . . | . . | . . | . . | . . | . . |

## TABLE 6: ALPHA= 0.025 POWER= 0.9    EXPECTED ACCRUAL THRU MINIMUM FOLLOW-UP= 7500

|  | FACT= | DEL=.01 1.0 .75 | .50 .25 | .00 BIN | DEL=.02 1.0 .75 | .50 .25 | .00 BIN | DEL=.05 1.0 .75 | .50 .25 | .00 BIN | DEL=.10 1.0 75 | .50 .25 | .00 BIN | DEL=.15 1.0 .75 | .50 .25 | .00 BIN |
|---|---|---|---|---|---|---|---|---|---|---|---|---|---|---|---|---|
| PCONT=*** | | | | | | REQUIRED | NUMBER | OF | PATIENTS | | | | | | |
| 0.01 | *** | 1606 | 1618 | 1618 | 593 | 593 | 593 | 193 | 193 | 193 | 99 | 99 | 99 | 68 | 68 | 68 |
| | *** | 1618 | 1618 | 6200 | 593 | 593 | 2049 | 193 | 193 | 558 | 99 | 99 | 227 | 68 | 68 | 135 |
| 0.02 | *** | 3568 | 3586 | 3612 | 1149 | 1149 | 1156 | 312 | 312 | 312 | 136 | 136 | 136 | 87 | 87 | 87 |
| | *** | 3575 | 3593 | 10235 | 1149 | 1149 | 3048 | 312 | 312 | 712 | 136 | 136 | 264 | 87 | 87 | 151 |
| 0.05 | *** | 10812 | 10925 | 11293 | 3087 | 3118 | 3162 | 661 | 668 | 668 | 237 | 237 | 237 | 136 | 136 | 136 |
| | *** | 10861 | 11049 | 21835 | 3099 | 3136 | 5916 | 668 | 668 | 1156 | 237 | 237 | 368 | 136 | 136 | 194 |
| 0.1 | *** | 23881 | 24211 | 26293 | 6511 | 6661 | 6950 | 1268 | 1280 | 1299 | 399 | 399 | 399 | 211 | 211 | 211 |
| | *** | 23993 | 24718 | 39487 | 6575 | 6774 | 10277 | 1268 | 1287 | 1829 | 399 | 399 | 526 | 211 | 211 | 260 |
| 0.15 | *** | 35724 | 36331 | 41536 | 9631 | 9961 | 10756 | 1824 | 1861 | 1899 | 537 | 537 | 549 | 275 | 275 | 275 |
| | *** | 35930 | 37343 | 55038 | 9762 | 10250 | 14112 | 1843 | 1880 | 2417 | 537 | 549 | 662 | 275 | 275 | 316 |
| 0.2 | *** | 45343 | 46287 | 55805 | 12218 | 12774 | 14293 | 2318 | 2375 | 2450 | 668 | 668 | 680 | 324 | 331 | 331 |
| | *** | 45661 | 47937 | 68488 | 12443 | 13306 | 17422 | 2337 | 2405 | 2922 | 668 | 680 | 778 | 331 | 331 | 362 |
| 0.25 | *** | 52437 | 53818 | 68506 | 14236 | 15043 | 17424 | 2724 | 2806 | 2930 | 774 | 781 | 793 | 368 | 368 | 380 |
| | *** | 52906 | 56206 | 79836 | 14555 | 15837 | 20206 | 2761 | 2862 | 3342 | 774 | 781 | 873 | 368 | 380 | 400 |
| 0.3 | *** | 57068 | 58955 | 79325 | 15668 | 16756 | 20075 | 3043 | 3162 | 3331 | 856 | 868 | 875 | 406 | 406 | 418 |
| | *** | 57706 | 62187 | 89082 | 16100 | 17843 | 22465 | 3099 | 3237 | 3678 | 856 | 875 | 946 | 406 | 406 | 428 |
| 0.35 | *** | 59393 | 61887 | 88081 | 16587 | 17949 | 22212 | 3286 | 3436 | 3650 | 912 | 931 | 950 | 436 | 436 | 436 |
| | *** | 60249 | 66050 | 96227 | 17131 | 19318 | 24199 | 3350 | 3530 | 3930 | 924 | 943 | 999 | 436 | 436 | 446 |
| 0.4 | *** | 59693 | 62900 | 94662 | 17049 | 18668 | 23806 | 3436 | 3624 | 3875 | 961 | 980 | 999 | 443 | 455 | 455 |
| | *** | 60793 | 68037 | 101271 | 17693 | 20300 | 25407 | 3518 | 3736 | 4098 | 968 | 987 | 1030 | 443 | 455 | 456 |
| 0.45 | *** | 58287 | 62300 | 99012 | 17105 | 18968 | 24837 | 3518 | 3725 | 4018 | 980 | 999 | 1018 | 455 | 455 | 462 |
| | *** | 59693 | 68424 | 104213 | 17855 | 20818 | 26090 | 3612 | 3849 | 4182 | 987 | 1006 | 1041 | 455 | 455 | 456 |
| 0.5 | *** | 55550 | 60418 | 101075 | 16824 | 18893 | 25299 | 3530 | 3743 | 4062 | 980 | 999 | 1018 | 443 | 455 | 455 |
| | *** | 57286 | 67437 | 105054 | 17668 | 20911 | 26248 | 3624 | 3886 | 4182 | 987 | 1006 | 1030 | 443 | 455 | 446 |
| 0.55 | *** | 51837 | 57549 | 100861 | 16268 | 18481 | 25186 | 3462 | 3687 | 4018 | 950 | 968 | 999 | 425 | 436 | 436 |
| | *** | 53918 | 65318 | 103793 | 17180 | 20600 | 25880 | 3568 | 3837 | 4098 | 961 | 987 | 999 | 436 | 436 | 428 |
| 0.6 | *** | 47518 | 53956 | 98368 | 15481 | 17761 | 24500 | 3331 | 3556 | 3875 | 905 | 931 | 950 | 406 | 406 | 418 |
| | *** | 49918 | 62243 | 100430 | 16418 | 19918 | 24987 | 3436 | 3706 | 3930 | 924 | 943 | 946 | 406 | 418 | 400 |
| 0.65 | *** | 42868 | 49812 | 93586 | 14480 | 16756 | 23255 | 3143 | 3350 | 3650 | 849 | 868 | 886 | 368 | 380 | 380 |
| | *** | 45511 | 58325 | 94967 | 15425 | 18868 | 23569 | 3237 | 3493 | 3678 | 856 | 875 | 873 | 368 | 380 | 362 |
| 0.7 | *** | 38093 | 45237 | 86536 | 13287 | 15474 | 21436 | 2881 | 3068 | 3331 | 762 | 774 | 793 | 331 | 331 | 331 |
| | *** | 40868 | 53656 | 87401 | 14199 | 17450 | 21625 | 2975 | 3193 | 3342 | 762 | 781 | 778 | 331 | 331 | 316 |
| 0.75 | *** | 33286 | 40280 | 77243 | 11911 | 13906 | 19055 | 2555 | 2712 | 2930 | 650 | 668 | 680 | 275 | 275 | 275 |
| | *** | 36031 | 48218 | 77734 | 12755 | 15668 | 19156 | 2630 | 2806 | 2922 | 661 | 668 | 662 | 275 | 275 | 260 |
| 0.8 | *** | 28418 | 34861 | 65731 | 10318 | 12024 | 16118 | 2150 | 2274 | 2431 | 530 | 537 | 549 | 211 | 211 | 211 |
| | *** | 30980 | 41937 | 65966 | 11049 | 13486 | 16161 | 2206 | 2349 | 2417 | 530 | 537 | 526 | 211 | 211 | 194 |
| 0.85 | *** | 23330 | 28824 | 52006 | 8461 | 9781 | 12643 | 1674 | 1749 | 1843 | 380 | 380 | 387 | . | . | . |
| | *** | 25543 | 34625 | 52096 | 9031 | 10850 | 12641 | 1711 | 1793 | 1829 | 380 | 387 | 368 | . | . | . |
| 0.9 | *** | 17712 | 21781 | 36118 | 6218 | 7055 | 8611 | 1100 | 1137 | 1175 | . | . | . | . | . | . |
| | *** | 19374 | 25831 | 36125 | 6586 | 7681 | 8596 | 1118 | 1156 | 1156 | . | . | . | . | . | . |
| 0.95 | *** | 10730 | 12800 | 18068 | 3324 | 3624 | 4043 | . | . | . | . | . | . | . | . | . |
| | *** | 11611 | 14618 | 18052 | 3462 | 3811 | 4025 | . | . | . | . | . | . | . | . | . |
| 0.98 | *** | 4737 | 5293 | 6218 | . | . | . | . | . | . | . | . | . | . | . | . |
| | *** | 4993 | 5686 | 6200 | . | . | . | . | . | . | . | . | . | . | . | . |

## TABLE 6: ALPHA= 0.025 POWER= 0.9    EXPECTED ACCRUAL THRU MINIMUM FOLLOW-UP= 8000

| | DEL=.01 | | | DEL=.02 | | | DEL=.05 | | | DEL=.10 | | | DEL=.15 | | |
|---|---|---|---|---|---|---|---|---|---|---|---|---|---|---|---|
| FACT= | 1.0 .75 | .50 .25 | .00 BIN | 1.0 .75 | .50 .25 | .00 BIN | 1.0 .75 | .50 .25 | .00 BIN | 1.0 75 | .50 .25 | .00 BIN | 1.0 .75 | .50 .25 | .00 BIN |
| PCONT=*** | | | | | REQUIRED NUMBER OF PATIENTS | | | | | | | | | | |
| 0.01 *** | 1613 1613 | 1613 1613 | 1625 6200 | 593 593 | 593 593 | 593 2049 | 193 193 | 193 193 | 193 558 | 93 93 | 93 93 | 93 227 | 65 65 | 65 65 | 65 135 |
| 0.02 *** | 3573 3573 | 3585 3605 | 3613 10235 | 1145 1145 | 1153 1153 | 1153 3048 | 313 313 | 313 313 | 313 712 | 133 133 | 133 133 | 133 264 | 85 85 | 85 85 | 85 151 |
| 0.05 *** | 10825 10865 | 10933 11053 | 11293 21835 | 3085 3105 | 3113 3145 | 3165 5916 | 665 665 | 665 665 | 673 1156 | 233 233 | 233 233 | 233 368 | 133 133 | 133 133 | 133 194 |
| 0.1 *** | 23905 24025 | 24253 24765 | 26293 39487 | 6525 6585 | 6673 6785 | 6953 10277 | 1265 1273 | 1285 1285 | 1293 1829 | 393 393 | 393 393 | 393 526 | 213 213 | 213 213 | 213 260 |
| 0.15 *** | 35765 35985 | 36413 37465 | 41533 55038 | 9653 9793 | 9985 10273 | 10753 14112 | 1833 1845 | 1865 1873 | 1893 2417 | 545 545 | 545 545 | 545 662 | 273 273 | 273 273 | 273 316 |
| 0.2 *** | 45405 45745 | 46413 48125 | 55805 68488 | 12273 12493 | 12825 13353 | 14285 17422 | 2325 2345 | 2373 2413 | 2445 2922 | 665 665 | 673 673 | 673 778 | 325 325 | 325 333 | 333 362 |
| 0.25 *** | 52533 53033 | 53993 56473 | 68505 79836 | 14305 14633 | 15113 15913 | 17425 20206 | 2733 2773 | 2813 2865 | 2925 3342 | 773 773 | 785 785 | 793 873 | 373 373 | 373 373 | 373 400 |
| 0.3 *** | 57193 57873 | 59193 62553 | 79325 89082 | 15765 16205 | 16865 17933 | 20085 22465 | 3053 3113 | 3173 3245 | 3333 3678 | 853 865 | 865 873 | 885 946 | 405 405 | 405 413 | 413 428 |
| 0.35 *** | 59565 60465 | 62205 66513 | 88085 96227 | 16705 17265 | 18085 19433 | 22213 24199 | 3293 3365 | 3445 3533 | 3645 3930 | 913 925 | 933 945 | 945 999 | 433 433 | 433 433 | 433 446 |
| 0.4 *** | 59913 61085 | 63305 68605 | 94665 101271 | 17185 17853 | 18833 20433 | 23805 25407 | 3453 3533 | 3633 3745 | 3873 4098 | 965 965 | 973 985 | 993 1030 | 445 445 | 453 453 | 453 456 |
| 0.45 *** | 58573 60053 | 62793 69073 | 99005 104213 | 17265 18033 | 19153 20973 | 24833 26090 | 3545 3633 | 3733 3865 | 4013 4182 | 973 985 | 993 1005 | 1013 1041 | 453 453 | 453 453 | 465 456 |
| 0.5 *** | 55905 57733 | 60993 68173 | 101085 105054 | 17013 17865 | 19093 21085 | 25293 26248 | 3553 3645 | 3765 3893 | 4065 4182 | 973 985 | 993 1005 | 1013 1030 | 445 445 | 453 453 | 453 446 |
| 0.55 *** | 52273 54445 | 58205 66113 | 100865 103793 | 16473 17385 | 18685 20785 | 25185 25880 | 3493 3593 | 3705 3845 | 4013 4098 | 953 965 | 973 985 | 993 999 | 433 433 | 433 433 | 445 428 |
| 0.6 *** | 48013 50513 | 54665 63073 | 98365 100430 | 15685 16633 | 17973 20093 | 24505 24987 | 3365 3465 | 3573 3713 | 3873 3930 | 913 925 | 933 945 | 953 946 | 405 405 | 413 413 | 413 400 |
| 0.65 *** | 43433 46153 | 50553 59173 | 93585 94967 | 14693 15633 | 16965 19045 | 23253 23569 | 3165 3265 | 3373 3493 | 3653 3678 | 845 853 | 865 873 | 885 873 | 373 373 | 373 373 | 373 362 |
| 0.7 *** | 38693 41525 | 45985 54473 | 86533 87401 | 13493 14405 | 15665 17613 | 21433 21625 | 2905 2985 | 3085 3193 | 3333 3342 | 765 765 | 773 785 | 793 778 | 325 333 | 333 333 | 333 316 |
| 0.75 *** | 33885 36685 | 40985 48985 | 77245 77734 | 12105 12933 | 14085 15813 | 19053 19156 | 2573 2645 | 2725 2813 | 2925 2922 | 653 665 | 665 673 | 685 662 | 273 273 | 273 273 | 273 260 |
| 0.8 *** | 28973 31573 | 35505 42605 | 65725 65966 | 10485 11205 | 12173 13605 | 16125 16161 | 2165 2225 | 2285 2353 | 2433 2417 | 525 533 | 533 545 | 545 526 | 213 213 | 213 213 | 213 194 |
| 0.85 *** | 23813 26053 | 29353 35153 | 52013 52096 | 8585 9153 | 9893 10933 | 12633 12641 | 1685 1713 | 1753 1793 | 1845 1829 | 385 385 | 385 385 | 385 368 | . . | . . | . . |
| 0.9 *** | 18073 19753 | 22165 26193 | 36113 36125 | 6305 6665 | 7125 7725 | 8605 8596 | 1105 1125 | 1133 1153 | 1173 1156 | . . | . . | . . | . . | . . | . . |
| 0.95 *** | 10925 11805 | 12985 14765 | 18065 18052 | 3353 3485 | 3645 3825 | 4045 4025 | . . | . . | . . | . . | . . | . . | . . | . . | . . |
| 0.98 *** | 4793 5045 | 5333 5713 | 6225 6200 | . . | . . | . . | . . | . . | . . | . . | . . | . . | . . | . . | . . |

## TABLE 6: ALPHA= 0.025 POWER= 0.9    EXPECTED ACCRUAL THRU MINIMUM FOLLOW-UP= 8500

| | | DEL=.01 | | | DEL=.02 | | | DEL=.05 | | | DEL=.10 | | | DEL=.15 | |
|---|---|---|---|---|---|---|---|---|---|---|---|---|---|---|---|---|
| FACT= | 1.0 .75 | .50 .25 | .00 BIN | 1.0 .75 | .50 .25 | .00 BIN | 1.0 .75 | .50 .25 | .00 BIN | 1.0 75 | .50 .25 | .00 BIN | 1.0 .75 | .50 .25 | .00 BIN |

PCONT=***           REQUIRED NUMBER OF PATIENTS

| PCONT | | DEL=.01 (1.0/.75) | DEL=.01 (.50/.25) | DEL=.01 (.00/BIN) | DEL=.02 (1.0/.75) | DEL=.02 (.50/.25) | DEL=.02 (.00/BIN) | DEL=.05 (1.0/.75) | DEL=.05 (.50/.25) | DEL=.05 (.00/BIN) | DEL=.10 (1.0/75) | DEL=.10 (.50/.25) | DEL=.10 (.00/BIN) | DEL=.15 (1.0/.75) | DEL=.15 (.50/.25) | DEL=.15 (.00/BIN) |
|---|---|---|---|---|---|---|---|---|---|---|---|---|---|---|---|---|
| 0.01 | *** | 1608 | 1621 | 1621 | 588 | 588 | 588 | 197 | 197 | 197 | 99 | 99 | 99 | 70 | 70 | 70 |
|  | *** | 1608 | 1621 | 6200 | 588 | 588 | 2049 | 197 | 197 | 558 | 99 | 99 | 227 | 70 | 70 | 135 |
| 0.02 | *** | 3576 | 3584 | 3618 | 1153 | 1153 | 1153 | 311 | 311 | 311 | 133 | 133 | 133 | 91 | 91 | 91 |
|  | *** | 3576 | 3597 | 10235 | 1153 | 1153 | 3048 | 311 | 311 | 712 | 133 | 133 | 264 | 91 | 91 | 151 |
| 0.05 | *** | 10830 | 10950 | 11298 | 3095 | 3116 | 3159 | 665 | 665 | 673 | 240 | 240 | 240 | 141 | 141 | 141 |
|  | *** | 10873 | 11064 | 21835 | 3108 | 3138 | 5916 | 665 | 673 | 1156 | 240 | 240 | 368 | 141 | 141 | 194 |
| 0.1 | *** | 23933 | 24295 | 26292 | 6538 | 6678 | 6955 | 1268 | 1281 | 1289 | 396 | 396 | 396 | 205 | 205 | 205 |
|  | *** | 24061 | 24813 | 39487 | 6601 | 6793 | 10277 | 1281 | 1289 | 1829 | 396 | 396 | 526 | 205 | 205 | 260 |
| 0.15 | *** | 35812 | 36492 | 41536 | 9683 | 10015 | 10758 | 1833 | 1863 | 1897 | 537 | 545 | 545 | 269 | 269 | 269 |
|  | *** | 36046 | 37563 | 55038 | 9823 | 10299 | 14112 | 1841 | 1876 | 2417 | 545 | 545 | 662 | 269 | 269 | 316 |
| 0.2 | *** | 45468 | 46530 | 55795 | 12318 | 12883 | 14286 | 2330 | 2386 | 2450 | 665 | 673 | 673 | 325 | 333 | 333 |
|  | *** | 45829 | 48294 | 68488 | 12543 | 13393 | 17422 | 2351 | 2415 | 2922 | 673 | 673 | 778 | 325 | 333 | 362 |
| 0.25 | *** | 52629 | 54172 | 68503 | 14371 | 15186 | 17418 | 2747 | 2819 | 2925 | 771 | 779 | 792 | 375 | 375 | 375 |
|  | *** | 53152 | 56730 | 79836 | 14698 | 15973 | 20206 | 2776 | 2875 | 3342 | 779 | 779 | 873 | 375 | 375 | 400 |
| 0.3 | *** | 57325 | 59442 | 79332 | 15858 | 16963 | 20074 | 3066 | 3180 | 3329 | 856 | 864 | 877 | 410 | 410 | 410 |
|  | *** | 58048 | 62906 | 89082 | 16305 | 18013 | 22465 | 3116 | 3244 | 3678 | 864 | 877 | 946 | 410 | 410 | 428 |
| 0.35 | *** | 59740 | 62523 | 88087 | 16823 | 18204 | 22220 | 3308 | 3456 | 3648 | 920 | 928 | 949 | 431 | 431 | 439 |
|  | *** | 60696 | 66965 | 96227 | 17388 | 19543 | 24199 | 3385 | 3541 | 3930 | 928 | 941 | 999 | 431 | 439 | 446 |
| 0.4 | *** | 60130 | 63692 | 94661 | 17325 | 18982 | 23806 | 3478 | 3640 | 3873 | 962 | 983 | 991 | 452 | 452 | 452 |
|  | *** | 61376 | 69140 | 101271 | 17991 | 20563 | 25407 | 3555 | 3746 | 4098 | 970 | 983 | 1030 | 452 | 452 | 456 |
| 0.45 | *** | 58855 | 63267 | 99010 | 17431 | 19322 | 24834 | 3563 | 3754 | 4009 | 983 | 1005 | 1013 | 452 | 452 | 460 |
|  | *** | 60420 | 69693 | 104213 | 18196 | 21115 | 26090 | 3648 | 3873 | 4182 | 991 | 1005 | 1041 | 452 | 460 | 456 |
| 0.5 | *** | 56255 | 61546 | 101079 | 17184 | 19266 | 25293 | 3576 | 3775 | 4065 | 983 | 1005 | 1013 | 452 | 452 | 452 |
|  | *** | 58167 | 68877 | 105054 | 18047 | 21243 | 26248 | 3669 | 3903 | 4182 | 991 | 1005 | 1030 | 452 | 452 | 446 |
| 0.55 | *** | 52693 | 58826 | 100866 | 16666 | 18876 | 25187 | 3512 | 3725 | 4009 | 962 | 970 | 991 | 431 | 439 | 439 |
|  | *** | 54958 | 66866 | 103793 | 17580 | 20945 | 25880 | 3605 | 3852 | 4098 | 962 | 983 | 999 | 431 | 439 | 428 |
| 0.6 | *** | 48506 | 55341 | 98359 | 15880 | 18161 | 24507 | 3385 | 3597 | 3881 | 906 | 928 | 949 | 410 | 410 | 418 |
|  | *** | 51091 | 63862 | 100430 | 16836 | 20265 | 24987 | 3478 | 3725 | 3930 | 920 | 941 | 946 | 410 | 410 | 400 |
| 0.65 | *** | 43972 | 51261 | 93578 | 14889 | 17155 | 23253 | 3193 | 3385 | 3648 | 843 | 864 | 885 | 375 | 375 | 375 |
|  | *** | 46777 | 59960 | 94967 | 15837 | 19203 | 23569 | 3278 | 3499 | 3678 | 856 | 877 | 873 | 375 | 375 | 362 |
| 0.7 | *** | 39263 | 46692 | 86536 | 13691 | 15845 | 21434 | 2925 | 3095 | 3329 | 758 | 779 | 792 | 325 | 333 | 333 |
|  | *** | 42166 | 55243 | 87401 | 14591 | 17771 | 21625 | 3002 | 3201 | 3342 | 771 | 779 | 778 | 333 | 333 | 316 |
| 0.75 | *** | 34452 | 41664 | 77250 | 12275 | 14243 | 19054 | 2585 | 2734 | 2925 | 651 | 665 | 686 | 269 | 282 | 282 |
|  | *** | 37300 | 49696 | 77734 | 13117 | 15943 | 19156 | 2662 | 2819 | 2922 | 665 | 673 | 662 | 282 | 282 | 260 |
| 0.8 | *** | 29509 | 36110 | 65732 | 10639 | 12310 | 16121 | 2181 | 2288 | 2428 | 524 | 537 | 545 | 205 | 218 | 218 |
|  | *** | 32144 | 43236 | 65966 | 11353 | 13712 | 16161 | 2237 | 2351 | 2417 | 537 | 537 | 526 | 218 | 218 | 194 |
| 0.85 | *** | 24281 | 29862 | 52013 | 8705 | 9993 | 12636 | 1693 | 1756 | 1841 | 375 | 388 | 388 | . | . | . |
|  | *** | 26534 | 35650 | 52096 | 9271 | 11013 | 12641 | 1727 | 1799 | 1829 | 375 | 388 | 368 | . | . | . |
| 0.9 | *** | 18430 | 22531 | 36118 | 6381 | 7188 | 8612 | 1111 | 1140 | 1175 | . | . | . | . | . | . |
|  | *** | 20108 | 26526 | 36125 | 6742 | 7770 | 8596 | 1119 | 1153 | 1156 | . | . | . | . | . | . |
| 0.95 | *** | 11120 | 13160 | 18068 | 3385 | 3661 | 4043 | . | . | . | . | . | . | . | . | . |
|  | *** | 11978 | 14902 | 18052 | 3512 | 3831 | 4025 | . | . | . | . | . | . | . | . | . |
| 0.98 | *** | 4851 | 5382 | 6219 | . | . | . | . | . | . | . | . | . | . | . | . |
|  | *** | 5093 | 5743 | 6200 | . | . | . | . | . | . | . | . | . | . | . | . |

TABLE 6: ALPHA= 0.025 POWER= 0.9   EXPECTED ACCRUAL THRU MINIMUM FOLLOW-UP= 9000

| | | DEL=.01 | | | DEL=.02 | | | DEL=.05 | | | DEL=.10 | | | DEL=.15 | | |
|---|---|---|---|---|---|---|---|---|---|---|---|---|---|---|---|---|---|
| FACT= | | 1.0 .75 | .50 .25 | .00 BIN | 1.0 .75 | .50 .25 | .00 BIN | 1.0 .75 | .50 .25 | .00 BIN | 1.0 75 | .50 .25 | .00 BIN | 1.0 .75 | .50 .25 | .00 BIN |
| PCONT=*** | | | | | REQUIRED NUMBER OF PATIENTS | | | | | | | | | | | |
| 0.01 | *** | 1612 | 1612 | 1626 | 591 | 591 | 591 | 195 | 195 | 195 | 96 | 96 | 96 | 74 | 74 | 74 |
| | *** | 1612 | 1612 | 6200 | 591 | 591 | 2049 | 195 | 195 | 558 | 96 | 96 | 227 | 74 | 74 | 135 |
| 0.02 | *** | 3570 | 3592 | 3615 | 1154 | 1154 | 1154 | 307 | 307 | 307 | 141 | 141 | 141 | 82 | 82 | 82 |
| | *** | 3584 | 3606 | 10235 | 1154 | 1154 | 3048 | 307 | 307 | 712 | 141 | 141 | 264 | 82 | 82 | 151 |
| 0.05 | *** | 10837 | 10964 | 11301 | 3097 | 3120 | 3165 | 667 | 667 | 667 | 240 | 240 | 240 | 141 | 141 | 141 |
| | *** | 10882 | 11076 | 21835 | 3111 | 3142 | 5916 | 667 | 667 | 1156 | 240 | 240 | 368 | 141 | 141 | 194 |
| 0.1 | *** | 23955 | 24329 | 26295 | 6554 | 6689 | 6959 | 1266 | 1275 | 1297 | 397 | 397 | 397 | 209 | 209 | 209 |
| | *** | 24090 | 24855 | 39487 | 6607 | 6801 | 10277 | 1275 | 1289 | 1829 | 397 | 397 | 526 | 209 | 209 | 260 |
| 0.15 | *** | 35849 | 36569 | 41527 | 9712 | 10041 | 10747 | 1837 | 1860 | 1896 | 546 | 546 | 546 | 276 | 276 | 276 |
| | *** | 36096 | 37671 | 55038 | 9847 | 10320 | 14112 | 1851 | 1882 | 2417 | 546 | 546 | 662 | 276 | 276 | 316 |
| 0.2 | *** | 45532 | 46657 | 55806 | 12359 | 12921 | 14294 | 2332 | 2377 | 2445 | 667 | 667 | 681 | 330 | 330 | 330 |
| | *** | 45915 | 48471 | 68488 | 12592 | 13425 | 17422 | 2355 | 2414 | 2922 | 667 | 681 | 778 | 330 | 330 | 362 |
| 0.25 | *** | 52724 | 54344 | 68505 | 14437 | 15261 | 17421 | 2751 | 2827 | 2931 | 771 | 780 | 794 | 375 | 375 | 375 |
| | *** | 53272 | 56985 | 79836 | 14775 | 16026 | 20206 | 2782 | 2872 | 3342 | 780 | 780 | 873 | 375 | 375 | 400 |
| 0.3 | *** | 57449 | 59676 | 79327 | 15945 | 17047 | 20076 | 3075 | 3187 | 3336 | 861 | 870 | 884 | 411 | 411 | 411 |
| | *** | 58214 | 63240 | 89082 | 16395 | 18096 | 22465 | 3134 | 3255 | 3678 | 861 | 870 | 946 | 411 | 411 | 428 |
| 0.35 | *** | 59901 | 62826 | 88080 | 16926 | 18321 | 22214 | 3322 | 3457 | 3651 | 915 | 937 | 951 | 434 | 434 | 442 |
| | *** | 60914 | 67380 | 96227 | 17497 | 19635 | 24199 | 3390 | 3547 | 3930 | 929 | 937 | 999 | 434 | 434 | 446 |
| 0.4 | *** | 60360 | 64072 | 94664 | 17452 | 19117 | 23811 | 3494 | 3651 | 3876 | 960 | 982 | 996 | 442 | 456 | 456 |
| | *** | 61656 | 69652 | 101271 | 18127 | 20684 | 25407 | 3570 | 3750 | 4098 | 974 | 982 | 1030 | 442 | 456 | 456 |
| 0.45 | *** | 59136 | 63726 | 99006 | 17579 | 19477 | 24832 | 3584 | 3764 | 4011 | 982 | 996 | 1019 | 456 | 456 | 456 |
| | *** | 60765 | 70296 | 104213 | 18352 | 21255 | 26090 | 3660 | 3876 | 4182 | 996 | 1005 | 1041 | 456 | 456 | 456 |
| 0.5 | *** | 56602 | 62084 | 101076 | 17354 | 19446 | 25296 | 3592 | 3786 | 4056 | 982 | 996 | 1019 | 442 | 456 | 456 |
| | *** | 58596 | 69540 | 105054 | 18217 | 21390 | 26248 | 3682 | 3907 | 4182 | 996 | 1005 | 1030 | 442 | 456 | 446 |
| 0.55 | *** | 53115 | 59429 | 100860 | 16836 | 19064 | 25184 | 3539 | 3741 | 4011 | 960 | 974 | 996 | 434 | 434 | 442 |
| | *** | 55455 | 67582 | 103793 | 17759 | 21097 | 25880 | 3629 | 3862 | 4098 | 974 | 982 | 999 | 434 | 434 | 428 |
| 0.6 | *** | 48989 | 55986 | 98362 | 16071 | 18352 | 24509 | 3404 | 3606 | 3876 | 915 | 929 | 951 | 411 | 411 | 411 |
| | *** | 51644 | 64612 | 100430 | 17025 | 20422 | 24987 | 3494 | 3727 | 3930 | 929 | 937 | 946 | 411 | 411 | 400 |
| 0.65 | *** | 44497 | 51936 | 93584 | 15081 | 17340 | 23249 | 3210 | 3390 | 3651 | 847 | 870 | 884 | 375 | 375 | 375 |
| | *** | 47369 | 60720 | 94967 | 16026 | 19356 | 23569 | 3291 | 3516 | 3678 | 861 | 870 | 873 | 375 | 375 | 362 |
| 0.7 | *** | 39817 | 47369 | 86541 | 13866 | 16026 | 21435 | 2940 | 3111 | 3336 | 771 | 780 | 794 | 330 | 330 | 330 |
| | *** | 42765 | 55972 | 87401 | 14775 | 17902 | 21625 | 3021 | 3210 | 3342 | 771 | 780 | 778 | 330 | 330 | 316 |
| 0.75 | *** | 35002 | 42306 | 77249 | 12449 | 14406 | 19050 | 2602 | 2751 | 2931 | 659 | 667 | 681 | 276 | 276 | 276 |
| | *** | 37896 | 50370 | 77734 | 13281 | 16071 | 19156 | 2670 | 2827 | 2922 | 667 | 667 | 662 | 276 | 276 | 260 |
| 0.8 | *** | 30021 | 36690 | 65729 | 10784 | 12435 | 16125 | 2189 | 2301 | 2436 | 532 | 532 | 546 | 209 | 209 | 217 |
| | *** | 32685 | 43822 | 65966 | 11490 | 13807 | 16161 | 2242 | 2355 | 2417 | 532 | 546 | 526 | 209 | 217 | 194 |
| 0.85 | *** | 24720 | 30345 | 52012 | 8826 | 10086 | 12637 | 1694 | 1770 | 1851 | 375 | 389 | 389 | . | . | . |
| | *** | 26992 | 36119 | 52096 | 9375 | 11085 | 12641 | 1725 | 1806 | 1829 | 389 | 389 | 368 | . | . | . |
| 0.9 | *** | 18757 | 22866 | 36119 | 6450 | 7237 | 8610 | 1109 | 1140 | 1176 | . | . | . | . | . | . |
| | *** | 20445 | 26835 | 36125 | 6801 | 7814 | 8596 | 1131 | 1154 | 1156 | . | . | . | . | . | . |
| 0.95 | *** | 11287 | 13312 | 18074 | 3412 | 3674 | 4042 | . | . | . | . | . | . | . | . | . |
| | *** | 12156 | 15022 | 18052 | 3539 | 3840 | 4025 | . | . | . | . | . | . | . | . | . |
| 0.98 | *** | 4897 | 5415 | 6216 | . | . | . | . | . | . | . | . | . | . | . | . |
| | *** | 5136 | 5766 | 6200 | . | . | . | . | . | . | . | . | . | . | . | . |

## TABLE 6: ALPHA= 0.025 POWER= 0.9    EXPECTED ACCRUAL THRU MINIMUM FOLLOW-UP= 9500

| | | DEL=.01 | | | DEL=.02 | | | DEL=.05 | | | DEL=.10 | | | DEL=.15 | | |
|---|---|---|---|---|---|---|---|---|---|---|---|---|---|---|---|---|
| FACT= | | 1.0 .75 | .50 .25 | .00 BIN | 1.0 .75 | .50 .25 | .00 BIN | 1.0 .75 | .50 .25 | .00 BIN | 1.0 75 | .50 .25 | .00 BIN | 1.0 .75 | .50 .25 | .00 BIN |
| PCONT=*** | | REQUIRED NUMBER OF PATIENTS | | | | | | | | | | | | | | |
| 0.01 | *** | 1607 1621 | 1621 | 585 585 | 585 | 196 196 | 196 | 101 101 | 101 | 63 63 | 63 | | | |
| | *** | 1607 1621 | 6200 | 585 585 | 2049 | 196 196 | 558 | 101 101 | 227 | 63 63 | 135 | | | |
| 0.02 | *** | 3578 3593 | 3616 | 1146 1146 | 1155 | 315 315 | 315 | 134 134 | 134 | 87 87 | 87 | | | |
| | *** | 3578 3602 | 10235 | 1146 1155 | 3048 | 315 315 | 712 | 134 134 | 264 | 87 87 | 151 | | | |
| 0.05 | *** | 10845 10964 | 11297 | 3094 3127 | 3165 | 671 671 | 671 | 244 244 | 244 | 134 134 | 134 | | | |
| | *** | 10893 11083 | 21835 | 3103 3141 | 5916 | 671 671 | 1156 | 244 244 | 368 | 134 134 | 194 | | | |
| 0.1 | *** | 23979 24374 | 26298 | 6561 6704 | 6950 | 1274 1274 | 1289 | 395 395 | 395 | 205 205 | 205 | | | |
| | *** | 24113 24896 | 39487 | 6618 6808 | 10277 | 1274 1289 | 1829 | 395 395 | 526 | 205 205 | 260 | | | |
| 0.15 | *** | 35893 36638 | 41530 | 9744 10062 | 10750 | 1835 1868 | 1892 | 538 538 | 553 | 277 277 | 277 | | | |
| | *** | 36154 37769 | 55038 | 9872 10338 | 14112 | 1844 1883 | 2417 | 538 538 | 662 | 277 277 | 316 | | | |
| 0.2 | *** | 45592 46770 | 55804 | 12404 12959 | 14289 | 2334 2390 | 2453 | 671 671 | 680 | 324 324 | 324 | | | |
| | *** | 45995 48632 | 68488 | 12641 13458 | 17422 | 2358 2414 | 2922 | 671 671 | 778 | 324 324 | 362 | | | |
| 0.25 | *** | 52812 54513 | 68501 | 14494 15325 | 17424 | 2761 2833 | 2928 | 775 775 | 790 | 372 372 | 372 | | | |
| | *** | 53396 57229 | 79836 | 14835 16085 | 20206 | 2794 2880 | 3342 | 775 790 | 873 | 372 372 | 400 | | | |
| 0.3 | *** | 57576 59904 | 79331 | 16023 17139 | 20084 | 3094 3198 | 3331 | 861 870 | 885 | 410 410 | 410 | | | |
| | *** | 58384 63561 | 89082 | 16474 18175 | 22465 | 3141 3260 | 3678 | 861 870 | 946 | 410 410 | 428 | | | |
| 0.35 | *** | 60070 63119 | 88080 | 17035 18436 | 22213 | 3340 3474 | 3649 | 918 933 | 942 | 434 434 | 434 | | | |
| | *** | 61139 67789 | 96227 | 17605 19728 | 24199 | 3403 3554 | 3930 | 933 942 | 999 | 434 434 | 446 | | | |
| 0.4 | *** | 60578 64449 | 94659 | 17581 19244 | 23804 | 3507 3664 | 3878 | 965 980 | 989 | 443 443 | 458 | | | |
| | *** | 61946 70149 | 101271 | 18270 20797 | 25407 | 3578 3759 | 4098 | 965 989 | 1030 | 443 458 | 456 | | | |
| 0.45 | *** | 59414 64179 | 99005 | 17724 19624 | 24834 | 3593 3768 | 4005 | 980 1004 | 1013 | 458 458 | 458 | | | |
| | *** | 61124 70862 | 104213 | 18508 21381 | 26090 | 3673 3887 | 4182 | 989 1013 | 1041 | 458 458 | 456 | | | |
| 0.5 | *** | 56944 62611 | 101086 | 17519 19600 | 25300 | 3616 3806 | 4053 | 980 1004 | 1013 | 443 458 | 458 | | | |
| | *** | 59010 70173 | 105054 | 18374 21524 | 26248 | 3697 3925 | 4182 | 989 1013 | 1030 | 443 458 | 446 | | | |
| 0.55 | *** | 53524 60008 | 100858 | 17011 19229 | 25190 | 3554 3744 | 4020 | 956 980 | 989 | 434 434 | 443 | | | |
| | *** | 55947 68273 | 103793 | 17938 21248 | 25880 | 3640 3863 | 4098 | 965 989 | 999 | 434 434 | 428 | | | |
| 0.6 | *** | 49463 56612 | 98364 | 16251 18517 | 24502 | 3426 3616 | 3878 | 918 933 | 956 | 410 410 | 410 | | | |
| | *** | 52185 65319 | 100430 | 17201 20559 | 24987 | 3507 3735 | 3930 | 918 942 | 946 | 410 410 | 400 | | | |
| 0.65 | *** | 45013 52574 | 93581 | 15254 17510 | 23258 | 3222 3412 | 3649 | 847 870 | 885 | 372 372 | 372 | | | |
| | *** | 47943 61433 | 94967 | 16204 19490 | 23569 | 3308 3521 | 3678 | 861 870 | 873 | 372 372 | 362 | | | |
| 0.7 | *** | 40358 48005 | 86537 | 14043 16180 | 21438 | 2960 3118 | 3331 | 766 775 | 790 | 324 324 | 339 | | | |
| | *** | 43359 56659 | 87401 | 14945 18033 | 21625 | 3032 3222 | 3342 | 775 790 | 778 | 324 339 | 316 | | | |
| 0.75 | *** | 35522 42908 | 77241 | 12603 14541 | 19054 | 2619 2747 | 2928 | 657 671 | 680 | 277 277 | 277 | | | |
| | *** | 38458 51007 | 77734 | 13434 16180 | 19156 | 2675 2833 | 2922 | 657 671 | 662 | 277 277 | 260 | | | |
| 0.8 | *** | 30510 37232 | 65732 | 10917 12555 | 16118 | 2200 2310 | 2429 | 529 538 | 538 | 205 205 | 220 | | | |
| | *** | 33209 44371 | 65966 | 11629 13900 | 16161 | 2248 2367 | 2417 | 538 538 | 526 | 205 220 | 194 | | | |
| 0.85 | *** | 25134 30795 | 52004 | 8922 10180 | 12641 | 1702 1773 | 1844 | 386 386 | 386 | . . | . | | | |
| | *** | 27438 36558 | 52096 | 9468 11145 | 12641 | 1740 1811 | 1829 | 386 386 | 368 | . . | . | | | |
| 0.9 | *** | 19078 23186 | 36115 | 6523 7298 | 8613 | 1108 1146 | 1179 | . . | . | . . | . | | | |
| | *** | 20773 27129 | 36125 | 6870 7844 | 8596 | 1132 1155 | 1156 | . . | . | . . | . | | | |
| 0.95 | *** | 11454 13458 | 18065 | 3435 3697 | 4044 | . . | . | . . | . | . . | . | | | |
| | *** | 12309 15144 | 18052 | 3554 3854 | 4025 | . . | . | . . | . | . . | . | | | |
| 0.98 | *** | 4946 5445 | 6214 | . . | . | . . | . | . . | . | . . | . | | | |
| | *** | 5169 5787 | 6200 | . . | . | . . | . | . . | . | . . | . | | | |

TABLE 6: ALPHA= 0.025 POWER= 0.9    EXPECTED ACCRUAL THRU MINIMUM FOLLOW-UP= 10000

| | | DEL=.01 | | | DEL=.02 | | | DEL=.05 | | | DEL=.10 | | | DEL=.15 | | |
|---|---|---|---|---|---|---|---|---|---|---|---|---|---|---|---|---|
| FACT= | | 1.0 .75 | .50 .25 | .00 BIN | 1.0 .75 | .50 .25 | .00 BIN | 1.0 .75 | .50 .25 | .00 BIN | 1.0 75 | .50 .25 | .00 BIN | 1.0 .75 | .50 .25 | .00 BIN |
| PCONT=*** | | | | | REQUIRED NUMBER OF PATIENTS | | | | | | | | | | | |
| 0.01 | *** | 1616 | 1616 | 1616 | 591 | 591 | 591 | 191 | 191 | 191 | 91 | 91 | 91 | 66 | 66 | 66 |
| | *** | 1616 | 1616 | 6200 | 591 | 591 | 2049 | 191 | 191 | 558 | 91 | 91 | 227 | 66 | 66 | 135 |
| 0.02 | *** | 3582 | 3591 | 3616 | 1141 | 1157 | 1157 | 307 | 307 | 307 | 132 | 132 | 132 | 91 | 91 | 91 |
| | *** | 3582 | 3607 | 10235 | 1157 | 1157 | 3048 | 307 | 307 | 712 | 132 | 132 | 264 | 91 | 91 | 151 |
| 0.05 | *** | 10857 | 10982 | 11291 | 3107 | 3132 | 3166 | 666 | 666 | 666 | 241 | 241 | 241 | 141 | 141 | 141 |
| | *** | 10907 | 11091 | 21835 | 3116 | 3141 | 5916 | 666 | 666 | 1156 | 241 | 241 | 368 | 141 | 141 | 194 |
| 0.1 | *** | 23991 | 24407 | 26291 | 6566 | 6707 | 6957 | 1266 | 1282 | 1291 | 391 | 391 | 391 | 207 | 207 | 207 |
| | *** | 24141 | 24941 | 39487 | 6632 | 6816 | 10277 | 1282 | 1291 | 1829 | 391 | 391 | 526 | 207 | 207 | 260 |
| 0.15 | *** | 35932 | 36707 | 41532 | 9766 | 10091 | 10757 | 1841 | 1866 | 1891 | 541 | 541 | 541 | 266 | 282 | 282 |
| | *** | 36207 | 37857 | 55038 | 9907 | 10357 | 14112 | 1857 | 1882 | 2417 | 541 | 541 | 662 | 266 | 282 | 316 |
| 0.2 | *** | 45657 | 46891 | 55807 | 12441 | 13007 | 14291 | 2341 | 2391 | 2441 | 666 | 666 | 682 | 332 | 332 | 332 |
| | *** | 46082 | 48791 | 68488 | 12682 | 13491 | 17422 | 2366 | 2416 | 2922 | 666 | 682 | 778 | 332 | 332 | 362 |
| 0.25 | *** | 52907 | 54682 | 68507 | 14557 | 15382 | 17416 | 2766 | 2832 | 2932 | 782 | 782 | 791 | 366 | 382 | 382 |
| | *** | 53516 | 57457 | 79836 | 14891 | 16132 | 20206 | 2791 | 2882 | 3342 | 782 | 782 | 873 | 366 | 382 | 400 |
| 0.3 | *** | 57707 | 60132 | 79332 | 16107 | 17216 | 20082 | 3107 | 3207 | 3332 | 857 | 866 | 882 | 407 | 407 | 416 |
| | *** | 58541 | 63866 | 89082 | 16566 | 18241 | 22465 | 3141 | 3257 | 3678 | 866 | 882 | 946 | 407 | 407 | 428 |
| 0.35 | *** | 60241 | 63416 | 88082 | 17132 | 18532 | 22216 | 3357 | 3482 | 3641 | 916 | 932 | 941 | 432 | 432 | 441 |
| | *** | 61357 | 68182 | 96227 | 17707 | 19816 | 24199 | 3407 | 3557 | 3930 | 932 | 941 | 999 | 432 | 432 | 446 |
| 0.4 | *** | 60791 | 64816 | 94666 | 17691 | 19366 | 23807 | 3516 | 3666 | 3882 | 966 | 982 | 991 | 441 | 457 | 457 |
| | *** | 62216 | 70616 | 101271 | 18391 | 20891 | 25407 | 3591 | 3766 | 4098 | 966 | 991 | 1030 | 441 | 457 | 456 |
| 0.45 | *** | 59691 | 64616 | 99007 | 17857 | 19757 | 24832 | 3616 | 3782 | 4016 | 982 | 1007 | 1016 | 457 | 457 | 457 |
| | *** | 61466 | 71407 | 104213 | 18641 | 21491 | 26090 | 3691 | 3891 | 4182 | 991 | 1007 | 1041 | 457 | 457 | 456 |
| 0.5 | *** | 57282 | 63107 | 101082 | 17666 | 19757 | 25291 | 3632 | 3816 | 4057 | 982 | 1007 | 1016 | 441 | 457 | 457 |
| | *** | 59432 | 70782 | 105054 | 18532 | 21657 | 26248 | 3716 | 3932 | 4182 | 991 | 1007 | 1030 | 441 | 457 | 446 |
| 0.55 | *** | 53916 | 60566 | 100866 | 17182 | 19391 | 25182 | 3566 | 3757 | 4016 | 966 | 982 | 991 | 432 | 432 | 441 |
| | *** | 56416 | 68916 | 103793 | 18107 | 21382 | 25880 | 3657 | 3882 | 4098 | 966 | 991 | 999 | 432 | 441 | 428 |
| 0.6 | *** | 49916 | 57216 | 98366 | 16416 | 18691 | 24507 | 3441 | 3632 | 3882 | 916 | 932 | 957 | 407 | 407 | 416 |
| | *** | 52707 | 65991 | 100430 | 17366 | 20691 | 24987 | 3532 | 3741 | 3930 | 932 | 941 | 946 | 407 | 416 | 400 |
| 0.65 | *** | 44516 | 53207 | 93582 | 15416 | 17666 | 23257 | 3241 | 3416 | 3657 | 857 | 866 | 882 | 366 | 382 | 382 |
| | *** | 48507 | 62107 | 94967 | 16366 | 19616 | 23569 | 3316 | 3532 | 3678 | 857 | 882 | 873 | 382 | 382 | 362 |
| 0.7 | *** | 40866 | 48616 | 86532 | 14207 | 16332 | 21432 | 2966 | 3132 | 3332 | 766 | 782 | 791 | 332 | 332 | 332 |
| | *** | 43916 | 57316 | 87401 | 15107 | 18157 | 21625 | 3041 | 3216 | 3342 | 766 | 782 | 778 | 332 | 332 | 316 |
| 0.75 | *** | 36032 | 43491 | 77241 | 12757 | 14682 | 19057 | 2632 | 2757 | 2932 | 657 | 666 | 682 | 282 | 282 | 282 |
| | *** | 39007 | 51607 | 77734 | 13582 | 16282 | 19156 | 2691 | 2841 | 2922 | 666 | 682 | 662 | 282 | 282 | 260 |
| 0.8 | *** | 30982 | 37757 | 65732 | 11041 | 12666 | 16116 | 2207 | 2307 | 2432 | 532 | 541 | 541 | 216 | 216 | 216 |
| | *** | 33707 | 44891 | 65966 | 11741 | 13982 | 16161 | 2257 | 2366 | 2417 | 532 | 541 | 526 | 216 | 216 | 194 |
| 0.85 | *** | 25541 | 31232 | 52007 | 9032 | 10257 | 12641 | 1707 | 1766 | 1841 | 382 | 382 | 391 | . | . | . |
| | *** | 27857 | 36966 | 52096 | 9566 | 11207 | 12641 | 1741 | 1807 | 1829 | 382 | 382 | 368 | . | . | . |
| 0.9 | *** | 19366 | 23491 | 36116 | 6582 | 7341 | 8607 | 1116 | 1141 | 1182 | . | . | . | . | . | . |
| | *** | 21082 | 27391 | 36125 | 6916 | 7882 | 8596 | 1132 | 1157 | 1156 | . | . | . | . | . | . |
| 0.95 | *** | 11607 | 13607 | 18066 | 3457 | 3707 | 4041 | . | . | . | . | . | . | . | . | . |
| | *** | 12457 | 15241 | 18052 | 3582 | 3866 | 4025 | . | . | . | . | . | . | . | . | . |
| 0.98 | *** | 4991 | 5482 | 6216 | . | . | . | . | . | . | . | . | . | . | . | . |
| | *** | 5207 | 5807 | 6200 | . | . | . | . | . | . | . | . | . | . | . | . |

## TABLE 6: ALPHA= 0.025 POWER= 0.9   EXPECTED ACCRUAL THRU MINIMUM FOLLOW-UP= 11000

| | | DEL=.01 | | | DEL=.02 | | | DEL=.05 | | | DEL=.10 | | | DEL=.15 | | |
|---|---|---|---|---|---|---|---|---|---|---|---|---|---|---|---|---|
| | FACT= | 1.0 .75 | .50 .25 | .00 BIN | 1.0 .75 | .50 .25 | .00 BIN | 1.0 .75 | .50 .25 | .00 BIN | 1.0 75 | .50 .25 | .00 BIN | 1.0 .75 | .50 .25 | .00 BIN |
| PCONT=*** | | | | REQUIRED NUMBER OF PATIENTS | | | | | | | | | | | | |
| 0.01 | *** | 1613 | 1613 | 1613 | 595 | 595 | 595 | 200 | 200 | 200 | 100 | 100 | 100 | 73 | 73 | 73 |
| | *** | 1613 | 1613 | 6200 | 595 | 595 | 2049 | 200 | 200 | 558 | 100 | 100 | 227 | 73 | 73 | 135 |
| 0.02 | *** | 3582 | 3593 | 3620 | 1145 | 1145 | 1162 | 310 | 310 | 310 | 128 | 128 | 128 | 90 | 90 | 90 |
| | *** | 3582 | 3610 | 10235 | 1145 | 1145 | 3048 | 310 | 310 | 712 | 128 | 128 | 264 | 90 | 90 | 151 |
| 0.05 | *** | 10870 | 10990 | 11293 | 3098 | 3125 | 3170 | 667 | 667 | 667 | 238 | 238 | 238 | 145 | 145 | 145 |
| | *** | 10925 | 11100 | 21835 | 3115 | 3142 | 5916 | 667 | 667 | 1156 | 238 | 238 | 368 | 145 | 145 | 194 |
| 0.1 | *** | 24042 | 24482 | 26297 | 6590 | 6728 | 6948 | 1272 | 1283 | 1300 | 392 | 392 | 403 | 210 | 210 | 210 |
| | *** | 24207 | 25015 | 39487 | 6645 | 6827 | 10277 | 1283 | 1283 | 1829 | 392 | 392 | 526 | 210 | 210 | 260 |
| 0.15 | *** | 36015 | 36840 | 41532 | 9808 | 10127 | 10760 | 1850 | 1860 | 1888 | 540 | 540 | 540 | 265 | 282 | 282 |
| | *** | 36307 | 38023 | 55038 | 9945 | 10385 | 14112 | 1860 | 1877 | 2417 | 540 | 540 | 662 | 265 | 282 | 316 |
| 0.2 | *** | 45795 | 47115 | 55805 | 12520 | 13080 | 14290 | 2345 | 2400 | 2455 | 667 | 678 | 678 | 320 | 320 | 337 |
| | *** | 46245 | 49078 | 68488 | 12750 | 13548 | 17422 | 2372 | 2427 | 2922 | 667 | 678 | 778 | 320 | 337 | 362 |
| 0.25 | *** | 53093 | 55007 | 68510 | 14665 | 15500 | 17425 | 2768 | 2840 | 2933 | 777 | 777 | 788 | 375 | 375 | 375 |
| | *** | 53753 | 57895 | 79836 | 15005 | 16215 | 20206 | 2812 | 2878 | 3342 | 777 | 788 | 873 | 375 | 375 | 400 |
| 0.3 | *** | 57960 | 60573 | 79328 | 16260 | 17370 | 20082 | 3115 | 3208 | 3335 | 860 | 870 | 887 | 403 | 403 | 420 |
| | *** | 58868 | 64450 | 89082 | 16710 | 18360 | 22465 | 3153 | 3263 | 3678 | 870 | 870 | 946 | 403 | 403 | 428 |
| 0.35 | *** | 60573 | 63983 | 88090 | 17315 | 18718 | 22210 | 3373 | 3500 | 3648 | 925 | 942 | 953 | 430 | 430 | 430 |
| | *** | 61783 | 68922 | 96227 | 17910 | 19972 | 24199 | 3428 | 3565 | 3930 | 925 | 942 | 999 | 430 | 430 | 446 |
| 0.4 | *** | 61233 | 65523 | 94662 | 17920 | 19587 | 23805 | 3538 | 3692 | 3868 | 970 | 980 | 997 | 447 | 447 | 458 |
| | *** | 62762 | 71507 | 101271 | 18625 | 21083 | 25407 | 3610 | 3775 | 4098 | 970 | 980 | 1030 | 447 | 447 | 456 |
| 0.45 | *** | 60232 | 65457 | 99007 | 18113 | 20010 | 24840 | 3637 | 3802 | 4005 | 980 | 1008 | 1025 | 447 | 458 | 458 |
| | *** | 62140 | 72425 | 104213 | 18910 | 21705 | 26090 | 3720 | 3895 | 4182 | 997 | 1008 | 1041 | 458 | 458 | 456 |
| 0.5 | *** | 57950 | 64082 | 101080 | 17948 | 20038 | 25290 | 3665 | 3830 | 4060 | 980 | 997 | 1025 | 447 | 447 | 458 |
| | *** | 60232 | 71920 | 105054 | 18828 | 21880 | 26248 | 3730 | 3940 | 4182 | 997 | 1008 | 1030 | 447 | 447 | 446 |
| 0.55 | *** | 54705 | 61645 | 100860 | 17480 | 19680 | 25180 | 3593 | 3775 | 4022 | 970 | 980 | 997 | 430 | 430 | 447 |
| | *** | 57328 | 70132 | 103793 | 18405 | 21622 | 25880 | 3692 | 3885 | 4098 | 970 | 980 | 999 | 430 | 430 | 428 |
| 0.6 | *** | 50800 | 58362 | 98358 | 16738 | 18982 | 24510 | 3472 | 3648 | 3885 | 925 | 942 | 953 | 403 | 403 | 420 |
| | *** | 53715 | 67255 | 100430 | 17690 | 20935 | 24987 | 3555 | 3758 | 3930 | 925 | 942 | 946 | 403 | 420 | 400 |
| 0.65 | *** | 46465 | 54375 | 93590 | 15737 | 17965 | 23255 | 3263 | 3428 | 3648 | 860 | 870 | 887 | 375 | 375 | 375 |
| | *** | 49562 | 63367 | 94967 | 16683 | 19862 | 23569 | 3345 | 3538 | 3678 | 860 | 870 | 873 | 375 | 375 | 362 |
| 0.7 | *** | 41845 | 49782 | 86533 | 14500 | 16600 | 21430 | 3005 | 3142 | 3335 | 777 | 777 | 788 | 337 | 337 | 337 |
| | *** | 44980 | 58527 | 87401 | 15407 | 18360 | 21625 | 3070 | 3235 | 3342 | 777 | 788 | 778 | 337 | 337 | 316 |
| 0.75 | *** | 36995 | 44595 | 77238 | 13025 | 14923 | 19048 | 2647 | 2768 | 2922 | 667 | 667 | 678 | 282 | 282 | 282 |
| | *** | 40030 | 52725 | 77734 | 13840 | 16463 | 19156 | 2713 | 2840 | 2922 | 667 | 678 | 662 | 282 | 282 | 260 |
| 0.8 | *** | 31863 | 38738 | 65732 | 11282 | 12877 | 16122 | 2235 | 2317 | 2427 | 530 | 540 | 540 | 210 | 210 | 210 |
| | *** | 34640 | 45860 | 65966 | 11970 | 14125 | 16161 | 2273 | 2372 | 2417 | 540 | 540 | 526 | 210 | 210 | 194 |
| 0.85 | *** | 26297 | 32028 | 52010 | 9203 | 10413 | 12640 | 1723 | 1778 | 1850 | 375 | 392 | 392 | . | . | . |
| | *** | 28635 | 37720 | 52096 | 9742 | 11310 | 12641 | 1750 | 1805 | 1829 | 375 | 392 | 368 | . | . | . |
| 0.9 | *** | 19928 | 24053 | 36115 | 6700 | 7432 | 8615 | 1118 | 1145 | 1173 | . | . | . | . | . | . |
| | *** | 21650 | 27892 | 36125 | 7030 | 7927 | 8596 | 1135 | 1162 | 1156 | . | . | . | . | . | . |
| 0.95 | *** | 11887 | 13850 | 18075 | 3500 | 3730 | 4050 | . | . | . | . | . | . | . | . | . |
| | *** | 12740 | 15435 | 18052 | 3610 | 3885 | 4025 | . | . | . | . | . | . | . | . | . |
| 0.98 | *** | 5067 | 5535 | 6222 | . | . | . | . | . | . | . | . | . | . | . | . |
| | *** | 5270 | 5837 | 6200 | . | . | . | . | . | . | . | . | . | . | . | . |

TABLE 6: ALPHA= 0.025 POWER= 0.9    EXPECTED ACCRUAL THRU MINIMUM FOLLOW-UP= 12000

| | | DEL=.01 | | | DEL=.02 | | | DEL=.05 | | | DEL=.10 | | | DEL=.15 | | |
|---|---|---|---|---|---|---|---|---|---|---|---|---|---|---|---|---|---|
| FACT= | | 1.0 .75 | .50 .25 | .00 BIN | 1.0 .75 | .50 .25 | .00 BIN | 1.0 .75 | .50 .25 | .00 BIN | 1.0 75 | .50 .25 | .00 BIN | 1.0 .75 | .50 .25 | .00 BIN |
| PCONT=*** | | | | | REQUIRED NUMBER OF PATIENTS | | | | | | | | | | | |
| 0.01 | *** | 1609 | 1609 | 1628 | 589 | 589 | 589 | 199 | 199 | 199 | 98 | 98 | 98 | 68 | 68 | 68 |
| | *** | 1609 | 1609 | 6200 | 589 | 589 | 2049 | 199 | 199 | 558 | 98 | 98 | 227 | 68 | 68 | 135 |
| 0.02 | *** | 3578 | 3589 | 3619 | 1148 | 1148 | 1159 | 308 | 308 | 308 | 139 | 139 | 139 | 79 | 79 | 79 |
| | *** | 3589 | 3608 | 10235 | 1148 | 1148 | 3048 | 308 | 308 | 712 | 139 | 139 | 264 | 79 | 79 | 151 |
| 0.05 | *** | 10879 | 11018 | 11299 | 3109 | 3128 | 3158 | 668 | 668 | 668 | 229 | 229 | 229 | 139 | 139 | 139 |
| | *** | 10939 | 11119 | 21835 | 3109 | 3139 | 5916 | 668 | 668 | 1156 | 229 | 229 | 368 | 139 | 139 | 194 |
| 0.1 | *** | 24079 | 24548 | 26288 | 6608 | 6739 | 6949 | 1279 | 1279 | 1298 | 398 | 398 | 398 | 218 | 218 | 218 |
| | *** | 24259 | 25088 | 39487 | 6668 | 6829 | 10277 | 1279 | 1279 | 1829 | 398 | 398 | 526 | 218 | 218 | 260 |
| 0.15 | *** | 36098 | 36979 | 41528 | 9848 | 10159 | 10748 | 1849 | 1868 | 1898 | 548 | 548 | 548 | 278 | 278 | 278 |
| | *** | 36409 | 38179 | 55038 | 9979 | 10399 | 14112 | 1868 | 1879 | 2417 | 548 | 548 | 662 | 278 | 278 | 316 |
| 0.2 | *** | 45919 | 47329 | 55808 | 12589 | 13148 | 14288 | 2359 | 2389 | 2449 | 668 | 668 | 679 | 319 | 338 | 338 |
| | *** | 46418 | 49358 | 68488 | 12829 | 13598 | 17422 | 2378 | 2419 | 2922 | 668 | 679 | 778 | 319 | 338 | 362 |
| 0.25 | *** | 53269 | 55328 | 68509 | 14768 | 15589 | 17419 | 2779 | 2858 | 2929 | 769 | 788 | 788 | 368 | 379 | 379 |
| | *** | 53989 | 58298 | 79836 | 15109 | 16298 | 20206 | 2809 | 2888 | 3342 | 788 | 788 | 873 | 368 | 379 | 400 |
| 0.3 | *** | 58208 | 60998 | 79328 | 16388 | 17509 | 20078 | 3128 | 3218 | 3338 | 859 | 878 | 878 | 409 | 409 | 409 |
| | *** | 59198 | 64999 | 89082 | 16868 | 18469 | 22465 | 3169 | 3278 | 3678 | 859 | 878 | 946 | 409 | 409 | 428 |
| 0.35 | *** | 60908 | 64538 | 88088 | 17498 | 18889 | 22219 | 3398 | 3499 | 3649 | 919 | 938 | 949 | 428 | 439 | 439 |
| | *** | 62209 | 69608 | 96227 | 18079 | 20108 | 24199 | 3439 | 3578 | 3930 | 938 | 938 | 999 | 439 | 439 | 446 |
| 0.4 | *** | 61658 | 66199 | 94669 | 18128 | 19789 | 23809 | 3559 | 3698 | 3878 | 968 | 979 | 998 | 439 | 458 | 458 |
| | *** | 63308 | 72319 | 101271 | 18829 | 21248 | 25407 | 3638 | 3788 | 4098 | 979 | 979 | 1030 | 458 | 458 | 456 |
| 0.45 | *** | 60769 | 66259 | 99008 | 18349 | 20239 | 24829 | 3668 | 3818 | 4009 | 998 | 1009 | 1009 | 458 | 458 | 458 |
| | *** | 62798 | 73369 | 104213 | 19148 | 21889 | 26090 | 3739 | 3908 | 4182 | 998 | 1009 | 1041 | 458 | 458 | 456 |
| 0.5 | *** | 58598 | 64988 | 101078 | 18218 | 20288 | 25298 | 3679 | 3848 | 4058 | 998 | 998 | 1009 | 439 | 458 | 458 |
| | *** | 60998 | 72949 | 105054 | 19088 | 22088 | 26248 | 3758 | 3949 | 4182 | 998 | 1009 | 1030 | 458 | 458 | 446 |
| 0.55 | *** | 55459 | 62648 | 100868 | 17768 | 19939 | 25189 | 3619 | 3799 | 4009 | 968 | 979 | 998 | 428 | 439 | 439 |
| | *** | 58208 | 71258 | 103793 | 18679 | 21829 | 25880 | 3709 | 3889 | 4098 | 979 | 979 | 999 | 439 | 439 | 428 |
| 0.6 | *** | 51638 | 59419 | 98359 | 17018 | 19249 | 24499 | 3499 | 3668 | 3878 | 919 | 938 | 949 | 409 | 409 | 409 |
| | *** | 54668 | 68408 | 100430 | 17978 | 21158 | 24987 | 3578 | 3758 | 3930 | 938 | 938 | 946 | 409 | 409 | 400 |
| 0.65 | *** | 47378 | 55459 | 93578 | 16028 | 18218 | 23258 | 3289 | 3458 | 3649 | 859 | 878 | 878 | 368 | 379 | 379 |
| | *** | 50558 | 64519 | 94967 | 16958 | 20059 | 23569 | 3368 | 3548 | 3678 | 859 | 878 | 873 | 379 | 379 | 362 |
| 0.7 | *** | 42769 | 50858 | 86539 | 14779 | 16849 | 21439 | 3019 | 3158 | 3338 | 769 | 788 | 788 | 338 | 338 | 338 |
| | *** | 45979 | 59629 | 87401 | 15668 | 18559 | 21625 | 3079 | 3248 | 3342 | 769 | 788 | 778 | 338 | 338 | 316 |
| 0.75 | *** | 37898 | 45608 | 77239 | 13279 | 15139 | 19058 | 2678 | 2779 | 2929 | 668 | 668 | 679 | 278 | 278 | 278 |
| | *** | 40988 | 53738 | 77734 | 14078 | 16628 | 19156 | 2719 | 2858 | 2922 | 668 | 679 | 662 | 278 | 278 | 260 |
| 0.8 | *** | 32689 | 39638 | 65719 | 11498 | 13058 | 16118 | 2239 | 2329 | 2438 | 529 | 529 | 548 | 218 | 218 | 218 |
| | *** | 35498 | 46729 | 65966 | 12169 | 14258 | 16161 | 2288 | 2378 | 2417 | 529 | 548 | 526 | 218 | 218 | 194 |
| 0.85 | *** | 26989 | 32749 | 52009 | 9379 | 10538 | 12638 | 1729 | 1789 | 1849 | 379 | 379 | 379 | . | . | . |
| | *** | 29359 | 38389 | 52096 | 9889 | 11389 | 12641 | 1759 | 1808 | 1829 | 379 | 379 | 368 | . | . | . |
| 0.9 | *** | 20449 | 24559 | 36109 | 6799 | 7508 | 8599 | 1129 | 1148 | 1178 | . | . | . | . | . | . |
| | *** | 22159 | 28328 | 36125 | 7118 | 7988 | 8596 | 1129 | 1159 | 1156 | . | . | . | . | . | . |
| 0.95 | *** | 12158 | 14078 | 18068 | 3529 | 3758 | 4039 | . | . | . | . | . | . | . | . | . |
| | *** | 12979 | 15608 | 18052 | 3638 | 3889 | 4025 | . | . | . | . | . | . | . | . | . |
| 0.98 | *** | 5138 | 5569 | 6218 | . | . | . | . | . | . | . | . | . | . | . | . |
| | *** | 5329 | 5869 | 6200 | . | . | . | . | . | . | . | . | . | . | . | . |

## TABLE 6: ALPHA= 0.025 POWER= 0.9    EXPECTED ACCRUAL THRU MINIMUM FOLLOW-UP= 13000

| | | DEL=.01 | | | DEL=.02 | | | DEL=.05 | | | DEL=.10 | | | DEL=.15 | | |
|---|---|---|---|---|---|---|---|---|---|---|---|---|---|---|---|---|
| FACT= | | 1.0 .75 | .50 .25 | .00 BIN | 1.0 .75 | .50 .25 | .00 BIN | 1.0 .75 | .50 .25 | .00 BIN | 1.0 75 | .50 .25 | .00 BIN | 1.0 .75 | .50 .25 | .00 BIN |
| PCONT=*** | | | | | REQUIRED NUMBER OF PATIENTS | | | | | | | | | | | |
| 0.01 | *** | 1613 | 1613 | 1613 | 594 | 594 | 594 | 204 | 204 | 204 | 106 | 106 | 106 | 74 | 74 | 74 |
| | *** | 1613 | 1613 | 6200 | 594 | 594 | 2049 | 204 | 204 | 558 | 106 | 106 | 227 | 74 | 74 | 135 |
| 0.02 | *** | 3584 | 3596 | 3616 | 1146 | 1146 | 1158 | 313 | 313 | 313 | 139 | 139 | 139 | 86 | 86 | 86 |
| | *** | 3584 | 3596 | 10235 | 1146 | 1158 | 3048 | 313 | 313 | 712 | 139 | 139 | 264 | 86 | 86 | 151 |
| 0.05 | *** | 10896 | 11026 | 11298 | 3108 | 3129 | 3161 | 671 | 671 | 671 | 236 | 236 | 236 | 139 | 139 | 139 |
| | *** | 10941 | 11124 | 21835 | 3129 | 3141 | 5916 | 671 | 671 | 1156 | 236 | 236 | 368 | 139 | 139 | 194 |
| 0.1 | *** | 24136 | 24591 | 26281 | 6618 | 6748 | 6943 | 1276 | 1288 | 1288 | 399 | 399 | 399 | 204 | 216 | 216 |
| | *** | 24298 | 25143 | 39487 | 6683 | 6846 | 10277 | 1276 | 1288 | 1829 | 399 | 399 | 526 | 204 | 216 | 260 |
| 0.15 | *** | 36181 | 37103 | 41523 | 9889 | 10193 | 10746 | 1861 | 1873 | 1894 | 541 | 541 | 541 | 269 | 269 | 269 |
| | *** | 36506 | 38326 | 55038 | 10019 | 10421 | 14112 | 1861 | 1894 | 2417 | 541 | 541 | 662 | 269 | 269 | 316 |
| 0.2 | *** | 46041 | 47536 | 55791 | 12651 | 13204 | 14288 | 2361 | 2393 | 2446 | 671 | 671 | 671 | 334 | 334 | 334 |
| | *** | 46581 | 49604 | 68488 | 12891 | 13638 | 17422 | 2381 | 2426 | 2922 | 671 | 671 | 778 | 334 | 334 | 362 |
| 0.25 | *** | 53451 | 55628 | 68498 | 14861 | 15686 | 17429 | 2804 | 2848 | 2934 | 768 | 789 | 789 | 378 | 378 | 378 |
| | *** | 54231 | 58671 | 79836 | 15219 | 16356 | 20206 | 2816 | 2881 | 3342 | 789 | 789 | 873 | 378 | 378 | 400 |
| 0.3 | *** | 58456 | 61413 | 79321 | 16519 | 17624 | 20073 | 3141 | 3226 | 3324 | 866 | 866 | 886 | 411 | 411 | 411 |
| | *** | 59516 | 65496 | 89082 | 16986 | 18566 | 22465 | 3173 | 3271 | 3678 | 866 | 866 | 946 | 411 | 411 | 428 |
| 0.35 | *** | 61239 | 65074 | 88084 | 17656 | 19054 | 22218 | 3401 | 3519 | 3649 | 931 | 931 | 951 | 431 | 431 | 443 |
| | *** | 62616 | 70241 | 96227 | 18241 | 20224 | 24199 | 3454 | 3584 | 3930 | 931 | 951 | 999 | 431 | 431 | 446 |
| 0.4 | *** | 62084 | 66841 | 94661 | 18318 | 19976 | 23811 | 3584 | 3714 | 3876 | 963 | 984 | 996 | 443 | 443 | 443 |
| | *** | 63818 | 73081 | 101271 | 19021 | 21394 | 25407 | 3649 | 3791 | 4098 | 984 | 984 | 1030 | 443 | 443 | 456 |
| 0.45 | *** | 61304 | 67003 | 99004 | 18578 | 20451 | 24839 | 3681 | 3823 | 4006 | 996 | 996 | 1016 | 443 | 464 | 464 |
| | *** | 63416 | 74251 | 104213 | 19379 | 22056 | 26090 | 3758 | 3921 | 4182 | 996 | 1016 | 1041 | 464 | 464 | 456 |
| 0.5 | *** | 59224 | 65854 | 101084 | 18469 | 20516 | 25294 | 3714 | 3856 | 4051 | 996 | 996 | 1016 | 443 | 443 | 464 |
| | *** | 61726 | 73926 | 105054 | 19326 | 22251 | 26248 | 3779 | 3953 | 4182 | 996 | 1016 | 1030 | 443 | 443 | 446 |
| 0.55 | *** | 56181 | 63591 | 100868 | 18014 | 20191 | 25176 | 3649 | 3811 | 4018 | 963 | 984 | 996 | 431 | 431 | 443 |
| | *** | 59029 | 72289 | 103793 | 18936 | 22011 | 25880 | 3726 | 3909 | 4098 | 984 | 984 | 999 | 431 | 443 | 428 |
| 0.6 | *** | 52443 | 60426 | 98366 | 17278 | 19488 | 24493 | 3519 | 3681 | 3876 | 919 | 931 | 951 | 411 | 411 | 411 |
| | *** | 55551 | 69461 | 100430 | 18221 | 21341 | 24987 | 3596 | 3779 | 3930 | 931 | 951 | 946 | 411 | 411 | 400 |
| 0.65 | *** | 48218 | 56494 | 93576 | 16291 | 18448 | 23246 | 3324 | 3466 | 3649 | 854 | 866 | 886 | 378 | 378 | 378 |
| | *** | 51489 | 65573 | 94967 | 17213 | 20236 | 23569 | 3389 | 3551 | 3678 | 866 | 886 | 873 | 378 | 378 | 362 |
| 0.7 | *** | 43636 | 51858 | 86536 | 15024 | 17071 | 21438 | 3043 | 3173 | 3336 | 768 | 789 | 789 | 334 | 334 | 334 |
| | *** | 46918 | 60633 | 87401 | 15913 | 18729 | 21625 | 3096 | 3238 | 3342 | 768 | 789 | 778 | 334 | 334 | 316 |
| 0.75 | *** | 38728 | 46528 | 77241 | 13508 | 15328 | 19054 | 2686 | 2804 | 2934 | 659 | 671 | 671 | 281 | 281 | 281 |
| | *** | 41881 | 54653 | 77734 | 14288 | 16779 | 19156 | 2739 | 2848 | 2922 | 671 | 671 | 662 | 281 | 281 | 260 |
| 0.8 | *** | 33451 | 40451 | 65724 | 11688 | 13216 | 16129 | 2251 | 2328 | 2426 | 529 | 541 | 541 | 216 | 216 | 216 |
| | *** | 36311 | 47524 | 65966 | 12359 | 14374 | 16161 | 2296 | 2381 | 2417 | 541 | 541 | 526 | 216 | 216 | 194 |
| 0.85 | *** | 27646 | 33431 | 52009 | 9531 | 10648 | 12631 | 1743 | 1796 | 1841 | 378 | 378 | 378 | . | . | . |
| | *** | 30018 | 39009 | 52096 | 10031 | 11481 | 12641 | 1764 | 1808 | 1829 | 378 | 378 | 368 | . | . | . |
| 0.9 | *** | 20918 | 25013 | 36116 | 6899 | 7561 | 8601 | 1126 | 1146 | 1179 | . | . | . | . | . | . |
| | *** | 22641 | 28718 | 36125 | 7203 | 8016 | 8596 | 1146 | 1158 | 1156 | . | . | . | . | . | . |
| 0.95 | *** | 12391 | 14276 | 18058 | 3563 | 3779 | 4039 | . | . | . | . | . | . | . | . | . |
| | *** | 13204 | 15751 | 18052 | 3661 | 3909 | 4025 | . | . | . | . | . | . | . | . | . |
| 0.98 | *** | 5188 | 5611 | 6216 | . | . | . | . | . | . | . | . | . | . | . | . |
| | *** | 5383 | 5891 | 6200 | . | . | . | . | . | . | . | . | . | . | . | . |

TABLE 6: ALPHA= 0.025 POWER= 0.9     EXPECTED ACCRUAL THRU MINIMUM FOLLOW-UP= 14000

| PCONT= | FACT= | DEL=.01 1.0/.75 | .50/.25 | .00 BIN | DEL=.02 1.0/.75 | .50/.25 | .00 BIN | DEL=.05 1.0/.75 | .50/.25 | .00 BIN | DEL=.10 1.0/75 | .50/.25 | .00 BIN | DEL=.15 1.0/.75 | .50/.25 | .00 BIN |
|---|---|---|---|---|---|---|---|---|---|---|---|---|---|---|---|---|
| | | | | | | | REQUIRED NUMBER OF PATIENTS | | | | | | | | |
| 0.01 | *** | 1619 | 1619 | 1619 | 582 | 582 | 582 | 197 | 197 | 197 | 92 | 92 | 92 | 57 | 57 | 57 |
| | *** | 1619 | 1619 | 6200 | 582 | 582 | 2049 | 197 | 197 | 558 | 92 | 92 | 227 | 57 | 57 | 135 |
| 0.02 | *** | 3579 | 3592 | 3614 | 1142 | 1142 | 1164 | 302 | 302 | 302 | 127 | 127 | 127 | 92 | 92 | 92 |
| | *** | 3592 | 3614 | 10235 | 1142 | 1142 | 3048 | 302 | 302 | 712 | 127 | 127 | 264 | 92 | 92 | 151 |
| 0.05 | *** | 10907 | 11034 | 11292 | 3102 | 3137 | 3159 | 674 | 674 | 674 | 232 | 232 | 232 | 127 | 127 | 127 |
| | *** | 10964 | 11139 | 21835 | 3124 | 3159 | 5916 | 674 | 674 | 1156 | 232 | 232 | 368 | 127 | 127 | 194 |
| 0.1 | *** | 24172 | 24662 | 26294 | 6637 | 6764 | 6952 | 1282 | 1282 | 1282 | 394 | 394 | 394 | 219 | 219 | 219 |
| | *** | 24347 | 25187 | 39487 | 6694 | 6847 | 10277 | 1282 | 1282 | 1829 | 394 | 394 | 526 | 219 | 219 | 260 |
| 0.15 | *** | 36247 | 37227 | 41532 | 9927 | 10229 | 10754 | 1864 | 1877 | 1899 | 547 | 547 | 547 | 267 | 267 | 267 |
| | *** | 36619 | 38452 | 55038 | 10054 | 10452 | 14112 | 1864 | 1877 | 2417 | 547 | 547 | 662 | 267 | 267 | 316 |
| 0.2 | *** | 46174 | 47749 | 55799 | 12714 | 13252 | 14289 | 2367 | 2402 | 2437 | 674 | 674 | 674 | 324 | 324 | 324 |
| | *** | 46734 | 49849 | 68488 | 12959 | 13672 | 17422 | 2389 | 2424 | 2922 | 674 | 674 | 778 | 324 | 324 | 362 |
| 0.25 | *** | 53642 | 55917 | 68504 | 14954 | 15772 | 17417 | 2809 | 2857 | 2927 | 779 | 779 | 792 | 372 | 372 | 372 |
| | *** | 54469 | 59019 | 79836 | 15304 | 16424 | 20206 | 2822 | 2892 | 3342 | 779 | 792 | 873 | 372 | 372 | 400 |
| 0.3 | *** | 58704 | 61797 | 79332 | 16647 | 17732 | 20077 | 3159 | 3229 | 3334 | 862 | 862 | 884 | 407 | 407 | 407 |
| | *** | 59824 | 65962 | 89082 | 17102 | 18642 | 22465 | 3194 | 3277 | 3678 | 862 | 884 | 946 | 407 | 407 | 428 |
| 0.35 | *** | 61574 | 65564 | 88082 | 17802 | 19189 | 22212 | 3417 | 3522 | 3649 | 932 | 932 | 954 | 429 | 429 | 442 |
| | *** | 63022 | 70827 | 96227 | 18397 | 20344 | 24199 | 3474 | 3579 | 3930 | 932 | 954 | 999 | 429 | 442 | 446 |
| 0.4 | *** | 62497 | 67454 | 94662 | 18502 | 20147 | 23809 | 3592 | 3719 | 3872 | 967 | 989 | 989 | 442 | 442 | 442 |
| | *** | 64317 | 73789 | 101271 | 19202 | 21512 | 25407 | 3662 | 3789 | 4098 | 967 | 989 | 1030 | 442 | 442 | 456 |
| 0.45 | *** | 61797 | 67734 | 99002 | 18782 | 20637 | 24837 | 3697 | 3837 | 4012 | 989 | 1002 | 1024 | 442 | 464 | 464 |
| | *** | 64024 | 75062 | 104213 | 19574 | 22199 | 26090 | 3767 | 3929 | 4182 | 1002 | 1002 | 1041 | 464 | 464 | 456 |
| 0.5 | *** | 59824 | 66662 | 101089 | 18677 | 20707 | 25292 | 3719 | 3872 | 4069 | 989 | 1002 | 1024 | 442 | 442 | 464 |
| | *** | 62427 | 74817 | 105054 | 19552 | 22422 | 26248 | 3802 | 3964 | 4182 | 1002 | 1002 | 1030 | 442 | 442 | 446 |
| 0.55 | *** | 56884 | 64479 | 100857 | 18257 | 20392 | 25187 | 3662 | 3824 | 4012 | 967 | 989 | 989 | 429 | 442 | 442 |
| | *** | 59824 | 73229 | 103793 | 19167 | 22177 | 25880 | 3754 | 3907 | 4098 | 967 | 989 | 999 | 429 | 442 | 428 |
| 0.6 | *** | 53222 | 61364 | 98359 | 17522 | 19714 | 24509 | 3544 | 3697 | 3872 | 932 | 932 | 954 | 407 | 407 | 407 |
| | *** | 56407 | 70442 | 100430 | 18467 | 21499 | 24987 | 3614 | 3789 | 3930 | 932 | 954 | 946 | 407 | 407 | 400 |
| 0.65 | *** | 49044 | 57444 | 93577 | 16529 | 18664 | 23249 | 3334 | 3474 | 3649 | 862 | 862 | 884 | 372 | 372 | 372 |
| | *** | 52369 | 66544 | 94967 | 17452 | 20392 | 23569 | 3404 | 3557 | 3678 | 862 | 884 | 873 | 372 | 372 | 362 |
| 0.7 | *** | 44459 | 52789 | 86529 | 15247 | 17264 | 21429 | 3054 | 3172 | 3334 | 779 | 779 | 792 | 324 | 337 | 337 |
| | *** | 47797 | 61574 | 87401 | 16122 | 18874 | 21625 | 3124 | 3242 | 3342 | 779 | 792 | 778 | 324 | 337 | 316 |
| 0.75 | *** | 39524 | 47412 | 77254 | 13707 | 15514 | 19049 | 2704 | 2809 | 2927 | 674 | 674 | 674 | 267 | 267 | 267 |
| | *** | 42709 | 55497 | 77734 | 14499 | 16892 | 19156 | 2752 | 2857 | 2922 | 674 | 674 | 662 | 267 | 267 | 260 |
| 0.8 | *** | 34182 | 41217 | 65717 | 11874 | 13357 | 16122 | 2262 | 2332 | 2424 | 534 | 534 | 547 | 219 | 219 | 219 |
| | *** | 37052 | 48239 | 65966 | 12517 | 14477 | 16161 | 2297 | 2389 | 2417 | 534 | 547 | 526 | 219 | 219 | 194 |
| 0.85 | *** | 28254 | 34042 | 52019 | 9647 | 10754 | 12644 | 1737 | 1794 | 1842 | 372 | 394 | 394 | . | . | . |
| | *** | 30647 | 39559 | 52096 | 10159 | 11537 | 12641 | 1772 | 1807 | 1829 | 372 | 394 | 368 | . | . | . |
| 0.9 | *** | 21372 | 25454 | 36107 | 6974 | 7617 | 8597 | 1129 | 1142 | 1177 | . | . | . | . | . | . |
| | *** | 23087 | 29059 | 36125 | 7267 | 8059 | 8596 | 1142 | 1164 | 1156 | . | . | . | . | . | . |
| 0.95 | *** | 12609 | 14442 | 18069 | 3592 | 3789 | 4047 | . | . | . | . | . | . | . | . | . |
| | *** | 13414 | 15877 | 18052 | 3684 | 3907 | 4025 | . | . | . | . | . | . | . | . | . |
| 0.98 | *** | 5237 | 5657 | 6217 | . | . | . | . | . | . | . | . | . | . | . | . |
| | *** | 5434 | 5902 | 6200 | . | . | . | . | . | . | . | . | . | . | . | . |

## TABLE 6: ALPHA= 0.025 POWER= 0.9    EXPECTED ACCRUAL THRU MINIMUM FOLLOW-UP= 15000

PCONT=***                          REQUIRED NUMBER OF PATIENTS

| PCONT | FACT= | DEL=.01 1.0/.75 | DEL=.01 .50/.25 | DEL=.01 .00/BIN | DEL=.02 1.0/.75 | DEL=.02 .50/.25 | DEL=.02 .00/BIN | DEL=.05 1.0/.75 | DEL=.05 .50/.25 | DEL=.05 .00/BIN | DEL=.10 1.0/75 | DEL=.10 .50/.25 | DEL=.10 .00/BIN | DEL=.15 1.0/.75 | DEL=.15 .50/.25 | DEL=.15 .00/BIN |
|---|---|---|---|---|---|---|---|---|---|---|---|---|---|---|---|---|
| 0.01 | *** | 1622 | 1622 | 1622 | 586 | 586 | 586 | 197 | 197 | 197 | 99 | 99 | 99 | 61 | 61 | 61 |
|  | *** | 1622 | 1622 | 6200 | 586 | 586 | 2049 | 197 | 197 | 558 | 99 | 99 | 227 | 61 | 61 | 135 |
| 0.02 | *** | 3586 | 3586 | 3610 | 1149 | 1149 | 1149 | 310 | 310 | 310 | 136 | 136 | 136 | 85 | 85 | 85 |
|  | *** | 3586 | 3610 | 10235 | 1149 | 1149 | 3048 | 310 | 310 | 712 | 136 | 136 | 264 | 85 | 85 | 151 |
| 0.05 | *** | 10922 | 11049 | 11297 | 3122 | 3136 | 3160 | 661 | 661 | 661 | 235 | 235 | 235 | 136 | 136 | 136 |
|  | *** | 10974 | 11147 | 21835 | 3122 | 3160 | 5916 | 661 | 661 | 1156 | 235 | 235 | 368 | 136 | 136 | 194 |
| 0.1 | *** | 24211 | 24722 | 26297 | 6661 | 6774 | 6947 | 1285 | 1285 | 1299 | 399 | 399 | 399 | 211 | 211 | 211 |
|  | *** | 24399 | 25247 | 39487 | 6699 | 6849 | 10277 | 1285 | 1285 | 1829 | 399 | 399 | 526 | 211 | 211 | 260 |
| 0.15 | *** | 36324 | 37336 | 41536 | 9961 | 10247 | 10749 | 1861 | 1885 | 1899 | 535 | 549 | 549 | 272 | 272 | 272 |
|  | *** | 36699 | 38574 | 55038 | 10097 | 10472 | 14112 | 1861 | 1885 | 2417 | 549 | 549 | 662 | 272 | 272 | 316 |
| 0.2 | *** | 46285 | 47935 | 55810 | 12774 | 13299 | 14297 | 2372 | 2410 | 2447 | 661 | 685 | 685 | 324 | 324 | 324 |
|  | *** | 46885 | 50049 |  | 12999 | 13711 | 17422 | 2386 | 2424 | 2922 | 661 | 685 | 778 | 324 | 324 | 362 |
| 0.25 | *** | 53822 | 56199 | 68499 | 15047 | 15835 | 17424 | 2799 | 2860 | 2935 | 774 | 774 | 797 | 361 | 385 | 385 |
|  | *** | 54685 | 59335 | 79836 | 15385 | 16472 | 20206 | 2836 | 2897 | 3342 | 774 | 797 | 873 | 385 | 385 | 400 |
| 0.3 | *** | 58960 | 62185 | 79322 | 16749 | 17836 | 20072 | 3160 | 3235 | 3324 | 872 | 872 | 872 | 399 | 399 | 422 |
|  | *** | 60136 | 66399 | 89082 | 17222 | 18722 | 22465 | 3197 | 3286 | 3678 | 872 | 872 | 946 | 399 | 399 | 428 |
| 0.35 | *** | 61885 | 66047 | 88074 | 17949 | 19322 | 22210 | 3436 | 3535 | 3647 | 924 | 947 | 947 | 436 | 436 | 436 |
|  | *** | 63422 | 71386 | 96227 | 18535 | 20424 | 24199 | 3474 | 3586 | 3930 | 924 | 947 | 999 | 436 | 436 | 446 |
| 0.4 | *** | 62897 | 68035 | 94660 | 18661 | 20297 | 23799 | 3624 | 3736 | 3872 | 985 | 985 | 999 | 460 | 460 | 460 |
|  | *** | 64810 | 74461 | 101271 | 19360 | 21624 | 25407 | 3661 | 3797 | 4098 | 985 | 985 | 1030 | 460 | 460 | 456 |
| 0.45 | *** | 62297 | 68424 | 99010 | 18961 | 20822 | 24835 | 3722 | 3849 | 4022 | 999 | 999 | 1022 | 460 | 460 | 460 |
|  | *** | 64622 | 75811 | 104213 | 19749 | 22336 | 26090 | 3774 | 3924 | 4182 | 999 | 1022 | 1041 | 460 | 460 | 456 |
| 0.5 | *** | 60422 | 67435 | 101072 | 18886 | 20911 | 25299 | 3736 | 3886 | 4060 | 999 | 999 | 1022 | 460 | 460 | 460 |
|  | *** | 63099 | 75647 | 105054 | 19749 | 22561 | 26248 | 3811 | 3961 | 4182 | 999 | 1022 | 1030 | 460 | 460 | 446 |
| 0.55 | *** | 57549 | 65311 | 100861 | 18474 | 20597 | 25186 | 3685 | 3835 | 4022 | 961 | 985 | 999 | 436 | 436 | 436 |
|  | *** | 60572 | 74110 | 103793 | 19397 | 22322 | 25880 | 3760 | 3924 | 4098 | 985 | 985 | 999 | 436 | 436 | 428 |
| 0.6 | *** | 53949 | 62236 | 98372 | 17761 | 19922 | 24497 | 3549 | 3699 | 3872 | 924 | 947 | 947 | 399 | 422 | 422 |
|  | *** | 57211 | 71349 | 100430 | 18685 | 21661 | 24987 | 3624 | 3774 | 3930 | 924 | 947 | 946 | 399 | 422 | 400 |
| 0.65 | *** | 49810 | 58322 | 93586 | 16749 | 18872 | 23260 | 3347 | 3497 | 3647 | 872 | 872 | 886 | 385 | 385 | 385 |
|  | *** | 53199 | 67435 | 94967 | 17672 | 20536 | 23569 | 3422 | 3572 | 3678 | 872 | 872 | 873 | 385 | 385 | 362 |
| 0.7 | *** | 45235 | 53649 | 86536 | 15474 | 17447 | 21436 | 3061 | 3197 | 3324 | 774 | 774 | 797 | 324 | 324 | 324 |
|  | *** | 48624 | 62424 | 87401 | 16336 | 18999 | 21625 | 3122 | 3249 | 3342 | 774 | 797 | 778 | 324 | 324 | 316 |
| 0.75 | *** | 40285 | 48211 | 77236 | 13899 | 15661 | 19060 | 2710 | 2799 | 2935 | 661 | 661 | 685 | 272 | 272 | 272 |
|  | *** | 43486 | 56274 | 77734 | 14672 | 17011 | 19156 | 2761 | 2860 | 2922 | 661 | 685 | 662 | 272 | 272 | 260 |
| 0.8 | *** | 34861 | 41935 | 65724 | 12024 | 13486 | 16111 | 2274 | 2349 | 2424 | 535 | 535 | 549 | 211 | 211 | 211 |
|  | *** | 37749 | 48886 | 65966 | 12661 | 14560 | 16161 | 2311 | 2386 | 2417 | 535 | 535 | 526 | 211 | 211 | 194 |
| 0.85 | *** | 28824 | 34622 | 51999 | 9774 | 10847 | 12647 | 1749 | 1786 | 1847 | 385 | 385 | 385 | . | . | . |
|  | *** | 31224 | 40074 | 52096 | 10261 | 11611 | 12641 | 1772 | 1824 | 1829 | 385 | 385 | 368 | . | . | . |
| 0.9 | *** | 21774 | 25824 | 36122 | 7060 | 7674 | 8611 | 1135 | 1149 | 1172 | . | . | . | . | . | . |
|  | *** | 23499 | 29386 | 36125 | 7336 | 8086 | 8596 | 1149 | 1172 | 1156 | . | . | . | . | . | . |
| 0.95 | *** | 12797 | 14611 | 18061 | 3624 | 3811 | 4036 | . | . | . | . | . | . | . | . | . |
|  | *** | 13599 | 15999 | 18052 | 3699 | 3924 | 4025 | . | . | . | . | . | . | . | . | . |
| 0.98 | *** | 5297 | 5686 | 6211 | . | . | . | . | . | . | . | . | . | . | . | . |
|  | *** | 5485 | 5935 | 6200 | . | . | . | . | . | . | . | . | . | . | . | . |

TABLE 6: ALPHA= 0.025 POWER= 0.9    EXPECTED ACCRUAL THRU MINIMUM FOLLOW-UP= 17000

| FACT= | DEL=.01 1.0 .75 | .50 .25 | .00 BIN | DEL=.02 1.0 .75 | .50 .25 | .00 BIN | DEL=.05 1.0 .75 | .50 .25 | .00 BIN | DEL=.10 1.0 75 | .50 .25 | .00 BIN | DEL=.15 1.0 .75 | .50 .25 | .00 BIN |
|---|---|---|---|---|---|---|---|---|---|---|---|---|---|---|---|
| PCONT=*** | | | | | | REQUIRED NUMBER OF PATIENTS | | | | | | | | | |
| 0.01 *** | 1626 | 1626 | 1626 | 580 | 580 | 580 | 197 | 197 | 197 | 96 | 96 | 96 | 70 | 70 | 70 |
| *** | 1626 | 1626 | 6200 | 580 | 580 | 2049 | 197 | 197 | 558 | 96 | 96 | 227 | 70 | 70 | 135 |
| 0.02 *** | 3581 | 3597 | 3624 | 1159 | 1159 | 1159 | 309 | 309 | 309 | 139 | 139 | 139 | 96 | 96 | 96 |
| *** | 3597 | 3597 | 10235 | 1159 | 1159 | 3048 | 309 | 309 | 712 | 139 | 139 | 264 | 96 | 96 | 151 |
| 0.05 *** | 10950 | 11061 | 11290 | 3114 | 3130 | 3156 | 665 | 665 | 665 | 240 | 240 | 240 | 139 | 139 | 139 |
| *** | 10992 | 11162 | 21835 | 3130 | 3156 | 5916 | 665 | 665 | 1156 | 240 | 240 | 368 | 139 | 139 | 194 |
| 0.1 *** | 24295 | 24805 | 26292 | 6684 | 6785 | 6955 | 1286 | 1286 | 1286 | 394 | 394 | 394 | 197 | 197 | 197 |
| *** | 24491 | 25341 | 39487 | 6726 | 6870 | 10277 | 1286 | 1286 | 1829 | 394 | 394 | 526 | 197 | 197 | 260 |
| 0.15 *** | 36492 | 37555 | 41534 | 10015 | 10296 | 10764 | 1855 | 1881 | 1897 | 537 | 537 | 537 | 266 | 266 | 266 |
| *** | 36901 | 38787 | 55038 | 10142 | 10482 | 14112 | 1881 | 1881 | 2417 | 537 | 537 | 662 | 266 | 266 | 316 |
| 0.2 *** | 46522 | 48291 | 55787 | 12889 | 13399 | 14291 | 2391 | 2407 | 2450 | 665 | 665 | 665 | 325 | 325 | 325 |
| *** | 47186 | 50432 | 68488 | 13101 | 13755 | 17422 | 2391 | 2434 | 2922 | 665 | 665 | 778 | 325 | 325 | 362 |
| 0.25 *** | 54172 | 56722 | 68495 | 15184 | 15965 | 17410 | 2816 | 2875 | 2917 | 776 | 776 | 792 | 367 | 367 | 367 |
| *** | 55107 | 59910 | 79836 | 15524 | 16560 | 20206 | 2832 | 2901 | 3342 | 776 | 792 | 873 | 367 | 367 | 400 |
| 0.3 *** | 59442 | 62911 | 79332 | 16969 | 18005 | 20071 | 3172 | 3241 | 3326 | 861 | 877 | 877 | 410 | 410 | 410 |
| *** | 60717 | 67204 | 89082 | 17410 | 18839 | 22465 | 3215 | 3284 | 3678 | 877 | 877 | 946 | 410 | 410 | 428 |
| 0.35 *** | 62529 | 66965 | 88087 | 18201 | 19535 | 22212 | 3454 | 3539 | 3640 | 920 | 946 | 946 | 436 | 436 | 436 |
| *** | 64186 | 72389 | 96227 | 18770 | 20597 | 24199 | 3496 | 3597 | 3930 | 946 | 946 | 999 | 436 | 436 | 446 |
| 0.4 *** | 63692 | 69132 | 94659 | 18982 | 20555 | 23811 | 3640 | 3751 | 3879 | 989 | 989 | 989 | 452 | 452 | 452 |
| *** | 65759 | 75661 | 101271 | 19662 | 21830 | 25407 | 3682 | 3810 | 4098 | 989 | 989 | 1030 | 452 | 452 | 456 |
| 0.45 *** | 63267 | 69685 | 99010 | 19322 | 21107 | 24831 | 3751 | 3879 | 4006 | 1005 | 1005 | 1005 | 452 | 452 | 452 |
| *** | 65732 | 77165 | 104213 | 20087 | 22552 | 26090 | 3810 | 3937 | 4182 | 1005 | 1005 | 1041 | 452 | 452 | 456 |
| 0.5 *** | 61551 | 68877 | 101076 | 19264 | 21235 | 25299 | 3767 | 3895 | 4065 | 1005 | 1005 | 1005 | 452 | 452 | 452 |
| *** | 64399 | 77149 | 105054 | 20114 | 22807 | 26248 | 3836 | 3980 | 4182 | 1005 | 1005 | 1030 | 452 | 452 | 446 |
| 0.55 *** | 58831 | 66864 | 100864 | 18881 | 20937 | 25187 | 3725 | 3852 | 4006 | 962 | 989 | 989 | 436 | 436 | 436 |
| *** | 61976 | 75704 | 103793 | 19774 | 22595 | 25880 | 3794 | 3937 | 4098 | 989 | 989 | 999 | 436 | 436 | 428 |
| 0.6 *** | 55346 | 63862 | 98356 | 18159 | 20257 | 24507 | 3597 | 3725 | 3879 | 920 | 946 | 946 | 410 | 410 | 410 |
| *** | 58720 | 72984 | 100430 | 19067 | 21915 | 24987 | 3640 | 3794 | 3930 | 946 | 946 | 946 | 410 | 410 | 400 |
| 0.65 *** | 51266 | 59952 | 93570 | 17155 | 19195 | 23259 | 3385 | 3496 | 3640 | 861 | 877 | 877 | 367 | 367 | 367 |
| *** | 54751 | 69047 | 94967 | 18047 | 20794 | 23569 | 3454 | 3581 | 3678 | 861 | 877 | 873 | 367 | 367 | 362 |
| 0.7 *** | 46692 | 55235 | 86541 | 15837 | 17776 | 21431 | 3087 | 3199 | 3326 | 776 | 776 | 792 | 325 | 325 | 325 |
| *** | 50161 | 63947 | 87401 | 16687 | 19221 | 21625 | 3156 | 3257 | 3342 | 776 | 792 | 778 | 325 | 325 | 316 |
| 0.75 *** | 41661 | 49694 | 77250 | 14249 | 15949 | 19051 | 2731 | 2816 | 2917 | 665 | 665 | 691 | 282 | 282 | 282 |
| *** | 44934 | 57657 | 77734 | 14987 | 17197 | 19156 | 2774 | 2875 | 2922 | 665 | 665 | 662 | 282 | 282 | 260 |
| 0.8 *** | 36110 | 43234 | 65732 | 12310 | 13712 | 16119 | 2280 | 2349 | 2434 | 537 | 537 | 537 | 224 | 224 | 224 |
| *** | 39042 | 50076 | 65966 | 12931 | 14716 | 16161 | 2322 | 2391 | 2417 | 537 | 537 | 526 | 224 | 224 | 194 |
| 0.85 *** | 29862 | 35642 | 52005 | 9999 | 11019 | 12634 | 1754 | 1796 | 1839 | 394 | 394 | 394 | . | . | . |
| *** | 32285 | 40955 | 52096 | 10466 | 11715 | 12641 | 1770 | 1812 | 1829 | 394 | 394 | 368 | . | . | . |
| 0.9 *** | 22536 | 26531 | 36110 | 7194 | 7762 | 8612 | 1132 | 1159 | 1175 | . | . | . | . | . | . |
| *** | 24236 | 29931 | 36125 | 7449 | 8145 | 8596 | 1159 | 1159 | 1156 | . | . | . | . | . | . |
| 0.95 *** | 13160 | 14902 | 18074 | 3666 | 3836 | 4049 | . | . | . | . | . | . | . | . | . |
| *** | 13925 | 16204 | 18052 | 3751 | 3937 | 4025 | . | . | . | . | . | . | . | . | . |
| 0.98 *** | 5382 | 5749 | 6216 | . | . | . | . | . | . | . | . | . | . | . | . |
| *** | 5552 | 5961 | 6200 | . | . | . | . | . | . | . | . | . | . | . | . |

## TABLE 6: ALPHA= 0.025 POWER= 0.9     EXPECTED ACCRUAL THRU MINIMUM FOLLOW-UP= 20000

| | | DEL=.01 | | | DEL=.02 | | | DEL=.05 | | | DEL=.10 | | | DEL=.15 | | |
|---|---|---|---|---|---|---|---|---|---|---|---|---|---|---|---|---|
| FACT= | | 1.0 .75 | .50 .25 | .00 BIN | 1.0 .75 | .50 .25 | .00 BIN | 1.0 .75 | .50 .25 | .00 BIN | 1.0 75 | .50 .25 | .00 BIN | 1.0 .75 | .50 .25 | .00 BIN |
| PCONT=*** | | | | | | REQUIRED NUMBER OF PATIENTS | | | | | | | | | | |
| 0.01 | *** | 1613 | 1613 | 1613 | 582 | 582 | 582 | 182 | 182 | 182 | 82 | 82 | 82 | 63 | 63 | 63 |
| | *** | 1613 | 1613 | 6200 | 582 | 582 | 2049 | 182 | 182 | 558 | 82 | 82 | 227 | 63 | 63 | 135 |
| 0.02 | *** | 3582 | 3613 | 3613 | 1163 | 1163 | 1163 | 313 | 313 | 313 | 132 | 132 | 132 | 82 | 82 | 82 |
| | *** | 3582 | 3613 | 10235 | 1163 | 1163 | 3048 | 313 | 313 | 712 | 132 | 132 | 264 | 82 | 82 | 151 |
| 0.05 | *** | 10982 | 11082 | 11282 | 3132 | 3132 | 3163 | 663 | 663 | 663 | 232 | 232 | 232 | 132 | 132 | 132 |
| | *** | 11032 | 11182 | 21835 | 3132 | 3163 | 5916 | 663 | 663 | 1156 | 232 | 232 | 368 | 132 | 132 | 194 |
| 0.1 | *** | 24413 | 24932 | 26282 | 6713 | 6813 | 6963 | 1282 | 1282 | 1282 | 382 | 382 | 382 | 213 | 213 | 213 |
| | *** | 24613 | 25432 | 39487 | 6763 | 6882 | 10277 | 1282 | 1282 | 1829 | 382 | 382 | 526 | 213 | 213 | 260 |
| 0.15 | *** | 36713 | 37863 | 41532 | 10082 | 10363 | 10763 | 1863 | 1882 | 1882 | 532 | 532 | 532 | 282 | 282 | 282 |
| | *** | 37163 | 39063 | 55038 | 10213 | 10532 | 14112 | 1863 | 1882 | 2417 | 532 | 532 | 662 | 282 | 282 | 316 |
| 0.2 | *** | 46882 | 48782 | 55813 | 13013 | 13482 | 14282 | 2382 | 2413 | 2432 | 663 | 682 | 682 | 332 | 332 | 332 |
| | *** | 47613 | 50932 | 68488 | 13213 | 13832 | 17422 | 2413 | 2432 | 2922 | 663 | 682 | 778 | 332 | 332 | 362 |
| 0.25 | *** | 54682 | 57463 | 68513 | 15382 | 16132 | 17413 | 2832 | 2882 | 2932 | 782 | 782 | 782 | 382 | 382 | 382 |
| | *** | 55732 | 60663 | 79836 | 15713 | 16663 | 20206 | 2863 | 2913 | 3342 | 782 | 782 | 873 | 382 | 382 | 400 |
| 0.3 | *** | 60132 | 63863 | 79332 | 17213 | 18232 | 20082 | 3213 | 3263 | 3332 | 863 | 882 | 882 | 413 | 413 | 413 |
| | *** | 61532 | 68213 | 89082 | 17663 | 18982 | 22465 | 3232 | 3282 | 3678 | 863 | 882 | 946 | 413 | 413 | 428 |
| 0.35 | *** | 63413 | 68182 | 88082 | 18532 | 19813 | 22213 | 3482 | 3563 | 3632 | 932 | 932 | 932 | 432 | 432 | 432 |
| | *** | 65232 | 73682 | 96227 | 19082 | 20782 | 24199 | 3513 | 3613 | 3930 | 932 | 932 | 999 | 432 | 432 | 446 |
| 0.4 | *** | 64813 | 70613 | 94663 | 19363 | 20882 | 23813 | 3663 | 3763 | 3882 | 982 | 982 | 982 | 463 | 463 | 463 |
| | *** | 67032 | 77182 | 101271 | 20032 | 22063 | 25407 | 3713 | 3813 | 4098 | 982 | 982 | 1030 | 463 | 463 | 456 |
| 0.45 | *** | 64613 | 71413 | 99013 | 19763 | 21482 | 24832 | 3782 | 3882 | 4013 | 1013 | 1013 | 1013 | 463 | 463 | 463 |
| | *** | 67263 | 78932 | 104213 | 20513 | 22832 | 26090 | 3832 | 3932 | 4182 | 1013 | 1013 | 1041 | 463 | 463 | 456 |
| 0.5 | *** | 63113 | 70782 | 101082 | 19763 | 21663 | 25282 | 3813 | 3932 | 4063 | 1013 | 1013 | 1013 | 463 | 463 | 463 |
| | *** | 66132 | 79063 | 105054 | 20582 | 23113 | 26248 | 3863 | 3982 | 4182 | 1013 | 1013 | 1030 | 463 | 463 | 446 |
| 0.55 | *** | 60563 | 68913 | 100863 | 19382 | 21382 | 25182 | 3763 | 3882 | 4013 | 982 | 982 | 982 | 432 | 432 | 432 |
| | *** | 63882 | 77732 | 103793 | 20263 | 22882 | 25880 | 3813 | 3932 | 4098 | 982 | 982 | 999 | 432 | 432 | 428 |
| 0.6 | *** | 57213 | 65982 | 98363 | 18682 | 20682 | 24513 | 3632 | 3732 | 3882 | 932 | 932 | 963 | 413 | 413 | 413 |
| | *** | 60732 | 75063 | 100430 | 19563 | 22213 | 24987 | 3682 | 3813 | 3930 | 932 | 932 | 946 | 413 | 413 | 400 |
| 0.65 | *** | 53213 | 62113 | 93582 | 17663 | 19613 | 23263 | 3413 | 3532 | 3663 | 863 | 882 | 882 | 382 | 382 | 382 |
| | *** | 56813 | 71113 | 94967 | 18532 | 21082 | 23569 | 3463 | 3582 | 3678 | 863 | 882 | 873 | 382 | 382 | 362 |
| 0.7 | *** | 48613 | 57313 | 86532 | 16332 | 18163 | 21432 | 3132 | 3213 | 3332 | 782 | 782 | 782 | 332 | 332 | 332 |
| | *** | 52163 | 65882 | 87401 | 17132 | 19482 | 21625 | 3182 | 3282 | 3342 | 782 | 782 | 778 | 332 | 332 | 316 |
| 0.75 | *** | 43482 | 51613 | 77232 | 14682 | 16282 | 19063 | 2763 | 2832 | 2932 | 663 | 682 | 682 | 282 | 282 | 282 |
| | *** | 46832 | 59413 | 77734 | 15382 | 17432 | 19156 | 2782 | 2882 | 2922 | 663 | 682 | 662 | 282 | 282 | 260 |
| 0.8 | *** | 37763 | 44882 | 65732 | 12663 | 13982 | 16113 | 2313 | 2363 | 2432 | 532 | 532 | 532 | 213 | 213 | 213 |
| | *** | 40713 | 51532 | 65966 | 13263 | 14882 | 16161 | 2332 | 2382 | 2417 | 532 | 532 | 526 | 213 | 213 | 194 |
| 0.85 | *** | 31232 | 36963 | 52013 | 10263 | 11213 | 12632 | 1763 | 1813 | 1832 | 382 | 382 | 382 | . | . | . |
| | *** | 33632 | 42063 | 52096 | 10682 | 11832 | 12641 | 1782 | 1832 | 1829 | 382 | 382 | 368 | . | . | . |
| 0.9 | *** | 23482 | 27382 | 36113 | 7332 | 7882 | 8613 | 1132 | 1163 | 1182 | . | . | . | . | . | . |
| | *** | 25163 | 30613 | 36125 | 7582 | 8213 | 8596 | 1163 | 1163 | 1156 | . | . | . | . | . | . |
| 0.95 | *** | 13613 | 15232 | 18063 | 3713 | 3863 | 4032 | . | . | . | . | . | . | . | . | . |
| | *** | 14332 | 16432 | 18052 | 3782 | 3932 | 4025 | . | . | . | . | . | . | . | . | . |
| 0.98 | *** | 5482 | 5813 | 6213 | . | . | . | . | . | . | . | . | . | . | . | . |
| | *** | 5632 | 5982 | 6200 | . | . | . | . | . | . | . | . | . | . | . | . |

TABLE 6: ALPHA= 0.025 POWER= 0.9    EXPECTED ACCRUAL THRU MINIMUM FOLLOW-UP= 25000

| | | DEL=.01 | | | DEL=.02 | | | DEL=.05 | | | DEL=.10 | | | DEL=.15 | | |
|---|---|---|---|---|---|---|---|---|---|---|---|---|---|---|---|---|---|
| FACT= | | 1.0<br>.75 | .50<br>.25 | .00<br>BIN | 1.0<br>.75 | .50<br>.25 | .00<br>BIN | 1.0<br>.75 | .50<br>.25 | .00<br>BIN | 1.0<br>75 | .50<br>.25 | .00<br>BIN | 1.0<br>.75 | .50<br>.25 | .00<br>BIN |
| PCONT=*** | | | | | REQUIRED NUMBER OF PATIENTS | | | | | | | | | | | |
| 0.01 | *** | 1602 | 1602 | 1602 | 579 | 579 | 579 | 204 | 204 | 204 | 102 | 102 | 102 | 79 | 79 | 79 |
| | *** | 1602 | 1602 | 6200 | 579 | 579 | 2049 | 204 | 204 | 558 | 102 | 102 | 227 | 79 | 79 | 135 |
| 0.02 | *** | 3602 | 3602 | 3602 | 1141 | 1141 | 1141 | 290 | 290 | 290 | 141 | 141 | 141 | 79 | 79 | 79 |
| | *** | 3602 | 3602 | 10235 | 1141 | 1141 | 3048 | 290 | 290 | 712 | 141 | 141 | 264 | 79 | 79 | 151 |
| 0.05 | *** | 11016 | 11141 | 11290 | 3141 | 3141 | 3165 | 665 | 665 | 665 | 227 | 227 | 227 | 141 | 141 | 141 |
| | *** | 11079 | 11204 | 21835 | 3141 | 3165 | 5916 | 665 | 665 | 1156 | 227 | 227 | 368 | 141 | 141 | 194 |
| 0.1 | *** | 24579 | 25102 | 26290 | 6727 | 6829 | 6954 | 1290 | 1290 | 1290 | 391 | 391 | 391 | 204 | 204 | 204 |
| | *** | 24790 | 25579 | 39487 | 6790 | 6891 | 10277 | 1290 | 1290 | 1829 | 391 | 391 | 526 | 204 | 204 | 260 |
| 0.15 | *** | 37040 | 38266 | 41540 | 10165 | 10415 | 10766 | 1852 | 1891 | 1891 | 540 | 540 | 540 | 266 | 266 | 266 |
| | *** | 37540 | 39415 | 55038 | 10290 | 10579 | 14112 | 1891 | 1891 | 2417 | 540 | 540 | 662 | 266 | 266 | 316 |
| 0.2 | *** | 47454 | 49477 | 55790 | 13165 | 13602 | 14290 | 2391 | 2415 | 2454 | 665 | 665 | 665 | 329 | 329 | 329 |
| | *** | 48227 | 51579 | 68488 | 13391 | 13915 | 17422 | 2415 | 2415 | 2922 | 665 | 665 | 778 | 329 | 329 | 362 |
| 0.25 | *** | 55477 | 58477 | 68516 | 15641 | 16329 | 17415 | 2852 | 2891 | 2915 | 790 | 790 | 790 | 391 | 391 | 391 |
| | *** | 56641 | 61665 | 79836 | 15954 | 16790 | 20206 | 2852 | 2915 | 3342 | 790 | 790 | 873 | 391 | 391 | 400 |
| 0.3 | *** | 61204 | 65266 | 79329 | 17579 | 18516 | 20079 | 3227 | 3266 | 3329 | 852 | 891 | 891 | 415 | 415 | 415 |
| | *** | 62790 | 69579 | 89082 | 17977 | 19165 | 22465 | 3227 | 3290 | 3678 | 852 | 891 | 946 | 415 | 415 | 428 |
| 0.35 | *** | 64790 | 69915 | 88079 | 18977 | 20165 | 22204 | 3516 | 3579 | 3641 | 954 | 954 | 954 | 415 | 454 | 454 |
| | *** | 66829 | 75391 | 96227 | 19516 | 21040 | 24199 | 3540 | 3602 | 3930 | 954 | 954 | 999 | 415 | 454 | 446 |
| 0.4 | *** | 66516 | 72704 | 94665 | 19891 | 21329 | 23790 | 3704 | 3790 | 3891 | 977 | 977 | 977 | 454 | 454 | 454 |
| | *** | 68954 | 79227 | 101271 | 20516 | 22352 | 25407 | 3727 | 3829 | 4098 | 977 | 977 | 1030 | 454 | 454 | 456 |
| 0.45 | *** | 66641 | 73829 | 99016 | 20352 | 21977 | 24829 | 3829 | 3915 | 4016 | 1016 | 1016 | 1016 | 454 | 454 | 454 |
| | *** | 69477 | 81266 | 104213 | 21079 | 23165 | 26090 | 3852 | 3954 | 4182 | 1016 | 1016 | 1041 | 454 | 454 | 456 |
| 0.5 | *** | 65415 | 73454 | 101079 | 20391 | 22165 | 25290 | 3852 | 3954 | 4040 | 1016 | 1016 | 1016 | 454 | 454 | 454 |
| | *** | 68641 | 81641 | 105054 | 21204 | 23454 | 26248 | 3891 | 4016 | 4182 | 1016 | 1016 | 1030 | 454 | 454 | 446 |
| 0.55 | *** | 63141 | 71766 | 100852 | 20079 | 21915 | 25165 | 3790 | 3915 | 4016 | 977 | 977 | 977 | 415 | 454 | 454 |
| | *** | 66602 | 80454 | 103793 | 20891 | 23266 | 25880 | 3852 | 3954 | 4098 | 977 | 977 | 999 | 454 | 454 | 428 |
| 0.6 | *** | 59915 | 68954 | 98352 | 19391 | 21227 | 24516 | 3665 | 3766 | 3891 | 954 | 954 | 954 | 415 | 415 | 415 |
| | *** | 63602 | 77829 | 100430 | 20204 | 22602 | 24987 | 3727 | 3829 | 3930 | 954 | 954 | 946 | 415 | 415 | 400 |
| 0.65 | *** | 55977 | 65040 | 93579 | 18329 | 20141 | 23266 | 3454 | 3540 | 3641 | 852 | 891 | 891 | 391 | 391 | 391 |
| | *** | 59704 | 73829 | 94967 | 19141 | 21454 | 23569 | 3516 | 3602 | 3678 | 852 | 891 | 873 | 391 | 391 | 362 |
| 0.7 | *** | 51352 | 60141 | 86540 | 16954 | 18641 | 21415 | 3165 | 3227 | 3329 | 790 | 790 | 790 | 329 | 329 | 329 |
| | *** | 54977 | 68454 | 87401 | 17704 | 19829 | 21625 | 3204 | 3290 | 3342 | 790 | 790 | 778 | 329 | 329 | 316 |
| 0.75 | *** | 46079 | 54204 | 77227 | 15227 | 16704 | 19040 | 2790 | 2852 | 2915 | 665 | 665 | 665 | 266 | 266 | 266 |
| | *** | 49454 | 61665 | 77734 | 15891 | 17704 | 19156 | 2829 | 2891 | 2922 | 665 | 665 | 662 | 266 | 266 | 260 |
| 0.8 | *** | 40040 | 47141 | 65727 | 13141 | 14329 | 16102 | 2329 | 2391 | 2415 | 540 | 540 | 540 | 204 | 204 | 204 |
| | *** | 43016 | 53415 | 65966 | 13665 | 15102 | 16161 | 2352 | 2391 | 2417 | 540 | 540 | 526 | 204 | 204 | 194 |
| 0.85 | *** | 33102 | 38704 | 52016 | 10602 | 11454 | 12641 | 1790 | 1829 | 1852 | 391 | 391 | 391 | . | . | . |
| | *** | 35477 | 43477 | 52096 | 10977 | 11977 | 12641 | 1790 | 1829 | 1829 | 391 | 391 | 368 | . | . | . |
| 0.9 | *** | 24790 | 28516 | 36102 | 7540 | 8016 | 8602 | 1141 | 1165 | 1165 | . | . | . | . | . | . |
| | *** | 26415 | 31454 | 36125 | 7766 | 8290 | 8596 | 1165 | 1165 | 1156 | . | . | . | . | . | . |
| 0.95 | *** | 14165 | 15665 | 18079 | 3766 | 3891 | 4040 | . | . | . | . | . | . | . | . | . |
| | *** | 14852 | 16704 | 18052 | 3829 | 3954 | 4025 | . | . | . | . | . | . | . | . | . |
| 0.98 | *** | 5602 | 5891 | 6227 | . | . | . | . | . | . | . | . | . | . | . | . |
| | *** | 5727 | 6040 | 6200 | . | . | . | . | . | . | . | . | . | . | . | . |

## TABLE 7: ALPHA= 0.05 POWER= 0.8    EXPECTED ACCRUAL THRU MINIMUM FOLLOW-UP= 30

| | | DEL=.10 | | | DEL=.15 | | | DEL=.20 | | | DEL=.25 | | | DEL=.30 | | |
|---|---|---|---|---|---|---|---|---|---|---|---|---|---|---|---|---|---|
| FACT= | | 1.0 .75 | .50 .25 | .00 BIN | 1.0 .75 | .50 .25 | .00 BIN | 1.0 .75 | .50 .25 | .00 BIN | 1.0 75 | .50 .25 | .00 BIN | 1.0 .75 | .50 .25 | .00 BIN |
| PCONT=*** | | REQUIRED NUMBER OF PATIENTS | | | | | | | | | | | | | | |
| 0.05 | *** | 130 | 131 | 141 | 76 | 77 | 82 | 54 | 55 | 58 | 42 | 43 | 45 | 35 | 35 | 37 |
| | *** | 131 | 133 | 217 | 77 | 79 | 115 | 54 | 56 | 73 | 42 | 44 | 51 | 35 | 36 | 38 |
| 0.1 | *** | 206 | 208 | 235 | 109 | 112 | 125 | 72 | 74 | 82 | 54 | 55 | 60 | 43 | 44 | 47 |
| | *** | 206 | 212 | 310 | 110 | 115 | 153 | 73 | 77 | 93 | 54 | 57 | 63 | 43 | 45 | 46 |
| 0.15 | *** | 266 | 269 | 323 | 134 | 138 | 163 | 86 | 89 | 103 | 62 | 64 | 73 | 48 | 50 | 56 |
| | *** | 267 | 276 | 390 | 136 | 143 | 186 | 87 | 93 | 110 | 63 | 67 | 73 | 49 | 52 | 52 |
| 0.2 | *** | 309 | 315 | 400 | 152 | 157 | 195 | 95 | 99 | 120 | 67 | 71 | 83 | 51 | 54 | 62 |
| | *** | 311 | 324 | 458 | 154 | 165 | 213 | 96 | 105 | 124 | 69 | 75 | 81 | 53 | 57 | 57 |
| 0.25 | *** | 338 | 345 | 466 | 163 | 170 | 222 | 100 | 106 | 134 | 70 | 75 | 91 | 53 | 57 | 67 |
| | *** | 340 | 358 | 514 | 165 | 181 | 235 | 103 | 114 | 135 | 72 | 80 | 87 | 55 | 61 | 60 |
| 0.3 | *** | 352 | 362 | 519 | 168 | 177 | 243 | 103 | 110 | 144 | 72 | 78 | 97 | 54 | 59 | 71 |
| | *** | 355 | 379 | 557 | 171 | 191 | 252 | 106 | 119 | 143 | 74 | 84 | 91 | 56 | 63 | 62 |
| 0.35 | *** | 354 | 366 | 559 | 168 | 180 | 259 | 102 | 112 | 151 | 71 | 78 | 100 | 54 | 59 | 72 |
| | *** | 358 | 389 | 588 | 172 | 196 | 263 | 106 | 122 | 147 | 74 | 85 | 93 | 56 | 63 | 63 |
| 0.4 | *** | 345 | 361 | 587 | 164 | 178 | 268 | 100 | 111 | 155 | 70 | 78 | 102 | 52 | 58 | 72 |
| | *** | 350 | 389 | 606 | 169 | 197 | 268 | 104 | 123 | 149 | 73 | 85 | 93 | 55 | 63 | 62 |
| 0.45 | *** | 327 | 347 | 600 | 156 | 173 | 271 | 96 | 108 | 155 | 67 | 75 | 101 | 50 | 56 | 71 |
| | *** | 334 | 380 | 613 | 163 | 194 | 268 | 101 | 121 | 147 | 71 | 83 | 91 | 53 | 61 | 60 |
| 0.5 | *** | 303 | 327 | 601 | 147 | 165 | 268 | 91 | 104 | 152 | 64 | 72 | 98 | 48 | 54 | 68 |
| | *** | 311 | 366 | 606 | 154 | 188 | 263 | 96 | 117 | 143 | 67 | 80 | 87 | 50 | 59 | 57 |
| 0.55 | *** | 275 | 304 | 587 | 136 | 156 | 260 | 85 | 98 | 145 | 59 | 68 | 92 | 44 | 50 | 64 |
| | *** | 285 | 346 | 588 | 144 | 179 | 252 | 90 | 111 | 135 | 63 | 76 | 81 | 47 | 55 | 52 |
| 0.6 | *** | 245 | 278 | 561 | 124 | 144 | 245 | 78 | 91 | 135 | 54 | 63 | 85 | 40 | 46 | 58 |
| | *** | 257 | 323 | 557 | 132 | 168 | 235 | 83 | 104 | 124 | 58 | 70 | 73 | 43 | 50 | 46 |
| 0.65 | *** | 214 | 250 | 521 | 111 | 131 | 224 | 70 | 82 | 122 | 49 | 56 | 75 | 36 | 41 | 51 |
| | *** | 228 | 296 | 514 | 119 | 154 | 213 | 75 | 94 | 110 | 52 | 63 | 63 | 38 | 44 | 38 |
| 0.7 | *** | 185 | 221 | 467 | 97 | 117 | 197 | 62 | 72 | 105 | 42 | 49 | 64 | . | . | . |
| | *** | 199 | 265 | 458 | 105 | 137 | 186 | 66 | 83 | 93 | 45 | 54 | 51 | . | . | . |
| 0.75 | *** | 156 | 191 | 401 | 83 | 100 | 165 | 52 | 61 | 85 | . | . | . | . | . | . |
| | *** | 170 | 232 | 390 | 90 | 118 | 153 | 56 | 69 | 73 | . | . | . | . | . | . |
| 0.8 | *** | 128 | 159 | 321 | 68 | 81 | 127 | . | . | . | . | . | . | . | . | . |
| | *** | 140 | 193 | 310 | 73 | 95 | 115 | . | . | . | . | . | . | . | . | . |
| 0.85 | *** | 99 | 123 | 229 | . | . | . | . | . | . | . | . | . | . | . | . |
| | *** | 108 | 148 | 217 | . | . | . | . | . | . | . | . | . | . | . | . |

TABLE 7: ALPHA= 0.05  POWER= 0.8    EXPECTED ACCRUAL THRU MINIMUM FOLLOW-UP= 40

| | | DEL=.10 | | | DEL=.15 | | | DEL=.20 | | | DEL=.25 | | | DEL=.30 | | |
|---|---|---|---|---|---|---|---|---|---|---|---|---|---|---|---|---|---|
| FACT= | | 1.0 .75 | .50 .25 | .00 BIN | 1.0 .75 | .50 .25 | .00 BIN | 1.0 .75 | .50 .25 | .00 BIN | 1.0 75 | .50 .25 | .00 BIN | 1.0 .75 | .50 .25 | .00 BIN |
| PCONT=*** | | REQUIRED NUMBER OF PATIENTS | | | | | | | | | | | | | | |
| 0.05 | *** | 131 | 132 | 141 | 77 | 78 | 82 | 54 | 55 | 58 | 42 | 43 | 45 | 35 | 36 | 37 |
| | *** | 131 | 134 | 217 | 77 | 79 | 115 | 55 | 56 | 73 | 43 | 44 | 51 | 35 | 36 | 38 |
| 0.1 | *** | 206 | 209 | 235 | 110 | 113 | 125 | 73 | 75 | 82 | 54 | 56 | 60 | 43 | 45 | 47 |
| | *** | 207 | 214 | 310 | 111 | 116 | 153 | 74 | 78 | 93 | 55 | 58 | 63 | 44 | 46 | 46 |
| 0.15 | *** | 267 | 271 | 323 | 136 | 140 | 163 | 87 | 90 | 103 | 63 | 66 | 73 | 49 | 51 | 56 |
| | *** | 268 | 279 | 390 | 137 | 146 | 186 | 88 | 94 | 110 | 64 | 68 | 73 | 50 | 53 | 52 |
| 0.2 | *** | 311 | 318 | 400 | 154 | 160 | 195 | 97 | 102 | 120 | 69 | 73 | 83 | 53 | 56 | 62 |
| | *** | 313 | 330 | 458 | 156 | 169 | 213 | 99 | 107 | 124 | 70 | 76 | 81 | 54 | 58 | 57 |
| 0.25 | *** | 340 | 350 | 466 | 165 | 174 | 222 | 103 | 109 | 134 | 72 | 77 | 91 | 55 | 59 | 67 |
| | *** | 343 | 366 | 514 | 169 | 186 | 235 | 105 | 117 | 135 | 74 | 82 | 87 | 57 | 62 | 60 |
| 0.3 | *** | 355 | 368 | 519 | 171 | 182 | 243 | 106 | 114 | 144 | 74 | 80 | 97 | 56 | 60 | 71 |
| | *** | 360 | 390 | 557 | 175 | 197 | 252 | 109 | 123 | 143 | 77 | 86 | 91 | 58 | 64 | 62 |
| 0.35 | *** | 358 | 374 | 559 | 172 | 186 | 259 | 106 | 116 | 151 | 74 | 81 | 100 | 56 | 61 | 72 |
| | *** | 363 | 402 | 588 | 177 | 203 | 263 | 110 | 127 | 147 | 77 | 88 | 93 | 58 | 65 | 63 |
| 0.4 | *** | 350 | 371 | 587 | 169 | 185 | 268 | 104 | 116 | 155 | 73 | 81 | 102 | 55 | 60 | 72 |
| | *** | 357 | 404 | 606 | 175 | 205 | 268 | 109 | 127 | 149 | 76 | 88 | 93 | 57 | 65 | 62 |
| 0.45 | *** | 334 | 359 | 600 | 163 | 181 | 271 | 101 | 113 | 155 | 71 | 79 | 101 | 53 | 59 | 71 |
| | *** | 343 | 398 | 613 | 170 | 203 | 268 | 106 | 126 | 147 | 74 | 86 | 91 | 55 | 63 | 60 |
| 0.5 | *** | 311 | 342 | 601 | 154 | 175 | 268 | 96 | 109 | 152 | 67 | 76 | 98 | 50 | 56 | 68 |
| | *** | 322 | 385 | 606 | 162 | 198 | 263 | 102 | 122 | 143 | 71 | 83 | 87 | 53 | 61 | 57 |
| 0.55 | *** | 285 | 320 | 587 | 144 | 165 | 260 | 90 | 104 | 145 | 63 | 71 | 92 | 47 | 52 | 64 |
| | *** | 298 | 367 | 588 | 152 | 189 | 252 | 96 | 116 | 135 | 67 | 79 | 81 | 49 | 57 | 52 |
| 0.6 | *** | 257 | 295 | 561 | 132 | 154 | 245 | 83 | 96 | 135 | 58 | 66 | 85 | 43 | 48 | 58 |
| | *** | 271 | 344 | 557 | 141 | 178 | 235 | 89 | 109 | 124 | 61 | 73 | 73 | 45 | 52 | 46 |
| 0.65 | *** | 228 | 268 | 521 | 119 | 141 | 224 | 75 | 87 | 122 | 52 | 59 | 75 | 38 | 42 | 51 |
| | *** | 243 | 317 | 514 | 128 | 163 | 213 | 80 | 99 | 110 | 55 | 65 | 63 | 40 | 46 | 38 |
| 0.7 | *** | 199 | 239 | 467 | 105 | 125 | 197 | 66 | 77 | 105 | 45 | 51 | 64 | . | . | . |
| | *** | 214 | 285 | 458 | 113 | 146 | 186 | 71 | 86 | 93 | 48 | 56 | 51 | . | . | . |
| 0.75 | *** | 170 | 207 | 401 | 90 | 108 | 165 | 56 | 64 | 85 | . | . | . | . | . | . |
| | *** | 185 | 249 | 390 | 97 | 125 | 153 | 59 | 72 | 73 | . | . | . | . | . | . |
| 0.8 | *** | 140 | 173 | 321 | 73 | 87 | 127 | . | . | . | . | . | . | . | . | . |
| | *** | 153 | 208 | 310 | 79 | 100 | 115 | . | . | . | . | . | . | . | . | . |
| 0.85 | *** | 108 | 133 | 229 | . | . | . | . | . | . | . | . | . | . | . | . |
| | *** | 119 | 159 | 217 | . | . | . | . | . | . | . | . | . | . | . | . |

## TABLE 7: ALPHA= 0.05  POWER= 0.8    EXPECTED ACCRUAL THRU MINIMUM FOLLOW-UP= 50

|  |  | DEL=.10 | | | DEL=.15 | | | DEL=.20 | | | DEL=.25 | | | DEL=.30 | | |
|---|---|---|---|---|---|---|---|---|---|---|---|---|---|---|---|---|
| FACT= | | 1.0 .75 | .50 .25 | .00 BIN | 1.0 .75 | .50 .25 | .00 BIN | 1.0 .75 | .50 .25 | .00 BIN | 1.0 75 | .50 .25 | .00 BIN | 1.0 .75 | .50 .25 | .00 BIN |
| PCONT=*** | | | | | REQUIRED NUMBER OF PATIENTS | | | | | | | | | | | |
| 0.05 | *** | 131 | 133 | 141 | 77 | 78 | 82 | 55 | 56 | 58 | 43 | 43 | 45 | 35 | 36 | 37 |
|  | *** | 132 | 135 | 217 | 77 | 80 | 115 | 55 | 56 | 73 | 43 | 44 | 51 | 35 | 36 | 38 |
| 0.1 | *** | 207 | 211 | 235 | 111 | 114 | 125 | 74 | 76 | 82 | 55 | 57 | 60 | 44 | 45 | 47 |
|  | *** | 208 | 216 | 310 | 112 | 117 | 153 | 75 | 78 | 93 | 56 | 58 | 63 | 44 | 46 | 46 |
| 0.15 | *** | 268 | 273 | 323 | 137 | 142 | 163 | 88 | 92 | 103 | 64 | 67 | 73 | 50 | 52 | 56 |
|  | *** | 270 | 283 | 390 | 139 | 148 | 186 | 89 | 95 | 110 | 65 | 69 | 73 | 50 | 53 | 52 |
| 0.2 | *** | 313 | 321 | 400 | 156 | 163 | 195 | 98 | 104 | 120 | 70 | 74 | 83 | 54 | 57 | 62 |
|  | *** | 316 | 335 | 458 | 158 | 172 | 213 | 100 | 109 | 124 | 72 | 77 | 81 | 55 | 59 | 57 |
| 0.25 | *** | 343 | 354 | 466 | 168 | 178 | 222 | 105 | 112 | 134 | 74 | 79 | 91 | 56 | 60 | 67 |
|  | *** | 347 | 373 | 514 | 172 | 190 | 235 | 108 | 119 | 135 | 76 | 83 | 87 | 58 | 63 | 60 |
| 0.3 | *** | 358 | 374 | 519 | 174 | 187 | 243 | 108 | 117 | 144 | 76 | 82 | 97 | 57 | 62 | 71 |
|  | *** | 364 | 399 | 557 | 179 | 202 | 252 | 112 | 126 | 143 | 79 | 87 | 91 | 59 | 65 | 62 |
| 0.35 | *** | 362 | 382 | 559 | 176 | 191 | 259 | 109 | 120 | 151 | 76 | 83 | 100 | 57 | 62 | 72 |
|  | *** | 369 | 413 | 588 | 182 | 209 | 263 | 113 | 130 | 147 | 79 | 90 | 93 | 60 | 66 | 63 |
| 0.4 | *** | 355 | 380 | 587 | 174 | 192 | 268 | 108 | 120 | 155 | 75 | 83 | 102 | 57 | 62 | 72 |
|  | *** | 364 | 417 | 606 | 181 | 212 | 268 | 113 | 131 | 149 | 79 | 90 | 93 | 59 | 66 | 62 |
| 0.45 | *** | 340 | 370 | 600 | 168 | 188 | 271 | 105 | 118 | 155 | 73 | 81 | 101 | 55 | 60 | 71 |
|  | *** | 351 | 412 | 613 | 176 | 210 | 268 | 110 | 130 | 147 | 77 | 88 | 91 | 57 | 64 | 60 |
| 0.5 | *** | 320 | 354 | 601 | 160 | 182 | 268 | 100 | 114 | 152 | 70 | 78 | 98 | 52 | 58 | 68 |
|  | *** | 332 | 401 | 606 | 169 | 205 | 263 | 106 | 126 | 143 | 74 | 85 | 87 | 54 | 62 | 57 |
| 0.55 | *** | 295 | 334 | 587 | 150 | 173 | 260 | 94 | 108 | 145 | 66 | 74 | 92 | 49 | 54 | 64 |
|  | *** | 309 | 384 | 588 | 159 | 197 | 252 | 100 | 120 | 135 | 69 | 81 | 81 | 51 | 58 | 52 |
| 0.6 | *** | 268 | 310 | 561 | 139 | 162 | 245 | 87 | 100 | 135 | 61 | 68 | 85 | 44 | 49 | 58 |
|  | *** | 284 | 361 | 557 | 148 | 185 | 235 | 93 | 112 | 124 | 64 | 75 | 73 | 47 | 53 | 46 |
| 0.65 | *** | 239 | 283 | 521 | 126 | 148 | 224 | 79 | 91 | 122 | 54 | 61 | 75 | 39 | 43 | 51 |
|  | *** | 256 | 333 | 514 | 135 | 170 | 213 | 84 | 102 | 110 | 57 | 67 | 63 | 41 | 46 | 38 |
| 0.7 | *** | 211 | 253 | 467 | 112 | 132 | 197 | 70 | 80 | 105 | 47 | 53 | 64 | . | . | . |
|  | *** | 227 | 301 | 458 | 120 | 152 | 186 | 74 | 89 | 93 | 50 | 57 | 51 | . | . | . |
| 0.75 | *** | 181 | 221 | 401 | 96 | 113 | 165 | 59 | 67 | 85 | . | . | . | . | . | . |
|  | *** | 197 | 263 | 390 | 103 | 130 | 153 | 62 | 74 | 73 | . | . | . | . | . | . |
| 0.8 | *** | 150 | 184 | 321 | 78 | 91 | 127 | . | . | . | . | . | . | . | . | . |
|  | *** | 164 | 219 | 310 | 83 | 103 | 115 | . | . | . | . | . | . | . | . | . |
| 0.85 | *** | 116 | 142 | 229 | . | . | . | . | . | . | . | . | . | . | . | . |
|  | *** | 127 | 167 | 217 | . | . | . | . | . | . | . | . | . | . | . | . |

TABLE 7: ALPHA= 0.05  POWER= 0.8    EXPECTED ACCRUAL THRU MINIMUM FOLLOW-UP= 60

| | | DEL=.10 | | | DEL=.15 | | | DEL=.20 | | | DEL=.25 | | | DEL=.30 | | |
|---|---|---|---|---|---|---|---|---|---|---|---|---|---|---|---|---|---|
| FACT= | | 1.0 .75 | .50 .25 | .00 BIN | 1.0 .75 | .50 .25 | .00 BIN | 1.0 .75 | .50 .25 | .00 BIN | 1.0 75 | .50 .25 | .00 BIN | 1.0 .75 | .50 .25 | .00 BIN |
| PCONT=*** | | REQUIRED NUMBER OF PATIENTS | | | | | | | | | | | | | | |
| 0.05 | *** | 131 | 133 | 141 | 77 | 79 | 82 | 55 | 56 | 58 | 43 | 44 | 45 | 35 | 36 | 37 |
| | *** | 132 | 135 | 217 | 78 | 80 | 115 | 55 | 57 | 73 | 43 | 44 | 51 | 36 | 36 | 38 |
| 0.1 | *** | 208 | 212 | 235 | 112 | 115 | 125 | 74 | 77 | 82 | 55 | 57 | 60 | 44 | 45 | 47 |
| | *** | 209 | 217 | 310 | 113 | 118 | 153 | 75 | 79 | 93 | 56 | 58 | 63 | 45 | 46 | 46 |
| 0.15 | *** | 269 | 276 | 323 | 138 | 143 | 163 | 89 | 93 | 103 | 64 | 67 | 73 | 50 | 52 | 56 |
| | *** | 271 | 286 | 390 | 140 | 149 | 186 | 90 | 96 | 110 | 66 | 69 | 73 | 51 | 54 | 52 |
| 0.2 | *** | 314 | 324 | 400 | 157 | 165 | 195 | 99 | 105 | 120 | 71 | 75 | 83 | 54 | 57 | 62 |
| | *** | 318 | 339 | 458 | 160 | 174 | 213 | 102 | 110 | 124 | 73 | 78 | 81 | 56 | 59 | 57 |
| 0.25 | *** | 345 | 358 | 466 | 170 | 181 | 222 | 106 | 114 | 134 | 75 | 80 | 91 | 57 | 61 | 67 |
| | *** | 350 | 379 | 514 | 174 | 193 | 235 | 109 | 121 | 135 | 77 | 84 | 87 | 59 | 63 | 60 |
| 0.3 | *** | 362 | 379 | 519 | 177 | 191 | 243 | 110 | 119 | 144 | 78 | 84 | 97 | 59 | 63 | 71 |
| | *** | 368 | 406 | 557 | 182 | 206 | 252 | 114 | 128 | 143 | 80 | 89 | 91 | 60 | 66 | 62 |
| 0.35 | *** | 366 | 389 | 559 | 180 | 196 | 259 | 112 | 122 | 151 | 78 | 85 | 100 | 59 | 63 | 72 |
| | *** | 374 | 422 | 588 | 186 | 214 | 263 | 116 | 132 | 147 | 81 | 91 | 93 | 61 | 67 | 63 |
| 0.4 | *** | 361 | 389 | 587 | 178 | 197 | 268 | 111 | 123 | 155 | 78 | 85 | 102 | 58 | 63 | 72 |
| | *** | 371 | 428 | 606 | 185 | 217 | 268 | 116 | 134 | 149 | 81 | 91 | 93 | 60 | 67 | 62 |
| 0.45 | *** | 347 | 380 | 600 | 173 | 194 | 271 | 108 | 121 | 155 | 75 | 83 | 101 | 56 | 61 | 71 |
| | *** | 359 | 425 | 613 | 181 | 216 | 268 | 113 | 132 | 147 | 79 | 90 | 91 | 59 | 65 | 60 |
| 0.5 | *** | 327 | 366 | 601 | 165 | 188 | 268 | 104 | 117 | 152 | 72 | 80 | 98 | 54 | 59 | 68 |
| | *** | 342 | 414 | 606 | 175 | 211 | 263 | 109 | 129 | 143 | 76 | 87 | 87 | 56 | 63 | 57 |
| 0.55 | *** | 304 | 346 | 587 | 156 | 179 | 260 | 98 | 111 | 145 | 68 | 76 | 92 | 50 | 55 | 64 |
| | *** | 320 | 398 | 588 | 165 | 203 | 252 | 104 | 123 | 135 | 71 | 82 | 81 | 52 | 59 | 52 |
| 0.6 | *** | 278 | 323 | 561 | 144 | 168 | 245 | 91 | 104 | 135 | 63 | 70 | 85 | 46 | 50 | 58 |
| | *** | 295 | 375 | 557 | 154 | 191 | 235 | 96 | 115 | 124 | 66 | 76 | 73 | 48 | 53 | 46 |
| 0.65 | *** | 250 | 296 | 521 | 131 | 154 | 224 | 82 | 94 | 122 | 56 | 63 | 75 | 41 | 44 | 51 |
| | *** | 268 | 347 | 514 | 141 | 175 | 213 | 87 | 104 | 110 | 59 | 68 | 63 | 42 | 47 | 38 |
| 0.7 | *** | 221 | 265 | 467 | 117 | 137 | 197 | 72 | 83 | 105 | 49 | 54 | 64 | . | . | . |
| | *** | 239 | 314 | 458 | 125 | 157 | 186 | 77 | 91 | 93 | 51 | 58 | 51 | . | . | . |
| 0.75 | *** | 191 | 232 | 401 | 100 | 118 | 165 | 61 | 69 | 85 | . | . | . | . | . | . |
| | *** | 207 | 275 | 390 | 108 | 134 | 153 | 64 | 75 | 73 | . | . | . | . | . | . |
| 0.8 | *** | 159 | 193 | 321 | 81 | 95 | 127 | . | . | . | . | . | . | . | . | . |
| | *** | 173 | 228 | 310 | 87 | 106 | 115 | . | . | . | . | . | . | . | . | . |
| 0.85 | *** | 123 | 148 | 229 | . | . | . | . | . | . | . | . | . | . | . | . |
| | *** | 133 | 173 | 217 | . | . | . | . | . | . | . | . | . | . | . | . |

## TABLE 7: ALPHA= 0.05  POWER= 0.8   EXPECTED ACCRUAL THRU MINIMUM FOLLOW-UP= 70

| | | DEL=.10 | | | DEL=.15 | | | DEL=.20 | | | DEL=.25 | | | DEL=.30 | |
|---|---|---|---|---|---|---|---|---|---|---|---|---|---|---|---|
| FACT= | 1.0 .75 | .50 .25 | .00 BIN | 1.0 .75 | .50 .25 | .00 BIN | 1.0 .75 | .50 .25 | .00 BIN | 1.0 75 | .50 .25 | .00 BIN | 1.0 .75 | .50 .25 | .00 BIN |

PCONT=***    REQUIRED NUMBER OF PATIENTS

| PCONT | DEL=.10 1.0/.75 | .50/.25 | .00/BIN | DEL=.15 1.0/.75 | .50/.25 | .00/BIN | DEL=.20 1.0/.75 | .50/.25 | .00/BIN | DEL=.25 1.0/.75 | .50/.25 | .00/BIN | DEL=.30 1.0/.75 | .50/.25 | .00/BIN |
|---|---|---|---|---|---|---|---|---|---|---|---|---|---|---|---|
| 0.05 *** | 132 | 134 | 141 | 77 | 79 | 82 | 55 | 56 | 58 | 43 | 44 | 45 | 36 | 36 | 37 |
| *** | 132 | 136 | 217 | 78 | 80 | 115 | 55 | 57 | 73 | 43 | 44 | 51 | 36 | 36 | 38 |
| 0.1 *** | 208 | 213 | 235 | 112 | 116 | 125 | 75 | 77 | 82 | 56 | 57 | 60 | 44 | 45 | 47 |
| *** | 210 | 219 | 310 | 114 | 119 | 153 | 76 | 79 | 93 | 56 | 59 | 63 | 45 | 46 | 46 |
| 0.15 *** | 270 | 278 | 323 | 139 | 145 | 163 | 90 | 94 | 103 | 65 | 68 | 73 | 51 | 52 | 56 |
| *** | 273 | 288 | 390 | 141 | 151 | 186 | 91 | 97 | 110 | 66 | 70 | 73 | 51 | 54 | 52 |
| 0.2 *** | 316 | 327 | 400 | 159 | 167 | 195 | 101 | 106 | 120 | 72 | 76 | 83 | 55 | 58 | 62 |
| *** | 320 | 343 | 458 | 162 | 176 | 213 | 103 | 111 | 124 | 73 | 79 | 81 | 56 | 60 | 57 |
| 0.25 *** | 347 | 362 | 466 | 172 | 183 | 222 | 108 | 115 | 134 | 76 | 81 | 91 | 58 | 61 | 67 |
| *** | 353 | 385 | 514 | 177 | 195 | 235 | 111 | 122 | 135 | 78 | 85 | 87 | 59 | 64 | 60 |
| 0.3 *** | 365 | 385 | 519 | 180 | 194 | 243 | 112 | 121 | 144 | 79 | 85 | 97 | 60 | 64 | 71 |
| *** | 372 | 413 | 557 | 186 | 209 | 252 | 116 | 130 | 143 | 81 | 90 | 91 | 61 | 66 | 62 |
| 0.35 *** | 370 | 395 | 559 | 183 | 200 | 259 | 114 | 125 | 151 | 80 | 87 | 100 | 60 | 64 | 72 |
| *** | 379 | 430 | 588 | 190 | 218 | 263 | 118 | 134 | 147 | 83 | 92 | 93 | 62 | 68 | 63 |
| 0.4 *** | 366 | 396 | 587 | 182 | 201 | 268 | 113 | 125 | 155 | 79 | 87 | 102 | 59 | 64 | 72 |
| *** | 377 | 437 | 606 | 190 | 221 | 268 | 118 | 136 | 149 | 82 | 92 | 93 | 61 | 67 | 62 |
| 0.45 *** | 353 | 389 | 600 | 177 | 199 | 271 | 111 | 124 | 155 | 77 | 85 | 101 | 57 | 62 | 71 |
| *** | 367 | 435 | 613 | 186 | 221 | 268 | 116 | 135 | 147 | 81 | 91 | 91 | 60 | 66 | 60 |
| 0.5 *** | 335 | 376 | 601 | 170 | 193 | 268 | 107 | 120 | 152 | 74 | 82 | 98 | 55 | 60 | 68 |
| *** | 350 | 426 | 606 | 180 | 216 | 263 | 112 | 131 | 143 | 78 | 88 | 87 | 57 | 63 | 57 |
| 0.55 *** | 312 | 357 | 587 | 161 | 185 | 260 | 101 | 114 | 145 | 70 | 77 | 92 | 51 | 56 | 64 |
| *** | 329 | 409 | 588 | 171 | 208 | 252 | 106 | 125 | 135 | 73 | 83 | 81 | 53 | 59 | 52 |
| 0.6 *** | 287 | 334 | 561 | 149 | 173 | 245 | 94 | 106 | 135 | 64 | 72 | 85 | 47 | 51 | 58 |
| *** | 305 | 387 | 557 | 159 | 195 | 235 | 99 | 117 | 124 | 68 | 77 | 73 | 49 | 54 | 46 |
| 0.65 *** | 259 | 307 | 521 | 136 | 159 | 224 | 85 | 97 | 122 | 58 | 64 | 75 | 41 | 45 | 51 |
| *** | 278 | 359 | 514 | 146 | 180 | 213 | 90 | 106 | 110 | 61 | 69 | 63 | 43 | 47 | 38 |
| 0.7 *** | 230 | 276 | 467 | 121 | 142 | 197 | 75 | 85 | 105 | 50 | 55 | 64 | . | . | . |
| *** | 249 | 324 | 458 | 130 | 160 | 186 | 79 | 93 | 93 | 52 | 59 | 51 | . | . | . |
| 0.75 *** | 200 | 241 | 401 | 104 | 122 | 165 | 63 | 71 | 85 | . | . | . | . | . | . |
| *** | 216 | 284 | 390 | 112 | 137 | 153 | 66 | 76 | 73 | . | . | . | . | . | . |
| 0.8 *** | 166 | 201 | 321 | 84 | 98 | 127 | . | . | . | . | . | . | . | . | . |
| *** | 181 | 236 | 310 | 90 | 108 | 115 | . | . | . | . | . | . | . | . | . |
| 0.85 *** | 128 | 154 | 229 | . | . | . | . | . | . | . | . | . | . | . | . |
| *** | 139 | 178 | 217 | . | . | . | . | . | . | . | . | . | . | . | . |

## TABLE 7: ALPHA= 0.05  POWER= 0.8    EXPECTED ACCRUAL THRU MINIMUM FOLLOW-UP= 80

| | | DEL=.10 | | | DEL=.15 | | | DEL=.20 | | | DEL=.25 | | | DEL=.30 | |
|---|---|---|---|---|---|---|---|---|---|---|---|---|---|---|---|---|
| FACT= | | 1.0 .75 | .50 .25 | .00 BIN | 1.0 .75 | .50 .25 | .00 BIN | 1.0 .75 | .50 .25 | .00 BIN | 1.0 75 | .50 .25 | .00 BIN | 1.0 .75 | .50 .25 | .00 BIN |
| PCONT=*** | | REQUIRED NUMBER OF PATIENTS | | | | | | | | | | | | | | |
| 0.05 | *** | 132 134 141 | | | 78 79 82 | | | 55 56 58 | | | 43 44 45 | | | 36 36 37 | | |
| | *** | 133 136 217 | | | 78 80 115 | | | 56 57 73 | | | 43 44 51 | | | 36 36 38 | | |
| 0.1 | *** | 209 214 235 | | | 113 116 125 | | | 75 78 82 | | | 56 58 60 | | | 45 46 47 | | |
| | *** | 211 220 310 | | | 114 119 153 | | | 76 79 93 | | | 57 59 63 | | | 45 46 46 | | |
| 0.15 | *** | 271 279 323 | | | 140 146 163 | | | 90 94 103 | | | 66 68 73 | | | 51 53 56 | | |
| | *** | 274 290 390 | | | 142 152 186 | | | 92 98 110 | | | 67 70 73 | | | 52 54 52 | | |
| 0.2 | *** | 318 330 400 | | | 160 169 195 | | | 102 107 120 | | | 73 76 83 | | | 56 58 62 | | |
| | *** | 322 347 458 | | | 164 178 213 | | | 104 112 124 | | | 74 79 81 | | | 57 60 57 | | |
| 0.25 | *** | 350 366 466 | | | 174 186 222 | | | 109 117 134 | | | 77 82 91 | | | 59 62 67 | | |
| | *** | 356 389 514 | | | 179 198 235 | | | 113 123 135 | | | 79 86 87 | | | 60 64 60 | | |
| 0.3 | *** | 368 390 519 | | | 182 197 243 | | | 114 123 144 | | | 80 86 97 | | | 60 64 71 | | |
| | *** | 376 419 557 | | | 188 212 252 | | | 118 131 143 | | | 83 90 91 | | | 62 67 62 | | |
| 0.35 | *** | 374 402 559 | | | 186 203 259 | | | 116 127 151 | | | 81 88 100 | | | 61 65 72 | | |
| | *** | 384 437 588 | | | 193 221 263 | | | 121 136 147 | | | 84 93 93 | | | 63 68 63 | | |
| 0.4 | *** | 371 404 587 | | | 185 205 268 | | | 116 127 155 | | | 81 88 102 | | | 60 65 72 | | |
| | *** | 383 446 606 | | | 193 225 268 | | | 121 137 149 | | | 84 93 93 | | | 62 68 62 | | |
| 0.45 | *** | 359 398 600 | | | 181 203 271 | | | 113 126 155 | | | 79 86 101 | | | 59 63 71 | | |
| | *** | 374 445 613 | | | 190 225 268 | | | 119 137 147 | | | 82 92 91 | | | 61 67 60 | | |
| 0.5 | *** | 342 385 601 | | | 175 198 268 | | | 109 122 152 | | | 76 83 98 | | | 56 61 68 | | |
| | *** | 358 436 606 | | | 184 220 263 | | | 115 133 143 | | | 79 89 87 | | | 58 64 57 | | |
| 0.55 | *** | 320 367 587 | | | 165 189 260 | | | 104 116 145 | | | 71 79 92 | | | 52 57 64 | | |
| | *** | 338 420 588 | | | 175 212 252 | | | 109 127 135 | | | 75 84 81 | | | 54 60 52 | | |
| 0.6 | *** | 295 344 561 | | | 154 178 245 | | | 96 109 135 | | | 66 73 85 | | | 48 52 58 | | |
| | *** | 314 397 557 | | | 164 199 235 | | | 102 119 124 | | | 69 78 73 | | | 50 54 46 | | |
| 0.65 | *** | 268 317 521 | | | 141 163 224 | | | 87 99 122 | | | 59 65 75 | | | 42 46 51 | | |
| | *** | 287 369 514 | | | 150 183 213 | | | 92 108 110 | | | 62 69 63 | | | 44 48 38 | | |
| 0.7 | *** | 239 285 467 | | | 125 146 197 | | | 77 86 105 | | | 51 56 64 | | | . . . | | |
| | *** | 257 334 458 | | | 134 163 186 | | | 81 94 93 | | | 53 59 51 | | | . . . | | |
| 0.75 | *** | 207 249 401 | | | 108 125 165 | | | 64 72 85 | | | . . . | | | . . . | | |
| | *** | 224 292 390 | | | 115 139 153 | | | 68 77 73 | | | . . . | | | . . . | | |
| 0.8 | *** | 173 208 321 | | | 87 100 127 | | | . . . | | | . . . | | | . . . | | |
| | *** | 187 242 310 | | | 93 110 115 | | | . . . | | | . . . | | | . . . | | |
| 0.85 | *** | 133 159 229 | | | . . . | | | . . . | | | . . . | | | . . . | | |
| | *** | 144 182 217 | | | . . . | | | . . . | | | . . . | | | . . . | | |

## TABLE 7: ALPHA= 0.05  POWER= 0.8    EXPECTED ACCRUAL THRU MINIMUM FOLLOW-UP= 90

| | | DEL=.10 | | | DEL=.15 | | | DEL=.20 | | | DEL=.25 | | | DEL=.30 | | |
|---|---|---|---|---|---|---|---|---|---|---|---|---|---|---|---|---|
| FACT= | | 1.0 .75 | .50 .25 | .00 BIN | 1.0 .75 | .50 .25 | .00 BIN | 1.0 .75 | .50 .25 | .00 BIN | 1.0 75 | .50 .25 | .00 BIN | 1.0 .75 | .50 .25 | .00 BIN |
| PCONT=*** | | REQUIRED NUMBER OF PATIENTS | | | | | | | | | | | | | | |
| 0.05 | *** | 132 | 134 | 141 | 78 | 79 | 82 | 55 | 56 | 58 | 43 | 44 | 45 | 36 | 36 | 37 |
| | *** | 133 | 137 | 217 | 79 | 80 | 115 | 56 | 57 | 73 | 44 | 44 | 51 | 36 | 37 | 38 |
| 0.1 | *** | 210 | 215 | 235 | 113 | 117 | 125 | 76 | 78 | 82 | 56 | 58 | 60 | 45 | 46 | 47 |
| | *** | 212 | 221 | 310 | 115 | 120 | 153 | 77 | 80 | 93 | 57 | 59 | 63 | 45 | 47 | 46 |
| 0.15 | *** | 272 | 281 | 323 | 141 | 147 | 163 | 91 | 95 | 103 | 66 | 69 | 73 | 51 | 53 | 56 |
| | *** | 276 | 292 | 390 | 143 | 153 | 186 | 93 | 98 | 110 | 67 | 70 | 73 | 52 | 54 | 52 |
| 0.2 | *** | 319 | 333 | 400 | 162 | 170 | 195 | 103 | 108 | 120 | 73 | 77 | 83 | 56 | 58 | 62 |
| | *** | 324 | 350 | 458 | 165 | 179 | 213 | 105 | 113 | 124 | 75 | 79 | 81 | 57 | 60 | 57 |
| 0.25 | *** | 352 | 370 | 466 | 176 | 188 | 222 | 111 | 118 | 134 | 78 | 83 | 91 | 59 | 62 | 67 |
| | *** | 358 | 393 | 514 | 181 | 199 | 235 | 114 | 124 | 135 | 80 | 86 | 87 | 61 | 64 | 60 |
| 0.3 | *** | 371 | 394 | 519 | 185 | 200 | 243 | 116 | 125 | 144 | 81 | 87 | 97 | 61 | 65 | 71 |
| | *** | 379 | 424 | 557 | 191 | 214 | 252 | 119 | 132 | 143 | 84 | 91 | 91 | 63 | 67 | 62 |
| 0.35 | *** | 378 | 407 | 559 | 189 | 206 | 259 | 118 | 128 | 151 | 82 | 89 | 100 | 62 | 66 | 72 |
| | *** | 389 | 444 | 588 | 196 | 223 | 263 | 122 | 137 | 147 | 85 | 93 | 93 | 63 | 69 | 63 |
| 0.4 | *** | 375 | 410 | 587 | 189 | 209 | 268 | 118 | 129 | 155 | 82 | 89 | 102 | 61 | 65 | 72 |
| | *** | 389 | 453 | 606 | 197 | 228 | 268 | 123 | 139 | 149 | 85 | 94 | 93 | 63 | 68 | 62 |
| 0.45 | *** | 365 | 405 | 600 | 185 | 207 | 271 | 116 | 128 | 155 | 80 | 87 | 101 | 59 | 64 | 71 |
| | *** | 380 | 453 | 613 | 194 | 228 | 268 | 121 | 138 | 147 | 83 | 93 | 91 | 61 | 67 | 60 |
| 0.5 | *** | 348 | 393 | 601 | 178 | 202 | 268 | 112 | 124 | 152 | 77 | 84 | 98 | 57 | 61 | 68 |
| | *** | 366 | 445 | 606 | 188 | 223 | 263 | 117 | 135 | 143 | 80 | 90 | 87 | 59 | 64 | 57 |
| 0.55 | *** | 327 | 376 | 587 | 169 | 193 | 259 | 106 | 118 | 145 | 73 | 80 | 92 | 53 | 57 | 64 |
| | *** | 346 | 429 | 588 | 179 | 215 | 252 | 111 | 129 | 135 | 76 | 85 | 81 | 55 | 60 | 52 |
| 0.6 | *** | 303 | 353 | 561 | 158 | 182 | 245 | 98 | 110 | 135 | 67 | 74 | 85 | 48 | 52 | 58 |
| | *** | 323 | 406 | 557 | 168 | 203 | 235 | 104 | 120 | 124 | 70 | 78 | 73 | 50 | 55 | 46 |
| 0.65 | *** | 276 | 325 | 521 | 145 | 167 | 224 | 89 | 100 | 122 | 60 | 66 | 75 | 43 | 46 | 51 |
| | *** | 296 | 377 | 514 | 154 | 186 | 213 | 94 | 109 | 110 | 63 | 70 | 63 | 44 | 48 | 38 |
| 0.7 | *** | 246 | 294 | 467 | 129 | 149 | 197 | 79 | 88 | 105 | 52 | 57 | 64 | . | . | . |
| | *** | 265 | 342 | 458 | 137 | 166 | 186 | 83 | 95 | 93 | 54 | 60 | 51 | . | . | . |
| 0.75 | *** | 214 | 257 | 401 | 111 | 127 | 165 | 66 | 73 | 85 | . | . | . | . | . | . |
| | *** | 232 | 299 | 390 | 118 | 141 | 153 | 69 | 78 | 73 | . | . | . | . | . | . |
| 0.8 | *** | 179 | 214 | 321 | 89 | 102 | 127 | . | . | . | . | . | . | . | . | . |
| | *** | 193 | 247 | 310 | 95 | 112 | 115 | . | . | . | . | . | . | . | . | . |
| 0.85 | *** | 138 | 163 | 229 | . | . | . | . | . | . | . | . | . | . | . | . |
| | *** | 148 | 186 | 217 | . | . | . | . | . | . | . | . | . | . | . | . |

TABLE 7: ALPHA= 0.05  POWER= 0.8    EXPECTED ACCRUAL THRU MINIMUM FOLLOW-UP= 100

| | | DEL=.10 | | | DEL=.15 | | | DEL=.20 | | | DEL=.25 | | | DEL=.30 | |
|---|---|---|---|---|---|---|---|---|---|---|---|---|---|---|---|
| FACT= | 1.0 .75 | .50 .25 | .00 BIN | 1.0 .75 | .50 .25 | .00 BIN | 1.0 .75 | .50 .25 | .00 BIN | 1.0 75 | .50 .25 | .00 BIN | 1.0 .75 | .50 .25 | .00 BIN |
| PCONT=*** | | | | REQUIRED NUMBER OF PATIENTS | | | | | | | | | | | |
| 0.05 *** | 133 | 135 | 141 | 78 | 80 | 82 | 56 | 56 | 58 | 43 | 44 | 45 | 36 | 36 | 37 |
| *** | 133 | 137 | 217 | 79 | 81 | 115 | 56 | 57 | 73 | 44 | 44 | 51 | 36 | 37 | 38 |
| 0.1 *** | 211 | 216 | 235 | 114 | 117 | 125 | 76 | 78 | 82 | 57 | 58 | 60 | 45 | 46 | 47 |
| *** | 213 | 222 | 310 | 115 | 120 | 153 | 77 | 80 | 93 | 57 | 59 | 63 | 45 | 47 | 46 |
| 0.15 *** | 273 | 283 | 323 | 142 | 148 | 163 | 92 | 95 | 103 | 67 | 69 | 73 | 52 | 53 | 56 |
| *** | 277 | 294 | 390 | 144 | 153 | 186 | 93 | 98 | 110 | 68 | 71 | 73 | 52 | 54 | 52 |
| 0.2 *** | 321 | 335 | 400 | 163 | 172 | 195 | 104 | 109 | 120 | 74 | 77 | 83 | 57 | 59 | 62 |
| *** | 326 | 352 | 458 | 167 | 180 | 213 | 106 | 113 | 124 | 75 | 80 | 81 | 58 | 60 | 57 |
| 0.25 *** | 354 | 373 | 466 | 178 | 190 | 222 | 112 | 119 | 134 | 79 | 83 | 91 | 60 | 63 | 67 |
| *** | 361 | 397 | 514 | 183 | 201 | 235 | 115 | 125 | 135 | 81 | 87 | 87 | 61 | 65 | 60 |
| 0.3 *** | 374 | 399 | 519 | 187 | 202 | 243 | 117 | 126 | 144 | 82 | 87 | 97 | 62 | 65 | 71 |
| *** | 383 | 429 | 557 | 193 | 216 | 252 | 121 | 133 | 143 | 84 | 91 | 91 | 63 | 68 | 62 |
| 0.35 *** | 382 | 413 | 559 | 191 | 209 | 259 | 120 | 130 | 151 | 83 | 90 | 100 | 62 | 66 | 72 |
| *** | 393 | 450 | 588 | 199 | 226 | 263 | 124 | 138 | 147 | 86 | 94 | 93 | 64 | 69 | 63 |
| 0.4 *** | 380 | 417 | 587 | 192 | 212 | 268 | 120 | 131 | 155 | 83 | 90 | 102 | 62 | 66 | 72 |
| *** | 394 | 460 | 606 | 200 | 231 | 268 | 124 | 140 | 149 | 86 | 95 | 93 | 64 | 69 | 62 |
| 0.45 *** | 370 | 412 | 600 | 188 | 210 | 271 | 118 | 130 | 155 | 81 | 88 | 101 | 60 | 64 | 71 |
| *** | 387 | 460 | 613 | 197 | 231 | 268 | 123 | 139 | 147 | 85 | 94 | 91 | 62 | 67 | 60 |
| 0.5 *** | 354 | 401 | 601 | 182 | 205 | 268 | 114 | 126 | 152 | 78 | 85 | 98 | 58 | 62 | 68 |
| *** | 373 | 452 | 606 | 192 | 227 | 263 | 119 | 136 | 143 | 82 | 91 | 87 | 59 | 65 | 57 |
| 0.55 *** | 334 | 384 | 587 | 173 | 197 | 260 | 108 | 120 | 145 | 74 | 81 | 92 | 54 | 58 | 64 |
| *** | 354 | 437 | 588 | 183 | 218 | 252 | 113 | 130 | 135 | 77 | 86 | 81 | 56 | 60 | 52 |
| 0.6 *** | 310 | 361 | 561 | 162 | 185 | 245 | 100 | 112 | 135 | 68 | 75 | 85 | 49 | 53 | 58 |
| *** | 330 | 414 | 557 | 171 | 206 | 235 | 105 | 121 | 124 | 71 | 79 | 73 | 51 | 55 | 46 |
| 0.65 *** | 283 | 333 | 521 | 148 | 170 | 224 | 91 | 102 | 122 | 61 | 67 | 75 | 43 | 46 | 51 |
| *** | 303 | 385 | 514 | 157 | 189 | 213 | 96 | 110 | 110 | 64 | 70 | 63 | 45 | 48 | 38 |
| 0.7 *** | 253 | 301 | 467 | 132 | 152 | 197 | 80 | 89 | 105 | 53 | 57 | 64 | . | . | . |
| *** | 273 | 349 | 458 | 140 | 168 | 186 | 84 | 96 | 93 | 55 | 60 | 51 | . | . | . |
| 0.75 *** | 221 | 263 | 401 | 113 | 130 | 165 | 67 | 74 | 85 | . | . | . | . | . | . |
| *** | 238 | 305 | 390 | 120 | 143 | 153 | 70 | 79 | 73 | . | . | . | . | . | . |
| 0.8 *** | 184 | 219 | 321 | 91 | 103 | 127 | . | . | . | . | . | . | . | . | . |
| *** | 199 | 252 | 310 | 97 | 113 | 115 | . | . | . | . | . | . | . | . | . |
| 0.85 *** | 142 | 167 | 229 | . | . | . | . | . | . | . | . | . | . | . | . |
| *** | 152 | 189 | 217 | . | . | . | . | . | . | . | . | . | . | . | . |

| TABLE 7: ALPHA= 0.05  POWER= 0.8 | | | EXPECTED ACCRUAL THRU MINIMUM FOLLOW-UP= 110 | | | | | | | | | | | |

| | | DEL=.05 | | | DEL=.10 | | | DEL=.15 | | | DEL=.20 | | | DEL=.25 | | |
|---|---|---|---|---|---|---|---|---|---|---|---|---|---|---|---|---|
| FACT= | | 1.0 .75 | .50 .25 | .00 BIN | 1.0 .75 | .50 .25 | .00 BIN | 1.0 .75 | .50 .25 | .00 BIN | 1.0 75 | .50 .25 | .00 BIN | 1.0 .75 | .50 .25 | .00 BIN |
| PCONT=*** | | | | | REQUIRED | NUMBER | OF PATIENTS | | | | | | | | | |
| 0.05 | *** | 371 | 374 | 395 | 133 | 135 | 141 | 78 | 80 | 82 | 56 | 56 | 58 | 43 | 44 | 45 |
| | *** | 372 | 378 | 681 | 134 | 137 | 217 | 79 | 81 | 115 | 56 | 57 | 73 | 44 | 44 | 51 |
| 0.1 | *** | 676 | 683 | 762 | 211 | 217 | 235 | 114 | 118 | 125 | 76 | 78 | 82 | 57 | 58 | 60 |
| | *** | 678 | 694 | 1076 | 213 | 223 | 310 | 116 | 121 | 153 | 77 | 80 | 93 | 57 | 59 | 63 |
| 0.15 | *** | 936 | 947 | 1117 | 274 | 284 | 323 | 143 | 149 | 163 | 92 | 96 | 103 | 67 | 69 | 73 |
| | *** | 940 | 967 | 1422 | 278 | 296 | 390 | 145 | 154 | 186 | 94 | 99 | 110 | 68 | 71 | 73 |
| 0.2 | *** | 1137 | 1154 | 1441 | 323 | 337 | 400 | 164 | 173 | 195 | 104 | 110 | 120 | 74 | 78 | 83 |
| | *** | 1143 | 1185 | 1719 | 328 | 355 | 458 | 168 | 181 | 213 | 107 | 114 | 124 | 76 | 80 | 81 |
| 0.25 | *** | 1278 | 1301 | 1724 | 356 | 376 | 466 | 179 | 191 | 222 | 113 | 120 | 134 | 80 | 84 | 91 |
| | *** | 1285 | 1345 | 1967 | 364 | 401 | 514 | 184 | 202 | 235 | 116 | 125 | 135 | 82 | 87 | 87 |
| 0.3 | *** | 1360 | 1391 | 1960 | 377 | 403 | 519 | 189 | 204 | 243 | 118 | 127 | 144 | 83 | 88 | 97 |
| | *** | 1370 | 1451 | 2164 | 386 | 434 | 557 | 195 | 218 | 252 | 122 | 134 | 143 | 85 | 92 | 91 |
| 0.35 | *** | 1389 | 1430 | 2147 | 385 | 417 | 559 | 194 | 212 | 259 | 121 | 131 | 151 | 84 | 90 | 100 |
| | *** | 1402 | 1508 | 2313 | 398 | 455 | 588 | 201 | 228 | 263 | 125 | 139 | 147 | 87 | 95 | 93 |
| 0.4 | *** | 1371 | 1425 | 2281 | 384 | 422 | 587 | 194 | 214 | 268 | 121 | 132 | 155 | 84 | 91 | 102 |
| | *** | 1389 | 1522 | 2412 | 399 | 466 | 606 | 203 | 233 | 268 | 126 | 141 | 149 | 87 | 95 | 93 |
| 0.45 | *** | 1315 | 1384 | 2362 | 375 | 419 | 600 | 191 | 213 | 271 | 119 | 131 | 155 | 83 | 89 | 101 |
| | *** | 1338 | 1502 | 2461 | 392 | 467 | 613 | 200 | 233 | 268 | 124 | 141 | 147 | 86 | 94 | 91 |
| 0.5 | *** | 1230 | 1315 | 2390 | 360 | 408 | 601 | 185 | 208 | 268 | 115 | 128 | 152 | 79 | 86 | 98 |
| | *** | 1259 | 1454 | 2461 | 379 | 459 | 606 | 195 | 229 | 263 | 121 | 137 | 143 | 82 | 91 | 87 |
| 0.55 | *** | 1123 | 1226 | 2363 | 340 | 391 | 587 | 176 | 200 | 259 | 110 | 122 | 145 | 75 | 82 | 92 |
| | *** | 1159 | 1384 | 2412 | 360 | 444 | 588 | 186 | 221 | 252 | 115 | 131 | 135 | 78 | 86 | 81 |
| 0.6 | *** | 1005 | 1126 | 2283 | 316 | 368 | 561 | 165 | 188 | 245 | 102 | 113 | 135 | 69 | 75 | 85 |
| | *** | 1049 | 1297 | 2313 | 337 | 422 | 557 | 175 | 208 | 235 | 107 | 122 | 124 | 72 | 79 | 73 |
| 0.65 | *** | 884 | 1018 | 2149 | 289 | 340 | 521 | 151 | 173 | 224 | 93 | 103 | 122 | 62 | 67 | 75 |
| | *** | 933 | 1197 | 2164 | 310 | 392 | 514 | 160 | 191 | 213 | 97 | 111 | 110 | 64 | 71 | 63 |
| 0.7 | *** | 765 | 906 | 1962 | 259 | 308 | 467 | 135 | 154 | 197 | 82 | 90 | 105 | 53 | 58 | 64 |
| | *** | 818 | 1084 | 1967 | 279 | 355 | 458 | 143 | 170 | 186 | 85 | 97 | 93 | 55 | 60 | 51 |
| 0.75 | *** | 651 | 791 | 1722 | 226 | 269 | 401 | 116 | 132 | 165 | 68 | 75 | 85 | . | . | . |
| | *** | 705 | 959 | 1719 | 244 | 310 | 390 | 123 | 145 | 153 | 71 | 79 | 73 | . | . | . |
| 0.8 | *** | 541 | 670 | 1431 | 189 | 224 | 321 | 93 | 105 | 127 | . | . | . | . | . | . |
| | *** | 591 | 819 | 1422 | 204 | 256 | 310 | 98 | 114 | 115 | . | . | . | . | . | . |
| 0.85 | *** | 430 | 539 | 1087 | 145 | 170 | 229 | . | . | . | . | . | . | . | . | . |
| | *** | 473 | 659 | 1076 | 156 | 191 | 217 | . | . | . | . | . | . | . | . | . |
| 0.9 | *** | 310 | 386 | 693 | . | . | . | . | . | . | . | . | . | . | . | . |
| | *** | 340 | 465 | 681 | . | . | . | . | . | . | . | . | . | . | . | . |

TABLE 7: ALPHA= 0.05  POWER= 0.8    EXPECTED ACCRUAL THRU MINIMUM FOLLOW-UP= 120

| | | DEL=.05 | | | DEL=.10 | | | DEL=.15 | | | DEL=.20 | | | DEL=.25 | | |
|---|---|---|---|---|---|---|---|---|---|---|---|---|---|---|---|---|---|
| FACT= | | 1.0 .75 | .50 .25 | .00 BIN | 1.0 .75 | .50 .25 | .00 BIN | 1.0 .75 | .50 .25 | .00 BIN | 1.0 75 | .50 .25 | .00 BIN | 1.0 .75 | .50 .25 | .00 BIN |
| PCONT=*** | | REQUIRED NUMBER OF PATIENTS | | | | | | | | | | | | | | |
| 0.05 | *** | 371 | 374 | 395 | 133 | 135 | 141 | 79 | 80 | 82 | 56 | 57 | 58 | 43 | 44 | 45 |
| | *** | 372 | 379 | 681 | 134 | 137 | 217 | 79 | 81 | 115 | 56 | 57 | 73 | 44 | 44 | 51 |
| 0.1 | *** | 677 | 684 | 762 | 212 | 217 | 235 | 115 | 118 | 125 | 77 | 79 | 82 | 57 | 58 | 60 |
| | *** | 679 | 696 | 1076 | 214 | 223 | 310 | 116 | 121 | 153 | 78 | 80 | 93 | 58 | 59 | 63 |
| 0.15 | *** | 937 | 949 | 1117 | 276 | 286 | 323 | 143 | 149 | 163 | 93 | 96 | 103 | 67 | 69 | 73 |
| | *** | 941 | 971 | 1422 | 279 | 297 | 390 | 146 | 154 | 186 | 94 | 99 | 110 | 68 | 71 | 73 |
| 0.2 | *** | 1139 | 1157 | 1441 | 324 | 339 | 400 | 165 | 174 | 195 | 105 | 110 | 120 | 75 | 78 | 83 |
| | *** | 1145 | 1190 | 1719 | 330 | 357 | 458 | 169 | 182 | 213 | 107 | 114 | 124 | 76 | 80 | 81 |
| 0.25 | *** | 1280 | 1305 | 1724 | 358 | 379 | 466 | 181 | 193 | 222 | 114 | 121 | 134 | 80 | 84 | 91 |
| | *** | 1288 | 1353 | 1967 | 366 | 404 | 514 | 186 | 203 | 235 | 117 | 126 | 135 | 82 | 87 | 87 |
| 0.3 | *** | 1363 | 1397 | 1960 | 379 | 406 | 519 | 191 | 206 | 243 | 119 | 128 | 144 | 84 | 89 | 97 |
| | *** | 1374 | 1461 | 2164 | 390 | 437 | 557 | 197 | 219 | 252 | 123 | 134 | 143 | 86 | 92 | 91 |
| 0.35 | *** | 1392 | 1438 | 2147 | 389 | 422 | 559 | 196 | 214 | 259 | 122 | 132 | 151 | 85 | 91 | 100 |
| | *** | 1408 | 1521 | 2313 | 402 | 460 | 588 | 203 | 230 | 263 | 127 | 140 | 147 | 88 | 95 | 93 |
| 0.4 | *** | 1376 | 1435 | 2281 | 389 | 428 | 587 | 197 | 217 | 268 | 123 | 134 | 155 | 85 | 91 | 102 |
| | *** | 1396 | 1538 | 2412 | 404 | 471 | 606 | 205 | 235 | 268 | 127 | 142 | 149 | 88 | 96 | 93 |
| 0.45 | *** | 1322 | 1396 | 2362 | 380 | 425 | 600 | 194 | 216 | 271 | 121 | 132 | 155 | 83 | 90 | 101 |
| | *** | 1347 | 1521 | 2461 | 398 | 473 | 613 | 203 | 235 | 268 | 126 | 141 | 147 | 86 | 95 | 91 |
| 0.5 | *** | 1238 | 1329 | 2390 | 366 | 414 | 601 | 188 | 211 | 268 | 117 | 129 | 152 | 80 | 87 | 98 |
| | *** | 1269 | 1475 | 2461 | 385 | 466 | 606 | 198 | 231 | 263 | 122 | 138 | 143 | 83 | 91 | 87 |
| 0.55 | *** | 1133 | 1243 | 2363 | 346 | 397 | 587 | 179 | 203 | 259 | 111 | 123 | 145 | 76 | 82 | 92 |
| | *** | 1172 | 1407 | 2412 | 367 | 451 | 588 | 189 | 223 | 252 | 116 | 132 | 135 | 79 | 87 | 81 |
| 0.6 | *** | 1017 | 1145 | 2283 | 323 | 375 | 561 | 168 | 191 | 245 | 104 | 115 | 135 | 70 | 76 | 85 |
| | *** | 1064 | 1322 | 2313 | 344 | 428 | 557 | 178 | 210 | 235 | 109 | 123 | 124 | 73 | 80 | 73 |
| 0.65 | *** | 898 | 1038 | 2149 | 296 | 347 | 521 | 154 | 175 | 224 | 94 | 104 | 122 | 63 | 68 | 75 |
| | *** | 950 | 1222 | 2164 | 317 | 398 | 514 | 163 | 193 | 213 | 99 | 111 | 110 | 65 | 71 | 63 |
| 0.7 | *** | 780 | 927 | 1962 | 265 | 314 | 467 | 137 | 157 | 197 | 83 | 91 | 105 | 54 | 58 | 64 |
| | *** | 836 | 1108 | 1967 | 285 | 360 | 458 | 146 | 172 | 186 | 86 | 97 | 93 | 56 | 61 | 51 |
| 0.75 | *** | 666 | 810 | 1722 | 232 | 275 | 401 | 118 | 134 | 165 | 69 | 75 | 85 | . | . | . |
| | *** | 722 | 981 | 1719 | 249 | 315 | 390 | 125 | 146 | 153 | 72 | 80 | 73 | . | . | . |
| 0.8 | *** | 556 | 688 | 1430 | 193 | 228 | 321 | 95 | 106 | 127 | . | . | . | . | . | . |
| | *** | 607 | 839 | 1422 | 208 | 260 | 310 | 100 | 115 | 115 | . | . | . | . | . | . |
| 0.85 | *** | 443 | 553 | 1087 | 148 | 173 | 229 | . | . | . | . | . | . | . | . | . |
| | *** | 487 | 674 | 1076 | 159 | 193 | 217 | . | . | . | . | . | . | . | . | . |
| 0.9 | *** | 319 | 396 | 693 | . | . | . | . | . | . | . | . | . | . | . | . |
| | *** | 350 | 475 | 681 | . | . | . | . | . | . | . | . | . | . | . | . |

## TABLE 7: ALPHA= 0.05  POWER= 0.8    EXPECTED ACCRUAL THRU MINIMUM FOLLOW-UP= 130

| | | DEL=.05 | | | DEL=.10 | | | DEL=.15 | | | DEL=.20 | | | DEL=.25 | | |
|---|---|---|---|---|---|---|---|---|---|---|---|---|---|---|---|---|
| FACT= | | 1.0 .75 | .50 .25 | .00 BIN | 1.0 .75 | .50 .25 | .00 BIN | 1.0 .75 | .50 .25 | .00 BIN | 1.0 75 | .50 .25 | .00 BIN | 1.0 .75 | .50 .25 | .00 BIN |
| PCONT=*** | | | | | | REQUIRED | NUMBER | OF PATIENTS | | | | | | | | |
| 0.05 | *** | 371 | 375 | 395 | 133 | 136 | 141 | 79 | 80 | 82 | 56 | 57 | 58 | 44 | 44 | 45 |
| | *** | 373 | 380 | 681 | 134 | 138 | 217 | 79 | 81 | 115 | 56 | 57 | 73 | 44 | 44 | 51 |
| 0.1 | *** | 678 | 685 | 762 | 212 | 218 | 235 | 115 | 119 | 125 | 77 | 79 | 82 | 57 | 58 | 60 |
| | *** | 680 | 698 | 1076 | 215 | 224 | 310 | 117 | 121 | 153 | 78 | 80 | 93 | 58 | 59 | 63 |
| 0.15 | *** | 938 | 951 | 1117 | 277 | 287 | 323 | 144 | 150 | 163 | 93 | 97 | 103 | 67 | 70 | 73 |
| | *** | 942 | 974 | 1422 | 281 | 298 | 390 | 147 | 155 | 186 | 95 | 99 | 110 | 68 | 71 | 73 |
| 0.2 | *** | 1140 | 1159 | 1441 | 326 | 341 | 400 | 166 | 175 | 195 | 106 | 111 | 120 | 75 | 78 | 83 |
| | *** | 1147 | 1196 | 1719 | 332 | 359 | 458 | 170 | 183 | 213 | 108 | 115 | 124 | 77 | 80 | 81 |
| 0.25 | *** | 1282 | 1309 | 1724 | 360 | 382 | 466 | 182 | 194 | 222 | 115 | 121 | 134 | 81 | 85 | 91 |
| | *** | 1291 | 1360 | 1967 | 369 | 406 | 514 | 187 | 205 | 235 | 118 | 126 | 135 | 83 | 88 | 87 |
| 0.3 | *** | 1365 | 1402 | 1960 | 382 | 410 | 519 | 192 | 207 | 243 | 120 | 129 | 144 | 84 | 89 | 97 |
| | *** | 1378 | 1471 | 2164 | 393 | 441 | 557 | 199 | 221 | 252 | 124 | 135 | 143 | 87 | 93 | 91 |
| 0.35 | *** | 1396 | 1445 | 2147 | 392 | 426 | 559 | 198 | 216 | 259 | 124 | 133 | 151 | 86 | 91 | 100 |
| | *** | 1413 | 1533 | 2313 | 405 | 464 | 588 | 205 | 231 | 263 | 128 | 140 | 147 | 88 | 95 | 93 |
| 0.4 | *** | 1381 | 1444 | 2281 | 393 | 433 | 587 | 199 | 219 | 268 | 124 | 135 | 155 | 86 | 92 | 102 |
| | *** | 1402 | 1553 | 2412 | 408 | 476 | 606 | 208 | 237 | 268 | 129 | 143 | 149 | 89 | 96 | 93 |
| 0.45 | *** | 1328 | 1407 | 2362 | 385 | 430 | 600 | 197 | 218 | 271 | 122 | 134 | 155 | 84 | 91 | 101 |
| | *** | 1355 | 1538 | 2461 | 403 | 478 | 613 | 206 | 237 | 268 | 127 | 142 | 147 | 87 | 95 | 91 |
| 0.5 | *** | 1246 | 1343 | 2390 | 371 | 420 | 601 | 191 | 214 | 268 | 119 | 130 | 152 | 81 | 88 | 98 |
| | *** | 1280 | 1495 | 2461 | 391 | 472 | 606 | 200 | 233 | 263 | 124 | 139 | 143 | 84 | 92 | 87 |
| 0.55 | *** | 1143 | 1260 | 2363 | 352 | 404 | 587 | 182 | 205 | 259 | 113 | 124 | 145 | 77 | 83 | 92 |
| | *** | 1185 | 1429 | 2412 | 373 | 457 | 588 | 192 | 225 | 252 | 118 | 133 | 135 | 80 | 87 | 81 |
| 0.6 | *** | 1029 | 1163 | 2283 | 328 | 381 | 561 | 171 | 193 | 245 | 105 | 116 | 135 | 71 | 76 | 85 |
| | *** | 1078 | 1345 | 2313 | 350 | 434 | 557 | 180 | 212 | 235 | 110 | 124 | 124 | 73 | 80 | 73 |
| 0.65 | *** | 911 | 1058 | 2149 | 301 | 353 | 521 | 156 | 178 | 224 | 95 | 105 | 122 | 63 | 68 | 75 |
| | *** | 966 | 1245 | 2164 | 323 | 403 | 514 | 166 | 195 | 213 | 100 | 112 | 110 | 66 | 71 | 63 |
| 0.7 | *** | 795 | 946 | 1962 | 271 | 319 | 467 | 140 | 158 | 197 | 84 | 92 | 105 | 55 | 58 | 64 |
| | *** | 853 | 1131 | 1967 | 291 | 365 | 458 | 148 | 173 | 186 | 87 | 98 | 93 | 56 | 61 | 51 |
| 0.75 | *** | 681 | 829 | 1722 | 237 | 279 | 401 | 120 | 135 | 165 | 70 | 76 | 85 | . | . | . |
| | *** | 739 | 1002 | 1719 | 254 | 319 | 390 | 127 | 147 | 153 | 73 | 80 | 73 | . | . | . |
| 0.8 | *** | 570 | 704 | 1431 | 197 | 232 | 321 | 96 | 107 | 127 | . | . | . | . | . | . |
| | *** | 623 | 857 | 1422 | 212 | 263 | 310 | 101 | 115 | 115 | . | . | . | . | . | . |
| 0.85 | *** | 455 | 567 | 1087 | 151 | 176 | 229 | . | . | . | . | . | . | . | . | . |
| | *** | 500 | 688 | 1076 | 162 | 196 | 217 | . | . | . | . | . | . | . | . | . |
| 0.9 | *** | 327 | 405 | 693 | . | . | . | . | . | . | . | . | . | . | . | . |
| | *** | 359 | 484 | 681 | . | . | . | . | . | . | . | . | . | . | . | . |

TABLE 7: ALPHA= 0.05  POWER= 0.8     EXPECTED ACCRUAL THRU MINIMUM FOLLOW-UP= 140

| | | DEL=.05 | | | DEL=.10 | | | DEL=.15 | | | DEL=.20 | | | DEL=.25 | | |
|---|---|---|---|---|---|---|---|---|---|---|---|---|---|---|---|---|---|
| FACT= | | 1.0 .75 | .50 .25 | .00 BIN | 1.0 .75 | .50 .25 | .00 BIN | 1.0 .75 | .50 .25 | .00 BIN | 1.0 75 | .50 .25 | .00 BIN | 1.0 .75 | .50 .25 | .00 BIN |
| PCONT=*** | | | | | REQUIRED | NUMBER OF | PATIENTS | | | | | | | | | |
| 0.05 | *** | 372 | 375 | 395 | 134 | 136 | 141 | 79 | 80 | 82 | 56 | 57 | 58 | 44 | 44 | 45 |
| | *** | 373 | 380 | 681 | 134 | 138 | 217 | 79 | 81 | 115 | 56 | 57 | 73 | 44 | 44 | 51 |
| 0.1 | *** | 678 | 686 | 762 | 213 | 219 | 235 | 116 | 119 | 125 | 77 | 79 | 82 | 57 | 59 | 60 |
| | *** | 681 | 700 | 1076 | 215 | 225 | 310 | 117 | 121 | 153 | 78 | 80 | 93 | 58 | 59 | 63 |
| 0.15 | *** | 939 | 953 | 1117 | 278 | 288 | 323 | 145 | 151 | 163 | 94 | 97 | 103 | 68 | 70 | 73 |
| | *** | 944 | 978 | 1422 | 282 | 299 | 390 | 147 | 155 | 186 | 95 | 99 | 110 | 69 | 71 | 73 |
| 0.2 | *** | 1142 | 1162 | 1441 | 327 | 343 | 400 | 167 | 176 | 195 | 106 | 111 | 120 | 76 | 79 | 83 |
| | *** | 1149 | 1201 | 1719 | 333 | 361 | 458 | 171 | 183 | 213 | 109 | 115 | 124 | 77 | 81 | 81 |
| 0.25 | *** | 1284 | 1313 | 1724 | 363 | 385 | 466 | 183 | 195 | 222 | 115 | 122 | 134 | 81 | 85 | 91 |
| | *** | 1294 | 1367 | 1967 | 371 | 409 | 514 | 188 | 205 | 235 | 118 | 127 | 135 | 83 | 88 | 87 |
| 0.3 | *** | 1368 | 1408 | 1960 | 385 | 413 | 519 | 194 | 209 | 243 | 121 | 130 | 144 | 85 | 90 | 97 |
| | *** | 1382 | 1480 | 2164 | 396 | 444 | 557 | 200 | 222 | 252 | 125 | 136 | 143 | 87 | 93 | 91 |
| 0.35 | *** | 1400 | 1452 | 2147 | 396 | 430 | 559 | 200 | 218 | 259 | 125 | 134 | 151 | 87 | 92 | 100 |
| | *** | 1418 | 1545 | 2313 | 409 | 468 | 588 | 207 | 233 | 263 | 129 | 141 | 147 | 89 | 96 | 93 |
| 0.4 | *** | 1386 | 1453 | 2281 | 396 | 437 | 587 | 201 | 221 | 268 | 125 | 136 | 155 | 87 | 92 | 102 |
| | *** | 1409 | 1568 | 2412 | 413 | 480 | 606 | 210 | 238 | 268 | 130 | 144 | 149 | 89 | 97 | 93 |
| 0.45 | *** | 1334 | 1419 | 2362 | 389 | 435 | 600 | 199 | 221 | 271 | 124 | 135 | 155 | 85 | 91 | 101 |
| | *** | 1363 | 1555 | 2461 | 408 | 483 | 613 | 208 | 239 | 268 | 129 | 143 | 147 | 88 | 95 | 91 |
| 0.5 | *** | 1254 | 1357 | 2390 | 376 | 426 | 601 | 193 | 216 | 268 | 120 | 131 | 152 | 82 | 88 | 98 |
| | *** | 1290 | 1514 | 2461 | 396 | 477 | 606 | 203 | 235 | 263 | 125 | 140 | 143 | 85 | 92 | 87 |
| 0.55 | *** | 1153 | 1275 | 2363 | 357 | 409 | 587 | 185 | 208 | 260 | 114 | 125 | 145 | 77 | 83 | 92 |
| | *** | 1197 | 1450 | 2412 | 378 | 462 | 588 | 194 | 227 | 252 | 119 | 133 | 135 | 80 | 87 | 81 |
| 0.6 | *** | 1041 | 1180 | 2283 | 334 | 387 | 561 | 173 | 195 | 245 | 106 | 117 | 135 | 71 | 77 | 85 |
| | *** | 1092 | 1366 | 2313 | 356 | 439 | 557 | 183 | 214 | 235 | 111 | 125 | 124 | 74 | 80 | 73 |
| 0.65 | *** | 925 | 1076 | 2149 | 307 | 359 | 521 | 159 | 180 | 224 | 97 | 106 | 122 | 64 | 69 | 75 |
| | *** | 982 | 1267 | 2164 | 328 | 408 | 514 | 168 | 197 | 213 | 101 | 113 | 110 | 66 | 72 | 63 |
| 0.7 | *** | 809 | 964 | 1962 | 276 | 324 | 467 | 142 | 160 | 197 | 85 | 93 | 105 | 55 | 59 | 64 |
| | *** | 869 | 1152 | 1967 | 296 | 370 | 458 | 150 | 175 | 186 | 88 | 98 | 93 | 57 | 61 | 51 |
| 0.75 | *** | 696 | 846 | 1722 | 241 | 284 | 401 | 122 | 137 | 165 | 71 | 76 | 85 | . | . | . |
| | *** | 755 | 1022 | 1719 | 259 | 323 | 390 | 128 | 148 | 153 | 73 | 80 | 73 | . | . | . |
| 0.8 | *** | 583 | 720 | 1430 | 201 | 236 | 321 | 98 | 108 | 127 | . | . | . | . | . | . |
| | *** | 637 | 874 | 1422 | 216 | 266 | 310 | 102 | 116 | 115 | . | . | . | . | . | . |
| 0.85 | *** | 466 | 580 | 1087 | 154 | 178 | 229 | . | . | . | . | . | . | . | . | . |
| | *** | 512 | 701 | 1076 | 165 | 197 | 217 | . | . | . | . | . | . | . | . | . |
| 0.9 | *** | 335 | 413 | 693 | . | . | . | . | . | . | . | . | . | . | . | . |
| | *** | 367 | 492 | 681 | . | . | . | . | . | . | . | . | . | . | . | . |

TABLE 7: ALPHA= 0.05  POWER= 0.8     EXPECTED ACCRUAL THRU MINIMUM FOLLOW-UP= 150

| | | DEL=.05 | | | DEL=.10 | | | DEL=.15 | | | DEL=.20 | | | DEL=.25 | | |
|---|---|---|---|---|---|---|---|---|---|---|---|---|---|---|---|---|
| FACT= | | 1.0 .75 | .50 .25 | .00 BIN | 1.0 .75 | .50 .25 | .00 BIN | 1.0 .75 | .50 .25 | .00 BIN | 1.0 75 | .50 .25 | .00 BIN | 1.0 .75 | .50 .25 | .00 BIN |
| PCONT=*** | | REQUIRED NUMBER OF PATIENTS | | | | | | | | | | | | | | |
| 0.05 | *** | 372 | 376 | 395 | 134 | 136 | 141 | 79 | 80 | 82 | 56 | 57 | 58 | 44 | 44 | 45 |
| | *** | 373 | 381 | 681 | 135 | 138 | 217 | 80 | 81 | 115 | 56 | 57 | 73 | 44 | 44 | 51 |
| 0.1 | *** | 679 | 687 | 762 | 213 | 219 | 235 | 116 | 119 | 125 | 77 | 79 | 82 | 57 | 59 | 60 |
| | *** | 682 | 702 | 1076 | 216 | 225 | 310 | 117 | 122 | 153 | 78 | 80 | 93 | 58 | 59 | 63 |
| 0.15 | *** | 940 | 955 | 1117 | 278 | 289 | 323 | 145 | 151 | 163 | 94 | 97 | 103 | 68 | 70 | 73 |
| | *** | 945 | 981 | 1422 | 283 | 300 | 390 | 148 | 156 | 186 | 95 | 100 | 110 | 69 | 71 | 73 |
| 0.2 | *** | 1143 | 1165 | 1441 | 329 | 345 | 400 | 168 | 177 | 195 | 107 | 112 | 120 | 76 | 79 | 83 |
| | *** | 1151 | 1205 | 1719 | 335 | 362 | 458 | 172 | 184 | 213 | 109 | 115 | 124 | 77 | 81 | 81 |
| 0.25 | *** | 1286 | 1317 | 1724 | 364 | 387 | 466 | 185 | 196 | 222 | 116 | 123 | 134 | 82 | 85 | 91 |
| | *** | 1297 | 1374 | 1967 | 373 | 411 | 514 | 190 | 206 | 235 | 119 | 127 | 135 | 83 | 88 | 87 |
| 0.3 | *** | 1371 | 1414 | 1960 | 387 | 416 | 519 | 196 | 210 | 243 | 122 | 130 | 144 | 85 | 90 | 97 |
| | *** | 1385 | 1489 | 2164 | 399 | 447 | 557 | 202 | 223 | 252 | 126 | 136 | 143 | 87 | 93 | 91 |
| 0.35 | *** | 1404 | 1460 | 2147 | 399 | 434 | 559 | 202 | 219 | 259 | 126 | 135 | 151 | 87 | 92 | 100 |
| | *** | 1423 | 1556 | 2313 | 413 | 471 | 588 | 209 | 234 | 263 | 130 | 142 | 147 | 90 | 96 | 93 |
| 0.4 | *** | 1391 | 1462 | 2281 | 400 | 442 | 587 | 203 | 223 | 268 | 126 | 137 | 155 | 87 | 93 | 102 |
| | *** | 1415 | 1582 | 2412 | 417 | 485 | 606 | 212 | 240 | 268 | 131 | 144 | 149 | 90 | 97 | 93 |
| 0.45 | *** | 1341 | 1430 | 2362 | 394 | 440 | 600 | 201 | 223 | 271 | 125 | 136 | 155 | 86 | 92 | 101 |
| | *** | 1372 | 1571 | 2461 | 412 | 488 | 613 | 210 | 241 | 268 | 130 | 144 | 147 | 88 | 96 | 91 |
| 0.5 | *** | 1261 | 1370 | 2390 | 381 | 431 | 601 | 196 | 218 | 268 | 121 | 132 | 152 | 83 | 89 | 98 |
| | *** | 1300 | 1532 | 2461 | 401 | 482 | 606 | 205 | 237 | 263 | 126 | 140 | 143 | 85 | 93 | 87 |
| 0.55 | *** | 1163 | 1291 | 2363 | 362 | 415 | 587 | 187 | 210 | 259 | 115 | 126 | 145 | 78 | 84 | 92 |
| | *** | 1209 | 1469 | 2412 | 383 | 467 | 588 | 197 | 228 | 252 | 120 | 134 | 135 | 81 | 88 | 81 |
| 0.6 | *** | 1052 | 1197 | 2283 | 339 | 392 | 561 | 175 | 198 | 245 | 107 | 118 | 135 | 72 | 77 | 85 |
| | *** | 1106 | 1387 | 2313 | 361 | 444 | 557 | 185 | 215 | 235 | 112 | 125 | 124 | 74 | 81 | 73 |
| 0.65 | *** | 938 | 1093 | 2149 | 312 | 364 | 521 | 161 | 182 | 224 | 98 | 107 | 122 | 65 | 69 | 75 |
| | *** | 997 | 1287 | 2164 | 333 | 413 | 514 | 170 | 198 | 213 | 102 | 113 | 110 | 67 | 72 | 63 |
| 0.7 | *** | 823 | 982 | 1962 | 281 | 329 | 467 | 144 | 162 | 197 | 86 | 93 | 105 | 55 | 59 | 64 |
| | *** | 884 | 1172 | 1967 | 301 | 374 | 458 | 152 | 176 | 186 | 89 | 98 | 93 | 57 | 61 | 51 |
| 0.75 | *** | 709 | 863 | 1722 | 245 | 288 | 401 | 123 | 138 | 165 | 71 | 77 | 85 | . | . | . |
| | *** | 770 | 1040 | 1719 | 263 | 326 | 390 | 130 | 149 | 153 | 74 | 81 | 73 | . | . | . |
| 0.8 | *** | 595 | 735 | 1430 | 205 | 239 | 321 | 99 | 109 | 127 | . | . | . | . | . | . |
| | *** | 651 | 889 | 1422 | 219 | 268 | 310 | 103 | 117 | 115 | . | . | . | . | . | . |
| 0.85 | *** | 477 | 592 | 1087 | 157 | 180 | 229 | . | . | . | . | . | . | . | . | . |
| | *** | 523 | 713 | 1076 | 167 | 199 | 217 | . | . | . | . | . | . | . | . | . |
| 0.9 | *** | 343 | 421 | 693 | . | . | . | . | . | . | . | . | . | . | . | . |
| | *** | 375 | 499 | 681 | . | . | . | . | . | . | . | . | . | . | . | . |

TABLE 7: ALPHA= 0.05  POWER= 0.8    EXPECTED ACCRUAL THRU MINIMUM FOLLOW-UP= 160

| | | DEL=.05 | | | DEL=.10 | | | DEL=.15 | | | DEL=.20 | | | DEL=.25 | | |
|---|---|---|---|---|---|---|---|---|---|---|---|---|---|---|---|---|---|
| FACT= | | 1.0 .75 | .50 .25 | .00 BIN | 1.0 .75 | .50 .25 | .00 BIN | 1.0 .75 | .50 .25 | .00 BIN | 1.0 75 | .50 .25 | .00 BIN | 1.0 .75 | .50 .25 | .00 BIN |
| PCONT=*** | | | | | | | REQUIRED NUMBER OF PATIENTS | | | | | | | | | |
| 0.05 | *** | 372 | 376 | 395 | 134 | 136 | 141 | 79 | 80 | 82 | 56 | 57 | 58 | 44 | 44 | 45 |
| | *** | 374 | 381 | 681 | 135 | 138 | 217 | 80 | 81 | 115 | 56 | 57 | 73 | 44 | 45 | 51 |
| 0.1 | *** | 679 | 688 | 762 | 214 | 220 | 235 | 116 | 119 | 125 | 78 | 79 | 82 | 58 | 59 | 60 |
| | *** | 682 | 703 | 1076 | 216 | 226 | 310 | 118 | 122 | 153 | 78 | 81 | 93 | 58 | 59 | 63 |
| 0.15 | *** | 941 | 956 | 1117 | 279 | 290 | 323 | 146 | 152 | 163 | 94 | 98 | 103 | 68 | 70 | 73 |
| | *** | 946 | 984 | 1422 | 284 | 301 | 390 | 148 | 156 | 186 | 96 | 100 | 110 | 69 | 71 | 73 |
| 0.2 | *** | 1145 | 1168 | 1441 | 330 | 347 | 400 | 169 | 178 | 195 | 107 | 112 | 120 | 76 | 79 | 83 |
| | *** | 1153 | 1210 | 1719 | 337 | 364 | 458 | 173 | 185 | 213 | 109 | 115 | 124 | 78 | 81 | 81 |
| 0.25 | *** | 1288 | 1322 | 1724 | 366 | 389 | 466 | 186 | 198 | 222 | 117 | 123 | 134 | 82 | 86 | 91 |
| | *** | 1299 | 1381 | 1967 | 375 | 413 | 514 | 191 | 207 | 235 | 120 | 128 | 135 | 84 | 88 | 87 |
| 0.3 | *** | 1374 | 1419 | 1960 | 390 | 419 | 519 | 197 | 212 | 243 | 123 | 131 | 144 | 86 | 90 | 97 |
| | *** | 1389 | 1498 | 2164 | 401 | 450 | 557 | 203 | 224 | 252 | 127 | 136 | 143 | 88 | 93 | 91 |
| 0.35 | *** | 1408 | 1467 | 2147 | 402 | 437 | 559 | 203 | 221 | 259 | 127 | 136 | 151 | 88 | 93 | 100 |
| | *** | 1428 | 1567 | 2313 | 416 | 475 | 588 | 211 | 235 | 263 | 131 | 142 | 147 | 90 | 96 | 93 |
| 0.4 | *** | 1396 | 1472 | 2281 | 404 | 446 | 587 | 205 | 225 | 268 | 127 | 137 | 155 | 88 | 93 | 102 |
| | *** | 1422 | 1595 | 2412 | 420 | 488 | 606 | 214 | 241 | 268 | 132 | 145 | 149 | 90 | 97 | 93 |
| 0.45 | *** | 1347 | 1441 | 2362 | 398 | 445 | 600 | 203 | 225 | 271 | 126 | 137 | 155 | 86 | 92 | 101 |
| | *** | 1380 | 1587 | 2461 | 417 | 492 | 613 | 212 | 242 | 268 | 131 | 144 | 147 | 89 | 96 | 91 |
| 0.5 | *** | 1269 | 1383 | 2390 | 385 | 436 | 601 | 198 | 220 | 268 | 122 | 133 | 152 | 83 | 89 | 98 |
| | *** | 1310 | 1550 | 2461 | 406 | 486 | 606 | 207 | 238 | 263 | 127 | 141 | 143 | 86 | 93 | 87 |
| 0.55 | *** | 1172 | 1305 | 2363 | 367 | 420 | 587 | 189 | 212 | 260 | 116 | 127 | 145 | 79 | 84 | 92 |
| | *** | 1221 | 1488 | 2412 | 388 | 471 | 588 | 199 | 230 | 252 | 121 | 135 | 135 | 81 | 88 | 81 |
| 0.6 | *** | 1064 | 1213 | 2283 | 344 | 397 | 561 | 178 | 199 | 245 | 109 | 119 | 135 | 73 | 78 | 85 |
| | *** | 1119 | 1406 | 2313 | 366 | 448 | 557 | 187 | 217 | 235 | 113 | 126 | 124 | 75 | 81 | 73 |
| 0.65 | *** | 950 | 1110 | 2149 | 317 | 369 | 521 | 163 | 183 | 224 | 99 | 108 | 122 | 65 | 69 | 75 |
| | *** | 1011 | 1306 | 2164 | 338 | 417 | 514 | 172 | 199 | 213 | 103 | 114 | 110 | 67 | 72 | 63 |
| 0.7 | *** | 836 | 998 | 1962 | 285 | 334 | 467 | 146 | 163 | 197 | 86 | 94 | 105 | 56 | 59 | 64 |
| | *** | 899 | 1190 | 1967 | 305 | 378 | 458 | 153 | 177 | 186 | 90 | 99 | 93 | 57 | 61 | 51 |
| 0.75 | *** | 722 | 879 | 1722 | 249 | 292 | 401 | 125 | 139 | 165 | 72 | 77 | 85 | . | . | . |
| | *** | 784 | 1057 | 1719 | 267 | 329 | 390 | 131 | 150 | 153 | 74 | 81 | 73 | . | . | . |
| 0.8 | *** | 608 | 749 | 1431 | 208 | 242 | 321 | 100 | 110 | 127 | . | . | . | . | . | . |
| | *** | 664 | 904 | 1422 | 223 | 271 | 310 | 104 | 117 | 115 | . | . | . | . | . | . |
| 0.85 | *** | 487 | 603 | 1087 | 159 | 182 | 229 | . | . | . | . | . | . | . | . | . |
| | *** | 533 | 725 | 1076 | 169 | 200 | 217 | . | . | . | . | . | . | . | . | . |
| 0.9 | *** | 350 | 429 | 693 | . | . | . | . | . | . | . | . | . | . | . | . |
| | *** | 382 | 506 | 681 | . | . | . | . | . | . | . | . | . | . | . | . |

## TABLE 7: ALPHA= 0.05  POWER= 0.8    EXPECTED ACCRUAL THRU MINIMUM FOLLOW-UP= 170

|  | | DEL=.05 | | | DEL=.10 | | | DEL=.15 | | | DEL=.20 | | | DEL=.25 | | |
|---|---|---|---|---|---|---|---|---|---|---|---|---|---|---|---|---|---|
| FACT= | | 1.0 .75 | .50 .25 | .00 BIN | 1.0 .75 | .50 .25 | .00 BIN | 1.0 .75 | .50 .25 | .00 BIN | 1.0 75 | .50 .25 | .00 BIN | 1.0 .75 | .50 .25 | .00 BIN |
| PCONT=*** | | | | | | | REQUIRED NUMBER OF PATIENTS | | | | | | | | | |
| 0.05 | *** | 372 | 376 | 395 | 134 | 136 | 141 | 79 | 80 | 82 | 56 | 57 | 58 | 44 | 44 | 45 |
|  | *** | 374 | 382 | 681 | 135 | 138 | 217 | 80 | 81 | 115 | 57 | 57 | 73 | 44 | 45 | 51 |
| 0.1 | *** | 680 | 689 | 762 | 214 | 221 | 235 | 116 | 120 | 125 | 78 | 79 | 82 | 58 | 59 | 60 |
|  | *** | 683 | 705 | 1076 | 217 | 226 | 310 | 118 | 122 | 153 | 79 | 81 | 93 | 58 | 59 | 63 |
| 0.15 | *** | 942 | 958 | 1117 | 280 | 291 | 323 | 146 | 152 | 163 | 95 | 98 | 103 | 68 | 70 | 73 |
|  | *** | 947 | 987 | 1422 | 285 | 302 | 390 | 149 | 157 | 186 | 96 | 100 | 110 | 69 | 72 | 73 |
| 0.2 | *** | 1146 | 1171 | 1441 | 331 | 348 | 400 | 170 | 178 | 195 | 108 | 112 | 120 | 77 | 79 | 83 |
|  | *** | 1155 | 1215 | 1719 | 338 | 365 | 458 | 173 | 185 | 213 | 110 | 116 | 124 | 78 | 81 | 81 |
| 0.25 | *** | 1290 | 1326 | 1724 | 368 | 391 | 466 | 187 | 198 | 222 | 117 | 124 | 134 | 82 | 86 | 91 |
|  | *** | 1302 | 1387 | 1967 | 377 | 415 | 514 | 192 | 208 | 235 | 120 | 128 | 135 | 84 | 88 | 87 |
| 0.3 | *** | 1377 | 1425 | 1960 | 392 | 422 | 519 | 198 | 213 | 243 | 124 | 131 | 144 | 86 | 91 | 97 |
|  | *** | 1393 | 1507 | 2164 | 404 | 453 | 557 | 205 | 225 | 252 | 127 | 137 | 143 | 88 | 93 | 91 |
| 0.35 | *** | 1411 | 1474 | 2147 | 405 | 441 | 559 | 205 | 222 | 259 | 127 | 136 | 151 | 88 | 93 | 100 |
|  | *** | 1433 | 1578 | 2313 | 419 | 478 | 588 | 212 | 236 | 263 | 131 | 143 | 147 | 91 | 96 | 93 |
| 0.4 | *** | 1401 | 1480 | 2281 | 407 | 449 | 587 | 207 | 226 | 268 | 128 | 138 | 155 | 88 | 94 | 102 |
|  | *** | 1428 | 1608 | 2412 | 424 | 492 | 606 | 215 | 242 | 268 | 133 | 145 | 149 | 91 | 97 | 93 |
| 0.45 | *** | 1353 | 1452 | 2362 | 402 | 449 | 600 | 205 | 226 | 271 | 127 | 137 | 155 | 87 | 93 | 101 |
|  | *** | 1388 | 1602 | 2461 | 421 | 496 | 613 | 214 | 243 | 268 | 132 | 145 | 147 | 90 | 96 | 91 |
| 0.5 | *** | 1277 | 1396 | 2390 | 389 | 440 | 601 | 200 | 222 | 268 | 123 | 134 | 152 | 84 | 89 | 98 |
|  | *** | 1320 | 1566 | 2461 | 410 | 490 | 606 | 209 | 240 | 263 | 128 | 141 | 143 | 86 | 93 | 87 |
| 0.55 | *** | 1182 | 1320 | 2363 | 371 | 424 | 587 | 191 | 213 | 259 | 117 | 128 | 145 | 79 | 85 | 92 |
|  | *** | 1232 | 1506 | 2412 | 393 | 476 | 588 | 201 | 231 | 252 | 122 | 135 | 135 | 82 | 88 | 81 |
| 0.6 | *** | 1075 | 1228 | 2283 | 348 | 402 | 561 | 180 | 201 | 245 | 110 | 119 | 135 | 73 | 78 | 85 |
|  | *** | 1132 | 1424 | 2313 | 371 | 453 | 557 | 189 | 218 | 235 | 114 | 126 | 124 | 75 | 81 | 73 |
| 0.65 | *** | 962 | 1126 | 2149 | 321 | 373 | 521 | 165 | 185 | 224 | 99 | 108 | 122 | 66 | 70 | 75 |
|  | *** | 1025 | 1325 | 2164 | 343 | 421 | 514 | 174 | 200 | 213 | 103 | 114 | 110 | 67 | 72 | 63 |
| 0.7 | *** | 849 | 1014 | 1962 | 289 | 338 | 467 | 147 | 165 | 197 | 87 | 94 | 105 | 56 | 59 | 64 |
|  | *** | 913 | 1208 | 1967 | 310 | 381 | 458 | 155 | 178 | 186 | 91 | 99 | 93 | 58 | 61 | 51 |
| 0.75 | *** | 735 | 894 | 1722 | 253 | 295 | 401 | 126 | 140 | 165 | 72 | 78 | 85 | . | . | . |
|  | *** | 797 | 1073 | 1719 | 271 | 332 | 390 | 133 | 151 | 153 | 75 | 81 | 73 | . | . | . |
| 0.8 | *** | 619 | 762 | 1430 | 211 | 245 | 321 | 101 | 111 | 127 | . | . | . | . | . | . |
|  | *** | 676 | 918 | 1422 | 226 | 273 | 310 | 105 | 118 | 115 | . | . | . | . | . | . |
| 0.85 | *** | 496 | 613 | 1087 | 161 | 184 | 229 | . | . | . | . | . | . | . | . | . |
|  | *** | 544 | 735 | 1076 | 171 | 202 | 217 | . | . | . | . | . | . | . | . | . |
| 0.9 | *** | 357 | 436 | 693 | . | . | . | . | . | . | . | . | . | . | . | . |
|  | *** | 389 | 512 | 681 | . | . | . | . | . | . | . | . | . | . | . | . |

TABLE 7: ALPHA= 0.05  POWER= 0.8     EXPECTED ACCRUAL THRU MINIMUM FOLLOW-UP= 180

| PCONT | | DEL=.05 | | | DEL=.10 | | | DEL=.15 | | | DEL=.20 | | | DEL=.25 | | |
|---|---|---|---|---|---|---|---|---|---|---|---|---|---|---|---|---|
| FACT= | | 1.0 / .75 | .50 / .25 | .00 / BIN | 1.0 / .75 | .50 / .25 | .00 / BIN | 1.0 / .75 | .50 / .25 | .00 / BIN | 1.0 / 75 | .50 / .25 | .00 / BIN | 1.0 / .75 | .50 / .25 | .00 / BIN |
| PCONT=*** | | | | | REQUIRED NUMBER OF PATIENTS | | | | | | | | | | | |
| 0.05 | *** | 373 | 377 | 395 | 134 | 137 | 141 | 79 | 80 | 82 | 56 | 57 | 58 | 44 | 44 | 45 |
|  | *** | 374 | 382 | 681 | 135 | 138 | 217 | 80 | 81 | 115 | 57 | 57 | 73 | 44 | 45 | 51 |
| 0.1 | *** | 680 | 690 | 762 | 215 | 221 | 235 | 117 | 120 | 125 | 78 | 80 | 82 | 58 | 59 | 60 |
|  | *** | 684 | 706 | 1076 | 217 | 226 | 310 | 118 | 122 | 153 | 79 | 81 | 93 | 58 | 60 | 63 |
| 0.15 | *** | 943 | 960 | 1117 | 281 | 292 | 323 | 147 | 153 | 163 | 95 | 98 | 103 | 69 | 70 | 73 |
|  | *** | 949 | 989 | 1422 | 286 | 303 | 390 | 149 | 157 | 186 | 96 | 100 | 110 | 69 | 72 | 73 |
| 0.2 | *** | 1148 | 1174 | 1441 | 333 | 350 | 400 | 170 | 179 | 195 | 108 | 113 | 120 | 77 | 80 | 83 |
|  | *** | 1157 | 1219 | 1719 | 339 | 367 | 458 | 174 | 186 | 213 | 110 | 116 | 124 | 78 | 81 | 81 |
| 0.25 | *** | 1292 | 1330 | 1724 | 370 | 393 | 465 | 188 | 199 | 222 | 118 | 124 | 134 | 83 | 86 | 91 |
|  | *** | 1305 | 1394 | 1967 | 379 | 417 | 514 | 193 | 208 | 235 | 121 | 128 | 135 | 84 | 89 | 87 |
| 0.3 | *** | 1380 | 1430 | 1960 | 394 | 424 | 519 | 200 | 214 | 243 | 125 | 132 | 144 | 87 | 91 | 97 |
|  | *** | 1397 | 1515 | 2164 | 406 | 455 | 557 | 206 | 226 | 252 | 128 | 137 | 143 | 89 | 94 | 91 |
| 0.35 | *** | 1415 | 1481 | 2147 | 407 | 444 | 559 | 206 | 223 | 259 | 128 | 137 | 151 | 89 | 93 | 100 |
|  | *** | 1438 | 1588 | 2313 | 422 | 481 | 588 | 214 | 237 | 263 | 132 | 143 | 147 | 91 | 97 | 93 |
| 0.4 | *** | 1406 | 1489 | 2281 | 410 | 453 | 587 | 209 | 228 | 268 | 129 | 139 | 155 | 89 | 94 | 102 |
|  | *** | 1434 | 1620 | 2412 | 428 | 495 | 606 | 217 | 243 | 268 | 134 | 146 | 149 | 91 | 98 | 93 |
| 0.45 | *** | 1359 | 1462 | 2362 | 405 | 453 | 600 | 207 | 228 | 271 | 128 | 138 | 155 | 87 | 93 | 101 |
|  | *** | 1396 | 1616 | 2461 | 425 | 499 | 613 | 216 | 245 | 268 | 132 | 145 | 147 | 90 | 96 | 91 |
| 0.5 | *** | 1285 | 1408 | 2390 | 393 | 445 | 601 | 202 | 224 | 268 | 124 | 135 | 152 | 84 | 90 | 98 |
|  | *** | 1329 | 1582 | 2461 | 414 | 494 | 606 | 211 | 241 | 263 | 129 | 142 | 143 | 87 | 93 | 87 |
| 0.55 | *** | 1191 | 1333 | 2363 | 375 | 429 | 587 | 193 | 215 | 260 | 118 | 129 | 145 | 80 | 85 | 92 |
|  | *** | 1243 | 1522 | 2412 | 398 | 479 | 588 | 203 | 232 | 252 | 123 | 136 | 135 | 82 | 88 | 81 |
| 0.6 | *** | 1085 | 1243 | 2283 | 353 | 406 | 561 | 182 | 203 | 245 | 110 | 120 | 135 | 74 | 78 | 85 |
|  | *** | 1145 | 1442 | 2313 | 375 | 456 | 557 | 191 | 219 | 235 | 115 | 127 | 124 | 76 | 81 | 73 |
| 0.65 | *** | 974 | 1141 | 2149 | 325 | 377 | 521 | 167 | 186 | 224 | 100 | 109 | 122 | 66 | 70 | 75 |
|  | *** | 1038 | 1342 | 2164 | 347 | 425 | 514 | 175 | 201 | 213 | 104 | 114 | 110 | 68 | 72 | 63 |
| 0.7 | *** | 861 | 1029 | 1962 | 294 | 342 | 467 | 149 | 166 | 197 | 88 | 95 | 105 | 57 | 60 | 64 |
|  | *** | 927 | 1225 | 1967 | 314 | 384 | 458 | 156 | 179 | 186 | 91 | 100 | 93 | 58 | 62 | 51 |
| 0.75 | *** | 747 | 908 | 1722 | 257 | 299 | 401 | 127 | 141 | 165 | 73 | 78 | 85 | . | . | . |
|  | *** | 810 | 1088 | 1719 | 275 | 335 | 390 | 134 | 151 | 153 | 75 | 81 | 73 | . | . | . |
| 0.8 | *** | 630 | 774 | 1431 | 214 | 247 | 321 | 102 | 112 | 127 | . | . | . | . | . | . |
|  | *** | 688 | 931 | 1422 | 228 | 275 | 310 | 106 | 118 | 115 | . | . | . | . | . | . |
| 0.85 | *** | 506 | 623 | 1087 | 163 | 186 | 229 | . | . | . | . | . | . | . | . | . |
|  | *** | 553 | 745 | 1076 | 173 | 203 | 217 | . | . | . | . | . | . | . | . | . |
| 0.9 | *** | 363 | 442 | 693 | . | . | . | . | . | . | . | . | . | . | . | . |
|  | *** | 396 | 518 | 681 | . | . | . | . | . | . | . | . | . | . | . | . |

## TABLE 7: ALPHA= 0.05 POWER= 0.8 EXPECTED ACCRUAL THRU MINIMUM FOLLOW-UP= 190

| | | DEL=.05 | | | DEL=.10 | | | DEL=.15 | | | DEL=.20 | | | DEL=.25 | | |
|---|---|---|---|---|---|---|---|---|---|---|---|---|---|---|---|---|
| FACT= | | 1.0 .75 | .50 .25 | .00 BIN | 1.0 .75 | .50 .25 | .00 BIN | 1.0 .75 | .50 .25 | .00 BIN | 1.0 75 | .50 .25 | .00 BIN | 1.0 .75 | .50 .25 | .00 BIN |

PCONT=***    REQUIRED NUMBER OF PATIENTS

| PCONT | | DEL=.05 1.0/.75 | .50/.25 | .00/BIN | DEL=.10 1.0/.75 | .50/.25 | .00/BIN | DEL=.15 1.0/.75 | .50/.25 | .00/BIN | DEL=.20 1.0/.75 | .50/.25 | .00/BIN | DEL=.25 1.0/.75 | .50/.25 | .00/BIN |
|---|---|---|---|---|---|---|---|---|---|---|---|---|---|---|---|---|
| 0.05 | *** | 373 | 377 | 395 | 135 | 137 | 141 | 79 | 80 | 82 | 56 | 57 | 58 | 44 | 44 | 45 |
| | *** | 374 | 383 | 681 | 135 | 138 | 217 | 80 | 81 | 115 | 57 | 57 | 73 | 44 | 45 | 51 |
| 0.1 | *** | 681 | 691 | 762 | 215 | 222 | 235 | 117 | 120 | 125 | 78 | 80 | 82 | 58 | 59 | 60 |
| | *** | 685 | 708 | 1076 | 218 | 227 | 310 | 118 | 122 | 153 | 79 | 81 | 93 | 58 | 60 | 63 |
| 0.15 | *** | 944 | 962 | 1117 | 282 | 293 | 323 | 147 | 153 | 163 | 95 | 98 | 103 | 69 | 70 | 73 |
| | *** | 950 | 992 | 1422 | 287 | 304 | 390 | 150 | 157 | 186 | 97 | 100 | 110 | 70 | 72 | 73 |
| 0.2 | *** | 1149 | 1177 | 1441 | 334 | 351 | 400 | 171 | 179 | 195 | 109 | 113 | 120 | 77 | 80 | 83 |
| | *** | 1158 | 1224 | 1719 | 341 | 368 | 458 | 175 | 186 | 213 | 111 | 116 | 124 | 78 | 81 | 81 |
| 0.25 | *** | 1294 | 1334 | 1724 | 372 | 395 | 466 | 189 | 200 | 222 | 118 | 124 | 134 | 83 | 87 | 91 |
| | *** | 1308 | 1400 | 1967 | 381 | 419 | 514 | 194 | 209 | 235 | 121 | 128 | 135 | 85 | 89 | 87 |
| 0.3 | *** | 1383 | 1435 | 1960 | 396 | 427 | 519 | 201 | 215 | 243 | 125 | 132 | 144 | 87 | 91 | 97 |
| | *** | 1401 | 1523 | 2164 | 409 | 457 | 557 | 207 | 226 | 252 | 128 | 137 | 143 | 89 | 94 | 91 |
| 0.35 | *** | 1419 | 1488 | 2147 | 410 | 447 | 559 | 208 | 225 | 259 | 129 | 137 | 151 | 89 | 94 | 100 |
| | *** | 1443 | 1598 | 2313 | 425 | 483 | 588 | 215 | 238 | 263 | 133 | 143 | 147 | 91 | 97 | 93 |
| 0.4 | *** | 1410 | 1498 | 2281 | 414 | 456 | 587 | 210 | 229 | 268 | 130 | 139 | 155 | 89 | 94 | 102 |
| | *** | 1441 | 1632 | 2412 | 431 | 498 | 606 | 218 | 244 | 268 | 134 | 146 | 149 | 92 | 98 | 93 |
| 0.45 | *** | 1365 | 1473 | 2362 | 409 | 457 | 600 | 209 | 229 | 271 | 129 | 139 | 155 | 88 | 93 | 101 |
| | *** | 1403 | 1629 | 2461 | 428 | 503 | 613 | 218 | 246 | 268 | 133 | 146 | 147 | 90 | 97 | 91 |
| 0.5 | *** | 1292 | 1420 | 2390 | 397 | 449 | 601 | 203 | 225 | 268 | 125 | 135 | 152 | 85 | 90 | 98 |
| | *** | 1339 | 1597 | 2461 | 418 | 497 | 606 | 213 | 242 | 263 | 130 | 142 | 143 | 87 | 94 | 87 |
| 0.55 | *** | 1200 | 1347 | 2363 | 380 | 433 | 587 | 195 | 217 | 260 | 119 | 129 | 145 | 80 | 85 | 92 |
| | *** | 1254 | 1538 | 2412 | 402 | 483 | 588 | 204 | 234 | 252 | 124 | 136 | 135 | 83 | 89 | 81 |
| 0.6 | *** | 1096 | 1257 | 2283 | 357 | 411 | 561 | 183 | 204 | 245 | 111 | 121 | 135 | 74 | 79 | 85 |
| | *** | 1157 | 1458 | 2313 | 379 | 460 | 557 | 192 | 220 | 235 | 116 | 127 | 124 | 76 | 82 | 73 |
| 0.65 | *** | 986 | 1156 | 2149 | 329 | 381 | 521 | 168 | 188 | 224 | 101 | 109 | 122 | 66 | 70 | 75 |
| | *** | 1051 | 1359 | 2164 | 351 | 428 | 514 | 177 | 202 | 213 | 105 | 115 | 110 | 68 | 73 | 63 |
| 0.7 | *** | 873 | 1044 | 1962 | 297 | 345 | 467 | 150 | 167 | 197 | 89 | 95 | 105 | 57 | 60 | 64 |
| | *** | 940 | 1240 | 1967 | 317 | 387 | 458 | 158 | 180 | 186 | 92 | 100 | 93 | 58 | 62 | 51 |
| 0.75 | *** | 758 | 921 | 1722 | 260 | 302 | 401 | 129 | 142 | 165 | 73 | 78 | 85 | . | . | . |
| | *** | 823 | 1103 | 1719 | 278 | 337 | 390 | 135 | 152 | 153 | 76 | 82 | 73 | . | . | . |
| 0.8 | *** | 640 | 786 | 1431 | 217 | 250 | 321 | 103 | 112 | 127 | . | . | . | . | . | . |
| | *** | 699 | 943 | 1422 | 231 | 277 | 310 | 107 | 119 | 115 | . | . | . | . | . | . |
| 0.85 | *** | 514 | 633 | 1087 | 165 | 187 | 229 | . | . | . | . | . | . | . | . | . |
| | *** | 562 | 754 | 1076 | 175 | 204 | 217 | . | . | . | . | . | . | . | . | . |
| 0.9 | *** | 369 | 448 | 693 | . | . | . | . | . | . | . | . | . | . | . | . |
| | *** | 402 | 524 | 681 | . | . | . | . | . | . | . | . | . | . | . | . |

TABLE 7: ALPHA= 0.05  POWER= 0.8     EXPECTED ACCRUAL THRU MINIMUM FOLLOW-UP= 200

| | DEL=.05 | | | DEL=.10 | | | DEL=.15 | | | DEL=.20 | | | DEL=.25 | | |
|---|---|---|---|---|---|---|---|---|---|---|---|---|---|---|---|---|
| FACT= | 1.0 .75 | .50 .25 | .00 BIN | 1.0 .75 | .50 .25 | .00 BIN | 1.0 .75 | .50 .25 | .00 BIN | 1.0 75 | .50 .25 | .00 BIN | 1.0 .75 | .50 .25 | .00 BIN |
| PCONT=*** | | | | REQUIRED NUMBER OF PATIENTS | | | | | | | | | | | |
| 0.05 *** | 373 | 378 | 395 | 135 | 137 | 141 | 80 | 81 | 82 | 56 | 57 | 58 | 44 | 44 | 45 |
| *** | 375 | 383 | 681 | 136 | 138 | 217 | 80 | 81 | 115 | 57 | 57 | 73 | 44 | 45 | 51 |
| 0.1 *** | 682 | 692 | 762 | 216 | 222 | 235 | 117 | 120 | 125 | 78 | 80 | 82 | 58 | 59 | 60 |
| *** | 685 | 709 | 1076 | 218 | 227 | 310 | 119 | 122 | 153 | 79 | 81 | 93 | 58 | 60 | 63 |
| 0.15 *** | 945 | 964 | 1117 | 283 | 294 | 323 | 148 | 153 | 163 | 95 | 98 | 103 | 69 | 71 | 73 |
| *** | 951 | 995 | 1422 | 287 | 304 | 390 | 150 | 157 | 186 | 97 | 100 | 110 | 70 | 72 | 73 |
| 0.2 *** | 1151 | 1180 | 1441 | 335 | 352 | 400 | 172 | 180 | 195 | 109 | 113 | 120 | 77 | 80 | 83 |
| *** | 1160 | 1228 | 1719 | 342 | 369 | 458 | 175 | 186 | 213 | 111 | 116 | 124 | 78 | 81 | 81 |
| 0.25 *** | 1297 | 1338 | 1724 | 373 | 397 | 466 | 190 | 201 | 222 | 119 | 125 | 134 | 83 | 87 | 91 |
| *** | 1311 | 1405 | 1967 | 383 | 420 | 514 | 195 | 210 | 235 | 122 | 129 | 135 | 85 | 89 | 87 |
| 0.3 *** | 1385 | 1441 | 1960 | 399 | 429 | 519 | 202 | 216 | 243 | 126 | 133 | 144 | 87 | 91 | 97 |
| *** | 1404 | 1530 | 2164 | 411 | 459 | 557 | 208 | 227 | 252 | 129 | 138 | 143 | 89 | 94 | 91 |
| 0.35 *** | 1423 | 1495 | 2147 | 413 | 450 | 559 | 209 | 226 | 259 | 130 | 138 | 151 | 90 | 94 | 100 |
| *** | 1447 | 1608 | 2313 | 428 | 486 | 588 | 216 | 239 | 263 | 133 | 144 | 147 | 92 | 97 | 93 |
| 0.4 *** | 1415 | 1506 | 2281 | 417 | 460 | 587 | 212 | 231 | 268 | 131 | 140 | 155 | 90 | 95 | 102 |
| *** | 1447 | 1643 | 2412 | 434 | 501 | 606 | 220 | 245 | 268 | 135 | 146 | 149 | 92 | 98 | 93 |
| 0.45 *** | 1372 | 1483 | 2362 | 412 | 460 | 600 | 210 | 231 | 271 | 130 | 139 | 155 | 88 | 94 | 101 |
| *** | 1411 | 1642 | 2461 | 432 | 506 | 613 | 219 | 247 | 268 | 134 | 146 | 147 | 91 | 97 | 91 |
| 0.5 *** | 1300 | 1432 | 2390 | 401 | 452 | 601 | 205 | 227 | 268 | 126 | 136 | 152 | 85 | 91 | 98 |
| *** | 1348 | 1611 | 2461 | 422 | 501 | 606 | 214 | 243 | 263 | 131 | 143 | 143 | 88 | 94 | 87 |
| 0.55 *** | 1209 | 1360 | 2363 | 384 | 437 | 587 | 197 | 218 | 260 | 120 | 130 | 145 | 81 | 86 | 92 |
| *** | 1265 | 1554 | 2412 | 406 | 486 | 588 | 206 | 235 | 252 | 125 | 136 | 135 | 83 | 89 | 81 |
| 0.6 *** | 1106 | 1271 | 2283 | 361 | 414 | 561 | 185 | 206 | 245 | 112 | 121 | 135 | 75 | 79 | 85 |
| *** | 1169 | 1474 | 2313 | 383 | 463 | 557 | 194 | 221 | 235 | 116 | 127 | 124 | 77 | 82 | 73 |
| 0.65 *** | 997 | 1170 | 2149 | 333 | 385 | 521 | 170 | 189 | 224 | 102 | 110 | 122 | 67 | 70 | 75 |
| *** | 1064 | 1374 | 2164 | 355 | 431 | 514 | 178 | 203 | 213 | 105 | 115 | 110 | 68 | 73 | 63 |
| 0.7 *** | 884 | 1058 | 1962 | 301 | 349 | 467 | 152 | 168 | 197 | 89 | 96 | 105 | 57 | 60 | 64 |
| *** | 952 | 1255 | 1967 | 321 | 390 | 458 | 159 | 180 | 186 | 92 | 100 | 93 | 58 | 62 | 51 |
| 0.75 *** | 770 | 935 | 1722 | 263 | 305 | 401 | 130 | 143 | 165 | 74 | 79 | 85 | . | . | . |
| *** | 835 | 1116 | 1719 | 281 | 339 | 390 | 136 | 152 | 153 | 76 | 82 | 73 | . | . | . |
| 0.8 *** | 651 | 798 | 1431 | 219 | 252 | 321 | 103 | 113 | 127 | . | . | . | . | . | . |
| *** | 710 | 954 | 1422 | 234 | 278 | 310 | 108 | 119 | 115 | . | . | . | . | . | . |
| 0.85 *** | 523 | 642 | 1087 | 167 | 189 | 229 | . | . | . | . | . | . | . | . | . |
| *** | 571 | 763 | 1076 | 176 | 205 | 217 | . | . | . | . | . | . | . | . | . |
| 0.9 *** | 375 | 454 | 693 | . | . | . | . | . | . | . | . | . | . | . | . |
| *** | 408 | 529 | 681 | . | . | . | . | . | . | . | . | . | . | . | . |

## TABLE 7: ALPHA= 0.05  POWER= 0.8    EXPECTED ACCRUAL THRU MINIMUM FOLLOW-UP= 225

| | | DEL=.05 | | | DEL=.10 | | | DEL=.15 | | | DEL=.20 | | | DEL=.25 | | |
|---|---|---|---|---|---|---|---|---|---|---|---|---|---|---|---|---|---|
| **FACT=** | | 1.0 .75 | .50 .25 | .00 BIN | 1.0 .75 | .50 .25 | .00 BIN | 1.0 .75 | .50 .25 | .00 BIN | 1.0 75 | .50 .25 | .00 BIN | 1.0 .75 | .50 .25 | .00 BIN |
| **PCONT=*** ** | | | | REQUIRED | NUMBER OF | PATIENTS | | | | | | | | | | |
| 0.05 | *** | 374 | 379 | 395 | 135 | 137 | 141 | 80 | 81 | 82 | 57 | 57 | 58 | 44 | 44 | 45 |
| | *** | 376 | 384 | 681 | 136 | 139 | 217 | 80 | 81 | 115 | 57 | 57 | 73 | 44 | 45 | 51 |
| 0.1 | *** | 683 | 695 | 762 | 217 | 223 | 235 | 118 | 121 | 125 | 78 | 80 | 82 | 58 | 59 | 60 |
| | *** | 687 | 712 | 1076 | 219 | 228 | 310 | 119 | 123 | 153 | 79 | 81 | 93 | 59 | 60 | 63 |
| 0.15 | *** | 947 | 968 | 1117 | 285 | 296 | 323 | 149 | 154 | 163 | 96 | 99 | 103 | 69 | 71 | 73 |
| | *** | 955 | 1001 | 1422 | 289 | 306 | 390 | 151 | 158 | 186 | 97 | 101 | 110 | 70 | 72 | 73 |
| 0.2 | *** | 1154 | 1186 | 1441 | 338 | 355 | 400 | 173 | 181 | 195 | 110 | 114 | 120 | 78 | 80 | 83 |
| | *** | 1165 | 1237 | 1719 | 345 | 372 | 458 | 177 | 187 | 213 | 112 | 117 | 124 | 79 | 82 | 81 |
| 0.25 | *** | 1302 | 1347 | 1724 | 377 | 401 | 466 | 192 | 203 | 222 | 120 | 126 | 134 | 84 | 87 | 91 |
| | *** | 1317 | 1419 | 1967 | 387 | 424 | 514 | 196 | 211 | 235 | 123 | 129 | 135 | 86 | 89 | 87 |
| 0.3 | *** | 1393 | 1454 | 1960 | 404 | 435 | 519 | 204 | 218 | 243 | 127 | 134 | 144 | 88 | 92 | 97 |
| | *** | 1414 | 1548 | 2164 | 416 | 464 | 557 | 210 | 228 | 252 | 130 | 138 | 143 | 90 | 94 | 91 |
| 0.35 | *** | 1432 | 1511 | 2147 | 419 | 456 | 559 | 212 | 228 | 259 | 131 | 139 | 151 | 90 | 95 | 100 |
| | *** | 1460 | 1630 | 2313 | 434 | 491 | 588 | 219 | 241 | 263 | 135 | 144 | 147 | 92 | 97 | 93 |
| 0.4 | *** | 1427 | 1526 | 2281 | 424 | 467 | 587 | 215 | 233 | 268 | 133 | 141 | 155 | 91 | 95 | 102 |
| | *** | 1463 | 1670 | 2412 | 442 | 507 | 606 | 223 | 247 | 268 | 137 | 147 | 149 | 93 | 98 | 93 |
| 0.45 | *** | 1387 | 1507 | 2362 | 420 | 468 | 600 | 214 | 234 | 271 | 131 | 141 | 155 | 89 | 94 | 101 |
| | *** | 1430 | 1673 | 2461 | 440 | 513 | 613 | 223 | 249 | 268 | 136 | 147 | 147 | 92 | 97 | 91 |
| 0.5 | *** | 1319 | 1460 | 2390 | 410 | 461 | 601 | 209 | 230 | 268 | 128 | 137 | 152 | 86 | 91 | 98 |
| | *** | 1370 | 1644 | 2461 | 431 | 508 | 606 | 218 | 245 | 263 | 132 | 144 | 143 | 89 | 94 | 87 |
| 0.55 | *** | 1231 | 1390 | 2363 | 392 | 446 | 587 | 201 | 221 | 259 | 122 | 131 | 145 | 82 | 86 | 92 |
| | *** | 1291 | 1589 | 2412 | 415 | 494 | 588 | 210 | 237 | 252 | 126 | 137 | 135 | 84 | 89 | 81 |
| 0.6 | *** | 1131 | 1304 | 2283 | 370 | 423 | 561 | 189 | 209 | 245 | 114 | 122 | 135 | 75 | 79 | 85 |
| | *** | 1197 | 1511 | 2313 | 392 | 471 | 557 | 198 | 223 | 235 | 118 | 128 | 124 | 77 | 82 | 73 |
| 0.65 | *** | 1023 | 1203 | 2149 | 342 | 393 | 521 | 174 | 192 | 224 | 103 | 111 | 122 | 68 | 71 | 75 |
| | *** | 1093 | 1410 | 2164 | 364 | 438 | 514 | 182 | 205 | 213 | 107 | 116 | 110 | 69 | 73 | 63 |
| 0.7 | *** | 911 | 1090 | 1962 | 309 | 356 | 467 | 155 | 171 | 197 | 90 | 97 | 105 | 58 | 60 | 64 |
| | *** | 982 | 1290 | 1967 | 329 | 396 | 458 | 162 | 182 | 186 | 93 | 101 | 93 | 59 | 62 | 51 |
| 0.75 | *** | 796 | 965 | 1722 | 271 | 311 | 401 | 132 | 145 | 165 | 75 | 79 | 85 | . | . | . |
| | *** | 863 | 1148 | 1719 | 288 | 345 | 390 | 138 | 154 | 153 | 77 | 82 | 73 | . | . | . |
| 0.8 | *** | 674 | 824 | 1430 | 225 | 257 | 321 | 105 | 114 | 127 | . | . | . | . | . | . |
| | *** | 735 | 981 | 1422 | 239 | 282 | 310 | 109 | 120 | 115 | . | . | . | . | . | . |
| 0.85 | *** | 542 | 663 | 1087 | 171 | 192 | 229 | . | . | . | . | . | . | . | . | . |
| | *** | 591 | 783 | 1076 | 180 | 207 | 217 | . | . | . | . | . | . | . | . | . |
| 0.9 | *** | 388 | 468 | 693 | . | . | . | . | . | . | . | . | . | . | . | . |
| | *** | 421 | 540 | 681 | . | . | . | . | . | . | . | . | . | . | . | . |

TABLE 7: ALPHA= 0.05  POWER= 0.8    EXPECTED ACCRUAL THRU MINIMUM FOLLOW-UP= 250

| | DEL=.05 | | | DEL=.10 | | | DEL=.15 | | | DEL=.20 | | | DEL=.25 | | |
|---|---|---|---|---|---|---|---|---|---|---|---|---|---|---|---|
| FACT= | 1.0 .75 | .50 .25 | .00 BIN | 1.0 .75 | .50 .25 | .00 BIN | 1.0 .75 | .50 .25 | .00 BIN | 1.0 75 | .50 .25 | .00 BIN | 1.0 .75 | .50 .25 | .00 BIN |
| PCONT=*** | | | | REQUIRED NUMBER OF PATIENTS | | | | | | | | | | | |
| 0.05 *** | 374 | 379 | 395 | 135 | 137 | 141 | 80 | 81 | 82 | 57 | 57 | 58 | 44 | 44 | 45 |
| *** | 376 | 385 | 681 | 136 | 139 | 217 | 80 | 82 | 115 | 57 | 57 | 73 | 44 | 45 | 51 |
| 0.1 *** | 684 | 697 | 762 | 218 | 224 | 235 | 118 | 121 | 125 | 79 | 80 | 82 | 58 | 59 | 60 |
| *** | 689 | 715 | 1076 | 220 | 229 | 310 | 119 | 123 | 153 | 79 | 81 | 93 | 59 | 60 | 63 |
| 0.15 *** | 950 | 973 | 1117 | 286 | 298 | 323 | 150 | 155 | 163 | 97 | 99 | 103 | 70 | 71 | 73 |
| *** | 958 | 1006 | 1422 | 291 | 307 | 390 | 152 | 158 | 186 | 98 | 101 | 110 | 70 | 72 | 73 |
| 0.2 *** | 1158 | 1193 | 1441 | 340 | 358 | 400 | 175 | 182 | 195 | 111 | 114 | 120 | 78 | 80 | 83 |
| *** | 1170 | 1246 | 1719 | 348 | 374 | 458 | 178 | 188 | 213 | 112 | 117 | 124 | 79 | 82 | 81 |
| 0.25 *** | 1307 | 1357 | 1724 | 381 | 405 | 466 | 194 | 204 | 222 | 121 | 126 | 134 | 85 | 87 | 91 |
| *** | 1324 | 1432 | 1967 | 391 | 427 | 514 | 198 | 212 | 235 | 123 | 130 | 135 | 86 | 89 | 87 |
| 0.3 *** | 1400 | 1466 | 1960 | 408 | 439 | 519 | 207 | 220 | 243 | 128 | 135 | 144 | 89 | 92 | 97 |
| *** | 1423 | 1565 | 2164 | 421 | 467 | 557 | 213 | 230 | 252 | 131 | 139 | 143 | 91 | 94 | 91 |
| 0.35 *** | 1441 | 1527 | 2147 | 424 | 462 | 559 | 215 | 230 | 259 | 133 | 140 | 151 | 91 | 95 | 100 |
| *** | 1472 | 1651 | 2313 | 440 | 496 | 588 | 222 | 242 | 263 | 136 | 145 | 147 | 93 | 98 | 93 |
| 0.4 *** | 1439 | 1546 | 2281 | 430 | 474 | 587 | 218 | 236 | 268 | 134 | 142 | 155 | 92 | 96 | 102 |
| *** | 1477 | 1694 | 2412 | 448 | 513 | 606 | 226 | 249 | 268 | 138 | 148 | 149 | 94 | 99 | 93 |
| 0.45 *** | 1402 | 1530 | 2362 | 427 | 476 | 600 | 217 | 236 | 271 | 133 | 142 | 155 | 90 | 95 | 101 |
| *** | 1448 | 1700 | 2461 | 448 | 519 | 613 | 226 | 251 | 268 | 137 | 148 | 147 | 92 | 98 | 91 |
| 0.5 *** | 1336 | 1485 | 2390 | 417 | 469 | 601 | 212 | 232 | 268 | 129 | 139 | 152 | 87 | 92 | 98 |
| *** | 1392 | 1675 | 2461 | 439 | 514 | 606 | 221 | 247 | 263 | 134 | 144 | 143 | 89 | 94 | 87 |
| 0.55 *** | 1252 | 1418 | 2363 | 401 | 454 | 587 | 204 | 224 | 259 | 124 | 132 | 145 | 83 | 87 | 92 |
| *** | 1315 | 1622 | 2412 | 423 | 500 | 588 | 213 | 239 | 252 | 128 | 138 | 135 | 84 | 89 | 81 |
| 0.6 *** | 1154 | 1333 | 2283 | 378 | 431 | 561 | 192 | 211 | 245 | 115 | 123 | 135 | 76 | 80 | 85 |
| *** | 1223 | 1544 | 2313 | 400 | 477 | 557 | 201 | 225 | 235 | 119 | 129 | 124 | 78 | 82 | 73 |
| 0.65 *** | 1048 | 1233 | 2149 | 350 | 401 | 521 | 177 | 194 | 224 | 105 | 112 | 122 | 68 | 71 | 75 |
| *** | 1121 | 1443 | 2164 | 372 | 444 | 514 | 184 | 207 | 213 | 108 | 116 | 110 | 70 | 73 | 63 |
| 0.7 *** | 937 | 1120 | 1962 | 317 | 363 | 467 | 158 | 173 | 197 | 92 | 97 | 105 | 58 | 61 | 64 |
| *** | 1009 | 1321 | 1967 | 336 | 401 | 458 | 164 | 183 | 186 | 94 | 101 | 93 | 59 | 62 | 51 |
| 0.75 *** | 820 | 992 | 1722 | 277 | 317 | 401 | 134 | 147 | 165 | 76 | 80 | 85 | . | . | . |
| *** | 889 | 1175 | 1719 | 294 | 349 | 390 | 140 | 155 | 153 | 78 | 82 | 73 | . | . | . |
| 0.8 *** | 696 | 848 | 1431 | 230 | 261 | 321 | 107 | 115 | 127 | . | . | . | . | . | . |
| *** | 758 | 1004 | 1422 | 244 | 285 | 310 | 111 | 120 | 115 | . | . | . | . | . | . |
| 0.85 *** | 560 | 681 | 1087 | 174 | 194 | 229 | . | . | . | . | . | . | . | . | . |
| *** | 610 | 800 | 1076 | 183 | 209 | 217 | . | . | . | . | . | . | . | . | . |
| 0.9 *** | 400 | 479 | 693 | . | . | . | . | . | . | . | . | . | . | . | . |
| *** | 434 | 550 | 681 | . | . | . | . | . | . | . | . | . | . | . | . |

## TABLE 7: ALPHA= 0.05 POWER= 0.8     EXPECTED ACCRUAL THRU MINIMUM FOLLOW-UP= 275

| | | DEL=.05 | | | DEL=.10 | | | DEL=.15 | | | DEL=.20 | | | DEL=.25 | |
|---|---|---|---|---|---|---|---|---|---|---|---|---|---|---|---|
| FACT= | 1.0 .75 | .50 .25 | .00 BIN | 1.0 .75 | .50 .25 | .00 BIN | 1.0 .75 | .50 .25 | .00 BIN | 1.0 75 | .50 .25 | .00 BIN | 1.0 .75 | .50 .25 | .00 BIN |

PCONT=***  REQUIRED NUMBER OF PATIENTS

| PCONT | | DEL=.05 1.0/.75 | .50/.25 | .00/BIN | DEL=.10 1.0/.75 | .50/.25 | .00/BIN | DEL=.15 1.0/.75 | .50/.25 | .00/BIN | DEL=.20 1.0/75 | .50/.25 | .00/BIN | DEL=.25 1.0/.75 | .50/.25 | .00/BIN |
|---|---|---|---|---|---|---|---|---|---|---|---|---|---|---|---|---|
| 0.05 | *** | 375 | 380 | 395 | 136 | 138 | 141 | 80 | 81 | 82 | 57 | 57 | 58 | 44 | 44 | 45 |
| | *** | 377 | 385 | 681 | 136 | 139 | 217 | 80 | 81 | 115 | 57 | 57 | 73 | 44 | 45 | 51 |
| 0.1 | *** | 686 | 700 | 762 | 219 | 224 | 235 | 119 | 121 | 125 | 79 | 80 | 82 | 58 | 59 | 60 |
| | *** | 691 | 717 | 1076 | 221 | 229 | 310 | 120 | 123 | 153 | 80 | 81 | 93 | 59 | 60 | 63 |
| 0.15 | *** | 952 | 977 | 1117 | 288 | 299 | 322 | 150 | 155 | 163 | 97 | 99 | 103 | 70 | 71 | 73 |
| | *** | 961 | 1011 | 1422 | 293 | 308 | 390 | 153 | 158 | 186 | 98 | 101 | 110 | 70 | 72 | 73 |
| 0.2 | *** | 1162 | 1199 | 1441 | 343 | 360 | 400 | 176 | 183 | 195 | 111 | 115 | 120 | 79 | 81 | 83 |
| | *** | 1175 | 1254 | 1719 | 350 | 375 | 458 | 179 | 188 | 213 | 113 | 117 | 124 | 79 | 82 | 81 |
| 0.25 | *** | 1312 | 1365 | 1724 | 384 | 408 | 465 | 195 | 205 | 222 | 122 | 127 | 134 | 85 | 88 | 91 |
| | *** | 1331 | 1443 | 1967 | 394 | 430 | 514 | 200 | 212 | 235 | 124 | 130 | 135 | 86 | 89 | 87 |
| 0.3 | *** | 1407 | 1478 | 1960 | 412 | 443 | 519 | 209 | 221 | 243 | 129 | 135 | 144 | 89 | 93 | 97 |
| | *** | 1432 | 1580 | 2164 | 425 | 471 | 557 | 214 | 231 | 252 | 132 | 139 | 143 | 91 | 95 | 91 |
| 0.35 | *** | 1451 | 1542 | 2147 | 429 | 467 | 559 | 217 | 232 | 259 | 134 | 141 | 151 | 92 | 96 | 100 |
| | *** | 1483 | 1670 | 2313 | 445 | 500 | 588 | 224 | 243 | 263 | 137 | 145 | 147 | 94 | 98 | 93 |
| 0.4 | *** | 1451 | 1564 | 2281 | 436 | 479 | 587 | 221 | 238 | 268 | 135 | 143 | 155 | 92 | 96 | 102 |
| | *** | 1492 | 1716 | 2412 | 454 | 518 | 606 | 228 | 250 | 268 | 139 | 148 | 149 | 94 | 99 | 93 |
| 0.45 | *** | 1416 | 1551 | 2362 | 434 | 482 | 600 | 220 | 239 | 271 | 134 | 143 | 155 | 91 | 95 | 101 |
| | *** | 1466 | 1726 | 2461 | 454 | 524 | 613 | 228 | 252 | 268 | 138 | 148 | 147 | 93 | 98 | 91 |
| 0.5 | *** | 1354 | 1510 | 2390 | 424 | 475 | 601 | 215 | 235 | 268 | 131 | 139 | 152 | 88 | 92 | 98 |
| | *** | 1412 | 1702 | 2461 | 446 | 520 | 606 | 224 | 249 | 263 | 135 | 145 | 143 | 90 | 95 | 87 |
| 0.55 | *** | 1272 | 1445 | 2363 | 408 | 461 | 587 | 207 | 226 | 260 | 125 | 133 | 145 | 83 | 87 | 92 |
| | *** | 1338 | 1651 | 2412 | 430 | 506 | 588 | 216 | 240 | 252 | 129 | 139 | 135 | 85 | 90 | 81 |
| 0.6 | *** | 1176 | 1361 | 2283 | 386 | 438 | 561 | 195 | 213 | 245 | 117 | 124 | 135 | 77 | 80 | 85 |
| | *** | 1248 | 1573 | 2313 | 408 | 482 | 557 | 203 | 227 | 235 | 120 | 129 | 124 | 78 | 83 | 73 |
| 0.65 | *** | 1071 | 1261 | 2149 | 357 | 407 | 520 | 179 | 196 | 224 | 106 | 113 | 122 | 69 | 72 | 75 |
| | *** | 1146 | 1472 | 2164 | 379 | 449 | 514 | 187 | 208 | 213 | 109 | 117 | 110 | 70 | 73 | 63 |
| 0.7 | *** | 960 | 1147 | 1962 | 323 | 369 | 467 | 160 | 175 | 197 | 92 | 98 | 105 | 59 | 61 | 64 |
| | *** | 1034 | 1348 | 1967 | 343 | 406 | 458 | 166 | 184 | 186 | 95 | 101 | 93 | 60 | 62 | 51 |
| 0.75 | *** | 842 | 1017 | 1722 | 283 | 322 | 401 | 136 | 148 | 165 | 76 | 80 | 85 | . | . | . |
| | *** | 913 | 1200 | 1719 | 300 | 352 | 390 | 142 | 155 | 153 | 78 | 83 | 73 | . | . | . |
| 0.8 | *** | 716 | 870 | 1431 | 235 | 265 | 321 | 108 | 116 | 127 | . | . | . | . | . | . |
| | *** | 778 | 1025 | 1422 | 248 | 288 | 310 | 112 | 121 | 115 | . | . | . | . | . | . |
| 0.85 | *** | 576 | 698 | 1087 | 177 | 197 | 229 | . | . | . | . | . | . | . | . | . |
| | *** | 627 | 815 | 1076 | 186 | 211 | 217 | . | . | . | . | . | . | . | . | . |
| 0.9 | *** | 411 | 490 | 693 | . | . | . | . | . | . | . | . | . | . | . | . |
| | *** | 444 | 559 | 681 | . | . | . | . | . | . | . | . | . | . | . | . |

TABLE 7: ALPHA= 0.05  POWER= 0.8    EXPECTED ACCRUAL THRU MINIMUM FOLLOW-UP= 300

|        |       | DEL=.05 |     |      | DEL=.10 |     |      | DEL=.15 |     |      | DEL=.20 |     |      | DEL=.25 |     |      |
|--------|-------|------|------|------|------|------|------|------|------|------|------|------|------|------|------|------|
| FACT=  |       | 1.0 | .50 | .00 | 1.0 | .50 | .00 | 1.0 | .50 | .00 | 1.0 | .50 | .00 | 1.0 | .50 | .00 |
|        |       | .75 | .25 | BIN | .75 | .25 | BIN | .75 | .25 | BIN | 75 | .25 | BIN | .75 | .25 | BIN |
| PCONT= | ***   |     |     |     | REQUIRED NUMBER OF PATIENTS | | | | | | | | | | | |
| 0.05 | *** | 376 | 381 | 395 | 136 | 138 | 141 | 80 | 81 | 82 | 57 | 57 | 58 | 44 | 44 | 45 |
|      | *** | 378 | 386 | 681 | 137 | 139 | 217 | 81 | 82 | 115 | 57 | 58 | 73 | 44 | 45 | 51 |
| 0.1 | *** | 687 | 702 | 762 | 219 | 225 | 235 | 119 | 121 | 125 | 79 | 80 | 82 | 59 | 59 | 60 |
|     | *** | 692 | 719 | 1076 | 222 | 229 | 310 | 120 | 123 | 153 | 80 | 81 | 93 | 59 | 60 | 63 |
| 0.15 | *** | 955 | 981 | 1117 | 289 | 300 | 322 | 151 | 156 | 163 | 97 | 100 | 103 | 70 | 71 | 73 |
|      | *** | 964 | 1016 | 1422 | 294 | 309 | 390 | 153 | 159 | 186 | 98 | 101 | 110 | 71 | 72 | 73 |
| 0.2 | *** | 1165 | 1205 | 1441 | 345 | 362 | 400 | 177 | 184 | 195 | 112 | 115 | 120 | 79 | 81 | 83 |
|     | *** | 1180 | 1262 | 1719 | 352 | 377 | 458 | 180 | 189 | 213 | 113 | 117 | 124 | 80 | 82 | 81 |
| 0.25 | *** | 1317 | 1374 | 1724 | 387 | 411 | 466 | 196 | 206 | 222 | 123 | 127 | 134 | 85 | 88 | 91 |
|      | *** | 1337 | 1454 | 1967 | 397 | 432 | 514 | 201 | 213 | 235 | 125 | 130 | 135 | 87 | 89 | 87 |
| 0.3 | *** | 1414 | 1489 | 1960 | 416 | 447 | 519 | 210 | 223 | 243 | 130 | 136 | 144 | 90 | 93 | 97 |
|     | *** | 1441 | 1594 | 2164 | 429 | 474 | 557 | 216 | 232 | 252 | 133 | 140 | 143 | 91 | 95 | 91 |
| 0.35 | *** | 1459 | 1556 | 2147 | 434 | 471 | 559 | 219 | 234 | 259 | 135 | 142 | 151 | 92 | 96 | 100 |
|      | *** | 1495 | 1687 | 2313 | 450 | 504 | 588 | 226 | 244 | 263 | 138 | 146 | 147 | 94 | 98 | 93 |
| 0.4 | *** | 1462 | 1582 | 2281 | 442 | 484 | 586 | 223 | 240 | 268 | 136 | 144 | 155 | 93 | 97 | 102 |
|     | *** | 1506 | 1737 | 2412 | 460 | 522 | 606 | 231 | 252 | 268 | 140 | 149 | 149 | 95 | 99 | 93 |
| 0.45 | *** | 1430 | 1571 | 2362 | 440 | 488 | 600 | 223 | 241 | 271 | 136 | 144 | 155 | 92 | 96 | 101 |
|      | *** | 1483 | 1749 | 2461 | 460 | 529 | 613 | 231 | 253 | 268 | 139 | 149 | 147 | 94 | 98 | 91 |
| 0.5 | *** | 1370 | 1532 | 2389 | 431 | 481 | 601 | 218 | 237 | 268 | 132 | 140 | 152 | 89 | 93 | 98 |
|     | *** | 1432 | 1728 | 2461 | 452 | 525 | 606 | 226 | 250 | 263 | 136 | 145 | 143 | 91 | 95 | 87 |
| 0.55 | *** | 1291 | 1469 | 2363 | 415 | 467 | 587 | 210 | 228 | 259 | 126 | 134 | 145 | 84 | 88 | 92 |
|      | *** | 1360 | 1677 | 2412 | 437 | 511 | 588 | 218 | 241 | 252 | 130 | 139 | 135 | 86 | 90 | 81 |
| 0.6 | *** | 1197 | 1387 | 2283 | 392 | 444 | 561 | 198 | 215 | 245 | 118 | 125 | 135 | 77 | 81 | 85 |
|     | *** | 1271 | 1600 | 2313 | 414 | 487 | 557 | 206 | 228 | 235 | 121 | 130 | 124 | 79 | 83 | 73 |
| 0.65 | *** | 1093 | 1287 | 2149 | 364 | 413 | 520 | 182 | 198 | 224 | 107 | 113 | 122 | 69 | 72 | 75 |
|      | *** | 1170 | 1499 | 2164 | 385 | 453 | 514 | 189 | 209 | 213 | 110 | 117 | 110 | 70 | 73 | 63 |
| 0.7 | *** | 982 | 1172 | 1962 | 329 | 374 | 467 | 162 | 176 | 197 | 93 | 98 | 105 | 59 | 61 | 64 |
|     | *** | 1058 | 1373 | 1967 | 349 | 410 | 458 | 168 | 185 | 186 | 96 | 102 | 93 | 60 | 62 | 51 |
| 0.75 | *** | 863 | 1040 | 1722 | 288 | 326 | 401 | 138 | 149 | 165 | 77 | 81 | 85 | . | . | . |
|      | *** | 934 | 1222 | 1719 | 305 | 355 | 390 | 143 | 156 | 153 | 79 | 83 | 73 | . | . | . |
| 0.8 | *** | 735 | 889 | 1430 | 239 | 268 | 321 | 109 | 117 | 127 | . | . | . | . | . | . |
|     | *** | 798 | 1043 | 1422 | 252 | 290 | 310 | 113 | 121 | 115 | . | . | . | . | . | . |
| 0.85 | *** | 592 | 713 | 1087 | 180 | 199 | 229 | . | . | . | . | . | . | . | . | . |
|      | *** | 642 | 829 | 1076 | 189 | 212 | 217 | . | . | . | . | . | . | . | . | . |
| 0.9 | *** | 421 | 499 | 693 | . | . | . | . | . | . | . | . | . | . | . | . |
|     | *** | 454 | 567 | 681 | . | . | . | . | . | . | . | . | . | . | . | . |

## TABLE 7: ALPHA= 0.05  POWER= 0.8    EXPECTED ACCRUAL THRU MINIMUM FOLLOW-UP= 325

|  |  | DEL=.05 | | | DEL=.10 | | | DEL=.15 | | | DEL=.20 | | | DEL=.25 | | |
|---|---|---|---|---|---|---|---|---|---|---|---|---|---|---|---|---|
| FACT= | | 1.0 .75 | .50 .25 | .00 BIN | 1.0 .75 | .50 .25 | .00 BIN | 1.0 .75 | .50 .25 | .00 BIN | 1.0 75 | .50 .25 | .00 BIN | 1.0 .75 | .50 .25 | .00 BIN |
| PCONT=*** | | | | | REQUIRED NUMBER OF PATIENTS | | | | | | | | | | | |
| 0.05 | *** | 376 | 381 | 395 | 136 | 138 | 141 | 80 | 81 | 82 | 57 | 57 | 58 | 44 | 44 | 45 |
|  | *** | 378 | 387 | 681 | 137 | 139 | 217 | 81 | 82 | 115 | 57 | 57 | 73 | 44 | 45 | 51 |
| 0.1 | *** | 689 | 704 | 762 | 220 | 226 | 235 | 119 | 122 | 125 | 79 | 81 | 82 | 59 | 60 | 60 |
|  | *** | 694 | 721 | 1076 | 223 | 230 | 310 | 120 | 123 | 153 | 80 | 81 | 93 | 59 | 60 | 63 |
| 0.15 | *** | 957 | 985 | 1117 | 291 | 302 | 323 | 152 | 156 | 163 | 98 | 100 | 103 | 70 | 71 | 73 |
|  | *** | 967 | 1020 | 1422 | 295 | 310 | 390 | 154 | 159 | 186 | 99 | 101 | 110 | 71 | 72 | 73 |
| 0.2 | *** | 1169 | 1211 | 1441 | 347 | 364 | 400 | 178 | 185 | 195 | 112 | 116 | 120 | 79 | 81 | 83 |
|  | *** | 1184 | 1269 | 1719 | 354 | 378 | 458 | 181 | 189 | 213 | 114 | 117 | 124 | 80 | 82 | 81 |
| 0.25 | *** | 1323 | 1382 | 1724 | 390 | 414 | 466 | 198 | 207 | 222 | 123 | 128 | 134 | 86 | 88 | 91 |
|  | *** | 1344 | 1464 | 1967 | 400 | 434 | 514 | 202 | 214 | 235 | 125 | 130 | 135 | 87 | 90 | 87 |
| 0.3 | *** | 1420 | 1500 | 1960 | 420 | 451 | 519 | 212 | 224 | 244 | 131 | 136 | 144 | 90 | 93 | 97 |
|  | *** | 1449 | 1607 | 2164 | 433 | 476 | 557 | 218 | 232 | 252 | 134 | 140 | 143 | 92 | 95 | 91 |
| 0.35 | *** | 1469 | 1570 | 2147 | 438 | 476 | 559 | 221 | 235 | 259 | 136 | 142 | 151 | 93 | 96 | 100 |
|  | *** | 1506 | 1703 | 2313 | 454 | 507 | 588 | 227 | 245 | 263 | 139 | 146 | 147 | 94 | 98 | 93 |
| 0.4 | *** | 1474 | 1598 | 2281 | 447 | 489 | 587 | 225 | 242 | 268 | 138 | 145 | 155 | 93 | 97 | 102 |
|  | *** | 1520 | 1756 | 2412 | 465 | 525 | 606 | 233 | 253 | 268 | 141 | 149 | 149 | 95 | 99 | 93 |
| 0.45 | *** | 1444 | 1591 | 2362 | 446 | 493 | 600 | 225 | 242 | 271 | 137 | 144 | 155 | 92 | 96 | 101 |
|  | *** | 1499 | 1770 | 2461 | 466 | 533 | 613 | 233 | 255 | 268 | 140 | 149 | 147 | 94 | 98 | 91 |
| 0.5 | *** | 1387 | 1554 | 2390 | 437 | 487 | 601 | 221 | 239 | 268 | 133 | 141 | 152 | 89 | 93 | 98 |
|  | *** | 1451 | 1751 | 2461 | 458 | 529 | 606 | 229 | 251 | 263 | 137 | 146 | 143 | 91 | 95 | 87 |
| 0.55 | *** | 1309 | 1492 | 2363 | 421 | 472 | 587 | 212 | 230 | 260 | 127 | 135 | 145 | 84 | 88 | 92 |
|  | *** | 1380 | 1702 | 2412 | 443 | 515 | 588 | 220 | 243 | 252 | 131 | 140 | 135 | 86 | 90 | 81 |
| 0.6 | *** | 1217 | 1411 | 2283 | 398 | 450 | 561 | 200 | 217 | 245 | 119 | 126 | 135 | 78 | 81 | 85 |
|  | *** | 1293 | 1625 | 2313 | 420 | 491 | 557 | 208 | 229 | 235 | 122 | 130 | 124 | 79 | 83 | 73 |
| 0.65 | *** | 1114 | 1311 | 2149 | 370 | 418 | 521 | 184 | 200 | 224 | 108 | 114 | 122 | 69 | 72 | 75 |
|  | *** | 1192 | 1523 | 2164 | 391 | 457 | 514 | 191 | 210 | 213 | 110 | 118 | 110 | 71 | 74 | 63 |
| 0.7 | *** | 1002 | 1195 | 1962 | 335 | 379 | 467 | 164 | 177 | 197 | 94 | 99 | 105 | 59 | 61 | 64 |
|  | *** | 1080 | 1396 | 1967 | 354 | 413 | 458 | 170 | 186 | 186 | 96 | 102 | 93 | 60 | 63 | 51 |
| 0.75 | *** | 883 | 1061 | 1722 | 293 | 330 | 401 | 140 | 150 | 165 | 78 | 81 | 85 | . | . | . |
|  | *** | 955 | 1243 | 1719 | 309 | 358 | 390 | 144 | 157 | 153 | 79 | 83 | 73 | . | . | . |
| 0.8 | *** | 752 | 908 | 1431 | 243 | 271 | 321 | 110 | 117 | 127 | . | . | . | . | . | . |
|  | *** | 816 | 1060 | 1422 | 255 | 292 | 310 | 114 | 122 | 115 | . | . | . | . | . | . |
| 0.85 | *** | 606 | 727 | 1087 | 183 | 201 | 229 | . | . | . | . | . | . | . | . | . |
|  | *** | 656 | 841 | 1076 | 191 | 213 | 217 | . | . | . | . | . | . | . | . | . |
| 0.9 | *** | 431 | 508 | 693 | . | . | . | . | . | . | . | . | . | . | . | . |
|  | *** | 463 | 573 | 681 | . | . | . | . | . | . | . | . | . | . | . | . |

**TABLE 7: ALPHA= 0.05  POWER= 0.8    EXPECTED ACCRUAL THRU MINIMUM FOLLOW-UP= 350**

| | DEL=.05 | | | DEL=.10 | | | DEL=.15 | | | DEL=.20 | | | DEL=.25 | | |
|---|---|---|---|---|---|---|---|---|---|---|---|---|---|---|---|
| FACT= | 1.0 | .50 | .00 | 1.0 | .50 | .00 | 1.0 | .50 | .00 | 1.0 | .50 | .00 | 1.0 | .50 | .00 |
| | .75 | .25 | BIN | .75 | .25 | BIN | .75 | .25 | BIN | 75 | .25 | BIN | .75 | .25 | BIN |
| PCONT=*** | REQUIRED NUMBER OF PATIENTS | | | | | | | | | | | | | | |
| 0.05  *** | 377 | 382 | 395 | 136 | 138 | 141 | 80 | 81 | 82 | 57 | 57 | 58 | 44 | 45 | 45 |
| *** | 379 | 387 | 681 | 137 | 139 | 217 | 81 | 82 | 115 | 57 | 57 | 73 | 44 | 45 | 51 |
| 0.1  *** | 690 | 705 | 762 | 221 | 226 | 236 | 120 | 122 | 125 | 80 | 81 | 82 | 59 | 59 | 60 |
| *** | 696 | 723 | 1076 | 223 | 230 | 310 | 121 | 123 | 153 | 80 | 81 | 93 | 59 | 60 | 63 |
| 0.15  *** | 959 | 988 | 1117 | 292 | 303 | 323 | 152 | 157 | 163 | 98 | 100 | 103 | 70 | 71 | 73 |
| *** | 970 | 1024 | 1422 | 297 | 311 | 390 | 154 | 159 | 186 | 99 | 101 | 110 | 71 | 72 | 73 |
| 0.2  *** | 1172 | 1217 | 1441 | 349 | 366 | 400 | 179 | 185 | 195 | 113 | 116 | 120 | 79 | 81 | 83 |
| *** | 1189 | 1275 | 1719 | 356 | 379 | 458 | 182 | 190 | 213 | 114 | 118 | 124 | 80 | 82 | 81 |
| 0.25  *** | 1328 | 1390 | 1724 | 392 | 416 | 465 | 199 | 208 | 222 | 124 | 128 | 134 | 86 | 88 | 91 |
| *** | 1350 | 1473 | 1967 | 403 | 435 | 514 | 203 | 214 | 235 | 126 | 131 | 135 | 87 | 90 | 87 |
| 0.3  *** | 1427 | 1511 | 1960 | 423 | 454 | 519 | 213 | 225 | 243 | 132 | 137 | 144 | 91 | 94 | 97 |
| *** | 1458 | 1620 | 2164 | 436 | 479 | 557 | 219 | 233 | 252 | 134 | 140 | 143 | 92 | 95 | 91 |
| 0.35  *** | 1477 | 1583 | 2147 | 442 | 479 | 559 | 223 | 237 | 259 | 137 | 143 | 151 | 93 | 96 | 100 |
| *** | 1516 | 1718 | 2313 | 458 | 510 | 588 | 229 | 246 | 263 | 139 | 147 | 147 | 95 | 98 | 93 |
| 0.4  *** | 1485 | 1614 | 2281 | 451 | 493 | 587 | 227 | 243 | 268 | 139 | 145 | 155 | 94 | 97 | 102 |
| *** | 1533 | 1774 | 2412 | 469 | 529 | 606 | 234 | 254 | 268 | 142 | 150 | 149 | 96 | 99 | 93 |
| 0.45  *** | 1457 | 1609 | 2362 | 451 | 498 | 600 | 227 | 244 | 271 | 138 | 145 | 155 | 93 | 96 | 101 |
| *** | 1515 | 1790 | 2461 | 471 | 536 | 613 | 235 | 256 | 268 | 141 | 150 | 147 | 94 | 98 | 91 |
| 0.5  *** | 1402 | 1574 | 2390 | 442 | 492 | 601 | 223 | 240 | 268 | 134 | 142 | 152 | 90 | 93 | 98 |
| *** | 1468 | 1773 | 2461 | 464 | 533 | 606 | 231 | 252 | 263 | 138 | 146 | 143 | 91 | 95 | 87 |
| 0.55  *** | 1327 | 1514 | 2363 | 427 | 478 | 587 | 214 | 232 | 260 | 128 | 135 | 145 | 85 | 88 | 92 |
| *** | 1400 | 1725 | 2412 | 449 | 519 | 588 | 222 | 244 | 252 | 132 | 140 | 135 | 87 | 90 | 81 |
| 0.6  *** | 1236 | 1433 | 2283 | 404 | 454 | 561 | 202 | 219 | 245 | 120 | 126 | 135 | 78 | 81 | 85 |
| *** | 1314 | 1648 | 2313 | 426 | 495 | 557 | 209 | 230 | 235 | 123 | 130 | 124 | 80 | 83 | 73 |
| 0.65  *** | 1133 | 1333 | 2149 | 375 | 423 | 521 | 186 | 201 | 224 | 108 | 114 | 122 | 70 | 72 | 75 |
| *** | 1213 | 1546 | 2164 | 396 | 461 | 514 | 193 | 211 | 213 | 111 | 118 | 110 | 71 | 74 | 63 |
| 0.7  *** | 1022 | 1216 | 1962 | 340 | 383 | 467 | 166 | 178 | 197 | 95 | 99 | 105 | 59 | 61 | 64 |
| *** | 1100 | 1417 | 1967 | 358 | 416 | 458 | 171 | 187 | 186 | 97 | 102 | 93 | 61 | 62 | 51 |
| 0.75  *** | 901 | 1081 | 1722 | 297 | 334 | 401 | 141 | 151 | 165 | 78 | 81 | 85 | . | . | . |
| *** | 974 | 1261 | 1719 | 313 | 361 | 390 | 145 | 157 | 153 | 80 | 83 | 73 | . | . | . |
| 0.8  *** | 768 | 924 | 1431 | 246 | 274 | 321 | 111 | 118 | 127 | . | . | . | . | . | . |
| *** | 832 | 1076 | 1422 | 258 | 294 | 310 | 114 | 122 | 115 | . | . | . | . | . | . |
| 0.85  *** | 618 | 740 | 1087 | 185 | 202 | 229 | . | . | . | . | . | . | . | . | . |
| *** | 669 | 852 | 1076 | 193 | 214 | 217 | . | . | . | . | . | . | . | . | . |
| 0.9  *** | 439 | 515 | 693 | . | . | . | . | . | . | . | . | . | . | . | . |
| *** | 472 | 579 | 681 | . | . | . | . | . | . | . | . | . | . | . | . |

## TABLE 7: ALPHA= 0.05  POWER= 0.8    EXPECTED ACCRUAL THRU MINIMUM FOLLOW-UP= 375

|  |  | DEL=.05 | | | DEL=.10 | | | DEL=.15 | | | DEL=.20 | | | DEL=.25 | | |
|---|---|---|---|---|---|---|---|---|---|---|---|---|---|---|---|---|
| FACT= | | 1.0 .75 | .50 .25 | .00 BIN | 1.0 .75 | .50 .25 | .00 BIN | 1.0 .75 | .50 .25 | .00 BIN | 1.0 75 | .50 .25 | .00 BIN | 1.0 .75 | .50 .25 | .00 BIN |
| PCONT=*** | | | | | REQUIRED NUMBER OF PATIENTS | | | | | | | | | | | |
| 0.05 | *** | 377 | 383 | 395 | 137 | 138 | 141 | 80 | 81 | 82 | 57 | 57 | 58 | 44 | 45 | 45 |
|  | *** | 379 | 387 | 681 | 137 | 139 | 217 | 81 | 82 | 115 | 57 | 58 | 73 | 44 | 45 | 51 |
| 0.1 | *** | 691 | 707 | 762 | 221 | 227 | 235 | 120 | 122 | 125 | 80 | 81 | 82 | 59 | 59 | 60 |
|  | *** | 697 | 725 | 1076 | 224 | 230 | 310 | 121 | 123 | 153 | 80 | 81 | 93 | 59 | 60 | 63 |
| 0.15 | *** | 962 | 992 | 1117 | 293 | 304 | 323 | 153 | 157 | 163 | 98 | 100 | 103 | 70 | 72 | 73 |
|  | *** | 973 | 1028 | 1422 | 298 | 312 | 390 | 155 | 160 | 186 | 99 | 101 | 110 | 71 | 72 | 73 |
| 0.2 | *** | 1176 | 1222 | 1441 | 351 | 368 | 400 | 179 | 186 | 195 | 113 | 116 | 120 | 80 | 81 | 83 |
|  | *** | 1193 | 1281 | 1719 | 358 | 380 | 458 | 182 | 190 | 213 | 114 | 118 | 124 | 80 | 82 | 81 |
| 0.25 | *** | 1333 | 1398 | 1724 | 395 | 418 | 466 | 200 | 209 | 222 | 124 | 128 | 134 | 86 | 88 | 91 |
|  | *** | 1356 | 1482 | 1967 | 405 | 437 | 514 | 204 | 215 | 235 | 126 | 131 | 135 | 88 | 90 | 87 |
| 0.3 | *** | 1434 | 1521 | 1960 | 426 | 456 | 519 | 215 | 226 | 243 | 132 | 137 | 144 | 91 | 94 | 97 |
|  | *** | 1466 | 1631 | 2164 | 439 | 481 | 557 | 220 | 234 | 252 | 135 | 140 | 143 | 92 | 95 | 91 |
| 0.35 | *** | 1486 | 1596 | 2147 | 446 | 482 | 559 | 224 | 238 | 259 | 137 | 143 | 151 | 94 | 97 | 100 |
|  | *** | 1527 | 1732 | 2313 | 462 | 512 | 588 | 230 | 247 | 263 | 140 | 147 | 147 | 95 | 99 | 93 |
| 0.4 | *** | 1495 | 1629 | 2281 | 455 | 497 | 587 | 229 | 244 | 268 | 139 | 146 | 155 | 94 | 98 | 102 |
|  | *** | 1546 | 1790 | 2412 | 474 | 531 | 606 | 236 | 254 | 268 | 142 | 150 | 149 | 96 | 100 | 93 |
| 0.45 | *** | 1470 | 1626 | 2362 | 456 | 502 | 600 | 229 | 245 | 271 | 139 | 146 | 155 | 93 | 97 | 101 |
|  | *** | 1530 | 1809 | 2461 | 475 | 539 | 613 | 236 | 257 | 268 | 142 | 150 | 147 | 95 | 99 | 91 |
| 0.5 | *** | 1417 | 1593 | 2390 | 448 | 497 | 601 | 225 | 242 | 268 | 135 | 142 | 152 | 90 | 93 | 98 |
|  | *** | 1485 | 1793 | 2461 | 469 | 536 | 606 | 232 | 253 | 263 | 138 | 147 | 143 | 92 | 95 | 87 |
| 0.55 | *** | 1343 | 1535 | 2363 | 432 | 482 | 587 | 216 | 233 | 260 | 129 | 136 | 145 | 85 | 88 | 92 |
|  | *** | 1418 | 1745 | 2412 | 454 | 523 | 588 | 224 | 245 | 252 | 132 | 140 | 135 | 87 | 90 | 81 |
| 0.6 | *** | 1254 | 1454 | 2283 | 410 | 459 | 560 | 204 | 220 | 245 | 120 | 127 | 135 | 79 | 81 | 85 |
|  | *** | 1333 | 1670 | 2313 | 431 | 498 | 557 | 211 | 231 | 235 | 123 | 131 | 124 | 80 | 83 | 73 |
| 0.65 | *** | 1152 | 1355 | 2149 | 380 | 427 | 520 | 187 | 202 | 224 | 109 | 115 | 122 | 70 | 73 | 75 |
|  | *** | 1233 | 1566 | 2164 | 401 | 464 | 514 | 194 | 212 | 213 | 112 | 118 | 110 | 71 | 74 | 63 |
| 0.7 | *** | 1040 | 1236 | 1962 | 344 | 387 | 467 | 167 | 179 | 197 | 95 | 100 | 105 | 60 | 62 | 64 |
|  | *** | 1120 | 1437 | 1967 | 363 | 419 | 458 | 173 | 187 | 186 | 97 | 102 | 93 | 61 | 63 | 51 |
| 0.75 | *** | 918 | 1099 | 1722 | 301 | 337 | 401 | 142 | 152 | 165 | 78 | 81 | 85 | . | . | . |
|  | *** | 992 | 1279 | 1719 | 317 | 363 | 390 | 146 | 158 | 153 | 80 | 83 | 73 | . | . | . |
| 0.8 | *** | 783 | 940 | 1430 | 249 | 276 | 321 | 112 | 118 | 127 | . | . | . | . | . | . |
|  | *** | 848 | 1090 | 1422 | 261 | 295 | 310 | 115 | 122 | 115 | . | . | . | . | . | . |
| 0.85 | *** | 631 | 752 | 1087 | 187 | 204 | 229 | . | . | . | . | . | . | . | . | . |
|  | *** | 681 | 862 | 1076 | 194 | 215 | 217 | . | . | . | . | . | . | . | . | . |
| 0.9 | *** | 447 | 522 | 693 | . | . | . | . | . | . | . | . | . | . | . | . |
|  | *** | 479 | 585 | 681 | . | . | . | . | . | . | . | . | . | . | . | . |

## TABLE 7: ALPHA= 0.05  POWER= 0.8    EXPECTED ACCRUAL THRU MINIMUM FOLLOW-UP= 400

| | | DEL=.05 | | | DEL=.10 | | | DEL=.15 | | | DEL=.20 | | | DEL=.25 | | |
|---|---|---|---|---|---|---|---|---|---|---|---|---|---|---|---|---|---|
| FACT= | | 1.0 .75 | .50 .25 | .00 BIN | 1.0 .75 | .50 .25 | .00 BIN | 1.0 .75 | .50 .25 | .00 BIN | 1.0 75 | .50 .25 | .00 BIN | 1.0 .75 | .50 .25 | .00 BIN |
| PCONT=*** | | | | | REQUIRED NUMBER OF PATIENTS | | | | | | | | | | | |
| 0.05 | *** | 378 | 383 | 395 | 137 | 138 | 141 | 81 | 81 | 82 | 57 | 57 | 58 | 44 | 45 | 45 |
| | *** | 380 | 388 | 681 | 138 | 139 | 217 | 81 | 82 | 115 | 57 | 58 | 73 | 44 | 45 | 51 |
| 0.1 | *** | 692 | 709 | 762 | 222 | 227 | 235 | 120 | 122 | 125 | 80 | 81 | 82 | 59 | 60 | 60 |
| | *** | 699 | 727 | 1076 | 224 | 231 | 310 | 121 | 124 | 153 | 80 | 81 | 93 | 59 | 60 | 63 |
| 0.15 | *** | 964 | 995 | 1117 | 294 | 304 | 323 | 153 | 157 | 163 | 98 | 100 | 103 | 71 | 72 | 73 |
| | *** | 975 | 1031 | 1422 | 299 | 312 | 390 | 155 | 160 | 186 | 99 | 101 | 110 | 71 | 72 | 73 |
| 0.2 | *** | 1180 | 1228 | 1441 | 352 | 369 | 400 | 180 | 186 | 195 | 113 | 116 | 120 | 80 | 81 | 83 |
| | *** | 1197 | 1287 | 1719 | 360 | 382 | 458 | 183 | 190 | 213 | 115 | 118 | 124 | 81 | 82 | 81 |
| 0.25 | *** | 1338 | 1405 | 1724 | 397 | 420 | 466 | 201 | 210 | 222 | 125 | 129 | 134 | 87 | 89 | 91 |
| | *** | 1363 | 1490 | 1967 | 407 | 439 | 514 | 205 | 215 | 235 | 127 | 131 | 135 | 88 | 90 | 87 |
| 0.3 | *** | 1441 | 1530 | 1960 | 429 | 459 | 519 | 216 | 227 | 243 | 133 | 138 | 144 | 91 | 94 | 97 |
| | *** | 1474 | 1642 | 2164 | 442 | 483 | 557 | 221 | 234 | 252 | 135 | 141 | 143 | 93 | 95 | 91 |
| 0.35 | *** | 1495 | 1608 | 2147 | 450 | 486 | 559 | 226 | 239 | 259 | 138 | 144 | 151 | 94 | 97 | 100 |
| | *** | 1537 | 1745 | 2313 | 465 | 514 | 588 | 232 | 248 | 263 | 141 | 147 | 147 | 95 | 99 | 93 |
| 0.4 | *** | 1506 | 1643 | 2281 | 460 | 501 | 587 | 231 | 245 | 268 | 140 | 146 | 155 | 95 | 98 | 102 |
| | *** | 1558 | 1805 | 2412 | 477 | 534 | 606 | 237 | 255 | 268 | 143 | 150 | 149 | 96 | 100 | 93 |
| 0.45 | *** | 1483 | 1642 | 2362 | 460 | 506 | 600 | 231 | 247 | 271 | 139 | 146 | 155 | 94 | 97 | 101 |
| | *** | 1544 | 1826 | 2461 | 480 | 542 | 613 | 238 | 257 | 268 | 143 | 150 | 147 | 95 | 99 | 91 |
| 0.5 | *** | 1432 | 1611 | 2390 | 452 | 501 | 601 | 227 | 243 | 268 | 136 | 143 | 152 | 91 | 94 | 98 |
| | *** | 1502 | 1812 | 2461 | 473 | 539 | 606 | 234 | 254 | 263 | 139 | 147 | 143 | 92 | 96 | 87 |
| 0.55 | *** | 1360 | 1554 | 2363 | 437 | 486 | 587 | 218 | 235 | 260 | 130 | 136 | 145 | 86 | 89 | 92 |
| | *** | 1436 | 1765 | 2412 | 458 | 526 | 588 | 226 | 246 | 252 | 133 | 140 | 135 | 87 | 90 | 81 |
| 0.6 | *** | 1271 | 1474 | 2283 | 414 | 463 | 561 | 206 | 221 | 245 | 121 | 127 | 135 | 79 | 82 | 85 |
| | *** | 1352 | 1689 | 2313 | 436 | 501 | 557 | 213 | 232 | 235 | 124 | 131 | 124 | 80 | 83 | 73 |
| 0.65 | *** | 1170 | 1374 | 2149 | 385 | 431 | 521 | 189 | 203 | 224 | 110 | 115 | 122 | 70 | 73 | 75 |
| | *** | 1252 | 1586 | 2164 | 405 | 467 | 514 | 196 | 213 | 213 | 112 | 118 | 110 | 72 | 74 | 63 |
| 0.7 | *** | 1058 | 1255 | 1962 | 349 | 390 | 467 | 168 | 180 | 197 | 96 | 100 | 105 | 60 | 62 | 64 |
| | *** | 1138 | 1455 | 1967 | 367 | 421 | 458 | 174 | 188 | 186 | 98 | 102 | 93 | 61 | 63 | 51 |
| 0.75 | *** | 935 | 1116 | 1722 | 305 | 339 | 401 | 143 | 152 | 165 | 79 | 82 | 85 | . | . | . |
| | *** | 1009 | 1295 | 1719 | 320 | 365 | 390 | 147 | 158 | 153 | 80 | 84 | 73 | . | . | . |
| 0.8 | *** | 798 | 954 | 1431 | 252 | 278 | 321 | 113 | 119 | 127 | . | . | . | . | . | . |
| | *** | 863 | 1102 | 1422 | 264 | 297 | 310 | 116 | 123 | 115 | . | . | . | . | . | . |
| 0.85 | *** | 642 | 763 | 1087 | 189 | 205 | 229 | . | . | . | . | . | . | . | . | . |
| | *** | 693 | 872 | 1076 | 196 | 216 | 217 | . | . | . | . | . | . | . | . | . |
| 0.9 | *** | 454 | 529 | 693 | . | . | . | . | . | . | . | . | . | . | . | . |
| | *** | 486 | 590 | 681 | . | . | . | . | . | . | . | . | . | . | . | . |

TABLE 7: ALPHA= 0.05  POWER= 0.8    EXPECTED ACCRUAL THRU MINIMUM FOLLOW-UP= 425

REQUIRED NUMBER OF PATIENTS

| PCONT | FACT= | DEL=.05 1.0/.75 | .50/.25 | .00/BIN | DEL=.10 1.0/.75 | .50/.25 | .00/BIN | DEL=.15 1.0/.75 | .50/.25 | .00/BIN | DEL=.20 1.0/75 | .50/.25 | .00/BIN | DEL=.25 1.0/.75 | .50/.25 | .00/BIN |
|---|---|---|---|---|---|---|---|---|---|---|---|---|---|---|---|---|
| 0.05 | *** | 378 | 383 | 395 | 137 | 138 | 141 | 81 | 81 | 82 | 57 | 57 | 58 | 44 | 45 | 45 |
|  | *** | 380 | 388 | 681 | 138 | 139 | 217 | 81 | 82 | 115 | 57 | 58 | 73 | 44 | 45 | 51 |
| 0.1 | *** | 694 | 711 | 762 | 222 | 227 | 235 | 120 | 122 | 125 | 80 | 81 | 82 | 59 | 60 | 60 |
|  | *** | 700 | 728 | 1076 | 225 | 231 | 310 | 121 | 124 | 153 | 80 | 81 | 93 | 59 | 60 | 63 |
| 0.15 | *** | 966 | 998 | 1117 | 295 | 305 | 323 | 154 | 158 | 163 | 99 | 101 | 103 | 71 | 72 | 73 |
|  | *** | 978 | 1034 | 1422 | 299 | 313 | 390 | 155 | 160 | 186 | 99 | 102 | 110 | 71 | 72 | 73 |
| 0.2 | *** | 1183 | 1233 | 1441 | 354 | 370 | 400 | 181 | 187 | 195 | 113 | 116 | 120 | 80 | 81 | 83 |
|  | *** | 1201 | 1292 | 1719 | 361 | 383 | 458 | 184 | 190 | 213 | 115 | 118 | 124 | 81 | 82 | 81 |
| 0.25 | *** | 1342 | 1412 | 1724 | 399 | 422 | 465 | 202 | 210 | 222 | 125 | 129 | 134 | 87 | 89 | 91 |
|  | *** | 1368 | 1498 | 1967 | 409 | 440 | 514 | 206 | 215 | 235 | 127 | 131 | 135 | 88 | 90 | 87 |
| 0.3 | *** | 1447 | 1540 | 1960 | 432 | 461 | 519 | 217 | 228 | 243 | 133 | 138 | 144 | 92 | 94 | 97 |
|  | *** | 1482 | 1651 | 2164 | 450 | 484 | 557 | 222 | 235 | 252 | 136 | 141 | 143 | 93 | 95 | 91 |
| 0.35 | *** | 1503 | 1619 | 2147 | 453 | 489 | 560 | 227 | 240 | 259 | 138 | 144 | 151 | 94 | 97 | 101 |
|  | *** | 1547 | 1757 | 2313 | 468 | 516 | 588 | 233 | 248 | 263 | 141 | 147 | 147 | 96 | 99 | 93 |
| 0.4 | *** | 1516 | 1657 | 2281 | 463 | 504 | 587 | 232 | 246 | 268 | 141 | 147 | 155 | 95 | 98 | 102 |
|  | *** | 1570 | 1820 | 2412 | 481 | 537 | 606 | 239 | 256 | 268 | 144 | 150 | 149 | 96 | 100 | 93 |
| 0.45 | *** | 1495 | 1658 | 2362 | 464 | 510 | 600 | 232 | 248 | 271 | 140 | 146 | 155 | 94 | 97 | 101 |
|  | *** | 1558 | 1842 | 2461 | 484 | 545 | 613 | 239 | 258 | 268 | 143 | 150 | 147 | 95 | 99 | 91 |
| 0.5 | *** | 1446 | 1628 | 2390 | 457 | 504 | 601 | 228 | 244 | 268 | 137 | 143 | 152 | 91 | 94 | 98 |
|  | *** | 1517 | 1829 | 2461 | 478 | 542 | 606 | 235 | 255 | 263 | 140 | 147 | 143 | 92 | 96 | 87 |
| 0.55 | *** | 1375 | 1572 | 2363 | 442 | 490 | 587 | 220 | 236 | 260 | 130 | 137 | 145 | 86 | 89 | 92 |
|  | *** | 1453 | 1784 | 2412 | 463 | 528 | 588 | 227 | 246 | 252 | 134 | 141 | 135 | 87 | 91 | 81 |
| 0.6 | *** | 1288 | 1493 | 2283 | 419 | 467 | 561 | 207 | 222 | 245 | 122 | 128 | 135 | 79 | 82 | 85 |
|  | *** | 1370 | 1708 | 2313 | 440 | 504 | 557 | 214 | 232 | 235 | 125 | 131 | 124 | 81 | 83 | 73 |
| 0.65 | *** | 1187 | 1393 | 2149 | 389 | 435 | 520 | 190 | 204 | 224 | 110 | 115 | 122 | 71 | 73 | 75 |
|  | *** | 1270 | 1604 | 2164 | 409 | 469 | 514 | 197 | 213 | 213 | 113 | 119 | 110 | 72 | 74 | 63 |
| 0.7 | *** | 1074 | 1273 | 1962 | 353 | 393 | 467 | 170 | 181 | 197 | 96 | 100 | 105 | 60 | 62 | 64 |
|  | *** | 1155 | 1471 | 1967 | 371 | 424 | 458 | 175 | 188 | 186 | 98 | 103 | 93 | 61 | 63 | 51 |
| 0.75 | *** | 950 | 1132 | 1722 | 308 | 342 | 401 | 144 | 153 | 165 | 79 | 82 | 85 | . | . | . |
|  | *** | 1025 | 1309 | 1719 | 323 | 367 | 390 | 148 | 158 | 153 | 81 | 84 | 73 | . | . | . |
| 0.8 | *** | 811 | 968 | 1430 | 255 | 280 | 321 | 113 | 119 | 127 | . | . | . | . | . | . |
|  | *** | 876 | 1114 | 1422 | 266 | 298 | 310 | 116 | 123 | 115 | . | . | . | . | . | . |
| 0.85 | *** | 653 | 773 | 1087 | 190 | 206 | 229 | . | . | . | . | . | . | . | . | . |
|  | *** | 703 | 880 | 1076 | 198 | 216 | 217 | . | . | . | . | . | . | . | . | . |
| 0.9 | *** | 461 | 535 | 693 | . | . | . | . | . | . | . | . | . | . | . | . |
|  | *** | 493 | 594 | 681 | . | . | . | . | . | . | . | . | . | . | . | . |

TABLE 7: ALPHA= 0.05  POWER= 0.8    EXPECTED ACCRUAL THRU MINIMUM FOLLOW-UP= 450

| | DEL=.05 | | | DEL=.10 | | | DEL=.15 | | | DEL=.20 | | | DEL=.25 | | |
|---|---|---|---|---|---|---|---|---|---|---|---|---|---|---|---|
| FACT= | 1.0 .75 | .50 .25 | .00 BIN | 1.0 .75 | .50 .25 | .00 BIN | 1.0 .75 | .50 .25 | .00 BIN | 1.0 75 | .50 .25 | .00 BIN | 1.0 .75 | .50 .25 | .00 BIN |
| PCONT=*** | | | | REQUIRED NUMBER OF PATIENTS | | | | | | | | | | | |
| 0.05 *** | 379 381 | 384 388 | 395 681 | 137 138 | 139 140 | 141 217 | 81 81 | 81 82 | 82 115 | 57 57 | 57 58 | 58 73 | 45 45 | 45 45 | 45 51 |
| 0.1 *** | 695 702 | 712 729 | 762 1076 | 223 225 | 228 231 | 235 310 | 121 122 | 123 124 | 125 153 | 80 81 | 81 81 | 82 93 | 59 59 | 60 60 | 60 63 |
| 0.15 *** | 968 981 | 1001 1037 | 1117 1422 | 296 300 | 306 313 | 323 390 | 154 156 | 158 160 | 163 186 | 99 100 | 100 102 | 103 110 | 71 71 | 72 72 | 73 73 |
| 0.2 *** | 1186 1206 | 1237 1297 | 1441 1719 | 355 363 | 372 383 | 400 458 | 181 184 | 187 191 | 195 213 | 114 115 | 117 118 | 120 124 | 80 81 | 82 82 | 83 81 |
| 0.25 *** | 1347 1374 | 1419 1504 | 1724 1967 | 401 411 | 424 441 | 465 514 | 203 206 | 211 216 | 222 235 | 126 127 | 129 131 | 134 135 | 87 88 | 89 90 | 91 87 |
| 0.3 *** | 1454 1489 | 1548 1661 | 1960 2164 | 435 447 | 464 486 | 519 557 | 218 223 | 228 235 | 243 252 | 134 136 | 138 141 | 144 143 | 92 93 | 94 95 | 97 91 |
| 0.35 *** | 1511 1556 | 1630 1769 | 2147 2313 | 456 471 | 491 518 | 559 588 | 228 234 | 240 249 | 259 263 | 139 141 | 144 147 | 151 147 | 95 96 | 97 99 | 100 93 |
| 0.4 *** | 1526 1581 | 1670 1833 | 2281 2412 | 467 485 | 507 539 | 586 606 | 234 240 | 247 257 | 268 268 | 141 144 | 147 151 | 155 149 | 95 97 | 98 100 | 102 93 |
| 0.45 *** | 1507 1571 | 1673 1857 | 2362 2461 | 468 488 | 513 547 | 600 613 | 234 240 | 249 259 | 271 268 | 141 144 | 147 151 | 155 147 | 94 96 | 97 99 | 101 91 |
| 0.5 *** | 1459 1532 | 1644 1845 | 2390 2461 | 461 482 | 508 545 | 600 606 | 230 237 | 245 255 | 268 263 | 137 140 | 144 147 | 152 143 | 91 93 | 94 96 | 98 87 |
| 0.55 *** | 1390 1469 | 1589 1800 | 2363 2412 | 446 467 | 494 531 | 587 588 | 221 228 | 237 247 | 259 252 | 131 134 | 137 141 | 145 135 | 86 87 | 89 91 | 92 81 |
| 0.6 *** | 1304 1387 | 1511 1725 | 2283 2313 | 423 444 | 471 507 | 561 557 | 209 216 | 223 233 | 245 235 | 122 125 | 128 131 | 135 124 | 79 81 | 82 83 | 85 73 |
| 0.65 *** | 1203 1287 | 1410 1620 | 2149 2164 | 393 413 | 438 471 | 521 514 | 192 198 | 205 213 | 224 213 | 111 113 | 116 119 | 122 110 | 71 72 | 73 74 | 75 63 |
| 0.7 *** | 1090 1172 | 1290 1487 | 1962 1967 | 356 374 | 396 425 | 467 458 | 171 176 | 182 189 | 197 186 | 96 99 | 100 103 | 105 93 | 60 61 | 62 63 | 64 51 |
| 0.75 *** | 965 1040 | 1148 1323 | 1722 1719 | 311 326 | 345 368 | 401 390 | 145 149 | 154 159 | 165 153 | 79 81 | 82 84 | 85 73 | . . | . . | . . |
| 0.8 *** | 824 889 | 981 1125 | 1431 1422 | 257 268 | 282 299 | 321 310 | 114 117 | 120 123 | 127 115 | . . | . . | . . | . . | . . | . . |
| 0.85 *** | 663 714 | 783 888 | 1087 1076 | 192 199 | 207 217 | 229 217 | . . | . . | . . | . . | . . | . . | . . | . . | . . |
| 0.9 *** | 468 499 | 540 599 | 693 681 | . . | . . | . . | . . | . . | . . | . . | . . | . . | . . | . . | . . |

## TABLE 7: ALPHA= 0.05  POWER= 0.8    EXPECTED ACCRUAL THRU MINIMUM FOLLOW-UP= 475

| | | DEL=.05 | | | DEL=.10 | | | DEL=.15 | | | DEL=.20 | | | DEL=.25 | | |
|---|---|---|---|---|---|---|---|---|---|---|---|---|---|---|---|---|---|
| FACT= | | 1.0 .75 | .50 .25 | .00 BIN | 1.0 .75 | .50 .25 | .00 BIN | 1.0 .75 | .50 .25 | .00 BIN | 1.0 75 | .50 .25 | .00 BIN | 1.0 .75 | .50 .25 | .00 BIN |
| PCONT=*** | | | | | REQUIRED | NUMBER OF | PATIENTS | | | | | | | | | |
| 0.05 | *** | 379 | 384 | 395 | 137 | 139 | 141 | 81 | 81 | 82 | 57 | 57 | 58 | 45 | 45 | 45 |
| | *** | 381 | 389 | 681 | 138 | 140 | 217 | 81 | 82 | 115 | 57 | 58 | 73 | 45 | 45 | 51 |
| 0.1 | *** | 696 | 713 | 762 | 223 | 228 | 235 | 121 | 123 | 125 | 80 | 81 | 82 | 59 | 60 | 60 |
| | *** | 703 | 731 | 1076 | 226 | 231 | 310 | 122 | 124 | 153 | 80 | 81 | 93 | 59 | 60 | 63 |
| 0.15 | *** | 970 | 1004 | 1117 | 297 | 307 | 322 | 154 | 158 | 163 | 99 | 101 | 103 | 71 | 72 | 73 |
| | *** | 983 | 1040 | 1422 | 301 | 314 | 390 | 156 | 160 | 186 | 100 | 102 | 110 | 71 | 72 | 73 |
| 0.2 | *** | 1190 | 1242 | 1441 | 357 | 373 | 400 | 182 | 188 | 195 | 114 | 117 | 120 | 80 | 82 | 83 |
| | *** | 1210 | 1302 | 1719 | 364 | 384 | 458 | 184 | 191 | 213 | 115 | 118 | 124 | 81 | 82 | 81 |
| 0.25 | *** | 1352 | 1426 | 1724 | 403 | 425 | 466 | 203 | 211 | 222 | 126 | 129 | 134 | 87 | 89 | 91 |
| | *** | 1380 | 1511 | 1967 | 413 | 442 | 514 | 207 | 216 | 235 | 127 | 131 | 135 | 88 | 90 | 87 |
| 0.3 | *** | 1460 | 1557 | 1960 | 437 | 466 | 519 | 219 | 229 | 243 | 134 | 139 | 144 | 92 | 94 | 97 |
| | *** | 1497 | 1670 | 2164 | 450 | 487 | 557 | 224 | 235 | 252 | 136 | 141 | 143 | 93 | 96 | 91 |
| 0.35 | *** | 1519 | 1641 | 2147 | 459 | 494 | 559 | 229 | 241 | 259 | 140 | 145 | 151 | 95 | 97 | 100 |
| | *** | 1565 | 1780 | 2313 | 474 | 520 | 588 | 235 | 249 | 263 | 142 | 148 | 147 | 96 | 99 | 93 |
| 0.4 | *** | 1536 | 1682 | 2281 | 470 | 510 | 587 | 235 | 248 | 268 | 142 | 148 | 155 | 96 | 98 | 102 |
| | *** | 1592 | 1846 | 2412 | 488 | 541 | 606 | 241 | 257 | 268 | 145 | 151 | 149 | 97 | 100 | 93 |
| 0.45 | *** | 1518 | 1687 | 2362 | 472 | 516 | 600 | 235 | 250 | 271 | 141 | 147 | 155 | 94 | 97 | 101 |
| | *** | 1584 | 1872 | 2461 | 491 | 549 | 613 | 242 | 259 | 268 | 144 | 151 | 147 | 96 | 99 | 91 |
| 0.5 | *** | 1473 | 1660 | 2390 | 465 | 511 | 601 | 231 | 246 | 268 | 138 | 144 | 152 | 91 | 94 | 98 |
| | *** | 1547 | 1860 | 2461 | 485 | 547 | 606 | 238 | 256 | 263 | 141 | 148 | 143 | 93 | 96 | 87 |
| 0.55 | *** | 1404 | 1606 | 2363 | 450 | 497 | 587 | 223 | 238 | 260 | 132 | 138 | 145 | 86 | 89 | 92 |
| | *** | 1485 | 1816 | 2412 | 471 | 533 | 588 | 229 | 247 | 252 | 134 | 141 | 135 | 88 | 91 | 81 |
| 0.6 | *** | 1319 | 1527 | 2283 | 427 | 474 | 561 | 210 | 224 | 245 | 123 | 128 | 135 | 80 | 82 | 85 |
| | *** | 1403 | 1741 | 2313 | 448 | 509 | 557 | 217 | 233 | 235 | 126 | 131 | 124 | 81 | 83 | 73 |
| 0.65 | *** | 1218 | 1427 | 2149 | 397 | 441 | 520 | 193 | 206 | 224 | 111 | 116 | 122 | 71 | 73 | 75 |
| | *** | 1303 | 1636 | 2164 | 416 | 473 | 514 | 199 | 214 | 213 | 114 | 119 | 110 | 72 | 74 | 63 |
| 0.7 | *** | 1105 | 1305 | 1962 | 359 | 399 | 467 | 172 | 183 | 197 | 97 | 101 | 105 | 61 | 62 | 64 |
| | *** | 1187 | 1501 | 1967 | 377 | 427 | 458 | 177 | 189 | 186 | 99 | 103 | 93 | 61 | 63 | 51 |
| 0.75 | *** | 979 | 1162 | 1722 | 314 | 347 | 401 | 146 | 154 | 165 | 80 | 82 | 85 | . | . | . |
| | *** | 1054 | 1335 | 1719 | 329 | 370 | 390 | 150 | 159 | 153 | 81 | 84 | 73 | . | . | . |
| 0.8 | *** | 836 | 993 | 1430 | 259 | 283 | 321 | 115 | 120 | 127 | . | . | . | . | . | . |
| | *** | 902 | 1136 | 1422 | 270 | 300 | 310 | 117 | 123 | 115 | . | . | . | . | . | . |
| 0.85 | *** | 672 | 792 | 1087 | 193 | 208 | 229 | . | . | . | . | . | . | . | . | . |
| | *** | 723 | 895 | 1076 | 200 | 218 | 217 | . | . | . | . | . | . | . | . | . |
| 0.9 | *** | 473 | 545 | 693 | . | . | . | . | . | . | . | . | . | . | . | . |
| | *** | 505 | 602 | 681 | . | . | . | . | . | . | . | . | . | . | . | . |

TABLE 7: ALPHA= 0.05  POWER= 0.8    EXPECTED ACCRUAL THRU MINIMUM FOLLOW-UP= 500

| | DEL=.05 | | | DEL=.10 | | | DEL=.15 | | | DEL=.20 | | | DEL=.25 | | |
|---|---|---|---|---|---|---|---|---|---|---|---|---|---|---|---|
| FACT= | 1.0 .75 | .50 .25 | .00 BIN | 1.0 .75 | .50 .25 | .00 BIN | 1.0 .75 | .50 .25 | .00 BIN | 1.0 75 | .50 .25 | .00 BIN | 1.0 .75 | .50 .25 | .00 BIN |
| PCONT=*** | | | | REQUIRED NUMBER OF PATIENTS | | | | | | | | | | | |
| 0.05 *** | 379 | 385 | 395 | 138 | 139 | 141 | 81 | 82 | 82 | 57 | 58 | 58 | 44 | 45 | 45 |
| *** | 382 | 389 | 681 | 138 | 140 | 217 | 81 | 82 | 115 | 57 | 58 | 73 | 44 | 45 | 51 |
| 0.1 *** | 697 | 715 | 762 | 224 | 228 | 235 | 121 | 123 | 125 | 80 | 81 | 82 | 59 | 60 | 60 |
| *** | 704 | 732 | 1076 | 226 | 232 | 310 | 122 | 124 | 153 | 81 | 82 | 93 | 59 | 60 | 63 |
| 0.15 *** | 973 | 1006 | 1117 | 298 | 307 | 323 | 155 | 158 | 163 | 99 | 101 | 103 | 71 | 72 | 73 |
| *** | 986 | 1043 | 1422 | 302 | 314 | 390 | 156 | 160 | 186 | 100 | 102 | 110 | 72 | 73 | 73 |
| 0.2 *** | 1193 | 1246 | 1441 | 358 | 373 | 400 | 183 | 188 | 195 | 114 | 117 | 120 | 80 | 82 | 83 |
| *** | 1213 | 1306 | 1719 | 365 | 385 | 458 | 185 | 191 | 213 | 116 | 118 | 124 | 81 | 83 | 81 |
| 0.25 *** | 1357 | 1432 | 1724 | 405 | 427 | 466 | 204 | 212 | 222 | 126 | 130 | 134 | 88 | 89 | 91 |
| *** | 1385 | 1518 | 1967 | 415 | 443 | 514 | 208 | 217 | 235 | 128 | 132 | 135 | 88 | 90 | 87 |
| 0.3 *** | 1466 | 1565 | 1960 | 439 | 468 | 519 | 220 | 230 | 243 | 135 | 139 | 144 | 92 | 94 | 97 |
| *** | 1504 | 1678 | 2164 | 452 | 489 | 557 | 224 | 236 | 252 | 137 | 141 | 143 | 93 | 96 | 91 |
| 0.35 *** | 1527 | 1651 | 2147 | 462 | 496 | 559 | 230 | 242 | 259 | 140 | 145 | 151 | 95 | 98 | 100 |
| *** | 1574 | 1790 | 2313 | 477 | 522 | 588 | 236 | 250 | 263 | 143 | 148 | 147 | 96 | 99 | 93 |
| 0.4 *** | 1546 | 1694 | 2281 | 473 | 513 | 587 | 236 | 249 | 268 | 143 | 148 | 155 | 96 | 98 | 102 |
| *** | 1603 | 1858 | 2412 | 491 | 543 | 606 | 242 | 258 | 268 | 145 | 151 | 149 | 97 | 100 | 93 |
| 0.45 *** | 1530 | 1700 | 2362 | 476 | 519 | 600 | 236 | 251 | 271 | 142 | 148 | 155 | 95 | 98 | 101 |
| *** | 1597 | 1885 | 2461 | 494 | 552 | 613 | 243 | 260 | 268 | 145 | 151 | 147 | 96 | 99 | 91 |
| 0.5 *** | 1485 | 1675 | 2390 | 469 | 514 | 601 | 233 | 247 | 268 | 138 | 144 | 152 | 92 | 94 | 98 |
| *** | 1561 | 1875 | 2461 | 489 | 549 | 606 | 239 | 257 | 263 | 141 | 148 | 143 | 93 | 96 | 87 |
| 0.55 *** | 1418 | 1622 | 2363 | 454 | 500 | 587 | 224 | 239 | 259 | 132 | 138 | 145 | 87 | 89 | 93 |
| *** | 1500 | 1832 | 2412 | 474 | 536 | 588 | 231 | 248 | 252 | 135 | 141 | 135 | 88 | 91 | 81 |
| 0.6 *** | 1333 | 1543 | 2283 | 431 | 477 | 561 | 211 | 225 | 245 | 123 | 129 | 135 | 80 | 82 | 85 |
| *** | 1418 | 1756 | 2313 | 451 | 511 | 557 | 218 | 234 | 235 | 126 | 132 | 124 | 81 | 83 | 73 |
| 0.65 *** | 1233 | 1443 | 2149 | 401 | 444 | 521 | 194 | 207 | 224 | 112 | 116 | 122 | 71 | 73 | 75 |
| *** | 1319 | 1651 | 2164 | 420 | 475 | 514 | 200 | 215 | 213 | 114 | 119 | 110 | 72 | 74 | 63 |
| 0.7 *** | 1120 | 1321 | 1962 | 363 | 401 | 467 | 173 | 183 | 197 | 97 | 101 | 105 | 61 | 62 | 64 |
| *** | 1202 | 1515 | 1967 | 380 | 429 | 458 | 178 | 190 | 186 | 99 | 103 | 93 | 61 | 63 | 51 |
| 0.75 *** | 992 | 1175 | 1722 | 317 | 349 | 401 | 147 | 155 | 165 | 80 | 83 | 85 | . | . | . |
| *** | 1068 | 1348 | 1719 | 331 | 371 | 390 | 150 | 159 | 153 | 81 | 84 | 73 | . | . | . |
| 0.8 *** | 848 | 1004 | 1431 | 261 | 285 | 321 | 115 | 120 | 127 | . | . | . | . | . | . |
| *** | 913 | 1145 | 1422 | 272 | 301 | 310 | 118 | 123 | 115 | . | . | . | . | . | . |
| 0.85 *** | 681 | 800 | 1087 | 194 | 209 | 229 | . | . | . | . | . | . | . | . | . |
| *** | 732 | 902 | 1076 | 201 | 218 | 217 | . | . | . | . | . | . | . | . | . |
| 0.9 *** | 479 | 550 | 693 | . | . | . | . | . | . | . | . | . | . | . | . |
| *** | 510 | 606 | 681 | . | . | . | . | . | . | . | . | . | . | . | . |

## TABLE 7: ALPHA= 0.05 POWER= 0.8     EXPECTED ACCRUAL THRU MINIMUM FOLLOW-UP= 550

| | | DEL=.02 | | | DEL=.05 | | | DEL=.10 | | | DEL=.15 | | | DEL=.20 | | |
|---|---|---|---|---|---|---|---|---|---|---|---|---|---|---|---|---|
| FACT= | | 1.0 | .50 | .00 | 1.0 | .50 | .00 | 1.0 | .50 | .00 | 1.0 | .50 | .00 | 1.0 | .50 | .00 |
| | | .75 | .25 | BIN | .75 | .25 | BIN | .75 | .25 | BIN | 75 | .25 | BIN | .75 | .25 | BIN |

PCONT=***      REQUIRED NUMBER OF PATIENTS

| PCONT | | .02 | | | .05 | | | .10 | | | .15 | | | .20 | | |
|---|---|---|---|---|---|---|---|---|---|---|---|---|---|---|---|---|
| 0.05 | *** | 1764 | 1776 | 1863 | 380 | 385 | 395 | 138 | 139 | 140 | 81 | 81 | 82 | 57 | 57 | 58 |
| | *** | 1768 | 1794 | 3481 | 382 | 389 | 681 | 138 | 140 | 217 | 81 | 82 | 115 | 57 | 58 | 73 |
| 0.1 | *** | 3672 | 3699 | 4092 | 699 | 717 | 762 | 224 | 229 | 235 | 121 | 123 | 125 | 80 | 81 | 82 |
| | *** | 3681 | 3751 | 6047 | 707 | 734 | 1076 | 226 | 232 | 310 | 122 | 124 | 153 | 81 | 81 | 93 |
| 0.15 | *** | 5367 | 5415 | 6328 | 976 | 1011 | 1117 | 299 | 308 | 322 | 155 | 158 | 163 | 99 | 101 | 103 |
| | *** | 5383 | 5509 | 8304 | 990 | 1047 | 1422 | 303 | 314 | 390 | 157 | 160 | 186 | 100 | 102 | 110 |
| 0.2 | *** | 6721 | 6795 | 8409 | 1199 | 1254 | 1441 | 360 | 375 | 400 | 183 | 188 | 195 | 115 | 117 | 120 |
| | *** | 6745 | 6940 | 10251 | 1221 | 1314 | 1719 | 367 | 386 | 458 | 186 | 192 | 213 | 116 | 118 | 124 |
| 0.25 | *** | 7697 | 7803 | 10253 | 1365 | 1443 | 1724 | 408 | 430 | 465 | 205 | 212 | 222 | 127 | 130 | 134 |
| | *** | 7733 | 8012 | 11890 | 1396 | 1529 | 1967 | 418 | 445 | 514 | 209 | 217 | 235 | 128 | 132 | 135 |
| 0.3 | *** | 8303 | 8449 | 11816 | 1478 | 1581 | 1960 | 443 | 471 | 519 | 221 | 231 | 243 | 135 | 139 | 144 |
| | *** | 8352 | 8734 | 13219 | 1518 | 1693 | 2164 | 455 | 491 | 557 | 226 | 236 | 252 | 137 | 142 | 143 |
| 0.35 | *** | 8566 | 8759 | 13073 | 1542 | 1669 | 2147 | 467 | 500 | 559 | 232 | 243 | 259 | 141 | 145 | 151 |
| | *** | 8630 | 9135 | 14239 | 1592 | 1809 | 2313 | 481 | 525 | 588 | 237 | 250 | 263 | 143 | 148 | 147 |
| 0.4 | *** | 8523 | 8775 | 14009 | 1564 | 1716 | 2281 | 479 | 518 | 587 | 238 | 250 | 268 | 143 | 148 | 155 |
| | *** | 8607 | 9257 | 14950 | 1624 | 1880 | 2412 | 496 | 546 | 606 | 244 | 258 | 268 | 146 | 151 | 149 |
| 0.45 | *** | 8223 | 8547 | 14614 | 1551 | 1726 | 2362 | 482 | 524 | 600 | 239 | 252 | 271 | 143 | 148 | 155 |
| | *** | 8331 | 9147 | 15352 | 1620 | 1909 | 2461 | 500 | 555 | 613 | 245 | 261 | 268 | 145 | 151 | 147 |
| 0.5 | *** | 7716 | 8126 | 14886 | 1510 | 1702 | 2390 | 475 | 520 | 600 | 235 | 249 | 268 | 140 | 145 | 152 |
| | *** | 7854 | 8853 | 15445 | 1587 | 1902 | 2461 | 495 | 553 | 606 | 241 | 257 | 263 | 142 | 148 | 143 |
| 0.55 | *** | 7057 | 7568 | 14820 | 1445 | 1651 | 2363 | 461 | 506 | 587 | 226 | 240 | 259 | 133 | 138 | 145 |
| | *** | 7232 | 8418 | 15228 | 1528 | 1859 | 2412 | 481 | 539 | 588 | 233 | 249 | 252 | 136 | 142 | 135 |
| 0.6 | *** | 6305 | 6924 | 14419 | 1361 | 1573 | 2283 | 438 | 482 | 561 | 213 | 226 | 245 | 124 | 129 | 135 |
| | *** | 6522 | 7879 | 14703 | 1447 | 1784 | 2313 | 457 | 514 | 557 | 220 | 235 | 235 | 127 | 132 | 124 |
| 0.65 | *** | 5517 | 6237 | 13682 | 1261 | 1472 | 2149 | 407 | 449 | 520 | 196 | 208 | 224 | 113 | 117 | 122 |
| | *** | 5777 | 7262 | 13868 | 1348 | 1677 | 2164 | 426 | 479 | 514 | 202 | 215 | 213 | 114 | 119 | 110 |
| 0.7 | *** | 4743 | 5534 | 12613 | 1147 | 1348 | 1962 | 369 | 406 | 467 | 175 | 184 | 197 | 98 | 101 | 105 |
| | *** | 5037 | 6584 | 12724 | 1230 | 1540 | 1967 | 385 | 432 | 458 | 179 | 190 | 186 | 100 | 103 | 93 |
| 0.75 | *** | 4012 | 4826 | 11213 | 1017 | 1200 | 1722 | 322 | 352 | 401 | 148 | 155 | 165 | 80 | 83 | 85 |
| | *** | 4322 | 5847 | 11271 | 1093 | 1369 | 1719 | 335 | 373 | 390 | 151 | 160 | 153 | 81 | 84 | 73 |
| 0.8 | *** | 3328 | 4107 | 9486 | 870 | 1025 | 1431 | 265 | 288 | 321 | 116 | 121 | 127 | . | . | . |
| | *** | 3630 | 5043 | 9509 | 935 | 1163 | 1422 | 276 | 302 | 310 | 118 | 124 | 115 | . | . | . |
| 0.85 | *** | 2671 | 3355 | 7436 | 698 | 815 | 1087 | 197 | 211 | 229 | . | . | . | . | . | . |
| | *** | 2939 | 4144 | 7438 | 748 | 914 | 1076 | 203 | 219 | 217 | . | . | . | . | . | . |
| 0.9 | *** | 1993 | 2516 | 5066 | 490 | 559 | 693 | . | . | . | . | . | . | . | . | . |
| | *** | 2201 | 3090 | 5058 | 520 | 612 | 681 | . | . | . | . | . | . | . | . | . |
| 0.95 | *** | 1180 | 1456 | 2380 | . | . | . | . | . | . | . | . | . | . | . | . |
| | *** | 1293 | 1726 | 2368 | . | . | . | . | . | . | . | . | . | . | . | . |

TABLE 7: ALPHA= 0.05  POWER= 0.8    EXPECTED ACCRUAL THRU MINIMUM FOLLOW-UP= 600

| | | DEL=.02 | | | DEL=.05 | | | DEL=.10 | | | DEL=.15 | | | DEL=.20 | | |
|---|---|---|---|---|---|---|---|---|---|---|---|---|---|---|---|---|---|
| FACT= | | 1.0 .75 | .50 .25 | .00 BIN | 1.0 .75 | .50 .25 | .00 BIN | 1.0 .75 | .50 .25 | .00 BIN | 1.0 75 | .50 .25 | .00 BIN | 1.0 .75 | .50 .25 | .00 BIN |
| PCONT=*** | | REQUIRED NUMBER OF PATIENTS | | | | | | | | | | | | | | |
| 0.05 | *** | 1765 | 1778 | 1863 | 381 | 386 | 395 | 138 | 139 | 140 | 81 | 82 | 82 | 57 | 58 | 58 |
|  | *** | 1770 | 1797 | 3481 | 383 | 390 | 681 | 138 | 140 | 217 | 81 | 82 | 115 | 57 | 58 | 73 |
| 0.1 | *** | 3674 | 3704 | 4092 | 701 | 719 | 762 | 225 | 229 | 235 | 121 | 123 | 125 | 80 | 81 | 82 |
|  | *** | 3685 | 3760 | 6047 | 709 | 736 | 1076 | 227 | 232 | 310 | 122 | 124 | 153 | 81 | 82 | 93 |
| 0.15 | *** | 5372 | 5424 | 6328 | 980 | 1016 | 1117 | 300 | 309 | 322 | 156 | 159 | 163 | 100 | 101 | 103 |
|  | *** | 5389 | 5525 | 8304 | 995 | 1051 | 1422 | 304 | 315 | 390 | 157 | 161 | 186 | 100 | 102 | 110 |
| 0.2 | *** | 6727 | 6808 | 8408 | 1205 | 1262 | 1441 | 362 | 377 | 400 | 184 | 189 | 195 | 115 | 117 | 120 |
|  | *** | 6754 | 6965 | 10251 | 1228 | 1321 | 1719 | 369 | 387 | 458 | 186 | 192 | 213 | 116 | 118 | 124 |
| 0.25 | *** | 7707 | 7822 | 10252 | 1374 | 1454 | 1724 | 411 | 432 | 466 | 206 | 213 | 222 | 127 | 130 | 134 |
|  | *** | 7745 | 8048 | 11890 | 1405 | 1539 | 1967 | 420 | 446 | 514 | 209 | 217 | 235 | 128 | 132 | 135 |
| 0.3 | *** | 8316 | 8475 | 11816 | 1489 | 1594 | 1960 | 447 | 474 | 519 | 223 | 232 | 243 | 136 | 140 | 144 |
|  | *** | 8369 | 8783 | 13219 | 1530 | 1706 | 2164 | 459 | 493 | 557 | 227 | 237 | 252 | 138 | 142 | 143 |
| 0.35 | *** | 8583 | 8794 | 13073 | 1556 | 1687 | 2147 | 471 | 503 | 559 | 234 | 244 | 259 | 142 | 146 | 151 |
|  | *** | 8653 | 9199 | 14239 | 1607 | 1825 | 2313 | 485 | 527 | 588 | 239 | 251 | 263 | 143 | 148 | 147 |
| 0.4 | *** | 8546 | 8821 | 14009 | 1582 | 1737 | 2281 | 484 | 521 | 586 | 240 | 251 | 268 | 144 | 149 | 155 |
|  | *** | 8638 | 9338 | 14950 | 1643 | 1899 | 2412 | 501 | 548 | 606 | 245 | 259 | 268 | 146 | 152 | 149 |
| 0.45 | *** | 8252 | 8605 | 14614 | 1571 | 1749 | 2362 | 488 | 529 | 600 | 241 | 253 | 271 | 143 | 149 | 155 |
|  | *** | 8371 | 9246 | 15352 | 1642 | 1931 | 2461 | 506 | 558 | 613 | 247 | 262 | 268 | 146 | 152 | 147 |
| 0.5 | *** | 7753 | 8198 | 14886 | 1532 | 1728 | 2389 | 481 | 525 | 601 | 237 | 250 | 268 | 140 | 145 | 152 |
|  | *** | 7904 | 8968 | 15445 | 1611 | 1925 | 2461 | 501 | 556 | 606 | 243 | 258 | 263 | 143 | 148 | 143 |
| 0.55 | *** | 7105 | 7655 | 14821 | 1469 | 1677 | 2363 | 467 | 511 | 587 | 228 | 241 | 259 | 134 | 139 | 145 |
|  | *** | 7295 | 8548 | 15228 | 1554 | 1884 | 2412 | 486 | 542 | 588 | 235 | 250 | 252 | 136 | 142 | 135 |
| 0.6 | *** | 6365 | 7026 | 14419 | 1387 | 1600 | 2283 | 444 | 487 | 560 | 215 | 228 | 245 | 125 | 130 | 135 |
|  | *** | 6598 | 8020 | 14703 | 1474 | 1808 | 2313 | 463 | 518 | 557 | 221 | 236 | 235 | 127 | 132 | 124 |
| 0.65 | *** | 5590 | 6350 | 13682 | 1287 | 1499 | 2149 | 413 | 453 | 520 | 198 | 209 | 224 | 113 | 117 | 122 |
|  | *** | 5866 | 7409 | 13868 | 1374 | 1701 | 2164 | 431 | 482 | 514 | 203 | 216 | 213 | 115 | 119 | 110 |
| 0.7 | *** | 4826 | 5653 | 12613 | 1172 | 1373 | 1962 | 374 | 410 | 467 | 176 | 185 | 197 | 98 | 101 | 105 |
|  | *** | 5135 | 6731 | 12724 | 1255 | 1561 | 1967 | 390 | 434 | 458 | 180 | 191 | 186 | 100 | 103 | 93 |
| 0.75 | *** | 4101 | 4943 | 11213 | 1040 | 1222 | 1722 | 326 | 355 | 401 | 149 | 156 | 165 | 80 | 83 | 85 |
|  | *** | 4424 | 5987 | 11271 | 1116 | 1388 | 1719 | 339 | 375 | 390 | 152 | 160 | 153 | 82 | 84 | 73 |
| 0.8 | *** | 3416 | 4217 | 9487 | 889 | 1043 | 1430 | 268 | 290 | 321 | 116 | 121 | 127 | . | . | . |
|  | *** | 3727 | 5169 | 9509 | 954 | 1178 | 1422 | 278 | 304 | 310 | 119 | 124 | 115 | . | . | . |
| 0.85 | *** | 2750 | 3449 | 7436 | 713 | 829 | 1087 | 199 | 212 | 229 | . | . | . | . | . | . |
|  | *** | 3025 | 4248 | 7438 | 763 | 924 | 1076 | 205 | 220 | 217 | . | . | . | . | . | . |
| 0.9 | *** | 2054 | 2586 | 5066 | 499 | 566 | 692 | . | . | . | . | . | . | . | . | . |
|  | *** | 2267 | 3162 | 5058 | 529 | 617 | 681 | . | . | . | . | . | . | . | . | . |
| 0.95 | *** | 1214 | 1491 | 2380 | . | . | . | . | . | . | . | . | . | . | . | . |
|  | *** | 1328 | 1757 | 2368 | . | . | . | . | . | . | . | . | . | . | . | . |

## TABLE 7: ALPHA= 0.05  POWER= 0.8    EXPECTED ACCRUAL THRU MINIMUM FOLLOW-UP= 650

| | | DEL=.02 | | | DEL=.05 | | | DEL=.10 | | | DEL=.15 | | | DEL=.20 | | |
|---|---|---|---|---|---|---|---|---|---|---|---|---|---|---|---|---|
| FACT= | | 1.0 .75 | .50 .25 | .00 BIN | 1.0 .75 | .50 .25 | .00 BIN | 1.0 .75 | .50 .25 | .00 BIN | 1.0 75 | .50 .25 | .00 BIN | 1.0 .75 | .50 .25 | .00 BIN |
| PCONT=*** | | | | | | REQUIRED NUMBER OF PATIENTS | | | | | | | | | | |
| 0.05 | *** | 1767 | 1780 | 1863 | 381 | 387 | 395 | 138 | 139 | 141 | 81 | 81 | 82 | 57 | 58 | 58 |
| | *** | 1771 | 1800 | 3481 | 384 | 390 | 681 | 138 | 140 | 217 | 81 | 82 | 115 | 58 | 58 | 73 |
| 0.1 | *** | 3677 | 3709 | 4092 | 704 | 721 | 762 | 226 | 230 | 236 | 122 | 123 | 125 | 81 | 81 | 82 |
| | *** | 3688 | 3768 | 6047 | 711 | 737 | 1076 | 228 | 232 | 310 | 123 | 124 | 153 | 81 | 81 | 93 |
| 0.15 | *** | 5376 | 5433 | 6328 | 985 | 1020 | 1117 | 302 | 310 | 322 | 156 | 159 | 163 | 100 | 101 | 103 |
| | *** | 5395 | 5541 | 8304 | 999 | 1055 | 1422 | 305 | 315 | 390 | 158 | 161 | 186 | 101 | 102 | 110 |
| 0.2 | *** | 6734 | 6821 | 8409 | 1211 | 1269 | 1441 | 364 | 379 | 400 | 185 | 189 | 195 | 116 | 117 | 120 |
| | *** | 6763 | 6991 | 10251 | 1234 | 1327 | 1719 | 371 | 388 | 458 | 187 | 192 | 213 | 116 | 119 | 124 |
| 0.25 | *** | 7717 | 7842 | 10252 | 1382 | 1464 | 1724 | 414 | 434 | 465 | 207 | 214 | 222 | 128 | 130 | 133 |
| | *** | 7758 | 8085 | 11890 | 1414 | 1548 | 1967 | 423 | 448 | 514 | 210 | 218 | 235 | 129 | 132 | 135 |
| 0.3 | *** | 8330 | 8501 | 11816 | 1500 | 1607 | 1960 | 451 | 476 | 519 | 224 | 232 | 244 | 136 | 140 | 144 |
| | *** | 8387 | 8832 | 13219 | 1543 | 1719 | 2164 | 462 | 495 | 557 | 228 | 237 | 252 | 138 | 142 | 143 |
| 0.35 | *** | 8601 | 8829 | 13073 | 1570 | 1703 | 2147 | 476 | 507 | 559 | 236 | 245 | 259 | 142 | 146 | 151 |
| | *** | 8677 | 9263 | 14239 | 1623 | 1841 | 2313 | 489 | 529 | 588 | 240 | 251 | 263 | 144 | 149 | 147 |
| 0.4 | *** | 8569 | 8866 | 14009 | 1598 | 1756 | 2281 | 489 | 525 | 587 | 242 | 253 | 268 | 145 | 149 | 155 |
| | *** | 8668 | 9417 | 14950 | 1661 | 1917 | 2412 | 505 | 551 | 606 | 247 | 260 | 268 | 147 | 152 | 149 |
| 0.45 | *** | 8282 | 8662 | 14615 | 1591 | 1770 | 2362 | 493 | 532 | 600 | 242 | 255 | 271 | 145 | 149 | 155 |
| | *** | 8410 | 9341 | 15352 | 1663 | 1952 | 2461 | 510 | 561 | 613 | 248 | 262 | 268 | 146 | 152 | 147 |
| 0.5 | *** | 7791 | 8270 | 14886 | 1554 | 1751 | 2389 | 487 | 529 | 601 | 239 | 251 | 268 | 141 | 146 | 152 |
| | *** | 7954 | 9079 | 15445 | 1634 | 1947 | 2461 | 506 | 559 | 606 | 244 | 259 | 263 | 143 | 149 | 143 |
| 0.55 | *** | 7153 | 7741 | 14821 | 1492 | 1702 | 2363 | 472 | 515 | 587 | 230 | 243 | 259 | 135 | 140 | 145 |
| | *** | 7357 | 8672 | 15228 | 1578 | 1906 | 2412 | 491 | 545 | 588 | 236 | 250 | 252 | 137 | 142 | 135 |
| 0.6 | *** | 6424 | 7125 | 14419 | 1411 | 1625 | 2283 | 450 | 491 | 561 | 217 | 229 | 245 | 126 | 130 | 135 |
| | *** | 6674 | 8154 | 14703 | 1499 | 1831 | 2313 | 468 | 521 | 557 | 223 | 236 | 235 | 128 | 132 | 124 |
| 0.65 | *** | 5661 | 6458 | 13682 | 1311 | 1523 | 2149 | 418 | 457 | 521 | 200 | 210 | 224 | 114 | 118 | 122 |
| | *** | 5953 | 7548 | 13868 | 1399 | 1723 | 2164 | 436 | 484 | 514 | 205 | 216 | 213 | 116 | 120 | 110 |
| 0.7 | *** | 4907 | 5765 | 12613 | 1195 | 1396 | 1962 | 379 | 413 | 467 | 177 | 186 | 197 | 99 | 102 | 105 |
| | *** | 5230 | 6868 | 12724 | 1279 | 1581 | 1967 | 394 | 437 | 458 | 181 | 191 | 186 | 100 | 103 | 93 |
| 0.75 | *** | 4187 | 5055 | 11213 | 1061 | 1243 | 1722 | 330 | 358 | 401 | 150 | 157 | 165 | 81 | 83 | 85 |
| | *** | 4520 | 6118 | 11271 | 1137 | 1405 | 1719 | 343 | 377 | 390 | 153 | 161 | 153 | 82 | 84 | 73 |
| 0.8 | *** | 3500 | 4320 | 9487 | 907 | 1060 | 1431 | 271 | 292 | 321 | 117 | 122 | 127 | . | . | . |
| | *** | 3819 | 5286 | 9509 | 972 | 1191 | 1422 | 281 | 305 | 310 | 119 | 124 | 115 | . | . | . |
| 0.85 | *** | 2824 | 3537 | 7436 | 727 | 841 | 1087 | 201 | 213 | 229 | . | . | . | . | . | . |
| | *** | 3106 | 4344 | 7438 | 777 | 934 | 1076 | 207 | 220 | 217 | . | . | . | . | . | . |
| 0.9 | *** | 2112 | 2651 | 5067 | 508 | 574 | 692 | . | . | . | . | . | . | . | . | . |
| | *** | 2328 | 3230 | 5058 | 537 | 622 | 681 | . | . | . | . | . | . | . | . | . |
| 0.95 | *** | 1245 | 1523 | 2381 | . | . | . | . | . | . | . | . | . | . | . | . |
| | *** | 1360 | 1786 | 2368 | . | . | . | . | . | . | . | . | . | . | . | . |

TABLE 7: ALPHA= 0.05 POWER= 0.8    EXPECTED ACCRUAL THRU MINIMUM FOLLOW-UP= 700

| | | DEL=.02 | | | DEL=.05 | | | DEL=.10 | | | DEL=.15 | | | DEL=.20 | | |
|---|---|---|---|---|---|---|---|---|---|---|---|---|---|---|---|---|---|
| FACT= | | 1.0 .75 | .50 .25 | .00 BIN | 1.0 .75 | .50 .25 | .00 BIN | 1.0 .75 | .50 .25 | .00 BIN | 1.0 75 | .50 .25 | .00 BIN | 1.0 .75 | .50 .25 | .00 BIN |
| PCONT=*** | | REQUIRED NUMBER OF PATIENTS | | | | | | | | | | | | | | | |
| 0.05 | *** | 1768 | 1781 | 1863 | 382 | 387 | 395 | 138 | 139 | 141 | 81 | 82 | 82 | 57 | 58 | 58 |
| | *** | 1773 | 1802 | 3481 | 384 | 390 | 681 | 138 | 140 | 217 | 81 | 82 | 115 | 58 | 58 | 73 |
| 0.1 | *** | 3680 | 3714 | 4092 | 705 | 723 | 762 | 226 | 230 | 236 | 122 | 123 | 125 | 81 | 81 | 82 |
| | *** | 3691 | 3776 | 6047 | 713 | 738 | 1076 | 228 | 233 | 310 | 123 | 124 | 153 | 81 | 82 | 93 |
| 0.15 | *** | 5380 | 5441 | 6328 | 988 | 1024 | 1117 | 303 | 311 | 323 | 156 | 159 | 163 | 100 | 101 | 103 |
| | *** | 5401 | 5556 | 8304 | 1003 | 1058 | 1422 | 306 | 316 | 390 | 158 | 161 | 186 | 100 | 102 | 110 |
| 0.2 | *** | 6741 | 6835 | 8409 | 1217 | 1276 | 1441 | 366 | 380 | 400 | 185 | 190 | 195 | 116 | 117 | 120 |
| | *** | 6772 | 7015 | 10251 | 1241 | 1332 | 1719 | 372 | 388 | 458 | 187 | 192 | 213 | 117 | 119 | 124 |
| 0.25 | *** | 7726 | 7861 | 10253 | 1390 | 1473 | 1724 | 416 | 436 | 465 | 208 | 214 | 222 | 128 | 131 | 134 |
| | *** | 7771 | 8120 | 11890 | 1423 | 1556 | 1967 | 425 | 449 | 514 | 211 | 218 | 235 | 129 | 132 | 135 |
| 0.3 | *** | 8343 | 8528 | 11816 | 1511 | 1620 | 1960 | 453 | 479 | 519 | 225 | 233 | 243 | 137 | 140 | 144 |
| | *** | 8405 | 8880 | 13219 | 1554 | 1730 | 2164 | 465 | 496 | 557 | 229 | 238 | 252 | 138 | 142 | 143 |
| 0.35 | *** | 8618 | 8864 | 13073 | 1583 | 1718 | 2147 | 479 | 509 | 559 | 236 | 246 | 259 | 143 | 147 | 151 |
| | *** | 8700 | 9324 | 14239 | 1637 | 1854 | 2313 | 493 | 531 | 588 | 241 | 252 | 263 | 145 | 149 | 147 |
| 0.4 | *** | 8592 | 8911 | 14009 | 1614 | 1773 | 2281 | 493 | 529 | 586 | 243 | 254 | 268 | 145 | 150 | 155 |
| | *** | 8699 | 9494 | 14950 | 1678 | 1933 | 2412 | 509 | 553 | 606 | 248 | 260 | 268 | 147 | 152 | 149 |
| 0.45 | *** | 8311 | 8719 | 14614 | 1609 | 1790 | 2362 | 498 | 536 | 600 | 244 | 256 | 271 | 145 | 149 | 155 |
| | *** | 8449 | 9433 | 15352 | 1682 | 1969 | 2461 | 515 | 563 | 613 | 250 | 263 | 268 | 147 | 152 | 147 |
| 0.5 | *** | 7829 | 8339 | 14886 | 1574 | 1773 | 2389 | 492 | 533 | 600 | 240 | 252 | 268 | 142 | 146 | 152 |
| | *** | 8003 | 9185 | 15445 | 1655 | 1966 | 2461 | 510 | 562 | 606 | 246 | 260 | 263 | 144 | 149 | 143 |
| 0.55 | *** | 7200 | 7824 | 14821 | 1514 | 1724 | 2363 | 478 | 519 | 587 | 232 | 244 | 260 | 135 | 140 | 145 |
| | *** | 7418 | 8790 | 15228 | 1601 | 1926 | 2412 | 496 | 548 | 588 | 237 | 251 | 252 | 138 | 142 | 135 |
| 0.6 | *** | 6483 | 7220 | 14419 | 1433 | 1648 | 2283 | 454 | 495 | 561 | 219 | 230 | 245 | 126 | 130 | 135 |
| | *** | 6747 | 8280 | 14703 | 1522 | 1851 | 2313 | 473 | 523 | 557 | 224 | 237 | 235 | 128 | 133 | 124 |
| 0.65 | *** | 5731 | 6562 | 13682 | 1333 | 1546 | 2149 | 423 | 460 | 520 | 201 | 211 | 224 | 114 | 118 | 122 |
| | *** | 6037 | 7678 | 13868 | 1422 | 1742 | 2164 | 440 | 486 | 514 | 206 | 217 | 213 | 116 | 120 | 110 |
| 0.7 | *** | 4986 | 5873 | 12613 | 1216 | 1417 | 1962 | 383 | 416 | 467 | 178 | 187 | 197 | 99 | 102 | 105 |
| | *** | 5321 | 6998 | 12724 | 1300 | 1599 | 1967 | 398 | 438 | 458 | 182 | 192 | 186 | 101 | 103 | 93 |
| 0.75 | *** | 4269 | 5160 | 11213 | 1081 | 1262 | 1722 | 334 | 361 | 401 | 151 | 157 | 165 | 81 | 83 | 86 |
| | *** | 4612 | 6240 | 11271 | 1157 | 1420 | 1719 | 346 | 378 | 390 | 154 | 161 | 153 | 82 | 84 | 73 |
| 0.8 | *** | 3579 | 4418 | 9487 | 924 | 1076 | 1430 | 274 | 294 | 321 | 118 | 122 | 127 | . | . | . |
| | *** | 3907 | 5395 | 9509 | 989 | 1203 | 1422 | 283 | 306 | 310 | 120 | 124 | 115 | . | . | . |
| 0.85 | *** | 2895 | 3620 | 7436 | 740 | 852 | 1087 | 202 | 214 | 229 | . | . | . | . | . | . |
| | *** | 3181 | 4433 | 7438 | 789 | 942 | 1076 | 208 | 221 | 217 | . | . | . | . | . | . |
| 0.9 | *** | 2166 | 2712 | 5066 | 515 | 579 | 693 | . | . | . | . | . | . | . | . | . |
| | *** | 2385 | 3291 | 5058 | 544 | 626 | 681 | . | . | . | . | . | . | . | . | . |
| 0.95 | *** | 1275 | 1552 | 2380 | . | . | . | . | . | . | . | . | . | . | . | . |
| | *** | 1390 | 1812 | 2368 | . | . | . | . | . | . | . | . | . | . | . | . |

## TABLE 7: ALPHA= 0.05 POWER= 0.8    EXPECTED ACCRUAL THRU MINIMUM FOLLOW-UP= 750

|  |  | DEL=.02 | | | DEL=.05 | | | DEL=.10 | | | DEL=.15 | | | DEL=.20 | | |
|---|---|---|---|---|---|---|---|---|---|---|---|---|---|---|---|---|
| FACT= | | 1.0 .75 | .50 .25 | .00 BIN | 1.0 .75 | .50 .25 | .00 BIN | 1.0 .75 | .50 .25 | .00 BIN | 1.0 75 | .50 .25 | .00 BIN | 1.0 .75 | .50 .25 | .00 BIN |
| PCONT=*** | | REQUIRED NUMBER OF PATIENTS | | | | | | | | | | | | | | |
| 0.05 | *** | 1769 | 1783 | 1863 | 383 | 387 | 395 | 139 | 139 | 141 | 81 | 82 | 82 | 57 | 57 | 58 |
|  | *** | 1774 | 1804 | 3481 | 385 | 391 | 681 | 139 | 140 | 217 | 81 | 82 | 115 | 57 | 58 | 73 |
| 0.1 | *** | 3682 | 3719 | 4092 | 707 | 725 | 762 | 227 | 230 | 235 | 122 | 124 | 125 | 81 | 81 | 82 |
|  | *** | 3694 | 3784 | 6047 | 715 | 740 | 1076 | 229 | 233 | 310 | 123 | 124 | 153 | 81 | 82 | 93 |
| 0.15 | *** | 5385 | 5450 | 6328 | 992 | 1028 | 1117 | 304 | 311 | 323 | 157 | 160 | 163 | 100 | 101 | 102 |
|  | *** | 5406 | 5572 | 8304 | 1006 | 1061 | 1422 | 307 | 317 | 390 | 158 | 161 | 186 | 100 | 102 | 110 |
| 0.2 | *** | 6747 | 6848 | 8409 | 1222 | 1281 | 1441 | 368 | 380 | 400 | 186 | 190 | 195 | 116 | 118 | 120 |
|  | *** | 6781 | 7039 | 10251 | 1246 | 1338 | 1719 | 373 | 389 | 458 | 188 | 192 | 213 | 117 | 119 | 124 |
| 0.25 | *** | 7736 | 7880 | 10253 | 1398 | 1482 | 1724 | 418 | 437 | 466 | 209 | 215 | 222 | 128 | 131 | 134 |
|  | *** | 7784 | 8154 | 11890 | 1432 | 1564 | 1967 | 427 | 450 | 514 | 212 | 218 | 235 | 130 | 132 | 135 |
| 0.3 | *** | 8356 | 8554 | 11816 | 1521 | 1631 | 1960 | 456 | 481 | 519 | 226 | 234 | 244 | 138 | 140 | 144 |
|  | *** | 8422 | 8926 | 13219 | 1565 | 1740 | 2164 | 468 | 498 | 557 | 229 | 238 | 252 | 139 | 142 | 143 |
| 0.35 | *** | 8636 | 8899 | 13073 | 1596 | 1732 | 2147 | 483 | 512 | 559 | 238 | 247 | 259 | 143 | 147 | 151 |
|  | *** | 8724 | 9384 | 14239 | 1651 | 1867 | 2313 | 496 | 533 | 588 | 242 | 252 | 263 | 145 | 149 | 147 |
| 0.4 | *** | 8615 | 8956 | 14009 | 1629 | 1790 | 2281 | 498 | 531 | 587 | 244 | 254 | 268 | 146 | 150 | 155 |
|  | *** | 8730 | 9568 | 14950 | 1694 | 1948 | 2412 | 513 | 555 | 606 | 249 | 261 | 268 | 148 | 152 | 149 |
| 0.45 | *** | 8341 | 8775 | 14614 | 1626 | 1809 | 2362 | 502 | 539 | 600 | 245 | 257 | 271 | 145 | 150 | 155 |
|  | *** | 8488 | 9521 | 15352 | 1700 | 1986 | 2461 | 519 | 565 | 613 | 250 | 263 | 268 | 147 | 152 | 147 |
| 0.5 | *** | 7867 | 8408 | 14886 | 1593 | 1793 | 2389 | 497 | 536 | 601 | 242 | 253 | 268 | 142 | 146 | 152 |
|  | *** | 8053 | 9287 | 15445 | 1675 | 1984 | 2461 | 514 | 564 | 606 | 247 | 260 | 263 | 144 | 149 | 143 |
| 0.55 | *** | 7248 | 7906 | 14821 | 1534 | 1745 | 2363 | 482 | 522 | 587 | 233 | 244 | 259 | 136 | 140 | 145 |
|  | *** | 7479 | 8903 | 15228 | 1622 | 1945 | 2412 | 500 | 550 | 588 | 239 | 251 | 252 | 138 | 143 | 135 |
| 0.6 | *** | 6541 | 7312 | 14419 | 1454 | 1669 | 2283 | 459 | 499 | 560 | 220 | 231 | 244 | 127 | 130 | 135 |
|  | *** | 6819 | 8401 | 14703 | 1543 | 1870 | 2313 | 477 | 525 | 557 | 225 | 237 | 235 | 129 | 133 | 124 |
| 0.65 | *** | 5800 | 6661 | 13683 | 1354 | 1566 | 2149 | 427 | 464 | 520 | 202 | 212 | 224 | 115 | 118 | 122 |
|  | *** | 6119 | 7802 | 13868 | 1443 | 1760 | 2164 | 444 | 489 | 514 | 207 | 217 | 213 | 116 | 120 | 110 |
| 0.7 | *** | 5062 | 5975 | 12613 | 1236 | 1436 | 1962 | 386 | 419 | 467 | 179 | 187 | 197 | 100 | 102 | 105 |
|  | *** | 5409 | 7120 | 12724 | 1321 | 1615 | 1967 | 401 | 440 | 458 | 183 | 192 | 186 | 101 | 104 | 93 |
| 0.75 | *** | 4348 | 5260 | 11213 | 1099 | 1279 | 1722 | 337 | 363 | 400 | 152 | 158 | 165 | 81 | 83 | 85 |
|  | *** | 4700 | 6355 | 11271 | 1175 | 1434 | 1719 | 349 | 380 | 390 | 154 | 161 | 153 | 82 | 84 | 73 |
| 0.8 | *** | 3655 | 4510 | 9486 | 940 | 1090 | 1430 | 276 | 295 | 321 | 118 | 122 | 127 | . | . | . |
|  | *** | 3990 | 5497 | 9509 | 1004 | 1214 | 1422 | 285 | 307 | 310 | 120 | 124 | 115 | . | . | . |
| 0.85 | *** | 2961 | 3698 | 7436 | 752 | 862 | 1087 | 204 | 215 | 229 | . | . | . | . | . | . |
|  | *** | 3253 | 4516 | 7438 | 800 | 949 | 1076 | 209 | 221 | 217 | . | . | . | . | . | . |
| 0.9 | *** | 2218 | 2769 | 5066 | 522 | 585 | 693 | . | . | . | . | . | . | . | . | . |
|  | *** | 2440 | 3348 | 5058 | 550 | 630 | 681 | . | . | . | . | . | . | . | . | . |
| 0.95 | *** | 1302 | 1579 | 2380 | . | . | . | . | . | . | . | . | . | . | . | . |
|  | *** | 1418 | 1836 | 2368 | . | . | . | . | . | . | . | . | . | . | . | . |

TABLE 7: ALPHA= 0.05  POWER= 0.8     EXPECTED ACCRUAL THRU MINIMUM FOLLOW-UP= 800

| | | DEL=.02 | | | DEL=.05 | | | DEL=.10 | | | DEL=.15 | | | DEL=.20 | | |
|---|---|---|---|---|---|---|---|---|---|---|---|---|---|---|---|---|---|
| FACT= | | 1.0 .75 | .50 .25 | .00 BIN | 1.0 .75 | .50 .25 | .00 BIN | 1.0 .75 | .50 .25 | .00 BIN | 1.0 75 | .50 .25 | .00 BIN | 1.0 .75 | .50 .25 | .00 BIN |
| PCONT=*** | | | | | REQUIRED NUMBER OF PATIENTS | | | | | | | | | | | |
| 0.05 | *** | 1770 | 1785 | 1863 | 383 | 388 | 395 | 138 | 139 | 141 | 81 | 82 | 82 | 57 | 58 | 58 |
| | *** | 1775 | 1806 | 3481 | 385 | 391 | 681 | 139 | 140 | 217 | 81 | 82 | 115 | 58 | 58 | 73 |
| 0.1 | *** | 3685 | 3724 | 4092 | 709 | 727 | 762 | 227 | 231 | 235 | 122 | 124 | 125 | 81 | 81 | 82 |
| | *** | 3698 | 3792 | 6047 | 716 | 741 | 1076 | 229 | 233 | 310 | 123 | 124 | 153 | 81 | 82 | 93 |
| 0.15 | *** | 5389 | 5458 | 6328 | 995 | 1031 | 1117 | 304 | 312 | 323 | 157 | 160 | 163 | 100 | 101 | 103 |
| | *** | 5412 | 5586 | 8304 | 1010 | 1064 | 1422 | 308 | 317 | 390 | 159 | 161 | 186 | 101 | 102 | 110 |
| 0.2 | *** | 6754 | 6861 | 8409 | 1228 | 1287 | 1441 | 369 | 382 | 400 | 186 | 190 | 195 | 116 | 118 | 120 |
| | *** | 6790 | 7063 | 10251 | 1252 | 1342 | 1719 | 375 | 390 | 458 | 188 | 193 | 213 | 117 | 119 | 124 |
| 0.25 | *** | 7746 | 7899 | 10253 | 1405 | 1490 | 1724 | 420 | 439 | 466 | 210 | 215 | 222 | 129 | 131 | 134 |
| | *** | 7797 | 8188 | 11890 | 1440 | 1571 | 1967 | 429 | 451 | 514 | 212 | 219 | 235 | 130 | 132 | 135 |
| 0.3 | *** | 8369 | 8580 | 11816 | 1530 | 1642 | 1960 | 459 | 483 | 519 | 227 | 234 | 243 | 138 | 141 | 144 |
| | *** | 8440 | 8972 | 13219 | 1575 | 1749 | 2164 | 470 | 499 | 557 | 230 | 239 | 252 | 139 | 142 | 143 |
| 0.35 | *** | 8653 | 8933 | 13073 | 1608 | 1745 | 2147 | 486 | 514 | 559 | 239 | 248 | 259 | 144 | 147 | 151 |
| | *** | 8747 | 9442 | 14239 | 1664 | 1878 | 2313 | 499 | 534 | 588 | 243 | 253 | 263 | 145 | 149 | 147 |
| 0.4 | *** | 8638 | 9000 | 14009 | 1643 | 1805 | 2281 | 501 | 534 | 587 | 245 | 255 | 268 | 146 | 150 | 155 |
| | *** | 8760 | 9640 | 14950 | 1709 | 1961 | 2412 | 516 | 557 | 606 | 250 | 261 | 268 | 148 | 152 | 149 |
| 0.45 | *** | 8371 | 8831 | 14615 | 1642 | 1826 | 2362 | 506 | 542 | 600 | 247 | 257 | 271 | 146 | 150 | 155 |
| | *** | 8527 | 9607 | 15352 | 1718 | 2001 | 2461 | 522 | 567 | 613 | 252 | 264 | 268 | 148 | 152 | 147 |
| 0.5 | *** | 7904 | 8476 | 14886 | 1611 | 1812 | 2390 | 501 | 539 | 601 | 243 | 254 | 268 | 143 | 147 | 152 |
| | *** | 8102 | 9384 | 15445 | 1694 | 2000 | 2461 | 518 | 566 | 606 | 248 | 261 | 263 | 145 | 149 | 143 |
| 0.55 | *** | 7295 | 7985 | 14821 | 1554 | 1765 | 2363 | 486 | 526 | 587 | 235 | 246 | 260 | 136 | 140 | 145 |
| | *** | 7539 | 9010 | 15228 | 1641 | 1962 | 2412 | 504 | 552 | 588 | 240 | 252 | 252 | 138 | 143 | 135 |
| 0.6 | *** | 6599 | 7401 | 14419 | 1474 | 1689 | 2283 | 463 | 501 | 561 | 221 | 232 | 245 | 127 | 131 | 135 |
| | *** | 6890 | 8515 | 14703 | 1564 | 1886 | 2313 | 481 | 527 | 557 | 226 | 238 | 235 | 129 | 133 | 124 |
| 0.65 | *** | 5867 | 6757 | 13682 | 1374 | 1586 | 2149 | 431 | 467 | 521 | 203 | 213 | 224 | 115 | 118 | 122 |
| | *** | 6198 | 7919 | 13868 | 1463 | 1776 | 2164 | 447 | 490 | 514 | 208 | 218 | 213 | 117 | 120 | 110 |
| 0.7 | *** | 5136 | 6073 | 12613 | 1255 | 1455 | 1962 | 390 | 421 | 467 | 180 | 188 | 197 | 100 | 102 | 105 |
| | *** | 5493 | 7235 | 12724 | 1339 | 1630 | 1967 | 404 | 442 | 458 | 184 | 192 | 186 | 101 | 104 | 93 |
| 0.75 | *** | 4424 | 5356 | 11213 | 1116 | 1295 | 1722 | 339 | 365 | 401 | 152 | 158 | 165 | 82 | 84 | 85 |
| | *** | 4785 | 6463 | 11271 | 1192 | 1447 | 1719 | 351 | 381 | 390 | 155 | 161 | 153 | 83 | 84 | 73 |
| 0.8 | *** | 3728 | 4597 | 9487 | 954 | 1102 | 1431 | 278 | 297 | 321 | 119 | 123 | 127 | . | . | . |
| | *** | 4069 | 5593 | 9509 | 1018 | 1224 | 1422 | 287 | 308 | 310 | 121 | 125 | 115 | . | . | . |
| 0.85 | *** | 3025 | 3771 | 7436 | 763 | 872 | 1087 | 205 | 216 | 229 | . | . | . | . | . | . |
| | *** | 3322 | 4594 | 7438 | 811 | 956 | 1076 | 210 | 222 | 217 | . | . | . | . | . | . |
| 0.9 | *** | 2267 | 2823 | 5066 | 529 | 590 | 693 | . | . | . | . | . | . | . | . | . |
| | *** | 2491 | 3401 | 5058 | 556 | 633 | 681 | . | . | . | . | . | . | . | . | . |
| 0.95 | *** | 1328 | 1605 | 2380 | . | . | . | . | . | . | . | . | . | . | . | . |
| | *** | 1444 | 1858 | 2368 | . | . | . | . | . | . | . | . | . | . | . | . |

TABLE 7: ALPHA= 0.05  POWER= 0.8     EXPECTED ACCRUAL THRU MINIMUM FOLLOW-UP= 850

| | | DEL=.02 | | | DEL=.05 | | | DEL=.10 | | | DEL=.15 | | | DEL=.20 | | |
|---|---|---|---|---|---|---|---|---|---|---|---|---|---|---|---|---|---|
| FACT= | | 1.0 .75 | .50 .25 | .00 BIN | 1.0 .75 | .50 .25 | .00 BIN | 1.0 .75 | .50 .25 | .00 BIN | 1.0 75 | .50 .25 | .00 BIN | 1.0 .75 | .50 .25 | .00 BIN |
| PCONT=*** | | | | | REQUIRED NUMBER OF PATIENTS | | | | | | | | | | | |
| 0.05 | *** | 1771 | 1787 | 1863 | 383 | 388 | 395 | 138 | 139 | 140 | 82 | 82 | 82 | 57 | 57 | 57 |
| | *** | 1777 | 1808 | 3481 | 385 | 391 | 681 | 139 | 140 | 217 | 82 | 82 | 115 | 57 | 57 | 73 |
| 0.1 | *** | 3687 | 3728 | 4092 | 711 | 728 | 762 | 227 | 231 | 236 | 122 | 123 | 125 | 81 | 82 | 82 |
| | *** | 3701 | 3799 | 6047 | 718 | 742 | 1076 | 229 | 233 | 310 | 123 | 124 | 153 | 81 | 82 | 93 |
| 0.15 | *** | 5393 | 5467 | 6328 | 998 | 1035 | 1117 | 305 | 312 | 323 | 157 | 160 | 163 | 101 | 102 | 103 |
| | *** | 5418 | 5601 | 8304 | 1013 | 1066 | 1422 | 309 | 317 | 390 | 158 | 161 | 186 | 101 | 102 | 110 |
| 0.2 | *** | 6761 | 6874 | 8409 | 1233 | 1292 | 1441 | 371 | 383 | 400 | 187 | 190 | 195 | 117 | 118 | 120 |
| | *** | 6799 | 7086 | 10251 | 1257 | 1346 | 1719 | 376 | 390 | 458 | 189 | 193 | 213 | 117 | 119 | 124 |
| 0.25 | *** | 7755 | 7919 | 10253 | 1412 | 1498 | 1724 | 422 | 440 | 465 | 210 | 215 | 222 | 129 | 131 | 134 |
| | *** | 7809 | 8221 | 11890 | 1447 | 1577 | 1967 | 430 | 451 | 514 | 213 | 219 | 235 | 130 | 133 | 135 |
| 0.3 | *** | 8382 | 8606 | 11816 | 1540 | 1651 | 1960 | 461 | 484 | 519 | 227 | 235 | 243 | 138 | 141 | 144 |
| | *** | 8457 | 9016 | 13219 | 1585 | 1757 | 2164 | 472 | 499 | 557 | 231 | 239 | 252 | 139 | 142 | 143 |
| 0.35 | *** | 8671 | 8967 | 13073 | 1619 | 1757 | 2146 | 488 | 516 | 560 | 240 | 248 | 259 | 144 | 147 | 151 |
| | *** | 8771 | 9499 | 14239 | 1676 | 1889 | 2313 | 501 | 535 | 588 | 243 | 253 | 263 | 146 | 149 | 147 |
| 0.4 | *** | 8661 | 9044 | 14009 | 1657 | 1820 | 2281 | 504 | 537 | 587 | 246 | 256 | 268 | 147 | 151 | 155 |
| | *** | 8790 | 9709 | 14950 | 1723 | 1974 | 2412 | 519 | 559 | 606 | 251 | 261 | 268 | 148 | 153 | 149 |
| 0.45 | *** | 8400 | 8886 | 14614 | 1658 | 1842 | 2362 | 510 | 545 | 600 | 248 | 258 | 271 | 146 | 151 | 155 |
| | *** | 8566 | 9689 | 15352 | 1734 | 2015 | 2461 | 526 | 569 | 613 | 253 | 264 | 268 | 148 | 153 | 147 |
| 0.5 | *** | 7941 | 8542 | 14886 | 1628 | 1829 | 2390 | 504 | 542 | 600 | 244 | 255 | 269 | 143 | 147 | 152 |
| | *** | 8150 | 9478 | 15445 | 1711 | 2015 | 2461 | 521 | 567 | 606 | 249 | 261 | 263 | 145 | 150 | 143 |
| 0.55 | *** | 7341 | 8062 | 14821 | 1572 | 1784 | 2363 | 491 | 528 | 587 | 236 | 246 | 259 | 137 | 141 | 145 |
| | *** | 7598 | 9113 | 15228 | 1660 | 1977 | 2412 | 508 | 554 | 588 | 241 | 253 | 252 | 139 | 142 | 135 |
| 0.6 | *** | 6655 | 7486 | 14419 | 1493 | 1708 | 2283 | 467 | 504 | 561 | 222 | 232 | 244 | 128 | 131 | 135 |
| | *** | 6959 | 8624 | 14703 | 1583 | 1902 | 2313 | 484 | 529 | 557 | 227 | 238 | 235 | 129 | 133 | 124 |
| 0.65 | *** | 5932 | 6849 | 13683 | 1393 | 1603 | 2149 | 435 | 469 | 520 | 204 | 213 | 224 | 116 | 119 | 122 |
| | *** | 6275 | 8030 | 13868 | 1481 | 1790 | 2164 | 450 | 492 | 514 | 208 | 218 | 213 | 117 | 120 | 110 |
| 0.7 | *** | 5207 | 6167 | 12613 | 1273 | 1471 | 1962 | 393 | 424 | 467 | 181 | 188 | 197 | 100 | 103 | 105 |
| | *** | 5574 | 7344 | 12724 | 1357 | 1643 | 1967 | 407 | 443 | 458 | 185 | 192 | 186 | 102 | 104 | 93 |
| 0.75 | *** | 4497 | 5446 | 11213 | 1132 | 1309 | 1722 | 342 | 367 | 401 | 153 | 158 | 165 | 82 | 84 | 85 |
| | *** | 4866 | 6565 | 11271 | 1208 | 1459 | 1719 | 354 | 382 | 390 | 156 | 162 | 153 | 83 | 85 | 73 |
| 0.8 | *** | 3797 | 4680 | 9487 | 968 | 1114 | 1430 | 280 | 298 | 321 | 119 | 123 | 127 | . | . | . |
| | *** | 4145 | 5683 | 9509 | 1031 | 1233 | 1422 | 289 | 309 | 310 | 121 | 124 | 115 | . | . | . |
| 0.85 | *** | 3086 | 3841 | 7437 | 773 | 880 | 1087 | 206 | 216 | 229 | . | . | . | . | . | . |
| | *** | 3387 | 4667 | 7438 | 820 | 962 | 1076 | 211 | 222 | 217 | . | . | . | . | . | . |
| 0.9 | *** | 2313 | 2873 | 5066 | 535 | 594 | 692 | . | . | . | . | . | . | . | . | . |
| | *** | 2539 | 3451 | 5058 | 562 | 636 | 681 | . | . | . | . | . | . | . | . | . |
| 0.95 | *** | 1352 | 1629 | 2380 | . | . | . | . | . | . | . | . | . | . | . | . |
| | *** | 1468 | 1878 | 2368 | . | . | . | . | . | . | . | . | . | . | . | . |

TABLE 7: ALPHA= 0.05  POWER= 0.8    EXPECTED ACCRUAL THRU MINIMUM FOLLOW-UP= 900

| | | DEL=.02 | | | DEL=.05 | | | DEL=.10 | | | DEL=.15 | | | DEL=.20 | | |
|---|---|---|---|---|---|---|---|---|---|---|---|---|---|---|---|---|
| FACT= | | 1.0 .75 | .50 .25 | .00 BIN | 1.0 .75 | .50 .25 | .00 BIN | 1.0 .75 | .50 .25 | .00 BIN | 1.0 75 | .50 .25 | .00 BIN | 1.0 .75 | .50 .25 | .00 BIN |
| PCONT=*** | | | | REQUIRED NUMBER OF PATIENTS | | | | | | | | | | | | |
| 0.05 | *** | 1772 | 1788 | 1863 | 384 | 388 | 395 | 138 | 140 | 141 | 81 | 82 | 82 | 57 | 57 | 57 |
| | *** | 1778 | 1810 | 3481 | 386 | 392 | 681 | 139 | 140 | 217 | 82 | 82 | 115 | 57 | 57 | 73 |
| 0.1 | *** | 3690 | 3733 | 4092 | 712 | 729 | 762 | 228 | 231 | 235 | 123 | 124 | 125 | 81 | 81 | 82 |
| | *** | 3704 | 3806 | 6047 | 720 | 743 | 1076 | 230 | 233 | 310 | 123 | 125 | 153 | 81 | 82 | 93 |
| 0.15 | *** | 5398 | 5475 | 6328 | 1001 | 1037 | 1117 | 306 | 313 | 323 | 158 | 160 | 163 | 100 | 101 | 102 |
| | *** | 5424 | 5615 | 8304 | 1016 | 1068 | 1422 | 309 | 317 | 390 | 159 | 162 | 186 | 101 | 102 | 110 |
| 0.2 | *** | 6768 | 6888 | 8408 | 1237 | 1297 | 1441 | 371 | 383 | 399 | 187 | 191 | 195 | 117 | 118 | 120 |
| | *** | 6808 | 7108 | 10251 | 1262 | 1350 | 1719 | 377 | 390 | 458 | 189 | 193 | 213 | 117 | 119 | 124 |
| 0.25 | *** | 7765 | 7937 | 10252 | 1419 | 1504 | 1724 | 424 | 441 | 465 | 210 | 216 | 222 | 129 | 131 | 134 |
| | *** | 7822 | 8253 | 11890 | 1454 | 1583 | 1967 | 432 | 452 | 514 | 213 | 219 | 235 | 130 | 132 | 135 |
| 0.3 | *** | 8396 | 8632 | 11816 | 1548 | 1661 | 1961 | 464 | 486 | 519 | 228 | 235 | 243 | 138 | 141 | 144 |
| | *** | 8475 | 9059 | 13219 | 1594 | 1765 | 2164 | 474 | 501 | 557 | 231 | 239 | 252 | 140 | 143 | 143 |
| 0.35 | *** | 8688 | 9001 | 13073 | 1630 | 1769 | 2147 | 491 | 518 | 559 | 240 | 249 | 259 | 144 | 147 | 151 |
| | *** | 8794 | 9554 | 14239 | 1687 | 1899 | 2313 | 504 | 536 | 588 | 244 | 253 | 263 | 146 | 149 | 147 |
| 0.4 | *** | 8684 | 9088 | 14009 | 1670 | 1833 | 2281 | 507 | 539 | 586 | 247 | 257 | 268 | 147 | 151 | 155 |
| | *** | 8821 | 9777 | 14950 | 1737 | 1985 | 2412 | 522 | 560 | 606 | 252 | 262 | 268 | 149 | 153 | 149 |
| 0.45 | *** | 8429 | 8940 | 14615 | 1673 | 1857 | 2362 | 513 | 548 | 600 | 249 | 259 | 271 | 147 | 151 | 155 |
| | *** | 8605 | 9768 | 15352 | 1749 | 2027 | 2461 | 528 | 570 | 613 | 253 | 264 | 268 | 149 | 153 | 147 |
| 0.5 | *** | 7979 | 8607 | 14886 | 1644 | 1845 | 2390 | 508 | 545 | 600 | 245 | 255 | 269 | 144 | 147 | 152 |
| | *** | 8198 | 9568 | 15445 | 1728 | 2029 | 2461 | 525 | 569 | 606 | 250 | 262 | 263 | 145 | 149 | 143 |
| 0.55 | *** | 7388 | 8137 | 14820 | 1589 | 1800 | 2363 | 494 | 531 | 587 | 237 | 247 | 260 | 137 | 141 | 145 |
| | *** | 7656 | 9212 | 15228 | 1677 | 1991 | 2412 | 511 | 556 | 588 | 242 | 253 | 252 | 139 | 143 | 135 |
| 0.6 | *** | 6711 | 7570 | 14419 | 1511 | 1725 | 2283 | 470 | 506 | 560 | 224 | 233 | 245 | 128 | 131 | 135 |
| | *** | 7026 | 8728 | 14703 | 1601 | 1916 | 2313 | 487 | 531 | 557 | 228 | 239 | 235 | 129 | 133 | 124 |
| 0.65 | *** | 5996 | 6938 | 13682 | 1410 | 1620 | 2149 | 438 | 471 | 521 | 205 | 213 | 224 | 116 | 119 | 122 |
| | *** | 6350 | 8136 | 13868 | 1499 | 1804 | 2164 | 453 | 493 | 514 | 209 | 218 | 213 | 117 | 120 | 110 |
| 0.7 | *** | 5276 | 6257 | 12612 | 1289 | 1487 | 1962 | 396 | 425 | 467 | 182 | 189 | 197 | 100 | 102 | 105 |
| | *** | 5653 | 7448 | 12724 | 1373 | 1656 | 1967 | 410 | 444 | 458 | 185 | 193 | 186 | 101 | 104 | 93 |
| 0.75 | *** | 4567 | 5534 | 11213 | 1148 | 1323 | 1722 | 344 | 368 | 401 | 154 | 159 | 165 | 82 | 83 | 85 |
| | *** | 4943 | 6662 | 11271 | 1223 | 1469 | 1719 | 356 | 383 | 390 | 156 | 162 | 153 | 83 | 84 | 73 |
| 0.8 | *** | 3864 | 4759 | 9487 | 981 | 1125 | 1431 | 282 | 299 | 321 | 119 | 123 | 127 | . | . | . |
| | *** | 4217 | 5769 | 9509 | 1043 | 1242 | 1422 | 290 | 309 | 310 | 121 | 125 | 115 | . | . | . |
| 0.85 | *** | 3144 | 3908 | 7436 | 783 | 888 | 1087 | 207 | 217 | 229 | . | . | . | . | . | . |
| | *** | 3449 | 4735 | 7438 | 829 | 968 | 1076 | 212 | 223 | 217 | . | . | . | . | . | . |
| 0.9 | *** | 2357 | 2921 | 5067 | 540 | 599 | 693 | . | . | . | . | . | . | . | . | . |
| | *** | 2586 | 3497 | 5058 | 567 | 639 | 681 | . | . | . | . | . | . | . | . | . |
| 0.95 | *** | 1376 | 1650 | 2381 | . | . | . | . | . | . | . | . | . | . | . | . |
| | *** | 1491 | 1896 | 2368 | . | . | . | . | . | . | . | . | . | . | . | . |

# TABLE 7: ALPHA= 0.05 POWER= 0.8    EXPECTED ACCRUAL THRU MINIMUM FOLLOW-UP= 950

| | | DEL=.02 | | | DEL=.05 | | | DEL=.10 | | | DEL=.15 | | | DEL=.20 | | |
|---|---|---|---|---|---|---|---|---|---|---|---|---|---|---|---|---|
| FACT= | | 1.0 .75 | .50 .25 | .00 BIN | 1.0 .75 | .50 .25 | .00 BIN | 1.0 .75 | .50 .25 | .00 BIN | 1.0 75 | .50 .25 | .00 BIN | 1.0 .75 | .50 .25 | .00 BIN |
| PCONT=*** | | | | | REQUIRED | NUMBER OF | PATIENTS | | | | | | | | | |
| 0.05 | *** | 1773 | 1790 | 1863 | 384 | 388 | 395 | 139 | 140 | 141 | 82 | 82 | 82 | 57 | 58 | 58 |
| | *** | 1779 | 1812 | 3481 | 386 | 391 | 681 | 139 | 140 | 217 | 82 | 82 | 115 | 58 | 58 | 73 |
| 0.1 | *** | 3692 | 3738 | 4092 | 713 | 730 | 762 | 228 | 231 | 235 | 122 | 124 | 125 | 81 | 82 | 82 |
| | *** | 3707 | 3813 | 6047 | 721 | 743 | 1076 | 230 | 234 | 310 | 123 | 124 | 153 | 82 | 82 | 93 |
| 0.15 | *** | 5402 | 5484 | 6328 | 1003 | 1040 | 1117 | 306 | 314 | 323 | 158 | 160 | 163 | 101 | 102 | 103 |
| | *** | 5429 | 5628 | 8304 | 1019 | 1070 | 1422 | 310 | 318 | 390 | 159 | 162 | 186 | 101 | 102 | 110 |
| 0.2 | *** | 6774 | 6901 | 8409 | 1242 | 1302 | 1440 | 372 | 384 | 400 | 188 | 191 | 196 | 116 | 118 | 120 |
| | *** | 6817 | 7129 | 10251 | 1267 | 1354 | 1719 | 378 | 391 | 458 | 189 | 193 | 213 | 117 | 119 | 124 |
| 0.25 | *** | 7774 | 7956 | 10252 | 1426 | 1511 | 1724 | 425 | 442 | 466 | 211 | 216 | 222 | 129 | 131 | 134 |
| | *** | 7835 | 8284 | 11890 | 1461 | 1588 | 1967 | 433 | 452 | 514 | 213 | 219 | 235 | 130 | 133 | 135 |
| 0.3 | *** | 8409 | 8658 | 11816 | 1557 | 1670 | 1960 | 466 | 487 | 519 | 229 | 235 | 243 | 139 | 141 | 144 |
| | *** | 8493 | 9101 | 13219 | 1603 | 1773 | 2164 | 476 | 501 | 557 | 232 | 239 | 252 | 140 | 143 | 143 |
| 0.35 | *** | 8706 | 9035 | 13073 | 1641 | 1780 | 2147 | 494 | 520 | 559 | 241 | 249 | 258 | 144 | 148 | 151 |
| | *** | 8817 | 9608 | 14239 | 1698 | 1907 | 2313 | 506 | 538 | 588 | 245 | 254 | 263 | 146 | 149 | 147 |
| 0.4 | *** | 8707 | 9131 | 14009 | 1682 | 1845 | 2281 | 510 | 540 | 587 | 248 | 257 | 268 | 147 | 151 | 154 |
| | *** | 8851 | 9842 | 14950 | 1750 | 1996 | 2412 | 524 | 561 | 606 | 253 | 262 | 268 | 149 | 153 | 149 |
| 0.45 | *** | 8459 | 8993 | 14615 | 1687 | 1872 | 2362 | 516 | 549 | 600 | 249 | 259 | 271 | 147 | 151 | 155 |
| | *** | 8643 | 9844 | 15352 | 1763 | 2040 | 2461 | 531 | 572 | 613 | 254 | 265 | 268 | 149 | 153 | 147 |
| 0.5 | *** | 8016 | 8670 | 14885 | 1660 | 1860 | 2389 | 511 | 547 | 600 | 246 | 256 | 268 | 144 | 147 | 152 |
| | *** | 8246 | 9654 | 15445 | 1743 | 2042 | 2461 | 527 | 571 | 606 | 251 | 262 | 263 | 146 | 150 | 143 |
| 0.55 | *** | 7433 | 8210 | 14821 | 1606 | 1816 | 2363 | 497 | 533 | 587 | 238 | 247 | 260 | 138 | 141 | 145 |
| | *** | 7713 | 9306 | 15228 | 1694 | 2005 | 2412 | 514 | 557 | 588 | 242 | 253 | 252 | 139 | 143 | 135 |
| 0.6 | *** | 6765 | 7651 | 14419 | 1527 | 1741 | 2282 | 474 | 509 | 561 | 224 | 234 | 245 | 128 | 131 | 135 |
| | *** | 7093 | 8827 | 14703 | 1617 | 1929 | 2313 | 490 | 532 | 557 | 229 | 239 | 235 | 130 | 133 | 124 |
| 0.65 | *** | 6058 | 7023 | 13682 | 1427 | 1636 | 2149 | 441 | 473 | 520 | 206 | 214 | 224 | 116 | 119 | 122 |
| | *** | 6423 | 8237 | 13868 | 1515 | 1817 | 2164 | 456 | 495 | 514 | 210 | 219 | 213 | 117 | 120 | 110 |
| 0.7 | *** | 5343 | 6343 | 12612 | 1305 | 1501 | 1962 | 399 | 427 | 467 | 182 | 190 | 197 | 101 | 103 | 105 |
| | *** | 5729 | 7546 | 12724 | 1389 | 1667 | 1967 | 412 | 445 | 458 | 186 | 193 | 186 | 102 | 104 | 93 |
| 0.75 | *** | 4635 | 5617 | 11213 | 1161 | 1336 | 1722 | 347 | 369 | 401 | 154 | 159 | 165 | 82 | 84 | 85 |
| | *** | 5018 | 6755 | 11271 | 1236 | 1478 | 1719 | 357 | 384 | 390 | 156 | 162 | 153 | 83 | 84 | 73 |
| 0.8 | *** | 3928 | 4835 | 9487 | 993 | 1135 | 1431 | 283 | 300 | 321 | 120 | 123 | 127 | . | . | . |
| | *** | 4286 | 5850 | 9509 | 1055 | 1249 | 1422 | 291 | 310 | 310 | 121 | 125 | 115 | . | . | . |
| 0.85 | *** | 3200 | 3971 | 7436 | 792 | 895 | 1087 | 208 | 217 | 229 | . | . | . | . | . | . |
| | *** | 3508 | 4801 | 7438 | 837 | 973 | 1076 | 213 | 223 | 217 | . | . | . | . | . | . |
| 0.9 | *** | 2400 | 2966 | 5067 | 545 | 602 | 692 | . | . | . | . | . | . | . | . | . |
| | *** | 2630 | 3541 | 5058 | 571 | 641 | 681 | . | . | . | . | . | . | . | . | . |
| 0.95 | *** | 1397 | 1671 | 2381 | . | . | . | . | . | . | . | . | . | . | . | . |
| | *** | 1512 | 1913 | 2368 | . | . | . | . | . | . | . | . | . | . | . | . |

TABLE 7: ALPHA= 0.05  POWER= 0.8    EXPECTED ACCRUAL THRU MINIMUM FOLLOW-UP= 1000

| | DEL=.02 | | | DEL=.05 | | | DEL=.10 | | | DEL=.15 | | | DEL=.20 | | |
|---|---|---|---|---|---|---|---|---|---|---|---|---|---|---|---|
| FACT= | 1.0 .75 | .50 .25 | .00 BIN | 1.0 .75 | .50 .25 | .00 BIN | 1.0 .75 | .50 .25 | .00 BIN | 1.0 75 | .50 .25 | .00 BIN | 1.0 .75 | .50 .25 | .00 BIN |
| PCONT=*** | | | | | | REQUIRED NUMBER OF PATIENTS | | | | | | | | | |
| 0.05 *** | 1774 | 1791 | 1863 | 385 | 389 | 395 | 139 | 140 | 141 | 81 | 82 | 82 | 58 | 58 | 58 |
| *** | 1780 | 1813 | 3481 | 386 | 392 | 681 | 140 | 140 | 217 | 81 | 82 | 115 | 58 | 58 | 73 |
| 0.1 *** | 3695 | 3742 | 4092 | 715 | 731 | 762 | 228 | 231 | 235 | 123 | 124 | 125 | 81 | 81 | 82 |
| *** | 3711 | 3819 | 6047 | 722 | 745 | 1076 | 230 | 233 | 310 | 123 | 125 | 153 | 81 | 82 | 93 |
| 0.15 *** | 5406 | 5492 | 6328 | 1006 | 1043 | 1117 | 307 | 314 | 323 | 158 | 160 | 163 | 101 | 101 | 103 |
| *** | 5435 | 5641 | 8304 | 1021 | 1072 | 1422 | 310 | 318 | 390 | 160 | 161 | 186 | 101 | 102 | 110 |
| 0.2 *** | 6781 | 6914 | 8409 | 1246 | 1306 | 1441 | 373 | 385 | 400 | 188 | 191 | 195 | 117 | 118 | 120 |
| *** | 6826 | 7151 | 10251 | 1271 | 1357 | 1719 | 379 | 391 | 458 | 190 | 193 | 213 | 118 | 119 | 124 |
| 0.25 *** | 7784 | 7975 | 10253 | 1431 | 1518 | 1724 | 427 | 443 | 466 | 211 | 216 | 222 | 130 | 131 | 134 |
| *** | 7848 | 8315 | 11890 | 1467 | 1593 | 1967 | 435 | 453 | 514 | 214 | 219 | 235 | 131 | 133 | 135 |
| 0.3 *** | 8422 | 8683 | 11816 | 1565 | 1678 | 1960 | 468 | 489 | 519 | 230 | 236 | 243 | 139 | 141 | 144 |
| *** | 8510 | 9142 | 13219 | 1612 | 1779 | 2164 | 477 | 502 | 557 | 233 | 240 | 252 | 140 | 143 | 143 |
| 0.35 *** | 8724 | 9069 | 13073 | 1651 | 1790 | 2146 | 496 | 521 | 560 | 242 | 250 | 259 | 145 | 148 | 151 |
| *** | 8840 | 9660 | 14239 | 1708 | 1916 | 2313 | 508 | 538 | 588 | 246 | 254 | 263 | 146 | 150 | 147 |
| 0.4 *** | 8730 | 9173 | 14009 | 1694 | 1858 | 2281 | 513 | 543 | 586 | 249 | 258 | 268 | 148 | 151 | 155 |
| *** | 8881 | 9905 | 14950 | 1762 | 2005 | 2412 | 526 | 562 | 606 | 253 | 263 | 268 | 150 | 153 | 149 |
| 0.45 *** | 8488 | 9045 | 14615 | 1700 | 1885 | 2362 | 519 | 551 | 600 | 251 | 260 | 271 | 148 | 151 | 155 |
| *** | 8681 | 9919 | 15352 | 1777 | 2051 | 2461 | 534 | 573 | 613 | 255 | 265 | 268 | 150 | 153 | 147 |
| 0.5 *** | 8053 | 8733 | 14886 | 1675 | 1875 | 2390 | 515 | 549 | 601 | 247 | 256 | 268 | 145 | 148 | 152 |
| *** | 8293 | 9738 | 15445 | 1759 | 2054 | 2461 | 530 | 572 | 606 | 251 | 262 | 263 | 146 | 150 | 143 |
| 0.55 *** | 7479 | 8281 | 14821 | 1621 | 1831 | 2363 | 500 | 536 | 587 | 239 | 248 | 260 | 138 | 141 | 145 |
| *** | 7769 | 9397 | 15228 | 1710 | 2017 | 2412 | 516 | 558 | 588 | 243 | 253 | 252 | 140 | 143 | 135 |
| 0.6 *** | 6820 | 7730 | 14419 | 1543 | 1756 | 2283 | 477 | 511 | 561 | 225 | 234 | 245 | 129 | 131 | 135 |
| *** | 7157 | 8923 | 14703 | 1633 | 1941 | 2313 | 493 | 533 | 557 | 230 | 239 | 235 | 130 | 133 | 124 |
| 0.65 *** | 6119 | 7106 | 13683 | 1443 | 1651 | 2149 | 444 | 475 | 521 | 207 | 215 | 224 | 116 | 119 | 122 |
| *** | 6493 | 8334 | 13868 | 1531 | 1828 | 2164 | 458 | 496 | 514 | 211 | 219 | 213 | 118 | 120 | 110 |
| 0.7 *** | 5409 | 6426 | 12613 | 1321 | 1515 | 1962 | 401 | 429 | 467 | 183 | 190 | 197 | 101 | 103 | 105 |
| *** | 5801 | 7641 | 12724 | 1403 | 1678 | 1967 | 414 | 446 | 458 | 186 | 193 | 186 | 102 | 104 | 93 |
| 0.75 *** | 4701 | 5697 | 11213 | 1175 | 1348 | 1722 | 349 | 371 | 401 | 155 | 160 | 165 | 83 | 84 | 85 |
| *** | 5091 | 6842 | 11271 | 1250 | 1488 | 1719 | 359 | 385 | 390 | 157 | 162 | 153 | 83 | 85 | 73 |
| 0.8 *** | 3990 | 4907 | 9486 | 1004 | 1145 | 1431 | 285 | 301 | 321 | 120 | 123 | 127 | . | . | . |
| *** | 4353 | 5926 | 9509 | 1065 | 1256 | 1422 | 293 | 310 | 310 | 122 | 125 | 115 | . | . | . |
| 0.85 *** | 3253 | 4031 | 7436 | 800 | 902 | 1087 | 209 | 218 | 229 | . | . | . | . | . | . |
| *** | 3565 | 4862 | 7438 | 845 | 977 | 1076 | 213 | 223 | 217 | . | . | . | . | . | . |
| 0.9 *** | 2440 | 3010 | 5066 | 550 | 606 | 693 | . | . | . | . | . | . | . | . | . |
| *** | 2672 | 3581 | 5058 | 575 | 643 | 681 | . | . | . | . | . | . | . | . | . |
| 0.95 *** | 1418 | 1690 | 2380 | . | . | . | . | . | . | . | . | . | . | . | . |
| *** | 1533 | 1929 | 2368 | . | . | . | . | . | . | . | . | . | . | . | . |

# TABLE 7: ALPHA= 0.05  POWER= 0.8    EXPECTED ACCRUAL THRU MINIMUM FOLLOW-UP= 1100

|  |  | DEL=.02 |  |  | DEL=.05 |  |  | DEL=.10 |  |  | DEL=.15 |  |  | DEL=.20 |  |
|---|---|---|---|---|---|---|---|---|---|---|---|---|---|---|---|
| FACT= | | 1.0 .75 | .50 .25 | .00 BIN | 1.0 .75 | .50 .25 | .00 BIN | 1.0 .75 | .50 .25 | .00 BIN | 1.0 75 | .50 .25 | .00 BIN | 1.0 .75 | .50 .25 | .00 BIN |
| PCONT=*** | | | | | REQUIRED | NUMBER OF | PATIENTS | | | | | | | | | |
| 0.05 | *** | 1776 | 1794 | 1863 | 385 | 389 | 395 | 139 | 140 | 140 | 81 | 82 | 82 | 57 | 58 | 58 |
|  | *** | 1783 | 1816 | 3481 | 387 | 392 | 681 | 139 | 140 | 217 | 82 | 82 | 115 | 58 | 58 | 73 |
| 0.1 | *** | 3700 | 3751 | 4092 | 717 | 734 | 762 | 229 | 232 | 235 | 123 | 124 | 125 | 81 | 81 | 82 |
|  | *** | 3717 | 3831 | 6047 | 725 | 746 | 1076 | 230 | 234 | 310 | 123 | 125 | 153 | 81 | 82 | 93 |
| 0.15 | *** | 5415 | 5509 | 6329 | 1011 | 1047 | 1116 | 308 | 314 | 323 | 158 | 160 | 163 | 101 | 102 | 103 |
|  | *** | 5447 | 5666 | 8304 | 1027 | 1075 | 1422 | 312 | 318 | 390 | 159 | 162 | 186 | 101 | 102 | 110 |
| 0.2 | *** | 6795 | 6940 | 8409 | 1254 | 1314 | 1441 | 375 | 386 | 400 | 188 | 192 | 195 | 117 | 118 | 120 |
|  | *** | 6843 | 7191 | 10251 | 1280 | 1363 | 1719 | 380 | 392 | 458 | 190 | 193 | 213 | 118 | 119 | 124 |
| 0.25 | *** | 7803 | 8012 | 10253 | 1443 | 1529 | 1724 | 430 | 445 | 466 | 213 | 217 | 222 | 130 | 131 | 133 |
|  | *** | 7873 | 8374 | 11890 | 1479 | 1602 | 1967 | 437 | 455 | 514 | 214 | 219 | 235 | 131 | 133 | 135 |
| 0.3 | *** | 8449 | 8733 | 11816 | 1581 | 1693 | 1960 | 471 | 491 | 519 | 230 | 236 | 243 | 139 | 142 | 144 |
|  | *** | 8545 | 9220 | 13219 | 1627 | 1791 | 2164 | 480 | 503 | 557 | 233 | 240 | 252 | 140 | 143 | 143 |
| 0.35 | *** | 8759 | 9135 | 13073 | 1669 | 1809 | 2146 | 500 | 525 | 559 | 243 | 250 | 258 | 145 | 148 | 151 |
|  | *** | 8887 | 9759 | 14239 | 1728 | 1930 | 2313 | 511 | 540 | 588 | 247 | 254 | 263 | 147 | 149 | 147 |
| 0.4 | *** | 8775 | 9257 | 14008 | 1716 | 1880 | 2281 | 518 | 546 | 587 | 250 | 258 | 268 | 148 | 151 | 155 |
|  | *** | 8941 | 10026 | 14950 | 1785 | 2023 | 2412 | 531 | 564 | 606 | 254 | 263 | 268 | 150 | 153 | 149 |
| 0.45 | *** | 8546 | 9147 | 14614 | 1726 | 1909 | 2362 | 524 | 555 | 600 | 252 | 261 | 271 | 148 | 151 | 155 |
|  | *** | 8757 | 10059 | 15352 | 1803 | 2070 | 2461 | 538 | 576 | 613 | 257 | 265 | 268 | 150 | 153 | 147 |
| 0.5 | *** | 8126 | 8853 | 14886 | 1702 | 1902 | 2390 | 520 | 553 | 600 | 249 | 257 | 268 | 145 | 148 | 152 |
|  | *** | 8386 | 9896 | 15445 | 1786 | 2075 | 2461 | 535 | 574 | 606 | 253 | 263 | 263 | 147 | 150 | 143 |
| 0.55 | *** | 7568 | 8418 | 14821 | 1651 | 1859 | 2363 | 506 | 539 | 587 | 240 | 249 | 259 | 138 | 142 | 145 |
|  | *** | 7879 | 9569 | 15228 | 1739 | 2039 | 2412 | 521 | 561 | 588 | 244 | 254 | 252 | 140 | 143 | 135 |
| 0.6 | *** | 6924 | 7879 | 14419 | 1573 | 1784 | 2282 | 482 | 514 | 560 | 226 | 235 | 245 | 129 | 132 | 135 |
|  | *** | 7281 | 9102 | 14703 | 1662 | 1963 | 2313 | 497 | 535 | 557 | 230 | 239 | 235 | 131 | 133 | 124 |
| 0.65 | *** | 6237 | 7262 | 13682 | 1472 | 1677 | 2149 | 449 | 478 | 521 | 208 | 215 | 224 | 117 | 119 | 122 |
|  | *** | 6628 | 8515 | 13868 | 1560 | 1849 | 2164 | 463 | 498 | 514 | 212 | 219 | 213 | 118 | 120 | 110 |
| 0.7 | *** | 5534 | 6584 | 12613 | 1348 | 1539 | 1962 | 406 | 432 | 467 | 184 | 191 | 197 | 101 | 103 | 105 |
|  | *** | 5941 | 7816 | 12724 | 1430 | 1697 | 1967 | 418 | 448 | 458 | 187 | 194 | 186 | 103 | 104 | 93 |
| 0.75 | *** | 4826 | 5847 | 11213 | 1200 | 1369 | 1722 | 352 | 373 | 401 | 155 | 159 | 165 | 82 | 84 | 85 |
|  | *** | 5228 | 7006 | 11271 | 1273 | 1504 | 1719 | 362 | 386 | 390 | 158 | 162 | 153 | 83 | 85 | 73 |
| 0.8 | *** | 4107 | 5043 | 9486 | 1024 | 1163 | 1431 | 287 | 302 | 321 | 121 | 124 | 126 | . | . | . |
|  | *** | 4479 | 6069 | 9509 | 1085 | 1269 | 1422 | 295 | 312 | 310 | 122 | 125 | 115 | . | . | . |
| 0.85 | *** | 3354 | 4144 | 7436 | 815 | 914 | 1087 | 210 | 219 | 229 | . | . | . | . | . | . |
|  | *** | 3672 | 4975 | 7438 | 859 | 985 | 1076 | 214 | 224 | 217 | . | . | . | . | . | . |
| 0.9 | *** | 2516 | 3090 | 5066 | 559 | 612 | 692 | . | . | . | . | . | . | . | . | . |
|  | *** | 2750 | 3656 | 5058 | 583 | 647 | 681 | . | . | . | . | . | . | . | . | . |
| 0.95 | *** | 1456 | 1726 | 2380 | . | . | . | . | . | . | . | . | . | . | . | . |
|  | *** | 1570 | 1957 | 2368 | . | . | . | . | . | . | . | . | . | . | . | . |

TABLE 7: ALPHA= 0.05  POWER= 0.8    EXPECTED ACCRUAL THRU MINIMUM FOLLOW-UP= 1200

| | DEL=.02 | | | DEL=.05 | | | DEL=.10 | | | DEL=.15 | | | DEL=.20 | | |
|---|---|---|---|---|---|---|---|---|---|---|---|---|---|---|---|
| FACT= | 1.0 .75 | .50 .25 | .00 BIN | 1.0 .75 | .50 .25 | .00 BIN | 1.0 .75 | .50 .25 | .00 BIN | 1.0 75 | .50 .25 | .00 BIN | 1.0 .75 | .50 .25 | .00 BIN |
| PCONT=*** | | | | REQUIRED NUMBER OF PATIENTS | | | | | | | | | | | |
| 0.05 *** | 1777 | 1797 | 1863 | 385 | 390 | 395 | 139 | 139 | 140 | 82 | 82 | 82 | 58 | 58 | 58 |
| *** | 1785 | 1819 | 3481 | 388 | 392 | 681 | 139 | 140 | 217 | 82 | 82 | 115 | 58 | 58 | 73 |
| 0.1 *** | 3704 | 3760 | 4092 | 719 | 736 | 762 | 229 | 232 | 235 | 123 | 124 | 124 | 81 | 82 | 82 |
| *** | 3724 | 3841 | 6047 | 727 | 747 | 1076 | 231 | 234 | 310 | 124 | 124 | 153 | 81 | 82 | 93 |
| 0.15 *** | 5424 | 5525 | 6328 | 1016 | 1051 | 1117 | 309 | 315 | 322 | 159 | 160 | 163 | 101 | 102 | 103 |
| *** | 5458 | 5689 | 8304 | 1031 | 1078 | 1422 | 312 | 319 | 390 | 160 | 161 | 186 | 101 | 102 | 110 |
| 0.2 *** | 6808 | 6965 | 8408 | 1261 | 1321 | 1441 | 376 | 387 | 400 | 189 | 192 | 195 | 117 | 118 | 120 |
| *** | 6861 | 7229 | 10251 | 1287 | 1368 | 1719 | 382 | 393 | 458 | 190 | 193 | 213 | 118 | 119 | 124 |
| 0.25 *** | 7822 | 8048 | 10252 | 1454 | 1539 | 1723 | 432 | 446 | 466 | 213 | 217 | 222 | 130 | 132 | 133 |
| *** | 7899 | 8429 | 11890 | 1490 | 1609 | 1967 | 439 | 455 | 514 | 215 | 220 | 235 | 131 | 133 | 135 |
| 0.3 *** | 8475 | 8783 | 11815 | 1594 | 1706 | 1960 | 474 | 493 | 519 | 232 | 237 | 243 | 139 | 142 | 144 |
| *** | 8580 | 9295 | 13219 | 1642 | 1801 | 2164 | 482 | 505 | 557 | 234 | 240 | 252 | 140 | 142 | 143 |
| 0.35 *** | 8794 | 9199 | 13073 | 1687 | 1825 | 2146 | 503 | 526 | 559 | 244 | 250 | 259 | 145 | 148 | 151 |
| *** | 8932 | 9853 | 14239 | 1745 | 1944 | 2313 | 514 | 541 | 588 | 247 | 254 | 263 | 147 | 150 | 147 |
| 0.4 *** | 8821 | 9338 | 14008 | 1737 | 1899 | 2281 | 521 | 548 | 586 | 251 | 259 | 268 | 148 | 151 | 154 |
| *** | 9000 | 10139 | 14950 | 1805 | 2038 | 2412 | 534 | 565 | 606 | 255 | 263 | 268 | 150 | 153 | 149 |
| 0.45 *** | 8605 | 9246 | 14614 | 1749 | 1931 | 2362 | 529 | 558 | 600 | 253 | 262 | 271 | 148 | 151 | 154 |
| *** | 8830 | 10191 | 15352 | 1826 | 2088 | 2461 | 542 | 577 | 613 | 257 | 266 | 268 | 150 | 153 | 147 |
| 0.5 *** | 8198 | 8968 | 14886 | 1728 | 1925 | 2389 | 525 | 556 | 601 | 250 | 258 | 268 | 145 | 148 | 151 |
| *** | 8476 | 10043 | 15445 | 1811 | 2094 | 2461 | 539 | 576 | 606 | 254 | 263 | 263 | 147 | 150 | 143 |
| 0.55 *** | 7655 | 8548 | 14821 | 1677 | 1884 | 2363 | 511 | 542 | 587 | 241 | 250 | 259 | 139 | 142 | 145 |
| *** | 7984 | 9727 | 15228 | 1765 | 2058 | 2412 | 526 | 562 | 588 | 245 | 254 | 252 | 140 | 143 | 135 |
| 0.6 *** | 7026 | 8020 | 14419 | 1600 | 1808 | 2283 | 487 | 517 | 560 | 228 | 235 | 244 | 130 | 132 | 135 |
| *** | 7400 | 9268 | 14703 | 1689 | 1983 | 2313 | 501 | 537 | 557 | 232 | 240 | 235 | 130 | 133 | 124 |
| 0.65 *** | 6350 | 7409 | 13682 | 1498 | 1701 | 2149 | 453 | 481 | 520 | 209 | 216 | 223 | 117 | 119 | 121 |
| *** | 6757 | 8682 | 13868 | 1585 | 1867 | 2164 | 466 | 499 | 514 | 212 | 220 | 213 | 118 | 121 | 110 |
| 0.7 *** | 5653 | 6730 | 12613 | 1373 | 1561 | 1962 | 409 | 434 | 467 | 185 | 190 | 197 | 101 | 103 | 105 |
| *** | 6073 | 7978 | 12724 | 1454 | 1713 | 1967 | 421 | 449 | 458 | 188 | 194 | 186 | 102 | 104 | 93 |
| 0.75 *** | 4943 | 5987 | 11213 | 1222 | 1388 | 1722 | 355 | 375 | 400 | 156 | 160 | 165 | 82 | 84 | 85 |
| *** | 5356 | 7155 | 11271 | 1294 | 1518 | 1719 | 364 | 387 | 390 | 158 | 163 | 153 | 83 | 85 | 73 |
| 0.8 *** | 4217 | 5169 | 9487 | 1043 | 1177 | 1430 | 290 | 304 | 321 | 121 | 124 | 127 | . | . | . |
| *** | 4597 | 6199 | 9509 | 1102 | 1279 | 1422 | 296 | 312 | 310 | 122 | 125 | 115 | . | . | . |
| 0.85 *** | 3448 | 4248 | 7436 | 829 | 924 | 1087 | 211 | 220 | 229 | . | . | . | . | . | . |
| *** | 3771 | 5077 | 7438 | 871 | 992 | 1076 | 215 | 224 | 217 | . | . | . | . | . | . |
| 0.9 *** | 2586 | 3162 | 5066 | 566 | 617 | 692 | . | . | . | . | . | . | . | . | . |
| *** | 2822 | 3724 | 5058 | 589 | 650 | 681 | . | . | . | . | . | . | . | . | . |
| 0.95 *** | 1491 | 1757 | 2380 | . | . | . | . | . | . | . | . | . | . | . | . |
| *** | 1605 | 1982 | 2368 | . | . | . | . | . | . | . | . | . | . | . | . |

## TABLE 7: ALPHA= 0.05  POWER= 0.8    EXPECTED ACCRUAL THRU MINIMUM FOLLOW-UP= 1300

| | DEL=.02 | | | DEL=.05 | | | DEL=.10 | | | DEL=.15 | | | DEL=.20 | | |
|---|---|---|---|---|---|---|---|---|---|---|---|---|---|---|---|
| FACT= | 1.0 .75 | .50 .25 | .00 BIN | 1.0 .75 | .50 .25 | .00 BIN | 1.0 .75 | .50 .25 | .00 BIN | 1.0 75 | .50 .25 | .00 BIN | 1.0 .75 | .50 .25 | .00 BIN |

PCONT=***  REQUIRED NUMBER OF PATIENTS

| PCONT=*** | 1.0/.75 | .50/.25 | .00/BIN | 1.0/.75 | .50/.25 | .00/BIN | 1.0/.75 | .50/.25 | .00/BIN | 1.0/75 | .50/.25 | .00/BIN | 1.0/.75 | .50/.25 | .00/BIN |
|---|---|---|---|---|---|---|---|---|---|---|---|---|---|---|---|
| 0.05 *** | 1779 | 1800 | 1863 | 387 | 390 | 395 | 139 | 140 | 141 | 81 | 82 | 82 | 58 | 58 | 58 |
| *** | 1787 | 1821 | 3481 | 388 | 393 | 681 | 140 | 141 | 217 | 81 | 82 | 115 | 58 | 58 | 73 |
| 0.1 *** | 3709 | 3768 | 4092 | 721 | 737 | 762 | 230 | 232 | 236 | 123 | 124 | 125 | 81 | 81 | 82 |
| *** | 3730 | 3852 | 6047 | 728 | 747 | 1076 | 231 | 234 | 310 | 123 | 124 | 153 | 81 | 82 | 93 |
| 0.15 *** | 5432 | 5541 | 6329 | 1020 | 1055 | 1117 | 310 | 315 | 323 | 159 | 161 | 162 | 101 | 102 | 102 |
| *** | 5470 | 5711 | 8304 | 1035 | 1081 | 1422 | 313 | 318 | 390 | 160 | 162 | 186 | 102 | 102 | 110 |
| 0.2 *** | 6821 | 6991 | 8409 | 1269 | 1327 | 1441 | 379 | 388 | 400 | 189 | 192 | 195 | 117 | 119 | 120 |
| *** | 6879 | 7266 | 10251 | 1293 | 1372 | 1719 | 383 | 393 | 458 | 191 | 193 | 213 | 118 | 120 | 124 |
| 0.25 *** | 7842 | 8084 | 10252 | 1464 | 1548 | 1724 | 434 | 448 | 466 | 214 | 218 | 222 | 130 | 132 | 133 |
| *** | 7924 | 8482 | 11890 | 1500 | 1617 | 1967 | 440 | 456 | 514 | 215 | 220 | 235 | 131 | 133 | 135 |
| 0.3 *** | 8501 | 8832 | 11816 | 1607 | 1719 | 1961 | 476 | 495 | 519 | 232 | 237 | 244 | 140 | 142 | 144 |
| *** | 8614 | 9365 | 13219 | 1655 | 1811 | 2164 | 485 | 505 | 557 | 235 | 240 | 252 | 141 | 143 | 143 |
| 0.35 *** | 8829 | 9262 | 13073 | 1703 | 1840 | 2147 | 507 | 529 | 559 | 245 | 251 | 258 | 146 | 149 | 151 |
| *** | 8979 | 9942 | 14239 | 1761 | 1956 | 2313 | 517 | 543 | 588 | 249 | 255 | 263 | 147 | 149 | 147 |
| 0.4 *** | 8866 | 9417 | 14009 | 1756 | 1917 | 2281 | 525 | 551 | 587 | 253 | 260 | 268 | 149 | 152 | 154 |
| *** | 9059 | 10247 | 14950 | 1824 | 2052 | 2412 | 537 | 567 | 606 | 256 | 263 | 268 | 150 | 154 | 149 |
| 0.45 *** | 8662 | 9341 | 14615 | 1771 | 1952 | 2362 | 532 | 561 | 601 | 254 | 263 | 271 | 149 | 152 | 155 |
| *** | 8903 | 10315 | 15352 | 1848 | 2104 | 2461 | 546 | 578 | 613 | 258 | 266 | 268 | 150 | 154 | 147 |
| 0.5 *** | 8270 | 9079 | 14886 | 1751 | 1947 | 2390 | 529 | 559 | 601 | 251 | 259 | 268 | 146 | 149 | 152 |
| *** | 8564 | 10181 | 15445 | 1835 | 2111 | 2461 | 543 | 578 | 606 | 255 | 263 | 263 | 147 | 150 | 143 |
| 0.55 *** | 7741 | 8672 | 14821 | 1702 | 1906 | 2363 | 515 | 545 | 588 | 243 | 250 | 259 | 140 | 142 | 146 |
| *** | 8087 | 9875 | 15228 | 1789 | 2076 | 2412 | 529 | 565 | 588 | 246 | 254 | 252 | 141 | 144 | 135 |
| 0.6 *** | 7125 | 8154 | 14419 | 1625 | 1831 | 2283 | 491 | 521 | 561 | 229 | 237 | 245 | 130 | 133 | 135 |
| *** | 7515 | 9422 | 14703 | 1714 | 2000 | 2313 | 505 | 539 | 557 | 232 | 240 | 235 | 131 | 134 | 124 |
| 0.65 *** | 6458 | 7548 | 13682 | 1524 | 1722 | 2149 | 458 | 484 | 521 | 211 | 216 | 224 | 118 | 120 | 122 |
| *** | 6879 | 8836 | 13868 | 1610 | 1884 | 2164 | 470 | 500 | 514 | 213 | 220 | 213 | 119 | 120 | 110 |
| 0.7 *** | 5765 | 6868 | 12613 | 1396 | 1581 | 1962 | 413 | 436 | 467 | 186 | 191 | 198 | 102 | 103 | 105 |
| *** | 6197 | 8127 | 12724 | 1476 | 1728 | 1967 | 424 | 451 | 458 | 188 | 194 | 186 | 102 | 104 | 93 |
| 0.75 *** | 5055 | 6118 | 11213 | 1243 | 1405 | 1722 | 358 | 377 | 401 | 157 | 161 | 165 | 83 | 84 | 85 |
| *** | 5476 | 7292 | 11271 | 1314 | 1530 | 1719 | 367 | 388 | 390 | 159 | 162 | 153 | 84 | 84 | 73 |
| 0.8 *** | 4320 | 5286 | 9487 | 1060 | 1191 | 1431 | 292 | 305 | 321 | 122 | 124 | 127 | . | . | . |
| *** | 4707 | 6318 | 9509 | 1118 | 1289 | 1422 | 298 | 313 | 310 | 123 | 125 | 115 | . | . | . |
| 0.85 *** | 3537 | 4344 | 7436 | 841 | 934 | 1087 | 213 | 220 | 229 | . | . | . | . | . | . |
| *** | 3864 | 5172 | 7438 | 882 | 999 | 1076 | 216 | 224 | 217 | . | . | . | . | . | . |
| 0.9 *** | 2651 | 3230 | 5067 | 574 | 622 | 692 | . | . | . | . | . | . | . | . | . |
| *** | 2889 | 3785 | 5058 | 596 | 653 | 681 | . | . | . | . | . | . | . | . | . |
| 0.95 *** | 1523 | 1786 | 2381 | . | . | . | . | . | . | . | . | . | . | . | . |
| *** | 1636 | 2005 | 2368 | . | . | . | . | . | . | . | . | . | . | . | . |

TABLE 7: ALPHA= 0.05  POWER= 0.8    EXPECTED ACCRUAL THRU MINIMUM FOLLOW-UP= 1400

| | | DEL=.02 | | | DEL=.05 | | | DEL=.10 | | | DEL=.15 | | | DEL=.20 | | |
|---|---|---|---|---|---|---|---|---|---|---|---|---|---|---|---|---|---|
| FACT= | | 1.0 .75 | .50 .25 | .00 BIN | 1.0 .75 | .50 .25 | .00 BIN | 1.0 .75 | .50 .25 | .00 BIN | 1.0 75 | .50 .25 | .00 BIN | 1.0 .75 | .50 .25 | .00 BIN |
| PCONT=*** | | | | | REQUIRED NUMBER OF PATIENTS | | | | | | | | | | | |
| 0.05 | *** | 1781 | 1802 | 1863 | 387 | 390 | 395 | 139 | 140 | 141 | 81 | 81 | 82 | 58 | 58 | 58 |
| | *** | 1789 | 1823 | 3481 | 388 | 393 | 681 | 139 | 140 | 217 | 81 | 82 | 115 | 58 | 58 | 73 |
| 0.1 | *** | 3714 | 3776 | 4092 | 724 | 738 | 762 | 230 | 233 | 235 | 123 | 124 | 125 | 81 | 81 | 82 |
| | *** | 3736 | 3861 | 6047 | 730 | 749 | 1076 | 231 | 234 | 310 | 123 | 124 | 153 | 81 | 82 | 93 |
| 0.15 | *** | 5441 | 5556 | 6328 | 1025 | 1058 | 1116 | 311 | 316 | 323 | 159 | 161 | 163 | 101 | 101 | 102 |
| | *** | 5481 | 5732 | 8304 | 1039 | 1082 | 1422 | 313 | 319 | 390 | 160 | 162 | 186 | 101 | 102 | 110 |
| 0.2 | *** | 6835 | 7015 | 8409 | 1276 | 1333 | 1441 | 380 | 388 | 400 | 190 | 192 | 195 | 117 | 119 | 120 |
| | *** | 6897 | 7300 | 10251 | 1300 | 1376 | 1719 | 384 | 394 | 458 | 191 | 193 | 213 | 118 | 119 | 124 |
| 0.25 | *** | 7861 | 8120 | 10252 | 1473 | 1557 | 1724 | 436 | 449 | 465 | 214 | 218 | 222 | 130 | 132 | 134 |
| | *** | 7949 | 8531 | 11890 | 1509 | 1623 | 1967 | 442 | 457 | 514 | 216 | 220 | 235 | 131 | 133 | 135 |
| 0.3 | *** | 8528 | 8879 | 11816 | 1620 | 1730 | 1960 | 479 | 496 | 519 | 233 | 238 | 243 | 140 | 142 | 144 |
| | *** | 8648 | 9432 | 13219 | 1667 | 1819 | 2164 | 486 | 507 | 557 | 235 | 241 | 252 | 141 | 143 | 143 |
| 0.35 | *** | 8864 | 9324 | 13073 | 1718 | 1854 | 2146 | 509 | 531 | 559 | 246 | 252 | 259 | 147 | 149 | 151 |
| | *** | 9024 | 10026 | 14239 | 1776 | 1966 | 2313 | 520 | 544 | 588 | 248 | 255 | 263 | 148 | 150 | 147 |
| 0.4 | *** | 8911 | 9494 | 14009 | 1774 | 1933 | 2281 | 528 | 553 | 586 | 254 | 260 | 268 | 150 | 152 | 155 |
| | *** | 9117 | 10347 | 14950 | 1842 | 2065 | 2412 | 540 | 569 | 606 | 256 | 264 | 268 | 150 | 153 | 149 |
| 0.45 | *** | 8719 | 9432 | 14614 | 1790 | 1970 | 2362 | 536 | 563 | 600 | 255 | 262 | 271 | 150 | 152 | 155 |
| | *** | 8975 | 10431 | 15352 | 1867 | 2117 | 2461 | 549 | 580 | 613 | 259 | 267 | 268 | 150 | 153 | 147 |
| 0.5 | *** | 8340 | 9185 | 14885 | 1773 | 1966 | 2390 | 533 | 562 | 600 | 252 | 260 | 269 | 146 | 149 | 151 |
| | *** | 8649 | 10310 | 15445 | 1856 | 2125 | 2461 | 546 | 579 | 606 | 255 | 263 | 263 | 148 | 150 | 143 |
| 0.55 | *** | 7824 | 8790 | 14821 | 1725 | 1926 | 2363 | 519 | 548 | 587 | 244 | 251 | 260 | 140 | 143 | 145 |
| | *** | 8186 | 10013 | 15228 | 1811 | 2091 | 2412 | 533 | 566 | 588 | 248 | 255 | 252 | 141 | 143 | 135 |
| 0.6 | *** | 7220 | 8280 | 14419 | 1648 | 1851 | 2283 | 495 | 523 | 561 | 230 | 237 | 245 | 130 | 133 | 135 |
| | *** | 7624 | 9565 | 14703 | 1736 | 2015 | 2313 | 508 | 540 | 557 | 234 | 241 | 235 | 131 | 134 | 124 |
| 0.65 | *** | 6562 | 7678 | 13682 | 1546 | 1742 | 2149 | 460 | 486 | 521 | 211 | 217 | 224 | 118 | 120 | 122 |
| | *** | 6995 | 8980 | 13868 | 1631 | 1899 | 2164 | 472 | 502 | 514 | 213 | 220 | 213 | 119 | 121 | 110 |
| 0.7 | *** | 5873 | 6997 | 12613 | 1417 | 1599 | 1962 | 416 | 438 | 467 | 186 | 192 | 197 | 102 | 103 | 105 |
| | *** | 6315 | 8265 | 12724 | 1496 | 1740 | 1967 | 426 | 451 | 458 | 189 | 194 | 186 | 102 | 104 | 93 |
| 0.75 | *** | 5160 | 6240 | 11213 | 1262 | 1420 | 1722 | 360 | 378 | 401 | 157 | 161 | 164 | 83 | 84 | 86 |
| | *** | 5589 | 7419 | 11271 | 1332 | 1541 | 1719 | 369 | 388 | 390 | 159 | 163 | 153 | 84 | 85 | 73 |
| 0.8 | *** | 4418 | 5395 | 9487 | 1075 | 1203 | 1431 | 294 | 306 | 321 | 122 | 124 | 127 | . | . | . |
| | *** | 4810 | 6428 | 9509 | 1132 | 1297 | 1422 | 299 | 313 | 310 | 123 | 125 | 115 | . | . | . |
| 0.85 | *** | 3620 | 4433 | 7437 | 852 | 941 | 1087 | 214 | 221 | 229 | . | . | . | . | . | . |
| | *** | 3950 | 5257 | 7438 | 892 | 1004 | 1076 | 217 | 225 | 217 | . | . | . | . | . | . |
| 0.9 | *** | 2712 | 3291 | 5066 | 579 | 626 | 693 | . | . | . | . | . | . | . | . | . |
| | *** | 2951 | 3839 | 5058 | 601 | 656 | 681 | . | . | . | . | . | . | . | . | . |
| 0.95 | *** | 1552 | 1812 | 2380 | . | . | . | . | . | . | . | . | . | . | . | . |
| | *** | 1664 | 2025 | 2368 | . | . | . | . | . | . | . | . | . | . | . | . |

## TABLE 7: ALPHA= 0.05  POWER= 0.8    EXPECTED ACCRUAL THRU MINIMUM FOLLOW-UP= 1500

| | | DEL=.02 | | | DEL=.05 | | | DEL=.10 | | | DEL=.15 | | | DEL=.20 | | |
|---|---|---|---|---|---|---|---|---|---|---|---|---|---|---|---|---|
| FACT= | | 1.0 / .75 | .50 / .25 | .00 / BIN | 1.0 / .75 | .50 / .25 | .00 / BIN | 1.0 / .75 | .50 / .25 | .00 / BIN | 1.0 / 75 | .50 / .25 | .00 / BIN | 1.0 / .75 | .50 / .25 | .00 / BIN |
| PCONT=*** | | REQUIRED NUMBER OF PATIENTS | | | | | | | | | | | | | | |
| 0.05 | *** | 1783 | 1805 | 1863 | 387 | 391 | 395 | 140 | 140 | 140 | 82 | 82 | 82 | 57 | 58 | 58 |
| | *** | 1792 | 1825 | 3481 | 389 | 393 | 681 | 140 | 140 | 217 | 82 | 82 | 115 | 57 | 58 | 73 |
| 0.1 | *** | 3719 | 3784 | 4092 | 725 | 740 | 762 | 230 | 232 | 235 | 124 | 124 | 125 | 82 | 82 | 82 |
| | *** | 3742 | 3870 | 6047 | 731 | 750 | 1076 | 232 | 234 | 310 | 124 | 125 | 153 | 82 | 82 | 93 |
| 0.15 | *** | 5450 | 5572 | 6328 | 1027 | 1061 | 1117 | 311 | 317 | 322 | 159 | 161 | 163 | 101 | 102 | 102 |
| | *** | 5492 | 5752 | 8304 | 1042 | 1085 | 1422 | 314 | 320 | 390 | 160 | 162 | 186 | 101 | 102 | 110 |
| 0.2 | *** | 6848 | 7039 | 8408 | 1282 | 1338 | 1441 | 380 | 389 | 399 | 190 | 192 | 195 | 118 | 119 | 120 |
| | *** | 6914 | 7332 | 10251 | 1306 | 1380 | 1719 | 384 | 394 | 458 | 191 | 194 | 213 | 118 | 119 | 124 |
| 0.25 | *** | 7880 | 8154 | 10252 | 1482 | 1564 | 1724 | 437 | 450 | 466 | 215 | 218 | 222 | 131 | 132 | 134 |
| | *** | 7974 | 8579 | 11890 | 1518 | 1628 | 1967 | 443 | 457 | 514 | 217 | 220 | 235 | 131 | 133 | 135 |
| 0.3 | *** | 8554 | 8926 | 11816 | 1631 | 1740 | 1960 | 481 | 498 | 519 | 233 | 238 | 244 | 140 | 142 | 144 |
| | *** | 8683 | 9495 | 13219 | 1678 | 1826 | 2164 | 488 | 507 | 557 | 236 | 241 | 252 | 142 | 143 | 143 |
| 0.35 | *** | 8899 | 9384 | 13073 | 1732 | 1867 | 2147 | 512 | 532 | 560 | 247 | 252 | 259 | 147 | 149 | 151 |
| | *** | 9068 | 10105 | 14239 | 1790 | 1975 | 2313 | 521 | 545 | 588 | 249 | 255 | 263 | 148 | 150 | 147 |
| 0.4 | *** | 8956 | 9568 | 14009 | 1790 | 1948 | 2281 | 532 | 555 | 587 | 254 | 260 | 268 | 150 | 152 | 155 |
| | *** | 9173 | 10442 | 14950 | 1858 | 2075 | 2412 | 543 | 570 | 606 | 258 | 264 | 268 | 151 | 154 | 149 |
| 0.45 | *** | 8775 | 9521 | 14615 | 1808 | 1985 | 2362 | 539 | 565 | 600 | 257 | 263 | 271 | 150 | 152 | 155 |
| | *** | 9045 | 10540 | 15352 | 1885 | 2130 | 2461 | 551 | 581 | 613 | 260 | 267 | 268 | 151 | 154 | 147 |
| 0.5 | *** | 8408 | 9287 | 14885 | 1792 | 1984 | 2390 | 536 | 563 | 601 | 253 | 260 | 268 | 146 | 149 | 152 |
| | *** | 8733 | 10430 | 15445 | 1875 | 2138 | 2461 | 549 | 580 | 606 | 257 | 264 | 263 | 148 | 150 | 143 |
| 0.55 | *** | 7906 | 8902 | 14821 | 1745 | 1944 | 2363 | 522 | 550 | 587 | 245 | 251 | 260 | 140 | 142 | 145 |
| | *** | 8281 | 10144 | 15228 | 1832 | 2105 | 2412 | 535 | 567 | 588 | 248 | 255 | 252 | 142 | 143 | 135 |
| 0.6 | *** | 7312 | 8401 | 14419 | 1670 | 1869 | 2283 | 499 | 525 | 560 | 230 | 237 | 245 | 130 | 133 | 135 |
| | *** | 7730 | 9699 | 14703 | 1756 | 2029 | 2313 | 511 | 542 | 557 | 234 | 241 | 235 | 131 | 134 | 124 |
| 0.65 | *** | 6661 | 7802 | 13683 | 1567 | 1760 | 2149 | 464 | 488 | 520 | 212 | 217 | 224 | 118 | 120 | 122 |
| | *** | 7105 | 9113 | 13868 | 1651 | 1912 | 2164 | 475 | 503 | 514 | 215 | 220 | 213 | 119 | 121 | 110 |
| 0.7 | *** | 5975 | 7119 | 12613 | 1436 | 1615 | 1962 | 419 | 440 | 467 | 187 | 192 | 197 | 102 | 104 | 105 |
| | *** | 6427 | 8393 | 12724 | 1515 | 1752 | 1967 | 428 | 453 | 458 | 189 | 195 | 186 | 103 | 104 | 93 |
| 0.75 | *** | 5260 | 6355 | 11213 | 1279 | 1434 | 1722 | 363 | 380 | 400 | 157 | 161 | 165 | 83 | 84 | 85 |
| | *** | 5697 | 7537 | 11271 | 1347 | 1550 | 1719 | 371 | 390 | 390 | 159 | 163 | 153 | 83 | 85 | 73 |
| 0.8 | *** | 4509 | 5497 | 9487 | 1089 | 1214 | 1430 | 295 | 307 | 322 | 122 | 125 | 127 | . | . | . |
| | *** | 4907 | 6529 | 9509 | 1145 | 1304 | 1422 | 301 | 314 | 310 | 124 | 125 | 115 | . | . | . |
| 0.85 | *** | 3697 | 4516 | 7436 | 862 | 950 | 1087 | 215 | 221 | 229 | . | . | . | . | . | . |
| | *** | 4031 | 5335 | 7438 | 902 | 1009 | 1076 | 218 | 225 | 217 | . | . | . | . | . | . |
| 0.9 | *** | 2769 | 3348 | 5066 | 585 | 630 | 693 | . | . | . | . | . | . | . | . | . |
| | *** | 3009 | 3890 | 5058 | 605 | 658 | 681 | . | . | . | . | . | . | . | . | . |
| 0.95 | *** | 1580 | 1835 | 2380 | . | . | . | . | . | . | . | . | . | . | . | . |
| | *** | 1690 | 2042 | 2368 | . | . | . | . | . | . | . | . | . | . | . | . |

TABLE 7: ALPHA= 0.05  POWER= 0.8    EXPECTED ACCRUAL THRU MINIMUM FOLLOW-UP= 1600

| | DEL=.02 | | | DEL=.05 | | | DEL=.10 | | | DEL=.15 | | | DEL=.20 | | |
|---|---|---|---|---|---|---|---|---|---|---|---|---|---|---|---|
| FACT= | 1.0 .75 | .50 .25 | .00 BIN | 1.0 .75 | .50 .25 | .00 BIN | 1.0 .75 | .50 .25 | .00 BIN | 1.0 75 | .50 .25 | .00 BIN | 1.0 .75 | .50 .25 | .00 BIN |
| PCONT=*** | | | | | REQUIRED | NUMBER | OF PATIENTS | | | | | | | | |
| 0.05 *** | 1785 | 1806 | 1863 | 388 | 391 | 395 | 139 | 140 | 141 | 82 | 82 | 82 | 58 | 58 | 58 |
| *** | 1793 | 1827 | 3481 | 389 | 393 | 681 | 140 | 140 | 217 | 82 | 82 | 115 | 58 | 58 | 73 |
| 0.1 *** | 3724 | 3792 | 4092 | 727 | 741 | 762 | 231 | 233 | 235 | 124 | 124 | 125 | 81 | 82 | 82 |
| *** | 3748 | 3879 | 6047 | 733 | 750 | 1076 | 232 | 234 | 310 | 124 | 125 | 153 | 82 | 82 | 93 |
| 0.15 *** | 5458 | 5586 | 6328 | 1031 | 1064 | 1117 | 312 | 317 | 323 | 160 | 161 | 163 | 101 | 102 | 103 |
| *** | 5503 | 5769 | 8304 | 1046 | 1086 | 1422 | 314 | 320 | 390 | 160 | 162 | 186 | 102 | 102 | 110 |
| 0.2 *** | 6861 | 7063 | 8409 | 1287 | 1342 | 1441 | 382 | 390 | 400 | 190 | 193 | 195 | 118 | 119 | 120 |
| *** | 6931 | 7363 | 10251 | 1311 | 1383 | 1719 | 386 | 395 | 458 | 192 | 194 | 213 | 118 | 119 | 124 |
| 0.25 *** | 7899 | 8188 | 10253 | 1490 | 1571 | 1724 | 439 | 451 | 466 | 215 | 219 | 222 | 131 | 132 | 134 |
| *** | 8000 | 8623 | 11890 | 1525 | 1633 | 1967 | 444 | 458 | 514 | 217 | 220 | 235 | 132 | 133 | 135 |
| 0.3 *** | 8580 | 8972 | 11816 | 1642 | 1749 | 1960 | 483 | 499 | 519 | 234 | 239 | 243 | 141 | 142 | 144 |
| *** | 8717 | 9555 | 13219 | 1688 | 1833 | 2164 | 490 | 508 | 557 | 236 | 241 | 252 | 142 | 143 | 143 |
| 0.35 *** | 8933 | 9442 | 13073 | 1745 | 1878 | 2147 | 514 | 534 | 559 | 248 | 253 | 259 | 147 | 149 | 151 |
| *** | 9113 | 10180 | 14239 | 1803 | 1984 | 2313 | 524 | 546 | 588 | 250 | 256 | 263 | 148 | 150 | 147 |
| 0.4 *** | 9000 | 9640 | 14009 | 1805 | 1961 | 2281 | 534 | 557 | 587 | 255 | 261 | 268 | 150 | 152 | 155 |
| *** | 9230 | 10532 | 14950 | 1873 | 2086 | 2412 | 545 | 571 | 606 | 258 | 264 | 268 | 151 | 154 | 149 |
| 0.45 *** | 8831 | 9607 | 14615 | 1826 | 2001 | 2362 | 542 | 567 | 600 | 257 | 264 | 271 | 150 | 152 | 155 |
| *** | 9114 | 10643 | 15352 | 1902 | 2141 | 2461 | 554 | 583 | 613 | 260 | 267 | 268 | 151 | 154 | 147 |
| 0.5 *** | 8476 | 9384 | 14886 | 1812 | 2000 | 2390 | 539 | 566 | 601 | 254 | 261 | 268 | 147 | 149 | 152 |
| *** | 8813 | 10545 | 15445 | 1893 | 2151 | 2461 | 552 | 582 | 606 | 257 | 264 | 263 | 148 | 150 | 143 |
| 0.55 *** | 7985 | 9010 | 14821 | 1765 | 1962 | 2363 | 526 | 552 | 587 | 246 | 252 | 260 | 140 | 143 | 145 |
| *** | 8373 | 10265 | 15228 | 1850 | 2117 | 2412 | 538 | 569 | 588 | 249 | 256 | 252 | 142 | 144 | 135 |
| 0.6 *** | 7401 | 8515 | 14419 | 1689 | 1886 | 2283 | 501 | 527 | 561 | 232 | 238 | 245 | 131 | 133 | 135 |
| *** | 7830 | 9825 | 14703 | 1775 | 2041 | 2313 | 513 | 543 | 557 | 235 | 241 | 235 | 132 | 134 | 124 |
| 0.65 *** | 6757 | 7919 | 13682 | 1586 | 1776 | 2149 | 467 | 490 | 521 | 213 | 218 | 224 | 118 | 120 | 122 |
| *** | 7211 | 9239 | 13868 | 1669 | 1923 | 2164 | 478 | 504 | 514 | 215 | 221 | 213 | 119 | 121 | 110 |
| 0.7 *** | 6073 | 7235 | 12613 | 1455 | 1630 | 1962 | 421 | 442 | 467 | 188 | 192 | 197 | 102 | 104 | 105 |
| *** | 6533 | 8514 | 12724 | 1532 | 1763 | 1967 | 431 | 454 | 458 | 190 | 195 | 186 | 103 | 105 | 93 |
| 0.75 *** | 5356 | 6463 | 11213 | 1295 | 1447 | 1722 | 365 | 381 | 401 | 158 | 161 | 165 | 84 | 84 | 85 |
| *** | 5799 | 7647 | 11271 | 1362 | 1560 | 1719 | 373 | 390 | 390 | 160 | 163 | 153 | 84 | 85 | 73 |
| 0.8 *** | 4597 | 5593 | 9487 | 1102 | 1224 | 1431 | 297 | 308 | 321 | 123 | 125 | 127 | . | . | . |
| *** | 4999 | 6623 | 9509 | 1157 | 1311 | 1422 | 302 | 314 | 310 | 124 | 126 | 115 | . | . | . |
| 0.85 *** | 3771 | 4594 | 7436 | 872 | 956 | 1087 | 216 | 222 | 229 | . | . | . | . | . | . |
| *** | 4108 | 5408 | 7438 | 910 | 1013 | 1076 | 219 | 225 | 217 | . | . | . | . | . | . |
| 0.9 *** | 2823 | 3401 | 5066 | 590 | 633 | 693 | . | . | . | . | . | . | . | . | . |
| *** | 3064 | 3936 | 5058 | 610 | 660 | 681 | . | . | . | . | . | . | . | . | . |
| 0.95 *** | 1605 | 1858 | 2380 | . | . | . | . | . | . | . | . | . | . | . | . |
| *** | 1715 | 2058 | 2368 | . | . | . | . | . | . | . | . | . | . | . | . |

## TABLE 7: ALPHA= 0.05  POWER= 0.8    EXPECTED ACCRUAL THRU MINIMUM FOLLOW-UP= 1700

|  | | DEL=.02 | | | DEL=.05 | | | DEL=.10 | | | DEL=.15 | | | DEL=.20 | | |
|---|---|---|---|---|---|---|---|---|---|---|---|---|---|---|---|---|
| FACT= | | 1.0 .75 | .50 .25 | .00 BIN | 1.0 .75 | .50 .25 | .00 BIN | 1.0 .75 | .50 .25 | .00 BIN | 1.0 75 | .50 .25 | .00 BIN | 1.0 .75 | .50 .25 | .00 BIN |
| PCONT=*** | | | | REQUIRED NUMBER OF PATIENTS | | | | | | | | | | | | |
| 0.05 | *** | 1787 | 1808 | 1863 | 388 | 391 | 395 | 139 | 140 | 140 | 82 | 82 | 82 | 57 | 57 | 57 |
|  | *** | 1795 | 1829 | 3481 | 390 | 393 | 681 | 140 | 140 | 217 | 82 | 82 | 115 | 57 | 57 | 73 |
| 0.1 | *** | 3728 | 3798 | 4092 | 728 | 741 | 762 | 231 | 233 | 236 | 123 | 124 | 125 | 82 | 82 | 82 |
|  | *** | 3754 | 3886 | 6047 | 734 | 751 | 1076 | 231 | 233 | 310 | 124 | 124 | 153 | 82 | 82 | 93 |
| 0.15 | *** | 5467 | 5600 | 6328 | 1035 | 1066 | 1117 | 312 | 318 | 323 | 160 | 161 | 163 | 102 | 102 | 103 |
|  | *** | 5514 | 5786 | 8304 | 1049 | 1088 | 1422 | 314 | 320 | 390 | 160 | 163 | 186 | 102 | 102 | 110 |
| 0.2 | *** | 6874 | 7086 | 8408 | 1292 | 1346 | 1440 | 382 | 390 | 399 | 190 | 193 | 195 | 118 | 119 | 120 |
|  | *** | 6948 | 7392 | 10251 | 1316 | 1387 | 1719 | 386 | 395 | 458 | 191 | 194 | 213 | 119 | 119 | 124 |
| 0.25 | *** | 7919 | 8221 | 10253 | 1498 | 1576 | 1724 | 440 | 452 | 465 | 216 | 219 | 222 | 131 | 133 | 134 |
|  | *** | 8024 | 8665 | 11890 | 1532 | 1637 | 1967 | 445 | 458 | 514 | 216 | 221 | 235 | 131 | 133 | 135 |
| 0.3 | *** | 8606 | 9016 | 11816 | 1651 | 1757 | 1960 | 484 | 499 | 518 | 235 | 239 | 243 | 141 | 142 | 144 |
|  | *** | 8750 | 9611 | 13219 | 1698 | 1839 | 2164 | 492 | 509 | 557 | 237 | 241 | 252 | 141 | 143 | 143 |
| 0.35 | *** | 8967 | 9498 | 13073 | 1757 | 1889 | 2146 | 516 | 535 | 560 | 248 | 253 | 259 | 148 | 148 | 151 |
|  | *** | 9156 | 10252 | 14239 | 1814 | 1991 | 2313 | 526 | 546 | 588 | 250 | 256 | 263 | 148 | 150 | 147 |
| 0.4 | *** | 9044 | 9709 | 14009 | 1820 | 1974 | 2281 | 537 | 559 | 586 | 256 | 261 | 267 | 151 | 153 | 155 |
|  | *** | 9284 | 10618 | 14950 | 1886 | 2095 | 2412 | 547 | 571 | 606 | 258 | 265 | 268 | 152 | 154 | 149 |
| 0.45 | *** | 8886 | 9689 | 14615 | 1842 | 2014 | 2362 | 545 | 569 | 600 | 258 | 265 | 271 | 151 | 153 | 155 |
|  | *** | 9181 | 10741 | 15352 | 1916 | 2150 | 2461 | 556 | 583 | 613 | 261 | 267 | 268 | 152 | 154 | 147 |
| 0.5 | *** | 8542 | 9479 | 14885 | 1829 | 2016 | 2390 | 542 | 567 | 600 | 255 | 261 | 269 | 148 | 150 | 152 |
|  | *** | 8892 | 10652 | 15445 | 1910 | 2162 | 2461 | 554 | 583 | 606 | 258 | 265 | 263 | 148 | 151 | 143 |
| 0.55 | *** | 8062 | 9113 | 14821 | 1784 | 1977 | 2363 | 528 | 554 | 588 | 246 | 253 | 259 | 141 | 142 | 146 |
|  | *** | 8463 | 10380 | 15228 | 1868 | 2128 | 2412 | 541 | 569 | 588 | 250 | 256 | 252 | 141 | 144 | 135 |
| 0.6 | *** | 7486 | 8624 | 14419 | 1707 | 1902 | 2283 | 503 | 529 | 561 | 233 | 238 | 244 | 131 | 133 | 135 |
|  | *** | 7927 | 9943 | 14703 | 1792 | 2052 | 2313 | 515 | 544 | 557 | 235 | 241 | 235 | 131 | 134 | 124 |
| 0.65 | *** | 6849 | 8030 | 13683 | 1603 | 1790 | 2149 | 469 | 492 | 520 | 214 | 218 | 224 | 119 | 120 | 122 |
|  | *** | 7312 | 9356 | 13868 | 1686 | 1933 | 2164 | 480 | 505 | 514 | 216 | 221 | 213 | 119 | 121 | 110 |
| 0.7 | *** | 6166 | 7344 | 12613 | 1472 | 1644 | 1962 | 424 | 443 | 467 | 188 | 192 | 197 | 103 | 104 | 105 |
|  | *** | 6634 | 8626 | 12724 | 1547 | 1772 | 1967 | 432 | 454 | 458 | 190 | 195 | 186 | 103 | 104 | 93 |
| 0.75 | *** | 5446 | 6565 | 11213 | 1309 | 1459 | 1722 | 367 | 382 | 401 | 158 | 161 | 165 | 84 | 85 | 85 |
|  | *** | 5894 | 7749 | 11271 | 1376 | 1567 | 1719 | 374 | 391 | 390 | 160 | 163 | 153 | 84 | 85 | 73 |
| 0.8 | *** | 4680 | 5683 | 9487 | 1115 | 1234 | 1430 | 297 | 309 | 321 | 123 | 124 | 126 | . | . | . |
|  | *** | 5086 | 6710 | 9509 | 1168 | 1316 | 1422 | 303 | 314 | 310 | 123 | 125 | 115 | . | . | . |
| 0.85 | *** | 3841 | 4666 | 7436 | 879 | 962 | 1087 | 216 | 222 | 229 | . | . | . | . | . | . |
|  | *** | 4180 | 5476 | 7438 | 918 | 1017 | 1076 | 219 | 225 | 217 | . | . | . | . | . | . |
| 0.9 | *** | 2873 | 3451 | 5066 | 594 | 636 | 692 | . | . | . | . | . | . | . | . | . |
|  | *** | 3114 | 3978 | 5058 | 614 | 662 | 681 | . | . | . | . | . | . | . | . | . |
| 0.95 | *** | 1629 | 1877 | 2380 | . | . | . | . | . | . | . | . | . | . | . | . |
|  | *** | 1737 | 2073 | 2368 | . | . | . | . | . | . | . | . | . | . | . | . |

TABLE 7: ALPHA= 0.05  POWER= 0.8    EXPECTED ACCRUAL THRU MINIMUM FOLLOW-UP= 1800

| | | DEL=.02 | | | DEL=.05 | | | DEL=.10 | | | DEL=.15 | | | DEL=.20 | | |
|---|---|---|---|---|---|---|---|---|---|---|---|---|---|---|---|---|---|
| FACT= | | 1.0 .75 | .50 .25 | .00 BIN | 1.0 .75 | .50 .25 | .00 BIN | 1.0 .75 | .50 .25 | .00 BIN | 1.0 75 | .50 .25 | .00 BIN | 1.0 .75 | .50 .25 | .00 BIN |
| PCONT=*** | | | | | REQUIRED NUMBER OF PATIENTS | | | | | | | | | | | |
| 0.05 | *** | 1788 | 1810 | 1863 | 388 | 391 | 395 | 139 | 141 | 141 | 82 | 82 | 82 | 57 | 57 | 57 |
| | *** | 1797 | 1830 | 3481 | 390 | 393 | 681 | 139 | 141 | 217 | 82 | 82 | 115 | 57 | 57 | 73 |
| 0.1 | *** | 3732 | 3806 | 4092 | 729 | 742 | 762 | 231 | 233 | 235 | 123 | 125 | 125 | 81 | 82 | 82 |
| | *** | 3759 | 3894 | 6047 | 735 | 751 | 1076 | 231 | 234 | 310 | 123 | 125 | 153 | 82 | 82 | 93 |
| 0.15 | *** | 5475 | 5615 | 6328 | 1037 | 1068 | 1117 | 312 | 317 | 323 | 159 | 162 | 163 | 101 | 102 | 102 |
| | *** | 5525 | 5802 | 8304 | 1050 | 1089 | 1422 | 315 | 319 | 390 | 161 | 162 | 186 | 102 | 102 | 110 |
| 0.2 | *** | 6888 | 7107 | 8408 | 1297 | 1350 | 1441 | 384 | 390 | 399 | 191 | 193 | 195 | 118 | 119 | 120 |
| | *** | 6966 | 7419 | 10251 | 1320 | 1388 | 1719 | 387 | 395 | 458 | 192 | 195 | 213 | 118 | 119 | 124 |
| 0.25 | *** | 7937 | 8253 | 10252 | 1504 | 1583 | 1723 | 441 | 452 | 465 | 216 | 219 | 222 | 132 | 132 | 134 |
| | *** | 8048 | 8706 | 11890 | 1539 | 1641 | 1967 | 447 | 459 | 514 | 217 | 220 | 235 | 132 | 132 | 135 |
| 0.3 | *** | 8632 | 9060 | 11816 | 1660 | 1765 | 1961 | 486 | 501 | 519 | 235 | 240 | 243 | 141 | 143 | 144 |
| | *** | 8783 | 9666 | 13219 | 1707 | 1845 | 2164 | 492 | 510 | 557 | 237 | 240 | 252 | 141 | 143 | 143 |
| 0.35 | *** | 9001 | 9555 | 13074 | 1770 | 1899 | 2146 | 519 | 537 | 559 | 249 | 253 | 258 | 147 | 150 | 150 |
| | *** | 9199 | 10320 | 14239 | 1826 | 1998 | 2313 | 526 | 546 | 588 | 251 | 256 | 263 | 148 | 150 | 147 |
| 0.4 | *** | 9087 | 9777 | 14008 | 1833 | 1986 | 2281 | 539 | 560 | 586 | 256 | 262 | 267 | 150 | 153 | 155 |
| | *** | 9339 | 10698 | 14950 | 1899 | 2103 | 2412 | 549 | 573 | 606 | 258 | 264 | 268 | 152 | 154 | 149 |
| 0.45 | *** | 8940 | 9768 | 14615 | 1857 | 2027 | 2362 | 548 | 570 | 600 | 258 | 264 | 271 | 150 | 153 | 155 |
| | *** | 9246 | 10833 | 15352 | 1932 | 2160 | 2461 | 558 | 585 | 613 | 262 | 267 | 268 | 152 | 154 | 147 |
| 0.5 | *** | 8607 | 9568 | 14886 | 1845 | 2029 | 2389 | 544 | 569 | 600 | 255 | 262 | 269 | 147 | 150 | 152 |
| | *** | 8968 | 10755 | 15445 | 1926 | 2171 | 2461 | 555 | 584 | 606 | 258 | 264 | 263 | 148 | 150 | 143 |
| 0.55 | *** | 8137 | 9211 | 14820 | 1800 | 1991 | 2364 | 531 | 555 | 587 | 247 | 253 | 260 | 141 | 143 | 145 |
| | *** | 8549 | 10488 | 15228 | 1884 | 2139 | 2412 | 542 | 570 | 588 | 249 | 256 | 252 | 141 | 144 | 135 |
| 0.6 | *** | 7570 | 8727 | 14419 | 1725 | 1916 | 2283 | 506 | 531 | 560 | 233 | 238 | 245 | 132 | 132 | 135 |
| | *** | 8020 | 10055 | 14703 | 1809 | 2062 | 2313 | 517 | 544 | 557 | 236 | 242 | 235 | 132 | 134 | 124 |
| 0.65 | *** | 6938 | 8136 | 13682 | 1620 | 1804 | 2148 | 471 | 492 | 521 | 213 | 218 | 224 | 119 | 120 | 121 |
| | *** | 7409 | 9467 | 13868 | 1701 | 1943 | 2164 | 481 | 506 | 514 | 216 | 222 | 213 | 119 | 121 | 110 |
| 0.7 | *** | 6257 | 7447 | 12612 | 1487 | 1656 | 1962 | 425 | 444 | 467 | 189 | 193 | 197 | 102 | 103 | 105 |
| | *** | 6731 | 8732 | 12724 | 1561 | 1781 | 1967 | 434 | 456 | 458 | 191 | 195 | 186 | 103 | 105 | 93 |
| 0.75 | *** | 5534 | 6662 | 11213 | 1323 | 1469 | 1722 | 368 | 382 | 400 | 159 | 162 | 165 | 83 | 84 | 85 |
| | *** | 5987 | 7845 | 11271 | 1388 | 1575 | 1719 | 375 | 391 | 390 | 161 | 163 | 153 | 84 | 85 | 73 |
| 0.8 | *** | 4758 | 5769 | 9487 | 1125 | 1242 | 1431 | 299 | 309 | 321 | 123 | 125 | 127 | . | . | . |
| | *** | 5169 | 6792 | 9509 | 1178 | 1322 | 1422 | 303 | 315 | 310 | 123 | 126 | 115 | . | . | . |
| 0.85 | *** | 3908 | 4735 | 7436 | 888 | 967 | 1086 | 217 | 222 | 229 | . | . | . | . | . | . |
| | *** | 4248 | 5538 | 7438 | 924 | 1020 | 1076 | 219 | 226 | 217 | . | . | . | . | . | . |
| 0.9 | *** | 2922 | 3498 | 5067 | 598 | 639 | 693 | . | . | . | . | . | . | . | . | . |
| | *** | 3162 | 4017 | 5058 | 618 | 663 | 681 | . | . | . | . | . | . | . | . | . |
| 0.95 | *** | 1650 | 1896 | 2380 | . | . | . | . | . | . | . | . | . | . | . | . |
| | *** | 1757 | 2085 | 2368 | . | . | . | . | . | . | . | . | . | . | . | . |

## TABLE 7: ALPHA= 0.05  POWER= 0.8    EXPECTED ACCRUAL THRU MINIMUM FOLLOW-UP= 1900

|         |       | DEL=.02 | | | DEL=.05 | | | DEL=.10 | | | DEL=.15 | | | DEL=.20 | | |
|---------|-------|------|------|------|------|------|------|------|------|------|------|------|------|------|------|------|
| FACT=   |       | 1.0<br>.75 | .50<br>.25 | .00<br>BIN | 1.0<br>.75 | .50<br>.25 | .00<br>BIN | 1.0<br>.75 | .50<br>.25 | .00<br>BIN | 1.0<br>75 | .50<br>.25 | .00<br>BIN | 1.0<br>.75 | .50<br>.25 | .00<br>BIN |
| PCONT=*** | | | | | REQUIRED NUMBER OF PATIENTS | | | | | | | | | | | |
| 0.05 | *** | 1789 | 1812 | 1863 | 388 | 391 | 395 | 140 | 140 | 141 | 82 | 82 | 82 | 58 | 58 | 58 |
|      | *** | 1799 | 1831 | 3481 | 391 | 393 | 681 | 140 | 140 | 217 | 82 | 82 | 115 | 58 | 58 | 73 |
| 0.1 | *** | 3738 | 3813 | 4092 | 730 | 743 | 762 | 231 | 234 | 235 | 123 | 125 | 125 | 82 | 82 | 82 |
|     | *** | 3765 | 3899 | 6047 | 736 | 752 | 1076 | 232 | 234 | 310 | 125 | 125 | 153 | 82 | 82 | 93 |
| 0.15 | *** | 5483 | 5627 | 6328 | 1040 | 1070 | 1117 | 313 | 318 | 323 | 160 | 161 | 163 | 102 | 102 | 103 |
|      | *** | 5536 | 5817 | 8304 | 1053 | 1091 | 1422 | 315 | 320 | 390 | 161 | 163 | 186 | 102 | 102 | 110 |
| 0.2 | *** | 6901 | 7129 | 8409 | 1301 | 1353 | 1440 | 383 | 391 | 400 | 191 | 193 | 196 | 118 | 118 | 120 |
|     | *** | 6982 | 7445 | 10251 | 1325 | 1390 | 1719 | 387 | 395 | 458 | 192 | 194 | 213 | 118 | 120 | 124 |
| 0.25 | *** | 7956 | 8284 | 10252 | 1512 | 1588 | 1724 | 441 | 452 | 465 | 216 | 220 | 222 | 132 | 133 | 134 |
|      | *** | 8072 | 8744 | 11890 | 1545 | 1645 | 1967 | 448 | 458 | 514 | 217 | 220 | 235 | 132 | 133 | 135 |
| 0.3 | *** | 8658 | 9101 | 11815 | 1669 | 1773 | 1960 | 486 | 501 | 519 | 235 | 239 | 243 | 141 | 142 | 144 |
|     | *** | 8816 | 9717 | 13219 | 1714 | 1850 | 2164 | 494 | 509 | 557 | 237 | 241 | 252 | 142 | 144 | 143 |
| 0.35 | *** | 9036 | 9608 | 13073 | 1780 | 1907 | 2147 | 520 | 538 | 559 | 249 | 254 | 258 | 148 | 149 | 151 |
|      | *** | 9242 | 10383 | 14239 | 1835 | 2004 | 2313 | 528 | 547 | 588 | 251 | 256 | 263 | 148 | 151 | 147 |
| 0.4 | *** | 9131 | 9842 | 14009 | 1845 | 1996 | 2281 | 540 | 562 | 586 | 258 | 262 | 268 | 151 | 153 | 154 |
|     | *** | 9390 | 10775 | 14950 | 1911 | 2110 | 2412 | 551 | 573 | 606 | 260 | 265 | 268 | 152 | 154 | 149 |
| 0.45 | *** | 8993 | 9844 | 14614 | 1871 | 2040 | 2362 | 550 | 572 | 600 | 258 | 265 | 270 | 151 | 153 | 155 |
|      | *** | 9310 | 10921 | 15352 | 1945 | 2168 | 2461 | 560 | 585 | 613 | 262 | 268 | 268 | 152 | 154 | 147 |
| 0.5 | *** | 8670 | 9654 | 14885 | 1861 | 2042 | 2389 | 547 | 571 | 600 | 256 | 262 | 268 | 147 | 149 | 152 |
|     | *** | 9043 | 10851 | 15445 | 1940 | 2180 | 2461 | 558 | 584 | 606 | 258 | 265 | 263 | 148 | 151 | 143 |
| 0.55 | *** | 8210 | 9306 | 14821 | 1816 | 2004 | 2363 | 533 | 557 | 588 | 247 | 253 | 260 | 141 | 144 | 144 |
|      | *** | 8632 | 10591 | 15228 | 1899 | 2148 | 2412 | 545 | 571 | 588 | 250 | 256 | 252 | 142 | 144 | 135 |
| 0.6 | *** | 7651 | 8827 | 14418 | 1740 | 1930 | 2282 | 509 | 532 | 560 | 234 | 239 | 244 | 132 | 133 | 135 |
|     | *** | 8110 | 10160 | 14703 | 1824 | 2072 | 2313 | 520 | 545 | 557 | 236 | 242 | 235 | 133 | 134 | 124 |
| 0.65 | *** | 7022 | 8238 | 13682 | 1636 | 1816 | 2149 | 474 | 495 | 520 | 213 | 218 | 224 | 118 | 120 | 122 |
|      | *** | 7502 | 9571 | 13868 | 1716 | 1952 | 2164 | 483 | 507 | 514 | 216 | 220 | 213 | 120 | 121 | 110 |
| 0.7 | *** | 6343 | 7546 | 12612 | 1501 | 1667 | 1961 | 427 | 445 | 467 | 190 | 193 | 197 | 103 | 104 | 106 |
|     | *** | 6823 | 8831 | 12724 | 1574 | 1788 | 1967 | 436 | 456 | 458 | 191 | 194 | 186 | 103 | 104 | 93 |
| 0.75 | *** | 5616 | 6754 | 11213 | 1336 | 1478 | 1721 | 369 | 383 | 401 | 159 | 161 | 165 | 84 | 84 | 85 |
|      | *** | 6075 | 7936 | 11271 | 1400 | 1580 | 1719 | 376 | 391 | 390 | 160 | 163 | 153 | 84 | 85 | 73 |
| 0.8 | *** | 4835 | 5849 | 9487 | 1135 | 1249 | 1431 | 300 | 310 | 322 | 123 | 125 | 127 | . | . | . |
|     | *** | 5247 | 6870 | 9509 | 1187 | 1327 | 1422 | 305 | 315 | 310 | 125 | 125 | 115 | . | . | . |
| 0.85 | *** | 3971 | 4801 | 7436 | 895 | 972 | 1087 | 217 | 223 | 229 | . | . | . | . | . | . |
|      | *** | 4313 | 5597 | 7438 | 931 | 1023 | 1076 | 220 | 225 | 217 | . | . | . | . | . | . |
| 0.9 | *** | 2966 | 3541 | 5067 | 602 | 641 | 692 | . | . | . | . | . | . | . | . | . |
|     | *** | 3207 | 4054 | 5058 | 621 | 665 | 681 | . | . | . | . | . | . | . | . | . |
| 0.95 | *** | 1671 | 1913 | 2381 | . | . | . | . | . | . | . | . | . | . | . | . |
|      | *** | 1778 | 2098 | 2368 | . | . | . | . | . | . | . | . | . | . | . | . |

## TABLE 7: ALPHA= 0.05  POWER= 0.8    EXPECTED ACCRUAL THRU MINIMUM FOLLOW-UP= 2000

| | | DEL=.02 | | | DEL=.05 | | | DEL=.10 | | | DEL=.15 | | | DEL=.20 | | |
|---|---|---|---|---|---|---|---|---|---|---|---|---|---|---|---|---|---|
| FACT= | | 1.0 .75 | .50 .25 | .00 BIN | 1.0 .75 | .50 .25 | .00 BIN | 1.0 .75 | .50 .25 | .00 BIN | 1.0 75 | .50 .25 | .00 BIN | 1.0 .75 | .50 .25 | .00 BIN |
| PCONT=*** | | | | | REQUIRED | NUMBER | OF PATIENTS | | | | | | | | | |
| 0.05 | *** | 1791 | 1814 | 1862 | 389 | 392 | 395 | 140 | 140 | 141 | 82 | 82 | 82 | 57 | 57 | 57 |
| | *** | 1800 | 1832 | 3481 | 390 | 394 | 681 | 140 | 140 | 217 | 82 | 82 | 115 | 57 | 57 | 73 |
| 0.1 | *** | 3742 | 3819 | 4092 | 731 | 745 | 762 | 231 | 234 | 235 | 124 | 125 | 125 | 81 | 82 | 82 |
| | *** | 3771 | 3906 | 6047 | 737 | 752 | 1076 | 232 | 235 | 310 | 124 | 125 | 153 | 81 | 82 | 93 |
| 0.15 | *** | 5492 | 5641 | 6329 | 1042 | 1072 | 1117 | 314 | 317 | 322 | 160 | 161 | 162 | 101 | 102 | 102 |
| | *** | 5546 | 5832 | 8304 | 1056 | 1092 | 1422 | 316 | 320 | 390 | 161 | 162 | 186 | 102 | 102 | 110 |
| 0.2 | *** | 6914 | 7151 | 8409 | 1306 | 1357 | 1441 | 385 | 391 | 400 | 191 | 194 | 195 | 119 | 119 | 120 |
| | *** | 6999 | 7471 | 10251 | 1329 | 1394 | 1719 | 389 | 396 | 458 | 192 | 194 | 213 | 119 | 120 | 124 |
| 0.25 | *** | 7975 | 8315 | 10252 | 1517 | 1594 | 1724 | 444 | 454 | 466 | 216 | 219 | 222 | 131 | 132 | 134 |
| | *** | 8096 | 8781 | 11890 | 1551 | 1649 | 1967 | 447 | 459 | 514 | 217 | 221 | 235 | 132 | 134 | 135 |
| 0.3 | *** | 8684 | 9142 | 11816 | 1677 | 1779 | 1960 | 489 | 502 | 519 | 236 | 240 | 244 | 141 | 142 | 144 |
| | *** | 8847 | 9766 | 13219 | 1722 | 1855 | 2164 | 495 | 510 | 557 | 237 | 241 | 252 | 142 | 144 | 143 |
| 0.35 | *** | 9069 | 9660 | 13074 | 1790 | 1916 | 2146 | 521 | 539 | 560 | 250 | 254 | 259 | 147 | 150 | 151 |
| | *** | 9284 | 10445 | 14239 | 1845 | 2010 | 2313 | 530 | 549 | 588 | 251 | 256 | 263 | 149 | 150 | 147 |
| 0.4 | *** | 9174 | 9905 | 14009 | 1857 | 2005 | 2281 | 542 | 562 | 586 | 257 | 262 | 267 | 151 | 152 | 155 |
| | *** | 9442 | 10847 | 14950 | 1922 | 2117 | 2412 | 552 | 574 | 606 | 260 | 265 | 268 | 152 | 154 | 149 |
| 0.45 | *** | 9045 | 9919 | 14615 | 1885 | 2051 | 2362 | 551 | 574 | 600 | 260 | 265 | 271 | 151 | 152 | 155 |
| | *** | 9372 | 11004 | 15352 | 1957 | 2176 | 2461 | 562 | 586 | 613 | 262 | 269 | 268 | 152 | 154 | 147 |
| 0.5 | *** | 8732 | 9739 | 14886 | 1875 | 2054 | 2390 | 549 | 572 | 601 | 256 | 262 | 269 | 147 | 150 | 152 |
| | *** | 9115 | 10942 | 15445 | 1954 | 2189 | 2461 | 560 | 585 | 606 | 260 | 265 | 263 | 149 | 151 | 143 |
| 0.55 | *** | 8281 | 9397 | 14821 | 1831 | 2017 | 2364 | 536 | 559 | 587 | 249 | 254 | 260 | 141 | 144 | 145 |
| | *** | 8712 | 10689 | 15228 | 1914 | 2156 | 2412 | 546 | 572 | 588 | 251 | 256 | 252 | 142 | 144 | 135 |
| 0.6 | *** | 7730 | 8922 | 14419 | 1756 | 1941 | 2282 | 511 | 534 | 561 | 234 | 239 | 245 | 131 | 134 | 135 |
| | *** | 8196 | 10260 | 14703 | 1837 | 2080 | 2313 | 521 | 546 | 557 | 236 | 242 | 235 | 132 | 135 | 124 |
| 0.65 | *** | 7106 | 8334 | 13682 | 1651 | 1829 | 2149 | 475 | 496 | 521 | 215 | 219 | 224 | 119 | 120 | 122 |
| | *** | 7592 | 9670 | 13868 | 1730 | 1960 | 2164 | 485 | 507 | 514 | 217 | 221 | 213 | 120 | 121 | 110 |
| 0.7 | *** | 6426 | 7641 | 12612 | 1515 | 1677 | 1962 | 429 | 446 | 467 | 190 | 194 | 197 | 104 | 104 | 105 |
| | *** | 6912 | 8925 | 12724 | 1587 | 1796 | 1967 | 437 | 456 | 458 | 191 | 195 | 186 | 104 | 105 | 93 |
| 0.75 | *** | 5697 | 6842 | 11214 | 1347 | 1487 | 1722 | 371 | 385 | 401 | 160 | 162 | 165 | 84 | 85 | 85 |
| | *** | 6160 | 8021 | 11271 | 1410 | 1587 | 1719 | 377 | 392 | 390 | 161 | 164 | 153 | 84 | 85 | 73 |
| 0.8 | *** | 4907 | 5926 | 9486 | 1145 | 1256 | 1431 | 301 | 310 | 321 | 124 | 125 | 127 | . | . | . |
| | *** | 5324 | 6941 | 9509 | 1195 | 1331 | 1422 | 306 | 316 | 310 | 124 | 126 | 115 | . | . | . |
| 0.85 | *** | 4031 | 4862 | 7436 | 902 | 977 | 1087 | 219 | 224 | 229 | . | . | . | . | . | . |
| | *** | 4375 | 5652 | 7438 | 936 | 1026 | 1076 | 221 | 226 | 217 | . | . | . | . | . | . |
| 0.9 | *** | 3010 | 3581 | 5066 | 606 | 644 | 692 | . | . | . | . | . | . | . | . | . |
| | *** | 3251 | 4087 | 5058 | 624 | 666 | 681 | . | . | . | . | . | . | . | . | . |
| 0.95 | *** | 1690 | 1929 | 2380 | . | . | . | . | . | . | . | . | . | . | . | . |
| | *** | 1795 | 2110 | 2368 | . | . | . | . | . | . | . | . | . | . | . | . |

TABLE 7: ALPHA= 0.05  POWER= 0.8    EXPECTED ACCRUAL THRU MINIMUM FOLLOW-UP= 2250

| | | DEL=.02 | | | DEL=.05 | | | DEL=.10 | | | DEL=.15 | | | DEL=.20 | |
|---|---|---|---|---|---|---|---|---|---|---|---|---|---|---|---|---|
| FACT= | 1.0 .75 | .50 .25 | .00 BIN | 1.0 .75 | .50 .25 | .00 BIN | 1.0 .75 | .50 .25 | .00 BIN | 1.0 75 | .50 .25 | .00 BIN | 1.0 .75 | .50 .25 | .00 BIN |
| PCONT=*** | | | | REQUIRED NUMBER OF PATIENTS | | | | | | | | | | | |
| 0.05 *** | 1796 | 1816 | 1863 | 389 | 392 | 395 | 140 | 140 | 140 | 81 | 81 | 83 | 57 | 57 | 57 |
| *** | 1804 | 1835 | 3481 | 390 | 393 | 681 | 140 | 140 | 217 | 81 | 81 | 115 | 57 | 57 | 73 |
| 0.1 *** | 3753 | 3833 | 4092 | 734 | 747 | 762 | 232 | 233 | 236 | 123 | 125 | 125 | 81 | 81 | 83 |
| *** | 3784 | 3920 | 6047 | 739 | 753 | 1076 | 233 | 235 | 310 | 123 | 125 | 153 | 81 | 81 | 93 |
| 0.15 *** | 5512 | 5672 | 6328 | 1047 | 1076 | 1116 | 314 | 319 | 323 | 160 | 162 | 163 | 101 | 102 | 102 |
| *** | 5571 | 5865 | 8304 | 1062 | 1094 | 1422 | 316 | 320 | 390 | 162 | 162 | 186 | 102 | 102 | 110 |
| 0.2 *** | 6946 | 7201 | 8409 | 1316 | 1364 | 1441 | 387 | 392 | 399 | 191 | 194 | 195 | 118 | 119 | 119 |
| *** | 7039 | 7527 | 10251 | 1337 | 1397 | 1719 | 389 | 396 | 458 | 192 | 194 | 213 | 119 | 119 | 124 |
| 0.25 *** | 8021 | 8388 | 10253 | 1531 | 1604 | 1724 | 446 | 454 | 465 | 218 | 219 | 222 | 132 | 133 | 133 |
| *** | 8155 | 8864 | 11890 | 1563 | 1655 | 1967 | 449 | 460 | 514 | 218 | 221 | 235 | 132 | 133 | 135 |
| 0.3 *** | 8746 | 9239 | 11817 | 1697 | 1794 | 1960 | 492 | 505 | 519 | 236 | 240 | 243 | 142 | 143 | 145 |
| *** | 8926 | 9879 | 13219 | 1739 | 1864 | 2164 | 497 | 511 | 557· | 239 | 241 | 252 | 142 | 143 | 143 |
| 0.35 *** | 9151 | 9783 | 13074 | 1812 | 1934 | 2147 | 525 | 541 | 559 | 250 | 254 | 258 | 149 | 150 | 151 |
| *** | 9384 | 10586 | 14239 | 1867 | 2023 | 2313 | 533 | 550 | 588 | 253 | 257 | 263 | 149 | 150 | 147 |
| 0.4 *** | 9278 | 10054 | 14009 | 1884 | 2027 | 2280 | 547 | 565 | 586 | 258 | 263 | 268 | 151 | 153 | 154 |
| *** | 9568 | 11016 | 14950 | 1947 | 2131 | 2412 | 555 | 575 | 606 | 261 | 266 | 268 | 151 | 154 | 149 |
| 0.45 *** | 9173 | 10094 | 14615 | 1915 | 2075 | 2362 | 556 | 576 | 600 | 261 | 266 | 271 | 151 | 153 | 154 |
| *** | 9522 | 11196 | 15352 | 1985 | 2193 | 2461 | 565 | 587 | 613 | 263 | 268 | 268 | 151 | 154 | 147 |
| 0.5 *** | 8883 | 9933 | 14886 | 1908 | 2080 | 2389 | 554 | 575 | 600 | 257 | 263 | 268 | 149 | 150 | 151 |
| *** | 9286 | 11153 | 15445 | 1984 | 2207 | 2461 | 564 | 587 | 606 | 260 | 266 | 263 | 149 | 150 | 143 |
| 0.55 *** | 8451 | 9610 | 14820 | 1866 | 2044 | 2364 | 539 | 561 | 587 | 249 | 254 | 260 | 142 | 143 | 145 |
| *** | 8903 | 10911 | 15228 | 1945 | 2175 | 2412 | 550 | 573 | 588 | 252 | 257 | 252 | 143 | 145 | 135 |
| 0.6 *** | 7916 | 9145 | 14419 | 1790 | 1968 | 2282 | 516 | 536 | 561 | 235 | 240 | 244 | 132 | 133 | 134 |
| *** | 8400 | 10487 | 14703 | 1870 | 2098 | 2313 | 525 | 548 | 557 | 237 | 241 | 235 | 133 | 134 | 124 |
| 0.65 *** | 7300 | 8558 | 13682 | 1683 | 1855 | 2148 | 479 | 497 | 520 | 215 | 219 | 223 | 119 | 120 | 122 |
| *** | 7801 | 9896 | 13868 | 1760 | 1977 | 2164 | 489 | 509 | 514 | 218 | 222 | 213 | 119 | 120 | 110 |
| 0.7 *** | 6622 | 7858 | 12612 | 1545 | 1701 | 1962 | 433 | 448 | 466 | 191 | 194 | 196 | 104 | 104 | 105 |
| *** | 7120 | 9139 | 12724 | 1616 | 1811 | 1967 | 440 | 457 | 458 | 192 | 195 | 186 | 104 | 105 | 93 |
| 0.75 *** | 5883 | 7044 | 11213 | 1374 | 1507 | 1722 | 374 | 387 | 401 | 160 | 163 | 164 | 84 | 84 | 86 |
| *** | 6355 | 8214 | 11271 | 1434 | 1600 | 1719 | 379 | 393 | 390 | 162 | 164 | 153 | 84 | 86 | 73 |
| 0.8 *** | 5075 | 6103 | 9486 | 1167 | 1271 | 1430 | 303 | 312 | 322 | 123 | 125 | 126 | . | . | . |
| *** | 5497 | 7104 | 9509 | 1214 | 1341 | 1422 | 308 | 316 | 310 | 125 | 126 | 115 | . | . | . |
| 0.85 *** | 4170 | 5002 | 7436 | 916 | 987 | 1087 | 219 | 223 | 229 | . | . | . | . | . | . |
| *** | 4516 | 5775 | 7438 | 949 | 1032 | 1076 | 222 | 226 | 217 | . | . | . | . | . | . |
| 0.9 *** | 3109 | 3674 | 5067 | 613 | 648 | 693 | . | . | . | . | . | . | . | . | . |
| *** | 3348 | 4162 | 5058 | 629 | 669 | 681 | . | . | . | . | . | . | . | . | . |
| 0.95 *** | 1734 | 1964 | 2381 | . | . | . | . | . | . | . | . | . | . | . | . |
| *** | 1836 | 2134 | 2368 | . | . | . | . | . | . | . | . | . | . | . | . |

TABLE 7: ALPHA= 0.05  POWER= 0.8     EXPECTED ACCRUAL THRU MINIMUM FOLLOW-UP= 2500

| | | DEL=.02 | | | DEL=.05 | | | DEL=.10 | | | DEL=.15 | | | DEL=.20 | | |
|---|---|---|---|---|---|---|---|---|---|---|---|---|---|---|---|---|
| FACT= | | 1.0 .75 | .50 .25 | .00 BIN | 1.0 .75 | .50 .25 | .00 BIN | 1.0 .75 | .50 .25 | .00 BIN | 1.0 75 | .50 .25 | .00 BIN | 1.0 .75 | .50 .25 | .00 BIN |
| PCONT=*** | | | | | REQUIRED | NUMBER OF | PATIENTS | | | | | | | | | |
| 0.05 | *** | 1798 | 1820 | 1862 | 390 | 392 | 395 | 140 | 140 | 140 | 83 | 83 | 83 | 58 | 58 | 58 |
| | *** | 1808 | 1837 | 3481 | 392 | 393 | 681 | 140 | 140 | 217 | 83 | 83 | 115 | 58 | 58 | 73 |
| 0.1 | *** | 3764 | 3846 | 4092 | 736 | 748 | 762 | 233 | 234 | 236 | 124 | 124 | 124 | 81 | 83 | 83 |
| | *** | 3796 | 3933 | 6047 | 742 | 754 | 1076 | 233 | 234 | 310 | 124 | 124 | 153 | 83 | 83 | 93 |
| 0.15 | *** | 5533 | 5699 | 6327 | 1052 | 1079 | 1117 | 315 | 318 | 323 | 161 | 162 | 162 | 101 | 102 | 102 |
| | *** | 5596 | 5893 | 8304 | 1065 | 1096 | 1422 | 317 | 320 | 390 | 161 | 162 | 186 | 101 | 102 | 110 |
| 0.2 | *** | 6977 | 7248 | 8409 | 1323 | 1370 | 1440 | 387 | 393 | 399 | 192 | 193 | 195 | 118 | 118 | 120 |
| | *** | 7077 | 7577 | 10251 | 1345 | 1401 | 1719 | 390 | 396 | 458 | 193 | 195 | 213 | 118 | 120 | 124 |
| 0.25 | *** | 8067 | 8456 | 10252 | 1543 | 1614 | 1724 | 446 | 456 | 465 | 217 | 220 | 221 | 133 | 133 | 134 |
| | *** | 8211 | 8940 | 11890 | 1574 | 1662 | 1967 | 451 | 461 | 514 | 218 | 221 | 235 | 133 | 133 | 135 |
| 0.3 | *** | 8808 | 9331 | 11815 | 1712 | 1806 | 1961 | 493 | 506 | 518 | 237 | 240 | 243 | 142 | 143 | 143 |
| | *** | 9001 | 9979 | 13219 | 1754 | 1873 | 2164 | 499 | 512 | 557 | 239 | 242 | 252 | 142 | 143 | 143 |
| 0.35 | *** | 9231 | 9898 | 13073 | 1833 | 1949 | 2146 | 527 | 542 | 559 | 251 | 254 | 259 | 148 | 149 | 151 |
| | *** | 9481 | 10712 | 14239 | 1886 | 2034 | 2313 | 536 | 549 | 588 | 252 | 256 | 263 | 149 | 151 | 147 |
| 0.4 | *** | 9377 | 10193 | 14009 | 1909 | 2046 | 2281 | 549 | 567 | 587 | 259 | 264 | 268 | 151 | 152 | 154 |
| | *** | 9687 | 11167 | 14950 | 1970 | 2145 | 2412 | 558 | 576 | 606 | 261 | 265 | 268 | 152 | 154 | 149 |
| 0.45 | *** | 9293 | 10254 | 14615 | 1942 | 2096 | 2362 | 559 | 577 | 599 | 262 | 267 | 271 | 151 | 152 | 154 |
| | *** | 9662 | 11367 | 15352 | 2011 | 2208 | 2461 | 568 | 589 | 613 | 264 | 268 | 268 | 152 | 154 | 147 |
| 0.5 | *** | 9024 | 10114 | 14886 | 1936 | 2102 | 2390 | 558 | 577 | 601 | 259 | 264 | 268 | 148 | 149 | 151 |
| | *** | 9446 | 11340 | 15445 | 2011 | 2223 | 2461 | 567 | 589 | 606 | 261 | 265 | 263 | 149 | 151 | 143 |
| 0.55 | *** | 8611 | 9802 | 14820 | 1895 | 2067 | 2364 | 543 | 564 | 587 | 249 | 254 | 259 | 142 | 143 | 145 |
| | *** | 9079 | 11109 | 15228 | 1971 | 2190 | 2412 | 552 | 574 | 588 | 252 | 258 | 252 | 143 | 145 | 135 |
| 0.6 | *** | 8087 | 9346 | 14418 | 1820 | 1992 | 2283 | 520 | 539 | 561 | 236 | 240 | 245 | 133 | 134 | 136 |
| | *** | 8589 | 10690 | 14703 | 1896 | 2114 | 2313 | 527 | 548 | 557 | 239 | 242 | 235 | 133 | 134 | 124 |
| 0.65 | *** | 7479 | 8761 | 13683 | 1712 | 1876 | 2149 | 483 | 499 | 520 | 217 | 220 | 224 | 120 | 120 | 121 |
| | *** | 7993 | 10095 | 13868 | 1786 | 1992 | 2164 | 492 | 511 | 514 | 218 | 221 | 213 | 120 | 121 | 110 |
| 0.7 | *** | 6801 | 8054 | 12612 | 1571 | 1721 | 1962 | 436 | 449 | 467 | 192 | 193 | 196 | 102 | 104 | 106 |
| | *** | 7308 | 9327 | 12724 | 1639 | 1824 | 1967 | 442 | 458 | 458 | 192 | 195 | 186 | 104 | 104 | 93 |
| 0.75 | *** | 6054 | 7224 | 11214 | 1396 | 1524 | 1721 | 376 | 387 | 401 | 161 | 162 | 165 | 84 | 84 | 86 |
| | *** | 6533 | 8383 | 11271 | 1454 | 1611 | 1719 | 381 | 393 | 390 | 162 | 164 | 153 | 84 | 86 | 73 |
| 0.8 | *** | 5227 | 6259 | 9487 | 1184 | 1284 | 1431 | 304 | 312 | 321 | 124 | 124 | 126 | . | . | . |
| | *** | 5654 | 7245 | 9509 | 1231 | 1349 | 1422 | 309 | 317 | 310 | 124 | 126 | 115 | . | . | . |
| 0.85 | *** | 4296 | 5126 | 7436 | 929 | 995 | 1087 | 220 | 224 | 229 | . | . | . | . | . | . |
| | *** | 4643 | 5881 | 7438 | 961 | 1037 | 1076 | 221 | 226 | 217 | . | . | . | . | . | . |
| 0.9 | *** | 3196 | 3754 | 5067 | 620 | 652 | 692 | . | . | . | . | . | . | . | . | . |
| | *** | 3434 | 4226 | 5058 | 636 | 671 | 681 | . | . | . | . | . | . | . | . | . |
| 0.95 | *** | 1773 | 1993 | 2381 | . | . | . | . | . | . | . | . | . | . | . | . |
| | *** | 1871 | 2154 | 2368 | . | . | . | . | . | . | . | . | . | . | . | . |

TABLE 7: ALPHA= 0.05 POWER= 0.8    EXPECTED ACCRUAL THRU MINIMUM FOLLOW-UP= 2750

| | | DEL=.02 | | | DEL=.05 | | | DEL=.10 | | | DEL=.15 | | | DEL=.20 | |
|---|---|---|---|---|---|---|---|---|---|---|---|---|---|---|---|---|
| FACT= | 1.0 .75 | .50 .25 | .00 BIN | 1.0 .75 | .50 .25 | .00 BIN | 1.0 .75 | .50 .25 | .00 BIN | 1.0 75 | .50 .25 | .00 BIN | 1.0 .75 | .50 .25 | .00 BIN |
| PCONT=*** | | | | | | REQUIRED NUMBER OF PATIENTS | | | | | | | | | |
| 0.05 *** | 1800 1811 | 1823 1838 | 1862 3481 | 390 391 | 393 393 | 395 681 | 140 140 | 140 140 | 140 217 | 82 82 | 82 82 | 82 115 | 58 58 | 58 58 | 58 73 |
| 0.1 *** | 3774 3808 | 3860 3942 | 4092 6047 | 738 744 | 749 754 | 762 1076 | 233 233 | 233 235 | 235 310 | 123 125 | 125 125 | 125 153 | 82 82 | 82 82 | 82 93 |
| 0.15 *** | 5553 5620 | 5726 5919 | 6328 8304 | 1057 1068 | 1082 1098 | 1116 1422 | 315 318 | 319 321 | 322 390 | 161 161 | 161 163 | 163 186 | 101 102 | 102 102 | 102 110 |
| 0.2 *** | 7008 7115 | 7292 7622 | 8409 10251 | 1332 1352 | 1376 1405 | 1442 1719 | 388 391 | 393 397 | 400 458 | 192 194 | 194 194 | 195 213 | 118 118 | 120 120 | 120 124 |
| 0.25 *** | 8110 8263 | 8519 9008 | 10252 11890 | 1555 1584 | 1622 1666 | 1724 1967 | 448 452 | 456 460 | 465 514 | 218 219 | 219 221 | 223 235 | 132 132 | 133 133 | 133 135 |
| 0.3 *** | 8868 9073 | 9415 10070 | 11816 13219 | 1727 1768 | 1818 1880 | 1961 2164 | 496 501 | 507 511 | 518 557 | 239 239 | 240 242 | 243 252 | 142 142 | 142 144 | 144 143 |
| 0.35 *** | 9308 9573 | 10004 10826 | 13072 14239 | 1851 1902 | 1964 2041 | 2146 2313 | 531 538 | 544 551 | 560 588 | 252 254 | 256 257 | 259 263 | 149 149 | 149 150 | 150 147 |
| 0.4 *** | 9475 9798 | 10322 11300 | 14009 14950 | 1930 1988 | 2062 2155 | 2280 2412 | 553 560 | 569 577 | 587 606 | 260 263 | 264 266 | 267 268 | 153 153 | 153 154 | 154 149 |
| 0.45 *** | 9410 9795 | 10401 11520 | 14614 15352 | 1965 2031 | 2113 2219 | 2363 2461 | 563 570 | 580 589 | 601 613 | 263 264 | 266 269 | 271 268 | 153 153 | 154 154 | 154 147 |
| 0.5 *** | 9159 9597 | 10277 11508 | 14886 15445 | 1961 2033 | 2122 2236 | 2390 2461 | 562 570 | 579 589 | 601 606 | 259 260 | 264 266 | 267 263 | 149 149 | 150 150 | 153 143 |
| 0.55 *** | 8761 9245 | 9980 11285 | 14820 15228 | 1921 1995 | 2088 2205 | 2363 2412 | 548 556 | 565 575 | 587 588 | 250 252 | 256 257 | 259 252 | 142 142 | 144 144 | 146 135 |
| 0.6 *** | 8249 8761 | 9530 10871 | 14418 14703 | 1845 1921 | 2012 2127 | 2282 2313 | 522 531 | 539 549 | 560 557 | 236 239 | 240 242 | 245 235 | 132 133 | 133 133 | 135 124 |
| 0.65 *** | 7646 8170 | 8946 10273 | 13683 13868 | 1737 1807 | 1895 2003 | 2150 2164 | 486 493 | 501 510 | 520 514 | 216 218 | 219 221 | 225 213 | 120 120 | 120 122 | 122 110 |
| 0.7 *** | 6966 7481 | 8231 9494 | 12614 12724 | 1594 1660 | 1737 1835 | 1962 1967 | 438 445 | 452 459 | 467 458 | 192 194 | 194 195 | 197 186 | 102 104 | 104 104 | 104 93 |
| 0.75 *** | 6209 6694 | 7389 8533 | 11212 11271 | 1418 1473 | 1538 1618 | 1721 1719 | 377 383 | 388 395 | 400 390 | 161 161 | 163 164 | 164 153 | 84 84 | 85 85 | 85 73 |
| 0.8 *** | 5369 5797 | 6400 7371 | 9487 9509 | 1201 1244 | 1295 1356 | 1431 1422 | 305 309 | 312 318 | 321 310 | 125 125 | 125 126 | 126 115 | . . | . . | . . |
| 0.85 *** | 4412 4757 | 5237 5974 | 7437 7438 | 940 969 | 1003 1041 | 1088 1076 | 221 223 | 225 226 | 228 217 | . . | . . | . . | . . | . . | . . |
| 0.9 *** | 3275 3512 | 3825 4282 | 5066 5058 | 625 639 | 656 673 | 692 681 | . . | . . | . . | . . | . . | . . | . . | . . | . . |
| 0.95 *** | 1806 1902 | 2019 2172 | 2380 2368 | . . | . . | . . | . . | . . | . . | . . | . . | . . | . . | . . | . . |

TABLE 7: ALPHA= 0.05  POWER= 0.8    EXPECTED ACCRUAL THRU MINIMUM FOLLOW-UP= 3000

| | | DEL=.01 | | | DEL=.02 | | | DEL=.05 | | | DEL=.10 | | | DEL=.15 | | |
|---|---|---|---|---|---|---|---|---|---|---|---|---|---|---|---|---|---|
| FACT= | | 1.0 .75 | .50 .25 | .00 BIN | 1.0 .75 | .50 .25 | .00 BIN | 1.0 .75 | .50 .25 | .00 BIN | 1.0 75 | .50 .25 | .00 BIN | 1.0 .75 | .50 .25 | .00 BIN |
| PCONT=*** | | | | | | | REQUIRED | NUMBER OF | PATIENTS | | | | | | |
| 0.01 | *** | 947 | 950 | 955 | 347 | 347 | 350 | 115 | 115 | 115 | 58 | 58 | 58 | 40 | 40 | 40 |
| | *** | 947 | 950 | 3648 | 347 | 350 | 1206 | 115 | 115 | 328 | 58 | 58 | 134 | 40 | 40 | 80 |
| 0.02 | *** | 2095 | 2105 | 2128 | 673 | 677 | 680 | 182 | 182 | 182 | 80 | 80 | 80 | 50 | 50 | 50 |
| | *** | 2098 | 2113 | 6022 | 673 | 677 | 1793 | 182 | 182 | 419 | 80 | 80 | 155 | 50 | 50 | 89 |
| 0.05 | *** | 6340 | 6392 | 6647 | 1805 | 1825 | 1862 | 392 | 392 | 395 | 140 | 140 | 140 | 80 | 80 | 80 |
| | *** | 6358 | 6463 | 12848 | 1813 | 1840 | 3481 | 392 | 392 | 681 | 140 | 140 | 217 | 80 | 80 | 115 |
| 0.1 | *** | 13990 | 14128 | 15470 | 3782 | 3868 | 4093 | 740 | 748 | 763 | 230 | 235 | 235 | 122 | 125 | 125 |
| | *** | 14035 | 14368 | 23235 | 3820 | 3950 | 6047 | 745 | 755 | 1076 | 235 | 235 | 310 | 125 | 125 | 153 |
| 0.15 | *** | 20905 | 21152 | 24437 | 5570 | 5750 | 6328 | 1060 | 1085 | 1115 | 317 | 320 | 320 | 160 | 163 | 163 |
| | *** | 20987 | 21617 | 32385 | 5642 | 5942 | 8304 | 1070 | 1100 | 1422 | 317 | 320 | 390 | 160 | 163 | 186 |
| 0.2 | *** | 26495 | 26882 | 32833 | 7037 | 7333 | 8410 | 1337 | 1378 | 1442 | 388 | 392 | 400 | 193 | 193 | 193 |
| | *** | 26623 | 27617 | 40298 | 7150 | 7663 | 10251 | 1355 | 1408 | 1719 | 392 | 395 | 458 | 193 | 193 | 213 |
| 0.25 | *** | 30595 | 31153 | 40310 | 8155 | 8578 | 10250 | 1562 | 1630 | 1723 | 448 | 455 | 467 | 220 | 220 | 223 |
| | *** | 30782 | 32215 | 46976 | 8315 | 9065 | 11890 | 1592 | 1670 | 1967 | 452 | 460 | 514 | 220 | 220 | 235 |
| 0.3 | *** | 33215 | 33985 | 46678 | 8927 | 9493 | 11815 | 1738 | 1825 | 1960 | 497 | 508 | 520 | 238 | 242 | 242 |
| | *** | 33475 | 35435 | 52416 | 9140 | 10150 | 13219 | 1780 | 1885 | 2164 | 500 | 512 | 557 | 238 | 242 | 252 |
| 0.35 | *** | 34465 | 35488 | 51830 | 9385 | 10105 | 13075 | 1865 | 1975 | 2147 | 530 | 545 | 560 | 253 | 253 | 257 |
| | *** | 34805 | 37385 | 56620 | 9658 | 10930 | 14239 | 1915 | 2050 | 2313 | 538 | 553 | 588 | 253 | 257 | 263 |
| 0.4 | *** | 34490 | 35822 | 55700 | 9568 | 10442 | 14008 | 1948 | 2075 | 2282 | 553 | 568 | 587 | 260 | 265 | 268 |
| | *** | 34940 | 38222 | 59588 | 9905 | 11425 | 14950 | 2005 | 2162 | 2412 | 560 | 575 | 606 | 260 | 265 | 268 |
| 0.45 | *** | 33490 | 35188 | 58258 | 9520 | 10540 | 14615 | 1985 | 2128 | 2360 | 565 | 580 | 598 | 265 | 268 | 272 |
| | *** | 34063 | 38120 | 61319 | 9917 | 11657 | 15352 | 2050 | 2230 | 2461 | 572 | 590 | 613 | 265 | 268 | 268 |
| 0.5 | *** | 31660 | 33785 | 59477 | 9287 | 10430 | 14885 | 1982 | 2140 | 2390 | 565 | 580 | 602 | 260 | 265 | 268 |
| | *** | 32390 | 37250 | 61814 | 9737 | 11660 | 15445 | 2053 | 2245 | 2461 | 572 | 590 | 606 | 260 | 265 | 263 |
| 0.55 | *** | 29233 | 31820 | 59350 | 8900 | 10142 | 14822 | 1945 | 2105 | 2365 | 550 | 568 | 587 | 250 | 253 | 268 |
| | *** | 30140 | 35770 | 61072 | 9395 | 11443 | 15228 | 2015 | 2215 | 2412 | 557 | 575 | 588 | 253 | 257 | 252 |
| 0.6 | *** | 26435 | 29477 | 57875 | 8402 | 9700 | 14417 | 1870 | 2027 | 2282 | 523 | 542 | 560 | 238 | 242 | 245 |
| | *** | 27530 | 33805 | 59093 | 8923 | 11030 | 14703 | 1940 | 2140 | 2313 | 535 | 550 | 557 | 238 | 242 | 235 |
| 0.65 | *** | 23477 | 26893 | 55063 | 7802 | 9115 | 13682 | 1760 | 1910 | 2147 | 490 | 505 | 520 | 215 | 220 | 223 |
| | *** | 24740 | 31445 | 55878 | 8335 | 10430 | 13868 | 1828 | 2015 | 2164 | 497 | 512 | 514 | 220 | 223 | 213 |
| 0.7 | *** | 20522 | 24163 | 50920 | 7120 | 8395 | 12613 | 1615 | 1753 | 1963 | 440 | 452 | 467 | 193 | 193 | 197 |
| | *** | 21902 | 28750 | 51427 | 7640 | 9643 | 12724 | 1678 | 1843 | 1967 | 445 | 460 | 458 | 193 | 197 | 186 |
| 0.75 | *** | 17657 | 21317 | 45452 | 6355 | 7535 | 11215 | 1435 | 1550 | 1723 | 380 | 388 | 400 | 160 | 163 | 163 |
| | *** | 19070 | 25727 | 45739 | 6842 | 8665 | 11271 | 1487 | 1625 | 1719 | 385 | 395 | 390 | 163 | 163 | 153 |
| 0.8 | *** | 14882 | 18332 | 38675 | 5495 | 6527 | 9485 | 1213 | 1303 | 1430 | 305 | 313 | 320 | 125 | 125 | 125 |
| | *** | 16232 | 22337 | 38815 | 5927 | 7480 | 9509 | 1255 | 1360 | 1422 | 310 | 317 | 310 | 125 | 125 | 115 |
| 0.85 | *** | 12115 | 15118 | 30602 | 4517 | 5335 | 7435 | 950 | 1007 | 1085 | 220 | 223 | 227 | . | . | . |
| | *** | 13303 | 18470 | 30654 | 4862 | 6055 | 7438 | 977 | 1045 | 1076 | 223 | 227 | 217 | . | . | . |
| 0.9 | *** | 9175 | 11465 | 21250 | 3347 | 3890 | 5065 | 628 | 658 | 692 | . | . | . | . | . | . |
| | *** | 10097 | 13892 | 21256 | 3580 | 4330 | 5058 | 643 | 673 | 681 | . | . | . | . | . | . |
| 0.95 | *** | 5627 | 6865 | 10633 | 1835 | 2042 | 2380 | . | . | . | . | . | . | . | . | . |
| | *** | 6137 | 8035 | 10622 | 1930 | 2185 | 2368 | . | . | . | . | . | . | . | . | . |
| 0.98 | *** | 2570 | 2945 | 3662 | . | . | . | . | . | . | . | . | . | . | . | . |
| | *** | 2735 | 3230 | 3648 | . | . | . | . | . | . | . | . | . | . | . | . |

## TABLE 7: ALPHA= 0.05  POWER= 0.8    EXPECTED ACCRUAL THRU MINIMUM FOLLOW-UP= 3250

| | | DEL=.01 | | | DEL=.02 | | | DEL=.05 | | | DEL=.10 | | | DEL=.15 | | |
|---|---|---|---|---|---|---|---|---|---|---|---|---|---|---|---|---|
| FACT= | | 1.0 .75 | .50 .25 | .00 BIN | 1.0 .75 | .50 .25 | .00 BIN | 1.0 .75 | .50 .25 | .00 BIN | 1.0 75 | .50 .25 | .00 BIN | 1.0 .75 | .50 .25 | .00 BIN |
| PCONT=*** | | | | | REQUIRED NUMBER OF PATIENTS | | | | | | | | | | | |
| 0.01 | *** | 948 | 948 | 953 | 347 | 347 | 347 | 116 | 116 | 116 | 59 | 59 | 59 | 43 | 43 | 43 |
| | *** | 948 | 953 | 3648 | 347 | 347 | 1206 | 116 | 116 | 328 | 59 | 59 | 134 | 43 | 43 | 80 |
| 0.02 | *** | 2094 | 2107 | 2126 | 672 | 677 | 680 | 181 | 181 | 184 | 79 | 79 | 79 | 51 | 51 | 51 |
| | *** | 2099 | 2115 | 6022 | 677 | 677 | 1793 | 181 | 181 | 419 | 79 | 79 | 155 | 51 | 51 | 89 |
| 0.05 | *** | 6343 | 6397 | 6649 | 1806 | 1826 | 1863 | 393 | 393 | 396 | 141 | 141 | 141 | 84 | 84 | 84 |
| | *** | 6364 | 6470 | 12848 | 1814 | 1842 | 3481 | 393 | 393 | 681 | 141 | 141 | 217 | 84 | 84 | 115 |
| 0.1 | *** | 14002 | 14148 | 15473 | 3792 | 3881 | 4092 | 742 | 750 | 761 | 233 | 233 | 233 | 124 | 124 | 124 |
| | *** | 14051 | 14403 | 23235 | 3829 | 3959 | 6047 | 745 | 753 | 1076 | 233 | 233 | 310 | 124 | 124 | 153 |
| 0.15 | *** | 20924 | 21193 | 24437 | 5587 | 5774 | 6327 | 1062 | 1086 | 1116 | 314 | 319 | 322 | 160 | 160 | 160 |
| | *** | 21014 | 21688 | 32385 | 5661 | 5961 | 8304 | 1075 | 1099 | 1422 | 319 | 319 | 390 | 160 | 160 | 186 |
| 0.2 | *** | 26526 | 26945 | 32836 | 7066 | 7372 | 8407 | 1343 | 1384 | 1441 | 387 | 396 | 401 | 192 | 192 | 192 |
| | *** | 26669 | 27728 | 40298 | 7185 | 7700 | 10251 | 1362 | 1408 | 1719 | 393 | 396 | 458 | 192 | 192 | 213 |
| 0.25 | *** | 30642 | 31246 | 40311 | 8196 | 8634 | 10251 | 1571 | 1636 | 1725 | 449 | 458 | 466 | 217 | 222 | 222 |
| | *** | 30845 | 32381 | 46976 | 8363 | 9122 | 11890 | 1598 | 1676 | 1967 | 452 | 461 | 514 | 217 | 222 | 235 |
| 0.3 | *** | 33283 | 34111 | 46676 | 8984 | 9569 | 11816 | 1749 | 1834 | 1961 | 498 | 506 | 517 | 238 | 241 | 241 |
| | *** | 33559 | 35655 | 52416 | 9208 | 10227 | 13219 | 1790 | 1891 | 2164 | 501 | 514 | 557 | 238 | 241 | 252 |
| 0.35 | *** | 34550 | 35655 | 51832 | 9455 | 10199 | 13071 | 1879 | 1985 | 2148 | 534 | 547 | 558 | 254 | 254 | 257 |
| | *** | 34919 | 37670 | 56620 | 9744 | 11023 | 14239 | 1928 | 2058 | 2313 | 539 | 550 | 588 | 254 | 257 | 263 |
| 0.4 | *** | 34602 | 36040 | 55702 | 9658 | 10552 | 14010 | 1964 | 2086 | 2281 | 558 | 571 | 588 | 263 | 263 | 266 |
| | *** | 35086 | 38572 | 59588 | 10007 | 11535 | 14950 | 2021 | 2172 | 2412 | 563 | 579 | 606 | 263 | 266 | 268 |
| 0.45 | *** | 33632 | 35460 | 58259 | 9626 | 10666 | 14614 | 2004 | 2142 | 2362 | 566 | 582 | 599 | 263 | 266 | 271 |
| | *** | 34252 | 38539 | 61319 | 10037 | 11784 | 15352 | 2066 | 2237 | 2461 | 574 | 591 | 613 | 266 | 271 | 268 |
| 0.5 | *** | 31844 | 34114 | 59478 | 9406 | 10573 | 14888 | 2004 | 2151 | 2391 | 566 | 582 | 599 | 263 | 263 | 266 |
| | *** | 32627 | 37730 | 61814 | 9869 | 11795 | 15445 | 2069 | 2256 | 2461 | 574 | 591 | 606 | 263 | 266 | 263 |
| 0.55 | *** | 29464 | 32210 | 59351 | 9038 | 10292 | 14823 | 1964 | 2118 | 2362 | 550 | 566 | 588 | 249 | 254 | 257 |
| | *** | 30434 | 36300 | 61072 | 9541 | 11589 | 15228 | 2034 | 2224 | 2412 | 558 | 579 | 588 | 254 | 257 | 252 |
| 0.6 | *** | 26718 | 29914 | 57877 | 8542 | 9853 | 14419 | 1891 | 2042 | 2281 | 526 | 542 | 558 | 238 | 241 | 246 |
| | *** | 27874 | 34371 | 59093 | 9073 | 11177 | 14703 | 1961 | 2148 | 2313 | 534 | 550 | 557 | 238 | 241 | 235 |
| 0.65 | *** | 23804 | 27368 | 55066 | 7949 | 9268 | 13680 | 1777 | 1923 | 2148 | 490 | 506 | 523 | 217 | 222 | 225 |
| | *** | 25133 | 32026 | 55878 | 8485 | 10573 | 13868 | 1847 | 2021 | 2164 | 498 | 509 | 514 | 217 | 222 | 213 |
| 0.7 | *** | 20887 | 24649 | 50917 | 7261 | 8542 | 12613 | 1631 | 1766 | 1961 | 441 | 452 | 466 | 192 | 192 | 198 |
| | *** | 22317 | 29326 | 51427 | 7786 | 9780 | 12724 | 1693 | 1850 | 1967 | 449 | 461 | 458 | 192 | 198 | 186 |
| 0.75 | *** | 18032 | 21794 | 45449 | 6489 | 7673 | 11215 | 1449 | 1563 | 1720 | 379 | 387 | 401 | 160 | 165 | 165 |
| | *** | 19489 | 26266 | 45739 | 6977 | 8786 | 11271 | 1501 | 1631 | 1719 | 384 | 396 | 390 | 160 | 165 | 153 |
| 0.8 | *** | 15245 | 18771 | 38672 | 5617 | 6644 | 9487 | 1224 | 1311 | 1433 | 306 | 314 | 319 | 124 | 124 | 127 |
| | *** | 16629 | 22821 | 38815 | 6048 | 7578 | 9509 | 1265 | 1368 | 1422 | 311 | 319 | 310 | 124 | 124 | 115 |
| 0.85 | *** | 12437 | 15492 | 30604 | 4612 | 5425 | 7437 | 956 | 1013 | 1086 | 222 | 225 | 230 | . | . | . |
| | *** | 13653 | 18869 | 30654 | 4959 | 6129 | 7438 | 986 | 1046 | 1076 | 222 | 225 | 217 | . | . | . |
| 0.9 | *** | 9428 | 11743 | 21249 | 3415 | 3946 | 5067 | 631 | 661 | 693 | . | . | . | . | . | . |
| | *** | 10362 | 14167 | 21256 | 3646 | 4374 | 5058 | 647 | 677 | 681 | . | . | . | . | . | . |
| 0.95 | *** | 5766 | 7006 | 10633 | 1863 | 2061 | 2378 | . | . | . | . | . | . | . | . | . |
| | *** | 6283 | 8155 | 10622 | 1953 | 2199 | 2368 | . | . | . | . | . | . | . | . | . |
| 0.98 | *** | 2619 | 2984 | 3659 | . | . | . | . | . | . | . | . | . | . | . | . |
| | *** | 2781 | 3256 | 3648 | . | . | . | . | . | . | . | . | . | . | . | . |

TABLE 7: ALPHA= 0.05  POWER= 0.8     EXPECTED ACCRUAL THRU MINIMUM FOLLOW-UP= 3500

| | | DEL=.01 | | | DEL=.02 | | | DEL=.05 | | | DEL=.10 | | | DEL=.15 | | |
|---|---|---|---|---|---|---|---|---|---|---|---|---|---|---|---|---|
| FACT= | | 1.0 .75 | .50 .25 | .00 BIN | 1.0 .75 | .50 .25 | .00 BIN | 1.0 .75 | .50 .25 | .00 BIN | 1.0 75 | .50 .25 | .00 BIN | 1.0 .75 | .50 .25 | .00 BIN |
| PCONT=*** | | | | | REQUIRED NUMBER OF PATIENTS | | | | | | | | | | | |
| 0.01 | *** | 948 | 951 | 951 | 347 | 347 | 347 | 116 | 116 | 116 | 58 | 58 | 58 | 41 | 41 | 41 |
| | *** | 948 | 951 | 3648 | 347 | 347 | 1206 | 116 | 116 | 328 | 58 | 58 | 134 | 41 | 41 | 80 |
| 0.02 | *** | 2097 | 2106 | 2129 | 676 | 676 | 680 | 181 | 181 | 181 | 81 | 81 | 81 | 50 | 50 | 50 |
| | *** | 2103 | 2115 | 6022 | 676 | 676 | 1793 | 181 | 181 | 419 | 81 | 81 | 155 | 50 | 50 | 89 |
| 0.05 | *** | 6350 | 6408 | 6647 | 1808 | 1831 | 1861 | 391 | 391 | 396 | 137 | 137 | 143 | 81 | 81 | 81 |
| | *** | 6367 | 6478 | 12848 | 1817 | 1843 | 3481 | 391 | 391 | 681 | 137 | 143 | 217 | 81 | 81 | 115 |
| 0.1 | *** | 14011 | 14172 | 15473 | 3803 | 3888 | 4092 | 741 | 750 | 764 | 233 | 233 | 233 | 125 | 125 | 125 |
| | *** | 14064 | 14435 | 23235 | 3838 | 3966 | 6047 | 746 | 755 | 1076 | 233 | 233 | 310 | 125 | 125 | 153 |
| 0.15 | *** | 20945 | 21233 | 24436 | 5606 | 5795 | 6329 | 1065 | 1088 | 1117 | 318 | 318 | 321 | 160 | 160 | 163 |
| | *** | 21041 | 21755 | 32385 | 5681 | 5979 | 8304 | 1079 | 1100 | 1422 | 318 | 321 | 390 | 160 | 163 | 186 |
| 0.2 | *** | 26559 | 27008 | 32833 | 7099 | 7405 | 8406 | 1350 | 1388 | 1441 | 391 | 396 | 400 | 190 | 195 | 195 |
| | *** | 26711 | 27840 | 40298 | 7216 | 7732 | 10251 | 1368 | 1411 | 1719 | 391 | 396 | 458 | 195 | 195 | 213 |
| 0.25 | *** | 30689 | 31336 | 40308 | 8236 | 8686 | 10252 | 1581 | 1639 | 1721 | 452 | 458 | 466 | 216 | 221 | 221 |
| | *** | 30902 | 32535 | 46976 | 8411 | 9173 | 11890 | 1607 | 1677 | 1967 | 452 | 461 | 514 | 221 | 221 | 235 |
| 0.3 | *** | 33343 | 34236 | 46678 | 9036 | 9640 | 11815 | 1761 | 1840 | 1957 | 501 | 510 | 519 | 239 | 242 | 242 |
| | *** | 33641 | 35869 | 52416 | 9269 | 10293 | 13219 | 1796 | 1893 | 2164 | 505 | 513 | 557 | 239 | 242 | 252 |
| 0.35 | *** | 34635 | 35820 | 51829 | 9526 | 10284 | 13075 | 1893 | 1992 | 2146 | 536 | 545 | 557 | 251 | 256 | 260 |
| | *** | 35032 | 37943 | 56620 | 9823 | 11106 | 14239 | 1940 | 2062 | 2313 | 540 | 554 | 588 | 256 | 256 | 263 |
| 0.4 | *** | 34714 | 36254 | 55700 | 9741 | 10660 | 14006 | 1980 | 2097 | 2281 | 557 | 571 | 583 | 260 | 265 | 268 |
| | *** | 35233 | 38908 | 59588 | 10103 | 11635 | 14950 | 2033 | 2176 | 2412 | 566 | 580 | 606 | 265 | 265 | 268 |
| 0.45 | *** | 33778 | 35723 | 58255 | 9727 | 10786 | 14615 | 2018 | 2155 | 2360 | 571 | 583 | 601 | 265 | 268 | 268 |
| | *** | 34443 | 38935 | 61319 | 10147 | 11897 | 15352 | 2080 | 2246 | 2461 | 575 | 592 | 613 | 265 | 268 | 268 |
| 0.5 | *** | 32028 | 34437 | 59476 | 9523 | 10704 | 14886 | 2024 | 2167 | 2391 | 566 | 583 | 601 | 260 | 265 | 268 |
| | *** | 32868 | 38188 | 61814 | 9995 | 11923 | 15445 | 2088 | 2263 | 2461 | 575 | 592 | 606 | 265 | 265 | 263 |
| 0.55 | *** | 29691 | 32588 | 59348 | 9164 | 10436 | 14820 | 1983 | 2132 | 2365 | 554 | 571 | 589 | 251 | 256 | 260 |
| | *** | 30724 | 36800 | 61072 | 9675 | 11722 | 15228 | 2050 | 2234 | 2412 | 563 | 580 | 588 | 256 | 256 | 252 |
| 0.6 | *** | 26991 | 30339 | 57878 | 8677 | 9998 | 14417 | 1910 | 2059 | 2281 | 528 | 545 | 563 | 239 | 242 | 242 |
| | *** | 28213 | 34901 | 59093 | 9211 | 11311 | 14703 | 1975 | 2155 | 2313 | 536 | 554 | 557 | 239 | 242 | 235 |
| 0.65 | *** | 24126 | 27819 | 55066 | 8082 | 9412 | 13682 | 1796 | 1936 | 2150 | 493 | 505 | 519 | 216 | 221 | 225 |
| | *** | 25509 | 32573 | 55878 | 8625 | 10704 | 13868 | 1861 | 2033 | 2164 | 496 | 513 | 514 | 221 | 221 | 213 |
| 0.7 | *** | 21239 | 25110 | 50919 | 7396 | 8677 | 12611 | 1648 | 1773 | 1963 | 443 | 452 | 466 | 190 | 195 | 195 |
| | *** | 22718 | 29861 | 51427 | 7925 | 9902 | 12724 | 1709 | 1858 | 1967 | 449 | 461 | 458 | 195 | 195 | 186 |
| 0.75 | *** | 18395 | 22245 | 45450 | 6612 | 7799 | 11211 | 1464 | 1569 | 1721 | 382 | 391 | 400 | 160 | 163 | 163 |
| | *** | 19891 | 26772 | 45739 | 7108 | 8896 | 11271 | 1511 | 1639 | 1719 | 388 | 396 | 390 | 163 | 163 | 153 |
| 0.8 | *** | 15590 | 19186 | 38672 | 5725 | 6752 | 9488 | 1236 | 1318 | 1429 | 309 | 312 | 321 | 125 | 125 | 125 |
| | *** | 17004 | 23269 | 38815 | 6157 | 7671 | 9509 | 1275 | 1371 | 1422 | 312 | 318 | 310 | 125 | 125 | 115 |
| 0.85 | *** | 12743 | 15843 | 30601 | 4701 | 5506 | 7435 | 965 | 1018 | 1088 | 221 | 225 | 230 | . | . | . |
| | *** | 13976 | 19235 | 30654 | 5043 | 6192 | 7438 | 991 | 1053 | 1076 | 225 | 225 | 217 | . | . | . |
| 0.9 | *** | 9663 | 12002 | 21251 | 3476 | 3996 | 5063 | 636 | 662 | 694 | . | . | . | . | . | . |
| | *** | 10608 | 14423 | 21256 | 3704 | 4413 | 5058 | 650 | 676 | 681 | . | . | . | . | . | . |
| 0.95 | *** | 5900 | 7134 | 10634 | 1887 | 2080 | 2377 | . | . | . | . | . | . | . | . | . |
| | *** | 6416 | 8266 | 10622 | 1975 | 2211 | 2368 | . | . | . | . | . | . | . | . | . |
| 0.98 | *** | 2663 | 3016 | 3660 | . | . | . | . | . | . | . | . | . | . | . | . |
| | *** | 2820 | 3278 | 3648 | . | . | . | . | . | . | . | . | . | . | . | . |

TABLE 7: ALPHA= 0.05  POWER= 0.8    EXPECTED ACCRUAL THRU MINIMUM FOLLOW-UP= 3750

| | | DEL=.01 | | | DEL=.02 | | | DEL=.05 | | | DEL=.10 | | | DEL=.15 | | |
|---|---|---|---|---|---|---|---|---|---|---|---|---|---|---|---|---|---|
| FACT= | | 1.0 .75 | .50 .25 | .00 BIN | 1.0 .75 | .50 .25 | .00 BIN | 1.0 .75 | .50 .25 | .00 BIN | 1.0 75 | .50 .25 | .00 BIN | 1.0 .75 | .50 .25 | .00 BIN |
| PCONT=*** | | | | | REQUIRED NUMBER OF PATIENTS | | | | | | | | | | | |
| 0.01 | *** | 950 | 950 | 953 | 350 | 350 | 350 | 115 | 115 | 115 | 59 | 59 | 59 | 40 | 40 | 40 |
| | *** | 950 | 950 | 3648 | 350 | 350 | 1206 | 115 | 115 | 328 | 59 | 59 | 134 | 40 | 40 | 80 |
| 0.02 | *** | 2097 | 2106 | 2125 | 672 | 678 | 678 | 181 | 181 | 184 | 81 | 81 | 81 | 53 | 53 | 53 |
| | *** | 2103 | 2116 | 6022 | 678 | 678 | 1793 | 181 | 184 | 419 | 81 | 81 | 155 | 53 | 53 | 89 |
| 0.05 | *** | 6353 | 6409 | 6644 | 1812 | 1831 | 1863 | 391 | 391 | 397 | 138 | 138 | 138 | 81 | 81 | 81 |
| | *** | 6372 | 6484 | 12848 | 1822 | 1844 | 3481 | 391 | 397 | 681 | 138 | 138 | 217 | 81 | 81 | 115 |
| 0.1 | *** | 14022 | 14191 | 15472 | 3809 | 3897 | 4090 | 743 | 753 | 762 | 231 | 231 | 237 | 125 | 125 | 125 |
| | *** | 14078 | 14468 | 23235 | 3847 | 3972 | 6047 | 747 | 756 | 1076 | 231 | 237 | 310 | 125 | 125 | 153 |
| 0.15 | *** | 20965 | 21275 | 24438 | 5622 | 5815 | 6325 | 1072 | 1090 | 1118 | 316 | 322 | 322 | 162 | 162 | 162 |
| | *** | 21068 | 21818 | 32385 | 5697 | 5997 | 8304 | 1081 | 1103 | 1422 | 316 | 322 | 390 | 162 | 162 | 186 |
| 0.2 | *** | 26590 | 27072 | 32834 | 7122 | 7437 | 8406 | 1353 | 1390 | 1441 | 391 | 397 | 400 | 194 | 194 | 194 |
| | *** | 26753 | 27944 | 40298 | 7250 | 7759 | 10251 | 1372 | 1413 | 1719 | 391 | 397 | 458 | 194 | 194 | 213 |
| 0.25 | *** | 30734 | 31428 | 40309 | 8275 | 8734 | 10253 | 1587 | 1643 | 1722 | 453 | 456 | 466 | 218 | 218 | 222 |
| | *** | 30968 | 32688 | 46976 | 8453 | 9218 | 11890 | 1615 | 1681 | 1967 | 456 | 462 | 514 | 218 | 222 | 235 |
| 0.3 | *** | 33409 | 34362 | 46675 | 9091 | 9706 | 11815 | 1769 | 1850 | 1962 | 500 | 509 | 518 | 237 | 241 | 241 |
| | *** | 33728 | 36078 | 52416 | 9331 | 10356 | 13219 | 1806 | 1897 | 2164 | 503 | 513 | 557 | 241 | 241 | 252 |
| 0.35 | *** | 34718 | 35988 | 51831 | 9593 | 10366 | 13072 | 1906 | 2003 | 2144 | 537 | 547 | 559 | 250 | 256 | 259 |
| | *** | 35150 | 38206 | 56620 | 9897 | 11187 | 14239 | 1947 | 2065 | 2313 | 541 | 550 | 588 | 256 | 256 | 263 |
| 0.4 | *** | 34825 | 36466 | 55703 | 9828 | 10756 | 14009 | 1994 | 2106 | 2281 | 559 | 575 | 588 | 259 | 265 | 269 |
| | *** | 35384 | 39237 | 59588 | 10193 | 11731 | 14950 | 2047 | 2187 | 2412 | 565 | 578 | 606 | 265 | 265 | 268 |
| 0.45 | *** | 33922 | 35988 | 58259 | 9828 | 10900 | 14613 | 2037 | 2168 | 2359 | 569 | 584 | 597 | 265 | 269 | 269 |
| | *** | 34634 | 39322 | 61319 | 10253 | 12006 | 15352 | 2097 | 2253 | 2461 | 578 | 593 | 613 | 265 | 269 | 268 |
| 0.5 | *** | 32209 | 34756 | 59478 | 9634 | 10825 | 14884 | 2037 | 2178 | 2388 | 569 | 584 | 603 | 259 | 265 | 269 |
| | *** | 33100 | 38622 | 61814 | 10113 | 12040 | 15445 | 2103 | 2272 | 2461 | 578 | 593 | 606 | 265 | 265 | 263 |
| 0.55 | *** | 29918 | 32950 | 59350 | 9284 | 10563 | 14819 | 2000 | 2144 | 2365 | 556 | 569 | 588 | 250 | 256 | 259 |
| | *** | 31006 | 37278 | 61072 | 9803 | 11843 | 15228 | 2065 | 2243 | 2412 | 565 | 578 | 588 | 256 | 256 | 252 |
| 0.6 | *** | 27265 | 30743 | 57878 | 8800 | 10131 | 14416 | 1925 | 2069 | 2281 | 531 | 547 | 559 | 237 | 241 | 247 |
| | *** | 28544 | 35406 | 59093 | 9344 | 11434 | 14703 | 1990 | 2163 | 2313 | 537 | 550 | 557 | 241 | 241 | 235 |
| 0.65 | *** | 24438 | 28250 | 55062 | 8209 | 9547 | 13681 | 1812 | 1947 | 2150 | 494 | 503 | 518 | 218 | 222 | 222 |
| | *** | 25872 | 33087 | 55878 | 8759 | 10825 | 13868 | 1878 | 2037 | 2164 | 500 | 513 | 514 | 218 | 222 | 213 |
| 0.7 | *** | 21575 | 25553 | 50918 | 7522 | 8806 | 12612 | 1662 | 1788 | 1962 | 443 | 456 | 466 | 194 | 194 | 194 |
| | *** | 23103 | 30368 | 51427 | 8056 | 10015 | 12724 | 1722 | 1863 | 1967 | 447 | 462 | 458 | 194 | 194 | 186 |
| 0.75 | *** | 18738 | 22672 | 45453 | 6734 | 7915 | 11215 | 1475 | 1578 | 1722 | 381 | 391 | 400 | 162 | 162 | 166 |
| | *** | 20272 | 27247 | 45739 | 7225 | 8993 | 11271 | 1525 | 1643 | 1719 | 387 | 397 | 390 | 162 | 162 | 153 |
| 0.8 | *** | 15916 | 19572 | 38675 | 5828 | 6850 | 9484 | 1244 | 1325 | 1431 | 306 | 316 | 322 | 125 | 125 | 125 |
| | *** | 17359 | 23688 | 38815 | 6259 | 7750 | 9509 | 1281 | 1375 | 1422 | 312 | 316 | 310 | 125 | 125 | 115 |
| 0.85 | *** | 13028 | 16175 | 30603 | 4784 | 5581 | 7437 | 972 | 1025 | 1084 | 222 | 228 | 228 | . | . | . |
| | *** | 14284 | 19572 | 30654 | 5125 | 6256 | 7438 | 997 | 1053 | 1076 | 222 | 228 | 217 | . | . | . |
| 0.9 | *** | 9884 | 12247 | 21250 | 3528 | 4043 | 5065 | 640 | 663 | 691 | . | . | . | . | . | . |
| | *** | 10840 | 14659 | 21256 | 3753 | 4447 | 5058 | 653 | 678 | 681 | . | . | . | . | . | . |
| 0.95 | *** | 6022 | 7253 | 10634 | 1909 | 2093 | 2378 | . | . | . | . | . | . | . | . | . |
| | *** | 6537 | 8369 | 10622 | 1994 | 2219 | 2368 | . | . | . | . | . | . | . | . | . |
| 0.98 | *** | 2703 | 3050 | 3659 | . | . | . | . | . | . | . | . | . | . | . | . |
| | *** | 2853 | 3303 | 3648 | . | . | . | . | . | . | . | . | . | . | . | . |

TABLE 7: ALPHA= 0.05  POWER= 0.8    EXPECTED ACCRUAL THRU MINIMUM FOLLOW-UP= 4000

| | | DEL=.01 | | | DEL=.02 | | | DEL=.05 | | | DEL=.10 | | | DEL=.15 | | |
|---|---|---|---|---|---|---|---|---|---|---|---|---|---|---|---|---|---|
| FACT= | | 1.0 .75 | .50 .25 | .00 BIN | 1.0 .75 | .50 .25 | .00 BIN | 1.0 .75 | .50 .25 | .00 BIN | 1.0 75 | .50 .25 | .00 BIN | 1.0 .75 | .50 .25 | .00 BIN |
| PCONT=*** | | | | REQUIRED NUMBER OF PATIENTS | | | | | | | | | | | | |
| 0.01 | *** | 947 947 | 953 953 | 953 3648 | 347 347 | 347 347 | 347 1206 | 113 113 | 113 113 | 113 328 | 57 57 | 57 57 | 57 134 | 43 43 | 43 43 | 43 80 |
| 0.02 | *** | 2097 2103 | 2107 2117 | 2127 6022 | 673 677 | 677 677 | 677 1793 | 183 183 | 183 183 | 183 419 | 77 77 | 77 77 | 77 155 | 53 53 | 53 53 | 53 89 |
| 0.05 | *** | 6357 6383 | 6417 6493 | 6647 12848 | 1813 1823 | 1833 1847 | 1863 3481 | 393 393 | 393 393 | 393 681 | 137 137 | 137 143 | 143 217 | 83 83 | 83 83 | 83 115 |
| 0.1 | *** | 14033 14097 | 14213 14497 | 15473 23235 | 3817 3853 | 3907 3977 | 4093 6047 | 743 747 | 753 757 | 763 1076 | 233 233 | 233 233 | 233 310 | 123 123 | 123 123 | 123 153 |
| 0.15 | *** | 20987 21097 | 21313 21877 | 24437 32385 | 5643 5717 | 5833 6013 | 6327 8304 | 1073 1083 | 1093 1103 | 1117 1422 | 317 317 | 317 323 | 323 390 | 163 163 | 163 163 | 163 186 |
| 0.2 | *** | 26623 26797 | 27137 28047 | 32833 40298 | 7153 7277 | 7473 7787 | 8407 10251 | 1357 1373 | 1393 1413 | 1443 1719 | 393 393 | 397 397 | 397 458 | 193 193 | 193 193 | 193 213 |
| 0.25 | *** | 30783 31027 | 31517 32837 | 40307 46976 | 8313 8497 | 8783 9257 | 10253 11890 | 1593 1617 | 1647 1683 | 1723 1967 | 453 457 | 457 463 | 467 514 | 217 217 | 223 223 | 223 235 |
| 0.3 | *** | 33473 33813 | 34487 36277 | 46677 52416 | 9143 9387 | 9767 10413 | 11817 13219 | 1777 1813 | 1853 1903 | 1957 2164 | 503 507 | 507 513 | 517 557 | 237 237 | 243 243 | 243 252 |
| 0.35 | *** | 34807 35263 | 36153 38463 | 51833 56620 | 9657 9967 | 10443 11257 | 13073 14239 | 1917 1957 | 2007 2073 | 2147 2313 | 537 543 | 547 553 | 557 588 | 253 253 | 257 257 | 257 263 |
| 0.4 | *** | 34937 35533 | 36673 39547 | 55703 59588 | 9903 10283 | 10847 11813 | 14007 14950 | 2003 2057 | 2117 2187 | 2283 2412 | 563 567 | 573 577 | 587 606 | 263 263 | 263 267 | 267 268 |
| 0.45 | *** | 34063 34817 | 36247 39687 | 58257 61319 | 9917 10353 | 11003 12103 | 14613 15352 | 2053 2107 | 2177 2257 | 2363 2461 | 573 577 | 587 593 | 597 613 | 263 267 | 267 267 | 273 268 |
| 0.5 | *** | 32387 33333 | 35063 39037 | 59477 61814 | 9737 10223 | 10943 12143 | 14887 15445 | 2053 2117 | 2187 2277 | 2387 2461 | 573 577 | 583 593 | 603 606 | 263 263 | 263 267 | 267 263 |
| 0.55 | *** | 30143 31283 | 33303 37733 | 59347 61072 | 9397 9923 | 10687 11953 | 14823 15228 | 2017 2083 | 2157 2247 | 2363 2412 | 557 563 | 573 577 | 587 588 | 253 253 | 257 257 | 257 252 |
| 0.6 | *** | 27527 28863 | 31133 35887 | 57877 59093 | 8923 9473 | 10257 11547 | 14417 14703 | 1943 2003 | 2077 2167 | 2283 2313 | 533 537 | 547 553 | 563 557 | 237 237 | 243 243 | 243 235 |
| 0.65 | *** | 24743 26227 | 28663 33573 | 55063 55878 | 8333 8883 | 9667 10937 | 13683 13868 | 1827 1887 | 1957 2043 | 2147 2164 | 497 503 | 507 513 | 523 514 | 217 217 | 223 223 | 223 213 |
| 0.7 | *** | 21903 23467 | 25973 30843 | 50917 51427 | 7643 8173 | 8923 10117 | 12613 12724 | 1677 1733 | 1797 1873 | 1963 1967 | 447 453 | 457 463 | 467 458 | 193 193 | 193 197 | 197 186 |
| 0.75 | *** | 19067 20637 | 23073 27693 | 45453 45739 | 6843 7337 | 8023 9083 | 11213 11271 | 1487 1533 | 1587 1647 | 1723 1719 | 383 387 | 393 397 | 403 390 | 163 163 | 163 163 | 163 153 |
| 0.8 | *** | 16233 17703 | 19943 24083 | 38673 38815 | 5927 6353 | 6943 7827 | 9487 9509 | 1257 1293 | 1333 1377 | 1433 1422 | 307 313 | 317 317 | 323 310 | 123 123 | 127 127 | 127 115 |
| 0.85 | *** | 13303 14577 | 16483 19893 | 30603 30654 | 4863 5203 | 5653 6307 | 7437 7438 | 977 1003 | 1027 1053 | 1087 1076 | 223 223 | 227 227 | 227 217 | . . | . . | . . |
| 0.9 | *** | 10097 11063 | 12473 14877 | 21253 21256 | 3583 3803 | 4087 4473 | 5067 5058 | 643 653 | 667 677 | 693 681 | . . | . . | . . | . . | . . | . . |
| 0.95 | *** | 6137 6653 | 7367 8463 | 10633 10622 | 1927 2013 | 2107 2227 | 2377 2368 | . . | . . | . . | . . | . . | . . | . . | . . | . . |
| 0.98 | *** | 2737 2887 | 3077 3317 | 3663 3648 | . . | . . | . . | . . | . . | . . | . . | . . | . . | . . | . . | . . |

## TABLE 7: ALPHA= 0.05  POWER= 0.8    EXPECTED ACCRUAL THRU MINIMUM FOLLOW-UP= 4250

| | FACT= | DEL=.01 | | | DEL=.02 | | | DEL=.05 | | | DEL=.10 | | | DEL=.15 | | |
|---|---|---|---|---|---|---|---|---|---|---|---|---|---|---|---|---|
| | | 1.0 .75 | .50 .25 | .00 BIN | 1.0 .75 | .50 .25 | .00 BIN | 1.0 .75 | .50 .25 | .00 BIN | 1.0 75 | .50 .25 | .00 BIN | 1.0 .75 | .50 .25 | .00 BIN |
| PCONT=*** | | | | | REQUIRED NUMBER OF PATIENTS | | | | | | | | | | | |
| 0.01 | *** | 949 949 | 949 953 | 953 3648 | 347 347 | 347 347 | 347 1206 | 113 113 | 113 113 | 113 328 | 56 56 | 56 56 | 56 134 | 39 39 | 39 39 | 39 80 |
| 0.02 | *** | 2100 2107 | 2111 2118 | 2128 6022 | 677 677 | 677 677 | 677 1793 | 184 184 | 184 184 | 184 419 | 82 82 | 82 82 | 82 155 | 50 50 | 50 50 | 50 89 |
| 0.05 | *** | 6361 6382 | 6425 6499 | 6648 12848 | 1813 1824 | 1835 1845 | 1863 3481 | 390 390 | 390 396 | 396 681 | 141 141 | 141 141 | 141 217 | 82 82 | 82 82 | 82 115 |
| 0.1 | *** | 14043 14113 | 14234 14521 | 15473 23235 | 3828 3864 | 3913 3981 | 4094 6047 | 747 747 | 751 758 | 762 1076 | 230 230 | 237 237 | 237 310 | 124 124 | 124 124 | 124 153 |
| 0.15 | *** | 21009 21126 | 21353 21937 | 24441 32385 | 5656 5734 | 5847 6028 | 6329 8304 | 1076 1080 | 1091 1102 | 1119 1422 | 315 315 | 322 322 | 322 390 | 163 163 | 163 163 | 163 186 |
| 0.2 | *** | 26655 26835 | 27197 28142 | 32834 40298 | 7175 7307 | 7498 7813 | 8408 10251 | 1363 1378 | 1395 1416 | 1442 1719 | 390 396 | 396 396 | 400 458 | 194 194 | 194 194 | 194 213 |
| 0.25 | *** | 30826 31092 | 31613 32983 | 40308 46976 | 8354 8539 | 8822 9300 | 10250 11890 | 1597 1622 | 1650 1686 | 1724 1967 | 453 453 | 460 460 | 464 514 | 220 220 | 220 220 | 220 235 |
| 0.3 | *** | 33536 33901 | 34609 36468 | 46679 52416 | 9194 9442 | 9825 10462 | 11818 13219 | 1788 1820 | 1856 1905 | 1958 2164 | 503 507 | 513 513 | 517 557 | 241 241 | 241 241 | 241 252 |
| 0.35 | *** | 34889 35374 | 36313 38710 | 51832 56620 | 9725 10037 | 10515 11323 | 13072 14239 | 1926 1969 | 2015 2075 | 2143 2313 | 538 545 | 549 556 | 560 588 | 252 252 | 258 258 | 258 263 |
| 0.4 | *** | 35048 35675 | 36883 39847 | 55703 59588 | 9980 10363 | 10936 11893 | 14007 14950 | 2015 2064 | 2122 2196 | 2281 2412 | 560 566 | 577 581 | 588 606 | 262 262 | 262 269 | 269 268 |
| 0.45 | *** | 34205 35002 | 36500 40038 | 58260 61319 | 10005 10448 | 11100 12194 | 14613 15352 | 2064 2118 | 2185 2266 | 2362 2461 | 577 581 | 588 592 | 598 613 | 262 269 | 269 269 | 269 268 |
| 0.5 | *** | 32569 33561 | 35363 39433 | 59475 61814 | 9835 10331 | 11053 12243 | 14882 15445 | 2068 2128 | 2196 2281 | 2387 2461 | 570 581 | 588 592 | 598 606 | 262 262 | 262 269 | 269 263 |
| 0.55 | *** | 30363 31553 | 33646 38162 | 59348 61072 | 9506 10037 | 10802 12056 | 14818 15228 | 2033 2090 | 2164 2256 | 2362 2412 | 560 566 | 570 581 | 588 588 | 252 252 | 258 258 | 258 252 |
| 0.6 | *** | 27792 29173 | 31510 36341 | 57878 59093 | 9034 9587 | 10377 11652 | 14421 14703 | 1958 2015 | 2090 2175 | 2281 2313 | 534 538 | 545 556 | 560 557 | 237 241 | 241 241 | 241 235 |
| 0.65 | *** | 25036 26566 | 29063 34035 | 55062 55878 | 8450 9003 | 9789 11036 | 13682 13868 | 1841 1898 | 1969 2047 | 2149 2164 | 496 503 | 507 513 | 517 514 | 220 220 | 220 220 | 226 213 |
| 0.7 | *** | 22213 23824 | 26368 31294 | 50918 51427 | 7753 8284 | 9034 10207 | 12615 12724 | 1693 1739 | 1803 1873 | 1962 1967 | 449 449 | 453 460 | 464 458 | 194 194 | 194 194 | 198 186 |
| 0.75 | *** | 19387 20981 | 23457 28110 | 45450 45739 | 6945 7441 | 8121 9166 | 11213 11271 | 1495 1544 | 1590 1650 | 1724 1719 | 386 390 | 390 396 | 400 390 | 163 163 | 163 163 | 163 153 |
| 0.8 | *** | 16529 18023 | 20290 24451 | 38672 38815 | 6017 6446 | 7026 7891 | 9485 9509 | 1261 1299 | 1335 1378 | 1431 1422 | 311 311 | 315 315 | 322 310 | 124 124 | 124 124 | 124 115 |
| 0.85 | *** | 13565 14850 | 16773 20191 | 30603 30654 | 4933 5267 | 5713 6357 | 7434 7438 | 981 1006 | 1027 1055 | 1087 1076 | 226 226 | 226 226 | 230 217 | . . | . . | . . |
| 0.9 | *** | 10299 11270 | 12683 15080 | 21253 21256 | 3630 3849 | 4126 4502 | 5065 5058 | 645 655 | 666 677 | 694 681 | . . | . . | . . | . . | . . | . . |
| 0.95 | *** | 6244 6761 | 7473 8550 | 10632 10622 | 1948 2026 | 2122 2234 | 2377 2368 | . . | . . | . . | . . | . . | . . | . . | . . | . . |
| 0.98 | *** | 2770 2918 | 3099 3333 | 3658 3648 | . . | . . | . . | . . | . . | . . | . . | . . | . . | . . | . . | . . |

## TABLE 7: ALPHA= 0.05  POWER= 0.8   EXPECTED ACCRUAL THRU MINIMUM FOLLOW-UP= 4500

| | | DEL=.01 | | | DEL=.02 | | | DEL=.05 | | | DEL=.10 | | | DEL=.15 | | |
|---|---|---|---|---|---|---|---|---|---|---|---|---|---|---|---|---|
| FACT= | | 1.0 | .50 | .00 | 1.0 | .50 | .00 | 1.0 | .50 | .00 | 1.0 | .50 | .00 | 1.0 | .50 | .00 |
| | | .75 | .25 | BIN | .75 | .25 | BIN | .75 | .25 | BIN | 75 | .25 | BIN | .75 | .25 | BIN |
| PCONT= | *** | | | | REQUIRED NUMBER OF PATIENTS | | | | | | | | | | | |
| 0.01 | *** | 948 | 948 | 953 | 345 | 352 | 352 | 116 | 116 | 116 | 60 | 60 | 60 | 41 | 41 | 41 |
| | *** | 948 | 953 | 3648 | 345 | 352 | 1206 | 116 | 116 | 328 | 60 | 60 | 134 | 41 | 41 | 80 |
| 0.02 | *** | 2100 | 2111 | 2130 | 678 | 678 | 678 | 183 | 183 | 183 | 82 | 82 | 82 | 53 | 53 | 53 |
| | *** | 2107 | 2118 | 6022 | 678 | 678 | 1793 | 183 | 183 | 419 | 82 | 82 | 155 | 53 | 53 | 89 |
| 0.05 | *** | 6364 | 6431 | 6645 | 1815 | 1837 | 1864 | 390 | 390 | 397 | 138 | 138 | 138 | 82 | 82 | 82 |
| | *** | 6393 | 6506 | 12848 | 1826 | 1848 | 3481 | 390 | 397 | 681 | 138 | 138 | 217 | 82 | 82 | 115 |
| 0.1 | *** | 14059 | 14257 | 15472 | 3833 | 3918 | 4091 | 746 | 750 | 761 | 233 | 233 | 233 | 127 | 127 | 127 |
| | *** | 14126 | 14550 | 23235 | 3866 | 3990 | 6047 | 750 | 757 | 1076 | 233 | 233 | 310 | 127 | 127 | 153 |
| 0.15 | *** | 21030 | 21394 | 24438 | 5673 | 5865 | 6326 | 1076 | 1095 | 1117 | 318 | 318 | 323 | 161 | 161 | 161 |
| | *** | 21153 | 21997 | 32385 | 5752 | 6038 | 8304 | 1083 | 1106 | 1422 | 318 | 323 | 390 | 161 | 161 | 186 |
| 0.2 | *** | 26688 | 27262 | 32835 | 7203 | 7530 | 8407 | 1365 | 1398 | 1443 | 390 | 397 | 397 | 195 | 195 | 195 |
| | *** | 26880 | 28241 | 40298 | 7331 | 7838 | 10251 | 1380 | 1414 | 1719 | 390 | 397 | 458 | 195 | 195 | 213 |
| 0.25 | *** | 30873 | 31699 | 40312 | 8389 | 8861 | 10252 | 1605 | 1657 | 1725 | 453 | 458 | 465 | 217 | 221 | 221 |
| | *** | 31155 | 33123 | 46976 | 8580 | 9334 | 11890 | 1628 | 1684 | 1967 | 458 | 465 | 514 | 221 | 221 | 235 |
| 0.3 | *** | 33600 | 34732 | 46680 | 9240 | 9881 | 11816 | 1792 | 1864 | 1961 | 503 | 510 | 521 | 240 | 240 | 244 |
| | *** | 33983 | 36656 | 52416 | 9491 | 10515 | 13219 | 1826 | 1909 | 2164 | 510 | 514 | 557 | 240 | 244 | 252 |
| 0.35 | *** | 34980 | 36476 | 51832 | 9784 | 10583 | 13076 | 1931 | 2021 | 2145 | 543 | 548 | 559 | 255 | 255 | 255 |
| | *** | 35486 | 38944 | 56620 | 10106 | 11388 | 14239 | 1976 | 2078 | 2313 | 543 | 555 | 588 | 255 | 255 | 263 |
| 0.4 | *** | 35164 | 37083 | 55702 | 10054 | 11017 | 14010 | 2028 | 2130 | 2280 | 566 | 577 | 588 | 262 | 266 | 266 |
| | *** | 35823 | 40136 | 59588 | 10443 | 11966 | 14950 | 2073 | 2197 | 2412 | 570 | 581 | 606 | 262 | 266 | 268 |
| 0.45 | *** | 34350 | 36746 | 58256 | 10095 | 11197 | 14617 | 2073 | 2190 | 2359 | 577 | 588 | 600 | 266 | 266 | 273 |
| | *** | 35186 | 40373 | 61319 | 10538 | 12277 | 15352 | 2130 | 2269 | 2461 | 581 | 593 | 613 | 266 | 266 | 268 |
| 0.5 | *** | 32745 | 35655 | 59475 | 9930 | 11152 | 14887 | 2078 | 2208 | 2388 | 577 | 588 | 600 | 262 | 266 | 266 |
| | *** | 33787 | 39810 | 61814 | 10432 | 12333 | 15445 | 2141 | 2287 | 2461 | 581 | 593 | 606 | 262 | 266 | 263 |
| 0.55 | *** | 30581 | 33978 | 59347 | 9611 | 10909 | 14820 | 2044 | 2175 | 2366 | 559 | 570 | 588 | 255 | 255 | 262 |
| | *** | 31823 | 38573 | 61072 | 10144 | 12153 | 15228 | 2107 | 2258 | 2412 | 566 | 581 | 588 | 255 | 255 | 252 |
| 0.6 | *** | 28050 | 31875 | 57878 | 9143 | 10488 | 14419 | 1965 | 2096 | 2280 | 536 | 548 | 559 | 240 | 240 | 244 |
| | *** | 29478 | 36768 | 59093 | 9701 | 11748 | 14703 | 2028 | 2179 | 2313 | 543 | 555 | 557 | 240 | 244 | 235 |
| 0.65 | *** | 25320 | 29438 | 55065 | 8558 | 9896 | 13683 | 1853 | 1976 | 2145 | 498 | 510 | 521 | 217 | 221 | 221 |
| | *** | 26895 | 34473 | 55878 | 9116 | 11130 | 13868 | 1909 | 2055 | 2164 | 503 | 514 | 514 | 221 | 221 | 213 |
| 0.7 | *** | 22519 | 26749 | 50921 | 7856 | 9138 | 12615 | 1702 | 1808 | 1961 | 446 | 458 | 465 | 195 | 195 | 195 |
| | *** | 24161 | 31717 | 51427 | 8396 | 10297 | 12724 | 1751 | 1882 | 1967 | 453 | 465 | 458 | 195 | 195 | 186 |
| 0.75 | *** | 19691 | 23824 | 45453 | 7046 | 8216 | 11213 | 1504 | 1601 | 1725 | 386 | 390 | 401 | 161 | 165 | 165 |
| | *** | 21315 | 28511 | 45739 | 7534 | 9244 | 11271 | 1549 | 1657 | 1719 | 390 | 397 | 390 | 161 | 165 | 153 |
| 0.8 | *** | 16822 | 20625 | 38674 | 6101 | 7102 | 9487 | 1268 | 1342 | 1432 | 311 | 318 | 323 | 127 | 127 | 127 |
| | *** | 18334 | 24798 | 38815 | 6528 | 7957 | 9509 | 1301 | 1380 | 1422 | 311 | 318 | 310 | 127 | 127 | 115 |
| 0.85 | *** | 13818 | 17051 | 30603 | 5003 | 5775 | 7433 | 986 | 1031 | 1088 | 221 | 228 | 228 | . | . | . |
| | *** | 15116 | 20467 | 30654 | 5336 | 6398 | 7438 | 1009 | 1061 | 1076 | 221 | 228 | 217 | . | . | . |
| 0.9 | *** | 10488 | 12885 | 21248 | 3675 | 4159 | 5066 | 649 | 667 | 694 | . | . | . | . | . | . |
| | *** | 11467 | 15263 | 21256 | 3889 | 4526 | 5058 | 656 | 678 | 681 | . | . | . | . | . | . |
| 0.95 | *** | 6348 | 7568 | 10635 | 1965 | 2134 | 2381 | . | . | . | . | . | . | . | . | . |
| | *** | 6866 | 8625 | 10622 | 2040 | 2242 | 2368 | . | . | . | . | . | . | . | . | . |
| 0.98 | *** | 2798 | 3124 | 3660 | . | . | . | . | . | . | . | . | . | . | . | . |
| | *** | 2944 | 3349 | 3648 | . | . | . | . | . | . | . | . | . | . | . | . |

## TABLE 7: ALPHA= 0.05  POWER= 0.8    EXPECTED ACCRUAL THRU MINIMUM FOLLOW-UP= 4750

| | | DEL=.01 | | | DEL=.02 | | | DEL=.05 | | | DEL=.10 | | | DEL=.15 | | |
|---|---|---|---|---|---|---|---|---|---|---|---|---|---|---|---|---|---|
| FACT= | | 1.0 .75 | .50 .25 | .00 BIN | 1.0 .75 | .50 .25 | .00 BIN | 1.0 .75 | .50 .25 | .00 BIN | 1.0 75 | .50 .25 | .00 BIN | 1.0 .75 | .50 .25 | .00 BIN |
| PCONT=*** | | | | | REQUIRED NUMBER OF PATIENTS | | | | | | | | | | | |
| 0.01 | *** | 946 | 953 | 953 | 348 | 348 | 348 | 115 | 115 | 115 | 55 | 55 | 55 | 39 | 39 | 39 |
| | *** | 946 | 953 | 3648 | 348 | 348 | 1206 | 115 | 115 | 328 | 55 | 55 | 134 | 39 | 39 | 80 |
| 0.02 | *** | 2098 | 2110 | 2129 | 673 | 680 | 680 | 182 | 182 | 182 | 79 | 79 | 79 | 51 | 51 | 51 |
| | *** | 2105 | 2117 | 6022 | 673 | 680 | 1793 | 182 | 182 | 419 | 79 | 79 | 155 | 51 | 51 | 89 |
| 0.05 | *** | 6368 | 6440 | 6646 | 1820 | 1837 | 1860 | 388 | 395 | 395 | 139 | 139 | 139 | 79 | 79 | 79 |
| | *** | 6397 | 6511 | 12848 | 1825 | 1849 | 3481 | 395 | 395 | 681 | 139 | 139 | 217 | 79 | 79 | 115 |
| 0.1 | *** | 14068 | 14277 | 15469 | 3839 | 3927 | 4093 | 744 | 752 | 763 | 234 | 234 | 234 | 122 | 122 | 122 |
| | *** | 14139 | 14574 | 23235 | 3875 | 3993 | 6047 | 752 | 756 | 1076 | 234 | 234 | 310 | 122 | 122 | 153 |
| 0.15 | *** | 21050 | 21430 | 24435 | 5684 | 5882 | 6325 | 1077 | 1096 | 1120 | 317 | 317 | 324 | 162 | 162 | 162 |
| | *** | 21181 | 22048 | 32385 | 5767 | 6048 | 8304 | 1084 | 1108 | 1422 | 317 | 324 | 390 | 162 | 162 | 186 |
| 0.2 | *** | 26722 | 27320 | 32830 | 7223 | 7556 | 8411 | 1369 | 1397 | 1440 | 395 | 395 | 400 | 193 | 193 | 193 |
| | *** | 26924 | 28330 | 40298 | 7359 | 7857 | 10251 | 1381 | 1417 | 1719 | 395 | 395 | 458 | 193 | 193 | 213 |
| 0.25 | *** | 30919 | 31785 | 40307 | 8423 | 8902 | 10252 | 1607 | 1659 | 1725 | 455 | 459 | 467 | 217 | 222 | 222 |
| | *** | 31215 | 33253 | 46976 | 8617 | 9365 | 11890 | 1630 | 1690 | 1967 | 455 | 459 | 514 | 222 | 222 | 235 |
| 0.3 | *** | 33662 | 34857 | 46677 | 9282 | 9931 | 11812 | 1801 | 1868 | 1963 | 502 | 514 | 519 | 241 | 241 | 241 |
| | *** | 34065 | 36832 | 52416 | 9544 | 10560 | 13219 | 1832 | 1908 | 2164 | 507 | 514 | 557 | 241 | 241 | 252 |
| 0.35 | *** | 35063 | 36630 | 51830 | 9840 | 10648 | 13070 | 1944 | 2027 | 2145 | 542 | 550 | 562 | 253 | 257 | 257 |
| | *** | 35597 | 39179 | 56620 | 10168 | 11444 | 14239 | 1979 | 2082 | 2313 | 542 | 554 | 588 | 253 | 257 | 263 |
| 0.4 | *** | 35272 | 37279 | 55702 | 10125 | 11095 | 14009 | 2034 | 2141 | 2283 | 566 | 573 | 585 | 265 | 265 | 269 |
| | *** | 35965 | 40414 | 59588 | 10517 | 12037 | 14950 | 2082 | 2200 | 2412 | 566 | 578 | 606 | 265 | 265 | 268 |
| 0.45 | *** | 34488 | 36987 | 58255 | 10173 | 11285 | 14614 | 2086 | 2200 | 2359 | 578 | 585 | 602 | 265 | 269 | 269 |
| | *** | 35367 | 40699 | 61319 | 10624 | 12353 | 15352 | 2141 | 2272 | 2461 | 585 | 590 | 613 | 265 | 269 | 268 |
| 0.5 | *** | 32925 | 35937 | 59473 | 10026 | 11249 | 14883 | 2093 | 2212 | 2390 | 573 | 585 | 602 | 265 | 265 | 269 |
| | *** | 34006 | 40177 | 61814 | 10525 | 12417 | 15445 | 2145 | 2295 | 2461 | 578 | 590 | 606 | 265 | 265 | 263 |
| 0.55 | *** | 30795 | 34298 | 59347 | 9705 | 11012 | 14823 | 2058 | 2181 | 2359 | 562 | 573 | 585 | 253 | 257 | 257 |
| | *** | 32082 | 38970 | 61072 | 10244 | 12239 | 15228 | 2117 | 2264 | 2412 | 566 | 578 | 588 | 253 | 257 | 252 |
| 0.6 | *** | 28294 | 32220 | 57875 | 9247 | 10589 | 14420 | 1979 | 2105 | 2283 | 538 | 550 | 562 | 241 | 241 | 245 |
| | *** | 29774 | 37184 | 59093 | 9805 | 11843 | 14703 | 2039 | 2188 | 2313 | 542 | 554 | 557 | 241 | 241 | 235 |
| 0.65 | *** | 25599 | 29810 | 55060 | 8660 | 9995 | 13683 | 1868 | 1987 | 2145 | 495 | 507 | 519 | 217 | 222 | 222 |
| | *** | 27214 | 34885 | 55878 | 9218 | 11218 | 13868 | 1920 | 2058 | 2164 | 502 | 514 | 514 | 222 | 222 | 213 |
| 0.7 | *** | 22815 | 27119 | 50916 | 7960 | 9235 | 12615 | 1713 | 1820 | 1963 | 447 | 459 | 467 | 193 | 193 | 198 |
| | *** | 24490 | 32118 | 51427 | 8494 | 10375 | 12724 | 1761 | 1884 | 1967 | 455 | 459 | 458 | 193 | 198 | 186 |
| 0.75 | *** | 19989 | 24174 | 45449 | 7133 | 8297 | 11213 | 1516 | 1607 | 1718 | 388 | 395 | 400 | 162 | 162 | 162 |
| | *** | 21640 | 28883 | 45739 | 7627 | 9313 | 11271 | 1559 | 1659 | 1719 | 388 | 395 | 390 | 162 | 162 | 153 |
| 0.8 | *** | 17096 | 20944 | 38673 | 6183 | 7176 | 9484 | 1279 | 1345 | 1428 | 312 | 317 | 324 | 127 | 127 | 127 |
| | *** | 18628 | 25124 | 38815 | 6606 | 8012 | 9509 | 1310 | 1385 | 1422 | 312 | 317 | 310 | 127 | 127 | 115 |
| 0.85 | *** | 14056 | 17317 | 30605 | 5067 | 5827 | 7437 | 989 | 1037 | 1089 | 222 | 229 | 229 | . | . | . |
| | *** | 15370 | 20730 | 30654 | 5395 | 6440 | 7438 | 1013 | 1060 | 1076 | 222 | 229 | 217 | . | . | . |
| 0.9 | *** | 10667 | 13078 | 21252 | 3713 | 4195 | 5067 | 649 | 668 | 692 | . | . | . | . | . | . |
| | *** | 11653 | 15441 | 21256 | 3927 | 4552 | 5058 | 661 | 680 | 681 | . | . | . | . | . | . |
| 0.95 | *** | 6444 | 7655 | 10632 | 1979 | 2145 | 2378 | . | . | . | . | . | . | . | . | . |
| | *** | 6962 | 8700 | 10622 | 2058 | 2248 | 2368 | . | . | . | . | . | . | . | . | . |
| 0.98 | *** | 2830 | 3143 | 3661 | . | . | . | . | . | . | . | . | . | . | . | . |
| | *** | 2972 | 3364 | 3648 | . | . | . | . | . | . | . | . | . | . | . | . |

TABLE 7: ALPHA= 0.05  POWER= 0.8    EXPECTED ACCRUAL THRU MINIMUM FOLLOW-UP= 5000

| | | DEL=.01 | | | DEL=.02 | | | DEL=.05 | | | DEL=.10 | | | DEL=.15 | | |
|---|---|---|---|---|---|---|---|---|---|---|---|---|---|---|---|---|
| FACT= | | 1.0 .75 | .50 .25 | .00 BIN | 1.0 .75 | .50 .25 | .00 BIN | 1.0 .75 | .50 .25 | .00 BIN | 1.0 75 | .50 .25 | .00 BIN | 1.0 .75 | .50 .25 | .00 BIN |
| PCONT=*** | | | | | REQUIRED | NUMBER OF | PATIENTS | | | | | | | | | |
| 0.01 | *** | 946 | 954 | 954 | 346 | 346 | 346 | 116 | 116 | 116 | 58 | 58 | 58 | 41 | 41 | 41 |
| | *** | 946 | 954 | 3648 | 346 | 346 | 1206 | 116 | 116 | 328 | 58 | 58 | 134 | 41 | 41 | 80 |
| 0.02 | *** | 2104 | 2108 | 2129 | 679 | 679 | 679 | 183 | 183 | 183 | 79 | 79 | 79 | 54 | 54 | 54 |
| | *** | 2108 | 2121 | 6022 | 679 | 679 | 1793 | 183 | 183 | 419 | 79 | 79 | 155 | 54 | 54 | 89 |
| 0.05 | *** | 6371 | 6441 | 6646 | 1821 | 1833 | 1858 | 391 | 391 | 396 | 141 | 141 | 141 | 83 | 83 | 83 |
| | *** | 6404 | 6516 | 12848 | 1829 | 1846 | 3481 | 391 | 396 | 681 | 141 | 141 | 217 | 83 | 83 | 115 |
| 0.1 | *** | 14079 | 14296 | 15471 | 3846 | 3933 | 4091 | 746 | 754 | 758 | 233 | 233 | 233 | 121 | 121 | 121 |
| | *** | 14154 | 14596 | 23235 | 3883 | 3996 | 6047 | 754 | 758 | 1076 | 233 | 233 | 310 | 121 | 121 | 153 |
| 0.15 | *** | 21071 | 21471 | 24441 | 5696 | 5891 | 6329 | 1079 | 1096 | 1116 | 316 | 321 | 321 | 158 | 158 | 158 |
| | *** | 21208 | 22104 | 32385 | 5779 | 6058 | 8304 | 1083 | 1104 | 1422 | 321 | 321 | 390 | 158 | 158 | 186 |
| 0.2 | *** | 26754 | 27383 | 32833 | 7246 | 7579 | 8408 | 1371 | 1404 | 1441 | 391 | 396 | 396 | 191 | 196 | 196 |
| | *** | 26966 | 28421 | 40298 | 7383 | 7879 | 10251 | 1383 | 1421 | 1719 | 396 | 396 | 458 | 191 | 196 | 213 |
| 0.25 | *** | 30966 | 31879 | 40308 | 8454 | 8941 | 10254 | 1616 | 1658 | 1721 | 454 | 458 | 466 | 221 | 221 | 221 |
| | *** | 31279 | 33383 | 46976 | 8654 | 9396 | 11890 | 1633 | 1691 | 1967 | 458 | 458 | 514 | 221 | 221 | 235 |
| 0.3 | *** | 33729 | 34971 | 46679 | 9329 | 9979 | 11816 | 1804 | 1871 | 1958 | 504 | 508 | 516 | 241 | 241 | 241 |
| | *** | 34154 | 37008 | 52416 | 9591 | 10604 | 13219 | 1833 | 1908 | 2164 | 508 | 516 | 557 | 241 | 241 | 252 |
| 0.35 | *** | 35146 | 36783 | 51829 | 9896 | 10708 | 13071 | 1946 | 2033 | 2146 | 541 | 546 | 558 | 254 | 254 | 258 |
| | *** | 35708 | 39396 | 56620 | 10229 | 11496 | 14239 | 1991 | 2083 | 2313 | 546 | 554 | 588 | 254 | 258 | 263 |
| 0.4 | *** | 35383 | 37479 | 55704 | 10191 | 11166 | 14008 | 2046 | 2146 | 2279 | 566 | 579 | 583 | 266 | 266 | 266 |
| | *** | 36108 | 40683 | 59588 | 10591 | 12104 | 14950 | 2091 | 2204 | 2412 | 571 | 579 | 606 | 266 | 266 | 268 |
| 0.45 | *** | 34633 | 37221 | 58258 | 10254 | 11366 | 14616 | 2096 | 2208 | 2358 | 579 | 591 | 596 | 266 | 266 | 271 |
| | *** | 35546 | 41008 | 61319 | 10708 | 12429 | 15352 | 2146 | 2279 | 2461 | 583 | 596 | 613 | 266 | 271 | 268 |
| 0.5 | *** | 33104 | 36216 | 59479 | 10116 | 11341 | 14883 | 2104 | 2221 | 2391 | 579 | 591 | 604 | 266 | 266 | 266 |
| | *** | 34221 | 40521 | 61814 | 10616 | 12496 | 15445 | 2158 | 2296 | 2461 | 583 | 596 | 606 | 266 | 266 | 263 |
| 0.55 | *** | 31004 | 34608 | 59346 | 9804 | 11108 | 14821 | 2066 | 2191 | 2366 | 566 | 571 | 583 | 254 | 258 | 258 |
| | *** | 32333 | 39346 | 61072 | 10341 | 12329 | 15228 | 2121 | 2266 | 2412 | 566 | 579 | 588 | 254 | 258 | 252 |
| 0.6 | *** | 28541 | 32558 | 57879 | 9346 | 10691 | 14416 | 1991 | 2116 | 2283 | 541 | 546 | 558 | 241 | 241 | 246 |
| | *** | 30058 | 37571 | 59093 | 9904 | 11921 | 14703 | 2046 | 2191 | 2313 | 541 | 554 | 557 | 241 | 241 | 235 |
| 0.65 | *** | 25871 | 30158 | 55066 | 8758 | 10096 | 13683 | 1879 | 1991 | 2146 | 496 | 508 | 521 | 221 | 221 | 221 |
| | *** | 27521 | 35283 | 55878 | 9316 | 11296 | 13868 | 1929 | 2066 | 2164 | 504 | 516 | 514 | 221 | 221 | 213 |
| 0.7 | *** | 23104 | 27471 | 50916 | 8054 | 9329 | 12608 | 1721 | 1821 | 1958 | 446 | 458 | 466 | 191 | 196 | 196 |
| | *** | 24808 | 32504 | 51427 | 8591 | 10454 | 12724 | 1766 | 1883 | 1967 | 454 | 458 | 458 | 196 | 196 | 186 |
| 0.75 | *** | 20271 | 24508 | 45454 | 7221 | 8383 | 11216 | 1521 | 1608 | 1721 | 383 | 391 | 404 | 158 | 166 | 166 |
| | *** | 21946 | 29241 | 45739 | 7716 | 9379 | 11271 | 1566 | 1658 | 1719 | 391 | 396 | 390 | 166 | 166 | 153 |
| 0.8 | *** | 17358 | 21246 | 38671 | 6258 | 7246 | 9483 | 1283 | 1346 | 1429 | 308 | 316 | 321 | 121 | 129 | 129 |
| | *** | 18908 | 25433 | 38815 | 6683 | 8066 | 9509 | 1316 | 1383 | 1422 | 316 | 316 | 310 | 129 | 129 | 115 |
| 0.85 | *** | 14283 | 17571 | 30604 | 5129 | 5879 | 7433 | 996 | 1033 | 1083 | 221 | 229 | 229 | . | . | . |
| | *** | 15608 | 20979 | 30654 | 5454 | 6479 | 7438 | 1016 | 1058 | 1076 | 229 | 229 | 217 | . | . | . |
| 0.9 | *** | 10841 | 13254 | 21254 | 3754 | 4229 | 5066 | 654 | 671 | 691 | . | . | . | . | . | . |
| | *** | 11833 | 15608 | 21256 | 3966 | 4571 | 5058 | 658 | 679 | 681 | . | . | . | . | . | . |
| 0.95 | *** | 6541 | 7741 | 10633 | 1991 | 2154 | 2379 | . | . | . | . | . | . | . | . | . |
| | *** | 7046 | 8766 | 10622 | 2066 | 2254 | 2368 | . | . | . | . | . | . | . | . | . |
| 0.98 | *** | 2854 | 3166 | 3658 | . | . | . | . | . | . | . | . | . | . | . | . |
| | *** | 2996 | 3379 | 3648 | . | . | . | . | . | . | . | . | . | . | . | . |

## TABLE 7: ALPHA= 0.05  POWER= 0.8     EXPECTED ACCRUAL THRU MINIMUM FOLLOW-UP= 5500

| | | DEL=.01 | | | DEL=.02 | | | DEL=.05 | | | DEL=.10 | | | DEL=.15 | | |
|---|---|---|---|---|---|---|---|---|---|---|---|---|---|---|---|---|
| FACT= | | 1.0 .75 | .50 .25 | .00 BIN | 1.0 .75 | .50 .25 | .00 BIN | 1.0 .75 | .50 .25 | .00 BIN | 1.0 75 | .50 .25 | .00 BIN | 1.0 .75 | .50 .25 | .00 BIN |
| PCONT=*** | | | | | REQUIRED NUMBER OF PATIENTS | | | | | | | | | | | |
| 0.01 | *** | 953 | 953 | 953 | 348 | 348 | 348 | 114 | 114 | 114 | 59 | 59 | 59 | 37 | 37 | 37 |
| | *** | 953 | 953 | 3648 | 348 | 348 | 1206 | 114 | 114 | 328 | 59 | 59 | 134 | 37 | 37 | 80 |
| 0.02 | *** | 2099 | 2113 | 2127 | 678 | 678 | 678 | 183 | 183 | 183 | 78 | 78 | 78 | 50 | 50 | 50 |
| | *** | 2108 | 2121 | 6022 | 678 | 678 | 1793 | 183 | 183 | 419 | 78 | 78 | 155 | 50 | 50 | 89 |
| 0.05 | *** | 6384 | 6453 | 6645 | 1824 | 1838 | 1860 | 394 | 394 | 394 | 141 | 141 | 141 | 78 | 78 | 78 |
| | *** | 6411 | 6521 | 12848 | 1833 | 1852 | 3481 | 394 | 394 | 681 | 141 | 141 | 217 | 78 | 78 | 115 |
| 0.1 | *** | 14103 | 14331 | 15473 | 3859 | 3942 | 4093 | 746 | 752 | 760 | 229 | 238 | 238 | 128 | 128 | 128 |
| | *** | 14185 | 14639 | 23235 | 3895 | 4005 | 6047 | 752 | 760 | 1076 | 238 | 238 | 310 | 128 | 128 | 153 |
| 0.15 | *** | 21110 | 21542 | 24438 | 5724 | 5916 | 6329 | 1082 | 1095 | 1118 | 320 | 320 | 320 | 160 | 160 | 160 |
| | *** | 21261 | 22202 | 32385 | 5806 | 6081 | 8304 | 1090 | 1104 | 1422 | 320 | 320 | 390 | 160 | 160 | 186 |
| 0.2 | *** | 26816 | 27504 | 32830 | 7291 | 7621 | 8410 | 1379 | 1406 | 1439 | 394 | 394 | 403 | 196 | 196 | 196 |
| | *** | 27050 | 28590 | 40298 | 7429 | 7915 | 10251 | 1393 | 1420 | 1719 | 394 | 394 | 458 | 196 | 196 | 213 |
| 0.25 | *** | 31057 | 32047 | 40310 | 8520 | 9010 | 10253 | 1618 | 1668 | 1723 | 458 | 458 | 463 | 215 | 224 | 224 |
| | *** | 31400 | 33628 | 46976 | 8721 | 9455 | 11890 | 1640 | 1695 | 1967 | 458 | 463 | 514 | 224 | 224 | 235 |
| 0.3 | *** | 33856 | 35204 | 46677 | 9414 | 10069 | 11815 | 1819 | 1879 | 1962 | 504 | 513 | 518 | 238 | 243 | 243 |
| | *** | 34324 | 37340 | 52416 | 9684 | 10679 | 13219 | 1846 | 1915 | 2164 | 513 | 513 | 557 | 243 | 243 | 252 |
| 0.35 | *** | 35319 | 37088 | 51828 | 10005 | 10825 | 13072 | 1962 | 2039 | 2149 | 545 | 554 | 559 | 257 | 257 | 257 |
| | *** | 35933 | 39815 | 56620 | 10344 | 11595 | 14239 | 1998 | 2085 | 2313 | 545 | 554 | 588 | 257 | 257 | 263 |
| 0.4 | *** | 35603 | 37858 | 55705 | 10322 | 11298 | 14007 | 2058 | 2154 | 2278 | 568 | 573 | 587 | 265 | 265 | 265 |
| | *** | 36392 | 41185 | 59588 | 10720 | 12214 | 14950 | 2108 | 2209 | 2412 | 573 | 581 | 606 | 265 | 265 | 268 |
| 0.45 | *** | 34907 | 37679 | 58254 | 10399 | 11518 | 14612 | 2113 | 2218 | 2360 | 581 | 587 | 600 | 265 | 270 | 270 |
| | *** | 35905 | 41598 | 61319 | 10858 | 12558 | 15352 | 2163 | 2286 | 2461 | 581 | 595 | 613 | 265 | 270 | 268 |
| 0.5 | *** | 33444 | 36744 | 59478 | 10275 | 11504 | 14887 | 2121 | 2237 | 2388 | 581 | 587 | 600 | 265 | 265 | 265 |
| | *** | 34645 | 41177 | 61814 | 10784 | 12640 | 15445 | 2176 | 2305 | 2461 | 581 | 595 | 606 | 265 | 265 | 263 |
| 0.55 | *** | 31423 | 35204 | 59349 | 9978 | 11284 | 14818 | 2085 | 2204 | 2360 | 568 | 573 | 587 | 257 | 257 | 257 |
| | *** | 32830 | 40049 | 61072 | 10523 | 12475 | 15228 | 2140 | 2278 | 2412 | 568 | 581 | 588 | 257 | 257 | 252 |
| 0.6 | *** | 29016 | 33202 | 57878 | 9533 | 10872 | 14419 | 2011 | 2127 | 2278 | 540 | 545 | 559 | 238 | 243 | 243 |
| | *** | 30611 | 38311 | 59093 | 10088 | 12076 | 14703 | 2066 | 2195 | 2313 | 545 | 554 | 557 | 243 | 243 | 235 |
| 0.65 | *** | 26395 | 30823 | 55064 | 8947 | 10275 | 13685 | 1893 | 2003 | 2149 | 499 | 513 | 518 | 215 | 224 | 224 |
| | *** | 28109 | 36020 | 55878 | 9505 | 11444 | 13868 | 1943 | 2072 | 2164 | 504 | 513 | 514 | 224 | 224 | 213 |
| 0.7 | *** | 23645 | 28136 | 50920 | 8232 | 9491 | 12613 | 1736 | 1833 | 1962 | 449 | 458 | 463 | 196 | 196 | 196 |
| | *** | 25405 | 33215 | 51427 | 8763 | 10591 | 12724 | 1783 | 1893 | 1967 | 458 | 463 | 458 | 196 | 196 | 186 |
| 0.75 | *** | 20813 | 25144 | 45453 | 7388 | 8534 | 11210 | 1535 | 1618 | 1723 | 389 | 394 | 403 | 160 | 160 | 160 |
| | *** | 22532 | 29902 | 45739 | 7874 | 9497 | 11271 | 1577 | 1668 | 1719 | 389 | 394 | 390 | 160 | 160 | 153 |
| 0.8 | *** | 17865 | 21811 | 38674 | 6398 | 7374 | 9483 | 1296 | 1357 | 1434 | 312 | 320 | 320 | 128 | 128 | 128 |
| | *** | 19446 | 26010 | 38815 | 6815 | 8163 | 9509 | 1324 | 1393 | 1422 | 312 | 320 | 310 | 128 | 128 | 115 |
| 0.85 | *** | 14716 | 18044 | 30603 | 5234 | 5971 | 7434 | 999 | 1040 | 1090 | 224 | 224 | 229 | . | . | . |
| | *** | 16064 | 21432 | 30654 | 5559 | 6549 | 7438 | 1021 | 1063 | 1076 | 224 | 229 | 217 | . | . | . |
| 0.9 | *** | 11169 | 13589 | 21248 | 3826 | 4280 | 5064 | 655 | 669 | 691 | . | . | . | . | . | . |
| | *** | 12164 | 15913 | 21256 | 4033 | 4610 | 5058 | 664 | 683 | 681 | . | . | . | . | . | . |
| 0.95 | *** | 6705 | 7896 | 10633 | 2017 | 2168 | 2383 | . | . | . | . | . | . | . | . | . |
| | *** | 7214 | 8886 | 10622 | 2085 | 2264 | 2368 | . | . | . | . | . | . | . | . | . |
| 0.98 | *** | 2905 | 3199 | 3661 | . | . | . | . | . | . | . | . | . | . | . | . |
| | *** | 3034 | 3400 | 3648 | . | . | . | . | . | . | . | . | . | . | . | . |

TABLE 7: ALPHA= 0.05 POWER= 0.8 EXPECTED ACCRUAL THRU MINIMUM FOLLOW-UP= 6000

| | | DEL=.01 | | | DEL=.02 | | | DEL=.05 | | | DEL=.10 | | | DEL=.15 | | |
|---|---|---|---|---|---|---|---|---|---|---|---|---|---|---|---|---|
| FACT= | | 1.0 .75 | .50 .25 | .00 BIN | 1.0 .75 | .50 .25 | .00 BIN | 1.0 .75 | .50 .25 | .00 BIN | 1.0 75 | .50 .25 | .00 BIN | 1.0 .75 | .50 .25 | .00 BIN |
| PCONT=*** | | | | REQUIRED NUMBER OF PATIENTS | | | | | | | | | | | | |
| 0.01 | *** | 949 | 949 | 955 | 349 | 349 | 349 | 115 | 115 | 115 | 55 | 55 | 55 | 40 | 40 | 40 |
| | *** | 949 | 949 | 3648 | 349 | 349 | 1206 | 115 | 115 | 328 | 55 | 55 | 134 | 40 | 40 | 80 |
| 0.02 | *** | 2104 | 2110 | 2125 | 679 | 679 | 679 | 184 | 184 | 184 | 79 | 79 | 79 | 49 | 49 | 49 |
| | *** | 2110 | 2119 | 6022 | 679 | 679 | 1793 | 184 | 184 | 419 | 79 | 79 | 155 | 49 | 49 | 89 |
| 0.05 | *** | 6394 | 6460 | 6649 | 1825 | 1840 | 1864 | 394 | 394 | 394 | 139 | 139 | 139 | 79 | 79 | 79 |
| | *** | 6415 | 6529 | 12848 | 1834 | 1849 | 3481 | 394 | 394 | 681 | 139 | 139 | 217 | 79 | 79 | 115 |
| 0.1 | *** | 14125 | 14365 | 15469 | 3865 | 3949 | 4090 | 745 | 754 | 760 | 235 | 235 | 235 | 124 | 124 | 124 |
| | *** | 14215 | 14680 | 23235 | 3904 | 4009 | 6047 | 754 | 760 | 1076 | 235 | 235 | 310 | 124 | 124 | 153 |
| 0.15 | *** | 21154 | 21619 | 24439 | 5749 | 5944 | 6325 | 1084 | 1099 | 1114 | 319 | 319 | 319 | 160 | 160 | 160 |
| | *** | 21310 | 22294 | 32385 | 5830 | 6094 | 8304 | 1090 | 1105 | 1422 | 319 | 319 | 390 | 160 | 160 | 186 |
| 0.2 | *** | 26884 | 27619 | 32830 | 7330 | 7660 | 8410 | 1375 | 1405 | 1444 | 394 | 394 | 400 | 190 | 190 | 190 |
| | *** | 27139 | 28744 | 40298 | 7474 | 7945 | 10251 | 1390 | 1420 | 1719 | 394 | 400 | 458 | 190 | 190 | 213 |
| 0.25 | *** | 31150 | 32215 | 40309 | 8575 | 9064 | 10249 | 1630 | 1669 | 1720 | 454 | 460 | 469 | 220 | 220 | 220 |
| | *** | 31519 | 33859 | 46976 | 8779 | 9499 | 11890 | 1645 | 1699 | 1967 | 460 | 460 | 514 | 220 | 220 | 235 |
| 0.3 | *** | 33985 | 35434 | 46675 | 9490 | 10150 | 11815 | 1825 | 1885 | 1960 | 505 | 514 | 520 | 244 | 244 | 244 |
| | *** | 34489 | 37654 | 52416 | 9769 | 10744 | 13219 | 1855 | 1915 | 2164 | 505 | 514 | 557 | 244 | 244 | 252 |
| 0.35 | *** | 35485 | 37384 | 51829 | 10105 | 10930 | 13075 | 1975 | 2050 | 2149 | 544 | 550 | 559 | 250 | 259 | 259 |
| | *** | 36154 | 40210 | 56620 | 10444 | 11680 | 14239 | 2005 | 2095 | 2313 | 550 | 559 | 588 | 259 | 259 | 263 |
| 0.4 | *** | 35824 | 38224 | 55699 | 10444 | 11425 | 14005 | 2074 | 2164 | 2265 | 565 | 574 | 589 | 265 | 265 | 265 |
| | *** | 36670 | 41659 | 59588 | 10849 | 12319 | 14950 | 2119 | 2215 | 2412 | 574 | 580 | 606 | 265 | 265 | 268 |
| 0.45 | *** | 35185 | 38119 | 58255 | 10540 | 11659 | 14614 | 2125 | 2230 | 2359 | 580 | 589 | 595 | 265 | 265 | 274 |
| | *** | 36244 | 42139 | 61319 | 11005 | 12679 | 15352 | 2179 | 2290 | 2461 | 589 | 595 | 613 | 265 | 265 | 268 |
| 0.5 | *** | 33784 | 37249 | 59479 | 10429 | 11659 | 14884 | 2140 | 2245 | 2389 | 580 | 589 | 604 | 265 | 265 | 265 |
| | *** | 35059 | 41779 | 61814 | 10939 | 12769 | 15445 | 2185 | 2314 | 2461 | 580 | 595 | 606 | 265 | 265 | 263 |
| 0.55 | *** | 31819 | 35770 | 59350 | 10144 | 11440 | 14824 | 2104 | 2215 | 2365 | 565 | 574 | 589 | 250 | 259 | 259 |
| | *** | 33304 | 40699 | 61072 | 10690 | 12610 | 15228 | 2155 | 2284 | 2412 | 574 | 580 | 588 | 259 | 259 | 252 |
| 0.6 | *** | 29479 | 33805 | 57874 | 9700 | 11029 | 14419 | 2029 | 2140 | 2284 | 544 | 550 | 559 | 244 | 244 | 244 |
| | *** | 31135 | 38980 | 59093 | 10255 | 12205 | 14703 | 2080 | 2200 | 2313 | 544 | 559 | 557 | 244 | 244 | 235 |
| 0.65 | *** | 26890 | 31444 | 55060 | 9115 | 10429 | 13684 | 1909 | 2014 | 2149 | 505 | 514 | 520 | 220 | 220 | 220 |
| | *** | 28660 | 36694 | 55878 | 9670 | 11575 | 13868 | 1960 | 2074 | 2164 | 505 | 514 | 514 | 220 | 220 | 213 |
| 0.7 | *** | 24160 | 28750 | 50920 | 8395 | 9640 | 12610 | 1750 | 1840 | 1960 | 454 | 460 | 469 | 190 | 199 | 199 |
| | *** | 25969 | 33874 | 51427 | 8920 | 10705 | 12727 | 1795 | 1900 | 1967 | 454 | 460 | 458 | 190 | 199 | 186 |
| 0.75 | *** | 21319 | 25729 | 45454 | 7534 | 8665 | 11215 | 1549 | 1624 | 1720 | 385 | 394 | 400 | 160 | 160 | 160 |
| | *** | 23074 | 30499 | 45739 | 8020 | 9604 | 11271 | 1585 | 1669 | 1719 | 394 | 394 | 390 | 160 | 160 | 153 |
| 0.8 | *** | 18334 | 22339 | 38674 | 6529 | 7480 | 9484 | 1300 | 1360 | 1429 | 310 | 319 | 319 | 124 | 124 | 124 |
| | *** | 19945 | 26530 | 38815 | 6940 | 8245 | 9509 | 1330 | 1390 | 1422 | 319 | 319 | 310 | 124 | 124 | 115 |
| 0.85 | *** | 15115 | 18469 | 30604 | 5335 | 6055 | 7435 | 1009 | 1045 | 1084 | 220 | 229 | 229 | . | . | . |
| | *** | 16480 | 21844 | 30654 | 5650 | 6604 | 7438 | 1024 | 1060 | 1076 | 229 | 229 | 217 | . | . | . |
| 0.9 | *** | 11464 | 13894 | 21250 | 3889 | 4330 | 5065 | 655 | 670 | 694 | . | . | . | . | . | . |
| | *** | 12469 | 16180 | 21256 | 4084 | 4639 | 5058 | 664 | 685 | 681 | . | . | . | . | . | . |
| 0.95 | *** | 6865 | 8035 | 10630 | 2044 | 2185 | 2380 | . | . | . | . | . | . | . | . | . |
| | *** | 7369 | 8995 | 10622 | 2110 | 2275 | 2368 | . | . | . | . | . | . | . | . | . |
| 0.98 | *** | 2944 | 3229 | 3664 | . | . | . | . | . | . | . | . | . | . | . | . |
| | *** | 3079 | 3415 | 3648 | . | . | . | . | . | . | . | . | . | . | . | . |

TABLE 7: ALPHA= 0.05 POWER= 0.8     EXPECTED ACCRUAL THRU MINIMUM FOLLOW-UP= 6500

| | | DEL=.01 | | | DEL=.02 | | | DEL=.05 | | | DEL=.10 | | | DEL=.15 | | |
|---|---|---|---|---|---|---|---|---|---|---|---|---|---|---|---|---|
| FACT= | | 1.0 .75 | .50 .25 | .00 BIN | 1.0 .75 | .50 .25 | .00 BIN | 1.0 .75 | .50 .25 | .00 BIN | 1.0 75 | .50 .25 | .00 BIN | 1.0 .75 | .50 .25 | .00 BIN |
| PCONT=*** | | | | | REQUIRED NUMBER OF PATIENTS | | | | | | | | | | | |
| 0.01 | *** | 947 | 953 | 953 | 346 | 346 | 346 | 118 | 118 | 118 | 59 | 59 | 59 | 43 | 43 | 43 |
| | *** | 947 | 953 | 3648 | 346 | 346 | 1206 | 118 | 118 | 328 | 59 | 59 | 134 | 43 | 43 | 80 |
| 0.02 | *** | 2107 | 2117 | 2123 | 677 | 677 | 677 | 183 | 183 | 183 | 76 | 76 | 76 | 53 | 53 | 53 |
| | *** | 2107 | 2123 | 6022 | 677 | 677 | 1793 | 183 | 183 | 419 | 76 | 76 | 155 | 53 | 53 | 89 |
| 0.05 | *** | 6397 | 6472 | 6651 | 1825 | 1841 | 1863 | 395 | 395 | 395 | 141 | 141 | 141 | 86 | 86 | 86 |
| | *** | 6429 | 6537 | 12848 | 1831 | 1847 | 3481 | 395 | 395 | 681 | 141 | 141 | 217 | 86 | 86 | 115 |
| 0.1 | *** | 14148 | 14402 | 15475 | 3878 | 3959 | 4089 | 752 | 752 | 758 | 232 | 232 | 232 | 124 | 124 | 124 |
| | *** | 14240 | 14717 | 23235 | 3911 | 4018 | 6047 | 752 | 758 | 1076 | 232 | 232 | 310 | 124 | 124 | 153 |
| 0.15 | *** | 21195 | 21688 | 24434 | 5773 | 5958 | 6326 | 1083 | 1099 | 1116 | 319 | 319 | 319 | 157 | 157 | 157 |
| | *** | 21363 | 22381 | 32385 | 5855 | 6115 | 8304 | 1093 | 1110 | 1422 | 319 | 319 | 390 | 157 | 157 | 186 |
| 0.2 | *** | 26947 | 27727 | 32836 | 7372 | 7697 | 8406 | 1386 | 1408 | 1441 | 395 | 395 | 401 | 189 | 189 | 189 |
| | *** | 27223 | 28887 | 40298 | 7512 | 7973 | 10251 | 1392 | 1424 | 1719 | 395 | 395 | 458 | 189 | 189 | 213 |
| 0.25 | *** | 31243 | 32381 | 40311 | 8633 | 9121 | 10248 | 1636 | 1678 | 1727 | 460 | 460 | 466 | 222 | 222 | 222 |
| | *** | 31643 | 34071 | 46976 | 8834 | 9543 | 11890 | 1652 | 1695 | 1967 | 460 | 460 | 514 | 222 | 222 | 235 |
| 0.3 | *** | 34113 | 35657 | 46675 | 9566 | 10226 | 11818 | 1831 | 1890 | 1961 | 508 | 514 | 514 | 238 | 238 | 238 |
| | *** | 34650 | 37938 | 52416 | 9842 | 10801 | 13219 | 1857 | 1922 | 2164 | 508 | 514 | 557 | 238 | 238 | 252 |
| 0.35 | *** | 35657 | 37672 | 51832 | 10199 | 11022 | 13070 | 1987 | 2058 | 2150 | 547 | 547 | 557 | 254 | 254 | 254 |
| | *** | 36362 | 40571 | 56620 | 10541 | 11753 | 14239 | 2020 | 2101 | 2313 | 547 | 557 | 588 | 254 | 254 | 263 |
| 0.4 | *** | 36037 | 38572 | 55699 | 10551 | 11532 | 14012 | 2085 | 2172 | 2280 | 573 | 579 | 590 | 265 | 265 | 265 |
| | *** | 36947 | 42098 | 59588 | 10963 | 12409 | 14950 | 2123 | 2221 | 2412 | 573 | 579 | 606 | 265 | 265 | 268 |
| 0.45 | *** | 35462 | 38539 | 58261 | 10665 | 11786 | 14613 | 2139 | 2237 | 2361 | 579 | 590 | 596 | 265 | 271 | 271 |
| | *** | 36583 | 42645 | 61319 | 11136 | 12777 | 15352 | 2188 | 2296 | 2461 | 590 | 596 | 613 | 265 | 271 | 268 |
| 0.5 | *** | 34113 | 37727 | 59480 | 10573 | 11792 | 14890 | 2150 | 2253 | 2393 | 579 | 590 | 596 | 265 | 265 | 265 |
| | *** | 35462 | 42342 | 61814 | 11087 | 12881 | 15445 | 2198 | 2318 | 2461 | 590 | 596 | 606 | 265 | 265 | 263 |
| 0.55 | *** | 32212 | 36297 | 59350 | 10291 | 11591 | 14825 | 2117 | 2221 | 2361 | 563 | 579 | 590 | 254 | 254 | 254 |
| | *** | 33756 | 41302 | 61072 | 10843 | 12728 | 15228 | 2166 | 2286 | 2412 | 573 | 579 | 588 | 254 | 254 | 252 |
| 0.6 | *** | 29911 | 34373 | 57877 | 9852 | 11174 | 14418 | 2042 | 2150 | 2280 | 541 | 547 | 557 | 238 | 238 | 248 |
| | *** | 31633 | 39606 | 59093 | 10411 | 12328 | 14703 | 2091 | 2204 | 2313 | 547 | 557 | 557 | 238 | 238 | 235 |
| 0.65 | *** | 27370 | 32023 | 55066 | 9267 | 10573 | 13677 | 1922 | 2020 | 2150 | 508 | 508 | 525 | 222 | 222 | 222 |
| | *** | 29190 | 37321 | 55878 | 9826 | 11688 | 13868 | 1971 | 2085 | 2164 | 508 | 514 | 514 | 222 | 222 | 213 |
| 0.7 | *** | 24646 | 29326 | 50916 | 8542 | 9777 | 12615 | 1766 | 1847 | 1961 | 449 | 460 | 466 | 189 | 200 | 200 |
| | *** | 26498 | 34471 | 51427 | 9072 | 10811 | 12724 | 1808 | 1906 | 1967 | 460 | 466 | 458 | 189 | 200 | 186 |
| 0.75 | *** | 21796 | 26265 | 45446 | 7675 | 8786 | 11217 | 1565 | 1630 | 1717 | 384 | 395 | 401 | 167 | 167 | 167 |
| | *** | 23583 | 31048 | 45739 | 8152 | 9696 | 11271 | 1597 | 1678 | 1719 | 395 | 395 | 390 | 167 | 167 | 153 |
| 0.8 | *** | 18773 | 22820 | 38669 | 6641 | 7577 | 9484 | 1311 | 1370 | 1435 | 313 | 319 | 319 | 124 | 124 | 124 |
| | *** | 20404 | 27012 | 38815 | 7047 | 8314 | 9509 | 1337 | 1392 | 1422 | 313 | 319 | 310 | 124 | 124 | 115 |
| 0.85 | *** | 15491 | 18871 | 30603 | 5422 | 6131 | 7437 | 1012 | 1045 | 1083 | 222 | 222 | 232 | . | . | . |
| | *** | 16872 | 22218 | 30654 | 5731 | 6657 | 7438 | 1028 | 1067 | 1076 | 222 | 232 | 217 | . | . | . |
| 0.9 | *** | 11743 | 14164 | 21249 | 3943 | 4376 | 5064 | 661 | 677 | 693 | . | . | . | . | . | . |
| | *** | 12751 | 16423 | 21256 | 4138 | 4668 | 5058 | 671 | 687 | 681 | . | . | . | . | . | . |
| 0.95 | *** | 7008 | 8152 | 10632 | 2058 | 2198 | 2377 | . | . | . | . | . | . | . | . | . |
| | *** | 7502 | 9088 | 10622 | 2123 | 2280 | 2368 | . | . | . | . | . | . | . | . | . |
| 0.98 | *** | 2984 | 3255 | 3661 | . | . | . | . | . | . | . | . | . | . | . | . |
| | *** | 3108 | 3433 | 3648 | . | . | . | . | . | . | . | . | . | . | . | . |

TABLE 7: ALPHA= 0.05  POWER= 0.8  EXPECTED ACCRUAL THRU MINIMUM FOLLOW-UP= 7000

| | | DEL=.01 | | | DEL=.02 | | | DEL=.05 | | | DEL=.10 | | | DEL=.15 | | |
|---|---|---|---|---|---|---|---|---|---|---|---|---|---|---|---|---|---|
| FACT= | | 1.0 .75 | .50 .25 | .00 BIN | 1.0 .75 | .50 .25 | .00 BIN | 1.0 .75 | .50 .25 | .00 BIN | 1.0 75 | .50 .25 | .00 BIN | 1.0 .75 | .50 .25 | .00 BIN |
| PCONT=*** | | | | REQUIRED NUMBER OF PATIENTS | | | | | | | | | | | | |
| 0.01 | *** | 950 | 950 | 950 | 344 | 344 | 344 | 116 | 116 | 116 | 57 | 57 | 57 | 40 | 40 | 40 |
| | *** | 950 | 950 | 3648 | 344 | 344 | 1206 | 116 | 116 | 328 | 57 | 57 | 134 | 40 | 40 | 80 |
| 0.02 | *** | 2105 | 2111 | 2129 | 676 | 676 | 676 | 180 | 180 | 180 | 81 | 81 | 81 | 46 | 46 | 46 |
| | *** | 2111 | 2122 | 6022 | 676 | 676 | 1793 | 180 | 180 | 419 | 81 | 81 | 155 | 46 | 46 | 89 |
| 0.05 | *** | 6410 | 6480 | 6644 | 1831 | 1842 | 1860 | 390 | 390 | 396 | 134 | 145 | 145 | 81 | 81 | 81 |
| | *** | 6434 | 6539 | 12848 | 1831 | 1849 | 3481 | 390 | 396 | 681 | 134 | 145 | 217 | 81 | 81 | 115 |
| 0.1 | *** | 14169 | 14431 | 15475 | 3890 | 3966 | 4089 | 746 | 757 | 764 | 232 | 232 | 232 | 127 | 127 | 127 |
| | *** | 14267 | 14757 | 23235 | 3925 | 4019 | 6047 | 757 | 757 | 1076 | 232 | 232 | 310 | 127 | 127 | 153 |
| 0.15 | *** | 21232 | 21757 | 24435 | 5797 | 5979 | 6329 | 1090 | 1096 | 1114 | 320 | 320 | 320 | 162 | 162 | 162 |
| | *** | 21414 | 22457 | 32385 | 5874 | 6119 | 8304 | 1096 | 1107 | 1422 | 320 | 320 | 390 | 162 | 162 | 186 |
| 0.2 | *** | 27007 | 27836 | 32835 | 7407 | 7729 | 8405 | 1387 | 1411 | 1440 | 396 | 396 | 396 | 197 | 197 | 197 |
| | *** | 27305 | 29026 | 40298 | 7547 | 8002 | 10251 | 1394 | 1422 | 1719 | 396 | 396 | 458 | 197 | 197 | 213 |
| 0.25 | *** | 31336 | 32537 | 40307 | 8685 | 9175 | 10249 | 1639 | 1674 | 1720 | 460 | 460 | 466 | 221 | 221 | 221 |
| | *** | 31756 | 34276 | 46976 | 8895 | 9584 | 11890 | 1656 | 1702 | 1967 | 460 | 460 | 514 | 221 | 221 | 235 |
| 0.3 | *** | 34235 | 35869 | 46677 | 9636 | 10295 | 11817 | 1842 | 1895 | 1954 | 512 | 512 | 519 | 239 | 239 | 239 |
| | *** | 34812 | 38214 | 52416 | 9910 | 10861 | 13219 | 1866 | 1930 | 2164 | 512 | 512 | 557 | 239 | 239 | 252 |
| 0.35 | *** | 35816 | 37945 | 51829 | 10284 | 11106 | 13077 | 1989 | 2059 | 2146 | 547 | 554 | 554 | 256 | 256 | 256 |
| | *** | 36580 | 40920 | 56620 | 10627 | 11824 | 14239 | 2024 | 2105 | 2313 | 547 | 554 | 588 | 256 | 256 | 263 |
| 0.4 | *** | 36254 | 38907 | 55696 | 10662 | 11631 | 14005 | 2094 | 2175 | 2280 | 571 | 582 | 582 | 267 | 267 | 267 |
| | *** | 37216 | 42512 | 59588 | 11065 | 12489 | 14950 | 2140 | 2227 | 2412 | 571 | 582 | 606 | 267 | 267 | 268 |
| 0.45 | *** | 35722 | 38931 | 58251 | 10785 | 11894 | 14617 | 2157 | 2245 | 2356 | 582 | 589 | 600 | 267 | 267 | 267 |
| | *** | 36901 | 43114 | 61319 | 11257 | 12874 | 15352 | 2199 | 2297 | 2461 | 589 | 600 | 613 | 267 | 267 | 268 |
| 0.5 | *** | 34434 | 38190 | 59476 | 10704 | 11922 | 14886 | 2164 | 2262 | 2391 | 582 | 589 | 600 | 267 | 267 | 267 |
| | *** | 35845 | 42869 | 61814 | 11211 | 12979 | 15445 | 2210 | 2321 | 2461 | 589 | 600 | 606 | 267 | 267 | 263 |
| 0.55 | *** | 32590 | 36796 | 59347 | 10435 | 11719 | 14816 | 2129 | 2234 | 2367 | 571 | 582 | 589 | 256 | 256 | 256 |
| | *** | 34189 | 41865 | 61072 | 10977 | 12832 | 15228 | 2181 | 2297 | 2412 | 571 | 582 | 588 | 256 | 256 | 252 |
| 0.6 | *** | 30339 | 34900 | 57877 | 9997 | 11310 | 14414 | 2059 | 2157 | 2280 | 547 | 554 | 565 | 239 | 239 | 239 |
| | *** | 32106 | 40185 | 59093 | 10557 | 12430 | 14703 | 2105 | 2216 | 2313 | 547 | 554 | 557 | 239 | 239 | 235 |
| 0.65 | *** | 27819 | 32572 | 55066 | 9409 | 10704 | 13679 | 1936 | 2035 | 2146 | 501 | 512 | 519 | 221 | 221 | 221 |
| | *** | 29685 | 37892 | 55878 | 9962 | 11789 | 13868 | 1982 | 2087 | 2164 | 512 | 512 | 514 | 221 | 221 | 213 |
| 0.7 | *** | 25106 | 29860 | 50919 | 8674 | 9899 | 12611 | 1772 | 1860 | 1965 | 449 | 460 | 466 | 197 | 197 | 197 |
| | *** | 26996 | 35022 | 51427 | 9199 | 10907 | 12724 | 1814 | 1901 | 1967 | 460 | 460 | 458 | 197 | 197 | 186 |
| 0.75 | *** | 22247 | 26769 | 45452 | 7799 | 8895 | 11211 | 1569 | 1639 | 1720 | 390 | 396 | 396 | 162 | 162 | 162 |
| | *** | 24056 | 31557 | 45739 | 8271 | 9776 | 11271 | 1604 | 1674 | 1719 | 390 | 396 | 390 | 162 | 162 | 153 |
| 0.8 | *** | 19185 | 23269 | 38669 | 6749 | 7670 | 9490 | 1317 | 1370 | 1429 | 309 | 320 | 320 | 127 | 127 | 127 |
| | *** | 20836 | 27445 | 38815 | 7151 | 8387 | 9509 | 1341 | 1394 | 1422 | 320 | 320 | 310 | 127 | 127 | 115 |
| 0.85 | *** | 15842 | 19237 | 30601 | 5506 | 6189 | 7431 | 1020 | 1055 | 1090 | 221 | 221 | 232 | . | . | . |
| | *** | 17231 | 22551 | 30654 | 5815 | 6696 | 7438 | 1037 | 1072 | 1076 | 221 | 232 | 217 | . | . | . |
| 0.9 | *** | 11999 | 14425 | 21250 | 3995 | 4415 | 5062 | 659 | 676 | 694 | . | . | . | . | . | . |
| | *** | 13014 | 16636 | 21256 | 4187 | 4695 | 5058 | 670 | 687 | 681 | . | . | . | . | . | . |
| 0.95 | *** | 7134 | 8265 | 10634 | 2076 | 2210 | 2374 | . | . | . | . | . | . | . | . | . |
| | *** | 7624 | 9175 | 10622 | 2140 | 2286 | 2368 | . | . | . | . | . | . | . | . | . |
| 0.98 | *** | 3015 | 3277 | 3662 | . | . | . | . | . | . | . | . | . | . | . | . |
| | *** | 3137 | 3452 | 3648 | . | . | . | . | . | . | . | . | . | . | . | . |

TABLE 7: ALPHA= 0.05  POWER= 0.8    EXPECTED ACCRUAL THRU MINIMUM FOLLOW-UP= 7500

REQUIRED NUMBER OF PATIENTS

| PCONT=*** | FACT= | DEL=.01 1.0/.75 | DEL=.01 .50/.25 | DEL=.01 .00/BIN | DEL=.02 1.0/.75 | DEL=.02 .50/.25 | DEL=.02 .00/BIN | DEL=.05 1.0/.75 | DEL=.05 .50/.25 | DEL=.05 .00/BIN | DEL=.10 1.0/75 | DEL=.10 .50/.25 | DEL=.10 .00/BIN | DEL=.15 1.0/.75 | DEL=.15 .50/.25 | DEL=.15 .00/BIN |
|---|---|---|---|---|---|---|---|---|---|---|---|---|---|---|---|---|
| 0.01 | *** | 950 | 950 | 950 | 350 | 350 | 350 | 118 | 118 | 118 | 61 | 61 | 61 | 43 | 43 | 43 |
|  | *** | 950 | 950 | 3648 | 350 | 350 | 1206 | 118 | 118 | 328 | 61 | 61 | 134 | 43 | 43 | 80 |
| 0.02 | *** | 2105 | 2112 | 2124 | 680 | 680 | 680 | 181 | 181 | 181 | 80 | 80 | 80 | 50 | 50 | 50 |
|  | *** | 2112 | 2124 | 6022 | 680 | 680 | 1793 | 181 | 181 | 419 | 80 | 80 | 155 | 50 | 50 | 89 |
| 0.05 | *** | 6406 | 6481 | 6643 | 1831 | 1843 | 1861 | 387 | 399 | 399 | 136 | 136 | 136 | 80 | 80 | 80 |
|  | *** | 6443 | 6549 | 12848 | 1831 | 1850 | 3481 | 387 | 399 | 681 | 136 | 136 | 217 | 80 | 80 | 115 |
| 0.1 | *** | 14187 | 14468 | 15474 | 3893 | 3968 | 4093 | 755 | 755 | 762 | 230 | 237 | 237 | 125 | 125 | 125 |
|  | *** | 14293 | 14780 | 23235 | 3931 | 4025 | 6047 | 755 | 755 | 1076 | 230 | 237 | 310 | 125 | 125 | 153 |
| 0.15 | *** | 21275 | 21818 | 24436 | 5818 | 5993 | 6324 | 1093 | 1100 | 1118 | 324 | 324 | 324 | 162 | 162 | 162 |
|  | *** | 21474 | 22531 | 32385 | 5893 | 6136 | 8304 | 1093 | 1111 | 1422 | 324 | 324 | 390 | 162 | 162 | 186 |
| 0.2 | *** | 27068 | 27943 | 32836 | 7437 | 7756 | 8405 | 1393 | 1411 | 1437 | 399 | 399 | 399 | 193 | 193 | 193 |
|  | *** | 27380 | 29150 | 40298 | 7580 | 8018 | 10251 | 1400 | 1430 | 1719 | 399 | 399 | 458 | 193 | 193 | 213 |
| 0.25 | *** | 31430 | 32686 | 40306 | 8731 | 9218 | 10250 | 1643 | 1681 | 1718 | 455 | 462 | 462 | 218 | 218 | 218 |
|  | *** | 31880 | 34468 | 46976 | 8937 | 9612 | 11890 | 1662 | 1700 | 1967 | 462 | 462 | 514 | 218 | 218 | 235 |
| 0.3 | *** | 34362 | 36080 | 46674 | 9706 | 10355 | 11818 | 1850 | 1899 | 1962 | 511 | 511 | 518 | 237 | 237 | 237 |
|  | *** | 34974 | 38468 | 52416 | 9980 | 10906 | 13219 | 1868 | 1925 | 2164 | 511 | 518 | 557 | 237 | 237 | 252 |
| 0.35 | *** | 35986 | 38206 | 51830 | 10362 | 11187 | 13074 | 2000 | 2068 | 2143 | 549 | 549 | 556 | 256 | 256 | 256 |
|  | *** | 36781 | 41236 | 56620 | 10711 | 11881 | 14239 | 2030 | 2105 | 2313 | 549 | 556 | 588 | 256 | 256 | 263 |
| 0.4 | *** | 36462 | 39237 | 55700 | 10756 | 11731 | 14011 | 2105 | 2187 | 2281 | 575 | 575 | 586 | 268 | 268 | 268 |
|  | *** | 37475 | 42893 | 59588 | 11168 | 12568 | 14950 | 2143 | 2225 | 2412 | 575 | 586 | 606 | 268 | 268 | 268 |
| 0.45 | *** | 35986 | 39324 | 58261 | 10899 | 12005 | 14611 | 2168 | 2255 | 2356 | 586 | 593 | 593 | 268 | 268 | 268 |
|  | *** | 37224 | 43561 | 61319 | 11368 | 12950 | 15352 | 2206 | 2300 | 2461 | 586 | 593 | 613 | 268 | 268 | 268 |
| 0.5 | *** | 34756 | 38618 | 59480 | 10824 | 12043 | 14881 | 2180 | 2274 | 2386 | 586 | 593 | 605 | 268 | 268 | 268 |
|  | *** | 36211 | 43355 | 61814 | 11337 | 13074 | 15445 | 2225 | 2330 | 2461 | 586 | 593 | 606 | 268 | 268 | 263 |
| 0.55 | *** | 32949 | 37280 | 59349 | 10561 | 11843 | 14818 | 2143 | 2243 | 2368 | 568 | 575 | 586 | 256 | 256 | 256 |
|  | *** | 34606 | 42380 | 61072 | 11105 | 12924 | 15228 | 2187 | 2300 | 2412 | 575 | 586 | 588 | 256 | 256 | 252 |
| 0.6 | *** | 30743 | 35405 | 57875 | 10130 | 11431 | 14412 | 2068 | 2161 | 2281 | 549 | 549 | 556 | 237 | 237 | 249 |
|  | *** | 32555 | 40718 | 59093 | 10693 | 12530 | 14703 | 2112 | 2218 | 2313 | 549 | 556 | 557 | 237 | 237 | 235 |
| 0.65 | *** | 28250 | 33087 | 55062 | 9549 | 10824 | 13681 | 1943 | 2037 | 2150 | 500 | 511 | 518 | 218 | 218 | 218 |
|  | *** | 30155 | 38431 | 55878 | 10093 | 11881 | 13868 | 1993 | 2086 | 2164 | 511 | 518 | 514 | 218 | 218 | 213 |
| 0.7 | *** | 25550 | 30368 | 50918 | 8806 | 10018 | 12612 | 1786 | 1861 | 1962 | 455 | 462 | 462 | 193 | 193 | 193 |
|  | *** | 27474 | 35536 | 51427 | 9324 | 10993 | 12724 | 1824 | 1906 | 1967 | 455 | 462 | 458 | 193 | 193 | 186 |
| 0.75 | *** | 22674 | 27249 | 45455 | 7918 | 8993 | 11218 | 1580 | 1643 | 1718 | 387 | 399 | 399 | 162 | 162 | 162 |
|  | *** | 24511 | 32030 | 45739 | 8386 | 9849 | 11271 | 1606 | 1681 | 1719 | 387 | 399 | 390 | 162 | 162 | 153 |
| 0.8 | *** | 19568 | 23686 | 38675 | 6849 | 7749 | 9481 | 1325 | 1374 | 1430 | 312 | 312 | 324 | 125 | 125 | 125 |
|  | *** | 21249 | 27849 | 38815 | 7243 | 8443 | 9509 | 1343 | 1400 | 1422 | 312 | 324 | 310 | 125 | 125 | 115 |
| 0.85 | *** | 16175 | 19568 | 30605 | 5581 | 6256 | 7437 | 1025 | 1055 | 1081 | 230 | 230 | 230 | . | . | . |
|  | *** | 17574 | 22868 | 30654 | 5881 | 6743 | 7438 | 1036 | 1074 | 1076 | 230 | 230 | 217 | . | . | . |
| 0.9 | *** | 12249 | 14656 | 21249 | 4043 | 4449 | 5068 | 661 | 680 | 687 | . | . | . | . | . | . |
|  | *** | 13250 | 16843 | 21256 | 4224 | 4711 | 5058 | 668 | 687 | 681 | . | . | . | . | . | . |
| 0.95 | *** | 7250 | 8368 | 10636 | 2093 | 2218 | 2375 | . | . | . | . | . | . | . | . | . |
|  | *** | 7737 | 9249 | 10622 | 2150 | 2293 | 2368 | . | . | . | . | . | . | . | . | . |
| 0.98 | *** | 3050 | 3305 | 3661 | . | . | . | . | . | . | . | . | . | . | . | . |
|  | *** | 3162 | 3462 | 3648 | . | . | . | . | . | . | . | . | . | . | . | . |

TABLE 7: ALPHA= 0.05  POWER= 0.8    EXPECTED ACCRUAL THRU MINIMUM FOLLOW-UP= 8000

| | | DEL=.01 | | | DEL=.02 | | | DEL=.05 | | | DEL=.10 | | | DEL=.15 | | |
|---|---|---|---|---|---|---|---|---|---|---|---|---|---|---|---|---|---|
| FACT= | | 1.0 .75 | .50 .25 | .00 BIN | 1.0 .75 | .50 .25 | .00 BIN | 1.0 .75 | .50 .25 | .00 BIN | 1.0 75 | .50 .25 | .00 BIN | 1.0 .75 | .50 .25 | .00 BIN |
| PCONT=*** | | | | REQUIRED NUMBER OF PATIENTS | | | | | | | | | | | | |
| 0.01 | *** | 953 | 953 | 953 | 345 | 345 | 345 | 113 | 113 | 113 | 53 | 53 | 53 | 45 | 45 | 45 |
| | *** | 953 | 953 | 3648 | 345 | 345 | 1206 | 113 | 113 | 328 | 53 | 53 | 134 | 45 | 45 | 80 |
| 0.02 | *** | 2105 | 2113 | 2125 | 673 | 673 | 673 | 185 | 185 | 185 | 73 | 73 | 73 | 53 | 53 | 53 |
| | *** | 2113 | 2125 | 6022 | 673 | 673 | 1793 | 185 | 185 | 419 | 73 | 73 | 155 | 53 | 53 | 89 |
| 0.05 | *** | 6413 | 6493 | 6645 | 1833 | 1845 | 1865 | 393 | 393 | 393 | 133 | 145 | 145 | 85 | 85 | 85 |
| | *** | 6445 | 6553 | 12848 | 1833 | 1853 | 3481 | 393 | 393 | 681 | 133 | 145 | 217 | 85 | 85 | 115 |
| 0.1 | *** | 14213 | 14493 | 15473 | 3905 | 3973 | 4093 | 753 | 753 | 765 | 233 | 233 | 233 | 125 | 125 | 125 |
| | *** | 14325 | 14813 | 23235 | 3933 | 4025 | 6047 | 753 | 753 | 1076 | 233 | 233 | 310 | 125 | 125 | 153 |
| 0.15 | *** | 21313 | 21873 | 24433 | 5833 | 6013 | 6325 | 1093 | 1105 | 1113 | 313 | 325 | 325 | 165 | 165 | 165 |
| | *** | 21513 | 22593 | 32385 | 5913 | 6145 | 8304 | 1093 | 1105 | 1422 | 325 | 325 | 390 | 165 | 165 | 186 |
| 0.2 | *** | 27133 | 28045 | 32833 | 7473 | 7785 | 8405 | 1393 | 1413 | 1445 | 393 | 393 | 393 | 193 | 193 | 193 |
| | *** | 27465 | 29273 | 40298 | 7605 | 8033 | 10251 | 1405 | 1425 | 1719 | 393 | 393 | 458 | 193 | 193 | 213 |
| 0.25 | *** | 31513 | 32833 | 40305 | 8785 | 9253 | 10253 | 1645 | 1685 | 1725 | 453 | 465 | 465 | 225 | 225 | 225 |
| | *** | 31993 | 34645 | 46976 | 8985 | 9645 | 11890 | 1665 | 1705 | 1967 | 465 | 465 | 514 | 225 | 225 | 235 |
| 0.3 | *** | 34485 | 36273 | 46673 | 9765 | 10413 | 11813 | 1853 | 1905 | 1953 | 505 | 513 | 513 | 245 | 245 | 245 |
| | *** | 35125 | 38705 | 52416 | 10045 | 10953 | 13219 | 1873 | 1925 | 2164 | 513 | 513 | 557 | 245 | 245 | 252 |
| 0.35 | *** | 36153 | 38465 | 51833 | 10445 | 11253 | 13073 | 2005 | 2073 | 2145 | 545 | 553 | 553 | 253 | 253 | 253 |
| | *** | 36985 | 41545 | 56620 | 10785 | 11945 | 14239 | 2033 | 2105 | 2313 | 553 | 553 | 588 | 253 | 253 | 263 |
| 0.4 | *** | 36673 | 39545 | 55705 | 10845 | 11813 | 14005 | 2113 | 2185 | 2285 | 573 | 573 | 585 | 265 | 265 | 265 |
| | *** | 37733 | 43253 | 59588 | 11253 | 12633 | 14950 | 2153 | 2233 | 2412 | 573 | 585 | 606 | 265 | 265 | 268 |
| 0.45 | *** | 36245 | 39685 | 58253 | 11005 | 12105 | 14613 | 2173 | 2253 | 2365 | 585 | 593 | 593 | 265 | 265 | 273 |
| | *** | 37533 | 43973 | 61319 | 11473 | 13033 | 15352 | 2213 | 2305 | 2461 | 585 | 593 | 613 | 265 | 265 | 268 |
| 0.5 | *** | 35065 | 39033 | 59473 | 10945 | 12145 | 14885 | 2185 | 2273 | 2385 | 585 | 593 | 605 | 265 | 265 | 265 |
| | *** | 36573 | 43813 | 61814 | 11453 | 13153 | 15445 | 2233 | 2325 | 2461 | 585 | 593 | 606 | 265 | 265 | 263 |
| 0.55 | *** | 33305 | 37733 | 59345 | 10685 | 11953 | 14825 | 2153 | 2245 | 2365 | 573 | 573 | 585 | 253 | 253 | 253 |
| | *** | 35013 | 42865 | 61072 | 11225 | 13013 | 15228 | 2193 | 2305 | 2412 | 573 | 585 | 588 | 253 | 253 | 252 |
| 0.6 | *** | 31133 | 35885 | 57873 | 10253 | 11545 | 14413 | 2073 | 2165 | 2285 | 545 | 553 | 565 | 245 | 245 | 245 |
| | *** | 32993 | 41225 | 59093 | 10813 | 12613 | 14703 | 2125 | 2225 | 2313 | 545 | 553 | 557 | 245 | 245 | 235 |
| 0.65 | *** | 28665 | 33573 | 55065 | 9665 | 10933 | 13685 | 1953 | 2045 | 2145 | 505 | 513 | 525 | 225 | 225 | 225 |
| | *** | 30605 | 38925 | 55878 | 10213 | 11965 | 13868 | 1993 | 2093 | 2164 | 513 | 513 | 514 | 225 | 225 | 213 |
| 0.7 | *** | 25973 | 30845 | 50913 | 8925 | 10113 | 12613 | 1793 | 1873 | 1965 | 453 | 465 | 465 | 193 | 193 | 193 |
| | *** | 27913 | 36013 | 51427 | 9445 | 11065 | 12724 | 1833 | 1913 | 1967 | 453 | 465 | 458 | 193 | 193 | 186 |
| 0.75 | *** | 23073 | 27693 | 45453 | 8025 | 9085 | 11213 | 1585 | 1645 | 1725 | 393 | 393 | 405 | 165 | 165 | 165 |
| | *** | 24933 | 32453 | 45739 | 8485 | 9913 | 11271 | 1613 | 1685 | 1719 | 393 | 393 | 390 | 165 | 165 | 153 |
| 0.8 | *** | 19945 | 24085 | 38673 | 6945 | 7825 | 9485 | 1333 | 1373 | 1433 | 313 | 313 | 325 | 125 | 125 | 125 |
| | *** | 21625 | 28213 | 38815 | 7333 | 8493 | 9509 | 1353 | 1405 | 1422 | 313 | 313 | 310 | 125 | 125 | 115 |
| 0.85 | *** | 16485 | 19893 | 30605 | 5653 | 6305 | 7433 | 1025 | 1053 | 1085 | 225 | 225 | 225 | . | . | . |
| | *** | 17885 | 23153 | 30654 | 5945 | 6773 | 7438 | 1033 | 1065 | 1076 | 225 | 225 | 217 | . | . | . |
| 0.9 | *** | 12473 | 14873 | 21253 | 4085 | 4473 | 5065 | 665 | 673 | 693 | . | . | . | . | . | . |
| | *** | 13485 | 17025 | 21256 | 4265 | 4733 | 5058 | 673 | 685 | 681 | . | . | . | . | . | . |
| 0.95 | *** | 7365 | 8465 | 10633 | 2105 | 2225 | 2373 | . | . | . | . | . | . | . | . | . |
| | *** | 7845 | 9313 | 10622 | 2165 | 2293 | 2368 | . | . | . | . | . | . | . | . | . |
| 0.98 | *** | 3073 | 3313 | 3665 | . | . | . | . | . | . | . | . | . | . | . | . |
| | *** | 3185 | 3473 | 3648 | . | . | . | . | . | . | . | . | . | . | . | . |

## TABLE 7: ALPHA= 0.05  POWER= 0.8     EXPECTED ACCRUAL THRU MINIMUM FOLLOW-UP= 8500

| | | DEL=.01 | | | DEL=.02 | | | DEL=.05 | | | DEL=.10 | | | DEL=.15 | | |
|---|---|---|---|---|---|---|---|---|---|---|---|---|---|---|---|---|
| FACT= | | 1.0 .75 | .50 .25 | .00 BIN | 1.0 .75 | .50 .25 | .00 BIN | 1.0 .75 | .50 .25 | .00 BIN | 1.0 75 | .50 .25 | .00 BIN | 1.0 .75 | .50 .25 | .00 BIN |
| PCONT=*** | | | | | REQUIRED NUMBER OF PATIENTS | | | | | | | | | | | |
| 0.01 | *** | 949 | 949 | 949 | 346 | 346 | 346 | 112 | 112 | 112 | 56 | 56 | 56 | 35 | 35 | 35 |
| | *** | 949 | 949 | 3648 | 346 | 346 | 1206 | 112 | 112 | 328 | 56 | 56 | 134 | 35 | 35 | 80 |
| 0.02 | *** | 2110 | 2118 | 2131 | 673 | 673 | 673 | 184 | 184 | 184 | 78 | 78 | 78 | 48 | 48 | 48 |
| | *** | 2110 | 2118 | 6022 | 673 | 673 | 1793 | 184 | 184 | 419 | 78 | 78 | 155 | 48 | 48 | 89 |
| 0.05 | *** | 6423 | 6495 | 6644 | 1833 | 1841 | 1863 | 388 | 396 | 396 | 141 | 141 | 141 | 78 | 78 | 78 |
| | *** | 6453 | 6559 | 12848 | 1841 | 1855 | 3481 | 396 | 396 | 681 | 141 | 141 | 217 | 78 | 78 | 115 |
| 0.1 | *** | 14230 | 14520 | 15476 | 3916 | 3980 | 4094 | 750 | 758 | 758 | 240 | 240 | 240 | 120 | 120 | 120 |
| | *** | 14350 | 14838 | 23235 | 3945 | 4030 | 6047 | 758 | 758 | 1076 | 240 | 240 | 310 | 120 | 120 | 153 |
| 0.15 | *** | 21349 | 21936 | 24443 | 5850 | 6028 | 6325 | 1090 | 1098 | 1119 | 325 | 325 | 325 | 163 | 163 | 163 |
| | *** | 21561 | 22658 | 32385 | 5921 | 6155 | 8304 | 1098 | 1111 | 1422 | 325 | 325 | 390 | 163 | 163 | 186 |
| 0.2 | *** | 27193 | 28141 | 32837 | 7494 | 7813 | 8408 | 1395 | 1416 | 1438 | 396 | 396 | 396 | 197 | 197 | 197 |
| | *** | 27546 | 29381 | 40298 | 7635 | 8060 | 10251 | 1408 | 1430 | 1719 | 396 | 396 | 458 | 197 | 197 | 213 |
| 0.25 | *** | 31613 | 32986 | 40304 | 8825 | 9300 | 10248 | 1650 | 1685 | 1727 | 460 | 460 | 460 | 218 | 218 | 218 |
| | *** | 32101 | 34813 | 46976 | 9024 | 9675 | 11890 | 1663 | 1706 | 1967 | 460 | 460 | 514 | 218 | 218 | 235 |
| 0.3 | *** | 34609 | 36471 | 46679 | 9823 | 10461 | 11821 | 1855 | 1905 | 1961 | 516 | 516 | 516 | 240 | 240 | 240 |
| | *** | 35281 | 38936 | 52416 | 10100 | 10992 | 13219 | 1884 | 1926 | 2164 | 516 | 516 | 557 | 240 | 240 | 252 |
| 0.35 | *** | 36309 | 38710 | 51835 | 10511 | 11319 | 13075 | 2011 | 2075 | 2139 | 545 | 558 | 558 | 261 | 261 | 261 |
| | *** | 37193 | 41826 | 56620 | 10865 | 11991 | 14239 | 2046 | 2110 | 2313 | 545 | 558 | 588 | 261 | 261 | 263 |
| 0.4 | *** | 36883 | 39850 | 55702 | 10936 | 11893 | 14010 | 2118 | 2195 | 2280 | 580 | 580 | 588 | 261 | 269 | 269 |
| | *** | 37980 | 43598 | 59588 | 11340 | 12692 | 14950 | 2160 | 2237 | 2412 | 580 | 580 | 606 | 261 | 269 | 268 |
| 0.45 | *** | 36500 | 40041 | 58260 | 11098 | 12190 | 14613 | 2181 | 2266 | 2365 | 588 | 588 | 601 | 269 | 269 | 269 |
| | *** | 37831 | 44363 | 61319 | 11566 | 13096 | 15352 | 2224 | 2309 | 2461 | 588 | 601 | 613 | 269 | 269 | 268 |
| 0.5 | *** | 35366 | 39433 | 59471 | 11056 | 12246 | 14881 | 2195 | 2280 | 2386 | 588 | 588 | 601 | 261 | 269 | 269 |
| | *** | 36917 | 44248 | 61814 | 11553 | 13231 | 15445 | 2237 | 2330 | 2461 | 588 | 601 | 606 | 261 | 269 | 263 |
| 0.55 | *** | 33645 | 38158 | 59344 | 10801 | 12055 | 14817 | 2160 | 2258 | 2365 | 566 | 580 | 588 | 261 | 261 | 261 |
| | *** | 35395 | 43321 | 61072 | 11340 | 13096 | 15228 | 2203 | 2301 | 2412 | 580 | 580 | 588 | 261 | 261 | 252 |
| 0.6 | *** | 31506 | 36343 | 57878 | 10376 | 11651 | 14421 | 2088 | 2173 | 2280 | 545 | 558 | 558 | 240 | 240 | 240 |
| | *** | 33411 | 41698 | 59093 | 10928 | 12692 | 14703 | 2131 | 2224 | 2313 | 545 | 558 | 557 | 240 | 240 | 235 |
| 0.65 | *** | 29063 | 34035 | 55065 | 9789 | 11035 | 13678 | 1969 | 2046 | 2152 | 503 | 516 | 516 | 218 | 218 | 226 |
| | *** | 31039 | 39390 | 55878 | 10320 | 12041 | 13868 | 2003 | 2096 | 2164 | 516 | 516 | 514 | 218 | 218 | 213 |
| 0.7 | *** | 26364 | 31294 | 50921 | 9037 | 10206 | 12615 | 1799 | 1876 | 1961 | 452 | 460 | 460 | 197 | 197 | 197 |
| | *** | 28340 | 36458 | 51427 | 9547 | 11141 | 12724 | 1833 | 1918 | 1967 | 460 | 460 | 458 | 197 | 197 | 186 |
| 0.75 | *** | 23453 | 28106 | 45446 | 8123 | 9165 | 11213 | 1586 | 1650 | 1727 | 388 | 396 | 396 | 163 | 163 | 163 |
| | *** | 25344 | 32866 | 45739 | 8578 | 9972 | 11271 | 1621 | 1685 | 1719 | 396 | 396 | 390 | 163 | 163 | 153 |
| 0.8 | *** | 20286 | 24451 | 38668 | 7026 | 7890 | 9483 | 1331 | 1374 | 1430 | 311 | 311 | 325 | 120 | 120 | 120 |
| | *** | 21986 | 28553 | 38815 | 7409 | 8535 | 9509 | 1353 | 1408 | 1422 | 311 | 325 | 310 | 120 | 120 | 115 |
| 0.85 | *** | 16772 | 20193 | 30606 | 5709 | 6360 | 7430 | 1026 | 1055 | 1090 | 226 | 226 | 226 | . | . | . |
| | *** | 18183 | 23410 | 30654 | 5998 | 6814 | 7438 | 1047 | 1068 | 1076 | 226 | 226 | 217 | . | . | . |
| 0.9 | *** | 12679 | 15080 | 21256 | 4128 | 4498 | 5063 | 665 | 673 | 694 | . | . | . | . | . | . |
| | *** | 13691 | 17184 | 21256 | 4298 | 4753 | 5058 | 673 | 686 | 681 | . | . | . | . | . | . |
| 0.95 | *** | 7473 | 8548 | 10631 | 2118 | 2237 | 2373 | . | . | . | . | . | . | . | . | . |
| | *** | 7940 | 9377 | 10622 | 2173 | 2301 | 2368 | . | . | . | . | . | . | . | . | . |
| 0.98 | *** | 3095 | 3329 | 3661 | . | . | . | . | . | . | . | . | . | . | . | . |
| | *** | 3215 | 3478 | 3648 | . | . | . | . | . | . | . | . | . | . | . | . |

TABLE 7: ALPHA= 0.05  POWER= 0.8     EXPECTED ACCRUAL THRU MINIMUM FOLLOW-UP= 9000

| | DEL=.01 | | | DEL=.02 | | | DEL=.05 | | | DEL=.10 | | | DEL=.15 | | |
|---|---|---|---|---|---|---|---|---|---|---|---|---|---|---|---|
| FACT= | 1.0 .75 | .50 .25 | .00 BIN | 1.0 .75 | .50 .25 | .00 BIN | 1.0 .75 | .50 .25 | .00 BIN | 1.0 75 | .50 .25 | .00 BIN | 1.0 .75 | .50 .25 | .00 BIN |
| PCONT=*** | | | | REQUIRED NUMBER OF PATIENTS | | | | | | | | | | | |
| 0.01 *** | 951 | 951 | 951 | 352 | 352 | 352 | 119 | 119 | 119 | 60 | 60 | 60 | 37 | 37 | 37 |
| *** | 951 | 951 | 3648 | 352 | 352 | 1206 | 119 | 119 | 328 | 60 | 60 | 134 | 37 | 37 | 80 |
| 0.02 *** | 2107 | 2121 | 2130 | 681 | 681 | 681 | 186 | 186 | 186 | 82 | 82 | 82 | 51 | 51 | 51 |
| *** | 2107 | 2121 | 6022 | 681 | 681 | 1793 | 186 | 186 | 419 | 82 | 82 | 155 | 51 | 51 | 89 |
| 0.05 *** | 6427 | 6509 | 6644 | 1837 | 1851 | 1860 | 389 | 397 | 397 | 141 | 141 | 141 | 82 | 82 | 82 |
| *** | 6464 | 6562 | 12848 | 1837 | 1851 | 3481 | 389 | 397 | 681 | 141 | 141 | 217 | 82 | 82 | 115 |
| 0.1 *** | 14257 | 14550 | 15472 | 3921 | 3989 | 4087 | 749 | 757 | 757 | 231 | 231 | 231 | 127 | 127 | 127 |
| *** | 14370 | 14865 | 23235 | 3952 | 4034 | 6047 | 757 | 757 | 1076 | 231 | 231 | 310 | 127 | 127 | 153 |
| 0.15 *** | 21390 | 21997 | 24441 | 5865 | 6036 | 6329 | 1095 | 1109 | 1117 | 321 | 321 | 321 | 164 | 164 | 164 |
| *** | 21615 | 22717 | 32385 | 5946 | 6157 | 8304 | 1095 | 1109 | 1422 | 321 | 321 | 390 | 164 | 164 | 186 |
| 0.2 *** | 27262 | 28244 | 32834 | 7530 | 7836 | 8407 | 1401 | 1410 | 1446 | 397 | 397 | 397 | 195 | 195 | 195 |
| *** | 27614 | 29490 | 40298 | 7665 | 8070 | 10251 | 1410 | 1424 | 1719 | 397 | 397 | 458 | 195 | 195 | 213 |
| 0.25 *** | 31695 | 33126 | 40312 | 8857 | 9330 | 10252 | 1657 | 1680 | 1725 | 456 | 465 | 465 | 217 | 217 | 217 |
| *** | 32212 | 34971 | 46976 | 9060 | 9704 | 11890 | 1671 | 1702 | 1967 | 456 | 465 | 514 | 217 | 217 | 235 |
| 0.3 *** | 34732 | 36659 | 46680 | 9884 | 10514 | 11819 | 1860 | 1905 | 1964 | 510 | 510 | 524 | 240 | 240 | 240 |
| *** | 35430 | 39142 | 52416 | 10154 | 11031 | 13219 | 1882 | 1927 | 2164 | 510 | 510 | 557 | 240 | 240 | 252 |
| 0.35 *** | 36479 | 38940 | 51832 | 10581 | 11391 | 13079 | 2017 | 2076 | 2144 | 546 | 555 | 555 | 254 | 254 | 254 |
| *** | 37387 | 42090 | 56620 | 10927 | 12044 | 14239 | 2054 | 2107 | 2313 | 555 | 555 | 588 | 254 | 254 | 263 |
| 0.4 *** | 37086 | 40132 | 55702 | 11017 | 11962 | 14010 | 2130 | 2197 | 2279 | 577 | 577 | 591 | 262 | 262 | 262 |
| *** | 38220 | 43926 | 59588 | 11422 | 12750 | 14950 | 2166 | 2234 | 2412 | 577 | 577 | 606 | 262 | 262 | 268 |
| 0.45 *** | 36749 | 40371 | 58259 | 11197 | 12277 | 14617 | 2189 | 2265 | 2355 | 591 | 591 | 600 | 262 | 262 | 276 |
| *** | 38121 | 44736 | 61319 | 11661 | 13169 | 15352 | 2234 | 2310 | 2461 | 591 | 600 | 613 | 262 | 262 | 268 |
| 0.5 *** | 35655 | 39809 | 59474 | 11152 | 12336 | 14887 | 2211 | 2287 | 2391 | 591 | 591 | 600 | 262 | 262 | 262 |
| *** | 37252 | 44646 | 61814 | 11661 | 13304 | 15445 | 2242 | 2332 | 2461 | 591 | 600 | 606 | 262 | 262 | 263 |
| 0.55 *** | 33981 | 38571 | 59347 | 10905 | 12156 | 14820 | 2175 | 2256 | 2369 | 569 | 577 | 591 | 254 | 254 | 262 |
| *** | 35767 | 43755 | 61072 | 11445 | 13169 | 15228 | 2211 | 2310 | 2412 | 577 | 577 | 588 | 254 | 254 | 252 |
| 0.6 *** | 31875 | 36771 | 57876 | 10491 | 11751 | 14415 | 2099 | 2175 | 2279 | 546 | 555 | 555 | 240 | 240 | 240 |
| *** | 33801 | 42135 | 59093 | 11031 | 12764 | 14703 | 2144 | 2234 | 2313 | 546 | 555 | 557 | 240 | 240 | 235 |
| 0.65 *** | 29436 | 34476 | 55064 | 9892 | 11130 | 13686 | 1972 | 2054 | 2144 | 510 | 510 | 524 | 217 | 217 | 217 |
| *** | 31447 | 39831 | 55878 | 10432 | 12111 | 13868 | 2017 | 2099 | 2164 | 510 | 510 | 514 | 217 | 217 | 213 |
| 0.7 *** | 26745 | 31717 | 50924 | 9141 | 10297 | 12615 | 1806 | 1882 | 1964 | 456 | 465 | 465 | 195 | 195 | 195 |
| *** | 28747 | 36870 | 51427 | 9645 | 11197 | 12724 | 1837 | 1919 | 1967 | 456 | 465 | 458 | 195 | 195 | 186 |
| 0.75 *** | 23820 | 28514 | 45456 | 8219 | 9240 | 11211 | 1604 | 1657 | 1725 | 389 | 397 | 397 | 164 | 164 | 164 |
| *** | 25724 | 33239 | 45739 | 8669 | 10027 | 11271 | 1626 | 1680 | 1719 | 397 | 397 | 390 | 164 | 164 | 153 |
| 0.8 *** | 20625 | 24801 | 38670 | 7102 | 7957 | 9487 | 1342 | 1379 | 1432 | 321 | 321 | 321 | 127 | 127 | 127 |
| *** | 22335 | 28882 | 38815 | 7476 | 8579 | 9509 | 1356 | 1401 | 1422 | 321 | 321 | 310 | 127 | 127 | 115 |
| 0.85 *** | 17047 | 20467 | 30606 | 5775 | 6396 | 7431 | 1027 | 1064 | 1086 | 231 | 231 | 231 | . | . | . |
| *** | 18465 | 23662 | 30654 | 6059 | 6832 | 7438 | 1041 | 1072 | 1076 | 231 | 231 | 217 | . | . | . |
| 0.9 *** | 12885 | 15261 | 21246 | 4155 | 4529 | 5069 | 667 | 681 | 690 | . | . | . | . | . | . |
| *** | 13889 | 17340 | 21256 | 4326 | 4762 | 5058 | 667 | 681 | 681 | . | . | . | . | . | . |
| 0.95 *** | 7566 | 8624 | 10635 | 2130 | 2242 | 2377 | . | . | . | . | . | . | . | . | . |
| *** | 8039 | 9434 | 10622 | 2189 | 2310 | 2368 | . | . | . | . | . | . | . | . | . |
| 0.98 *** | 3120 | 3345 | 3660 | . | . | . | . | . | . | . | . | . | . | . | . |
| *** | 3232 | 3494 | 3648 | . | . | . | . | . | . | . | . | . | . | . | . |

TABLE 7: ALPHA= 0.05  POWER= 0.8     EXPECTED ACCRUAL THRU MINIMUM FOLLOW-UP= 9500

| | DEL=.01 | | | DEL=.02 | | | DEL=.05 | | | DEL=.10 | | | DEL=.15 | | |
|---|---|---|---|---|---|---|---|---|---|---|---|---|---|---|---|
| FACT= | 1.0 .75 | .50 .25 | .00 BIN | 1.0 .75 | .50 .25 | .00 BIN | 1.0 .75 | .50 .25 | .00 BIN | 1.0 75 | .50 .25 | .00 BIN | 1.0 .75 | .50 .25 | .00 BIN |
| PCONT=*** | | | | REQUIRED NUMBER OF PATIENTS | | | | | | | | | | | |
| 0.01  *** | 956 | 956 | 956 | 348 | 348 | 348 | 110 | 110 | 110 | 54 | 54 | 54 | 39 | 39 | 39 |
|        *** | 956 | 956 | 3648 | 348 | 348 | 1206 | 110 | 110 | 328 | 54 | 54 | 134 | 39 | 39 | 80 |
| 0.02  *** | 2105 | 2120 | 2129 | 680 | 680 | 680 | 182 | 182 | 182 | 78 | 78 | 78 | 54 | 54 | 54 |
|        *** | 2120 | 2120 | 6022 | 680 | 680 | 1793 | 182 | 182 | 419 | 78 | 78 | 155 | 54 | 54 | 89 |
| 0.05  *** | 6443 | 6514 | 6642 | 1835 | 1844 | 1859 | 395 | 395 | 395 | 134 | 134 | 134 | 78 | 78 | 78 |
|        *** | 6466 | 6561 | 12848 | 1844 | 1859 | 3481 | 395 | 395 | 681 | 134 | 134 | 217 | 78 | 78 | 115 |
| 0.1  *** | 14280 | 14574 | 15468 | 3925 | 3996 | 4091 | 752 | 752 | 766 | 229 | 229 | 229 | 125 | 125 | 125 |
|        *** | 14384 | 14883 | 23235 | 3958 | 4044 | 6047 | 752 | 752 | 1076 | 229 | 229 | 310 | 125 | 125 | 153 |
| 0.15  *** | 21429 | 22046 | 24430 | 5882 | 6048 | 6324 | 1099 | 1108 | 1123 | 315 | 324 | 324 | 158 | 158 | 158 |
|        *** | 21666 | 22783 | 32385 | 5953 | 6167 | 8304 | 1099 | 1108 | 1422 | 315 | 324 | 390 | 158 | 158 | 186 |
| 0.2  *** | 27319 | 28325 | 32829 | 7559 | 7853 | 8414 | 1393 | 1417 | 1440 | 395 | 395 | 395 | 196 | 196 | 196 |
|        *** | 27699 | 29584 | 40298 | 7687 | 8090 | 10251 | 1408 | 1431 | 1719 | 395 | 395 | 458 | 196 | 196 | 213 |
| 0.25  *** | 31784 | 33256 | 40310 | 8898 | 9364 | 10252 | 1654 | 1693 | 1725 | 458 | 458 | 467 | 220 | 220 | 220 |
|        *** | 32330 | 35118 | 46976 | 9103 | 9729 | 11890 | 1669 | 1702 | 1967 | 458 | 467 | 514 | 220 | 220 | 235 |
| 0.3  *** | 34857 | 36828 | 46675 | 9934 | 10560 | 11810 | 1868 | 1906 | 1963 | 514 | 514 | 514 | 244 | 244 | 244 |
|        *** | 35584 | 39345 | 52416 | 10204 | 11059 | 13219 | 1892 | 1930 | 2164 | 514 | 514 | 557 | 244 | 244 | 252 |
| 0.35  *** | 36629 | 39179 | 51829 | 10646 | 11439 | 13069 | 2025 | 2082 | 2144 | 553 | 553 | 562 | 253 | 253 | 253 |
|        *** | 37579 | 42353 | 56620 | 10988 | 12080 | 14239 | 2049 | 2105 | 2313 | 553 | 553 | 588 | 253 | 253 | 263 |
| 0.4  *** | 37279 | 40414 | 55700 | 11098 | 12033 | 14004 | 2144 | 2200 | 2286 | 576 | 576 | 585 | 268 | 268 | 268 |
|        *** | 38458 | 44229 | 59588 | 11501 | 12793 | 14950 | 2168 | 2239 | 2412 | 576 | 585 | 606 | 268 | 268 | 268 |
| 0.45  *** | 36985 | 40699 | 58250 | 11288 | 12356 | 14613 | 2200 | 2272 | 2358 | 585 | 585 | 600 | 268 | 268 | 268 |
|        *** | 38395 | 45084 | 61319 | 11739 | 13220 | 15352 | 2239 | 2310 | 2461 | 585 | 600 | 613 | 268 | 268 | 268 |
| 0.5  *** | 35940 | 40177 | 59476 | 11249 | 12413 | 14883 | 2215 | 2295 | 2390 | 585 | 585 | 600 | 268 | 268 | 268 |
|        *** | 37564 | 45022 | 61814 | 11748 | 13363 | 15445 | 2248 | 2334 | 2461 | 585 | 600 | 606 | 268 | 268 | 263 |
| 0.55  *** | 34301 | 38965 | 59343 | 11012 | 12238 | 14826 | 2177 | 2263 | 2358 | 576 | 576 | 585 | 253 | 253 | 253 |
|        *** | 36130 | 44158 | 61072 | 11549 | 13235 | 15228 | 2224 | 2310 | 2412 | 576 | 585 | 588 | 253 | 253 | 252 |
| 0.6  *** | 32220 | 37184 | 57870 | 10584 | 11843 | 14423 | 2105 | 2191 | 2286 | 553 | 553 | 562 | 244 | 244 | 244 |
|        *** | 34183 | 42552 | 59093 | 11130 | 12831 | 14703 | 2144 | 2224 | 2313 | 553 | 553 | 557 | 244 | 244 | 235 |
| 0.65  *** | 29813 | 34880 | 55059 | 9990 | 11216 | 13686 | 1987 | 2058 | 2144 | 505 | 514 | 514 | 220 | 220 | 220 |
|        *** | 31840 | 40239 | 55878 | 10528 | 12175 | 13868 | 2025 | 2096 | 2164 | 514 | 514 | 514 | 220 | 220 | 213 |
| 0.7  *** | 27114 | 32116 | 50912 | 9230 | 10370 | 12618 | 1820 | 1883 | 1963 | 458 | 458 | 467 | 196 | 196 | 196 |
|        *** | 29133 | 37255 | 51427 | 9729 | 11264 | 12724 | 1844 | 1915 | 1967 | 458 | 467 | 458 | 196 | 196 | 186 |
| 0.75  *** | 24169 | 28886 | 45449 | 8295 | 9316 | 11216 | 1607 | 1654 | 1716 | 395 | 395 | 395 | 158 | 158 | 158 |
|        *** | 26093 | 33589 | 45739 | 8746 | 10076 | 11271 | 1630 | 1693 | 1719 | 395 | 395 | 390 | 158 | 158 | 153 |
| 0.8  *** | 20939 | 25119 | 38671 | 7179 | 8010 | 9483 | 1345 | 1384 | 1431 | 315 | 315 | 324 | 125 | 125 | 125 |
|        *** | 22664 | 29180 | 38815 | 7544 | 8628 | 9509 | 1360 | 1408 | 1422 | 315 | 315 | 310 | 125 | 125 | 115 |
| 0.85  *** | 17320 | 20725 | 30605 | 5825 | 6443 | 7440 | 1037 | 1060 | 1084 | 229 | 229 | 229 | . | . | . |
|        *** | 18730 | 23884 | 30654 | 6110 | 6870 | 7438 | 1051 | 1075 | 1076 | 229 | 229 | 217 | . | . | . |
| 0.9  *** | 13078 | 15444 | 21248 | 4195 | 4552 | 5065 | 671 | 680 | 695 | . | . | . | . | . | . |
|        *** | 14075 | 17486 | 21256 | 4362 | 4780 | 5058 | 671 | 680 | 681 | . | . | . | . | . | . |
| 0.95  *** | 7654 | 8699 | 10632 | 2144 | 2248 | 2381 | . | . | . | . | . | . | . | . | . |
|        *** | 8114 | 9483 | 10622 | 2191 | 2310 | 2368 | . | . | . | . | . | . | . | . | . |
| 0.98  *** | 3141 | 3364 | 3664 | . | . | . | . | . | . | . | . | . | . | . | . |
|        *** | 3245 | 3498 | 3648 | . | . | . | . | . | . | . | . | . | . | . | . |

TABLE 7: ALPHA= 0.05  POWER= 0.8     EXPECTED ACCRUAL THRU MINIMUM FOLLOW-UP= 10000

| | | DEL=.01 | | | DEL=.02 | | | DEL=.05 | | | DEL=.10 | | | DEL=.15 | | |
|---|---|---|---|---|---|---|---|---|---|---|---|---|---|---|---|---|
| FACT= | | 1.0 .75 | .50 .25 | .00 BIN | 1.0 .75 | .50 .25 | .00 BIN | 1.0 .75 | .50 .25 | .00 BIN | 1.0 75 | .50 .25 | .00 BIN | 1.0 .75 | .50 .25 | .00 BIN |
| PCONT=*** | | | | | | | REQUIRED NUMBER OF PATIENTS | | | | | | | | |
| 0.01 | *** | 957 | 957 | 957 | 341 | 341 | 341 | 116 | 116 | 116 | 57 | 57 | 57 | 41 | 41 | 41 |
| | *** | 957 | 957 | 3648 | 341 | 341 | 1206 | 116 | 116 | 328 | 57 | 57 | 134 | 41 | 41 | 80 |
| 0.02 | *** | 2107 | 2116 | 2132 | 682 | 682 | 682 | 182 | 182 | 182 | 82 | 82 | 82 | 57 | 57 | 57 |
| | *** | 2116 | 2116 | 6022 | 682 | 682 | 1793 | 182 | 182 | 419 | 82 | 82 | 155 | 57 | 57 | 89 |
| 0.05 | *** | 6441 | 6516 | 6641 | 1832 | 1841 | 1857 | 391 | 391 | 391 | 141 | 141 | 141 | 82 | 82 | 82 |
| | *** | 6466 | 6566 | 12848 | 1841 | 1857 | 3481 | 391 | 391 | 681 | 141 | 141 | 217 | 82 | 82 | 115 |
| 0.1 | *** | 14291 | 14591 | 15466 | 3932 | 3991 | 4091 | 757 | 757 | 757 | 232 | 232 | 232 | 116 | 116 | 116 |
| | *** | 14416 | 14907 | 23235 | 3957 | 4041 | 6047 | 757 | 757 | 1076 | 232 | 232 | 310 | 116 | 116 | 153 |
| 0.15 | *** | 21466 | 22107 | 24441 | 5891 | 6057 | 6332 | 1091 | 1107 | 1116 | 316 | 316 | 316 | 157 | 157 | 157 |
| | *** | 21707 | 22832 | 32385 | 5966 | 6182 | 8304 | 1107 | 1107 | 1422 | 316 | 316 | 390 | 157 | 157 | 186 |
| 0.2 | *** | 27382 | 28416 | 32832 | 7582 | 7882 | 8407 | 1407 | 1416 | 1441 | 391 | 391 | 391 | 191 | 191 | 191 |
| | *** | 27766 | 29682 | 40298 | 7707 | 8107 | 10251 | 1407 | 1432 | 1719 | 391 | 391 | 458 | 191 | 191 | 213 |
| 0.25 | *** | 31882 | 33382 | 40307 | 8941 | 9391 | 10257 | 1657 | 1691 | 1716 | 457 | 457 | 466 | 216 | 216 | 216 |
| | *** | 32432 | 35257 | 46976 | 9141 | 9741 | 11890 | 1666 | 1707 | 1967 | 457 | 466 | 514 | 216 | 216 | 235 |
| 0.3 | *** | 34966 | 37007 | 46682 | 9982 | 10607 | 11816 | 1866 | 1907 | 1957 | 507 | 516 | 516 | 241 | 241 | 241 |
| | *** | 35732 | 39541 | 52416 | 10241 | 11091 | 13219 | 1891 | 1932 | 2164 | 516 | 516 | 557 | 241 | 241 | 252 |
| 0.35 | *** | 36782 | 39391 | 51832 | 10707 | 11491 | 13066 | 2032 | 2082 | 2141 | 541 | 557 | 557 | 257 | 257 | 257 |
| | *** | 37757 | 42591 | 56620 | 11057 | 12116 | 14239 | 2057 | 2116 | 2313 | 557 | 557 | 588 | 257 | 257 | 263 |
| 0.4 | *** | 37482 | 40682 | 55707 | 11166 | 12107 | 14007 | 2141 | 2207 | 2282 | 582 | 582 | 582 | 266 | 266 | 266 |
| | *** | 38682 | 44507 | 59588 | 11566 | 12841 | 14950 | 2166 | 2241 | 2412 | 582 | 582 | 606 | 266 | 266 | 268 |
| 0.45 | *** | 37216 | 41007 | 58257 | 11366 | 12432 | 14616 | 2207 | 2282 | 2357 | 591 | 591 | 591 | 266 | 266 | 266 |
| | *** | 38666 | 45407 | 61319 | 11816 | 13282 | 15352 | 2241 | 2316 | 2461 | 591 | 591 | 613 | 266 | 266 | 268 |
| 0.5 | *** | 36216 | 40516 | 59482 | 11341 | 12491 | 14882 | 2216 | 2291 | 2391 | 591 | 591 | 607 | 266 | 266 | 266 |
| | *** | 37882 | 45391 | 61814 | 11841 | 13416 | 15445 | 2257 | 2341 | 2461 | 591 | 591 | 606 | 266 | 266 | 263 |
| 0.55 | *** | 34607 | 39341 | 59341 | 11107 | 12332 | 14816 | 2191 | 2266 | 2366 | 566 | 582 | 582 | 257 | 257 | 257 |
| | *** | 36466 | 44541 | 61072 | 11632 | 13291 | 15228 | 2232 | 2316 | 2412 | 582 | 582 | 588 | 257 | 257 | 252 |
| 0.6 | *** | 32557 | 37566 | 57882 | 10691 | 11916 | 14416 | 2116 | 2191 | 2282 | 541 | 557 | 557 | 241 | 241 | 241 |
| | *** | 34557 | 42941 | 59093 | 11232 | 12891 | 14703 | 2157 | 2232 | 2313 | 557 | 557 | 557 | 241 | 241 | 235 |
| 0.65 | *** | 30157 | 35282 | 55066 | 10091 | 11291 | 13682 | 1991 | 2066 | 2141 | 507 | 516 | 516 | 216 | 216 | 216 |
| | *** | 32216 | 40632 | 55878 | 10616 | 12232 | 13868 | 2032 | 2107 | 2164 | 507 | 516 | 514 | 216 | 216 | 213 |
| 0.7 | *** | 27466 | 32507 | 50916 | 9332 | 10457 | 12607 | 1816 | 1882 | 1957 | 457 | 457 | 466 | 191 | 191 | 191 |
| | *** | 29507 | 37632 | 51427 | 9816 | 11316 | 12724 | 1857 | 1916 | 1967 | 457 | 466 | 458 | 191 | 191 | 185 |
| 0.75 | *** | 24507 | 29241 | 45457 | 8382 | 9382 | 11216 | 1607 | 1657 | 1716 | 391 | 391 | 407 | 166 | 166 | 166 |
| | *** | 26441 | 33932 | 45739 | 8816 | 10116 | 11271 | 1632 | 1691 | 1719 | 391 | 391 | 390 | 166 | 166 | 153 |
| 0.8 | *** | 21241 | 25432 | 38666 | 7241 | 8066 | 9482 | 1341 | 1382 | 1432 | 316 | 316 | 316 | 132 | 132 | 132 |
| | *** | 22966 | 29457 | 38815 | 7607 | 8657 | 9509 | 1366 | 1407 | 1422 | 316 | 316 | 310 | 132 | 132 | 115 |
| 0.85 | *** | 17566 | 20982 | 30607 | 5882 | 6482 | 7432 | 1032 | 1057 | 1082 | 232 | 232 | 232 | . | . | . |
| | *** | 18991 | 24107 | 30654 | 6157 | 6891 | 7438 | 1041 | 1066 | 1076 | 232 | 232 | 217 | . | . | . |
| 0.9 | *** | 13257 | 15607 | 21257 | 4232 | 4566 | 5066 | 666 | 682 | 691 | . | . | . | . | . | . |
| | *** | 14257 | 17616 | 21256 | 4382 | 4791 | 5058 | 682 | 682 | 681 | . | . | . | . | . | . |
| 0.95 | *** | 7741 | 8766 | 10632 | 2157 | 2257 | 2382 | . | . | . | . | . | . | . | . | . |
| | *** | 8191 | 9532 | 10622 | 2207 | 2316 | 2368 | . | . | . | . | . | . | . | . | . |
| 0.98 | *** | 3166 | 3382 | 3657 | . | . | . | . | . | . | . | . | . | . | . | . |
| | *** | 3266 | 3507 | 3648 | . | . | . | . | . | . | . | . | . | . | . | . |

## TABLE 7: ALPHA= 0.05  POWER= 0.8    EXPECTED ACCRUAL THRU MINIMUM FOLLOW-UP= 11000

| | DEL=.01 | | | DEL=.02 | | | DEL=.05 | | | DEL=.10 | | | DEL=.15 | | |
|---|---|---|---|---|---|---|---|---|---|---|---|---|---|---|---|
| FACT= | 1.0 .75 | .50 .25 | .00 BIN | 1.0 .75 | .50 .25 | .00 BIN | 1.0 .75 | .50 .25 | .00 BIN | 1.0 75 | .50 .25 | .00 BIN | 1.0 .75 | .50 .25 | .00 BIN |

PCONT=***                    REQUIRED NUMBER OF PATIENTS

| PCONT | 1.0 | .50 | .00 | 1.0 | .50 | .00 | 1.0 | .50 | .00 | 1.0 | .50 | .00 | 1.0 | .50 | .00 |
|---|---|---|---|---|---|---|---|---|---|---|---|---|---|---|---|
| 0.01 *** | 953 | 953 | 953 | 348 | 348 | 348 | 117 | 117 | 117 | 62 | 62 | 62 | 35 | 35 | 35 |
| *** | 953 | 953 | 3648 | 348 | 348 | 1206 | 117 | 117 | 328 | 62 | 62 | 134 | 35 | 35 | 80 |
| 0.02 *** | 2108 | 2125 | 2125 | 678 | 678 | 678 | 183 | 183 | 183 | 73 | 73 | 73 | 45 | 45 | 45 |
| *** | 2108 | 2125 | 6022 | 678 | 678 | 1793 | 183 | 183 | 419 | 73 | 73 | 155 | 45 | 45 | 89 |
| 0.05 *** | 6453 | 6525 | 6645 | 1833 | 1850 | 1860 | 392 | 392 | 392 | 145 | 145 | 145 | 73 | 73 | 73 |
| *** | 6480 | 6580 | 12848 | 1850 | 1850 | 3481 | 392 | 392 | 681 | 145 | 145 | 217 | 73 | 73 | 115 |
| 0.1 *** | 14335 | 14637 | 15473 | 3940 | 4005 | 4088 | 750 | 760 | 760 | 238 | 238 | 238 | 128 | 128 | 128 |
| *** | 14455 | 14940 | 23235 | 3967 | 4050 | 6047 | 750 | 760 | 1076 | 238 | 238 | 310 | 128 | 128 | 153 |
| 0.15 *** | 21540 | 22200 | 24438 | 5920 | 6085 | 6332 | 1090 | 1107 | 1118 | 320 | 320 | 320 | 155 | 155 | 155 |
| *** | 21798 | 22925 | 32385 | 5985 | 6195 | 8304 | 1107 | 1107 | 1422 | 320 | 320 | 390 | 155 | 155 | 186 |
| 0.2 *** | 27507 | 28590 | 32825 | 7625 | 7910 | 8405 | 1410 | 1420 | 1437 | 392 | 392 | 403 | 200 | 200 | 200 |
| *** | 27903 | 29855 | 40298 | 7745 | 8120 | 10251 | 1410 | 1437 | 1719 | 392 | 392 | 458 | 200 | 200 | 213 |
| 0.25 *** | 32045 | 33623 | 40305 | 9010 | 9450 | 10248 | 1668 | 1695 | 1723 | 458 | 458 | 458 | 227 | 227 | 227 |
| *** | 32633 | 35520 | 46976 | 9203 | 9780 | 11890 | 1685 | 1712 | 1967 | 458 | 458 | 514 | 227 | 227 | 235 |
| 0.3 *** | 35207 | 37335 | 46675 | 10072 | 10677 | 11815 | 1877 | 1915 | 1960 | 513 | 513 | 513 | 238 | 238 | 238 |
| *** | 36005 | 39893 | 52416 | 10330 | 11145 | 13219 | 1888 | 1932 | 2164 | 513 | 513 | 557 | 238 | 238 | 252 |
| 0.35 *** | 37088 | 39810 | 51828 | 10825 | 11595 | 13070 | 2042 | 2080 | 2152 | 557 | 557 | 557 | 255 | 255 | 255 |
| *** | 38122 | 43028 | 56620 | 11155 | 12190 | 14239 | 2070 | 2108 | 2313 | 557 | 557 | 588 | 255 | 255 | 263 |
| 0.4 *** | 37858 | 41185 | 55705 | 11293 | 12217 | 14005 | 2152 | 2207 | 2273 | 568 | 585 | 585 | 265 | 265 | 265 |
| *** | 39123 | 45035 | 59588 | 11695 | 12932 | 14950 | 2180 | 2245 | 2412 | 585 | 585 | 606 | 265 | 265 | 268 |
| 0.45 *** | 37682 | 41598 | 58252 | 11513 | 12558 | 14610 | 2218 | 2290 | 2355 | 585 | 595 | 595 | 265 | 265 | 265 |
| *** | 39195 | 46015 | 61319 | 11970 | 13372 | 15352 | 2245 | 2317 | 2461 | 595 | 595 | 613 | 265 | 265 | 268 |
| 0.5 *** | 36747 | 41175 | 59473 | 11502 | 12640 | 14885 | 2235 | 2300 | 2383 | 585 | 595 | 595 | 265 | 265 | 265 |
| *** | 38480 | 46053 | 61814 | 11997 | 13520 | 15445 | 2262 | 2345 | 2461 | 595 | 595 | 606 | 265 | 265 | 263 |
| 0.55 *** | 35207 | 40047 | 59352 | 11282 | 12475 | 14813 | 2207 | 2273 | 2355 | 568 | 585 | 585 | 255 | 255 | 255 |
| *** | 37115 | 45245 | 61072 | 11805 | 13400 | 15228 | 2235 | 2317 | 2412 | 585 | 585 | 588 | 255 | 255 | 252 |
| 0.6 *** | 33200 | 38315 | 57878 | 10870 | 12080 | 14417 | 2125 | 2190 | 2273 | 540 | 557 | 557 | 238 | 238 | 238 |
| *** | 35245 | 43660 | 59093 | 11392 | 12998 | 14703 | 2163 | 2235 | 2313 | 557 | 557 | 557 | 238 | 238 | 235 |
| 0.65 *** | 30818 | 36015 | 55062 | 10275 | 11447 | 13685 | 1998 | 2070 | 2152 | 513 | 513 | 513 | 227 | 227 | 227 |
| *** | 32925 | 41340 | 55878 | 10787 | 12338 | 13868 | 2042 | 2108 | 2164 | 513 | 513 | 514 | 227 | 227 | 213 |
| 0.7 *** | 28140 | 33210 | 50920 | 9495 | 10595 | 12613 | 1833 | 1888 | 1960 | 458 | 458 | 458 | 200 | 200 | 200 |
| *** | 30202 | 38298 | 51427 | 9973 | 11403 | 12724 | 1860 | 1932 | 1967 | 458 | 458 | 458 | 200 | 200 | 186 |
| 0.75 *** | 25142 | 29900 | 45448 | 8532 | 9495 | 11210 | 1613 | 1668 | 1723 | 392 | 392 | 403 | 155 | 155 | 155 |
| *** | 27095 | 34530 | 45739 | 8955 | 10210 | 11271 | 1640 | 1695 | 1719 | 392 | 392 | 390 | 155 | 155 | 153 |
| 0.8 *** | 21815 | 26005 | 38672 | 7377 | 8158 | 9478 | 1355 | 1393 | 1437 | 320 | 320 | 320 | 128 | 128 | 128 |
| *** | 23547 | 29965 | 38815 | 7718 | 8725 | 9509 | 1365 | 1410 | 1422 | 320 | 320 | 310 | 128 | 128 | 115 |
| 0.85 *** | 18047 | 21430 | 30598 | 5975 | 6552 | 7432 | 1035 | 1063 | 1090 | 227 | 227 | 227 | . | . | . |
| *** | 19460 | 24482 | 30654 | 6233 | 6937 | 7438 | 1052 | 1080 | 1076 | 227 | 227 | 217 | . | . | . |
| 0.9 *** | 13592 | 15913 | 21248 | 4280 | 4610 | 5067 | 667 | 678 | 695 | . | . | . | . | . | . |
| *** | 14582 | 17855 | 21256 | 4435 | 4820 | 5058 | 678 | 678 | 681 | . | . | . | . | . | . |
| 0.95 *** | 7900 | 8890 | 10633 | 2163 | 2262 | 2383 | . | . | . | . | . | . | . | . | . |
| *** | 8340 | 9605 | 10622 | 2218 | 2317 | 2368 | . | . | . | . | . | . | . | . | . |
| 0.98 *** | 3197 | 3400 | 3665 | . | . | . | . | . | . | . | . | . | . | . | . |
| *** | 3290 | 3527 | 3648 | . | . | . | . | . | . | . | . | . | . | . | . |

TABLE 7: ALPHA= 0.05  POWER= 0.8     EXPECTED ACCRUAL THRU MINIMUM FOLLOW-UP= 12000

| | DEL=.01 | | | DEL=.02 | | | DEL=.05 | | | DEL=.10 | | | DEL=.15 | | |
|---|---|---|---|---|---|---|---|---|---|---|---|---|---|---|---|
| FACT= | 1.0 .75 | .50 .25 | .00 BIN | 1.0 .75 | .50 .25 | .00 BIN | 1.0 .75 | .50 .25 | .00 BIN | 1.0 75 | .50 .25 | .00 BIN | 1.0 .75 | .50 .25 | .00 BIN |
| PCONT=*** | | | | REQUIRED NUMBER OF PATIENTS | | | | | | | | | | | |
| 0.01 *** | 949 949 | 949 949 | 949 3648 | 349 349 | 349 349 | 349 1206 | 109 109 | 109 109 | 109 328 | 49 49 | 49 49 | 49 134 | 38 38 | 38 38 | 38 80 |
| 0.02 *** | 2108 2119 | 2119 2119 | 2119 6022 | 679 679 | 679 679 | 679 1793 | 188 188 | 188 188 | 188 419 | 79 79 | 79 79 | 79 155 | 49 49 | 49 49 | 49 89 |
| 0.05 *** | 6458 6488 | 6529 6578 | 6649 12848 | 1838 1849 | 1849 1849 | 1868 3481 | 398 398 | 398 398 | 398 681 | 139 139 | 139 139 | 139 217 | 79 79 | 79 79 | 79 115 |
| 0.1 *** | 14359 14498 | 14678 14978 | 15469 23235 | 3949 3979 | 4009 4039 | 4088 6047 | 758 758 | 758 758 | 758 1076 | 229 229 | 229 229 | 229 310 | 128 128 | 128 128 | 128 153 |
| 0.15 *** | 21619 21878 | 22298 22999 | 24439 32385 | 5948 6008 | 6098 6199 | 6319 8304 | 1099 1099 | 1099 1118 | 1118 1422 | 319 319 | 319 319 | 319 390 | 158 158 | 158 158 | 158 186 |
| 0.2 *** | 27619 28039 | 28748 30008 | 32828 40298 | 7658 7789 | 7939 8149 | 8408 10251 | 1399 1418 | 1418 1429 | 1448 1719 | 398 398 | 398 398 | 398 458 | 188 188 | 188 188 | 188 213 |
| 0.25 *** | 32209 32839 | 33859 35749 | 40309 46976 | 9068 9259 | 9499 9818 | 10249 11890 | 1669 1688 | 1699 1699 | 1718 1967 | 458 458 | 458 458 | 469 514 | 218 218 | 218 218 | 218 235 |
| 0.3 *** | 35438 36278 | 37658 40208 | 46669 52416 | 10148 10418 | 10748 11179 | 11809 13219 | 1879 1898 | 1909 1939 | 1958 2164 | 518 518 | 518 518 | 518 557 | 248 248 | 248 248 | 248 252 |
| 0.35 *** | 37388 38468 | 40208 43448 | 51829 56620 | 10928 11258 | 11678 12248 | 13069 14239 | 2048 2078 | 2089 2119 | 2149 2313 | 548 548 | 559 559 | 559 588 | 259 259 | 259 259 | 259 263 |
| 0.4 *** | 38228 39548 | 41659 45529 | 55699 59588 | 11419 11809 | 12319 12998 | 13999 14950 | 2168 2179 | 2209 2239 | 2288 2412 | 578 578 | 578 578 | 589 606 | 259 259 | 259 259 | 259 268 |
| 0.45 *** | 38119 39679 | 42139 46568 | 58249 61319 | 11659 12098 | 12679 13448 | 14618 15352 | 2228 2258 | 2288 2318 | 2359 2461 | 589 589 | 589 589 | 589 613 | 259 259 | 259 278 | 278 268 |
| 0.5 *** | 37249 39038 | 41779 46658 | 59479 61814 | 11659 12139 | 12769 13609 | 14888 15445 | 2239 2269 | 2318 2348 | 2389 2461 | 589 589 | 589 589 | 608 606 | 259 259 | 259 259 | 259 263 |
| 0.55 *** | 35768 37729 | 40699 45889 | 59348 61072 | 11438 11948 | 12608 13489 | 14828 15228 | 2209 2239 | 2288 2318 | 2359 2412 | 578 578 | 578 578 | 589 588 | 259 259 | 259 259 | 259 252 |
| 0.6 *** | 33799 35888 | 38978 44318 | 57878 59093 | 11029 11539 | 12199 13099 | 14419 14703 | 2138 2168 | 2198 2239 | 2288 2313 | 548 548 | 559 559 | 559 557 | 248 248 | 248 248 | 248 235 |
| 0.65 *** | 31448 33578 | 36698 41978 | 55058 55878 | 10429 10939 | 11569 12428 | 13688 13868 | 2018 2048 | 2078 2108 | 2149 2164 | 518 518 | 518 518 | 518 514 | 218 218 | 218 218 | 218 213 |
| 0.7 *** | 28748 30848 | 33878 38899 | 50918 51427 | 9638 10118 | 10699 11498 | 12608 12724 | 1838 1868 | 1898 1928 | 1958 1967 | 458 458 | 458 458 | 469 458 | 199 199 | 199 199 | 199 186 |
| 0.75 *** | 25729 27698 | 30499 35078 | 45458 45739 | 8659 9079 | 9608 10279 | 11209 11271 | 1628 1639 | 1669 1699 | 1718 1719 | 398 398 | 398 398 | 398 390 | 158 158 | 158 158 | 158 153 |
| 0.8 *** | 22339 24079 | 26528 30428 | 38678 38815 | 7478 7819 | 8239 8779 | 9488 9509 | 1358 1369 | 1388 1418 | 1429 1422 | 319 319 | 319 319 | 319 310 | 128 128 | 128 128 | 128 115 |
| 0.85 *** | 18469 19898 | 21848 24829 | 30608 30654 | 6049 6308 | 6608 6968 | 7429 7438 | 1039 1058 | 1058 1069 | 1088 1076 | 229 229 | 229 229 | 229 217 | . . | . . | . . |
| 0.9 *** | 13898 14869 | 16178 18068 | 21248 21256 | 4328 4478 | 4639 4838 | 5059 5058 | 668 679 | 679 679 | 698 681 | . . | . . | . . | . . | . . | . . |
| 0.95 *** | 8029 8468 | 8989 9679 | 10628 10622 | 2179 2228 | 2269 2318 | 2378 2368 | . . | . . | . . | . . | . . | . . | . . | . . | . . |
| 0.98 *** | 3229 3319 | 3409 3529 | 3668 3648 | . . | . . | . . | . . | . . | . . | . . | . . | . . | . . | . . | . . |

## TABLE 7: ALPHA= 0.05  POWER= 0.8     EXPECTED ACCRUAL THRU MINIMUM FOLLOW-UP= 13000

| | | DEL=.01 | | | DEL=.02 | | | DEL=.05 | | | DEL=.10 | | | DEL=.15 | | |
|---|---|---|---|---|---|---|---|---|---|---|---|---|---|---|---|---|---|
| FACT= | | 1.0 .75 | .50 .25 | .00 BIN | 1.0 .75 | .50 .25 | .00 BIN | 1.0 .75 | .50 .25 | .00 BIN | 1.0 75 | .50 .25 | .00 BIN | 1.0 .75 | .50 .25 | .00 BIN |
| PCONT=*** | | | | | REQUIRED NUMBER OF PATIENTS | | | | | | | | | | | |
| 0.01 | *** | 951 | 951 | 951 | 346 | 346 | 346 | 118 | 118 | 118 | 53 | 53 | 53 | 41 | 41 | 41 |
| | *** | 951 | 951 | 3648 | 346 | 346 | 1206 | 118 | 118 | 328 | 53 | 53 | 134 | 41 | 41 | 80 |
| 0.02 | *** | 2121 | 2121 | 2121 | 671 | 671 | 671 | 183 | 183 | 183 | 74 | 74 | 74 | 53 | 53 | 53 |
| | *** | 2121 | 2121 | 6022 | 671 | 671 | 1793 | 183 | 183 | 419 | 74 | 74 | 155 | 53 | 53 | 89 |
| 0.05 | *** | 6476 | 6541 | 6651 | 1841 | 1841 | 1861 | 399 | 399 | 399 | 139 | 139 | 139 | 86 | 86 | 86 |
| | *** | 6488 | 6586 | 12848 | 1841 | 1861 | 3481 | 399 | 399 | 681 | 139 | 139 | 217 | 86 | 86 | 115 |
| 0.1 | *** | 14406 | 14711 | 15479 | 3953 | 4018 | 4083 | 756 | 756 | 756 | 236 | 236 | 236 | 118 | 118 | 118 |
| | *** | 14536 | 15003 | 23235 | 3986 | 4051 | 6047 | 756 | 756 | 1076 | 236 | 236 | 310 | 118 | 118 | 153 |
| 0.15 | *** | 21686 | 22381 | 24428 | 5956 | 6119 | 6326 | 1093 | 1114 | 1114 | 313 | 313 | 313 | 151 | 151 | 151 |
| | *** | 21958 | 23084 | 32385 | 6033 | 6216 | 8304 | 1093 | 1114 | 1422 | 313 | 313 | 390 | 151 | 151 | 186 |
| 0.2 | *** | 27731 | 28881 | 32834 | 7691 | 7971 | 8406 | 1406 | 1418 | 1439 | 399 | 399 | 399 | 183 | 183 | 183 |
| | *** | 28166 | 30148 | 40298 | 7821 | 8166 | 10251 | 1418 | 1439 | 1719 | 399 | 399 | 458 | 183 | 183 | 213 |
| 0.25 | *** | 32379 | 34069 | 40309 | 9121 | 9543 | 10246 | 1678 | 1699 | 1731 | 464 | 464 | 464 | 216 | 216 | 216 |
| | *** | 33029 | 35966 | 46976 | 9304 | 9836 | 11890 | 1678 | 1711 | 1967 | 464 | 464 | 514 | 216 | 216 | 235 |
| 0.3 | *** | 35661 | 37936 | 46679 | 10226 | 10799 | 11818 | 1894 | 1926 | 1959 | 508 | 508 | 508 | 236 | 236 | 236 |
| | *** | 36539 | 40504 | 52416 | 10486 | 11221 | 13219 | 1906 | 1938 | 2164 | 508 | 508 | 557 | 236 | 236 | 252 |
| 0.35 | *** | 37676 | 40569 | 51826 | 11026 | 11753 | 13074 | 2056 | 2101 | 2154 | 541 | 561 | 561 | 248 | 248 | 248 |
| | *** | 38793 | 43798 | 56620 | 11351 | 12294 | 14239 | 2068 | 2121 | 2313 | 561 | 561 | 588 | 248 | 248 | 263 |
| 0.4 | *** | 38566 | 42096 | 55693 | 11526 | 12403 | 14016 | 2166 | 2219 | 2284 | 573 | 573 | 594 | 269 | 269 | 269 |
| | *** | 39951 | 45964 | 59588 | 11916 | 13053 | 14950 | 2198 | 2251 | 2412 | 573 | 573 | 606 | 269 | 269 | 268 |
| 0.45 | *** | 38533 | 42649 | 58261 | 11786 | 12781 | 14613 | 2231 | 2296 | 2361 | 594 | 594 | 594 | 269 | 269 | 269 |
| | *** | 40146 | 47069 | 61319 | 12229 | 13529 | 15352 | 2263 | 2328 | 2461 | 594 | 594 | 613 | 269 | 269 | 268 |
| 0.5 | *** | 37721 | 42336 | 59484 | 11786 | 12879 | 14894 | 2251 | 2316 | 2393 | 594 | 594 | 594 | 269 | 269 | 269 |
| | *** | 39561 | 47199 | 61814 | 12273 | 13691 | 15445 | 2284 | 2349 | 2461 | 594 | 594 | 606 | 269 | 269 | 263 |
| 0.55 | *** | 36291 | 41296 | 59354 | 11591 | 12728 | 14829 | 2219 | 2284 | 2361 | 573 | 573 | 594 | 248 | 248 | 248 |
| | *** | 38306 | 46463 | 61072 | 12099 | 13573 | 15228 | 2251 | 2328 | 2412 | 573 | 573 | 588 | 248 | 248 | 252 |
| 0.6 | *** | 34373 | 39606 | 57871 | 11168 | 12326 | 14418 | 2154 | 2198 | 2284 | 541 | 561 | 561 | 236 | 236 | 248 |
| | *** | 36486 | 44903 | 59093 | 11688 | 13183 | 14703 | 2186 | 2251 | 2313 | 561 | 561 | 557 | 236 | 248 | 235 |
| 0.65 | *** | 32021 | 37319 | 55064 | 10571 | 11688 | 13671 | 2024 | 2089 | 2154 | 508 | 508 | 529 | 216 | 216 | 216 |
| | *** | 34178 | 42563 | 55878 | 11071 | 12501 | 13868 | 2056 | 2121 | 2164 | 508 | 508 | 514 | 216 | 216 | 213 |
| 0.7 | *** | 29324 | 34471 | 50916 | 9771 | 10811 | 12619 | 1841 | 1906 | 1959 | 464 | 464 | 464 | 204 | 204 | 204 |
| | *** | 31436 | 39443 | 51427 | 10246 | 11558 | 12724 | 1873 | 1926 | 1967 | 464 | 464 | 458 | 204 | 204 | 186 |
| 0.75 | *** | 26269 | 31046 | 45444 | 8784 | 9694 | 11221 | 1634 | 1678 | 1711 | 399 | 399 | 399 | 171 | 171 | 171 |
| | *** | 28251 | 35564 | 45739 | 9186 | 10344 | 11271 | 1646 | 1699 | 1719 | 399 | 399 | 390 | 171 | 171 | 153 |
| 0.8 | *** | 22824 | 27016 | 38663 | 7581 | 8308 | 9478 | 1374 | 1386 | 1439 | 313 | 313 | 313 | 118 | 118 | 118 |
| | *** | 24558 | 30831 | 38815 | 7918 | 8816 | 9509 | 1374 | 1406 | 1422 | 313 | 313 | 310 | 118 | 118 | 115 |
| 0.85 | *** | 18871 | 22218 | 30603 | 6131 | 6651 | 7431 | 1049 | 1061 | 1081 | 216 | 236 | 236 | . | . | . |
| | *** | 20289 | 25131 | 30654 | 6379 | 6996 | 7438 | 1061 | 1081 | 1076 | 216 | 236 | 217 | . | . | . |
| 0.9 | *** | 14158 | 16421 | 21243 | 4376 | 4668 | 5058 | 671 | 691 | 691 | . | . | . | . | . | . |
| | *** | 15133 | 18241 | 21256 | 4506 | 4851 | 5058 | 671 | 691 | 681 | . | . | . | . | . | . |
| 0.95 | *** | 8146 | 9088 | 10636 | 2198 | 2284 | 2381 | . | . | . | . | . | . | . | . | . |
| | *** | 8568 | 9738 | 10622 | 2231 | 2328 | 2368 | . | . | . | . | . | . | . | . | . |
| 0.98 | *** | 3259 | 3433 | 3661 | . | . | . | . | . | . | . | . | . | . | . | . |
| | *** | 3336 | 3531 | 3648 | . | . | . | . | . | . | . | . | . | . | . | . |

TABLE 7: ALPHA= 0.05  POWER= 0.8     EXPECTED ACCRUAL THRU MINIMUM FOLLOW-UP= 14000

| | DEL=.01 | | | DEL=.02 | | | DEL=.05 | | | DEL=.10 | | | DEL=.15 | | |
|---|---|---|---|---|---|---|---|---|---|---|---|---|---|---|---|
| FACT= | 1.0 .75 | .50 .25 | .00 BIN | 1.0 .75 | .50 .25 | .00 BIN | 1.0 .75 | .50 .25 | .00 BIN | 1.0 75 | .50 .25 | .00 BIN | 1.0 .75 | .50 .25 | .00 BIN |
| PCONT=*** | | | | REQUIRED NUMBER OF PATIENTS | | | | | | | | | | | |
| 0.01 *** | 954 | 954 | 954 | 337 | 337 | 337 | 114 | 114 | 114 | 57 | 57 | 57 | 44 | 44 | 44 |
| *** | 954 | 954 | 3648 | 337 | 337 | 1206 | 114 | 114 | 328 | 57 | 57 | 134 | 44 | 44 | 80 |
| 0.02 *** | 2109 | 2122 | 2122 | 674 | 674 | 674 | 184 | 184 | 184 | 79 | 79 | 79 | 44 | 44 | 44 |
| *** | 2122 | 2122 | 6022 | 674 | 674 | 1793 | 184 | 184 | 419 | 79 | 79 | 155 | 44 | 44 | 89 |
| 0.05 *** | 6484 | 6532 | 6637 | 1842 | 1842 | 1864 | 394 | 394 | 394 | 149 | 149 | 149 | 79 | 79 | 79 |
| *** | 6497 | 6589 | 12848 | 1842 | 1864 | 3481 | 394 | 394 | 681 | 149 | 149 | 217 | 79 | 79 | 115 |
| 0.1 *** | 14429 | 14757 | 15479 | 3964 | 4012 | 4082 | 757 | 757 | 757 | 232 | 232 | 232 | 127 | 127 | 127 |
| *** | 14569 | 15024 | 23235 | 3999 | 4047 | 6047 | 757 | 757 | 1076 | 232 | 232 | 310 | 127 | 127 | 153 |
| 0.15 *** | 21757 | 22457 | 24439 | 5972 | 6112 | 6322 | 1094 | 1107 | 1107 | 324 | 324 | 324 | 162 | 162 | 162 |
| *** | 22037 | 23157 | 32385 | 6042 | 6217 | 8304 | 1107 | 1107 | 1422 | 324 | 324 | 390 | 162 | 162 | 186 |
| 0.2 *** | 27834 | 29024 | 32839 | 7722 | 8002 | 8409 | 1409 | 1422 | 1444 | 394 | 394 | 394 | 197 | 197 | 197 |
| *** | 28302 | 30262 | 40298 | 7849 | 8177 | 10251 | 1422 | 1422 | 1719 | 394 | 394 | 458 | 197 | 197 | 213 |
| 0.25 *** | 32537 | 34274 | 40307 | 9179 | 9577 | 10242 | 1667 | 1702 | 1724 | 464 | 464 | 464 | 219 | 219 | 219 |
| *** | 33202 | 36164 | 46976 | 9354 | 9879 | 11890 | 1689 | 1702 | 1967 | 464 | 464 | 514 | 219 | 219 | 235 |
| 0.3 *** | 35862 | 38207 | 46677 | 10299 | 10859 | 11817 | 1899 | 1934 | 1947 | 512 | 512 | 512 | 232 | 232 | 232 |
| *** | 36772 | 40762 | 52416 | 10544 | 11257 | 13219 | 1912 | 1934 | 2164 | 512 | 512 | 557 | 232 | 232 | 252 |
| 0.35 *** | 37949 | 40924 | 51822 | 11104 | 11817 | 13077 | 2052 | 2109 | 2144 | 547 | 547 | 547 | 254 | 254 | 254 |
| *** | 39104 | 44144 | 56620 | 11419 | 12342 | 14239 | 2074 | 2122 | 2313 | 547 | 547 | 588 | 254 | 254 | 263 |
| 0.4 *** | 38907 | 42512 | 55694 | 11629 | 12482 | 14009 | 2179 | 2227 | 2284 | 582 | 582 | 582 | 267 | 267 | 267 |
| *** | 40329 | 46362 | 59588 | 12014 | 13112 | 14950 | 2192 | 2249 | 2412 | 582 | 582 | 606 | 267 | 267 | 268 |
| 0.45 *** | 38929 | 43107 | 58249 | 11887 | 12867 | 14617 | 2249 | 2297 | 2354 | 582 | 604 | 604 | 267 | 267 | 267 |
| *** | 40587 | 47517 | 61319 | 12329 | 13589 | 15352 | 2262 | 2332 | 2461 | 582 | 604 | 613 | 267 | 267 | 268 |
| 0.5 *** | 38194 | 42862 | 59474 | 11922 | 12972 | 14884 | 2262 | 2319 | 2389 | 582 | 604 | 604 | 267 | 267 | 267 |
| *** | 40049 | 47714 | 61814 | 12399 | 13764 | 15445 | 2284 | 2354 | 2461 | 582 | 604 | 606 | 267 | 267 | 263 |
| 0.55 *** | 36794 | 41869 | 59347 | 11712 | 12832 | 14814 | 2227 | 2297 | 2367 | 582 | 582 | 582 | 254 | 254 | 254 |
| *** | 38837 | 46992 | 61072 | 12202 | 13637 | 15228 | 2262 | 2319 | 2412 | 582 | 582 | 588 | 254 | 254 | 252 |
| 0.6 *** | 34904 | 40189 | 57877 | 11314 | 12434 | 14407 | 2157 | 2214 | 2284 | 547 | 547 | 569 | 232 | 232 | 232 |
| *** | 37039 | 45439 | 59093 | 11804 | 13252 | 14703 | 2179 | 2249 | 2313 | 547 | 547 | 557 | 232 | 232 | 235 |
| 0.65 *** | 32572 | 37892 | 55064 | 10697 | 11782 | 13672 | 2039 | 2087 | 2144 | 512 | 512 | 512 | 219 | 219 | 219 |
| *** | 34742 | 43094 | 55878 | 11187 | 12574 | 13868 | 2052 | 2109 | 2164 | 512 | 512 | 514 | 219 | 219 | 213 |
| 0.7 *** | 29864 | 35022 | 50912 | 9892 | 10907 | 12609 | 1864 | 1899 | 1969 | 464 | 464 | 464 | 197 | 197 | 197 |
| *** | 31977 | 39944 | 51427 | 10347 | 11629 | 12724 | 1877 | 1934 | 1967 | 464 | 464 | 458 | 197 | 197 | 186 |
| 0.75 *** | 26762 | 31557 | 45452 | 8899 | 9774 | 11209 | 1632 | 1667 | 1724 | 394 | 394 | 394 | 162 | 162 | 162 |
| *** | 28757 | 36002 | 45739 | 9284 | 10382 | 11271 | 1654 | 1702 | 1719 | 394 | 394 | 390 | 162 | 162 | 153 |
| 0.8 *** | 23262 | 27449 | 38662 | 7674 | 8387 | 9494 | 1374 | 1387 | 1422 | 324 | 324 | 324 | 127 | 127 | 127 |
| *** | 25012 | 31194 | 38815 | 7989 | 8864 | 9509 | 1387 | 1409 | 1422 | 324 | 324 | 310 | 127 | 127 | 115 |
| 0.85 *** | 19237 | 22549 | 30599 | 6182 | 6694 | 7429 | 1059 | 1072 | 1094 | 219 | 232 | 232 | . | . | . |
| *** | 20637 | 25397 | 30654 | 6427 | 7022 | 7438 | 1059 | 1072 | 1076 | 219 | 232 | 217 | . | . | . |
| 0.9 *** | 14429 | 16634 | 21254 | 4419 | 4699 | 5062 | 674 | 687 | 687 | . | . | . | . | . | . |
| *** | 15387 | 18397 | 21256 | 4537 | 4874 | 5058 | 674 | 687 | 681 | . | . | . | . | . | . |
| 0.95 *** | 8269 | 9179 | 10627 | 2214 | 2284 | 2367 | . | . | . | . | . | . | . | . | . |
| *** | 8667 | 9787 | 10622 | 2249 | 2332 | 2368 | . | . | . | . | . | . | . | . | . |
| 0.98 *** | 3277 | 3452 | 3662 | . | . | . | . | . | . | . | . | . | . | . | . |
| *** | 3369 | 3544 | 3648 | . | . | . | . | . | . | . | . | . | . | . | . |

TABLE 7: ALPHA= 0.05 POWER= 0.8     EXPECTED ACCRUAL THRU MINIMUM FOLLOW-UP= 15000

PCONT=***      REQUIRED NUMBER OF PATIENTS

| PCONT | | DEL=.01 1.0/.75 | .50/.25 | .00/BIN | DEL=.02 1.0/.75 | .50/.25 | .00/BIN | DEL=.05 1.0/.75 | .50/.25 | .00/BIN | DEL=.10 1.0/75 | .50/.25 | .00/BIN | DEL=.15 1.0/.75 | .50/.25 | .00/BIN |
|---|---|---|---|---|---|---|---|---|---|---|---|---|---|---|---|---|
| 0.01 | *** | 947 | 947 | 947 | 347 | 347 | 347 | 122 | 122 | 122 | 61 | 61 | 61 | 47 | 47 | 47 |
|      | *** | 947 | 947 | 3648 | 347 | 347 | 1206 | 122 | 122 | 328 | 61 | 61 | 134 | 47 | 47 | 80 |
| 0.02 | *** | 2110 | 2124 | 2124 | 685 | 685 | 685 | 174 | 174 | 174 | 85 | 85 | 85 | 47 | 47 | 47 |
|      | *** | 2124 | 2124 | 6022 | 685 | 685 | 1793 | 174 | 174 | 419 | 85 | 85 | 155 | 47 | 47 | 89 |
| 0.05 | *** | 6474 | 6549 | 6647 | 1847 | 1847 | 1861 | 399 | 399 | 399 | 136 | 136 | 136 | 85 | 85 | 85 |
|      | *** | 6511 | 6586 | 12848 | 1847 | 1861 | 3481 | 399 | 399 | 681 | 136 | 136 | 217 | 85 | 85 | 115 |
| 0.1 | *** | 14461 | 14785 | 15474 | 3961 | 4022 | 4097 | 760 | 760 | 760 | 235 | 235 | 235 | 122 | 122 | 122 |
|     | *** | 14597 | 15047 | 23235 | 3999 | 4060 | 6047 | 760 | 760 | 1076 | 235 | 235 | 310 | 122 | 122 | 153 |
| 0.15 | *** | 21811 | 22524 | 24436 | 5986 | 6136 | 6324 | 1097 | 1111 | 1111 | 324 | 324 | 324 | 160 | 160 | 160 |
|      | *** | 22097 | 23222 | 32385 | 6061 | 6211 | 8304 | 1097 | 1111 | 1422 | 324 | 324 | 390 | 160 | 160 | 186 |
| 0.2 | *** | 27947 | 29147 | 32836 | 7749 | 8011 | 8410 | 1411 | 1435 | 1435 | 399 | 399 | 399 | 197 | 197 | 197 |
|     | *** | 28411 | 30385 | 40298 | 7885 | 8185 | 10251 | 1411 | 1435 | 1719 | 399 | 399 | 458 | 197 | 197 | 213 |
| 0.25 | *** | 32686 | 34472 | 40299 | 9211 | 9610 | 10247 | 1674 | 1697 | 1711 | 460 | 460 | 460 | 211 | 211 | 211 |
|      | *** | 33385 | 36324 | 46976 | 9399 | 9886 | 11890 | 1697 | 1711 | 1967 | 460 | 460 | 514 | 211 | 211 | 235 |
| 0.3 | *** | 36085 | 38461 | 46674 | 10360 | 10899 | 11822 | 1899 | 1922 | 1960 | 511 | 511 | 511 | 235 | 235 | 235 |
|     | *** | 36999 | 41011 | 52416 | 10599 | 11297 | 13219 | 1899 | 1936 | 2164 | 511 | 511 | 557 | 235 | 235 | 252 |
| 0.35 | *** | 38199 | 41236 | 51835 | 11185 | 11874 | 13074 | 2072 | 2110 | 2147 | 549 | 549 | 549 | 249 | 249 | 249 |
|      | *** | 39399 | 44447 | 56620 | 11499 | 12385 | 14239 | 2086 | 2124 | 2313 | 549 | 549 | 588 | 249 | 249 | 263 |
| 0.4 | *** | 39235 | 42886 | 55697 | 11724 | 12572 | 14011 | 2185 | 2222 | 2274 | 572 | 586 | 586 | 272 | 272 | 272 |
|     | *** | 40674 | 46735 | 59588 | 12099 | 13172 | 14950 | 2199 | 2260 | 2412 | 572 | 586 | 606 | 272 | 272 | 268 |
| 0.45 | *** | 39324 | 43561 | 58261 | 12010 | 12947 | 14611 | 2260 | 2297 | 2349 | 586 | 586 | 586 | 272 | 272 | 272 |
|      | *** | 41011 | 47935 | 61319 | 12422 | 13636 | 15352 | 2274 | 2335 | 2461 | 586 | 586 | 613 | 272 | 272 | 268 |
| 0.5 | *** | 38611 | 43360 | 59485 | 12047 | 13074 | 14874 | 2274 | 2335 | 2386 | 586 | 586 | 610 | 272 | 272 | 272 |
|     | *** | 40524 | 48160 | 61814 | 12497 | 13824 | 15445 | 2297 | 2349 | 2461 | 586 | 586 | 606 | 272 | 272 | 263 |
| 0.55 | *** | 37285 | 42385 | 59349 | 11836 | 12924 | 14822 | 2236 | 2297 | 2372 | 572 | 586 | 586 | 249 | 249 | 249 |
|      | *** | 39347 | 47461 | 61072 | 12324 | 13711 | 15228 | 2260 | 2335 | 2412 | 572 | 586 | 588 | 249 | 249 | 252 |
| 0.6 | *** | 35410 | 40711 | 57872 | 11424 | 12535 | 14410 | 2161 | 2222 | 2274 | 549 | 549 | 549 | 235 | 235 | 249 |
|     | *** | 37561 | 45924 | 59093 | 11911 | 13322 | 14703 | 2185 | 2236 | 2313 | 549 | 549 | 557 | 235 | 249 | 235 |
| 0.65 | *** | 33085 | 38424 | 55060 | 10824 | 11874 | 13674 | 2035 | 2086 | 2147 | 511 | 511 | 511 | 211 | 211 | 211 |
|      | *** | 35274 | 43561 | 55878 | 11297 | 12647 | 13868 | 2072 | 2110 | 2164 | 511 | 511 | 514 | 211 | 211 | 213 |
| 0.7 | *** | 30361 | 35536 | 50911 | 10022 | 10997 | 12610 | 1861 | 1899 | 1960 | 460 | 460 | 460 | 197 | 197 | 197 |
|     | *** | 32499 | 40397 | 51427 | 10449 | 11672 | 12724 | 1885 | 1936 | 1967 | 460 | 460 | 458 | 197 | 197 | 186 |
| 0.75 | *** | 27249 | 32035 | 45460 | 8986 | 9849 | 11222 | 1636 | 1674 | 1711 | 399 | 399 | 399 | 160 | 160 | 160 |
|      | *** | 29236 | 36399 | 45739 | 9385 | 10435 | 11271 | 1660 | 1697 | 1719 | 399 | 399 | 390 | 160 | 160 | 153 |
| 0.8 | *** | 23686 | 27849 | 38672 | 7749 | 8447 | 9474 | 1374 | 1397 | 1435 | 310 | 324 | 324 | 122 | 122 | 122 |
|     | *** | 25435 | 31524 | 38815 | 8072 | 8897 | 9509 | 1374 | 1411 | 1422 | 310 | 324 | 310 | 122 | 122 | 115 |
| 0.85 | *** | 19561 | 22861 | 30610 | 6249 | 6736 | 7435 | 1060 | 1074 | 1074 | 235 | 235 | 235 | . | . | . |
|      | *** | 20972 | 25660 | 30654 | 6474 | 7060 | 7438 | 1060 | 1074 | 1076 | 235 | 235 | 217 | . | . | . |
| 0.9 | *** | 14649 | 16847 | 21249 | 4449 | 4711 | 5072 | 685 | 685 | 685 | . | . | . | . | . | . |
|     | *** | 15610 | 18549 | 21256 | 4561 | 4885 | 5058 | 685 | 685 | 681 | . | . | . | . | . | . |
| 0.95 | *** | 8372 | 9249 | 10636 | 2222 | 2297 | 2372 | . | . | . | . | . | . | . | . | . |
|      | *** | 8761 | 9849 | 10622 | 2260 | 2335 | 2368 | . | . | . | . | . | . | . | . | . |
| 0.98 | *** | 3310 | 3460 | 3661 | . | . | . | . | . | . | . | . | . | . | . | . |
|      | *** | 3385 | 3549 | 3648 | . | . | . | . | . | . | . | . | . | . | . | . |

TABLE 7: ALPHA= 0.05  POWER= 0.8    EXPECTED ACCRUAL THRU MINIMUM FOLLOW-UP= 17000

| | | DEL=.01 | | | DEL=.02 | | | DEL=.05 | | | DEL=.10 | | | DEL=.15 | | |
|---|---|---|---|---|---|---|---|---|---|---|---|---|---|---|---|---|
| FACT= | | 1.0 .75 | .50 .25 | .00 BIN | 1.0 .75 | .50 .25 | .00 BIN | 1.0 .75 | .50 .25 | .00 BIN | 1.0 75 | .50 .25 | .00 BIN | 1.0 .75 | .50 .25 | .00 BIN |
| PCONT=*** | | | | REQUIRED NUMBER OF PATIENTS | | | | | | | | | | | |
| 0.01 | *** | 946 | 946 | 946 | 351 | 351 | 351 | 112 | 112 | 112 | 54 | 54 | 54 | 27 | 27 | 27 |
| | *** | 946 | 946 | 3648 | 351 | 351 | 1206 | 112 | 112 | 328 | 54 | 54 | 134 | 27 | 27 | 80 |
| 0.02 | *** | 2110 | 2110 | 2136 | 665 | 665 | 665 | 181 | 181 | 181 | 70 | 70 | 70 | 54 | 54 | 54 |
| | *** | 2110 | 2110 | 6022 | 665 | 665 | 1793 | 181 | 181 | 419 | 70 | 70 | 155 | 54 | 54 | 89 |
| 0.05 | *** | 6487 | 6556 | 6641 | 1839 | 1855 | 1855 | 394 | 394 | 394 | 139 | 139 | 139 | 70 | 70 | 70 |
| | *** | 6530 | 6599 | 12848 | 1855 | 1855 | 3481 | 394 | 394 | 681 | 139 | 139 | 217 | 70 | 70 | 115 |
| 0.1 | *** | 14520 | 14844 | 15481 | 3980 | 4022 | 4091 | 750 | 750 | 750 | 240 | 240 | 240 | 112 | 112 | 112 |
| | *** | 14647 | 15099 | 23235 | 4006 | 4065 | 6047 | 750 | 750 | 1076 | 240 | 240 | 310 | 112 | 112 | 153 |
| 0.15 | *** | 21941 | 22664 | 24449 | 6020 | 6147 | 6317 | 1090 | 1116 | 1116 | 325 | 325 | 325 | 155 | 155 | 155 |
| | *** | 22239 | 23317 | 32385 | 6089 | 6232 | 8304 | 1116 | 1116 | 1422 | 325 | 325 | 390 | 155 | 155 | 186 |
| 0.2 | *** | 28146 | 29379 | 32837 | 7805 | 8060 | 8400 | 1414 | 1430 | 1430 | 394 | 394 | 394 | 197 | 197 | 197 |
| | *** | 28630 | 30585 | 40298 | 7916 | 8214 | 10251 | 1414 | 1430 | 1719 | 394 | 394 | 458 | 197 | 197 | 213 |
| 0.25 | *** | 32991 | 34819 | 40301 | 9292 | 9675 | 10254 | 1685 | 1711 | 1727 | 452 | 452 | 452 | 224 | 224 | 224 |
| | *** | 33714 | 36646 | 46976 | 9462 | 9930 | 11890 | 1685 | 1711 | 1967 | 452 | 452 | 514 | 224 | 224 | 235 |
| 0.3 | *** | 36476 | 38941 | 46676 | 10466 | 10992 | 11826 | 1897 | 1924 | 1966 | 521 | 521 | 521 | 240 | 240 | 240 |
| | *** | 37454 | 41422 | 52416 | 10695 | 11359 | 13219 | 1924 | 1940 | 2164 | 521 | 521 | 557 | 240 | 240 | 252 |
| 0.35 | *** | 38702 | 41831 | 51835 | 11316 | 11996 | 13075 | 2067 | 2110 | 2136 | 564 | 564 | 564 | 266 | 266 | 266 |
| | *** | 39961 | 44992 | 56620 | 11630 | 12464 | 14239 | 2094 | 2136 | 2313 | 564 | 564 | 588 | 266 | 266 | 263 |
| 0.4 | *** | 39850 | 43590 | 55702 | 11885 | 12692 | 14010 | 2195 | 2237 | 2280 | 580 | 580 | 580 | 266 | 266 | 266 |
| | *** | 41337 | 47372 | 59588 | 12251 | 13245 | 14950 | 2221 | 2264 | 2412 | 580 | 580 | 606 | 266 | 266 | 268 |
| 0.45 | *** | 40046 | 44355 | 58252 | 12182 | 13101 | 14605 | 2264 | 2306 | 2365 | 580 | 606 | 606 | 266 | 266 | 266 |
| | *** | 41789 | 48674 | 61319 | 12591 | 13739 | 15352 | 2280 | 2322 | 2461 | 580 | 606 | 613 | 266 | 266 | 268 |
| 0.5 | *** | 39425 | 44254 | 59469 | 12251 | 13229 | 14886 | 2280 | 2322 | 2391 | 580 | 606 | 606 | 266 | 266 | 266 |
| | *** | 41380 | 48971 | 61814 | 12676 | 13925 | 15445 | 2306 | 2365 | 2461 | 580 | 606 | 606 | 266 | 266 | 263 |
| 0.55 | *** | 38150 | 43319 | 59341 | 12055 | 13101 | 14817 | 2264 | 2306 | 2365 | 580 | 580 | 580 | 266 | 266 | 266 |
| | *** | 40275 | 48334 | 61072 | 12522 | 13824 | 15228 | 2280 | 2322 | 2412 | 580 | 580 | 588 | 266 | 266 | 252 |
| 0.6 | *** | 36349 | 41704 | 57870 | 11656 | 12692 | 14419 | 2179 | 2221 | 2280 | 564 | 564 | 564 | 240 | 240 | 240 |
| | *** | 38532 | 46804 | 59093 | 12124 | 13415 | 14703 | 2195 | 2264 | 2313 | 564 | 564 | 557 | 240 | 240 | 235 |
| 0.65 | *** | 34027 | 39382 | 55065 | 11035 | 12039 | 13670 | 2051 | 2094 | 2152 | 521 | 521 | 521 | 224 | 224 | 224 |
| | *** | 36237 | 44424 | 55878 | 11486 | 12735 | 13868 | 2067 | 2110 | 2164 | 521 | 521 | 514 | 224 | 224 | 213 |
| 0.7 | *** | 31291 | 36450 | 50926 | 10211 | 11146 | 12607 | 1881 | 1924 | 1966 | 452 | 452 | 452 | 197 | 197 | 197 |
| | *** | 33432 | 41194 | 51427 | 10636 | 11784 | 12724 | 1897 | 1940 | 1967 | 452 | 452 | 458 | 197 | 197 | 186 |
| 0.75 | *** | 28104 | 32864 | 45444 | 9165 | 9972 | 11205 | 1642 | 1685 | 1727 | 394 | 394 | 394 | 155 | 155 | 155 |
| | *** | 30101 | 37114 | 45739 | 9531 | 10509 | 11271 | 1669 | 1711 | 1719 | 394 | 394 | 390 | 155 | 155 | 153 |
| 0.8 | *** | 24449 | 28545 | 38660 | 7890 | 8527 | 9489 | 1371 | 1414 | 1430 | 309 | 325 | 325 | 112 | 112 | 112 |
| | *** | 26191 | 32115 | 38815 | 8187 | 8952 | 9509 | 1387 | 1414 | 1422 | 325 | 325 | 310 | 112 | 112 | 115 |
| 0.85 | *** | 20199 | 23402 | 30611 | 6360 | 6811 | 7422 | 1047 | 1074 | 1090 | 224 | 224 | 224 | . | . | . |
| | *** | 21575 | 26080 | 30654 | 6572 | 7082 | 7438 | 1074 | 1074 | 1076 | 224 | 224 | 217 | . | . | . |
| 0.9 | *** | 15072 | 17181 | 21261 | 4490 | 4745 | 5069 | 665 | 691 | 691 | . | . | . | . | . | . |
| | *** | 16007 | 18796 | 21256 | 4617 | 4899 | 5058 | 691 | 691 | 681 | . | . | . | . | . | . |
| 0.95 | *** | 8554 | 9377 | 10636 | 2237 | 2306 | 2365 | . | . | . | . | . | . | . | . | . |
| | *** | 8936 | 9930 | 10622 | 2264 | 2349 | 2368 | . | . | . | . | . | . | . | . | . |
| 0.98 | *** | 3326 | 3470 | 3666 | . | . | . | . | . | . | . | . | . | . | . | . |
| | *** | 3411 | 3555 | 3648 | . | . | . | . | . | . | . | . | . | . | . | . |

TABLE 7: ALPHA= 0.05  POWER= 0.8    EXPECTED ACCRUAL THRU MINIMUM FOLLOW-UP= 20000

| | | DEL=.01 | | | DEL=.02 | | | DEL=.05 | | | DEL=.10 | | | DEL=.15 | | |
|---|---|---|---|---|---|---|---|---|---|---|---|---|---|---|---|---|
| | FACT= | 1.0 .75 | .50 .25 | .00 BIN | 1.0 .75 | .50 .25 | .00 BIN | 1.0 .75 | .50 .25 | .00 BIN | 1.0 75 | .50 .25 | .00 BIN | 1.0 .75 | .50 .25 | .00 BIN |
| PCONT=*** | | REQUIRED NUMBER OF PATIENTS | | | | | | | | | | | | | | |
| 0.01 | *** | 963 963 | 963 | 332 332 | 332 | 113 113 | 113 | 63 63 | 63 | 32 32 | 32 | | | | | |

| PCONT | | DEL.01 1.0/.75 | DEL.01 .50/.25 | DEL.01 .00 BIN | DEL.02 1.0/.75 | DEL.02 .50/.25 | DEL.02 .00 BIN | DEL.05 1.0/.75 | DEL.05 .50/.25 | DEL.05 .00 BIN | DEL.10 1.0/75 | DEL.10 .50/.25 | DEL.10 .00 BIN | DEL.15 1.0/.75 | DEL.15 .50/.25 | DEL.15 .00 BIN |
|---|---|---|---|---|---|---|---|---|---|---|---|---|---|---|---|---|
| 0.01 | *** | 963 | 963 | 963 | 332 | 332 | 332 | 113 | 113 | 113 | 63 | 63 | 63 | 32 | 32 | 32 |
| | *** | 963 | 963 | 3648 | 332 | 332 | 1206 | 113 | 113 | 328 | 63 | 63 | 134 | 32 | 32 | 80 |
| 0.02 | *** | 2113 | 2113 | 2132 | 682 | 682 | 682 | 182 | 182 | 182 | 82 | 82 | 82 | 63 | 63 | 63 |
| | *** | 2113 | 2132 | 6022 | 682 | 682 | 1793 | 182 | 182 | 419 | 82 | 82 | 155 | 63 | 63 | 89 |
| 0.05 | *** | 6513 | 6563 | 6632 | 1832 | 1863 | 1863 | 382 | 382 | 382 | 132 | 132 | 132 | 82 | 82 | 82 |
| | *** | 6532 | 6613 | 12848 | 1863 | 1863 | 3481 | 382 | 382 | 681 | 132 | 132 | 217 | 82 | 82 | 115 |
| 0.1 | *** | 14582 | 14913 | 15463 | 3982 | 4032 | 4082 | 763 | 763 | 763 | 232 | 232 | 232 | 113 | 113 | 113 |
| | *** | 14732 | 15132 | 23235 | 4013 | 4063 | 6047 | 763 | 763 | 1076 | 232 | 232 | 310 | 113 | 113 | 153 |
| 0.15 | *** | 22113 | 22832 | 24432 | 6063 | 6182 | 6332 | 1113 | 1113 | 1113 | 313 | 313 | 313 | 163 | 163 | 163 |
| | *** | 22413 | 23463 | 32385 | 6113 | 6232 | 8304 | 1113 | 1113 | 1422 | 313 | 313 | 390 | 163 | 163 | 186 |
| 0.2 | *** | 28413 | 29682 | 32832 | 7882 | 8113 | 8413 | 1413 | 1432 | 1432 | 382 | 382 | 382 | 182 | 182 | 182 |
| | *** | 28932 | 30832 | 40298 | 7982 | 8232 | 10251 | 1413 | 1432 | 1719 | 382 | 382 | 458 | 182 | 182 | 213 |
| 0.25 | *** | 33382 | 35263 | 40313 | 9382 | 9732 | 10263 | 1682 | 1713 | 1713 | 463 | 463 | 463 | 213 | 213 | 213 |
| | *** | 34132 | 37032 | 46976 | 9563 | 9963 | 11890 | 1682 | 1713 | 1967 | 463 | 463 | 514 | 213 | 213 | 235 |
| 0.3 | *** | 37013 | 39532 | 46682 | 10613 | 11082 | 11813 | 1913 | 1932 | 1963 | 513 | 513 | 513 | 232 | 232 | 232 |
| | *** | 38032 | 41963 | 52416 | 10813 | 11413 | 13219 | 1913 | 1932 | 2164 | 513 | 513 | 557 | 232 | 232 | 252 |
| 0.35 | *** | 39382 | 42582 | 51832 | 11482 | 12113 | 13063 | 2082 | 2113 | 2132 | 563 | 563 | 563 | 263 | 263 | 263 |
| | *** | 40682 | 45663 | 56620 | 11782 | 12532 | 14239 | 2082 | 2132 | 2313 | 563 | 563 | 588 | 263 | 263 | 263 |
| 0.4 | *** | 40682 | 44513 | 55713 | 12113 | 12832 | 14013 | 2213 | 2232 | 2282 | 582 | 582 | 582 | 263 | 263 | 263 |
| | *** | 42232 | 48182 | 59588 | 12432 | 13363 | 14950 | 2213 | 2263 | 2412 | 582 | 582 | 606 | 263 | 263 | 268 |
| 0.45 | *** | 41013 | 45413 | 58263 | 12432 | 13282 | 14613 | 2282 | 2313 | 2363 | 582 | 582 | 582 | 263 | 263 | 263 |
| | *** | 42813 | 49613 | 61319 | 12813 | 13863 | 15352 | 2282 | 2332 | 2461 | 582 | 582 | 613 | 263 | 263 | 268 |
| 0.5 | *** | 40513 | 45382 | 59482 | 12482 | 13413 | 14882 | 2282 | 2332 | 2382 | 582 | 582 | 613 | 263 | 263 | 263 |
| | *** | 42513 | 49982 | 61814 | 12913 | 14063 | 15445 | 2313 | 2363 | 2461 | 582 | 582 | 606 | 263 | 263 | 263 |
| 0.55 | *** | 39332 | 44532 | 59332 | 12332 | 13282 | 14813 | 2263 | 2313 | 2363 | 582 | 582 | 582 | 263 | 263 | 263 |
| | *** | 41482 | 49382 | 61072 | 12763 | 13963 | 15228 | 2282 | 2332 | 2412 | 582 | 582 | 588 | 263 | 263 | 252 |
| 0.6 | *** | 37563 | 42932 | 57882 | 11913 | 12882 | 14413 | 2182 | 2232 | 2282 | 563 | 563 | 563 | 232 | 232 | 232 |
| | *** | 39813 | 47882 | 59093 | 12363 | 13563 | 14703 | 2213 | 2263 | 2313 | 563 | 563 | 557 | 232 | 232 | 235 |
| 0.65 | *** | 35282 | 40632 | 55063 | 11282 | 12232 | 13682 | 2063 | 2113 | 2132 | 513 | 513 | 513 | 213 | 213 | 213 |
| | *** | 37513 | 45463 | 55878 | 11713 | 12863 | 13868 | 2082 | 2132 | 2164 | 513 | 513 | 514 | 213 | 213 | 213 |
| 0.7 | *** | 32513 | 37632 | 50913 | 10463 | 11313 | 12613 | 1882 | 1913 | 1963 | 463 | 463 | 463 | 182 | 182 | 182 |
| | *** | 34663 | 42182 | 51427 | 10832 | 11882 | 12724 | 1913 | 1932 | 1967 | 463 | 463 | 458 | 182 | 182 | 186 |
| 0.75 | *** | 29232 | 33932 | 45463 | 9382 | 10113 | 11213 | 1663 | 1682 | 1713 | 382 | 382 | 413 | 163 | 163 | 163 |
| | *** | 31213 | 37982 | 45739 | 9713 | 10613 | 11271 | 1682 | 1713 | 1719 | 382 | 382 | 390 | 163 | 163 | 153 |
| 0.8 | *** | 25432 | 29463 | 38663 | 8063 | 8663 | 9482 | 1382 | 1413 | 1432 | 313 | 313 | 313 | 132 | 132 | 132 |
| | *** | 27163 | 32813 | 38815 | 8332 | 9032 | 9509 | 1382 | 1413 | 1422 | 313 | 313 | 310 | 132 | 132 | 115 |
| 0.85 | *** | 20982 | 24113 | 30613 | 6482 | 6882 | 7432 | 1063 | 1063 | 1082 | 232 | 232 | 232 | . | . | . |
| | *** | 22332 | 26582 | 30654 | 6663 | 7132 | 7438 | 1063 | 1082 | 1076 | 232 | 232 | 217 | . | . | . |
| 0.9 | *** | 15613 | 17613 | 21263 | 4563 | 4782 | 5063 | 682 | 682 | 682 | . | . | . | . | . | . |
| | *** | 16482 | 19082 | 21256 | 4682 | 4913 | 5058 | 682 | 682 | 681 | . | . | . | . | . | . |
| 0.95 | *** | 8763 | 9532 | 10632 | 2263 | 2313 | 2382 | . | . | . | . | . | . | . | . | . |
| | *** | 9113 | 10013 | 10622 | 2282 | 2332 | 2368 | . | . | . | . | . | . | . | . | . |
| 0.98 | *** | 3382 | 3513 | 3663 | . | . | . | . | . | . | . | . | . | . | . | . |
| | *** | 3432 | 3582 | 3648 | . | . | . | . | . | . | . | . | . | . | . | . |

TABLE 7: ALPHA= 0.05  POWER= 0.8    EXPECTED ACCRUAL THRU MINIMUM FOLLOW-UP= 25000

| | | DEL=.01 | | | DEL=.02 | | | DEL=.05 | | | DEL=.10 | | | DEL=.15 | | |
|---|---|---|---|---|---|---|---|---|---|---|---|---|---|---|---|---|
| FACT= | | 1.0 .75 | .50 .25 | .00 BIN | 1.0 .75 | .50 .25 | .00 BIN | 1.0 .75 | .50 .25 | .00 BIN | 1.0 75 | .50 .25 | .00 BIN | 1.0 .75 | .50 .25 | .00 BIN |
| PCONT=*** | | | | REQUIRED | NUMBER | OF PATIENTS | | | | | | | | | | |
| 0.01 | *** | 954 | 954 | 954 | 352 | 352 | 352 | 102 | 102 | 102 | 40 | 40 | 40 | 40 | 40 | 40 |
| | *** | 954 | 954 | 3648 | 352 | 352 | 1206 | 102 | 102 | 328 | 40 | 40 | 134 | 40 | 40 | 80 |
| 0.02 | *** | 2102 | 2102 | 2141 | 665 | 665 | 665 | 165 | 165 | 165 | 79 | 79 | 79 | 40 | 40 | 40 |
| | *** | 2102 | 2141 | 6022 | 665 | 665 | 1793 | 165 | 165 | 419 | 79 | 79 | 155 | 40 | 40 | 89 |
| 0.05 | *** | 6540 | 6579 | 6641 | 1852 | 1852 | 1852 | 391 | 391 | 391 | 141 | 141 | 141 | 79 | 79 | 79 |
| | *** | 6540 | 6602 | 12848 | 1852 | 1852 | 3481 | 391 | 391 | 681 | 141 | 141 | 217 | 79 | 79 | 115 |
| 0.1 | *** | 14704 | 14977 | 15477 | 4016 | 4040 | 4079 | 766 | 766 | 766 | 227 | 227 | 227 | 102 | 102 | 102 |
| | *** | 14829 | 15204 | 23235 | 4016 | 4079 | 6047 | 766 | 766 | 1076 | 227 | 227 | 310 | 102 | 102 | 153 |
| 0.15 | *** | 22329 | 23040 | 24454 | 6102 | 6204 | 6329 | 1102 | 1102 | 1102 | 329 | 329 | 329 | 165 | 165 | 165 |
| | *** | 22641 | 23602 | 32385 | 6141 | 6266 | 8304 | 1102 | 1102 | 1422 | 329 | 329 | 390 | 165 | 165 | 186 |
| 0.2 | *** | 28829 | 30079 | 32829 | 7954 | 8141 | 8415 | 1415 | 1415 | 1454 | 391 | 391 | 391 | 204 | 204 | 204 |
| | *** | 29352 | 31141 | 40298 | 8040 | 8266 | 10251 | 1415 | 1415 | 1719 | 391 | 391 | 458 | 204 | 204 | 213 |
| 0.25 | *** | 33977 | 35852 | 40290 | 9516 | 9829 | 10266 | 1704 | 1704 | 1727 | 454 | 454 | 454 | 227 | 227 | 227 |
| | *** | 34766 | 37516 | 46976 | 9665 | 10016 | 11890 | 1704 | 1704 | 1967 | 454 | 454 | 514 | 227 | 227 | 235 |
| 0.3 | *** | 37790 | 40352 | 46665 | 10766 | 11204 | 11829 | 1915 | 1954 | 1954 | 516 | 516 | 516 | 227 | 227 | 227 |
| | *** | 38852 | 42641 | 52416 | 10977 | 11477 | 13219 | 1915 | 1954 | 2164 | 516 | 516 | 557 | 227 | 227 | 252 |
| 0.35 | *** | 40391 | 43641 | 51829 | 11727 | 12266 | 13079 | 2102 | 2102 | 2141 | 540 | 540 | 540 | 266 | 266 | 266 |
| | *** | 41727 | 46540 | 56620 | 11977 | 12641 | 14239 | 2102 | 2141 | 2313 | 540 | 540 | 588 | 266 | 266 | 263 |
| 0.4 | *** | 41891 | 45727 | 55704 | 12352 | 13040 | 14016 | 2227 | 2227 | 2266 | 579 | 579 | 579 | 266 | 266 | 266 |
| | *** | 43477 | 49227 | 59588 | 12665 | 13454 | 14950 | 2227 | 2266 | 2412 | 579 | 579 | 606 | 266 | 266 | 268 |
| 0.45 | *** | 42391 | 46829 | 58266 | 12727 | 13477 | 14602 | 2290 | 2329 | 2352 | 602 | 602 | 602 | 266 | 266 | 266 |
| | *** | 44227 | 50790 | 61319 | 13079 | 13977 | 15352 | 2290 | 2329 | 2461 | 602 | 602 | 613 | 266 | 266 | 268 |
| 0.5 | *** | 42079 | 46954 | 59477 | 12829 | 13641 | 14891 | 2329 | 2352 | 2391 | 602 | 602 | 602 | 266 | 266 | 266 |
| | *** | 44102 | 51290 | 61814 | 13204 | 14204 | 15445 | 2329 | 2352 | 2461 | 602 | 602 | 606 | 266 | 266 | 263 |
| 0.55 | *** | 41016 | 46165 | 59352 | 12665 | 13540 | 14829 | 2290 | 2329 | 2352 | 579 | 579 | 579 | 266 | 266 | 266 |
| | *** | 43165 | 50766 | 61072 | 13079 | 14102 | 15228 | 2290 | 2329 | 2412 | 579 | 579 | 588 | 266 | 266 | 252 |
| 0.6 | *** | 39290 | 44602 | 57891 | 12266 | 13141 | 14415 | 2204 | 2227 | 2290 | 540 | 540 | 540 | 227 | 227 | 227 |
| | *** | 41540 | 49266 | 59093 | 12665 | 13704 | 14703 | 2227 | 2266 | 2313 | 540 | 540 | 557 | 227 | 227 | 235 |
| 0.65 | *** | 37016 | 42266 | 55079 | 11641 | 12477 | 13665 | 2079 | 2102 | 2141 | 516 | 516 | 516 | 227 | 227 | 227 |
| | *** | 39227 | 46829 | 55878 | 12016 | 13016 | 13868 | 2102 | 2141 | 2164 | 516 | 516 | 514 | 227 | 227 | 213 |
| 0.7 | *** | 34165 | 39165 | 50915 | 10766 | 11516 | 12602 | 1891 | 1915 | 1954 | 454 | 454 | 454 | 204 | 204 | 204 |
| | *** | 36290 | 43415 | 51427 | 11102 | 12016 | 12724 | 1915 | 1954 | 1967 | 454 | 454 | 458 | 204 | 204 | 186 |
| 0.75 | *** | 30790 | 35329 | 45454 | 9641 | 10290 | 11204 | 1665 | 1704 | 1727 | 391 | 391 | 391 | 165 | 165 | 165 |
| | *** | 32727 | 39079 | 45739 | 9954 | 10704 | 11271 | 1665 | 1704 | 1719 | 391 | 391 | 390 | 165 | 165 | 153 |
| 0.8 | *** | 26766 | 30641 | 38665 | 8290 | 8790 | 9477 | 1391 | 1415 | 1415 | 329 | 329 | 329 | 141 | 141 | 141 |
| | *** | 28454 | 33704 | 38815 | 8516 | 9102 | 9509 | 1391 | 1415 | 1422 | 329 | 329 | 310 | 141 | 141 | 115 |
| 0.85 | *** | 22040 | 24977 | 30602 | 6641 | 6977 | 7415 | 1079 | 1079 | 1079 | 227 | 227 | 227 | . | . | . |
| | *** | 23329 | 27227 | 30654 | 6790 | 7204 | 7438 | 1079 | 1079 | 1076 | 227 | 227 | 217 | . | . | . |
| 0.9 | *** | 16290 | 18141 | 21266 | 4641 | 4829 | 5079 | 665 | 704 | 704 | . | . | . | . | . | . |
| | *** | 17141 | 19454 | 21256 | 4727 | 4954 | 5058 | 665 | 704 | 681 | . | . | . | . | . | . |
| 0.95 | *** | 9040 | 9704 | 10641 | 2266 | 2329 | 2391 | . | . | . | . | . | . | . | . | . |
| | *** | 9352 | 10141 | 10622 | 2290 | 2352 | 2368 | . | . | . | . | . | . | . | . | . |
| 0.98 | *** | 3415 | 3540 | 3665 | . | . | . | . | . | . | . | . | . | . | . | . |
| | *** | 3477 | 3602 | 3648 | . | . | . | . | . | . | . | . | . | . | . | . |

TABLE 8: ALPHA= 0.05 POWER= 0.9    EXPECTED ACCRUAL THRU MINIMUM FOLLOW-UP= 30

| | | DEL=.10 | | | DEL=.15 | | | DEL=.20 | | | DEL=.25 | | | DEL=.30 | | |
|---|---|---|---|---|---|---|---|---|---|---|---|---|---|---|---|---|
| FACT= | | 1.0 .75 | .50 .25 | .00 BIN | 1.0 .75 | .50 .25 | .00 BIN | 1.0 .75 | .50 .25 | .00 BIN | 1.0 75 | .50 .25 | .00 BIN | 1.0 .75 | .50 .25 | .00 BIN |
| PCONT=*** | | | | | REQUIRED NUMBER OF PATIENTS | | | | | | | | | | | |
| 0.05 | *** | 180 | 181 | 195 | 105 | 106 | 114 | 74 | 75 | 80 | 58 | 59 | 62 | 48 | 48 | 51 |
| | *** | 180 | 183 | 300 | 105 | 108 | 158 | 74 | 76 | 101 | 58 | 60 | 71 | 48 | 49 | 53 |
| 0.1 | *** | 284 | 286 | 326 | 150 | 153 | 173 | 99 | 101 | 113 | 73 | 75 | 83 | 58 | 60 | 65 |
| | *** | 285 | 290 | 429 | 151 | 157 | 212 | 100 | 104 | 129 | 74 | 78 | 88 | 59 | 62 | 63 |
| 0.15 | *** | 366 | 370 | 447 | 184 | 188 | 225 | 117 | 121 | 142 | 84 | 87 | 101 | 65 | 68 | 77 |
| | *** | 367 | 377 | 540 | 186 | 195 | 257 | 118 | 126 | 153 | 85 | 91 | 101 | 66 | 71 | 72 |
| 0.2 | *** | 426 | 432 | 554 | 208 | 214 | 270 | 129 | 134 | 166 | 91 | 96 | 115 | 69 | 73 | 86 |
| | *** | 428 | 442 | 634 | 210 | 223 | 295 | 131 | 142 | 172 | 93 | 101 | 112 | 71 | 77 | 79 |
| 0.25 | *** | 465 | 472 | 645 | 222 | 230 | 308 | 136 | 143 | 185 | 95 | 101 | 126 | 72 | 77 | 93 |
| | *** | 467 | 486 | 711 | 225 | 243 | 326 | 138 | 153 | 187 | 97 | 108 | 120 | 74 | 82 | 83 |
| 0.3 | *** | 484 | 493 | 719 | 228 | 238 | 337 | 138 | 147 | 199 | 96 | 103 | 134 | 72 | 78 | 98 |
| | *** | 487 | 512 | 771 | 232 | 255 | 349 | 142 | 159 | 197 | 99 | 112 | 126 | 74 | 84 | 86 |
| 0.35 | *** | 485 | 497 | 775 | 227 | 240 | 358 | 137 | 148 | 209 | 95 | 104 | 139 | 71 | 78 | 100 |
| | *** | 489 | 522 | 814 | 232 | 260 | 364 | 141 | 162 | 204 | 98 | 113 | 129 | 74 | 85 | 87 |
| 0.4 | *** | 471 | 487 | 812 | 220 | 236 | 371 | 133 | 146 | 214 | 92 | 102 | 141 | 69 | 77 | 100 |
| | *** | 476 | 518 | 840 | 226 | 260 | 372 | 138 | 162 | 206 | 96 | 113 | 129 | 72 | 84 | 86 |
| 0.45 | *** | 445 | 465 | 831 | 209 | 228 | 375 | 127 | 142 | 214 | 88 | 99 | 139 | 66 | 74 | 98 |
| | *** | 451 | 503 | 848 | 216 | 254 | 372 | 132 | 159 | 204 | 92 | 110 | 126 | 69 | 82 | 83 |
| 0.5 | *** | 409 | 435 | 832 | 194 | 216 | 372 | 119 | 135 | 210 | 83 | 94 | 135 | 62 | 70 | 94 |
| | *** | 418 | 479 | 840 | 202 | 245 | 364 | 125 | 153 | 197 | 87 | 106 | 120 | 65 | 78 | 79 |
| 0.55 | *** | 367 | 399 | 813 | 177 | 202 | 359 | 110 | 127 | 201 | 77 | 88 | 128 | 57 | 66 | 88 |
| | *** | 378 | 450 | 814 | 187 | 232 | 349 | 117 | 145 | 187 | 82 | 100 | 112 | 61 | 73 | 72 |
| 0.6 | *** | 323 | 361 | 776 | 160 | 186 | 339 | 100 | 117 | 187 | 70 | 81 | 117 | 52 | 60 | 80 |
| | *** | 337 | 416 | 771 | 170 | 217 | 326 | 107 | 135 | 172 | 75 | 92 | 101 | 55 | 67 | 63 |
| 0.65 | *** | 279 | 321 | 721 | 142 | 168 | 310 | 90 | 106 | 169 | 63 | 73 | 104 | 46 | 53 | 70 |
| | *** | 294 | 378 | 711 | 152 | 198 | 295 | 96 | 123 | 153 | 67 | 83 | 88 | 49 | 59 | 53 |
| 0.7 | *** | 237 | 281 | 647 | 124 | 149 | 273 | 78 | 93 | 146 | 54 | 63 | 88 | . | . | . |
| | *** | 253 | 337 | 634 | 133 | 177 | 257 | 84 | 108 | 129 | 58 | 71 | 71 | . | . | . |
| 0.75 | *** | 197 | 241 | 555 | 105 | 127 | 228 | 66 | 78 | 118 | . | . | . | . | . | . |
| | *** | 214 | 293 | 540 | 114 | 152 | 212 | 71 | 90 | 101 | . | . | . | . | . | . |
| 0.8 | *** | 160 | 199 | 445 | 85 | 103 | 175 | . | . | . | . | . | . | . | . | . |
| | *** | 175 | 245 | 429 | 92 | 123 | 158 | . | . | . | . | . | . | . | . | . |
| 0.85 | *** | 123 | 154 | 317 | . | . | . | . | . | . | . | . | . | . | . | . |
| | *** | 135 | 189 | 300 | . | . | . | . | . | . | . | . | . | . | . | . |

TABLE 8: ALPHA= 0.05  POWER= 0.9    EXPECTED ACCRUAL THRU MINIMUM FOLLOW-UP= 40

| | DEL=.10 | | | DEL=.15 | | | DEL=.20 | | | DEL=.25 | | | DEL=.30 | | |
|---|---|---|---|---|---|---|---|---|---|---|---|---|---|---|---|
| FACT= | 1.0 .75 | .50 .25 | .00 BIN | 1.0 .75 | .50 .25 | .00 BIN | 1.0 .75 | .50 .25 | .00 BIN | 1.0 75 | .50 .25 | .00 BIN | 1.0 .75 | .50 .25 | .00 BIN |
| PCONT=*** | | | | REQUIRED NUMBER OF PATIENTS | | | | | | | | | | | |
| 0.05 *** | 180 | 182 | 195 | 105 | 107 | 114 | 74 | 76 | 80 | 58 | 59 | 62 | 48 | 49 | 51 |
| *** | 181 | 184 | 300 | 106 | 109 | 158 | 75 | 77 | 101 | 58 | 60 | 71 | 48 | 50 | 53 |
| 0.1 *** | 285 | 287 | 326 | 151 | 154 | 173 | 100 | 103 | 113 | 74 | 76 | 83 | 59 | 61 | 65 |
| *** | 286 | 293 | 429 | 152 | 158 | 212 | 101 | 106 | 129 | 75 | 79 | 88 | 60 | 62 | 63 |
| 0.15 *** | 367 | 372 | 447 | 186 | 191 | 225 | 118 | 123 | 142 | 85 | 89 | 101 | 66 | 69 | 77 |
| *** | 369 | 381 | 540 | 187 | 198 | 257 | 120 | 128 | 153 | 87 | 93 | 101 | 67 | 72 | 72 |
| 0.2 *** | 428 | 435 | 554 | 210 | 217 | 270 | 131 | 137 | 166 | 93 | 98 | 115 | 71 | 75 | 86 |
| *** | 430 | 448 | 634 | 212 | 228 | 295 | 133 | 145 | 172 | 95 | 103 | 112 | 73 | 79 | 79 |
| 0.25 *** | 467 | 477 | 645 | 225 | 235 | 308 | 138 | 147 | 185 | 97 | 104 | 126 | 74 | 79 | 93 |
| *** | 471 | 495 | 711 | 228 | 249 | 326 | 141 | 157 | 187 | 100 | 111 | 120 | 76 | 84 | 83 |
| 0.3 *** | 487 | 500 | 719 | 232 | 244 | 337 | 142 | 152 | 199 | 99 | 107 | 134 | 74 | 81 | 98 |
| *** | 491 | 524 | 771 | 236 | 263 | 349 | 146 | 165 | 197 | 102 | 115 | 126 | 77 | 86 | 86 |
| 0.35 *** | 489 | 506 | 775 | 232 | 248 | 358 | 141 | 154 | 209 | 98 | 108 | 139 | 74 | 81 | 100 |
| *** | 495 | 536 | 814 | 237 | 270 | 364 | 146 | 168 | 204 | 102 | 117 | 129 | 77 | 87 | 87 |
| 0.4 *** | 476 | 498 | 812 | 226 | 245 | 371 | 138 | 153 | 214 | 96 | 107 | 141 | 72 | 80 | 100 |
| *** | 483 | 536 | 840 | 233 | 271 | 372 | 144 | 169 | 206 | 100 | 117 | 129 | 75 | 87 | 86 |
| 0.45 *** | 451 | 478 | 831 | 216 | 238 | 375 | 132 | 149 | 215 | 92 | 104 | 139 | 69 | 77 | 98 |
| *** | 461 | 524 | 848 | 224 | 267 | 372 | 139 | 166 | 204 | 97 | 115 | 126 | 73 | 85 | 83 |
| 0.5 *** | 418 | 451 | 832 | 202 | 227 | 372 | 125 | 143 | 210 | 87 | 99 | 135 | 65 | 74 | 94 |
| *** | 429 | 503 | 840 | 212 | 258 | 364 | 132 | 161 | 197 | 92 | 111 | 120 | 69 | 81 | 79 |
| 0.55 *** | 379 | 418 | 813 | 187 | 214 | 359 | 117 | 134 | 201 | 82 | 93 | 128 | 61 | 69 | 88 |
| *** | 393 | 476 | 814 | 197 | 246 | 349 | 124 | 153 | 187 | 86 | 104 | 112 | 64 | 76 | 72 |
| 0.6 *** | 337 | 381 | 776 | 170 | 198 | 339 | 107 | 125 | 187 | 75 | 86 | 117 | 55 | 63 | 80 |
| *** | 353 | 443 | 771 | 181 | 230 | 326 | 114 | 142 | 172 | 79 | 96 | 101 | 59 | 69 | 63 |
| 0.65 *** | 294 | 343 | 721 | 152 | 180 | 310 | 96 | 113 | 169 | 67 | 77 | 104 | 49 | 56 | 70 |
| *** | 313 | 406 | 711 | 163 | 211 | 295 | 103 | 129 | 153 | 71 | 86 | 88 | 52 | 61 | 53 |
| 0.7 *** | 253 | 303 | 647 | 133 | 160 | 273 | 84 | 99 | 146 | 58 | 67 | 88 | . | . | . |
| *** | 272 | 364 | 634 | 144 | 189 | 257 | 90 | 114 | 129 | 62 | 74 | 71 | . | . | . |
| 0.75 *** | 214 | 262 | 555 | 114 | 137 | 228 | 71 | 83 | 118 | . | . | . | . | . | . |
| *** | 233 | 317 | 540 | 123 | 162 | 212 | 76 | 95 | 101 | . | . | . | . | . | . |
| 0.8 *** | 175 | 217 | 445 | 92 | 111 | 175 | . | . | . | . | . | . | . | . | . |
| *** | 192 | 265 | 429 | 100 | 130 | 158 | . | . | . | . | . | . | . | . | . |
| 0.85 *** | 135 | 168 | 317 | . | . | . | . | . | . | . | . | . | . | . | . |
| *** | 148 | 204 | 300 | . | . | . | . | . | . | . | . | . | . | . | . |

| TABLE 8: ALPHA= 0.05  POWER= 0.9 | | | | | | EXPECTED ACCRUAL THRU MINIMUM FOLLOW-UP= 50 | | | | | | | | |

|  |  | DEL=.10 | | | DEL=.15 | | | DEL=.20 | | | DEL=.25 | | | DEL=.30 | | |
|---|---|---|---|---|---|---|---|---|---|---|---|---|---|---|---|---|
| FACT= |  | 1.0 .75 | .50 .25 | .00 BIN | 1.0 .75 | .50 .25 | .00 BIN | 1.0 .75 | .50 .25 | .00 BIN | 1.0 75 | .50 .25 | .00 BIN | 1.0 .75 | .50 .25 | .00 BIN |
| PCONT=*** |  |  |  |  | REQUIRED NUMBER OF PATIENTS | | | | | | | | | | | |
| 0.05 | *** | 181 | 182 | 195 | 106 | 107 | 114 | 75 | 76 | 80 | 58 | 59 | 62 | 48 | 49 | 51 |
|  | *** | 181 | 185 | 300 | 106 | 109 | 158 | 75 | 77 | 101 | 59 | 60 | 71 | 49 | 50 | 53 |
| 0.1 | *** | 285 | 289 | 326 | 152 | 155 | 173 | 101 | 104 | 113 | 75 | 77 | 83 | 59 | 61 | 65 |
|  | *** | 287 | 295 | 429 | 153 | 160 | 212 | 102 | 107 | 129 | 76 | 79 | 88 | 60 | 63 | 63 |
| 0.15 | *** | 369 | 374 | 447 | 187 | 193 | 225 | 119 | 124 | 142 | 86 | 90 | 101 | 67 | 70 | 77 |
|  | *** | 371 | 385 | 540 | 189 | 201 | 257 | 121 | 130 | 153 | 88 | 94 | 101 | 68 | 73 | 72 |
| 0.2 | *** | 430 | 438 | 554 | 212 | 220 | 270 | 133 | 140 | 166 | 94 | 100 | 115 | 72 | 76 | 86 |
|  | *** | 433 | 454 | 634 | 215 | 232 | 295 | 135 | 147 | 172 | 96 | 105 | 112 | 74 | 80 | 79 |
| 0.25 | *** | 470 | 482 | 645 | 228 | 239 | 308 | 141 | 150 | 185 | 99 | 106 | 126 | 75 | 80 | 93 |
|  | *** | 474 | 503 | 711 | 232 | 255 | 326 | 144 | 160 | 187 | 102 | 113 | 120 | 77 | 85 | 83 |
| 0.3 | *** | 490 | 506 | 719 | 235 | 250 | 337 | 145 | 156 | 199 | 101 | 110 | 134 | 76 | 83 | 98 |
|  | *** | 496 | 534 | 771 | 241 | 270 | 349 | 149 | 169 | 197 | 105 | 118 | 126 | 79 | 88 | 86 |
| 0.35 | *** | 493 | 514 | 775 | 236 | 254 | 358 | 145 | 158 | 209 | 101 | 111 | 139 | 76 | 83 | 100 |
|  | *** | 500 | 550 | 814 | 243 | 278 | 364 | 150 | 173 | 204 | 105 | 120 | 129 | 79 | 89 | 87 |
| 0.4 | *** | 482 | 508 | 812 | 231 | 253 | 371 | 142 | 158 | 214 | 99 | 110 | 141 | 75 | 82 | 100 |
|  | *** | 491 | 551 | 840 | 239 | 280 | 372 | 148 | 174 | 206 | 104 | 120 | 129 | 78 | 89 | 86 |
| 0.45 | *** | 458 | 491 | 831 | 222 | 247 | 375 | 137 | 154 | 215 | 96 | 107 | 139 | 72 | 80 | 98 |
|  | *** | 470 | 542 | 848 | 231 | 277 | 372 | 144 | 172 | 204 | 101 | 118 | 126 | 75 | 87 | 83 |
| 0.5 | *** | 427 | 466 | 832 | 209 | 237 | 372 | 130 | 148 | 210 | 91 | 103 | 135 | 68 | 76 | 94 |
|  | *** | 440 | 523 | 840 | 220 | 269 | 364 | 138 | 167 | 197 | 96 | 114 | 120 | 72 | 83 | 79 |
| 0.55 | *** | 389 | 435 | 813 | 195 | 224 | 359 | 122 | 140 | 201 | 85 | 97 | 128 | 63 | 71 | 88 |
|  | *** | 406 | 497 | 814 | 206 | 257 | 349 | 130 | 159 | 187 | 90 | 108 | 112 | 67 | 78 | 72 |
| 0.6 | *** | 349 | 400 | 776 | 178 | 208 | 339 | 112 | 130 | 187 | 78 | 90 | 117 | 58 | 65 | 80 |
|  | *** | 368 | 465 | 771 | 190 | 241 | 326 | 120 | 148 | 172 | 83 | 99 | 101 | 61 | 71 | 63 |
| 0.65 | *** | 308 | 362 | 721 | 161 | 190 | 310 | 101 | 118 | 169 | 70 | 80 | 104 | 51 | 58 | 70 |
|  | *** | 329 | 428 | 711 | 172 | 221 | 295 | 108 | 134 | 153 | 75 | 89 | 88 | 54 | 62 | 53 |
| 0.7 | *** | 268 | 322 | 647 | 142 | 169 | 273 | 89 | 104 | 146 | 61 | 69 | 88 | . | . | . |
|  | *** | 289 | 385 | 634 | 153 | 198 | 257 | 95 | 118 | 129 | 64 | 76 | 71 | . | . | . |
| 0.75 | *** | 228 | 279 | 555 | 121 | 145 | 228 | 75 | 87 | 118 | . | . | . | . | . | . |
|  | *** | 248 | 337 | 540 | 131 | 169 | 212 | 80 | 98 | 101 | . | . | . | . | . | . |
| 0.8 | *** | 188 | 232 | 445 | 98 | 118 | 175 | . | . | . | . | . | . | . | . | . |
|  | *** | 206 | 281 | 429 | 106 | 136 | 158 | . | . | . | . | . | . | . | . | . |
| 0.85 | *** | 145 | 179 | 317 | . | . | . | . | . | . | . | . | . | . | . | . |
|  | *** | 159 | 215 | 300 | . | . | . | . | . | . | . | . | . | . | . | . |

TABLE 8: ALPHA= 0.05  POWER= 0.9     EXPECTED ACCRUAL THRU MINIMUM FOLLOW-UP= 60

| | DEL=.10 | | | DEL=.15 | | | DEL=.20 | | | DEL=.25 | | | DEL=.30 | | |
|---|---|---|---|---|---|---|---|---|---|---|---|---|---|---|---|
| FACT= | 1.0 .75 | .50 .25 | .00 BIN | 1.0 .75 | .50 .25 | .00 BIN | 1.0 .75 | .50 .25 | .00 BIN | 1.0 75 | .50 .25 | .00 BIN | 1.0 .75 | .50 .25 | .00 BIN |

PCONT=***  REQUIRED NUMBER OF PATIENTS

| PCONT | DEL=.10 1.0/.75 | .50/.25 | .00/BIN | DEL=.15 1.0/.75 | .50/.25 | .00/BIN | DEL=.20 1.0/.75 | .50/.25 | .00/BIN | DEL=.25 1.0/.75 | .50/.25 | .00/BIN | DEL=.30 1.0/.75 | .50/.25 | .00/BIN |
|---|---|---|---|---|---|---|---|---|---|---|---|---|---|---|---|
| 0.05 *** | 181 | 183 | 195 | 106 | 108 | 114 | 75 | 76 | 80 | 59 | 60 | 62 | 48 | 49 | 51 |
| *** | 182 | 186 | 300 | 107 | 110 | 158 | 76 | 78 | 101 | 59 | 61 | 71 | 49 | 50 | 53 |
| 0.1 *** | 286 | 290 | 326 | 153 | 157 | 173 | 101 | 104 | 113 | 75 | 78 | 83 | 60 | 62 | 65 |
| *** | 287 | 297 | 429 | 154 | 161 | 212 | 103 | 108 | 129 | 76 | 80 | 88 | 61 | 63 | 63 |
| 0.15 *** | 370 | 377 | 447 | 188 | 195 | 225 | 121 | 126 | 142 | 87 | 91 | 101 | 68 | 71 | 77 |
| *** | 372 | 388 | 540 | 191 | 203 | 257 | 123 | 131 | 153 | 89 | 95 | 101 | 69 | 73 | 72 |
| 0.2 *** | 432 | 442 | 554 | 214 | 223 | 270 | 134 | 142 | 166 | 96 | 101 | 115 | 73 | 77 | 86 |
| *** | 435 | 459 | 634 | 217 | 235 | 295 | 137 | 149 | 172 | 98 | 106 | 112 | 75 | 81 | 79 |
| 0.25 *** | 472 | 486 | 645 | 230 | 243 | 308 | 143 | 153 | 185 | 101 | 108 | 126 | 77 | 82 | 93 |
| *** | 477 | 511 | 711 | 235 | 259 | 326 | 147 | 163 | 187 | 104 | 114 | 120 | 79 | 86 | 83 |
| 0.3 *** | 493 | 512 | 719 | 238 | 255 | 337 | 147 | 159 | 199 | 103 | 112 | 134 | 78 | 84 | 98 |
| *** | 500 | 544 | 771 | 244 | 275 | 349 | 152 | 172 | 197 | 107 | 120 | 126 | 81 | 89 | 86 |
| 0.35 *** | 497 | 522 | 775 | 240 | 260 | 358 | 148 | 162 | 209 | 104 | 113 | 139 | 78 | 85 | 100 |
| *** | 506 | 561 | 814 | 248 | 284 | 364 | 154 | 177 | 204 | 108 | 122 | 129 | 81 | 91 | 87 |
| 0.4 *** | 487 | 518 | 812 | 236 | 260 | 371 | 146 | 162 | 214 | 102 | 113 | 141 | 77 | 84 | 100 |
| *** | 498 | 565 | 840 | 245 | 287 | 372 | 153 | 178 | 206 | 107 | 123 | 129 | 80 | 90 | 86 |
| 0.45 *** | 465 | 503 | 831 | 228 | 254 | 375 | 142 | 159 | 214 | 99 | 110 | 139 | 74 | 82 | 98 |
| *** | 478 | 558 | 848 | 238 | 285 | 372 | 149 | 176 | 204 | 104 | 121 | 126 | 77 | 88 | 83 |
| 0.5 *** | 435 | 479 | 832 | 216 | 245 | 371 | 135 | 153 | 210 | 94 | 106 | 135 | 70 | 78 | 94 |
| *** | 451 | 541 | 840 | 227 | 277 | 364 | 143 | 171 | 197 | 99 | 116 | 120 | 74 | 84 | 79 |
| 0.55 *** | 399 | 450 | 813 | 202 | 232 | 359 | 127 | 145 | 201 | 88 | 100 | 128 | 66 | 73 | 88 |
| *** | 418 | 516 | 814 | 214 | 266 | 349 | 134 | 163 | 187 | 93 | 110 | 112 | 69 | 79 | 72 |
| 0.6 *** | 361 | 416 | 776 | 186 | 217 | 339 | 117 | 135 | 187 | 81 | 92 | 117 | 60 | 67 | 80 |
| *** | 381 | 484 | 771 | 198 | 249 | 326 | 125 | 152 | 172 | 86 | 101 | 101 | 63 | 72 | 63 |
| 0.65 *** | 321 | 378 | 721 | 168 | 198 | 310 | 106 | 123 | 169 | 73 | 83 | 104 | 53 | 59 | 70 |
| *** | 343 | 446 | 711 | 180 | 229 | 295 | 113 | 138 | 153 | 77 | 91 | 88 | 56 | 63 | 53 |
| 0.7 *** | 281 | 337 | 647 | 149 | 177 | 273 | 93 | 108 | 146 | 63 | 71 | 88 | . | . | . |
| *** | 303 | 403 | 634 | 160 | 205 | 257 | 99 | 121 | 129 | 67 | 78 | 71 | . | . | . |
| 0.75 *** | 241 | 293 | 555 | 127 | 152 | 228 | 78 | 90 | 118 | . | . | . | . | . | . |
| *** | 262 | 352 | 540 | 137 | 175 | 212 | 83 | 100 | 101 | . | . | . | . | . | . |
| 0.8 *** | 199 | 245 | 445 | 103 | 123 | 175 | . | . | . | . | . | . | . | . | . |
| *** | 217 | 294 | 429 | 111 | 140 | 158 | . | . | . | . | . | . | . | . | . |
| 0.85 *** | 154 | 189 | 317 | . | . | . | . | . | . | . | . | . | . | . | . |
| *** | 168 | 224 | 300 | . | . | . | . | . | . | . | . | . | . | . | . |

TABLE 8: ALPHA= 0.05  POWER= 0.9     EXPECTED ACCRUAL THRU MINIMUM FOLLOW-UP= 70

| | DEL=.10 | | | DEL=.15 | | | DEL=.20 | | | DEL=.25 | | | DEL=.30 | | |
|---|---|---|---|---|---|---|---|---|---|---|---|---|---|---|---|
| FACT= | 1.0 .75 | .50 .25 | .00 BIN | 1.0 .75 | .50 .25 | .00 BIN | 1.0 .75 | .50 .25 | .00 BIN | 1.0 75 | .50 .25 | .00 BIN | 1.0 .75 | .50 .25 | .00 BIN |
| PCONT=*** | | | | REQUIRED NUMBER OF PATIENTS | | | | | | | | | | | |
| 0.05 *** | 181 | 184 | 195 | 106 | 108 | 114 | 75 | 77 | 80 | 59 | 60 | 62 | 49 | 49 | 51 |
| *** | 182 | 186 | 300 | 107 | 110 | 158 | 76 | 78 | 101 | 59 | 61 | 71 | 49 | 50 | 53 |
| 0.1 *** | 287 | 291 | 326 | 153 | 158 | 173 | 102 | 105 | 113 | 76 | 78 | 83 | 60 | 62 | 65 |
| *** | 288 | 299 | 429 | 155 | 162 | 212 | 103 | 108 | 129 | 77 | 80 | 88 | 61 | 63 | 63 |
| 0.15 *** | 371 | 379 | 447 | 189 | 196 | 225 | 122 | 127 | 142 | 88 | 92 | 101 | 68 | 71 | 77 |
| *** | 374 | 392 | 540 | 192 | 205 | 257 | 124 | 132 | 153 | 90 | 95 | 101 | 70 | 74 | 72 |
| 0.2 *** | 433 | 445 | 554 | 215 | 226 | 270 | 136 | 143 | 166 | 97 | 102 | 115 | 74 | 78 | 86 |
| *** | 437 | 464 | 634 | 219 | 238 | 295 | 139 | 151 | 172 | 99 | 107 | 112 | 76 | 81 | 79 |
| 0.25 *** | 475 | 491 | 645 | 232 | 246 | 308 | 145 | 155 | 185 | 102 | 109 | 126 | 78 | 83 | 93 |
| *** | 480 | 517 | 711 | 238 | 263 | 326 | 149 | 165 | 187 | 105 | 115 | 120 | 80 | 87 | 83 |
| 0.3 *** | 497 | 518 | 719 | 242 | 259 | 337 | 150 | 162 | 199 | 105 | 114 | 134 | 79 | 85 | 98 |
| *** | 504 | 552 | 771 | 248 | 280 | 349 | 155 | 174 | 197 | 109 | 121 | 126 | 82 | 90 | 86 |
| 0.35 *** | 502 | 529 | 775 | 244 | 265 | 358 | 151 | 166 | 209 | 106 | 116 | 139 | 80 | 86 | 100 |
| *** | 511 | 572 | 814 | 252 | 290 | 364 | 157 | 180 | 204 | 110 | 124 | 129 | 82 | 92 | 87 |
| 0.4 *** | 492 | 527 | 812 | 241 | 265 | 371 | 149 | 166 | 214 | 104 | 115 | 141 | 78 | 86 | 100 |
| *** | 505 | 578 | 840 | 250 | 293 | 372 | 156 | 181 | 206 | 109 | 124 | 129 | 81 | 91 | 86 |
| 0.45 *** | 472 | 514 | 831 | 233 | 261 | 375 | 145 | 163 | 214 | 101 | 113 | 139 | 76 | 83 | 98 |
| *** | 487 | 572 | 848 | 244 | 292 | 372 | 153 | 180 | 204 | 106 | 122 | 126 | 79 | 89 | 83 |
| 0.5 *** | 443 | 492 | 832 | 222 | 252 | 372 | 139 | 157 | 210 | 97 | 109 | 135 | 72 | 80 | 94 |
| *** | 461 | 556 | 840 | 234 | 285 | 364 | 147 | 175 | 197 | 102 | 118 | 120 | 75 | 85 | 79 |
| 0.55 *** | 409 | 463 | 813 | 208 | 240 | 359 | 131 | 149 | 201 | 91 | 102 | 128 | 67 | 74 | 88 |
| *** | 429 | 532 | 814 | 221 | 273 | 349 | 139 | 166 | 187 | 96 | 112 | 112 | 70 | 80 | 72 |
| 0.6 *** | 371 | 430 | 776 | 192 | 224 | 339 | 121 | 139 | 187 | 84 | 94 | 117 | 61 | 68 | 80 |
| *** | 394 | 501 | 771 | 205 | 256 | 326 | 129 | 155 | 172 | 88 | 103 | 101 | 64 | 73 | 63 |
| 0.65 *** | 332 | 393 | 721 | 174 | 205 | 310 | 110 | 126 | 169 | 75 | 85 | 104 | 54 | 60 | 70 |
| *** | 356 | 463 | 711 | 187 | 236 | 295 | 117 | 141 | 153 | 79 | 92 | 88 | 57 | 64 | 53 |
| 0.7 *** | 292 | 351 | 647 | 155 | 183 | 273 | 96 | 111 | 146 | 65 | 73 | 88 | . | . | . |
| *** | 316 | 418 | 634 | 166 | 210 | 257 | 103 | 123 | 129 | 69 | 79 | 71 | . | . | . |
| 0.75 *** | 252 | 306 | 555 | 133 | 157 | 228 | 81 | 93 | 118 | . | . | . | . | . | . |
| *** | 273 | 365 | 540 | 143 | 180 | 212 | 86 | 102 | 101 | . | . | . | . | . | . |
| 0.8 *** | 209 | 256 | 445 | 108 | 127 | 175 | . | . | . | . | . | . | . | . | . |
| *** | 228 | 304 | 429 | 116 | 143 | 158 | . | . | . | . | . | . | . | . | . |
| 0.85 *** | 161 | 197 | 317 | . | . | . | . | . | . | . | . | . | . | . | . |
| *** | 176 | 231 | 300 | . | . | . | . | . | . | . | . | . | . | . | . |

TABLE 8: ALPHA= 0.05  POWER= 0.9     EXPECTED ACCRUAL THRU MINIMUM FOLLOW-UP= 80

| | | DEL=.10 | | | DEL=.15 | | | DEL=.20 | | | DEL=.25 | | | DEL=.30 | | |
|---|---|---|---|---|---|---|---|---|---|---|---|---|---|---|---|---|---|
| FACT= | | 1.0 .75 | .50 .25 | .00 BIN | 1.0 .75 | .50 .25 | .00 BIN | 1.0 .75 | .50 .25 | .00 BIN | 1.0 75 | .50 .25 | .00 BIN | 1.0 .75 | .50 .25 | .00 BIN |
| PCONT=*** | | | | | REQUIRED NUMBER OF PATIENTS | | | | | | | | | | | |
| 0.05 | *** | 182 | 184 | 195 | 107 | 109 | 114 | 76 | 77 | 80 | 59 | 60 | 62 | 49 | 50 | 51 |
| | *** | 183 | 187 | 300 | 107 | 110 | 158 | 76 | 78 | 101 | 59 | 61 | 71 | 49 | 50 | 53 |
| 0.1 | *** | 287 | 293 | 326 | 154 | 158 | 173 | 103 | 106 | 113 | 76 | 79 | 83 | 61 | 62 | 65 |
| | *** | 289 | 301 | 429 | 156 | 163 | 212 | 104 | 109 | 129 | 77 | 81 | 88 | 61 | 64 | 63 |
| 0.15 | *** | 372 | 381 | 447 | 191 | 198 | 225 | 123 | 128 | 142 | 89 | 93 | 101 | 69 | 72 | 77 |
| | *** | 375 | 395 | 540 | 193 | 206 | 257 | 125 | 133 | 153 | 90 | 96 | 101 | 70 | 74 | 72 |
| 0.2 | *** | 435 | 448 | 554 | 217 | 228 | 270 | 137 | 145 | 166 | 98 | 103 | 115 | 75 | 79 | 86 |
| | *** | 439 | 469 | 634 | 221 | 240 | 295 | 140 | 152 | 172 | 100 | 108 | 112 | 77 | 82 | 79 |
| 0.25 | *** | 477 | 495 | 645 | 235 | 249 | 308 | 147 | 157 | 185 | 104 | 111 | 126 | 79 | 84 | 93 |
| | *** | 483 | 523 | 711 | 240 | 266 | 326 | 151 | 166 | 187 | 107 | 116 | 120 | 81 | 87 | 83 |
| 0.3 | *** | 500 | 524 | 719 | 244 | 263 | 337 | 152 | 165 | 199 | 107 | 115 | 134 | 81 | 86 | 98 |
| | *** | 508 | 560 | 771 | 252 | 284 | 349 | 157 | 176 | 197 | 110 | 122 | 126 | 83 | 91 | 86 |
| 0.35 | *** | 506 | 536 | 775 | 248 | 270 | 358 | 154 | 168 | 209 | 108 | 117 | 139 | 81 | 87 | 100 |
| | *** | 517 | 582 | 814 | 256 | 295 | 364 | 160 | 182 | 204 | 112 | 125 | 129 | 84 | 92 | 87 |
| 0.4 | *** | 498 | 536 | 812 | 245 | 271 | 371 | 153 | 169 | 214 | 107 | 117 | 141 | 80 | 87 | 100 |
| | *** | 511 | 589 | 840 | 255 | 299 | 372 | 159 | 184 | 206 | 111 | 126 | 129 | 83 | 92 | 86 |
| 0.45 | *** | 478 | 524 | 831 | 238 | 267 | 375 | 149 | 166 | 215 | 104 | 115 | 139 | 77 | 85 | 98 |
| | *** | 495 | 584 | 848 | 249 | 297 | 372 | 156 | 183 | 204 | 108 | 124 | 126 | 80 | 90 | 83 |
| 0.5 | *** | 451 | 503 | 832 | 227 | 258 | 372 | 143 | 161 | 210 | 99 | 111 | 135 | 74 | 81 | 94 |
| | *** | 470 | 570 | 840 | 240 | 291 | 364 | 150 | 178 | 197 | 104 | 120 | 120 | 77 | 86 | 79 |
| 0.55 | *** | 418 | 476 | 813 | 214 | 246 | 359 | 134 | 153 | 201 | 93 | 104 | 128 | 69 | 76 | 88 |
| | *** | 440 | 546 | 814 | 227 | 279 | 349 | 142 | 169 | 187 | 98 | 113 | 112 | 72 | 81 | 72 |
| 0.6 | *** | 381 | 443 | 776 | 198 | 230 | 339 | 125 | 142 | 187 | 86 | 96 | 117 | 63 | 69 | 80 |
| | *** | 405 | 515 | 771 | 211 | 262 | 326 | 132 | 158 | 172 | 91 | 105 | 101 | 66 | 74 | 63 |
| 0.65 | *** | 343 | 406 | 721 | 180 | 211 | 310 | 113 | 129 | 169 | 77 | 86 | 104 | 56 | 61 | 70 |
| | *** | 367 | 477 | 711 | 193 | 241 | 295 | 120 | 143 | 153 | 81 | 93 | 88 | 58 | 65 | 53 |
| 0.7 | *** | 303 | 364 | 647 | 160 | 189 | 273 | 99 | 114 | 146 | 67 | 74 | 88 | . | . | . |
| | *** | 327 | 431 | 634 | 172 | 215 | 257 | 105 | 125 | 129 | 70 | 80 | 71 | . | . | . |
| 0.75 | *** | 262 | 317 | 555 | 137 | 162 | 228 | 83 | 95 | 118 | . | . | . | . | . | . |
| | *** | 284 | 377 | 540 | 148 | 184 | 212 | 88 | 104 | 101 | . | . | . | . | . | . |
| 0.8 | *** | 217 | 265 | 445 | 111 | 130 | 175 | . | . | . | . | . | . | . | . | . |
| | *** | 237 | 314 | 429 | 119 | 146 | 158 | . | . | . | . | . | . | . | . | . |
| 0.85 | *** | 168 | 204 | 317 | . | . | . | . | . | . | . | . | . | . | . | . |
| | *** | 183 | 238 | 300 | . | . | . | . | . | . | . | . | . | . | . | . |

## TABLE 8: ALPHA= 0.05  POWER= 0.9    EXPECTED ACCRUAL THRU MINIMUM FOLLOW-UP= 90

| | | DEL=.10 | | | DEL=.15 | | | DEL=.20 | | | DEL=.25 | | | DEL=.30 | | |
|---|---|---|---|---|---|---|---|---|---|---|---|---|---|---|---|---|
| FACT= | | 1.0 | .50 | .00 | 1.0 | .50 | .00 | 1.0 | .50 | .00 | 1.0 | .50 | .00 | 1.0 | .50 | .00 |
| | | .75 | .25 | BIN | .75 | .25 | BIN | .75 | .25 | BIN | 75 | .25 | BIN | .75 | .25 | BIN |
| PCONT=*** | | | | | REQUIRED NUMBER OF PATIENTS | | | | | | | | | | | |
| 0.05 | *** | 182 | 185 | 195 | 107 | 109 | 114 | 76 | 77 | 80 | 59 | 60 | 62 | 49 | 50 | 51 |
| | *** | 183 | 188 | 300 | 108 | 111 | 158 | 76 | 78 | 101 | 60 | 61 | 71 | 49 | 50 | 53 |
| 0.1 | *** | 288 | 294 | 326 | 155 | 159 | 173 | 103 | 106 | 113 | 77 | 79 | 83 | 61 | 63 | 65 |
| | *** | 290 | 302 | 429 | 157 | 164 | 212 | 104 | 109 | 129 | 78 | 81 | 88 | 62 | 64 | 63 |
| 0.15 | *** | 373 | 383 | 447 | 192 | 199 | 225 | 123 | 129 | 142 | 90 | 93 | 101 | 70 | 72 | 77 |
| | *** | 377 | 397 | 540 | 195 | 208 | 257 | 126 | 134 | 153 | 91 | 96 | 101 | 71 | 74 | 72 |
| 0.2 | *** | 437 | 451 | 554 | 219 | 230 | 270 | 138 | 146 | 166 | 99 | 104 | 115 | 76 | 79 | 86 |
| | *** | 442 | 473 | 634 | 223 | 242 | 295 | 142 | 153 | 172 | 101 | 108 | 112 | 77 | 82 | 79 |
| 0.25 | *** | 479 | 499 | 645 | 237 | 252 | 308 | 148 | 159 | 185 | 105 | 112 | 126 | 80 | 84 | 93 |
| | *** | 486 | 529 | 711 | 243 | 269 | 326 | 153 | 168 | 187 | 108 | 117 | 120 | 82 | 88 | 83 |
| 0.3 | *** | 503 | 529 | 719 | 247 | 266 | 337 | 154 | 167 | 199 | 108 | 117 | 134 | 82 | 87 | 98 |
| | *** | 512 | 568 | 771 | 255 | 287 | 349 | 159 | 178 | 197 | 112 | 123 | 126 | 84 | 91 | 86 |
| 0.35 | *** | 510 | 543 | 775 | 251 | 274 | 358 | 156 | 171 | 209 | 109 | 119 | 139 | 82 | 88 | 100 |
| | *** | 522 | 590 | 814 | 260 | 299 | 364 | 162 | 184 | 204 | 113 | 127 | 129 | 85 | 93 | 87 |
| 0.4 | *** | 503 | 544 | 812 | 249 | 276 | 371 | 155 | 172 | 214 | 108 | 119 | 141 | 81 | 88 | 100 |
| | *** | 518 | 599 | 840 | 260 | 303 | 372 | 162 | 186 | 206 | 113 | 127 | 129 | 84 | 93 | 86 |
| 0.45 | *** | 485 | 533 | 831 | 243 | 272 | 375 | 152 | 169 | 214 | 106 | 117 | 139 | 79 | 86 | 98 |
| | *** | 503 | 596 | 848 | 254 | 302 | 372 | 159 | 185 | 204 | 110 | 125 | 126 | 82 | 91 | 83 |
| 0.5 | *** | 459 | 514 | 832 | 232 | 264 | 371 | 146 | 164 | 210 | 101 | 112 | 135 | 75 | 82 | 94 |
| | *** | 479 | 582 | 840 | 245 | 296 | 364 | 153 | 180 | 197 | 106 | 121 | 120 | 78 | 87 | 79 |
| 0.55 | *** | 427 | 487 | 813 | 219 | 252 | 359 | 138 | 156 | 201 | 95 | 106 | 128 | 70 | 77 | 88 |
| | *** | 450 | 559 | 814 | 232 | 284 | 349 | 145 | 172 | 187 | 100 | 115 | 112 | 73 | 81 | 72 |
| 0.6 | *** | 391 | 455 | 776 | 203 | 236 | 339 | 128 | 145 | 187 | 88 | 98 | 117 | 64 | 70 | 80 |
| | *** | 416 | 528 | 771 | 217 | 267 | 326 | 135 | 160 | 172 | 92 | 106 | 101 | 67 | 74 | 63 |
| 0.65 | *** | 353 | 417 | 721 | 185 | 217 | 310 | 116 | 132 | 169 | 79 | 88 | 104 | 57 | 62 | 70 |
| | *** | 378 | 489 | 711 | 198 | 246 | 295 | 123 | 145 | 153 | 83 | 94 | 88 | 59 | 65 | 53 |
| 0.7 | *** | 313 | 375 | 647 | 165 | 193 | 273 | 102 | 116 | 146 | 68 | 75 | 88 | . | . | . |
| | *** | 337 | 442 | 634 | 177 | 219 | 257 | 108 | 127 | 129 | 71 | 81 | 71 | . | . | . |
| 0.75 | *** | 271 | 327 | 555 | 142 | 166 | 228 | 85 | 97 | 118 | . | . | . | . | . | . |
| | *** | 293 | 387 | 540 | 152 | 187 | 212 | 90 | 105 | 101 | . | . | . | . | . | . |
| 0.8 | *** | 225 | 273 | 445 | 115 | 133 | 175 | . | . | . | . | . | . | . | . | . |
| | *** | 245 | 322 | 429 | 123 | 148 | 158 | . | . | . | . | . | . | . | . | . |
| 0.85 | *** | 174 | 210 | 317 | . | . | . | . | . | . | . | . | . | . | . | . |
| | *** | 189 | 243 | 300 | . | . | . | . | . | . | . | . | . | . | . | . |

## TABLE 8: ALPHA= 0.05  POWER= 0.9    EXPECTED ACCRUAL THRU MINIMUM FOLLOW-UP= 100

| | | DEL=.10 | | | DEL=.15 | | | DEL=.20 | | | DEL=.25 | | | DEL=.30 | | |
|---|---|---|---|---|---|---|---|---|---|---|---|---|---|---|---|---|
| FACT= | | 1.0 .75 | .50 .25 | .00 BIN | 1.0 .75 | .50 .25 | .00 BIN | 1.0 .75 | .50 .25 | .00 BIN | 1.0 75 | .50 .25 | .00 BIN | 1.0 .75 | .50 .25 | .00 BIN |
| PCONT=*** | | | | | REQUIRED NUMBER OF PATIENTS | | | | | | | | | | | |
| 0.05 | *** | 182 | 185 | 195 | 107 | 109 | 114 | 76 | 77 | 80 | 59 | 60 | 62 | 49 | 50 | 51 |
| | *** | 183 | 188 | 300 | 108 | 111 | 158 | 77 | 78 | 101 | 60 | 61 | 71 | 49 | 50 | 53 |
| 0.1 | *** | 289 | 295 | 326 | 155 | 160 | 173 | 104 | 107 | 113 | 77 | 79 | 83 | 61 | 63 | 65 |
| | *** | 291 | 303 | 429 | 157 | 165 | 212 | 105 | 109 | 129 | 78 | 81 | 88 | 62 | 64 | 63 |
| 0.15 | *** | 374 | 385 | 447 | 193 | 201 | 225 | 124 | 130 | 142 | 90 | 94 | 101 | 70 | 73 | 77 |
| | *** | 378 | 400 | 540 | 196 | 209 | 257 | 127 | 134 | 153 | 92 | 97 | 101 | 71 | 75 | 72 |
| 0.2 | *** | 438 | 454 | 554 | 220 | 232 | 270 | 140 | 147 | 166 | 100 | 105 | 115 | 76 | 80 | 86 |
| | *** | 444 | 476 | 634 | 225 | 244 | 295 | 143 | 154 | 172 | 102 | 109 | 112 | 78 | 83 | 79 |
| 0.25 | *** | 482 | 503 | 645 | 239 | 255 | 308 | 150 | 160 | 185 | 106 | 113 | 126 | 80 | 85 | 93 |
| | *** | 489 | 534 | 711 | 245 | 271 | 326 | 154 | 169 | 187 | 109 | 118 | 120 | 82 | 88 | 83 |
| 0.3 | *** | 506 | 534 | 719 | 250 | 270 | 337 | 156 | 169 | 199 | 110 | 118 | 134 | 83 | 88 | 98 |
| | *** | 516 | 574 | 771 | 258 | 290 | 349 | 161 | 180 | 197 | 113 | 124 | 126 | 85 | 92 | 86 |
| 0.35 | *** | 514 | 550 | 775 | 254 | 278 | 358 | 158 | 173 | 209 | 111 | 120 | 139 | 83 | 89 | 100 |
| | *** | 527 | 598 | 814 | 264 | 302 | 364 | 165 | 186 | 204 | 115 | 127 | 129 | 86 | 94 | 87 |
| 0.4 | *** | 508 | 551 | 812 | 253 | 280 | 371 | 158 | 174 | 214 | 110 | 120 | 141 | 82 | 89 | 100 |
| | *** | 524 | 608 | 840 | 264 | 307 | 372 | 165 | 188 | 206 | 114 | 128 | 129 | 85 | 93 | 86 |
| 0.45 | *** | 491 | 542 | 831 | 247 | 277 | 375 | 154 | 172 | 215 | 107 | 118 | 139 | 80 | 87 | 98 |
| | *** | 510 | 606 | 848 | 259 | 307 | 372 | 162 | 187 | 204 | 112 | 126 | 126 | 83 | 91 | 83 |
| 0.5 | *** | 466 | 523 | 832 | 237 | 269 | 372 | 148 | 167 | 210 | 103 | 114 | 135 | 76 | 83 | 94 |
| | *** | 488 | 593 | 840 | 250 | 300 | 364 | 156 | 182 | 197 | 108 | 122 | 120 | 79 | 88 | 79 |
| 0.55 | *** | 435 | 497 | 813 | 224 | 257 | 359 | 140 | 159 | 201 | 97 | 108 | 128 | 71 | 78 | 88 |
| | *** | 459 | 570 | 814 | 237 | 289 | 349 | 148 | 174 | 187 | 102 | 116 | 112 | 74 | 82 | 72 |
| 0.6 | *** | 400 | 465 | 776 | 208 | 241 | 339 | 130 | 148 | 187 | 90 | 99 | 117 | 65 | 71 | 80 |
| | *** | 425 | 539 | 771 | 222 | 272 | 326 | 138 | 162 | 172 | 94 | 107 | 101 | 68 | 75 | 63 |
| 0.65 | *** | 362 | 428 | 721 | 190 | 221 | 310 | 118 | 134 | 169 | 80 | 89 | 104 | 58 | 62 | 70 |
| | *** | 388 | 500 | 711 | 203 | 250 | 295 | 125 | 147 | 153 | 84 | 95 | 88 | 60 | 66 | 53 |
| 0.7 | *** | 322 | 385 | 647 | 169 | 198 | 273 | 104 | 118 | 146 | 69 | 76 | 88 | . | . | . |
| | *** | 347 | 452 | 634 | 181 | 223 | 257 | 110 | 129 | 129 | 72 | 81 | 71 | . | . | . |
| 0.75 | *** | 279 | 337 | 555 | 145 | 169 | 228 | 87 | 98 | 118 | . | . | . | . | . | . |
| | *** | 302 | 396 | 540 | 156 | 190 | 212 | 92 | 106 | 101 | . | . | . | . | . | . |
| 0.8 | *** | 232 | 281 | 445 | 118 | 136 | 175 | . | . | . | . | . | . | . | . | . |
| | *** | 252 | 329 | 429 | 125 | 151 | 158 | . | . | . | . | . | . | . | . | . |
| 0.85 | *** | 179 | 215 | 317 | . | . | . | . | . | . | . | . | . | . | . | . |
| | *** | 194 | 248 | 300 | . | . | . | . | . | . | . | . | . | . | . | . |

## TABLE 8: ALPHA= 0.05  POWER= 0.9    EXPECTED ACCRUAL THRU MINIMUM FOLLOW-UP= 110

| | | DEL=.05 | | | DEL=.10 | | | DEL=.15 | | | DEL=.20 | | | DEL=.25 | | |
|---|---|---|---|---|---|---|---|---|---|---|---|---|---|---|---|---|---|
| FACT= | | 1.0 .75 | .50 .25 | .00 BIN | 1.0 .75 | .50 .25 | .00 BIN | 1.0 .75 | .50 .25 | .00 BIN | 1.0 75 | .50 .25 | .00 BIN | 1.0 .75 | .50 .25 | .00 BIN |
| PCONT=*** | | REQUIRED NUMBER OF PATIENTS | | | | | | | | | | | | | | |
| 0.05 | *** | 512 | 515 | 547 | 183 | 185 | 195 | 108 | 109 | 114 | 76 | 78 | 80 | 60 | 60 | 62 |
| | *** | 513 | 521 | 943 | 184 | 188 | 300 | 108 | 111 | 158 | 77 | 79 | 101 | 60 | 61 | 71 |
| 0.1 | *** | 934 | 941 | 1055 | 290 | 296 | 326 | 156 | 161 | 173 | 104 | 107 | 113 | 77 | 80 | 83 |
| | *** | 936 | 953 | 1491 | 292 | 304 | 429 | 158 | 165 | 212 | 105 | 110 | 129 | 78 | 81 | 88 |
| 0.15 | *** | 1292 | 1303 | 1547 | 375 | 387 | 447 | 194 | 202 | 225 | 125 | 130 | 142 | 91 | 94 | 101 |
| | *** | 1296 | 1324 | 1970 | 379 | 402 | 540 | 197 | 210 | 257 | 127 | 135 | 153 | 92 | 97 | 101 |
| 0.2 | *** | 1569 | 1585 | 1996 | 440 | 457 | 554 | 222 | 234 | 270 | 141 | 148 | 166 | 100 | 105 | 115 |
| | *** | 1574 | 1618 | 2381 | 446 | 480 | 634 | 226 | 246 | 295 | 144 | 155 | 172 | 103 | 109 | 112 |
| 0.25 | *** | 1761 | 1784 | 2388 | 484 | 507 | 645 | 241 | 257 | 308 | 151 | 161 | 185 | 107 | 113 | 126 |
| | *** | 1768 | 1830 | 2724 | 492 | 539 | 711 | 247 | 273 | 326 | 156 | 170 | 187 | 110 | 119 | 120 |
| 0.3 | *** | 1871 | 1903 | 2715 | 509 | 539 | 719 | 252 | 273 | 337 | 158 | 170 | 199 | 111 | 119 | 134 |
| | *** | 1882 | 1965 | 2998 | 520 | 580 | 771 | 260 | 293 | 349 | 163 | 181 | 197 | 114 | 125 | 126 |
| 0.35 | *** | 1907 | 1949 | 2973 | 518 | 556 | 775 | 257 | 281 | 358 | 160 | 175 | 209 | 112 | 121 | 139 |
| | *** | 1921 | 2030 | 3203 | 532 | 605 | 814 | 267 | 305 | 364 | 167 | 188 | 204 | 116 | 128 | 129 |
| 0.4 | *** | 1878 | 1932 | 3159 | 513 | 559 | 812 | 256 | 284 | 371 | 160 | 176 | 214 | 112 | 121 | 141 |
| | *** | 1896 | 2037 | 3340 | 530 | 616 | 840 | 267 | 311 | 372 | 167 | 190 | 206 | 116 | 129 | 129 |
| 0.45 | *** | 1795 | 1864 | 3272 | 497 | 550 | 831 | 251 | 281 | 375 | 157 | 174 | 214 | 109 | 119 | 139 |
| | *** | 1818 | 1994 | 3409 | 517 | 615 | 848 | 263 | 311 | 372 | 164 | 189 | 204 | 114 | 127 | 126 |
| 0.5 | *** | 1669 | 1757 | 3310 | 473 | 532 | 832 | 241 | 273 | 372 | 151 | 169 | 210 | 105 | 115 | 135 |
| | *** | 1699 | 1914 | 3409 | 496 | 603 | 840 | 254 | 304 | 364 | 159 | 184 | 197 | 109 | 123 | 120 |
| 0.55 | *** | 1512 | 1622 | 3273 | 442 | 507 | 813 | 228 | 261 | 359 | 143 | 161 | 201 | 99 | 109 | 128 |
| | *** | 1550 | 1806 | 3340 | 468 | 581 | 814 | 242 | 293 | 349 | 151 | 176 | 187 | 103 | 116 | 112 |
| 0.6 | *** | 1338 | 1471 | 3162 | 408 | 475 | 776 | 213 | 245 | 339 | 133 | 150 | 187 | 91 | 100 | 117 |
| | *** | 1385 | 1677 | 3203 | 434 | 549 | 771 | 226 | 276 | 326 | 140 | 164 | 172 | 95 | 107 | 101 |
| 0.65 | *** | 1160 | 1314 | 2976 | 370 | 438 | 721 | 194 | 225 | 310 | 121 | 136 | 169 | 82 | 90 | 104 |
| | *** | 1215 | 1535 | 2998 | 397 | 510 | 711 | 207 | 254 | 295 | 127 | 149 | 153 | 85 | 96 | 88 |
| 0.7 | *** | 987 | 1156 | 2718 | 330 | 394 | 647 | 173 | 201 | 273 | 106 | 119 | 146 | 70 | 77 | 88 |
| | *** | 1050 | 1380 | 2724 | 356 | 461 | 634 | 185 | 226 | 257 | 112 | 130 | 129 | 73 | 82 | 71 |
| 0.75 | *** | 826 | 998 | 2386 | 286 | 345 | 555 | 149 | 172 | 228 | 89 | 99 | 118 | . | . | . |
| | *** | 892 | 1215 | 2381 | 310 | 403 | 540 | 159 | 192 | 212 | 94 | 107 | 101 | . | . | . |
| 0.8 | *** | 677 | 839 | 1981 | 239 | 288 | 445 | 120 | 138 | 175 | . | . | . | . | . | . |
| | *** | 740 | 1035 | 1970 | 259 | 335 | 429 | 128 | 152 | 158 | . | . | . | . | . | . |
| 0.85 | *** | 534 | 673 | 1506 | 184 | 220 | 317 | . | . | . | . | . | . | . | . | . |
| | *** | 588 | 833 | 1491 | 199 | 252 | 300 | . | . | . | . | . | . | . | . | . |
| 0.9 | *** | 383 | 483 | 959 | . | . | . | . | . | . | . | . | . | . | . | . |
| | *** | 423 | 593 | 943 | . | . | . | . | . | . | . | . | . | . | . | . |

TABLE 8: ALPHA= 0.05   POWER= 0.9   EXPECTED ACCRUAL THRU MINIMUM FOLLOW-UP= 120

| | | DEL=.05 | | | DEL=.10 | | | DEL=.15 | | | DEL=.20 | | | DEL=.25 | | |
|---|---|---|---|---|---|---|---|---|---|---|---|---|---|---|---|---|---|
| FACT= | | 1.0 .75 | .50 .25 | .00 BIN | 1.0 .75 | .50 .25 | .00 BIN | 1.0 .75 | .50 .25 | .00 BIN | 1.0 75 | .50 .25 | .00 BIN | 1.0 .75 | .50 .25 | .00 BIN |
| PCONT=*** | | | | REQUIRED NUMBER OF PATIENTS | | | | | | | | | | | | |
| 0.05 | *** | 513 | 516 | 547 | 183 | 186 | 195 | 108 | 110 | 114 | 76 | 78 | 80 | 60 | 61 | 62 |
| | *** | 514 | 521 | 943 | 184 | 189 | 300 | 109 | 111 | 158 | 77 | 79 | 101 | 60 | 61 | 71 |
| 0.1 | *** | 935 | 942 | 1055 | 290 | 297 | 326 | 157 | 161 | 173 | 104 | 108 | 113 | 78 | 80 | 83 |
| | *** | 937 | 955 | 1491 | 293 | 306 | 429 | 158 | 166 | 212 | 106 | 110 | 129 | 79 | 81 | 88 |
| 0.15 | *** | 1293 | 1305 | 1547 | 377 | 388 | 447 | 195 | 203 | 225 | 126 | 131 | 142 | 91 | 95 | 101 |
| | *** | 1297 | 1328 | 1970 | 381 | 404 | 540 | 198 | 211 | 257 | 128 | 135 | 153 | 93 | 97 | 101 |
| 0.2 | *** | 1570 | 1588 | 1996 | 442 | 459 | 554 | 223 | 235 | 270 | 142 | 149 | 166 | 101 | 106 | 115 |
| | *** | 1576 | 1623 | 2381 | 448 | 483 | 634 | 228 | 247 | 295 | 145 | 156 | 172 | 103 | 110 | 112 |
| 0.25 | *** | 1763 | 1788 | 2388 | 486 | 511 | 645 | 243 | 259 | 308 | 153 | 163 | 185 | 108 | 114 | 126 |
| | *** | 1771 | 1838 | 2724 | 495 | 543 | 711 | 249 | 275 | 326 | 157 | 171 | 187 | 111 | 119 | 120 |
| 0.3 | *** | 1874 | 1908 | 2715 | 512 | 544 | 719 | 255 | 275 | 337 | 159 | 172 | 199 | 112 | 120 | 134 |
| | *** | 1885 | 1976 | 2998 | 524 | 585 | 771 | 263 | 295 | 349 | 165 | 182 | 197 | 115 | 125 | 126 |
| 0.35 | *** | 1911 | 1956 | 2973 | 522 | 561 | 775 | 260 | 284 | 358 | 162 | 177 | 209 | 113 | 122 | 139 |
| | *** | 1926 | 2044 | 3203 | 536 | 612 | 814 | 270 | 308 | 364 | 168 | 189 | 204 | 117 | 129 | 129 |
| 0.4 | *** | 1883 | 1942 | 3159 | 518 | 565 | 812 | 260 | 287 | 371 | 162 | 178 | 214 | 113 | 123 | 141 |
| | *** | 1903 | 2054 | 3340 | 535 | 624 | 840 | 271 | 314 | 372 | 169 | 192 | 206 | 117 | 130 | 129 |
| 0.45 | *** | 1801 | 1877 | 3272 | 503 | 558 | 831 | 254 | 285 | 375 | 159 | 176 | 214 | 110 | 121 | 139 |
| | *** | 1827 | 2016 | 3409 | 524 | 623 | 848 | 267 | 314 | 372 | 166 | 190 | 204 | 115 | 128 | 126 |
| 0.5 | *** | 1677 | 1772 | 3310 | 479 | 541 | 832 | 245 | 277 | 371 | 153 | 171 | 210 | 106 | 116 | 135 |
| | *** | 1709 | 1939 | 3409 | 503 | 612 | 840 | 258 | 308 | 364 | 161 | 186 | 197 | 111 | 124 | 120 |
| 0.55 | *** | 1523 | 1641 | 3273 | 450 | 516 | 813 | 232 | 266 | 359 | 145 | 163 | 201 | 100 | 110 | 128 |
| | *** | 1563 | 1834 | 3340 | 476 | 590 | 814 | 246 | 296 | 349 | 153 | 177 | 187 | 104 | 117 | 112 |
| 0.6 | *** | 1351 | 1493 | 3162 | 416 | 484 | 776 | 217 | 249 | 339 | 135 | 152 | 187 | 92 | 101 | 117 |
| | *** | 1401 | 1708 | 3203 | 443 | 559 | 771 | 230 | 279 | 326 | 142 | 165 | 172 | 96 | 108 | 101 |
| 0.65 | *** | 1175 | 1338 | 2977 | 378 | 446 | 721 | 198 | 229 | 310 | 123 | 138 | 169 | 83 | 91 | 104 |
| | *** | 1235 | 1566 | 2998 | 406 | 519 | 711 | 211 | 257 | 295 | 129 | 150 | 153 | 86 | 96 | 88 |
| 0.7 | *** | 1005 | 1181 | 2718 | 337 | 403 | 647 | 177 | 205 | 273 | 108 | 121 | 146 | 71 | 78 | 88 |
| | *** | 1071 | 1412 | 2724 | 364 | 469 | 634 | 189 | 229 | 257 | 114 | 131 | 129 | 74 | 82 | 71 |
| 0.75 | *** | 845 | 1023 | 2386 | 293 | 352 | 555 | 152 | 175 | 228 | 90 | 100 | 118 | . | . | . |
| | *** | 913 | 1244 | 2381 | 317 | 410 | 540 | 162 | 195 | 212 | 95 | 108 | 101 | . | . | . |
| 0.8 | *** | 696 | 862 | 1981 | 245 | 294 | 445 | 123 | 140 | 175 | . | . | . | . | . | . |
| | *** | 760 | 1061 | 1970 | 265 | 340 | 429 | 130 | 154 | 158 | . | . | . | . | . | . |
| 0.85 | *** | 550 | 692 | 1506 | 189 | 224 | 317 | . | . | . | . | . | . | . | . | . |
| | *** | 606 | 854 | 1491 | 204 | 255 | 300 | . | . | . | . | . | . | . | . | . |
| 0.9 | *** | 395 | 497 | 959 | . | . | . | . | . | . | . | . | . | . | . | . |
| | *** | 436 | 606 | 943 | . | . | . | . | . | . | . | . | . | . | . | . |

TABLE 8: ALPHA= 0.05  POWER= 0.9     EXPECTED ACCRUAL THRU MINIMUM FOLLOW-UP= 130

| | | DEL=.05 | | | DEL=.10 | | | DEL=.15 | | | DEL=.20 | | | DEL=.25 | | |
|---|---|---|---|---|---|---|---|---|---|---|---|---|---|---|---|---|---|
| FACT= | | 1.0 .75 | .50 .25 | .00 BIN | 1.0 .75 | .50 .25 | .00 BIN | 1.0 .75 | .50 .25 | .00 BIN | 1.0 75 | .50 .25 | .00 BIN | 1.0 .75 | .50 .25 | .00 BIN |
| PCONT=*** | | | | REQUIRED NUMBER OF PATIENTS | | | | | | | | | | | | |
| 0.05 | *** | 513 | 516 | 547 | 183 | 186 | 195 | 108 | 110 | 114 | 77 | 78 | 80 | 60 | 61 | 62 |
| | *** | 514 | 522 | 943 | 184 | 189 | 300 | 109 | 111 | 158 | 77 | 79 | 101 | 60 | 61 | 71 |
| 0.1 | *** | 935 | 943 | 1055 | 291 | 298 | 326 | 157 | 162 | 173 | 105 | 108 | 113 | 78 | 80 | 83 |
| | *** | 938 | 957 | 1491 | 294 | 307 | 429 | 159 | 166 | 212 | 106 | 110 | 129 | 79 | 81 | 88 |
| 0.15 | *** | 1294 | 1307 | 1547 | 378 | 390 | 447 | 196 | 204 | 225 | 126 | 132 | 142 | 92 | 95 | 101 |
| | *** | 1298 | 1332 | 1970 | 382 | 406 | 540 | 199 | 212 | 257 | 129 | 136 | 153 | 93 | 97 | 101 |
| 0.2 | *** | 1572 | 1591 | 1996 | 443 | 462 | 554 | 224 | 237 | 270 | 142 | 150 | 166 | 102 | 106 | 115 |
| | *** | 1578 | 1629 | 2381 | 450 | 486 | 634 | 229 | 248 | 295 | 146 | 156 | 172 | 104 | 110 | 112 |
| 0.25 | *** | 1765 | 1792 | 2388 | 488 | 514 | 645 | 245 | 261 | 308 | 154 | 164 | 185 | 109 | 115 | 126 |
| | *** | 1774 | 1846 | 2724 | 498 | 547 | 711 | 251 | 277 | 326 | 158 | 172 | 187 | 111 | 120 | 120 |
| 0.3 | *** | 1877 | 1914 | 2715 | 515 | 548 | 719 | 257 | 278 | 337 | 161 | 173 | 200 | 113 | 120 | 134 |
| | *** | 1889 | 1986 | 2998 | 527 | 590 | 771 | 265 | 297 | 349 | 166 | 183 | 197 | 116 | 126 | 126 |
| 0.35 | *** | 1915 | 1964 | 2973 | 525 | 567 | 775 | 263 | 287 | 358 | 164 | 178 | 209 | 115 | 123 | 139 |
| | *** | 1931 | 2058 | 3203 | 541 | 618 | 814 | 273 | 311 | 364 | 170 | 190 | 204 | 118 | 130 | 129 |
| 0.4 | *** | 1888 | 1952 | 3159 | 522 | 572 | 812 | 263 | 291 | 371 | 164 | 180 | 214 | 114 | 124 | 141 |
| | *** | 1909 | 2072 | 3340 | 541 | 631 | 840 | 274 | 317 | 372 | 171 | 193 | 206 | 118 | 131 | 129 |
| 0.45 | *** | 1808 | 1889 | 3272 | 508 | 565 | 831 | 258 | 288 | 375 | 161 | 178 | 214 | 112 | 122 | 139 |
| | *** | 1835 | 2037 | 3409 | 530 | 631 | 848 | 270 | 317 | 372 | 168 | 192 | 204 | 116 | 129 | 126 |
| 0.5 | *** | 1685 | 1788 | 3310 | 486 | 549 | 832 | 249 | 281 | 372 | 155 | 173 | 210 | 107 | 117 | 135 |
| | *** | 1720 | 1963 | 3409 | 510 | 620 | 840 | 262 | 311 | 364 | 163 | 187 | 197 | 112 | 125 | 120 |
| 0.55 | *** | 1533 | 1659 | 3273 | 457 | 524 | 813 | 236 | 269 | 359 | 148 | 165 | 201 | 101 | 111 | 128 |
| | *** | 1577 | 1861 | 3340 | 483 | 598 | 814 | 250 | 299 | 349 | 155 | 179 | 187 | 106 | 118 | 112 |
| 0.6 | *** | 1364 | 1514 | 3162 | 423 | 493 | 776 | 221 | 253 | 339 | 137 | 154 | 187 | 93 | 102 | 117 |
| | *** | 1417 | 1737 | 3203 | 451 | 567 | 771 | 234 | 282 | 326 | 144 | 167 | 172 | 97 | 109 | 101 |
| 0.65 | *** | 1191 | 1361 | 2977 | 386 | 455 | 721 | 202 | 233 | 310 | 125 | 140 | 169 | 84 | 92 | 104 |
| | *** | 1253 | 1596 | 2998 | 413 | 527 | 711 | 215 | 260 | 295 | 131 | 151 | 153 | 87 | 97 | 88 |
| 0.7 | *** | 1022 | 1205 | 2718 | 345 | 410 | 647 | 180 | 208 | 273 | 110 | 122 | 146 | 72 | 78 | 88 |
| | *** | 1091 | 1441 | 2724 | 371 | 477 | 634 | 192 | 231 | 257 | 115 | 132 | 129 | 75 | 83 | 71 |
| 0.75 | *** | 863 | 1047 | 2386 | 300 | 359 | 555 | 155 | 178 | 228 | 92 | 101 | 118 | . | . | . |
| | *** | 934 | 1272 | 2381 | 324 | 417 | 540 | 165 | 197 | 212 | 96 | 108 | 101 | . | . | . |
| 0.8 | *** | 713 | 884 | 1981 | 250 | 299 | 445 | 125 | 142 | 175 | . | . | . | . | . | . |
| | *** | 779 | 1085 | 1970 | 271 | 345 | 429 | 132 | 155 | 158 | . | . | . | . | . | . |
| 0.85 | *** | 565 | 710 | 1506 | 193 | 228 | 317 | . | . | . | . | . | . | . | . | . |
| | *** | 622 | 873 | 1491 | 208 | 259 | 300 | . | . | . | . | . | . | . | . | . |
| 0.9 | *** | 406 | 509 | 959 | . | . | . | . | . | . | . | . | . | . | . | . |
| | *** | 447 | 619 | 943 | . | . | . | . | . | . | . | . | . | . | . | . |

TABLE 8: ALPHA= 0.05  POWER= 0.9     EXPECTED ACCRUAL THRU MINIMUM FOLLOW-UP= 140

| PCONT | FACT= | DEL=.05 1.0 .75 | .50 .25 | .00 BIN | DEL=.10 1.0 .75 | .50 .25 | .00 BIN | DEL=.15 1.0 .75 | .50 .25 | .00 BIN | DEL=.20 1.0 75 | .50 .25 | .00 BIN | DEL=.25 1.0 .75 | .50 .25 | .00 BIN |
|---|---|---|---|---|---|---|---|---|---|---|---|---|---|---|---|---|
| | | REQUIRED NUMBER OF PATIENTS | | | | | | | | | | | | | | |
| 0.05 | *** | 513 | 517 | 547 | 183 | 186 | 195 | 108 | 110 | 113 | 77 | 78 | 80 | 60 | 61 | 62 |
| | *** | 514 | 523 | 943 | 185 | 189 | 300 | 109 | 111 | 158 | 77 | 79 | 101 | 60 | 61 | 71 |
| 0.1 | *** | 936 | 944 | 1055 | 291 | 299 | 326 | 158 | 162 | 173 | 105 | 108 | 113 | 78 | 80 | 83 |
| | *** | 939 | 959 | 1491 | 294 | 307 | 429 | 160 | 166 | 212 | 106 | 110 | 129 | 79 | 82 | 88 |
| 0.15 | *** | 1295 | 1309 | 1547 | 379 | 392 | 447 | 196 | 205 | 225 | 127 | 132 | 142 | 92 | 95 | 101 |
| | *** | 1300 | 1335 | 1970 | 384 | 407 | 540 | 200 | 212 | 257 | 129 | 136 | 153 | 93 | 98 | 101 |
| 0.2 | *** | 1573 | 1594 | 1996 | 445 | 464 | 554 | 226 | 238 | 270 | 143 | 151 | 166 | 102 | 107 | 115 |
| | *** | 1580 | 1635 | 2381 | 452 | 488 | 634 | 231 | 249 | 295 | 147 | 157 | 172 | 104 | 110 | 112 |
| 0.25 | *** | 1767 | 1796 | 2388 | 491 | 517 | 645 | 246 | 263 | 308 | 155 | 165 | 185 | 109 | 115 | 126 |
| | *** | 1777 | 1854 | 2724 | 501 | 551 | 711 | 253 | 278 | 326 | 159 | 173 | 187 | 112 | 120 | 120 |
| 0.3 | *** | 1880 | 1920 | 2715 | 518 | 552 | 719 | 259 | 280 | 337 | 162 | 174 | 200 | 114 | 121 | 134 |
| | *** | 1893 | 1997 | 2998 | 531 | 595 | 771 | 267 | 299 | 349 | 167 | 184 | 197 | 117 | 126 | 126 |
| 0.35 | *** | 1919 | 1971 | 2973 | 529 | 572 | 775 | 265 | 290 | 358 | 166 | 180 | 209 | 116 | 124 | 139 |
| | *** | 1936 | 2072 | 3203 | 545 | 624 | 814 | 275 | 313 | 364 | 172 | 191 | 204 | 119 | 130 | 129 |
| 0.4 | *** | 1893 | 1962 | 3159 | 527 | 578 | 812 | 265 | 293 | 371 | 166 | 181 | 214 | 115 | 124 | 141 |
| | *** | 1916 | 2088 | 3340 | 546 | 637 | 840 | 277 | 320 | 372 | 172 | 194 | 206 | 119 | 131 | 129 |
| 0.45 | *** | 1814 | 1901 | 3272 | 514 | 572 | 831 | 261 | 292 | 375 | 163 | 180 | 214 | 113 | 123 | 139 |
| | *** | 1843 | 2057 | 3409 | 536 | 638 | 848 | 274 | 320 | 372 | 170 | 193 | 204 | 117 | 130 | 126 |
| 0.5 | *** | 1693 | 1803 | 3310 | 492 | 556 | 832 | 252 | 285 | 372 | 157 | 175 | 210 | 109 | 118 | 135 |
| | *** | 1730 | 1987 | 3409 | 517 | 628 | 840 | 266 | 314 | 364 | 165 | 188 | 197 | 113 | 125 | 120 |
| 0.55 | *** | 1543 | 1677 | 3273 | 463 | 532 | 813 | 240 | 273 | 359 | 149 | 167 | 201 | 102 | 112 | 128 |
| | *** | 1590 | 1887 | 3340 | 491 | 606 | 814 | 254 | 302 | 349 | 157 | 180 | 187 | 107 | 118 | 112 |
| 0.6 | *** | 1377 | 1535 | 3162 | 430 | 501 | 776 | 224 | 256 | 339 | 139 | 155 | 187 | 95 | 103 | 117 |
| | *** | 1433 | 1765 | 3203 | 458 | 575 | 771 | 238 | 285 | 326 | 146 | 168 | 172 | 98 | 109 | 101 |
| 0.65 | *** | 1206 | 1384 | 2976 | 393 | 463 | 721 | 205 | 236 | 310 | 126 | 141 | 169 | 85 | 92 | 104 |
| | *** | 1271 | 1624 | 2998 | 421 | 534 | 711 | 218 | 262 | 295 | 133 | 152 | 153 | 88 | 97 | 88 |
| 0.7 | *** | 1039 | 1228 | 2717 | 351 | 418 | 647 | 183 | 210 | 273 | 111 | 123 | 146 | 73 | 79 | 88 |
| | *** | 1110 | 1469 | 2724 | 378 | 484 | 634 | 195 | 233 | 257 | 117 | 133 | 129 | 76 | 83 | 71 |
| 0.75 | *** | 881 | 1069 | 2386 | 306 | 365 | 555 | 157 | 180 | 228 | 93 | 102 | 118 | . | . | . |
| | *** | 953 | 1298 | 2381 | 331 | 423 | 540 | 167 | 198 | 212 | 97 | 109 | 101 | . | . | . |
| 0.8 | *** | 729 | 904 | 1981 | 256 | 304 | 445 | 127 | 143 | 175 | . | . | . | . | . | . |
| | *** | 798 | 1108 | 1970 | 276 | 350 | 429 | 134 | 156 | 158 | . | . | . | . | . | . |
| 0.85 | *** | 579 | 726 | 1506 | 197 | 231 | 317 | . | . | . | . | . | . | . | . | . |
| | *** | 637 | 892 | 1491 | 211 | 262 | 300 | . | . | . | . | . | . | . | . | . |
| 0.9 | *** | 416 | 521 | 959 | . | . | . | . | . | . | . | . | . | . | . | . |
| | *** | 458 | 631 | 943 | . | . | . | . | . | . | . | . | . | . | . | . |

## TABLE 8: ALPHA= 0.05 POWER= 0.9     EXPECTED ACCRUAL THRU MINIMUM FOLLOW-UP= 150

| | | DEL=.05 | | | DEL=.10 | | | DEL=.15 | | | DEL=.20 | | | DEL=.25 | | |
|---|---|---|---|---|---|---|---|---|---|---|---|---|---|---|---|---|
| FACT= | | 1.0 .75 | .50 .25 | .00 BIN | 1.0 .75 | .50 .25 | .00 BIN | 1.0 .75 | .50 .25 | .00 BIN | 1.0 75 | .50 .25 | .00 BIN | 1.0 .75 | .50 .25 | .00 BIN |

PCONT=***  REQUIRED NUMBER OF PATIENTS

| PCONT | FACT | 1.0/.75 | .50/.25 | .00/BIN | 1.0/.75 | .50/.25 | .00/BIN | 1.0/.75 | .50/.25 | .00/BIN | 1.0/75 | .50/.25 | .00/BIN | 1.0/.75 | .50/.25 | .00/BIN |
|---|---|---|---|---|---|---|---|---|---|---|---|---|---|---|---|---|
| 0.05 | *** | 513 | 517 | 547 | 184 | 187 | 195 | 108 | 110 | 113 | 77 | 78 | 80 | 60 | 61 | 62 |
| | *** | 515 | 524 | 943 | 185 | 190 | 300 | 109 | 112 | 158 | 77 | 79 | 101 | 60 | 61 | 71 |
| 0.1 | *** | 937 | 945 | 1055 | 292 | 300 | 326 | 158 | 163 | 173 | 105 | 108 | 113 | 78 | 80 | 83 |
| | *** | 939 | 961 | 1491 | 295 | 308 | 429 | 160 | 167 | 212 | 107 | 111 | 129 | 79 | 82 | 88 |
| 0.15 | *** | 1296 | 1311 | 1547 | 380 | 393 | 447 | 197 | 206 | 225 | 127 | 133 | 142 | 92 | 96 | 101 |
| | *** | 1301 | 1339 | 1970 | 385 | 409 | 540 | 201 | 213 | 257 | 130 | 136 | 153 | 94 | 98 | 101 |
| 0.2 | *** | 1575 | 1597 | 1996 | 446 | 466 | 554 | 227 | 239 | 270 | 144 | 152 | 166 | 103 | 107 | 115 |
| | *** | 1582 | 1640 | 2381 | 454 | 491 | 634 | 232 | 250 | 295 | 147 | 157 | 172 | 105 | 111 | 112 |
| 0.25 | *** | 1769 | 1801 | 2388 | 493 | 520 | 645 | 248 | 264 | 308 | 156 | 166 | 185 | 110 | 116 | 126 |
| | *** | 1780 | 1861 | 2724 | 503 | 554 | 711 | 255 | 280 | 326 | 160 | 173 | 187 | 113 | 120 | 120 |
| 0.3 | *** | 1883 | 1925 | 2715 | 521 | 557 | 719 | 261 | 282 | 337 | 163 | 175 | 199 | 114 | 122 | 134 |
| | *** | 1897 | 2007 | 2998 | 534 | 599 | 771 | 270 | 301 | 349 | 169 | 185 | 197 | 118 | 127 | 126 |
| 0.35 | *** | 1922 | 1979 | 2973 | 533 | 577 | 775 | 268 | 292 | 358 | 167 | 181 | 209 | 116 | 125 | 139 |
| | *** | 1941 | 2085 | 3203 | 550 | 629 | 814 | 278 | 315 | 364 | 173 | 192 | 204 | 120 | 131 | 129 |
| 0.4 | *** | 1898 | 1971 | 3159 | 531 | 583 | 812 | 268 | 296 | 371 | 167 | 183 | 214 | 116 | 125 | 141 |
| | *** | 1923 | 2105 | 3340 | 551 | 643 | 840 | 280 | 322 | 372 | 174 | 195 | 206 | 120 | 132 | 129 |
| 0.45 | *** | 1820 | 1914 | 3272 | 519 | 578 | 831 | 264 | 295 | 375 | 165 | 181 | 214 | 114 | 123 | 139 |
| | *** | 1852 | 2076 | 3409 | 542 | 645 | 848 | 277 | 322 | 372 | 172 | 194 | 204 | 118 | 130 | 126 |
| 0.5 | *** | 1701 | 1817 | 3310 | 497 | 563 | 832 | 255 | 288 | 371 | 159 | 176 | 210 | 110 | 119 | 135 |
| | *** | 1741 | 2009 | 3409 | 523 | 635 | 840 | 269 | 317 | 364 | 167 | 189 | 197 | 114 | 126 | 120 |
| 0.55 | *** | 1553 | 1695 | 3273 | 470 | 539 | 813 | 243 | 276 | 359 | 151 | 168 | 201 | 103 | 113 | 128 |
| | *** | 1603 | 1912 | 3340 | 497 | 613 | 814 | 257 | 305 | 349 | 159 | 181 | 187 | 108 | 119 | 112 |
| 0.6 | *** | 1389 | 1555 | 3162 | 437 | 508 | 776 | 227 | 260 | 339 | 141 | 157 | 187 | 95 | 104 | 117 |
| | *** | 1449 | 1791 | 3203 | 465 | 582 | 771 | 241 | 287 | 326 | 148 | 169 | 172 | 99 | 110 | 101 |
| 0.65 | *** | 1220 | 1405 | 2977 | 399 | 470 | 721 | 208 | 239 | 310 | 128 | 142 | 169 | 86 | 93 | 104 |
| | *** | 1289 | 1651 | 2998 | 428 | 541 | 711 | 221 | 264 | 295 | 134 | 153 | 153 | 89 | 98 | 88 |
| 0.7 | *** | 1055 | 1250 | 2717 | 358 | 424 | 647 | 186 | 213 | 273 | 112 | 125 | 146 | 74 | 79 | 88 |
| | *** | 1129 | 1495 | 2724 | 385 | 490 | 634 | 197 | 235 | 257 | 118 | 133 | 129 | 76 | 83 | 71 |
| 0.75 | *** | 897 | 1090 | 2386 | 312 | 371 | 555 | 160 | 182 | 228 | 94 | 103 | 118 | . | . | . |
| | *** | 972 | 1322 | 2381 | 337 | 428 | 540 | 169 | 200 | 212 | 98 | 109 | 101 | . | . | . |
| 0.8 | *** | 745 | 923 | 1981 | 260 | 309 | 445 | 128 | 145 | 175 | . | . | . | . | . | . |
| | *** | 815 | 1130 | 1970 | 281 | 354 | 429 | 136 | 157 | 158 | . | . | . | . | . | . |
| 0.85 | *** | 593 | 742 | 1506 | 200 | 235 | 317 | . | . | . | . | . | . | . | . | . |
| | *** | 652 | 908 | 1491 | 215 | 264 | 300 | . | . | . | . | . | . | . | . | . |
| 0.9 | *** | 426 | 532 | 959 | . | . | . | . | . | . | . | . | . | . | . | . |
| | *** | 469 | 642 | 943 | . | . | . | . | . | . | . | . | . | . | . | . |

TABLE 8: ALPHA= 0.05  POWER= 0.9    EXPECTED ACCRUAL THRU MINIMUM FOLLOW-UP= 160

| PCONT | DEL=.05 1.0/.75 | DEL=.05 .50/.25 | DEL=.05 .00/BIN | DEL=.10 1.0/.75 | DEL=.10 .50/.25 | DEL=.10 .00/BIN | DEL=.15 1.0/.75 | DEL=.15 .50/.25 | DEL=.15 .00/BIN | DEL=.20 1.0/75 | DEL=.20 .50/.25 | DEL=.20 .00/BIN | DEL=.25 1.0/.75 | DEL=.25 .50/.25 | DEL=.25 .00/BIN |
|---|---|---|---|---|---|---|---|---|---|---|---|---|---|---|---|
| 0.05 | 514 | 518 | 547 | 184 | 187 | 195 | 109 | 110 | 114 | 77 | 78 | 80 | 60 | 61 | 62 |
|       | 515 | 524 | 943 | 185 | 190 | 300 | 109 | 112 | 158 | 78 | 79 | 101 | 60 | 61 | 71 |
| 0.1  | 937 | 946 | 1055 | 293 | 301 | 326 | 158 | 163 | 173 | 106 | 109 | 113 | 79 | 81 | 83 |
|       | 940 | 963 | 1491 | 296 | 309 | 429 | 160 | 167 | 212 | 107 | 111 | 129 | 79 | 82 | 88 |
| 0.15 | 1297 | 1313 | 1547 | 381 | 395 | 447 | 198 | 206 | 225 | 128 | 133 | 142 | 93 | 96 | 101 |
|       | 1302 | 1343 | 1970 | 386 | 410 | 540 | 201 | 214 | 257 | 130 | 137 | 153 | 94 | 98 | 101 |
| 0.2  | 1576 | 1600 | 1996 | 448 | 469 | 554 | 228 | 240 | 270 | 145 | 152 | 166 | 103 | 108 | 115 |
|       | 1584 | 1645 | 2381 | 456 | 493 | 634 | 233 | 251 | 295 | 148 | 158 | 172 | 105 | 111 | 112 |
| 0.25 | 1771 | 1805 | 2388 | 495 | 523 | 645 | 249 | 266 | 308 | 157 | 166 | 185 | 111 | 116 | 126 |
|       | 1782 | 1869 | 2724 | 506 | 557 | 711 | 256 | 281 | 326 | 161 | 174 | 187 | 113 | 121 | 120 |
| 0.3  | 1885 | 1931 | 2715 | 524 | 560 | 719 | 263 | 284 | 337 | 165 | 176 | 199 | 115 | 122 | 134 |
|       | 1901 | 2017 | 2998 | 538 | 603 | 771 | 272 | 303 | 349 | 170 | 186 | 197 | 118 | 127 | 126 |
| 0.35 | 1926 | 1986 | 2973 | 536 | 582 | 775 | 270 | 295 | 358 | 168 | 182 | 209 | 117 | 125 | 139 |
|       | 1946 | 2098 | 3203 | 554 | 634 | 814 | 280 | 317 | 364 | 174 | 193 | 204 | 121 | 131 | 129 |
| 0.4  | 1903 | 1981 | 3159 | 536 | 589 | 812 | 271 | 299 | 371 | 169 | 184 | 214 | 117 | 126 | 141 |
|       | 1929 | 2121 | 3340 | 556 | 649 | 840 | 282 | 324 | 372 | 176 | 196 | 206 | 121 | 132 | 129 |
| 0.45 | 1827 | 1926 | 3272 | 524 | 584 | 831 | 267 | 297 | 375 | 166 | 183 | 215 | 115 | 124 | 139 |
|       | 1860 | 2095 | 3409 | 547 | 651 | 848 | 280 | 325 | 372 | 173 | 195 | 204 | 119 | 131 | 126 |
| 0.5  | 1709 | 1832 | 3310 | 503 | 570 | 832 | 258 | 291 | 372 | 161 | 178 | 210 | 111 | 120 | 135 |
|       | 1752 | 2030 | 3409 | 529 | 641 | 840 | 272 | 319 | 364 | 168 | 190 | 197 | 115 | 126 | 120 |
| 0.55 | 1563 | 1712 | 3273 | 476 | 546 | 813 | 246 | 279 | 359 | 153 | 169 | 201 | 104 | 113 | 128 |
|       | 1616 | 1935 | 3340 | 504 | 620 | 814 | 260 | 307 | 349 | 160 | 182 | 187 | 108 | 120 | 112 |
| 0.6  | 1401 | 1574 | 3162 | 443 | 515 | 776 | 230 | 262 | 339 | 142 | 158 | 187 | 96 | 105 | 117 |
|       | 1464 | 1816 | 3203 | 472 | 589 | 771 | 244 | 290 | 326 | 149 | 170 | 172 | 100 | 110 | 101 |
| 0.65 | 1235 | 1426 | 2977 | 406 | 477 | 721 | 211 | 241 | 310 | 129 | 143 | 169 | 86 | 93 | 104 |
|       | 1306 | 1677 | 2998 | 434 | 547 | 711 | 224 | 266 | 295 | 136 | 154 | 153 | 90 | 98 | 88 |
| 0.7  | 1071 | 1271 | 2718 | 364 | 431 | 647 | 189 | 215 | 273 | 114 | 125 | 146 | 74 | 80 | 88 |
|       | 1147 | 1520 | 2724 | 391 | 496 | 634 | 200 | 237 | 257 | 119 | 134 | 129 | 77 | 84 | 71 |
| 0.75 | 913 | 1110 | 2386 | 317 | 377 | 555 | 162 | 184 | 228 | 95 | 104 | 118 | . | . | . |
|       | 990 | 1346 | 2381 | 342 | 433 | 540 | 171 | 201 | 212 | 99 | 110 | 101 | . | . | . |
| 0.8  | 760 | 941 | 1981 | 265 | 314 | 445 | 130 | 146 | 175 | . | . | . | . | . | . |
|       | 831 | 1150 | 1970 | 285 | 357 | 429 | 137 | 158 | 158 | . | . | . | . | . | . |
| 0.85 | 606 | 757 | 1506 | 204 | 238 | 317 | . | . | . | . | . | . | . | . | . |
|       | 666 | 924 | 1491 | 218 | 267 | 300 | . | . | . | . | . | . | . | . | . |
| 0.9  | 436 | 542 | 959 | . | . | . | . | . | . | . | . | . | . | . | . |
|       | 479 | 652 | 943 | . | . | . | . | . | . | . | . | . | . | . | . |

PCONT=***    REQUIRED NUMBER OF PATIENTS

TABLE 8: ALPHA= 0.05  POWER= 0.9    EXPECTED ACCRUAL THRU MINIMUM FOLLOW-UP= 170

| | | DEL=.05 | | | DEL=.10 | | | DEL=.15 | | | DEL=.20 | | | DEL=.25 | | |
|---|---|---|---|---|---|---|---|---|---|---|---|---|---|---|---|---|
| FACT= | | 1.0 .75 | .50 .25 | .00 BIN | 1.0 .75 | .50 .25 | .00 BIN | 1.0 .75 | .50 .25 | .00 BIN | 1.0 75 | .50 .25 | .00 BIN | 1.0 .75 | .50 .25 | .00 BIN |
| PCONT=*** | | | | | | | REQUIRED NUMBER OF PATIENTS | | | | | | | | | |
| 0.05 | *** | 514 | 518 | 547 | 184 | 187 | 195 | 109 | 110 | 113 | 77 | 78 | 80 | 60 | 61 | 62 |
| | *** | 515 | 525 | 943 | 186 | 190 | 300 | 109 | 112 | 158 | 78 | 79 | 101 | 60 | 61 | 71 |
| 0.1 | *** | 938 | 947 | 1055 | 293 | 301 | 326 | 159 | 164 | 173 | 106 | 109 | 113 | 79 | 81 | 83 |
| | *** | 941 | 965 | 1491 | 296 | 310 | 429 | 161 | 167 | 212 | 107 | 111 | 129 | 80 | 82 | 88 |
| 0.15 | *** | 1298 | 1315 | 1547 | 382 | 396 | 447 | 199 | 207 | 225 | 128 | 133 | 142 | 93 | 96 | 101 |
| | *** | 1304 | 1346 | 1970 | 387 | 412 | 540 | 202 | 214 | 257 | 131 | 137 | 153 | 94 | 98 | 101 |
| 0.2 | *** | 1578 | 1603 | 1996 | 450 | 471 | 554 | 229 | 241 | 270 | 146 | 153 | 166 | 104 | 108 | 115 |
| | *** | 1586 | 1651 | 2381 | 458 | 495 | 634 | 234 | 252 | 295 | 149 | 158 | 172 | 106 | 111 | 112 |
| 0.25 | *** | 1773 | 1809 | 2388 | 497 | 526 | 645 | 251 | 267 | 308 | 158 | 167 | 185 | 111 | 117 | 126 |
| | *** | 1785 | 1877 | 2724 | 508 | 560 | 711 | 258 | 282 | 326 | 162 | 174 | 187 | 114 | 121 | 120 |
| 0.3 | *** | 1888 | 1937 | 2715 | 526 | 564 | 719 | 265 | 286 | 337 | 166 | 177 | 199 | 116 | 123 | 134 |
| | *** | 1904 | 2027 | 2998 | 541 | 607 | 771 | 273 | 304 | 349 | 171 | 186 | 197 | 119 | 128 | 126 |
| 0.35 | *** | 1930 | 1994 | 2973 | 540 | 586 | 775 | 272 | 297 | 358 | 170 | 183 | 209 | 118 | 126 | 139 |
| | *** | 1951 | 2111 | 3203 | 558 | 638 | 814 | 282 | 319 | 364 | 176 | 194 | 204 | 122 | 132 | 129 |
| 0.4 | *** | 1908 | 1990 | 3159 | 540 | 594 | 812 | 273 | 301 | 371 | 170 | 185 | 214 | 118 | 127 | 141 |
| | *** | 1936 | 2136 | 3340 | 561 | 654 | 840 | 285 | 326 | 372 | 177 | 197 | 206 | 122 | 133 | 129 |
| 0.45 | *** | 1833 | 1937 | 3272 | 528 | 590 | 831 | 269 | 300 | 375 | 168 | 184 | 215 | 116 | 125 | 139 |
| | *** | 1869 | 2113 | 3409 | 553 | 657 | 848 | 282 | 327 | 372 | 175 | 196 | 204 | 120 | 131 | 126 |
| 0.5 | *** | 1717 | 1846 | 3310 | 508 | 576 | 832 | 261 | 293 | 371 | 162 | 179 | 210 | 111 | 120 | 135 |
| | *** | 1762 | 2051 | 3409 | 535 | 647 | 840 | 275 | 321 | 364 | 170 | 191 | 197 | 116 | 127 | 120 |
| 0.55 | *** | 1573 | 1728 | 3273 | 481 | 553 | 813 | 249 | 282 | 359 | 154 | 171 | 201 | 105 | 114 | 128 |
| | *** | 1628 | 1958 | 3340 | 510 | 626 | 814 | 263 | 309 | 349 | 162 | 183 | 187 | 109 | 120 | 112 |
| 0.6 | *** | 1413 | 1592 | 3162 | 449 | 522 | 776 | 233 | 265 | 339 | 144 | 159 | 187 | 97 | 105 | 117 |
| | *** | 1479 | 1840 | 3203 | 478 | 595 | 771 | 247 | 292 | 326 | 151 | 171 | 172 | 101 | 110 | 101 |
| 0.65 | *** | 1249 | 1445 | 2976 | 412 | 483 | 721 | 214 | 244 | 310 | 131 | 144 | 169 | 87 | 94 | 104 |
| | *** | 1322 | 1701 | 2998 | 441 | 553 | 711 | 227 | 268 | 295 | 137 | 154 | 153 | 90 | 99 | 88 |
| 0.7 | *** | 1086 | 1291 | 2718 | 370 | 436 | 647 | 191 | 217 | 273 | 115 | 126 | 146 | 75 | 80 | 88 |
| | *** | 1164 | 1544 | 2724 | 397 | 501 | 634 | 202 | 239 | 257 | 120 | 135 | 129 | 77 | 84 | 71 |
| 0.75 | *** | 929 | 1130 | 2386 | 323 | 382 | 555 | 164 | 186 | 228 | 96 | 104 | 118 | . | . | . |
| | *** | 1007 | 1367 | 2381 | 347 | 437 | 540 | 173 | 202 | 212 | 100 | 110 | 101 | . | . | . |
| 0.8 | *** | 775 | 959 | 1981 | 269 | 318 | 445 | 132 | 147 | 175 | . | . | . | . | . | . |
| | *** | 847 | 1169 | 1970 | 290 | 361 | 429 | 139 | 159 | 158 | . | . | . | . | . | . |
| 0.85 | *** | 618 | 771 | 1506 | 207 | 241 | 317 | . | . | . | . | . | . | . | . | . |
| | *** | 679 | 939 | 1491 | 221 | 269 | 300 | . | . | . | . | . | . | . | . | . |
| 0.9 | *** | 445 | 552 | 959 | . | . | . | . | . | . | . | . | . | . | . | . |
| | *** | 488 | 661 | 943 | . | . | . | . | . | . | . | . | . | . | . | . |

TABLE 8: ALPHA= 0.05  POWER= 0.9    EXPECTED ACCRUAL THRU MINIMUM FOLLOW-UP= 180

| | | DEL=.05 | | | DEL=.10 | | | DEL=.15 | | | DEL=.20 | | | DEL=.25 | | |
|---|---|---|---|---|---|---|---|---|---|---|---|---|---|---|---|---|
| FACT= | | 1.0 .75 | .50 .25 | .00 BIN | 1.0 .75 | .50 .25 | .00 BIN | 1.0 .75 | .50 .25 | .00 BIN | 1.0 75 | .50 .25 | .00 BIN | 1.0 .75 | .50 .25 | .00 BIN |
| PCONT=*** | | | | | REQUIRED NUMBER OF PATIENTS | | | | | | | | | | | |
| 0.05 | *** | 514 | 519 | 547 | 185 | 188 | 195 | 109 | 111 | 114 | 77 | 78 | 80 | 60 | 61 | 62 |
| | *** | 516 | 526 | 943 | 186 | 190 | 300 | 110 | 112 | 158 | 78 | 79 | 101 | 60 | 61 | 71 |
| 0.1 | *** | 938 | 949 | 1055 | 294 | 302 | 326 | 159 | 164 | 173 | 106 | 109 | 114 | 79 | 81 | 83 |
| | *** | 942 | 967 | 1491 | 297 | 310 | 429 | 161 | 168 | 212 | 108 | 111 | 129 | 80 | 82 | 88 |
| 0.15 | *** | 1299 | 1317 | 1547 | 383 | 397 | 447 | 199 | 208 | 225 | 129 | 134 | 142 | 93 | 96 | 101 |
| | *** | 1305 | 1349 | 1970 | 388 | 413 | 540 | 203 | 215 | 257 | 131 | 137 | 153 | 95 | 98 | 101 |
| 0.2 | *** | 1579 | 1606 | 1996 | 451 | 473 | 554 | 230 | 242 | 270 | 146 | 153 | 166 | 104 | 108 | 115 |
| | *** | 1588 | 1656 | 2381 | 459 | 497 | 634 | 235 | 253 | 295 | 149 | 159 | 172 | 106 | 111 | 112 |
| 0.25 | *** | 1775 | 1813 | 2388 | 499 | 529 | 645 | 252 | 269 | 308 | 159 | 168 | 185 | 112 | 117 | 126 |
| | *** | 1788 | 1884 | 2724 | 510 | 563 | 711 | 259 | 283 | 326 | 163 | 175 | 187 | 114 | 121 | 120 |
| 0.3 | *** | 1891 | 1942 | 2715 | 529 | 568 | 719 | 266 | 287 | 337 | 167 | 178 | 199 | 117 | 123 | 134 |
| | *** | 1908 | 2037 | 2998 | 544 | 611 | 771 | 275 | 305 | 349 | 172 | 187 | 197 | 120 | 128 | 126 |
| 0.35 | *** | 1934 | 2001 | 2973 | 543 | 590 | 775 | 274 | 299 | 358 | 171 | 184 | 209 | 119 | 127 | 139 |
| | *** | 1956 | 2123 | 3203 | 561 | 642 | 814 | 284 | 320 | 364 | 177 | 194 | 204 | 122 | 132 | 129 |
| 0.4 | *** | 1913 | 2000 | 3159 | 544 | 599 | 812 | 276 | 303 | 371 | 172 | 186 | 214 | 119 | 127 | 141 |
| | *** | 1942 | 2151 | 3340 | 565 | 659 | 840 | 287 | 328 | 372 | 178 | 198 | 206 | 123 | 133 | 129 |
| 0.45 | *** | 1839 | 1949 | 3272 | 533 | 596 | 831 | 272 | 302 | 375 | 169 | 185 | 215 | 117 | 125 | 139 |
| | *** | 1877 | 2131 | 3409 | 558 | 662 | 848 | 285 | 329 | 372 | 176 | 197 | 204 | 121 | 131 | 126 |
| 0.5 | *** | 1725 | 1860 | 3310 | 514 | 582 | 832 | 264 | 296 | 371 | 164 | 180 | 210 | 112 | 121 | 135 |
| | *** | 1772 | 2071 | 3409 | 541 | 653 | 840 | 277 | 323 | 364 | 171 | 192 | 197 | 116 | 127 | 120 |
| 0.55 | *** | 1583 | 1745 | 3273 | 487 | 559 | 813 | 252 | 284 | 359 | 156 | 172 | 201 | 106 | 114 | 128 |
| | *** | 1641 | 1979 | 3340 | 516 | 632 | 814 | 266 | 311 | 349 | 163 | 184 | 187 | 110 | 120 | 112 |
| 0.6 | *** | 1425 | 1610 | 3162 | 455 | 528 | 776 | 236 | 267 | 339 | 145 | 160 | 187 | 98 | 106 | 117 |
| | *** | 1493 | 1862 | 3203 | 484 | 601 | 771 | 249 | 294 | 326 | 152 | 171 | 172 | 101 | 111 | 101 |
| 0.65 | *** | 1262 | 1464 | 2976 | 417 | 489 | 721 | 217 | 246 | 310 | 132 | 145 | 169 | 88 | 94 | 104 |
| | *** | 1338 | 1724 | 2998 | 447 | 559 | 711 | 229 | 270 | 295 | 138 | 155 | 153 | 91 | 99 | 88 |
| 0.7 | *** | 1101 | 1310 | 2718 | 375 | 442 | 647 | 193 | 219 | 273 | 116 | 127 | 146 | 75 | 81 | 88 |
| | *** | 1181 | 1566 | 2724 | 403 | 506 | 634 | 205 | 240 | 257 | 121 | 135 | 129 | 78 | 84 | 71 |
| 0.75 | *** | 944 | 1148 | 2386 | 327 | 387 | 555 | 166 | 187 | 228 | 96 | 105 | 118 | . | . | . |
| | *** | 1023 | 1388 | 2381 | 352 | 441 | 540 | 175 | 204 | 212 | 100 | 111 | 101 | . | . | . |
| 0.8 | *** | 789 | 975 | 1981 | 273 | 322 | 445 | 133 | 148 | 175 | . | . | . | . | . | . |
| | *** | 862 | 1187 | 1970 | 294 | 364 | 429 | 140 | 160 | 158 | . | . | . | . | . | . |
| 0.85 | *** | 630 | 785 | 1506 | 210 | 243 | 317 | . | . | . | . | . | . | . | . | . |
| | *** | 692 | 953 | 1491 | 224 | 271 | 300 | . | . | . | . | . | . | . | . | . |
| 0.9 | *** | 453 | 561 | 959 | . | . | . | . | . | . | . | . | . | . | . | . |
| | *** | 497 | 670 | 943 | . | . | . | . | . | . | . | . | . | . | . | . |

# TABLE 8: ALPHA= 0.05  POWER= 0.9    EXPECTED ACCRUAL THRU MINIMUM FOLLOW-UP= 190

|  |  | DEL=.05 | | | DEL=.10 | | | DEL=.15 | | | DEL=.20 | | | DEL=.25 | | |
|---|---|---|---|---|---|---|---|---|---|---|---|---|---|---|---|---|
| FACT= | | 1.0 .75 | .50 .25 | .00 BIN | 1.0 .75 | .50 .25 | .00 BIN | 1.0 .75 | .50 .25 | .00 BIN | 1.0 75 | .50 .25 | .00 BIN | 1.0 .75 | .50 .25 | .00 BIN |
| PCONT=*** | | REQUIRED NUMBER OF PATIENTS | | | | | | | | | | | | | | |
| 0.05 | *** | 515 | 519 | 547 | 185 | 188 | 195 | 109 | 111 | 113 | 77 | 78 | 80 | 60 | 61 | 62 |
| | *** | 516 | 526 | 943 | 186 | 191 | 300 | 110 | 112 | 158 | 78 | 79 | 101 | 61 | 61 | 71 |
| 0.1 | *** | 939 | 950 | 1055 | 294 | 303 | 326 | 160 | 164 | 173 | 107 | 109 | 113 | 79 | 81 | 83 |
| | *** | 942 | 969 | 1491 | 298 | 311 | 429 | 162 | 168 | 212 | 108 | 111 | 129 | 80 | 82 | 88 |
| 0.15 | *** | 1300 | 1319 | 1547 | 384 | 398 | 447 | 200 | 208 | 225 | 129 | 134 | 142 | 94 | 97 | 101 |
| | *** | 1306 | 1353 | 1970 | 390 | 414 | 540 | 203 | 215 | 257 | 131 | 137 | 153 | 95 | 98 | 101 |
| 0.2 | *** | 1581 | 1609 | 1996 | 453 | 475 | 554 | 231 | 243 | 270 | 147 | 154 | 166 | 104 | 109 | 115 |
| | *** | 1590 | 1661 | 2381 | 461 | 499 | 634 | 236 | 254 | 295 | 150 | 159 | 172 | 106 | 111 | 112 |
| 0.25 | *** | 1778 | 1817 | 2388 | 501 | 532 | 645 | 253 | 270 | 308 | 159 | 169 | 185 | 112 | 118 | 126 |
| | *** | 1791 | 1891 | 2724 | 513 | 565 | 711 | 260 | 284 | 326 | 163 | 175 | 187 | 115 | 121 | 120 |
| 0.3 | *** | 1894 | 1948 | 2715 | 532 | 571 | 719 | 268 | 289 | 337 | 168 | 179 | 199 | 117 | 124 | 134 |
| | *** | 1912 | 2046 | 2998 | 547 | 614 | 771 | 277 | 307 | 349 | 173 | 187 | 197 | 120 | 128 | 126 |
| 0.35 | *** | 1937 | 2009 | 2973 | 546 | 594 | 775 | 276 | 300 | 358 | 172 | 185 | 209 | 120 | 127 | 139 |
| | *** | 1961 | 2135 | 3203 | 565 | 646 | 814 | 286 | 322 | 364 | 178 | 195 | 204 | 123 | 132 | 129 |
| 0.4 | *** | 1918 | 2009 | 3159 | 548 | 604 | 812 | 278 | 306 | 371 | 173 | 187 | 214 | 120 | 128 | 141 |
| | *** | 1949 | 2166 | 3340 | 570 | 664 | 840 | 289 | 329 | 372 | 179 | 198 | 206 | 123 | 133 | 129 |
| 0.45 | *** | 1846 | 1961 | 3272 | 538 | 601 | 831 | 274 | 305 | 375 | 171 | 186 | 215 | 117 | 126 | 139 |
| | *** | 1885 | 2148 | 3409 | 563 | 667 | 848 | 287 | 330 | 372 | 177 | 198 | 204 | 121 | 132 | 126 |
| 0.5 | *** | 1733 | 1874 | 3310 | 519 | 588 | 832 | 267 | 298 | 372 | 165 | 181 | 210 | 113 | 122 | 135 |
| | *** | 1783 | 2090 | 3409 | 546 | 658 | 840 | 280 | 325 | 364 | 172 | 193 | 197 | 117 | 127 | 120 |
| 0.55 | *** | 1593 | 1760 | 3273 | 492 | 565 | 813 | 254 | 287 | 359 | 157 | 173 | 201 | 107 | 115 | 128 |
| | *** | 1653 | 2000 | 3340 | 522 | 638 | 814 | 268 | 313 | 349 | 164 | 184 | 187 | 111 | 121 | 112 |
| 0.6 | *** | 1437 | 1628 | 3162 | 460 | 534 | 776 | 239 | 270 | 339 | 147 | 161 | 187 | 99 | 106 | 117 |
| | *** | 1507 | 1884 | 3203 | 490 | 606 | 771 | 252 | 296 | 326 | 153 | 172 | 172 | 102 | 111 | 101 |
| 0.65 | *** | 1276 | 1483 | 2977 | 423 | 494 | 721 | 219 | 248 | 310 | 133 | 146 | 169 | 88 | 95 | 104 |
| | *** | 1354 | 1746 | 2998 | 452 | 564 | 711 | 231 | 272 | 295 | 139 | 156 | 153 | 91 | 99 | 88 |
| 0.7 | *** | 1115 | 1329 | 2718 | 380 | 447 | 647 | 195 | 221 | 273 | 117 | 128 | 146 | 76 | 81 | 88 |
| | *** | 1197 | 1587 | 2724 | 408 | 510 | 634 | 207 | 241 | 257 | 122 | 135 | 129 | 78 | 84 | 71 |
| 0.75 | *** | 958 | 1166 | 2386 | 332 | 391 | 555 | 168 | 189 | 228 | 97 | 106 | 118 | . | . | . |
| | *** | 1039 | 1408 | 2381 | 357 | 445 | 540 | 177 | 205 | 212 | 101 | 111 | 101 | . | . | . |
| 0.8 | *** | 802 | 991 | 1981 | 277 | 325 | 445 | 135 | 150 | 175 | . | . | . | . | . | . |
| | *** | 877 | 1203 | 1970 | 298 | 367 | 429 | 141 | 160 | 158 | . | . | . | . | . | . |
| 0.85 | *** | 641 | 798 | 1506 | 212 | 246 | 317 | . | . | . | . | . | . | . | . | . |
| | *** | 704 | 966 | 1491 | 227 | 272 | 300 | . | . | . | . | . | . | . | . | . |
| 0.9 | *** | 461 | 569 | 959 | . | . | . | . | . | . | . | . | . | . | . | . |
| | *** | 505 | 678 | 943 | . | . | . | . | . | . | . | . | . | . | . | . |

TABLE 8: ALPHA= 0.05  POWER= 0.9    EXPECTED ACCRUAL THRU MINIMUM FOLLOW-UP= 200

| | | DEL=.05 | | | DEL=.10 | | | DEL=.15 | | | DEL=.20 | | | DEL=.25 | |
|---|---|---|---|---|---|---|---|---|---|---|---|---|---|---|---|---|
| FACT= | | 1.0 .75 | .50 .25 | .00 BIN | 1.0 .75 | .50 .25 | .00 BIN | 1.0 .75 | .50 .25 | .00 BIN | 1.0 75 | .50 .25 | .00 BIN | 1.0 .75 | .50 .25 | .00 BIN |
| PCONT=*** | | | | REQUIRED | NUMBER | OF PATIENTS | | | | | | | | | | |
| 0.05 | *** | 515 | 520 | 547 | 185 | 188 | 195 | 109 | 111 | 114 | 77 | 78 | 80 | 60 | 61 | 62 |
| | *** | 516 | 527 | 943 | 186 | 191 | 300 | 110 | 112 | 158 | 78 | 79 | 101 | 61 | 61 | 71 |
| 0.1 | *** | 939 | 951 | 1055 | 295 | 303 | 326 | 160 | 165 | 173 | 107 | 109 | 113 | 79 | 81 | 83 |
| | *** | 943 | 970 | 1491 | 298 | 311 | 429 | 162 | 168 | 212 | 108 | 111 | 129 | 80 | 82 | 88 |
| 0.15 | *** | 1301 | 1321 | 1547 | 385 | 400 | 447 | 201 | 209 | 225 | 130 | 134 | 142 | 94 | 97 | 101 |
| | *** | 1308 | 1356 | 1970 | 391 | 415 | 540 | 204 | 215 | 257 | 132 | 138 | 153 | 95 | 99 | 101 |
| 0.2 | *** | 1582 | 1612 | 1996 | 454 | 476 | 554 | 232 | 244 | 270 | 147 | 154 | 166 | 105 | 109 | 115 |
| | *** | 1592 | 1666 | 2381 | 463 | 501 | 634 | 237 | 254 | 295 | 150 | 159 | 172 | 107 | 112 | 112 |
| 0.25 | *** | 1780 | 1821 | 2388 | 503 | 534 | 645 | 255 | 271 | 308 | 160 | 169 | 185 | 113 | 118 | 126 |
| | *** | 1794 | 1898 | 2724 | 515 | 568 | 711 | 262 | 285 | 326 | 164 | 176 | 187 | 115 | 122 | 120 |
| 0.3 | *** | 1897 | 1954 | 2715 | 534 | 574 | 719 | 270 | 290 | 337 | 169 | 180 | 199 | 118 | 124 | 134 |
| | *** | 1916 | 2056 | 2998 | 550 | 617 | 771 | 278 | 308 | 349 | 173 | 188 | 197 | 121 | 128 | 126 |
| 0.35 | *** | 1941 | 2016 | 2973 | 550 | 598 | 775 | 278 | 302 | 358 | 173 | 186 | 209 | 120 | 127 | 139 |
| | *** | 1966 | 2147 | 3203 | 569 | 650 | 814 | 288 | 323 | 364 | 179 | 196 | 204 | 123 | 132 | 129 |
| 0.4 | *** | 1923 | 2018 | 3159 | 551 | 608 | 812 | 280 | 307 | 371 | 174 | 188 | 214 | 120 | 128 | 141 |
| | *** | 1955 | 2180 | 3340 | 574 | 668 | 840 | 292 | 331 | 372 | 180 | 199 | 206 | 124 | 134 | 129 |
| 0.45 | *** | 1852 | 1972 | 3272 | 542 | 606 | 831 | 277 | 307 | 375 | 172 | 187 | 215 | 118 | 126 | 139 |
| | *** | 1893 | 2164 | 3409 | 567 | 672 | 848 | 289 | 332 | 372 | 179 | 198 | 204 | 122 | 132 | 126 |
| 0.5 | *** | 1741 | 1888 | 3310 | 523 | 593 | 832 | 269 | 300 | 372 | 167 | 182 | 210 | 114 | 122 | 135 |
| | *** | 1793 | 2108 | 3409 | 551 | 663 | 840 | 282 | 327 | 364 | 174 | 194 | 197 | 118 | 128 | 120 |
| 0.55 | *** | 1603 | 1776 | 3273 | 497 | 570 | 813 | 257 | 289 | 359 | 159 | 174 | 201 | 108 | 116 | 128 |
| | *** | 1665 | 2020 | 3340 | 527 | 643 | 814 | 271 | 315 | 349 | 165 | 185 | 187 | 111 | 121 | 112 |
| 0.6 | *** | 1449 | 1645 | 3162 | 465 | 539 | 776 | 241 | 272 | 339 | 148 | 162 | 187 | 99 | 107 | 117 |
| | *** | 1521 | 1905 | 3203 | 496 | 611 | 771 | 254 | 297 | 326 | 154 | 173 | 172 | 103 | 111 | 101 |
| 0.65 | *** | 1289 | 1501 | 2977 | 428 | 500 | 721 | 221 | 250 | 310 | 134 | 147 | 169 | 89 | 95 | 104 |
| | *** | 1369 | 1767 | 2998 | 457 | 568 | 711 | 234 | 273 | 295 | 140 | 156 | 153 | 92 | 99 | 88 |
| 0.7 | *** | 1129 | 1346 | 2718 | 385 | 452 | 647 | 198 | 223 | 273 | 118 | 129 | 146 | 76 | 81 | 88 |
| | *** | 1213 | 1608 | 2724 | 413 | 515 | 634 | 209 | 243 | 257 | 123 | 136 | 129 | 79 | 84 | 71 |
| 0.75 | *** | 972 | 1183 | 2386 | 337 | 396 | 555 | 169 | 190 | 228 | 98 | 106 | 118 | . | . | . |
| | *** | 1054 | 1426 | 2381 | 361 | 449 | 540 | 178 | 206 | 212 | 102 | 111 | 101 | . | . | . |
| 0.8 | *** | 815 | 1006 | 1981 | 281 | 329 | 445 | 136 | 151 | 175 | . | . | . | . | . | . |
| | *** | 891 | 1220 | 1970 | 301 | 370 | 429 | 142 | 161 | 158 | . | . | . | . | . | . |
| 0.85 | *** | 652 | 810 | 1506 | 215 | 248 | 317 | . | . | . | . | . | . | . | . | . |
| | *** | 715 | 979 | 1491 | 229 | 274 | 300 | . | . | . | . | . | . | . | . | . |
| 0.9 | *** | 469 | 577 | 959 | . | . | . | . | . | . | . | . | . | . | . | . |
| | *** | 513 | 686 | 943 | . | . | . | . | . | . | . | . | . | . | . | . |

## TABLE 8: ALPHA= 0.05 POWER= 0.9    EXPECTED ACCRUAL THRU MINIMUM FOLLOW-UP= 225

|  |  | DEL=.05 | | | DEL=.10 | | | DEL=.15 | | | DEL=.20 | | | DEL=.25 | | |
|---|---|---|---|---|---|---|---|---|---|---|---|---|---|---|---|---|
| FACT= | | 1.0 .75 | .50 .25 | .00 BIN | 1.0 .75 | .50 .25 | .00 BIN | 1.0 .75 | .50 .25 | .00 BIN | 1.0 75 | .50 .25 | .00 BIN | 1.0 .75 | .50 .25 | .00 BIN |
| PCONT=*** | | | | | REQUIRED NUMBER OF PATIENTS | | | | | | | | | | | |
| 0.05 | *** | 515 | 521 | 547 | 185 | 189 | 195 | 109 | 111 | 113 | 78 | 79 | 80 | 60 | 61 | 62 |
|  | *** | 517 | 528 | 943 | 187 | 191 | 300 | 110 | 112 | 158 | 78 | 79 | 101 | 61 | 61 | 71 |
| 0.1 | *** | 941 | 954 | 1055 | 296 | 305 | 326 | 161 | 165 | 173 | 107 | 110 | 113 | 80 | 81 | 83 |
|  | *** | 945 | 974 | 1491 | 300 | 313 | 429 | 163 | 168 | 212 | 108 | 111 | 129 | 80 | 82 | 88 |
| 0.15 | *** | 1303 | 1325 | 1547 | 387 | 402 | 447 | 202 | 210 | 225 | 131 | 135 | 142 | 94 | 97 | 101 |
|  | *** | 1311 | 1363 | 1970 | 393 | 417 | 540 | 206 | 216 | 257 | 133 | 138 | 153 | 96 | 99 | 101 |
| 0.2 | *** | 1586 | 1619 | 1996 | 457 | 480 | 554 | 234 | 246 | 270 | 149 | 155 | 166 | 106 | 109 | 115 |
|  | *** | 1597 | 1678 | 2381 | 466 | 505 | 634 | 239 | 256 | 295 | 152 | 160 | 172 | 107 | 112 | 112 |
| 0.25 | *** | 1785 | 1832 | 2388 | 508 | 540 | 645 | 257 | 274 | 308 | 162 | 170 | 185 | 114 | 119 | 126 |
|  | *** | 1801 | 1915 | 2724 | 520 | 573 | 711 | 264 | 287 | 326 | 166 | 177 | 187 | 116 | 122 | 120 |
| 0.3 | *** | 1904 | 1967 | 2715 | 540 | 581 | 719 | 273 | 293 | 337 | 171 | 181 | 200 | 119 | 125 | 134 |
|  | *** | 1925 | 2078 | 2998 | 557 | 624 | 771 | 282 | 310 | 349 | 175 | 189 | 197 | 122 | 129 | 126 |
| 0.35 | *** | 1951 | 2034 | 2973 | 557 | 607 | 775 | 282 | 306 | 358 | 176 | 188 | 209 | 122 | 129 | 139 |
|  | *** | 1979 | 2174 | 3203 | 577 | 658 | 814 | 292 | 326 | 364 | 181 | 197 | 204 | 125 | 133 | 129 |
| 0.4 | *** | 1935 | 2041 | 3159 | 560 | 618 | 812 | 285 | 312 | 371 | 177 | 190 | 214 | 122 | 129 | 141 |
|  | *** | 1971 | 2213 | 3340 | 583 | 678 | 840 | 296 | 334 | 372 | 183 | 200 | 206 | 125 | 134 | 129 |
| 0.45 | *** | 1868 | 2000 | 3272 | 552 | 617 | 831 | 282 | 311 | 375 | 175 | 189 | 214 | 120 | 128 | 139 |
|  | *** | 1914 | 2203 | 3409 | 578 | 682 | 848 | 295 | 336 | 372 | 181 | 200 | 204 | 123 | 133 | 126 |
| 0.5 | *** | 1761 | 1920 | 3310 | 535 | 605 | 832 | 275 | 305 | 372 | 169 | 185 | 210 | 115 | 123 | 135 |
|  | *** | 1818 | 2152 | 3409 | 563 | 674 | 840 | 288 | 330 | 364 | 176 | 195 | 197 | 119 | 129 | 120 |
| 0.55 | *** | 1627 | 1813 | 3273 | 509 | 583 | 813 | 263 | 294 | 359 | 161 | 176 | 201 | 109 | 117 | 128 |
|  | *** | 1695 | 2067 | 3340 | 539 | 654 | 814 | 276 | 319 | 349 | 168 | 187 | 187 | 113 | 122 | 112 |
| 0.6 | *** | 1477 | 1685 | 3162 | 478 | 552 | 776 | 246 | 277 | 339 | 150 | 164 | 187 | 101 | 108 | 117 |
|  | *** | 1555 | 1954 | 3203 | 508 | 622 | 771 | 260 | 301 | 326 | 157 | 174 | 172 | 104 | 112 | 101 |
| 0.65 | *** | 1320 | 1543 | 2976 | 440 | 512 | 721 | 226 | 254 | 310 | 137 | 149 | 169 | 90 | 96 | 104 |
|  | *** | 1405 | 1816 | 2998 | 470 | 579 | 711 | 239 | 276 | 295 | 142 | 158 | 153 | 93 | 100 | 88 |
| 0.7 | *** | 1162 | 1388 | 2718 | 396 | 463 | 647 | 202 | 227 | 273 | 120 | 130 | 146 | 77 | 82 | 88 |
|  | *** | 1250 | 1655 | 2724 | 424 | 524 | 634 | 213 | 245 | 257 | 125 | 137 | 129 | 79 | 85 | 71 |
| 0.75 | *** | 1005 | 1222 | 2386 | 347 | 405 | 555 | 173 | 193 | 228 | 100 | 107 | 118 | . | . | . |
|  | *** | 1090 | 1470 | 2381 | 371 | 457 | 540 | 182 | 208 | 212 | 103 | 112 | 101 | . | . | . |
| 0.8 | *** | 845 | 1041 | 1981 | 289 | 336 | 445 | 138 | 153 | 175 | . | . | . | . | . | . |
|  | *** | 923 | 1257 | 1970 | 309 | 376 | 429 | 145 | 162 | 158 | . | . | . | . | . | . |
| 0.85 | *** | 678 | 838 | 1506 | 221 | 253 | 317 | . | . | . | . | . | . | . | . | . |
|  | *** | 742 | 1007 | 1491 | 235 | 278 | 300 | . | . | . | . | . | . | . | . | . |
| 0.9 | *** | 487 | 596 | 959 | . | . | . | . | . | . | . | . | . | . | . | . |
|  | *** | 532 | 703 | 943 | . | . | . | . | . | . | . | . | . | . | . | . |

TABLE 8: ALPHA= 0.05  POWER= 0.9    EXPECTED ACCRUAL THRU MINIMUM FOLLOW-UP= 250

| PCONT=*** | DEL=.05 | | | DEL=.10 | | | DEL=.15 | | | DEL=.20 | | | DEL=.25 | | |
|---|---|---|---|---|---|---|---|---|---|---|---|---|---|---|---|
| FACT= | 1.0 .75 | .50 .25 | .00 BIN | 1.0 .75 | .50 .25 | .00 BIN | 1.0 .75 | .50 .25 | .00 BIN | 1.0 75 | .50 .25 | .00 BIN | 1.0 .75 | .50 .25 | .00 BIN |
| | | | | REQUIRED NUMBER OF PATIENTS | | | | | | | | | | | |
| 0.05 *** | 516 | 522 | 547 | 186 | 189 | 195 | 110 | 111 | 114 | 78 | 79 | 80 | 61 | 61 | 62 |
| *** | 518 | 529 | 943 | 187 | 191 | 300 | 110 | 112 | 158 | 78 | 79 | 101 | 61 | 62 | 71 |
| 0.1 *** | 942 | 956 | 1055 | 298 | 306 | 326 | 162 | 166 | 173 | 108 | 110 | 114 | 80 | 81 | 83 |
| *** | 947 | 978 | 1491 | 301 | 314 | 429 | 163 | 169 | 212 | 109 | 112 | 129 | 81 | 82 | 88 |
| 0.15 *** | 1306 | 1330 | 1547 | 389 | 405 | 447 | 203 | 211 | 225 | 131 | 136 | 142 | 95 | 97 | 101 |
| *** | 1314 | 1371 | 1970 | 396 | 420 | 540 | 207 | 217 | 257 | 133 | 138 | 153 | 96 | 99 | 101 |
| 0.2 *** | 1590 | 1626 | 1996 | 461 | 484 | 554 | 236 | 248 | 270 | 150 | 156 | 166 | 106 | 110 | 115 |
| *** | 1602 | 1689 | 2381 | 470 | 508 | 634 | 241 | 257 | 295 | 153 | 160 | 172 | 108 | 112 | 112 |
| 0.25 *** | 1790 | 1842 | 2388 | 512 | 545 | 645 | 260 | 276 | 308 | 163 | 172 | 185 | 115 | 119 | 126 |
| *** | 1808 | 1930 | 2724 | 525 | 578 | 711 | 267 | 289 | 326 | 167 | 177 | 187 | 117 | 122 | 120 |
| 0.3 *** | 1911 | 1981 | 2715 | 546 | 588 | 719 | 276 | 296 | 337 | 172 | 183 | 199 | 120 | 126 | 134 |
| *** | 1935 | 2099 | 2998 | 563 | 630 | 771 | 285 | 312 | 349 | 177 | 190 | 197 | 123 | 129 | 126 |
| 0.35 *** | 1960 | 2052 | 2973 | 564 | 615 | 775 | 286 | 309 | 358 | 177 | 189 | 209 | 123 | 129 | 139 |
| *** | 1991 | 2201 | 3203 | 584 | 666 | 814 | 296 | 328 | 364 | 183 | 198 | 204 | 126 | 134 | 129 |
| 0.4 *** | 1947 | 2063 | 3159 | 569 | 628 | 812 | 289 | 316 | 371 | 179 | 192 | 214 | 123 | 130 | 141 |
| *** | 1987 | 2244 | 3340 | 592 | 686 | 840 | 300 | 337 | 372 | 185 | 202 | 206 | 126 | 135 | 129 |
| 0.45 *** | 1883 | 2026 | 3272 | 562 | 627 | 831 | 287 | 316 | 375 | 177 | 191 | 214 | 121 | 129 | 139 |
| *** | 1934 | 2239 | 3409 | 588 | 692 | 848 | 299 | 339 | 372 | 183 | 201 | 204 | 124 | 133 | 126 |
| 0.5 *** | 1780 | 1951 | 3310 | 545 | 616 | 832 | 279 | 309 | 372 | 172 | 186 | 210 | 117 | 124 | 135 |
| *** | 1842 | 2192 | 3409 | 574 | 684 | 840 | 292 | 334 | 364 | 178 | 196 | 197 | 120 | 129 | 120 |
| 0.55 *** | 1650 | 1848 | 3273 | 520 | 594 | 813 | 267 | 298 | 359 | 164 | 178 | 201 | 110 | 118 | 128 |
| *** | 1723 | 2110 | 3340 | 551 | 664 | 814 | 281 | 322 | 349 | 170 | 188 | 187 | 114 | 122 | 112 |
| 0.6 *** | 1504 | 1723 | 3162 | 489 | 563 | 776 | 251 | 281 | 339 | 153 | 166 | 187 | 102 | 108 | 117 |
| *** | 1586 | 1998 | 3203 | 519 | 632 | 771 | 264 | 304 | 326 | 159 | 175 | 172 | 105 | 112 | 101 |
| 0.65 *** | 1350 | 1582 | 2977 | 451 | 523 | 721 | 231 | 258 | 310 | 139 | 151 | 169 | 91 | 97 | 104 |
| *** | 1439 | 1860 | 2998 | 481 | 588 | 711 | 243 | 279 | 295 | 144 | 158 | 153 | 94 | 100 | 88 |
| 0.7 *** | 1193 | 1427 | 2718 | 407 | 473 | 647 | 206 | 230 | 273 | 122 | 131 | 146 | 78 | 82 | 88 |
| *** | 1284 | 1697 | 2724 | 435 | 532 | 634 | 217 | 248 | 257 | 126 | 138 | 129 | 80 | 85 | 71 |
| 0.75 *** | 1035 | 1258 | 2386 | 356 | 414 | 555 | 177 | 196 | 228 | 101 | 108 | 118 | . | . | . |
| *** | 1123 | 1508 | 2381 | 380 | 464 | 540 | 185 | 209 | 212 | 104 | 113 | 101 | . | . | . |
| 0.8 *** | 873 | 1073 | 1981 | 297 | 343 | 445 | 141 | 154 | 175 | . | . | . | . | . | . |
| *** | 953 | 1290 | 1970 | 316 | 381 | 429 | 147 | 164 | 158 | . | . | . | . | . | . |
| 0.85 *** | 701 | 864 | 1506 | 226 | 257 | 317 | . | . | . | . | . | . | . | . | . |
| *** | 767 | 1033 | 1491 | 240 | 281 | 300 | . | . | . | . | . | . | . | . | . |
| 0.9 *** | 503 | 613 | 959 | . | . | . | . | . | . | . | . | . | . | . | . |
| *** | 548 | 718 | 943 | . | . | . | . | . | . | . | . | . | . | . | . |

TABLE 8: ALPHA= 0.05  POWER= 0.9     EXPECTED ACCRUAL THRU MINIMUM FOLLOW-UP= 275

|  |  | DEL=.05 | | | DEL=.10 | | | DEL=.15 | | | DEL=.20 | | | DEL=.25 | | |
|---|---|---|---|---|---|---|---|---|---|---|---|---|---|---|---|---|
| FACT= | | 1.0<br>.75 | .50<br>.25 | .00<br>BIN | 1.0<br>.75 | .50<br>.25 | .00<br>BIN | 1.0<br>.75 | .50<br>.25 | .00<br>BIN | 1.0<br>75 | .50<br>.25 | .00<br>BIN | 1.0<br>.75 | .50<br>.25 | .00<br>BIN |
| PCONT=*** | | | | REQUIRED | NUMBER | OF | PATIENTS | | | | | | | | | |
| 0.05 | *** | 517 | 523 | 547 | 186 | 189 | 195 | 110 | 111 | 113 | 78 | 79 | 80 | 61 | 61 | 62 |
|  | *** | 519 | 530 | 943 | 188 | 191 | 300 | 111 | 112 | 158 | 78 | 79 | 101 | 61 | 62 | 71 |
| 0.1 | *** | 944 | 959 | 1055 | 299 | 307 | 326 | 162 | 166 | 173 | 108 | 110 | 113 | 80 | 81 | 83 |
|  | *** | 949 | 981 | 1491 | 302 | 314 | 429 | 164 | 169 | 212 | 109 | 112 | 129 | 81 | 82 | 88 |
| 0.15 | *** | 1308 | 1334 | 1547 | 391 | 407 | 447 | 204 | 212 | 225 | 132 | 136 | 142 | 95 | 98 | 101 |
|  | *** | 1317 | 1377 | 1970 | 398 | 421 | 540 | 208 | 218 | 257 | 134 | 139 | 153 | 96 | 99 | 101 |
| 0.2 | *** | 1593 | 1633 | 1996 | 464 | 488 | 553 | 238 | 249 | 270 | 151 | 157 | 166 | 107 | 110 | 115 |
|  | *** | 1607 | 1699 | 2381 | 473 | 511 | 634 | 243 | 258 | 295 | 153 | 161 | 172 | 109 | 112 | 112 |
| 0.25 | *** | 1795 | 1852 | 2388 | 517 | 550 | 645 | 262 | 278 | 308 | 165 | 172 | 185 | 115 | 120 | 126 |
|  | *** | 1815 | 1945 | 2724 | 530 | 582 | 711 | 269 | 290 | 326 | 168 | 178 | 187 | 117 | 123 | 120 |
| 0.3 | *** | 1918 | 1994 | 2715 | 551 | 594 | 719 | 279 | 299 | 337 | 174 | 184 | 199 | 121 | 126 | 134 |
|  | *** | 1944 | 2118 | 2998 | 569 | 635 | 771 | 288 | 314 | 349 | 178 | 191 | 197 | 123 | 130 | 126 |
| 0.35 | *** | 1970 | 2069 | 2973 | 571 | 622 | 775 | 289 | 312 | 358 | 179 | 191 | 209 | 124 | 130 | 139 |
|  | *** | 2004 | 2225 | 3203 | 591 | 672 | 814 | 299 | 330 | 364 | 184 | 199 | 204 | 127 | 134 | 129 |
| 0.4 | *** | 1959 | 2084 | 3159 | 576 | 636 | 812 | 293 | 319 | 371 | 181 | 194 | 214 | 124 | 131 | 141 |
|  | *** | 2003 | 2273 | 3340 | 601 | 693 | 840 | 304 | 339 | 372 | 187 | 202 | 206 | 127 | 135 | 129 |
| 0.45 | *** | 1898 | 2052 | 3272 | 570 | 637 | 831 | 291 | 319 | 375 | 179 | 193 | 215 | 122 | 129 | 139 |
|  | *** | 1953 | 2272 | 3409 | 597 | 700 | 848 | 303 | 341 | 372 | 185 | 202 | 204 | 125 | 134 | 126 |
| 0.5 | *** | 1799 | 1981 | 3310 | 554 | 626 | 832 | 284 | 313 | 371 | 174 | 188 | 210 | 118 | 125 | 135 |
|  | *** | 1865 | 2229 | 3409 | 584 | 693 | 840 | 297 | 336 | 364 | 180 | 198 | 197 | 121 | 130 | 120 |
| 0.55 | *** | 1673 | 1881 | 3273 | 530 | 604 | 813 | 272 | 302 | 359 | 166 | 179 | 201 | 112 | 118 | 128 |
|  | *** | 1750 | 2149 | 3340 | 561 | 673 | 814 | 285 | 325 | 349 | 172 | 189 | 187 | 115 | 123 | 112 |
| 0.6 | *** | 1530 | 1758 | 3162 | 499 | 573 | 776 | 256 | 284 | 339 | 155 | 167 | 187 | 103 | 109 | 117 |
|  | *** | 1616 | 2038 | 3203 | 530 | 641 | 771 | 268 | 306 | 326 | 161 | 176 | 172 | 106 | 113 | 101 |
| 0.65 | *** | 1378 | 1618 | 2977 | 461 | 532 | 721 | 235 | 261 | 310 | 141 | 152 | 169 | 92 | 97 | 104 |
|  | *** | 1471 | 1900 | 2998 | 491 | 596 | 711 | 247 | 281 | 295 | 146 | 159 | 153 | 95 | 100 | 88 |
| 0.7 | *** | 1222 | 1462 | 2718 | 416 | 482 | 647 | 210 | 233 | 273 | 123 | 132 | 146 | 79 | 83 | 88 |
|  | *** | 1316 | 1736 | 2724 | 444 | 540 | 634 | 220 | 249 | 257 | 127 | 138 | 129 | 81 | 85 | 71 |
| 0.75 | *** | 1063 | 1292 | 2386 | 364 | 421 | 555 | 179 | 198 | 228 | 102 | 109 | 118 | . | . | . |
|  | *** | 1154 | 1543 | 2381 | 388 | 470 | 540 | 188 | 211 | 212 | 105 | 113 | 101 | . | . | . |
| 0.8 | *** | 899 | 1103 | 1981 | 303 | 349 | 445 | 143 | 156 | 175 | . | . | . | . | . | . |
|  | *** | 981 | 1320 | 1970 | 323 | 385 | 429 | 149 | 164 | 158 | . | . | . | . | . | . |
| 0.85 | *** | 722 | 887 | 1506 | 231 | 261 | 317 | . | . | . | . | . | . | . | . | . |
|  | *** | 789 | 1055 | 1491 | 244 | 283 | 300 | . | . | . | . | . | . | . | . | . |
| 0.9 | *** | 518 | 628 | 959 | . | . | . | . | . | . | . | . | . | . | . | . |
|  | *** | 564 | 731 | 943 | . | . | . | . | . | . | . | . | . | . | . | . |

TABLE 8: ALPHA= 0.05  POWER= 0.9     EXPECTED ACCRUAL THRU MINIMUM FOLLOW-UP= 300

| | | DEL=.05 | | | DEL=.10 | | | DEL=.15 | | | DEL=.20 | | | DEL=.25 | | |
|---|---|---|---|---|---|---|---|---|---|---|---|---|---|---|---|---|---|
| FACT= | | 1.0 .75 | .50 .25 | .00 BIN | 1.0 .75 | .50 .25 | .00 BIN | 1.0 .75 | .50 .25 | .00 BIN | 1.0 75 | .50 .25 | .00 BIN | 1.0 .75 | .50 .25 | .00 BIN |
| PCONT=*** | | | | | REQUIRED NUMBER OF PATIENTS | | | | | | | | | | | |
| 0.05 | *** | 517 | 524 | 547 | 187 | 190 | 195 | 110 | 112 | 113 | 78 | 79 | 80 | 61 | 61 | 62 |
| | *** | 520 | 531 | 943 | 188 | 192 | 300 | 111 | 112 | 158 | 78 | 79 | 101 | 61 | 61 | 71 |
| 0.1 | *** | 945 | 961 | 1055 | 300 | 308 | 326 | 163 | 167 | 173 | 108 | 111 | 113 | 80 | 82 | 83 |
| | *** | 951 | 985 | 1491 | 303 | 315 | 429 | 165 | 169 | 212 | 109 | 112 | 129 | 81 | 82 | 88 |
| 0.15 | *** | 1311 | 1339 | 1547 | 393 | 409 | 447 | 205 | 213 | 225 | 133 | 136 | 142 | 96 | 98 | 101 |
| | *** | 1321 | 1383 | 1970 | 400 | 423 | 540 | 209 | 218 | 257 | 134 | 139 | 153 | 97 | 99 | 101 |
| 0.2 | *** | 1597 | 1640 | 1996 | 466 | 491 | 553 | 239 | 250 | 270 | 151 | 157 | 166 | 107 | 111 | 115 |
| | *** | 1612 | 1709 | 2381 | 476 | 513 | 634 | 244 | 259 | 295 | 154 | 161 | 172 | 109 | 113 | 112 |
| 0.25 | *** | 1801 | 1861 | 2388 | 520 | 554 | 645 | 264 | 280 | 308 | 166 | 173 | 185 | 116 | 120 | 126 |
| | *** | 1821 | 1959 | 2724 | 534 | 585 | 711 | 271 | 291 | 326 | 169 | 178 | 187 | 118 | 123 | 120 |
| 0.3 | *** | 1925 | 2007 | 2715 | 556 | 599 | 719 | 282 | 301 | 337 | 175 | 185 | 199 | 122 | 127 | 134 |
| | *** | 1954 | 2137 | 2998 | 574 | 640 | 771 | 290 | 316 | 349 | 180 | 191 | 197 | 124 | 130 | 126 |
| 0.35 | *** | 1979 | 2085 | 2973 | 577 | 629 | 775 | 292 | 315 | 358 | 181 | 192 | 209 | 125 | 131 | 139 |
| | *** | 2016 | 2248 | 3203 | 598 | 678 | 814 | 302 | 332 | 364 | 186 | 199 | 204 | 127 | 134 | 129 |
| 0.4 | *** | 1971 | 2105 | 3159 | 583 | 643 | 812 | 296 | 322 | 371 | 183 | 195 | 214 | 125 | 132 | 141 |
| | *** | 2018 | 2301 | 3340 | 608 | 700 | 840 | 307 | 341 | 372 | 188 | 203 | 206 | 128 | 136 | 129 |
| 0.45 | *** | 1914 | 2076 | 3272 | 578 | 645 | 831 | 295 | 322 | 375 | 181 | 194 | 214 | 123 | 130 | 139 |
| | *** | 1972 | 2303 | 3409 | 606 | 707 | 848 | 307 | 343 | 372 | 187 | 203 | 204 | 126 | 134 | 126 |
| 0.5 | *** | 1817 | 2009 | 3310 | 563 | 635 | 832 | 288 | 316 | 371 | 176 | 189 | 210 | 119 | 126 | 135 |
| | *** | 1888 | 2263 | 3409 | 593 | 700 | 840 | 300 | 339 | 364 | 182 | 198 | 197 | 122 | 130 | 120 |
| 0.55 | *** | 1695 | 1912 | 3273 | 539 | 613 | 813 | 276 | 305 | 359 | 168 | 181 | 201 | 112 | 119 | 128 |
| | *** | 1776 | 2185 | 3340 | 570 | 681 | 814 | 289 | 327 | 349 | 174 | 190 | 187 | 115 | 123 | 112 |
| 0.6 | *** | 1555 | 1791 | 3162 | 508 | 582 | 776 | 259 | 287 | 339 | 157 | 169 | 187 | 104 | 110 | 117 |
| | *** | 1645 | 2076 | 3203 | 539 | 648 | 771 | 272 | 308 | 326 | 162 | 177 | 172 | 107 | 113 | 101 |
| 0.65 | *** | 1405 | 1651 | 2977 | 470 | 541 | 721 | 239 | 264 | 310 | 142 | 153 | 169 | 93 | 98 | 104 |
| | *** | 1501 | 1937 | 2998 | 500 | 603 | 711 | 250 | 283 | 295 | 147 | 160 | 153 | 95 | 101 | 88 |
| 0.7 | *** | 1250 | 1495 | 2717 | 424 | 490 | 647 | 213 | 235 | 273 | 124 | 133 | 145 | 79 | 83 | 88 |
| | *** | 1346 | 1771 | 2724 | 452 | 546 | 634 | 223 | 251 | 257 | 129 | 139 | 129 | 81 | 85 | 71 |
| 0.75 | *** | 1090 | 1322 | 2386 | 371 | 428 | 555 | 182 | 200 | 228 | 103 | 109 | 118 | . | . | . |
| | *** | 1183 | 1575 | 2381 | 396 | 475 | 540 | 190 | 212 | 212 | 106 | 113 | 101 | . | . | . |
| 0.8 | *** | 923 | 1129 | 1981 | 309 | 354 | 445 | 145 | 157 | 175 | . | . | . | . | . | . |
| | *** | 1006 | 1346 | 1970 | 328 | 389 | 429 | 151 | 165 | 158 | . | . | . | . | . | . |
| 0.85 | *** | 742 | 908 | 1506 | 235 | 264 | 317 | . | . | . | . | . | . | . | . | . |
| | *** | 810 | 1075 | 1491 | 248 | 286 | 300 | . | . | . | . | . | . | . | . | . |
| 0.9 | *** | 532 | 642 | 959 | . | . | . | . | . | . | . | . | . | . | . | . |
| | *** | 577 | 743 | 943 | . | . | . | . | . | . | . | . | . | . | . | . |

TABLE 8: ALPHA= 0.05  POWER= 0.9    EXPECTED ACCRUAL THRU MINIMUM FOLLOW-UP= 325

| | | DEL=.05 | | | DEL=.10 | | | DEL=.15 | | | DEL=.20 | | | DEL=.25 | | |
|---|---|---|---|---|---|---|---|---|---|---|---|---|---|---|---|---|---|
| FACT= | | 1.0 .75 | .50 .25 | .00 BIN | 1.0 .75 | .50 .25 | .00 BIN | 1.0 .75 | .50 .25 | .00 BIN | 1.0 75 | .50 .25 | .00 BIN | 1.0 .75 | .50 .25 | .00 BIN |
| PCONT=*** | | | | | REQUIRED NUMBER OF PATIENTS | | | | | | | | | | | |
| 0.05 | *** | 518 | 525 | 547 | 187 | 190 | 195 | 110 | 112 | 114 | 78 | 79 | 80 | 61 | 61 | 62 |
| | *** | 520 | 532 | 943 | 188 | 192 | 300 | 111 | 112 | 158 | 79 | 79 | 101 | 61 | 62 | 71 |
| 0.1 | *** | 947 | 964 | 1055 | 301 | 309 | 326 | 163 | 167 | 173 | 109 | 111 | 114 | 81 | 82 | 83 |
| | *** | 953 | 988 | 1491 | 304 | 316 | 429 | 165 | 170 | 212 | 110 | 112 | 129 | 81 | 82 | 88 |
| 0.15 | *** | 1313 | 1343 | 1547 | 395 | 411 | 447 | 207 | 214 | 225 | 133 | 137 | 142 | 96 | 98 | 101 |
| | *** | 1324 | 1389 | 1970 | 402 | 424 | 540 | 210 | 219 | 257 | 135 | 139 | 153 | 97 | 99 | 101 |
| 0.2 | *** | 1601 | 1647 | 1996 | 469 | 494 | 554 | 241 | 252 | 270 | 152 | 158 | 166 | 108 | 111 | 115 |
| | *** | 1617 | 1719 | 2381 | 479 | 515 | 634 | 246 | 260 | 295 | 155 | 161 | 172 | 109 | 113 | 112 |
| 0.25 | *** | 1806 | 1871 | 2388 | 524 | 558 | 645 | 266 | 281 | 308 | 167 | 174 | 185 | 117 | 121 | 126 |
| | *** | 1828 | 1972 | 2724 | 538 | 589 | 711 | 273 | 292 | 326 | 170 | 179 | 187 | 118 | 123 | 120 |
| 0.3 | *** | 1932 | 2020 | 2715 | 561 | 604 | 719 | 284 | 303 | 337 | 177 | 186 | 199 | 122 | 127 | 134 |
| | *** | 1963 | 2154 | 2998 | 579 | 644 | 771 | 292 | 317 | 349 | 181 | 192 | 197 | 125 | 130 | 126 |
| 0.35 | *** | 1988 | 2101 | 2973 | 583 | 635 | 775 | 295 | 317 | 358 | 182 | 193 | 209 | 125 | 131 | 139 |
| | *** | 2028 | 2269 | 3203 | 604 | 683 | 814 | 305 | 334 | 364 | 187 | 200 | 204 | 128 | 135 | 129 |
| 0.4 | *** | 1983 | 2125 | 3159 | 590 | 650 | 812 | 299 | 324 | 371 | 184 | 196 | 214 | 126 | 132 | 141 |
| | *** | 2034 | 2326 | 3340 | 615 | 706 | 840 | 310 | 343 | 372 | 190 | 204 | 206 | 129 | 136 | 129 |
| 0.45 | *** | 1928 | 2099 | 3272 | 586 | 653 | 831 | 298 | 325 | 375 | 183 | 195 | 214 | 124 | 131 | 139 |
| | *** | 1991 | 2332 | 3409 | 614 | 713 | 848 | 310 | 346 | 372 | 188 | 204 | 204 | 127 | 135 | 126 |
| 0.5 | *** | 1836 | 2036 | 3310 | 571 | 643 | 832 | 291 | 320 | 372 | 178 | 191 | 210 | 120 | 127 | 135 |
| | *** | 1910 | 2294 | 3409 | 601 | 707 | 840 | 304 | 341 | 364 | 184 | 199 | 197 | 123 | 130 | 120 |
| 0.55 | *** | 1716 | 1941 | 3273 | 548 | 622 | 813 | 279 | 308 | 359 | 170 | 182 | 201 | 114 | 120 | 128 |
| | *** | 1801 | 2219 | 3340 | 579 | 688 | 814 | 292 | 329 | 349 | 175 | 190 | 187 | 116 | 123 | 112 |
| 0.6 | *** | 1578 | 1822 | 3162 | 517 | 590 | 776 | 263 | 290 | 339 | 158 | 170 | 187 | 105 | 110 | 117 |
| | *** | 1672 | 2110 | 3203 | 548 | 655 | 771 | 275 | 310 | 326 | 164 | 177 | 172 | 107 | 114 | 101 |
| 0.65 | *** | 1431 | 1683 | 2977 | 478 | 549 | 721 | 242 | 267 | 310 | 144 | 154 | 169 | 94 | 98 | 104 |
| | *** | 1529 | 1971 | 2998 | 508 | 610 | 711 | 253 | 285 | 295 | 148 | 160 | 153 | 96 | 101 | 88 |
| 0.7 | *** | 1276 | 1526 | 2718 | 432 | 497 | 647 | 216 | 237 | 273 | 126 | 134 | 146 | 80 | 84 | 88 |
| | *** | 1375 | 1803 | 2724 | 460 | 551 | 634 | 225 | 253 | 257 | 130 | 139 | 129 | 82 | 86 | 71 |
| 0.75 | *** | 1115 | 1351 | 2385 | 378 | 434 | 555 | 184 | 201 | 228 | 104 | 110 | 118 | . | . | . |
| | *** | 1209 | 1604 | 2381 | 402 | 479 | 540 | 192 | 213 | 212 | 107 | 114 | 101 | . | . | . |
| 0.8 | *** | 946 | 1155 | 1981 | 315 | 358 | 445 | 146 | 158 | 175 | . | . | . | . | . | . |
| | *** | 1030 | 1371 | 1970 | 334 | 392 | 429 | 152 | 166 | 158 | . | . | . | . | . | . |
| 0.85 | *** | 761 | 928 | 1506 | 238 | 267 | 317 | . | . | . | . | . | . | . | . | . |
| | *** | 829 | 1094 | 1491 | 251 | 288 | 300 | . | . | . | . | . | . | . | . | . |
| 0.9 | *** | 544 | 654 | 959 | . | . | . | . | . | . | . | . | . | . | . | . |
| | *** | 590 | 754 | 943 | . | . | . | . | . | . | . | . | . | . | . | . |

TABLE 8: ALPHA= 0.05 POWER= 0.9    EXPECTED ACCRUAL THRU MINIMUM FOLLOW-UP= 350

| PCONT | FACT | DEL=.05 1.0 .75 | DEL=.05 .50 .25 | DEL=.05 .00 BIN | DEL=.10 1.0 .75 | DEL=.10 .50 .25 | DEL=.10 .00 BIN | DEL=.15 1.0 .75 | DEL=.15 .50 .25 | DEL=.15 .00 BIN | DEL=.20 1.0 75 | DEL=.20 .50 .25 | DEL=.20 .00 BIN | DEL=.25 1.0 .75 | DEL=.25 .50 .25 | DEL=.25 .00 BIN |
|---|---|---|---|---|---|---|---|---|---|---|---|---|---|---|---|---|
| | | REQUIRED NUMBER OF PATIENTS | | | | | | | | | | | | | | |
| 0.05 | *** | 519 | 525 | 547 | 187 | 190 | 195 | 111 | 112 | 113 | 78 | 79 | 80 | 61 | 61 | 62 |
| | *** | 521 | 533 | 943 | 189 | 192 | 300 | 111 | 113 | 158 | 79 | 79 | 101 | 61 | 62 | 71 |
| 0.1 | *** | 948 | 966 | 1055 | 302 | 310 | 326 | 164 | 167 | 173 | 109 | 111 | 113 | 81 | 82 | 83 |
| | *** | 954 | 990 | 1491 | 305 | 316 | 429 | 166 | 170 | 212 | 110 | 112 | 129 | 81 | 83 | 88 |
| 0.15 | *** | 1316 | 1348 | 1547 | 397 | 412 | 447 | 207 | 214 | 225 | 134 | 137 | 142 | 96 | 98 | 101 |
| | *** | 1327 | 1394 | 1970 | 403 | 426 | 540 | 210 | 219 | 257 | 135 | 139 | 153 | 97 | 99 | 101 |
| 0.2 | *** | 1604 | 1653 | 1996 | 472 | 496 | 554 | 242 | 253 | 270 | 153 | 158 | 166 | 108 | 111 | 115 |
| | *** | 1621 | 1727 | 2381 | 482 | 517 | 634 | 247 | 260 | 295 | 155 | 162 | 172 | 110 | 113 | 112 |
| 0.25 | *** | 1811 | 1880 | 2388 | 528 | 561 | 645 | 268 | 283 | 308 | 167 | 175 | 185 | 117 | 121 | 126 |
| | *** | 1835 | 1985 | 2724 | 542 | 592 | 711 | 274 | 293 | 326 | 171 | 179 | 187 | 119 | 123 | 120 |
| 0.3 | *** | 1940 | 2032 | 2715 | 566 | 609 | 719 | 286 | 305 | 337 | 178 | 187 | 199 | 123 | 128 | 134 |
| | *** | 1972 | 2170 | 2998 | 584 | 648 | 771 | 294 | 318 | 349 | 182 | 192 | 197 | 125 | 131 | 126 |
| 0.35 | *** | 1998 | 2117 | 2973 | 588 | 640 | 775 | 298 | 319 | 358 | 184 | 194 | 209 | 126 | 132 | 139 |
| | *** | 2040 | 2289 | 3203 | 610 | 687 | 814 | 307 | 335 | 364 | 188 | 201 | 204 | 129 | 135 | 129 |
| 0.4 | *** | 1995 | 2144 | 3159 | 596 | 657 | 812 | 302 | 327 | 371 | 186 | 197 | 214 | 127 | 133 | 141 |
| | *** | 2049 | 2350 | 3340 | 621 | 711 | 840 | 313 | 345 | 372 | 191 | 205 | 206 | 130 | 136 | 129 |
| 0.45 | *** | 1943 | 2122 | 3272 | 593 | 659 | 831 | 301 | 328 | 375 | 184 | 196 | 215 | 125 | 131 | 139 |
| | *** | 2009 | 2359 | 3409 | 621 | 719 | 848 | 313 | 347 | 372 | 190 | 204 | 204 | 128 | 135 | 126 |
| 0.5 | *** | 1853 | 2061 | 3310 | 579 | 650 | 832 | 295 | 322 | 372 | 180 | 192 | 210 | 121 | 127 | 135 |
| | *** | 1931 | 2324 | 3409 | 609 | 713 | 840 | 307 | 342 | 364 | 185 | 200 | 197 | 124 | 131 | 120 |
| 0.55 | *** | 1737 | 1969 | 3273 | 556 | 629 | 813 | 283 | 310 | 359 | 171 | 183 | 201 | 114 | 120 | 128 |
| | *** | 1825 | 2250 | 3340 | 587 | 694 | 814 | 295 | 331 | 349 | 177 | 191 | 187 | 117 | 124 | 112 |
| 0.6 | *** | 1602 | 1851 | 3162 | 525 | 598 | 776 | 266 | 293 | 339 | 160 | 171 | 187 | 105 | 111 | 117 |
| | *** | 1698 | 2142 | 3203 | 556 | 661 | 771 | 278 | 312 | 326 | 165 | 178 | 172 | 108 | 114 | 101 |
| 0.65 | *** | 1455 | 1713 | 2976 | 486 | 556 | 721 | 245 | 269 | 310 | 145 | 155 | 169 | 94 | 99 | 104 |
| | *** | 1556 | 2003 | 2998 | 516 | 615 | 711 | 256 | 286 | 295 | 150 | 161 | 153 | 96 | 101 | 88 |
| 0.7 | *** | 1301 | 1555 | 2717 | 439 | 503 | 647 | 218 | 239 | 273 | 127 | 135 | 146 | 80 | 84 | 88 |
| | *** | 1401 | 1833 | 2724 | 467 | 556 | 634 | 228 | 254 | 257 | 131 | 140 | 129 | 82 | 86 | 71 |
| 0.75 | *** | 1139 | 1378 | 2386 | 384 | 439 | 555 | 186 | 203 | 228 | 105 | 111 | 118 | . | . | . |
| | *** | 1235 | 1632 | 2381 | 408 | 483 | 540 | 194 | 214 | 212 | 108 | 114 | 101 | . | . | . |
| 0.8 | *** | 967 | 1178 | 1981 | 320 | 362 | 445 | 148 | 159 | 175 | . | . | . | . | . | . |
| | *** | 1052 | 1394 | 1970 | 338 | 395 | 429 | 153 | 167 | 158 | . | . | . | . | . | . |
| 0.85 | *** | 778 | 946 | 1506 | 242 | 270 | 317 | . | . | . | . | . | . | . | . | . |
| | *** | 847 | 1111 | 1491 | 254 | 290 | 300 | . | . | . | . | . | . | . | . | . |
| 0.9 | *** | 556 | 665 | 959 | . | . | . | . | . | . | . | . | . | . | . | . |
| | *** | 602 | 763 | 943 | . | . | . | . | . | . | . | . | . | . | . | . |

## TABLE 8: ALPHA= 0.05  POWER= 0.9     EXPECTED ACCRUAL THRU MINIMUM FOLLOW-UP= 375

| | | DEL=.05 | | | DEL=.10 | | | DEL=.15 | | | DEL=.20 | | | DEL=.25 | | |
|---|---|---|---|---|---|---|---|---|---|---|---|---|---|---|---|---|
| FACT= | | 1.0 .75 | .50 .25 | .00 BIN | 1.0 .75 | .50 .25 | .00 BIN | 1.0 .75 | .50 .25 | .00 BIN | 1.0 75 | .50 .25 | .00 BIN | 1.0 .75 | .50 .25 | .00 BIN |
| PCONT=*** | | | | | REQUIRED NUMBER OF PATIENTS | | | | | | | | | | | |
| 0.05 | *** | 519 | 526 | 547 | 188 | 190 | 195 | 111 | 112 | 114 | 78 | 79 | 80 | 61 | 61 | 62 |
| | *** | 522 | 533 | 943 | 189 | 192 | 300 | 111 | 113 | 158 | 79 | 79 | 101 | 61 | 62 | 71 |
| 0.1 | *** | 949 | 968 | 1055 | 302 | 311 | 326 | 164 | 168 | 173 | 109 | 111 | 114 | 81 | 82 | 83 |
| | *** | 956 | 993 | 1491 | 306 | 317 | 429 | 166 | 170 | 212 | 110 | 112 | 129 | 81 | 83 | 88 |
| 0.15 | *** | 1318 | 1352 | 1547 | 398 | 414 | 447 | 208 | 215 | 225 | 134 | 137 | 142 | 96 | 98 | 101 |
| | *** | 1330 | 1400 | 1970 | 405 | 427 | 540 | 211 | 220 | 257 | 136 | 140 | 153 | 97 | 100 | 101 |
| 0.2 | *** | 1608 | 1660 | 1996 | 474 | 498 | 553 | 243 | 253 | 270 | 154 | 159 | 166 | 109 | 111 | 115 |
| | *** | 1626 | 1735 | 2381 | 484 | 519 | 634 | 248 | 261 | 295 | 156 | 162 | 172 | 110 | 113 | 112 |
| 0.25 | *** | 1816 | 1889 | 2388 | 531 | 565 | 645 | 270 | 284 | 308 | 168 | 175 | 185 | 118 | 121 | 126 |
| | *** | 1842 | 1997 | 2724 | 545 | 594 | 711 | 276 | 294 | 326 | 171 | 180 | 187 | 119 | 123 | 120 |
| 0.3 | *** | 1947 | 2044 | 2715 | 570 | 613 | 719 | 288 | 306 | 337 | 179 | 187 | 200 | 124 | 128 | 134 |
| | *** | 1981 | 2185 | 2998 | 588 | 651 | 771 | 296 | 319 | 349 | 183 | 193 | 197 | 126 | 131 | 126 |
| 0.35 | *** | 2007 | 2132 | 2973 | 593 | 645 | 775 | 300 | 321 | 358 | 185 | 195 | 209 | 127 | 132 | 139 |
| | *** | 2051 | 2308 | 3203 | 615 | 692 | 814 | 309 | 337 | 364 | 190 | 201 | 204 | 129 | 135 | 129 |
| 0.4 | *** | 2007 | 2162 | 3160 | 602 | 662 | 812 | 305 | 329 | 371 | 187 | 198 | 214 | 128 | 133 | 141 |
| | *** | 2063 | 2372 | 3340 | 628 | 716 | 840 | 316 | 346 | 372 | 192 | 205 | 206 | 130 | 137 | 129 |
| 0.45 | *** | 1958 | 2143 | 3272 | 600 | 666 | 831 | 304 | 330 | 375 | 186 | 197 | 215 | 126 | 132 | 139 |
| | *** | 2026 | 2384 | 3409 | 627 | 724 | 848 | 316 | 349 | 372 | 191 | 205 | 204 | 129 | 135 | 126 |
| 0.5 | *** | 1871 | 2085 | 3310 | 586 | 657 | 832 | 298 | 325 | 372 | 181 | 193 | 210 | 122 | 127 | 135 |
| | *** | 1951 | 2352 | 3409 | 616 | 719 | 840 | 310 | 344 | 364 | 186 | 200 | 197 | 124 | 131 | 120 |
| 0.55 | *** | 1757 | 1995 | 3273 | 563 | 636 | 813 | 286 | 313 | 359 | 173 | 184 | 201 | 115 | 121 | 128 |
| | *** | 1848 | 2280 | 3340 | 594 | 700 | 814 | 298 | 332 | 349 | 178 | 192 | 187 | 118 | 124 | 112 |
| 0.6 | *** | 1624 | 1879 | 3162 | 532 | 605 | 776 | 269 | 295 | 339 | 161 | 172 | 187 | 106 | 111 | 118 |
| | *** | 1723 | 2172 | 3203 | 563 | 667 | 771 | 281 | 313 | 326 | 166 | 179 | 172 | 108 | 114 | 101 |
| 0.65 | *** | 1478 | 1740 | 2976 | 493 | 562 | 721 | 248 | 271 | 310 | 146 | 155 | 169 | 95 | 99 | 104 |
| | *** | 1581 | 2032 | 2998 | 523 | 620 | 711 | 258 | 288 | 295 | 151 | 161 | 153 | 97 | 101 | 88 |
| 0.7 | *** | 1324 | 1582 | 2717 | 446 | 509 | 647 | 221 | 241 | 273 | 128 | 135 | 146 | 81 | 84 | 88 |
| | *** | 1427 | 1861 | 2724 | 473 | 561 | 634 | 230 | 255 | 257 | 131 | 140 | 129 | 82 | 86 | 71 |
| 0.75 | *** | 1161 | 1403 | 2386 | 390 | 444 | 555 | 188 | 204 | 228 | 105 | 111 | 118 | . | . | . |
| | *** | 1258 | 1656 | 2381 | 414 | 487 | 540 | 196 | 215 | 212 | 108 | 114 | 101 | . | . | . |
| 0.8 | *** | 987 | 1199 | 1981 | 324 | 366 | 445 | 149 | 160 | 175 | . | . | . | . | . | . |
| | *** | 1073 | 1414 | 1970 | 343 | 398 | 429 | 154 | 167 | 158 | . | . | . | . | . | . |
| 0.85 | *** | 795 | 963 | 1505 | 245 | 272 | 317 | . | . | . | . | . | . | . | . | . |
| | *** | 864 | 1126 | 1491 | 257 | 291 | 300 | . | . | . | . | . | . | . | . | . |
| 0.9 | *** | 567 | 676 | 959 | . | . | . | . | . | . | . | . | . | . | . | . |
| | *** | 613 | 772 | 943 | . | . | . | . | . | . | . | . | . | . | . | . |

TABLE 8: ALPHA= 0.05  POWER= 0.9    EXPECTED ACCRUAL THRU MINIMUM FOLLOW-UP= 400

| | | DEL=.05 | | | DEL=.10 | | | DEL=.15 | | | DEL=.20 | | | DEL=.25 | | |
|---|---|---|---|---|---|---|---|---|---|---|---|---|---|---|---|---|---|
| FACT= | | 1.0 .75 | .50 .25 | .00 BIN | 1.0 .75 | .50 .25 | .00 BIN | 1.0 .75 | .50 .25 | .00 BIN | 1.0 75 | .50 .25 | .00 BIN | 1.0 .75 | .50 .25 | .00 BIN |
| PCONT=*** | | | | | REQUIRED | NUMBER OF | PATIENTS | | | | | | | | | |
| 0.05 | *** | 520 | 527 | 547 | 188 | 191 | 195 | 111 | 112 | 114 | 78 | 79 | 80 | 61 | 61 | 62 |
| | *** | 523 | 534 | 943 | 189 | 192 | 300 | 111 | 113 | 158 | 79 | 79 | 101 | 61 | 62 | 71 |
| 0.1 | *** | 951 | 970 | 1055 | 303 | 311 | 326 | 165 | 168 | 173 | 109 | 111 | 113 | 81 | 82 | 83 |
| | *** | 958 | 995 | 1491 | 307 | 317 | 429 | 166 | 170 | 212 | 110 | 112 | 129 | 81 | 83 | 88 |
| 0.15 | *** | 1321 | 1356 | 1547 | 400 | 415 | 447 | 209 | 215 | 225 | 134 | 138 | 142 | 97 | 99 | 101 |
| | *** | 1333 | 1404 | 1970 | 406 | 428 | 540 | 212 | 220 | 257 | 136 | 140 | 153 | 98 | 100 | 101 |
| 0.2 | *** | 1612 | 1666 | 1996 | 476 | 501 | 554 | 244 | 254 | 270 | 154 | 159 | 166 | 109 | 112 | 115 |
| | *** | 1631 | 1743 | 2381 | 487 | 521 | 634 | 249 | 261 | 295 | 156 | 162 | 172 | 110 | 113 | 112 |
| 0.25 | *** | 1821 | 1898 | 2388 | 534 | 568 | 645 | 271 | 285 | 308 | 169 | 176 | 185 | 118 | 122 | 126 |
| | *** | 1848 | 2008 | 2724 | 548 | 597 | 711 | 277 | 295 | 326 | 172 | 180 | 187 | 120 | 124 | 120 |
| 0.3 | *** | 1954 | 2056 | 2715 | 574 | 617 | 719 | 290 | 308 | 337 | 180 | 188 | 199 | 124 | 128 | 134 |
| | *** | 1990 | 2200 | 2998 | 592 | 654 | 771 | 298 | 320 | 349 | 183 | 193 | 197 | 126 | 131 | 126 |
| 0.35 | *** | 2016 | 2147 | 2973 | 598 | 650 | 775 | 302 | 323 | 358 | 186 | 196 | 209 | 127 | 132 | 139 |
| | *** | 2063 | 2326 | 3203 | 620 | 695 | 814 | 311 | 338 | 364 | 190 | 202 | 204 | 130 | 135 | 129 |
| 0.4 | *** | 2018 | 2180 | 3159 | 608 | 668 | 812 | 307 | 331 | 371 | 188 | 199 | 214 | 128 | 134 | 141 |
| | *** | 2077 | 2393 | 3340 | 633 | 720 | 840 | 318 | 348 | 372 | 193 | 206 | 206 | 131 | 137 | 129 |
| 0.45 | *** | 1972 | 2164 | 3272 | 606 | 672 | 831 | 307 | 332 | 375 | 187 | 198 | 215 | 126 | 132 | 139 |
| | *** | 2043 | 2408 | 3409 | 634 | 729 | 848 | 318 | 350 | 372 | 192 | 206 | 204 | 129 | 135 | 126 |
| 0.5 | *** | 1888 | 2108 | 3310 | 593 | 663 | 832 | 300 | 327 | 372 | 182 | 194 | 210 | 122 | 128 | 135 |
| | *** | 1971 | 2378 | 3409 | 623 | 724 | 840 | 312 | 345 | 364 | 187 | 201 | 197 | 125 | 131 | 120 |
| 0.55 | *** | 1776 | 2020 | 3273 | 570 | 643 | 813 | 289 | 315 | 359 | 174 | 185 | 201 | 116 | 121 | 128 |
| | *** | 1870 | 2307 | 3340 | 601 | 705 | 814 | 300 | 334 | 349 | 179 | 192 | 187 | 118 | 124 | 112 |
| 0.6 | *** | 1645 | 1905 | 3162 | 539 | 611 | 776 | 272 | 297 | 339 | 162 | 173 | 187 | 107 | 111 | 117 |
| | *** | 1746 | 2200 | 3203 | 570 | 672 | 771 | 283 | 315 | 326 | 167 | 179 | 172 | 109 | 114 | 101 |
| 0.65 | *** | 1501 | 1767 | 2977 | 500 | 568 | 721 | 250 | 273 | 310 | 147 | 156 | 169 | 95 | 99 | 104 |
| | *** | 1606 | 2060 | 2998 | 529 | 625 | 711 | 260 | 289 | 295 | 151 | 162 | 153 | 97 | 102 | 88 |
| 0.7 | *** | 1346 | 1608 | 2718 | 452 | 515 | 647 | 223 | 243 | 273 | 129 | 136 | 146 | 81 | 84 | 88 |
| | *** | 1451 | 1887 | 2724 | 479 | 565 | 634 | 232 | 256 | 257 | 132 | 140 | 129 | 83 | 86 | 71 |
| 0.75 | *** | 1183 | 1426 | 2386 | 396 | 449 | 555 | 190 | 206 | 228 | 106 | 111 | 118 | . | . | . |
| | *** | 1281 | 1680 | 2381 | 419 | 490 | 540 | 197 | 216 | 212 | 109 | 115 | 101 | . | . | . |
| 0.8 | *** | 1006 | 1220 | 1981 | 329 | 370 | 445 | 151 | 161 | 175 | . | . | . | . | . | . |
| | *** | 1093 | 1434 | 1970 | 347 | 400 | 429 | 155 | 168 | 158 | . | . | . | . | . | . |
| 0.85 | *** | 810 | 979 | 1506 | 248 | 274 | 317 | . | . | . | . | . | . | . | . | . |
| | *** | 880 | 1140 | 1491 | 260 | 292 | 300 | . | . | . | . | . | . | . | . | . |
| 0.9 | *** | 577 | 686 | 959 | . | . | . | . | . | . | . | . | . | . | . | . |
| | *** | 623 | 780 | 943 | . | . | . | . | . | . | . | . | . | . | . | . |

## TABLE 8: ALPHA= 0.05  POWER= 0.9     EXPECTED ACCRUAL THRU MINIMUM FOLLOW-UP= 425

| | | DEL=.05 | | | DEL=.10 | | | DEL=.15 | | | DEL=.20 | | | DEL=.25 | | |
|---|---|---|---|---|---|---|---|---|---|---|---|---|---|---|---|---|---|
| FACT= | | 1.0 .75 | .50 .25 | .00 BIN | 1.0 .75 | .50 .25 | .00 BIN | 1.0 .75 | .50 .25 | .00 BIN | 1.0 75 | .50 .25 | .00 BIN | 1.0 .75 | .50 .25 | .00 BIN |
| PCONT=*** | | | | | REQUIRED NUMBER OF PATIENTS | | | | | | | | | | | |
| 0.05 | *** | 520 | 528 | 547 | 188 | 191 | 195 | 111 | 112 | 113 | 78 | 79 | 80 | 61 | 61 | 62 |
| | *** | 523 | 535 | 943 | 189 | 192 | 300 | 111 | 113 | 158 | 79 | 79 | 101 | 61 | 62 | 71 |
| 0.1 | *** | 952 | 972 | 1055 | 304 | 312 | 326 | 165 | 168 | 173 | 110 | 111 | 113 | 81 | 82 | 83 |
| | *** | 960 | 997 | 1491 | 307 | 318 | 429 | 166 | 170 | 212 | 110 | 112 | 129 | 82 | 83 | 88 |
| 0.15 | *** | 1323 | 1360 | 1547 | 401 | 416 | 447 | 209 | 216 | 225 | 135 | 138 | 142 | 97 | 99 | 101 |
| | *** | 1336 | 1409 | 1970 | 408 | 428 | 540 | 212 | 220 | 257 | 136 | 140 | 153 | 98 | 100 | 101 |
| 0.2 | *** | 1615 | 1672 | 1996 | 478 | 503 | 554 | 245 | 255 | 270 | 155 | 159 | 166 | 109 | 112 | 115 |
| | *** | 1635 | 1751 | 2381 | 489 | 523 | 634 | 249 | 262 | 295 | 157 | 162 | 172 | 110 | 113 | 112 |
| 0.25 | *** | 1827 | 1906 | 2388 | 537 | 570 | 645 | 272 | 286 | 308 | 170 | 176 | 185 | 118 | 122 | 126 |
| | *** | 1855 | 2018 | 2724 | 551 | 598 | 711 | 278 | 295 | 326 | 173 | 180 | 187 | 120 | 124 | 120 |
| 0.3 | *** | 1960 | 2067 | 2715 | 578 | 621 | 719 | 292 | 309 | 337 | 180 | 188 | 200 | 125 | 129 | 134 |
| | *** | 1999 | 2213 | 2998 | 596 | 657 | 771 | 299 | 321 | 349 | 184 | 193 | 197 | 127 | 131 | 126 |
| 0.35 | *** | 2025 | 2161 | 2974 | 603 | 654 | 775 | 304 | 324 | 358 | 187 | 196 | 209 | 128 | 133 | 139 |
| | *** | 2074 | 2343 | 3203 | 624 | 699 | 814 | 313 | 339 | 364 | 191 | 202 | 204 | 130 | 136 | 129 |
| 0.4 | *** | 2030 | 2197 | 3159 | 613 | 673 | 812 | 310 | 333 | 371 | 189 | 200 | 214 | 129 | 134 | 141 |
| | *** | 2091 | 2413 | 3340 | 638 | 724 | 840 | 320 | 349 | 372 | 194 | 206 | 206 | 131 | 137 | 129 |
| 0.45 | *** | 1986 | 2184 | 3272 | 612 | 677 | 832 | 309 | 334 | 375 | 188 | 199 | 214 | 127 | 132 | 139 |
| | *** | 2060 | 2431 | 3409 | 639 | 733 | 848 | 320 | 351 | 372 | 193 | 206 | 204 | 130 | 136 | 126 |
| 0.5 | *** | 1904 | 2131 | 3310 | 599 | 669 | 832 | 303 | 329 | 371 | 183 | 195 | 210 | 123 | 128 | 135 |
| | *** | 1990 | 2402 | 3409 | 629 | 728 | 840 | 314 | 347 | 364 | 188 | 201 | 197 | 125 | 131 | 120 |
| 0.55 | *** | 1795 | 2044 | 3273 | 577 | 649 | 813 | 291 | 317 | 359 | 175 | 186 | 201 | 116 | 121 | 128 |
| | *** | 1891 | 2333 | 3340 | 608 | 709 | 814 | 303 | 335 | 349 | 180 | 193 | 187 | 119 | 124 | 112 |
| 0.6 | *** | 1665 | 1930 | 3162 | 546 | 617 | 776 | 274 | 299 | 339 | 163 | 173 | 187 | 107 | 112 | 118 |
| | *** | 1769 | 2227 | 3203 | 576 | 676 | 771 | 285 | 316 | 326 | 168 | 180 | 172 | 109 | 114 | 101 |
| 0.65 | *** | 1522 | 1792 | 2976 | 506 | 574 | 721 | 252 | 275 | 310 | 148 | 157 | 169 | 96 | 99 | 104 |
| | *** | 1629 | 2086 | 2998 | 535 | 629 | 711 | 263 | 290 | 295 | 152 | 162 | 153 | 98 | 102 | 88 |
| 0.7 | *** | 1368 | 1632 | 2717 | 458 | 520 | 647 | 225 | 244 | 273 | 129 | 136 | 146 | 82 | 85 | 88 |
| | *** | 1473 | 1911 | 2724 | 485 | 569 | 634 | 234 | 257 | 257 | 133 | 141 | 129 | 83 | 86 | 71 |
| 0.75 | *** | 1203 | 1448 | 2385 | 401 | 453 | 555 | 192 | 206 | 228 | 107 | 112 | 118 | . | . | . |
| | *** | 1302 | 1701 | 2381 | 424 | 493 | 540 | 198 | 216 | 212 | 109 | 115 | 101 | . | . | . |
| 0.8 | *** | 1024 | 1239 | 1981 | 332 | 373 | 445 | 152 | 162 | 175 | . | . | . | . | . | . |
| | *** | 1112 | 1451 | 1970 | 350 | 402 | 429 | 156 | 168 | 158 | . | . | . | . | . | . |
| 0.85 | *** | 825 | 994 | 1506 | 250 | 276 | 317 | . | . | . | . | . | . | . | . | . |
| | *** | 894 | 1153 | 1491 | 262 | 294 | 300 | . | . | . | . | . | . | . | . | . |
| 0.9 | *** | 587 | 694 | 959 | . | . | . | . | . | . | . | . | . | . | . | . |
| | *** | 632 | 787 | 943 | . | . | . | . | . | . | . | . | . | . | . | . |

TABLE 8: ALPHA= 0.05  POWER= 0.9     EXPECTED ACCRUAL THRU MINIMUM FOLLOW-UP= 450

| | DEL=.05 | | | DEL=.10 | | | DEL=.15 | | | DEL=.20 | | | DEL=.25 | | |
|---|---|---|---|---|---|---|---|---|---|---|---|---|---|---|---|
| FACT= | 1.0 .75 | .50 .25 | .00 BIN | 1.0 .75 | .50 .25 | .00 BIN | 1.0 .75 | .50 .25 | .00 BIN | 1.0 75 | .50 .25 | .00 BIN | 1.0 .75 | .50 .25 | .00 BIN |
| PCONT=*** | | | | REQUIRED NUMBER OF PATIENTS | | | | | | | | | | | |
| 0.05 *** | 521 524 | 528 535 | 547 943 | 189 190 | 191 193 | 195 300 | 111 111 | 112 113 | 113 158 | 78 79 | 79 80 | 80 101 | 61 61 | 61 62 | 62 71 |
| 0.1 *** | 954 961 | 974 999 | 1055 1491 | 305 308 | 312 318 | 326 429 | 165 167 | 168 171 | 173 212 | 110 111 | 111 112 | 113 129 | 81 82 | 82 83 | 83 88 |
| 0.15 *** | 1325 1339 | 1363 1413 | 1547 1970 | 402 409 | 417 429 | 447 540 | 210 213 | 216 220 | 225 257 | 135 136 | 138 140 | 142 153 | 97 98 | 99 100 | 101 101 |
| 0.2 *** | 1619 1640 | 1678 1757 | 1995 2381 | 480 491 | 505 524 | 554 634 | 246 250 | 256 262 | 270 295 | 155 157 | 160 163 | 166 172 | 109 111 | 112 113 | 115 112 |
| 0.25 *** | 1832 1861 | 1914 2028 | 2388 2724 | 540 554 | 573 600 | 645 711 | 274 280 | 287 296 | 308 326 | 171 173 | 177 180 | 185 187 | 119 120 | 122 124 | 126 120 |
| 0.3 *** | 1967 2007 | 2078 2226 | 2715 2998 | 581 599 | 624 660 | 719 771 | 293 301 | 310 322 | 337 349 | 181 185 | 189 194 | 199 197 | 125 127 | 129 131 | 134 126 |
| 0.35 *** | 2034 2085 | 2174 2359 | 2973 3203 | 607 629 | 658 702 | 775 814 | 306 315 | 326 339 | 358 364 | 188 192 | 197 203 | 209 204 | 129 131 | 133 136 | 139 129 |
| 0.4 *** | 2041 2105 | 2213 2432 | 3159 3340 | 618 643 | 678 727 | 812 840 | 312 322 | 334 350 | 371 372 | 190 195 | 200 207 | 214 206 | 129 132 | 134 137 | 141 129 |
| 0.45 *** | 2000 2076 | 2203 2452 | 3272 3409 | 617 645 | 682 738 | 831 848 | 311 322 | 336 352 | 375 372 | 189 194 | 200 207 | 214 204 | 127 130 | 133 136 | 139 126 |
| 0.5 *** | 1920 2009 | 2152 2425 | 3310 3409 | 605 635 | 675 733 | 832 840 | 305 316 | 330 348 | 372 364 | 185 189 | 195 202 | 210 197 | 123 126 | 129 132 | 135 120 |
| 0.55 *** | 1813 1911 | 2067 2357 | 3273 3340 | 583 613 | 654 713 | 813 814 | 294 305 | 319 336 | 359 349 | 176 181 | 186 193 | 201 187 | 117 119 | 122 124 | 128 112 |
| 0.6 *** | 1685 1791 | 1954 2251 | 3162 3203 | 552 582 | 622 680 | 776 771 | 277 288 | 301 317 | 339 326 | 164 169 | 174 180 | 187 172 | 108 110 | 112 114 | 117 101 |
| 0.65 *** | 1543 1651 | 1816 2110 | 2976 2998 | 512 541 | 579 633 | 721 711 | 254 264 | 276 291 | 310 295 | 149 153 | 158 163 | 168 153 | 96 98 | 100 102 | 104 88 |
| 0.7 *** | 1388 1495 | 1655 1934 | 2718 2724 | 463 490 | 524 572 | 647 634 | 227 235 | 245 258 | 273 257 | 130 133 | 137 141 | 145 129 | 82 83 | 85 86 | 88 71 |
| 0.75 *** | 1222 1323 | 1470 1721 | 2386 2381 | 405 428 | 457 496 | 555 540 | 193 200 | 208 217 | 228 212 | 107 109 | 112 115 | 118 101 | . . | . . | . . |
| 0.8 *** | 1041 1130 | 1257 1468 | 1981 1970 | 336 354 | 375 404 | 445 429 | 153 157 | 162 168 | 175 158 | . . | . . | . . | . . | . . | . . |
| 0.85 *** | 838 909 | 1007 1165 | 1506 1491 | 253 264 | 278 295 | 317 300 | . . | . . | . . | . . | . . | . . | . . | . . | . . |
| 0.9 *** | 596 642 | 703 794 | 959 943 | . . | . . | . . | . . | . . | . . | . . | . . | . . | . . | . . | . . |

TABLE 8: ALPHA= 0.05  POWER= 0.9     EXPECTED ACCRUAL THRU MINIMUM FOLLOW-UP= 475

|  |  | DEL=.05 | | | DEL=.10 | | | DEL=.15 | | | DEL=.20 | | | DEL=.25 | | |
|---|---|---|---|---|---|---|---|---|---|---|---|---|---|---|---|---|
| FACT= | | 1.0 | .50 | .00 | 1.0 | .50 | .00 | 1.0 | .50 | .00 | 1.0 | .50 | .00 | 1.0 | .50 | .00 |
| | | .75 | .25 | BIN | .75 | .25 | BIN | .75 | .25 | BIN | 75 | .25 | BIN | .75 | .25 | BIN |

PCONT=***            REQUIRED NUMBER OF PATIENTS

| PCONT | | DEL=.05 1.0/.75 | .50/.25 | .00/BIN | DEL=.10 1.0/.75 | .50/.25 | .00/BIN | DEL=.15 1.0/.75 | .50/.25 | .00/BIN | DEL=.20 1.0/75 | .50/.25 | .00/BIN | DEL=.25 1.0/.75 | .50/.25 | .00/BIN |
|---|---|---|---|---|---|---|---|---|---|---|---|---|---|---|---|---|
| 0.05 | *** | 521 | 529 | 547 | 189 | 191 | 194 | 111 | 112 | 113 | 79 | 79 | 80 | 61 | 61 | 62 |
| | *** | 524 | 536 | 943 | 190 | 193 | 300 | 112 | 113 | 158 | 79 | 80 | 101 | 61 | 62 | 71 |
| 0.1 | *** | 955 | 976 | 1055 | 305 | 313 | 326 | 165 | 169 | 173 | 110 | 112 | 113 | 81 | 82 | 83 |
| | *** | 963 | 1001 | 1491 | 309 | 319 | 429 | 167 | 171 | 212 | 111 | 112 | 129 | 82 | 83 | 88 |
| 0.15 | *** | 1328 | 1367 | 1547 | 403 | 419 | 447 | 210 | 217 | 225 | 135 | 138 | 142 | 97 | 99 | 101 |
| | *** | 1342 | 1417 | 1970 | 410 | 430 | 540 | 213 | 221 | 257 | 137 | 140 | 153 | 98 | 100 | 101 |
| 0.2 | *** | 1622 | 1683 | 1996 | 482 | 506 | 553 | 247 | 256 | 270 | 156 | 160 | 166 | 110 | 112 | 115 |
| | *** | 1644 | 1764 | 2381 | 492 | 525 | 634 | 251 | 262 | 295 | 158 | 163 | 172 | 111 | 113 | 112 |
| 0.25 | *** | 1837 | 1923 | 2388 | 542 | 575 | 644 | 275 | 288 | 308 | 171 | 177 | 185 | 119 | 122 | 126 |
| | *** | 1868 | 2037 | 2724 | 557 | 602 | 711 | 281 | 297 | 326 | 174 | 181 | 187 | 121 | 124 | 120 |
| 0.3 | *** | 1974 | 2088 | 2715 | 585 | 627 | 719 | 295 | 311 | 337 | 182 | 189 | 200 | 125 | 129 | 134 |
| | *** | 2016 | 2239 | 2998 | 603 | 662 | 771 | 302 | 322 | 349 | 186 | 194 | 197 | 127 | 131 | 126 |
| 0.35 | *** | 2043 | 2188 | 2973 | 611 | 662 | 775 | 308 | 327 | 358 | 188 | 197 | 209 | 129 | 133 | 139 |
| | *** | 2096 | 2374 | 3203 | 633 | 704 | 814 | 317 | 340 | 364 | 193 | 203 | 204 | 131 | 136 | 129 |
| 0.4 | *** | 2052 | 2229 | 3159 | 623 | 682 | 812 | 314 | 336 | 371 | 191 | 201 | 214 | 130 | 134 | 141 |
| | *** | 2118 | 2450 | 3340 | 648 | 731 | 840 | 324 | 351 | 372 | 196 | 207 | 206 | 132 | 137 | 129 |
| 0.45 | *** | 2013 | 2221 | 3272 | 623 | 687 | 831 | 314 | 337 | 375 | 190 | 200 | 214 | 128 | 133 | 139 |
| | *** | 2092 | 2472 | 3409 | 650 | 741 | 848 | 324 | 354 | 372 | 195 | 207 | 204 | 130 | 136 | 126 |
| 0.5 | *** | 1936 | 2172 | 3310 | 611 | 680 | 832 | 308 | 332 | 371 | 185 | 196 | 210 | 124 | 129 | 135 |
| | *** | 2027 | 2447 | 3409 | 640 | 737 | 840 | 319 | 349 | 364 | 190 | 202 | 197 | 126 | 132 | 120 |
| 0.55 | *** | 1831 | 2089 | 3273 | 589 | 659 | 813 | 296 | 320 | 359 | 177 | 187 | 201 | 117 | 122 | 128 |
| | *** | 1931 | 2380 | 3340 | 619 | 717 | 814 | 307 | 337 | 349 | 182 | 193 | 187 | 119 | 125 | 112 |
| 0.6 | *** | 1704 | 1976 | 3162 | 558 | 628 | 776 | 279 | 302 | 339 | 165 | 175 | 187 | 108 | 112 | 117 |
| | *** | 1812 | 2274 | 3203 | 588 | 684 | 771 | 289 | 318 | 326 | 169 | 180 | 172 | 110 | 115 | 101 |
| 0.65 | *** | 1562 | 1838 | 2977 | 517 | 584 | 721 | 256 | 278 | 310 | 150 | 158 | 169 | 96 | 100 | 104 |
| | *** | 1673 | 2132 | 2998 | 546 | 637 | 711 | 266 | 292 | 295 | 153 | 163 | 153 | 98 | 102 | 88 |
| 0.7 | *** | 1408 | 1676 | 2718 | 469 | 528 | 647 | 228 | 246 | 273 | 131 | 137 | 146 | 82 | 85 | 88 |
| | *** | 1516 | 1955 | 2724 | 495 | 575 | 634 | 237 | 258 | 257 | 134 | 141 | 129 | 83 | 86 | 71 |
| 0.75 | *** | 1241 | 1489 | 2385 | 410 | 460 | 555 | 194 | 208 | 228 | 108 | 112 | 118 | . | . | . |
| | *** | 1342 | 1740 | 2381 | 432 | 498 | 540 | 201 | 217 | 212 | 110 | 115 | 101 | . | . | . |
| 0.8 | *** | 1058 | 1274 | 1981 | 340 | 378 | 445 | 153 | 163 | 175 | . | . | . | . | . | . |
| | *** | 1146 | 1484 | 1970 | 357 | 406 | 429 | 158 | 169 | 158 | . | . | . | . | . | . |
| 0.85 | *** | 851 | 1020 | 1505 | 255 | 279 | 317 | . | . | . | . | . | . | . | . | . |
| | *** | 922 | 1176 | 1491 | 266 | 296 | 300 | . | . | . | . | . | . | . | . | . |
| 0.9 | *** | 605 | 711 | 959 | . | . | . | . | . | . | . | . | . | . | . | . |
| | *** | 650 | 800 | 943 | . | . | . | . | . | . | . | . | . | . | . | . |

## TABLE 8: ALPHA= 0.05  POWER= 0.9    EXPECTED ACCRUAL THRU MINIMUM FOLLOW-UP= 500

| | DEL=.05 | | | DEL=.10 | | | DEL=.15 | | | DEL=.20 | | | DEL=.25 | | |
|---|---|---|---|---|---|---|---|---|---|---|---|---|---|---|---|
| FACT= | 1.0 | .50 | .00 | 1.0 | .50 | .00 | 1.0 | .50 | .00 | 1.0 | .50 | .00 | 1.0 | .50 | .00 |
| | .75 | .25 | BIN | .75 | .25 | BIN | .75 | .25 | BIN | 75 | .25 | BIN | .75 | .25 | BIN |

PCONT=***                     REQUIRED NUMBER OF PATIENTS

| PCONT | DEL=.05 1.0/.75 | .50/.25 | .00/BIN | DEL=.10 1.0/.75 | .50/.25 | .00/BIN | DEL=.15 1.0/.75 | .50/.25 | .00/BIN | DEL=.20 1.0/75 | .50/.25 | .00/BIN | DEL=.25 1.0/.75 | .50/.25 | .00/BIN |
|---|---|---|---|---|---|---|---|---|---|---|---|---|---|---|---|
| 0.05 *** | 522 | 529 | 547 | 189 | 191 | 195 | 111 | 112 | 113 | 79 | 79 | 80 | 61 | 62 | 62 |
| *** | 525 | 536 | 943 | 190 | 193 | 300 | 112 | 113 | 158 | 79 | 80 | 101 | 61 | 62 | 71 |
| 0.1 *** | 956 | 978 | 1055 | 306 | 313 | 326 | 166 | 169 | 173 | 110 | 112 | 113 | 81 | 82 | 83 |
| *** | 964 | 1003 | 1491 | 309 | 319 | 429 | 167 | 171 | 212 | 111 | 113 | 129 | 82 | 83 | 88 |
| 0.15 *** | 1330 | 1371 | 1547 | 405 | 420 | 447 | 211 | 217 | 225 | 136 | 138 | 142 | 97 | 99 | 101 |
| *** | 1345 | 1421 | 1970 | 411 | 431 | 540 | 214 | 221 | 257 | 137 | 140 | 153 | 98 | 100 | 101 |
| 0.2 *** | 1626 | 1689 | 1996 | 484 | 508 | 553 | 248 | 257 | 270 | 156 | 160 | 166 | 110 | 112 | 115 |
| *** | 1649 | 1770 | 2381 | 494 | 526 | 634 | 252 | 263 | 295 | 158 | 163 | 172 | 111 | 113 | 112 |
| 0.25 *** | 1842 | 1930 | 2388 | 545 | 578 | 645 | 276 | 288 | 308 | 172 | 178 | 185 | 119 | 123 | 126 |
| *** | 1874 | 2046 | 2724 | 559 | 604 | 711 | 282 | 297 | 326 | 174 | 181 | 187 | 121 | 124 | 120 |
| 0.3 *** | 1981 | 2099 | 2715 | 588 | 630 | 719 | 296 | 312 | 337 | 183 | 190 | 199 | 126 | 129 | 134 |
| *** | 2024 | 2250 | 2998 | 606 | 664 | 771 | 303 | 323 | 349 | 186 | 194 | 197 | 128 | 132 | 126 |
| 0.35 *** | 2052 | 2201 | 2973 | 615 | 666 | 775 | 309 | 328 | 358 | 189 | 198 | 209 | 129 | 134 | 139 |
| *** | 2107 | 2389 | 3203 | 637 | 707 | 814 | 318 | 341 | 364 | 193 | 203 | 204 | 131 | 136 | 129 |
| 0.4 *** | 2063 | 2244 | 3159 | 628 | 686 | 812 | 316 | 337 | 371 | 192 | 202 | 214 | 130 | 135 | 141 |
| *** | 2131 | 2467 | 3340 | 653 | 734 | 840 | 325 | 352 | 372 | 197 | 207 | 206 | 133 | 138 | 129 |
| 0.45 *** | 2026 | 2239 | 3272 | 628 | 692 | 831 | 316 | 339 | 375 | 191 | 201 | 214 | 128 | 133 | 139 |
| *** | 2107 | 2491 | 3409 | 655 | 744 | 848 | 326 | 354 | 372 | 196 | 207 | 204 | 131 | 136 | 126 |
| 0.5 *** | 1951 | 2192 | 3310 | 616 | 684 | 832 | 309 | 333 | 372 | 186 | 196 | 210 | 124 | 129 | 135 |
| *** | 2044 | 2468 | 3409 | 645 | 740 | 840 | 320 | 350 | 364 | 191 | 203 | 197 | 127 | 132 | 120 |
| 0.55 *** | 1848 | 2110 | 3273 | 594 | 664 | 813 | 298 | 322 | 359 | 178 | 188 | 201 | 118 | 122 | 128 |
| *** | 1950 | 2402 | 3340 | 624 | 721 | 814 | 309 | 338 | 349 | 183 | 194 | 187 | 120 | 125 | 112 |
| 0.6 *** | 1723 | 1998 | 3162 | 563 | 632 | 776 | 281 | 303 | 339 | 166 | 175 | 187 | 108 | 113 | 118 |
| *** | 1832 | 2296 | 3203 | 593 | 688 | 771 | 291 | 319 | 326 | 170 | 181 | 172 | 110 | 115 | 101 |
| 0.65 *** | 1582 | 1860 | 2977 | 523 | 588 | 721 | 258 | 279 | 310 | 151 | 158 | 168 | 97 | 100 | 104 |
| *** | 1693 | 2154 | 2998 | 551 | 640 | 711 | 268 | 293 | 295 | 154 | 163 | 153 | 98 | 102 | 88 |
| 0.7 *** | 1427 | 1697 | 2718 | 473 | 533 | 647 | 230 | 248 | 273 | 131 | 138 | 146 | 83 | 85 | 88 |
| *** | 1536 | 1975 | 2724 | 499 | 578 | 634 | 238 | 259 | 257 | 134 | 141 | 129 | 84 | 87 | 71 |
| 0.75 *** | 1258 | 1508 | 2386 | 414 | 464 | 555 | 196 | 209 | 228 | 108 | 113 | 118 | . | . | . |
| *** | 1360 | 1758 | 2381 | 436 | 501 | 540 | 202 | 218 | 212 | 110 | 115 | 101 | . | . | . |
| 0.8 *** | 1073 | 1290 | 1981 | 343 | 381 | 445 | 154 | 163 | 175 | . | . | . | . | . | . |
| *** | 1163 | 1498 | 1970 | 360 | 408 | 429 | 159 | 169 | 158 | . | . | . | . | . | . |
| 0.85 *** | 864 | 1033 | 1506 | 257 | 281 | 317 | . | . | . | . | . | . | . | . | . |
| *** | 934 | 1187 | 1491 | 268 | 297 | 300 | . | . | . | . | . | . | . | . | . |
| 0.9 *** | 613 | 718 | 959 | . | . | . | . | . | . | . | . | . | . | . | . |
| *** | 658 | 806 | 943 | . | . | . | . | . | . | . | . | . | . | . | . |

TABLE 8: ALPHA= 0.05  POWER= 0.9    EXPECTED ACCRUAL THRU MINIMUM FOLLOW-UP= 550

|  |  | DEL=.02 | | | DEL=.05 | | | DEL=.10 | | | DEL=.15 | | | DEL=.20 | | |
|---|---|---|---|---|---|---|---|---|---|---|---|---|---|---|---|---|
| FACT= | | 1.0 .75 | .50 .25 | .00 BIN | 1.0 .75 | .50 .25 | .00 BIN | 1.0 .75 | .50 .25 | .00 BIN | 1.0 75 | .50 .25 | .00 BIN | 1.0 .75 | .50 .25 | .00 BIN |
| PCONT=*** | | | | | REQUIRED NUMBER OF PATIENTS | | | | | | | | | | | |
| 0.05 | *** | 2439 | 2451 | 2580 | 523 | 530 | 547 | 189 | 191 | 195 | 111 | 112 | 113 | 79 | 79 | 80 |
| | *** | 2443 | 2472 | 4822 | 526 | 537 | 943 | 190 | 193 | 300 | 112 | 113 | 158 | 79 | 80 | 101 |
| 0.1 | *** | 5076 | 5103 | 5668 | 959 | 981 | 1055 | 307 | 314 | 326 | 166 | 169 | 173 | 110 | 112 | 113 |
| | *** | 5085 | 5157 | 8376 | 968 | 1006 | 1491 | 310 | 319 | 429 | 168 | 171 | 212 | 111 | 113 | 129 |
| 0.15 | *** | 7416 | 7464 | 8766 | 1334 | 1377 | 1547 | 407 | 421 | 446 | 212 | 217 | 225 | 136 | 139 | 142 |
| | *** | 7432 | 7559 | 11502 | 1350 | 1427 | 1970 | 413 | 432 | 540 | 215 | 221 | 257 | 137 | 140 | 153 |
| 0.2 | *** | 9281 | 9354 | 11647 | 1633 | 1699 | 1996 | 488 | 511 | 553 | 249 | 258 | 270 | 157 | 161 | 166 |
| | *** | 9305 | 9502 | 14199 | 1658 | 1782 | 2381 | 498 | 528 | 634 | 253 | 264 | 295 | 158 | 163 | 172 |
| 0.25 | *** | 10621 | 10727 | 14201 | 1852 | 1945 | 2388 | 550 | 582 | 644 | 278 | 290 | 308 | 173 | 178 | 185 |
| | *** | 10656 | 10938 | 16469 | 1886 | 2062 | 2724 | 564 | 607 | 711 | 283 | 298 | 326 | 175 | 181 | 187 |
| 0.3 | *** | 11445 | 11591 | 16367 | 1994 | 2118 | 2715 | 594 | 635 | 719 | 299 | 314 | 337 | 184 | 191 | 199 |
| | *** | 11494 | 11880 | 18310 | 2040 | 2272 | 2998 | 612 | 668 | 771 | 306 | 324 | 349 | 187 | 195 | 197 |
| 0.35 | *** | 11790 | 11983 | 18108 | 2069 | 2225 | 2973 | 622 | 672 | 775 | 312 | 330 | 358 | 191 | 199 | 209 |
| | *** | 11854 | 12368 | 19723 | 2127 | 2415 | 3203 | 643 | 712 | 814 | 321 | 343 | 364 | 195 | 203 | 204 |
| 0.4 | *** | 11708 | 11961 | 19404 | 2084 | 2274 | 3159 | 636 | 693 | 812 | 319 | 339 | 371 | 194 | 202 | 214 |
| | *** | 11793 | 12460 | 20708 | 2156 | 2498 | 3340 | 661 | 739 | 840 | 328 | 353 | 372 | 198 | 208 | 206 |
| 0.45 | *** | 11265 | 11589 | 20243 | 2052 | 2272 | 3272 | 637 | 700 | 831 | 319 | 341 | 375 | 193 | 202 | 214 |
| | *** | 11373 | 12223 | 21265 | 2136 | 2527 | 3409 | 664 | 750 | 848 | 329 | 356 | 372 | 197 | 208 | 204 |
| 0.5 | *** | 10527 | 10942 | 20619 | 1981 | 2228 | 3310 | 626 | 693 | 832 | 313 | 336 | 371 | 188 | 198 | 210 |
| | *** | 10666 | 11729 | 21393 | 2077 | 2506 | 3409 | 655 | 746 | 840 | 324 | 352 | 364 | 192 | 203 | 197 |
| 0.55 | *** | 9571 | 10097 | 20529 | 1881 | 2149 | 3273 | 604 | 673 | 813 | 302 | 324 | 359 | 179 | 189 | 201 |
| | *** | 9748 | 11047 | 21093 | 1986 | 2442 | 3340 | 634 | 727 | 814 | 312 | 340 | 349 | 184 | 195 | 187 |
| 0.6 | *** | 8475 | 9131 | 19973 | 1758 | 2038 | 3162 | 573 | 641 | 776 | 284 | 306 | 339 | 167 | 176 | 187 |
| | *** | 8698 | 10237 | 20365 | 1870 | 2337 | 3203 | 602 | 694 | 771 | 294 | 321 | 326 | 171 | 181 | 172 |
| 0.65 | *** | 7321 | 8115 | 18952 | 1618 | 1900 | 2976 | 532 | 596 | 721 | 261 | 281 | 310 | 152 | 159 | 169 |
| | *** | 7599 | 9344 | 19209 | 1731 | 2193 | 2998 | 560 | 646 | 711 | 270 | 294 | 295 | 155 | 164 | 153 |
| 0.7 | *** | 6189 | 7102 | 17471 | 1462 | 1735 | 2718 | 482 | 540 | 647 | 233 | 250 | 273 | 132 | 138 | 146 |
| | *** | 6520 | 8396 | 17625 | 1573 | 2012 | 2724 | 507 | 583 | 634 | 241 | 260 | 257 | 135 | 142 | 129 |
| 0.75 | *** | 5139 | 6115 | 15532 | 1292 | 1543 | 2386 | 421 | 470 | 555 | 198 | 211 | 228 | 109 | 113 | 118 |
| | *** | 5504 | 7403 | 15612 | 1394 | 1790 | 2381 | 443 | 505 | 540 | 204 | 219 | 212 | 111 | 115 | 101 |
| 0.8 | *** | 4190 | 5151 | 13140 | 1103 | 1320 | 1981 | 349 | 385 | 445 | 156 | 164 | 175 | . | . | . |
| | *** | 4558 | 6353 | 13172 | 1192 | 1525 | 1970 | 365 | 410 | 429 | 160 | 169 | 158 | . | . | . |
| 0.85 | *** | 3318 | 4180 | 10300 | 887 | 1055 | 1506 | 261 | 283 | 317 | . | . | . | . | . | . |
| | *** | 3653 | 5212 | 10303 | 958 | 1206 | 1491 | 271 | 298 | 300 | . | . | . | . | . | . |
| 0.9 | *** | 2458 | 3132 | 7018 | 628 | 731 | 959 | . | . | . | . | . | . | . | . | . |
| | *** | 2723 | 3901 | 7006 | 672 | 816 | 943 | . | . | . | . | . | . | . | . | . |
| 0.95 | *** | 1464 | 1835 | 3297 | . | . | . | . | . | . | . | . | . | . | . | . |
| | *** | 1614 | 2219 | 3280 | . | . | . | . | . | . | . | . | . | . | . | . |

TABLE 8: ALPHA= 0.05  POWER= 0.9     EXPECTED ACCRUAL THRU MINIMUM FOLLOW-UP= 600

| | | DEL=.02 | | | DEL=.05 | | | DEL=.10 | | | DEL=.15 | | | DEL=.20 | | |
|---|---|---|---|---|---|---|---|---|---|---|---|---|---|---|---|---|---|
| FACT= | | 1.0 .75 | .50 .25 | .00 BIN | 1.0 .75 | .50 .25 | .00 BIN | 1.0 .75 | .50 .25 | .00 BIN | 1.0 75 | .50 .25 | .00 BIN | 1.0 .75 | .50 .25 | .00 BIN |
| PCONT=*** | | REQUIRED NUMBER OF PATIENTS | | | | | | | | | | | | | | |
| 0.05 | *** | 2440 | 2453 | 2580 | 524 | 531 | 547 | 190 | 192 | 194 | 112 | 112 | 113 | 79 | 79 | 80 |
| | *** | 2445 | 2476 | 4822 | 527 | 538 | 943 | 191 | 193 | 300 | 112 | 113 | 158 | 79 | 79 | 101 |
| 0.1 | *** | 5078 | 5108 | 5668 | 961 | 985 | 1055 | 308 | 315 | 326 | 167 | 169 | 173 | 110 | 112 | 113 |
| | *** | 5088 | 5166 | 8376 | 970 | 1009 | 1491 | 311 | 320 | 429 | 168 | 171 | 212 | 111 | 113 | 129 |
| 0.15 | *** | 7420 | 7472 | 8766 | 1339 | 1383 | 1547 | 409 | 423 | 446 | 213 | 218 | 225 | 136 | 139 | 142 |
| | *** | 7438 | 7576 | 11502 | 1356 | 1434 | 1970 | 415 | 433 | 540 | 215 | 221 | 257 | 137 | 140 | 153 |
| 0.2 | *** | 9287 | 9368 | 11647 | 1640 | 1709 | 1996 | 491 | 513 | 553 | 250 | 259 | 270 | 157 | 161 | 166 |
| | *** | 9314 | 9528 | 14199 | 1666 | 1792 | 2381 | 500 | 530 | 634 | 254 | 264 | 295 | 159 | 163 | 172 |
| 0.25 | *** | 10631 | 10746 | 14201 | 1861 | 1959 | 2388 | 554 | 585 | 644 | 280 | 291 | 308 | 173 | 178 | 185 |
| | *** | 10669 | 10976 | 16469 | 1898 | 2077 | 2724 | 568 | 610 | 711 | 285 | 298 | 326 | 176 | 181 | 187 |
| 0.3 | *** | 11458 | 11617 | 16367 | 2007 | 2137 | 2715 | 599 | 640 | 719 | 301 | 316 | 337 | 185 | 191 | 199 |
| | *** | 11511 | 11932 | 18310 | 2056 | 2292 | 2998 | 617 | 671 | 771 | 308 | 325 | 349 | 188 | 195 | 197 |
| 0.35 | *** | 11807 | 12018 | 18108 | 2085 | 2248 | 2973 | 629 | 678 | 775 | 315 | 332 | 358 | 192 | 199 | 209 |
| | *** | 11878 | 12436 | 19723 | 2147 | 2440 | 3203 | 650 | 716 | 814 | 323 | 344 | 364 | 196 | 204 | 204 |
| 0.4 | *** | 11731 | 12007 | 19404 | 2105 | 2300 | 3159 | 643 | 700 | 812 | 322 | 341 | 371 | 195 | 203 | 214 |
| | *** | 11823 | 12547 | 20708 | 2180 | 2527 | 3340 | 668 | 744 | 840 | 331 | 355 | 372 | 199 | 208 | 206 |
| 0.45 | *** | 11294 | 11648 | 20243 | 2076 | 2303 | 3272 | 645 | 707 | 831 | 322 | 343 | 375 | 194 | 203 | 214 |
| | *** | 11412 | 12332 | 21265 | 2164 | 2558 | 3409 | 672 | 756 | 848 | 332 | 358 | 372 | 198 | 208 | 204 |
| 0.5 | *** | 10565 | 11017 | 20619 | 2009 | 2263 | 3310 | 635 | 700 | 832 | 316 | 338 | 371 | 189 | 198 | 210 |
| | *** | 10716 | 11861 | 21393 | 2108 | 2541 | 3409 | 663 | 752 | 840 | 326 | 353 | 364 | 194 | 204 | 197 |
| 0.55 | *** | 9619 | 10190 | 20528 | 1912 | 2185 | 3273 | 613 | 680 | 813 | 305 | 327 | 359 | 181 | 190 | 201 |
| | *** | 9812 | 11201 | 21093 | 2020 | 2478 | 3340 | 643 | 733 | 814 | 315 | 341 | 349 | 185 | 195 | 187 |
| 0.6 | *** | 8536 | 9243 | 19972 | 1791 | 2076 | 3162 | 582 | 648 | 776 | 287 | 308 | 339 | 169 | 177 | 187 |
| | *** | 8779 | 10408 | 20365 | 1905 | 2373 | 3203 | 611 | 699 | 771 | 297 | 322 | 326 | 173 | 181 | 172 |
| 0.65 | *** | 7398 | 8245 | 18952 | 1651 | 1937 | 2977 | 541 | 603 | 721 | 264 | 283 | 310 | 153 | 160 | 169 |
| | *** | 7697 | 9527 | 19209 | 1767 | 2229 | 2998 | 568 | 650 | 711 | 273 | 295 | 295 | 156 | 164 | 153 |
| 0.7 | *** | 6282 | 7244 | 17471 | 1495 | 1771 | 2717 | 490 | 546 | 647 | 235 | 251 | 273 | 133 | 139 | 145 |
| | *** | 6634 | 8583 | 17625 | 1607 | 2045 | 2724 | 515 | 587 | 634 | 242 | 261 | 257 | 136 | 142 | 129 |
| 0.75 | *** | 5243 | 6260 | 15532 | 1322 | 1575 | 2386 | 428 | 475 | 555 | 200 | 212 | 228 | 109 | 113 | 118 |
| | *** | 5626 | 7584 | 15612 | 1426 | 1819 | 2381 | 449 | 508 | 540 | 205 | 219 | 212 | 111 | 116 | 101 |
| 0.8 | *** | 4297 | 5290 | 13140 | 1129 | 1346 | 1981 | 353 | 389 | 445 | 157 | 165 | 175 | . | . | . |
| | *** | 4678 | 6518 | 13172 | 1220 | 1548 | 1970 | 370 | 413 | 429 | 161 | 170 | 158 | . | . | . |
| 0.85 | *** | 3416 | 4301 | 10300 | 908 | 1075 | 1505 | 264 | 286 | 317 | . | . | . | . | . | . |
| | *** | 3761 | 5351 | 10303 | 979 | 1222 | 1491 | 274 | 300 | 300 | . | . | . | . | . | . |
| 0.9 | *** | 2536 | 3224 | 7018 | 641 | 743 | 959 | . | . | . | . | . | . | . | . | . |
| | *** | 2808 | 4002 | 7006 | 685 | 825 | 943 | . | . | . | . | . | . | . | . | . |
| 0.95 | *** | 1508 | 1883 | 3297 | . | . | . | . | . | . | . | . | . | . | . | . |
| | *** | 1661 | 2266 | 3280 | . | . | . | . | . | . | . | . | . | . | . | . |

## TABLE 8: ALPHA= 0.05 POWER= 0.9    EXPECTED ACCRUAL THRU MINIMUM FOLLOW-UP= 650

| | DEL=.02 | | | DEL=.05 | | | DEL=.10 | | | DEL=.15 | | | DEL=.20 | | |
|---|---|---|---|---|---|---|---|---|---|---|---|---|---|---|---|
| FACT= | 1.0 .75 | .50 .25 | .00 BIN | 1.0 .75 | .50 .25 | .00 BIN | 1.0 .75 | .50 .25 | .00 BIN | 1.0 75 | .50 .25 | .00 BIN | 1.0 .75 | .50 .25 | .00 BIN |
| PCONT=*** | | | | REQUIRED NUMBER OF PATIENTS | | | | | | | | | | | |
| 0.05 *** | 2442 | 2455 | 2580 | 525 | 532 | 547 | 190 | 192 | 194 | 112 | 112 | 114 | 79 | 80 | 80 |
| *** | 2446 | 2479 | 4822 | 528 | 538 | 943 | 191 | 193 | 300 | 112 | 113 | 158 | 79 | 80 | 101 |
| 0.1 *** | 5081 | 5113 | 5668 | 964 | 987 | 1055 | 309 | 316 | 326 | 167 | 170 | 173 | 111 | 112 | 114 |
| *** | 5091 | 5176 | 8376 | 973 | 1011 | 1491 | 312 | 320 | 429 | 168 | 171 | 212 | 111 | 113 | 129 |
| 0.15 *** | 7425 | 7481 | 8766 | 1343 | 1389 | 1547 | 411 | 424 | 447 | 214 | 219 | 225 | 137 | 139 | 142 |
| *** | 7444 | 7593 | 11502 | 1361 | 1440 | 1970 | 417 | 434 | 540 | 216 | 222 | 257 | 138 | 140 | 153 |
| 0.2 *** | 9294 | 9381 | 11647 | 1647 | 1719 | 1996 | 493 | 515 | 554 | 252 | 259 | 270 | 158 | 162 | 166 |
| *** | 9323 | 9555 | 14199 | 1674 | 1801 | 2381 | 503 | 532 | 634 | 255 | 264 | 295 | 159 | 164 | 172 |
| 0.25 *** | 10640 | 10766 | 14201 | 1871 | 1972 | 2388 | 558 | 588 | 645 | 281 | 292 | 308 | 174 | 179 | 185 |
| *** | 10682 | 11014 | 16469 | 1909 | 2091 | 2724 | 571 | 612 | 711 | 286 | 299 | 326 | 176 | 182 | 187 |
| 0.3 *** | 11472 | 11643 | 16367 | 2020 | 2154 | 2715 | 604 | 644 | 718 | 303 | 317 | 337 | 186 | 192 | 199 |
| *** | 11529 | 11984 | 18310 | 2070 | 2310 | 2998 | 622 | 674 | 771 | 309 | 326 | 349 | 189 | 195 | 197 |
| 0.35 *** | 11825 | 12054 | 18108 | 2101 | 2269 | 2973 | 635 | 683 | 775 | 317 | 334 | 358 | 193 | 200 | 209 |
| *** | 11901 | 12504 | 19723 | 2166 | 2462 | 3203 | 656 | 720 | 814 | 325 | 345 | 364 | 197 | 204 | 204 |
| 0.4 *** | 11754 | 12053 | 19404 | 2125 | 2326 | 3159 | 650 | 705 | 812 | 324 | 343 | 371 | 196 | 204 | 214 |
| *** | 11854 | 12634 | 20708 | 2202 | 2553 | 3340 | 674 | 748 | 840 | 333 | 356 | 372 | 200 | 209 | 206 |
| 0.45 *** | 11324 | 11708 | 20243 | 2099 | 2332 | 3272 | 653 | 713 | 831 | 325 | 346 | 375 | 195 | 204 | 214 |
| *** | 11452 | 12440 | 21265 | 2190 | 2588 | 3409 | 679 | 760 | 848 | 335 | 359 | 372 | 199 | 209 | 204 |
| 0.5 *** | 10603 | 11091 | 20619 | 2036 | 2294 | 3310 | 643 | 707 | 832 | 320 | 341 | 372 | 191 | 199 | 210 |
| *** | 10767 | 11989 | 21393 | 2138 | 2572 | 3409 | 671 | 757 | 840 | 329 | 354 | 364 | 195 | 204 | 197 |
| 0.55 *** | 9667 | 10282 | 20529 | 1941 | 2219 | 3273 | 622 | 688 | 813 | 308 | 329 | 359 | 182 | 190 | 201 |
| *** | 9875 | 11349 | 21093 | 2052 | 2511 | 3340 | 651 | 738 | 814 | 318 | 342 | 349 | 186 | 195 | 187 |
| 0.6 *** | 8597 | 9354 | 19972 | 1822 | 2110 | 3162 | 591 | 655 | 776 | 290 | 310 | 339 | 170 | 177 | 187 |
| *** | 8859 | 10572 | 20365 | 1938 | 2407 | 3203 | 619 | 704 | 771 | 300 | 323 | 326 | 174 | 182 | 172 |
| 0.65 *** | 7474 | 8372 | 18952 | 1683 | 1971 | 2976 | 549 | 610 | 721 | 267 | 285 | 310 | 154 | 160 | 168 |
| *** | 7794 | 9701 | 19209 | 1800 | 2261 | 2998 | 576 | 655 | 711 | 275 | 296 | 295 | 157 | 164 | 153 |
| 0.7 *** | 6373 | 7380 | 17471 | 1526 | 1803 | 2718 | 497 | 552 | 647 | 237 | 253 | 273 | 134 | 139 | 146 |
| *** | 6743 | 8759 | 17625 | 1640 | 2075 | 2724 | 521 | 591 | 634 | 244 | 262 | 257 | 137 | 142 | 129 |
| 0.75 *** | 5344 | 6399 | 15532 | 1351 | 1605 | 2385 | 434 | 479 | 555 | 201 | 213 | 228 | 110 | 114 | 118 |
| *** | 5743 | 7754 | 15612 | 1456 | 1846 | 2381 | 454 | 511 | 540 | 207 | 220 | 212 | 112 | 116 | 101 |
| 0.8 *** | 4398 | 5420 | 13140 | 1154 | 1371 | 1981 | 358 | 392 | 445 | 158 | 166 | 175 | . | . | . |
| *** | 4792 | 6673 | 13172 | 1245 | 1570 | 1970 | 374 | 415 | 429 | 162 | 171 | 158 | . | . | . |
| 0.85 *** | 3509 | 4415 | 10300 | 928 | 1094 | 1505 | 267 | 288 | 317 | . | . | . | . | . | . |
| *** | 3863 | 5481 | 10303 | 998 | 1237 | 1491 | 276 | 301 | 300 | . | . | . | . | . | . |
| 0.9 *** | 2610 | 3310 | 7018 | 654 | 754 | 959 | . | . | . | . | . | . | . | . | . |
| *** | 2887 | 4094 | 7006 | 697 | 833 | 943 | . | . | . | . | . | . | . | . | . |
| 0.95 *** | 1550 | 1928 | 3297 | . | . | . | . | . | . | . | . | . | . | . | . |
| *** | 1705 | 2308 | 3280 | . | . | . | . | . | . | . | . | . | . | . | . |

TABLE 8: ALPHA= 0.05  POWER= 0.9    EXPECTED ACCRUAL THRU MINIMUM FOLLOW-UP= 700

| | | DEL=.02 | | | DEL=.05 | | | DEL=.10 | | | DEL=.15 | | | DEL=.20 | | |
|---|---|---|---|---|---|---|---|---|---|---|---|---|---|---|---|---|
| FACT= | | 1.0 .75 | .50 .25 | .00 BIN | 1.0 .75 | .50 .25 | .00 BIN | 1.0 .75 | .50 .25 | .00 BIN | 1.0 75 | .50 .25 | .00 BIN | 1.0 .75 | .50 .25 | .00 BIN |
| PCONT=*** | | | | | REQUIRED | NUMBER OF | PATIENTS | | | | | | | | | |
| 0.05 | *** | 2443 | 2457 | 2580 | 525 | 533 | 547 | 190 | 192 | 194 | 112 | 113 | 114 | 79 | 79 | 80 |
| | *** | 2448 | 2482 | 4822 | 528 | 539 | 943 | 191 | 193 | 300 | 112 | 113 | 158 | 79 | 79 | 101 |
| 0.1 | *** | 5083 | 5118 | 5668 | 966 | 990 | 1055 | 310 | 317 | 326 | 167 | 170 | 173 | 111 | 112 | 114 |
| | *** | 5095 | 5185 | 8376 | 976 | 1013 | 1491 | 313 | 320 | 429 | 169 | 171 | 212 | 111 | 113 | 129 |
| 0.15 | *** | 7429 | 7490 | 8766 | 1348 | 1395 | 1547 | 412 | 425 | 446 | 214 | 219 | 225 | 137 | 139 | 142 |
| | *** | 7450 | 7610 | 11502 | 1366 | 1444 | 1970 | 418 | 435 | 540 | 216 | 222 | 257 | 138 | 141 | 153 |
| 0.2 | *** | 9301 | 9395 | 11647 | 1653 | 1727 | 1996 | 496 | 517 | 554 | 253 | 260 | 270 | 158 | 162 | 166 |
| | *** | 9332 | 9581 | 14199 | 1682 | 1810 | 2381 | 506 | 533 | 634 | 256 | 265 | 295 | 160 | 163 | 172 |
| 0.25 | *** | 10650 | 10785 | 14201 | 1880 | 1985 | 2388 | 561 | 592 | 645 | 282 | 293 | 308 | 175 | 179 | 185 |
| | *** | 10695 | 11052 | 16469 | 1920 | 2103 | 2724 | 575 | 614 | 711 | 288 | 300 | 326 | 177 | 182 | 187 |
| 0.3 | *** | 11485 | 11670 | 16367 | 2032 | 2170 | 2715 | 609 | 648 | 719 | 305 | 318 | 337 | 187 | 192 | 199 |
| | *** | 11546 | 12035 | 18310 | 2085 | 2326 | 2998 | 626 | 677 | 771 | 311 | 327 | 349 | 189 | 196 | 197 |
| 0.35 | *** | 11842 | 12089 | 18108 | 2117 | 2289 | 2973 | 640 | 688 | 775 | 319 | 335 | 358 | 194 | 201 | 209 |
| | *** | 11925 | 12571 | 19723 | 2183 | 2482 | 3203 | 661 | 723 | 814 | .327 | 345 | 364 | 197 | 205 | 204 |
| 0.4 | *** | 11777 | 12098 | 19404 | 2144 | 2350 | 3159 | 656 | 711 | 812 | 327 | 345 | 371 | 197 | 205 | 214 |
| | *** | 11884 | 12719 | 20708 | 2224 | 2576 | 3340 | 681 | 752 | 840 | 335 | 357 | 372 | 201 | 209 | 206 |
| 0.45 | *** | 11353 | 11766 | 20243 | 2122 | 2359 | 3272 | 660 | 719 | 831 | 327 | 347 | 375 | 196 | 205 | 215 |
| | *** | 11491 | 12544 | 21265 | 2215 | 2614 | 3409 | 686 | 765 | 848 | 337 | 360 | 372 | 200 | 209 | 204 |
| 0.5 | *** | 10641 | 11165 | 20619 | 2061 | 2324 | 3310 | 650 | 713 | 831 | 322 | 342 | 372 | 192 | 200 | 210 |
| | *** | 10817 | 12114 | 21393 | 2165 | 2601 | 3409 | 678 | 761 | 840 | 331 | 355 | 364 | 195 | 205 | 197 |
| 0.55 | *** | 9716 | 10372 | 20529 | 1969 | 2250 | 3273 | 629 | 694 | 813 | 310 | 331 | 359 | 183 | 191 | 201 |
| | *** | 9939 | 11491 | 21093 | 2081 | 2541 | 3340 | 658 | 742 | 814 | 320 | 344 | 349 | 187 | 196 | 187 |
| 0.6 | *** | 8658 | 9462 | 19973 | 1851 | 2142 | 3162 | 598 | 661 | 776 | 293 | 312 | 339 | 171 | 178 | 187 |
| | *** | 8937 | 10729 | 20365 | 1969 | 2437 | 3203 | 626 | 708 | 771 | 302 | 324 | 326 | 174 | 182 | 172 |
| 0.65 | *** | 7550 | 8494 | 18952 | 1713 | 2003 | 2977 | 556 | 615 | 721 | 269 | 286 | 310 | 155 | 161 | 169 |
| | *** | 7888 | 9866 | 19209 | 1831 | 2291 | 2998 | 582 | 659 | 711 | 277 | 297 | 295 | 158 | 165 | 153 |
| 0.7 | *** | 6462 | 7511 | 17470 | 1555 | 1833 | 2718 | 503 | 556 | 647 | 239 | 254 | 273 | 135 | 140 | 145 |
| | *** | 6850 | 8926 | 17625 | 1669 | 2102 | 2724 | 527 | 594 | 634 | 246 | 263 | 257 | 137 | 142 | 129 |
| 0.75 | *** | 5441 | 6530 | 15532 | 1378 | 1632 | 2385 | 439 | 483 | 555 | 203 | 214 | 228 | 110 | 114 | 118 |
| | *** | 5854 | 7914 | 15612 | 1483 | 1870 | 2381 | 459 | 514 | 540 | 208 | 221 | 212 | 112 | 116 | 101 |
| 0.8 | *** | 4496 | 5544 | 13140 | 1178 | 1394 | 1981 | 362 | 395 | 445 | 159 | 166 | 175 | . | . | . |
| | *** | 4901 | 6818 | 13172 | 1268 | 1589 | 1970 | 377 | 417 | 429 | 163 | 171 | 158 | . | . | . |
| 0.85 | *** | 3596 | 4522 | 10300 | 946 | 1111 | 1506 | 270 | 289 | 317 | . | . | . | . | . | . |
| | *** | 3959 | 5601 | 10303 | 1016 | 1251 | 1491 | 279 | 302 | 300 | . | . | . | . | . | . |
| 0.9 | *** | 2679 | 3391 | 7018 | 665 | 763 | 959 | . | . | . | . | . | . | . | . | . |
| | *** | 2962 | 4181 | 7006 | 708 | 840 | 943 | . | . | . | . | . | . | . | . | . |
| 0.95 | *** | 1589 | 1969 | 3297 | . | . | . | . | . | . | . | . | . | . | . | . |
| | *** | 1745 | 2347 | 3280 | . | . | . | . | . | . | . | . | . | . | . | . |

## TABLE 8: ALPHA= 0.05  POWER= 0.9    EXPECTED ACCRUAL THRU MINIMUM FOLLOW-UP= 750

| | | DEL=.02 | | | DEL=.05 | | | DEL=.10 | | | DEL=.15 | | | DEL=.20 | | |
|---|---|---|---|---|---|---|---|---|---|---|---|---|---|---|---|---|
| | FACT= | 1.0 .75 | .50 .25 | .00 BIN | 1.0 .75 | .50 .25 | .00 BIN | 1.0 .75 | .50 .25 | .00 BIN | 1.0 75 | .50 .25 | .00 BIN | 1.0 .75 | .50 .25 | .00 BIN |
| PCONT=*** | | | | | REQUIRED NUMBER OF PATIENTS | | | | | | | | | | | |
| 0.05 | *** | 2444 | 2459 | 2580 | 526 | 533 | 547 | 190 | 192 | 195 | 112 | 113 | 114 | 79 | 79 | 80 |
| | *** | 2449 | 2485 | 4822 | 529 | 539 | 943 | 191 | 193 | 300 | 112 | 113 | 158 | 79 | 79 | 101 |
| 0.1 | *** | 5086 | 5123 | 5668 | 968 | 993 | 1055 | 310 | 317 | 326 | 168 | 170 | 173 | 111 | 112 | 114 |
| | *** | 5098 | 5194 | 8376 | 978 | 1015 | 1491 | 313 | 321 | 429 | 169 | 171 | 212 | 112 | 113 | 129 |
| 0.15 | *** | 7433 | 7499 | 8766 | 1352 | 1399 | 1547 | 414 | 427 | 446 | 215 | 220 | 225 | 138 | 139 | 142 |
| | *** | 7455 | 7627 | 11502 | 1370 | 1449 | 1970 | 420 | 435 | 540 | 217 | 222 | 257 | 139 | 141 | 153 |
| 0.2 | *** | 9308 | 9408 | 11647 | 1660 | 1735 | 1996 | 499 | 519 | 553 | 253 | 261 | 270 | 159 | 162 | 166 |
| | *** | 9341 | 9607 | 14199 | 1689 | 1818 | 2381 | 508 | 534 | 634 | 257 | 265 | 295 | 160 | 164 | 172 |
| 0.25 | *** | 10660 | 10804 | 14201 | 1889 | 1997 | 2388 | 565 | 594 | 645 | 284 | 294 | 308 | 175 | 180 | 185 |
| | *** | 10708 | 11089 | 16469 | 1930 | 2115 | 2724 | 578 | 615 | 711 | 289 | 300 | 326 | 177 | 182 | 187 |
| 0.3 | *** | 11498 | 11696 | 16367 | 2044 | 2185 | 2715 | 613 | 651 | 719 | 306 | 319 | 337 | 187 | 193 | 199 |
| | *** | 11564 | 12085 | 18310 | 2099 | 2341 | 2998 | 630 | 679 | 771 | 312 | 327 | 349 | 190 | 196 | 197 |
| 0.35 | *** | 11860 | 12124 | 18108 | 2132 | 2308 | 2974 | 645 | 692 | 775 | 321 | 337 | 358 | 195 | 201 | 209 |
| | *** | 11948 | 12637 | 19723 | 2200 | 2501 | 3203 | 666 | 726 | 814 | 328 | 346 | 364 | 198 | 205 | 204 |
| 0.4 | *** | 11800 | 12144 | 19404 | 2162 | 2372 | 3160 | 663 | 715 | 812 | 329 | 346 | 371 | 198 | 205 | 214 |
| | *** | 11915 | 12803 | 20708 | 2245 | 2599 | 3340 | 686 | 755 | 840 | 337 | 357 | 372 | 201 | 209 | 206 |
| 0.45 | *** | 11383 | 11824 | 20243 | 2143 | 2384 | 3272 | 666 | 724 | 831 | 330 | 349 | 375 | 198 | 205 | 214 |
| | *** | 11530 | 12647 | 21265 | 2239 | 2639 | 3409 | 692 | 768 | 848 | 339 | 361 | 372 | 201 | 209 | 204 |
| 0.5 | *** | 10678 | 11239 | 20619 | 2085 | 2352 | 3310 | 657 | 719 | 832 | 325 | 344 | 371 | 193 | 200 | 210 |
| | *** | 10867 | 12235 | 21393 | 2192 | 2628 | 3409 | 684 | 765 | 840 | 334 | 356 | 364 | 196 | 205 | 197 |
| 0.55 | *** | 9764 | 10462 | 20529 | 1995 | 2280 | 3273 | 636 | 700 | 814 | 313 | 332 | 359 | 184 | 191 | 201 |
| | *** | 10002 | 11629 | 21093 | 2110 | 2569 | 3340 | 664 | 746 | 814 | 322 | 344 | 349 | 188 | 196 | 187 |
| 0.6 | *** | 8719 | 9567 | 19972 | 1879 | 2172 | 3162 | 605 | 667 | 776 | 295 | 313 | 339 | 172 | 179 | 187 |
| | *** | 9015 | 10879 | 20365 | 1998 | 2464 | 3203 | 632 | 712 | 771 | 304 | 325 | 326 | 175 | 183 | 172 |
| 0.65 | *** | 7624 | 8612 | 18952 | 1740 | 2032 | 2976 | 562 | 620 | 721 | 271 | 288 | 310 | 155 | 161 | 169 |
| | *** | 7980 | 10024 | 18952 | 1860 | 2317 | 2998 | 589 | 662 | 711 | 279 | 298 | 295 | 158 | 165 | 153 |
| 0.7 | *** | 6549 | 7636 | 17470 | 1582 | 1861 | 2718 | 509 | 561 | 647 | 241 | 255 | 273 | 135 | 140 | 145 |
| | *** | 6953 | 9084 | 17625 | 1697 | 2126 | 2724 | 532 | 597 | 634 | 248 | 263 | 257 | 138 | 143 | 129 |
| 0.75 | *** | 5535 | 6655 | 15532 | 1403 | 1656 | 2386 | 444 | 487 | 555 | 204 | 215 | 228 | 111 | 114 | 118 |
| | *** | 5962 | 8065 | 15612 | 1508 | 1891 | 2381 | 464 | 516 | 540 | 209 | 221 | 212 | 113 | 116 | 101 |
| 0.8 | *** | 4589 | 5662 | 13140 | 1199 | 1414 | 1981 | 366 | 398 | 445 | 160 | 167 | 175 | . | . | . |
| | *** | 5004 | 6955 | 13172 | 1290 | 1606 | 1970 | 381 | 419 | 429 | 163 | 171 | 158 | . | . | . |
| 0.85 | *** | 3680 | 4623 | 10300 | 963 | 1126 | 1505 | 272 | 291 | 317 | . | . | . | . | . | . |
| | *** | 4050 | 5714 | 10303 | 1032 | 1263 | 1491 | 281 | 303 | 300 | . | . | . | . | . | . |
| 0.9 | *** | 2745 | 3467 | 7018 | 676 | 772 | 959 | . | . | . | . | . | . | . | . | . |
| | *** | 3033 | 4261 | 7006 | 718 | 846 | 943 | . | . | . | . | . | . | . | . | . |
| 0.95 | *** | 1626 | 2008 | 3297 | . | . | . | . | . | . | . | . | . | . | . | . |
| | *** | 1783 | 2382 | 3280 | . | . | . | . | . | . | . | . | . | . | . | . |

TABLE 8: ALPHA= 0.05  POWER= 0.9     EXPECTED ACCRUAL THRU MINIMUM FOLLOW-UP= 800

| | DEL=.02 | | | DEL=.05 | | | DEL=.10 | | | DEL=.15 | | | DEL=.20 | | |
|---|---|---|---|---|---|---|---|---|---|---|---|---|---|---|---|
| FACT= | 1.0 .75 | .50 .25 | .00 BIN | 1.0 .75 | .50 .25 | .00 BIN | 1.0 .75 | .50 .25 | .00 BIN | 1.0 75 | .50 .25 | .00 BIN | 1.0 .75 | .50 .25 | .00 BIN |

PCONT=***                    REQUIRED NUMBER OF PATIENTS

| PCONT | | .02 1.0/.75 | .02 .50/.25 | .02 .00/BIN | .05 1.0/.75 | .05 .50/.25 | .05 .00/BIN | .10 1.0/.75 | .10 .50/.25 | .10 .00/BIN | .15 1.0/.75 | .15 .50/.25 | .15 .00/BIN | .20 1.0/.75 | .20 .50/.25 | .20 .00/BIN |
|---|---|---|---|---|---|---|---|---|---|---|---|---|---|---|---|---|
| 0.05 | *** | 2445 | 2461 | 2580 | 527 | 534 | 547 | 191 | 192 | 195 | 112 | 113 | 114 | 79 | 79 | 80 |
| | *** | 2450 | 2488 | 4822 | 530 | 540 | 943 | 191 | 193 | 300 | 112 | 113 | 158 | 79 | 80 | 101 |
| 0.1 | *** | 5088 | 5128 | 5668 | 970 | 995 | 1055 | 311 | 317 | 326 | 168 | 170 | 173 | 111 | 112 | 113 |
| | *** | 5101 | 5203 | 8376 | 980 | 1018 | 1491 | 314 | 321 | 429 | 169 | 172 | 212 | 112 | 113 | 129 |
| 0.15 | *** | 7438 | 7507 | 8766 | 1356 | 1404 | 1547 | 415 | 428 | 447 | 215 | 220 | 225 | 138 | 140 | 142 |
| | *** | 7461 | 7643 | 11502 | 1375 | 1453 | 1970 | 421 | 436 | 540 | 217 | 222 | 257 | 139 | 141 | 153 |
| 0.2 | *** | 9314 | 9422 | 11647 | 1666 | 1743 | 1996 | 501 | 521 | 554 | 254 | 261 | 270 | 159 | 162 | 166 |
| | *** | 9350 | 9632 | 14199 | 1696 | 1825 | 2381 | 510 | 535 | 634 | 258 | 265 | 295 | 161 | 164 | 172 |
| 0.25 | *** | 10669 | 10823 | 14201 | 1898 | 2008 | 2388 | 568 | 597 | 645 | 285 | 295 | 308 | 176 | 180 | 185 |
| | *** | 10721 | 11126 | 16469 | 1940 | 2125 | 2724 | 581 | 617 | 711 | 290 | 301 | 326 | 178 | 182 | 187 |
| 0.3 | *** | 11511 | 11723 | 16367 | 2056 | 2200 | 2715 | 617 | 654 | 719 | 308 | 320 | 337 | 188 | 193 | 199 |
| | *** | 11582 | 12135 | 18310 | 2112 | 2355 | 2998 | 634 | 681 | 771 | 314 | 328 | 349 | 190 | 196 | 197 |
| 0.35 | *** | 11878 | 12159 | 18108 | 2147 | 2326 | 2973 | 650 | 695 | 775 | 323 | 338 | 358 | 196 | 202 | 209 |
| | *** | 11972 | 12703 | 19723 | 2217 | 2518 | 3203 | 670 | 728 | 814 | 330 | 347 | 364 | 198 | 205 | 204 |
| 0.4 | *** | 11823 | 12190 | 19404 | 2180 | 2393 | 3159 | 668 | 720 | 812 | 331 | 348 | 371 | 199 | 206 | 214 |
| | *** | 11946 | 12885 | 20708 | 2264 | 2619 | 3340 | 691 | 758 | 840 | 339 | 358 | 372 | 202 | 210 | 206 |
| 0.45 | *** | 11412 | 11883 | 20243 | 2164 | 2408 | 3272 | 672 | 729 | 831 | 332 | 350 | 375 | 198 | 206 | 215 |
| | *** | 11570 | 12746 | 21265 | 2261 | 2662 | 3409 | 697 | 771 | 848 | 340 | 362 | 372 | 202 | 210 | 204 |
| 0.5 | *** | 10716 | 11311 | 20619 | 2108 | 2378 | 3310 | 663 | 724 | 832 | 327 | 345 | 372 | 194 | 201 | 210 |
| | *** | 10917 | 12352 | 21393 | 2217 | 2652 | 3409 | 690 | 768 | 840 | 335 | 357 | 364 | 197 | 205 | 197 |
| 0.55 | *** | 9812 | 10550 | 20529 | 2020 | 2307 | 3273 | 643 | 705 | 813 | 315 | 334 | 359 | 185 | 192 | 201 |
| | *** | 10065 | 11761 | 21093 | 2136 | 2594 | 3340 | 670 | 750 | 814 | 324 | 345 | 349 | 188 | 196 | 187 |
| 0.6 | *** | 8779 | 9670 | 19973 | 1905 | 2200 | 3162 | 611 | 672 | 776 | 297 | 315 | 339 | 173 | 179 | 187 |
| | *** | 9092 | 11023 | 20365 | 2025 | 2490 | 3203 | 638 | 715 | 771 | 305 | 326 | 326 | 176 | 183 | 172 |
| 0.65 | *** | 7697 | 8726 | 18952 | 1767 | 2060 | 2977 | 568 | 625 | 721 | 273 | 289 | 310 | 156 | 162 | 169 |
| | *** | 8071 | 10173 | 19209 | 1887 | 2342 | 2998 | 594 | 665 | 711 | 280 | 299 | 295 | 159 | 165 | 153 |
| 0.7 | *** | 6634 | 7757 | 17471 | 1608 | 1887 | 2718 | 515 | 565 | 647 | 243 | 256 | 273 | 136 | 140 | 146 |
| | *** | 7053 | 9234 | 17625 | 1723 | 2149 | 2724 | 537 | 600 | 634 | 249 | 264 | 257 | 138 | 143 | 129 |
| 0.75 | *** | 5626 | 6776 | 15532 | 1426 | 1680 | 2386 | 449 | 490 | 555 | 206 | 216 | 228 | 111 | 115 | 118 |
| | *** | 6065 | 8208 | 15612 | 1532 | 1911 | 2381 | 468 | 518 | 540 | 210 | 222 | 212 | 113 | 116 | 101 |
| 0.8 | *** | 4678 | 5774 | 13140 | 1220 | 1434 | 1981 | 370 | 400 | 445 | 161 | 168 | 175 | . | . | . |
| | *** | 5104 | 7083 | 13172 | 1310 | 1622 | 1970 | 384 | 420 | 429 | 164 | 171 | 158 | . | . | . |
| 0.85 | *** | 3761 | 4720 | 10300 | 979 | 1140 | 1506 | 274 | 292 | 317 | . | . | . | . | . | . |
| | *** | 4138 | 5821 | 10303 | 1048 | 1274 | 1491 | 283 | 304 | 300 | . | . | . | . | . | . |
| 0.9 | *** | 2808 | 3539 | 7018 | 686 | 780 | 959 | . | . | . | . | . | . | . | . | . |
| | *** | 3099 | 4336 | 7006 | 727 | 852 | 943 | . | . | . | . | . | . | . | . | . |
| 0.95 | *** | 1661 | 2044 | 3297 | . | . | . | . | . | . | . | . | . | . | . | . |
| | *** | 1818 | 2415 | 3280 | . | . | . | . | . | . | . | . | . | . | . | . |

TABLE 8: ALPHA= 0.05  POWER= 0.9     EXPECTED ACCRUAL THRU MINIMUM FOLLOW-UP= 850

| | | DEL=.02 | | | DEL=.05 | | | DEL=.10 | | | DEL=.15 | | | DEL=.20 | | |
|---|---|---|---|---|---|---|---|---|---|---|---|---|---|---|---|---|---|
| FACT= | | 1.0 .75 | .50 .25 | .00 BIN | 1.0 .75 | .50 .25 | .00 BIN | 1.0 .75 | .50 .25 | .00 BIN | 1.0 75 | .50 .25 | .00 BIN | 1.0 .75 | .50 .25 | .00 BIN |
| PCONT=*** | | REQUIRED NUMBER OF PATIENTS | | | | | | | | | | | | | | |
| 0.05 | *** | 2446 | 2463 | 2580 | 528 | 535 | 547 | 191 | 192 | 195 | 112 | 113 | 113 | 79 | 79 | 80 |
| | *** | 2452 | 2490 | 4822 | 530 | 540 | 943 | 191 | 193 | 300 | 112 | 113 | 158 | 79 | 80 | 101 |
| 0.1 | *** | 5091 | 5133 | 5668 | 972 | 997 | 1055 | 312 | 318 | 326 | 168 | 170 | 173 | 111 | 112 | 113 |
| | *** | 5105 | 5211 | 8376 | 983 | 1019 | 1491 | 315 | 322 | 429 | 169 | 172 | 212 | 112 | 113 | 129 |
| 0.15 | *** | 7442 | 7516 | 8766 | 1360 | 1409 | 1547 | 416 | 428 | 446 | 216 | 220 | 225 | 138 | 140 | 142 |
| | *** | 7467 | 7659 | 11502 | 1379 | 1457 | 1970 | 422 | 436 | 540 | 218 | 222 | 257 | 139 | 141 | 153 |
| 0.2 | *** | 9321 | 9435 | 11647 | 1672 | 1751 | 1995 | 503 | 522 | 554 | 255 | 261 | 270 | 159 | 162 | 166 |
| | *** | 9359 | 9658 | 14199 | 1703 | 1831 | 2381 | 512 | 536 | 634 | 258 | 266 | 295 | 161 | 164 | 172 |
| 0.25 | *** | 10679 | 10843 | 14201 | 1906 | 2018 | 2388 | 570 | 598 | 645 | 286 | 295 | 308 | 176 | 180 | 185 |
| | *** | 10733 | 11162 | 16469 | 1950 | 2135 | 2724 | 583 | 618 | 711 | 290 | 301 | 326 | 178 | 182 | 187 |
| 0.3 | *** | 11525 | 11749 | 16367 | 2067 | 2213 | 2715 | 621 | 657 | 718 | 309 | 321 | 337 | 188 | 193 | 199 |
| | *** | 11599 | 12184 | 18310 | 2124 | 2368 | 2998 | 637 | 683 | 771 | 315 | 328 | 349 | 191 | 196 | 197 |
| 0.35 | *** | 11895 | 12194 | 18108 | 2161 | 2343 | 2974 | 654 | 699 | 775 | 324 | 339 | 358 | 196 | 202 | 209 |
| | *** | 11995 | 12767 | 19723 | 2232 | 2534 | 3203 | 674 | 731 | 814 | 331 | 348 | 364 | 199 | 205 | 204 |
| 0.4 | *** | 11846 | 12235 | 19404 | 2197 | 2413 | 3160 | 673 | 724 | 813 | 333 | 349 | 371 | 200 | 206 | 214 |
| | *** | 11976 | 12965 | 20708 | 2282 | 2637 | 3340 | 696 | 761 | 840 | 340 | 359 | 372 | 203 | 210 | 206 |
| 0.45 | *** | 11442 | 11940 | 20244 | 2184 | 2431 | 3272 | 678 | 733 | 832 | 334 | 351 | 375 | 199 | 206 | 214 |
| | *** | 11609 | 12843 | 21265 | 2282 | 2683 | 3409 | 702 | 774 | 848 | 342 | 362 | 372 | 203 | 210 | 204 |
| 0.5 | *** | 10754 | 11383 | 20619 | 2130 | 2402 | 3310 | 669 | 729 | 832 | 328 | 346 | 372 | 195 | 202 | 210 |
| | *** | 10967 | 12465 | 21393 | 2240 | 2675 | 3409 | 696 | 771 | 840 | 337 | 358 | 364 | 198 | 205 | 197 |
| 0.55 | *** | 9860 | 10637 | 20529 | 2044 | 2333 | 3273 | 649 | 709 | 814 | 317 | 335 | 359 | 186 | 192 | 201 |
| | *** | 10127 | 11888 | 21093 | 2161 | 2618 | 3340 | 675 | 752 | 814 | 325 | 346 | 349 | 189 | 197 | 187 |
| 0.6 | *** | 8839 | 9770 | 19973 | 1930 | 2227 | 3162 | 617 | 676 | 776 | 299 | 316 | 339 | 173 | 180 | 187 |
| | *** | 9168 | 11161 | 20365 | 2051 | 2514 | 3203 | 644 | 718 | 771 | 307 | 326 | 326 | 176 | 183 | 172 |
| 0.65 | *** | 7770 | 8837 | 18952 | 1792 | 2086 | 2976 | 574 | 629 | 720 | 275 | 290 | 310 | 157 | 162 | 169 |
| | *** | 8159 | 10317 | 19209 | 1913 | 2365 | 2998 | 599 | 668 | 711 | 282 | 299 | 295 | 159 | 165 | 153 |
| 0.7 | *** | 6716 | 7873 | 17471 | 1632 | 1911 | 2718 | 520 | 569 | 647 | 244 | 257 | 273 | 136 | 140 | 146 |
| | *** | 7150 | 9376 | 17625 | 1748 | 2170 | 2724 | 542 | 602 | 634 | 250 | 264 | 257 | 138 | 143 | 129 |
| 0.75 | *** | 5714 | 6890 | 15532 | 1448 | 1701 | 2385 | 453 | 493 | 555 | 206 | 216 | 228 | 112 | 115 | 118 |
| | *** | 6164 | 8344 | 15612 | 1554 | 1929 | 2381 | 471 | 520 | 540 | 211 | 222 | 212 | 113 | 117 | 101 |
| 0.8 | *** | 4764 | 5881 | 13140 | 1239 | 1451 | 1981 | 373 | 402 | 445 | 162 | 168 | 175 | . | . | . |
| | *** | 5199 | 7205 | 13172 | 1329 | 1636 | 1970 | 386 | 422 | 429 | 165 | 171 | 158 | . | . | . |
| 0.85 | *** | 3837 | 4811 | 10301 | 994 | 1153 | 1506 | 276 | 293 | 317 | . | . | . | . | . | . |
| | *** | 4221 | 5921 | 10303 | 1062 | 1284 | 1491 | 284 | 305 | 300 | . | . | . | . | . | . |
| 0.9 | *** | 2868 | 3607 | 7018 | 695 | 787 | 959 | . | . | . | . | . | . | . | . | . |
| | *** | 3163 | 4406 | 7006 | 735 | 856 | 943 | . | . | . | . | . | . | . | . | . |
| 0.95 | *** | 1694 | 2077 | 3297 | . | . | . | . | . | . | . | . | . | . | . | . |
| | *** | 1852 | 2446 | 3280 | . | . | . | . | . | . | . | . | . | . | . | . |

TABLE 8: ALPHA= 0.05  POWER= 0.9    EXPECTED ACCRUAL THRU MINIMUM FOLLOW-UP= 900

| | | DEL=.02 | | | DEL=.05 | | | DEL=.10 | | | DEL=.15 | | | DEL=.20 | | |
|---|---|---|---|---|---|---|---|---|---|---|---|---|---|---|---|---|---|
| FACT= | | 1.0 | .50 | .00 | 1.0 | .50 | .00 | 1.0 | .50 | .00 | 1.0 | .50 | .00 | 1.0 | .50 | .00 |
| | | .75 | .25 | BIN | .75 | .25 | BIN | .75 | .25 | BIN | 75 | .25 | BIN | .75 | .25 | BIN |
| PCONT=*** | | | | REQUIRED NUMBER OF PATIENTS | | | | | | | | | | | | |
| 0.05 | *** | 2447 | 2465 | 2580 | 528 | 535 | 548 | 191 | 192 | 195 | 112 | 113 | 113 | 79 | 80 | 80 |
| | *** | 2453 | 2493 | 4822 | 531 | 540 | 943 | 192 | 194 | 300 | 113 | 113 | 158 | 80 | 80 | 101 |
| 0.1 | *** | 5093 | 5138 | 5668 | 974 | 999 | 1055 | 312 | 318 | 326 | 168 | 171 | 173 | 111 | 112 | 113 |
| | *** | 5108 | 5220 | 8376 | 984 | 1020 | 1491 | 315 | 322 | 429 | 170 | 172 | 212 | 112 | 113 | 129 |
| 0.15 | *** | 7446 | 7525 | 8766 | 1363 | 1413 | 1547 | 417 | 429 | 447 | 216 | 220 | 225 | 138 | 140 | 142 |
| | *** | 7472 | 7675 | 11502 | 1383 | 1460 | 1970 | 423 | 437 | 540 | 218 | 222 | 257 | 139 | 141 | 153 |
| 0.2 | *** | 9327 | 9449 | 11647 | 1677 | 1757 | 1995 | 505 | 524 | 554 | 255 | 262 | 270 | 160 | 163 | 165 |
| | *** | 9368 | 9683 | 14199 | 1709 | 1837 | 2381 | 513 | 537 | 634 | 259 | 266 | 295 | 161 | 164 | 172 |
| 0.25 | *** | 10689 | 10862 | 14201 | 1914 | 2028 | 2388 | 573 | 600 | 645 | 287 | 296 | 308 | 177 | 180 | 185 |
| | *** | 10746 | 11198 | 16469 | 1959 | 2144 | 2724 | 585 | 620 | 711 | 291 | 301 | 326 | 179 | 182 | 187 |
| 0.3 | *** | 11538 | 11775 | 16367 | 2078 | 2226 | 2715 | 624 | 660 | 719 | 310 | 322 | 337 | 189 | 194 | 199 |
| | *** | 11617 | 12233 | 18310 | 2136 | 2380 | 2998 | 640 | 685 | 771 | 316 | 329 | 349 | 191 | 197 | 197 |
| 0.35 | *** | 11913 | 12229 | 18108 | 2174 | 2359 | 2973 | 658 | 702 | 775 | 326 | 339 | 358 | 197 | 203 | 209 |
| | *** | 12018 | 12830 | 19723 | 2248 | 2549 | 3203 | 678 | 732 | 814 | 332 | 348 | 364 | 199 | 206 | 204 |
| 0.4 | *** | 11870 | 12281 | 19404 | 2213 | 2432 | 3159 | 677 | 728 | 812 | 334 | 350 | 371 | 200 | 207 | 214 |
| | *** | 12007 | 13043 | 20708 | 2301 | 2655 | 3340 | 700 | 763 | 840 | 342 | 360 | 372 | 203 | 210 | 206 |
| 0.45 | *** | 11471 | 11998 | 20243 | 2203 | 2452 | 3272 | 683 | 738 | 831 | 335 | 352 | 375 | 200 | 207 | 215 |
| | *** | 11648 | 12938 | 21265 | 2303 | 2702 | 3409 | 707 | 777 | 848 | 343 | 363 | 372 | 203 | 210 | 204 |
| 0.5 | *** | 10792 | 11454 | 20619 | 2152 | 2425 | 3310 | 675 | 732 | 831 | 330 | 348 | 371 | 195 | 202 | 210 |
| | *** | 11017 | 12575 | 21393 | 2262 | 2696 | 3409 | 701 | 774 | 840 | 339 | 359 | 364 | 198 | 206 | 197 |
| 0.55 | *** | 9908 | 10722 | 20529 | 2067 | 2357 | 3273 | 654 | 713 | 813 | 318 | 336 | 359 | 186 | 193 | 201 |
| | *** | 10190 | 12011 | 21093 | 2186 | 2640 | 3340 | 681 | 756 | 814 | 327 | 347 | 349 | 190 | 197 | 187 |
| 0.6 | *** | 8898 | 9868 | 19972 | 1954 | 2251 | 3162 | 622 | 680 | 776 | 300 | 317 | 339 | 174 | 180 | 187 |
| | *** | 9243 | 11293 | 20365 | 2076 | 2536 | 3203 | 648 | 721 | 771 | 308 | 327 | 326 | 177 | 183 | 172 |
| 0.65 | *** | 7841 | 8945 | 18952 | 1816 | 2109 | 2976 | 579 | 633 | 721 | 276 | 291 | 310 | 158 | 163 | 168 |
| | *** | 8245 | 10454 | 19209 | 1937 | 2386 | 2998 | 603 | 671 | 711 | 283 | 300 | 295 | 160 | 165 | 153 |
| 0.7 | *** | 6797 | 7985 | 17471 | 1655 | 1934 | 2718 | 524 | 572 | 647 | 245 | 258 | 273 | 137 | 141 | 145 |
| | *** | 7244 | 9513 | 17625 | 1771 | 2190 | 2724 | 546 | 604 | 634 | 251 | 265 | 257 | 138 | 143 | 129 |
| 0.75 | *** | 5799 | 7001 | 15532 | 1469 | 1721 | 2386 | 457 | 496 | 555 | 208 | 217 | 228 | 112 | 115 | 118 |
| | *** | 6260 | 8473 | 15612 | 1575 | 1946 | 2381 | 475 | 522 | 540 | 212 | 222 | 212 | 113 | 117 | 101 |
| 0.8 | *** | 4847 | 5984 | 13140 | 1257 | 1468 | 1981 | 375 | 404 | 445 | 162 | 168 | 175 | . | . | . |
| | *** | 5290 | 7320 | 13172 | 1346 | 1649 | 1970 | 389 | 423 | 429 | 165 | 172 | 158 | . | . | . |
| 0.85 | *** | 3911 | 4898 | 10301 | 1007 | 1165 | 1505 | 278 | 295 | 317 | . | . | . | . | . | . |
| | *** | 4301 | 6016 | 10303 | 1075 | 1293 | 1491 | 286 | 305 | 300 | . | . | . | . | . | . |
| 0.9 | *** | 2925 | 3672 | 7018 | 703 | 794 | 959 | . | . | . | . | . | . | . | . | . |
| | *** | 3224 | 4473 | 7006 | 743 | 861 | 943 | . | . | . | . | . | . | . | . | . |
| 0.95 | *** | 1725 | 2109 | 3297 | . | . | . | . | . | . | . | . | . | . | . | . |
| | *** | 1883 | 2474 | 3280 | . | . | . | . | . | . | . | . | . | . | . | . |

TABLE 8: ALPHA= 0.05  POWER= 0.9    EXPECTED ACCRUAL THRU MINIMUM FOLLOW-UP= 950

| | | DEL=.02 | | | DEL=.05 | | | DEL=.10 | | | DEL=.15 | | | DEL=.20 | |
|---|---|---|---|---|---|---|---|---|---|---|---|---|---|---|---|---|
| FACT= | 1.0 .75 | .50 .25 | .00 BIN | 1.0 .75 | .50 .25 | .00 BIN | 1.0 .75 | .50 .25 | .00 BIN | 1.0 75 | .50 .25 | .00 BIN | 1.0 .75 | .50 .25 | .00 BIN |
| PCONT=*** | | | | | REQUIRED NUMBER OF PATIENTS | | | | | | | | | | |
| 0.05 *** | 2448 | 2466 | 2580 | 528 | 536 | 547 | 191 | 192 | 194 | 112 | 113 | 114 | 79 | 80 | 80 |
| *** | 2454 | 2495 | 4822 | 532 | 540 | 943 | 192 | 194 | 300 | 112 | 113 | 158 | 79 | 80 | 101 |
| 0.1 *** | 5096 | 5143 | 5668 | 976 | 1001 | 1055 | 313 | 318 | 326 | 169 | 171 | 173 | 112 | 112 | 114 |
| *** | 5111 | 5227 | 8376 | 986 | 1022 | 1491 | 315 | 322 | 429 | 169 | 172 | 212 | 112 | 113 | 129 |
| 0.15 *** | 7450 | 7533 | 8766 | 1367 | 1417 | 1547 | 419 | 430 | 447 | 217 | 220 | 225 | 139 | 140 | 142 |
| *** | 7478 | 7690 | 11502 | 1387 | 1464 | 1970 | 424 | 438 | 540 | 219 | 223 | 257 | 139 | 141 | 153 |
| 0.2 *** | 9335 | 9462 | 11647 | 1683 | 1764 | 1996 | 506 | 525 | 553 | 256 | 262 | 270 | 160 | 163 | 166 |
| *** | 9377 | 9707 | 14199 | 1716 | 1843 | 2381 | 515 | 538 | 634 | 259 | 266 | 295 | 161 | 164 | 172 |
| 0.25 *** | 10698 | 10881 | 14201 | 1923 | 2037 | 2388 | 576 | 602 | 644 | 287 | 296 | 308 | 177 | 181 | 185 |
| *** | 10759 | 11233 | 16469 | 1968 | 2153 | 2724 | 587 | 621 | 711 | 292 | 302 | 326 | 179 | 182 | 187 |
| 0.3 *** | 11551 | 11801 | 16367 | 2088 | 2238 | 2715 | 627 | 662 | 718 | 311 | 323 | 337 | 190 | 194 | 200 |
| *** | 11635 | 12281 | 18310 | 2148 | 2392 | 2998 | 642 | 686 | 771 | 317 | 329 | 349 | 191 | 197 | 197 |
| 0.35 *** | 11930 | 12264 | 18108 | 2187 | 2374 | 2973 | 662 | 704 | 774 | 327 | 340 | 358 | 197 | 203 | 209 |
| *** | 12042 | 12891 | 19723 | 2262 | 2563 | 3203 | 681 | 735 | 814 | 333 | 349 | 364 | 200 | 205 | 204 |
| 0.4 *** | 11892 | 12326 | 19405 | 2229 | 2450 | 3160 | 682 | 730 | 812 | 336 | 351 | 371 | 201 | 207 | 214 |
| *** | 12037 | 13120 | 20708 | 2318 | 2671 | 3340 | 704 | 766 | 840 | 343 | 360 | 372 | 204 | 210 | 206 |
| 0.45 *** | 11501 | 12055 | 20243 | 2221 | 2472 | 3272 | 687 | 741 | 831 | 337 | 353 | 375 | 200 | 207 | 215 |
| *** | 11687 | 13030 | 21265 | 2322 | 2721 | 3409 | 711 | 779 | 848 | 345 | 363 | 372 | 203 | 210 | 204 |
| 0.5 *** | 10830 | 11524 | 20619 | 2172 | 2447 | 3310 | 679 | 736 | 831 | 332 | 349 | 371 | 196 | 202 | 210 |
| *** | 11066 | 12681 | 21393 | 2284 | 2716 | 3409 | 705 | 777 | 840 | 340 | 359 | 364 | 199 | 206 | 197 |
| 0.55 *** | 9955 | 10805 | 20528 | 2089 | 2380 | 3273 | 659 | 717 | 813 | 320 | 337 | 359 | 187 | 193 | 201 |
| *** | 10251 | 12130 | 21093 | 2208 | 2660 | 3340 | 685 | 758 | 814 | 328 | 348 | 349 | 190 | 197 | 187 |
| 0.6 *** | 8957 | 9963 | 19973 | 1976 | 2274 | 3162 | 628 | 684 | 776 | 302 | 318 | 338 | 175 | 180 | 187 |
| *** | 9317 | 11421 | 20365 | 2099 | 2556 | 3203 | 653 | 723 | 771 | 310 | 328 | 326 | 177 | 184 | 172 |
| 0.65 *** | 7911 | 9049 | 18952 | 1838 | 2132 | 2977 | 584 | 637 | 721 | 277 | 292 | 310 | 158 | 163 | 169 |
| *** | 8330 | 10585 | 19209 | 1960 | 2405 | 2998 | 608 | 673 | 711 | 285 | 300 | 295 | 160 | 166 | 153 |
| 0.7 *** | 6876 | 8093 | 17471 | 1676 | 1955 | 2718 | 528 | 575 | 647 | 247 | 258 | 273 | 137 | 141 | 146 |
| *** | 7335 | 9643 | 17625 | 1793 | 2208 | 2724 | 549 | 606 | 634 | 252 | 266 | 257 | 139 | 143 | 129 |
| 0.75 *** | 5881 | 7107 | 15532 | 1489 | 1740 | 2385 | 460 | 498 | 555 | 209 | 217 | 228 | 112 | 115 | 118 |
| *** | 6353 | 8596 | 15612 | 1595 | 1961 | 2381 | 478 | 523 | 540 | 213 | 222 | 212 | 114 | 116 | 101 |
| 0.8 *** | 4927 | 6081 | 13140 | 1274 | 1484 | 1982 | 378 | 406 | 445 | 163 | 169 | 175 | . | . | . |
| *** | 5378 | 7431 | 13172 | 1363 | 1662 | 1970 | 391 | 424 | 429 | 166 | 172 | 158 | . | . | . |
| 0.85 *** | 3982 | 4982 | 10300 | 1020 | 1176 | 1505 | 279 | 296 | 317 | . | . | . | . | . | . |
| *** | 4377 | 6106 | 10303 | 1088 | 1302 | 1491 | 287 | 306 | 300 | . | . | . | . | . | . |
| 0.9 *** | 2979 | 3733 | 7018 | 711 | 800 | 959 | . | . | . | . | . | . | . | . | . |
| *** | 3282 | 4535 | 7006 | 751 | 866 | 943 | . | . | . | . | . | . | . | . | . |
| 0.95 *** | 1755 | 2139 | 3297 | . | . | . | . | . | . | . | . | . | . | . | . |
| *** | 1914 | 2500 | 3280 | . | . | . | . | . | . | . | . | . | . | . | . |

## TABLE 8: ALPHA= 0.05  POWER= 0.9    EXPECTED ACCRUAL THRU MINIMUM FOLLOW-UP= 1000

| | DEL=.02 | | | DEL=.05 | | | DEL=.10 | | | DEL=.15 | | | DEL=.20 | | |
|---|---|---|---|---|---|---|---|---|---|---|---|---|---|---|---|
| FACT= | 1.0 / .75 | .50 / .25 | .00 / BIN | 1.0 / .75 | .50 / .25 | .00 / BIN | 1.0 / .75 | .50 / .25 | .00 / BIN | 1.0 / 75 | .50 / .25 | .00 / BIN | 1.0 / .75 | .50 / .25 | .00 / BIN |
| PCONT=*** | | | | | | | REQUIRED NUMBER OF PATIENTS | | | | | | | | |
| 0.05 *** | 2449 | 2469 | 2580 | 530 | 536 | 547 | 191 | 193 | 195 | 112 | 113 | 113 | 80 | 80 | 80 |
|      *** | 2456 | 2497 | 4822 | 532 | 541 | 943 | 192 | 194 | 300 | 113 | 113 | 158 | 80 | 80 | 101 |
| 0.1 *** | 5098 | 5147 | 5668 | 978 | 1003 | 1055 | 313 | 319 | 326 | 169 | 171 | 173 | 111 | 113 | 113 |
|     *** | 5115 | 5236 | 8376 | 988 | 1023 | 1491 | 316 | 322 | 429 | 170 | 172 | 212 | 112 | 113 | 129 |
| 0.15 *** | 7455 | 7542 | 8766 | 1371 | 1421 | 1547 | 420 | 431 | 446 | 217 | 221 | 225 | 138 | 140 | 142 |
|      *** | 7484 | 7706 | 11502 | 1391 | 1467 | 1970 | 425 | 438 | 540 | 219 | 223 | 257 | 139 | 141 | 153 |
| 0.2 *** | 9341 | 9475 | 11647 | 1689 | 1770 | 1996 | 508 | 526 | 553 | 257 | 263 | 270 | 160 | 163 | 166 |
|     *** | 9386 | 9731 | 14199 | 1721 | 1848 | 2381 | 516 | 538 | 634 | 260 | 266 | 295 | 161 | 165 | 172 |
| 0.25 *** | 10708 | 10900 | 14201 | 1930 | 2046 | 2388 | 578 | 604 | 645 | 288 | 297 | 308 | 178 | 181 | 185 |
|      *** | 10772 | 11268 | 16469 | 1976 | 2160 | 2724 | 590 | 622 | 711 | 293 | 302 | 326 | 179 | 183 | 187 |
| 0.3 *** | 11564 | 11828 | 16367 | 2099 | 2250 | 2715 | 630 | 665 | 719 | 312 | 323 | 337 | 190 | 195 | 200 |
|     *** | 11652 | 12328 | 18310 | 2160 | 2402 | 2998 | 645 | 688 | 771 | 318 | 330 | 349 | 192 | 197 | 197 |
| 0.35 *** | 11948 | 12299 | 18108 | 2201 | 2389 | 2973 | 666 | 707 | 775 | 328 | 341 | 358 | 198 | 203 | 209 |
|      *** | 12065 | 12952 | 19723 | 2276 | 2576 | 3203 | 685 | 736 | 814 | 335 | 349 | 364 | 200 | 206 | 204 |
| 0.4 *** | 11915 | 12371 | 19405 | 2245 | 2467 | 3160 | 686 | 734 | 812 | 337 | 351 | 371 | 201 | 207 | 214 |
|     *** | 12068 | 13196 | 20708 | 2334 | 2686 | 3340 | 708 | 768 | 840 | 344 | 361 | 372 | 205 | 211 | 206 |
| 0.45 *** | 11531 | 12111 | 20243 | 2239 | 2491 | 3272 | 691 | 745 | 831 | 339 | 355 | 375 | 201 | 207 | 215 |
|      *** | 11727 | 13120 | 21265 | 2341 | 2738 | 3409 | 715 | 781 | 848 | 346 | 364 | 372 | 204 | 211 | 204 |
| 0.5 *** | 10867 | 11593 | 20619 | 2191 | 2468 | 3310 | 685 | 740 | 831 | 333 | 350 | 371 | 196 | 203 | 210 |
|     *** | 11116 | 12785 | 21393 | 2305 | 2735 | 3409 | 710 | 779 | 840 | 341 | 360 | 364 | 200 | 206 | 197 |
| 0.55 *** | 10002 | 10888 | 20529 | 2110 | 2401 | 3273 | 665 | 721 | 813 | 322 | 338 | 360 | 188 | 194 | 201 |
|      *** | 10312 | 12245 | 21093 | 2230 | 2680 | 3340 | 690 | 760 | 814 | 330 | 348 | 349 | 191 | 197 | 187 |
| 0.6 *** | 9015 | 10057 | 19973 | 1998 | 2296 | 3162 | 632 | 688 | 776 | 303 | 319 | 339 | 175 | 181 | 187 |
|     *** | 9390 | 11543 | 20365 | 2121 | 2575 | 3203 | 657 | 726 | 771 | 311 | 328 | 326 | 178 | 184 | 172 |
| 0.65 *** | 7980 | 9150 | 18952 | 1860 | 2154 | 2976 | 588 | 640 | 721 | 279 | 293 | 310 | 158 | 163 | 168 |
|      *** | 8413 | 10712 | 19209 | 1982 | 2424 | 2998 | 611 | 675 | 711 | 285 | 301 | 295 | 161 | 166 | 153 |
| 0.7 *** | 6953 | 8198 | 17471 | 1697 | 1975 | 2718 | 533 | 578 | 647 | 248 | 259 | 273 | 138 | 141 | 146 |
|     *** | 7425 | 9768 | 17625 | 1813 | 2225 | 2724 | 553 | 608 | 634 | 253 | 266 | 257 | 140 | 143 | 129 |
| 0.75 *** | 5961 | 7210 | 15532 | 1508 | 1758 | 2386 | 464 | 501 | 555 | 210 | 218 | 228 | 113 | 115 | 118 |
|      *** | 6443 | 8715 | 15612 | 1614 | 1976 | 2381 | 481 | 525 | 540 | 213 | 223 | 212 | 114 | 116 | 101 |
| 0.8 *** | 5005 | 6176 | 13140 | 1290 | 1498 | 1981 | 381 | 408 | 445 | 163 | 169 | 175 | . | . | . |
|     *** | 5463 | 7536 | 13172 | 1379 | 1673 | 1970 | 393 | 425 | 429 | 166 | 172 | 158 | . | . | . |
| 0.85 *** | 4050 | 5062 | 10300 | 1033 | 1187 | 1506 | 281 | 297 | 317 | . | . | . | . | . | . |
|      *** | 4451 | 6191 | 10303 | 1100 | 1309 | 1491 | 288 | 306 | 300 | . | . | . | . | . | . |
| 0.9 *** | 3033 | 3791 | 7018 | 718 | 806 | 959 | . | . | . | . | . | . | . | . | . |
|     *** | 3338 | 4594 | 7006 | 757 | 870 | 943 | . | . | . | . | . | . | . | . | . |
| 0.95 *** | 1783 | 2167 | 3297 | . | . | . | . | . | . | . | . | . | . | . | . |
|      *** | 1943 | 2525 | 3280 | . | . | . | . | . | . | . | . | . | . | . | . |

# TABLE 8: ALPHA= 0.05  POWER= 0.9    EXPECTED ACCRUAL THRU MINIMUM FOLLOW-UP= 1100

| | | DEL=.02 | | | DEL=.05 | | | DEL=.10 | | | DEL=.15 | | | DEL=.20 | | |
|---|---|---|---|---|---|---|---|---|---|---|---|---|---|---|---|---|
| FACT= | | 1.0 .75 | .50 .25 | .00 BIN | 1.0 .75 | .50 .25 | .00 BIN | 1.0 .75 | .50 .25 | .00 BIN | 1.0 75 | .50 .25 | .00 BIN | 1.0 .75 | .50 .25 | .00 BIN |

PCONT=***    REQUIRED NUMBER OF PATIENTS

| PCONT | DEL.02 a | b | c | DEL.05 a | b | c | DEL.10 a | b | c | DEL.15 a | b | c | DEL.20 a | b | c |
|---|---|---|---|---|---|---|---|---|---|---|---|---|---|---|---|
| 0.05 | 2451 | 2472 | 2580 | 530 | 537 | 547 | 191 | 192 | 195 | 112 | 113 | 114 | 79 | 80 | 80 |
| | 2458 | 2501 | 4822 | 533 | 541 | 943 | 192 | 194 | 300 | 113 | 113 | 158 | 79 | 80 | 101 |
| 0.1 | 5103 | 5157 | 5668 | 981 | 1006 | 1055 | 314 | 319 | 326 | 169 | 170 | 173 | 111 | 113 | 114 |
| | 5121 | 5251 | 8376 | 992 | 1026 | 1491 | 317 | 323 | 429 | 170 | 172 | 212 | 112 | 113 | 129 |
| 0.15 | 7463 | 7559 | 8766 | 1377 | 1427 | 1547 | 422 | 432 | 446 | 217 | 221 | 225 | 139 | 140 | 142 |
| | 7496 | 7735 | 11502 | 1398 | 1473 | 1970 | 426 | 439 | 540 | 219 | 223 | 257 | 140 | 141 | 153 |
| 0.2 | 9354 | 9502 | 11647 | 1699 | 1781 | 1996 | 511 | 528 | 554 | 258 | 263 | 270 | 161 | 163 | 166 |
| | 9404 | 9779 | 14199 | 1732 | 1858 | 2381 | 518 | 540 | 634 | 261 | 267 | 295 | 162 | 164 | 172 |
| 0.25 | 10727 | 10938 | 14201 | 1945 | 2062 | 2388 | 582 | 607 | 644 | 290 | 298 | 307 | 178 | 181 | 185 |
| | 10798 | 11336 | 16469 | 1992 | 2175 | 2724 | 593 | 624 | 711 | 294 | 302 | 326 | 180 | 183 | 187 |
| 0.3 | 11591 | 11880 | 16367 | 2118 | 2272 | 2715 | 635 | 668 | 719 | 314 | 324 | 337 | 191 | 195 | 199 |
| | 11687 | 12420 | 18310 | 2180 | 2421 | 2998 | 650 | 690 | 771 | 319 | 330 | 349 | 192 | 197 | 197 |
| 0.35 | 11983 | 12368 | 18108 | 2225 | 2415 | 2974 | 672 | 712 | 775 | 330 | 342 | 358 | 199 | 203 | 209 |
| | 12112 | 13069 | 19723 | 2302 | 2600 | 3203 | 690 | 739 | 814 | 336 | 350 | 364 | 201 | 206 | 204 |
| 0.4 | 11961 | 12460 | 19404 | 2274 | 2498 | 3159 | 693 | 739 | 812 | 339 | 353 | 371 | 202 | 208 | 214 |
| | 12129 | 13341 | 20708 | 2365 | 2714 | 3340 | 714 | 771 | 840 | 346 | 362 | 372 | 205 | 211 | 206 |
| 0.45 | 11589 | 12223 | 20244 | 2272 | 2527 | 3272 | 700 | 750 | 831 | 341 | 356 | 375 | 202 | 208 | 214 |
| | 11805 | 13293 | 21265 | 2376 | 2769 | 3409 | 723 | 785 | 848 | 348 | 365 | 372 | 205 | 211 | 204 |
| 0.5 | 10942 | 11730 | 20619 | 2228 | 2506 | 3310 | 693 | 746 | 832 | 336 | 351 | 371 | 197 | 203 | 210 |
| | 11214 | 12983 | 21393 | 2342 | 2768 | 3409 | 717 | 783 | 840 | 343 | 361 | 364 | 200 | 206 | 197 |
| 0.55 | 10097 | 11047 | 20529 | 2149 | 2441 | 3273 | 673 | 727 | 813 | 324 | 340 | 359 | 188 | 195 | 201 |
| | 10432 | 12464 | 21093 | 2270 | 2714 | 3340 | 698 | 764 | 814 | 331 | 349 | 349 | 191 | 197 | 187 |
| 0.6 | 9131 | 10237 | 19973 | 2039 | 2337 | 3162 | 641 | 694 | 776 | 306 | 320 | 339 | 176 | 181 | 187 |
| | 9532 | 11776 | 20365 | 2162 | 2610 | 3203 | 665 | 730 | 771 | 313 | 329 | 326 | 178 | 184 | 172 |
| 0.65 | 8115 | 9344 | 18952 | 1900 | 2193 | 2976 | 596 | 646 | 720 | 281 | 294 | 310 | 159 | 164 | 169 |
| | 8573 | 10950 | 19209 | 2023 | 2457 | 2998 | 619 | 679 | 711 | 287 | 301 | 295 | 161 | 166 | 153 |
| 0.7 | 7102 | 8397 | 17471 | 1735 | 2012 | 2718 | 540 | 583 | 647 | 250 | 260 | 273 | 138 | 142 | 146 |
| | 7595 | 10003 | 17625 | 1852 | 2255 | 2724 | 559 | 611 | 634 | 254 | 266 | 257 | 140 | 144 | 129 |
| 0.75 | 6115 | 7403 | 15532 | 1544 | 1790 | 2386 | 470 | 505 | 555 | 210 | 219 | 228 | 113 | 115 | 118 |
| | 6615 | 8936 | 15612 | 1648 | 2002 | 2381 | 486 | 527 | 540 | 214 | 224 | 212 | 114 | 117 | 101 |
| 0.8 | 5152 | 6353 | 13140 | 1319 | 1525 | 1981 | 385 | 411 | 445 | 164 | 169 | 175 | . | . | . |
| | 5623 | 7732 | 13172 | 1407 | 1694 | 1970 | 397 | 426 | 429 | 167 | 172 | 158 | . | . | . |
| 0.85 | 4180 | 5212 | 10300 | 1055 | 1206 | 1506 | 283 | 298 | 317 | . | . | . | . | . | . |
| | 4590 | 6351 | 10303 | 1121 | 1323 | 1491 | 290 | 307 | 300 | . | . | . | . | . | . |
| 0.9 | 3132 | 3901 | 7017 | 731 | 816 | 959 | . | . | . | . | . | . | . | . | . |
| | 3442 | 4702 | 7006 | 769 | 876 | 943 | . | . | . | . | . | . | . | . | . |
| 0.95 | 1835 | 2219 | 3297 | . | . | . | . | . | . | . | . | . | . | . | . |
| | 1995 | 2569 | 3280 | . | . | . | . | . | . | . | . | . | . | . | . |

TABLE 8: ALPHA= 0.05  POWER= 0.9     EXPECTED ACCRUAL THRU MINIMUM FOLLOW-UP= 1200

| | DEL=.02 | | | DEL=.05 | | | DEL=.10 | | | DEL=.15 | | | DEL=.20 | | |
|---|---|---|---|---|---|---|---|---|---|---|---|---|---|---|---|
| FACT= | 1.0 .75 | .50 .25 | .00 BIN | 1.0 .75 | .50 .25 | .00 BIN | 1.0 .75 | .50 .25 | .00 BIN | 1.0 75 | .50 .25 | .00 BIN | 1.0 .75 | .50 .25 | .00 BIN |
| PCONT=*** | | | | REQUIRED NUMBER OF PATIENTS | | | | | | | | | | | |
| 0.05 *** | 2453 | 2476 | 2580 | 531 | 538 | 547 | 192 | 193 | 194 | 112 | 112 | 113 | 79 | 79 | 79 |
| *** | 2461 | 2505 | 4822 | 534 | 541 | 943 | 192 | 193 | 300 | 112 | 113 | 158 | 79 | 79 | 101 |
| 0.1 *** | 5108 | 5166 | 5668 | 985 | 1009 | 1055 | 315 | 319 | 325 | 169 | 171 | 172 | 112 | 112 | 113 |
| *** | 5128 | 5265 | 8376 | 995 | 1027 | 1491 | 317 | 322 | 429 | 170 | 172 | 212 | 112 | 113 | 129 |
| 0.15 *** | 7472 | 7576 | 8766 | 1383 | 1434 | 1546 | 423 | 433 | 446 | 218 | 221 | 225 | 139 | 140 | 142 |
| *** | 7507 | 7764 | 11502 | 1404 | 1477 | 1970 | 427 | 439 | 540 | 220 | 223 | 257 | 139 | 141 | 153 |
| 0.2 *** | 9368 | 9528 | 11647 | 1709 | 1792 | 1996 | 513 | 530 | 553 | 259 | 264 | 270 | 161 | 163 | 166 |
| *** | 9421 | 9824 | 14199 | 1743 | 1867 | 2381 | 521 | 541 | 634 | 261 | 267 | 295 | 162 | 164 | 172 |
| 0.25 *** | 10746 | 10976 | 14201 | 1959 | 2077 | 2388 | 585 | 610 | 644 | 291 | 298 | 307 | 178 | 181 | 185 |
| *** | 10823 | 11401 | 16469 | 2008 | 2187 | 2724 | 596 | 625 | 711 | 295 | 303 | 326 | 180 | 183 | 187 |
| 0.3 *** | 11617 | 11932 | 16366 | 2137 | 2292 | 2715 | 640 | 671 | 718 | 316 | 325 | 337 | 191 | 195 | 199 |
| *** | 11722 | 12508 | 18310 | 2200 | 2437 | 2998 | 654 | 692 | 771 | 320 | 331 | 349 | 193 | 197 | 197 |
| 0.35 *** | 12018 | 12436 | 18108 | 2248 | 2440 | 2973 | 678 | 716 | 775 | 332 | 343 | 358 | 199 | 204 | 209 |
| *** | 12159 | 13183 | 19723 | 2326 | 2620 | 3203 | 695 | 742 | 814 | 337 | 350 | 364 | 202 | 206 | 204 |
| 0.4 *** | 12007 | 12547 | 19404 | 2300 | 2527 | 3159 | 700 | 744 | 812 | 341 | 355 | 370 | 203 | 208 | 214 |
| *** | 12190 | 13480 | 20708 | 2393 | 2739 | 3340 | 720 | 774 | 840 | 347 | 362 | 372 | 205 | 211 | 206 |
| 0.45 *** | 11648 | 12332 | 20243 | 2303 | 2558 | 3271 | 707 | 756 | 831 | 343 | 358 | 375 | 202 | 208 | 214 |
| *** | 11882 | 13456 | 21265 | 2408 | 2797 | 3409 | 729 | 789 | 848 | 350 | 366 | 372 | 205 | 211 | 204 |
| 0.5 *** | 11017 | 11861 | 20619 | 2263 | 2541 | 3310 | 700 | 751 | 832 | 338 | 353 | 371 | 198 | 204 | 210 |
| *** | 11311 | 13169 | 21393 | 2377 | 2797 | 3409 | 724 | 787 | 840 | 345 | 361 | 364 | 201 | 207 | 197 |
| 0.55 *** | 10189 | 11200 | 20528 | 2185 | 2478 | 3273 | 680 | 733 | 813 | 327 | 341 | 359 | 190 | 195 | 201 |
| *** | 10550 | 12668 | 21093 | 2307 | 2745 | 3340 | 704 | 768 | 814 | 334 | 349 | 349 | 192 | 198 | 187 |
| 0.6 *** | 9243 | 10408 | 19972 | 2076 | 2373 | 3162 | 648 | 699 | 776 | 308 | 322 | 339 | 177 | 181 | 187 |
| *** | 9670 | 11993 | 20365 | 2200 | 2641 | 3203 | 671 | 733 | 771 | 315 | 330 | 326 | 179 | 184 | 172 |
| 0.65 *** | 8245 | 9527 | 18952 | 1937 | 2229 | 2977 | 603 | 650 | 721 | 283 | 295 | 310 | 160 | 164 | 169 |
| *** | 8726 | 11172 | 19209 | 2059 | 2486 | 2998 | 625 | 682 | 711 | 289 | 302 | 295 | 162 | 166 | 153 |
| 0.7 *** | 7244 | 8583 | 17470 | 1771 | 2044 | 2717 | 546 | 587 | 646 | 251 | 261 | 273 | 139 | 142 | 145 |
| *** | 7756 | 10220 | 17625 | 1887 | 2281 | 2724 | 565 | 613 | 634 | 256 | 267 | 257 | 140 | 144 | 129 |
| 0.75 *** | 6260 | 7584 | 15532 | 1575 | 1819 | 2386 | 475 | 508 | 555 | 212 | 219 | 228 | 113 | 115 | 118 |
| *** | 6775 | 9139 | 15612 | 1679 | 2025 | 2381 | 490 | 529 | 540 | 215 | 223 | 212 | 115 | 117 | 101 |
| 0.8 *** | 5290 | 6518 | 13140 | 1346 | 1548 | 1981 | 388 | 413 | 445 | 165 | 170 | 175 | . | . | . |
| *** | 5774 | 7911 | 13172 | 1433 | 1711 | 1970 | 400 | 427 | 429 | 167 | 172 | 158 | . | . | . |
| 0.85 *** | 4300 | 5351 | 10300 | 1075 | 1222 | 1505 | 286 | 300 | 317 | . | . | . | . | . | . |
| *** | 4720 | 6496 | 10303 | 1140 | 1335 | 1491 | 292 | 307 | 300 | . | . | . | . | . | . |
| 0.9 *** | 3223 | 4002 | 7018 | 743 | 825 | 959 | . | . | . | . | . | . | . | . | . |
| *** | 3538 | 4801 | 7006 | 780 | 882 | 943 | . | . | . | . | . | . | . | . | . |
| 0.95 *** | 1883 | 2266 | 3297 | . | . | . | . | . | . | . | . | . | . | . | . |
| *** | 2044 | 2609 | 3280 | . | . | . | . | . | . | . | . | . | . | . | . |

## TABLE 8: ALPHA= 0.05  POWER= 0.9     EXPECTED ACCRUAL THRU MINIMUM FOLLOW-UP= 1300

| | | DEL=.02 | | | DEL=.05 | | | DEL=.10 | | | DEL=.15 | | | DEL=.20 | | |
|---|---|---|---|---|---|---|---|---|---|---|---|---|---|---|---|---|
| FACT= | | 1.0 .75 | .50 .25 | .00 BIN | 1.0 .75 | .50 .25 | .00 BIN | 1.0 .75 | .50 .25 | .00 BIN | 1.0 75 | .50 .25 | .00 BIN | 1.0 .75 | .50 .25 | .00 BIN |
| PCONT=*** | | | | REQUIRED NUMBER OF PATIENTS | | | | | | | | | | | | |
| 0.05 | *** | 2455 | 2479 | 2580 | 532 | 538 | 547 | 192 | 193 | 194 | 112 | 113 | 114 | 80 | 80 | 80 |
| | *** | 2463 | 2509 | 4822 | 535 | 542 | 943 | 193 | 194 | 300 | 113 | 113 | 158 | 80 | 80 | 101 |
| 0.1 | *** | 5113 | 5176 | 5668 | 987 | 1012 | 1056 | 316 | 320 | 326 | 170 | 172 | 173 | 112 | 113 | 114 |
| | *** | 5134 | 5279 | 8376 | 998 | 1030 | 1491 | 318 | 323 | 429 | 171 | 172 | 212 | 112 | 113 | 129 |
| 0.15 | *** | 7481 | 7593 | 8766 | 1389 | 1440 | 1547 | 424 | 434 | 447 | 219 | 222 | 225 | 139 | 141 | 142 |
| | *** | 7519 | 7791 | 11502 | 1410 | 1481 | 1970 | 429 | 440 | 540 | 220 | 224 | 257 | 140 | 141 | 153 |
| 0.2 | *** | 9381 | 9555 | 11647 | 1719 | 1801 | 1995 | 515 | 531 | 553 | 259 | 264 | 271 | 162 | 163 | 166 |
| | *** | 9440 | 9869 | 14199 | 1753 | 1874 | 2381 | 523 | 541 | 634 | 262 | 267 | 295 | 162 | 164 | 172 |
| 0.25 | *** | 10766 | 11014 | 14201 | 1972 | 2091 | 2388 | 588 | 612 | 644 | 292 | 299 | 308 | 179 | 182 | 185 |
| | *** | 10848 | 11465 | 16469 | 2021 | 2198 | 2724 | 600 | 627 | 711 | 296 | 303 | 326 | 180 | 184 | 187 |
| 0.3 | *** | 11643 | 11984 | 16367 | 2154 | 2310 | 2715 | 644 | 674 | 718 | 317 | 326 | 337 | 192 | 195 | 199 |
| | *** | 11758 | 12593 | 18310 | 2218 | 2453 | 2998 | 658 | 694 | 771 | 321 | 331 | 349 | 193 | 198 | 197 |
| 0.35 | *** | 12054 | 12504 | 18108 | 2269 | 2462 | 2973 | 682 | 720 | 774 | 334 | 344 | 358 | 200 | 204 | 209 |
| | *** | 12205 | 13292 | 19723 | 2348 | 2639 | 3203 | 700 | 744 | 814 | 339 | 351 | 364 | 202 | 206 | 204 |
| 0.4 | *** | 12053 | 12634 | 19404 | 2326 | 2553 | 3159 | 705 | 748 | 812 | 343 | 356 | 370 | 204 | 209 | 214 |
| | *** | 12250 | 13613 | 20708 | 2420 | 2761 | 3340 | 725 | 777 | 840 | 349 | 362 | 372 | 206 | 211 | 206 |
| 0.45 | *** | 11707 | 12439 | 20244 | 2332 | 2588 | 3272 | 713 | 760 | 831 | 345 | 359 | 375 | 204 | 209 | 214 |
| | *** | 11959 | 13613 | 21265 | 2438 | 2821 | 3409 | 734 | 791 | 848 | 352 | 367 | 372 | 206 | 211 | 204 |
| 0.5 | *** | 11092 | 11989 | 20619 | 2294 | 2572 | 3309 | 707 | 757 | 832 | 341 | 354 | 371 | 199 | 204 | 210 |
| | *** | 11407 | 13346 | 21393 | 2410 | 2824 | 3409 | 730 | 790 | 840 | 347 | 362 | 364 | 201 | 207 | 197 |
| 0.55 | *** | 10281 | 11349 | 20529 | 2219 | 2511 | 3273 | 687 | 738 | 813 | 329 | 342 | 359 | 190 | 195 | 201 |
| | *** | 10665 | 12861 | 21093 | 2341 | 2772 | 3340 | 710 | 771 | 814 | 336 | 350 | 349 | 193 | 198 | 187 |
| 0.6 | *** | 9353 | 10572 | 19972 | 2110 | 2407 | 3162 | 655 | 704 | 776 | 310 | 323 | 339 | 177 | 182 | 187 |
| | *** | 9803 | 12197 | 20365 | 2235 | 2668 | 3203 | 678 | 736 | 771 | 316 | 331 | 326 | 180 | 185 | 172 |
| 0.65 | *** | 8372 | 9701 | 18952 | 1971 | 2261 | 2976 | 609 | 655 | 721 | 285 | 297 | 310 | 160 | 164 | 168 |
| | *** | 8873 | 11378 | 19209 | 2094 | 2512 | 2998 | 630 | 684 | 711 | 290 | 303 | 295 | 162 | 167 | 153 |
| 0.7 | *** | 7380 | 8760 | 17470 | 1803 | 2074 | 2718 | 552 | 591 | 647 | 253 | 262 | 273 | 139 | 142 | 146 |
| | *** | 7910 | 10422 | 17625 | 1918 | 2305 | 2724 | 570 | 616 | 634 | 257 | 267 | 257 | 141 | 144 | 129 |
| 0.75 | *** | 6399 | 7754 | 15532 | 1605 | 1846 | 2385 | 479 | 511 | 555 | 213 | 220 | 228 | 114 | 115 | 118 |
| | *** | 6927 | 9327 | 15612 | 1708 | 2045 | 2381 | 494 | 531 | 540 | 216 | 224 | 212 | 115 | 117 | 101 |
| 0.8 | *** | 5420 | 6673 | 13140 | 1371 | 1570 | 1981 | 393 | 415 | 445 | 166 | 171 | 175 | . | . | . |
| | *** | 5916 | 8077 | 13172 | 1457 | 1727 | 1970 | 403 | 429 | 429 | 168 | 173 | 158 | . | . | . |
| 0.85 | *** | 4414 | 5480 | 10300 | 1094 | 1238 | 1506 | 288 | 301 | 317 | . | . | . | . | . | . |
| | *** | 4841 | 6629 | 10303 | 1157 | 1345 | 1491 | 294 | 309 | 300 | . | . | . | . | . | . |
| 0.9 | *** | 3310 | 4094 | 7018 | 754 | 833 | 959 | . | . | . | . | . | . | . | . | . |
| | *** | 3629 | 4891 | 7006 | 790 | 887 | 943 | . | . | . | . | . | . | . | . | . |
| 0.95 | *** | 1928 | 2308 | 3297 | . | . | . | . | . | . | . | . | . | . | . | . |
| | *** | 2088 | 2645 | 3280 | . | . | . | . | . | . | . | . | . | . | . | . |

TABLE 8: ALPHA= 0.05  POWER= 0.9     EXPECTED ACCRUAL THRU MINIMUM FOLLOW-UP= 1400

| | | DEL=.02 | | | DEL=.05 | | | DEL=.10 | | | DEL=.15 | | | DEL=.20 | |
|---|---|---|---|---|---|---|---|---|---|---|---|---|---|---|---|---|
| FACT= | 1.0 .75 | .50 .25 | .00 BIN | 1.0 .75 | .50 .25 | .00 BIN | 1.0 .75 | .50 .25 | .00 BIN | 1.0 75 | .50 .25 | .00 BIN | 1.0 .75 | .50 .25 | .00 BIN |
| PCONT=*** | | | REQUIRED NUMBER OF PATIENTS | | | | | | | | | | | | |
| 0.05 *** | 2457 | 2481 | 2580 | 533 | 539 | 547 | 192 | 193 | 194 | 113 | 113 | 114 | 80 | 80 | 80 |
| *** | 2466 | 2512 | 4822 | 535 | 542 | 943 | 192 | 194 | 300 | 113 | 113 | 158 | 80 | 80 | 101 |
| 0.1 *** | 5118 | 5185 | 5668 | 990 | 1013 | 1055 | 317 | 320 | 325 | 170 | 171 | 173 | 112 | 113 | 114 |
| *** | 5141 | 5291 | 8376 | 1000 | 1031 | 1491 | 318 | 323 | 429 | 171 | 172 | 212 | 112 | 113 | 129 |
| 0.15 *** | 7490 | 7610 | 8766 | 1395 | 1445 | 1547 | 425 | 435 | 446 | 219 | 222 | 225 | 139 | 141 | 142 |
| *** | 7530 | 7817 | 11502 | 1416 | 1485 | 1970 | 430 | 440 | 540 | 220 | 223 | 257 | 140 | 141 | 153 |
| 0.2 *** | 9395 | 9581 | 11647 | 1727 | 1809 | 1996 | 517 | 533 | 554 | 260 | 265 | 270 | 162 | 164 | 165 |
| *** | 9457 | 9911 | 14199 | 1761 | 1880 | 2381 | 525 | 542 | 634 | 262 | 268 | 295 | 163 | 164 | 172 |
| 0.25 *** | 10784 | 11052 | 14201 | 1984 | 2103 | 2388 | 591 | 613 | 645 | 293 | 300 | 308 | 179 | 182 | 185 |
| *** | 10874 | 11526 | 16469 | 2034 | 2208 | 2724 | 602 | 627 | 711 | 297 | 304 | 326 | 180 | 184 | 187 |
| 0.3 *** | 11670 | 12035 | 16367 | 2170 | 2327 | 2715 | 647 | 677 | 718 | 318 | 326 | 337 | 192 | 196 | 199 |
| *** | 11792 | 12675 | 18310 | 2235 | 2466 | 2998 | 661 | 696 | 771 | 322 | 332 | 349 | 194 | 198 | 197 |
| 0.35 *** | 12089 | 12571 | 18108 | 2289 | 2482 | 2973 | 688 | 723 | 774 | 335 | 346 | 358 | 200 | 205 | 209 |
| *** | 12252 | 13395 | 19723 | 2369 | 2656 | 3203 | 703 | 746 | 814 | 340 | 352 | 364 | 203 | 206 | 204 |
| 0.4 *** | 12099 | 12719 | 19404 | 2349 | 2576 | 3160 | 710 | 752 | 812 | 345 | 357 | 371 | 205 | 209 | 214 |
| *** | 12310 | 13739 | 20708 | 2444 | 2781 | 3340 | 730 | 779 | 840 | 351 | 363 | 372 | 206 | 212 | 206 |
| 0.45 *** | 11766 | 12544 | 20243 | 2359 | 2614 | 3272 | 719 | 765 | 831 | 347 | 360 | 375 | 205 | 209 | 214 |
| *** | 12036 | 13760 | 21265 | 2466 | 2844 | 3409 | 740 | 794 | 848 | 353 | 367 | 372 | 206 | 212 | 204 |
| 0.5 *** | 11165 | 12114 | 20619 | 2324 | 2601 | 3310 | 713 | 761 | 831 | 342 | 355 | 372 | 199 | 205 | 210 |
| *** | 11501 | 13513 | 21393 | 2440 | 2848 | 3409 | 735 | 793 | 840 | 348 | 363 | 364 | 202 | 207 | 197 |
| 0.55 *** | 10372 | 11491 | 20528 | 2250 | 2541 | 3273 | 694 | 742 | 813 | 331 | 344 | 360 | 191 | 196 | 200 |
| *** | 10777 | 13043 | 21093 | 2372 | 2796 | 3340 | 716 | 773 | 814 | 337 | 351 | 349 | 193 | 198 | 187 |
| 0.6 *** | 9461 | 10729 | 19973 | 2142 | 2437 | 3162 | 661 | 708 | 776 | 311 | 324 | 339 | 178 | 182 | 187 |
| *** | 9932 | 12387 | 20365 | 2267 | 2692 | 3203 | 682 | 738 | 771 | 318 | 331 | 326 | 180 | 185 | 172 |
| 0.65 *** | 8494 | 9866 | 18952 | 2003 | 2291 | 2977 | 615 | 659 | 721 | 286 | 297 | 310 | 161 | 164 | 169 |
| *** | 9014 | 11572 | 19209 | 2125 | 2536 | 2998 | 635 | 687 | 711 | 291 | 304 | 295 | 163 | 166 | 153 |
| 0.7 *** | 7511 | 8926 | 17470 | 1833 | 2102 | 2718 | 556 | 594 | 647 | 254 | 262 | 273 | 140 | 143 | 145 |
| *** | 8057 | 10610 | 17625 | 1948 | 2327 | 2724 | 574 | 618 | 634 | 258 | 268 | 257 | 141 | 144 | 129 |
| 0.75 *** | 6530 | 7913 | 15532 | 1632 | 1870 | 2385 | 483 | 514 | 555 | 214 | 220 | 228 | 114 | 116 | 118 |
| *** | 7072 | 9502 | 15612 | 1734 | 2063 | 2381 | 498 | 533 | 540 | 217 | 224 | 212 | 115 | 117 | 101 |
| 0.8 *** | 5544 | 6818 | 13140 | 1394 | 1589 | 1981 | 395 | 417 | 444 | 166 | 171 | 175 | . | . | . |
| *** | 6049 | 8231 | 13172 | 1479 | 1741 | 1970 | 405 | 430 | 429 | 169 | 173 | 158 | . | . | . |
| 0.85 *** | 4522 | 5601 | 10300 | 1110 | 1250 | 1506 | 290 | 302 | 317 | . | . | . | . | . | . |
| *** | 4954 | 6751 | 10303 | 1172 | 1354 | 1491 | 296 | 309 | 300 | . | . | . | . | . | . |
| 0.9 *** | 3391 | 4181 | 7017 | 763 | 840 | 959 | . | . | . | . | . | . | . | . | . |
| *** | 3713 | 4973 | 7006 | 798 | 892 | 943 | . | . | . | . | . | . | . | . | . |
| 0.95 *** | 1970 | 2347 | 3297 | . | . | . | . | . | . | . | . | . | . | . | . |
| *** | 2129 | 2676 | 3280 | . | . | . | . | . | . | . | . | . | . | . | . |

## TABLE 8: ALPHA= 0.05  POWER= 0.9    EXPECTED ACCRUAL THRU MINIMUM FOLLOW-UP= 1500

|  |  | DEL=.02 | | | DEL=.05 | | | DEL=.10 | | | DEL=.15 | | | DEL=.20 | | |
|---|---|---|---|---|---|---|---|---|---|---|---|---|---|---|---|---|
| FACT= | | 1.0 .75 | .50 .25 | .00 BIN | 1.0 .75 | .50 .25 | .00 BIN | 1.0 .75 | .50 .25 | .00 BIN | 1.0 75 | .50 .25 | .00 BIN | 1.0 .75 | .50 .25 | .00 BIN |
| PCONT=*** | | | | | REQUIRED NUMBER OF PATIENTS | | | | | | | | | | | |
| 0.05 | *** | 2459 | 2484 | 2580 | 533 | 539 | 547 | 192 | 193 | 195 | 112 | 113 | 113 | 80 | 80 | 80 |
|  | *** | 2468 | 2515 | 4822 | 536 | 543 | 943 | 193 | 194 | 300 | 112 | 113 | 158 | 80 | 80 | 101 |
| 0.1 | *** | 5122 | 5194 | 5668 | 993 | 1015 | 1055 | 317 | 320 | 326 | 170 | 172 | 172 | 112 | 112 | 113 |
|  | *** | 5147 | 5303 | 8376 | 1003 | 1032 | 1491 | 319 | 323 | 429 | 170 | 172 | 212 | 112 | 113 | 129 |
| 0.15 | *** | 7499 | 7627 | 8765 | 1400 | 1449 | 1547 | 427 | 435 | 446 | 219 | 222 | 225 | 140 | 140 | 142 |
|  | *** | 7542 | 7842 | 11502 | 1421 | 1489 | 1970 | 431 | 440 | 540 | 220 | 224 | 257 | 140 | 142 | 153 |
| 0.2 | *** | 9408 | 9607 | 11647 | 1735 | 1818 | 1996 | 519 | 534 | 553 | 260 | 265 | 270 | 162 | 164 | 166 |
|  | *** | 9475 | 9952 | 14199 | 1770 | 1886 | 2381 | 526 | 543 | 634 | 262 | 267 | 295 | 163 | 165 | 172 |
| 0.25 | *** | 10804 | 11089 | 14201 | 1997 | 2115 | 2388 | 594 | 615 | 645 | 294 | 300 | 307 | 180 | 182 | 185 |
|  | *** | 10900 | 11585 | 16469 | 2045 | 2217 | 2724 | 604 | 629 | 711 | 297 | 304 | 326 | 181 | 184 | 187 |
| 0.3 | *** | 11696 | 12085 | 16367 | 2185 | 2341 | 2715 | 652 | 680 | 719 | 319 | 327 | 337 | 193 | 196 | 200 |
|  | *** | 11827 | 12754 | 18310 | 2250 | 2478 | 2998 | 665 | 697 | 771 | 323 | 332 | 349 | 194 | 198 | 197 |
| 0.35 | *** | 12124 | 12637 | 18108 | 2308 | 2501 | 2974 | 692 | 725 | 774 | 337 | 346 | 358 | 202 | 205 | 209 |
|  | *** | 12299 | 13495 | 19723 | 2389 | 2671 | 3203 | 707 | 748 | 814 | 341 | 352 | 364 | 203 | 207 | 204 |
| 0.4 | *** | 12144 | 12802 | 19404 | 2372 | 2599 | 3159 | 715 | 755 | 812 | 346 | 357 | 371 | 205 | 209 | 214 |
|  | *** | 12370 | 13860 | 20708 | 2467 | 2798 | 3340 | 734 | 781 | 840 | 352 | 364 | 372 | 207 | 212 | 206 |
| 0.45 | *** | 11825 | 12647 | 20243 | 2384 | 2639 | 3272 | 725 | 768 | 832 | 349 | 361 | 375 | 205 | 209 | 215 |
|  | *** | 12112 | 13901 | 21265 | 2491 | 2863 | 3409 | 744 | 796 | 848 | 354 | 367 | 372 | 207 | 212 | 204 |
| 0.5 | *** | 11239 | 12234 | 20619 | 2352 | 2628 | 3309 | 719 | 765 | 832 | 344 | 356 | 371 | 200 | 205 | 210 |
|  | *** | 11593 | 13672 | 21393 | 2467 | 2870 | 3409 | 740 | 795 | 840 | 350 | 364 | 364 | 202 | 207 | 197 |
| 0.55 | *** | 10462 | 11629 | 20528 | 2280 | 2569 | 3273 | 699 | 746 | 814 | 332 | 344 | 359 | 191 | 196 | 200 |
|  | *** | 10887 | 13215 | 21093 | 2402 | 2819 | 3340 | 721 | 776 | 814 | 338 | 352 | 349 | 194 | 199 | 187 |
| 0.6 | *** | 9567 | 10879 | 19972 | 2172 | 2465 | 3162 | 667 | 712 | 776 | 313 | 325 | 338 | 179 | 183 | 187 |
|  | *** | 10057 | 12567 | 20365 | 2296 | 2715 | 3203 | 687 | 740 | 771 | 319 | 332 | 326 | 181 | 185 | 172 |
| 0.65 | *** | 8612 | 10024 | 18952 | 2032 | 2317 | 2977 | 620 | 662 | 721 | 288 | 298 | 310 | 161 | 165 | 169 |
|  | *** | 9150 | 11753 | 19209 | 2153 | 2557 | 2998 | 640 | 689 | 711 | 292 | 304 | 295 | 163 | 167 | 153 |
| 0.7 | *** | 7636 | 9083 | 17470 | 1861 | 2126 | 2718 | 560 | 597 | 647 | 255 | 263 | 273 | 140 | 142 | 145 |
|  | *** | 8197 | 10787 | 17625 | 1975 | 2345 | 2724 | 577 | 620 | 634 | 259 | 268 | 257 | 142 | 144 | 129 |
| 0.75 | *** | 6655 | 8065 | 15532 | 1657 | 1891 | 2386 | 487 | 517 | 555 | 215 | 221 | 228 | 114 | 116 | 118 |
|  | *** | 7209 | 9667 | 15612 | 1758 | 2079 | 2381 | 500 | 534 | 540 | 217 | 225 | 212 | 115 | 117 | 101 |
| 0.8 | *** | 5662 | 6954 | 13140 | 1415 | 1606 | 1981 | 397 | 419 | 445 | 167 | 170 | 175 | . | . | . |
|  | *** | 6175 | 8374 | 13172 | 1498 | 1754 | 1970 | 408 | 431 | 429 | 169 | 173 | 158 | . | . | . |
| 0.85 | *** | 4623 | 5714 | 10300 | 1126 | 1263 | 1505 | 290 | 303 | 317 | . | . | . | . | . | . |
|  | *** | 5062 | 6865 | 10303 | 1187 | 1363 | 1491 | 297 | 309 | 300 | . | . | . | . | . | . |
| 0.9 | *** | 3467 | 4261 | 7018 | 772 | 847 | 959 | . | . | . | . | . | . | . | . | . |
|  | *** | 3791 | 5047 | 7006 | 806 | 895 | 943 | . | . | . | . | . | . | . | . | . |
| 0.95 | *** | 2008 | 2382 | 3297 | . | . | . | . | . | . | . | . | . | . | . | . |
|  | *** | 2167 | 2705 | 3280 | . | . | . | . | . | . | . | . | . | . | . | . |

TABLE 8: ALPHA= 0.05  POWER= 0.9     EXPECTED ACCRUAL THRU MINIMUM FOLLOW-UP= 1600

| | | DEL=.02 | | | DEL=.05 | | | DEL=.10 | | | DEL=.15 | | | DEL=.20 | | |
|---|---|---|---|---|---|---|---|---|---|---|---|---|---|---|---|---|---|
| FACT= | | 1.0<br>.75 | .50<br>.25 | .00<br>BIN | 1.0<br>.75 | .50<br>.25 | .00<br>BIN | 1.0<br>.75 | .50<br>.25 | .00<br>BIN | 1.0<br>75 | .50<br>.25 | .00<br>BIN | 1.0<br>.75 | .50<br>.25 | .00<br>BIN |
| PCONT=*** | | | | | REQUIRED NUMBER OF PATIENTS | | | | | | | | | | | |
| 0.05 | ***<br>*** | 2461<br>2471 | 2488<br>2518 | 2580<br>4822 | 534<br>537 | 540<br>543 | 547<br>943 | 192<br>193 | 193<br>194 | 195<br>300 | 113<br>113 | 113<br>113 | 114<br>158 | 79<br>80 | 80<br>80 | 80<br>101 |
| 0.1 | ***<br>*** | 5128<br>5154 | 5203<br>5315 | 5668<br>8376 | 995<br>1005 | 1018<br>1034 | 1055<br>1491 | 317<br>319 | 321<br>324 | 326<br>429 | 170<br>171 | 172<br>172 | 173<br>212 | 112<br>113 | 113<br>113 | 113<br>129 |
| 0.15 | ***<br>*** | 7507<br>7553 | 7643<br>7866 | 8766<br>11502 | 1404<br>1426 | 1453<br>1491 | 1547<br>1970 | 428<br>432 | 436<br>441 | 447<br>540 | 220<br>221 | 222<br>224 | 225<br>257 | 140<br>140 | 141<br>141 | 142<br>153 |
| 0.2 | ***<br>*** | 9422<br>9493 | 9632<br>9991 | 11647<br>14199 | 1743<br>1778 | 1825<br>1892 | 1996<br>2381 | 521<br>528 | 535<br>544 | 554<br>634 | 261<br>263 | 265<br>268 | 270<br>295 | 162<br>163 | 164<br>165 | 166<br>172 |
| 0.25 | ***<br>*** | 10823<br>10926 | 11126<br>11641 | 14201<br>16469 | 2008<br>2057 | 2125<br>2225 | 2388<br>2724 | 597<br>606 | 617<br>630 | 645<br>711 | 295<br>298 | 301<br>304 | 308<br>326 | 180<br>181 | 182<br>184 | 185<br>187 |
| 0.3 | ***<br>*** | 11723<br>11863 | 12135<br>12829 | 16367<br>18310 | 2200<br>2265 | 2355<br>2489 | 2715<br>2998 | 654<br>667 | 681<br>698 | 719<br>771 | 320<br>324 | 328<br>332 | 337<br>349 | 193<br>195 | 196<br>198 | 199<br>197 |
| 0.35 | ***<br>*** | 12159<br>12345 | 12703<br>13591 | 18108<br>19723 | 2326<br>2407 | 2518<br>2685 | 2973<br>3203 | 695<br>711 | 728<br>749 | 775<br>814 | 338<br>342 | 347<br>352 | 358<br>364 | 202<br>203 | 205<br>207 | 209<br>204 |
| 0.4 | ***<br>*** | 12190<br>12430 | 12885<br>13975 | 19404<br>20708 | 2393<br>2488 | 2619<br>2815 | 3159<br>3340 | 720<br>738 | 758<br>783 | 812<br>840 | 348<br>353 | 358<br>364 | 371<br>372 | 206<br>208 | 210<br>212 | 214<br>206 |
| 0.45 | ***<br>*** | 11883<br>12186 | 12746<br>14036 | 20243<br>21265 | 2408<br>2515 | 2662<br>2882 | 3272<br>3409 | 729<br>749 | 771<br>798 | 831<br>848 | 350<br>356 | 362<br>368 | 375<br>372 | 206<br>208 | 210<br>212 | 215<br>204 |
| 0.5 | ***<br>*** | 11311<br>11684 | 12352<br>13822 | 20619<br>21393 | 2378<br>2494 | 2652<br>2889 | 3310<br>3409 | 724<br>744 | 768<br>797 | 832<br>840 | 345<br>351 | 357<br>364 | 372<br>364 | 201<br>203 | 205<br>208 | 210<br>197 |
| 0.55 | ***<br>*** | 10550<br>10995 | 11761<br>13377 | 20529<br>21093 | 2307<br>2429 | 2594<br>2839 | 3273<br>3340 | 705<br>725 | 750<br>778 | 813<br>814 | 334<br>339 | 345<br>352 | 359<br>349 | 192<br>194 | 196<br>199 | 201<br>187 |
| 0.6 | ***<br>*** | 9670<br>10178 | 11023<br>12737 | 19973<br>20365 | 2200<br>2324 | 2490<br>2735 | 3162<br>3203 | 672<br>692 | 715<br>743 | 776<br>771 | 315<br>320 | 326<br>332 | 339<br>326 | 179<br>181 | 183<br>185 | 187<br>172 |
| 0.65 | ***<br>*** | 8726<br>9281 | 10173<br>11924 | 18952<br>19209 | 2060<br>2181 | 2342<br>2576 | 2977<br>2998 | 625<br>644 | 665<br>691 | 721<br>711 | 289<br>294 | 299<br>304 | 310<br>295 | 162<br>163 | 165<br>167 | 169<br>153 |
| 0.7 | ***<br>*** | 7757<br>8332 | 9234<br>10952 | 17471<br>17625 | 1887<br>2000 | 2149<br>2363 | 2718<br>2724 | 565<br>581 | 600<br>621 | 647<br>634 | 256<br>260 | 264<br>268 | 273<br>257 | 140<br>142 | 143<br>144 | 146<br>129 |
| 0.75 | ***<br>*** | 6776<br>7340 | 8208<br>9820 | 15532<br>15612 | 1680<br>1780 | 1911<br>2094 | 2386<br>2381 | 490<br>504 | 518<br>535 | 555<br>540 | 216<br>218 | 222<br>225 | 228<br>212 | 115<br>115 | 116<br>117 | 118<br>101 |
| 0.8 | ***<br>*** | 5774<br>6296 | 7083<br>8508 | 13140<br>13172 | 1434<br>1516 | 1622<br>1765 | 1981<br>1970 | 400<br>410 | 420<br>432 | 445<br>429 | 168<br>169 | 171<br>173 | 175<br>158 | .<br>. | .<br>. | .<br>. |
| 0.85 | ***<br>*** | 4720<br>5163 | 5821<br>6971 | 10300<br>10303 | 1140<br>1200 | 1274<br>1370 | 1506<br>1491 | 292<br>298 | 304<br>310 | 317<br>300 | .<br>. | .<br>. | .<br>. | .<br>. | .<br>. | .<br>. |
| 0.9 | ***<br>*** | 3539<br>3866 | 4336<br>5117 | 7018<br>7006 | 780<br>813 | 852<br>899 | 959<br>943 | .<br>. | .<br>. | .<br>. | .<br>. | .<br>. | .<br>. | .<br>. | .<br>. | .<br>. |
| 0.95 | ***<br>*** | 2044<br>2202 | 2415<br>2731 | 3297<br>3280 | .<br>. | .<br>. | .<br>. | .<br>. | .<br>. | .<br>. | .<br>. | .<br>. | .<br>. | .<br>. | .<br>. | .<br>. |

## TABLE 8: ALPHA= 0.05 POWER= 0.9    EXPECTED ACCRUAL THRU MINIMUM FOLLOW-UP= 1700

| | | DEL=.02 | | | DEL=.05 | | | DEL=.10 | | | DEL=.15 | | | DEL=.20 | | |
|---|---|---|---|---|---|---|---|---|---|---|---|---|---|---|---|---|
| FACT= | | 1.0 .75 | .50 .25 | .00 BIN | 1.0 .75 | .50 .25 | .00 BIN | 1.0 .75 | .50 .25 | .00 BIN | 1.0 75 | .50 .25 | .00 BIN | 1.0 .75 | .50 .25 | .00 BIN |
| PCONT=*** | | | | | | | | REQUIRED NUMBER OF PATIENTS | | | | | | | | |
| 0.05 | *** | 2463 | 2490 | 2579 | 534 | 539 | 547 | 192 | 193 | 194 | 112 | 114 | 114 | 80 | 80 | 80 |
| | *** | 2473 | 2520 | 4822 | 537 | 543 | 943 | 193 | 194 | 300 | 112 | 114 | 158 | 80 | 80 | 101 |
| 0.1 | *** | 5133 | 5212 | 5668 | 998 | 1019 | 1055 | 318 | 322 | 326 | 170 | 172 | 173 | 112 | 112 | 114 |
| | *** | 5161 | 5325 | 8376 | 1007 | 1035 | 1491 | 320 | 324 | 429 | 171 | 172 | 212 | 112 | 114 | 129 |
| 0.15 | *** | 7516 | 7660 | 8765 | 1409 | 1457 | 1547 | 428 | 437 | 446 | 220 | 222 | 225 | 140 | 141 | 142 |
| | *** | 7565 | 7889 | 11502 | 1430 | 1494 | 1970 | 432 | 441 | 540 | 221 | 224 | 257 | 140 | 141 | 153 |
| 0.2 | *** | 9435 | 9658 | 11647 | 1751 | 1831 | 1995 | 522 | 537 | 554 | 261 | 265 | 270 | 163 | 163 | 165 |
| | *** | 9510 | 10028 | 14199 | 1785 | 1897 | 2381 | 529 | 544 | 634 | 263 | 267 | 295 | 163 | 165 | 172 |
| 0.25 | *** | 10843 | 11162 | 14201 | 2018 | 2135 | 2387 | 598 | 618 | 645 | 295 | 301 | 308 | 180 | 182 | 185 |
| | *** | 10951 | 11696 | 16469 | 2067 | 2232 | 2724 | 607 | 630 | 711 | 299 | 304 | 326 | 182 | 184 | 187 |
| 0.3 | *** | 11749 | 12184 | 16366 | 2213 | 2368 | 2715 | 658 | 683 | 718 | 321 | 328 | 337 | 193 | 197 | 199 |
| | *** | 11898 | 12902 | 18310 | 2279 | 2499 | 2998 | 669 | 699 | 771 | 324 | 333 | 349 | 194 | 197 | 197 |
| 0.35 | *** | 12194 | 12767 | 18108 | 2343 | 2534 | 2974 | 699 | 731 | 775 | 339 | 347 | 358 | 202 | 205 | 209 |
| | *** | 12391 | 13683 | 19723 | 2424 | 2698 | 3203 | 714 | 751 | 814 | 343 | 352 | 364 | 204 | 207 | 204 |
| 0.4 | *** | 12235 | 12964 | 19404 | 2413 | 2637 | 3160 | 724 | 760 | 813 | 348 | 359 | 371 | 206 | 210 | 214 |
| | *** | 12488 | 14086 | 20708 | 2507 | 2829 | 3340 | 741 | 784 | 840 | 354 | 364 | 372 | 208 | 212 | 206 |
| 0.45 | *** | 11940 | 12843 | 20244 | 2431 | 2683 | 3271 | 733 | 775 | 832 | 352 | 362 | 375 | 206 | 210 | 214 |
| | *** | 12260 | 14164 | 21265 | 2537 | 2898 | 3409 | 752 | 800 | 848 | 357 | 369 | 372 | 208 | 212 | 204 |
| 0.5 | *** | 11383 | 12465 | 20619 | 2402 | 2675 | 3310 | 729 | 771 | 832 | 346 | 358 | 372 | 202 | 205 | 210 |
| | *** | 11774 | 13964 | 21393 | 2518 | 2907 | 3409 | 748 | 799 | 840 | 352 | 364 | 364 | 204 | 208 | 197 |
| 0.55 | *** | 10637 | 11888 | 20529 | 2333 | 2618 | 3274 | 709 | 752 | 814 | 335 | 346 | 359 | 192 | 197 | 201 |
| | *** | 11099 | 13531 | 21093 | 2454 | 2858 | 3340 | 729 | 780 | 814 | 340 | 352 | 349 | 194 | 199 | 187 |
| 0.6 | *** | 9770 | 11160 | 19973 | 2227 | 2514 | 3162 | 675 | 718 | 777 | 316 | 326 | 339 | 180 | 182 | 187 |
| | *** | 10295 | 12898 | 20365 | 2349 | 2753 | 3203 | 696 | 745 | 771 | 321 | 333 | 326 | 182 | 185 | 172 |
| 0.65 | *** | 8837 | 10317 | 18952 | 2086 | 2365 | 2976 | 629 | 668 | 720 | 290 | 299 | 310 | 163 | 165 | 169 |
| | *** | 9406 | 12086 | 19209 | 2205 | 2594 | 2998 | 647 | 692 | 711 | 294 | 305 | 295 | 163 | 167 | 153 |
| 0.7 | *** | 7873 | 9377 | 17471 | 1911 | 2171 | 2718 | 568 | 602 | 647 | 257 | 265 | 273 | 140 | 143 | 146 |
| | *** | 8459 | 11108 | 17625 | 2023 | 2379 | 2724 | 584 | 622 | 634 | 260 | 269 | 257 | 142 | 144 | 129 |
| 0.75 | *** | 6890 | 8344 | 15531 | 1701 | 1929 | 2385 | 493 | 520 | 554 | 216 | 222 | 228 | 114 | 117 | 118 |
| | *** | 7465 | 9964 | 15612 | 1801 | 2107 | 2381 | 505 | 537 | 540 | 219 | 225 | 212 | 116 | 117 | 101 |
| 0.8 | *** | 5881 | 7205 | 13140 | 1451 | 1636 | 1982 | 403 | 422 | 445 | 168 | 171 | 175 | . | . | . |
| | *** | 6410 | 8633 | 13172 | 1533 | 1775 | 1970 | 411 | 432 | 429 | 170 | 173 | 158 | . | . | . |
| 0.85 | *** | 4811 | 5921 | 10301 | 1153 | 1283 | 1506 | 293 | 305 | 318 | . | . | . | . | . | . |
| | *** | 5259 | 7070 | 10303 | 1211 | 1377 | 1491 | 299 | 310 | 300 | . | . | . | . | . | . |
| 0.9 | *** | 3607 | 4406 | 7018 | 787 | 856 | 959 | . | . | . | . | . | . | . | . | . |
| | *** | 3935 | 5182 | 7006 | 819 | 902 | 943 | . | . | . | . | . | . | . | . | . |
| 0.95 | *** | 2077 | 2446 | 3297 | . | . | . | . | . | . | . | . | . | . | . | . |
| | *** | 2234 | 2755 | 3280 | . | . | . | . | . | . | . | . | . | . | . | . |

TABLE 8: ALPHA= 0.05  POWER= 0.9    EXPECTED ACCRUAL THRU MINIMUM FOLLOW-UP= 1800

| | | DEL=.02 | | | DEL=.05 | | | DEL=.10 | | | DEL=.15 | | | DEL=.20 | | |
|---|---|---|---|---|---|---|---|---|---|---|---|---|---|---|---|---|---|
| FACT= | | 1.0 .75 | .50 .25 | .00 BIN | 1.0 .75 | .50 .25 | .00 BIN | 1.0 .75 | .50 .25 | .00 BIN | 1.0 75 | .50 .25 | .00 BIN | 1.0 .75 | .50 .25 | .00 BIN |
| PCONT=*** | | | | | | REQUIRED NUMBER OF PATIENTS | | | | | | | | | | |
| 0.05 | *** | 2465 | 2493 | 2580 | 535 | 540 | 548 | 192 | 193 | 195 | 112 | 114 | 114 | 80 | 80 | 80 |
| | *** | 2476 | 2522 | 4822 | 537 | 543 | 943 | 193 | 195 | 300 | 112 | 114 | 158 | 80 | 80 | 101 |
| 0.1 | *** | 5138 | 5220 | 5667 | 999 | 1020 | 1055 | 318 | 321 | 326 | 171 | 172 | 173 | 112 | 112 | 114 |
| | *** | 5166 | 5336 | 8376 | 1009 | 1036 | 1491 | 319 | 324 | 429 | 171 | 172 | 212 | 112 | 114 | 129 |
| 0.15 | *** | 7525 | 7674 | 8766 | 1413 | 1460 | 1547 | 429 | 438 | 447 | 220 | 222 | 225 | 139 | 141 | 141 |
| | *** | 7577 | 7911 | 11502 | 1434 | 1496 | 1970 | 433 | 442 | 540 | 222 | 224 | 257 | 141 | 141 | 153 |
| 0.2 | *** | 9449 | 9683 | 11647 | 1757 | 1837 | 1995 | 524 | 537 | 553 | 262 | 265 | 270 | 163 | 164 | 165 |
| | *** | 9528 | 10064 | 14199 | 1792 | 1901 | 2381 | 530 | 544 | 634 | 264 | 267 | 295 | 163 | 165 | 172 |
| 0.25 | *** | 10862 | 11198 | 14201 | 2028 | 2144 | 2388 | 600 | 620 | 645 | 296 | 301 | 308 | 180 | 182 | 186 |
| | *** | 10977 | 11748 | 16469 | 2078 | 2240 | 2724 | 609 | 631 | 711 | 298 | 305 | 326 | 181 | 183 | 187 |
| 0.3 | *** | 11775 | 12233 | 16366 | 2226 | 2380 | 2715 | 660 | 685 | 719 | 321 | 328 | 337 | 193 | 197 | 199 |
| | *** | 11931 | 12971 | 18310 | 2292 | 2508 | 2998 | 672 | 701 | 771 | 325 | 333 | 349 | 195 | 198 | 197 |
| 0.35 | *** | 12228 | 12829 | 18108 | 2359 | 2549 | 2973 | 702 | 732 | 775 | 339 | 348 | 357 | 202 | 206 | 209 |
| | *** | 12437 | 13770 | 19723 | 2440 | 2709 | 3203 | 717 | 751 | 814 | 344 | 353 | 364 | 204 | 207 | 204 |
| 0.4 | *** | 12280 | 13043 | 19404 | 2432 | 2655 | 3159 | 728 | 762 | 812 | 350 | 360 | 371 | 207 | 210 | 213 |
| | *** | 12547 | 14192 | 20708 | 2526 | 2843 | 3340 | 744 | 785 | 840 | 354 | 366 | 372 | 208 | 213 | 206 |
| 0.45 | *** | 11998 | 12939 | 20243 | 2452 | 2702 | 3271 | 738 | 777 | 831 | 352 | 363 | 375 | 207 | 210 | 215 |
| | *** | 12332 | 14286 | 21265 | 2558 | 2913 | 3409 | 756 | 802 | 848 | 357 | 369 | 372 | 208 | 213 | 204 |
| 0.5 | *** | 11454 | 12575 | 20619 | 2425 | 2697 | 3309 | 732 | 774 | 831 | 348 | 359 | 371 | 202 | 206 | 210 |
| | *** | 11862 | 14100 | 21393 | 2541 | 2922 | 3409 | 751 | 800 | 840 | 353 | 364 | 364 | 204 | 208 | 197 |
| 0.55 | *** | 10722 | 12012 | 20529 | 2357 | 2640 | 3273 | 713 | 756 | 813 | 336 | 346 | 359 | 193 | 197 | 201 |
| | *** | 11200 | 13677 | 21093 | 2478 | 2874 | 3340 | 733 | 782 | 814 | 341 | 353 | 349 | 195 | 199 | 187 |
| 0.6 | *** | 9868 | 11292 | 19972 | 2251 | 2535 | 3162 | 681 | 721 | 776 | 317 | 327 | 339 | 180 | 183 | 186 |
| | *** | 10408 | 13050 | 20365 | 2373 | 2769 | 3203 | 699 | 746 | 771 | 321 | 333 | 326 | 181 | 186 | 172 |
| 0.65 | *** | 8945 | 10455 | 18951 | 2109 | 2386 | 2976 | 633 | 670 | 721 | 291 | 300 | 310 | 163 | 165 | 168 |
| | *** | 9528 | 12239 | 19209 | 2229 | 2610 | 2998 | 650 | 694 | 711 | 294 | 305 | 295 | 164 | 168 | 153 |
| 0.7 | *** | 7985 | 9513 | 17471 | 1934 | 2190 | 2718 | 571 | 604 | 647 | 258 | 265 | 273 | 141 | 143 | 145 |
| | *** | 8583 | 11256 | 17625 | 2045 | 2393 | 2724 | 587 | 624 | 634 | 261 | 269 | 257 | 141 | 144 | 129 |
| 0.75 | *** | 7001 | 8473 | 15531 | 1721 | 1946 | 2386 | 496 | 522 | 555 | 217 | 222 | 228 | 114 | 117 | 118 |
| | *** | 7584 | 10100 | 15612 | 1819 | 2119 | 2381 | 508 | 537 | 540 | 219 | 225 | 212 | 116 | 117 | 101 |
| 0.8 | *** | 5984 | 7320 | 13140 | 1468 | 1649 | 1981 | 404 | 423 | 445 | 168 | 172 | 175 | . | . | . |
| | *** | 6518 | 8750 | 13172 | 1548 | 1784 | 1970 | 413 | 433 | 429 | 170 | 173 | 158 | . | . | . |
| 0.85 | *** | 4898 | 6016 | 10300 | 1165 | 1293 | 1505 | 294 | 305 | 317 | . | . | . | . | . | . |
| | *** | 5352 | 7161 | 10303 | 1223 | 1383 | 1491 | 300 | 310 | 300 | . | . | . | . | . | . |
| 0.9 | *** | 3672 | 4473 | 7017 | 794 | 861 | 960 | . | . | . | . | . | . | . | . | . |
| | *** | 4002 | 5241 | 7006 | 825 | 906 | 943 | . | . | . | . | . | . | . | . | . |
| 0.95 | *** | 2109 | 2474 | 3297 | . | . | . | . | . | . | . | . | . | . | . | . |
| | *** | 2265 | 2776 | 3280 | . | . | . | . | . | . | . | . | . | . | . | . |

## TABLE 8: ALPHA= 0.05 POWER= 0.9     EXPECTED ACCRUAL THRU MINIMUM FOLLOW-UP= 1900

| PCONT | FACT= | DEL=.02 1.0 / .75 | .50 / .25 | .00 BIN | DEL=.05 1.0 / .75 | .50 / .25 | .00 BIN | DEL=.10 1.0 / .75 | .50 / .25 | .00 BIN | DEL=.15 1.0 / 75 | .50 / .25 | .00 BIN | DEL=.20 1.0 / .75 | .50 / .25 | .00 BIN |
|---|---|---|---|---|---|---|---|---|---|---|---|---|---|---|---|---|
| | | REQUIRED NUMBER OF PATIENTS | | | | | | | | | | | | | | |
| 0.05 | *** | 2466 | 2495 | 2580 | 535 | 540 | 547 | 192 | 193 | 194 | 113 | 113 | 114 | 79 | 79 | 79 |
| | *** | 2478 | 2524 | 4822 | 538 | 543 | 943 | 193 | 194 | 300 | 113 | 114 | 158 | 79 | 79 | 101 |
| 0.1 | *** | 5143 | 5227 | 5668 | 1001 | 1022 | 1056 | 318 | 322 | 326 | 171 | 172 | 173 | 113 | 113 | 114 |
| | *** | 5172 | 5345 | 8376 | 1010 | 1037 | 1491 | 320 | 324 | 429 | 171 | 172 | 212 | 113 | 113 | 129 |
| 0.15 | *** | 7533 | 7690 | 8766 | 1417 | 1464 | 1547 | 429 | 438 | 446 | 220 | 223 | 225 | 140 | 141 | 142 |
| | *** | 7588 | 7931 | 11502 | 1438 | 1498 | 1970 | 433 | 441 | 540 | 222 | 224 | 257 | 140 | 141 | 153 |
| 0.2 | *** | 9462 | 9708 | 11647 | 1764 | 1843 | 1996 | 524 | 538 | 553 | 262 | 266 | 270 | 163 | 163 | 166 |
| | *** | 9546 | 10098 | 14199 | 1797 | 1904 | 2381 | 531 | 545 | 634 | 265 | 268 | 295 | 163 | 165 | 172 |
| 0.25 | *** | 10881 | 11233 | 14201 | 2037 | 2153 | 2388 | 602 | 621 | 645 | 296 | 301 | 307 | 180 | 182 | 185 |
| | *** | 11002 | 11798 | 16469 | 2086 | 2245 | 2724 | 611 | 631 | 711 | 299 | 305 | 326 | 182 | 184 | 187 |
| 0.3 | *** | 11801 | 12281 | 16367 | 2238 | 2391 | 2716 | 662 | 686 | 718 | 323 | 329 | 337 | 193 | 197 | 199 |
| | *** | 11966 | 13038 | 18310 | 2303 | 2516 | 2998 | 673 | 702 | 771 | 325 | 332 | 349 | 196 | 198 | 197 |
| 0.35 | *** | 12264 | 12891 | 18108 | 2374 | 2562 | 2973 | 704 | 735 | 774 | 341 | 349 | 358 | 203 | 205 | 209 |
| | *** | 12482 | 13854 | 19723 | 2454 | 2719 | 3203 | 718 | 752 | 814 | 344 | 353 | 364 | 204 | 208 | 204 |
| 0.4 | *** | 12326 | 13121 | 19405 | 2450 | 2671 | 3160 | 730 | 766 | 812 | 351 | 360 | 370 | 206 | 210 | 213 |
| | *** | 12605 | 14294 | 20708 | 2545 | 2856 | 3340 | 747 | 787 | 840 | 355 | 365 | 372 | 209 | 212 | 206 |
| 0.45 | *** | 12055 | 13030 | 20243 | 2472 | 2720 | 3271 | 741 | 779 | 831 | 353 | 363 | 375 | 206 | 210 | 215 |
| | *** | 12404 | 14403 | 21265 | 2578 | 2927 | 3409 | 759 | 802 | 848 | 358 | 369 | 372 | 209 | 212 | 204 |
| 0.5 | *** | 11525 | 12681 | 20618 | 2447 | 2716 | 3309 | 736 | 776 | 831 | 349 | 360 | 372 | 201 | 206 | 210 |
| | *** | 11947 | 14231 | 21393 | 2562 | 2937 | 3409 | 755 | 801 | 840 | 353 | 365 | 364 | 204 | 208 | 197 |
| 0.55 | *** | 10805 | 12130 | 20528 | 2379 | 2660 | 3272 | 717 | 757 | 813 | 337 | 348 | 360 | 193 | 197 | 201 |
| | *** | 11300 | 13817 | 21093 | 2500 | 2890 | 3340 | 736 | 783 | 814 | 342 | 353 | 349 | 194 | 199 | 187 |
| 0.6 | *** | 9963 | 11421 | 19972 | 2274 | 2557 | 3162 | 684 | 723 | 776 | 318 | 327 | 338 | 180 | 184 | 187 |
| | *** | 10518 | 13194 | 20365 | 2396 | 2785 | 3203 | 703 | 748 | 771 | 323 | 332 | 326 | 182 | 185 | 172 |
| 0.65 | *** | 9048 | 10585 | 18952 | 2132 | 2405 | 2977 | 636 | 673 | 721 | 292 | 300 | 310 | 163 | 166 | 168 |
| | *** | 9644 | 12383 | 19209 | 2250 | 2624 | 2998 | 654 | 695 | 711 | 296 | 305 | 295 | 163 | 167 | 153 |
| 0.7 | *** | 8093 | 9644 | 17470 | 1954 | 2207 | 2718 | 574 | 607 | 647 | 258 | 266 | 273 | 141 | 144 | 146 |
| | *** | 8702 | 11395 | 17625 | 2065 | 2405 | 2724 | 590 | 626 | 634 | 261 | 269 | 257 | 142 | 144 | 129 |
| 0.75 | *** | 7107 | 8596 | 15532 | 1740 | 1961 | 2386 | 498 | 524 | 554 | 217 | 222 | 228 | 115 | 116 | 118 |
| | *** | 7698 | 10228 | 15612 | 1837 | 2130 | 2381 | 510 | 538 | 540 | 220 | 225 | 212 | 116 | 117 | 101 |
| 0.8 | *** | 6081 | 7431 | 13140 | 1484 | 1662 | 1982 | 406 | 424 | 445 | 168 | 172 | 175 | . | . | . |
| | *** | 6623 | 8861 | 13172 | 1562 | 1793 | 1970 | 414 | 433 | 429 | 170 | 173 | 158 | . | . | . |
| 0.85 | *** | 4981 | 6106 | 10300 | 1177 | 1301 | 1505 | 296 | 306 | 317 | . | . | . | . | . | . |
| | *** | 5438 | 7248 | 10303 | 1232 | 1388 | 1491 | 300 | 311 | 300 | . | . | . | . | . | . |
| 0.9 | *** | 3733 | 4535 | 7018 | 800 | 866 | 959 | . | . | . | . | . | . | . | . | . |
| | *** | 4065 | 5297 | 7006 | 830 | 907 | 943 | . | . | . | . | . | . | . | . | . |
| 0.95 | *** | 2139 | 2500 | 3298 | . | . | . | . | . | . | . | . | . | . | . | . |
| | *** | 2294 | 2796 | 3280 | . | . | . | . | . | . | . | . | . | . | . | . |

TABLE 8: ALPHA= 0.05  POWER= 0.9     EXPECTED ACCRUAL THRU MINIMUM FOLLOW-UP= 2000

| | | DEL=.02 | | | DEL=.05 | | | DEL=.10 | | | DEL=.15 | | | DEL=.20 | | |
|---|---|---|---|---|---|---|---|---|---|---|---|---|---|---|---|---|
| FACT= | | 1.0 .75 | .50 .25 | .00 BIN | 1.0 .75 | .50 .25 | .00 BIN | 1.0 .75 | .50 .25 | .00 BIN | 1.0 75 | .50 .25 | .00 BIN | 1.0 .75 | .50 .25 | .00 BIN |
| PCONT=*** | | | | | | | REQUIRED NUMBER OF PATIENTS | | | | | | | | |
| 0.05 | *** | 2469 | 2497 | 2580 | 536 | 541 | 547 | 192 | 194 | 195 | 112 | 114 | 114 | 80 | 80 | 80 |
| | *** | 2480 | 2526 | 4822 | 539 | 544 | 943 | 194 | 194 | 300 | 114 | 114 | 158 | 80 | 80 | 101 |
| 0.1 | *** | 5147 | 5236 | 5669 | 1002 | 1024 | 1055 | 319 | 322 | 326 | 171 | 172 | 172 | 112 | 112 | 114 |
| | *** | 5179 | 5354 | 8376 | 1012 | 1037 | 1491 | 320 | 324 | 429 | 171 | 172 | 212 | 112 | 114 | 129 |
| 0.15 | *** | 7542 | 7706 | 8766 | 1421 | 1467 | 1547 | 431 | 437 | 446 | 221 | 222 | 225 | 140 | 141 | 142 |
| | *** | 7599 | 7951 | 11502 | 1441 | 1501 | 1970 | 435 | 442 | 540 | 222 | 224 | 257 | 141 | 141 | 153 |
| 0.2 | *** | 9475 | 9731 | 11647 | 1770 | 1849 | 1996 | 526 | 539 | 554 | 262 | 266 | 270 | 162 | 165 | 166 |
| | *** | 9564 | 10131 | 14199 | 1804 | 1909 | 2381 | 532 | 546 | 634 | 265 | 269 | 295 | 164 | 165 | 172 |
| 0.25 | *** | 10900 | 11269 | 14201 | 2046 | 2160 | 2387 | 604 | 622 | 645 | 297 | 302 | 307 | 181 | 182 | 185 |
| | *** | 11027 | 11846 | 16469 | 2095 | 2251 | 2724 | 612 | 632 | 711 | 300 | 305 | 326 | 182 | 184 | 187 |
| 0.3 | *** | 11827 | 12329 | 16367 | 2250 | 2402 | 2715 | 665 | 687 | 719 | 324 | 330 | 337 | 195 | 197 | 200 |
| | *** | 12001 | 13104 | 18310 | 2315 | 2525 | 2998 | 675 | 702 | 771 | 326 | 334 | 349 | 196 | 199 | 197 |
| 0.35 | *** | 12299 | 12952 | 18109 | 2389 | 2576 | 2974 | 707 | 736 | 775 | 341 | 349 | 359 | 204 | 206 | 209 |
| | *** | 12526 | 13936 | 19723 | 2469 | 2729 | 3203 | 721 | 754 | 814 | 345 | 354 | 364 | 205 | 207 | 204 |
| 0.4 | *** | 12371 | 13196 | 19405 | 2467 | 2686 | 3160 | 734 | 767 | 812 | 351 | 361 | 371 | 207 | 211 | 214 |
| | *** | 12662 | 14391 | 20708 | 2561 | 2867 | 3340 | 750 | 789 | 840 | 356 | 366 | 372 | 209 | 212 | 206 |
| 0.45 | *** | 12111 | 13120 | 20244 | 2491 | 2739 | 3272 | 745 | 781 | 831 | 355 | 364 | 375 | 207 | 211 | 215 |
| | *** | 12475 | 14515 | 21265 | 2597 | 2940 | 3409 | 762 | 805 | 848 | 359 | 370 | 372 | 209 | 212 | 204 |
| 0.5 | *** | 11594 | 12785 | 20619 | 2467 | 2735 | 3310 | 740 | 779 | 831 | 350 | 360 | 371 | 202 | 206 | 210 |
| | *** | 12031 | 14356 | 21393 | 2582 | 2952 | 3409 | 759 | 804 | 840 | 355 | 365 | 364 | 205 | 209 | 197 |
| 0.55 | *** | 10887 | 12245 | 20529 | 2401 | 2680 | 3274 | 721 | 760 | 814 | 339 | 347 | 360 | 194 | 197 | 201 |
| | *** | 11397 | 13951 | 21093 | 2521 | 2905 | 3340 | 740 | 785 | 814 | 342 | 354 | 349 | 195 | 199 | 187 |
| 0.6 | *** | 10057 | 11544 | 19972 | 2296 | 2575 | 3162 | 687 | 726 | 776 | 319 | 329 | 339 | 181 | 184 | 187 |
| | *** | 10625 | 13332 | 20365 | 2417 | 2800 | 3203 | 705 | 749 | 771 | 324 | 334 | 326 | 182 | 185 | 172 |
| 0.65 | *** | 9150 | 10712 | 18952 | 2154 | 2424 | 2976 | 640 | 675 | 721 | 292 | 301 | 310 | 164 | 166 | 169 |
| | *** | 9757 | 12521 | 19209 | 2271 | 2637 | 2998 | 656 | 696 | 711 | 296 | 305 | 295 | 165 | 167 | 153 |
| 0.7 | *** | 8197 | 9769 | 17471 | 1975 | 2225 | 2717 | 577 | 609 | 647 | 259 | 266 | 274 | 141 | 144 | 146 |
| | *** | 8816 | 11529 | 17625 | 2084 | 2419 | 2724 | 592 | 626 | 634 | 262 | 270 | 257 | 142 | 145 | 129 |
| 0.75 | *** | 7210 | 8715 | 15532 | 1757 | 1976 | 2386 | 501 | 525 | 555 | 217 | 222 | 229 | 115 | 116 | 119 |
| | *** | 7809 | 10350 | 15612 | 1854 | 2141 | 2381 | 512 | 539 | 540 | 220 | 225 | 212 | 116 | 117 | 101 |
| 0.8 | *** | 6176 | 7536 | 13140 | 1499 | 1674 | 1981 | 407 | 425 | 445 | 169 | 172 | 175 | . | . | . |
| | *** | 6722 | 8966 | 13172 | 1576 | 1801 | 1970 | 416 | 435 | 429 | 171 | 174 | 158 | . | . | . |
| 0.85 | *** | 5062 | 6191 | 10300 | 1187 | 1309 | 1506 | 297 | 306 | 317 | . | . | . | . | . | . |
| | *** | 5521 | 7330 | 10303 | 1242 | 1394 | 1491 | 301 | 311 | 300 | . | . | . | . | . | . |
| 0.9 | *** | 3791 | 4594 | 7017 | 806 | 870 | 959 | . | . | . | . | . | . | . | . | . |
| | *** | 4124 | 5350 | 7006 | 835 | 910 | 943 | . | . | . | . | . | . | . | . | . |
| 0.95 | *** | 2167 | 2525 | 3297 | . | . | . | . | . | . | . | . | . | . | . | . |
| | *** | 2321 | 2815 | 3280 | . | . | . | . | . | . | . | . | . | . | . | . |

TABLE 8: ALPHA= 0.05  POWER= 0.9    EXPECTED ACCRUAL THRU MINIMUM FOLLOW-UP= 2250

| | | DEL=.02 | | | DEL=.05 | | | DEL=.10 | | | DEL=.15 | | | DEL=.20 | | |
|---|---|---|---|---|---|---|---|---|---|---|---|---|---|---|---|---|---|
| FACT= | | 1.0 .75 | .50 .25 | .00 BIN | 1.0 .75 | .50 .25 | .00 BIN | 1.0 .75 | .50 .25 | .00 BIN | 1.0 75 | .50 .25 | .00 BIN | 1.0 .75 | .50 .25 | .00 BIN |
| PCONT=*** | | | | | | | REQUIRED NUMBER OF PATIENTS | | | | | | | | |
| 0.05 | *** | 2473 | 2503 | 2580 | 537 | 541 | 547 | 192 | 194 | 195 | 112 | 114 | 114 | 80 | 80 | 80 |
| | *** | 2485 | 2531 | 4822 | 539 | 544 | 943 | 194 | 194 | 300 | 114 | 114 | 158 | 80 | 80 | 101 |
| 0.1 | *** | 5159 | 5255 | 5668 | 1006 | 1026 | 1056 | 319 | 323 | 326 | 171 | 171 | 173 | 112 | 114 | 114 |
| | *** | 5194 | 5374 | 8376 | 1015 | 1039 | 1491 | 320 | 325 | 429 | 171 | 173 | 212 | 112 | 114 | 129 |
| 0.15 | *** | 7564 | 7742 | 8766 | 1430 | 1473 | 1546 | 433 | 438 | 447 | 221 | 223 | 224 | 140 | 140 | 142 |
| | *** | 7627 | 7997 | 11502 | 1450 | 1506 | 1970 | 435 | 443 | 540 | 222 | 224 | 257 | 140 | 142 | 153 |
| 0.2 | *** | 9509 | 9790 | 11648 | 1784 | 1860 | 1995 | 528 | 539 | 554 | 264 | 267 | 269 | 163 | 164 | 165 |
| | *** | 9607 | 10209 | 14199 | 1818 | 1917 | 2381 | 534 | 547 | 634 | 266 | 268 | 295 | 164 | 165 | 172 |
| 0.25 | *** | 10947 | 11352 | 14202 | 2067 | 2178 | 2387 | 607 | 624 | 645 | 298 | 302 | 308 | 181 | 182 | 185 |
| | *** | 11089 | 11958 | 16469 | 2114 | 2264 | 2724 | 615 | 634 | 711 | 300 | 305 | 326 | 182 | 184 | 187 |
| 0.3 | *** | 11892 | 12442 | 16367 | 2278 | 2426 | 2715 | 669 | 690 | 718 | 325 | 330 | 337 | 195 | 196 | 199 |
| | *** | 12085 | 13254 | 18310 | 2341 | 2541 | 2998 | 679 | 704 | 771 | 327 | 333 | 349 | 195 | 198 | 197 |
| 0.35 | *** | 12385 | 13099 | 18108 | 2421 | 2606 | 2974 | 713 | 739 | 775 | 343 | 350 | 358 | 204 | 207 | 209 |
| | *** | 12638 | 14126 | 19723 | 2502 | 2750 | 3203 | 725 | 756 | 814 | 345 | 354 | 364 | 205 | 208 | 204 |
| 0.4 | *** | 12481 | 13376 | 19405 | 2505 | 2721 | 3160 | 741 | 772 | 812 | 354 | 361 | 371 | 208 | 210 | 213 |
| | *** | 12802 | 14618 | 20708 | 2598 | 2892 | 3340 | 755 | 790 | 840 | 357 | 367 | 372 | 209 | 212 | 206 |
| 0.45 | *** | 12251 | 13335 | 20243 | 2535 | 2775 | 3272 | 752 | 786 | 831 | 357 | 365 | 375 | 208 | 210 | 215 |
| | *** | 12646 | 14775 | 21265 | 2639 | 2968 | 3409 | 767 | 807 | 848 | 361 | 370 | 372 | 209 | 212 | 204 |
| 0.5 | *** | 11763 | 13030 | 20620 | 2516 | 2775 | 3310 | 748 | 784 | 832 | 351 | 361 | 371 | 204 | 207 | 209 |
| | *** | 12234 | 14643 | 21393 | 2628 | 2982 | 3409 | 764 | 806 | 840 | 357 | 367 | 364 | 205 | 208 | 197 |
| 0.55 | *** | 11086 | 12515 | 20528 | 2451 | 2722 | 3273 | 728 | 766 | 814 | 340 | 348 | 359 | 194 | 198 | 201 |
| | *** | 11628 | 14258 | 21093 | 2569 | 2936 | 3340 | 747 | 787 | 814 | 344 | 354 | 349 | 196 | 199 | 187 |
| 0.6 | *** | 10281 | 11832 | 19973 | 2347 | 2618 | 3162 | 696 | 731 | 776 | 320 | 329 | 339 | 181 | 184 | 187 |
| | *** | 10878 | 13650 | 20365 | 2465 | 2831 | 3203 | 711 | 752 | 771 | 325 | 334 | 326 | 182 | 185 | 172 |
| 0.65 | *** | 9390 | 11008 | 18952 | 2202 | 2465 | 2977 | 646 | 679 | 721 | 294 | 302 | 311 | 164 | 165 | 168 |
| | *** | 10023 | 12837 | 19209 | 2317 | 2667 | 2998 | 662 | 699 | 711 | 298 | 306 | 295 | 164 | 167 | 153 |
| 0.7 | *** | 8444 | 10059 | 17471 | 2021 | 2262 | 2718 | 583 | 612 | 646 | 260 | 267 | 272 | 142 | 143 | 146 |
| | *** | 9084 | 11832 | 17625 | 2126 | 2445 | 2724 | 597 | 628 | 634 | 263 | 269 | 257 | 143 | 145 | 129 |
| 0.75 | *** | 7450 | 8987 | 15532 | 1798 | 2008 | 2386 | 506 | 528 | 555 | 219 | 223 | 227 | 115 | 117 | 118 |
| | *** | 8065 | 10627 | 15612 | 1891 | 2162 | 2381 | 516 | 541 | 540 | 221 | 226 | 212 | 117 | 118 | 101 |
| 0.8 | *** | 6395 | 7778 | 13139 | 1531 | 1698 | 1981 | 412 | 427 | 446 | 170 | 173 | 176 | . | . | . |
| | *** | 6955 | 9204 | 13172 | 1605 | 1818 | 1970 | 419 | 435 | 429 | 171 | 174 | 158 | . | . | . |
| 0.85 | *** | 5248 | 6388 | 10301 | 1211 | 1326 | 1506 | 299 | 308 | 317 | . | . | . | . | . | . |
| | *** | 5714 | 7514 | 10303 | 1262 | 1405 | 1491 | 303 | 312 | 300 | . | . | . | . | . | . |
| 0.9 | *** | 3927 | 4729 | 7018 | 818 | 877 | 959 | . | . | . | . | . | . | . | . | . |
| | *** | 4260 | 5466 | 7006 | 846 | 915 | 943 | . | . | . | . | . | . | . | . | . |
| 0.95 | *** | 2232 | 2580 | 3297 | . | . | . | . | . | . | . | . | . | . | . | . |
| | *** | 2382 | 2856 | 3280 | . | . | . | . | . | . | . | . | . | . | . | . |

## TABLE 8: ALPHA= 0.05  POWER= 0.9    EXPECTED ACCRUAL THRU MINIMUM FOLLOW-UP= 2500

| | | DEL=.02 | | | DEL=.05 | | | DEL=.10 | | | DEL=.15 | | | DEL=.20 | | |
|---|---|---|---|---|---|---|---|---|---|---|---|---|---|---|---|---|
| FACT= | | 1.0<br>.75 | .50<br>.25 | .00<br>BIN | 1.0<br>.75 | .50<br>.25 | .00<br>BIN | 1.0<br>.75 | .50<br>.25 | .00<br>BIN | 1.0<br>75 | .50<br>.25 | .00<br>BIN | 1.0<br>.75 | .50<br>.25 | .00<br>BIN |
| PCONT=*** | | | | REQUIRED | NUMBER | OF | PATIENTS | | | | | | | | | |
| 0.05 | *** | 2477 | 2508 | 2579 | 537 | 542 | 546 | 193 | 193 | 195 | 114 | 114 | 114 | 79 | 79 | 79 |
|  | *** | 2489 | 2534 | 4822 | 540 | 545 | 943 | 193 | 195 | 300 | 114 | 114 | 158 | 79 | 79 | 101 |
| 0.1 | *** | 5171 | 5271 | 5668 | 1011 | 1029 | 1056 | 320 | 323 | 326 | 171 | 171 | 173 | 112 | 114 | 114 |
|  | *** | 5209 | 5393 | 8376 | 1018 | 1040 | 1491 | 321 | 324 | 429 | 171 | 173 | 212 | 112 | 114 | 129 |
| 0.15 | *** | 7584 | 7777 | 8765 | 1437 | 1479 | 1546 | 434 | 440 | 446 | 221 | 223 | 224 | 140 | 142 | 142 |
|  | *** | 7654 | 8039 | 11502 | 1456 | 1509 | 1970 | 437 | 443 | 540 | 223 | 224 | 257 | 140 | 142 | 153 |
| 0.2 | *** | 9542 | 9846 | 11646 | 1796 | 1870 | 1995 | 531 | 542 | 552 | 264 | 267 | 270 | 164 | 165 | 165 |
|  | *** | 9649 | 10279 | 14199 | 1829 | 1923 | 2381 | 536 | 546 | 634 | 265 | 268 | 295 | 164 | 165 | 172 |
| 0.25 | *** | 10995 | 11434 | 14201 | 2084 | 2193 | 2387 | 611 | 626 | 645 | 298 | 302 | 308 | 181 | 183 | 186 |
|  | *** | 11149 | 12062 | 16469 | 2133 | 2273 | 2724 | 618 | 634 | 711 | 301 | 306 | 326 | 183 | 184 | 187 |
| 0.3 | *** | 11958 | 12551 | 16367 | 2301 | 2445 | 2715 | 673 | 693 | 718 | 326 | 331 | 337 | 195 | 196 | 199 |
|  | *** | 12168 | 13392 | 18310 | 2364 | 2556 | 2998 | 683 | 706 | 771 | 327 | 334 | 349 | 196 | 198 | 197 |
| 0.35 | *** | 12470 | 13237 | 18108 | 2451 | 2629 | 2973 | 718 | 743 | 774 | 345 | 351 | 358 | 204 | 206 | 209 |
|  | *** | 12745 | 14298 | 19723 | 2529 | 2768 | 3203 | 729 | 758 | 814 | 348 | 354 | 364 | 206 | 208 | 204 |
| 0.4 | *** | 12590 | 13546 | 19404 | 2540 | 2749 | 3159 | 746 | 774 | 812 | 354 | 362 | 371 | 209 | 211 | 214 |
|  | *** | 12939 | 14823 | 20708 | 2631 | 2914 | 3340 | 761 | 792 | 840 | 359 | 367 | 372 | 211 | 212 | 206 |
| 0.45 | *** | 12386 | 13536 | 20243 | 2573 | 2809 | 3271 | 758 | 790 | 831 | 358 | 367 | 374 | 209 | 211 | 214 |
|  | *** | 12811 | 15012 | 21265 | 2676 | 2992 | 3409 | 773 | 809 | 848 | 362 | 370 | 372 | 211 | 212 | 204 |
| 0.5 | *** | 11926 | 13259 | 20618 | 2558 | 2811 | 3309 | 754 | 789 | 831 | 354 | 362 | 371 | 204 | 208 | 211 |
|  | *** | 12427 | 14902 | 21393 | 2668 | 3009 | 3409 | 770 | 809 | 840 | 358 | 367 | 364 | 206 | 209 | 197 |
| 0.55 | *** | 11276 | 12767 | 20529 | 2495 | 2759 | 3273 | 736 | 770 | 814 | 342 | 349 | 359 | 195 | 198 | 201 |
|  | *** | 11846 | 14536 | 21093 | 2611 | 2962 | 3340 | 751 | 790 | 814 | 346 | 354 | 349 | 196 | 199 | 187 |
| 0.6 | *** | 10492 | 12096 | 19973 | 2390 | 2654 | 3162 | 701 | 734 | 776 | 323 | 329 | 339 | 183 | 184 | 187 |
|  | *** | 11115 | 13934 | 20365 | 2506 | 2858 | 3203 | 717 | 754 | 771 | 326 | 334 | 326 | 183 | 186 | 172 |
| 0.65 | *** | 9615 | 11276 | 18952 | 2245 | 2499 | 2976 | 652 | 683 | 721 | 295 | 302 | 311 | 164 | 167 | 168 |
|  | *** | 10270 | 13120 | 19209 | 2358 | 2692 | 2998 | 667 | 701 | 711 | 299 | 306 | 295 | 165 | 167 | 153 |
| 0.7 | *** | 8673 | 10323 | 17470 | 2061 | 2293 | 2717 | 589 | 615 | 646 | 262 | 267 | 273 | 142 | 143 | 145 |
|  | *** | 9329 | 12101 | 17625 | 2164 | 2467 | 2724 | 601 | 629 | 634 | 264 | 270 | 257 | 143 | 145 | 129 |
| 0.75 | *** | 7670 | 9234 | 15533 | 1833 | 2036 | 2386 | 509 | 531 | 554 | 220 | 223 | 227 | 115 | 117 | 118 |
|  | *** | 8299 | 10873 | 15612 | 1923 | 2181 | 2381 | 520 | 542 | 540 | 221 | 226 | 212 | 117 | 117 | 101 |
| 0.8 | *** | 6596 | 7996 | 13140 | 1559 | 1720 | 1981 | 414 | 427 | 445 | 170 | 173 | 174 | . | . | . |
|  | *** | 7165 | 9414 | 13172 | 1631 | 1831 | 1970 | 421 | 436 | 429 | 171 | 174 | 158 | . | . | . |
| 0.85 | *** | 5417 | 6564 | 10299 | 1231 | 1340 | 1506 | 299 | 309 | 317 | . | . | . | . | . | . |
|  | *** | 5889 | 7676 | 10303 | 1281 | 1414 | 1491 | 304 | 312 | 300 | . | . | . | . | . | . |
| 0.9 | *** | 4049 | 4846 | 7018 | 829 | 884 | 959 | . | . | . | . | . | . | . | . | . |
|  | *** | 4384 | 5567 | 7006 | 854 | 918 | 943 | . | . | . | . | . | . | . | . | . |
| 0.95 | *** | 2287 | 2627 | 3296 | . | . | . | . | . | . | . | . | . | . | . | . |
|  | *** | 2436 | 2890 | 3280 | . | . | . | . | . | . | . | . | . | . | . | . |

TABLE 8: ALPHA= 0.05 POWER= 0.9    EXPECTED ACCRUAL THRU MINIMUM FOLLOW-UP= 2750

| | | DEL=.02 | | | DEL=.05 | | | DEL=.10 | | | DEL=.15 | | | DEL=.20 | | |
|---|---|---|---|---|---|---|---|---|---|---|---|---|---|---|---|---|
| FACT= | | 1.0 .75 | .50 .25 | .00 BIN | 1.0 .75 | .50 .25 | .00 BIN | 1.0 .75 | .50 .25 | .00 BIN | 1.0 75 | .50 .25 | .00 BIN | 1.0 .75 | .50 .25 | .00 BIN |
| PCONT=*** | | | | | REQUIRED NUMBER OF PATIENTS | | | | | | | | | | | |
| 0.05 | *** | 2481 | 2511 | 2579 | 539 | 542 | 548 | 194 | 194 | 194 | 113 | 113 | 113 | 80 | 80 | 80 |
| | *** | 2494 | 2538 | 4822 | 541 | 544 | 943 | 194 | 194 | 300 | 113 | 113 | 158 | 80 | 80 | 101 |
| 0.1 | *** | 5183 | 5288 | 5668 | 1013 | 1030 | 1055 | 321 | 322 | 326 | 171 | 171 | 173 | 113 | 113 | 113 |
| | *** | 5223 | 5409 | 8376 | 1020 | 1041 | 1491 | 321 | 324 | 429 | 171 | 173 | 212 | 113 | 113 | 129 |
| 0.15 | *** | 7605 | 7811 | 8765 | 1443 | 1484 | 1546 | 434 | 439 | 446 | 221 | 223 | 225 | 140 | 140 | 142 |
| | *** | 7681 | 8076 | 11502 | 1462 | 1512 | 1970 | 438 | 443 | 540 | 223 | 225 | 257 | 140 | 142 | 153 |
| 0.2 | *** | 9575 | 9899 | 11648 | 1807 | 1878 | 1995 | 532 | 542 | 553 | 264 | 267 | 269 | 163 | 164 | 166 |
| | *** | 9692 | 10343 | 14199 | 1840 | 1930 | 2381 | 538 | 548 | 634 | 266 | 269 | 295 | 164 | 164 | 172 |
| 0.25 | *** | 11043 | 11511 | 14202 | 2100 | 2206 | 2387 | 613 | 627 | 644 | 300 | 304 | 307 | 181 | 184 | 185 |
| | *** | 11209 | 12156 | 16449 | 2146 | 2282 | 2724 | 620 | 635 | 711 | 302 | 305 | 326 | 181 | 184 | 187 |
| 0.3 | *** | 12022 | 12655 | 16367 | 2322 | 2463 | 2715 | 676 | 696 | 718 | 326 | 331 | 336 | 195 | 197 | 199 |
| | *** | 12249 | 13518 | 18310 | 2384 | 2567 | 2998 | 685 | 706 | 771 | 329 | 335 | 349 | 197 | 199 | 197 |
| 0.35 | *** | 12555 | 13370 | 18108 | 2478 | 2652 | 2973 | 721 | 745 | 775 | 345 | 352 | 359 | 204 | 208 | 209 |
| | *** | 12851 | 14456 | 19723 | 2553 | 2784 | 3203 | 734 | 759 | 814 | 349 | 355 | 364 | 205 | 208 | 204 |
| 0.4 | *** | 12697 | 13708 | 19404 | 2570 | 2775 | 3158 | 751 | 778 | 813 | 357 | 364 | 370 | 209 | 211 | 214 |
| | *** | 13069 | 15011 | 20708 | 2660 | 2931 | 3340 | 764 | 793 | 840 | 360 | 367 | 372 | 211 | 212 | 206 |
| 0.45 | *** | 12519 | 13724 | 20243 | 2608 | 2837 | 3272 | 762 | 793 | 831 | 359 | 367 | 376 | 209 | 211 | 214 |
| | *** | 12969 | 15226 | 21265 | 2708 | 3013 | 3409 | 778 | 810 | 848 | 364 | 370 | 372 | 211 | 212 | 204 |
| 0.5 | *** | 12084 | 13473 | 20619 | 2595 | 2842 | 3310 | 759 | 792 | 831 | 355 | 362 | 370 | 204 | 208 | 209 |
| | *** | 12611 | 15138 | 21393 | 2703 | 3030 | 3409 | 775 | 810 | 840 | 359 | 367 | 364 | 205 | 209 | 197 |
| 0.55 | *** | 11456 | 12999 | 20528 | 2533 | 2790 | 3274 | 740 | 773 | 813 | 343 | 350 | 359 | 195 | 197 | 201 |
| | *** | 12051 | 14786 | 21093 | 2646 | 2985 | 3340 | 755 | 792 | 814 | 346 | 355 | 349 | 197 | 199 | 187 |
| 0.6 | *** | 10690 | 12340 | 19973 | 2430 | 2686 | 3162 | 707 | 738 | 776 | 324 | 331 | 338 | 181 | 185 | 187 |
| | *** | 11336 | 14191 | 20365 | 2543 | 2879 | 3340 | 721 | 755 | 771 | 328 | 335 | 326 | 184 | 185 | 172 |
| 0.65 | *** | 9826 | 11524 | 18952 | 2284 | 2529 | 2976 | 658 | 685 | 721 | 297 | 304 | 311 | 164 | 166 | 168 |
| | *** | 10497 | 13375 | 19209 | 2392 | 2714 | 2998 | 672 | 703 | 711 | 300 | 307 | 295 | 166 | 168 | 153 |
| 0.7 | *** | 8885 | 10565 | 17471 | 2095 | 2322 | 2717 | 594 | 618 | 648 | 263 | 267 | 273 | 142 | 144 | 146 |
| | *** | 9558 | 12343 | 17625 | 2196 | 2485 | 2724 | 604 | 632 | 634 | 264 | 271 | 257 | 144 | 144 | 129 |
| 0.75 | *** | 7875 | 9459 | 15532 | 1864 | 2058 | 2385 | 514 | 532 | 555 | 221 | 225 | 228 | 116 | 116 | 118 |
| | *** | 8514 | 11092 | 15612 | 1952 | 2196 | 2381 | 522 | 542 | 540 | 223 | 226 | 212 | 116 | 118 | 101 |
| 0.8 | *** | 6781 | 8193 | 13139 | 1584 | 1737 | 1981 | 417 | 429 | 445 | 170 | 173 | 175 | . | . | . |
| | *** | 7358 | 9600 | 13172 | 1655 | 1844 | 1970 | 422 | 438 | 429 | 171 | 175 | 158 | . | . | . |
| 0.85 | *** | 5571 | 6722 | 10300 | 1247 | 1352 | 1505 | 302 | 309 | 318 | . | . | . | . | . | . |
| | *** | 6046 | 7818 | 10303 | 1295 | 1421 | 1491 | 305 | 312 | 300 | . | . | . | . | . | . |
| 0.9 | *** | 4159 | 4953 | 7017 | 838 | 890 | 958 | . | . | . | . | . | . | . | . | . |
| | *** | 4494 | 5654 | 7006 | 862 | 923 | 943 | . | . | . | . | . | . | . | . | . |
| 0.95 | *** | 2337 | 2669 | 3298 | . | . | . | . | . | . | . | . | . | . | . | . |
| | *** | 2483 | 2920 | 3280 | . | . | . | . | . | . | . | . | . | . | . | . |

TABLE 8: ALPHA= 0.05  POWER= 0.9    EXPECTED ACCRUAL THRU MINIMUM FOLLOW-UP= 3000

| | DEL=.01 | | | DEL=.02 | | | DEL=.05 | | | DEL=.10 | | | DEL=.15 | | |
|---|---|---|---|---|---|---|---|---|---|---|---|---|---|---|---|
| FACT= | 1.0 .75 | .50 .25 | .00 BIN | 1.0 .75 | .50 .25 | .00 BIN | 1.0 .75 | .50 .25 | .00 BIN | 1.0 75 | .50 .25 | .00 BIN | 1.0 .75 | .50 .25 | .00 BIN |

PCONT=***                      REQUIRED NUMBER OF PATIENTS

| PCONT | 1.0/.75 (.01) | .50/.25 (.01) | .00/BIN (.01) | 1.0/.75 (.02) | .50/.25 (.02) | .00/BIN (.02) | 1.0/.75 (.05) | .50/.25 (.05) | .00/BIN (.05) | 1.0/.75 (.10) | .50/.25 (.10) | .00/BIN (.10) | 1.0/.75 (.15) | .50/.25 (.15) | .00/BIN (.15) |
|---|---|---|---|---|---|---|---|---|---|---|---|---|---|---|---|
| 0.01 *** | 1310 | 1315 | 1322 | 482 | 482 | 485 | 160 | 160 | 160 | 80 | 80 | 80 | 58 | 58 | 58 |
| *** | 1310 | 1318 | 5053 | 482 | 482 | 1670 | 160 | 160 | 455 | 80 | 80 | 185 | 58 | 58 | 110 |
| 0.02 *** | 2893 | 2908 | 2950 | 932 | 935 | 943 | 253 | 253 | 253 | 110 | 110 | 110 | 73 | 73 | 73 |
| *** | 2900 | 2923 | 8342 | 932 | 940 | 2484 | 253 | 253 | 581 | 110 | 110 | 215 | 73 | 73 | 123 |
| 0.05 *** | 8758 | 8815 | 9205 | 2485 | 2515 | 2578 | 538 | 542 | 545 | 193 | 193 | 193 | 115 | 115 | 115 |
| *** | 8777 | 8905 | 17796 | 2495 | 2540 | 4822 | 542 | 545 | 943 | 193 | 193 | 300 | 115 | 115 | 158 |
| 0.1 *** | 19322 | 19460 | 21430 | 5192 | 5305 | 5668 | 1015 | 1033 | 1055 | 320 | 325 | 325 | 170 | 170 | 170 |
| *** | 19367 | 19727 | 32183 | 5237 | 5425 | 8376 | 1022 | 1045 | 1491 | 320 | 325 | 429 | 170 | 170 | 212 |
| 0.15 *** | 28858 | 29110 | 33853 | 7843 | 8765 | | 1450 | 1487 | 1547 | 433 | 440 | 445 | 223 | 223 | 223 |
| *** | 28940 | 29597 | 44858 | 7705 | 8110 | 11502 | 1468 | 1513 | 1970 | 437 | 445 | 540 | 223 | 223 | 257 |
| 0.2 *** | 36550 | 36935 | 45478 | 9605 | 9950 | 11645 | 1817 | 1885 | 1997 | 535 | 542 | 553 | 265 | 268 | 268 |
| *** | 36680 | 37700 | 55820 | 9730 | 10400 | 14199 | 1847 | 1933 | 2381 | 538 | 550 | 634 | 265 | 268 | 295 |
| 0.25 *** | 42163 | 42722 | 55835 | 11087 | 11585 | 14200 | 2113 | 2218 | 2387 | 613 | 628 | 643 | 298 | 302 | 305 |
| *** | 42350 | 43825 | 65069 | 11267 | 12242 | 16469 | 2158 | 2290 | 2724 | 620 | 635 | 711 | 302 | 305 | 326 |
| 0.3 *** | 45715 | 46483 | 64655 | 12085 | 12752 | 16367 | 2342 | 2477 | 2713 | 680 | 695 | 718 | 328 | 332 | 335 |
| *** | 45970 | 47998 | 72605 | 12328 | 13633 | 18310 | 2402 | 2578 | 2998 | 688 | 707 | 771 | 328 | 335 | 349 |
| 0.35 *** | 47342 | 48370 | 71792 | 12635 | 13495 | 18107 | 2500 | 2672 | 2972 | 725 | 748 | 775 | 347 | 350 | 358 |
| *** | 47683 | 50372 | 78428 | 12950 | 14600 | 19723 | 2575 | 2795 | 3203 | 737 | 760 | 814 | 347 | 355 | 364 |
| 0.4 *** | 47260 | 48602 | 77158 | 12800 | 13858 | 19405 | 2597 | 2800 | 3160 | 755 | 782 | 812 | 358 | 362 | 370 |
| *** | 47705 | 51178 | 82539 | 13195 | 15182 | 20708 | 2687 | 2945 | 3340 | 767 | 797 | 840 | 362 | 365 | 372 |
| 0.45 *** | 45718 | 47447 | 80695 | 12647 | 13900 | 20245 | 2638 | 2863 | 3272 | 767 | 797 | 830 | 362 | 365 | 373 |
| *** | 46295 | 50668 | 84937 | 13120 | 15422 | 21265 | 2740 | 3028 | 3409 | 782 | 812 | 848 | 362 | 370 | 372 |
| 0.5 *** | 43003 | 45197 | 82382 | 12235 | 13670 | 20620 | 2627 | 2870 | 3310 | 763 | 793 | 830 | 355 | 362 | 370 |
| *** | 43742 | 49112 | 85622 | 12785 | 15355 | 21393 | 2735 | 3050 | 3409 | 778 | 812 | 840 | 358 | 365 | 364 |
| 0.55 *** | 39415 | 42155 | 82210 | 11627 | 13213 | 20530 | 2567 | 2818 | 3272 | 745 | 775 | 812 | 343 | 350 | 358 |
| *** | 40348 | 46757 | 84594 | 12245 | 15013 | 21093 | 2680 | 3005 | 3340 | 760 | 793 | 814 | 347 | 355 | 349 |
| 0.6 *** | 35275 | 38612 | 80170 | 10877 | 12568 | 19970 | 2465 | 2713 | 3163 | 710 | 740 | 775 | 325 | 332 | 340 |
| *** | 36440 | 43810 | 81854 | 11545 | 14425 | 20365 | 2575 | 2897 | 3203 | 725 | 755 | 771 | 328 | 335 | 326 |
| 0.65 *** | 30905 | 34810 | 76273 | 10022 | 11755 | 18950 | 2315 | 2555 | 2975 | 662 | 688 | 722 | 298 | 302 | 310 |
| *** | 32308 | 40427 | 77401 | 10712 | 13607 | 19209 | 2425 | 2732 | 2998 | 673 | 703 | 711 | 302 | 305 | 295 |
| 0.7 *** | 26590 | 30913 | 70532 | 9085 | 10787 | 17470 | 2125 | 2345 | 2717 | 598 | 620 | 647 | 265 | 268 | 272 |
| *** | 28190 | 36703 | 71235 | 9767 | 12565 | 17625 | 2225 | 2503 | 2724 | 610 | 632 | 634 | 265 | 272 | 257 |
| 0.75 *** | 22510 | 26995 | 62957 | 8065 | 9665 | 15530 | 1892 | 2080 | 2387 | 515 | 535 | 553 | 220 | 223 | 227 |
| *** | 24212 | 32660 | 63356 | 8713 | 11290 | 15612 | 1975 | 2210 | 2381 | 523 | 542 | 540 | 223 | 227 | 212 |
| 0.8 *** | 18703 | 23030 | 53570 | 6955 | 8372 | 13138 | 1607 | 1753 | 1982 | 418 | 430 | 445 | 170 | 175 | 175 |
| *** | 20375 | 28262 | 53764 | 7535 | 9767 | 13172 | 1675 | 1855 | 1970 | 425 | 437 | 429 | 170 | 175 | 158 |
| 0.85 *** | 15065 | 18905 | 42392 | 5713 | 6865 | 10300 | 1262 | 1363 | 1505 | 302 | 310 | 317 | . | . | . |
| *** | 16570 | 23365 | 42460 | 6190 | 7945 | 10303 | 1307 | 1427 | 1491 | 305 | 313 | 300 | . | . | . |
| 0.9 *** | 11357 | 14350 | 29435 | 4262 | 5045 | 7018 | 845 | 895 | 958 | . | . | . | . | . | . |
| *** | 12545 | 17660 | 29443 | 4592 | 5732 | 7006 | 868 | 925 | 943 | . | . | . | . | . | . |
| 0.95 *** | 7010 | 8702 | 14728 | 2383 | 2705 | 3298 | . | . | . | . | . | . | . | . | . |
| *** | 7700 | 10390 | 14713 | 2525 | 2945 | 3280 | . | . | . | . | . | . | . | . | . |
| 0.98 *** | 3290 | 3850 | 5068 | . | . | . | . | . | . | . | . | . | . | . | . |
| *** | 3530 | 4307 | 5053 | . | . | . | . | . | . | . | . | . | . | . | . |

TABLE 8: ALPHA= 0.05  POWER= 0.9    EXPECTED ACCRUAL THRU MINIMUM FOLLOW-UP= 3250

| | | DEL=.01 | | | DEL=.02 | | | DEL=.05 | | | DEL=.10 | | | DEL=.15 | | |
|---|---|---|---|---|---|---|---|---|---|---|---|---|---|---|---|---|---|
| FACT= | | 1.0 .75 | .50 .25 | .00 BIN | 1.0 .75 | .50 .25 | .00 BIN | 1.0 .75 | .50 .25 | .00 BIN | 1.0 75 | .50 .25 | .00 BIN | 1.0 .75 | .50 .25 | .00 BIN |
| PCONT=*** | | | | | REQUIRED NUMBER OF PATIENTS | | | | | | | | | | | |
| 0.01 | *** | 1311 | 1314 | 1322 | 482 | 482 | 485 | 160 | 160 | 160 | 79 | 79 | 79 | 54 | 54 | 54 |
| | *** | 1311 | 1319 | 5053 | 482 | 482 | 1670 | 160 | 160 | 455 | 79 | 79 | 185 | 54 | 54 | 110 |
| 0.02 | *** | 2895 | 2911 | 2947 | 932 | 937 | 940 | 254 | 254 | 254 | 111 | 111 | 111 | 71 | 71 | 71 |
| | *** | 2903 | 2922 | 8342 | 932 | 937 | 2484 | 254 | 254 | 581 | 111 | 111 | 215 | 71 | 71 | 123 |
| 0.05 | *** | 8764 | 8821 | 9208 | 2489 | 2516 | 2578 | 539 | 542 | 547 | 192 | 192 | 192 | 111 | 111 | 111 |
| | *** | 8786 | 8916 | 17796 | 2500 | 2541 | 4822 | 542 | 547 | 943 | 192 | 192 | 300 | 111 | 111 | 158 |
| 0.1 | *** | 19335 | 19486 | 21428 | 5206 | 5316 | 5669 | 1018 | 1034 | 1054 | 319 | 322 | 328 | 173 | 173 | 173 |
| | *** | 19384 | 19766 | 32183 | 5246 | 5438 | 8376 | 1026 | 1043 | 1491 | 322 | 322 | 429 | 173 | 173 | 212 |
| 0.15 | *** | 28879 | 29150 | 33851 | 7648 | 7871 | 8764 | 1452 | 1492 | 1546 | 436 | 441 | 444 | 222 | 222 | 225 |
| | *** | 28968 | 29675 | 44858 | 7729 | 8139 | 11502 | 1473 | 1517 | 1970 | 436 | 444 | 540 | 222 | 225 | 257 |
| 0.2 | *** | 36581 | 37004 | 45478 | 9639 | 9999 | 11646 | 1826 | 1891 | 1996 | 534 | 542 | 555 | 266 | 266 | 271 |
| | *** | 36722 | 37824 | 55820 | 9772 | 10454 | 14199 | 1855 | 1936 | 2381 | 539 | 547 | 634 | 266 | 271 | 295 |
| 0.25 | *** | 42207 | 42816 | 55832 | 11134 | 11654 | 14200 | 2126 | 2229 | 2386 | 615 | 628 | 644 | 298 | 303 | 306 |
| | *** | 42410 | 44002 | 65069 | 11324 | 12320 | 16469 | 2172 | 2297 | 2724 | 623 | 636 | 711 | 303 | 306 | 326 |
| 0.3 | *** | 45779 | 46611 | 64656 | 12149 | 12848 | 16366 | 2359 | 2492 | 2716 | 680 | 696 | 718 | 328 | 331 | 336 |
| | *** | 46055 | 48241 | 72605 | 12404 | 13737 | 18310 | 2419 | 2586 | 2998 | 688 | 709 | 771 | 331 | 336 | 349 |
| 0.35 | *** | 47428 | 48541 | 71795 | 12718 | 13615 | 18108 | 2521 | 2687 | 2971 | 729 | 750 | 774 | 347 | 352 | 360 |
| | *** | 47797 | 50689 | 78428 | 13051 | 14733 | 19723 | 2594 | 2809 | 3203 | 737 | 761 | 814 | 347 | 355 | 364 |
| 0.4 | *** | 47371 | 48826 | 77158 | 12905 | 14002 | 19405 | 2622 | 2817 | 3158 | 758 | 783 | 810 | 360 | 363 | 371 |
| | *** | 47859 | 51575 | 82539 | 13314 | 15343 | 20708 | 2708 | 2960 | 3340 | 769 | 799 | 840 | 360 | 368 | 372 |
| 0.45 | *** | 45863 | 47729 | 80695 | 12770 | 14067 | 20242 | 2668 | 2887 | 3272 | 769 | 799 | 831 | 360 | 368 | 376 |
| | *** | 46489 | 51158 | 84937 | 13266 | 15603 | 21265 | 2765 | 3044 | 3409 | 786 | 815 | 848 | 363 | 371 | 372 |
| 0.5 | *** | 43190 | 45551 | 82385 | 12380 | 13859 | 20619 | 2659 | 2895 | 3309 | 769 | 799 | 831 | 355 | 363 | 371 |
| | *** | 43986 | 49687 | 85622 | 12949 | 15554 | 21393 | 2760 | 3066 | 3409 | 783 | 815 | 840 | 360 | 368 | 364 |
| 0.55 | *** | 39653 | 42586 | 82206 | 11792 | 13417 | 20529 | 2597 | 2841 | 3272 | 750 | 777 | 815 | 344 | 352 | 360 |
| | *** | 40655 | 47412 | 84594 | 12429 | 15221 | 21093 | 2708 | 3020 | 3340 | 761 | 794 | 814 | 347 | 355 | 349 |
| 0.6 | *** | 35569 | 39116 | 80167 | 11056 | 12778 | 19974 | 2497 | 2741 | 3163 | 718 | 742 | 774 | 328 | 331 | 339 |
| | *** | 36817 | 44522 | 81854 | 11738 | 14639 | 20365 | 2606 | 2914 | 3203 | 729 | 758 | 771 | 328 | 336 | 326 |
| 0.65 | *** | 31268 | 35374 | 76272 | 10211 | 11966 | 18953 | 2346 | 2581 | 2976 | 664 | 688 | 721 | 298 | 303 | 311 |
| | *** | 32754 | 41172 | 77401 | 10909 | 13815 | 19209 | 2451 | 2749 | 2998 | 677 | 704 | 711 | 303 | 306 | 295 |
| 0.7 | *** | 27005 | 31511 | 70531 | 9268 | 10991 | 17471 | 2156 | 2367 | 2716 | 599 | 620 | 647 | 263 | 266 | 274 |
| | *** | 28687 | 37451 | 71235 | 9964 | 12762 | 17625 | 2248 | 2516 | 2724 | 612 | 631 | 634 | 266 | 271 | 257 |
| 0.75 | *** | 22959 | 27595 | 62958 | 8241 | 9858 | 15532 | 1915 | 2099 | 2386 | 517 | 534 | 555 | 222 | 225 | 230 |
| | *** | 24727 | 33380 | 63356 | 8899 | 11470 | 15612 | 1996 | 2221 | 2381 | 526 | 547 | 540 | 222 | 225 | 212 |
| 0.8 | *** | 19153 | 23592 | 53571 | 7115 | 8537 | 13141 | 1628 | 1769 | 1980 | 420 | 433 | 444 | 173 | 173 | 176 |
| | *** | 20876 | 28911 | 53764 | 7700 | 9918 | 13172 | 1693 | 1863 | 1970 | 425 | 436 | 429 | 173 | 173 | 158 |
| 0.85 | *** | 15473 | 19392 | 42391 | 5844 | 6998 | 10300 | 1278 | 1371 | 1506 | 303 | 311 | 314 | . | . | . |
| | *** | 17011 | 23906 | 42460 | 6324 | 8057 | 10303 | 1322 | 1433 | 1491 | 306 | 314 | 300 | . | . | . |
| 0.9 | *** | 11678 | 14720 | 29434 | 4352 | 5132 | 7017 | 851 | 899 | 956 | . | . | . | . | . | . |
| | *** | 12889 | 18051 | 29443 | 4686 | 5799 | 7006 | 875 | 929 | 943 | . | . | . | . | . | . |
| 0.95 | *** | 7201 | 8899 | 14728 | 2424 | 2736 | 3296 | . | . | . | . | . | . | . | . | . |
| | *** | 7895 | 10576 | 14713 | 2562 | 2968 | 3280 | . | . | . | . | . | . | . | . | . |
| 0.98 | *** | 3358 | 3911 | 5067 | . | . | . | . | . | . | . | . | . | . | . | . |
| | *** | 3597 | 4349 | 5053 | . | . | . | . | . | . | . | . | . | . | . | . |

TABLE 8: ALPHA= 0.05　POWER= 0.9　　EXPECTED ACCRUAL THRU MINIMUM FOLLOW-UP= 3500

| | DEL=.01 | | | DEL=.02 | | | DEL=.05 | | | DEL=.10 | | | DEL=.15 | | |
|---|---|---|---|---|---|---|---|---|---|---|---|---|---|---|---|
| FACT= | 1.0 .75 | .50 .25 | .00 BIN | 1.0 .75 | .50 .25 | .00 BIN | 1.0 .75 | .50 .25 | .00 BIN | 1.0 75 | .50 .25 | .00 BIN | 1.0 .75 | .50 .25 | .00 BIN |
| PCONT=*** | | | | | REQUIRED NUMBER OF PATIENTS | | | | | | | | | | |
| 0.01 *** | 1310 | 1315 | 1318 | 484 | 484 | 484 | 160 | 160 | 160 | 81 | 81 | 81 | 55 | 55 | 55 |
| *** | 1315 | 1318 | 5053 | 484 | 484 | 1670 | 160 | 160 | 455 | 81 | 81 | 185 | 55 | 55 | 110 |
| 0.02 *** | 2899 | 2911 | 2946 | 933 | 933 | 942 | 251 | 251 | 251 | 111 | 111 | 111 | 73 | 73 | 73 |
| *** | 2902 | 2925 | 8342 | 933 | 939 | 2484 | 251 | 251 | 581 | 111 | 111 | 215 | 73 | 73 | 123 |
| 0.05 *** | 8770 | 8831 | 9208 | 2491 | 2523 | 2578 | 540 | 545 | 545 | 195 | 195 | 195 | 111 | 111 | 111 |
| *** | 8791 | 8922 | 17796 | 2505 | 2543 | 4822 | 540 | 545 | 943 | 195 | 195 | 300 | 111 | 111 | 158 |
| 0.1 *** | 19343 | 19506 | 21431 | 5212 | 5331 | 5667 | 1021 | 1035 | 1056 | 321 | 321 | 326 | 172 | 172 | 172 |
| *** | 19401 | 19807 | 32183 | 5261 | 5448 | 8376 | 1026 | 1044 | 1491 | 321 | 326 | 429 | 172 | 172 | 212 |
| 0.15 *** | 28898 | 29193 | 33851 | 7668 | 7898 | 8765 | 1458 | 1493 | 1546 | 435 | 440 | 443 | 221 | 225 | 225 |
| *** | 28995 | 29747 | 44858 | 7755 | 8166 | 11502 | 1476 | 1520 | 1970 | 440 | 443 | 540 | 221 | 225 | 257 |
| 0.2 *** | 36613 | 37068 | 45480 | 9671 | 10048 | 11649 | 1835 | 1896 | 1998 | 536 | 545 | 554 | 265 | 268 | 268 |
| *** | 36765 | 37946 | 55820 | 9811 | 10503 | 14199 | 1861 | 1940 | 2381 | 540 | 548 | 634 | 265 | 268 | 295 |
| 0.25 *** | 42256 | 42907 | 55836 | 11180 | 11722 | 14198 | 2138 | 2234 | 2386 | 618 | 633 | 645 | 300 | 303 | 309 |
| *** | 42475 | 44181 | 65069 | 11381 | 12393 | 16469 | 2181 | 2304 | 2724 | 624 | 636 | 711 | 303 | 303 | 326 |
| 0.3 *** | 45838 | 46740 | 64656 | 12209 | 12935 | 16365 | 2374 | 2505 | 2715 | 685 | 697 | 720 | 326 | 330 | 335 |
| *** | 46141 | 48478 | 72605 | 12480 | 13836 | 18310 | 2430 | 2593 | 2998 | 688 | 706 | 771 | 330 | 335 | 349 |
| 0.35 *** | 47515 | 48708 | 71791 | 12798 | 13726 | 18106 | 2540 | 2701 | 2972 | 732 | 750 | 773 | 347 | 353 | 356 |
| *** | 47912 | 51001 | 78428 | 13145 | 14855 | 19723 | 2613 | 2815 | 3203 | 741 | 764 | 814 | 347 | 356 | 364 |
| 0.4 *** | 47483 | 49046 | 77155 | 13005 | 14137 | 19405 | 2645 | 2838 | 3161 | 764 | 785 | 811 | 361 | 365 | 370 |
| *** | 48005 | 51969 | 82539 | 13434 | 15485 | 20708 | 2733 | 2972 | 3340 | 773 | 799 | 840 | 361 | 365 | 372 |
| 0.45 *** | 46010 | 48014 | 80695 | 12891 | 14225 | 20241 | 2692 | 2908 | 3270 | 776 | 799 | 828 | 361 | 370 | 373 |
| *** | 46678 | 51631 | 84937 | 13402 | 15770 | 21265 | 2788 | 3060 | 3409 | 785 | 816 | 848 | 365 | 370 | 372 |
| 0.5 *** | 43371 | 45900 | 82384 | 12518 | 14032 | 20618 | 2683 | 2916 | 3310 | 773 | 799 | 828 | 356 | 365 | 370 |
| *** | 44228 | 50240 | 85622 | 13110 | 15735 | 21393 | 2788 | 3077 | 3409 | 785 | 816 | 840 | 361 | 370 | 364 |
| 0.55 *** | 39885 | 43009 | 82209 | 11950 | 13603 | 20530 | 2628 | 2867 | 3275 | 755 | 781 | 811 | 347 | 353 | 361 |
| *** | 40961 | 48031 | 84594 | 12603 | 15415 | 21093 | 2736 | 3039 | 3340 | 767 | 793 | 814 | 347 | 356 | 349 |
| 0.6 *** | 35863 | 39608 | 80170 | 11229 | 12973 | 19973 | 2526 | 2762 | 3161 | 720 | 746 | 776 | 326 | 330 | 338 |
| *** | 37190 | 45196 | 81854 | 11923 | 14834 | 20365 | 2631 | 2928 | 3203 | 732 | 758 | 771 | 330 | 335 | 326 |
| 0.65 *** | 31620 | 35916 | 76271 | 10383 | 12165 | 18950 | 2374 | 2601 | 2978 | 668 | 694 | 720 | 300 | 303 | 309 |
| *** | 33186 | 41875 | 77401 | 11098 | 14011 | 19209 | 2479 | 2759 | 2998 | 680 | 706 | 711 | 300 | 309 | 295 |
| 0.7 *** | 27411 | 32083 | 70531 | 9444 | 11185 | 17471 | 2181 | 2386 | 2718 | 601 | 624 | 645 | 265 | 268 | 274 |
| *** | 29161 | 38153 | 71235 | 10147 | 12944 | 17625 | 2272 | 2526 | 2724 | 615 | 633 | 634 | 265 | 268 | 257 |
| 0.75 *** | 23395 | 28160 | 62959 | 8411 | 10033 | 15534 | 1936 | 2111 | 2386 | 522 | 536 | 554 | 221 | 225 | 230 |
| *** | 25220 | 34049 | 63356 | 9071 | 11635 | 15612 | 2018 | 2234 | 2381 | 528 | 545 | 540 | 221 | 225 | 212 |
| 0.8 *** | 19576 | 24126 | 53570 | 7265 | 8691 | 13140 | 1642 | 1779 | 1980 | 423 | 431 | 443 | 172 | 172 | 172 |
| *** | 21347 | 29516 | 53764 | 7851 | 10056 | 13172 | 1703 | 1870 | 1970 | 426 | 440 | 429 | 172 | 172 | 158 |
| 0.85 *** | 15858 | 19851 | 42391 | 5970 | 7116 | 10301 | 1289 | 1380 | 1508 | 303 | 309 | 318 | . | . | . |
| *** | 17433 | 24410 | 42460 | 6446 | 8161 | 10303 | 1333 | 1438 | 1491 | 309 | 312 | 300 | . | . | . |
| 0.9 *** | 11981 | 15070 | 29438 | 4439 | 5212 | 7015 | 860 | 904 | 960 | . | . | . | . | . | . |
| *** | 13215 | 18413 | 29443 | 4771 | 5865 | 7006 | 881 | 930 | 943 | . | . | . | . | . | . |
| 0.95 *** | 7379 | 9085 | 14729 | 2461 | 2768 | 3296 | . | . | . | . | . | . | . | . | . |
| *** | 8079 | 10748 | 14713 | 2596 | 2986 | 3280 | . | . | . | . | . | . | . | . | . |
| 0.98 *** | 3418 | 3961 | 5069 | . | . | . | . | . | . | . | . | . | . | . | . |
| *** | 3655 | 4390 | 5053 | . | . | . | . | . | . | . | . | . | . | . | . |

## TABLE 8: ALPHA= 0.05 POWER= 0.9 EXPECTED ACCRUAL THRU MINIMUM FOLLOW-UP= 3750

|  | FACT= | DEL=.01 1.0/.75 | .50/.25 | .00 BIN | DEL=.02 1.0/.75 | .50/.25 | .00 BIN | DEL=.05 1.0/.75 | .50/.25 | .00 BIN | DEL=.10 1.0/75 | .50/.25 | .00 BIN | DEL=.15 1.0/.75 | .50/.25 | .00 BIN |
|---|---|---|---|---|---|---|---|---|---|---|---|---|---|---|---|---|

PCONT=***      REQUIRED NUMBER OF PATIENTS

| PCONT | FACT | 1.0/.75 | .50/.25 | .00 BIN | 1.0/.75 | .50/.25 | .00 BIN | 1.0/.75 | .50/.25 | .00 BIN | 1.0/75 | .50/.25 | .00 BIN | 1.0/.75 | .50/.25 | .00 BIN |
|---|---|---|---|---|---|---|---|---|---|---|---|---|---|---|---|---|
| 0.01 | *** | 1309 | 1315 | 1319 | 481 | 484 | 484 | 156 | 156 | 156 | 81 | 81 | 81 | 59 | 59 | 59 |
|  | *** | 1315 | 1319 | 5053 | 481 | 484 | 1670 | 156 | 156 | 455 | 81 | 81 | 185 | 59 | 59 | 110 |
| 0.02 | *** | 2900 | 2913 | 2947 | 931 | 934 | 940 | 250 | 250 | 256 | 109 | 109 | 109 | 72 | 72 | 72 |
|  | *** | 2903 | 2928 | 8342 | 934 | 940 | 2484 | 250 | 256 | 581 | 109 | 109 | 215 | 72 | 72 | 123 |
| 0.05 | *** | 8772 | 8838 | 9203 | 2497 | 2525 | 2581 | 541 | 541 | 547 | 194 | 194 | 194 | 115 | 115 | 115 |
|  | *** | 8797 | 8937 | 17796 | 2506 | 2547 | 4822 | 541 | 547 | 943 | 194 | 194 | 300 | 115 | 115 | 158 |
| 0.1 | *** | 19356 | 19531 | 21428 | 5225 | 5341 | 5669 | 1019 | 1038 | 1056 | 322 | 322 | 325 | 172 | 172 | 172 |
|  | *** | 19413 | 19844 | 32183 | 5272 | 5459 | 8376 | 1028 | 1043 | 1491 | 322 | 325 | 429 | 172 | 172 | 212 |
| 0.15 | *** | 28919 | 29234 | 33850 | 7684 | 7925 | 8763 | 1465 | 1497 | 1544 | 438 | 443 | 447 | 222 | 222 | 222 |
|  | *** | 29022 | 29825 | 44858 | 7778 | 8191 | 11502 | 1478 | 1522 | 1970 | 438 | 443 | 540 | 222 | 222 | 257 |
| 0.2 | *** | 36644 | 37131 | 45481 | 9700 | 10090 | 11647 | 1840 | 1906 | 1994 | 537 | 547 | 550 | 265 | 269 | 269 |
|  | *** | 36809 | 38065 | 55820 | 9847 | 10550 | 14199 | 1868 | 1943 | 2381 | 541 | 550 | 634 | 265 | 269 | 295 |
| 0.25 | *** | 42303 | 43000 | 55834 | 11225 | 11787 | 14200 | 2150 | 2243 | 2388 | 622 | 631 | 644 | 303 | 303 | 306 |
|  | *** | 42537 | 44350 | 65069 | 11434 | 12462 | 16469 | 2191 | 2309 | 2724 | 625 | 634 | 711 | 303 | 306 | 326 |
| 0.3 | *** | 45906 | 46868 | 64656 | 12269 | 13019 | 16366 | 2388 | 2515 | 2716 | 687 | 700 | 719 | 331 | 331 | 334 |
|  | *** | 46225 | 48709 | 72605 | 12550 | 13928 | 18310 | 2444 | 2600 | 2998 | 691 | 709 | 771 | 331 | 334 | 349 |
| 0.35 | *** | 47600 | 48878 | 71791 | 12875 | 13834 | 18106 | 2556 | 2716 | 2975 | 734 | 753 | 775 | 350 | 353 | 359 |
|  | *** | 48025 | 51303 | 78428 | 13234 | 14969 | 19723 | 2628 | 2825 | 3203 | 743 | 762 | 814 | 350 | 353 | 364 |
| 0.4 | *** | 47594 | 49268 | 77159 | 13100 | 14266 | 19403 | 2665 | 2853 | 3156 | 766 | 784 | 813 | 359 | 363 | 372 |
|  | *** | 48153 | 52347 | 82539 | 13544 | 15622 | 20708 | 2750 | 2984 | 3340 | 775 | 800 | 840 | 363 | 368 | 372 |
| 0.45 | *** | 46150 | 48293 | 80697 | 13006 | 14375 | 20243 | 2716 | 2922 | 3269 | 781 | 803 | 831 | 363 | 368 | 372 |
|  | *** | 46872 | 52090 | 84937 | 13534 | 15922 | 21265 | 2809 | 3072 | 3409 | 790 | 818 | 848 | 368 | 372 | 372 |
| 0.5 | *** | 43559 | 46250 | 82384 | 12653 | 14200 | 20618 | 2712 | 2931 | 3306 | 775 | 800 | 831 | 359 | 363 | 372 |
|  | *** | 44472 | 50772 | 85622 | 13259 | 15903 | 21393 | 2809 | 3091 | 3409 | 790 | 813 | 840 | 363 | 368 | 364 |
| 0.55 | *** | 40118 | 43422 | 82206 | 12100 | 13784 | 20528 | 2656 | 2884 | 3275 | 756 | 781 | 813 | 344 | 353 | 359 |
|  | *** | 41266 | 48631 | 84594 | 12766 | 15593 | 21093 | 2759 | 3050 | 3340 | 772 | 800 | 814 | 350 | 353 | 349 |
| 0.6 | *** | 36153 | 40084 | 80168 | 11388 | 13159 | 19972 | 2553 | 2781 | 3162 | 725 | 747 | 775 | 325 | 331 | 340 |
|  | *** | 37553 | 45841 | 81854 | 12097 | 15016 | 20365 | 2656 | 2941 | 3203 | 734 | 762 | 771 | 331 | 334 | 326 |
| 0.65 | *** | 31966 | 36443 | 76272 | 10553 | 12350 | 18953 | 2403 | 2618 | 2975 | 672 | 697 | 719 | 297 | 303 | 312 |
|  | *** | 33606 | 42547 | 77401 | 11275 | 14187 | 19209 | 2500 | 2772 | 2998 | 681 | 706 | 711 | 303 | 306 | 295 |
| 0.7 | *** | 27809 | 32631 | 70531 | 9612 | 11359 | 17468 | 2200 | 2403 | 2716 | 606 | 625 | 644 | 265 | 269 | 275 |
|  | *** | 29622 | 38819 | 71235 | 10325 | 13113 | 17625 | 2294 | 2538 | 2724 | 616 | 634 | 634 | 265 | 269 | 257 |
| 0.75 | *** | 23809 | 28703 | 62956 | 8566 | 10197 | 15531 | 1956 | 2125 | 2384 | 522 | 537 | 556 | 222 | 222 | 228 |
|  | *** | 25690 | 34681 | 63356 | 9231 | 11787 | 15612 | 2037 | 2238 | 2381 | 531 | 547 | 540 | 222 | 228 | 212 |
| 0.8 | *** | 19984 | 24631 | 53572 | 7403 | 8834 | 13141 | 1656 | 1788 | 1981 | 425 | 434 | 443 | 172 | 172 | 175 |
|  | *** | 21794 | 30087 | 53764 | 7994 | 10178 | 13172 | 1718 | 1878 | 1970 | 428 | 438 | 429 | 172 | 175 | 158 |
| 0.85 | *** | 16222 | 20284 | 42391 | 6081 | 7225 | 10300 | 1300 | 1384 | 1506 | 306 | 312 | 316 | . | . | . |
|  | *** | 17825 | 24884 | 42460 | 6565 | 8253 | 10303 | 1338 | 1441 | 1491 | 306 | 312 | 300 | . | . | . |
| 0.9 | *** | 12269 | 15391 | 29434 | 4522 | 5284 | 7019 | 865 | 906 | 959 | . | . | . | . | . | . |
|  | *** | 13522 | 18747 | 29443 | 4844 | 5918 | 7006 | 884 | 931 | 943 | . | . | . | . | . | . |
| 0.95 | *** | 7544 | 9256 | 14725 | 2491 | 2791 | 3297 | . | . | . | . | . | . | . | . | . |
|  | *** | 8247 | 10900 | 14713 | 2628 | 3003 | 3280 | . | . | . | . | . | . | . | . | . |
| 0.98 | *** | 3481 | 4009 | 5069 | . | . | . | . | . | . | . | . | . | . | . | . |
|  | *** | 3709 | 4422 | 5053 | . | . | . | . | . | . | . | . | . | . | . | . |

**TABLE 8: ALPHA= 0.05  POWER= 0.9    EXPECTED ACCRUAL THRU MINIMUM FOLLOW-UP= 4000**

| | DEL=.01 | | | DEL=.02 | | | DEL=.05 | | | DEL=.10 | | | DEL=.15 | | |
|---|---|---|---|---|---|---|---|---|---|---|---|---|---|---|---|
| FACT= | 1.0 .75 | .50 .25 | .00 BIN | 1.0 .75 | .50 .25 | .00 BIN | 1.0 .75 | .50 .25 | .00 BIN | 1.0 75 | .50 .25 | .00 BIN | 1.0 .75 | .50 .25 | .00 BIN |
| **PCONT=*** | | | | REQUIRED NUMBER OF PATIENTS | | | | | | | | | | | |
| 0.01 *** | 1313 | 1317 | 1323 | 483 | 483 | 483 | 157 | 157 | 157 | 83 | 83 | 83 | 57 | 57 | 57 |
| *** | 1313 | 1317 | 5053 | 483 | 483 | 1670 | 157 | 157 | 455 | 83 | 83 | 185 | 57 | 57 | 110 |
| 0.02 *** | 2903 | 2913 | 2947 | 933 | 937 | 943 | 253 | 253 | 253 | 113 | 113 | 113 | 73 | 73 | 73 |
| *** | 2907 | 2927 | 8342 | 933 | 937 | 2484 | 253 | 253 | 581 | 113 | 113 | 215 | 73 | 73 | 123 |
| 0.05 *** | 8777 | 8847 | 9207 | 2497 | 2527 | 2577 | 543 | 543 | 547 | 193 | 193 | 193 | 113 | 113 | 113 |
| *** | 8803 | 8943 | 17796 | 2507 | 2547 | 4822 | 543 | 547 | 943 | 193 | 193 | 300 | 113 | 113 | 158 |
| 0.1 *** | 19367 | 19553 | 21427 | 5237 | 5353 | 5667 | 1023 | 1037 | 1053 | 323 | 323 | 327 | 173 | 173 | 173 |
| *** | 19433 | 19883 | 32183 | 5283 | 5467 | 8376 | 1027 | 1047 | 1491 | 323 | 323 | 429 | 173 | 173 | 212 |
| 0.15 *** | 28943 | 29273 | 33853 | 7707 | 7953 | 8767 | 1467 | 1503 | 1547 | 437 | 443 | 447 | 223 | 223 | 223 |
| *** | 29053 | 29897 | 44858 | 7797 | 8217 | 11502 | 1483 | 1523 | 1970 | 437 | 443 | 540 | 223 | 223 | 257 |
| 0.2 *** | 36677 | 37197 | 45477 | 9733 | 10133 | 11647 | 1847 | 1907 | 1997 | 537 | 547 | 553 | 267 | 267 | 267 |
| *** | 36853 | 38183 | 55820 | 9883 | 10587 | 14199 | 1877 | 1947 | 2381 | 543 | 547 | 634 | 267 | 267 | 295 |
| 0.25 *** | 42347 | 43093 | 55833 | 11267 | 11847 | 14203 | 2157 | 2253 | 2387 | 623 | 633 | 643 | 303 | 303 | 307 |
| *** | 42597 | 44523 | 65069 | 11487 | 12523 | 16469 | 2203 | 2313 | 2724 | 627 | 637 | 711 | 303 | 307 | 326 |
| 0.3 *** | 45967 | 46993 | 64657 | 12327 | 13103 | 16367 | 2403 | 2523 | 2713 | 687 | 703 | 717 | 327 | 333 | 337 |
| *** | 46313 | 48943 | 72605 | 12623 | 14013 | 18310 | 2457 | 2607 | 2998 | 693 | 707 | 771 | 333 | 333 | 349 |
| 0.35 *** | 47683 | 49047 | 71793 | 12953 | 13937 | 18107 | 2577 | 2727 | 2973 | 737 | 753 | 773 | 347 | 353 | 357 |
| *** | 48143 | 51603 | 78428 | 13327 | 15077 | 19723 | 2643 | 2833 | 3203 | 743 | 763 | 814 | 353 | 357 | 364 |
| 0.4 *** | 47707 | 49487 | 77157 | 13197 | 14393 | 19403 | 2687 | 2867 | 3157 | 767 | 787 | 813 | 363 | 367 | 373 |
| *** | 48303 | 52717 | 82539 | 13653 | 15747 | 20708 | 2767 | 2993 | 3340 | 777 | 797 | 840 | 363 | 367 | 372 |
| 0.45 *** | 46297 | 48567 | 80697 | 13117 | 14513 | 20243 | 2737 | 2937 | 3273 | 783 | 803 | 833 | 363 | 367 | 373 |
| *** | 47063 | 52533 | 84937 | 13663 | 16063 | 21265 | 2827 | 3083 | 3409 | 793 | 817 | 848 | 367 | 373 | 372 |
| 0.5 *** | 43743 | 46587 | 82383 | 12783 | 14357 | 20617 | 2733 | 2953 | 3307 | 777 | 803 | 833 | 357 | 363 | 373 |
| *** | 44717 | 51287 | 85622 | 13403 | 16057 | 21393 | 2833 | 3103 | 3409 | 793 | 817 | 840 | 363 | 367 | 364 |
| 0.55 *** | 40347 | 43827 | 82207 | 12243 | 13953 | 20527 | 2677 | 2903 | 3273 | 757 | 783 | 813 | 347 | 353 | 357 |
| *** | 41563 | 49203 | 84594 | 12923 | 15757 | 21093 | 2783 | 3063 | 3340 | 773 | 797 | 814 | 353 | 357 | 349 |
| 0.6 *** | 36437 | 40547 | 80167 | 11543 | 13333 | 19973 | 2573 | 2797 | 3163 | 727 | 747 | 777 | 327 | 333 | 337 |
| *** | 37913 | 46453 | 81854 | 12263 | 15183 | 20365 | 2677 | 2953 | 3203 | 737 | 763 | 771 | 333 | 337 | 326 |
| 0.65 *** | 32307 | 36947 | 76273 | 10713 | 12523 | 18953 | 2423 | 2637 | 2977 | 673 | 697 | 723 | 303 | 303 | 307 |
| *** | 34017 | 43177 | 77401 | 11443 | 14353 | 19209 | 2523 | 2783 | 2998 | 683 | 707 | 711 | 303 | 307 | 295 |
| 0.7 *** | 28193 | 33153 | 70533 | 9767 | 11527 | 17473 | 2223 | 2417 | 2717 | 607 | 627 | 647 | 267 | 267 | 273 |
| *** | 30067 | 39447 | 71235 | 10487 | 13267 | 17625 | 2313 | 2547 | 2724 | 617 | 637 | 634 | 267 | 273 | 257 |
| 0.75 *** | 24213 | 29217 | 62957 | 8713 | 10347 | 15533 | 1977 | 2143 | 2387 | 523 | 537 | 553 | 223 | 223 | 227 |
| *** | 26143 | 35277 | 63356 | 9387 | 11923 | 15612 | 2053 | 2247 | 2381 | 533 | 547 | 540 | 223 | 227 | 212 |
| 0.8 *** | 20377 | 25107 | 53573 | 7537 | 8967 | 13137 | 1673 | 1803 | 1983 | 423 | 433 | 443 | 173 | 173 | 173 |
| *** | 22227 | 30623 | 53764 | 8127 | 10297 | 13172 | 1733 | 1883 | 1970 | 427 | 437 | 429 | 173 | 173 | 158 |
| 0.85 *** | 16573 | 20697 | 42393 | 6193 | 7327 | 10297 | 1307 | 1393 | 1507 | 307 | 313 | 317 | . | . | . |
| *** | 18203 | 25323 | 42460 | 6673 | 8337 | 10303 | 1347 | 1443 | 1491 | 307 | 313 | 300 | . | . | . |
| 0.9 *** | 12547 | 15703 | 29437 | 4593 | 5347 | 7017 | 867 | 907 | 957 | . | . | . | . | . | . |
| *** | 13813 | 19057 | 29443 | 4917 | 5967 | 7006 | 887 | 933 | 943 | . | . | . | . | . | . |
| 0.95 *** | 7697 | 9413 | 14727 | 2523 | 2813 | 3297 | . | . | . | . | . | . | . | . | . |
| *** | 8407 | 11043 | 14713 | 2653 | 3017 | 3280 | . | . | . | . | . | . | . | . | . |
| 0.98 *** | 3533 | 4053 | 5067 | . | . | . | . | . | . | . | . | . | . | . | . |
| *** | 3763 | 4457 | 5053 | . | . | . | . | . | . | . | . | . | . | . | . |

## TABLE 8: ALPHA= 0.05  POWER= 0.9    EXPECTED ACCRUAL THRU MINIMUM FOLLOW-UP= 4250

| | | DEL=.01 | | | DEL=.02 | | | DEL=.05 | | | DEL=.10 | | | DEL=.15 | | |
|---|---|---|---|---|---|---|---|---|---|---|---|---|---|---|---|---|
| FACT= | | 1.0 .75 | .50 .25 | .00 BIN | 1.0 .75 | .50 .25 | .00 BIN | 1.0 .75 | .50 .25 | .00 BIN | 1.0 75 | .50 .25 | .00 BIN | 1.0 .75 | .50 .25 | .00 BIN |
| PCONT=*** | | | | | | | REQUIRED NUMBER OF PATIENTS | | | | | | | | |
| 0.01 | *** | 1310 | 1314 | 1321 | 481 | 481 | 485 | 156 | 156 | 156 | 82 | 82 | 82 | 56 | 56 | 56 |
| | *** | 1314 | 1321 | 5053 | 481 | 481 | 1670 | 156 | 156 | 455 | 82 | 82 | 185 | 56 | 56 | 110 |
| 0.02 | *** | 2904 | 2914 | 2946 | 932 | 938 | 942 | 252 | 252 | 252 | 109 | 109 | 109 | 71 | 71 | 71 |
| | *** | 2908 | 2929 | 8342 | 932 | 938 | 2484 | 252 | 252 | 581 | 109 | 109 | 215 | 71 | 71 | 123 |
| 0.05 | *** | 8783 | 8854 | 9204 | 2500 | 2525 | 2578 | 538 | 545 | 545 | 194 | 194 | 194 | 113 | 113 | 113 |
| | *** | 8811 | 8953 | 17796 | 2511 | 2553 | 4822 | 545 | 545 | 943 | 194 | 194 | 300 | 113 | 113 | 158 |
| 0.1 | *** | 19383 | 19574 | 21427 | 5245 | 5362 | 5666 | 1023 | 1038 | 1055 | 322 | 322 | 326 | 173 | 173 | 173 |
| | *** | 19447 | 19918 | 32183 | 5294 | 5475 | 8376 | 1034 | 1044 | 1491 | 322 | 326 | 429 | 173 | 173 | 212 |
| 0.15 | *** | 28960 | 29311 | 33854 | 7721 | 7976 | 8762 | 1469 | 1501 | 1548 | 439 | 443 | 443 | 220 | 226 | 226 |
| | *** | 29077 | 29970 | 44858 | 7823 | 8238 | 11502 | 1484 | 1523 | 1970 | 439 | 443 | 540 | 220 | 226 | 257 |
| 0.2 | *** | 36713 | 37258 | 45478 | 9761 | 10171 | 11648 | 1856 | 1916 | 1994 | 538 | 545 | 556 | 269 | 269 | 269 |
| | *** | 36893 | 38296 | 55820 | 9916 | 10628 | 14199 | 1884 | 1952 | 2381 | 545 | 549 | 634 | 269 | 269 | 295 |
| 0.25 | *** | 42397 | 43187 | 55838 | 11312 | 11903 | 14202 | 2171 | 2256 | 2387 | 623 | 634 | 645 | 301 | 305 | 305 |
| | *** | 42663 | 44685 | 65069 | 11535 | 12583 | 16469 | 2207 | 2313 | 2724 | 630 | 641 | 711 | 305 | 305 | 326 |
| 0.3 | *** | 46035 | 47118 | 64656 | 12385 | 13178 | 16366 | 2415 | 2532 | 2717 | 687 | 704 | 719 | 333 | 333 | 337 |
| | *** | 46396 | 49165 | 72605 | 12689 | 14092 | 18310 | 2468 | 2610 | 2998 | 694 | 708 | 771 | 333 | 333 | 349 |
| 0.35 | *** | 47767 | 49218 | 71790 | 13023 | 14032 | 18108 | 2589 | 2738 | 2972 | 736 | 758 | 772 | 347 | 354 | 358 |
| | *** | 48255 | 51889 | 78428 | 13412 | 15176 | 19723 | 2659 | 2840 | 3203 | 747 | 762 | 814 | 354 | 354 | 364 |
| 0.4 | *** | 47820 | 49700 | 77155 | 13288 | 14506 | 19404 | 2702 | 2883 | 3159 | 768 | 789 | 811 | 358 | 364 | 368 |
| | *** | 48453 | 53075 | 82539 | 13756 | 15866 | 20708 | 2780 | 2999 | 3340 | 779 | 800 | 840 | 364 | 368 | 372 |
| 0.45 | *** | 46438 | 48846 | 80693 | 13231 | 14648 | 20244 | 2759 | 2957 | 3269 | 783 | 804 | 832 | 364 | 368 | 375 |
| | *** | 47257 | 52962 | 84937 | 13784 | 16200 | 21265 | 2844 | 3088 | 3409 | 793 | 815 | 848 | 368 | 375 | 372 |
| 0.5 | *** | 43927 | 46923 | 82383 | 12913 | 14500 | 20620 | 2755 | 2968 | 3308 | 783 | 804 | 832 | 358 | 364 | 368 |
| | *** | 44958 | 51783 | 85622 | 13539 | 16206 | 21393 | 2851 | 3116 | 3409 | 793 | 815 | 840 | 364 | 368 | 364 |
| 0.55 | *** | 40580 | 44224 | 82209 | 12381 | 14107 | 20531 | 2702 | 2918 | 3276 | 762 | 783 | 815 | 347 | 354 | 358 |
| | *** | 41859 | 49749 | 84594 | 13072 | 15909 | 21093 | 2802 | 3074 | 3340 | 772 | 800 | 814 | 347 | 358 | 349 |
| 0.6 | *** | 36723 | 40998 | 80169 | 11691 | 13497 | 19972 | 2596 | 2812 | 3163 | 726 | 751 | 779 | 326 | 333 | 337 |
| | *** | 38264 | 47040 | 81854 | 12417 | 15339 | 20365 | 2695 | 2968 | 3203 | 740 | 762 | 771 | 333 | 337 | 326 |
| 0.65 | *** | 32643 | 37435 | 76273 | 10862 | 12683 | 18952 | 2447 | 2653 | 2978 | 677 | 698 | 719 | 301 | 305 | 311 |
| | *** | 34418 | 43782 | 77401 | 11599 | 14506 | 19209 | 2536 | 2791 | 2998 | 687 | 708 | 711 | 305 | 305 | 295 |
| 0.7 | *** | 28563 | 33657 | 70532 | 9916 | 11684 | 17471 | 2245 | 2430 | 2717 | 609 | 630 | 645 | 262 | 269 | 273 |
| | *** | 30497 | 40042 | 71235 | 10639 | 13412 | 17625 | 2330 | 2557 | 2724 | 619 | 634 | 634 | 269 | 269 | 257 |
| 0.75 | *** | 24600 | 29711 | 62956 | 8854 | 10494 | 15530 | 1994 | 2153 | 2383 | 528 | 538 | 556 | 220 | 226 | 226 |
| | *** | 26576 | 35845 | 63356 | 9527 | 12052 | 15612 | 2064 | 2256 | 2381 | 534 | 545 | 540 | 226 | 226 | 212 |
| 0.8 | *** | 20754 | 25567 | 53568 | 7657 | 9088 | 13140 | 1686 | 1809 | 1979 | 428 | 432 | 443 | 173 | 173 | 173 |
| | *** | 22638 | 31128 | 53764 | 8252 | 10398 | 13172 | 1746 | 1888 | 1970 | 428 | 439 | 429 | 173 | 173 | 158 |
| 0.85 | *** | 16908 | 21087 | 42390 | 6293 | 7423 | 10299 | 1321 | 1399 | 1505 | 305 | 311 | 315 | . | . | . |
| | *** | 18565 | 25737 | 42460 | 6771 | 8418 | 10303 | 1357 | 1448 | 1491 | 311 | 315 | 300 | . | . | . |
| 0.9 | *** | 12806 | 15994 | 29434 | 4661 | 5411 | 7016 | 874 | 910 | 959 | . | . | . | . | . | . |
| | *** | 14085 | 19351 | 29443 | 4986 | 6017 | 7006 | 889 | 932 | 943 | . | . | . | . | . | . |
| 0.95 | *** | 7848 | 9566 | 14729 | 2553 | 2833 | 3297 | . | . | . | . | . | . | . | . | . |
| | *** | 8560 | 11174 | 14713 | 2681 | 3031 | 3280 | . | . | . | . | . | . | . | . | . |
| 0.98 | *** | 3584 | 4094 | 5071 | . | . | . | . | . | . | . | . | . | . | . | . |
| | *** | 3807 | 4487 | 5053 | . | . | . | . | . | . | . | . | . | . | . | . |

TABLE 8: ALPHA= 0.05  POWER= 0.9    EXPECTED ACCRUAL THRU MINIMUM FOLLOW-UP= 4500

| | | DEL=.01 | | | DEL=.02 | | | DEL=.05 | | | DEL=.10 | | | DEL=.15 | | |
|---|---|---|---|---|---|---|---|---|---|---|---|---|---|---|---|---|---|
| FACT= | | 1.0 .75 | .50 .25 | .00 BIN | 1.0 .75 | .50 .25 | .00 BIN | 1.0 .75 | .50 .25 | .00 BIN | 1.0 75 | .50 .25 | .00 BIN | 1.0 .75 | .50 .25 | .00 BIN |
| PCONT=*** | | | | | REQUIRED NUMBER OF PATIENTS | | | | | | | | | | | |
| 0.01 | *** | 1313 | 1313 | 1320 | 480 | 480 | 487 | 161 | 161 | 161 | 82 | 82 | 82 | 60 | 60 | 60 |
| | *** | 1313 | 1320 | 5053 | 480 | 480 | 1670 | 161 | 161 | 455 | 82 | 82 | 185 | 60 | 60 | 110 |
| 0.02 | *** | 2906 | 2917 | 2951 | 930 | 937 | 941 | 251 | 251 | 255 | 109 | 109 | 109 | 71 | 71 | 71 |
| | *** | 2910 | 2928 | 8342 | 937 | 937 | 2484 | 251 | 255 | 581 | 109 | 109 | 215 | 71 | 71 | 123 |
| 0.05 | *** | 8790 | 8861 | 9206 | 2501 | 2528 | 2580 | 543 | 543 | 548 | 195 | 195 | 195 | 116 | 116 | 116 |
| | *** | 8812 | 8963 | 17796 | 2516 | 2550 | 4822 | 543 | 543 | 943 | 195 | 195 | 300 | 116 | 116 | 158 |
| 0.1 | *** | 19391 | 19601 | 21428 | 5257 | 5374 | 5666 | 1027 | 1038 | 1054 | 323 | 323 | 323 | 172 | 172 | 172 |
| | *** | 19459 | 19950 | 32183 | 5302 | 5482 | 8376 | 1031 | 1050 | 1491 | 323 | 323 | 429 | 172 | 172 | 212 |
| 0.15 | *** | 28983 | 29355 | 33855 | 7743 | 7995 | 8767 | 1470 | 1504 | 1545 | 435 | 442 | 446 | 221 | 221 | 221 |
| | *** | 29107 | 30041 | 44858 | 7845 | 8261 | 11502 | 1488 | 1522 | 1970 | 442 | 442 | 540 | 221 | 221 | 257 |
| 0.2 | *** | 36746 | 37324 | 45480 | 9791 | 10207 | 11647 | 1860 | 1916 | 1995 | 536 | 548 | 555 | 266 | 266 | 266 |
| | *** | 36937 | 38411 | 55820 | 9953 | 10661 | 14199 | 1886 | 1954 | 2381 | 543 | 548 | 634 | 266 | 266 | 295 |
| 0.25 | *** | 42443 | 43282 | 55837 | 11355 | 11955 | 14201 | 2179 | 2265 | 2388 | 622 | 633 | 645 | 300 | 307 | 307 |
| | *** | 42720 | 44850 | 65069 | 11584 | 12637 | 16469 | 2220 | 2321 | 2724 | 626 | 638 | 711 | 300 | 307 | 326 |
| 0.3 | *** | 46099 | 47246 | 64657 | 12439 | 13256 | 16365 | 2426 | 2539 | 2715 | 690 | 705 | 716 | 330 | 334 | 334 |
| | *** | 46481 | 49384 | 72605 | 12754 | 14160 | 18310 | 2478 | 2618 | 2998 | 694 | 712 | 771 | 330 | 334 | 349 |
| 0.35 | *** | 47854 | 49384 | 71794 | 13098 | 14126 | 18109 | 2606 | 2748 | 2973 | 739 | 757 | 773 | 352 | 352 | 356 |
| | *** | 48367 | 52174 | 78428 | 13496 | 15270 | 19723 | 2670 | 2850 | 3203 | 746 | 761 | 814 | 352 | 356 | 364 |
| 0.4 | *** | 47933 | 49920 | 77156 | 13373 | 14617 | 19403 | 2719 | 2895 | 3158 | 773 | 791 | 813 | 363 | 368 | 368 |
| | *** | 48603 | 53430 | 82539 | 13856 | 15978 | 20708 | 2798 | 3007 | 3340 | 780 | 802 | 840 | 363 | 368 | 372 |
| 0.45 | *** | 46583 | 49114 | 80693 | 13335 | 14775 | 20242 | 2775 | 2966 | 3270 | 784 | 806 | 829 | 363 | 368 | 375 |
| | *** | 47445 | 53378 | 84937 | 13901 | 16320 | 21265 | 2861 | 3101 | 3409 | 795 | 818 | 848 | 368 | 375 | 372 |
| 0.5 | *** | 44108 | 47253 | 82380 | 13031 | 14644 | 20618 | 2775 | 2985 | 3311 | 784 | 806 | 829 | 363 | 368 | 368 |
| | *** | 45195 | 52260 | 85622 | 13672 | 16338 | 21393 | 2872 | 3124 | 3409 | 795 | 818 | 840 | 363 | 368 | 364 |
| 0.55 | *** | 40811 | 44614 | 82207 | 12513 | 14257 | 20528 | 2719 | 2933 | 3270 | 768 | 784 | 813 | 345 | 352 | 356 |
| | *** | 42157 | 50280 | 84594 | 13215 | 16050 | 21093 | 2820 | 3079 | 3340 | 773 | 802 | 814 | 352 | 356 | 349 |
| 0.6 | *** | 37005 | 41437 | 80171 | 11831 | 13650 | 19972 | 2618 | 2831 | 3165 | 728 | 750 | 773 | 330 | 334 | 341 |
| | *** | 38613 | 47602 | 81854 | 12570 | 15483 | 20365 | 2715 | 2973 | 3203 | 739 | 761 | 771 | 330 | 334 | 326 |
| 0.65 | *** | 32970 | 37905 | 76271 | 11006 | 12840 | 18953 | 2467 | 2670 | 2978 | 678 | 701 | 723 | 300 | 307 | 311 |
| | *** | 34811 | 44362 | 77401 | 11753 | 14644 | 19209 | 2557 | 2805 | 2998 | 690 | 712 | 711 | 300 | 307 | 295 |
| 0.7 | *** | 28927 | 34140 | 70530 | 10061 | 11831 | 17468 | 2265 | 2445 | 2719 | 611 | 626 | 645 | 266 | 266 | 273 |
| | *** | 30911 | 40616 | 71235 | 10785 | 13541 | 17625 | 2343 | 2561 | 2724 | 622 | 638 | 634 | 266 | 273 | 257 |
| 0.75 | *** | 24978 | 30187 | 62958 | 8985 | 10628 | 15533 | 2006 | 2163 | 2388 | 525 | 543 | 555 | 221 | 228 | 228 |
| | *** | 26992 | 36379 | 63356 | 9667 | 12169 | 15612 | 2078 | 2265 | 2381 | 532 | 548 | 540 | 221 | 228 | 212 |
| 0.8 | *** | 21113 | 26002 | 53569 | 7777 | 9206 | 13136 | 1695 | 1819 | 1983 | 424 | 435 | 446 | 172 | 172 | 176 |
| | *** | 23032 | 31605 | 53764 | 8373 | 10500 | 13172 | 1751 | 1893 | 1970 | 431 | 442 | 429 | 172 | 172 | 158 |
| 0.85 | *** | 17227 | 21457 | 42393 | 6386 | 7511 | 10301 | 1324 | 1403 | 1504 | 307 | 311 | 318 | . | . | . |
| | *** | 18903 | 26130 | 42460 | 6866 | 8490 | 10303 | 1365 | 1448 | 1491 | 307 | 311 | 300 | . | . | . |
| 0.9 | *** | 13053 | 16264 | 29433 | 4728 | 5464 | 7016 | 874 | 915 | 960 | . | . | . | . | . | . |
| | *** | 14351 | 19623 | 29443 | 5048 | 6056 | 7006 | 896 | 937 | 943 | . | . | . | . | . | . |
| 0.95 | *** | 7991 | 9701 | 14730 | 2580 | 2854 | 3300 | . | . | . | . | . | . | . | . | . |
| | *** | 8700 | 11298 | 14713 | 2703 | 3045 | 3280 | . | . | . | . | . | . | . | . | . |
| 0.98 | *** | 3626 | 4132 | 5070 | . | . | . | . | . | . | . | . | . | . | . | . |
| | *** | 3851 | 4508 | 5053 | . | . | . | . | . | . | . | . | . | . | . | . |

## TABLE 8: ALPHA= 0.05  POWER= 0.9    EXPECTED ACCRUAL THRU MINIMUM FOLLOW-UP= 4750

| | | DEL=.01 | | | DEL=.02 | | | DEL=.05 | | | DEL=.10 | | | DEL=.15 | | |
|---|---|---|---|---|---|---|---|---|---|---|---|---|---|---|---|---|
| FACT= | | 1.0 .75 | .50 .25 | .00 BIN | 1.0 .75 | .50 .25 | .00 BIN | 1.0 .75 | .50 .25 | .00 BIN | 1.0 75 | .50 .25 | .00 BIN | 1.0 .75 | .50 .25 | .00 BIN |
| PCONT=*** | | REQUIRED NUMBER OF PATIENTS | | | | | | | | | | | | | | |
| 0.01 | *** | 1314 | 1314 | 1322 | 483 | 483 | 483 | 158 | 158 | 158 | 79 | 79 | 79 | 55 | 55 | 55 |
| | *** | 1314 | 1314 | 5053 | 483 | 483 | 1670 | 158 | 158 | 455 | 79 | 79 | 185 | 55 | 55 | 110 |
| 0.02 | *** | 2905 | 2917 | 2948 | 934 | 934 | 942 | 253 | 253 | 253 | 110 | 110 | 110 | 75 | 75 | 75 |
| | *** | 2913 | 2929 | 8342 | 934 | 942 | 2484 | 253 | 253 | 581 | 110 | 110 | 215 | 75 | 75 | 123 |
| 0.05 | *** | 8791 | 8867 | 9207 | 2502 | 2533 | 2580 | 542 | 542 | 550 | 193 | 193 | 193 | 110 | 115 | 115 |
| | *** | 8819 | 8969 | 17796 | 2514 | 2549 | 4822 | 542 | 542 | 943 | 193 | 193 | 300 | 115 | 115 | 158 |
| 0.1 | *** | 19400 | 19621 | 21430 | 5264 | 5383 | 5668 | 1025 | 1041 | 1053 | 324 | 324 | 324 | 170 | 170 | 174 |
| | *** | 19478 | 19982 | 32183 | 5312 | 5490 | 8376 | 1029 | 1048 | 1491 | 324 | 324 | 429 | 170 | 174 | 212 |
| 0.15 | *** | 29002 | 29394 | 33852 | 7758 | 8019 | 8767 | 1476 | 1504 | 1547 | 435 | 443 | 447 | 222 | 222 | 222 |
| | *** | 29133 | 30107 | 44858 | 7865 | 8273 | 11502 | 1492 | 1523 | 1970 | 443 | 443 | 540 | 222 | 222 | 257 |
| 0.2 | *** | 36773 | 37386 | 45477 | 9817 | 10244 | 11645 | 1868 | 1920 | 1998 | 538 | 542 | 554 | 265 | 269 | 269 |
| | *** | 36982 | 38519 | 55820 | 9983 | 10695 | 14199 | 1892 | 1955 | 2381 | 542 | 550 | 634 | 269 | 269 | 295 |
| 0.25 | *** | 42492 | 43371 | 55832 | 11392 | 12009 | 14199 | 2188 | 2272 | 2390 | 625 | 633 | 645 | 300 | 305 | 305 |
| | *** | 42782 | 45010 | 65069 | 11634 | 12686 | 16469 | 2224 | 2324 | 2724 | 625 | 637 | 711 | 305 | 305 | 326 |
| 0.3 | *** | 46162 | 47373 | 64655 | 12496 | 13327 | 16367 | 2438 | 2549 | 2715 | 692 | 704 | 716 | 329 | 336 | 336 |
| | *** | 46570 | 49598 | 72605 | 12817 | 14230 | 18310 | 2485 | 2620 | 2998 | 697 | 709 | 771 | 329 | 336 | 349 |
| 0.35 | *** | 47943 | 49550 | 71792 | 13165 | 14210 | 18105 | 2616 | 2758 | 2972 | 740 | 756 | 775 | 348 | 352 | 360 |
| | *** | 48482 | 52448 | 78428 | 13577 | 15350 | 19723 | 2680 | 2853 | 3203 | 752 | 763 | 814 | 352 | 352 | 364 |
| 0.4 | *** | 48042 | 50132 | 77155 | 13462 | 14721 | 19407 | 2735 | 2901 | 3162 | 775 | 792 | 811 | 360 | 364 | 372 |
| | *** | 48750 | 53766 | 82539 | 13957 | 16075 | 20708 | 2810 | 3012 | 3340 | 780 | 799 | 840 | 364 | 372 | 372 |
| 0.45 | *** | 46732 | 49384 | 80694 | 13434 | 14895 | 20243 | 2794 | 2977 | 3269 | 787 | 811 | 827 | 364 | 372 | 376 |
| | *** | 47634 | 53778 | 84937 | 14016 | 16438 | 21265 | 2877 | 3107 | 3409 | 799 | 815 | 848 | 364 | 372 | 372 |
| 0.5 | *** | 44290 | 47579 | 82385 | 13149 | 14776 | 20618 | 2794 | 2996 | 3309 | 787 | 804 | 827 | 360 | 364 | 372 |
| | *** | 45430 | 52717 | 85622 | 13795 | 16467 | 21393 | 2882 | 3131 | 3409 | 799 | 815 | 840 | 364 | 372 | 364 |
| 0.55 | *** | 41036 | 44990 | 82207 | 12643 | 14400 | 20528 | 2739 | 2948 | 3274 | 768 | 787 | 811 | 348 | 352 | 360 |
| | *** | 42445 | 50785 | 84594 | 13351 | 16189 | 21093 | 2834 | 3091 | 3340 | 775 | 799 | 814 | 352 | 352 | 349 |
| 0.6 | *** | 37279 | 41855 | 80172 | 11966 | 13795 | 19970 | 2640 | 2842 | 3162 | 732 | 752 | 775 | 329 | 336 | 336 |
| | *** | 38953 | 48137 | 81854 | 12710 | 15619 | 20365 | 2727 | 2984 | 3203 | 740 | 763 | 771 | 329 | 336 | 326 |
| 0.65 | *** | 33294 | 38360 | 76269 | 11142 | 12983 | 18949 | 2485 | 2680 | 2977 | 680 | 697 | 720 | 300 | 305 | 312 |
| | *** | 35189 | 44907 | 77401 | 11895 | 14780 | 19209 | 2573 | 2810 | 2998 | 692 | 709 | 711 | 305 | 305 | 295 |
| 0.7 | *** | 29280 | 34607 | 70529 | 10192 | 11966 | 17472 | 2276 | 2454 | 2715 | 614 | 625 | 645 | 265 | 269 | 269 |
| | *** | 31318 | 41155 | 71235 | 10921 | 13672 | 17625 | 2359 | 2573 | 2724 | 621 | 637 | 634 | 269 | 269 | 257 |
| 0.75 | *** | 25337 | 30641 | 62957 | 9112 | 10755 | 15529 | 2022 | 2169 | 2383 | 530 | 542 | 554 | 222 | 222 | 229 |
| | *** | 27399 | 36892 | 63356 | 9793 | 12282 | 15612 | 2093 | 2264 | 2381 | 538 | 550 | 540 | 222 | 229 | 212 |
| 0.8 | *** | 21462 | 26413 | 53572 | 7888 | 9313 | 13142 | 1706 | 1825 | 1979 | 424 | 435 | 443 | 170 | 174 | 174 |
| | *** | 23409 | 32059 | 53764 | 8487 | 10589 | 13172 | 1761 | 1896 | 1970 | 431 | 443 | 429 | 174 | 174 | 158 |
| 0.85 | *** | 17531 | 21810 | 42390 | 6480 | 7596 | 10299 | 1333 | 1409 | 1504 | 305 | 312 | 317 | . | . | . |
| | *** | 19234 | 26501 | 42460 | 6955 | 8558 | 10303 | 1369 | 1452 | 1491 | 312 | 312 | 300 | . | . | . |
| 0.9 | *** | 13292 | 16526 | 29434 | 4789 | 5518 | 7014 | 882 | 918 | 958 | . | . | . | . | . | . |
| | *** | 14598 | 19882 | 29443 | 5102 | 6095 | 7006 | 899 | 934 | 943 | . | . | . | . | . | . |
| 0.95 | *** | 8119 | 9836 | 14728 | 2604 | 2870 | 3297 | . | . | . | . | . | . | . | . | . |
| | *** | 8838 | 11408 | 14713 | 2727 | 3055 | 3280 | . | . | . | . | . | . | . | . | . |
| 0.98 | *** | 3673 | 4164 | 5067 | . | . | . | . | . | . | . | . | . | . | . | . |
| | *** | 3891 | 4532 | 5053 | . | . | . | . | . | . | . | . | . | . | . | . |

TABLE 8: ALPHA= 0.05  POWER= 0.9     EXPECTED ACCRUAL THRU MINIMUM FOLLOW-UP= 5000

| | DEL=.01 | | | DEL=.02 | | | DEL=.05 | | | DEL=.10 | | | DEL=.15 | | |
|---|---|---|---|---|---|---|---|---|---|---|---|---|---|---|---|
| FACT= | 1.0 .75 | .50 .25 | .00 BIN | 1.0 .75 | .50 .25 | .00 BIN | 1.0 .75 | .50 .25 | .00 BIN | 1.0 75 | .50 .25 | .00 BIN | 1.0 .75 | .50 .25 | .00 BIN |

PCONT=***  REQUIRED NUMBER OF PATIENTS

| PCONT | 1.0/.75 | .50/.25 | .00/BIN | 1.0/.75 | .50/.25 | .00/BIN | 1.0/.75 | .50/.25 | .00/BIN | 1.0/75 | .50/.25 | .00/BIN | 1.0/.75 | .50/.25 | .00/BIN |
|---|---|---|---|---|---|---|---|---|---|---|---|---|---|---|---|
| 0.01 *** | 1316 | 1316 | 1321 | 483 | 483 | 483 | 158 | 158 | 158 | 79 | 79 | 79 | 58 | 58 | 58 |
| *** | 1316 | 1316 | 5053 | 483 | 483 | 1670 | 158 | 158 | 455 | 79 | 79 | 185 | 58 | 58 | 110 |
| 0.02 *** | 2904 | 2921 | 2946 | 933 | 933 | 941 | 254 | 254 | 254 | 108 | 108 | 108 | 71 | 71 | 71 |
| *** | 2908 | 2929 | 8342 | 933 | 941 | 2484 | 254 | 254 | 581 | 108 | 108 | 215 | 71 | 71 | 123 |
| 0.05 *** | 8796 | 8879 | 9204 | 2508 | 2533 | 2579 | 541 | 546 | 546 | 191 | 196 | 196 | 116 | 116 | 116 |
| *** | 8829 | 8979 | 17796 | 2521 | 2554 | 4822 | 541 | 546 | 943 | 191 | 196 | 300 | 116 | 116 | 158 |
| 0.1 *** | 19416 | 19641 | 21429 | 5271 | 5391 | 5666 | 1029 | 1041 | 1054 | 321 | 321 | 329 | 171 | 171 | 171 |
| *** | 19491 | 20016 | 32183 | 5321 | 5496 | 8376 | 1033 | 1046 | 1491 | 321 | 321 | 429 | 171 | 171 | 212 |
| 0.15 *** | 29021 | 29433 | 33854 | 7779 | 8041 | 8766 | 1479 | 1508 | 1546 | 441 | 441 | 446 | 221 | 221 | 221 |
| *** | 29166 | 30171 | 44858 | 7879 | 8291 | 11502 | 1491 | 1529 | 1970 | 441 | 446 | 540 | 221 | 221 | 257 |
| 0.2 *** | 36808 | 37454 | 45479 | 9846 | 10279 | 11646 | 1871 | 1921 | 1996 | 541 | 546 | 554 | 266 | 266 | 271 |
| *** | 37021 | 38629 | 55820 | 10016 | 10729 | 14199 | 1896 | 1954 | 2381 | 541 | 546 | 634 | 266 | 271 | 295 |
| 0.25 *** | 42533 | 43466 | 55833 | 11433 | 12058 | 14204 | 2191 | 2271 | 2383 | 629 | 633 | 646 | 304 | 304 | 308 |
| *** | 42846 | 45158 | 65069 | 11679 | 12733 | 16469 | 2229 | 2321 | 2724 | 629 | 641 | 711 | 304 | 304 | 326 |
| 0.3 *** | 46229 | 47504 | 64654 | 12554 | 13391 | 16366 | 2446 | 2554 | 2716 | 691 | 704 | 716 | 329 | 333 | 333 |
| *** | 46654 | 49808 | 72605 | 12879 | 14296 | 18310 | 2496 | 2629 | 2998 | 696 | 708 | 771 | 333 | 333 | 349 |
| 0.35 *** | 48029 | 49721 | 71791 | 13233 | 14296 | 18108 | 2629 | 2766 | 2971 | 741 | 758 | 771 | 354 | 354 | 358 |
| *** | 48596 | 52721 | 78428 | 13654 | 15433 | 19723 | 2691 | 2858 | 3203 | 746 | 766 | 814 | 354 | 354 | 364 |
| 0.4 *** | 48154 | 50346 | 77158 | 13546 | 14821 | 19404 | 2746 | 2916 | 3158 | 771 | 791 | 808 | 358 | 366 | 371 |
| *** | 48896 | 54096 | 82539 | 14046 | 16179 | 20708 | 2821 | 3021 | 3340 | 783 | 804 | 840 | 366 | 366 | 372 |
| 0.45 *** | 46871 | 49646 | 80696 | 13533 | 15008 | 20241 | 2808 | 2991 | 3271 | 791 | 808 | 829 | 366 | 371 | 371 |
| *** | 47821 | 54171 | 84937 | 14121 | 16546 | 21265 | 2891 | 3116 | 3409 | 796 | 821 | 848 | 366 | 371 | 372 |
| 0.5 *** | 44471 | 47896 | 82383 | 13258 | 14904 | 20616 | 2808 | 3008 | 3308 | 791 | 808 | 829 | 358 | 366 | 371 |
| *** | 45666 | 53158 | 85622 | 13916 | 16583 | 21393 | 2904 | 3141 | 3409 | 796 | 821 | 840 | 366 | 366 | 364 |
| 0.55 *** | 41266 | 45358 | 82208 | 12766 | 14533 | 20529 | 2758 | 2958 | 3271 | 771 | 791 | 816 | 346 | 354 | 358 |
| *** | 42729 | 51271 | 84594 | 13479 | 16308 | 21093 | 2854 | 3096 | 3340 | 779 | 804 | 814 | 354 | 358 | 349 |
| 0.6 *** | 37554 | 42271 | 80171 | 12096 | 13933 | 19971 | 2654 | 2858 | 3158 | 733 | 754 | 779 | 329 | 333 | 341 |
| *** | 39283 | 48658 | 81854 | 12846 | 15746 | 20365 | 2746 | 2991 | 3203 | 741 | 766 | 771 | 333 | 333 | 326 |
| 0.65 *** | 33608 | 38804 | 76271 | 11279 | 13121 | 18954 | 2496 | 2691 | 2979 | 683 | 704 | 721 | 304 | 304 | 308 |
| *** | 35558 | 45433 | 77401 | 12033 | 14904 | 19209 | 2583 | 2816 | 2998 | 691 | 708 | 711 | 304 | 308 | 295 |
| 0.7 *** | 29621 | 35054 | 70529 | 10321 | 12104 | 17471 | 2291 | 2466 | 2716 | 616 | 629 | 646 | 266 | 271 | 271 |
| *** | 31704 | 41671 | 71235 | 11058 | 13783 | 17625 | 2371 | 2579 | 2724 | 621 | 641 | 634 | 266 | 271 | 257 |
| 0.75 *** | 25691 | 31071 | 62958 | 9233 | 10871 | 15533 | 2033 | 2179 | 2383 | 529 | 541 | 554 | 221 | 229 | 229 |
| *** | 27783 | 37379 | 63356 | 9916 | 12383 | 15612 | 2104 | 2271 | 2381 | 533 | 546 | 540 | 221 | 229 | 212 |
| 0.8 *** | 21796 | 26816 | 53571 | 7996 | 9416 | 13141 | 1721 | 1829 | 1979 | 429 | 433 | 446 | 171 | 171 | 171 |
| *** | 23771 | 32491 | 53764 | 8591 | 10679 | 13172 | 1771 | 1896 | 1970 | 433 | 441 | 429 | 171 | 171 | 158 |
| 0.85 *** | 17879 | 22146 | 42391 | 6566 | 7679 | 10296 | 1341 | 1416 | 1504 | 308 | 308 | 316 | . | . | . |
| *** | 19546 | 26854 | 42460 | 7033 | 8616 | 10303 | 1371 | 1454 | 1491 | 308 | 316 | 300 | . | . | . |
| 0.9 *** | 13521 | 16779 | 29433 | 4846 | 5566 | 7016 | 883 | 916 | 958 | . | . | . | . | . | . |
| *** | 14841 | 20121 | 29443 | 5158 | 6129 | 7006 | 904 | 941 | 943 | . | . | . | . | . | . |
| 0.95 *** | 8246 | 9958 | 14729 | 2629 | 2891 | 3296 | . | . | . | . | . | . | . | . | . |
| *** | 8966 | 11516 | 14713 | 2746 | 3066 | 3280 | . | . | . | . | . | . | . | . | . |
| 0.98 *** | 3708 | 4196 | 5071 | . | . | . | . | . | . | . | . | . | . | . | . |
| *** | 3929 | 4554 | 5053 | . | . | . | . | . | . | . | . | . | . | . | . |

| TABLE 8: ALPHA= 0.05  POWER= 0.9     EXPECTED ACCRUAL THRU MINIMUM FOLLOW-UP= 5500 |

| | DEL=.01 | | | DEL=.02 | | | DEL=.05 | | | DEL=.10 | | | DEL=.15 | | |
|---|---|---|---|---|---|---|---|---|---|---|---|---|---|---|---|
| FACT= | 1.0 .75 | .50 .25 | .00 BIN | 1.0 .75 | .50 .25 | .00 BIN | 1.0 .75 | .50 .25 | .00 BIN | 1.0 75 | .50 .25 | .00 BIN | 1.0 .75 | .50 .25 | .00 BIN |

PCONT=***                    REQUIRED NUMBER OF PATIENTS

| PCONT | DEL=.01 | | | DEL=.02 | | | DEL=.05 | | | DEL=.10 | | | DEL=.15 | | |
|---|---|---|---|---|---|---|---|---|---|---|---|---|---|---|---|
| 0.01 *** | 1315 1315 | 1315 1315 | 1324 5053 | 485 485 | 485 485 | 485 1670 | 160 160 | 160 160 | 160 455 | 78 78 | 78 78 | 78 185 | 59 59 | 59 59 | 59 110 |
| 0.02 *** | 2905 2910 | 2919 2933 | 2946 8342 | 930 939 | 939 939 | 939 2484 | 251 251 | 251 251 | 251 581 | 114 114 | 114 114 | 114 215 | 73 73 | 73 73 | 73 123 |
| 0.05 *** | 8804 8837 | 8892 8988 | 9208 17796 | 2512 2520 | 2539 2553 | 2580 4822 | 540 540 | 545 545 | 545 943 | 196 196 | 196 196 | 196 300 | 114 114 | 114 114 | 114 158 |
| 0.1 *** | 19438 19520 | 19685 20070 | 21426 32183 | 5289 5339 | 5408 5509 | 5669 8376 | 1027 1035 | 1040 1049 | 1054 1491 | 320 325 | 325 325 | 325 429 | 169 169 | 174 174 | 174 212 |
| 0.15 *** | 29063 29214 | 29517 30295 | 33848 44858 | 7814 7915 | 8075 8323 | 8763 11502 | 1480 1494 | 1508 1530 | 1544 1970 | 435 444 | 444 444 | 444 540 | 224 224 | 224 224 | 224 257 |
| 0.2 *** | 36873 37107 | 37574 38834 | 45480 55820 | 9895 10074 | 10344 10784 | 11650 14199 | 1879 1901 | 1929 1956 | 1998 2381 | 540 545 | 545 554 | 554 634 | 265 265 | 270 270 | 270 295 |
| 0.25 *** | 42629 42973 | 43646 45461 | 55834 65069 | 11513 11765 | 12159 12819 | 14199 16469 | 2204 2237 | 2278 2328 | 2388 2724 | 628 628 | 636 642 | 642 711 | 306 306 | 306 306 | 306 326 |
| 0.3 *** | 46355 46823 | 47749 50210 | 64656 72605 | 12654 12989 | 13520 14414 | 16366 18310 | 2465 2512 | 2567 2635 | 2713 2998 | 697 697 | 705 710 | 719 771 | 334 334 | 334 334 | 334 349 |
| 0.35 *** | 48198 48822 | 50045 53235 | 71793 78428 | 13369 13800 | 14455 15583 | 18104 19723 | 2649 2713 | 2781 2869 | 2974 3203 | 746 752 | 760 765 | 774 814 | 353 353 | 353 353 | 361 364 |
| 0.4 *** | 48376 49193 | 50769 54729 | 77155 82539 | 13704 14227 | 15010 16353 | 19405 20708 | 2773 2850 | 2933 3034 | 3158 3340 | 779 788 | 793 801 | 815 840 | 361 367 | 367 367 | 367 372 |
| 0.45 *** | 47158 48198 | 50164 54913 | 80694 84937 | 13726 14323 | 15225 16751 | 20244 21265 | 2836 2919 | 3015 3125 | 3268 3409 | 793 801 | 807 820 | 829 848 | 367 367 | 367 375 | 375 372 |
| 0.5 *** | 44834 46135 | 48514 54005 | 82385 85622 | 13470 14144 | 15134 16806 | 20620 21393 | 2842 2924 | 3029 3153 | 3309 3409 | 793 801 | 807 820 | 829 840 | 361 367 | 367 367 | 367 364 |
| 0.55 *** | 41713 43289 | 46072 52190 | 82207 84594 | 12998 13726 | 14785 16545 | 20524 21093 | 2787 2878 | 2988 3111 | 3276 3340 | 774 779 | 793 801 | 815 814 | 348 353 | 353 353 | 361 349 |
| 0.6 *** | 38091 39925 | 43060 49633 | 80166 81854 | 12338 13099 | 14194 15981 | 19974 20365 | 2685 2773 | 2878 3007 | 3158 3203 | 738 746 | 752 765 | 774 771 | 334 334 | 334 334 | 339 326 |
| 0.65 *** | 34219 36268 | 39637 46429 | 76275 77401 | 11526 12288 | 13374 15129 | 18951 19209 | 2525 2616 | 2713 2828 | 2974 2998 | 683 691 | 705 710 | 719 711 | 306 306 | 306 306 | 312 295 |
| 0.7 *** | 30287 32454 | 35905 42643 | 70528 71235 | 10564 11306 | 12343 13993 | 17472 17625 | 2319 2396 | 2484 2589 | 2718 2724 | 614 623 | 628 636 | 650 634 | 265 270 | 270 270 | 270 257 |
| 0.75 *** | 26363 28527 | 31895 38289 | 62957 63356 | 9455 10143 | 11092 12571 | 15533 15612 | 2058 2121 | 2195 2278 | 2383 2381 | 532 540 | 540 545 | 554 540 | 224 224 | 224 224 | 229 212 |
| 0.8 *** | 22435 24465 | 27564 33293 | 53574 53764 | 8190 8790 | 9601 10825 | 13140 13172 | 1736 1783 | 1846 1907 | 1984 1970 | 430 430 | 435 444 | 444 429 | 174 174 | 174 174 | 174 158 |
| 0.85 *** | 18388 20148 | 22779 27504 | 42387 42460 | 6719 7187 | 7819 8727 | 10303 10303 | 1351 1384 | 1420 1461 | 1503 1491 | 306 312 | 312 312 | 320 300 | . . | . . | . . |
| 0.9 *** | 13952 15285 | 17238 20574 | 29434 29443 | 4954 5262 | 5655 6191 | 7016 7006 | 889 903 | 925 939 | 958 943 | . . | . . | . . | . . | . . | . . |
| 0.95 *** | 8488 9203 | 10184 11710 | 14730 14713 | 2671 2781 | 2919 3084 | 3295 3280 | . . | . . | . . | . . | . . | . . | . . | . . | . . |
| 0.98 *** | 3785 3991 | 4253 4596 | 5069 5053 | . . | . . | . . | . . | . . | . . | . . | . . | . . | . . | . . | . . |

TABLE 8: ALPHA= 0.05  POWER= 0.9     EXPECTED ACCRUAL THRU MINIMUM FOLLOW-UP= 6000

| | | DEL=.01 | | | DEL=.02 | | | DEL=.05 | | | DEL=.10 | | | DEL=.15 | |
|---|---|---|---|---|---|---|---|---|---|---|---|---|---|---|---|---|
| FACT= | 1.0 .75 | .50 .25 | .00 BIN | 1.0 .75 | .50 .25 | .00 BIN | 1.0 .75 | .50 .25 | .00 BIN | 1.0 75 | .50 .25 | .00 BIN | 1.0 .75 | .50 .25 | .00 BIN |
| PCONT=*** | | | REQUIRED NUMBER OF PATIENTS | | | | | | | | | | | | | |
| 0.01 *** | 1315 | 1315 | 1324 | 484 | 484 | 484 | 160 | 160 | 160 | 79 | 79 | 79 | 55 | 55 | 55 |
| *** | 1315 | 1315 | 5053 | 484 | 484 | 1670 | 160 | 160 | 455 | 79 | 79 | 185 | 55 | 55 | 110 |
| 0.02 *** | 2905 | 2920 | 2950 | 934 | 940 | 940 | 250 | 250 | 250 | 109 | 109 | 109 | 70 | 70 | 70 |
| *** | 2914 | 2935 | 8342 | 934 | 940 | 2484 | 250 | 250 | 581 | 109 | 109 | 215 | 70 | 70 | 123 |
| 0.05 *** | 8815 | 8905 | 9205 | 2515 | 2539 | 2575 | 544 | 544 | 544 | 190 | 190 | 190 | 115 | 115 | 115 |
| *** | 8845 | 9004 | 17796 | 2524 | 2560 | 4822 | 544 | 544 | 943 | 190 | 190 | 300 | 115 | 115 | 158 |
| 0.1 *** | 19459 | 19729 | 21430 | 5305 | 5425 | 5665 | 1030 | 1045 | 1054 | 325 | 325 | 325 | 169 | 169 | 169 |
| *** | 19555 | 20134 | 32183 | 5350 | 5524 | 8376 | 1039 | 1045 | 1491 | 325 | 325 | 429 | 169 | 169 | 212 |
| 0.15 *** | 29110 | 29599 | 33850 | 7840 | 8110 | 8764 | 1489 | 1510 | 1549 | 439 | 445 | 445 | 220 | 220 | 220 |
| *** | 29275 | 30415 | 44858 | 7954 | 8350 | 11502 | 1504 | 1525 | 1970 | 439 | 445 | 540 | 220 | 220 | 257 |
| 0.2 *** | 36934 | 37699 | 45475 | 9949 | 10399 | 11644 | 1885 | 1930 | 1999 | 544 | 550 | 550 | 265 | 265 | 265 |
| *** | 37195 | 39025 | 55820 | 10129 | 10834 | 14199 | 1909 | 1960 | 2381 | 544 | 550 | 634 | 265 | 265 | 295 |
| 0.25 *** | 42724 | 43825 | 55834 | 11584 | 12244 | 14200 | 2215 | 2290 | 2389 | 625 | 634 | 640 | 304 | 304 | 304 |
| *** | 43090 | 45745 | 65069 | 11845 | 12895 | 16469 | 2254 | 2335 | 2724 | 634 | 640 | 711 | 304 | 304 | 326 |
| 0.3 *** | 46480 | 47995 | 64654 | 12754 | 13630 | 16369 | 2479 | 2575 | 2710 | 694 | 709 | 715 | 334 | 334 | 334 |
| *** | 46990 | 50599 | 72605 | 13105 | 14515 | 18310 | 2524 | 2635 | 2998 | 700 | 709 | 771 | 334 | 334 | 349 |
| 0.35 *** | 48370 | 50374 | 71794 | 13495 | 14599 | 18109 | 2674 | 2794 | 2974 | 745 | 760 | 775 | 349 | 355 | 355 |
| *** | 49045 | 53725 | 78428 | 13939 | 15715 | 19723 | 2725 | 2875 | 3203 | 754 | 769 | 814 | 355 | 355 | 364 |
| 0.4 *** | 48604 | 51175 | 77155 | 13855 | 15184 | 19405 | 2800 | 2944 | 3160 | 784 | 799 | 814 | 364 | 364 | 370 |
| *** | 49489 | 55324 | 82539 | 14389 | 16510 | 20708 | 2869 | 3040 | 3340 | 790 | 805 | 840 | 364 | 370 | 372 |
| 0.45 *** | 47449 | 50665 | 80695 | 13900 | 15424 | 20245 | 2860 | 3025 | 3274 | 799 | 814 | 829 | 364 | 370 | 370 |
| *** | 48565 | 55615 | 84937 | 14515 | 16930 | 21265 | 2935 | 3139 | 3409 | 805 | 820 | 848 | 370 | 370 | 372 |
| 0.5 *** | 45199 | 49114 | 82384 | 13669 | 15355 | 20620 | 2869 | 3049 | 3310 | 790 | 814 | 829 | 364 | 364 | 370 |
| *** | 46585 | 54790 | 85622 | 14359 | 16999 | 21393 | 2950 | 3169 | 3409 | 805 | 820 | 840 | 364 | 370 | 364 |
| 0.55 *** | 42154 | 46759 | 82210 | 13210 | 15010 | 20530 | 2815 | 3004 | 3274 | 775 | 790 | 814 | 349 | 355 | 355 |
| *** | 43825 | 53050 | 84594 | 13954 | 16744 | 21093 | 2905 | 3124 | 3340 | 784 | 805 | 814 | 355 | 355 | 349 |
| 0.6 *** | 38614 | 43810 | 80170 | 12565 | 14425 | 19969 | 2710 | 2899 | 3160 | 739 | 754 | 775 | 334 | 334 | 340 |
| *** | 40549 | 50530 | 81854 | 13330 | 16189 | 20365 | 2800 | 3019 | 3203 | 745 | 769 | 771 | 334 | 334 | 326 |
| 0.65 *** | 34810 | 40429 | 76270 | 11755 | 13609 | 18949 | 2554 | 2734 | 2974 | 685 | 700 | 724 | 304 | 304 | 310 |
| *** | 36949 | 47344 | 77401 | 12520 | 15334 | 19209 | 2635 | 2839 | 2998 | 694 | 709 | 711 | 304 | 310 | 295 |
| 0.7 *** | 30910 | 36700 | 70534 | 10789 | 12565 | 17470 | 2344 | 2500 | 2719 | 619 | 634 | 649 | 265 | 274 | 274 |
| *** | 33154 | 43540 | 71235 | 11530 | 14185 | 17625 | 2419 | 2599 | 2724 | 625 | 640 | 634 | 265 | 274 | 257 |
| 0.75 *** | 26995 | 32659 | 62959 | 9664 | 11290 | 15529 | 2080 | 2209 | 2389 | 535 | 544 | 550 | 220 | 229 | 229 |
| *** | 29215 | 39124 | 63356 | 10345 | 12730 | 15612 | 2140 | 2290 | 2381 | 535 | 550 | 540 | 220 | 229 | 212 |
| 0.8 *** | 23029 | 28264 | 53569 | 8374 | 9769 | 13135 | 1750 | 1855 | 1984 | 430 | 439 | 445 | 175 | 175 | 175 |
| *** | 25105 | 34030 | 53764 | 8965 | 10960 | 13172 | 1804 | 1909 | 1970 | 430 | 439 | 429 | 175 | 175 | 158 |
| 0.85 *** | 18904 | 23365 | 42394 | 6865 | 7945 | 10300 | 1360 | 1429 | 1504 | 310 | 310 | 319 | . | . | . |
| *** | 20695 | 28090 | 42460 | 7330 | 8824 | 10303 | 1390 | 1465 | 1491 | 310 | 310 | 300 | . | . | . |
| 0.9 *** | 14350 | 17659 | 29434 | 5044 | 5734 | 7015 | 895 | 925 | 955 | . | . | . | . | . | . |
| *** | 15700 | 20974 | 29443 | 5350 | 6250 | 7006 | 910 | 940 | 943 | . | . | . | . | . | . |
| 0.95 *** | 8704 | 10390 | 14725 | 2704 | 2944 | 3295 | . | . | . | . | . | . | . | . | . |
| *** | 9415 | 11875 | 14713 | 2815 | 3100 | 3280 | . | . | . | . | . | . | . | . | . |
| 0.98 *** | 3850 | 4309 | 5065 | . | . | . | . | . | . | . | . | . | . | . | . |
| *** | 4054 | 4630 | 5053 | . | . | . | . | . | . | . | . | . | . | . | . |

## TABLE 8: ALPHA= 0.05 POWER= 0.9    EXPECTED ACCRUAL THRU MINIMUM FOLLOW-UP= 6500

|  |  | DEL=.01 | | | DEL=.02 | | | DEL=.05 | | | DEL=.10 | | | DEL=.15 | | |
|---|---|---|---|---|---|---|---|---|---|---|---|---|---|---|---|---|
| FACT= | | 1.0 .75 | .50 .25 | .00 BIN | 1.0 .75 | .50 .25 | .00 BIN | 1.0 .75 | .50 .25 | .00 BIN | 1.0 75 | .50 .25 | .00 BIN | 1.0 .75 | .50 .25 | .00 BIN |

PCONT=***                              REQUIRED NUMBER OF PATIENTS

| PCONT | | 1.0/.75 | .50/.25 | .00/BIN | 1.0/.75 | .50/.25 | .00/BIN | 1.0/.75 | .50/.25 | .00/BIN | 1.0/.75 | .50/.25 | .00/BIN | 1.0/.75 | .50/.25 | .00/BIN |
|---|---|---|---|---|---|---|---|---|---|---|---|---|---|---|---|---|
| 0.01 | *** | 1311 | 1321 | 1321 | 482 | 482 | 482 | 157 | 157 | 157 | 76 | 76 | 76 | 53 | 53 | 53 |
|  | *** | 1311 | 1321 | 5053 | 482 | 482 | 1670 | 157 | 157 | 455 | 76 | 76 | 185 | 53 | 53 | 110 |
| 0.02 | *** | 2913 | 2919 | 2946 | 937 | 937 | 937 | 254 | 254 | 254 | 108 | 108 | 108 | 70 | 70 | 70 |
|  | *** | 2913 | 2936 | 8342 | 937 | 937 | 2484 | 254 | 254 | 581 | 108 | 108 | 215 | 70 | 70 | 123 |
| 0.05 | *** | 8818 | 8916 | 9208 | 2513 | 2540 | 2578 | 541 | 547 | 547 | 189 | 189 | 189 | 108 | 108 | 108 |
|  | *** | 8861 | 9013 | 17796 | 2529 | 2556 | 4822 | 541 | 547 | 943 | 189 | 189 | 300 | 108 | 108 | 158 |
| 0.1 | *** | 19488 | 19765 | 21428 | 5318 | 5438 | 5666 | 1034 | 1045 | 1051 | 319 | 319 | 330 | 173 | 173 | 173 |
|  | *** | 19586 | 20177 | 32183 | 5367 | 5530 | 8376 | 1034 | 1051 | 1491 | 319 | 319 | 429 | 173 | 173 | 212 |
| 0.15 | *** | 29147 | 29677 | 33853 | 7870 | 8136 | 8763 | 1489 | 1516 | 1548 | 443 | 443 | 443 | 222 | 222 | 222 |
|  | *** | 29326 | 30528 | 44858 | 7983 | 8373 | 11502 | 1506 | 1532 | 1970 | 443 | 443 | 540 | 222 | 222 | 257 |
| 0.2 | *** | 37006 | 37824 | 45478 | 9998 | 10453 | 11646 | 1890 | 1938 | 1993 | 541 | 547 | 557 | 265 | 271 | 271 |
|  | *** | 37282 | 39216 | 55820 | 10183 | 10882 | 14199 | 1912 | 1961 | 2381 | 547 | 547 | 634 | 265 | 271 | 295 |
| 0.25 | *** | 42813 | 43999 | 55829 | 11656 | 12322 | 14197 | 2231 | 2296 | 2383 | 628 | 638 | 644 | 303 | 303 | 303 |
|  | *** | 43219 | 46025 | 65069 | 11922 | 12962 | 16469 | 2263 | 2334 | 2724 | 628 | 638 | 711 | 303 | 303 | 326 |
| 0.3 | *** | 46610 | 48241 | 64653 | 12848 | 13736 | 16368 | 2491 | 2588 | 2718 | 693 | 709 | 720 | 330 | 336 | 336 |
|  | *** | 47162 | 50965 | 72605 | 13206 | 14613 | 18310 | 2540 | 2643 | 2998 | 703 | 709 | 771 | 330 | 336 | 349 |
| 0.35 | *** | 48543 | 50688 | 71797 | 13612 | 14733 | 18107 | 2686 | 2806 | 2968 | 752 | 758 | 774 | 352 | 352 | 362 |
|  | *** | 49275 | 54188 | 78428 | 14061 | 15832 | 19723 | 2741 | 2881 | 3203 | 752 | 768 | 814 | 352 | 352 | 364 |
| 0.4 | *** | 48826 | 51572 | 77160 | 14002 | 15345 | 19407 | 2816 | 2962 | 3157 | 785 | 801 | 807 | 362 | 368 | 368 |
|  | *** | 49778 | 55894 | 82539 | 14548 | 16651 | 20708 | 2881 | 3049 | 3340 | 791 | 801 | 840 | 362 | 368 | 372 |
| 0.45 | *** | 47731 | 51160 | 80692 | 14067 | 15605 | 20242 | 2887 | 3043 | 3271 | 801 | 817 | 833 | 368 | 368 | 378 |
|  | *** | 48933 | 56268 | 84937 | 14695 | 17089 | 21265 | 2962 | 3147 | 3409 | 807 | 823 | 848 | 368 | 368 | 372 |
| 0.5 | *** | 45553 | 49687 | 82382 | 13856 | 15556 | 20616 | 2897 | 3066 | 3309 | 801 | 817 | 833 | 362 | 368 | 368 |
|  | *** | 47032 | 55537 | 85622 | 14548 | 17171 | 21393 | 2968 | 3173 | 3409 | 807 | 823 | 840 | 362 | 368 | 364 |
| 0.55 | *** | 42586 | 47412 | 82203 | 13417 | 15221 | 20528 | 2838 | 3017 | 3271 | 774 | 791 | 817 | 352 | 352 | 362 |
|  | *** | 44357 | 53857 | 84594 | 14158 | 16927 | 21093 | 2930 | 3131 | 3340 | 785 | 801 | 814 | 352 | 352 | 349 |
| 0.6 | *** | 39118 | 44519 | 80166 | 12777 | 14636 | 19976 | 2741 | 2913 | 3163 | 742 | 758 | 774 | 330 | 336 | 336 |
|  | *** | 41150 | 51371 | 81854 | 13547 | 16374 | 20365 | 2822 | 3027 | 3203 | 752 | 768 | 771 | 336 | 336 | 326 |
| 0.65 | *** | 35371 | 41172 | 76272 | 11965 | 13817 | 18952 | 2578 | 2751 | 2978 | 687 | 703 | 720 | 303 | 303 | 313 |
|  | *** | 37591 | 48192 | 77401 | 12734 | 15513 | 19209 | 2659 | 2848 | 2998 | 693 | 709 | 711 | 303 | 303 | 295 |
| 0.7 | *** | 31513 | 37451 | 70530 | 10990 | 12761 | 17473 | 2367 | 2513 | 2718 | 622 | 628 | 644 | 265 | 271 | 271 |
|  | *** | 33821 | 44367 | 71235 | 11737 | 14353 | 17625 | 2432 | 2605 | 2724 | 628 | 638 | 634 | 271 | 271 | 257 |
| 0.75 | *** | 27597 | 33382 | 62957 | 9858 | 11467 | 15529 | 2101 | 2221 | 2383 | 531 | 547 | 557 | 222 | 222 | 232 |
|  | *** | 29872 | 39888 | 63356 | 10535 | 12881 | 15612 | 2156 | 2296 | 2381 | 541 | 547 | 540 | 222 | 222 | 212 |
| 0.8 | *** | 23589 | 28913 | 53571 | 8536 | 9917 | 13141 | 1766 | 1863 | 1977 | 433 | 433 | 443 | 173 | 173 | 173 |
|  | *** | 25712 | 34698 | 53764 | 9127 | 11077 | 13172 | 1808 | 1912 | 1970 | 433 | 443 | 429 | 173 | 173 | 158 |
| 0.85 | *** | 19391 | 23908 | 42391 | 6998 | 8054 | 10297 | 1370 | 1435 | 1506 | 313 | 313 | 313 | . | . | . |
|  | *** | 21211 | 28627 | 42460 | 7453 | 8910 | 10303 | 1402 | 1467 | 1491 | 313 | 313 | 300 | . | . | . |
| 0.9 | *** | 14717 | 18048 | 29433 | 5129 | 5796 | 7014 | 898 | 931 | 953 | . | . | . | . | . | . |
|  | *** | 16082 | 21331 | 29443 | 5432 | 6293 | 7006 | 915 | 937 | 943 | . | . | . | . | . | . |
| 0.95 | *** | 8899 | 10573 | 14727 | 2735 | 2968 | 3293 | . | . | . | . | . | . | . | . | . |
|  | *** | 9608 | 12030 | 14713 | 2838 | 3114 | 3280 | . | . | . | . | . | . | . | . | . |
| 0.98 | *** | 3911 | 4349 | 5064 | . | . | . | . | . | . | . | . | . | . | . | . |
|  | *** | 4106 | 4658 | 5053 | . | . | . | . | . | . | . | . | . | . | . | . |

TABLE 8: ALPHA= 0.05  POWER= 0.9    EXPECTED ACCRUAL THRU MINIMUM FOLLOW-UP= 7000

| FACT= | DEL=.01 1.0 / .75 | DEL=.01 .50 / .25 | DEL=.01 .00 / BIN | DEL=.02 1.0 / .75 | DEL=.02 .50 / .25 | DEL=.02 .00 / BIN | DEL=.05 1.0 / .75 | DEL=.05 .50 / .25 | DEL=.05 .00 / BIN | DEL=.10 1.0 / 75 | DEL=.10 .50 / .25 | DEL=.10 .00 / BIN | DEL=.15 1.0 / .75 | DEL=.15 .50 / .25 | DEL=.15 .00 / BIN |
|---|---|---|---|---|---|---|---|---|---|---|---|---|---|---|---|
| PCONT=*** | | | | | REQUIRED NUMBER OF PATIENTS | | | | | | | | | | |
| 0.01 *** | 1317 | 1317 | 1317 | 484 | 484 | 484 | 162 | 162 | 162 | 81 | 81 | 81 | 57 | 57 | 57 |
| *** | 1317 | 1317 | 5053 | 484 | 484 | 1670 | 162 | 162 | 455 | 81 | 81 | 185 | 57 | 57 | 110 |
| 0.02 *** | 2910 | 2927 | 2945 | 932 | 939 | 939 | 250 | 250 | 250 | 110 | 110 | 110 | 75 | 75 | 75 |
| *** | 2916 | 2934 | 8342 | 939 | 939 | 2484 | 250 | 250 | 581 | 110 | 110 | 215 | 75 | 75 | 123 |
| 0.05 *** | 8831 | 8919 | 9210 | 2525 | 2542 | 2577 | 547 | 547 | 547 | 197 | 197 | 197 | 110 | 110 | 110 |
| *** | 8866 | 9024 | 17796 | 2531 | 2560 | 4822 | 547 | 547 | 943 | 197 | 197 | 300 | 110 | 110 | 158 |
| 0.1 *** | 19506 | 19804 | 21431 | 5331 | 5447 | 5664 | 1037 | 1044 | 1055 | 320 | 326 | 326 | 169 | 169 | 169 |
| *** | 19611 | 20224 | 32183 | 5377 | 5535 | 8376 | 1037 | 1044 | 1491 | 320 | 326 | 429 | 169 | 169 | 212 |
| 0.15 *** | 29195 | 29744 | 33850 | 7897 | 8166 | 8761 | 1492 | 1516 | 1545 | 442 | 442 | 442 | 221 | 221 | 221 |
| *** | 29376 | 30630 | 44858 | 8009 | 8394 | 11502 | 1510 | 1534 | 1970 | 442 | 442 | 540 | 221 | 221 | 257 |
| 0.2 *** | 37070 | 37945 | 45476 | 10050 | 10505 | 11649 | 1895 | 1936 | 2000 | 547 | 547 | 554 | 267 | 267 | 267 |
| *** | 37367 | 39386 | 55820 | 10231 | 10914 | 14199 | 1919 | 1965 | 2381 | 547 | 547 | 634 | 267 | 267 | 295 |
| 0.25 *** | 42904 | 44181 | 55836 | 11719 | 12395 | 14197 | 2234 | 2304 | 2385 | 635 | 635 | 641 | 302 | 302 | 309 |
| *** | 43341 | 46281 | 65069 | 11992 | 13025 | 16469 | 2269 | 2339 | 2724 | 635 | 641 | 711 | 302 | 309 | 326 |
| 0.3 *** | 46736 | 48480 | 64656 | 12937 | 13836 | 16367 | 2507 | 2595 | 2717 | 694 | 705 | 722 | 326 | 337 | 337 |
| *** | 47331 | 51315 | 72605 | 13305 | 14694 | 18310 | 2542 | 2647 | 2998 | 705 | 711 | 771 | 337 | 337 | 349 |
| 0.35 *** | 48707 | 51000 | 71790 | 13725 | 14851 | 18106 | 2700 | 2811 | 2969 | 746 | 764 | 775 | 355 | 355 | 355 |
| *** | 49495 | 54640 | 78428 | 14186 | 15936 | 19723 | 2752 | 2892 | 3203 | 757 | 764 | 814 | 355 | 355 | 364 |
| 0.4 *** | 49046 | 51969 | 77151 | 14134 | 15481 | 19401 | 2840 | 2969 | 3161 | 781 | 799 | 810 | 361 | 361 | 372 |
| *** | 50061 | 56425 | 82539 | 14687 | 16776 | 20708 | 2899 | 3056 | 3340 | 792 | 799 | 840 | 361 | 372 | 372 |
| 0.45 *** | 48014 | 51630 | 80697 | 14221 | 15772 | 20241 | 2910 | 3056 | 3266 | 799 | 816 | 827 | 372 | 372 | 372 |
| *** | 49291 | 56897 | 84937 | 14851 | 17231 | 21265 | 2980 | 3155 | 3409 | 810 | 827 | 848 | 372 | 372 | 372 |
| 0.5 *** | 45896 | 50236 | 82384 | 14029 | 15737 | 20620 | 2916 | 3074 | 3312 | 799 | 816 | 827 | 361 | 372 | 372 |
| *** | 47471 | 56232 | 85622 | 14729 | 17330 | 21393 | 2986 | 3179 | 3409 | 810 | 827 | 840 | 361 | 372 | 364 |
| 0.55 *** | 43009 | 48031 | 82209 | 13602 | 15411 | 20532 | 2864 | 3039 | 3277 | 781 | 792 | 810 | 355 | 355 | 361 |
| *** | 44864 | 54605 | 84594 | 14355 | 17091 | 21093 | 2945 | 3144 | 3340 | 792 | 799 | 814 | 355 | 355 | 349 |
| 0.6 *** | 39607 | 45196 | 80172 | 12972 | 14834 | 19972 | 2759 | 2927 | 3161 | 746 | 757 | 775 | 326 | 337 | 337 |
| *** | 41714 | 52161 | 81854 | 13749 | 16542 | 20365 | 2840 | 3032 | 3203 | 746 | 764 | 771 | 337 | 337 | 326 |
| 0.65 *** | 35915 | 41871 | 76270 | 12167 | 14011 | 18946 | 2601 | 2759 | 2980 | 694 | 705 | 722 | 302 | 309 | 309 |
| *** | 38207 | 48987 | 77401 | 12937 | 15674 | 19209 | 2671 | 2857 | 2998 | 694 | 711 | 711 | 302 | 309 | 295 |
| 0.7 *** | 32082 | 38155 | 70530 | 11187 | 12944 | 17470 | 2385 | 2525 | 2717 | 624 | 635 | 641 | 267 | 267 | 274 |
| *** | 34451 | 45137 | 71235 | 11922 | 14501 | 17625 | 2455 | 2612 | 2724 | 624 | 641 | 634 | 267 | 274 | 257 |
| 0.75 *** | 28162 | 34049 | 62959 | 10032 | 11631 | 15534 | 2111 | 2234 | 2385 | 536 | 547 | 554 | 221 | 221 | 232 |
| *** | 30490 | 40605 | 63356 | 10715 | 13014 | 15612 | 2164 | 2304 | 2381 | 536 | 547 | 540 | 221 | 221 | 212 |
| 0.8 *** | 24126 | 29516 | 53572 | 8691 | 10056 | 13136 | 1779 | 1866 | 1982 | 431 | 442 | 442 | 169 | 169 | 169 |
| *** | 26279 | 35326 | 53764 | 9280 | 11187 | 13172 | 1825 | 1919 | 1970 | 431 | 442 | 429 | 169 | 169 | 158 |
| 0.85 *** | 19850 | 24406 | 42390 | 7116 | 8160 | 10301 | 1376 | 1440 | 1510 | 309 | 309 | 320 | . | . | . |
| *** | 21694 | 29125 | 42460 | 7571 | 8982 | 10303 | 1405 | 1464 | 1491 | 309 | 309 | 300 | . | . | . |
| 0.9 *** | 15072 | 18415 | 29440 | 5209 | 5867 | 7011 | 904 | 932 | 956 | . | . | . | . | . | . |
| *** | 16444 | 21670 | 29443 | 5500 | 6340 | 7006 | 915 | 939 | 943 | . | . | . | . | . | . |
| 0.95 *** | 9087 | 10750 | 14729 | 2770 | 2986 | 3295 | . | . | . | . | . | . | . | . | . |
| *** | 9787 | 12167 | 14713 | 2864 | 3126 | 3280 | . | . | . | . | . | . | . | . | . |
| 0.98 *** | 3960 | 4386 | 5069 | . | . | . | . | . | . | . | . | . | . | . | . |
| *** | 4152 | 4684 | 5053 | . | . | . | . | . | . | . | . | . | . | . | . |

TABLE 8: ALPHA= 0.05  POWER= 0.9    EXPECTED ACCRUAL THRU MINIMUM FOLLOW-UP= 7500

| PCONT= | FACT= | DEL=.01 | | | DEL=.02 | | | DEL=.05 | | | DEL=.10 | | | DEL=.15 | | |
|---|---|---|---|---|---|---|---|---|---|---|---|---|---|---|---|---|
| | | 1.0 .75 | .50 .25 | .00 BIN | 1.0 .75 | .50 .25 | .00 BIN | 1.0 .75 | .50 .25 | .00 BIN | 1.0 75 | .50 .25 | .00 BIN | 1.0 .75 | .50 .25 | .00 BIN |
| *** | | REQUIRED NUMBER OF PATIENTS | | | | | | | | | | | | | | |
| 0.01 | *** | 1318 | 1318 | 1318 | 481 | 481 | 481 | 155 | 155 | 155 | 80 | 80 | 80 | 61 | 61 | 61 |
| | *** | 1318 | 1318 | 5053 | 481 | 481 | 1670 | 155 | 155 | 455 | 80 | 80 | 185 | 61 | 61 | 110 |
| 0.02 | *** | 2911 | 2930 | 2949 | 931 | 943 | 943 | 249 | 256 | 256 | 106 | 106 | 106 | 68 | 68 | 68 |
| | *** | 2918 | 2937 | 8342 | 931 | 943 | 2484 | 249 | 256 | 581 | 106 | 106 | 215 | 68 | 68 | 123 |
| 0.05 | *** | 8836 | 8937 | 9200 | 2525 | 2543 | 2581 | 537 | 549 | 549 | 193 | 193 | 193 | 118 | 118 | 118 |
| | *** | 8874 | 9031 | 17796 | 2536 | 2562 | 4822 | 549 | 549 | 943 | 193 | 193 | 300 | 118 | 118 | 158 |
| 0.1 | *** | 19531 | 19843 | 21425 | 5337 | 5461 | 5668 | 1036 | 1043 | 1055 | 324 | 324 | 324 | 174 | 174 | 174 |
| | *** | 19643 | 20274 | 32183 | 5393 | 5543 | 8376 | 1036 | 1043 | 1491 | 324 | 324 | 429 | 174 | 174 | 212 |
| 0.15 | *** | 29236 | 29825 | 33849 | 7925 | 8187 | 8761 | 1493 | 1524 | 1543 | 443 | 443 | 443 | 218 | 218 | 218 |
| | *** | 29431 | 30736 | 44858 | 8037 | 8412 | 11502 | 1505 | 1531 | 1970 | 443 | 443 | 540 | 218 | 218 | 257 |
| 0.2 | *** | 37130 | 38068 | 45481 | 10093 | 10550 | 11649 | 1906 | 1943 | 1993 | 549 | 549 | 549 | 268 | 268 | 268 |
| | *** | 37449 | 39556 | 55820 | 10280 | 10955 | 14199 | 1925 | 1962 | 2381 | 549 | 549 | 634 | 268 | 268 | 295 |
| 0.25 | *** | 42999 | 44349 | 55831 | 11787 | 12462 | 14199 | 2243 | 2311 | 2386 | 631 | 631 | 643 | 305 | 305 | 305 |
| | *** | 43468 | 46524 | 65069 | 12061 | 13081 | 16469 | 2274 | 2349 | 2724 | 631 | 643 | 711 | 305 | 305 | 326 |
| 0.3 | *** | 46868 | 48706 | 64655 | 13018 | 13925 | 16362 | 2518 | 2600 | 2712 | 699 | 706 | 718 | 331 | 331 | 331 |
| | *** | 47499 | 51650 | 72605 | 13393 | 14768 | 18310 | 2555 | 2656 | 2998 | 706 | 718 | 771 | 331 | 331 | 349 |
| 0.35 | *** | 48875 | 51305 | 71787 | 13831 | 14968 | 18106 | 2712 | 2825 | 2975 | 755 | 762 | 774 | 350 | 350 | 361 |
| | *** | 49718 | 55055 | 78428 | 14300 | 16036 | 19723 | 2768 | 2893 | 3203 | 755 | 762 | 814 | 350 | 361 | 364 |
| 0.4 | *** | 49268 | 52343 | 77161 | 14262 | 15624 | 19400 | 2855 | 2986 | 3155 | 781 | 800 | 811 | 361 | 368 | 368 |
| | *** | 50349 | 56937 | 82539 | 14825 | 16899 | 20708 | 2911 | 3061 | 3340 | 793 | 800 | 840 | 368 | 368 | 372 |
| 0.45 | *** | 48293 | 52093 | 80693 | 14375 | 15924 | 20243 | 2918 | 3068 | 3268 | 800 | 818 | 830 | 368 | 368 | 368 |
| | *** | 49643 | 57481 | 84937 | 15012 | 17368 | 21265 | 2993 | 3162 | 3409 | 811 | 818 | 848 | 368 | 368 | 372 |
| 0.5 | *** | 46250 | 50768 | 82381 | 14199 | 15905 | 20618 | 2930 | 3087 | 3305 | 800 | 811 | 830 | 361 | 368 | 368 |
| | *** | 47893 | 56881 | 85622 | 14900 | 17480 | 21393 | 3005 | 3193 | 3409 | 811 | 818 | 840 | 368 | 368 | 364 |
| 0.55 | *** | 43418 | 48631 | 82205 | 13786 | 15593 | 20525 | 2881 | 3050 | 3275 | 781 | 800 | 811 | 350 | 350 | 361 |
| | *** | 45361 | 55318 | 84594 | 14536 | 17243 | 21093 | 2956 | 3155 | 3340 | 793 | 800 | 814 | 350 | 361 | 349 |
| 0.6 | *** | 40081 | 45837 | 80168 | 13156 | 15012 | 19974 | 2780 | 2937 | 3162 | 743 | 762 | 774 | 331 | 331 | 343 |
| | *** | 42268 | 52899 | 81854 | 13936 | 16693 | 20365 | 2855 | 3043 | 3203 | 755 | 762 | 771 | 331 | 331 | 326 |
| 0.65 | *** | 36443 | 42549 | 76268 | 12350 | 14187 | 18950 | 2618 | 2768 | 2975 | 699 | 706 | 718 | 305 | 305 | 312 |
| | *** | 38799 | 49730 | 77401 | 13118 | 15818 | 19209 | 2693 | 2862 | 2998 | 699 | 718 | 711 | 305 | 305 | 295 |
| 0.7 | *** | 32630 | 38818 | 70531 | 11356 | 13111 | 17468 | 2405 | 2536 | 2712 | 624 | 631 | 643 | 268 | 268 | 275 |
| | *** | 35056 | 45849 | 71235 | 12099 | 14637 | 17625 | 2468 | 2618 | 2724 | 631 | 643 | 634 | 268 | 268 | 257 |
| 0.75 | *** | 28700 | 34681 | 62956 | 10193 | 11787 | 15530 | 2124 | 2236 | 2386 | 537 | 549 | 556 | 218 | 230 | 230 |
| | *** | 31074 | 41262 | 63356 | 10868 | 13130 | 15612 | 2180 | 2311 | 2381 | 537 | 549 | 540 | 230 | 230 | 212 |
| 0.8 | *** | 24631 | 30087 | 53574 | 8836 | 10175 | 13137 | 1786 | 1880 | 1981 | 436 | 436 | 443 | 174 | 174 | 174 |
| | *** | 26818 | 35900 | 53764 | 9418 | 11281 | 13172 | 1831 | 1925 | 1970 | 436 | 443 | 429 | 174 | 174 | 158 |
| 0.85 | *** | 20281 | 24886 | 42387 | 7224 | 8255 | 10299 | 1381 | 1437 | 1505 | 312 | 312 | 312 | . | . | . |
| | *** | 22149 | 29581 | 42460 | 7674 | 9050 | 10303 | 1411 | 1468 | 1491 | 312 | 312 | 300 | . | . | . |
| 0.9 | *** | 15387 | 18743 | 29431 | 5281 | 5918 | 7018 | 905 | 931 | 961 | . | . | . | . | . | . |
| | *** | 16775 | 21968 | 29443 | 5562 | 6380 | 7006 | 912 | 943 | 943 | . | . | . | . | . | . |
| 0.95 | *** | 9256 | 10899 | 14724 | 2787 | 3005 | 3293 | . | . | . | . | . | . | . | . | . |
| | *** | 9961 | 12286 | 14713 | 2893 | 3136 | 3280 | . | . | . | . | . | . | . | . | . |
| 0.98 | *** | 4006 | 4418 | 5068 | . | . | . | . | . | . | . | . | . | . | . | . |
| | *** | 4193 | 4700 | 5053 | . | . | . | . | . | . | . | . | . | . | . | . |

TABLE 8: ALPHA= 0.05  POWER= 0.9    EXPECTED ACCRUAL THRU MINIMUM FOLLOW-UP= 8000

| | | DEL=.01 | | | DEL=.02 | | | DEL=.05 | | | DEL=.10 | | | DEL=.15 | |
|---|---|---|---|---|---|---|---|---|---|---|---|---|---|---|---|---|
| FACT= | 1.0 .75 | .50 .25 | .00 BIN | 1.0 .75 | .50 .25 | .00 BIN | 1.0 .75 | .50 .25 | .00 BIN | 1.0 75 | .50 .25 | .00 BIN | 1.0 .75 | .50 .25 | .00 BIN |
| PCONT=*** | | | | | REQUIRED NUMBER OF PATIENTS | | | | | | | | | | |
| 0.01 *** | 1313 | 1313 | 1325 | 485 | 485 | 485 | 153 | 153 | 153 | 85 | 85 | 85 | 53 | 53 | 53 |
| *** | 1313 | 1313 | 5053 | 485 | 485 | 1670 | 153 | 153 | 455 | 85 | 85 | 185 | 53 | 53 | 110 |
| 0.02 *** | 2913 | 2925 | 2945 | 933 | 933 | 945 | 253 | 253 | 253 | 113 | 113 | 113 | 73 | 73 | 73 |
| *** | 2925 | 2933 | 8342 | 933 | 945 | 2484 | 253 | 253 | 581 | 113 | 113 | 215 | 73 | 73 | 123 |
| 0.05 *** | 8845 | 8945 | 9205 | 2525 | 2545 | 2573 | 545 | 545 | 545 | 193 | 193 | 193 | 113 | 113 | 113 |
| *** | 8885 | 9045 | 17796 | 2533 | 2565 | 4822 | 545 | 545 | 943 | 193 | 193 | 300 | 113 | 113 | 158 |
| 0.1 *** | 19553 | 19885 | 21425 | 5353 | 5465 | 5665 | 1033 | 1045 | 1053 | 325 | 325 | 325 | 173 | 173 | 173 |
| *** | 19673 | 20313 | 32183 | 5405 | 5553 | 8376 | 1045 | 1045 | 1491 | 325 | 325 | 429 | 173 | 173 | 212 |
| 0.15 *** | 29273 | 29893 | 33853 | 7953 | 8213 | 8765 | 1505 | 1525 | 1545 | 445 | 445 | 445 | 225 | 225 | 225 |
| *** | 29493 | 30825 | 44858 | 8065 | 8433 | 11502 | 1513 | 1533 | 1970 | 445 | 445 | 540 | 225 | 225 | 257 |
| 0.2 *** | 37193 | 38185 | 45473 | 10133 | 10585 | 11645 | 1905 | 1945 | 1993 | 545 | 545 | 553 | 265 | 265 | 265 |
| *** | 37533 | 39713 | 55820 | 10325 | 10985 | 14199 | 1925 | 1965 | 2381 | 545 | 553 | 634 | 265 | 265 | 295 |
| 0.25 *** | 43093 | 44525 | 55833 | 11845 | 12525 | 14205 | 2253 | 2313 | 2385 | 633 | 633 | 645 | 305 | 305 | 305 |
| *** | 43585 | 46765 | 65069 | 12125 | 13133 | 16469 | 2273 | 2345 | 2724 | 633 | 645 | 711 | 305 | 305 | 326 |
| 0.3 *** | 46993 | 48945 | 64653 | 13105 | 14013 | 16365 | 2525 | 2605 | 2713 | 705 | 705 | 713 | 333 | 333 | 333 |
| *** | 47665 | 51965 | 72605 | 13473 | 14845 | 18310 | 2565 | 2653 | 2998 | 705 | 713 | 771 | 333 | 333 | 349 |
| 0.35 *** | 49045 | 51605 | 71793 | 13933 | 15073 | 18105 | 2725 | 2833 | 2973 | 753 | 765 | 773 | 353 | 353 | 353 |
| *** | 49933 | 55453 | 78428 | 14405 | 16125 | 19723 | 2773 | 2893 | 3203 | 753 | 765 | 814 | 353 | 353 | 364 |
| 0.4 *** | 49485 | 52713 | 77153 | 14393 | 15745 | 19405 | 2865 | 2993 | 3153 | 785 | 793 | 813 | 365 | 365 | 373 |
| *** | 50625 | 57413 | 82539 | 14953 | 17005 | 20708 | 2925 | 3065 | 3340 | 793 | 805 | 840 | 365 | 365 | 372 |
| 0.45 *** | 48565 | 52533 | 80693 | 14513 | 16065 | 20245 | 2933 | 3085 | 3273 | 805 | 813 | 833 | 365 | 373 | 373 |
| *** | 49993 | 58033 | 84937 | 15153 | 17485 | 21265 | 3005 | 3165 | 3409 | 813 | 825 | 848 | 373 | 373 | 372 |
| 0.5 *** | 46585 | 51285 | 82385 | 14353 | 16053 | 20613 | 2953 | 3105 | 3305 | 805 | 813 | 833 | 365 | 365 | 373 |
| *** | 48313 | 57505 | 85622 | 15065 | 17605 | 21393 | 3025 | 3193 | 3409 | 805 | 825 | 840 | 365 | 365 | 364 |
| 0.55 *** | 43825 | 49205 | 82205 | 13953 | 15753 | 20525 | 2905 | 3065 | 3273 | 785 | 793 | 813 | 353 | 353 | 353 |
| *** | 45845 | 55985 | 84594 | 14705 | 17385 | 21093 | 2973 | 3153 | 3340 | 793 | 805 | 814 | 353 | 353 | 349 |
| 0.6 *** | 40545 | 46453 | 80165 | 13333 | 15185 | 19973 | 2793 | 2953 | 3165 | 745 | 765 | 773 | 333 | 333 | 333 |
| *** | 42805 | 53585 | 81854 | 14105 | 16833 | 20365 | 2873 | 3045 | 3203 | 753 | 765 | 771 | 333 | 333 | 326 |
| 0.65 *** | 36945 | 43173 | 76273 | 12525 | 14353 | 18953 | 2633 | 2785 | 2973 | 693 | 705 | 725 | 305 | 305 | 305 |
| *** | 39365 | 50413 | 77401 | 13293 | 15953 | 19209 | 2705 | 2873 | 2998 | 705 | 713 | 711 | 305 | 305 | 295 |
| 0.7 *** | 33153 | 39445 | 70533 | 11525 | 13265 | 17473 | 2413 | 2545 | 2713 | 625 | 633 | 645 | 265 | 273 | 273 |
| *** | 35625 | 46525 | 71235 | 12265 | 14765 | 17625 | 2473 | 2625 | 2724 | 633 | 645 | 634 | 265 | 273 | 257 |
| 0.75 *** | 29213 | 35273 | 62953 | 10345 | 11925 | 15533 | 2145 | 2245 | 2385 | 533 | 545 | 553 | 225 | 225 | 225 |
| *** | 31625 | 41885 | 63356 | 11025 | 13233 | 15612 | 2193 | 2313 | 2381 | 545 | 553 | 540 | 225 | 225 | 212 |
| 0.8 *** | 25105 | 30625 | 53573 | 8965 | 10293 | 13133 | 1805 | 1885 | 1985 | 433 | 433 | 445 | 173 | 173 | 173 |
| *** | 27325 | 36433 | 53764 | 9533 | 11373 | 13172 | 1833 | 1925 | 1970 | 433 | 445 | 429 | 173 | 173 | 158 |
| 0.85 *** | 20693 | 25325 | 42393 | 7325 | 8333 | 10293 | 1393 | 1445 | 1505 | 313 | 313 | 313 | . | . | . |
| *** | 22573 | 30005 | 42460 | 7773 | 9113 | 10303 | 1413 | 1473 | 1491 | 313 | 313 | 300 | . | . | . |
| 0.9 *** | 15705 | 19053 | 29433 | 5345 | 5965 | 7013 | 905 | 933 | 953 | . | . | . | . | . | . |
| *** | 17085 | 22245 | 29443 | 5625 | 6405 | 7006 | 925 | 945 | 943 | . | . | . | . | . | . |
| 0.95 *** | 9413 | 11045 | 14725 | 2813 | 3013 | 3293 | . | . | . | . | . | . | . | . | . |
| *** | 10113 | 12393 | 14713 | 2905 | 3145 | 3280 | . | . | . | . | . | . | . | . | . |
| 0.98 *** | 4053 | 4453 | 5065 | . | . | . | . | . | . | . | . | . | . | . | . |
| *** | 4233 | 4725 | 5053 | . | . | . | . | . | . | . | . | . | . | . | . |

## TABLE 8: ALPHA= 0.05  POWER= 0.9    EXPECTED ACCRUAL THRU MINIMUM FOLLOW-UP= 8500

| | | DEL=.01 | | | DEL=.02 | | | DEL=.05 | | | DEL=.10 | | | DEL=.15 | | |
|---|---|---|---|---|---|---|---|---|---|---|---|---|---|---|---|---|
| **FACT=** | | 1.0 .75 | .50 .25 | .00 BIN | 1.0 .75 | .50 .25 | .00 BIN | 1.0 .75 | .50 .25 | .00 BIN | 1.0 75 | .50 .25 | .00 BIN | 1.0 .75 | .50 .25 | .00 BIN |
| **PCONT=\*\*\*** | | | | | REQUIRED | NUMBER OF | PATIENTS | | | | | | | | | |
| 0.01 | \*\*\* | 1310 | 1323 | 1323 | 481 | 481 | 481 | 155 | 155 | 155 | 78 | 78 | 78 | 56 | 56 | 56 |
| | \*\*\* | 1310 | 1323 | 5053 | 481 | 481 | 1670 | 155 | 155 | 455 | 78 | 78 | 185 | 56 | 56 | 110 |
| 0.02 | \*\*\* | 2917 | 2925 | 2946 | 941 | 941 | 941 | 248 | 248 | 248 | 112 | 112 | 112 | 70 | 70 | 70 |
| | \*\*\* | 2917 | 2938 | 8342 | 941 | 941 | 2484 | 248 | 248 | 581 | 112 | 112 | 215 | 70 | 70 | 123 |
| 0.05 | \*\*\* | 8854 | 8952 | 9207 | 2521 | 2556 | 2577 | 545 | 545 | 545 | 197 | 197 | 197 | 112 | 112 | 112 |
| | \*\*\* | 8896 | 9045 | 17796 | 2535 | 2564 | 4822 | 545 | 545 | 943 | 197 | 197 | 300 | 112 | 112 | 158 |
| 0.1 | \*\*\* | 19577 | 19917 | 21426 | 5361 | 5475 | 5666 | 1034 | 1047 | 1055 | 325 | 325 | 325 | 176 | 176 | 176 |
| | \*\*\* | 19705 | 20350 | 32183 | 5411 | 5560 | 8376 | 1047 | 1047 | 1491 | 325 | 325 | 429 | 176 | 176 | 212 |
| 0.15 | \*\*\* | 29310 | 29968 | 33857 | 7975 | 8238 | 8761 | 1501 | 1523 | 1544 | 439 | 439 | 439 | 226 | 226 | 226 |
| | \*\*\* | 29543 | 30911 | 44858 | 8089 | 8450 | 11502 | 1515 | 1536 | 1970 | 439 | 439 | 540 | 226 | 226 | 257 |
| 0.2 | \*\*\* | 37257 | 38298 | 45481 | 10171 | 10631 | 11651 | 1918 | 1948 | 1990 | 545 | 545 | 558 | 269 | 269 | 269 |
| | \*\*\* | 37618 | 39871 | 55820 | 10363 | 11013 | 14199 | 1926 | 1969 | 2381 | 545 | 545 | 634 | 269 | 269 | 295 |
| 0.25 | \*\*\* | 43186 | 44681 | 55838 | 11906 | 12586 | 14201 | 2258 | 2309 | 2386 | 630 | 643 | 643 | 303 | 303 | 303 |
| | \*\*\* | 43704 | 46990 | 65069 | 12182 | 13181 | 16469 | 2288 | 2351 | 2724 | 630 | 643 | 711 | 303 | 303 | 326 |
| 0.3 | \*\*\* | 47117 | 49165 | 64656 | 13181 | 14095 | 16368 | 2535 | 2606 | 2713 | 707 | 707 | 715 | 333 | 333 | 333 |
| | \*\*\* | 47826 | 52268 | 72605 | 13550 | 14910 | 18310 | 2564 | 2662 | 2998 | 707 | 715 | 771 | 333 | 333 | 349 |
| 0.35 | \*\*\* | 49221 | 51885 | 71788 | 14031 | 15178 | 18111 | 2734 | 2840 | 2968 | 758 | 758 | 771 | 354 | 354 | 354 |
| | \*\*\* | 50156 | 55838 | 78428 | 14506 | 16206 | 19723 | 2790 | 2904 | 3203 | 758 | 771 | 814 | 354 | 354 | 364 |
| 0.4 | \*\*\* | 49696 | 53075 | 77151 | 14506 | 15866 | 19407 | 2883 | 3002 | 3159 | 792 | 800 | 813 | 367 | 367 | 367 |
| | \*\*\* | 50900 | 57878 | 82539 | 15072 | 17099 | 20708 | 2938 | 3074 | 3340 | 792 | 800 | 840 | 367 | 367 | 372 |
| 0.45 | \*\*\* | 48846 | 52961 | 80692 | 14647 | 16198 | 20244 | 2960 | 3087 | 3265 | 800 | 813 | 835 | 367 | 375 | 375 |
| | \*\*\* | 50334 | 58571 | 84937 | 15293 | 17601 | 21265 | 3023 | 3172 | 3409 | 813 | 821 | 848 | 367 | 375 | 372 |
| 0.5 | \*\*\* | 46926 | 51779 | 82379 | 14498 | 16206 | 20618 | 2968 | 3116 | 3308 | 800 | 813 | 835 | 367 | 367 | 367 |
| | \*\*\* | 48719 | 58090 | 85622 | 15208 | 17728 | 21393 | 3031 | 3201 | 3409 | 813 | 821 | 840 | 367 | 367 | 364 |
| 0.55 | \*\*\* | 44227 | 49752 | 82209 | 14103 | 15909 | 20533 | 2917 | 3074 | 3278 | 779 | 800 | 813 | 354 | 354 | 354 |
| | \*\*\* | 46310 | 56603 | 84594 | 14860 | 17516 | 21093 | 2989 | 3159 | 3340 | 792 | 800 | 814 | 354 | 354 | 349 |
| 0.6 | \*\*\* | 40997 | 47040 | 80169 | 13500 | 15335 | 19968 | 2811 | 2968 | 3159 | 750 | 758 | 779 | 333 | 333 | 333 |
| | \*\*\* | 43313 | 54236 | 81854 | 14273 | 16950 | 20365 | 2883 | 3053 | 3203 | 758 | 771 | 771 | 333 | 333 | 326 |
| 0.65 | \*\*\* | 37435 | 43781 | 76272 | 12679 | 14506 | 18948 | 2649 | 2790 | 2981 | 694 | 707 | 715 | 303 | 303 | 311 |
| | \*\*\* | 39900 | 51070 | 77401 | 13457 | 16079 | 19209 | 2713 | 2875 | 2998 | 707 | 715 | 711 | 303 | 311 | 295 |
| 0.7 | \*\*\* | 33653 | 40041 | 70535 | 11680 | 13415 | 17473 | 2428 | 2556 | 2713 | 630 | 630 | 643 | 269 | 269 | 269 |
| | \*\*\* | 36173 | 47146 | 71235 | 12416 | 14868 | 17625 | 2492 | 2628 | 2724 | 630 | 643 | 634 | 269 | 269 | 257 |
| 0.75 | \*\*\* | 29713 | 35841 | 62956 | 10490 | 12055 | 15526 | 2152 | 2258 | 2386 | 537 | 545 | 558 | 226 | 226 | 226 |
| | \*\*\* | 32157 | 42463 | 63356 | 11162 | 13338 | 15612 | 2203 | 2322 | 2381 | 545 | 545 | 540 | 226 | 226 | 212 |
| 0.8 | \*\*\* | 25570 | 31124 | 53564 | 9088 | 10397 | 13138 | 1812 | 1884 | 1982 | 431 | 439 | 439 | 176 | 176 | 176 |
| | \*\*\* | 27801 | 36938 | 53764 | 9653 | 11446 | 13172 | 1841 | 1926 | 1970 | 439 | 439 | 429 | 176 | 176 | 158 |
| 0.85 | \*\*\* | 21086 | 25740 | 42386 | 7422 | 8421 | 10299 | 1395 | 1451 | 1501 | 311 | 311 | 311 | . | . | . |
| | \*\*\* | 22977 | 30401 | 42460 | 7855 | 9173 | 10303 | 1416 | 1472 | 1491 | 311 | 311 | 300 | . | . | . |
| 0.9 | \*\*\* | 15994 | 19351 | 29437 | 5411 | 6020 | 7018 | 906 | 928 | 962 | . | . | . | . | . | . |
| | \*\*\* | 17388 | 22510 | 29443 | 5680 | 6445 | 7006 | 920 | 949 | 943 | . | . | . | . | . | . |
| 0.95 | \*\*\* | 9568 | 11170 | 14732 | 2832 | 3031 | 3300 | . | . | . | . | . | . | . | . | . |
| | \*\*\* | 10256 | 12501 | 14713 | 2925 | 3151 | 3280 | . | . | . | . | . | . | . | . | . |
| 0.98 | \*\*\* | 4094 | 4490 | 5071 | . | . | . | . | . | . | . | . | . | . | . | . |
| | \*\*\* | 4277 | 4745 | 5053 | . | . | . | . | . | . | . | . | . | . | . | . |

TABLE 8: ALPHA= 0.05  POWER= 0.9     EXPECTED ACCRUAL THRU MINIMUM FOLLOW-UP= 9000

| | | DEL=.01 | | | DEL=.02 | | | DEL=.05 | | | DEL=.10 | | | DEL=.15 | | |
|---|---|---|---|---|---|---|---|---|---|---|---|---|---|---|---|---|---|
| FACT= | | 1.0 .75 | .50 .25 | .00 BIN | 1.0 .75 | .50 .25 | .00 BIN | 1.0 .75 | .50 .25 | .00 BIN | 1.0 75 | .50 .25 | .00 BIN | 1.0 .75 | .50 .25 | .00 BIN |
| PCONT=*** | | | | | | | REQUIRED NUMBER OF PATIENTS | | | | | | | | |
| 0.01 | *** | 1311 | 1320 | 1320 | 479 | 479 | 487 | 164 | 164 | 164 | 82 | 82 | 82 | 60 | 60 | 60 |
| | *** | 1320 | 1320 | 5053 | 479 | 479 | 1670 | 164 | 164 | 455 | 82 | 82 | 185 | 60 | 60 | 110 |
| 0.02 | *** | 2917 | 2931 | 2954 | 937 | 937 | 937 | 254 | 254 | 254 | 105 | 105 | 105 | 74 | 74 | 74 |
| | *** | 2917 | 2940 | 8342 | 937 | 937 | 2484 | 254 | 254 | 581 | 105 | 105 | 215 | 74 | 74 | 123 |
| 0.05 | *** | 8857 | 8961 | 9209 | 2526 | 2549 | 2580 | 546 | 546 | 546 | 195 | 195 | 195 | 119 | 119 | 119 |
| | *** | 8902 | 9051 | 17796 | 2535 | 2557 | 4822 | 546 | 546 | 943 | 195 | 195 | 300 | 119 | 119 | 158 |
| 0.1 | *** | 19604 | 19950 | 21426 | 5370 | 5482 | 5662 | 1041 | 1050 | 1050 | 321 | 321 | 321 | 172 | 172 | 172 |
| | *** | 19725 | 20391 | 32183 | 5429 | 5564 | 8376 | 1041 | 1050 | 1491 | 321 | 321 | 429 | 172 | 172 | 212 |
| 0.15 | *** | 29355 | 30044 | 33855 | 7994 | 8264 | 8767 | 1500 | 1522 | 1545 | 442 | 442 | 442 | 217 | 217 | 217 |
| | *** | 29594 | 30997 | 44858 | 8106 | 8466 | 11502 | 1514 | 1536 | 1970 | 442 | 442 | 540 | 217 | 217 | 257 |
| 0.2 | *** | 37320 | 38414 | 45479 | 10207 | 10657 | 11647 | 1919 | 1950 | 1995 | 546 | 546 | 555 | 262 | 262 | 262 |
| | *** | 37702 | 40011 | 55820 | 10401 | 11040 | 14199 | 1927 | 1972 | 2381 | 546 | 546 | 634 | 262 | 262 | 295 |
| 0.25 | *** | 43282 | 44849 | 55837 | 11954 | 12637 | 14204 | 2265 | 2324 | 2391 | 636 | 636 | 645 | 307 | 307 | 307 |
| | *** | 43822 | 47197 | 65069 | 12246 | 13222 | 16469 | 2287 | 2346 | 2724 | 636 | 645 | 711 | 307 | 307 | 326 |
| 0.3 | *** | 47242 | 49380 | 64657 | 13259 | 14159 | 16364 | 2535 | 2616 | 2715 | 704 | 712 | 712 | 330 | 330 | 330 |
| | *** | 47999 | 52552 | 72605 | 13627 | 14969 | 18310 | 2580 | 2661 | 2998 | 704 | 712 | 771 | 330 | 330 | 349 |
| 0.35 | *** | 49380 | 52170 | 71790 | 14122 | 15270 | 18105 | 2751 | 2850 | 2976 | 757 | 757 | 771 | 352 | 352 | 352 |
| | *** | 50370 | 56197 | 78428 | 14595 | 16282 | 19723 | 2796 | 2909 | 3203 | 757 | 771 | 814 | 352 | 352 | 364 |
| 0.4 | *** | 49920 | 53430 | 77159 | 14617 | 15981 | 19401 | 2895 | 3007 | 3156 | 794 | 802 | 816 | 366 | 366 | 366 |
| | *** | 51180 | 58312 | 82539 | 15180 | 17182 | 20708 | 2940 | 3075 | 3340 | 794 | 802 | 840 | 366 | 366 | 372 |
| 0.45 | *** | 49110 | 53376 | 80691 | 14775 | 16319 | 20242 | 2962 | 3097 | 3269 | 802 | 816 | 825 | 366 | 375 | 375 |
| | *** | 50662 | 59069 | 84937 | 15419 | 17700 | 21265 | 3030 | 3179 | 3409 | 816 | 825 | 848 | 366 | 375 | 372 |
| 0.5 | *** | 47256 | 52260 | 82379 | 14640 | 16341 | 20616 | 2985 | 3120 | 3314 | 802 | 816 | 825 | 366 | 366 | 366 |
| | *** | 49110 | 58650 | 85622 | 15351 | 17835 | 21393 | 3052 | 3210 | 3409 | 816 | 825 | 840 | 366 | 366 | 364 |
| 0.55 | *** | 44610 | 50280 | 82207 | 14257 | 16049 | 20526 | 2931 | 3075 | 3269 | 780 | 802 | 816 | 352 | 352 | 352 |
| | *** | 46761 | 57201 | 84594 | 15014 | 17624 | 21093 | 3007 | 3165 | 3340 | 794 | 802 | 814 | 352 | 352 | 349 |
| 0.6 | *** | 41437 | 47602 | 80174 | 13650 | 15486 | 19972 | 2827 | 2976 | 3165 | 749 | 757 | 771 | 330 | 330 | 344 |
| | *** | 43814 | 54861 | 81854 | 14429 | 17070 | 20365 | 2895 | 3066 | 3203 | 757 | 771 | 771 | 330 | 330 | 326 |
| 0.65 | *** | 37905 | 44362 | 76267 | 12840 | 14640 | 18951 | 2670 | 2805 | 2976 | 704 | 712 | 726 | 307 | 307 | 307 |
| | *** | 40425 | 51689 | 77401 | 13605 | 16192 | 19209 | 2729 | 2886 | 2998 | 704 | 712 | 711 | 307 | 307 | 295 |
| 0.7 | *** | 34139 | 40619 | 70530 | 11827 | 13537 | 17466 | 2445 | 2557 | 2715 | 622 | 636 | 645 | 262 | 276 | 276 |
| | *** | 36704 | 47737 | 71235 | 12561 | 14977 | 17625 | 2504 | 2639 | 2724 | 636 | 645 | 634 | 276 | 276 | 257 |
| 0.75 | *** | 30187 | 36375 | 62961 | 10626 | 12165 | 15531 | 2166 | 2265 | 2391 | 546 | 546 | 555 | 231 | 231 | 231 |
| | *** | 32662 | 43004 | 63356 | 11287 | 13425 | 15612 | 2211 | 2324 | 2381 | 546 | 546 | 540 | 231 | 231 | 212 |
| 0.8 | *** | 26002 | 31605 | 53565 | 9209 | 10500 | 13132 | 1815 | 1896 | 1986 | 434 | 442 | 442 | 172 | 172 | 172 |
| | *** | 28266 | 37410 | 53764 | 9771 | 11526 | 13172 | 1851 | 1927 | 1970 | 434 | 442 | 429 | 172 | 172 | 158 |
| 0.85 | *** | 21457 | 26129 | 42396 | 7507 | 8489 | 10297 | 1401 | 1446 | 1500 | 307 | 307 | 321 | . | . | . |
| | *** | 23361 | 30772 | 42460 | 7949 | 9217 | 10303 | 1424 | 1477 | 1491 | 307 | 321 | 300 | . | . | . |
| 0.9 | *** | 16260 | 19626 | 29436 | 5460 | 6059 | 7012 | 915 | 937 | 960 | . | . | . | . | . | . |
| | *** | 17655 | 22740 | 29443 | 5730 | 6464 | 7006 | 929 | 951 | 943 | . | . | . | . | . | . |
| 0.95 | *** | 9704 | 11301 | 14730 | 2850 | 3044 | 3300 | . | . | . | . | . | . | . | . | . |
| | *** | 10387 | 12592 | 14713 | 2940 | 3156 | 3280 | . | . | . | . | . | . | . | . | . |
| 0.98 | *** | 4132 | 4506 | 5069 | . | . | . | . | . | . | . | . | . | . | . | . |
| | *** | 4304 | 4754 | 5053 | . | . | . | . | . | . | . | . | . | . | . | . |

**TABLE 8: ALPHA= 0.05  POWER= 0.9    EXPECTED ACCRUAL THRU MINIMUM FOLLOW-UP= 9500**

| | | DEL=.01 | | | DEL=.02 | | | DEL=.05 | | | DEL=.10 | | | DEL=.15 | | |
|---|---|---|---|---|---|---|---|---|---|---|---|---|---|---|---|---|
| FACT= | | 1.0 .75 | .50 .25 | .00 BIN | 1.0 .75 | .50 .25 | .00 BIN | 1.0 .75 | .50 .25 | .00 BIN | 1.0 75 | .50 .25 | .00 BIN | 1.0 .75 | .50 .25 | .00 BIN |
| PCONT=*** | | | | | | REQUIRED NUMBER OF PATIENTS | | | | | | | | | | |
| 0.01 | *** | 1313 | 1313 | 1322 | 481 | 481 | 481 | 158 | 158 | 158 | 78 | 78 | 78 | 54 | 54 | 54 |
| | *** | 1313 | 1322 | 5053 | 481 | 481 | 1670 | 158 | 158 | 455 | 78 | 78 | 185 | 54 | 54 | 110 |
| 0.02 | *** | 2913 | 2928 | 2951 | 933 | 942 | 942 | 253 | 253 | 253 | 110 | 110 | 110 | 78 | 78 | 78 |
| | *** | 2928 | 2937 | 8342 | 942 | 942 | 2484 | 253 | 253 | 581 | 110 | 110 | 215 | 78 | 78 | 123 |
| 0.05 | *** | 8865 | 8969 | 9207 | 2533 | 2548 | 2580 | 538 | 538 | 553 | 196 | 196 | 196 | 110 | 110 | 110 |
| | *** | 8913 | 9055 | 17796 | 2548 | 2571 | 4822 | 538 | 538 | 943 | 196 | 196 | 300 | 110 | 110 | 158 |
| 0.1 | *** | 19624 | 19980 | 21429 | 5383 | 5493 | 5668 | 1037 | 1051 | 1051 | 324 | 324 | 324 | 173 | 173 | 173 |
| | *** | 19752 | 20417 | 32183 | 5430 | 5564 | 8376 | 1037 | 1051 | 1491 | 324 | 324 | 429 | 173 | 173 | 212 |
| 0.15 | *** | 29394 | 30107 | 33850 | 8019 | 8271 | 8770 | 1503 | 1526 | 1550 | 443 | 443 | 443 | 220 | 220 | 220 |
| | *** | 29646 | 31080 | 44858 | 8129 | 8470 | 11502 | 1512 | 1535 | 1970 | 443 | 443 | 540 | 220 | 220 | 257 |
| 0.2 | *** | 37389 | 38514 | 45473 | 10243 | 10694 | 11644 | 1915 | 1954 | 2001 | 538 | 553 | 553 | 268 | 268 | 268 |
| | *** | 37778 | 40153 | 55820 | 10433 | 11074 | 14199 | 1939 | 1978 | 2381 | 553 | 553 | 634 | 268 | 268 | 295 |
| 0.25 | *** | 43374 | 45013 | 55828 | 12009 | 12689 | 14194 | 2272 | 2319 | 2390 | 633 | 633 | 648 | 300 | 300 | 300 |
| | *** | 43944 | 47397 | 65069 | 12294 | 13259 | 16469 | 2295 | 2358 | 2724 | 633 | 648 | 711 | 300 | 300 | 326 |
| 0.3 | *** | 47373 | 49596 | 64654 | 13330 | 14233 | 16370 | 2548 | 2619 | 2714 | 704 | 704 | 719 | 339 | 339 | 339 |
| | *** | 48157 | 52826 | 72605 | 13695 | 15016 | 18310 | 2580 | 2666 | 2998 | 704 | 719 | 771 | 339 | 339 | 349 |
| 0.35 | *** | 49549 | 52446 | 71788 | 14209 | 15349 | 18104 | 2761 | 2856 | 2975 | 752 | 766 | 775 | 348 | 348 | 363 |
| | *** | 50579 | 56540 | 78428 | 14693 | 16355 | 19723 | 2809 | 2904 | 3203 | 766 | 766 | 814 | 348 | 363 | 364 |
| 0.4 | *** | 50128 | 53762 | 77155 | 14717 | 16070 | 19410 | 2904 | 3008 | 3165 | 790 | 799 | 814 | 363 | 372 | 372 |
| | *** | 51449 | 58725 | 82539 | 15287 | 17273 | 20708 | 2951 | 3079 | 3340 | 799 | 799 | 840 | 363 | 372 | 372 |
| 0.45 | *** | 49383 | 53776 | 80694 | 14898 | 16441 | 20241 | 2975 | 3103 | 3269 | 814 | 814 | 823 | 372 | 372 | 372 |
| | *** | 50998 | 59548 | 84937 | 15539 | 17795 | 21265 | 3046 | 3189 | 3409 | 814 | 823 | 848 | 372 | 372 | 372 |
| 0.5 | *** | 47578 | 52717 | 82380 | 14779 | 16465 | 20621 | 2999 | 3127 | 3308 | 799 | 814 | 823 | 363 | 372 | 372 |
| | *** | 49501 | 59177 | 85622 | 15491 | 17938 | 21393 | 3055 | 3213 | 3409 | 814 | 823 | 840 | 363 | 372 | 364 |
| 0.55 | *** | 44989 | 50784 | 82205 | 14399 | 16189 | 20526 | 2951 | 3094 | 3269 | 790 | 799 | 814 | 348 | 348 | 363 |
| | *** | 47198 | 57766 | 84594 | 15159 | 17733 | 21093 | 3008 | 3174 | 3340 | 790 | 799 | 814 | 348 | 363 | 349 |
| 0.6 | *** | 41854 | 48133 | 80172 | 13790 | 15619 | 19965 | 2842 | 2984 | 3165 | 752 | 766 | 775 | 339 | 339 | 339 |
| | *** | 44285 | 55439 | 81854 | 14565 | 17178 | 20365 | 2913 | 3070 | 3203 | 752 | 766 | 771 | 339 | 339 | 326 |
| 0.65 | *** | 38363 | 44903 | 76268 | 12983 | 14779 | 18944 | 2675 | 2809 | 2975 | 695 | 704 | 719 | 300 | 300 | 315 |
| | *** | 40928 | 52265 | 77401 | 13743 | 16299 | 19209 | 2738 | 2889 | 2998 | 704 | 719 | 711 | 300 | 300 | 295 |
| 0.7 | *** | 34610 | 41150 | 70529 | 11962 | 13672 | 17472 | 2453 | 2571 | 2714 | 624 | 633 | 648 | 268 | 268 | 268 |
| | *** | 37208 | 48299 | 71235 | 12698 | 15073 | 17625 | 2509 | 2643 | 2724 | 633 | 648 | 634 | 268 | 268 | 257 |
| 0.75 | *** | 30644 | 36890 | 62953 | 10750 | 12285 | 15524 | 2168 | 2263 | 2381 | 538 | 553 | 553 | 220 | 229 | 229 |
| | *** | 33147 | 43516 | 63356 | 11415 | 13505 | 15612 | 2215 | 2319 | 2381 | 538 | 553 | 540 | 229 | 229 | 212 |
| 0.8 | *** | 26416 | 32054 | 53572 | 9316 | 10584 | 13140 | 1820 | 1892 | 1978 | 434 | 443 | 443 | 173 | 173 | 173 |
| | *** | 28696 | 37849 | 53764 | 9872 | 11582 | 13172 | 1859 | 1939 | 1970 | 434 | 443 | 429 | 173 | 173 | 158 |
| 0.85 | *** | 21809 | 26497 | 42385 | 7592 | 8556 | 10299 | 1408 | 1455 | 1503 | 315 | 315 | 315 | . | . | . |
| | *** | 23733 | 31119 | 42460 | 8019 | 9269 | 10303 | 1431 | 1479 | 1491 | 315 | 315 | 300 | . | . | . |
| 0.9 | *** | 16522 | 19885 | 29433 | 5516 | 6095 | 7013 | 918 | 933 | 956 | . | . | . | . | . | . |
| | *** | 17923 | 22973 | 29443 | 5778 | 6490 | 7006 | 933 | 942 | 943 | . | . | . | . | . | . |
| 0.95 | *** | 9839 | 11406 | 14731 | 2865 | 3055 | 3293 | . | . | . | . | . | . | . | . | . |
| | *** | 10513 | 12674 | 14713 | 2960 | 3165 | 3280 | . | . | . | . | . | . | . | . | . |
| 0.98 | *** | 4163 | 4528 | 5065 | . | . | . | . | . | . | . | . | . | . | . | . |
| | *** | 4338 | 4765 | 5053 | . | . | . | . | . | . | . | . | . | . | . | . |

## TABLE 8: ALPHA= 0.05  POWER= 0.9    EXPECTED ACCRUAL THRU MINIMUM FOLLOW-UP= 10000

| | | DEL=.01 | | | DEL=.02 | | | DEL=.05 | | | DEL=.10 | | | DEL=.15 | | |
|---|---|---|---|---|---|---|---|---|---|---|---|---|---|---|---|---|
| FACT= | | 1.0<br>.75 | .50<br>.25 | .00<br>BIN | 1.0<br>.75 | .50<br>.25 | .00<br>BIN | 1.0<br>.75 | .50<br>.25 | .00<br>BIN | 1.0<br>75 | .50<br>.25 | .00<br>BIN | 1.0<br>.75 | .50<br>.25 | .00<br>BIN |
| PCONT=*** | | | | | | REQUIRED NUMBER OF PATIENTS | | | | | | | | | | |
| 0.01 | *** | 1316 | 1316 | 1316 | 482 | 482 | 482 | 157 | 157 | 157 | 82 | 82 | 82 | 57 | 57 | 57 |
| | *** | 1316 | 1316 | 5053 | 482 | 482 | 1670 | 157 | 157 | 455 | 82 | 82 | 185 | 57 | 57 | 110 |
| 0.02 | *** | 2916 | 2932 | 2941 | 932 | 941 | 941 | 257 | 257 | 257 | 107 | 107 | 107 | 66 | 66 | 66 |
| | *** | 2916 | 2941 | 8342 | 941 | 941 | 2484 | 257 | 257 | 581 | 107 | 107 | 215 | 66 | 66 | 123 |
| 0.05 | *** | 8882 | 8982 | 9207 | 2532 | 2557 | 2582 | 541 | 541 | 541 | 191 | 191 | 191 | 116 | 116 | 116 |
| | *** | 8916 | 9066 | 17796 | 2541 | 2566 | 4822 | 541 | 541 | 943 | 191 | 191 | 300 | 116 | 116 | 158 |
| 0.1 | *** | 19641 | 20016 | 21432 | 5391 | 5491 | 5666 | 1041 | 1041 | 1057 | 316 | 316 | 332 | 166 | 166 | 166 |
| | *** | 19782 | 20457 | 32183 | 5441 | 5566 | 8376 | 1041 | 1057 | 1491 | 316 | 332 | 429 | 166 | 166 | 212 |
| 0.15 | *** | 29432 | 30166 | 33857 | 8041 | 8291 | 8766 | 1507 | 1532 | 1541 | 441 | 441 | 441 | 216 | 216 | 216 |
| | *** | 29691 | 31157 | 44858 | 8141 | 8491 | 11502 | 1516 | 1532 | 1970 | 441 | 441 | 540 | 216 | 216 | 257 |
| 0.2 | *** | 37457 | 38632 | 45482 | 10282 | 10732 | 11641 | 1916 | 1957 | 1991 | 541 | 541 | 557 | 266 | 266 | 266 |
| | *** | 37866 | 40282 | 55820 | 10466 | 11091 | 14199 | 1941 | 1966 | 2381 | 541 | 557 | 634 | 266 | 266 | 295 |
| 0.25 | *** | 43466 | 45157 | 55832 | 12057 | 12732 | 14207 | 2266 | 2316 | 2382 | 632 | 641 | 641 | 307 | 307 | 307 |
| | *** | 44057 | 47591 | 65069 | 12341 | 13291 | 16469 | 2291 | 2357 | 2724 | 632 | 641 | 711 | 307 | 307 | 326 |
| 0.3 | *** | 47507 | 49807 | 64657 | 13391 | 14291 | 16366 | 2557 | 2632 | 2716 | 707 | 707 | 716 | 332 | 332 | 332 |
| | *** | 48316 | 53091 | 72605 | 13766 | 15066 | 18310 | 2591 | 2666 | 2998 | 707 | 716 | 771 | 332 | 332 | 349 |
| 0.35 | *** | 49716 | 52716 | 71791 | 14291 | 15432 | 18107 | 2766 | 2857 | 2966 | 757 | 766 | 766 | 357 | 357 | 357 |
| | *** | 50791 | 56882 | 78428 | 14782 | 16416 | 19723 | 2807 | 2907 | 3203 | 757 | 766 | 814 | 357 | 357 | 364 |
| 0.4 | *** | 50341 | 54091 | 77157 | 14816 | 16182 | 19407 | 2916 | 3016 | 3157 | 791 | 807 | 807 | 366 | 366 | 366 |
| | *** | 51707 | 59116 | 82539 | 15391 | 17341 | 20708 | 2966 | 3082 | 3340 | 791 | 807 | 840 | 366 | 366 | 372 |
| 0.45 | *** | 49641 | 54166 | 80691 | 15007 | 16541 | 20241 | 2991 | 3116 | 3266 | 807 | 816 | 832 | 366 | 366 | 366 |
| | *** | 51316 | 60007 | 84937 | 15657 | 17882 | 21265 | 3041 | 3191 | 3409 | 816 | 832 | 848 | 366 | 366 | 372 |
| 0.5 | *** | 47891 | 53157 | 82382 | 14907 | 16582 | 20616 | 3007 | 3141 | 3307 | 807 | 816 | 832 | 366 | 366 | 366 |
| | *** | 49866 | 59682 | 85622 | 15616 | 18041 | 21393 | 3066 | 3216 | 3409 | 816 | 832 | 840 | 366 | 366 | 364 |
| 0.55 | *** | 45357 | 51266 | 82207 | 14532 | 16307 | 20532 | 2957 | 3091 | 3266 | 791 | 807 | 816 | 357 | 357 | 357 |
| | *** | 47616 | 58307 | 84594 | 15291 | 17832 | 21093 | 3032 | 3182 | 3340 | 791 | 807 | 814 | 357 | 357 | 349 |
| 0.6 | *** | 42266 | 48657 | 80166 | 13932 | 15741 | 19966 | 2857 | 2991 | 3157 | 757 | 766 | 782 | 332 | 332 | 341 |
| | *** | 44757 | 55991 | 81854 | 14707 | 17282 | 20365 | 2916 | 3066 | 3203 | 757 | 766 | 771 | 332 | 332 | 326 |
| 0.65 | *** | 38807 | 45432 | 76266 | 13116 | 14907 | 18957 | 2691 | 2816 | 2982 | 707 | 707 | 716 | 307 | 307 | 307 |
| | *** | 41407 | 52816 | 77401 | 13882 | 16391 | 19209 | 2757 | 2891 | 2998 | 707 | 716 | 711 | 307 | 307 | 295 |
| 0.7 | *** | 35057 | 41666 | 70532 | 12107 | 13782 | 17466 | 2466 | 2582 | 2716 | 632 | 641 | 641 | 266 | 266 | 266 |
| | *** | 37691 | 48832 | 71235 | 12832 | 15166 | 17625 | 2516 | 2641 | 2724 | 632 | 641 | 634 | 266 | 266 | 257 |
| 0.75 | *** | 31066 | 37382 | 62957 | 10866 | 12382 | 15532 | 2182 | 2266 | 2382 | 541 | 541 | 557 | 232 | 232 | 232 |
| | *** | 33607 | 44007 | 63356 | 11532 | 13591 | 15612 | 2216 | 2332 | 2381 | 541 | 557 | 540 | 232 | 232 | 212 |
| 0.8 | *** | 26816 | 32491 | 53566 | 9416 | 10682 | 13141 | 1832 | 1891 | 1982 | 432 | 441 | 441 | 166 | 166 | 166 |
| | *** | 29116 | 38266 | 53764 | 9966 | 11641 | 13172 | 1866 | 1941 | 1970 | 441 | 441 | 429 | 166 | 166 | 158 |
| 0.85 | *** | 22141 | 26857 | 42391 | 7682 | 8616 | 10291 | 1416 | 1457 | 1507 | 307 | 316 | 316 | . | . | . |
| | *** | 24082 | 31432 | 42460 | 8091 | 9307 | 10303 | 1432 | 1482 | 1491 | 316 | 316 | 300 | . | . | . |
| 0.9 | *** | 16782 | 20116 | 29432 | 5566 | 6132 | 7016 | 916 | 941 | 957 | . | . | . | . | . | . |
| | *** | 18182 | 23166 | 29443 | 5816 | 6516 | 7006 | 932 | 941 | 943 | . | . | . | . | . | . |
| 0.95 | *** | 9957 | 11516 | 14732 | 2891 | 3066 | 3291 | . | . | . | . | . | . | . | . | . |
| | *** | 10632 | 12757 | 14713 | 2966 | 3166 | 3280 | . | . | . | . | . | . | . | . | . |
| 0.98 | *** | 4191 | 4557 | 5066 | . | . | . | . | . | . | . | . | . | . | . | . |
| | *** | 4366 | 4782 | 5053 | . | . | . | . | . | . | . | . | . | . | . | . |

## TABLE 8: ALPHA= 0.05  POWER= 0.9    EXPECTED ACCRUAL THRU MINIMUM FOLLOW-UP= 11000

|  | DEL=.01 | | | DEL=.02 | | | DEL=.05 | | | DEL=.10 | | | DEL=.15 | | |
|---|---|---|---|---|---|---|---|---|---|---|---|---|---|---|---|
| FACT= | 1.0 .75 | .50 .25 | .00 BIN | 1.0 .75 | .50 .25 | .00 BIN | 1.0 .75 | .50 .25 | .00 BIN | 1.0 75 | .50 .25 | .00 BIN | 1.0 .75 | .50 .25 | .00 BIN |

PCONT=***                            REQUIRED NUMBER OF PATIENTS

| PCONT | DEL=.01 1.0/.75 | .50/.25 | .00/BIN | DEL=.02 1.0/.75 | .50/.25 | .00/BIN | DEL=.05 1.0/.75 | .50/.25 | .00/BIN | DEL=.10 1.0/.75 | .50/.25 | .00/BIN | DEL=.15 1.0/.75 | .50/.25 | .00/BIN |
|---|---|---|---|---|---|---|---|---|---|---|---|---|---|---|---|
| 0.01 *** | 1310 | 1310 | 1327 | 485 | 485 | 485 | 155 | 155 | 155 | 73 | 73 | 73 | 62 | 62 | 62 |
| *** | 1310 | 1310 | 5053 | 485 | 485 | 1670 | 155 | 155 | 455 | 73 | 73 | 185 | 62 | 62 | 110 |
| 0.02 *** | 2922 | 2933 | 2950 | 942 | 942 | 942 | 255 | 255 | 255 | 117 | 117 | 117 | 73 | 73 | 73 |
| *** | 2922 | 2933 | 8342 | 942 | 942 | 2484 | 255 | 255 | 581 | 117 | 117 | 215 | 73 | 73 | 123 |
| 0.05 *** | 8890 | 8983 | 9203 | 2537 | 2548 | 2575 | 540 | 540 | 540 | 200 | 200 | 200 | 117 | 117 | 117 |
| *** | 8928 | 9082 | 17796 | 2548 | 2565 | 4822 | 540 | 540 | 943 | 200 | 200 | 300 | 117 | 117 | 158 |
| 0.1 *** | 19680 | 20065 | 21430 | 5408 | 5507 | 5672 | 1035 | 1052 | 1052 | 320 | 320 | 320 | 172 | 172 | 172 |
| *** | 19835 | 20505 | 32183 | 5452 | 5573 | 8376 | 1035 | 1052 | 1491 | 320 | 320 | 429 | 172 | 172 | 212 |
| 0.15 *** | 29515 | 30295 | 33843 | 8075 | 8323 | 8763 | 1503 | 1530 | 1547 | 447 | 447 | 447 | 227 | 227 | 227 |
| *** | 29800 | 31285 | 44858 | 8185 | 8505 | 11502 | 1520 | 1530 | 1970 | 447 | 447 | 540 | 227 | 227 | 257 |
| 0.2 *** | 37572 | 38837 | 45475 | 10347 | 10787 | 11650 | 1932 | 1960 | 1998 | 540 | 557 | 557 | 265 | 265 | 265 |
| *** | 38023 | 40525 | 55820 | 10540 | 11128 | 14199 | 1943 | 1970 | 2381 | 540 | 557 | 634 | 265 | 265 | 295 |
| 0.25 *** | 43650 | 45465 | 55832 | 12162 | 12822 | 14197 | 2273 | 2328 | 2383 | 640 | 640 | 640 | 310 | 310 | 310 |
| *** | 44293 | 47950 | 65069 | 12437 | 13355 | 16469 | 2300 | 2355 | 2724 | 640 | 640 | 711 | 310 | 310 | 326 |
| 0.3 *** | 47747 | 50205 | 64660 | 13520 | 14417 | 16370 | 2565 | 2630 | 2713 | 705 | 705 | 722 | 337 | 337 | 337 |
| *** | 48638 | 53577 | 72605 | 13895 | 15160 | 18310 | 2592 | 2675 | 2998 | 705 | 705 | 771 | 337 | 337 | 349 |
| 0.35 *** | 50040 | 53230 | 71793 | 14455 | 15583 | 18102 | 2785 | 2867 | 2977 | 760 | 760 | 777 | 348 | 348 | 365 |
| *** | 51195 | 57493 | 78428 | 14940 | 16535 | 19723 | 2823 | 2922 | 3203 | 760 | 777 | 814 | 348 | 348 | 364 |
| 0.4 *** | 50772 | 54732 | 77155 | 15005 | 16353 | 19405 | 2933 | 3032 | 3153 | 788 | 805 | 815 | 365 | 365 | 365 |
| *** | 52213 | 59858 | 82539 | 15572 | 17480 | 20708 | 2977 | 3087 | 3340 | 805 | 805 | 840 | 365 | 365 | 372 |
| 0.45 *** | 50167 | 54908 | 80692 | 15225 | 16755 | 20247 | 3015 | 3125 | 3263 | 805 | 815 | 832 | 365 | 375 | 375 |
| *** | 51938 | 60848 | 84937 | 15875 | 18030 | 21265 | 3070 | 3197 | 3409 | 815 | 832 | 848 | 375 | 375 | 372 |
| 0.5 *** | 48517 | 54000 | 82380 | 15132 | 16810 | 20615 | 3032 | 3153 | 3307 | 805 | 815 | 832 | 365 | 365 | 365 |
| *** | 50590 | 60617 | 85622 | 15847 | 18212 | 21393 | 3087 | 3225 | 3409 | 815 | 832 | 840 | 365 | 365 | 364 |
| 0.55 *** | 46070 | 52185 | 82205 | 14785 | 16545 | 20522 | 2988 | 3115 | 3280 | 788 | 805 | 815 | 348 | 348 | 365 |
| *** | 48435 | 59297 | 84594 | 15528 | 18003 | 21093 | 3043 | 3180 | 3340 | 788 | 805 | 814 | 348 | 365 | 349 |
| 0.6 *** | 43055 | 49628 | 80170 | 14197 | 15985 | 19972 | 2878 | 3005 | 3153 | 750 | 760 | 777 | 337 | 337 | 337 |
| *** | 45630 | 57015 | 81854 | 14950 | 17453 | 20365 | 2933 | 3070 | 3203 | 760 | 777 | 771 | 337 | 337 | 326 |
| 0.65 *** | 39635 | 46427 | 76275 | 13372 | 15132 | 18955 | 2713 | 2823 | 2977 | 705 | 705 | 722 | 310 | 310 | 310 |
| *** | 42330 | 53835 | 77401 | 14125 | 16562 | 19209 | 2768 | 2895 | 2998 | 705 | 722 | 711 | 310 | 310 | 295 |
| 0.7 *** | 35905 | 42643 | 70528 | 12338 | 13988 | 17470 | 2482 | 2592 | 2713 | 623 | 640 | 650 | 265 | 265 | 265 |
| *** | 38600 | 49810 | 71235 | 13053 | 15325 | 17625 | 2537 | 2647 | 2724 | 640 | 640 | 634 | 265 | 265 | 257 |
| 0.75 *** | 31890 | 38287 | 62955 | 11090 | 12575 | 15528 | 2190 | 2273 | 2383 | 540 | 540 | 557 | 227 | 227 | 227 |
| *** | 34475 | 44887 | 63356 | 11733 | 13730 | 15612 | 2235 | 2328 | 2381 | 540 | 557 | 540 | 227 | 227 | 212 |
| 0.8 *** | 27562 | 33293 | 53577 | 9605 | 10825 | 13135 | 1850 | 1905 | 1987 | 430 | 447 | 447 | 172 | 172 | 172 |
| *** | 29900 | 39030 | 53764 | 10138 | 11750 | 13172 | 1877 | 1943 | 1970 | 430 | 447 | 429 | 172 | 172 | 158 |
| 0.85 *** | 22777 | 27507 | 42385 | 7817 | 8725 | 10303 | 1420 | 1465 | 1503 | 310 | 310 | 320 | . | . | . |
| *** | 24730 | 32028 | 42460 | 8230 | 9385 | 10303 | 1437 | 1475 | 1491 | 310 | 310 | 300 | . | . | . |
| 0.9 *** | 17233 | 20577 | 29432 | 5655 | 6195 | 7020 | 925 | 942 | 953 | . | . | . | . | . | . |
| *** | 18635 | 23547 | 29443 | 5903 | 6552 | 7006 | 925 | 953 | 943 | . | . | . | . | . | . |
| 0.95 *** | 10182 | 11705 | 14730 | 2922 | 3087 | 3290 | . | . | . | . | . | . | . | . | . |
| *** | 10853 | 12888 | 14713 | 3005 | 3180 | 3280 | . | . | . | . | . | . | . | . | . |
| 0.98 *** | 4253 | 4600 | 5067 | . | . | . | . | . | . | . | . | . | . | . | . |
| *** | 4407 | 4803 | 5053 | . | . | . | . | . | . | . | . | . | . | . | . |

TABLE 8: ALPHA= 0.05 POWER= 0.9    EXPECTED ACCRUAL THRU MINIMUM FOLLOW-UP= 12000

| | DEL=.01 | | | DEL=.02 | | | DEL=.05 | | | DEL=.10 | | | DEL=.15 | | |
|---|---|---|---|---|---|---|---|---|---|---|---|---|---|---|---|
| FACT= | 1.0 .75 | .50 .25 | .00 BIN | 1.0 .75 | .50 .25 | .00 BIN | 1.0 .75 | .50 .25 | .00 BIN | 1.0 75 | .50 .25 | .00 BIN | 1.0 .75 | .50 .25 | .00 BIN |
| PCONT=*** | | | | REQUIRED | NUMBER OF | PATIENTS | | | | | | | | | |
| 0.01 *** | 1309 | 1309 | 1328 | 488 | 488 | 488 | 158 | 158 | 158 | 79 | 79 | 79 | 49 | 49 | 49 |
| *** | 1309 | 1309 | 5053 | 488 | 488 | 1670 | 158 | 158 | 455 | 79 | 79 | 185 | 49 | 49 | 110 |
| 0.02 *** | 2918 | 2929 | 2948 | 938 | 938 | 938 | 248 | 248 | 248 | 109 | 109 | 109 | 68 | 68 | 68 |
| *** | 2929 | 2929 | 8342 | 938 | 938 | 2484 | 248 | 248 | 581 | 109 | 109 | 215 | 68 | 68 | 123 |
| 0.05 *** | 8899 | 9008 | 9199 | 2539 | 2558 | 2569 | 548 | 548 | 548 | 188 | 188 | 188 | 109 | 109 | 109 |
| *** | 8948 | 9079 | 17796 | 2539 | 2569 | 4822 | 548 | 548 | 943 | 188 | 188 | 300 | 109 | 109 | 158 |
| 0.1 *** | 19729 | 20138 | 21428 | 5419 | 5528 | 5659 | 1039 | 1039 | 1058 | 319 | 319 | 319 | 169 | 169 | 169 |
| *** | 19879 | 20558 | 32183 | 5468 | 5588 | 8376 | 1039 | 1058 | 1491 | 319 | 319 | 429 | 169 | 169 | 212 |
| 0.15 *** | 29599 | 30409 | 33848 | 8108 | 8348 | 8768 | 1508 | 1519 | 1549 | 439 | 439 | 439 | 218 | 218 | 218 |
| *** | 29899 | 31418 | 44858 | 8209 | 8528 | 11502 | 1519 | 1538 | 1970 | 439 | 439 | 540 | 218 | 218 | 257 |
| 0.2 *** | 37699 | 39019 | 45469 | 10399 | 10838 | 11648 | 1928 | 1958 | 1999 | 548 | 548 | 548 | 259 | 259 | 259 |
| *** | 38179 | 40748 | 55820 | 10579 | 11168 | 14199 | 1939 | 1969 | 2381 | 548 | 548 | 634 | 259 | 259 | 295 |
| 0.25 *** | 43819 | 45739 | 55838 | 12248 | 12889 | 14198 | 2288 | 2329 | 2389 | 638 | 638 | 638 | 308 | 308 | 308 |
| *** | 44528 | 48289 | 65069 | 12518 | 13418 | 16469 | 2318 | 2359 | 2724 | 638 | 638 | 711 | 308 | 308 | 326 |
| 0.3 *** | 47989 | 50599 | 64658 | 13628 | 14509 | 16369 | 2569 | 2629 | 2708 | 709 | 709 | 709 | 338 | 338 | 338 |
| *** | 48938 | 54019 | 72605 | 14018 | 15229 | 18310 | 2599 | 2678 | 2998 | 709 | 709 | 771 | 338 | 338 | 349 |
| 0.35 *** | 50378 | 53719 | 71798 | 14599 | 15709 | 18109 | 2798 | 2869 | 2978 | 758 | 769 | 769 | 349 | 349 | 349 |
| *** | 51608 | 58058 | 78428 | 15079 | 16628 | 19723 | 2828 | 2918 | 3203 | 758 | 769 | 814 | 349 | 349 | 364 |
| 0.4 *** | 51169 | 55328 | 77149 | 15188 | 16508 | 19399 | 2948 | 3038 | 3158 | 799 | 799 | 818 | 368 | 368 | 368 |
| *** | 52718 | 60529 | 82539 | 15739 | 17599 | 20708 | 2989 | 3098 | 3340 | 799 | 799 | 840 | 368 | 368 | 372 |
| 0.45 *** | 50659 | 55609 | 80689 | 15428 | 16928 | 20239 | 3019 | 3139 | 3278 | 818 | 818 | 829 | 368 | 368 | 368 |
| *** | 52538 | 61628 | 84937 | 16058 | 18169 | 21265 | 3079 | 3199 | 3409 | 818 | 829 | 848 | 368 | 368 | 372 |
| 0.5 *** | 49118 | 54788 | 82388 | 15349 | 16999 | 20618 | 3049 | 3169 | 3308 | 818 | 818 | 829 | 368 | 368 | 368 |
| *** | 51289 | 61478 | 85622 | 16058 | 18349 | 21393 | 3098 | 3229 | 3409 | 818 | 829 | 840 | 368 | 368 | 364 |
| 0.55 *** | 46759 | 53048 | 82208 | 15008 | 16748 | 20528 | 3008 | 3128 | 3278 | 788 | 799 | 818 | 349 | 349 | 349 |
| *** | 49208 | 60218 | 84594 | 15758 | 18169 | 21093 | 3068 | 3188 | 3340 | 799 | 799 | 814 | 349 | 349 | 349 |
| 0.6 *** | 43808 | 50528 | 80168 | 14419 | 16189 | 19969 | 2899 | 3019 | 3158 | 758 | 769 | 769 | 338 | 338 | 338 |
| *** | 46448 | 57949 | 81854 | 15188 | 17618 | 20365 | 2948 | 3079 | 3203 | 758 | 769 | 771 | 338 | 338 | 326 |
| 0.65 *** | 40429 | 47348 | 76268 | 13609 | 15338 | 18949 | 2738 | 2839 | 2978 | 698 | 709 | 728 | 308 | 308 | 308 |
| *** | 43178 | 54769 | 77401 | 14348 | 16718 | 19209 | 2779 | 2899 | 2998 | 709 | 709 | 711 | 308 | 308 | 295 |
| 0.7 *** | 36698 | 43538 | 70538 | 12559 | 14179 | 17468 | 2498 | 2599 | 2719 | 638 | 638 | 649 | 278 | 278 | 278 |
| *** | 39439 | 50689 | 71235 | 13268 | 15458 | 17625 | 2539 | 2659 | 2724 | 638 | 638 | 634 | 278 | 278 | 257 |
| 0.75 *** | 32659 | 39128 | 62959 | 11288 | 12728 | 15529 | 2209 | 2288 | 2389 | 548 | 548 | 548 | 229 | 229 | 229 |
| *** | 35269 | 45698 | 63356 | 11918 | 13838 | 15612 | 2239 | 2329 | 2381 | 548 | 548 | 540 | 229 | 229 | 212 |
| 0.8 *** | 28268 | 34028 | 53569 | 9769 | 10958 | 13129 | 1849 | 1909 | 1988 | 439 | 439 | 439 | 169 | 169 | 169 |
| *** | 30619 | 39709 | 53764 | 10298 | 11839 | 13172 | 1879 | 1939 | 1970 | 439 | 439 | 429 | 169 | 169 | 158 |
| 0.85 *** | 23359 | 28088 | 42398 | 7939 | 8828 | 10298 | 1429 | 1459 | 1508 | 308 | 308 | 319 | . | . | . |
| *** | 25328 | 32539 | 42460 | 8329 | 9439 | 10303 | 1448 | 1478 | 1491 | 308 | 319 | 300 | . | . | . |
| 0.9 *** | 17659 | 20978 | 29438 | 5738 | 6248 | 7009 | 919 | 938 | 949 | . | . | . | . | . | . |
| *** | 19058 | 23888 | 29443 | 5959 | 6589 | 7006 | 938 | 949 | 943 | . | . | . | . | . | . |
| 0.95 *** | 10388 | 11869 | 14719 | 2948 | 3098 | 3289 | . | . | . | . | . | . | . | . | . |
| *** | 11048 | 13009 | 14713 | 3019 | 3188 | 3280 | . | . | . | . | . | . | . | . | . |
| 0.98 *** | 4309 | 4628 | 5059 | . | . | . | . | . | . | . | . | . | . | . | . |
| *** | 4459 | 4819 | 5053 | . | . | . | . | . | . | . | . | . | . | . | . |

## TABLE 8: ALPHA= 0.05  POWER= 0.9    EXPECTED ACCRUAL THRU MINIMUM FOLLOW-UP= 13000

| | | DEL=.01 | | | DEL=.02 | | | DEL=.05 | | | DEL=.10 | | | DEL=.15 | |
|---|---|---|---|---|---|---|---|---|---|---|---|---|---|---|---|---|
| FACT= | 1.0 .75 | .50 .25 | .00 BIN | 1.0 .75 | .50 .25 | .00 BIN | 1.0 .75 | .50 .25 | .00 BIN | 1.0 75 | .50 .25 | .00 BIN | 1.0 .75 | .50 .25 | .00 BIN |

PCONT=***                       REQUIRED NUMBER OF PATIENTS

| PCONT | | 1.0 | .50 | .00/BIN | 1.0 | .50 | .00/BIN | 1.0 | .50 | .00/BIN | 1.0 | .50 | .00/BIN | 1.0 | .50 | .00/BIN |
|---|---|---|---|---|---|---|---|---|---|---|---|---|---|---|---|---|
| | | .75 | .25 | | .75 | .25 | | .75 | .25 | | 75 | .25 | | .75 | .25 | |
| 0.01 | *** | 1321 | 1321 | 1321 | 476 | 476 | 476 | 151 | 151 | 151 | 74 | 74 | 74 | 53 | 53 | 53 |
| | *** | 1321 | 1321 | 5053 | 476 | 476 | 1670 | 151 | 151 | 455 | 74 | 74 | 185 | 53 | 53 | 110 |
| 0.02 | *** | 2913 | 2934 | 2946 | 931 | 931 | 931 | 248 | 248 | 248 | 106 | 106 | 106 | 74 | 74 | 74 |
| | *** | 2934 | 2934 | 8342 | 931 | 931 | 2484 | 248 | 248 | 581 | 106 | 106 | 215 | 74 | 74 | 123 |
| 0.05 | *** | 8914 | 9011 | 9206 | 2544 | 2556 | 2576 | 541 | 541 | 541 | 183 | 183 | 183 | 106 | 106 | 106 |
| | *** | 8958 | 9088 | 17796 | 2544 | 2576 | 4822 | 541 | 541 | 943 | 183 | 183 | 300 | 106 | 106 | 158 |
| 0.1 | *** | 19769 | 20171 | 21426 | 5436 | 5534 | 5664 | 1049 | 1049 | 1049 | 313 | 313 | 334 | 171 | 171 | 171 |
| | *** | 19931 | 20614 | 32183 | 5481 | 5599 | 8376 | 1049 | 1049 | 1491 | 313 | 334 | 429 | 171 | 171 | 212 |
| 0.15 | *** | 29681 | 30526 | 33853 | 8134 | 8373 | 8763 | 1516 | 1536 | 1548 | 443 | 443 | 443 | 216 | 216 | 216 |
| | *** | 29986 | 31534 | 44858 | 8243 | 8536 | 11502 | 1516 | 1536 | 1970 | 443 | 443 | 540 | 216 | 216 | 257 |
| 0.2 | *** | 37818 | 39216 | 45476 | 10453 | 10876 | 11644 | 1938 | 1959 | 1991 | 541 | 541 | 561 | 269 | 269 | 269 |
| | *** | 38338 | 40959 | 55820 | 10636 | 11201 | 14199 | 1959 | 1971 | 2381 | 541 | 541 | 634 | 269 | 269 | 295 |
| 0.25 | *** | 43993 | 46029 | 55823 | 12326 | 12956 | 14191 | 2296 | 2328 | 2381 | 638 | 638 | 638 | 301 | 301 | 301 |
| | *** | 44741 | 48596 | 65069 | 12598 | 13464 | 16469 | 2316 | 2361 | 2724 | 638 | 638 | 711 | 301 | 301 | 326 |
| 0.3 | *** | 48239 | 50969 | 64651 | 13736 | 14613 | 16368 | 2588 | 2641 | 2718 | 703 | 703 | 724 | 334 | 334 | 334 |
| | *** | 49246 | 54446 | 72605 | 14114 | 15296 | 18310 | 2609 | 2674 | 2998 | 703 | 724 | 771 | 334 | 334 | 349 |
| 0.35 | *** | 50688 | 54186 | 71801 | 14731 | 15836 | 18111 | 2804 | 2881 | 2966 | 756 | 768 | 768 | 346 | 346 | 366 |
| | *** | 51988 | 58586 | 78428 | 15198 | 16714 | 19723 | 2836 | 2934 | 3203 | 768 | 768 | 814 | 346 | 346 | 364 |
| 0.4 | *** | 51566 | 55888 | 77164 | 15349 | 16649 | 19411 | 2966 | 3043 | 3161 | 801 | 801 | 801 | 366 | 366 | 366 |
| | *** | 53191 | 61153 | 82539 | 15901 | 17701 | 20708 | 2999 | 3096 | 3340 | 801 | 801 | 840 | 366 | 366 | 372 |
| 0.45 | *** | 51164 | 56266 | 80686 | 15609 | 17083 | 20236 | 3043 | 3141 | 3271 | 821 | 821 | 833 | 366 | 366 | 378 |
| | *** | 53093 | 62344 | 84937 | 16238 | 18286 | 21265 | 3096 | 3206 | 3409 | 821 | 821 | 848 | 366 | 378 | 372 |
| 0.5 | *** | 49681 | 55531 | 82376 | 15556 | 17169 | 20614 | 3064 | 3173 | 3303 | 821 | 821 | 833 | 366 | 366 | 366 |
| | *** | 51944 | 62258 | 85622 | 16238 | 18481 | 21393 | 3108 | 3238 | 3409 | 821 | 821 | 840 | 366 | 366 | 364 |
| 0.55 | *** | 47406 | 53861 | 82201 | 15219 | 16921 | 20528 | 3011 | 3129 | 3271 | 789 | 801 | 821 | 346 | 346 | 366 |
| | *** | 49929 | 61044 | 84594 | 15966 | 18306 | 21093 | 3076 | 3194 | 3340 | 801 | 801 | 814 | 346 | 366 | 349 |
| 0.6 | *** | 44513 | 51371 | 80166 | 14634 | 16368 | 19976 | 2913 | 3031 | 3161 | 756 | 768 | 768 | 334 | 334 | 334 |
| | *** | 47231 | 58801 | 81854 | 15381 | 17754 | 20365 | 2966 | 3096 | 3203 | 756 | 768 | 771 | 334 | 334 | 326 |
| 0.65 | *** | 41166 | 48186 | 76266 | 13821 | 15511 | 18956 | 2751 | 2848 | 2978 | 703 | 703 | 724 | 301 | 301 | 313 |
| | *** | 43981 | 55616 | 77401 | 14548 | 16844 | 19209 | 2804 | 2913 | 2998 | 703 | 724 | 711 | 301 | 313 | 295 |
| 0.7 | *** | 37449 | 44371 | 70534 | 12761 | 14353 | 17473 | 2511 | 2609 | 2718 | 626 | 638 | 638 | 269 | 269 | 269 |
| | *** | 40244 | 51489 | 71235 | 13464 | 15576 | 17625 | 2556 | 2653 | 2724 | 638 | 638 | 634 | 269 | 269 | 257 |
| 0.75 | *** | 33386 | 39886 | 62961 | 11461 | 12879 | 15523 | 2219 | 2296 | 2381 | 541 | 541 | 561 | 216 | 216 | 236 |
| | *** | 36031 | 46419 | 63356 | 12099 | 13951 | 15612 | 2251 | 2328 | 2381 | 541 | 541 | 540 | 216 | 216 | 212 |
| 0.8 | *** | 28913 | 34698 | 53569 | 9921 | 11071 | 13139 | 1861 | 1906 | 1971 | 431 | 443 | 443 | 171 | 171 | 171 |
| | *** | 31286 | 40321 | 53764 | 10441 | 11936 | 13172 | 1894 | 1938 | 1970 | 443 | 443 | 429 | 171 | 171 | 158 |
| 0.85 | *** | 23908 | 28621 | 42389 | 8048 | 8914 | 10291 | 1439 | 1471 | 1504 | 313 | 313 | 313 | . | . | . |
| | *** | 25879 | 33029 | 42460 | 8438 | 9499 | 10303 | 1451 | 1483 | 1491 | 313 | 313 | 300 | . | . | . |
| 0.9 | *** | 18046 | 21329 | 29433 | 5794 | 6293 | 7008 | 931 | 931 | 951 | . | . | . | . | . | . |
| | *** | 19444 | 24168 | 29443 | 6033 | 6618 | 7006 | 931 | 951 | 943 | . | . | . | . | . | . |
| 0.95 | *** | 10571 | 12034 | 14731 | 2966 | 3108 | 3291 | . | . | . | . | . | . | . | . | . |
| | *** | 11221 | 13118 | 14713 | 3031 | 3194 | 3280 | . | . | . | . | . | . | . | . | . |
| 0.98 | *** | 4343 | 4656 | 5058 | . | . | . | . | . | . | . | . | . | . | . | . |
| | *** | 4494 | 4851 | 5053 | . | . | . | . | . | . | . | . | . | . | . | . |

TABLE 8: ALPHA= 0.05 POWER= 0.9     EXPECTED ACCRUAL THRU MINIMUM FOLLOW-UP= 14000

| | | DEL=.01 | | | DEL=.02 | | | DEL=.05 | | | DEL=.10 | | | DEL=.15 | | |
|---|---|---|---|---|---|---|---|---|---|---|---|---|---|---|---|---|
| FACT= | | 1.0 .75 | .50 .25 | .00 BIN | 1.0 .75 | .50 .25 | .00 BIN | 1.0 .75 | .50 .25 | .00 BIN | 1.0 75 | .50 .25 | .00 BIN | 1.0 .75 | .50 .25 | .00 BIN |
| PCONT=*** | | REQUIRED NUMBER OF PATIENTS | | | | | | | | | | | | | | |
| 0.01 | *** | 1317 1317 | 1317 | 477 477 | 477 | 162 162 | 162 | 79 79 | 79 | 57 57 | 57 |
| | *** | 1317 1317 | 5053 | 477 477 | 1670 | 162 162 | 455 | 79 79 | 185 | 57 57 | 110 |
| 0.02 | *** | 2927 2927 | 2949 | 932 932 | 932 | 254 254 | 254 | 114 114 | 114 | 79 79 | 79 |
| | *** | 2927 2949 | 8342 | 932 932 | 2484 | 254 254 | 581 | 114 114 | 215 | 79 79 | 123 |
| 0.05 | *** | 8912 9017 | 9214 | 2542 2564 | 2577 | 547 547 | 547 | 197 197 | 197 | 114 114 | 114 |
| | *** | 8969 9087 | 17796 | 2542 2564 | 4822 | 547 547 | 943 | 197 197 | 300 | 114 114 | 158 |
| 0.1 | *** | 19797 20217 | 21429 | 5447 5539 | 5657 | 1037 1037 | 1059 | 324 324 | 324 | 162 162 | 162 |
| | *** | 19972 20659 | 32183 | 5482 5587 | 8376 | 1037 1059 | 1491 | 324 324 | 429 | 162 162 | 212 |
| 0.15 | *** | 29737 30634 | 33854 | 8164 8387 | 8759 | 1514 1527 | 1549 | 442 442 | 442 | 219 219 | 219 |
| | *** | 30087 31627 | 44858 | 8269 8562 | 11502 | 1527 1527 | 1970 | 442 442 | 540 | 219 219 | 257 |
| 0.2 | *** | 37949 39384 | 45474 | 10509 10907 | 11642 | 1934 1969 | 2004 | 547 547 | 547 | 267 267 | 267 |
| | *** | 38487 41134 | 55820 | 10684 11222 | 14199 | 1947 1982 | 2381 | 547 547 | 634 | 267 267 | 295 |
| 0.25 | *** | 44179 46279 | 55834 | 12399 13029 | 14197 | 2297 2332 | 2389 | 639 639 | 639 | 302 302 | 302 |
| | *** | 44949 48882 | 65069 | 12657 13497 | 16469 | 2319 2367 | 2724 | 639 639 | 711 | 302 302 | 326 |
| 0.3 | *** | 48484 51319 | 64654 | 13834 14687 | 16367 | 2599 2647 | 2717 | 709 709 | 722 | 337 337 | 337 |
| | *** | 49534 54819 | 72605 | 14197 15374 | 18310 | 2612 2682 | 2998 | 709 709 | 771 | 337 337 | 349 |
| 0.35 | *** | 51004 54644 | 71794 | 14849 15934 | 18104 | 2809 2892 | 2962 | 757 757 | 779 | 359 359 | 359 |
| | *** | 52347 59067 | 78428 | 15317 16787 | 19723 | 2844 2927 | 3203 | 757 779 | 814 | 359 359 | 364 |
| 0.4 | *** | 51962 56429 | 77149 | 15479 16774 | 19399 | 2962 3054 | 3159 | 792 792 | 814 | 359 372 | 372 |
| | *** | 53642 61727 | 82539 | 16039 17802 | 20708 | 3019 3102 | 3340 | 792 814 | 840 | 372 372 | 372 |
| 0.45 | *** | 51634 56897 | 80697 | 15772 17229 | 20239 | 3054 3159 | 3264 | 814 827 | 827 | 372 372 | 372 |
| | *** | 53642 64937 | 84937 | 16402 18397 | 21265 | 3102 3207 | 3409 | 814 827 | 848 | 372 372 | 372 |
| 0.5 | *** | 50234 56232 | 82377 | 15737 17334 | 20624 | 3067 3172 | 3312 | 814 827 | 827 | 372 372 | 372 |
| | *** | 52557 62974 | 85622 | 16424 18607 | 21393 | 3124 3242 | 3409 | 814 827 | 840 | 372 372 | 364 |
| 0.55 | *** | 48029 54609 | 82202 | 15409 17089 | 20532 | 3032 3137 | 3277 | 792 792 | 814 | 359 359 | 359 |
| | *** | 50619 61819 | 84594 | 16144 18432 | 21093 | 3089 3207 | 3340 | 792 814 | 814 | 359 359 | 349 |
| 0.6 | *** | 45194 52159 | 80172 | 14827 16542 | 19972 | 2927 3032 | 3159 | 757 757 | 779 | 337 337 | 337 |
| | *** | 47959 59592 | 81854 | 15584 17872 | 20365 | 2984 3089 | 3203 | 757 779 | 771 | 337 337 | 326 |
| 0.65 | *** | 41869 48987 | 76274 | 14009 15667 | 18944 | 2752 2857 | 2984 | 709 709 | 722 | 302 302 | 302 |
| | *** | 44717 56394 | 77401 | 14744 16962 | 19209 | 2809 2914 | 2998 | 709 709 | 711 | 302 302 | 295 |
| 0.7 | *** | 38159 45137 | 70534 | 12937 14499 | 17474 | 2529 2612 | 2717 | 639 639 | 639 | 267 267 | 267 |
| | *** | 40972 52229 | 71235 | 13624 15689 | 17625 | 2564 2669 | 2724 | 639 639 | 634 | 267 267 | 257 |
| 0.75 | *** | 34042 40609 | 62952 | 11629 13007 | 15527 | 2227 2297 | 2389 | 547 547 | 547 | 219 219 | 232 |
| | *** | 36724 47084 | 63356 | 12237 14044 | 15612 | 2262 2332 | 2381 | 547 547 | 540 | 219 219 | 212 |
| 0.8 | *** | 29514 35324 | 53572 | 10054 11187 | 13134 | 1864 1912 | 1982 | 442 442 | 442 | 162 162 | 162 |
| | *** | 31907 40889 | 53764 | 10557 11992 | 13172 | 1899 1947 | 1970 | 442 442 | 429 | 162 162 | 158 |
| 0.85 | *** | 24404 29129 | 42394 | 8164 8982 | 10299 | 1444 1457 | 1514 | 302 302 | 324 | . . | . |
| | *** | 26377 33447 | 42460 | 8527 9542 | 10303 | 1457 1479 | 1491 | 302 324 | 300 | . . | . |
| 0.9 | *** | 18419 21674 | 29444 | 5867 6344 | 7009 | 932 932 | 954 | . . | . | . . | . |
| | *** | 19797 24439 | 29443 | 6077 6637 | 7006 | 932 954 | 943 | . . | . | . . | . |
| 0.95 | *** | 10754 12167 | 14722 | 2984 3124 | 3299 | . . | . | . . | . | . . | . |
| | *** | 11362 13204 | 14713 | 3054 3207 | 3280 | . . | . | . . | . | . . | . |
| 0.98 | *** | 4384 4677 | 5062 | . . | . | . . | . | . . | . | . . | . |
| | *** | 4524 4852 | 5053 | . . | . | . . | . | . . | . | . . | . |

TABLE 8: ALPHA= 0.05  POWER= 0.9    EXPECTED ACCRUAL THRU MINIMUM FOLLOW-UP= 15000

| | | DEL=.01 | | | DEL=.02 | | | DEL=.05 | | | DEL=.10 | | | DEL=.15 | | |
|---|---|---|---|---|---|---|---|---|---|---|---|---|---|---|---|---|---|
| FACT= | | 1.0 .75 | .50 .25 | .00 BIN | 1.0 .75 | .50 .25 | .00 BIN | 1.0 .75 | .50 .25 | .00 BIN | 1.0 75 | .50 .25 | .00 BIN | 1.0 .75 | .50 .25 | .00 BIN |
| PCONT=*** | | | | | REQUIRED NUMBER OF PATIENTS | | | | | | | | | | | |
| 0.01 | *** | 1322 | 1322 | 1322 | 474 | 474 | 474 | 160 | 160 | 160 | 85 | 85 | 85 | 61 | 61 | 61 |
| | *** | 1322 | 1322 | 5053 | 474 | 474 | 1670 | 160 | 160 | 455 | 85 | 85 | 185 | 61 | 61 | 110 |
| 0.02 | *** | 2935 | 2935 | 2949 | 947 | 947 | 947 | 249 | 249 | 249 | 99 | 99 | 99 | 61 | 61 | 61 |
| | *** | 2935 | 2935 | 8342 | 947 | 947 | 2484 | 249 | 249 | 581 | 99 | 99 | 215 | 61 | 61 | 123 |
| 0.05 | *** | 8935 | 9024 | 9197 | 2536 | 2560 | 2574 | 549 | 549 | 549 | 197 | 197 | 197 | 122 | 122 | 122 |
| | *** | 8972 | 9099 | 17796 | 2560 | 2574 | 4822 | 549 | 549 | 943 | 197 | 197 | 300 | 122 | 122 | 158 |
| 0.1 | *** | 19847 | 20274 | 21422 | 5461 | 5536 | 5672 | 1036 | 1036 | 1060 | 324 | 324 | 324 | 174 | 174 | 174 |
| | *** | 20011 | 20686 | 32183 | 5499 | 5597 | 8376 | 1036 | 1060 | 1491 | 324 | 324 | 429 | 174 | 174 | 212 |
| 0.15 | *** | 29822 | 30736 | 33849 | 8185 | 8410 | 8761 | 1524 | 1524 | 1547 | 436 | 436 | 436 | 211 | 211 | 211 |
| | *** | 30174 | 31735 | 44858 | 8297 | 8574 | 11502 | 1524 | 1547 | 1970 | 436 | 436 | 540 | 211 | 211 | 257 |
| 0.2 | *** | 38072 | 39549 | 45474 | 10547 | 10960 | 11649 | 1936 | 1960 | 1997 | 549 | 549 | 549 | 272 | 272 | 272 |
| | *** | 38635 | 41311 | 55820 | 10735 | 11236 | 14199 | 1960 | 1974 | 2381 | 549 | 549 | 634 | 272 | 272 | 295 |
| 0.25 | *** | 44349 | 46524 | 55824 | 12460 | 13074 | 14199 | 2311 | 2349 | 2386 | 624 | 647 | 647 | 310 | 310 | 310 |
| | *** | 45160 | 49135 | 65069 | 12736 | 13547 | 16469 | 2311 | 2372 | 2724 | 647 | 647 | 711 | 310 | 310 | 326 |
| 0.3 | *** | 48699 | 51647 | 64660 | 13922 | 14761 | 16360 | 2597 | 2649 | 2710 | 699 | 722 | 722 | 324 | 324 | 324 |
| | *** | 49810 | 55172 | 72605 | 14297 | 15422 | 18310 | 2635 | 2686 | 2998 | 699 | 722 | 771 | 324 | 324 | 349 |
| 0.35 | *** | 51310 | 55060 | 71785 | 14972 | 16036 | 18099 | 2822 | 2897 | 2972 | 760 | 760 | 774 | 347 | 361 | 361 |
| | *** | 52711 | 59522 | 78428 | 15436 | 16861 | 19723 | 2860 | 2935 | 3203 | 760 | 774 | 814 | 347 | 361 | 364 |
| 0.4 | *** | 52336 | 56935 | 77161 | 15624 | 16899 | 19397 | 2986 | 3061 | 3160 | 797 | 797 | 811 | 361 | 361 | 361 |
| | *** | 54099 | 62274 | 82539 | 16172 | 17897 | 20708 | 3024 | 3099 | 3340 | 797 | 811 | 840 | 361 | 361 | 372 |
| 0.45 | *** | 52097 | 57474 | 80686 | 15924 | 17372 | 20236 | 3061 | 3160 | 3272 | 811 | 811 | 835 | 361 | 361 | 361 |
| | *** | 54174 | 63610 | 84937 | 16547 | 18497 | 21265 | 3122 | 3211 | 3409 | 811 | 835 | 848 | 361 | 361 | 372 |
| 0.5 | *** | 50761 | 56874 | 82374 | 15910 | 17485 | 20611 | 3085 | 3197 | 3310 | 811 | 811 | 835 | 361 | 361 | 361 |
| | *** | 53161 | 63647 | 85622 | 16585 | 18699 | 21393 | 3136 | 3249 | 3409 | 811 | 835 | 840 | 361 | 361 | 364 |
| 0.55 | *** | 48624 | 55322 | 82210 | 15586 | 17236 | 20522 | 3047 | 3160 | 3272 | 797 | 797 | 811 | 347 | 361 | 361 |
| | *** | 51272 | 62522 | 84594 | 16299 | 18535 | 21093 | 3099 | 3211 | 3340 | 797 | 811 | 814 | 361 | 361 | 349 |
| 0.6 | *** | 45835 | 52899 | 80161 | 15010 | 16697 | 19974 | 2935 | 3047 | 3160 | 760 | 760 | 774 | 324 | 324 | 347 |
| | *** | 48661 | 60310 | 81854 | 15736 | 17986 | 20365 | 2986 | 3099 | 3203 | 760 | 774 | 771 | 324 | 347 | 326 |
| 0.65 | *** | 42549 | 49735 | 76261 | 14185 | 15811 | 18947 | 2761 | 2860 | 2972 | 699 | 722 | 722 | 310 | 310 | 310 |
| | *** | 45436 | 57099 | 77401 | 14897 | 17072 | 19209 | 2822 | 2911 | 2998 | 699 | 722 | 711 | 310 | 310 | 295 |
| 0.7 | *** | 38822 | 45849 | 70524 | 13111 | 14635 | 17461 | 2536 | 2611 | 2710 | 624 | 647 | 647 | 272 | 272 | 272 |
| | *** | 41672 | 52899 | 71235 | 13786 | 15774 | 17625 | 2574 | 2672 | 2724 | 647 | 647 | 634 | 272 | 272 | 257 |
| 0.75 | *** | 34674 | 41260 | 62949 | 11785 | 13135 | 15535 | 2236 | 2311 | 2386 | 549 | 549 | 549 | 235 | 235 | 235 |
| | *** | 37374 | 47686 | 63356 | 12385 | 14124 | 15612 | 2274 | 2349 | 2381 | 549 | 549 | 540 | 235 | 235 | 212 |
| 0.8 | *** | 30085 | 35897 | 53574 | 10172 | 11274 | 13135 | 1885 | 1922 | 1974 | 436 | 436 | 436 | 174 | 174 | 174 |
| | *** | 32485 | 41386 | 53764 | 10674 | 12061 | 13172 | 1899 | 1960 | 1970 | 436 | 436 | 429 | 174 | 174 | 158 |
| 0.85 | *** | 24886 | 29574 | 42385 | 8260 | 9047 | 10299 | 1435 | 1472 | 1510 | 310 | 310 | 310 | . | . | . |
| | *** | 26860 | 33835 | 42460 | 8611 | 9586 | 10303 | 1449 | 1486 | 1491 | 310 | 310 | 300 | . | . | . |
| 0.9 | *** | 18736 | 21961 | 29424 | 5911 | 6385 | 7022 | 924 | 947 | 961 | . | . | . | . | . | . |
| | *** | 20124 | 24685 | 29443 | 6122 | 6661 | 7006 | 947 | 947 | 943 | . | . | . | . | . | . |
| 0.95 | *** | 10899 | 12286 | 14724 | 3010 | 3136 | 3286 | . | . | . | . | . | . | . | . | . |
| | *** | 11522 | 13285 | 14713 | 3061 | 3211 | 3280 | . | . | . | . | . | . | . | . | . |
| 0.98 | *** | 4411 | 4697 | 5072 | . | . | . | . | . | . | . | . | . | . | . | . |
| | *** | 4547 | 4861 | 5053 | . | . | . | . | . | . | . | . | . | . | . | . |

TABLE 8: ALPHA= 0.05  POWER= 0.9    EXPECTED ACCRUAL THRU MINIMUM FOLLOW-UP= 17000

| | DEL=.01 | | | DEL=.02 | | | DEL=.05 | | | DEL=.10 | | | DEL=.15 | | |
|---|---|---|---|---|---|---|---|---|---|---|---|---|---|---|---|
| FACT= | 1.0 .75 | .50 .25 | .00 BIN | 1.0 .75 | .50 .25 | .00 BIN | 1.0 .75 | .50 .25 | .00 BIN | 1.0 75 | .50 .25 | .00 BIN | 1.0 .75 | .50 .25 | .00 BIN |
| PCONT=*** | | | | | REQUIRED NUMBER OF PATIENTS | | | | | | | | | | |
| 0.01 *** | 1329 | 1329 | 1329 | 479 | 479 | 479 | 155 | 155 | 155 | 70 | 70 | 70 | 54 | 54 | 54 |
| *** | 1329 | 1329 | 5053 | 479 | 479 | 1670 | 155 | 155 | 455 | 70 | 70 | 185 | 54 | 54 | 110 |
| 0.02 *** | 2917 | 2944 | 2944 | 946 | 946 | 946 | 240 | 240 | 240 | 112 | 112 | 112 | 70 | 70 | 70 |
| *** | 2917 | 2944 | 8342 | 946 | 946 | 2484 | 240 | 240 | 581 | 112 | 112 | 215 | 70 | 70 | 123 |
| 0.05 *** | 8952 | 9037 | 9207 | 2561 | 2561 | 2577 | 537 | 537 | 537 | 197 | 197 | 197 | 112 | 112 | 112 |
| *** | 8995 | 9106 | 17796 | 2561 | 2577 | 4822 | 537 | 537 | 943 | 197 | 197 | 300 | 112 | 112 | 158 |
| 0.1 *** | 19917 | 20342 | 21431 | 5467 | 5552 | 5664 | 1047 | 1047 | 1047 | 325 | 325 | 325 | 181 | 181 | 181 |
| *** | 20087 | 20751 | 32183 | 5510 | 5595 | 8376 | 1047 | 1047 | 1491 | 325 | 325 | 429 | 181 | 181 | 212 |
| 0.15 *** | 29974 | 30909 | 33857 | 8230 | 8442 | 8766 | 1515 | 1541 | 1541 | 436 | 436 | 436 | 224 | 224 | 224 |
| *** | 30330 | 31902 | 44858 | 8341 | 8596 | 11502 | 1515 | 1541 | 1970 | 436 | 436 | 540 | 224 | 224 | 257 |
| 0.2 *** | 38304 | 39876 | 45486 | 10636 | 11019 | 11656 | 1940 | 1966 | 1982 | 537 | 537 | 564 | 266 | 266 | 266 |
| *** | 38899 | 41619 | 55820 | 10806 | 11290 | 14199 | 1966 | 1982 | 2381 | 537 | 537 | 634 | 266 | 266 | 295 |
| 0.25 *** | 44679 | 46990 | 55830 | 12591 | 13186 | 14206 | 2306 | 2349 | 2391 | 649 | 649 | 649 | 309 | 309 | 309 |
| *** | 45545 | 49609 | 65069 | 12846 | 13611 | 16469 | 2322 | 2365 | 2724 | 649 | 649 | 711 | 309 | 309 | 326 |
| 0.3 *** | 49157 | 52260 | 64654 | 14095 | 14902 | 16374 | 2604 | 2662 | 2705 | 707 | 707 | 707 | 325 | 325 | 325 |
| *** | 50347 | 55814 | 72605 | 14461 | 15524 | 18310 | 2646 | 2689 | 2998 | 707 | 707 | 771 | 325 | 325 | 349 |
| 0.35 *** | 51877 | 55830 | 71794 | 15184 | 16204 | 18116 | 2832 | 2901 | 2960 | 750 | 776 | 776 | 351 | 351 | 351 |
| *** | 53407 | 60319 | 78428 | 15625 | 16985 | 19723 | 2875 | 2944 | 3203 | 776 | 776 | 814 | 351 | 351 | 364 |
| 0.4 *** | 53067 | 57870 | 77149 | 15864 | 17096 | 19407 | 3002 | 3071 | 3156 | 792 | 792 | 819 | 367 | 367 | 367 |
| *** | 54937 | 63225 | 82539 | 16416 | 18031 | 20708 | 3029 | 3114 | 3340 | 792 | 819 | 840 | 367 | 367 | 372 |
| 0.45 *** | 52966 | 58576 | 80692 | 16204 | 17606 | 20241 | 3087 | 3172 | 3257 | 819 | 819 | 835 | 367 | 367 | 367 |
| *** | 55150 | 64696 | 84937 | 16815 | 18669 | 21265 | 3130 | 3215 | 3409 | 819 | 819 | 848 | 367 | 367 | 372 |
| 0.5 *** | 51776 | 58082 | 82376 | 16204 | 17734 | 20624 | 3114 | 3199 | 3300 | 819 | 819 | 835 | 367 | 367 | 367 |
| *** | 54284 | 64840 | 85622 | 16857 | 18881 | 21393 | 3156 | 3257 | 3409 | 819 | 819 | 840 | 367 | 367 | 364 |
| 0.55 *** | 49752 | 56595 | 82206 | 15906 | 17521 | 20539 | 3071 | 3156 | 3284 | 792 | 792 | 819 | 351 | 351 | 351 |
| *** | 52472 | 63777 | 84594 | 16602 | 18727 | 21093 | 3114 | 3215 | 3340 | 792 | 819 | 814 | 351 | 351 | 349 |
| 0.6 *** | 47032 | 54241 | 80166 | 15327 | 16942 | 19960 | 2960 | 3045 | 3156 | 750 | 776 | 776 | 325 | 325 | 325 |
| *** | 49949 | 61610 | 81854 | 16050 | 18175 | 20365 | 3002 | 3114 | 3203 | 776 | 776 | 771 | 325 | 325 | 326 |
| 0.65 *** | 43786 | 51070 | 76272 | 14504 | 16076 | 18940 | 2790 | 2875 | 2986 | 707 | 707 | 707 | 309 | 309 | 309 |
| *** | 46735 | 58380 | 77401 | 15200 | 17240 | 19209 | 2832 | 2917 | 2998 | 707 | 707 | 711 | 309 | 309 | 295 |
| 0.7 *** | 40046 | 47144 | 70535 | 13415 | 14860 | 17479 | 2561 | 2620 | 2705 | 622 | 649 | 649 | 266 | 266 | 266 |
| *** | 42952 | 54114 | 71235 | 14052 | 15949 | 17625 | 2604 | 2662 | 2724 | 649 | 649 | 634 | 266 | 266 | 257 |
| 0.75 *** | 35839 | 42469 | 62954 | 12055 | 13330 | 15524 | 2264 | 2322 | 2391 | 537 | 537 | 564 | 224 | 224 | 224 |
| *** | 38575 | 48775 | 63356 | 12634 | 14249 | 15612 | 2280 | 2349 | 2381 | 537 | 537 | 540 | 224 | 224 | 212 |
| 0.8 *** | 31121 | 36944 | 53561 | 10397 | 11444 | 13144 | 1881 | 1924 | 1982 | 436 | 436 | 436 | 181 | 181 | 181 |
| *** | 33544 | 42299 | 53764 | 10865 | 12166 | 13172 | 1897 | 1966 | 1970 | 436 | 436 | 429 | 181 | 181 | 158 |
| 0.35 *** | 25740 | 30399 | 42384 | 8426 | 9165 | 10296 | 1456 | 1472 | 1499 | 309 | 309 | 309 | . | . | . |
| *** | 27695 | 34521 | 42460 | 8766 | 9659 | 10303 | 1456 | 1499 | 1491 | 309 | 309 | 300 | . | . | . |
| 0.9 *** | 19349 | 22510 | 29437 | 6020 | 6445 | 7024 | 920 | 946 | 962 | . | . | . | . | . | . |
| *** | 20709 | 25086 | 29443 | 6216 | 6700 | 7006 | 946 | 946 | 943 | . | . | . | . | . | . |
| 0.95 *** | 11162 | 12506 | 14732 | 3029 | 3156 | 3300 | . | . | . | . | . | . | . | . | . |
| *** | 11757 | 13441 | 14713 | 3087 | 3215 | 3280 | . | . | . | . | . | . | . | . | . |
| 0.98 *** | 4490 | 4745 | 5069 | . | . | . | . | . | . | . | . | . | . | . | . |
| *** | 4601 | 4899 | 5053 | . | . | . | . | . | . | . | . | . | . | . | . |

# TABLE 8: ALPHA= 0.05  POWER= 0.9    EXPECTED ACCRUAL THRU MINIMUM FOLLOW-UP= 20000

| | | DEL=.01 | | | DEL=.02 | | | DEL=.05 | | | DEL=.10 | | | DEL=.15 | | |
|---|---|---|---|---|---|---|---|---|---|---|---|---|---|---|---|---|---|
| FACT= | | 1.0 .75 | .50 .25 | .00 BIN | 1.0 .75 | .50 .25 | .00 BIN | 1.0 .75 | .50 .25 | .00 BIN | 1.0 75 | .50 .25 | .00 BIN | 1.0 .75 | .50 .25 | .00 BIN |
| PCONT=*** | | | | | REQUIRED NUMBER OF PATIENTS | | | | | | | | | | | |
| 0.01 | *** | 1313 | 1313 | 1313 | 482 | 482 | 482 | 163 | 163 | 163 | 82 | 82 | 82 | 63 | 63 | 63 |
| | *** | 1313 | 1313 | 5053 | 482 | 482 | 1670 | 163 | 163 | 455 | 82 | 82 | 185 | 63 | 63 | 110 |
| 0.02 | *** | 2932 | 2932 | 2932 | 932 | 932 | 932 | 263 | 263 | 263 | 113 | 113 | 113 | 63 | 63 | 63 |
| | *** | 2932 | 2932 | 8342 | 932 | 932 | 2484 | 263 | 263 | 581 | 113 | 113 | 215 | 63 | 63 | 123 |
| 0.05 | *** | 8982 | 9063 | 9213 | 2563 | 2563 | 2582 | 532 | 532 | 532 | 182 | 182 | 182 | 113 | 113 | 113 |
| | *** | 9013 | 9132 | 17796 | 2563 | 2563 | 4822 | 532 | 532 | 943 | 182 | 182 | 300 | 113 | 113 | 158 |
| 0.1 | *** | 20013 | 20463 | 21432 | 5482 | 5563 | 5663 | 1032 | 1063 | 1063 | 313 | 332 | 332 | 163 | 163 | 163 |
| | *** | 20182 | 20832 | 32183 | 5532 | 5613 | 8376 | 1032 | 1063 | 1491 | 313 | 332 | 429 | 163 | 163 | 212 |
| 0.15 | *** | 30163 | 31163 | 33863 | 8282 | 8482 | 8763 | 1532 | 1532 | 1532 | 432 | 432 | 432 | 213 | 213 | 213 |
| | *** | 30563 | 32113 | 44858 | 8382 | 8613 | 11502 | 1532 | 1532 | 1970 | 432 | 432 | 540 | 213 | 213 | 257 |
| 0.2 | *** | 38632 | 40282 | 45482 | 10732 | 11082 | 11632 | 1963 | 1963 | 1982 | 532 | 563 | 563 | 263 | 263 | 263 |
| | *** | 39263 | 42013 | 55820 | 10882 | 11332 | 14199 | 1963 | 1982 | 2381 | 563 | 563 | 634 | 263 | 263 | 295 |
| 0.25 | *** | 45163 | 47582 | 55832 | 12732 | 13282 | 14213 | 2313 | 2363 | 2382 | 632 | 632 | 632 | 313 | 313 | 313 |
| | *** | 46113 | 50182 | 65069 | 12982 | 13682 | 16469 | 2332 | 2363 | 2724 | 632 | 632 | 711 | 313 | 313 | 326 |
| 0.3 | *** | 49813 | 53082 | 64663 | 14282 | 15063 | 16363 | 2632 | 2663 | 2713 | 713 | 713 | 713 | 332 | 332 | 332 |
| | *** | 51082 | 56613 | 72605 | 14632 | 15613 | 18310 | 2632 | 2682 | 2998 | 713 | 713 | 771 | 332 | 332 | 349 |
| 0.35 | *** | 52713 | 56882 | 71782 | 15432 | 16413 | 18113 | 2863 | 2913 | 2963 | 763 | 763 | 763 | 363 | 363 | 363 |
| | *** | 54332 | 61332 | 78428 | 15863 | 17132 | 19723 | 2882 | 2932 | 3203 | 763 | 763 | 814 | 363 | 363 | 364 |
| 0.4 | *** | 54082 | 59113 | 77163 | 16182 | 17332 | 19413 | 3013 | 3082 | 3163 | 813 | 813 | 813 | 363 | 363 | 363 |
| | *** | 56063 | 64432 | 82539 | 16682 | 18213 | 20708 | 3063 | 3113 | 3340 | 813 | 813 | 840 | 363 | 363 | 372 |
| 0.45 | *** | 54163 | 60013 | 80682 | 16532 | 17882 | 20232 | 3113 | 3182 | 3263 | 813 | 832 | 832 | 363 | 363 | 363 |
| | *** | 56482 | 66082 | 84937 | 17132 | 18863 | 21265 | 3163 | 3232 | 3409 | 813 | 832 | 848 | 363 | 363 | 372 |
| 0.5 | *** | 53163 | 59682 | 82382 | 16582 | 18032 | 20613 | 3132 | 3213 | 3313 | 813 | 832 | 832 | 363 | 363 | 363 |
| | *** | 55763 | 66363 | 85622 | 17232 | 19113 | 21393 | 3182 | 3263 | 3409 | 813 | 832 | 840 | 363 | 363 | 364 |
| 0.55 | *** | 51263 | 58313 | 82213 | 16313 | 17832 | 20532 | 3082 | 3182 | 3263 | 813 | 813 | 813 | 363 | 363 | 363 |
| | *** | 54113 | 65382 | 84594 | 16982 | 18932 | 21093 | 3132 | 3213 | 3340 | 813 | 813 | 814 | 363 | 363 | 349 |
| 0.6 | *** | 48663 | 55982 | 80163 | 15732 | 17282 | 19963 | 2982 | 3063 | 3163 | 763 | 763 | 782 | 332 | 332 | 332 |
| | *** | 51632 | 63232 | 81854 | 16432 | 18382 | 20365 | 3032 | 3113 | 3203 | 763 | 763 | 771 | 332 | 332 | 326 |
| 0.65 | *** | 45432 | 52813 | 76263 | 14913 | 16382 | 18963 | 2813 | 2882 | 2982 | 713 | 713 | 713 | 313 | 313 | 313 |
| | *** | 48463 | 59982 | 77401 | 15563 | 17463 | 19209 | 2863 | 2932 | 2998 | 713 | 713 | 711 | 313 | 313 | 295 |
| 0.7 | *** | 41663 | 48832 | 70532 | 13782 | 15163 | 17463 | 2582 | 2632 | 2713 | 632 | 632 | 632 | 263 | 263 | 263 |
| | *** | 44632 | 55613 | 71235 | 14413 | 16132 | 17625 | 2613 | 2682 | 2724 | 632 | 632 | 634 | 263 | 263 | 257 |
| 0.75 | *** | 37382 | 44013 | 62963 | 12382 | 13582 | 15532 | 2263 | 2332 | 2382 | 532 | 563 | 563 | 232 | 232 | 232 |
| | *** | 40132 | 50113 | 63356 | 12932 | 14413 | 15612 | 2282 | 2363 | 2381 | 532 | 563 | 540 | 232 | 232 | 212 |
| 0.8 | *** | 32482 | 38263 | 53563 | 10682 | 11632 | 13132 | 1882 | 1932 | 1982 | 432 | 432 | 432 | 163 | 163 | 163 |
| | *** | 34413 | 43413 | 53764 | 11113 | 12282 | 13172 | 1913 | 1963 | 1970 | 432 | 432 | 429 | 163 | 163 | 158 |
| 0.85 | *** | 26863 | 31432 | 42382 | 8613 | 9313 | 10282 | 1463 | 1482 | 1513 | 313 | 313 | 313 | . | . | . |
| | *** | 28813 | 35332 | 42460 | 8932 | 9763 | 10303 | 1463 | 1482 | 1491 | 313 | 313 | 300 | . | . | . |
| 0.9 | *** | 20113 | 23163 | 29432 | 6132 | 6513 | 7013 | 932 | 932 | 963 | . | . | . | . | . | . |
| | *** | 21432 | 25582 | 29443 | 6313 | 6732 | 7006 | 932 | 963 | 943 | . | . | . | . | . | . |
| 0.95 | *** | 11513 | 12763 | 14732 | 3063 | 3163 | 3282 | . | . | . | . | . | . | . | . | . |
| | *** | 12082 | 13613 | 14713 | 3113 | 3232 | 3280 | . | . | . | . | . | . | . | . | . |
| 0.98 | *** | 4563 | 4782 | 5063 | . | . | . | . | . | . | . | . | . | . | . | . |
| | *** | 4663 | 4913 | 5053 | . | . | . | . | . | . | . | . | . | . | . | . |

## TABLE 8: ALPHA= 0.05  POWER= 0.9    EXPECTED ACCRUAL THRU MINIMUM FOLLOW-UP= 25000

REQUIRED NUMBER OF PATIENTS

| PCONT | DEL=.01 1.0/.75 | .50/.25 | .00/BIN | DEL=.02 1.0/.75 | .50/.25 | .00/BIN | DEL=.05 1.0/.75 | .50/.25 | .00/BIN | DEL=.10 1.0/75 | .50/.25 | .00/BIN | DEL=.15 1.0/.75 | .50/.25 | .00/BIN |
|---|---|---|---|---|---|---|---|---|---|---|---|---|---|---|---|
| 0.01 | 1329 | 1329 | 1329 | 477 | 477 | 477 | 165 | 165 | 165 | 79 | 79 | 79 | 40 | 40 | 40 |
|      | 1329 | 1329 | 5053 | 477 | 477 | 1670 | 165 | 165 | 455 | 79 | 79 | 185 | 40 | 40 | 110 |
| 0.02 | 2915 | 2954 | 2954 | 954 | 954 | 954 | 266 | 266 | 266 | 102 | 102 | 102 | 79 | 79 | 79 |
|      | 2915 | 2954 | 8342 | 954 | 954 | 2484 | 266 | 266 | 581 | 102 | 102 | 215 | 79 | 79 | 123 |
| 0.05 | 9016 | 9079 | 9204 | 2540 | 2579 | 2579 | 540 | 540 | 540 | 204 | 204 | 204 | 102 | 102 | 102 |
|      | 9040 | 9141 | 17796 | 2579 | 2579 | 4822 | 540 | 540 | 943 | 204 | 204 | 300 | 102 | 102 | 158 |
| 0.1 | 20165 | 20579 | 21415 | 5516 | 5579 | 5665 | 1040 | 1040 | 1040 | 329 | 329 | 329 | 165 | 165 | 165 |
|     | 20329 | 20915 | 32183 | 5540 | 5641 | 8376 | 1040 | 1040 | 1491 | 329 | 329 | 429 | 165 | 165 | 212 |
| 0.15 | 30477 | 31477 | 33852 | 8352 | 8540 | 8766 | 1516 | 1540 | 1540 | 454 | 454 | 454 | 227 | 227 | 227 |
|      | 30891 | 32352 | 44858 | 8454 | 8641 | 11502 | 1540 | 1540 | 1970 | 454 | 454 | 540 | 227 | 227 | 257 |
| 0.2 | 39102 | 40852 | 45477 | 10852 | 11165 | 11641 | 1954 | 1977 | 1977 | 540 | 540 | 540 | 266 | 266 | 266 |
|     | 39829 | 42477 | 55820 | 11016 | 11391 | 14199 | 1977 | 1977 | 2381 | 540 | 540 | 634 | 266 | 266 | 295 |
| 0.25 | 45891 | 48454 | 55829 | 12915 | 13454 | 14204 | 2329 | 2352 | 2391 | 641 | 641 | 641 | 290 | 290 | 290 |
|      | 46915 | 50954 | 65069 | 13165 | 13766 | 16469 | 2352 | 2352 | 2724 | 641 | 641 | 711 | 290 | 290 | 326 |
| 0.3 | 50790 | 54227 | 64641 | 14579 | 15266 | 16352 | 2641 | 2665 | 2704 | 704 | 704 | 704 | 329 | 329 | 329 |
|     | 52165 | 57665 | 72605 | 14891 | 15766 | 18310 | 2665 | 2704 | 2998 | 704 | 704 | 771 | 329 | 329 | 349 |
| 0.35 | 53954 | 58329 | 71790 | 15766 | 16665 | 18102 | 2891 | 2915 | 2977 | 766 | 766 | 766 | 352 | 352 | 352 |
|      | 55704 | 62665 | 78428 | 16165 | 17290 | 19723 | 2891 | 2954 | 3203 | 766 | 766 | 814 | 352 | 352 | 364 |
| 0.4 | 55602 | 60852 | 77165 | 16579 | 17665 | 19391 | 3040 | 3102 | 3165 | 790 | 790 | 790 | 352 | 352 | 352 |
|     | 57727 | 66040 | 82539 | 17079 | 18415 | 20708 | 3079 | 3141 | 3340 | 790 | 790 | 840 | 352 | 352 | 372 |
| 0.45 | 55954 | 61977 | 80704 | 17016 | 18227 | 20227 | 3141 | 3204 | 3266 | 829 | 829 | 829 | 352 | 352 | 352 |
|      | 58391 | 67915 | 84937 | 17540 | 19102 | 21265 | 3165 | 3227 | 3409 | 829 | 829 | 848 | 352 | 352 | 372 |
| 0.5 | 55165 | 61852 | 82391 | 17079 | 18415 | 20602 | 3165 | 3227 | 3290 | 829 | 829 | 829 | 352 | 352 | 352 |
|     | 57891 | 68352 | 85622 | 17704 | 19352 | 21393 | 3204 | 3266 | 3409 | 829 | 829 | 840 | 352 | 352 | 364 |
| 0.55 | 53454 | 60641 | 82204 | 16829 | 18227 | 20516 | 3141 | 3204 | 3266 | 790 | 790 | 829 | 352 | 352 | 352 |
|      | 56391 | 67477 | 84594 | 17477 | 19204 | 21093 | 3165 | 3227 | 3340 | 790 | 790 | 814 | 352 | 352 | 349 |
| 0.6 | 50954 | 58391 | 80165 | 16290 | 17704 | 19977 | 3016 | 3079 | 3165 | 766 | 766 | 766 | 329 | 329 | 329 |
|     | 54016 | 65391 | 81854 | 16915 | 18665 | 20365 | 3040 | 3102 | 3203 | 766 | 766 | 771 | 329 | 329 | 326 |
| 0.65 | 47766 | 55204 | 76266 | 15415 | 16790 | 18954 | 2852 | 2915 | 2977 | 704 | 704 | 727 | 290 | 290 | 290 |
|      | 50852 | 62079 | 77401 | 16040 | 17704 | 19209 | 2891 | 2954 | 2998 | 704 | 704 | 711 | 290 | 290 | 295 |
| 0.7 | 43954 | 51102 | 70516 | 14266 | 15516 | 17477 | 2602 | 2665 | 2704 | 641 | 641 | 641 | 266 | 266 | 266 |
|     | 46954 | 57579 | 71235 | 14829 | 16352 | 17625 | 2641 | 2665 | 2724 | 641 | 641 | 634 | 266 | 266 | 257 |
| 0.75 | 39516 | 46079 | 62954 | 12790 | 13891 | 15540 | 2290 | 2329 | 2391 | 540 | 540 | 540 | 227 | 227 | 227 |
|      | 42266 | 51852 | 63356 | 13290 | 14602 | 15612 | 2329 | 2352 | 2381 | 540 | 540 | 540 | 227 | 227 | 212 |
| 0.8 | 34352 | 40016 | 53579 | 11016 | 11891 | 13141 | 1915 | 1954 | 1977 | 454 | 454 | 454 | 165 | 165 | 165 |
|     | 36766 | 44852 | 53764 | 11415 | 12454 | 13172 | 1915 | 1954 | 1970 | 454 | 454 | 429 | 165 | 165 | 158 |
| 0.85 | 28352 | 32790 | 42391 | 8852 | 9477 | 10290 | 1454 | 1477 | 1516 | 329 | 329 | 329 | . | . | . |
|      | 30266 | 36391 | 42460 | 9141 | 9852 | 10303 | 1477 | 1477 | 1491 | 329 | 329 | 300 | . | . | . |
| 0.9 | 21165 | 24040 | 29415 | 6266 | 6602 | 7016 | 954 | 954 | 954 | . | . | . | . | . | . |
|     | 22415 | 26204 | 29443 | 6415 | 6790 | 7006 | 954 | 954 | 943 | . | . | . | . | . | . |
| 0.95 | 11954 | 13079 | 14727 | 3102 | 3204 | 3290 | . | . | . | . | . | . | . | . | . |
|      | 12454 | 13790 | 14713 | 3141 | 3227 | 3280 | . | . | . | . | . | . | . | . | . |
| 0.98 | 4641 | 4829 | 5079 | . | . | . | . | . | . | . | . | . | . | . | . |
|      | 4727 | 4954 | 5053 | . | . | . | . | . | . | . | . | . | . | . | . |

# INDEX